Brocklehurst's Textbook of Geriatric Medicine and Gerontology

EIGHTH EDITION

HOWARD M. FILLIT, MD
Founding Executive Director and Chief Science Officer
Alzheimers Drug Discovery Foundation
Clinical Professor of Geriatric Medicine, Palliative Care and Neuroscience
Icahn School of Medicine at Mount Sinai
New York, New York

KENNETH ROCKWOOD, MD, FRCPC, FRCP
Professor of Geriatric Medicine & Neurology
Kathryn Allen Weldon Professor of Alzheimer Research
Department of Medicine
Dalhousie University;
Consultant Physician
Department of Medicine
Nova Scotia Health Authority
Halifax, Nova Scotia, Canada;
Honorary Professor of Geriatric Medicine
University of Manchester
Manchester, United Kingdom

JOHN YOUNG, MBBS(Hons), FRCP
Professor of Elderly Care Medicine
Academic Unit of Elderly Care and Rehabilitation
University of Leeds, United Kingdom;
Honorary Consultant Geriatrician
Bradford Teaching Hospitals NHS Foundation Trust
Bradford, United Kingdom

ELSEVIER

ELSEVIER

1600 John F. Kennedy Blvd.
Ste 1800
Philadelphia, PA 19103-2899

BROCKLEHURST'S TEXTBOOK OF GERIATRIC MEDICINE AND GERONTOLOGY, EIGHTH EDITION
ISBN: 978-0-7020-6185-1

Notices

Knowledge and best practice in this field are constantly changing. As new research and experience broaden our understanding, changes in research methods, professional practices, or medical treatment may become necessary.

Practitioners and researchers must always rely on their own experience and knowledge in evaluating and using any information, methods, compounds, or experiments described herein. In using such information or methods they should be mindful of their own safety and the safety of others, including parties for whom they have a professional responsibility.

With respect to any drug or pharmaceutical products identified, readers are advised to check the most current information provided (i) on procedures featured or (ii) by the manufacturer of each product to be administered, to verify the recommended dose or formula, the method and duration of administration, and contraindications. It is the responsibility of practitioners, relying on their own experience and knowledge of their patients, to make diagnoses, to determine dosages and the best treatment for each individual patient, and to take all appropriate safety precautions.

To the fullest extent of the law, neither the Publisher nor the authors, contributors, or editors, assume any liability for any injury and/or damage to persons or property as a matter of products liability, negligence or otherwise, or from any use or operation of any methods, products, instructions, or ideas contained in the material herein.

Previous editions copyrighted 2010, 2003, 1998, 1992, 1985, 1978, and 1973.

Library of Congress Cataloging-in-Publication Data

Names: Fillit, Howard M., editor. | Rockwood, Kenneth, editor. | Young, John, 1953- , editor.
Title: Brocklehurst's textbook of geriatric medicine and gerontology / [edited by] Howard M. Fillit, Kenneth Rockwood, John Young.
Other titles: Textbook of geriatric medicine and gerontology
Description: Eighth edition. | Philadelphia, PA : Elsevier, Inc., [2017] | Includes bibliographical references and index.
Identifiers: LCCN 2016010546 | ISBN 9780702061851
Subjects: | MESH: Geriatrics | Aging
Classification: LCC RC952 | NLM WT 100 | DDC 618.97—dc23 LC record available at http://lccn.loc.gov/2016010546

Content Strategist: Suzanne Toppy
Content Development Specialist: Lisa Barnes
Publishing Services Manager: Catherine Jackson
Senior Project Manager: Rachel E. McMullen
Design Direction: Brian Salisbury
Cover Illustration Artist: Peggy Magovern (www.PMagovern.com)

Printed in China
Last digit is the print number: 9 8 7 6 5 4 3 2 1

Roberta Diaz Brinton, PhD
Department of Pharmacology and Pharmaceutical Sciences
University of Southern California, School of Pharmacy Pharmaceutical Sciences Center
The Program in Neuroscience
University of Southern California
Los Angeles, California

Scott E. Brodie, MD, PhD
Professor of Ophthalmology
Department of Ophthalmology
Icahn School of Medicine at Mount Sinai
New York, New York

Jared R. Brosch, MD, MSc
Neurologist
Department of Neurology
Indiana University Health
Indianapolis, Indiana

Gina Browne, PhD, RegN, Hon LLD, FCAHS
Founder and Director
Health and Social Service Utilization Research Unit
McMaster University;
Professor
Department of Nursing; Clinical Epidemiology & Biostatistics
McMaster University
Hamilton, Canada

Patricia Bruckenthal, PhD, APRN-BC, ANP
Chair, Graduate Studies in Advanced Practice Nursing
School of Nursing
Stony Brook University
Stony Brook, New York

Jeffrey A. Burr, PhD, MA, BA
Professor
Department of Gerontology
University of Massachusetts Boston
Boston, Massachusetts

Richard Camicioli, MSc, MD, CM, FRCP(C)
Professor of Medicine (Neurology)
Department of Medicine
University of Alberta
Edmonton, Alberta, Canada

Jill L. Cantelmo, MSc, PhD
Vice President
Department of Clinical Services
The Access Group
Berkeley Heights, New Jersey

Robert V. Cantu, MD, MS
Associate Professor
Department of Orthopaedic Surgery
Dartmouth Hitchcock Medical Center
Lebanon, New Hampshire

Margred M. Capel, MBBS, BSc, MRCP, MSc
Consultant in Palliative Medicine
George Thomas Hospice
Cardiff, Wales, United Kingdom

Matteo Cesari, MD, PhD
Professor
Université de Toulouse III Paul Sabatier;
Advisor
Institut du Vieillissement, Gérontopôle
Centre Hospitalier Universitaire de Toulouse
Toulouse, France

Sean D. Christie, MD, FRCSC
Associate Professor
Department of Surgery (Neurosurgery)
Dalhousie University
Halifax, Nova Scotia, Canada

Duncan Cole, PhD, MRCP, FRCPath
Clinical Senior Lecturer
Honorary Consultant in Medical Biochemistry and Metabolic Medicine
Centre for Medical Education
Cardiff University School of Medicine
Cardiff, Wales, United Kingdom

Philip G. Conaghan, MBBS, PhD, FRACP, FRCP
Professor of Musculoskeletal Medicine
Leeds Institute of Rheumatic and Musculoskeletal Medicine
University of Leeds;
Deputy Director
NIHR Leeds Musculoskeletal Biomedical Research Unit
Leeds, United Kingdom

Simon Conroy, MBChB, PhD
Department of Geriatric Medicine
University Hospitals of Leicester
Leicester, United Kingdom

Tara K. Cooper, MRCOG
Consultant
Department of Obstetrics and Gynecology
St. John's Hospital
Livingston, Scotland, United Kingdom

Richard Cowie, BSc(Hons) MBChB FRCS(Ed), FRCS(Ed) (SN)
Consultant Neurosurgeon
NHS Hope Hospital, Salford
Salford, United Kingdom;
The Royal Manchester Children's Hospital
Manchester, United Kingdom;
The Alexandra Hospital
Cheadle, United Kingdom

Peter Crome, MD, PhD, DSc, FRCP, FFPM
Honorary Professor
Department of Primary Care and Population Health
University College London
London, United Kingdom;
Emeritus Professor
Keele University
Keele, United Kingdom

William Cross, B Med Sci, BM BS, FRCS(Urol), PhD
Consultant Urological Surgeon
Department of Urology
Leeds Teaching Hospitals NHS Trust
Leeds, Great Britain

Carmen-Lucia Curcio, PhD
Department of Gerontology and Geriatrics Program
University of Caldas
Manizales, Caldas, Colombia

Gwyneth A. Davies, MB BCh, MD, FRCP
Clinical Associate Professor
College of Medicine
Swansea University
Swansea, United Kingdom

Daniel Davis, MB, PhD
Clinical Research Fellow
MRC Unit for Lifelong Health and Ageing
University College, London
London, United Kingdom

Jugdeep Kaur Dhesi, BSc MBChB, PhD, FRCP
Ageing and Health
Guy's and St. Thomas' NHS Trust
London, Great Britain

Sadhna Diwan, MSSA, PhD
Professor
School of Social Work
San Jose State University;
Director
Center for Healthy Aging in Multicultural Populations
San Jose State University
San Jose, California

Timothy J. Doherty, MD, PhD, FRCP(C)
Associate Profesor
Departments of Physical Medicine and Rehabilitation and Clinical Neurological Sciences
Western University
London, Ontario, Canada

Dawn Dolan, PharmD
Pharmacist Senior Adult Oncology Program
Moffitt Cancer Center
Tampa, Florida

Ligia J. Dominguez, MD
Department of Internal Medicine and Specialties (DIBIMIS)
University of Palermo
Palermo, Italy

Eamonn Eeles, MBBS, MRCP, MSc, FRCP
Senior Lecturer
Department of Internal Medicine
University of Queensland
Brisbane, Austrailia

William B. Ershler, MD
Virginia Associates in Adult and Geriatric Hematology—Oncology
Inova Fairfax Hospital
Falls Church, Virginia

Nazanene Helen Esfandiari, MD
Clinical Assistant Professor
Internal Medicine/Divsion of Metabolism, Endocrinology & Metabolism
University of Michigan
Ann Arbor, Michigan

Julian Falutz, MD, FRCPC
Director
Comprehensive HIV and Aging Initiative
Chronic Viral Illness Service;
Senior Physician
Division of Geriatrics
Department of Medicine
McGill University Health Center
Montreal, Quebec, Canada

Martin R. Farlow, MD
Professor
Department of Neurology
Indiana University
Indianapolis, Indiana

Richard Feldstein, MD, MS
Clinical Assistant Professor
Department of Internal Medicine
New York University School of Medicine
New York, New York

Howard M. Fillit, MD
Founding Executive Director and Chief Science Officer
Alzheimers Drug Discovery Foundation;
Clinical Professor of Geriatric Medicine, Palliative Care and Neuroscience
Icahn School of Medicine at Mount Sinai
New York, New York

Caleb E. Finch, PhD
ARCO-Kieschnick Professor of Gerontology
Davis School of Gerontology
University of Southern California
Los Angeles, California

Andrew Y. Finlay, CBE, FRCP
Professor
Department of Dermatology and Wound Healing
Division of Infection and Immunity
Cardiff University School of Medicine
Cardiff, Wales, United Kingdom

James M. Fisher, MBBS, MRCP, MD
Specialist Registrar in Geriatric and General Internal Medicine
Health Education North East
Newcastle Upon Tyne, United Kingdom

Anne Forster, PhD, BA, FCSP
Professor
Academic Unit of Elderly Care and Rehabilitation
University of Leeds and Bradford Teaching Hospitals NHS Foundation Trust
Bradford, United Kingdom

Chris Fox, MBBS, BSc, MMedSci, MRCPsych, MD
Reader/Consultant Old Age Psychiatry
Norwich Medical School
University of East Anglia
Norwich, Norfolk, United Kingdom

Roger Michael Francis, MBChB, FRCP
Emeritus Professor of Geriatric Medicine
Institute of Cellular Medicine
Newcastle University
Newcastle upon Tyne, United Kingdom

Jasmine H. Francis, MD
Assistant Attending
Ophthalmic Oncology Service
Department of Surgery
Memorial Sloan Kettering Cancer Center
New York, New York

Terry Fulmer, PhD, RN, FAAN
President
John A. Hartford Foundation
New York, New York

James E. Galvin, MD, MPH
Professor
Department of Neurology, Psychiatry, Nursing, Nutrition and Popualtion Health
New York University Langone Medical Center
New York, New York

Maristela B. Garcia, MD
Division of Geriatrics
Department of Medicine
David Geffen School of Medicine
University of California, Los Angeles
Los Angeles, California

Jim George, MBChB, MMEd, FRCP
Consultant Physician
Department of Medicine for the Elderly
Cumberland Infirmary
Carlisle, United Kingdom

Neil D. Gillespie, BSc(Hons), MBChB, MD, FRCP(Ed), FHEA.
Consultant
Medicine for the Elderly
NHS Tayside
Dundee, United Kingdom

Robert Glickman, DMD
Professor and Chair
Oral and Maxillofacial Surgery
New York University College of Dentistry
New York, New York

Judah Goldstein, PCP, MSc, PhD
Postdoctoral Fellow
Division of Emergency Medical Services
Dalhousie University
Halifax, Nova Scotia, Canada

Fernando Gomez, MD, MS
Geriatric Medicine Coordinator
Department of Geriatric Medicine
University of Caldas
Manizales, Caldas, Colombia

Leslie B. Gordon, MD, PhD
Medical Director
The Progeria Research Foundation
Peabody, Massachusetts;
Associate Professor
Department of Pediatrics
Alpert Medical School of Brown University and Hasbro Children's Hospital
Providence, Rhode Island;
Lecturer
Department of Anesthesia
Boston Children's Hospital and Harvard University
Boston, Massachusetts

Adam L. Gordon, PhD, MBChB, MMedSci(Clin Ed)
Consultant and Honorary Associate Professor in Medicine of Older People
Department of Health Care of Older People
Nottingham University Hospitals NHS Trust
Nottingham, United Kingdom

Margot A. Gosney, MD, FRCP
Professor
Department of Clinical Health Sciences
University of Reading;
Professor
Department of Elderly Care
Royal Berkshire NHS Foundation Trust
Reading, United Kingdom

Leonard C. Gray, MBBS, MMed, PhD
Professor in Geriatric Medicine
School of Medicine
Director
Centre for Research in Geriatric Medicine;
Director
Centre for Online Health
The University of Queensland
Brisbane, Queensland, Australia

John Trevor Green, MB BCh, MD, FRCP, PGCME
Consultant Gastroenterologist/Clinical Senior Lecturer
Department of Gastroenterology
University Hospital Llandough
Cardiff, Wales, United Kingdom

David A. Greenwald, MD
Professor of Clinical Medicine
Albert Einstein College of Medicine;
Associate Division Director
Department of Gastroenterology Fellowship Program Director
Division of Gastroenterology and Liver Diseases
Albert Einstein College of Medicine/Montefiore Medical Center
Bronx, New York

Celia L. Gregson, BMedSci, BM, BS, MRCP, MSc, PhD
Consultant Senior Lecturer
Musculoskeletal Research Unit
University of Bristol
Bristol, United Kingdom

Khalid Hamandi, MBBS MRCP, BSc PhD
Consultant Neurologist
The Alan Richens Welsh Epilepsy Centre
University Hospital of Wales
Cardiff, Wales, United Kingdom

Yasir Hameed, MBChB, MRCPsych
Honorary Lecturer
University of East Anglia,
Specialist Registrar
Norfolk and Suffolk NHS Foundation Trust
Norwich, Norfolk, United Kingdom;
Clinical Instructor (St. George's International School of Medicine
True Blue, Grenada

Joanna L. Hampton, DME
Consultant
Addenbrookes Hospital
Cambridge University Hospitals Foundation Trust
Cambridge, United Kingdom

Sae Hwang Han, MS
University of Massachusetts Boston
Department of Gerontology
Boston, Massachusetts

Steven M. Handler, MD, PhD
Assistant Professor
Division of Geriatric Medicine
University of Pittsburgh
Pittsburgh, Pennsylvania

Joseph T. Hanlon, PharmD, MS
Professor
Department of Geriatrics
University of Pittsburgh, Schools of Medicine;
Health Scientist
Center for Health Equity Research and Geriatric Research Education and Clinical Center
Veterans Affairs Pittsburgh Healthcare System
Pittsburgh, Pennsylvania

Malene Hansen, PhD
Associate Professor
Development, Aging and Regeneration Program
Sanford-Burnham Medical Research Institute
La Jolla, California

Vivak Hansrani, MBChB
Clinical Research Fellow
Department of Academic Surgery Unit
Institute of Cardiovascular Sciences
Manchester, United Kingdom

Caroline Happold, MD
Department of Neurology
University Hospital Zurich
Zurich, Switzerland

Danielle Harari, MBBS, FRCP
Consultant Physician in Geriatric Medicine
Department of Ageing and Health
Guy's and St. Thomas' NHS Foundation Trust;
Senior Lecturer (Hon)
Health and Social Care Research
Kings College London
London, United Kingdom

Carien G. Hartmans, MSc
Researcher
Department of Psychiatry
VU University Medical Center
Amsterdam, the Netherlands;
Clinical Neuropsychologist
Department of Psychiatry
Altrecht, Institute for Mental Health Care
Utrecht, the Netherlands

George A. Heckman, MD, MSc, FRCPC
Schlegel Research Chair in Geriatric Medicine
Schlegel-University of Waterloo Research Institute for Aging
School of Public Health and Health Systems
University of Waterloo
Waterloo, Ontario, Canada

Vinod S. Hegade, MBBS, MRCP(UK), MRCP(Gastro)
Clinical Research Fellow
Institute of Cellular Medicine;
Honorary Hepatology Registrar
Department of Hepatology
Freeman Hospital,
Newcastle upon Tyne, United Kingdom

Paul Hernandez, MDCM, FRCPC
Professor of Medicine
Division of Respirology
Dalhousie University Faculty of Medicine;
Respirologist
Department of Medicine
QEII Health Sciences Centre
Halifax, Nova Scotia, Canada

Paul Higgs, BSc, PhD
Professor of the Sociology of Ageing
Department of Psychiatry
University College London
London, United Kingdom

Andrea Hilton, BPharm, MSc, PhD, MRPharmS, PGCHE, FHEA
Senior Lecturer
Faculty of Health and Social Care
University of Hull
Hull, United Kingdom

David B. Hogan, MD, FACP, FRCPC
Professor and Brenda Strafford Foundation Chair in Geriatric Medicine
University of Calgary
Calgary, Alberta, Canada

Søren Holm, BA, MA, MD, PhD, DrMedSci
Professor of Bioethics
School of Law
University of Manchester
Manchester, United Kingdom;
Professor of Medical Ethics
Centre for Medical Ethics, HELSAM
Oslo University
Oslo, Norway;
Professor of Medical Ethics
Centre for Ethics in Practic
Aalborg University
Aalborg, Denmark

Ben Hope-Gill, MBChB, MD, FRCP
Consultant Respiratory Physician
Department Respiratory Medicine
Cardiff and Vale University Health Board
Cardiff, Wales, United Kingdom

Susan E. Howlett, BSc(Hons), MSc, PhD
Professor
Department of Pharmacology
Dalhousie University
Halifax, Nova Scotia, Canada;
Professor
Department of Cardiovascular Physiology
University of Manchester
Manchester, United Kingdom

Ruth E. Hubbard, BSc, MBBS, MRCP, MSc, MD, FRACP
Centre for Research in Geriatric Medicine
University of Queensland,
Brisbane, Queensland, Australia

Joanna Hurley, MD, MBBCh, MRCP
Consultant Gastroenterologist
Prince Charles Hospital
Merthyr Tydfil, United Kingdom

Steve Illiffe, BSc, MBBS, FRCGP, FRCP
Professor
Department of Primary Care & Population Health
University College London
London, United Kingdom

Carol Jagger, BSc, MSc, PhD
AXA Professor of Epidemiology of Ageing
Institute for Ageing and Health
Newcastle University
Newcastle upon Tyne, United Kingdom

C. Shanthi Johnson, PhD, RD
Professor
Faculty of Kinesiology and Health Studies
University of Regina
Regina, Saskatchewan, Canada

Larry E. Johnson, ND, PhD
Associate Professor
Department of Geriatric Medicine, and Family and Preventive Medcine
University of Arkansas for Medical Sciences
Little Rock, Arkansas;
Medical Director
Community Living Center
Central Arkansas Veterans Healthcare System
North Little Rock, Arkansas

Seymor Katz, MD
Clinical Professor of Medicine
New York University School of Medicine
New York, New York;
Attending Gastroenterologist
North Shore University Hospital
Long Island Jewish Medical Center
Manhasset, New York;
St. Francis Hospital
Roslyn, New York

Helen I. Keen, MBBS, FRACP, PhD
Senior Lecturer
Medicine and Pharmacology
University of Western Austrailia
Perth, Western Australia, Australia;
Consultant Rheumatologist
Department of Rheumatology
Fiona Stanley Hospital
Murdoch, Western Australia, Australia

Nicholas A. Kefalides, MD, PhD[†]
Former Professor Emeritus
Department of Medicine
The Perelman School of Medicine
University of Pennsylvania
Philadelphia, Pennsylvania

Heather H. Keller, RD, PhD, FCD
Professor
Department of Kinesiology
University of Waterloo
Waterloo, Ontario, Canada;
Schlegel Research Chair, Nutrition & Aging
Schlegel-University of Waterloo Research Institute for Aging
Kitchener, Ontario, Canada

Rose Anne Kenny, MD, FRCPI, FRCP, FRCPE, FTCD, MRIA
Head of Department
Department of Medical Gerontology
Trinity College, Dublin;
Consultant Physician
Medicine for the Elderly, Falls & Blackout Unit
St. James's Hospital
Dublin, Ireland

James L. Kirkland, MD, PhD
Noaber Foundation Professor of Aging Research
Director, Robert and Arlene Kogod Center on Aging
Mayo Clinic
Rochester, Minnesota

Thomas B.L. Kirkwood, PhD
Professor
Newcastle University Institute for Ageing
Newcastle University
Newcastle-upon-Tyne, United Kingdom

Naoko Kishita, PhD
Senior Post-Doctoral Research Associate
Clinical Psychotherapist
Department of Clinical Psychology
Norwich Medical School
University of East Anglia
Norwich, Norfolk, United Kingdom

Brandon Koretz, MD
Professor of Clinical Medicine
Division of Geriatrics
Department of Medicine
David Geffen School of Medicine at UCLA,
Co-Chief, UCLA Division of Geriatrics
Los Angeles, California

George A. Kuchel, MD
Professor and Citicorp Chair in Geriatrics and Gerontology
University of Connecticut Center on Aging
University of Connecticut
Farmington, Connecticut

Chao-Qiang Lai, PhD
Research Molecular Biologist
Department of Nutrition and Genomics
Jean Mayer USDA Human Nutrition Research Center on Aging at Tufts University
Boston, Massachusetts

Ken Laidlaw, PhD
Professor of Clinical Psychology
Head of Department of Clinical Psychology
Norwich Medical School
University of East Anglia
Norwich, Norfolk, United Kingdom

W. Clark Lambert, MD, PhD
Professor
Department of Dermatology,
Department of Pathology and Laboratory Medicine
Rutgers—New Jersey Medical School
Newark, New Jersey

Louis R. Lapierre, PhD
Assistant Professor
Department of Molecular Biology, Cell Biology, and Biochemistry
Brown University
Providence, Rhode Island

Alexander Lapin, MD, Dr Phil (Chem), Dr Theol
Associate Professor
Clinical Institute of Medical and Chemical Diagnosis
Medical University of Vienna;
Head of the Laboratory Department
Sozialmedizinisches Zentrum Sophienspital
Vienna, Austria

Jacques S. Lee, MD, MSc
Director of Research
Department of Emergency Services
Sunnybrook Health Sciences Center;
Scientist
Department of Clinical Epidemiology
Sunnybrook Research Institute;
Assistant Preofessor
Department of Medicine
University of Toronto
Toronto, Ontario, Canada

Clara Li, PhD
Fellow
Department of Psychiatry
Icahn School of Medicine at Mount Sinai Medical Center
Alzheimer's Disease Research Center
New York, New York

Stuart A. Lipton, MD, PhD
Professor
Department of Neuroscience and Aging Research Center
Sanford-Burnham Medical Research Institute
La Jolla, California

Christina Laronga, MD, FACS
Surgical Oncologist
Senior Member Moffitt Cancer Center and Professor
Departments of Surgery and Oncological Sciences
University of South Florida College of Medicine
Tampa, Florida

Nancy L. Low Choy, PhD, MPhty(Research), BPhty(Hons)
Professor of Physiotherapy (Aged & Neurological Rehabiitation)
School of Physiotherapy, Faculty Health Sciences
Australian Catholic University Limited
Brisbane, Queensland, Austria

Christopher Lowe, MBChB, BSc(Hons), MRCS
Registrar in Vascular Surgery
Department of Vascular and Endovascular Surgery
University Hospital of South Manchester;
Research Fellow
Institute of Cardiovascular Sciences
University of Manchester
Manchester, United Kingdom

[†]Deceased.

Edward J. Macarak, PhD
Professor
Department of Dermatology & Cutaneous Biology
Thomas Jefferson University
Philadelphia, Pennsylvania

Robert L. Maher, Jr., PharmD, CGP
Assistant Professor of Pharmacy Practice
Clinical, Social, and Administrative Sciences
Duquesne University Mylan School of Pharmacy
Pittsburgh, Pennsylvania;
Director of Clinical Services
Department of Pharmacy
Patton Pharmacy
Patton, Pennsylvania

Ian Maidment, PhD, MA
Senior Lecturer
Department of Pharmacy
Lead Course Tutor, Postgraduate Psychiatric Pharmacy Programme
School of Life and Health Sciences;
ARCHA, Medicines and Devices in Ageing Cluster Lead
Aston University
Birmingham, United Kingdom

Jill Manthorpe, MA
Professor of Social Work
Social Care Workforce Research Unit
King's Collge London
London, United Kingdom

Maureen F. Markle-Reid, RN, MScN, PhD
Associate Professor and Canada Research Chair in Aging, Chronic Disease and Health Promotion Interventions
School of Nursing;
Scientific Director, Aging, Community and Health Research Unit
School of Nursing
McMaster University
Hamilton, Ontario, Canada

Jane Martin, PhD
Assistant Professor
Director, Neuropsychology
Department of Psychiatry
Icahn School of Medicine at Mount Sinai Medical Center
New York, New York

Finbarr C. Martin, MD, MSc, FRCP
Consultant Geriatrician
Department of Ageing and Health
Guys and St. Thomas' NHS Foundation Trust;
Professor
Division of Health and Social Care Research
King's College London
London, United Kingdom

Charles McCollum, MBChB, FRCS (Lon), FRCS (Ed) MD
Professor of Surgery
Academic Surgery Unit
University of Manchester
Manchester, United Kingdom

Michael A. McDevitt, MD, PhD
Assistant Professor of Medicine and Oncology
Department of Hematology and Hematological Malignancy
Johns Hopkins University School of Medicine
Baltimore, Maryland

Bruce S. McEwen, PhD
Professor
Laboratory of Neuroendocrinology
The Rockefeller University
New York, New York

Alexis McKee, MD
Assistant Professor
Division of Endocrinology
Saint Louis University
St. Louis, Missouri

Jolyon Meara, MD FRCP
Senior Lecturer in Geriatric Medicine
Academic Department Geriatric Medicine
Cardiff University (North Wales)
Cardiff, Wales, United Kingdom;
Glan Clwyd Hospital
Denbighshire, United Kingdom

Hylton B. Menz, PhD, BPod(Hons)
NHMRC Senior Research Fellow
Department of Podiatry, School of Allied Health;
NHMRC Senior Research Fellow
Lower Extremity and Gait Studies Program
La Trobe University
Bundoora, Victoria, Austria

Alex Mihalidis, PhD, MASc, BASc
Associate Professor
Department of Occupational Science & Occupational Therapy
University of Toronto;
Barbara G. Stymiest Research Chair
Toronto Rehabilitation Institute
University Health Network
Toronto, Ontario, Canada

Amanda Miller, BSc, MD
Fellow
Department of Nephrology
Dalhousie Medicine
Halifax, Nova Scotia, Canada

Arnold Mitnitski, PhD
Professor
Department of Medicine
Dalhousie University
Halifax, Nova Scotia, Canada

Noor Mohammed, MBBS, MRCP
Clinical Research Fellow
Departement of Gastroenterology
St. James Universiy Hospital NHS Trust
Leeds, United Kingdom

Christopher Moran, MB BCh
Stroke and Aging Research Group
Monash University;
Department of Neurosciences
Monash Health;
Geriatrician
Department of Aged Care
Alfred Health
Melbourme, Australia

Sulleman Moreea, FRCS(Glasg), FRCP
Consultant Gastroenterologist/Hepatologist
Digestive Disease Centre
Bradford Teaching Hospitals Foundation Trust
Bradford, United Kingdom

John E. Morley, MB BCh
Dammert Professor of Gerontology
Director, Division of Geriatric Medicine and Division of Endocrinology
Saint Louis University Medical Center;
Acting Director
Division of Endocrinology at Saint Louis University School of Medicine
Saint Louis University
St. Louis, Missouri

Elisabeth Mueller, Cand Med
Clinical Institute of Medical and Chemical Diagnosis
Medical University of Vienna
Sozialmedizinisches Zentrum Sophienspital
Vienna, Austria

Latana A. Munang, MBChB, FRCP (Edin)
Consultant Physician and Geriatrician
Department of Medicine
St. John's Hospital
Livingston, United Kingdom

Jan E. Mutchler, PhD
Professor
Department of Gerontology
University of Massachusetts Boston
Boston, Massachusetts

Phyo Myint, MBBS, MD, FRCP(Edin), FRCP(Lond)
Professor of Old Age Medicine
School of Medicine and Dentistry
University of Aberdeen
Foresterhill
Aberdeen, Scotland, United Kingdom

Preeti Nair, MBBS, FRACP
Rheumatology and Geriatrics Dual Trainee
Department of Rheumatology
Royal Perth Hospital
Perth, Australia

Tomohiro Nakamura, PhD
Research Assistant Professor
Neuroscience and Aging Research Center
Sanford-Burnham Medical Research Institute
La Jolla, California

Jennifer Greene Naples, PharmD, BCPS
Postdoctoral Fellow, Geriatric Pharmacotherapy
Department Geriatrics
University of Pittsburgh, Schools of Medicine and Pharmacy;
Research Assistant
Center for Health Equity Research and Geriatric Research Education and Clinical Center
Veterans Affairs Pittsburgh Healthcare System
Pittsburgh, Pennsylvania

James Nazroo, BSc(Hons), MBBS, MSc, PhD
Professor of Sociology
Department of Sociology
University of Manchester
Manchester, United Kingdom

Michael W. Nicolle, MD, FRCPC, D.Phil.
Chief, Division of Neurology
Clinical Neurological Sciences
University of Western Ontario
London, Ontario, Canada

Alice Nieuwboer, MSc, PhD
Neuromotor Rehabilitation Research Unit
Rehabilitation Sciences
Katholieke universiteit Leuven
Leuven, Belgium

Kelechi C. Ogbonna, PharmD
Assistant Professor, Geriatrics
Department of Pharmacotherapy & Outcomes Science
Virginia Commonwealth University
School of Pharmacy
Richmond, Virginia

José M. Ordovás, PhD
Director Nutrition and Genomics
Professor Nutrition and Genetics
Tufts University
Boston, Massachussetts

Joseph G. Ouslander, MD
Professor and Senior Associate Dean for Geriatric Programs
Charles E. Schmidt College of Medicine,
Chair
Integrated Medical Science Department
Charles E. Schmidt College of Medicine
Florida Atlantic University
Boca Raton, Florida

Maria Papaleontiou, MD
Clinical Lecturer
Metabolism, Endocrinology and Diabetes
University of Michigan
Ann Arbor, Michigan

Laurence D. Parnell, PhD
Computational Biologist
Nutrition and Genomics Laboratory
Jean Mayer USDA Human Nutrition Research Center on
Aging at Tufts University
Boston, Massachusetts

Judith Partridge, MSc MRCP
Proactive care of Older People undergoing Surgery (POPS)
Department of Ageing and Health
Guy's and St. Thomas' NHS Foundation Trust
London, United Kingdom

Gopal A. Patel, MD, FAAD
Dermatologist
Aesthetic Dermatology Associates
Riddle Memorial Hospital
Media, Pennsylvania

Steven R. Peacey, MBChB, MD, FRCP
Department of Diabetes and Endocrinology
Bradford Teaching Hospitals NHS Foundation Trust
Bradford, United Kingdom

Kacper K. Pierwola, MD
Department of Dermatology
Rutgers New Jersey Medical School
Newark, New Jersey

Megan Rose Perdue, MSW
Volunteer Adjunct Faculty
School of Social Work
San Jose State University
San Jose, California

Thomas T. Perls, MD, MPH
Professor
Department Medicine
Boston University
Boston, Massachusetts

Emily P. Peron, PharmD, MS
Assistant Professor, Geriatrics
Department of Pharmacotherapy and Outcomes Science
Virginia Commonwealth University,
Richmond, Virginia

Thanh G. Phan, PhD
Professor
Department of Medicine
Monash University
Melbourne, Victoria, Australia;
Professor
Department of Neurosciences
Monash Health
Clayton, Victoria, Australia

Katie Pink, MBBCh, MRCP
Department of Respiratory Medicine
University Hospital of Wales
Cardiff, Wales, United Kingdom

Joanna Pleming, MBBS, MSc
Specialist Registrar
Department of Geriatric Medicine
Barnet Hospital
Hertfordshire, United Kingdom

John Potter, DM, FRCP
Professor
Department of Ageing and Stroke Medicine
Norwich Medical School
University of East Anglia;
Honorary Consultant Physician
Stroke and Older Persons Medicine
Norfolk and Norwich University Hospital, Norwich
Norwich, Norfolk, United Kingdom

Richard Pugh, BSc, MBChB, FRCA, FFICM, PGCM
Consultant in Anaesthetics and Intensive Care Medicine
Glan Clwyd Hospital
Bodelwyddan, Wales, United Kingdom;
Honorary Clinical Lecturer
School of Medicine
Cardiff University
Cardiff, Wales, United Kingdom

Stephen Prescott, MD, FRCSEd(Urol)
Consultant Urological Surgeon
St. James's University Hospital
Leeds Teaching Hospitals NHS Trust
Leeds, United Kingdom

Malcolm C.A. Puntis, PhD, FRCS
Senior Lecturer
Cardiff University;
Consultant Surgeon
University Hospital of Wales
Cardiff, Wales, United Kingdom

David B. Reuben, MD
Archston Professor and Chief
Division of Geriatrics
Department of Medicine
David Geffen School of Medicine
Los Angeles, California

Kenneth Rockwood, MD, FRCPC, FRCP
Professor of Geriatric Medicine & Neurology
Kathryn Allen Weldon Professor of Alzheimer Research
Department of Medicine
Dalhousie University,
Consultant Physician
Department of Medicine
Nova Scotia Health Authority
Halifax, Nova Scotia, Canada;
Honorary Professor of Geriatric Medicine
University of Manchester
Manchester, United Kingdom

Christopher A. Rodrigues, PhD, FRCP
Consultant Gastroenterologist
Department of Gastroenterology
Kingston Hospital
Kingston-upon-Thames, Surrey, United Kingdom

Yves Roland, MD, PhD
Gérontopôle, Centre Hospitalier Universitaire de Toulouse
INSERM Université de Toulouse III Paul Sabatier
Toulouse, France

Roman Romero-Ortuno, Lic Med, MSc, MRCP(UK), PhD
Consultant Geriatrician
Department of Medicine for the Elderly
Addenbrooke's Hospital
Cambridge, United Kingdom

Debra J. Rose, PhD, FNAK
Professor, Department of Kinesiology;
Director, Center for Successful Aging
California State University, Fullerton
Fullerton, California

Sonja Rosen, MD
Assistant Clinical Professor
UCLA Medical Center
UCLA Santa Monica Orthopedic Hospital;
Division of Geriatric Medicine
Department of Medicine
David Geffen School of Medicine at University of California Los Angeles
Los Angeles, California

Philip A. Routledge, OBE, MD, FRCP, FRCPE, FBTS
Professor of Clinical Pharmacology
Section of Pharmacology, Therapeutics and Toxicology
Cardiff University;
Department of Clinical Pharmacology
University Hospital Llandough
Cardiff and Vale University Health Board
Cardiff, Wales, United Kingdom

Laurence Z. Rubenstein, MD, MPH
Professor and Chairman
Donald W. Reynolds Department of Geriatric Medicine
University of Oklahoma College of Medicine
Oklahoma City, Oklahoma

Lisa V. Rubenstein, MD, MSPH
Professor of Medicine in Residence
Department of Medicine
University of California, Los Angeles David Geffen School of Medicine,
Professor of Medicine
Department of Medicine
Veterans Affairs Greater Los Angeles Healthcare System
Los Angeles, California;
Senior Scientist
Department of Health
RAND Corporation
Santa Monica, California

Benjamin Rusak, BA, PhD
Professor
Department of Psychiatry and Psychology & Neuroscience
Dalhousie University
Halifax, Nova Scotia, Canada

Perminder S. Sachdev, MBBS, MD, FRANZCP, PhD, AM
Scientia Professor of Neuropsychiatry and Co-Director of CHeBA
Centre for Healthy Brain Ageing (CHeBA), School of Psychiatry
University of New South Wales;
Clinical Director
Neuropsychiatric Institute
Prince of Wales Hospital
Randwick, North South Wales, Australia

Gordon Sacks, PharmD
Professor and Department Head
Pharmacy Practice
Auburn University Harrison School of Pharmacy
Auburn, Alabama;
Pharmacist
Pharmacy Department
East Alabama Medical Center
Opelika, Alabama

Gerry Saldanha, MA(Oxon), FRCP
Consultant Neurologist
Department of Neurology
Maidstone & Tunbridge Wells NHS Trust
Tunbridge Wells, United Kingdom;
Honorary Consultant Neurologist
Department of Neurology
King's College Hospital NHS Foundation Trust
London, United Kingdom

Mary Sano, PhD
Department of Psychiatry
Icahn School of Medicine at Mount Sinai
New York, New York

K. Warner Schaie, PhD, ScD(Hon), Dr.phil.(hon)
Affiliate Profesor
Department of Psychiatry & Behavioral Sciences
University of Washington
Seattle, Washinton

Kenneth E. Schmader, MD
Professor of Medicine
Chief, Division of Geriatrics
Duke University Medical Center;
Director
Geriatric Research Education and Clinical Center (GRECC)
Durham VA Medical Center
Durham, North Carolina

Edward L. Schneider, MD
Professor of Gerontology
Leonard Davis School of Gerontology;
Professor of Biological Sciences
Dornsife College of Letters, Arts and Sciences;
Professor of Medicine
Keck School of Medicine
University of Southern California
Los Angeles, California

Andrea Schreiber, DMD
Associate Dean for Post-Graduate and Graduate Programs
Clinical Professor of Oral and Maxillofacial Surgery
New York University College of Dentistry
New York, New York

Robert A. Schwartz, MD, MPH, DSc(Hon), FRCP(Edin), FAAD, FACP
Professor and Head, Dermatology
Professor of Pathology
Professor of Pediatrics
Professor of Medicine
Rutgers-New Jersey Medical School;
Visiting Professor, Rutgers University School of Public Affairs and Administration
Newark, New Jersey;
Honorary Professor, China Medical University
Shenyang, China

Margaret Sewell, PhD
Clinical Assistant Professor
Department of Psychiatry
Ichan School of Medicine at Mount Sinai
New York, New York

Krupa Shah, MD, MPH
Assistant Professor
Department of Medicine
University of Rochester
Rochester, New York

Hamsaraj G.M. Shetty, BSc, MBBS, FRCP(Lond & Edin)
Consultant Physician & Honorary Senior Lecturer
Department of Medicine
University Hospital of Wales
Cardiff, Wales, United Kingdom

Felipe Sierra, PhD
Director
Division of Aging Biology
National Institute on Aging
Bethesda, Maryland

Alan J. Sinclair, MSc, MD, FRCP
Professor of Metabolic Medicine (Hon)
University of Aston and Director
Foundation for Diabetes Research in Older People
Diabetes Frail Ltd.
Droitwich Spa, United Kingdom

Patricia W. Slattum, PharmD, PhD
Professor and Director
Geriatric Pharmacotherapy Program
Pharmacotherapy and Outcomes Science
Virginia Commonwealth University
Richmond, Virginia

Kristel Sleegers, PhD, DSc
Group Leader Neurodegenerative Brain Diseases
VIB
Department of Molecular Genetics
Research Director
Laboratory of Neurogenetics
Institute Born-Bunge;
Professor
University of Antwerp
Antwerp, Belgium

Oliver Milling Smith, MBChB, BSc (Med Sci), MD, MRCOG
Consultant Obstetrician and Gynecologist
Forth Valley Royal Hospital
Women & Children
Larbert, United Kingdom

Phillip P. Smith, MD
Associate Professor
Department of Urology and Gynecology, Center on Aging
University of Connecticut
Farmington, Connecticut

Velandai K. Srikanth, PhD
Associate Professor
Stroke and Ageing Research Group
Monash University,
Department of Neurosciences
Monash Health
Melbourne, Victoria, Australia;
Associate Professor
Department of Epidemiology
Menzies Research Institute
Hobart, Tasmania, Australia

John M. Starr, FRCPEd
Honorary Professor of Health & Ageing
Centre for Cognitive Ageing and Cognitive Epidemiology
University of Edinburgh
Edinburgh, Scotland, United Kingdom

Richard G. Stefanacci, DO, MGH, MBA
School of Population Health
Thomas Jefferson University,
Senior Physician
Mercy LIFE
Philadelphia, Pennsylvania;
Chief Medical Officer
The Access Group
Berkeley Heights, New Jersey;
President
Board
Go4theGoal Foundation
Cherry Hill, New Jersey

Roxanne Sterniczuk, PhD
Student
Department of Psychology and Neuroscience
Dalhousie University
Halifax, Nova Scotia, Canada

Paul Stolee, BA(Hon), MPA, MSc, PhD
Associate Professor
School of Public Health and Health Systems
University of Waterloo
Waterloo, Ontario, Canada

Michael Stone, MD, FRCP
Consultant Physician
Department of Geriatric Medicine
Cardiff and Vale University Health Board
Cardiff, Wales, United Kingdom

Bryan D. Struck, MD
Assosociate Professor
Reynolds Department of Geriatric Medicine
University of Oklahoma Health Sciences Center
Oklahoma City VA Medical Center
Oklahoma City, Oklahoma

Allan D. Struthers, MD, FRCP, FESC, FMedSci
Professor of Cardiovascular Medicine
Division of Cardiovascular and Diabetes Medicine
University Dundee, Dundee, United Kingdom

Stephanie Studenski, MD, MPH
Director
Longitudinal Studies Section
National Institute on Aging
Baltimore, Maryland

Christian Peter Subbe, DM, MRCP
Consultant Physician
Acute, Respiratory & Intensive Care Medicine
Ysbyty Gwynedd;
Senior Clinical Lecturer
School of Medical Sciences
Bangor University
Bangor, Wales, United Kingdom

Arjun Sugumaran, MBBS, MRCP
Specialist Registrar in Gastroenterology and Hepatology
Gastroenterology Department
Morriston Hospital
Swansea, United Kingdom

Dennis H. Sullivan, MD
Director
Geriatric Research, Education & Clinical Center
Central Arkansas Veterans Healthcare System
Little Rock, Arkansas;
Professor & Vice Chair
Donald W. Reynolds Department of Geriatrics
University of Arkansas for Medical Sciences
Little Rock, Arkansas

Dennis D. Taub, PhD
Senior Investigator
Clinical Immunology Section
Laboratory of Immunology
Gerontology Research Center
National Institute on Aging/National Institute of Health
Baltimore, Maryland

Karthik Tennankore, MD, SM, FRCPC
Assistant Professor of Medicine
Division of Nephrology, Department of Medicine
Dalhousie University
Halifax, Nova Scotia, Canada

J.C. Tham, MBChB, MRCSEd, MSc
Upper Gastrointestinal Surgery Department
Derriford Hospital
Plymouth, United Kingdom

Olga Theou, PhD
Banting Postdoctoral Fellow
Department of Geriatric Medicine
Dalhousie University;
Affiliated Scientist
Geriatric Medicine
Nova Scotia Health Authority
Halifax, Nova Scotia, Canada

Chris Thorpe, MBBS, FRCA, FFICM
Consultant in Anaesthetics and Intensive Care Medicine
Ysbyty Gwynedd Hospital
Bangor, Wales, United Kingdom

Amanda G. Thrift, BSc(Hons), PhD, PGDipBiostat
Professor
Stroke & Ageing Research Group
Department of Medicine
School of Clinical Sciences at Monash Health
Monash University
Melbourne, Victoria, Australia

Jiuan Ting, MBBS
Medical Registrar
General Medicine
Royal Perth Hospital
Perth, Western Australia, Australia

Anthea Tinker, BCom, PhD
Professor of Social Gerontology
Gerontology, Social Science Health and Medicine
King's College London
London, United Kingdom

Desmond J. Tobin, BSc, PhD, MCMI, FRCPath
Professor of Cell Biology, Director of Centre for Skin Sciences
Centre for Skin Sciences, Faculty of Life Sciences
University of Bradford
Bradford, West Yorkshire, United Kingdom

Mohan K. Tummala, MD
Mercy Hospital
Department of Oncology and Hematology
Springfield, Missouri

Jane Turton, MBChB, MRCGP
Associate Specialist Physician
Department of Geriatric Medicine
Cardiff and Vale University Health Board
Cardiff, Wales, United Kingdom

Christine Van Broeckhoven, PhD, DSc
Group Leader Neurodegenerative Brain Diseases
Department of Molecular Genetics
VIB;
Research Director
Laboratory of Neurogenetics
Institute Born-Bunge;
Professor
University of Antwerp
Antwerp, Belgium

Annick Van Gils, MSc, BSc
Occupational therapist
Stroke unit
University Hospitals Leuven
Leuven, Belgium;
Lecturer
Occupational Therapy
Artevelde University College
Ghent, Belgium

Jessie Van Swearingen, PhD, PT
Associate Professor
Department of Physical Therapy
University of Pittsburgh
Pittsburgh, Pennsylvania

Bruno Vellas, MD, PhD
Gérontopôle, Centre Hospitalier Universitaire de Toulouse
INSERM UMR1027
Université de Toulouse III Paul Sabatier
Toulouse, France

Emma C. Veysey, MBChB, MRCP
Consultant Dermatologist
St. Vincent's Hospital
Melbourne, Victoria, Australia

Geert Verheyden, PhD
Assistant Professor
Department of Rehabilitation Sciences
KU Leuven;
Faculty Consultant
Department of Physical Medicine and Rehabilitation
University Hospitals Leuven
Leuven, Belgium

Dennis T. Villareal, MD
Professor of Medicine
Department of Medicine
Baylor College of Medicine;
Staff Physician
Department of Medicine
Michael E. DeBakey VA Medical Center
Houston, Texas

Adrian S. Wagg, MB, FRCP, FRCP(E), FHEA
Professor of Healthy Aging
Department of Medicine
University of Alberta
Edmonton, Alberta, Canada

Arnold Wald, MD
Professor of Medicine
Department of Medicine
Division of Gastroenterology & Hepatology
University of Wisconsin School of Medicine & Public Health
Madison, Wisconsin

Rosalie Wang, BSc(Hon), BSc(OT), PhD
Assistant Professor
Department of Occupational Science and Occupational Therapy
University of Toronto;
Affiliate Scientist
Department of Research—AI and Robotics in Rehabilitation
Toronto Rehabilitation Institute—University Health Network
Toronto, Ontario, Canada

Barbara Weinstein, MA, MPhi, PhD
Professor and Founding Executive Officer
AuD Program,
Professor
Department of Speech, Language, Hearing Sciences
Graduate Center, CUNY
New York, New York

Michael Weller, MD
Professor and Chair
Department of Neurology
University Hospital Zurich
Zurich, Switzerland

Sherry L. Willis, PhD
Research Professor of Psychiatry and Behavioral Sciences
Department of Psychiatry and Behavioral Sciences
Co-director of the Seattle Longitudinal Study
University of Washington
Seattle, Washington

K. Jane Wilson, PhD, FRCP(Lond)
Consultant Physician
Department of Medicine for the Elderly
Addenbrooke's Hospital
Cambridge University Hospitals NHS Trust
Cambridge, United Kingdom

Miles D. Witham, BM BCh, PhD
Clinical Senior Lecturer in Ageing and Health
Department of Ageing and Health
University of Dundee
Dundee, United Kingdom

Henry J. Woodford, BSc, MBBS, FRCP
Consultant Physician
Department of Elderly Medicine
North Tyneside Hospital
North Shields, Tyne and Wear, United Kingdom

Jean Woo, MA, MB BChir, MD
Emeritus Professor of Medicine
Medicine & Therapeutics
The Chinese University of Hong Kong
Hong Kong, The People's Republic of China

Frederick Wu, MD, FRCP(Lond), FRCP (Edin)
Professor of Medicine and Endocrinology
Centre for Endocrinology and Diabetes, Institute of Human Development, Faculty of Medical & Human Sciences
University of Manchester
Manchester, United Kingdom

John Young, MBBS(Hons) FRCP
Professor of Elderly Care Medicine
Academic Unit of Elderly Care and Rehabilitation
University of Leeds, United Kingdom;
Honorary Consultant Geriatrician
Bradford Teaching Hospitals NHS Foundation Trust
Bradford, United Kingdom

Zahra Ziaie, BS
Laboratory Manager
Science Center Port at University City Science Center
Philadelphia, Pennsylvania

Contents

PART II
Geriatric Medicine

PART I Gerontology

SECTION A Introduction to Gerontology

1 Introduction: Aging, Frailty, and Geriatric Medicine

Howard M. Fillit, Kenneth Rockwood, John Young

The eighth edition of our text is the first since the death of John Brocklehurst, whose name it rightly bears, as its originator and longtime editor. In his *Guardian* obituary (http://www.theguardian.com/science/2013/jul/17/john-brocklehurst), Ray Tallis (himself a former editor of *Brocklehurst*, in its third to sixth editions) honored John as "the leading geriatrician of his generation," and a man who "brought scientific gerontology to bear on our understanding of the diseases of old age." With other early leaders, he organized training programs that helped define the specialty and guide geriatric medicine in its critical adolescent years. Those physicians laid the foundation that allowed geriatric medicine to consist of approaches and procedures that were well enough defined to be tested. This proved fortunate, because medicine was entering the evidence age, which soon demonstrated the merit of the approach. They had a view of geriatric medicine as more than "internal medicine with social work consult." Even so, understanding just the claim of geriatric medicine continues to evolve. In the seventh edition, and continued here in the eighth, we press ahead with the view of geriatric medicine as the care of frail older adults.[1] Anyone who knows the frailty literature will recognize that this is not entirely a settled claim. Still, several points are inarguable.

First, frailty refers to a state of increased risk compared with others of the same age. This same age comparison is necessary. The risk of adverse health outcomes increases with age, so without this, everyone past their fifth decade, when the increase in risk becomes noticeable, would be seen as frail.

Second, frailty is related to age. This is one point that all frailty measures have in common.[2] Frailty becomes more common with age; the absolute variability in risk increases, even as relative variability declines after menopause.[3] Both trends indicate systems that are moving closer to failure. The first (increase in absolute variability) shows that more people are at an increased risk; the second, a decline in relative variability, captured by a reduction in the coefficient of variation, is compatible with a decline in the response repertoire. Older adults have less to fight back with. In other words, their repair processes are less efficient, which is evidenced, among other things, in prolonged recovery times.[4]

Third, although the use of dichotomous cut points can obscure the extent of agreement, it is clear that the phenotype definition[4] and the deficit accumulation definition[5] bear much in common, as do most current operational definitions, because these typically depend on either or both approaches.[2,6-12] Each identifies people who are at increased risk. For example, when people have none of the five phenotype characteristics, they have fewer deficits than when one is present.[7] Likewise, people with all five phenotypic features present (e.g., weight loss, reduced higher order activities such as gardening and heavy housework, feeling exhausted, reduced grip strength, slower walking speed) have the highest number of deficits overall.[7] As ever, theses can be nuanced. Given that risk cannot exceed 1, and given that at some age, it becomes indistinguishable from 1, there must be an age at which everyone is frail. These details, like so much else, require elaboration. In consequence, there is no merit in abandoning the value of understanding frailty, even if there is disagreement about its precise operational definition.

The reason that frailty is so central to geriatric medicine is compelling. The challenge of aging to medical care lies in the complexity of frailty. As people age, it is not just that any given illness becomes more common—all illnesses become more common. Age-related change, whether it crosses a disease threshold or not, follows, on average, a trajectory of decline. Managing single illnesses is tricky enough, but the complexity imposed by frailty—managing illness in the presence of multiple interacting medical and social problems that each become more common with age—requires a specialized body of knowledge and skills. This is what constitutes geriatric medicine.

With this focus on frailty in mind, we have continued to revise and evolve the textbook. The current eighth edition includes new entries on gerontechnology, homelessness, emergency and prehospital care, HIV and aging, intensive treatment of older adult patients, telemedicine, and the built environment. We have also added a chapter on frailty, written by two authors with much experience in regard to the various ways to define frailty. Obtaining a nonpartisan view is important because all chapter authors have been encouraged to revise their chapters, not just in relation to developments in their area, but also to ensure a discussion on how it is affected by frailty. For our part, we have aimed to advocate for both types of changes, which often have resulted in mutually beneficial exchanges. This reflects how the field is evolving. It also is a pragmatic challenge for textbooks in the Internet era. The goal is less to be a compendium of all the latest information than to be an account of what is usefully known. We see the role of this text as providing context and some sense of the evolution of an area. This approach can provide value in ways that merely recitation of what is up to date at the moment might not always achieve. This has long been a goal of Brocklehurst, and one that we are keen to continue.

In the eighth edition, we recognize the stellar contributions of Professor Kenneth Woodhouse, who joined us in the seventh edition, as we began the more explicit shift in emphasis toward frailty. Now we are delighted to welcome Professor John Young. He has conducted much of the useful UK research on clinical geriatric medicine for the last decade, securing our discipline a solid evidence base, and pointing out where we need to build further. This direction has benefitted enormously from his long history of clinical practice in geriatric medicine. Those skill sets are now brought to bear in the National Health Service for

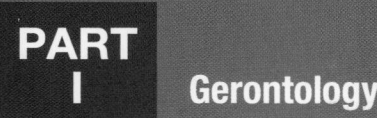

England and Wales, for which he is now the Clinical Service Director for Older Adults (or the "frailty czar," as this post otherwise is known). We feel privileged to have him join us.

As editors and chapter authors, we benefit from the engagement of the many readers who have taken time to let us know what they think of the text, both how it serves and how it might be improved. We thank them for this effort and hope that the dialogue remains ongoing. Providing health care for anyone is a special privilege; providing it for people in great need, even more so. It is not widely recognized enough that the care of frail older adults is a special challenge, requiring particular expertise. When it is done well, geriatric medicine is a thing of beauty, deeply rewarding to patient and practitioner. We wish our reader this joy of geriatrics.

KEY REFERENCES

1. Clegg A, Young J, Iliffe S, et al: Frailty in elderly people. Lancet 381:752–762, 2013.
2. Rodríguez-Mañas L, Féart C, Mann G, et al: Searching for an operational definition of frailty: a Delphi method–based consensus statement: the frailty operative definition-consensus conference project. J Gerontol A Biol Sci Med Sci 68:62–67, 2013.
3. Rockwood K, Mogilner A, Mitnitski A: Changes with age in the distribution of a frailty index. Mech Ageing Dev 125:517–519, 2004.
4. Mitnitski A, Song X, Rockwood K: Assessing biological aging: the origin of deficit accumulation. Biogerontology 14:709–717, 2013.
5. Fried LP, Tangen CM, Walston J: Frailty in older adults: evidence for a phenotype. J Gerontol A Biol Sci Med Sci 56:M146–M156, 2001.
6. Mitnitski AB, Mogilner AJ, Rockwood K: Accumulation of deficits as a proxy measure of aging. ScientificWorldJournal 1:323–336, 2001.
7. Rockwood K, Andrew M, Mitnitski A: A comparison of two approaches to measuring frailty in elderly people. J Gerontol A Biol Sci Med Sci 62:738–743, 2007.
8. Theou O, Brothers TD, Mitnitski A, et al: Operationalization of frailty using eight commonly used scales and comparison of their ability to predict all-cause mortality. J Am Geriatr Soc 61:1537–1551, 2013.
9. Theou O, Brothers TD, Peña FG, et al: Identifying common characteristics of frailty across seven scales. J Am Geriatr Soc 62:901–906, 2014.
10. Cesari M, Gambassi G, van Kan GA, et al: The frailty phenotype and the frailty index: different instruments for different purposes. Age Ageing 43:10–12, 2014.
11. Malmstrom TK, Miller DK, Morley JE: A comparison of four frailty models. J Am Geriatr Soc 62:721–726, 2014.
12. Clegg A, Rogers L, Young J: Diagnostic test accuracy of simple instruments for identifying frailty in community-dwelling older people: a systematic review. Age Ageing 44:148–152, 2015.

2 The Epidemiology of Aging

Carol Jagger

Age is not measured by years. Nature does not equally distribute energy. Some people are born old and tired while others are going strong at seventy.

Dorothy Thompson

INTRODUCTION

According to Wikipedia, epidemiology is defined as "the science that studies the patterns, causes, and effects of health and disease conditions in defined populations." Epidemiology was first concerned with epidemics of infectious diseases when these were the main cause of death. However, with what demographers termed the *epidemiologic transition*, when the main cause of death in most populations worldwide shifted from infectious to noninfectious disease, epidemiologists moved their attention to chronic diseases, as well as to aging, which is more a characteristic of the population as life expectancy increases.

The body of knowledge of the epidemiology of aging has evolved into concentrating on three main areas: the causes and consequences of the aging of populations, the natural history of diseases of old age, and the evaluation of services set up to assist older people. This chapter will concentrate on the first of these, with a discussion of the burden of disease in old age generally, rather than for specific disease, and the implications of this for health and care services; the other two sections will be covered more fully elsewhere in the text.

The Causes and Consequences of Population Aging

The early twenty-first century is unique in a number of aspects, but in relation to the people of the world, it is most remarkable as a time when humans live appreciably longer than ever before. Perhaps even more remarkably this rate of prolongation of average life expectancy shows little signs of abating. This extraordinary piece of good luck for those of us who live at this time is tempered a little by the knowledge that life insurers and those calculating pensions have been betting our money on our not living so long, so we may be poorer than we had hoped.

Longevity

The constancy of the increase in human life expectancy over the past decades, at around 2 years every decade, or 4 to 5 hours per day, has surprised scientists and the population generally. Before 1950, most of the gain in life expectancy was due to reductions in death rates at younger ages. Demographers were confidently predicting that once these gains, made by reducing mortality in early and middle life, had reached completion, growth in longevity would stop and we would see the fixed reality of the aging process. However, in the second half of the twentieth century, improvements in survival after the age of 65 years caused the increase in the length of people's lives and, indeed, mortality rates even in very old age have fallen. Experts who have repeatedly asserted that life expectancy is close to an ultimate ceiling have repeatedly been proven wrong, and most forecasts of the maximum possible life expectancy in recent years have been broken within 5 years of the forecast.[1,2]

The results of these remarkable increases in life expectancy have been the so-called graying of our populations. In 2010, around 8% of the world's population was aged 65 years or over, and this is expected to double, to 16%, by 2050—but these figures hide two facts. First, that the older population itself is aging; the fastest growing section of most populations worldwide is those aged 85 years and older, the very old, who are forecast to number 377 million worldwide by 2050. There has also been an exponential increase in the number of centenarians in countries such as Japan, France, and the United Kingdom (UK), as well as the emergence of another section of the population, supercentenarians, those aged 110 years and over. The modal age at death, a measure of average life span, has been increasing steadily in the UK (Figure 2-1), reaching 85 years for men and 89 years for women in 2010, and therefore already surpassing the upper limit for life span of 85 years to be reached by 2045 (theorized by Fries[3]).

Second, not all countries are aging at the same pace. It took France around 110 years for its older population (aged 65+ years) to rise from 7% of the population to 14%. Sweden took 80 years and the UK 50 years, but Brazil and South Korea are forecast to reach this level of demographic aging in less than 20 years. Thus, the political and societal accommodation to demographic aging will have to be made much more rapidly in developing countries.

The ratio of the dependent population to the economically active or working population is termed the *dependency ratio*. This has been commonly defined as the ratio of the population aged 65 years and over to those aged 15 to 64 years. For the European Union (EU) as a whole, the dependency ratio is 28.2 and it is projected to rise to 49.2 by 2050. However, the aging of the population and low fertility rates means that for some European countries, the dependency ratio is much higher. For example, the ratio in Spain is 27.2 but by 2050 will reach 60.5 (Table 2-1). Nevertheless, this ratio may become less useful in the future as the retirement age is increased, and indeed many people over the age of 65 remain in the workforce, whereas there are those under the age of 65 who are not part of the working population—children, students, housewives, husbands, and the unemployed. Being not formally employed does not mean that they are not contributing to the economy. Grandparents contribute hugely in terms of child care for working and retired people, especially women, and are one of the biggest groups caring for older disabled relatives, most often a spouse. Thus, the dependency ratio does not reflect the need for care, the more usual use of the term *dependency*. For this, the oldest old support ratio, the ratio of people aged 50 to 74 years to those aged 85 years and older, has been proposed.[4]

Because of the youthfulness of immigrants, immigration is often seen as a solution to the "problem" of population aging in countries with low fertility. Presently, the lack of people to take jobs in developed countries, for example in the care sector, draws young people from developing countries, lowering the average age of the population. There are, however, cohorts from the West Indies and Southeast Asia, predominantly India and Pakistan, who came to the UK in the 1960s and 1970s and who have now aged into the older population. Although their numbers are small, they will increase, and they are known to have higher risks of

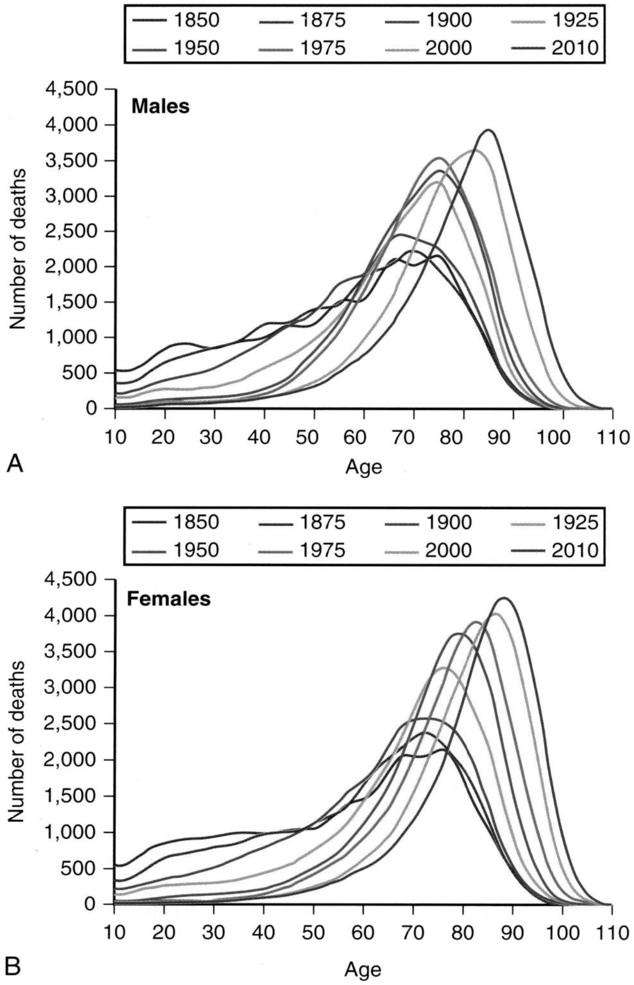

Figure 2-1. Modal age at death (United Kingdom), males (**A**) and females (**B**), selected years. *(From the Office for National Statistics: Mortality in England and Wales: Average Life Span, 2010, 2012.)*

TABLE 2-1 Old Age Dependency Ratio*

Country or Region	Year 2014	2025	2050
European Union (28 countries)	28.2	35.1	49.4
Austria	27.2	32.5	46.6
Belgium	27.3	31.8	37.9
Bulgaria	29.3	36.4	53.9
Croatia	27.5	35.7	49.1
Cyprus	19.5	27.9	42.3
Czech Republic	25.7	33.7	48.2
Denmark	28.3	33.6	39.4
Estonia	27.9	36.1	51.4
Finland	30.2	38.9	41.9
France	28.4	35.8	43.8
Germany	32.2	40.1	57.3
Greece	31.4	37.3	63.6
Hungary	25.8	33.5	47.3
Ireland	19.2	26.7	44.8
Italy	32.9	37.0	52.9
Latvia	28.6	36.6	50.5
Lithuania	27.5	38.6	51.9
Luxembourg	20.4	23.2	31.6
Malta	26.4	37.5	44.8
Netherlands	26.4	35.1	46.4
Poland	20.9	32.5	51.9
Portugal	30.2	38.1	64.3
Romania	24.3	31.8	48.5
Slovakia	19.0	28.9	54.2
Slovenia	25.7	36.4	53.9
Spain	27.2	34.2	62.5
Sweden	30.6	34.2	37.5
United Kingdom	26.9	31.7	40.6

*For population 65 years and older to population 15 to 64 years, 2014 to 2050.

From Eurostat: Population Projection 2014–2050, 2014, http://epp.eurostat.ec.europa.eu/portal/page/portal/population/data/database. Accessed 4 November 2014.

cardiovascular disease, stroke, and diabetes,[5] although little is known about their rates of cognitive impairment or disability.

Why Do We Age?

There now appears to be a reasonably clear consensus that the aging process is caused by an accumulation of molecular damage over time. The rate of aging in an individual is therefore a complex interaction among damage, maintenance, and repair. These interactions are, of course, influenced by genetic and environmental factors. It has been said that whoever created humans, whether nature or a creator, did a poor job but, being aware of it, put in a lot of backup systems. On the other hand, it may be a universal law that hyperefficiency is less effective in the long run than flexibility. This may be a useful lesson beyond the realms of longevity in a world seemingly more concerned about efficiency than effectiveness.

It is assumed that genetic changes are unlikely to alter appreciably, under evolutionary pressure, over the short period, during which longevity has dramatically increased. The reason for the increasing longevity is therefore said to be caused by the interplay of advances in income, nutrition, education, sanitation, and medicine, with the mix varying over age, period, cohort, place, and disease. It seems likely, then, that these changes are largely a result of a wide range of environmental factors.

The birth cohorts of the early 1900s experienced huge changes in socioeconomic conditions, hygiene, lifestyle, and medical care, leading to dramatic falls in infant mortality and infectious and respiratory disease rates. The main effects were improvements in housing, sanitation, and nutrition; the control of infectious diseases and maternal mortality; and the advent of antibiotics and vaccination.[6] In later years, it has been the survival of older people that has led to the extension of life expectancy, due predominantly to reductions in cardiovascular and stroke mortality and increasing survival for many cancers. Life expectancy at age 65 years in the UK has risen by 5.2 years for men and 3.8 years for women since 1981, equating to an increase of 40% for men and 20% for women.

HEALTHY AGING

The prevalence of the major chronic diseases—coronary heart disease (CHD), stroke, and dementia—which have grown in importance over the century, increases with age. This is particularly the case for dementia, where the prevalence approximately doubles for every 5-year increase in age.[7] Moreover, very old age is characterized by multiple, rather than single, diseases. In the Newcastle 85+ Study, none of the men and women aged 85 years were free of disease (Figure 2-2); on average, men and women had four and five diseases respectively, whereas around 30% had six or more diseases.[8] This accumulation of disease has implications for the delivery of health care because, at least in the UK, secondary care is organized predominantly around single diseases. However, the high level of multimorbidity is also a strong contributor to frailty, reflecting the accumulation of deficits inherent in the Frailty Index.[9]

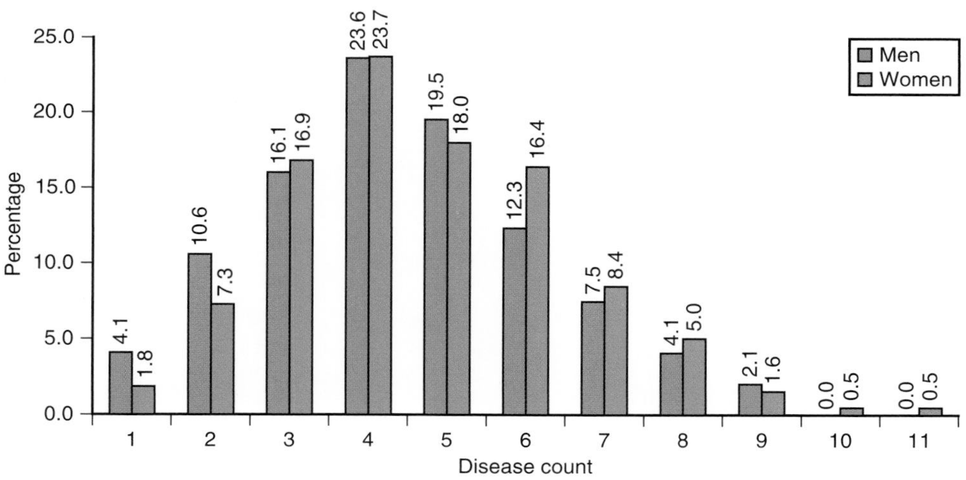

Figure 2-2. Multimorbidity in a population of 85-year-olds. *(From Kingston A, Davies K, Collerton J, et al: The contribution of diseases to the male-female disability-survival paradox in the very old: results from the Newcastle 85+ Study. Plos One 9:e88016, 2014.)*

In the past, life expectancy has been used as a surrogate measure of the health of populations and, even today, there are those who purport that we are healthier than previous cohorts simply because we are living longer. On the other hand, the burden of disease and increasing frailty and dependency in late old age would suggest the opposite. What is clear is that life expectancy itself does not equate with health, and we need to ensure that our extra years of life are healthy ones (or as Fries, termed it, *compression of morbidity*[3]) rather than unhealthy ones through extending the life of those already sick (expansion of morbidity).[10] To explore these opposing theories, the concept of health expectancy was developed. Health expectancy is a population health indicator combining information on the quantity of life (life expectancy) and quality of the remaining years (health).[11] Because there are many measures of health, there are many possible health expectancies, but the most common are based on self-reported general health (healthy life expectancy) and disability (disability-free life expectancy). Unlike quality-adjusted life-years (QALYs), health expectancies do not generally incorporate weighting of health states; they therefore give a more transparent picture of how the health of a population is evolving alongside increasing life expectancy.

More recently, the development of harmonized health measures across Europe has enabled comparative health expectancies between European countries. Indeed, the first health indicator for the EU was healthy life years (HLYs), a disability-free life expectancy. This indicator, computed annually across all EU countries, highlights the huge inequalities across Europe and that using life expectancy as the metric vastly underestimates inequalities. In 2011, male life expectancy at age 65 in the EU27 was 17.8 years, of which only 8.6 years (48%) were HLYs, but with a range of life expectancy across countries of 5.8 years (from 13.4 to 19.3 years) and a range of HLYs of 10.3 years (from 3.5 to 13.9 years; Table 2-2). More recently, frailty-free life expectancy has been computed for 13 countries who are part of the Survey of Health and Retirement in Europe (SHARE), showing considerable heterogeneity in the years spent as robust, prefrail, frail, or with severe activity limitation (Figure 2-3).[12]

Changes with Time

It is commonly believed that the new generations of older people are fitter than their past counterparts, but hard data to support this are scarce in countries other than the United States, where a meta-analysis concluded that there appeared to have been a significant reduction in the rate of functional decline over the last 3 decades.[13] In the UK, there have been two cohort studies of older people conducted identically over time, and their results reflect both views, with a worsening of disability in the young old (65 to 69 years),[14] although an apparent improvement in those aged 75 years and over.[15] What is also important is that to answer the question fully of whether we are living longer, healthier lives, health must be assessed alongside mortality. Trends in health expectancy are much less positive and vary considerably worldwide, even within Europe, with countries experiencing an expansion of disability, compression, and dynamic equilibrium.[16]

Turning to more specific problems that are common in older people, successive cohorts of older people appear to have a lower prevalence of vision and hearing impairment, high blood pressure, and cholesterol along with increasing obesity and mobility limitation.[17] Better levels of education seem to have gone some way to mitigate these increases, and they have certainly contributed to the reduction in the prevalence of dementia seen over the last 2 decades.[18] Nevertheless, the rising average body weight and body mass index (BMI) in all adult age groups in developed countries, and the increasing prevalence of obesity, is worrying.[19] Obesity is a risk factor for many conditions, but it has more of an impact on disability than mortality at older ages.[20] Thus, it seems unlikely that compression of disability will be achieved without large reductions in levels of obesity.

Trends in disability are highly sensitive in regard to whether milder levels, captured by instrumental activities of daily living (IADLs) are included or whether the focus is simply on basic self-care activities (ADLs). In the Netherlands, trends in the prevalence of limitation in most IADLs and ADLs for those aged 55 to 84 years was stable over the period 1990 to 2007.[21] Over approximately the same period (1987 to 2008), downward trends in the prevalence of mild disability and functional limitations were observed among older Norwegians.[22] Similarly, the prevalence of IADL difficulties decreased between 1988 and 2004 for Finnish young old (aged 65 to 69 years),[23] whereas Finnish nonagerians had a stable prevalence of ADL disability between 2001 and 2007.[24] In contrast, in the United States, between 2000 and 2008, the trends in prevalence of activity limitation were cohort-related, with prevalence decreases for those aged 85 years and over, stability for the 65- to 84-year-olds and increases, although

TABLE 2-2 Male and Female Life Expectancy (LE) and Healthy Life Years (HLYs)*

	Gender					
	Male			Female		
Country	*LE (Years)*	*HLYs (Years)*	*% HLY/LE*	*LE (Years)*	*HLYs (Years)*	*% HLYs/LE*
Austria	18.1	8.3	45.9	21.7	8.3	38.4
Belgium	18.0	9.8	54.5	21.6	10.3	47.5
Bulgaria	14.0	8.6	61.5	17.3	9.7	55.7
Cyprus	18.2	8.0	44.0	20.3	5.9	29.0
Czech Republic	15.6	8.4	53.8	19.2	8.7	45.4
Denmark	17.3	12.4	71.6	20.1	13.0	64.6
Estonia	14.8	5.6	37.9	20.1	5.7	28.6
Finland	17.7	8.4	47.3	21.7	8.6	39.8
France	19.3	9.7	50.5	23.8	9.9	41.8
Germany	18.2	6.7	36.7	21.2	7.3	34.2
Greece	18.2	9.0	49.6	21.2	7.9	37.2
Hungary	14.3	6.0	41.9	18.2	6.0	33.0
Ireland	17.9	10.9	60.8	20.9	11.8	56.5
Italy	18.6	8.1	43.4	22.4	7.0	31.1
Latvia	13.4	4.8	35.7	18.7	5.0	26.7
Lithuania	14.0	6.2	44.1	19.2	6.7	34.8
Luxembourg	17.8	11.5	64.6	21.6	11.8	54.8
Malta	17.7	11.8	67.0	21.0	11.0	52.3
Netherlands	18.1	10.4	57.7	21.2	9.9	46.8
Poland	15.4	7.6	49.7	19.9	8.3	41.8
Portugal	17.8	7.8	43.6	21.6	6.3	29.4
Romania	14.7	5.4	36.9	17.7	4.7	26.7
Slovakia	14.5	3.5	23.8	18.4	2.9	16.0
Slovenia	16.9	6.2	36.8	21.1	6.9	32.5
Spain	18.8	9.7	51.7	23.0	9.3	40.4
Sweden	18.5	13.9	75.0	21.3	15.2	71.3
United Kingdom	18.5	11.0	59.6	21.1	11.9	56.3
EU27	17.8	8.6	48.2	21.3	8.6	40.4
Minimum	13.4	3.5	23.8	17.3	2.9	16.0
Maximum	19.3	13.9	75.0	23.8	15.2	71.3
Range	5.8	10.4	51.2	6.4	12.3	55.4

*At age 65 years by European Union country, 2011.
From Eurohex: Expectancy Monitoring Unit, 2014, http://www.eurohex.eu/. Accessed 28 October 2014.

still low prevalence, for the preretirement age group aged 55 to 64 years.[25] What is most important in the comparison of cohort trends is the inclusion of older people in institutions, because many countries have now implemented policies to keep older people in their own homes. Thus, the proportion of the population in institutions has reduced over time, and this sector is more dependent than in the past.

Measuring Differences: Cross-sectional Versus Longitudinal Data

Much past research done on the aging process has been performed on cross-sectional data. Cross-sectional studies are easier and much less complicated to perform than longitudinal studies, and they are the best source of information for determining time trends. However, generally speaking, cross-sectional data indicate greater differences with age than longitudinal studies. Cross-sectional studies that originally were thought to show that smoking had a protective effect on Alzheimer disease were shown by longitudinal studies to be the opposite of the true effect, probably because smokers died before they had a chance to suffer from Alzheimer.[26] It is therefore important to distinguish between the types of data that are available when making judgments about populations of older people. Generally, cross-sectional data paint a bleaker picture of the impact of aging than longitudinal data. The process of aging for all of us is demonstrably longitudinal, so that wherever possible, we should be guided by such data. In recent years, there has been a rise in longitudinal studies of aging worldwide, with the U.S. HRS-AHEAD study providing a model for a growing number, including the English Longitudinal Study of Ageing (ELSA), the multicountry SHARE, and the Irish Longitudinal Study of Ageing (TILDA). Such multicountry studies of populations with varied histories of population aging afford a deeper understanding of the determinants of aging in individuals, as well as the interplay with socioeconomic and environmental factors.

Measuring Differences

Age Differences

The age distribution of older men and women is very different, especially in the oldest age groups. For example, there are approximately five female centenarians to every male centenarian, although this ratio has been steadily falling; in 2000, there were approximately nine female centenarians for every male centenarian and, in 2009, there were approximately six female centenarians for every male centenarian. The greater increases in male life expectancy are responsible for this fall, and gender differences according to age will become even less notable in the future.

Most measures of ill health increase with age, but a few do not. Levels of good or better self-rated general health are maintained, even to very old age.[8] Some of this effect is likely to be due to the form of the question; levels of comparative self-rated health (compared to peers) show less decline, and even an increase with age, whereas global self-rated health show declines with age.[27] Nevertheless, self-rated health is strongly predictive of

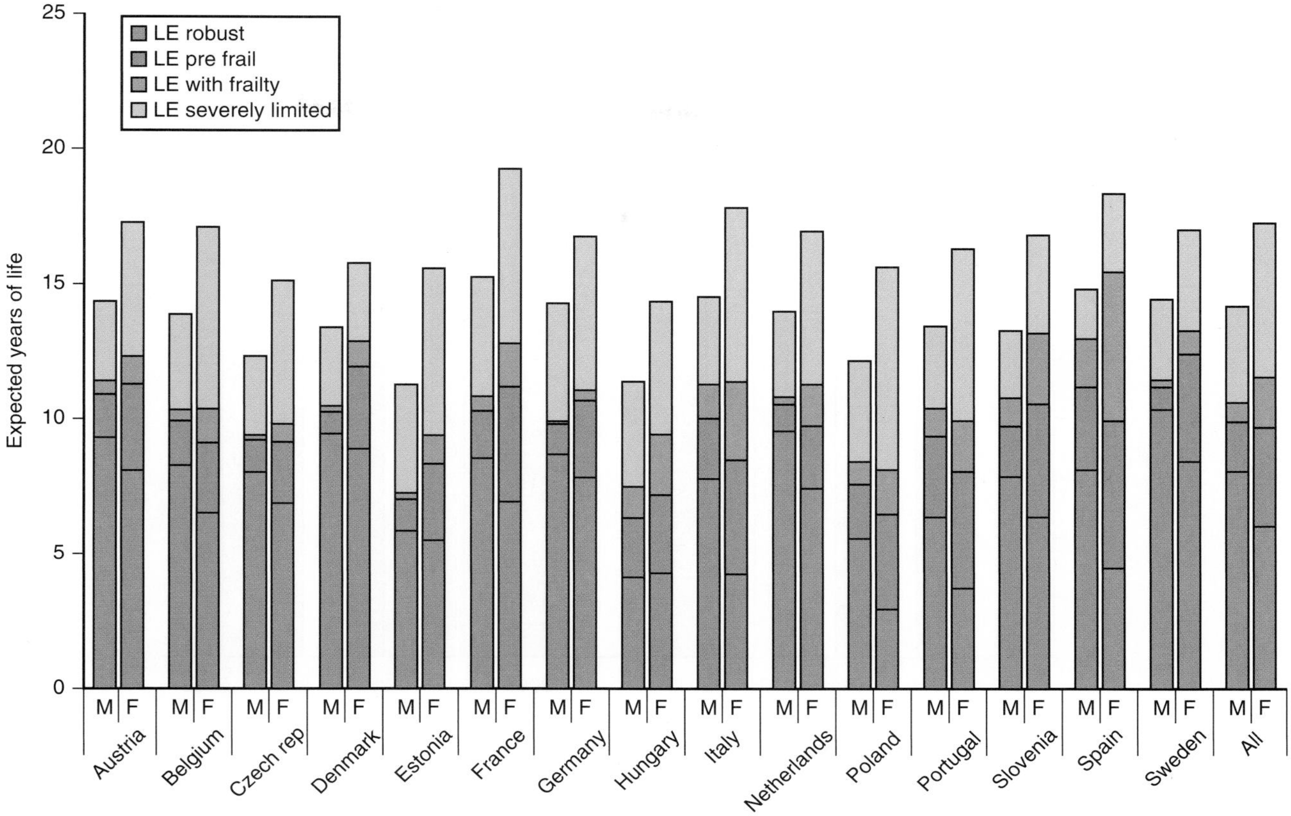

Figure 2-3. Frailty-free life expectancy (LE) at age 70 years by country. *(From Romero-Ortuno R, Fouweather T, Jagger C: Cross-national disparities in sex differences in life expectancy with and without frailty. Age Ageing 43:222-228, 2014.)*

mortality, institutionalization, and service use, even after accounting for morbidity and disability, although the underlying mechanisms are less well understood.[28] Similarly, the prevalence of depression does not rise with age. However, because depressive symptomatology is more prevalent at very old ages than physician-diagnosed depression,[8] it may be that depression is underdiagnosed or older people and health care professionals equate symptoms with aging.

When relationships among biologic parameters, lifestyle factors, and health outcomes are determined in studies, it is often assumed that they hold true across the whole age range. However, with the emergence of more very old individuals in studies, this supposition has been countered. Shorter telomeres were found to be predictive of mortality but, in populations of the very old, this relationship no longer holds.[29] Too often, studies of total populations simply adjust for age when exploring relationships between risk factors and outcomes and do not investigate possible interactions with age.

Gender Differences

The average life expectancy at birth of females born in the UK is 83 years compared with 79 years for males. However, 18 of these 83 years (22%) are years with disability, compared to 15 years (19%) for men. Therefore, women's extra years of life are mostly years with disability. Women are more likely than men to be living with high blood pressure, arthritis, back pain, mental illness, asthma, respiratory disease, and frailty. Men are more likely than women to be living with heart disease. This health-survival paradox, with men being more likely to die, but women become disabled, has been observed in many studies and countries but is not fully understood.[30,31]

Due to women's lower mortality rates, most studies of older populations have a larger proportion of women than men at any age, and this proportion increases with age. Because most health conditions are age-related, gender comparisons must account for age differences. Yet, even in studies of single birth cohorts, the health-survival paradox still exists,[32] despite women experiencing higher levels of most conditions, more frailty, and higher multimorbidity.

Although the gender differences in the structure by age of the older population is expected to persist in the future, things will slowly change. As a result of the faster increase in life expectancy of men, gender differences in the composition of the older age groups will most likely shrink over time. Thus, it is estimated that between 2012 and 2037, women will remain in the majority, but their share is due to decrease. For example, in the UK, the percentage of women aged 80 to 89 is expected to decrease, from 60.4% in 2012 to 55.0% in 2037 and to 50.5% in 2112.

Older men and women are very different with respect to their marital status; 69.5% of men are married, compared with 45% of women, whereas 14.4% of men are widowed compared with 40.2% of women. This gender imbalance varies by age, becoming more marked among older cohorts. In the future, these differences are expected to decrease dramatically. Figure 2-4 shows these changes.

There is predicted to be a dramatic increase in the share of divorced and separated individuals in the younger age groups of the older population between 2008 and 2033. Among the 65- to 74-year-olds, one in five women will belong to this group, whereas

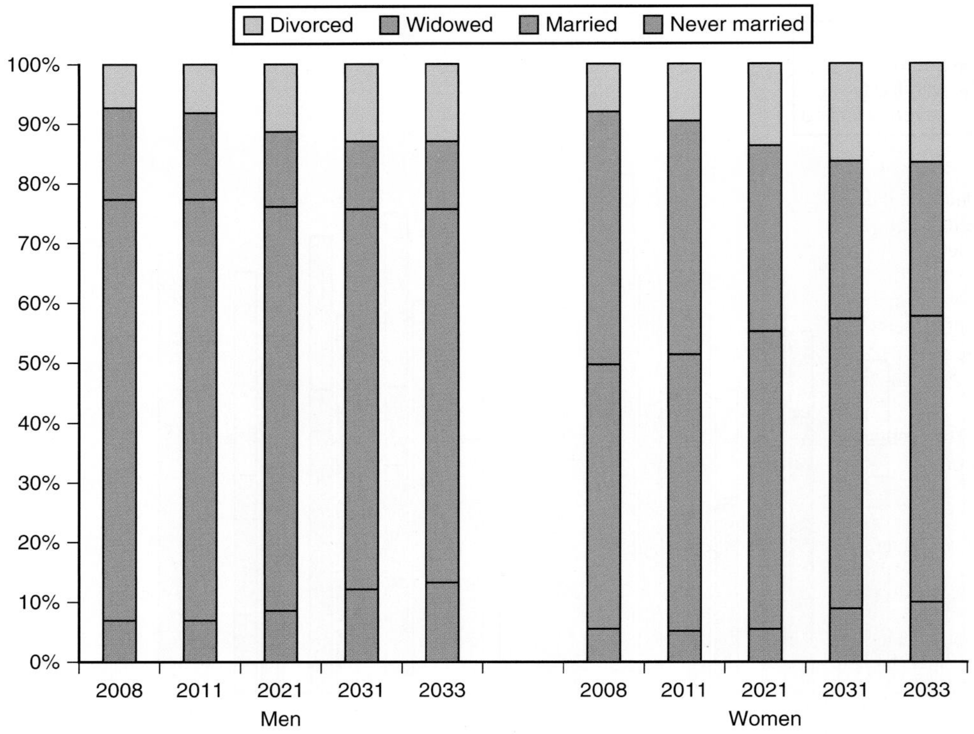

Figure 2-4. Projected percentage of older people by gender and marital status (England and Wales). (*Office for National Statistics: Statistical bulletin: 2008-based Marital Status Population Projections for England & Wales, 2010.*)

in 2008 the percentage stood at 12%. The increase in the proportion of divorced and separated men will not be as great because men have a higher propensity to remarry, but the proportion of single men will reach more than 16%. These changes will have implications for the provision of informal care because families, and predominantly women, have been the main carers.

The vast majority of those who live alone are widowed, although this percentage is much higher for women than men. Men are more likely to be married, perhaps living with a younger wife, whereas women in this group are for the most part widowed. Living alone is not directly related to loneliness, but the cause of living alone, especially widowhood, is closely related, so they are often associated. Changes in loneliness are not simply a result of changing marital status (e.g., widowhood), but have also been shown to be linked to changes in physical health.[33] Thus, improvements in health resulted in improvements in self-reported loneliness, suggesting that interventions to improve loneliness should not focus solely on improving social engagement.

Is Aging Inevitable?

The old joke says that "aging is inevitable, maturing is optional." However, lifestyle factors seem able to have an impact on aging. The best-known and obvious of these is smoking, which is related to a wide range of problems, some well known, as in lung disease, heart disease, and cancers, resulting in its being an important predictor for mortality[34] and functional decline.[35] Although smoking has a strong effect on life expectancy, other health behaviors have a greater effect on healthy life expectancy. In particular, normal weight (as opposed to obesity) resulted in the greatest reduction of years lived with cardiovascular disease (CVD).[36] There is increasing evidence of the effects of exercise and balance and strength training on mobility and the prevention of falls, even in older people in long-term care.[37-39]

Inequalities

Older people have tended to be neglected in research on health inequalities compared with people in other stages of life. One of the central reasons for this has been the difficulty of assigning people to social groupings after retirement because the approach has traditionally been based on occupational status, and this is difficult to attribute when older people are mainly retired. Nevertheless there is evidence that socioeconomic status groups, defined by education, social (occupational) class, or deprivation, have differential later life mortality and years with disability. At age 65, women with the highest education (12+ years) lived 1.7 years longer than women with the lowest education (0 to 9 years), but enjoyed 2.8 years more free of difficulties with mobility.[40] Furthermore, inequalities by socioeconomic group continue, even up to the end of life, with older people in the last year of life still being reluctant to take up their entitled benefits.[41] Primary health care professionals who see nearly all who die during their last year could play an important role in ensuring that older people who are less well-off are aware of the services and benefits available to them.

CONCLUSIONS

Epidemiology is about measuring and understanding the distribution of the characteristics of populations. In relation to aging, the early twenty-first century is unique in the span of human existence for the longevity of the human race. The aging of the population is a global phenomenon that requires international coordination nationally and locally, because there is a growing recognition that many countries are not yet ready for the future increase in the numbers of older people.

Although there has been a huge increase in research on aging, there are still large gaps in the jigsaw. More concerted efforts with comparative research, for example, with the multicountry longitudinal studies of aging in populations who are at different stages of the epidemiologic transition, will help us fill in more pieces of the puzzle and aid our understanding of how to age healthily.

KEY POINTS: THE EPIDEMIOLOGY OF AGING

- The world population is older than it has ever been.
- Measuring the effect of an aging population is not straightforward; longitudinal approaches more accurately describe people's experience than cross-sectional studies.
- Disability-free life expectancy is not increasing as fast as life expectancy in many countries.
- Inequalities in life and health expectancies between different social groups of older people appear to be increasing in the UK.

For a complete list of references, please visit www.expertconsult.com.

KEY REFERENCES

1. Oeppen J, Vaupel JW: Demography—broken limits to life expectancy. Science 296:1029–1031, 2002.
3. Fries JF: Aging, natural death, and the compression of morbidity. N Engl J Med 303:130–135, 1980.
4. Robine J-M, Michel J-P, Herrmann FR: Who will care for the oldest people? BMJ 334:570–571, 2007.
6. Cassel CK: Successful aging—how increased life expectancy and medical advances are changing geriatric care. Geriatrics 56:35–39, 2001.
8. Collerton J, Davies K, Jagger C, et al: Health and disease in 85 year olds: baseline findings from the Newcastle 85+cohort study. BMJ 339:b4904, 2009.
9. Rockwood K, Mitnitski A: Frailty in relation to the accumulation of deficits. J Gerontol A Biol Sci Med Sci 62:722–727, 2007.
11. Robine J-M, Ritchie K: Healthy life expectancy: Evaluation of a new global indicator of change in population health. BMJ 302:457–460, 1991.
18. Matthews FE, Arthur A, Barnes LE, et al: A two-decade comparison of prevalence of dementia in individuals aged 65 years and older from three geographical areas of England: results of the Cognitive Function and Ageing Study I and II. Lancet 382:1405–1412, 2013.
20. Reynolds SL, Saito Y, Crimmins EM: The impact of obesity on active life expectancy in older American men and women. Gerontologist 45:438–444, 2005.
21. van Gool CH, Picavet HSJ, Deeg DJH, et al: Trends in activity limitations: the Dutch older population between 1990 and 2007. Int J Epidemiol 40:1056–1067, 2011.
25. Freedman VA, Spillman BC, Andreski PM, et al: Trends in late-life activity limitations in the United States: an update from five national surveys. Demography 50:661–671, 2013.
28. Jylha M: What is self-rated health and why does it predict mortality? Towards a unified conceptual model. Soc Sci Med 69:307–316, 2009.
29. Martin-Ruiz CM, Gussekloo J, van Heemst D, et al: Telomere length in white blood cells is not associated with morbidity or mortality in the oldest old: a population-based study. Aging Cell 4:287–290, 2005.
32. Kingston A, Davies K, Collerton J, et al: The contribution of diseases to the male-female disability-survival paradox in the very old: results from the Newcastle 85+ Study. PLoS One 9:e88016, 2014.
33. Victor CR, Bowling A: A longitudinal analysis of loneliness among older people in Great Britain. J Psychol 146:313–331, 2012.
35. Stuck AE, Walthert JM, Nikolaus T, et al: Risk factors for functional status decline in community-living elderly people: a systematic literature review. Soc Sci Med 48:445–469, 1999.
36. Nusselder WJ, Franco OH, Peeters A, et al: Living healthier for longer: comparative effects of three heart-healthy behaviors on life expectancy with and without cardiovascular disease. BMC Public Health 9:487, 2009.
37. Pahor M, Guralnik J, Ambrosius W, et al: Effect of structured physical activity on prevention of major mobility disability in older adults. The LIFE Study Randomized Clinical Trial. JAMA 311:2387–2396, 2014.
40. Jagger C, Matthews R, Melzer D, et al: Educational differences in the dynamics of disability incidence, recovery and mortality: findings from the MRC Cognitive Function and Ageing Study (MRC CFAS). Int J Epidemiol 36:358–365, 2007.

3 The Future of Old Age

Caleb E. Finch, Edward L. Schneider

Biogerontology, the field of biologic aging research, is the final biomedical research frontier. The sequencing of the human genome and advancements in molecular technology have provided enormous potential for regenerative medicine. The list of readily replaceable body parts (e.g., eye lenses) and organs (e.g., hip joints, arterial transplants) will continue to grow. Even 30 years ago, little could be done to treat cataracts, but now lens replacements are routine surgical procedures. Advances in many disciplines have resulted in considerable insight into the diseases and disorders of aging. As we will discuss in this chapter, we propose that many more of the current common causes of morbidity and mortality can be eliminated in the upcoming decades. The final puzzle to be solved is the basic underlying cause of how we age. The exceptional life span of humans among primates may uncover aging changes that shorter lived species do not live long enough to incur. Human life span, already longer than any primate in premodern times, has more than doubled, whereas for those at age 70, the remaining life span has also more than doubled. Will this remarkable increase in longevity continue?

We have different backgrounds and have different expectations. CEF, as a molecular biologist, is more reserved about the pace of discovery on aging processes and demographic predictions for further increases than Edward Schneider LS who, as a physician-scientist, is more optimistic about the future benefits of biogerontology research. However, we agree on the challenges ahead from the current epidemic of obesity, as well as from antibiotic resistance and global environmental deterioration. Whatever the future of aging may be, we believe that a deeper understanding of aging will provide the gateway to extended life spans that are increasingly free of disease and disability. We have been debating these issues for several decades and hope that this chapter engages a broad audience of readers to explore the complexities of human aging along with us.

CHANGING LIFE SPANS

First, let us look at historical changes in the life span. Before 1800, life spans were very short, with life expectancies at birth of 30 to 40 years.[1,2] However, since 1800, human life expectancy has expanded in developing countries and has more than doubled, whether measured at birth or at age 70 years[1,3] (Figure 3-1).

About half of those born before 1800 did not reach the age of parenthood, and a mere 10%, at best, reached age 70. Then, during the industrial revolution, country after country developed better living conditions, with increased food distribution and improved hygiene, even before the understanding of infectious disease; after that came pasteurization and vaccination and finally, after WWII, antibiotics. Infectious disease dwindled from the major cause of death before 1900 to less than 5% of total deaths.[2,3] Now, most of us survive to older ages, where we accumulate the chronic diseases of aging, from atherosclerosis to cancer, and, if we live long enough, a rapidly increasing risk of Alzheimer disease (AD).[4,5]

These survival data can be further understood when plotted as mortality rates at each age of life (Figure 3-2). These are known as Gompertz curves, first described in 1825 by the Scottish actuary Benjamin Gompertz. After age 40, mortality rates accelerate, with a doubling every 7 to 8 years.[2,3,6] Sweden has the most comprehensive data obtained from nationwide household surveys that were initiated in the mid-eighteenth century (see Figure 3-2). The mortality rates in 1800 were high in the early years, starting with 10% to 30% infant mortality.[2,6] Even young adults in the eighteenth century had a 1% annual mortality rate. After about the age of 40, Sweden, like all other countries, shows accelerating (exponentially increasing) mortality rates, which are the basic manifestation of aging.

Note how the slope of the more recent population increases steadily with improving conditions, corresponding exactly to the increase in life expectancy shown in Figure 3-1. In fact, the curves get progressively steeper; paradoxically, as life spans have increased, the rates of mortality acceleration have also increased.[2,6] Note also that as infections were progressively minimized as a cause of early-age mortality, mortality at ages 10 to 40 years approached a minimum, below 0.1%/year. Those born most recently may now have an even lower mortality of 0.02%/year (2/10,000).[7] This historically unprecedented low baseline mortality represents deaths from conditions in which significant further reductions are unlikely (e.g., accidents, congenital defects, rare familial diseases). Across all ages, women have slightly lower mortality rates. Nonetheless, both genders incur mortality accelerations by the age of 40 years.

Maximum Life Spans: Have We Hit the Limit?

From these data on mortality rates, it can be calculated that the maximum human life spans are 120 for women and 113 for men,[6,7] which are very close to the reported records. Because world mortality data clearly show an approaching lower limit to baseline mortality without delay of the Gompertz mortality acceleration, we must consider that the continued expansion of human life span will soon reach a limit for the most populations. Since Jean Calment's record life span of 122 years in 1997, no one has exceeded 119 years, despite the avalanche of centenarians who are currently comprise the fastest growing age group. CF is thus reserved about predictions for 100-year life spans, based on forecasts[8] from the trends shown in Figure 3-1.

Compression of Morbidity

With increasing life spans came a new profile of disease. Instead of dying from infection, which was the norm before 1900, cancer, heart disease, and other chronic diseases of aging became increasingly prominent. Fries[9] hypothesized 3 decades ago that life expectancy had hit a barrier at age 85 years; as survival curves became more rectangular, the old age time of morbidity was hypothesized to become shorter before death. This compression of morbidity has the important implication that the shorter duration of morbidity would not increase health care costs for seniors, despite their longer life spans. The late Jacob Brody and ELS challenged this hypothesis.[10] Moreover, the recent analysis by Crimmins and Beltran-Sanchez[11] shows that increases in life expectancy have brought increased, not decreased, morbidity, with consequent skyrocketing increases in health care costs for seniors. Nonetheless, the faster acceleration of mortality has continued to rectangularize the survival curve, with little to no change in the maximum life span since 1980.

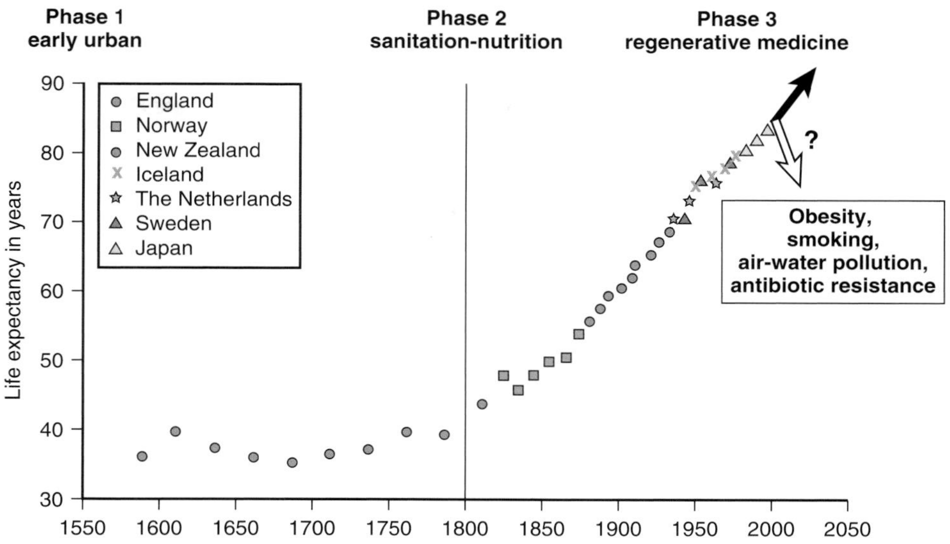

Figure 3-1. Life expectancy at birth, showing best practice countries from the human mortality database. *(Redrawn from Oeppen J, Vaupel JW: Demography. Broken limits to life expectancy. Science 296:1029-1031, 2002; additional information from Finch CE, Crimmins EM: Inflammatory exposure and historical changes in human life spans. Science 305:1736-1739, 2004.)*

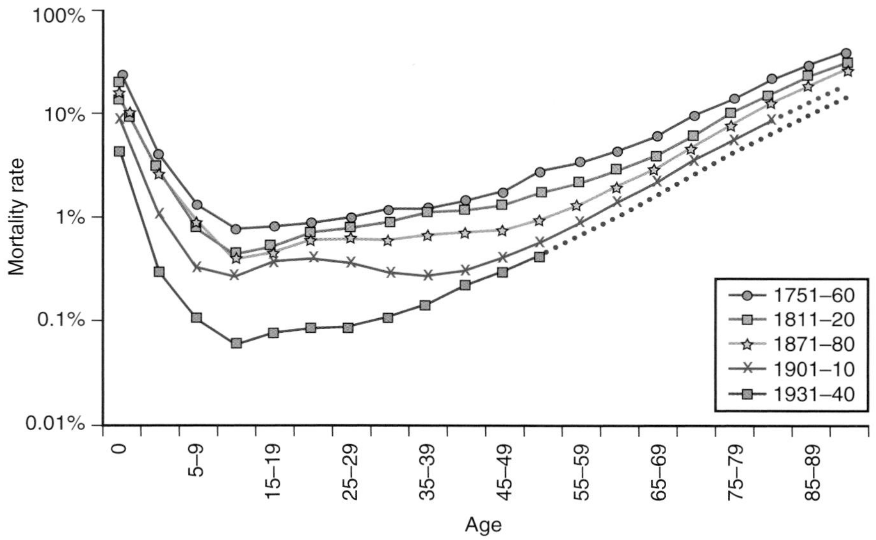

Figure 3-2. Annual mortality rates (% of age group dying per year) for Swedish birth cohorts across their life spans. *(Redrawn from Finch CE, Crimmins EM: Inflammatory exposure and historical changes in human life spans. Science 305:1736-1739, 2004.)*

What about future morbidity? To examine the future burden of disease, we must consider the major causes of death and disability at old ages. First, however, let's look at the potential impact of aging research, personalized medicine, artificial joints, and stem cells.

IMPACT OF BIOLOGICALLY ALTERING AGING PROCESSES

Almost all the diseases that we will discuss are diseases of older ages. The incidence of these conditions increases exponentially with aging, foreshadowing and anticipating the accelerating mortality rates of the Gompertz curve. Some diseases have been accelerating in regard to incidence even faster than the Gompertz curve. For example, AD incidence doubles every 5 years after age 60, and total mortality doubles every 7 to 8 years.[3,4] Longevity futurists are confronted with the depressing fact that most centenarians have clinical grade dementia.[5] Therefore, before considering expanding life expectancy, we must develop effective interventions to reduce or delay the incidence of AD and slow its course. For example, delaying the onset of AD by 5 years could cut its prevalence in half.[4] Biologists think this is possible because mice that are calorically restricted not only have increased life spans, but also have delayed onset of AD-like brain changes.[12]

Laboratory models have amply documented that every aspect of aging can be manipulated, from DNA damage to cross-linking of connective tissue collagen and elastin to ovarian egg cell loss to arterial lipids to brain amyloid levels.[3,12] In addition to food intake and exercise, aging processes can be manipulated by regulating gene activity without changing DNA sequence. We believe that it is within reach of the current younger generation of aging researchers to discover the molecular basis for aging fully.

However, it is unlikely that aging is controlled by a single gene or single biochemical or cellular mechanism.[3,13,14] Thus, we anticipate that multiple interventions will be developed for different aging pathways to slow or possibly reverse aging processes. Aging can be treated,[14] but interventions need to be initiated long before old age.

It is likely that antiaging interventions by specialized drugs and regenerative medicine for damaged organs is likely to be expensive. Already, even in nations with fully socialized medicine, older adults are given lower priority for major organ replacement. Drugs to slow AD and other dementias will be very expensive because of the huge costs in drug development However, those in poverty already age 10 years faster than the general U.S. population.[15] Thus, the so-called health elite, with ample private funds for medical treatment and potential rejuvenating therapy, may further deepen social disparities in health at later ages.

Personalized Aging Through Genome Sequencing

In the very near future, we anticipate that all initial health visits will include entire genome sequencing.[16] You and your physician will discuss potential genetic risk factors for various conditions and specific preventive measures. For example, carriers of genetic risk factors for type 2 diabetes would be counseled to avoid gaining substantial weight and exercise sufficiently. For cancer risk factors, frequent focused screening would be advised. Genome sequencing is already used to optimize cancer chemotherapy. In the future, there will be customized treatments for many other diseases and disorders that accompany aging, such as arthritis, hypertension, cardiovascular disease, and diabetes. DNA data will also decrease the incidence of adverse drug responses. For individuals with hypertension, the choice among antihypertensive treatments would be based on sequences that are most responsive to specific drugs.

Detrimental genes may also be removed, neutralized, or inactivated through targeted genetic therapies. Thus, the defective gene causing Huntington disease could theoretically be replaced after birth with the normal Huntington gene, even postnatally. Inherited disease–precipitating genes for hypercholesterolemia, hypertension, diabetes, and obesity could similarly be replaced by normal genes. Although personalized aging may permit the detection of probable causes of morbidity and mortality and lead to successful prevention, there will still be a need to repair damaged tissues and organs.

Artificial Joints and Repair of Compression Fractures

Osteoarthritis remains one of the leading causes of disability with aging. In the upcoming decades, we anticipate improvements in joint replacement and repair that will minimize the impact of this condition. Over the last few decades, knee and hip replacements have become commonplace, allowing relief from pain and increased function for those with severe arthritis of these joints.[17] We anticipate additional experience with shoulder, ankle, elbow, and wrist replacement surgeries that will make these procedures a viable approach to reduce pain and loss of functioning in these joints. Finally, vertebroplasty to restore compressed vertebrae to their original size can now effectively repair the vertebral compression fractures that occur commonly with aging.[18] We are optimistic about diminishing future disability from arthritis with the new technology for joint repair and replacement.

New Organs Through Stem Cells

In the near future, ES believes it likely that most organs can be regenerated or replaced. Thus, death and disability from organ failure, as well as organ transplantation, will be historical curiosities. Our old age–compromised immune systems will be able to be restored, and the increased mortality and morbidity associated with infectious diseases will be minimized. It may even be possible to infuse stem cell–derived neurons into the hippocampus and other areas to reverse age-related declines in memory and motor coordination. Infusion of neurons may also be an option for those suffering from AD and Parkinson disease. This may be more straightforward in Parkinson disease, where specific dopaminergic neurons degenerate, than in AD and other brain diseases with more diffuse neuron loss. CF, however, anticipates a very slow ascent up the steep slope of aging because of the enormous complexities of aging that must be unraveled, step by step.[13]

Figure 3-3 shows U.S. mortality trends by cause since 1960.[19] Heart disease continues to diminish, but only AD has increased, mostly due to greater survival to older ages.

Table 3-1 shows the top ten causes of death (in 2010).[20]

Cardiovascular Disease

We have witnessed extraordinary declines in heart disease over the last few decades that approach or even dip below mortality from cancer (see Figure 3-3). By 2008, the death rate for coronary heart disease was 72% lower than in 1950, and for stroke it was 78% lower.[21,22] By comparison, the death rate for all other conditions declined by just 15% during this time period.

What has caused this remarkable decline in mortality from heart disease and stroke? Having practiced medicine in 1960s, ES observed dramatic improvements in medical care during this era. In the 1960s, little could be done to prevent death from blocked coronary arteries beyond monitoring for arrhythmias and correcting them. Today, we can carry out rapid cardiac catheterization, enlarge narrowed coronary arteries with balloons, and place stents to restore blood flow and prevent death of heart muscle. Later, we can revascularize the heart through coronary artery bypass graft surgery. Treatment of congestive heart failure and heart arrhythmias has also improved dramatically. Rapid anticoagulation of stroke victims also prevents death and disability.

Declines in these conditions resulted from better scientific understanding of the risk factors, and also the development of new drugs to lower blood low-density lipoprotein (LDL) cholesterol levels and more effective antihypertensive agents. The continuing reduction in smoking[23] has also had a major role in the downward trends of atherosclerosis, hypertension, and cancer.

What will be available next in the upcoming decades? Although most low-hanging fruits may have already been plucked, we confidently anticipate improved diagnostic and therapeutic approaches to cardiovascular disease. Noninvasive diagnostic techniques may detect those individuals at risk for coronary and cerebral blood vessel occlusion.

Improvements in health behaviors by those detected to be at risk by genome sequencing could further reduce cardiovascular morbidity and mortality. The unknown in this equation is the expanding current obesity trend, which may limit the improvements in cardiovascular morbidity and mortality (see Figure 3-1).

Further discoveries on the aging process will yield new classes of drugs to maintain youthful vascular and myocardial health. Improved anticoagulants may more effectively lyse and remove blood clots in coronary and cerebral arteries. We anticipate that new drugs will reverse plaque formation and thus reverse cardiovascular disease. Statins may already prove to be shrinking atheromas. Nanotechnology and material sciences may produce nanoscale "roto-rooters" that crawl along arteries, chewing through arterial plaques. Backing up all these interventions will be the option to regenerate damaged heart tissues with stem cell–derived implants. It is highly likely that death from cardiovascular disease will diminish further as the leading cause of death.

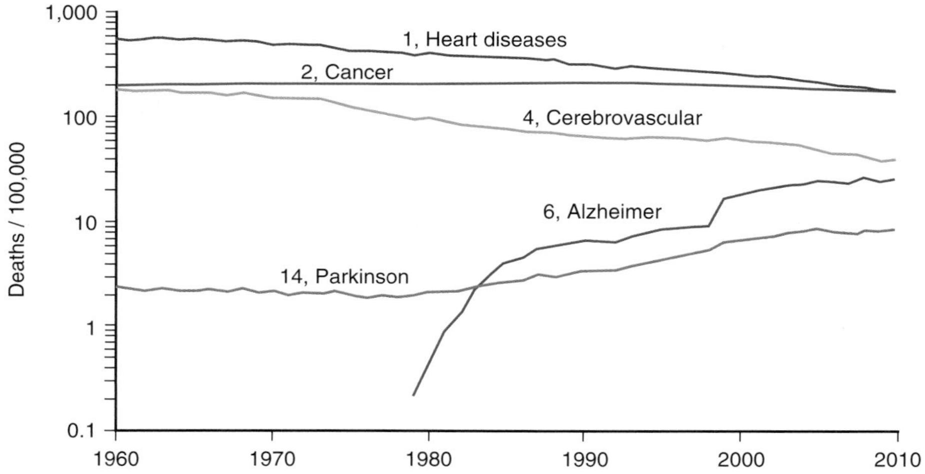

Figure 3-3. U.S. mortality by ranking cause. Not shown on the original graph, the third ranking cause of death is chronic lower respiratory disease, which had also decreased progressively to 5.6% of the total by 2010. *(Redrawn from National Institutes of Health; National Heart, Lung, and Blood Institute: Morbidity & mortality: chart book on cardiovascular, lung and blood diseases, 2012, p 25. http://www.nhlbi.nih.gov/files/docs/research/2012_ChartBook_508.pdf. Accessed September 7, 2015.)*

TABLE 3-1 Top Ten Leading Causes of Deaths in 2010, All Ages

Cause of Death	No. of Deaths
Heart disease	597,689
Cancer	574,743
Chronic lower respiratory disease	138,080
Stroke	129,476
Accidents	129,859
Alzheimer disease	83,494
Diabetes	69,071
Kidney disease	50,476
Influenza and pneumonia	50,097
Suicide	38,364

Data from

Cancer

Within the next few years, cancer will replace cardiovascular disease as the leading cause of death in the United States and other developed countries (see Figure 3-3). Although we have made some slight improvements in cancer mortality, they have not kept pace with the striking decline in cardiovascular mortality that has occurred since 1950. In our opinion, genome sequencing and tumor cell genome sequencing will change the course of cancers dramatically in the upcoming decades and cancer, like AIDS, will become a chronic condition that causes few deaths. Over the last decade, advances in cancer biology have transformed cancer therapy. DNA sequencing of cancer cells allows the design of drug treatments to target its mutant genes. The typical evolving mutations of cancer cells requires further DNA monitoring to optimize therapies. Thus, although overall morbidity from cancer may increase, we anticipate a substantial decrease in deaths from malignant diseases. Viruses are being developed that target and destroy specific tumor cells.[24] The micro-RNAs, whose dysregulation has been implicated in the development of many cancers, may soon be used in cancer therapy.[25]

Lung Disease

Chronic lung disease has surpassed stroke to assume its position as the third leading killer, after heart disease and cancer.[26] The future mortality related to this disorder will be linked to future smoking behaviors. Although U.S. smoking declined by half from 42% in 1965 to 19% in 2011, recent declines are less impressive.[23] The wild card is the expanding use of electronic cigarettes and legalization of marijuana, which produce potential carcinogens. It is unclear what impact electronic cigarettes will have on smoking habits or whether they will present a risk themselves. It is also not clear how increased use of marijuana will affect chronic obstructive pulmonary disease. We predict that because most current smokers have been smoking for decades, chronic lung disease will persist for several more decades as a leading cause of death. Stem cell–derived lungs may provide the option to smokers of replacing their damaged lungs.

Alzheimer Disease

The dementias of aging, once called senility, include AD as the majority core disorder, but also Lewy body dementia and frontotemporal dementia. Vascular damage often compounds the mental deterioration, especially at older ages. The total mortality from these disorders is unresolved. Often, death certificates will indicate pneumonia or cardiovascular disease as the cause of death in terminal AD patients. Unless an AD-modifying drug is developed,[4] the death rate from this condition will further escalate over the next few decades (see Figure 3-3) because, as described previously, the rate of AD increase with aging accelerates faster than mortality. Moreover, the successes in treating cancer and heart disease are allowing greater survival to later ages, with its greater risk of AD (see Figure 3-3). The pharmaceutical industry has spent several billions of dollars toward developing AD therapeutics without success; many promising candidate drugs and antibodies proved to have adverse side effects. We remain optimistic about the development of agents that will prevent or successfully treat the dementias of aging. However, we are depressed by the recent lack of government and private funding to combat this disease. In recognition of the enormous costs of AD, sustained increases in funding are warranted to develop effective interventions and attract the next generation of researchers.

Diabetes

Prediabetics can avoid becoming diabetics through exercise and proper diet. However, obesity, the biggest risk factor for type 2 diabetes, is increasing rapidly as a global epidemic that threatens to offset many medical advances to increase longevity. What will the future bring? The prevalence of type 2 diabetes will continue to increase until the so-called obesity epidemic is brought under control. Fortunately, we have new technology for monitoring blood sugar levels and the administration of insulin, which can ameliorate the presently widespread morbidity from blindness, heart and kidney disease, and peripheral vascular disease. The continuing declines in heart disease and cancer will probably soon elevate diabetes into one of the top three causes of morbidity. Again, replacement of damaged islet cells with stem cell–derived islet cells may restore normal glucose regulation in some diabetics.

Infectious Diseases

Infectious diseases were the most common causes of morbidity and mortality in adults until antibiotics became widely available by 1946 (see Figure 3-1). The new antiviral agents have been remarkably effective in combating human immunodeficiency virus infection and, most recently, hepatitis C. However, we fear the potential for explosive viral epidemics. Mutations in influenza, Middle East respiratory syndrome coronavirus (MERS-CoV), and Ebola and Marburg viruses, making them more transmissible, would cause substantial mortality.[27] We are still haunted by the 1919 influenza pandemic that killed 5% of the world's 1 billion population. We also worry about the development of multiple antibiotic-resistant conditions, such as tuberculosis and *Helicobacter pylori*. Rejuvenation of the immune system by stem cell therapy might reduce deaths from infections in older adults.

Accidents and Suicide

As death from various diseases declines, we expect deaths from accidents and suicides to result in proportionally more deaths. However, automobile accidents, which account for most accidental deaths, will certainly decline with the advent of technology to reduce driver error. The eventual introduction of driverless cars will have a great impact on reducing the incidence of driving deaths, most of which are related to alcohol consumption and/or sleep deprivation.

Kidney Disease

Kidney disease related to hypertension should decline with the increasing control of this disorder through medical treatment. However, the incidence of kidney disease related to diabetes will probably not change or even increase. Replacement of old and/or damaged kidneys by stem cell–derived organs will probably replace kidney transplantation and dialysis.

Environmental Concerns

We are deeply concerned about health consequences of the global changes in air pollution, warming, and rising coastal waters.[7] Global fossil fuel use continues as the main source of energy into the foreseeable future, and by 2040 is predicted to increase by 50%. Increased fossil fuel use for electric power and vehicular traffic portends further increases in air pollution, which has well-documented ill effects on lung and heart disorders. For example, household coal use in northern China since 1950 has shortened life expectancy by 5.5 years from cardiorespiratory mortality.[28] Surges in air pollution are associated with an increased risk of myocardial infarction (2.5%/100 $\mu g/m^3$ of particulate matter [PM]) 2.5 (airborne particles from fuel combustion, 2.5 μ in diameter[29]). Moreover, air pollution affects brain aging. Recent epidemiologic studies of large populations have shown that cognitive aging is accelerated by 2 to 3 years in association with gradients of ozone and PM2.5.[30,31] A study of the neurotoxic effects of urban air pollution found increased brain inflammation, but also altered glutamate receptors, which mediate memory.[32]

Global warming also affects older adults during heat waves, with higher mortality among men, as observed in the "killer summers" of 1995 and 2003. Most older adults live in cities, which are noted globally as heat islands. Here again we find a socioeconomic gradient, with higher mortality among older adults who cannot afford adequate ventilation or air conditioning. Increased infections are also likely because global warming favors insect expansion.[33] Furthermore, increased insect-borne infections are anticipated because the rising coastal water levels and flooding from extreme weather have expanded their breeding pools. Again, the health elites among older adults may be privileged to live in costly protected environments, as well as being able to afford the latest medical advances. (Some of these concerns for older adults as a vulnerable minority group were briefly addressed in 2010 by the National Academies of Science[33]). Thus, we predict that environmentally associated diseases will rise to the top by 2050 (Box 3-1).

BOX 3-1 Anticipated Top Five Causes of Death in 2050

1. Environmentally associated diseases—ischemic heart disease, stroke, cancer, chronic lower respiratory disease
2. Accidents
3. Diabetes
4. Multiple antibiotic-resistant infections—pneumonia, influenza, tuberculosis—and new pandemics
5. Suicide, homicide

FUTURE OF GERIATRICS

Despite the growth of the older population and future projections for acceleration in the growth rate of those over ages 65, 75, and 85 years, there is a shortage of geriatricians. We believe that this is related to the low pay that this group receives for its services, despite the increased complexity of their patients and increased time they spend with their patients. It is a challenge to attract medical students to geriatrics with the enormous debts that accumulate during their undergraduate and graduate education; medical students graduating in 2012 held average debts of $166,750. In 2012, the average compensation for an anesthesiologist was $432,000, for a general surgeon, $367,885, and for an obstetrician-gynecologist, $301,700.[34,35] The Bureau of Labor Statistics does not even list a salary for a geriatrician, which is usually the same or below that of a general practitioner, $184,000.[36] Thus, without enormous dedication to serving an aging population, it is hard for students to choose an underpaying specialty that makes it extremely hard for them to pay off their student loans.

Statistics also indicate that the number of residents choosing to enter geriatric residency programs decreased from 112 in 2005 to 75 in 2013.[36] Because so few medical students and fellows are choosing geriatrics, we have only about 7,500 geriatricians in the United States, despite the future need for 30,000.

We anticipate that the federal administration and Congress will, in the near future, recognize the importance of geriatricians to the future care and well-being of older Americans. Even if not motivated by altruism, U.S. congressional and individual state legislators will discover that efficient management of transitions in care is the key to constraining current and future health care costs. They may then move aggressively to increase reimbursement for geriatric care that, in turn, will encourage more physicians to choose careers in this important field.[37]

FUTURE OF FRAILTY

Since the valuable definition of frailty by Fried and colleagues,[38] considerable research has linked this phenotype with an increased risk of morbidity and higher health care costs.[39-42] Earlier in this chapter, we considered future biomedical advances that should reduce the impact of, or even eliminate, many current diseases and disorders that afflict older persons. However, we must ask whether the decreased impact of disease will necessarily reduce frailty or if frailty will increase as specific diseases are conquered. This is difficult to predict. What we can expect is the future development of assistive devices that range from driverless cars to programmable robots,[43-44] which should alleviate some burdens of frailty, as well as improve rehabilitation from falls and stroke, step by step.

Acknowledgments

CF is grateful for support from the National Institutes of Health (R21, AG-040683; P01 AG-026572, R. Brinton, PI; P01 ES-022845, R. McConnell, PI) and from the Cure Alzheimer's Fund.

KEY POINTS

1. Personalized aging strategies by identified genetic risk factors will have an impact on successful aging.
2. Artificial joints and stem cells will repair damaged joints and organs, reducing morbidity and mortality.
3. Deaths from cardiovascular disease and stroke will continue to decline.
4. Cancer will become the leading cause of death, pending future treatments.
5. Until reimbursement paradigms are changed, the shortage of geriatricians will continue, despite the urgent demand and diminishing numbers.
6. Biologic aging may be altered in the future by multiple interventions that target specific aging pathways.

For a complete list of references, please visit www.expertconsult.com.

KEY REFERENCES

3. Finch CE: The biology of human longevity. Inflammation, nutrition, and aging in the evolution of life spans, San Diego, 2007, Academic Press.
4. Khachaturian Z: Prevent Alzheimer's disease by 2020: a national strategic goal. Alzheimers Dement 5:81–84, 2009.
7. Finch CE, Beltran-Sanchez H, Crimmins EM: Uneven futures of human life spans: reckoning the realities of climate change with predictions from the Gompertz model. Gerontology 60:183–188, 2014.
10. Schneider EL, Brody JA: Aging, natural death, and the compression of morbidity: another view. N Engl J Med 309:854–856, 1983.
14. Fontana L, Kennedy BK, Longo VD, et al: Medical research: treat ageing. Nature 511:405–407, 2014.
15. Crimmins EM, Kim JK, Seeman TE: Poverty and biological risk: the earlier "aging" of the poor. J Gerontol A Biol Med Sci. 64:286–292, 2009.
32. Ailshire JA, Crimmins EM: Fine particulate matter air pollution and cognitive function among older US adults. Am J Epidemiol 180:359–366, 2014.
38. Fried LP, Tangen CM, Walston J, et al: Frailty in older adults: evidence for a phenotype. J Gerontol A Biol Med Sci 56:M146–M156, 2001.
39. Blodgett J, Theou O, Kirkland S, et al: The association between sedentary behaviour, moderate-vigorous physical activity and frailty in NHANES cohorts. Maturitas 80:187–191, 2015.
40. Cawthon PM, Marshall LM, Michael Y, et al: Frailty in older men: prevalence, progression and relationship with mortality. J Am Geriatr Soc 55:1216–1223, 2007.
41. Ensrud KE, Ewing SK, Taylor BC, et al: Frailty and risk of falls, fracture and mortality in older women: the study of osteoporotic fractures. J Gerontol A Biol Med Sci 62:744–751, 2007.
43. Massie CL, Kantak SS, Narayanan P, et al: Timing of motor cortical stimulation during planar robotic training differentially impacts neuroplasticity in older adults. Clin Neurophysiol 126:1024–1032, 2015.

4 Successful Aging: The Centenarians

Thomas T. Perls

DEMOGRAPHY OF CENTENARIANS

According to the U.S. Social Security Administration, in 2010, approximately 51,000 people aged 100 years and older collected Social Security benefits.[1] The U.S. census reported a similar number of 53,364 and an overall prevalence of 1.73 centenarians/10,000 people, with 80% of centenarians being women.[1] In the 1980s and 1990s, centenarians were deemed the fastest growing age group in the population (65.8% from 1980 to 2000) but, in 2007, the Census Bureau's Velkoff and Humes indicated that the earlier reported numbers were artificially too high.[2] In its 2010 report on centenarians, the U.S. Census indicated a 5.8% increase in centenarians from 2000 to 2010, whereas the overall population grew by 9.7%. On the other hand, octogerians and nonagerians are the fastest growing groups, with 21% and 30% growth, respectively, over the same period of time.

Figure 4-1 depicts the proportions of centenarians in other countries also noted by the census report on centenarians.[3] It is impressive that the proportion in Japan is twice that of the United States.

EXTRAORDINARY AGE CLAIMS

The oldest ever valid age claim is that of Jeanne Calment, who was from Southern France and died at the age of 122 years and 164 days in 1997.[4] The record for a man was recently established by a Japanese man named Jiroemon Kimura, who died at the age of 115 years and 253 days in 2013 (birth date, April 19, 1897). It is not unusual to hear of claims of people exceeding these ages, but 99% of claims of ages older than 115 years are false.[5] A clear tipoff that a claim is false is when someone is claimed to be the oldest person ever, and yet there was no mention of their age when they exceeded the current record of 122 years. For example, in 2009, the extraordinary age claim of Sakhan Dosova, of Kazakhstan, purported to be 130 years old (1879-2009), was published in a popular scientific journal, despite the fact that she never attracted attention when she surpassed 122 years and that there was no documentation supporting her being alive in the early 1880s.[6]

In 2014, according to the Gerontology Research Group (www.grg.org), there were approximately 62 supercentenarians (aged 110+ years) in the United States or a prevalence of about 1/5 million people. The Social Security Administration's Kestenbaum and Ferguson counted 325 supercentenarians who died in the period 1980 to 2003 and 90% of these were female.[7] In light of the above observations, the 2010 U.S. and Japanese census reports very likely list far too many supercentenarians, 330 (~1/400,000) and 711 (~1/180,000), respectively, speaking to the high false-positive rate for counts of supercentenarians in many national censuses.[8,9]

THE GENDER DISPARITY

Although female centenarians outnumber their male counterparts by approximately 8:1, male centenarians tend to have significantly better functional status than their female counterparts. The fact that male centenarians more frequently have better physical and cognitive function has been noted in most centenarian studies, most notably the Italian Centenarian Study.[10] A plausible hypothesis for why male centenarians fare better is that only those who are functionally independent are able to achieve such extreme old age. Women, on the other hand, appear to experience the double-edged sword of being able to live longer while also living more frequently with age-related illnesses and disability. This hypothesis is supported by a Danish study, in which 38% of men at age 98 years were functionally independent, but then this proportion rose to 53% among 100-year-olds. The proportion of women who were independent, however, continued to fall, from 30% of 98-year-olds to 28% of 100-year-olds.[11] Another paradox is that although the male centenarians might be exceptionally fit relative to the women, they appear to have higher age-related, disease-associated mortality rates, so that once they do develop a disease, such as dementia or stroke, their mortality risk probably is much higher than it might be for women. Such hypotheses point to the possibility that women are much more resilient than men with regard to aging and age-related diseases.

SUCCESSFUL AGING

In the New England Centenarian Study (NECS; http://www.bumc.bu.edu/centenarian), centenarians and their family members were studied primarily because of our long-held belief that these individuals are a model of successful aging. By determining environmental and genetic factors that are more or less common compared to those of other groups of people, we should be able to determine risk factors for premature versus healthy aging and to formulate strategies that enhance a person's ability to compress their disability toward the end of a longer life.

In 1980, James Fries proposed his "Compression of Morbidity" hypothesis.[12] This hypothesis states that as people approach the limit of their life span, they necessarily must compress the time that they experience diseases that affect mortality toward the end of their life. Previously, when the NECS investigated this hypothesis, with its sample of 424 centenarians, mean age 102 years, it was found that centenarians did not all exhibit this compression. Instead, a substantial proportion (43%), termed *survivors*, lived with at least one of 10 age-related diseases—heart disease, stroke, diabetes, cancer, dementia, chronic obstructive lung disease, osteoporosis, hypertension—for 20 years or more. Another 42%, termed *delayers*, lived with such a disease(s) between the ages of 80 and 99 years. Finally, those who had none of these diagnoses at the age of 100 years, or *escapers*, comprised 15% of the sample.[13] Of note, a study of the oldest subjects in the Health and Retirement Survey found a similar proportion of escapers.[14] Thus, our findings appeared to be inconsistent with the Compression of Morbidity hypothesis. On the other hand, it was also noted that on average, these subjects were disability-free until the age of 93 years.[15] Thus there appeared to generally be a compression of disability among centenarians, even despite a substantial incidence of age-related morbidities. Somehow, it seems that people who survive to 100 and older deal with these age-related diseases more effectively than other people with such diseases who die at a younger age. The ability to deal with stressors and, more generally, age-related diseases, leads to the as yet poorly defined notions of adaptive capacity, functional reserve, and resilience, which may be important distinguishing features of the ability to achieve exceptional old age.[16]

We suspected that to observe the compression of the morbidity phenomenon, we needed to include subjects who truly

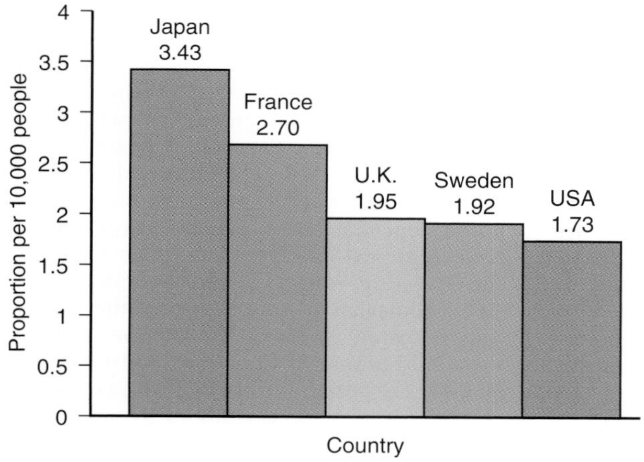

Figure 4-1. Proportion of centenarians/10,000 people in each of the countries noted.

survived near the limit of the human life span. There is a tremendous degree of selection (very large proportions of the sample die) that occurs between the ages of 100 to 104 years and 110+ years, and thus it would make sense that there could be a significant difference between these age groups in terms of determinants of survival. Thus, since 2007, we made a concerted effort to enroll and longitudinally follow as many people aged 105+ years as possible. With a total sample of 343 nonagerian siblings of centenarians, 884 100- to 104-year-olds, 430 105- to 109-year-olds, and 104 110+-year-olds, and 90% of the subjects deceased, we analyzed the ages of onset of cancer, cardiovascular disease, diabetes, dementia, and stroke.[17] We found that the ages of onset of numerous diseases were increasingly delayed with the older and older ages of the subjects in our NECS sample. For example, in Figure 4-2, Kaplan-Meyer survival curves show this progressive delay in age of onset for cancer, cardiovascular disease, and overall morbidity, where at least one of the following became clinically apparent—cardiovascular disease, cancer, diabetes, dementia, and/or stroke. Consistent with the Compression of Morbidity hypothesis, controls (spouses of the offspring of centenarians or the offspring of parents with an average life expectancy) experienced a mean 17.9% of their lives with one or more age-related diseases, centenarians (100 to 104 years) with 9%, semisupercentenarians (105 to 109 years) with 8.9%, and supercentenarians with 5.2%.

These findings have important implications for the study of the basic biology of aging. As Fries' article indicated, the compression of morbidity toward the end of life would implicate an overall exhaustion of organ reserve as the cause of death in these individuals.[12] Anecdotally, this is what we observed in most supercentenarians. Furthermore, this progressive rectangularization of the survival curve with older and older ages of death also suggests a limit to the human life span. Finally, the fact that most of the supercentenarians in our sample experienced morbidity and disability in only the last few years of their lives indicates substantial phenotypic homogeneity. This homogeneity suggests an increased power with these samples of oldest subjects to discover environmental and genetic determinants that they have in common that promote such exceptional survival.

PHENOTYPIC ASSOCIATIONS

There do not appear to be specific health behaviors that are consistently associated with exceptional longevity. However, that is not to say that for many people achieving these extreme ages, certain behaviors such as smoking would have caused their death

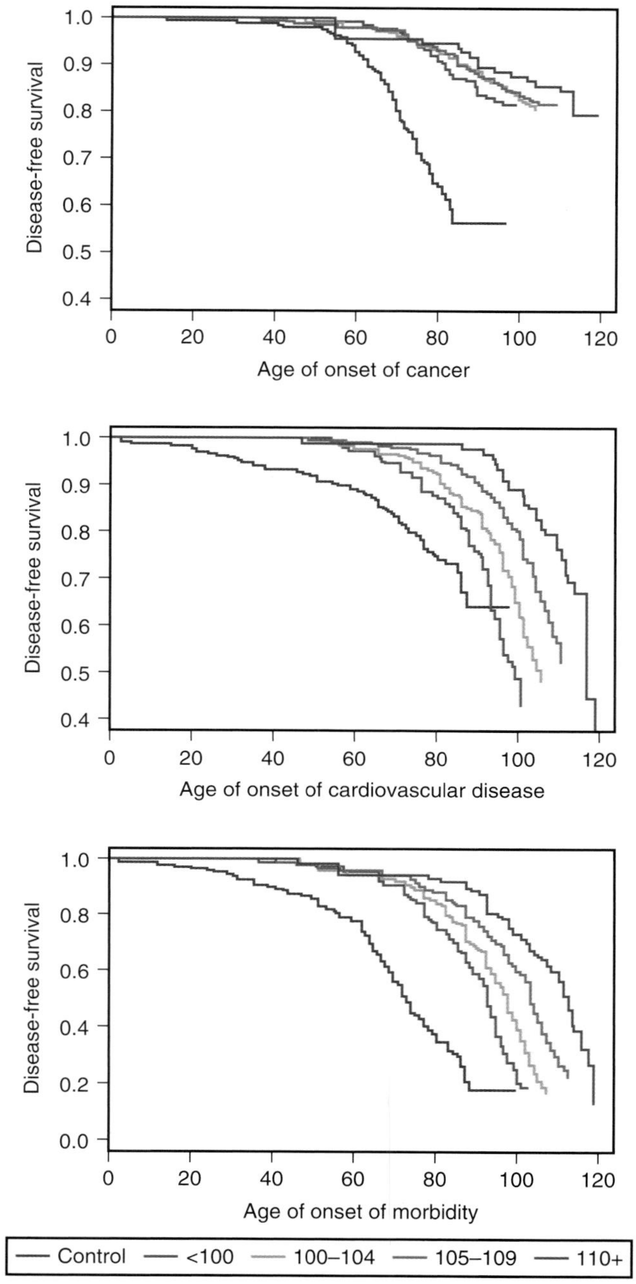

Figure 4-2. Kaplan-Meyer survival curves display disease-free survival for centenarians stratified by age (in years) at death and population controls: controls, *blue*; nonagerians, *red*; centenarians, *green*; semisupercentenarians, *yellow*; supercentenarians, *orange*.

at a substantially younger age. Alternatively, in some groups, healthy habits such as a Mediterranean diet may be an essential ingredient for exceptional longevity. It would make sense in terms of evolutionary theory that different ethnicities, environments, and cultures lead to different combinations of genetic and environmental variants that predispose to exceptional survival.

Personality

Some phenotypes have been associated with exceptional longevity, including certain personality types and maternal age. The

NECS assessed personality traits in the children of centenarians and found that both the males and females scored below normative values for neuroticism and above normal for extraversion. For the other personality domains of the NEO Five Factor Inventory, the offspring scored within normal range.[18] Similar findings were made with the offspring generation of the Long Life Family Study.[19] These findings make sense in light of the substantial literature demonstrating associations between elevated neuroticism and morbidities such as hypertension and cardiovascular disease.[20] Elevated extraversion could indicate a propensity to effectively establish social relationships conducive to better cognitive and psychological health. The Tokyo Centenarian Study, led by Hirose, found, however, that their centenarian subjects scored within the normal range for neuroticism but elevated openness, indicating the possibility that cultures and ethnicities can differ in regard to which personality traits are associated with exceptional longevity.[21]

Maternal Age

As discussed later, there is a growing body of evidence for a substantial genetic influence on survival to the most extreme ages. An important question is what would be the selection pressure(s) for the evolution of longevity-associated genetic variants. The pressure to have a longer period of time during which women can bear children and therefore have more of them, with greater success in passing one's genes down to subsequent generations, could be one such pressure.[22] This hypothesis is consistent with the disposable soma theory, in which the tradeoff in energy allocation between reproductive fitness and repair and maintenance functions can be delayed when longevity-associated variants facilitate slower aging and the delay or prevention of age-related diseases that also adversely affect fertility.[23]

Several studies have noted an association between older maternal age and increased odds of exceptional survival. The NECS assessed maternal age history in its sample of female centenarians and a birth cohort–matched referent sample of women who survived to the cohort's average life expectancy. Women who gave birth to a child after the age of 40 years (fertility assistance was not technologically available to this cohort) had four times greater odds of being a centenarian.[24] Other studies have noted such a correlation.[25-27] Numerous investigators are now searching for and investigating genes that influence reproductive fitness in terms of their ability also to influence rate of aging and susceptibility to age-related diseases.[28-30]

FAMILIAL ASSOCIATION AND HERITABILITY

Early on in the NECS, we discovered several families in which multiple siblings lived to such extreme ages that the probability of such clustering being observed would be fewer than one family per all the families existing in the world at the time.[31] Thus, for such families to exist, the family members with the trait must have some factors in common, and this could not be simply due to chance. Family members have genetic and nongenetic factors in common, and nongenetic factors have clearly been associated with increased probability of survival to older age, including education, socioeconomic status, access to health care, diet, environmental exposures (good and bad), refraining from tobacco use and excess alcohol, and others. Equally apparent is that some of these factors are not purely nongenetic because genetic associations have been noted for traits such as tobacco and alcohol use.

Sibling studies allow for the estimation of sibling recurrent risk for a trait expressed by another sibling. An initial study by the NECS found that siblings of centenarians had about a four times increased relative risk of living to 100 years compared to birth cohort–matched controls who did not have parental exceptional longevity.[32] That work was limited by a relatively small sample and the relatively young age of the centenarian probands. Similarly powered studies from Iceland and Utah have produced sibling relative risks in this range.[33,34] Later, when the New England study had many more centenarians who also had reached a substantially older age, the sibling relative risk for males was 18 and, for females, 8.5.[35] The increased relative risk noted in males has been observed in other studies and suggests that males are more dependent on a genetic component than females to achieve exceptional longevity.[36]

The heritability of aging, longevity, and life span has been noted by different Scandinavian twin studies and a study of Amish pedigrees to be approximately 25% to 30%. The ages at death of the subjects in these studies ranged from 73 (standard deviation [SD], 16) and 71 (SD, 17) years (52nd and 49th percentiles of survival).[37,38] In a 1998 Swedish twins study of longevity, which also interchangeably uses the term *life span*, no men in the sample lived past the age of 89 years and about 2% of the female sample lived to the age of 90+ years. This study estimated the genetic component of longevity to be about 33%.[39] In a 2001 study, "Heritability of Life Span in the Old Order Amish," the authors investigated Amish pedigrees for parental and offspring ages of death for subjects born prior to 1890 who survived to at least the age of 30 years. The mean age of death was 71 ± 16 years, and about 7% of the sample was aged 90+ years, with only a few subjects aged 95+ years, and they estimated the heritability of both to be 25 ± 5%.[40]

With percentiles of survival nowhere approaching those of centenarians (e.g., <1 percentile), the previously mentioned twin and other studies have little to do with exceptional longevity, and research and review articles continue misguidedly to promote the idea that the heritability of survival to an extreme age does not change with older and older ages and is relatively low, at about 25%. Furthermore, many people erroneously equate heritability with genetic contribution. Instead, heritability is a measure of familiality, which is due to genetic and environmental factors that family members have in common and that can influence the trait in question.[41] Consistent with these studies, the Seventh Day Adventist Health Study suggested that average humans can, in the setting of specific healthy behaviors, achieve an average life expectancy of 86 years.[42]

The NECS investigated sibling relative risk according to the proband's percentile of survival and the year in which they were born. Analyzing survival data from 1917 sibships in which at least one sibling survived to the age of 90 years or older, we found that sibling relative risk increases with older and older age of the proband and with earlier birth year of the proband at these ages. The siblings of males surviving to the fifth percentile (age 90 for those born in 1900) have themselves a 1.7 times greater chance of living to the same age compared to population controls. Siblings of males and females surviving to the oldest 0.01 percentile of survival have a 35.6 times greater chance of surviving to the same age.[43] It should be noted, however, that just because the chances are so much greater for these siblings than for the average person from the same birth cohort, it does not mean that they are assured of living to such an age because, after all, it remains an exceptionally rare phenotype. These findings also illustrate how very important it is for studies of the oldest old to describe precisely the phenotype they are studying by including the birth year cohort and the participants' percentile(s) of survival.

GENETIC DETERMINANTS

Sensitivity, Specificity, and Power

If one thing is clear, survival to extreme old age is a complex trait that survival to the 0.1 percentile (which for the 1900 birth cohort is about age 105) involves multiple subphenotypes, ranging from different rates and onsets of age-related diseases and different reactions to protective and destructive behavioral and environmental factors. For rarer survival, less than the 0.1 percentile, the survival phenotype, although still complex, may be more homogeneous, and therefore the power to discover underlying determinants may be greater than for less extreme survival.[44] For this reason, the Japanese and New England Centenarian Studies have for the past 5 years emphasized the recruitment of people aged 105+ years. Tan and colleagues found that the power to discover longevity-associated genetic variants significantly increases when studying centenarians instead of nonagerians.[43] Sebastiani and associates showed that the ability of a genetic model consisting of 281 single-nucleotide polymorphisms (SNPs) to distinguish between centenarians and average healthy people markedly improved with older age among the centenarians.[45] Along these lines, the failure of studies to discover associations with specific genetic variants could be due to the lack of power resulting from the sample not being phenotypically select enough (e.g., subjects who could be select enough are <0.1 percentile for survival or <1 percentile and being functionally independent, which would also be very rare). Similarly, lack of replication of many genetic findings may be the consequence of too much genetic background heterogeneity (e.g., statistically not accounting for multiple ethnicities).

Approaches to Gene Discovery

The major experimental designs for discovering genetic variants associated with exceptional survival or associated subphenotypes are genome-wide linkage mapping and association studies and candidate gene association studies.

Linkage Studies

A nonparametric linkage approach was used for the study of 137 NECS sibships (308 long-lived siblings), and a significant LOD (logarithm of odds) score was noted for a linkage peak on chromosome 4.[46] The linkage results were replicated by a study that used dizygous twins older than 90 years.[47] A subsequent study found that the likely gene responsible for the linkage was microsomal transfer protein (MTP).[48] Studies of nonagerians and, in one case, centenarians, declared that they could not replicate the association with MTP.[49-51] Subsequently, however, the Ashkenazi Jewish Centenarian Study noted that the CC genotype is significantly associated with the centenarian and offspring samples compared to controls. According to the authors, what might have led to negative findings in the younger sample studies was that in the Ashkenazi sample, there was an age-dependent, U-shaped distribution for this genotype, where its frequency declined from ages 50 to 85 years and then began to increase in the nonagerian years.[51,52] Additional nonparametric linkage analyses in centenarians have provided evidence for linkage in chromosomes 3, 9, 13, 14, and 19, but these results need to be followed up to identify specific loci implicated with exceptional longevity.[53-55]

Candidate Genes

Candidate gene association studies are hypothesis-driven selections of specific genes, which are then tested for association with the trait of interest, such as exceptional survival or its subphenotypes. These selection(s) can be based on their involvement in biologic pathways believed to influence life span or they could be gene(s) in or near a linkage peak previously associated with longevity. Several genes in the insulin signaling pathway (*AKT1, FOXO3, IGF1R*) have been the focus of attention in human longevity because of their dramatic effect on life span in lower organisms and other animal models.[56-59] Although the associations of many of these genes have been replicated in more than one study, the effects are small, and so far no gene associated with dramatic increase of life span in an animal model has reproduced a similar effect on human longevity. Other associations with exceptional longevity include genes involved with lipid metabolism (*CETP, APOC3*),[60,61] extreme variations of the human life span (*LMNA*,[61] *WRN*[44,62]), and neurologic disease (*APOE*,[63] *ADARB2*[64]). The first and most well-known genetic variant associated with being a centenarian is the E4 allele of apolipoprotein E, but this variant has a negative association with centenarians in that its frequency is much lower common compared to controls, presumably due to its association with vascular and Alzheimer disease.[63]

Genome-Wide Association Studies

Association studies typically include unrelated individuals and aim to identify genetic variants that correlate with the phenotype in a random sample of subjects. Genome-wide association studies (GWAS) are based on the assumption that the trait being investigated is influenced by common genetic variants (allele frequency > 5%), an assumption otherwise known as the common disease, common variant hypothesis.[65,66] The NECS conducted a unique analysis of GWAS data to discover combinations of genetic variants that are jointly associated with different chance of exceptional longevity.[45,67] The GWAS data was comprised of 801 centenarians (median age at death, 104 years) and genetically matched controls, genotyped at approximately 250K SNPs. The association of each SNP with exceptional longevity was first scored using a Bayesian method, and SNPs were ranked by the strength of these associations. Nested genetic risk prediction models were then determined, starting with the model that used only the most significant SNP for prediction, and adding one SNP at a time from the ordered list of SNPs until sensitivity and specificity of the model did not increase significantly. This approach identified 281 SNPs (and 281 genetic risk models) as being most predictive of exceptional longevity, and an ensemble of all these 281 models was then used for prediction. When evaluated in independent GWAS data of centenarians and controls, the ensemble of genetic models reached 60% specificity and a sensitivity ranging between 58% to predict nonagerians and centenarians and 85% to predict centenarians who lived to the age of 105 years and older. The greater sensitivity to recognize centenarians who lived to extremely old ages supports the hypothesis that the genetic component of survival to older and older ages becomes progressively stronger.[45]

The ensemble of genetic risk models was then used to generate genetic risk profiles of exceptional longevity that by cluster analysis, were used to group centenarians based on different genetic signatures of exceptional longevity. The genetic signatures represent combinations of genetic variants that produce a similar chance or probability for exceptional longevity and, interestingly, they correlated with different subphenotypes of extreme survival. For example, the signature that is most predictive of extreme longevity correlated with a significantly longer life span and delay of onset of dementia. Other examples include the first attempt to dissect the complex genetic base of exceptional longevity.[45]

The 281 SNPs identified with this analysis point to 130 genes and several regulatory regions. Some of the 130 genes are well-known longevity genes, such as *LMNA*, *WRN*, and *APOE*. Interestingly, one SNP in *TOMM40/APOE* reached genome-wide significance but had a very small genetic effect, and removing this SNP from the ensemble of genetic risk models did not affect the predictive accuracy. In addition to this SNP, no other SNP reached genome-wide significance by itself in the GWAS in the

NECS. This is consistent with results from other GWAS of aging and longevity that failed to discover SNPs that reached genome-wide significance, even with substantially larger sample sizes.[68-71] A meta-analysis determined that 128 of the 281 genetic variants were significantly associated with exceptional longevity in at least one of five centenarian studies.[72] These findings are consistent with the hypothesis that individual genes have modest effects on exceptional longevity, and therefore do not meet standard significance levels in a GWAS. However, combinations of many specific genes can have a very strong effect, especially for survival beyond the age of 105 years.

An additional secondary analysis of genetic data showed that centenarians from the NECS carry an average rate of disease variants discovered through GWAS as population controls. This result agrees with findings from the Leiden Longevity Study, which showed that the rate of disease-associated variants in their nonagerian sample was the same as in the general population.[73] Therefore, people who survive to extreme old age (with a few exceptions, such as apolipoprotein E-4) appear to have just as many disease variants as the general population. The genetic difference for these individuals is that they likely have higher frequencies of longevity or protective genetic variants that slow aging and decrease or delay the risk for age-related diseases.

WHOLE GENOME SEQUENCING

The lack of discovery of genes with major effects on human exceptional longevity suggests that many gene variants with individually modest effects contribute to this trait. Some of these gene variants may be rare in the population, and the recent technology of whole genome sequencing may provide additional discovery power. The NECS published the whole genome sequences of two supercentenarians and used the data to test some genetic models of human longevity.[74] These two sequences are a first step toward the generation of a reference panel of exceptionally long-lived individuals.

FUTURE DIRECTIONS

Research on human exceptional longevity has delivered many important discoveries about the genetic and nongenetic determinants of this trait. There is clear evidence that extreme human longevity has a strong genetic basis likely to be determined by many rare and common genetic variants interacting in synergistic and antagonistic ways. Genetic association studies have discovered possible modifiers but many remain to be discovered, and their roles in biologic mechanisms that link genotype to phenotype remain to be elucidated. Functional experiments that try to assess the individual effects of these variants with longevity may fail or be suboptimal because they would ignore other interacting genetic variants. A systems-based approach will be necessary to discover their roles in extending life span and health span, and new experimental models based, for example, on induced pluripotent stem cells may be useful. Also, several studies have shown that centenarians have many of the disease-associated variants found in the general population. This finding suggests that centenarians may carry protective variants that counter the effects of deleterious variants, slow the rate of aging, and decrease the risk for age-related diseases that contribute to premature mortality. Discovery of these protective variants and subsequent functional studies to determine the roles they play in slowing aging and decreasing the risk for age-related diseases will be major steps forward in the area of predictive and preventive medicine.

KEY POINTS: SUCCESSFUL AGING: THE CENTENARIANS

- Centenarians remain rare, at about 1.7/10,000 people. In 2015, there were about 50,000 centenarians in the United States. In 1980, the rate was about 1/10,000. Among the 1910 birth cohort, men ages 95+ years and women ages 100+ years fall into the top first percentile of survival. Supercentenarians, those who are 110+ years old, occur at a rate of about 1/5 million. There are currently about 50 "supers" in the United States and 350 worldwide.
- Compression of disability, rather than of morbidity, is common among centenarians, with over 90% having a history of being functionally independent at about age 93 years. However, most people who survive to ages older than 106 years essentially compress the time they experience disease and disability toward the relative ends of their lives, consistent with the compression of morbidity hypothesis.
- Although far fewer (≈15% of centenarians), male centenarians tend to have significantly better cognitive and physical function compared to female centenarians.
- Living beyond the top first percentile of survival runs strongly in families. Centenarians have just as many disease-associated genetic variants as the general population. What likely makes a survival difference for them is the presence of longevity or protective genetic variants. Single genetic variants have modest effects on the variation in survival to extreme ages, but many (hundreds) specific variants in specific combinations ("genetic signatures") can have a very strong influence, particularly to survive beyond age 105 years.

For a complete list of references, please visit www.expertconsult.com.

KEY REFERENCES

5. Young RD, Desjardins B, McLaughlin K, et al: Typologies of extreme longevity myths. Curr Gerontol Geriatr Res 2010:423087, 2010.
10. Franceschi C, Motta L, Valensin S, et al: Do men and women follow different trajectories to reach extreme longevity? Italian Multicenter Study on Centenarians (IMUSCE). Aging (Milano) 12:77–84, 2000.
11. Christensen K, McGue M, Petersen I, et al: Exceptional longevity does not result in excessive levels of disability. Proc Natl Acad Sci U S A 105:13274–13279, 2008.
13. Evert J, Lawler E, Bogan H, et al: Morbidity profiles of centenarians: survivors, delayers, and escapers. J Gerontol A Biol Sci Med Sci 58:232–237, 2003.
17. Andersen SL, Sebastiani P, Dworkis DA, et al: Health span approximates life span among many supercentenarians: compression of morbidity at the approximate limit of life span. J Gerontol A Biol Sci Med Sci 67:395–405, 2012.
18. Givens JL, Frederick M, Silverman L, et al: Personality traits of centenarians' offspring. J Am Geriatr Soc 57:683–685, 2009.
22. Perls TT, Fretts RC: The evolution of menopause and human life span. Ann Hum Biol 28:237–245, 2001.
24. Perls T, Alpert L, Fretts R: Middle-aged mothers live longer. Nature 389:133, 1997.
26. Smith KR, Gagnon A, Cawthon RM, et al: Familial aggregation of survival and late female reproduction. J Gerontol A Biol Sci Med Sci 64:740–744, 2009.
31. Perls T, Shea-Drinkwater M, Bowen-Flynn J, et al: Exceptional familial clustering for extreme longevity in humans. J Am Geriatr Soc 48:1483–1485, 2000.
34. Kerber RA, O'Brien E, Smith KR, et al: Familial excess longevity in Utah genealogies. J Gerontol A Biol Sci Med Sci 56:B130–B139, 2001.
35. Perls TT, Wilmoth J, Levenson R, et al: Life-long sustained mortality advantage of siblings of centenarians. Proc Natl Acad Sci U S A 99:8442–8447, 2002.
43. Sebastiani P, Nussbaum L, Andersen S, et al: Increasing sibling relative risk of survival to older and older ages and the importance of

precise definitions of "aging," "life span," and "longevity." J Gerontol A Biol Sci Med Sci Mar 26, 2015, doi:10.1093/gerona/glv020.
45. Sebastiani P, Solovieff N, DeWan AT, et al: Genetic signatures of exceptional longevity in humans. PLoS One 7:e29848, 2012.
46. Puca AA, Daly MJ, Brewster SJ, et al: A genome-wide scan for linkage to human exceptional longevity identifies a locus on chromosome 4. Proc Natl Acad Sci U S A 98:10505–10508, 2001.
52. Huffman DM, Deelen J, Ye K, et al: Distinguishing between longevity and buffered-deleterious genotypes for exceptional human longevity: the case of the MTP gene. J Gerontol A Biol Sci Med Sci 67:1153–1160, 2012.
60. Barzilai N, Atzmon G, Schechter C, et al: Unique lipoprotein phenotype and genotype associated with exceptional longevity. JAMA 290:2030–2040, 2003.
63. Schachter F, Faure-Delanef L, Guenot F, et al: Genetic associations with human longevity at the APOE and ACE loci. Nat Genet 6:29–32, 1994.
67. Sebastiani P, Perls TT: The genetics of extreme longevity: lessons from the new England centenarian study. Front Genet 3:277, 2012.
72. Sebastiani P, Bae H, Sun F, et al: Meta-analysis of genetic variants associated with human exceptional longevity. Aging (Albany NY) 5:653–661, 2013.

5 Evolution Theory and the Mechanisms of Aging

Thomas B.L. Kirkwood

The question "Why does aging occur?" calls for answers at the level of proximate physiologic mechanisms and at the level of ultimate evolutionary origins. This chapter provides an understanding of why aging has evolved and examines what evolution theory can tell us about the types of mechanisms we might regard as prime candidates to explain senescence.

Evolution theory is well recognized as a powerful tool with which to inquire about the genetic basis of the aging process.[1-4] Although human aging has its roots long ago in our past, the study of its evolution can throw important light on key present-day challenges. For example, a range of population-based studies, including one based on genealogic analysis of the entire population of Iceland, has shown consistent evidence for a genetic contribution to human longevity.[5] There is growing interest in knowing how many and what types of genes are likely to be involved in this heritability.[6,7] There is also interest in human genetic disorders such as Werner syndrome and Hutchinson-Gilford progeria, which are characterized by acceleration of many aspects of the senescent phenotype (see Chapter 11).

Before addressing questions about the evolutionary origin of aging, it is important to be precise about how the term *aging* is to be understood. In this chapter, aging is defined as "a progressive, generalized impairment of function, resulting in a loss of adaptive response to stress and in a growing risk of age-related disease." The overall effect of these changes is summed up in the increase in the probability of dying, or age-specific death rate, in the population.

This definition of aging—in terms of a mortality pattern showing progressive increase in age-specific mortality—allows comparisons to be made, even among species in which the detailed features of the aging process may differ markedly. In phylogenetic terms, aging is widespread but by no means universal.[8-12] The fact that not all species show an increase in age-specific mortality indicates that aging is not an inevitable consequence of wear and tear. On the other hand, the fact that very many species do show such an increase is evidence that the evolution of aging has occurred under rather general circumstances.

EVOLUTION OF AGING

Theories on the evolution of aging seek to explain why aging occurs through the action of natural selection. The decline in survivorship, which is often also accompanied by a decline in fertility, means that there is an age-associated loss of Darwinian fitness that is clearly deleterious to the organism in which it occurs. Natural selection acts to increase fitness, so it is at once clear that selection should be expected, other things being equal, to oppose aging. Thus, the challenge to evolution theory is to explain why aging occurs, in spite of its drawbacks.

Programmed, or "Adaptive," Aging

It is sometimes suggested that despite its disadvantages to the individual, aging is beneficial and even necessary at the species level, for example, to prevent overcrowding.[13,14] In this case, genes that actively cause aging might have evolved specifically to program the end of life in the same way as genes program development.

The difficulty with this view is that there is little evidence that intrinsic aging serves as a significant contributor to mortality in natural populations,[15] which means that it apparently does not play the adaptive role suggested for it. The theory also embodies the questionable supposition that selection for advantage at the species level will be more effective than selection among individuals for the advantages of a longer life. Aging is clearly a disadvantage to the individual, so any mutation that inactivates the hypothetical adaptive aging genes would confer a fitness advantage and, therefore, the nonaging mutation should spread through the population unless countered by selection at the species or group level. Conditions under which this so-called group selection can work successfully are highly restrictive,[16] especially when there is selection in the opposite direction acting at the level of the individual. Briefly, it is necessary that the population be divided among fairly isolated groups and that the introduction of a nonaging genotype into a group should rapidly lead to the group's extinction. The latter condition is necessary to provide the selection between groups that might, in principle, counter the tendency for selection at the level of individuals to favor the spread of nonaging mutants. Although theoretical special cases have been constructed that might permit the selection of genes to cause aging, it appears unlikely that the necessary conditions will be met with sufficient generality to explain the evolution of aging.[17]

Selection Weakens With Age

An observation of central importance to the evolution of aging is that the force of natural selection—that is, its ability to discriminate between alternative genotypes—weakens with age.[15,18-21] Because natural selection operates through the differential effects of genes on fitness, its discriminatory power must decline with age in proportion to the decline in the remaining fraction of the organism's lifetime expectation of reproduction. This is true whether or not the species exhibits aging.

The attenuation in the force of natural selection with age means inevitably that there is only loose genetic control over the later portions of the life span. For this reason, it has been suggested that aging might be due to an accumulation of mutations in the germline, which potentially are deleterious but are not expressed, or that produce no phenotypic effect until late in life.[15]

The idea is that if deleterious mutations are expressed so late that most individuals will already have died from some other cause, such as predation, even though the genes involved have the potential to cause harm, they will be subject to very little selection against them. Over the generations, a large number of such genes might accumulate. These would cause aging and death only when an individual is removed to a protected environment, away from the hazards of the wild, and so would live long enough to experience their negative effects.

A stronger version of this theory was proposed by Williams,[18] who suggested that because of the declining force of natural selection with age, any gene that conferred an advantage early in life would be favored by selection, even if the same gene had deleterious effects at older ages. Such "pleiotropic" genes could explain aging. The decline in the force of natural selection with age would ensure that even quite modest early benefits would outweigh severe harmful side effects, provided the latter occurred late enough.

Disposable Soma Theory

The disposable soma theory[1,4,21-23] explains aging by asking how an organism should allocate its metabolic resources best, primarily energy—on the one hand, keeping itself going from one day to the next and, on the other hand, growing its body and producing progeny to secure the continuance of its genes when it has itself died. No species is immune to hazards such as predation, starvation, and disease. All that is necessary by way of maintenance is that the body remains in sound condition until an age after which most individuals will have died from accidental causes. In fact, a greater investment in maintenance is a disadvantage because it eats into resources that in terms of natural selection, are better used for reproduction. The theory concludes that the optimum course is to invest fewer resources in the maintenance of somatic tissues than are necessary for indefinite survival (Figure 5-1). The result is that aging occurs through the gradual accumulation of unrepaired somatic defects, but the level of maintenance will be set, so that the deleterious effects do not become apparent until an age when survivorship in a wild environment would be extremely unlikely.

Comparison of Evolutionary Theories

The adaptive program theory is in a category of its own, and support for this theory is weak; it will not be considered further in this chapter. The disposable soma and pleiotropic genes theories are adaptive in the sense that aging is the result of positive selection for aspects of the organism's life history, but the essential difference is that aging itself is not adaptive, but is a negative trait, that arises only as a byproduct or tradeoff of some other benefit. The late-acting deleterious mutations theory assumes an essentially neutral evolutionary process, with the accumulation of mutations reflecting the inability of natural selection to maintain tight control over the later portions of the life span.

Among the nonadaptive theories, there is a common strand—namely, that old organisms count less. This is not due to any implicit assumption of frailty or obsolescence, which would render the theories circular, but to the simple mathematics of mortality. Even if old organisms retain exactly the same vigor as young ones, to the extent that old and young are physiologically indistinguishable, the fact that each cohort becomes numerically attenuated with age means that the selection force weakens. The nonadaptive theories are not mutually exclusive. Therefore, aging might in principle be due to a combination of any of them.

As regards the nature of gene action, the disposable soma theory is the most specific of the evolutionary theories because it suggests not only why aging occurs, but also predicts that the genetic basis of aging is to be found in the genes that regulate levels of somatic maintenance functions. Neither the pleiotropic genes theory nor the late-acting deleterious mutations theory is specific about the nature of the genes involved.

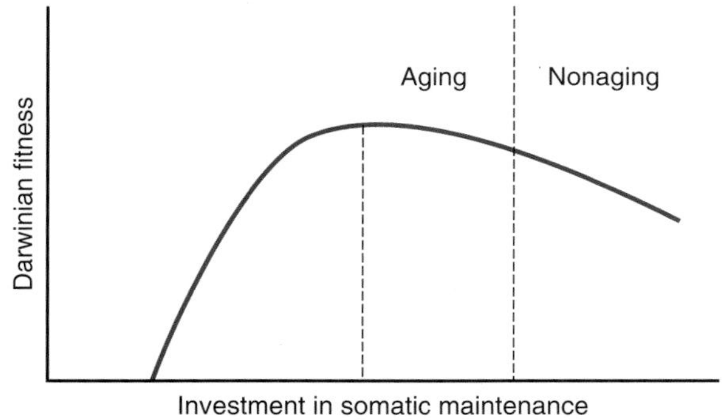

Figure 5-1. Relationship between Darwinian fitness and investment in somatic maintenance predicted by the disposable soma theory of aging. Fitness is maximized at a level that is less than that which would be required for indefinite longevity (nonaging).

GENETICS OF LIFE SPAN

This section discusses the genetics of life span, first from the point of view of interspecies comparisons. That is, it will ask "Why do species have the life spans they do?" It will then look at intraspecies variation and heritability of life span. Finally, there is a brief discussion of human progeroid syndromes, such as Werner and Hutchinson-Gilford progeria, as models of genetically accelerated senescence.

Species Differences in Longevity

In addition to explaining why aging occurs, evolution theory must also account for differences in species life spans. This raises basic questions about the genetic control of aging: specifically, how many genes are involved, and how are these modified by selection to produce changes in life span?

For each of the nonadaptive theories, the generality of the selection forces involved suggests that multiple genes will be implicated. If there is a very large number of independent genes causing aging, however, the life span may be slow to change, because modifying a single gene may have little effect by itself, and the probability of simultaneous independent modifications will be low. This suggests that a reasonably small number of primary genes are responsible for aging, or that there exists some mechanism for coordinate regulation.

The evolution of increased life span is most readily explained if it is assumed that an adaptation occurs that results in a general lowering of the accidental (age-independent) death rate. In the late-acting deleterious mutations theory, this may result in new pressure to eliminate or postpone the deleterious gene effects. In the pleiotropic genes theory, the balance between early benefit and late cost may be shifted in favor of reducing the harmful effects on late survival. In the disposable soma theory, there may be selection to adjust the optimum investment in maintenance to a higher level.

Variation Within Species

The variability in life span observed within a species or population clearly owes much to chance, but there is a significant heritable component as well.[5] Martin and colleagues[5] have applied the terms *public* and *private* to denote genetic factors related to aging that may be specific to individuals or shared across a population (perhaps even across species). Late-acting deleterious mutations are strong candidates for private genes because the fate of such alleles is determined largely by random genetic drift. Public genes are more likely to be those that arise through tradeoffs. In particular, the genes involved in regulating mechanisms of somatic maintenance are likely to be public genes of considerable importance. Although these genes are public in the sense that all individuals have them, there may nevertheless be

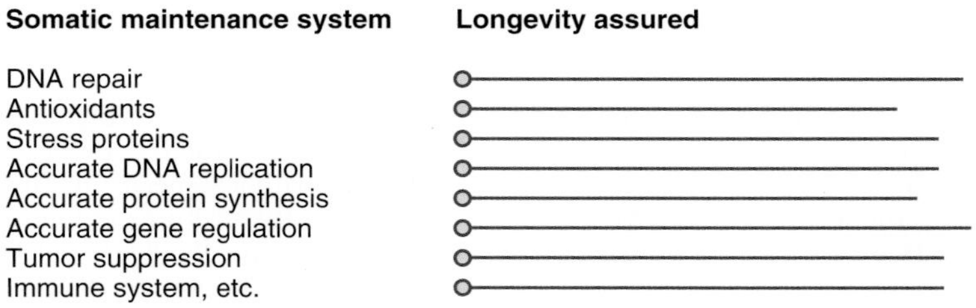

Figure 5-2. Polygenic control of longevity predicted by the disposable soma theory of aging. On average, the period of longevity assured by individual somatic maintenance systems is predicted to be similar, but some genetic variance about the average is also expected, as shown.

variations within a population in the precise levels at which these functions are set. These variations in setting may in turn be the cause of genetic variations in life expectancy.

As predicted by the disposable soma theory, the level of individual somatic maintenance systems should be set high enough so that the organism remains in sound condition through its natural expectation of life in a wild environment, but not much higher than this, or resources will be wasted. Numerous maintenance systems operate in parallel to preserve viability (Figure 5-2). Depending on the levels at which they are set, each maintenance system can be thought of as assuring a given span of life (see also Cutler[24] and Sacher[25] for earlier discussions of the concept of longevity assurance). When any one of these critical mechanisms has exhausted its potential for ensuring longevity, which happens because the accumulated defects threaten survival, the organism is liable to die.

If we now recall the shape of the fitness curve in Figure 5-1, we see that its peak—the point toward which natural selection is expected to exert evolutionary pressure—is rounded instead of sharp, so we can expect a fair amount of intrapopulation variance in the precise settings of maintenance processes. Selection is expected to direct these settings toward the peak, but once within the region of the peak, the fitness differences on which selection can operate become small.

Putting these ideas together generates the prediction summarized in Figure 5-2. On average, we expect the longevity assured by individual maintenance systems to be similar.[26,27] This is because if the setting of any one mechanism is so low that it consistently fails before any of the others, then selection will tend to increase the level at which it is set. Conversely, if any mechanism always tends to fail after the others, then there will be selection to tune down the level at which it is set to the extent that this mechanism involves a metabolic cost. In individuals, however, the genetic variance within the population is expected to result in variation in the extent to which the organism is predisposed to age from specific causes. For example, some individuals are likely to be less well protected against oxygen radicals than others, and these individuals will therefore experience greater oxidative damage.

Instances of extreme longevity, such as human centenarians, are of special interest because they are likely to be endowed with unusually high levels of each of the important ingredients of the cellular defense network.[6] Such individuals may also be distinguished by their freedom from alleles that predispose toward diseases that otherwise might shorten life expectancy. Schächter and associates[28] performed the first genetic study comparing centenarians with younger adult controls, which validated the general potential of this approach. Since then, a number of further studies have been conducted to examine the genetics of human longevity.

Recent years have seen the publication of results from several large investigations looking at individuals of extreme longevity (e.g., centenarians) or at families when there is reason to expect that family members share a genetic endowment predisposing them to above-average longevity. Examples of the latter design include studies that are recruiting nonagenarian siblings (i.e., cases in which two or more members of the same family are still alive past age 90).[29,30] The technologic advances that are presently being made in the capacity to assess DNA samples for possession of very large numbers of genetic markers at very high speed mean that the focus is now increasingly on genome-wide association studies and the linkage analyses that can be made using family groups. Herein lies both the strength of modern human genetics and a potential difficulty when studying a trait such as longevity, which is likely to prove highly polygenic. If large numbers of genetic loci contribute to the longevity phenotype, but these individually make only small contributions, the difficulty of extracting the signals from the statistical noise will be formidable.[31]

HUMAN PROGEROID SYNDROMES

A number of inherited human diseases have been characterized as showing a phenotype of accelerated aging. The best studied of these conditions is Werner syndrome, a rare autosomal recessive disorder affecting around 10 in 1 million people, who prematurely develop a variety of major age-related diseases, including arteriosclerosis, ocular cataracts, osteoporosis, malignant neoplasms, and type 2 diabetes. Cells grown from Werner syndrome patients show reduced division potential and increased chromosomal instability compared with age-matched controls, and there is evidence that the pathology associated with Werner syndrome may be related rather generally to impaired cell proliferation.

Yu and coworkers[32] have identified the gene responsible for Werner syndrome as a DNA helicase, an enzyme responsible for unwinding DNA for purposes of replication, repair, and expression of the genetic material. This discovery strongly supports the concept that accumulation of somatic defects is important in aging, and it well illustrates the predicted involvement of longevity assurance genes in determining the rate of aging. A defective helicase increases the rate of accumulation of DNA defects in actively dividing cell populations. A defect in this gene leads to accelerated aging, particularly in tissues in which cell division continues throughout life. In terms of the scheme shown in Figure 5-2, the mutation responsible for Werner syndrome can be considered equivalent to shortening the line for longevity assurance through DNA repair. However, as Figure 5-2 illustrates, DNA repair is only part of the network of longevity assurance mechanisms that determine the overall rate of aging. It is striking that Werner syndrome is not associated with accelerated aging in postmitotic tissues, such as brain and muscle, which is consistent with the fact that these tissues, by virtue of having little or no cell division during adult life, are relatively unaffected by having a defective DNA helicase.

Another striking example is Hutchinson-Gilford progeria. In this condition, features of aging develop even faster than in Werner syndrome. The discovery that Hutchinson-Gilford syndrome is associated with a mutation in the lamin A gene, which affects the integrity of the cell's nuclear membrane, has again confirmed the association between rapid aging and accelerated accumulation of molecular and cellular damage.[33]

TESTS OF THE EVOLUTIONARY THEORIES

A key prediction of the evolutionary theories is that altering the rate of decline in the force of natural selection will lead to the evolution of a concomitantly altered rate of aging. This has been tested by applying artificial selection on life history variables or by making comparisons within and between species on the effects of different levels of extrinsic mortality. For practical reasons, most studies have focused on short-lived species, in particular the fruit fly *Drosophila melanogaster* and the nematode worm *Caenorhabditis elegans*.

Evidence for tradeoffs between early and late fitness components, as predicted by the disposable soma and pleiotropic genes theories, comes from the success of artificial selection for increased longevity in *Drosophila*.[34-39] A general correlate of delayed senescence has been reduced fecundity in the long-lived flies. A similar tradeoff has also been reported for a human population, based on an analysis of birth and death records of British aristocrats.[40]

The nematode *C. elegans* has shown a growing number of long-lived mutants in which increased longevity has been consistently associated with increased resistance to biochemical and other stresses. Many of the affected genes are linked to pathways that control a switch between the normal developmental process of the worm and an alternative long-lived form called the dauer larva, which is invoked during times of food shortage. The emerging picture points to a fundamental link between metabolic control, growth and reproduction, and somatic maintenance.[41-43] These findings are directly consistent with the disposable soma theory, which predicts that at the heart of the evolutionary explanation of aging is the principle that organisms have been acted on by natural selection to optimize the use of metabolic resources (energy) between competing physiologic demands, such as growth, maintenance, and reproduction.

Consistent with this prediction, it is striking that insulin signaling pathways appear to have effects on aging that may be strongly conserved across the species range. Insulin signaling regulates responses to varying nutrient levels. Allied to the role of insulin signaling pathways is the discovery that a class of proteins called sirtuins and, in particular, the nutrient response pathway defined by the mechanistic target of rapamycin (mTOR), appear to be centrally involved in fine-tuning metabolic resources in response to variations in food supply.[44,45] Inhibition of the mTOR pathway extends the life span in model organisms and confers protection against a growing list of age-related pathologies. It has also long been known in laboratory rodents that restricted intake of calories simultaneously suppresses reproduction and upregulates a range of maintenance mechanisms, resulting in an extension of life span and the simultaneous postponement of age-related diseases. What is not at all clear, however, is whether the large effects on life span of modulating these pathways in very short-lived animals, such as nematodes and fruit flies, will be found to operate in longer lived species. On evolutionary grounds, it seems likely that there will have been greater evolutionary pressure to evolve a capacity to produce large responses to extreme environmental variation in small, short-lived animals. Therefore, the scope for such modulation in humans, including through dietary restriction, is expected to be much less. Nevertheless, it will be surprising if there are no metabolic consequences of a varying food supply.

From the comparative perspective, the evolutionary theories predict that in safe environments (those with low extrinsic mortality), aging will evolve to be retarded. Adaptations that reduce extrinsic mortality (e.g., wings, protective shells, large brains) are generally linked with increased longevity (e.g., bats, birds, turtles, humans). Field observations comparing a mainland population of opossums subject to significant predation by mammals with an island population not subject to mammalian predation found the predicted slower aging in the island population.[46]

At the molecular and cellular levels, the disposable soma theory predicts that the effort devoted to cellular maintenance and repair processes will vary directly with longevity. Numerous studies support this hypothesis. A direct relation between species longevity and rate of mitochondrial reactive oxygen species (ROS) production in captive mammals has been found,[47,48] as has a similar relationship between mammals and similarly sized but much longer-lived birds.[49] DNA repair capacity has been shown to correlate with mammalian life span in numerous comparative studies,[50] as has the level of poly(ADP-ribose) polymerase,[51] an enzyme that plays an important role in the maintenance of genomic integrity. The quality of maintenance and repair mechanisms may be revealed by the capability to cope with external stress. Comparisons of the functional capacity of cultured cells to withstand a variety of imposed stressors have shown that cells taken from long-lived species have superior stress resistance than that of cells from shorter lived species.[52,53]

Tests of the evolutionary theories support the idea that it is the evolved capacity of somatic cells to carry out effective maintenance and repair that mainly governs the time taken for damage to accumulate to levels where it interferes with the organism's viability, and hence regulates longevity.

CONCLUSIONS

Our answers to the question "Why does aging occur?" have broad implications for how we perceive the likely genetic basis of aging. First, evolution theory can illuminate a long-running debate about whether programmed or stochastic events, such as DNA damage, drive the aging process. The weakness of evolutionary support for the adaptive aging genes hypothesis calls the program theory into question. Any notion of an aging clock needs to be qualified by recognition of this fact. The existence of temporal controls in development and in cyclic processes such as diurnal and reproductive cycles does not provide a sufficient basis to suggest the existence of a clock that regulates aging, nor does the broad reproducibility of many features of aging provide any real evidence for an underlying active program. This is not to say, however, that the nature and rate of aging are not genetically determined. The issue that distinguishes programmed from stochastic theories of aging is not whether the factors that determine longevity are specified within the genome, but rather how this is arranged.

Second, evolution theory clearly indicates a polygenic basis for aging. Different mechanisms and even different types of genes may operate together. This presents a major challenge, and progress is likely to require a combination of approaches, including the following: (1) transgenic animal models in which candidate genetic factors are altered by genetic manipulation; (2) comparative studies to identify factors that correlate positively or negatively with species' life spans; (3) studies of the extremely long-lived (e.g., human centenarians) to identify factors associated with above-average expectation of life; and (4) selection experiments to investigate the response of life span to artificial selection pressures.

KEY POINTS: AGING

We are not programmed to die.

- Aging occurs because, in our evolutionary past, when life expectancy was much shorter, natural selection placed limited priority on long-term maintenance of the body.
- Aging is caused by a gradual accumulation of cell and tissue damage. Much of the damage arises as a side effect of essential biochemical processes, such as the use of oxygen to generate chemical energy through oxidative phosphorylation.
- Accumulation of damage begins early and continues progressively throughout life, resulting after several decades in the overt frailty, disability, and disease associated with aging.
- Multiple processes cause the damage that contributes to aging, and multiple genes regulate the efficacy of longevity assurance processes, such as DNA repair, that together influence the rate of aging.
- Nongenetic factors, such as nutrition and exercise, can have important effects in modulating the rate of buildup of damage within the body.

For a complete list of references, please visit www.expertconsult.com.

KEY REFERENCES

4. Kirkwood TBL, Austad SN: Why do we age? Nature 408:233–238, 2000.
7. Christensen K, Johnson TE, Vaupel JW: The quest for genetic determinants of human longevity: challenges and insights. Nat Rev Genet 7:436–448, 2006.
15. Medawar PB: An unsolved problem of biology, London, 1952, HK Lewis.
17. Kirkwood TB, Melov S: On the programmed/non-programmed nature of ageing within the life history. Curr Biol 21:R701–R707, 2011.
18. Williams GC: Pleiotropy, natural selection and the evolution of senescence. Evolution 11:398–411, 1957.
21. Kirkwood TBL: Evolution of ageing. Nature 270:301–304, 1977.
22. Kirkwood TBL, Holliday R: The evolution of ageing and longevity. Proc R Soc Lond B Biol Sci 205:531–546, 1979.
26. Kirkwood TBL: Understanding the odd science of aging. Cell 120:437–447, 2005.
27. Kirkwood TBL: A systematic look at an old problem. Nature 451:644–647, 2008.
28. Schächter F, FaureDelanef L, Guenot F, et al: Genetic associations with human longevity at the APOE and ACE loci. Nat Genet 6:29–32, 1994.
31. Deelen J, Beekman M, Uh HW, et al: Genome-wide association meta-analysis of human longevity identifies a novel locus conferring survival beyond 90 years of age. Hum Mol Genet 23:4420–4432, 2014.
42. Gems D, Partridge L: Insulin/IGF signaling and ageing: seeing the bigger picture. Curr Opin Genet Dev 11:287–292, 2001.
43. Kenyon C: The plasticity of aging: insights from long-lived mutants. Cell 120:449–460, 2005.
45. Johnson SC, Rabinovitch PS, Kaeberlein M: mTOR is a key modulator of ageing and age-related disease. Nature 493:338–345, 2013.
53. Kapahi P, Boulton ME, Kirkwood TBL: Positive correlation between mammalian life span and cellular resistance to stress. Free Radic Biol Med 26:495–500, 1999.

6 Methodologic Challenges of Research in Older People

Antony Bayer

INTRODUCTION

The difficulty of undertaking research involving older people tends to be exaggerated. It is wrongly assumed that too many will have significant comorbidity leading to a poor signal-to-noise ratio, an unacceptably high risk of adverse events, inability to complete necessary assessments, poor compliance, and high dropout rate. This can translate into arbitrary, unscientific, and unnecessary upper age limits. However, many of the changes commonly attributed to aging are typically due to reasons other than chronologic age, notably physical and cognitive comorbidities leading to frailty and psychosocial factors, such as relative lack of education and cigarette smoking. Furthermore, it is often older adults who have the greatest morbidity and mortality associated with the condition under study and who therefore will have the greatest absolute benefit from any effective intervention.

Ill-informed beliefs about the supposed high risk of developing mental incapacity and perceived low life expectancy after age 65 are sometimes used to justify the exclusion of older people from longitudinal studies because it is wrongly assumed that few will stay the course. In reality, the annual incidence of dementia in those older than 65 years is about 1%, and life expectancy at age 65 in England currently averages between 18 and 21 years.

Ethical concerns about experimenting on older populations, who are considered vulnerable only on the basis of chronologic age, demonstrate misguided paternalism of younger research workers and ignores the older person's right to autonomous decision making. Most of even the oldest old will have no significant cognitive impairment and will generally have the capacity to make an informed decision about participation. The consequences of excluding older people from therapeutic research, where they are left to receive treatment in the absence of evidence-based trials or are denied drugs because they have been untried in their age group, might be considered especially unethical[1] and imply that clinicians have a duty to encourage actively their inclusion in clinical trials.[2]

Guidance to promote research with older people has been developed by the European Forum for Good Clinical Practice,[3] and greater involvement of older people in clinical trials is also endorsed by regulatory authorities in Europe and the United States who evaluate drugs for registration.[4,5] All researchers should be careful, therefore, that ageist attitudes do not influence their research design and practice, and funding bodies and research ethics committees should challenge unnecessarily restrictive entry criteria, including inappropriate upper age limits.[6]

Study Designs

The optimum choice of design to study aging and age-related conditions and to understand the mechanisms underlying change and their consequences will depend on the research question to be answered (Figure 6-1). Qualitative studies, ecologic studies using available data, and quantitative studies using cross-sectional, case-control, and cohort designs will help generate hypotheses. These can then be tested in experimental studies using randomized controlled trial designs. Each design presents its own challenges and limitations.

Qualitative Methodologies

Qualitative research has its roots in anthropology and sociology and is an umbrella term for a heterogeneous group of methodologies with different theoretical underpinnings.[7] They aim to gain an in-depth understanding of peoples' behavior by exploring their knowledge, values, attitudes, beliefs, and fears. This allows subjects to give richer answers to real-world issues and allows the researcher to explore the full complexity of human behaviors, thus providing detailed insights that might be missed by other methods. For example, it may illuminate the reasons behind patients', carers', and clinicians' decisions about management, and therefore inform future policy developments,[8,9] or help characterize important issues such as abuse or risk management that may be difficult to quantify.[10,11]

Qualitative studies are hypothesis-generating rather than hypothesis-testing studies, but results can identify specific issues that need to be tested using quantitative methods or can help explain the outcomes of experimental studies. Thus, the two methods can usefully complement each other, and increasing numbers of studies are using mixed methodologies (e.g., a study trying to understand the attitudes of older adults toward enrollment into cancer clinical trials).[12]

Samples in qualitative research tend to be small and labor-intensive, with data collected usually by direct observation or active participation in the setting of interest, or by in-depth individual interviews (unstructured or semistructured), focus groups (guided group discussions), or examination of documents or other artifacts. Other methods used in qualitative research studies include diary methods, role playing and simulation, narrative analysis, and in-depth case studies. Although potential areas of interest may be identified beforehand, there is no predetermined set of questions, and subjects are encouraged to express their views and ideas at length. Rather than formal sample size calculations, numbers of participants may be decided by analyzing interviews alongside data collection, which is stopped when no new themes are emerging (saturation). Sampling tends to be purposive rather than comprehensive or random, deliberately aiming to reflect a specific range of experience and attitudes judged to be of likely relevance to the research question. The results are analyzed by exploring the content and identifying patterns or themes, often through an iterative process allowing meaning to emerge from the data, rather than by the deductive statistical approach of quantitative methods.

Critics of qualitative analysis are concerned that it is too influenced by the views and attitudes of the researchers when they are collecting and analyzing data, thus introducing unacceptable bias and problems with generalizability and reproducibility of findings. Qualitative research can be challenging with older people but, because it can be less intrusive than more structured quantitative methodologies, it may be especially suited to those who are frail. They may be unable or unwilling to take part in lengthy interviews because of communication deficits or fatigue, and several shorter interviews may be more practical. Focus groups may work best with just four or five older participants and need a skilled facilitator to ensure a high level of participant interaction. Extra effort is needed to ensure representative samples and

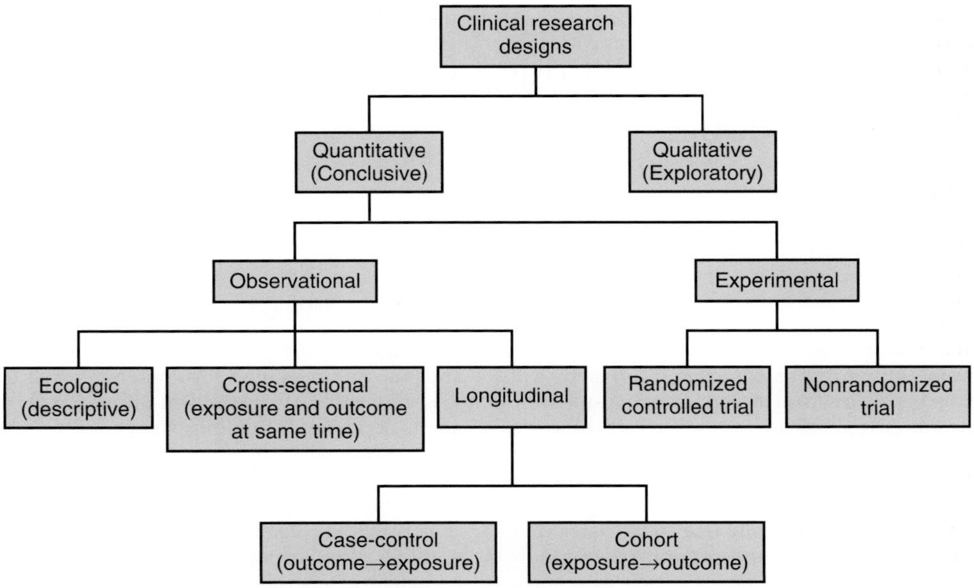

Figure 6-1. Research designs for clinical study.

support those who are less confident, easily fatigued, or have cognitive or physical deficits. Participant or nonparticipant observation may be especially useful in institutional settings, but time must be given to establish trust with the researcher if residents and staff are not to feel threatened. Assurances of confidentiality and commitment from management are essential. However, once trust has been established, attrition rates tend to be low, because participation tends not to be burdensome.[13]

Ecologic Studies

Ecologic studies use available data to characterize samples and generate hypotheses, although evidence for causality is generally weak. Data may be aggregated, such as census data and records of disease incidence by hospital, or individual, such as hospital discharge summaries or death certificates. Because the data are already available, there are advantages of speed and economy and the impact of factors operating at a population level (e.g., improved access to education, banning smoking in public places) may be difficult to measure at an individual level. However, measures may not be comparable over time or place, quality is always outside the researcher's control, and the available data may be selective. Many official statistics that are broken down by age will lump all those older than 65 years together or will only report information on adults of working age. When older people are included, they often exclude those not living in the community and those with cognitive impairment. Nevertheless, temporal data, such as the effect of daily variations in air pollution or temperature on mortality of older adults, where individual confounding factors remain constant over time, can provide robust evidence suggesting a causal effect. Ecologic data is also of value in studying the effects of early life factors on later health or disease on "life course epidemiology."[14]

Cross-Sectional Studies

Cross-sectional studies record information over a short period of time and are suited to report prevalence and the relationship between variables and age or dependency. They are relatively fast and simple to conduct because each subject is examined only once, and several outcomes or diseases can be studied simultaneously. For example, data from the Health and Retirement Study of 11,000 adults aged 65 years or older (representing the 34.5 million older Americans) highlighted the important finding that common geriatric conditions (e.g., cognitive impairment, falls, incontinence) were similar in prevalence to common chronic diseases in older adults, such as heart disease and diabetes, and were strongly and independently associated with dependency in activities of daily living.[15] However, cross-sectional studies give no information about incidence or causality and are of limited value when studying rare conditions or acute illness.

Data can be presented as the mean value for each age group, or age can be used as a continuous independent variable in a regression analysis, with the outcome of interest as the dependent variable. Associations can be confounded when the variable of interest affects the survival of subjects, with selective mortality leading to a survival bias. Misinterpretation can also arise from birth cohort effects, with associations and differences not arising due to age differences but due to the era in which people were born and brought up and to changes in exposure to environmental risk factors. Sometimes such differences from one generation to the next are of particular interest, and a time series design may then be appropriate, with sequential samples of a particular age group being studied every few years. The Cognitive Function and Ageing Studies (CFAS) 1 and 11, for example, were conducted 2 decades apart using the same diagnostic methods in the same older age group living in the same geographic areas and demonstrated a cohort effect in dementia prevalence, with later born populations having a lower risk than those born earlier in the past century.[16]

Selection of subjects needs to ensure that they are well matched at each time point, and methodologies need to be identical, to ensure that differences are solely due to temporal changes and not to selection bias.

Case-Control Studies

Case-control studies choose groups with (cases) and without (controls) the outcome of interest and look back at what different exposures they might have had to identify possible risk factors. They have been widely used in genetic epidemiologic studies (genome-wide association studies or GWAS) to identify susceptibility (risk) genes—for example, in Alzheimer disease.[17] They are the best design to study uncommon conditions. Because they are efficient in use of time and money and collect much relevant information on targeted individuals. Case-control studies may be nested within cohort studies, with a subset of matched controls being selected from within the cohort and compared to the incident cases of the condition of interest.

Bias can be introduced when cases and controls differ in ways other than just the outcome of interest (selection bias) or when cases are not typical (representativeness bias). Given the increasing heterogeneity characteristic of aging, bias can be a significant problem, and care needs to be taken to match cases and controls well. Recall bias may arise because cases are able to remember events better because of their significance or, unintentionally, they may be prompted to remember by investigators, who should therefore be blinded as to whether the person is a case or control when assessing exposures. People who have died do not make it into case-control studies, and their representatives are likely to be less reliable than people themselves at remembering exposures, introducing a potential survival bias. Although case-control studies can play a pivotal role in suggesting important associations, as in the original studies linking cigarette smoking and lung cancer,[18] confounding can also lead to highly misleading conclusions, as in the observational studies of combined hormone replacement therapy and cardiovascular disease in postmenopausal women.[19]

Cohort Studies

In a cohort or longitudinal study, a group of subjects are followed over time as they age to determine who develops a particular outcome or the rate at which a variable changes. In addition to risk, the number of people who actually develop the outcome of interest can be calculated (incidence). Inevitably, such studies take a long time and often require a large sample size—the rarer the outcome, the larger the sample needs to be—and are therefore expensive. The frequency of testing needs to be decided based on the rate of change, precision of the measures being used, available resources, and stamina of researchers and research subjects. Analysis of longitudinal data by slope analysis or other techniques requires specialist knowledge. Prominent cohort studies relevant to old people include the Baltimore Longitudinal Study of Aging,[20] Rotterdam Study,[21] and Caerphilly Cohort.[22] The UK Biobank has recently recruited a half-million people aged 40 to 69 years, all of whom have completed a very wide range of baseline assessments and who will now be followed long term (with some having state of the art imaging) to investigate risk factors for the major diseases of middle and old age. This resource is available for use by all bona fide researchers for all types of health-related research that is in the public interest.[22a]

Recall bias is avoided in cohort studies because subjects are enrolled before the outcome(s) and sequence of events can be more clearly established, although the possibility of reverse causality must always be considered. Cohort effects are minimal because all the subjects are generally from a single birth cohort. Ideally, longitudinal aging studies would follow subjects from birth to the grave but this is unlikely because they would then outlive the research team. When age range in a longitudinal study is wide, cohort effects can be identified by plotting rates of change within age groups and seeing if the plots join up smoothly (a true age effect), or are a disjointed group of line segments similar to that often seen in repeated cross-sectional studies.

Potential bias may arise when outcomes are not measured or not recorded in a consistent fashion over time, with small changes in methodology, such as new equipment, a change in assay technique, or differences in study personnel appearing to suggest age-related changes (detection bias). Ensuring a common period of training for all involved in the research, with periodic refresher courses and measures of inter- and intrarater reliability, can minimize problems, but researchers must stay alert to possible methodologic errors throughout data collection and analysis. Important outcomes may be missed if follow-up is too short or too long, so that subjects might die before they are reassessed. Inevitably, some subjects will drop out or be lost to follow-up (excursion bias), and there are various approaches to dealing with missing data by imputing values based on available records.

Clinical Trials

A clinical trial is the methodology of choice to examine causality, with the randomized controlled trial (RCT) acknowledged as the gold standard for experimental design. The Standard Protocol Items: Recommendations for Intervention Trials (SPIRIT 2013) provides a checklist and explanation of recommended items to include in trial protocols.[23]

In an RCT, the researcher controls exposure to a single variable, the risk or treatment, by randomly assigning subjects to one group (intervention) or another (control, often involving a placebo intervention), and all subjects are then followed up to determine the outcome. When an effective intervention exists already, a placebo control is unethical, and the new experimental intervention is then compared against an active control (the current standard of care). In rare cases, when the size of the treatment effect relative to the expected prognosis is dramatic, randomization may not be necessary, or ethical and historical controls (apparently similar former patients) may be used.[24]

Parallel group RCT designs are generally preferred, with intervention and control groups being treated simultaneously. Thus half the subjects receive treatment A (intervention) and the other half receives treatment B (control). In a crossover design, subjects swap groups halfway through the study (half the subjects receiving treatment A are followed by treatment B, with the other half receiving treatment B and then A), so each subject can act as his or her own control, assuming that there are no carryover or seasonal effects. In a factorial design, two (and occasionally more) interventions, each with their own control, are evaluated simultaneously in one study. For example, one group tests treatment A, another tests treatment B, a third group tests A and B combined, and the control group tests neither A nor B. Such designs are already used extensively in cancer and cardiovascular studies and are likely to be needed increasingly in other conditions with multiple therapeutic options. Although they are an efficient method to test therapies in combination, achieving two comparisons for little more than the price of one, interactions between the interventions can complicate analysis of the outcomes and their interpretation.

Bias in clinical trials is reduced by the use of random allocation and blinding. Randomization increases the likelihood (but does not ensure) that the groups will be well matched except for the intervention, distributing potential confounders both known and unknown between the intervention and control groups. Stratified randomization can be used to ensure that particular groups (e.g., the very old) are evenly distributed. Cluster randomization designs randomize groups of individuals (e.g., all those in a ward or nursing home) rather than individuals themselves and are increasingly common in health services research. Blinding means that the subject or investigator (single-blind) or both (double-blind) do not know to which group the subject is assigned. This prevents people from being treated differently in any way other than the intervention itself and helps ensure that outcome assessments are unbiased.

National regulatory authorities, such as the Food and Drug Administration (FDA) and European Medicines Agency (EMEA), require positive outcomes from RCTs before a drug or medical device is given marketing approval for patient use. They will have been preceded by extensive preclinical in vitro (laboratory) and in vivo (animal) testing that when appropriate, may include studies with nonhuman primate models of aging or transgenic animal models of disease. Clinical trials then progress through an orderly series of steps, commonly classified into phases I to IV. Recently the concept of preliminary phase 0 trials has also been introduced to describe exploratory, first in human studies using single subtherapeutic (microdoses) of the study drug or agent, designed to confirm that the drug broadly behaves in humans as predicted from preclinical testing.

In phase I trials, the study drug or agent is tested in a small group of subjects (20 to 80) in single ascending dose (SAD) and multiple ascending dose (MAD) studies to assess a safe dosage range, the best method of administration, and tolerance and safety (pharmacovigilance). Changes in the pharmacokinetics and pharmacodynamics of many drugs in older people, especially the frail, may significantly affect the choice of dose and dosing frequency for clinical use. A phase I trial usually recruits healthy young adults, so care must be taken when extrapolating results to older patients. When the study indication is common in older people, phase 1 trials may recruit older healthy volunteers or patients with the relevant condition—for example, as in initial studies of immunotherapy for Alzheimer disease.

In phase II trials, the study drug or agent is given to a larger group of subjects (100 to 300), generally patients with the study indication, to assess safety and dosing requirements further (phase IIA) and to undertake preliminary studies of efficacy (phase IIB). Usually, these proof of concept studies recruit a homogenous group of younger subjects to maximize the chances of success and minimize adverse events related to altered pharmacokinetics and pharmacodynamics, comorbid conditions, and drug interactions more characteristic of older patients. However, there have been calls for regulatory authorities to require phase II studies of new agents to be carried out in individuals aged 70 years and older.[25]

In phase III trials, the efficacy and safety of the study drug or agent is evaluated in RCTs; usually, two positive trials are required to gain approval from regulatory authorities. These require the recruitment of up to several thousand patients from multiple centers and can last for several years, depending on the study indication. It is at this phase that arbitrary exclusion criteria based on chronologic age is especially difficult to justify. Randomization stratified by age and predetermined subgroup analysis will allow any issues specific to older patients to become apparent. Phase IV (postmarketing) trials are designed to provide additional information about benefits and risks of treatment in long-term use in clinical practice. Serious adverse effects identified at this late stage in older patients have resulted in withdrawal or restricted use of several prominent drugs.

The carefully controlled nature of RCTs may themselves mean that they have limited generalizability, because subjects are often a very well-defined, highly selected group. Extensive lists of inclusion and exclusion criteria may exclude those with other comorbidities or who are taking other medications, and the resulting trial population might bear little resemblance to patients normally presenting in the clinic. For example, a minority of hospitalized older patients with heart failure fit the profile of populations of clinical trials,[26] with the result of unintended harm to patients when trial results were applied in clinical practice.[26-28] Certainly, perceived gains from narrow eligibility criteria (e.g., smaller, shorter, safer, less expensive trials) are often outweighed by the loss in generalizability and clinical applicability of the results and by less opportunity to test preplanned subgroup hypotheses (including any effect of age).[29] Pragmatic clinical trials tend to take all comers and best reflect the effectiveness rather than merely the efficacy of an intervention.

Exclusion of Older People from Research

Older people, especially the frail and very old, are too often excluded from RCTs, usually inappropriately and without justification.[30,31] This results in an inadequate evidence base to guide practice, so clinicians are left having to extrapolate trial findings to older patients who often carry the greatest burden of disease, but in whom available treatments have not been studied. The EMEA has stated that "there is no good basis for exclusion on basis of advanced age alone. … unless there is reason to believe that this will endanger the patient."[5] Studies have shown broad agreement among a range of health professionals that exclusion from clinical trials on age grounds alone is unjustified (87%), and that underrepresentation of older people in trials causes difficulties for prescribers (79%) and patients (73%).[32]

Fortunately, over time, there does seem to be a slow shift from exclusion based on age toward more justified exclusion based on failing organ function.[33] Nevertheless, a review of eligibility criteria of RCTs published in high-impact medical journals from 1994 to 2006 found that after inability to consent, age was the second most common exclusion criterion, with 38% of trials excluding those older than 65 years.[34] Age bias can be still be seen in clinical trials of the most common conditions of older people, including cancer,[35,36] cardiovascular disease,[37,38] Parkinson disease,[39] surgery,[40] type 2 diabetes,[41] osteoarthritis[42] and urinary incontinence.[43] In preauthorization phase II and III trials of recently approved medicines, upper age limits were applied in 30.7% of the trials, and a very small proportion of participants were aged 75 years and older, even for diseases characteristically associated with aging (e.g., venous thromboembolism, osteoporosis, atrial fibrillation).[44] Discrimination seems to be more common in Europe than in the United States and in drug trials sponsored by public institutions rather than private institutions.[33] However, a review of RCTs specifically involving very old subjects concluded that their methodologic quality did not differ from comparable trials in the general population.[45]

Reasons given for excluding older subjects from research include concerns about gaining consent, protocol eligibility criteria with restrictions on comorbidities and concomitant medications, worries about poor compliance and high attrition, and fears of an unacceptable level of adverse events limiting the ability to identify an effect of treatment. If relatively large numbers of very old patients need to be screened to enroll an eligible subject, then it may be considered to be inefficient in terms of money and time to try and recruit them.

Many of these concerns, however, are unfounded or can be easily overcome.[46,47] A systematic review[48] examining participation of older patients in phase III publicly funded RCTs in cancer between 1955 and 2000 found that in those trials with sufficient numbers of older enrollees, survival, event-free survival, and treatment-related mortality outcomes were similar to outcomes reported in the remainder of the studies. The authors concluded that the similarity in these two groups show that the enrollment of older adults in experimental RCTs is not associated with increased harm.

Informed Consent

Seeking truly informed and freely given consent is fundamental to all research involving human subjects. The research participant must be able to retain and understand the relevant facts explained to them, allowed sufficient time to weigh the benefits and risks to make a choice (without coercion), and then communicate their decision to the researcher.[49] Consent is more than getting a signature in triplicate on a consent form and should be regarded as a continuous process involving ongoing open dialogue between researchers and participants.

Older patients may have more difficulty comprehending consent information (mainly due to education differences rather than age itself), and particular attention should be given to compensating for communication and sensory deficits, improving readability of information sheets and consent forms, and considering the use of innovative consent procedures. However, most older people are cognitively intact and, in empirical studies of competency to consent to medical treatment, older control individuals were nearly all judged fully capable using various legal standards.[50,51] Gaining informed consent may require more time because of characteristics of the older person and her or his wish to involve family members in the decision.

Those with cognitive impairment and the institutionalized are especially vulnerable to exploitation and require special consideration and management although, even then, lack of capacity should not be assumed.[52-54] The MacArthur Competence Assessment Tool for Clinical Research (MacCAT-CR)[55] is a semistructured assessment of a potential research subject's decision making capacity to choose, understand, appreciate and reason through information needed to make an informed decision and can be a useful aid, although it is time-consuming to administer and requires specialist training. Briefer tools exist; for example, a three-item questionnaire has been successfully tested in patients with dementia and diabetes to determine their capacity to make informed decisions,[56] although their limitations need to be recognized.[57] If a prospective research participant is considered incapable of giving consent, the relevant legal procedure must be followed.[58,59]

Generally, research is allowed to go ahead unless the subject objects, an appropriate surrogate decision maker (usually the patient's next of kin) is providing proxy consent, there is ethics committee approval, and it has been determined whether the study has the potential to benefit the subject (so-called therapeutic research) or the research entails minimal risk and burden and cannot be undertaken with individuals able to consent (nontherapeutic research). An advanced consent model has been advocated for patients who may not be able to give their consent to participation at the time when the study intervention is to commence—for example, toward the end of life or in an emergency.[60] Research advance directives or advance decisions clearly document an individual's views on research participation, but have not been widely adopted.[61]

Recruitment

Research is dependent on recruiting and retaining sufficient numbers of suitable study subjects. There is no consistent evidence that chronologic age influences recruitment rate into trials, with agreement to participate depending more on health condition and gender rather than age.[62,63] Rather, the problem is that older patients are not given sufficient encouragement to take part. Thus, a study of breast cancer trials found that older age remained predictive of not being invited to take part after adjustment for comorbidity, cancer stage, functional status, and race, yet a similar proportion of younger and older patients were recruited when they were asked.[64] In addition to ageism, clinician apathy, and inexperience of the researcher may also contribute to the exclusion of older patients. A survey of French geriatricians found that nearly all considered that RCTs including very old subjects were scientifically necessary, but less than half participated actively in such studies, and many were never approached to do so.[65] Researchers have the greatest motivation and are therefore the most efficient recruiters. Older patients themselves do not appear to seek clinical trials actively, possibly due to a lack of knowledge, and are dependent on others to inform them of what is available.[12] Involving older people themselves as active partners in research design and conduct has become a policy requirement in the United Kingdom and may be helpful, although little is known about how involvement changes the research process.[66,67]

Although curiosity may prompt the initial interest of patients in research, anticipated personal benefits, such as health screening and regular monitoring and the possibility to help others, are the most important motivators for subsequent enrollment and for continued participation.[63,68] The main reasons for refusing enrollment are inconvenience and not wanting to be experimented on or a self-perception of not being a suitable research candidate. Older research participants are more motivated than younger ones by feelings of altruism and paying back those who treat them and are less concerned about financial compensation for volunteering.[69] Studies in which all patients receive the active treatment, as part of a crossover design or open label extension after a placebo control phase, seem to be preferred.

BOX 6-1 Barriers to Recruitment of Older People Into Research Studies[70,71]

PATIENT-BASED

- Lack of perceived benefits and relevance of the study, preferences for a particular treatment (or for no treatment); worry about uncertainty of treatment or outcome
- Difficulty understanding and reading consent form
- Fatigue, comorbidity, mobility problems
- Distrust of research assistant; fear of strangers; unfamiliarity with the research
- Refusal of relatives
- Length and number of sessions; additional procedures
- Cognitive assessment demanding or considered intrusive
- Delays prior to beginning the study; conflicting commitments
- Additional travel problems and cost for patient

CLINICIAN-BASED

- Time restraints and overload of the medical staff in charge of recruitment
- Lack of staff and training
- Worry about the impact on physician-patient relationship
- Loss of professional autonomy due to need to follow protocol
- Difficulty with the consent procedure; concerns about providing information to patients
- Lack of rewards and recognition

Adapted from Kemeny M, Muss HB, Komblith AB, et al: Barriers to participation of older women with breast cancer in clinical trials. J Clin Oncol 21:2268-2275, 2003; and Le Quintrec JL, Piette F, Hervé C: Clinical trials in very elderly people: the point of view of geriatricians. Therapie 60:109-115, 2005.

Challenges to successful recruitment of older people into research studies are patient- and clinician-based (Box 6-1).[70,71] The most common barriers to be overcome are lack of perceived benefit, distrust of research staff, poor health, and mobility problems. A Cochrane review of strategies to improve recruitment of participants (of all ages) to RCTs suggested that effective interventions are telephone reminders to nonrespondents, use of opt-out rather than opt-in procedures for contacting potential participants, and open designs where participants know which treatment they are receiving in the trial (although such a design is by definition unblinded).[72] An earlier literature review specific to older people had identified a number of factors open to modification to increase their participation in research studies. These included positive attitudes of staff toward research, acknowledgment of altruistic motives, gaining approval of family members, protocols designed for patient rather than staff convenience, and having a physician rather than a nurse approach the patient.[73] In a study of recruitment of frail older adults living at home into a RCT of geriatric assessment, yield (defined as the percentage of individuals contacted who later enrolled) was highest for community physician solicitations and presentations to religious or ethnic groups and lowest from media and mailing approaches (and often problematic because of frequent misunderstanding).[74]

Inclusion in research of people living in care homes is especially challenging given the particular issues around resident consent, loss of autonomy and confidentiality, and often negative staff attitudes and their poor compliance with intervention and data protection protocols. There are also practical difficulties of collecting data during the homes' busy schedule and issues of privacy (e.g., staff entering a resident's room during a research interview).[54,75,76] In the United Kingdom, a tool kit from the National Institute of Health Research has been developed to assist researchers with best practice on preparing and conducting research in care homes.[77]

Retention

Strategies to improve retention of older participants in research studies are listed in Box 6-2.[71] There is some evidence of higher dropout rates of older research subjects[78]; therefore, once entered into a study, maintaining good communication by regular face to face or telephone contacts with the researchers is of prime importance. Regular newsletters about study progress and lunchtime meetings to meet staff involved and other participants can also be useful.[68] Token gifts such as study-related calendars, refrigerator magnets, and pens and pads can also be given, but may be counterproductive if they appear too costly. Test sessions should aim to last no longer than 1 to 2 hours to avoid fatigue, and spacing data collection over multiple visits should be considered. Time must be allowed for social interaction and refreshments to prevent contacts from becoming too impersonal. It should be remembered that most older people (and their accompanying caregivers) have other commitments, and it is important to be flexible about the time and place of the study visits.

BOX 6-2 Strategies That Promote Recruitment and Retention of Older People in Research Studies

- Taking time to explain the goal of the study and how it can help others; frequent reminders of the aims of the study
- Using simple language and short consent form, with large print
- Provide feedback on performance; share results of study once completed
- Provide educational materials (documentation), gifts, or financial compensation
- Provide transportation; foster face to face and in-home interviews
- Partnerships with persons (family member, medical and community staff) or institutions that have knowledge of the participants and/or that participants know and trust physician's agreement or encouragement
- Conduct recruitment and study in natural gathering places (home, day care center)
- Provide oversight of medical condition and medical referral, if required
- Shorter sessions; frequent breaks; adapt tests and interviews
- Reminders (personalized letters), telephone reminders, regular contacts, and phone number of a contact person
- Phone call if absent to know the reasons and propose strategies to overcome them
- Gathering with other people with similar problems and socializing
- Importance of being flexible about the time and place of the interview
- Training and attitude of research staff; increase number of staff to allow more availability

Adapted from Le Quintrec JL, Piette F, Hervé C: Clinical trials in very elderly people: the point of view of geriatricians. Therapie 60:109-115, 2005.

Transport provision is critically important. Mobility and cognitive problems may make travel more difficult, and the distance from home to the research center influences recruitment of older persons more than younger ones.[79,80] A prepaid taxi to and from the research center has many advantages. When research participants make their own travel arrangements, they should be reimbursed and convenient car parking assured. Consideration should be given to easy access to the research office, which should be wheelchair-friendly and with suitable waiting areas for accompanying relatives or caregivers. Assessments that can be reliably performed by telephone or at the subject's home may be preferred to visits to the research center and are more likely to ensure that the subject is at ease. In an Alzheimer RCT, recruitment and retention of patients were significantly better when patients were assessed at home rather than at a clinic, and shorter recruitment periods and increased retention rates may offset the costs of these changes.[81] However, it is more difficult for researchers to set the agenda when they are guests in the subject's home, and ensuring that well-meaning relatives and pets do not interrupt testing sessions can be challenging. Regular mail delivery of study medication may reduce the number of necessary visits. A formal "thank you" when the study ends, and feedback of the final outcome, is appreciated and expected.

Outcomes

In addition to the standard outcome measures of morbidity and mortality, research in older people needs to consider broader issues such as functional capacity and ability to carry out activities of daily living, cognitive and social outcomes, burden of any intervention, and impact on caregivers. Certainly, quality is often considered a greater priority than quantity of life by those with limited life expectancy due to cancer, heart failure, or chronic obstructive pulmonary disease.[82] Chosen measurement instruments must be valid (recording the attribute that it purports to measure), reliable (recording consistent results under varying conditions of measurement), and responsive (able to detect change). Other factors to be considered when selecting an instrument are whether it is self-administered or researcher-administered, whether it measures capability (what can be done, relevant to experimental designs) or performance (what is done, relevant in pragmatic studies) and, perhaps most importantly, how long it takes to complete. Attention should also be given to the readability and style of self-completed questionnaires (Box 6-3).

The lack of validation of measurement instruments for use in older people is a problem. Scales must be able to encompass the heterogeneity characteristic of older populations, avoiding floor and ceiling effects, and they must be acceptable to the study subjects. Even an apparently simple measure such as height becomes an issue when the person cannot stand. Use of validated

BOX 6-3 Checklist When Choosing Outcome Measures

- Is the measure proven to be valid and reliable in the study population?
- Is the measure responsive to clinically significant change?
- Is it acceptable to research subject and user? Could presentation be improved?
- Who is administering the measure? Training needed? Can a proxy respondent complete it reliably?
- How long does it take to administer? Is the environment appropriate?
- Is scoring simple and results presented ready for analysis?
- Has the measure been piloted in the study population?

alternatives such as knee-floor height then need to be considered, perhaps even in those who can stand, to ensure consistency across the whole study population. Experience with measures in younger, more fit subjects cannot reliably be extrapolated to older patients, with their higher prevalence of mobility, sensory, and communication deficits. When norms for those older than 65 years are available, they may have been derived from small numbers of atypical, healthy, young old subjects and of little relevance to the frail octogenarian in a nursing home. Ideally, therefore, reliability should be established in each population sample where the measure is to be used. Certainly, all raters need to be trained to ensure consistency (inter- and intrarater reliability) and help minimize bias. Piloting of all outcome measures in the population to be studied will ensure that the final choice is feasible and will reduce the number of subsequent subject dropouts.

There are a growing number of measurement instruments that have established validity and reliability in older subjects, with some approaching the status of a gold standard. Examples are the Mini Mental State Examination (MMSE) for cognition,[83] Geriatric Depression Scale (GDS),[84] Barthel Index[85] and Katz Index[86] for basic activities of daily living, Lawton and Brody index for instrumental activities of daily living (IADLs),[87] Charlson Co-morbidity Index (CMI),[88] Mini Nutritional Assessment (MNA),[89] Timed Up-and-Go test (TUG) for risk of falls,[90] and Zarit Burden Scale for caregiver burden.[91] Clinical trials in dementia have their own extensive battery of assessment measures,[92] and expert groups have recommended suitable outcome measures for clinical trials for use in older people with frailty[93-95] and cancer.[96] Of the many generic quality of life measures available, the SF-36, EQ-5D and Nottingham Health Profile have good evidence of reliability, validity, and responsiveness when used with older people.[97]

CONCLUSIONS

The European research consortium PREDICT (Increasing the PaRticipation of the ElDerly In Clinical Trials) has compiled a charter for the rights of older people in clinical trials (Box 6-4).[98]

BOX 6-4 European Charter for the Rights of Older People in Clinical Trials

1. Older people have the right to access evidence-based treatments.
   - 1.1 Older people have the right to be offered evidence-based treatments.
     - 1.1.1 Older people should expect to be offered drugs and other treatments that have been properly evaluated in clinical trials and demonstrated to be effective in people of their age.
2. Clinical trials should promote the inclusion of older people in clinical trials and prevent discrimination.
   - 2.1 Older people should not be discriminated against in the recruitment for clinical trials.
     - 2.1.1 Older people should be informed about and invited to participate in clinical trials of treatments that are intended for use in older people.
     - 2.1.2 National and international regulators should ensure that older people are included in clinical trials without discrimination on grounds of age, gender, ethnicity, or social class.
     - 2.1.3 Research ethics committees, sponsors, medical journal editors, and regulators should review all studies critically for unjustified exclusions based on age, other illnesses, disability, and existing drug treatment. All such exclusions must be justified.
   - 2.2 The participation in clinical trials of people with multiple morbidities should be encouraged.
     - 2.2.1 National and international regulators should require that trials with drugs or other treatments intended for use in older people include those with multiple morbidities that are common in later life.
     - 2.2.2 National and international regulators should require that trials with drugs or other treatments intended for use in later life include older people who are taking commonly prescribed medications.
3. Clinical trials should be made as practicable as possible for older people.
   - 3.1 Clinical trials should be designed so that older people can participate easily.
     - 3.1.1 Older people should receive information about clinical trials that helps them make an informed decision about participation. Informed consent procedure should be adapted to the specific needs of older people, taking into account their level of literacy, any sensory deficits, and involving their family or caregiver, if needed.
     - 3.1.2 Specific training is needed to perform clinical trials in older people. Researchers should be trained to conduct clinical trials in people with communication, sensory, mobility, or cognitive problems.
     - 3.1.3 Researchers should be prepared to spend additional time with older people participating in a clinical trial to support their participation and adherence.
     - 3.1.4 Trial sponsors should recognize that older people may need extra support to take part in trials. Trial sponsors should provide support to enhance the inclusion and adherence of older people, especially those with mobility and communication problems and those who also have responsibilities caring for others.
     - 3.1.5 National and international regulators should encourage clinical trials that are designed to make the participation of older people easier.
4. Clinical trials in older people should be safe.
   - 4.1 Clinical trials in older people should be as safe as possible.
     - 4.1.1 Researchers should assess the benefits and risks of older people's participation in clinical trials.
5. Outcome measures should be relevant for older people.
   - 5.1 Clinical trials for common conditions in older people should use outcome measures that are relevant for older people.
     - 5.1.1 Researchers, trial sponsors and regulators should ensure that clinical trials for common conditions in older people use outcome measures that are relevant for older people, including quality of life measurements.
     - 5.1.2 Clinical trial sponsors should involve older people and carers in the design of clinical trials and in the choice of outcome measures for clinical trials of diseases of later life.
6. The values of older people participating in clinical trials should be respected.
   - 6.1 The individual values of each older person participating in clinical trials should be respected.
     - 6.1.1 Researchers should respect the values of each older person as an individual.
     - 6.1.2 Older people should be able to withdraw from clinical trials without detriment to other treatments and their overall care.

This incorporates the findings of empirical research involving a wide range of health professionals, ethicists, patients and their carers in nine European countries and highlights key principles. Given the accumulating evidence of past neglect, it is important that future RCTs reflect the older patient populations that will receive treatment in future clinical practice.[99]

KEY POINTS

- Older adults are still too often excluded from research because of concerns about gaining consent, unnecessarily strict protocol restrictions on comorbidities and concomitant medications, worries about poor compliance and high attrition, problems with assessments, and fears of an unacceptable level of adverse events. Many of these concerns are unfounded or may be easily overcome.
- The optimum choice of design to study aging and age-related conditions depends on the research question to be answered. Qualitative studies, ecologic studies using available data, and quantitative studies using cross-sectional, case-control and cohort designs will help generate hypotheses. These can then be tested in experimental studies, ideally using randomized controlled trial designs.
- Curiosity, anticipated personal health benefits, and the possibility to help others are the most important motivators for enrollment and for continued participation in research. The main reasons for refusing are inconvenience and not wanting to be experimented on or a self-perception of being unsuitable. Older research participants are more motivated than younger people by feelings of altruism and paying back those who treat them and are less concerned about financial compensation.
- Cognitively impaired older people may have more difficulty comprehending consent information, and special attention should be given to compensating for communication and sensory deficits, improving readability of information sheets, and allowing sufficient time for the consent process. People with cognitive impairment and those in institutions may require alternative consent procedures.
- Once entered into a study, retention is promoted by maintaining good communication, good transport provision, and test sessions no longer than necessary and arranged at times to suit the participant. Outcome measures must be acceptable, valid, reliable, and responsive and focus on quality of life, especially functional, cognitive, and social outcomes, as well as morbidity and mortality.

For a complete list of references, please visit www.expertconsult.com.

KEY REFERENCES

1. Watts G: Why the exclusion of older people from clinical research must stop. BMJ 344:e3445, 2012.
2. Bayer A, Fish M: The doctor's duty to the elderly patient in clinical trials. Drugs Aging 20:1087–1097, 2003.
3. Diener L, Hugonot-Diener L, et al: Guidance synthesis. Medical research for and with older people in Europe: proposed ethical guidance for good clinical practice: ethical considerations. J Nutr Health Aging 17:625–627, 2013.
4. Center for Drug Evaluation and Research: Guideline for the study of drugs likely to be used in the elderly. http://www.fda.gov/downloads/Drugs/GuidanceComplianceRegulatoryInformation/Guidances/ucm072048.pdf. Accessed October 8, 2014.
5. European Medicines Agency: ICH topic E7: studies in support of special populations: questions and answers. Available at <http://www.emea.europa.eu/pdfs/human/ich/60466109en.pdf>, (Accessed October 8, 2014).
6. Bayer A, Tadd W: Unjustified exclusion of elderly people from studies submitted to research ethics committee for approval: descriptive study. BMJ 321:992–993, 2000.
12. Townsley CA, Chan KK, Pond GR, et al: Understanding the attitudes of the elderly towards enrolment into cancer clinical trials. BMC Cancer 6:34, 2006.
13. Higgins I: Reflections on conducting qualitative research with elderly people. Qual Health Res 8:858–866, 1998.
31. Konrat C, Boutron I, Trinquart L, et al: Underrepresentation of elderly people in randomised controlled trials. The example of trials of 4 widely prescribed drugs. PLoS One 7:e33559, 2012.
32. Crome P, Lally F, Cherubini A, et al: Exclusion of older people from clinical trials: professional views from nine European countries participating in the PREDICT study. Drugs Aging 28:667–677, 2011.
33. Herrera AP, Snipes SA, King DW, et al: Disparate inclusion of older adults in clinical trials: priorities and opportunities for policy and practice change. Am J Public Health 100(Suppl 1):S105–S112, 2010.
62. Bloch F, Charasz N: Attitudes of older adults to their participation in clinical trials: a pilot study. Drugs Aging 31:373–377, 2014.
68. Tolmie EP, Mungall MM, Louden G, et al: Understanding why older people participate in clinical trials: the experience of the Scottish PROSPER participants. Age Ageing 33:374–378, 2004.
71. Provencher V, Mortenson WB, Tanguay-Garneau L, et al: Challenges and strategies pertaining to recruitment and retention of frail elderly in research studies: a systematic review. Arch Gerontol Geriatr 59:18–24, 2014.
73. Sugarman J, McCrory DC, Hubal RC: Getting meaningful informed consent from older adults: a structured literature review of empirical research. JAGS 46:517–524, 1998.
76. Wood F, Prout H, Bayer A, et al: Consent, including advanced consent, of older adults to research in care homes: a qualitative study of stakeholders' views. Trials 14:247, 2013.
77. NHS National Institute for Health Research: ENRICH (Enabling Research in Care Homes): a toolkit for care home research, London, 2011, Dementia and Neurodegenerative Diseases Research Network (DeNDRoN); NHS National Institute for Health Research.

7 Geroscience

Felipe Sierra

INTRODUCTION

From the biologic perspective, aging is a rather complex term to define. Aging is not a disease but, because aging is the main risk factor for so many chronic diseases and conditions, it is difficult to separate the two operationally. Richard Miller of the University of Michigan defines aging as the "process that progressively converts physiologically and cognitively fit healthy adults into less fit individuals with increasing vulnerability to injury, illness and death,"[1] and this seems like an adequate attempt. It separates aging from the associated chronic diseases (a domain best covered by geriatricians), but it also sets the stage for a recently blossoming new field linking the two areas, termed *geroscience* (http://en.wikipedia.org/wiki/Geroscience).

A "cure" for aging—a fountain of youth—has been a dream of humanity throughout history. And, although aging is inevitable, it is easy to accept that humans age at different rates, so not all 70-year-olds are similar to each other in terms of health. It is also easily acknowledged that life span and health span can be extended simply by adopting moderate changes in lifestyle, including diet and exercise. Unfortunately, this is not easy for most people. Indeed, although public policy has managed to change most people's behaviors in some domains (seatbelts, smoking, and putting babies on their backs represent successful recent examples), reversing behaviors concerning unhealthful habits in terms of diet and exercise is considerably more difficult. For example, it is known that in many laboratory animals, substantially reducing caloric intake extends life span and improves health in old age.[2,3] Yet, very few people would have the willpower to subject themselves to the harshness of that regimen, and the entire area of dietary restriction (DR) is more suitable for experimental investigations than would be useful as a practical approach to human health.

There is a significant urgency in our need to address the issues posed by the increasing number of older people in the world, including both developed and developing countries. The most dramatic rise in the population is in those 85 years of age and older, including centenarians, and this poses challenges that as a species, we are not equipped to handle. In fact, in addition to the biology, our health care systems, economy, and the very fabric of society will be put to a test to absorb and handle this unprecedented increase in the proportion of older adults in the human population.[4,5] In addition to the obvious need for more properly trained geriatricians and social workers, there is also a need to understand the biology driving the aging process better as a way to diminish the ravages of old age.

Research on aging biology has exploded in the last few decades, from a relatively backward field focused on descriptive work that catalogued the many changes that occur during aging—first to a highly mechanistic phase driven by genetics, molecular, and cellular studies, and now to the current stage where, without neglecting the still unfinished mechanistic and discovery work, some of the findings are poised for possible application in humans. Interestingly, although there is a pervasive notion that aging is bad, and therefore all changes observed with aging should be reversed, research has shown that this is not really the case. This is because some age-related changes actually represent adaptive positive responses from an organism that by being alive, must strive to maintain homeostasis in the face of multiple challenges. So, although some age-related phenomena appear to be involved in increasing the risk for age-related disease (e.g., the decrease in proteostasis leading to neurodegenerative diseases),[6,7] others are neutral (e.g., cosmetic changes like hair loss), and some appear to be beneficial to the health of the organism. Attempts to reverse them might have unexpectedly serious consequences (e.g., changes in some hormones, possibly in testosterone[8,9] or insulin-like growth factor [IGF]).[10] Other changes are the result of pathology and are therefore independent of the aging process per se, yet they are difficult to separate in the case of highly prevalent diseases and conditions.

The main initial drivers of research into the biology of aging included caloric restriction, cell senescence, and the free radical hypothesis.[11] These are still active areas of research, but some of these have undergone significant rethinking. On the other hand, it is generally acknowledged that the main transformative research leading to the current status of the field was the genetic work initially encouraged by the National Institute on Aging (NIA) Longevity Assurance Genes Initiative (LAG).[11,12] At present, there are several hundred genes that when modified, can increase the life span in animal models.[13] Many of these fall into well-defined (and well-studied) pathways, but many remain orphans and are poorly studied or understood. Interestingly, in some cases, variant alleles of these same genes have been associated with extended longevity in human centenarian studies.[14] Although there is wide recognition of the partially inheritable nature of longevity, the finding that individual genes, when manipulated, could lead to dramatic increases in longevity was not expected and was initially greeted with skepticism. Nevertheless, the finding of molecular drivers of the process brought aging biology research into the mainstream and has resulted in the current renaissance of the field. These events have been reviewed previously and will not be repeated here.[11,12] Rather, in this chapter I will focus on the following: (1) the main current areas of research; (2) a discussion of geroscience and the importance of studying aging at the most basic biologic level; and (3) a look into future prospects and needs, based on the current status of the field.

THE MAIN PILLARS OF RESEARCH ON AGING BIOLOGY

In October 2013, a group of experts convened in Bethesda, Maryland, to discuss the current status of research in geroscience, the intersection between basic aging research and chronic diseases.[15] Seven major areas were discussed, and these overlap significantly with the areas identified by López-Otín and colleagues in a recent opinion piece.[16] These represent apparent drivers of the process and will be the focus of this discussion. It should be mentioned, however, that we are still in dire need of markers that can be used for research purposes, independently of whether they are drivers or not. The field has traditionally shied away from looking at biomarkers under the assumption that markers of aging might be too elusive. However, new techniques, including a large set of *-omics* technologies, now open new possibilities that need to be explored; in the absence of such markers, progress in the field remains hindered. In addition to markers that can be used to test the effects of interventions, there is a need to define mechanistic drivers that can be targeted for these interventions, thus paving the way for possible therapeutics that might delay aging and concomitantly delay the onset and/or severity of multiple chronic diseases and conditions that affect primarily the older population. Major areas currently considered as potential drivers of the aging process include inflammation,[17] responsiveness to stress,[18] epigenetics,[19] metabolism,[20] macromolecular damage,[21] proteostasis,[22] and stem cells.[23] A brief overview of each of these topics follows.

Inflammation

Inflammation is a crucial early response that allows the organism to defend itself against aggression by pathogens or tissue damage. Inflammation has been associated with multiple chronic diseases of older adults[19,24]; yet, due to its protective role, dampening it might have serious deleterious effects, and it is important to preserve this response, even into old age. The molecular and cellular mechanisms involved in the inflammatory response have been well studied in young organisms, and a proper response is swift and short-lived. Aged organisms also often mount a vigorous response to challenges; in fact, in some aspects, it is an exacerbated response[25-27]; however, in many cases, they fail to turn off the response properly, leading to a low level inflammation termed *sterile inflammation*.[28] This is characterized by a mild chronic elevation in the serum levels of several cytokines and acute phase factors, some of which, such as interleukin 6 (IL-6), tumor necrosis factor-α (TNF-α), and C-reactive protein (CRP), are actively used in the clinical setting to assess inflammatory status.[29-31] This age-related, low-grade chronic inflammation might be a contributing factor to chronic diseases and conditions, and therefore efforts at curbing the inflammatory response are currently ongoing in the clinic. However, as mentioned earlier, interventions aimed at dampening the inflammatory response altogether (e.g., antiinflammatories) might be ill-advised for two reasons: (1) the main defect with aging appears to be in the shutting-off phase; and (2) dampening the response would leave older adults susceptible to disease from pathogens and injury. It really needs to be to clarified about whether sterile inflammation is really a maladaptive response before proceeding to the clinic. It is also entirely possible that the low-level inflammation is not really maladaptive, but might be an appropriate adaptive response to age- or disease-induced tissue damage or other injurious activities, such as changes in the microbiome and/or gut leakage. More focused research in this arena is needed.

Adaptation to Stress

In common parlance, stress refers primarily to psychological issues. In addition to the molecular underpinnings of psychological stress (e.g., cortisol), cells are also constantly exposed to stressors at the molecular level, including free radicals, environmental toxins, and UV light. Both types of stressors appear to accelerate the rate of aging, at least when they are chronic,[18,32] and recent work is beginning to show the interrelations between psychological stress and molecular responses, such as telomere shortening.[33-35] The similarities and differences between molecular and cellular responses to a variety of stresses have not been studied in detail, and it is possible, although still rather unproven, that the responses elicited by different sorts of stress might have commonalities at the subcellular level. If so, then the source of stress becomes less relevant, and a new focus on the mechanisms used by the cell to respond might become targets for future investigation. It might prove easier to intervene on the ability of the organism to respond to stress than to try to eliminate all sources of stress, something that is clearly unattainable. It has been observed that although powerful acute or mild chronic stresses are detrimental,[18,32] some mild stresses (both physiologic and psychological) appear to be beneficial, probably through a mechanism related to hormesis.[36] The mechanisms that control the switch between beneficial and detrimental are currently unknown, and they might relate to whether the stress is chronic or acute. Further understanding of this level of control could, in principle, allow researchers to manipulate that pivoting point in a manner that might allow us to increase the positive and decrease the negative.

Epigenetics

Efforts at understanding the genetic underpinnings of aging have been very fruitful in the past, and the discovery that individual genes and pathways can increase life span in many species was crucial in turning aging research from the descriptive to the mechanistic phase. Furthermore, some of the findings initially described in lower organisms (worms and flies) have been shown to correlate with extreme longevity in human populations (centenarians).[14] There has been a renewed interest in the epigenome, which is more malleable and might better reflect the role of additional modifiers of aging, including diet and the environment. In lower organisms, significant changes in the epigenome, including heterochromatin, transposable elements, and histone modifications, have been described to occur as a function of age.[37-40] Epigenetic changes have also been associated with a number of age-related diseases such as cancer[19] and, because aging is the major risk factor for most chronic conditions, including cancer, the cross-talk between epigenetic changes due to aging and those due to disease are being explored. Another active area of research, related to the previous section, "Adaptation to Stress," is the resolution between beneficial and deleterious adaptations to stress, because epigenetic marks might integrate complex responses to the environment. Thus, it is important to establish to what extent these epigenetic changes can drive pathology and to what extent those changes might be reversible. The origin of epigenetic changes and their downstream effects are currently the subject of intense study.

Metabolism

Aging is associated with many metabolic changes, and a challenge for researchers is to identify those that are causative factors of aging and disease susceptibility and differentiate those that simply correlate and those that represent adaptive responses. Changes in metabolism have been associated with age-related diseases, including diabetes, cardiovascular cancer, and neurodegenerative diseases. Although diabetes is considered primarily a metabolic disease, this is not the case for many others. Interestingly, many pathways that affect longevity have been shown to play critical roles in metabolism. This includes the first genetic pathway described as aging-related, the insulin-IGF pathway, as well as the mammalian target of rapamycin (mTOR) pathway. In addition, the best characterized way of extending life span, caloric restriction, should be considered primarily as a metabolic intervention. Sirtuins represent another pathway that affects aging, and it has also been shown to have dramatic effects on cellular metabolism, probably via regulation of NAD^+ (nicotinamide adenine dinucleotide, oxidized form) levels.[41] Sirtuin activators such as resveratrol have been shown to extend life span in several species but, at least in mice, resveratrol only extends life span if the animals are maintained under the severe metabolic stress imposed by a very high-fat diet.[42-44]

Mitochondria also represent a central hub in energy metabolism and have received considerable attention from researchers on aging. For a long time, the focus was on their role as potential sources of reactive oxygen species (ROS) and macromolecular damage[21,45] and, contrary to expectations, reducing the activity of the mitochondrial electron transport chain leads to increased longevity, perhaps because of reduced electron leakage, which results in reduced free radical production.[46-48] In addition to their role in producing free radicals, mitochondria have also been studied extensively because of their central role in intracellular energy production. In addition to these classical modifiers of metabolism, current interests include other factors, such as changes in the microbiome[49,50] and in circadian rhythms,[51,52] both of which have dramatic metabolic and proinflammatory effects.

Macromolecular Damage

The free radical theory of aging has been a major player in aging biology research for more than a half-century.[53] The original theory suggested that damage to macromolecules produced by free radicals in the mitochondria will result in the loss of cellular and tissue function observed during aging. Considerable circumstantial evidence in favor of that hypothesis has accumulated in the last few decades. However, a comprehensive attempt at testing this theory was provided in the form of a set of mouse models that were genetically manipulated to increase or decrease free radical scavenging capabilities. Most of these manipulations did lead to the expected changes in macromolecular damage (decrease or increase, depending on whether defenses were increased by transgenic technologies or decreased in knockout models) but, surprisingly, they did not affect mean or maximal life span.[45,54] A notable exception is the MCAT (mitochondrial catalase) mouse model, where expression of catalase in the mitochondria (but not other subcellular compartments) leads to increased longevity and a decrease in cardiovascular disease.[55] In spite of these results, the free radical theory remains a stalwart of research, because free radical damage has been repeatedly correlated with various age-related diseases, including cancer and cardiovascular diseases, the main killers in the Western world.[56] It seems likely that the negative results indicate that like resveratrol, free radicals only play a role in longevity under stressed conditions, but not under standard Institutional Animal Care and Use Committee (IACUC)–approved mouse housing. Importantly in that regard, controlling free radicals seems to play a role in health span, irrespective of their role in life span.

In addition to protein damage, DNA damage driven by manipulation of mitochondrial or nuclear DNA repair systems do lead to phenotypes that some authors call "accelerated aging."[57-59] In independent research studies, it has been found that many human accelerated aging syndromes, such as Hutchinson-Gilford, Werner, and Cockayne syndromes, the culprits for the disease have been identified as mutations in genes involved in DNA repair or other DNA transactions, including structural integrity of the nuclear lamina.[60,61] As discussed earlier ("Adaptation to Stress"), it is entirely possible that the apparent acceleration of aging phenotypes in these models and diseases might not be the direct result of DNA damage, but the phenotypes might be related to the cell's response to that damage, leading to cell senescence, stem cell depletion, or other outcomes.[62]

Finally, telomere integrity can also be considered as a subset of macromolecular damage, because there is evidence supporting the notion that telomere shortening leads to deleterious effects through activation of the DNA repair response[63,64] and activation of cellular senescence.[65] Epidemiologic studies have clearly associated telomere shortening with chronologic aging[66,67] and, perhaps more interestingly, it has been found that telomere shortening is accelerated by psychological stress.[68-71] Whether causative or solely a biomarker, these findings are exciting, and further research in this area is likely to shed light on these relationships in the next few years.

Proteostasis

Although damage and repair of DNA during aging have received considerable attention in the past, proteins are now sharing the limelight, based on the fact that proteins are responsible for actually carrying out most of the functions of a cell. Just as with other macromolecular damage, research has focused less on the source of damage and more on the mechanisms that control responses and preserve the health of the proteome. This includes quality control mechanisms, collectively termed *proteostasis*, which include mainly chaperones, autophagy, proteosomal degradations, and others, such as endoplasmic reticulum (ER) and mitochondrial unfolded protein responses (UPRs).[72-75] In addition to being implicated in the aging rate, at least in *Caenorhabditis elegans*,[76-78] proteostasis mechanisms have also been implicated in many age-related diseases, including neurodegeneration (e.g., Alzheimer, Parkinson diseases) and systemic diseases characterized by the accumulation of intracellular or extracellular protein aggregates.[79-81] Loss of proteostasis appears to play a double role in aging and related diseases. First, there is a general decline with age in the activity of several quality control pathways, including chaperone inducibility, autophagy, and proteasome functions.[76-78,82] In addition, there is an increased burden of damaged proteins that need to be considered as a result of accumulation of toxic aggregates and other entities. On the positive side, this means that the problems of protein aggregation can be attacked on two fronts—decrease the damage or increase the defenses. In the past, emphasis has been placed heavily on decreasing or precluding the damage (see earlier, "Macromolecular Damage'), but current efforts are shifting toward improving the defenses by activating otherwise depressed proteostasis pathways. Recent research suggests that the various protein quality control mechanisms can interact and compensate for each other, both within a given cell and, perhaps more exciting, even at a distance.[83,84] This might have important translational potential, because it might be possible to improve the entire system by intervening in focused (but yet to be determined) pathways and cells.

Stem Cells and Regeneration

The potential of stem cells as a panacea for all types of age-related diseases has been widely touted, especially in the media. However, these claims need to be tempered by a careful assessment of the possible roles of stem cells during aging and disease. The last decade has seen a set of elegant experiments using heterochronic parabiosis—the pairing of a young and old mouse so that the animals share a common circulatory system via a process called *anastomosis*—in which it has been shown that often the problem with aging resides less with the stem cells themselves, but rather with their niche and circulating activating factors.[85] Therefore, at least in the case of muscle[85] and perhaps the ovary,[86] stem cells are still present in older individuals, but their niche appears to be incapable of activating them. Further analyses have indicated the existence of circulating factors present in the serum of young mice, capable of activating stem cells in the tissue of the older parabiont partners,[87-89] as well as the opposite (factors in old serum capable of inhibiting stem cells in the younger animal).[90] It is crucial to gain a better understanding of stem cells and their niches in different tissues and their role (or not) in each age-related disease before rational therapeutic approaches can be devised. It might be easier to modify the niche than to inject actual young stem cells into old patients, which might not prove to be a useful strategy unless the aged niche can support the function of the injected young cells. Another exciting area of research in this area involves induced pluripotent stem cells (iPSCs),[91-93] which are already becoming important research tools, but might also have therapeutic potential (with the caveats described above for so-called standard young stem cells). This is a rapidly expanding field of research and much remains to be learned, both about stem cells in general and their aging characteristics and their possible roles in various age-related diseases.

Aging biology has undergone a revolutionary change in the last few decades, and there are many additional areas of exciting research that are not covered in the brief section just presented.

Notable among them are rather recent findings from comparative biology[94-96] or the use of novel animal models. Similarly, no discussion was included about the notable contributions of classical evolutionary biology or demography, fields, which certainly shape the theoretical and conceptual contexts within which aging biology research is conducted. With the advent of multiple *-omics* technologies, comprehensive approaches such as systems biology are gaining attention, although thus far little of substance has been produced.[21]

GEROSCIENCE

Epidemiologic studies suggest that aging might be the major risk factor for most age-related chronic diseases,[97] and much recent research aimed primarily at increasing life span has shown that this leads to a delay and softening of the diseases that normally accompany old age.[44,98,99] It should be emphasized that the goal of aging biology research is not to extend life span, but to increase health in later years, termed *health span*. Life span is merely used as a surrogate that is easier to measure, especially in genetically tractable low organisms such as *C. elegans*, *Drosophila melanogaster*, and yeast. The close relationship between aging biology and risk for age-related chronic diseases gave rise to the new field of geroscience, "an interdisciplinary field that aims to understand the relationship between aging and age-related diseases and disabilities"[15,100] (also see http://en.wikipedia.org/wiki/Geroscience; Figure 7-1).

That aging biology plays a role in age-related diseases is not a new concept. There is a wide consensus that the ultimate goal of biomedical research is to improve the quality of human life. Initial efforts were successful in eradicating or limiting the ravages of infectious diseases and, together with improvements in sanitation and public health, led to a dramatic increase in human longevity during the last century. Unfortunately, that triumph came with a price tag, because it is now known that chronic diseases and conditions of older adults represent the main hurdle toward reaching the goal of improving the quality of human life. Thus, the basic tenet of geroscience is that because aging is malleable, at least in many animal models, and aging is also the main risk factor for most diseases and conditions affecting humans, then addressing the basic biology of aging is likely to return a better payoff in terms of health than addressing diseases one at a time, as often done currently.

Conceptually, it is important to understand that unlike infectious diseases or genetic disorders, chronic diseases of aging are multifactorial and complex in nature. The current model used in biomedicine is focused on fighting disease-specific risk factors for different diseases (e.g., cholesterol for cardiovascular disease, glucose homeostasis for diabetes, amyloid deposits for Alzheimer disease). However, there is a growing realization that although important, those disease-specific factors are not sufficient, and overt disease often becomes apparent only after other elements are present, notably the environment and the receptive niche provided by aging itself[101] (Figure 7-2). For example, unless genetically driven, cancer often appears in humans in their 60s and 70s; the explanation often given is that it takes a long time for all the necessary mutations to accumulate in any given cell. However, most mice develop cancer by the age of 2 years. Mutation and repair rates are roughly comparable between mice and humans,[102-105] and the commonality is that in both cases, cancer strikes when individuals are well past midlife, when aging organisms become frail and lose resilience.

A separate issue that makes geroscience timely is the inadequacy of current efforts at addressing one disease at a time.

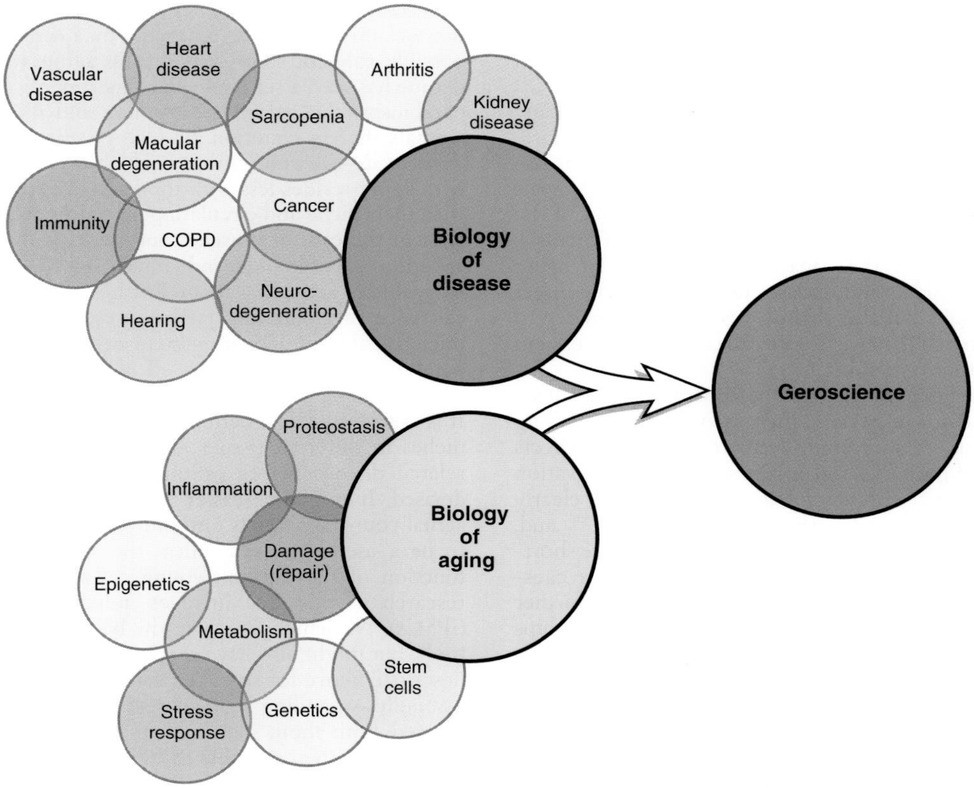

Figure 7-1. Geroscience is at the intersection between the biology of age-related chronic diseases and the basic biology of aging.

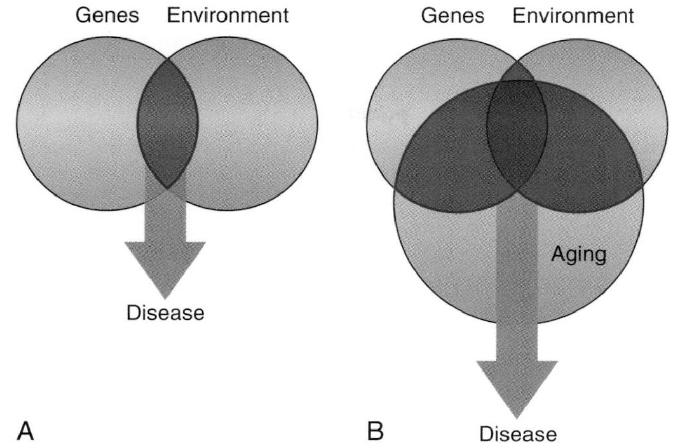

Figure 7-2. The major risk factors for disease. Disease can have multiple causes, grouped primarily into genes, environment, and aging and their interactions. **A,** When an individual is young, by definition, aging plays no role, and thus disease risk is determined solely by genetics, environment, and gene × environment interactions (shown by the *red-margined* intersection). **B,** In contrast, as an individual ages, the role of aging as a risk factor becomes ever more apparent until, at extreme age, it is the predominant risk factor for disease. Note that as this happens, the overall risk (the intersection containing at least two risk factors) becomes larger, which explains the age-related increase in overall morbidity. Centenarians are also subject to these variables, but appear to have a lower risk for disease as a result of a cohort effect—all other members of the cohort are dead, and survivors are those who are most resilient.

However, this is seldom seen in older adults, with comorbidities being the norm rather than the exception. Much current research in biomedicine is focused on preventing, curing, or managing one disease at a time, which is reflected at the level of the clinic, academia, and even funding agencies, such as the National Institutes of Health (NIH). This focus has further adverse effects; for example, clinical trials often exclude patients suffering from diseases other than the one being examined and often have an upper limit for age recruitment, thus effectively eliminating the very population for which the intervention is being tested from the trials—comorbid older adults. Because aging is the major risk factor for most chronic conditions, it follows logically that comorbidities are probably the direct result of that. Thus, by embracing that concept, geroscience aims at putting the emphasis on preventing or curing not one but all chronic diseases at once.

It has been known for centuries that aging is the major risk factor for disease and morbidity but is it true that nothing can be done about it? This is a major fallacy that has also been known to be incorrect for centuries. Chronologic age—the number of years humans have been on the globe—cannot be changed, but not everyone ages at the same rate, and there are large differences in the physiologic age of individuals in the same cohort. These differences are commonly believed to be driven by genetics and the environment so that in general, people who exercise, eat moderately, have a balanced diet, and avoid excessive stress tend to have a better physiologic makeup, even in their old age (although some "randomness" also plays a role). Such observations imply that the process of aging is not immutable but, on the contrary, is intrinsically malleable. In laboratory animals ranging from yeast to mice, aging can be delayed by behavioral (diet restriction),[2,3] genetic (more than 700 genes have been described that lead to extended life span),[13] and pharmacologic means (e.g., rapamycin, acarbose, metformin, and even resveratrol, under metabolically stressed conditions).[44,106-109] The significant advances in understanding the basic biology of aging that have been discussed indicate that the field is poised for further discoveries in the realm of pharmacologic means of extending life span. In most cases, these manipulations lead to significant resistance to disease and improvements in physiology; that is, the interventions also increase health span.

Most people, including older adults, do not consider extending life span to be a worthy goal unless accompanied by at least an extension of health span and, ideally, a compression of morbidity. As noted, this is also the goal of aging biology research and geroscience. Life span is simply used in research as an easy to measure binary surrogate. The issue of health is much more complex and should never be equated with absence of disease. The increased susceptibility to disease that occurs with age is primarily the result of an increase in physiologic frailty. Conversely, this frailty leaves us with a decreased ability to withstand stress. I have used the term *resilience* to refer to this ability to return to homeostasis as a response to a stress. Stress has many varieties including, in addition to the more easily recognizable psychological and environmental types, the stress caused directly or indirectly by disease or, in some cases, the interventions used to combat these same diseases (e.g., surgery, anesthesia, chemotherapy). The age-associated changes in frailty and resilience result in a decrease in the thresholds necessary for disease-specific insults to result in overt pathology. This explains, for example, why a prolonged period being bedridden is only a nuisance to a young individual, but could initiate a deadly cascade in an older adult. Age-related disease burdens can theoretically be alleviated by targeting any or all of these interrelated aspects—frailty, resilience, or the threshold at which insults become overt pathology.

The world as a whole is experiencing what has been called a *silver tsunami*, in which the convergence of lower birth rates and increased longevity is leading to a profound aging of most societies, including most developing countries. Thus, a concern is that if geroscience is successful, then most chronic diseases will be postponed as a group, life span will increase, and this will exacerbate the problem.[110] Although it is certainly true that life span will increase as a result of these efforts, two fallacies need to be considered: (1) although geroscience aims to postpone all chronic diseases at once, all biomedical research, in all domains, aims to extend life span by curing specific diseases; and (2) it is a mistake to think of these older adults, in current terms, as sick and frail. As discussed, multiple studies in mice and other species have indicated that addressing aging (as opposed to addressing one disease at a time) leads to robust older individuals, not sick ones. In fact, some studies have shown that it is our current approach that will lead to that dreaded outcome. It has been theorized that curing cancer, cardiovascular disease, or both would actually lead to a slight increase in the number of disabled people. This might occur because curing one fatal disease would allow a patient to live longer with other comorbid disabilities and conditions, including sarcopenia, osteoporosis, and sensory loss; although not life-threatening, this would considerably decrease the quality of life. If cured of only one of these diseases, individuals will keep on living with the other limitations until the next life-threatening disease (e.g., Alzheimer disease, diabetes, cancer) does kill them. (Actually, chronic diseases are not cured, they are simply managed.) In contrast, the same calculations have shown that delaying aging even minimally would produce the opposite effect, a decrease in the number of people with disabilities.[111,112] Therefore, under the scenario proposed by geroscience, the "new older adult" would not result in an undue burden on health or pension systems.

In summary, geroscience provides a new platform for thinking about an old problem. What are the molecular and cellular bases for the intersection between aging biology and chronic disease, and conditions that make the former the major risk factor for the latter? It is thought that by understanding this connection, we will be able to address and postpone all diseases and age-related disabilities at once, rather than one at a time, which is the current model.

A TENTATIVE LOOK INTO THE FUTURE

Based on the discussion in this chapter, it is clear that aging biology and geroscience are likely to become important areas of focus in biomedicine in the future. Although impressive scientific advances in the twentieth century have allowed the virtual obliteration of many infectious diseases, as well as significant advances in the detection, prevention, and treatment of many chronic and complex disorders, further advances in the coordinated attack on comorbidities of older adults remain a challenge. Furthermore, it is precisely those gains attained by biomedicine in the last century that are now allowing people to routinely live into their 80s and beyond, but with that apparent success comes the inevitable increase in chronic diseases and disabilities. Now is the time to work toward removing the word *inevitable* from that sentence. The advances in our understanding of the biology of aging, although still incomplete, give us a powerful tool in this regard. There is no time to lose; societal and health care systems are currently at or near their breaking point, and continuing the current trends will no longer be affordable.

There is therefore an urgent need to develop translational pathways that will allow the goals of aging biology and geroscience to be applied to the rapidly expanding older population. However, many hurdles remain and need to be addressed. Before discussing these, a review of prominent areas in which recent advances have been made will be presented (some have already been discussed in other contexts).

Questioning of Theories and Tenets of Aging

Some of the oldest theories and tenets of aging are currently being questioned, based on new empirical data. The free radical theory of aging has been a stalwart of aging biology research since the mid-1950s.[53] However, studies have shown that in most cases[45,54] (except as described by Schriner and associates[55]), genetic manipulation of free radical scavengers and their attendant damage to macromolecules has no effect on life span in mice, at least under the pristine environmental conditions in the laboratory. Another important tenet of aging biology research is the diet restriction paradigm. Diet restriction has been shown to increase life span and health span in many species.[43,113] However, studies in mice,[114,115] yeast,[116] and perhaps primates[117,118] have suggested that the efficacy of diet restriction is highly dependent on the genetic background of the individual, casting a shadow on our efforts to apply the paradigm (or interventions based on it) to very genetically heterogeneous humans. It should be noted, however, that these caveats are based solely on measurements of life span, but in the free radical and diet restriction paradigms, interventions do seem to improve health span, even when life span is not affected. Because health span is more desirable than merely life span, it would be irresponsible to ignore these areas of research as possibly being irrelevant within the context of aging research.

Interventions to Increase Life Span, Health Span, or Both

Several interventions have been shown to increase life span, health span, or both in several organisms. During the last decade, there has been a veritable explosion in the number of interventions purported to increase life span in mice and other species. Although much of the research has been based on genetic manipulations, these studies have pointed the way toward druggable targets. The best publicized of the pharmacologic interventions have been rapamycin and resveratrol, both of which extend life span and health span in a variety of organisms. Much controversy has focused on the fact that resveratrol only increases life span in mice subjected to metabolic stress.[44] In addition to the obvious fact that many people are under metabolic stress, these misgivings must be tempered based on two observations from the studies: (1) resveratrol improves health span, even in mice that do not benefit in terms of life span; and (2) resveratrol must be regarded as a first-generation drug, and second-generation sirtuin activators (STACs) have shown improvement of life span in mice under normal diets.

A second line of research is based on cellular (rather than molecular) aspects of aging. In the last decade, it has been found that senescent cells accumulate in various tissues and organs during aging to a larger extent than previously believed.[119-121] In addition, Campisi and coworkers have shown that senescent cells secrete many bioactive molecules, primarily proinflammatory and matrix-modifying factors, which can disrupt their immediate tissue vicinity, or perhaps even contribute to the organism-wide chronic inflammation of older adults.[101,122,123] Most importantly, using an elegant genetic trick, it has been recently shown directly that removing senescent cells leads to significant improvements in function in several systems, including adipose tissue, skeletal muscle, and the eye.[124] This is in spite of the fact that like resveratrol, the intervention did not lead to increased survival. Importantly, late life clearance of senescent cells attenuated the progression of already established age-related disorders and improved physiologic function (see next section).

Age-Related Pathology: Preventable and Perhaps Reversible

At least in some cases, age-related pathology is not only preventable, but might be reversible. As noted, removal of senescent cells leads to a reversal of already clinically observable pathology in several tissues.[124] In addition, there has been considerable recent excitement about the use of heterochronic parabiosis as a model to provide evidence for the existence of factors in the circulation of a young mouse that can reverse the aging phenotypes of an old mouse.[85,87-90] Parabiosis is a surgical technique to produce anastomosis and thus a sharing of circulatory systems between two individuals. This innovation has been to introduce heterochronism, in which the two animals differ primarily in their age. Using this system, laboratory studies have provided the first direct demonstration that a factor in the circulation of the young mouse (later identified as an activator of the notch-delta pathway) was capable of activating stem cells in old muscle.[85,125] More recently, others have been able to identify GDF-11, a member of the transforming growth factor (TGF) family, as a factor that can reverse already existing age-related cardiac hypertrophy in older mice.[87] GDF-11 also reverses aging phenotypes in several additional tissues, including the brain.[88-90]

These and many other pieces of data give credence to the belief that aging biology is poised to produce major breakthroughs in the way chronic diseases of older adults are viewed, both in the laboratory and in the clinic. However, many additional developments are needed before this promise can be brought to fruition. Without neglecting the need for continuous further discoveries in the areas of basic and preclinical translational research (see later), there are other major roadblocks beyond basic biology that will need to be addressed. First, potential interventions will need to be tested extensively for safety and pharmacokinetics in aged animal models before testing effects on multiple comorbidities in human clinical trials. This is particularly important because the interventions identified through research on the basic biology of aging are likely to have widespread effects on many organs and systems, and to be administered for extremely long periods, so there will be a need for very extensive analysis of these issues globally and longitudinally. Some of this work can be started already in those cases (e.g., with metformin, rapamycin, resveratrol) in which phase I or II clinical trials are already in progress for specific diseases or conditions. Ancillary additions to these studies to determine possible effects on diseases and conditions not primarily targeted would provide a fiscally conservative and effective means of obtaining preliminary information in this regard. In further studies, better-defined outcome measures need to be developed and validated.

A related roadblock is represented by the current status of clinical trial paradigms. The current model for clinical trials typically excludes subjects with morbidities unrelated to the one under study, as well as (more often than not) older adults.[126] However, these are exactly the populations being targeted for posttrial clinical purposes, older adults with multiple comorbidities. New paradigms will need to be developed to study the effectiveness of potential interventions in older animals and humans with multiple comorbidities. In animals, this involves testing interventions in aged animal models of the various diseases, preferably those that develop the disease naturally, rather than artificially through genetic manipulation. In the clinic, it will require a dramatic conceptual change to allow that although testing under the current sanitized conditions might allow for faster, cheaper, and cleaner analysis of the data, the onus is on trying to translate the findings into the real world—that is, the intervention needs to be effective in the clinic, rather than simply efficacious under tightly controlled conditions (refer to http://www.policymed.com/2014/02/fda-policies-and-procedures-for-proposed-trial-design-aimed-at-multiple-chronic-conditions.html#sthash.XqinSUlF.dpuf). In addition to testing effectiveness in clinically recognized diseases and conditions, many of the interventions currently under investigation might lead to accelerated recovery from clinical perturbations, such as chemotherapy or anesthesia. For example, research on diet restriction has led Raffaghello and Lee and colleagues to propose that a short period of fasting prior to chemotherapy is likely to decrease the notorious side effects of this treatment.[127,128] After encouraging preliminary data in models ranging from yeast to mice,[129] such hypotheses are currently in phase II clinical trials.

Exciting and promising as the current state of affairs appears, it is important to mention that although much emphasis has been placed on translating findings into clinical practice, scientists are well aware that many crucial developments in medicine have come from basic research that in itself was not meant to be translatable. Some of the findings described were not meant to be translated into humans, and yet clinical trials are being performed or are about to be initiated. Therefore, just as the translation, preclinical, and clinical paradigms need to be strengthened, this needs to be done without sacrificing basic research on the biology of aging. There have been many dreadful graphic depictions of the arduous road from "initial druggable hit" to U.S. Food and Drug Administration (FDA)–approved commercialization of drugs. Much effort has been devoted to strengthening the translation aspect of biomedical research. However, it is important to recognize that at the starting line of that graphic lies the initial discoveries that have come from basic research. If translation comes at the expense of basic research, soon there will be nothing new to translate; it is crucial that the spigot of basic biomedical research be kept open and flowing freely. In the specific area of aging, much more basic research remains to be done on molecular pathways (e.g., on known pathways such as the growth hormone–insulin–IGF-1–FOXO, mTOR, sirtuin, and AMPK [5′-adenosine monophosphate-activated protein kinase] networks and on new ones yet to be discovered), and on cell-based interventions such as stem and senescent cells, both of which show exceptional promise.

Thus, the potential impact of geroscience-based interventions is so broad that in parallel with the biomedical and population health aspects, it will be important to estimate the potential effects on health care and pension systems, as well as distribution of the workforce and other societal aspects. These will not be addressed here, but are no less important.

KEY POINTS

- Aging is the major risk factor for most chronic diseases and conditions affecting older adults.
- The rate of biologic aging can be manipulated (extended) by a variety of behavioral, genetic, and pharmacologic means in many animal models.
- When the rate of aging is decreased, it is most often accompanied by a delay in and decreased severity of naturally occurring diseases and conditions, as well as improved resistance to laboratory-induced diseases.
- At the molecular and cellular levels, a finite number of factors have been identified that control the rate of aging.
- The rapid pace of new discoveries makes it likely that additional pathways and drugs will be defined in the near future, thus making it likely that clinically relevant advances will occur as a result of studies on the biology of aging.
- A new field, geroscience, intends to bridge the gap and increase our understanding of the molecular and cellular underpinnings of aging that make it the main risk factor for disease and disability.

For a complete list of references, please visit www.expertconsult.com.

KEY REFERENCES

15. Kennedy BK, Berger SL, Brunet A, et al: Geroscience: linking aging to chronic disease. Cell 159:709–713, 2014.
16. López-Otín C, Blasco MA, Partridge L, et al: The hallmarks of aging. Cell 153:1194–1217, 2013.
33. Epel ES, Blackburn EH, Lin J, et al: Accelerated telomere shortening in response to life stress. Proc Natl Acad Sci U S A 101:17312–17315, 2004.
43. De Cabo R, Carmona-Gutierrez D, Bernier M, et al: The search for antiaging interventions: from elixirs to fasting regimens. Cell 157:1515–1526, 2014.
50. Heintz C, Mair W: You are what you host: microbiome modulation of the aging process. Cell 156:408–411, 2014.
77. Dillin A, Cohen E: Ageing and protein aggregation-mediated disorders: from invertebrates to mammals. Philos Trans R Soc Lond B Biol Sci 366:94–98, 2011.
82. Koga H, Kaushik S, Cuervo AM: Protein homeostasis and aging: the importance of exquisite quality control. Ageing Res Rev 10:205–215, 2011.
87. Loffredo FS, Steinhauser ML, Jay SM, et al: Growth differentiation factor 11 is a circulating factor that reverses age-related cardiac hypertrophy. Cell 153:828–839, 2013.
89. Villeda SA, Plambeck KE, Middeldorp J, et al: Young blood reverses age-related impairments in cognitive function and synaptic plasticity in mice. Nat Med 20:659–663, 2014.
95. Miller RA, Williams JB, Kiklevich JV, et al: Comparative cellular biogerontology: primer and prospectus. Ageing Res Rev 10:181–190, 2011.
100. Sierra F, Kohanski RA: Geroscience offers a new model for investigating the links between aging biology and susceptibility to aging-related chronic conditions. Public Policy Aging Rep 23:7–9, 2013.
108. Harrison DE, Strong R, Sharp ZD, et al: Rapamycin fed late in life extends lifespan in genetically heterogeneous mice. Nature 460:392–395, 2009.
112. Goldman DP, Cutler D, Rowe JW, et al: Substantial health and economic returns from delayed aging may warrant a new focus for medical research. Health Aff (Millwood) 32:1698–1705, 2013.

114. Liao CY, Rikke BA, Johnson TE, et al: Genetic variation in the murine lifespan response to dietary restriction: from life extension to life shortening. Aging Cell 9:92–95, 2010.
117. Colman RJ, Anderson RM, Johnson SC, et al: Caloric restriction delays disease onset and mortality in rhesus monkeys. Science 325:201–204, 2009.
118. Mattison JA, Roth GS, Beasley TM, et al: Impact of caloric restriction on health and survival in rhesus monkeys from the NIA study. Nature 489:318–321, 2012.
124. Baker DJ, Wijshake T, Tchkonia T, et al: Clearance of p16Ink4a-positive senescent cells delays ageing-associated disorders. Nature 479:232–236, 2011.
128. Lee C, Longo VD: Fasting vs dietary restriction in cellular protection and cancer treatment: from model organisms to patients. Oncogene 30:3305–3316, 2011.
130. Kirkland JL: Translating advances from the basic biology of aging into clinical application. Exp Gerontol 48:1–5, 2013.

8 Genetic Mechanisms of Aging

Chao-Qiang Lai, Laurence D. Parnell, José M. Ordovás

INTRODUCTION

Our society is experiencing unprecedented demographic changes where improvements in health care and living conditions together with decreased fertility rates have contributed to the aging of the population and a severe demographic redistribution.[1] Over the last 50 years, the ratio of people aged 60 years and over to children younger than 15 increased by about half, from 24 per hundred in 1950 to 33 per hundred in 2000. Worldwide by the year 2050, there will be 101 people 60 years and older for every 100 children 0 to 14 years old,[2] and many people over age 60 suffer from chronic illnesses or disabilities.[3] Therefore, to better understand the mechanisms of aging and the genetic and environmental factors that modulate the rate of aging, it is essential to cope with the impact of these demographic changes.[4] Aging can be defined as "a progressive, generalized impairment of function, resulting in an increased vulnerability to environmental challenge and a growing risk of disease and death."[5] It is generally assumed that accumulated damage to a variety of cellular systems is the underlying cause of aging.[5] To date, a large proportion of aging research has focused on individual age-related disorders compromising adult life expectancy and healthy aging, including cardiovascular disease (heart disease, hypertension), cerebrovascular diseases (stroke), cancer, chronic respiratory disease, diabetes, mental disorders, oral disease, and osteoarthritis and other bone/joint disorders. Environmental factors, such as diet, physical activity, smoking, and sunlight exposure, exert a direct impact on these disorders, whereas significant genetic components make separate contributions. Although individual genetic factors could be small differences in DNA sequences—single nucleotide polymorphisms or small insertions/deletions—in both the nuclear and mitochondrial genomes, the overall genetic contribution to aging processes is polygenic and complex.

The complexity of aging is reflected in that numerous models have been proposed to explain why and how organisms age and yet they address the problem only to a limited extent. The models that are more widely accepted include: (1) the oxidative stress theory implicating declines in mitochondrial function[6]; (2) the insulin/IGF-1 signaling (IIS) hypothesis suggesting that extended life span is associated with reduced IIS signaling[7]; (3) the somatic mutation/repair mechanisms focusing on the cellular capacity to respond to damage to cellular components, including DNA, proteins, and organelles[8]; (4) the immune system plays a central role in the process of aging[9]; (5) the telomere hypothesis of cell senescence, involving the loss of telomeric DNA and ultimately chromosomal instability[10]; and (6) inherited mutations associated with risk for common chronic and degenerative disorders.[11,12] In this work we will elaborate on the genetic component of each of these six hypotheses and the need for a more integrative approach to aging research.

MITOCHONDRIAL GENETICS, OXIDATIVE STRESS, AND AGING

The central role of mitochondria in aging, initially outlined by Harman,[13] proposed that aging, and associated chronic degenerative diseases, could be attributed to the deleterious effects of reactive oxygen species (ROS) on cell components. As the major site of ROS production, the mitochondrion is itself a prime target for oxidative damage. Moreover, this is the only organelle in animal cells with its own genome, (mtDNA), which is mostly unprotected, closely localized to the respiratory chain, and subject to irreversible damage by ROS. Specifically, accumulation of mtDNA somatic mutations, shown to occur with age,[14] often map within genes encoding 13 protein subunits of the electron transport chain (ETC) or 24 RNA components vital to mitochondrial protein synthesis. Not surprisingly, this mtDNA damage has been associated with deleterious functional alterations in the activity of ETC complexes. These mutations, whether single point mutations or deletions, have been shown in many studies to be associated with aging and with multiple chronic and degenerative disorders.[15] An early report examining the integrity of mtDNA found accumulated mtDNA damage more pronounced in senescent rats compared with young animals.[16] Other reports followed, including age-associated decreases in the respiratory chain capacity in various human tissues.[17] Hypotheses put forward stated that acquired mutations in mtDNA increase with time and segregate in mitotic tissues, eventually causing decline of respiratory chain function leading to age-associated degenerative disease and aging.[17] Furthermore, mtDNA haplotypes are associated with longevity in humans.[18,19] In sum, this mitochondrial genome–ROS production theory of aging is mechanistically sound and appealing.[20]

Deletions are the most commonly reported mtDNA mutations accumulating in aging tissues, and evidence for their role in aging is considered supporting.[21] In order to solidify the importance of mtDNA damage in aging, Trifunovic et al[22] developed a mouse model that indicated a causative link between mtDNA mutations and aging phenotypes in mammals. This "mtDNA mutator" mouse model was engineered with a defect in the proofreading function of mitochondrial DNA polymerase (Polg), leading to the progressive, random accumulation of mtDNA mutations during mitochondrial biogenesis. As mtDNA proofreading in these mice is efficiently curtailed, a phenotype develops with a threefold to fivefold increase in the levels of point mutations.[22] However, the abnormally higher rate of mutation took place during early embryonic stages, and mtDNA mutations continued to accumulate at a lower, near normal rate during subsequent life stages.[23] Although these mice display a completely normal phenotype at birth and in early adolescence, they subsequently acquire many features of premature aging, such as weight loss, reduced subcutaneous fat, alopecia, kyphosis, osteoporosis, anemia, reduced fertility, heart disease, sarcopenia, progressive hearing loss, and decreased spontaneous activity.[22] Such results confirm that mtDNA point mutations can cause aging phenotypes if present at high enough levels, but alone do not prove that the lower levels measured in normal aging are sufficient to cause aging phenotypes. Hence, attention turned to the focal distribution of mtDNA mutations rather than the overall amount as key in disrupting the efficiency of the respiratory chain and thus driving the observed aging phenotypes. To prove this hypothesis, Müller-Höcker examined hearts from individuals of different ages and reported focal respiratory chain deficiencies in a subset of cardiomyocytes in an age-dependent manner.[24] This was subsequently supported by evidence from a number of other cell types.[25-27] In sum, intracellular mosaicism, resulting from uneven distribution of acquired mtDNA mutations, can cause respiratory chain deficiency and lead to tissue dysfunction in the presence of low overall levels of mtDNA mutations.

The mitochondrial hypothesis of aging is conceptually straightforward, but in reality is much more complex[28] because a minimal threshold level of a pathogenic mtDNA mutation must be present in a cell to cause respiratory chain deficiency, and this threshold may vary between experimental models.[29] With 100 to 10,000 mtDNA copies per cell, mtDNAs that are mutated and normal at a given position coexist within a cell, tissue, or organ—a condition termed heteroplasmy. Different types of heteroplasmic mtDNA mutations have different thresholds for induction of respiratory chain dysfunction.[17] Moreover, subjects carrying heteroplasmic mtDNA mutations often display varying levels of mutated mtDNA in different organs and even in different cells of a single organ.[17] Furthermore, the intracellular distribution of mitochondria could play a role in the manifestation of the effects of mtDNA mutations.[30]

Although significant advances in our understanding of the role of mitochondria in aging have been made, it is likely that current theories will be revised as the link between mtDNA mutations and ROS production is more deeply probed.[31] Moreover, as the role of mitochondria in the response to caloric restriction is gaining relevance, available data are contradictory and not easily reconciled.[32] Thus research efforts will continue to describe the role of the mitochondrion in influencing the mechanisms of aging, but several boundaries should be heeded: (1) the difference in complexity between humans and model organisms at genetic, cellular, and organ levels; (2) the particular life span of each species, especially as medicine has allowed humans to live beyond a "normal" age of death; (3) the genetics of inbred animals often used in experiments contradicts humans who are highly outbred; and (4) the environmental conditions in which animals (highly standardized) and humans (quite different for anthropologic and cultural reasons) live.[33]

CHROMOSOMAL GENE MUTATIONS AND AGING

Genetic factors associated with human longevity and healthy aging remain largely unknown. Heritability estimates of longevity derived from twin registries and large population-based samples suggest a significant but modest genetic contribution to human life span of about 15% to 30%.[34] However, genetic influences on life span may be greater as an individual ages.[35] Moreover, the reported magnitude of the genetic contribution to other important aspects of aging such as healthy physical aging (wellness), physical performance, cognitive function, and bone aging are much larger.[34] Both exceptional longevity and a healthy aging phenotype have been linked to the same region on chromosome 4,[36,37] suggesting that although longevity per se and healthy aging are different phenotypes, they may share some common genetic pathways.

A number of potential candidate genes in a variety of biologic pathways have been associated with longevity in model organisms. Most of these genes have human orthologs and thus have potential to yield insights into human longevity.[38]

First, the most prominent hypothesis of aging states that mutants with decreased signaling through the insulin/IGF-1 signaling (IIS) pathway have extended life span. This pathway is evolutionarily conserved from nematodes to humans.[39] Thus genes of this pathway are promising candidate genes for influencing human longevity and healthy aging. Several studies have reported the association between genetic variants at *IGF1R* and *PI3KCB* and reduction of insulin-IGF-1 activation and longevity.[40,41] The finding that a nonsynonymous mutation in *IGF1R* was found to be overrepresented in centenarians of shorter stature when compared with controls[42] supports a role for the IIS pathway in life-span extension in humans, thus extending observations in model organisms.

Second, macromolecule repair mechanisms regulate the process of aging.[6] Dysfunctional systems for damage repair to cellular constituents, such as DNA, proteins, and organelles, could curtail life span. These repair mechanisms are evolutionarily conserved across species.[43] Many studies support the detrimental effects of defective repair on reduced life span. Examples are human premature aging patients with mutations in a RecQ helicase, a crucial enzyme responsible for DNA strand break repair.[44] Variation at this gene has shown association with cardiovascular diseases.[45] However, few studies have demonstrated that an enhanced repair ability increases life span.[46] In addition, the altered protein/waste accumulation in the process of aging could aggravate cellular damage.[10] Thus dysfunction in clearance of cellular waste, which is also called autophagy, would accelerate aging. Downregulation of autophagy gene expression, such as *Atg7* and *Atg12*, has shortened the life span of both wild type and *daf-2* mutant *Caenorhabditis elegans*.[47]

Third, the immune system plays a central role in the process of aging.[9] Although inflammation is an essential defense of immune systems, chronic inflammation often leads to premature aging and mortality.[48] One key player of inflammation is the cytokine interleukin 6 (*IL6*). *IL6* overexpression has been linked to many age-related that such as rheumatoid arthritis, osteoporosis, Alzheimer disease, cardiovascular diseases, and type 2 diabetes.[49,50] Human studies have also demonstrated that *IL6* genetic variation is associated with longevity.[51,52]

Finally, cardiovascular disease is the major cause of morbidity and mortality in industrialized countries and thus a major obstacle to healthy aging and longevity. Much attention has been placed on genes encoding proteins functioning in lipid metabolism. Plasma lipid levels are highly dependent on age, gender, nutritional status, and other behavioral factors. It is therefore difficult, at least in cross-sectional studies, to determine to what extent a particular lipoprotein phenotype is causally associated with aging. One way to circumvent this issue is to rely on long-term prospective studies or to perform family-based studies.[11] Well-designed case-control genetic studies may also be advantageous because identification of particular variants associated with longevity may provide some hints to the biologic pathways leading to exceptional longevity. To that end, a large number of allelic variants in genes encoding apolipoproteins (*APOE, APOB, APOC1, APOC2, APOC3, APOA1, and APOA5*), transfer proteins (microsomal transfer protein [MTP], cholesteryl ester transfer protein [CETP]), proteins associated with HDL particles (PON1), and transcription factors involved in lipid metabolism (peroxisome proliferator-activated receptor gamma [PPARG]) have been examined in elderly populations. Similar to many other aspects of lipoprotein metabolism and cardiovascular disease risk, the most explored locus in terms of associations with longevity has been that of the *apolipoprotein E* (*APOE*) gene. Since the initial observation by Davignon et al,[53] reports from different parts of the world have observed a higher frequency of the *APOE4* allele in middle-aged subjects compared with older subjects (octogenarians, nonagenarians, and centenarians), concluding that the presence of the *APOE4* allele was associated with decreased life span.[54]

To summarize, data accumulated so far illustrate that a variety of genes are involved in several mechanisms of aging, age-related diseases, and to a certain extent with longevity. Although thus far tenuous, there are a number of clues indicating that there is crosstalk between genes involved in longevity and those involved in age-related diseases that could be involved in longevity beyond effects on healthy aging.

Genetics is a valuable tool to expand our understanding of the molecular basis of aging. However, most studies published so far have been limited by design (e.g., cross-sectional study, small sample size, limited SNP coverage of a small number of candidate genes, interethnic differences) and so results have been inconsistent.[55] Most recently, genomewide association studies (GWAS) offer a more comprehensive and untargeted approach to detect genes with modest phenotypic effects that underlie common complex conditions.[56] Some notable findings are emerging from GWAS with a focus on aging-related phenotypes.[34,57,58] However, to benefit fully from the contribution of genetics, large prospective studies need to be undertaken and fully supported by extensive genotyping and analytical capacities to collect adequate phenotype data. Even more important is the urgent need for a reliable intermediate phenotype for aging, both for genetic studies and for therapeutic interventions.[57]

Telomeres and Aging

Telomeres are repetitive DNA sequences that are wrapped in specific protein complexes and located at the ends of linear chromosomes. Telomeres distinguish natural chromosome ends from DNA double-stranded breaks and thus promote genome stability.[59] Although traditionally considered as silent structural genomic regions, recent data suggest that telomeres are transcribed into RNA molecules, which remain associated with telomeric chromatin, suggesting RNA-mediated mechanisms in organizing telomere architecture.[60]

Telomere length has been proposed as a potentially reliable marker of biologic age, shorter telomeres reflecting more advanced age. Thus telomeres fit within mechanisms explaining the Hayflick limit[61] because they shorten progressively with each cell division. When a critical telomere length is reached, cells undergo senescence and subsequent apoptosis. Initial telomere length is mainly determined by genetic factors.[62,63] Although telomere shortening may be a normal biologic occurrence with each cell division, exposure to harmful environmental factors may affect its rate, accelerating telomere shortening.[64] To counter telomere shortening, telomerase, a cellular reverse transcriptase, promotes maintenance of telomere ends in human stem cells, reproductive cells, and cancer cells by adding TTAGGG repeats onto the telomeres. Moreover, recent studies suggest the existence of chromosome-specific mechanisms of telomere length regulation determining a telomere length profile, which is inherited and upheld throughout life.[65] Telomerases also may be involved in several essential cell signaling pathways without apparent involvement of well-established functions in telomere maintenance.[66] However, most normal human cells do not express telomerase and thus each time a cell divides some telomeric sequences are lost. When telomeres in a subset of cells become short (unprotected), cells enter an irreversible growth arrest state called replicative senescence.[67] The crucial role of telomeres in cell turnover and aging is highlighted by patients with 50% of normal telomerase levels resulting from a mutation in one of the telomerase genes. Short telomeres in such patients are implicated in a variety of disorders, including dyskeratosis congenita, aplastic anemia, pulmonary fibrosis, and cancer.[68] In addition to this manifestation in rare genetic disorders, short telomeres have been reported in the general population for several common chronic diseases, such as cardiovascular diseases,[69,70] hypertension,[71] diabetes,[72] and dementia.[73] With respect to cancer,[74] dysfunctional telomeres activate the oncoprotein p53 (TP53) to initiate cellular senescence or apoptosis to suppress tumorigenesis. However, in the absence of p53, telomere dysfunction is an important mechanism to generate chromosomal instability commonly found in human carcinomas.[75] Telomerase is expressed in the majority of human cancers, making it an attractive therapeutic target. Emerging antitelomerase therapies, currently in clinical trials, might prove useful against some human cancers.[76]

Based on current evidence, telomere shortening clearly accompanies human aging, and premature aging syndromes often are associated with short telomeres. These two observations are central to the hypothesis that telomere length directly influences longevity. If true, genetically determined mechanisms of telomere length homeostasis should significantly contribute to variations of longevity in the human population. Unraveling cause versus consequence of telomere shortening observed in the course of many aging-associated disorders is not an easy task. In addition, it remains unclear whether the biomarker value in a particular disease depends on shorter telomere length at birth or rather if it is merely a reflection of an accelerated telomere attrition during lifetime, or a combination of both. Although the importance of telomere attrition is supported by cross-sectional evidence associating shorter telomeres with oxidative stress and inflammation, longitudinal studies are required to accurately assess telomere attrition and its presumed link with accelerated aging.[77]

Epigenetics and Aging

There is wide recognition that the fetal environment may strongly influence the risk of cardiovascular diseases and diabetes, both age-related disorders, as supported by epidemiologic data in humans and experimental animal models. It has been widely assumed that these long-lasting consequences of early-life exposures depend on the same mechanisms as those underlying "cellular memory" (i.e., epigenetic inheritance systems). There is a growing body of evidence that environmentally induced perturbations in epigenetic processes (such as DNA methylation and histone modification) can determine different aspects of aging and the etiology and pathogenesis of age-related diseases.[78] Moreover, epigenetic alterations, such as global hypomethylation and CpG island hypermethylation, are progressively accumulated during aging and contribute to cell transformation, a hallmark of cancer.[79] Epigenetic tagging of genes controls expression of the genome and maintains cellular memory after many cellular divisions. Thus there is great importance in studying the epigenome to better comprehend genome health and the genetic mechanisms of aging. Moreover, tagging can be modulated by the environment, implying that environmentally induced changes in the epigenome could decrease or accelerate the process of unhealthy aging.[80]

An Integrative Approach to Aging Mechanisms

Caloric or dietary restriction (CR or DR)[81] is considered a universal mechanism that prolongs the life span of many organisms.[82] Although there is no unified explanation, multiple mechanisms and networks are thought to be involved. First, CR can extend life span through shifting energy metabolism. Although yeast under CR display enhanced respiration and decreased fermentation,[83] CR-mammals shift energy expenditure toward metabolizing fat and glycogen over glucose. One molecular mechanism potentially linking caloric restriction with longevity involves the PPARG pathway, possibly via lipid metabolism.[84] Picard et al[84] have shown that Sirt1 (sirtuin 1), the mammalian SIR2 ortholog, promotes fat mobilization in white adipocytes by repressing the effects of PPARG. Second, CR can extend life span by reducing ROS-mediated damage. Upon CR, SIRT1 also activates peroxisome proliferator-activated receptor gamma-coativator-1α (PPARGC1A), which regulates a series of nuclear receptors and controls mitochondrial function, oxidative phosphorylation, and cellular energy metabolism.[85] Upregulation of PPARGC1A reduces ROS production,[86] thus limiting mtDNA damage. PPARGC1A variants are associated with type 2 diabetes, CVD, DNA damage, and high blood pressure in humans.[87,88] Third, CR-animals are resistant to stress and inflammation through Foxo1 and Sirt1 inhibition of NF-κB signaling.[89] The most likely mechanism of CR-extension of life span adopts the hormesis hypothesis, a positive response of the organism to a low-intensity stressor.[90] CR is an evolutionarily conserved stress response using stress-responsive survival pathways that evolved long ago to provide for increased likelihood of survival in diverse environments.[82] Therefore, it is important to recognize the complexity of mechanisms involved in aging and the need to integrate several pathways and cellular mechanisms in understanding healthy aging. The term *network theory of aging* has been proposed[91] to overcome the reduction nature of individual models and to allow for interactions between individual contributing mechanisms. A proof of concept example is to consider interactions between two individual mechanisms that contribute to aging: DNA damage response and telomere maintenance. The key framework for considering these interactions is the integrative model, which predicts that telomere maintenance is an integral part of DNA damage response machinery. The integrative model predicts the dual phenotype, namely, dysfunctional DNA damage response and dysfunctional telomere maintenance, where one of these mechanisms is the cause of aging. In line with this prediction, between 87% and 90% of mouse models and human examples of premature aging show this dual phenotype. Hence the integrative model is consistent with the network theory of aging. Others have provided evidence suggesting the connection between DNA damage in telomeres and mitochondria during cellular senescence.[92] Accordingly, improvement of mitochondrial function results in less telomeric damage and slower telomere shortening, whereas telomere-dependent growth arrest is associated with increased mitochondrial dysfunction. Moreover, telomerase, the enzyme complex known to re-elongate shortened telomeres, also appears to function independently of telomeres to protect against oxidative stress. Together, these data suggest a self-amplifying cycle between the genetics of the mitochondrion and the telomere: DNA damage during cellular senescence promotes aging and age-related disorders.

KEY POINTS

- Important links between ROS production, mtDNA mutations, and aging, while strong, require further research.
- The mitochondrial role in the response to caloric restriction is coming to light.
- A number of nuclear encoded genes and their genetic variants affect any of several mechanisms of aging and longevity.
- Genomewide association studies hold promise to identify genetic variants pertinent to aging, but intermediate biomarkers of aging are critically needed.
- Shorter telomeres accompany human aging, and premature aging syndromes often associate with telomere shortening, but deciphering the causal role of telomere length in aging remains.
- The environment affects epigenetic processes and can influence the progression of aging and age-related diseases.
- The network theory of aging serves to link the genetic aspects of mtDNA damage, telomere maintenance with aging, and age-related disorders.

Acknowledgments

Supported by the National Institutes of Health, National Institute on Aging, Grant 5R03AG023914 and NIH/NHLBI Grant HL54776 and NIH/NIDDK DK075030 and contracts 53-K06-5-10 and 58-1950-9-001 from the U.S. Department of Agriculture Research Service.

For a complete list of references, please visit www.expertconsult.com.

KEY REFERENCES

8. Promislow DE: DNA repair and the evolution of longevity: a critical analysis. J Theor Biol 170:291–300, 1994.
9. Finch CE, Crimmins EM: Inflammatory exposure and historical changes in human life-spans. Science 305:1736–1739, 2004.
10. Collado M, Blasco MA, Serrano M: Cellular senescence in cancer and aging. Cell 130:223–233, 2007.
11. Martin GM, Bergman A, Barzilai N: Genetic determinants of human health span and life span: progress and new opportunities. PLoS Genet 3:e125, 2007.
17. Trifunovic A, Larsson NG: Mitochondrial dysfunction as a cause of ageing. J Intern Med 263:167–178, 2008.
28. Fukui H, Moraes CT: The mitochondrial impairment, oxidative stress and neurodegeneration connection: reality or just an attractive hypothesis? Trends Neurosci 31:251–256, 2008.
29. Dufour E, Terzioglu M, Sterky FH, et al: Age-associated mosaic respiratory chain deficiency causes trans-neuronal degeneration. Hum Mol Genet 17:1418–1426, 2008.
31. Meissner C: Mutations of mitochondrial DNA—cause or consequence of the ageing process? Z Gerontol Geriatr 40:325–333, 2007.
32. Masoro EJ: Overview of caloric restriction and ageing. Mech Ageing Dev 126:913–922, 2005.
35. Hjelmborg JvB, Iachine I, Skytthe A, et al: Genetic influence on human lifespan and longevity. Hum Genet 119:312–321, 2006.
38. Browner WS, Kahn AJ, Ziv E, et al: The genetics of human longevity. Am J Med 117:851–860, 2004.
41. van Heemst D, Beekman M, Mooijaart SP, et al: Reduced insulin/IGF-1 signalling and human longevity. Aging Cell 4:79–85, 2005.
50. Naugler WE, Karin M: The wolf in sheep's clothing: the role of interleukin-6 in immunity, inflammation and cancer. Trends Mol Med 14:109–119, 2008.
59. Shay JW, Wright WE: Hallmarks of telomeres in ageing research. J Pathol 211:114–123, 2007.
68. Aubert G, Lansdorp PM: Telomeres and aging. Physiol Rev 88:557–579, 2008.
78. Vaiserman AM: Epigenetic engineering and its possible role in anti-aging intervention. Rejuvenation Res 11:39–42, 2008.
82. Sinclair DA: Toward a unified theory of caloric restriction and longevity regulation. Mech Ageing Dev 126:987–1002, 2005.
91. Slijepcevic P: DNA damage response, telomere maintenance and ageing in light of the integrative model. Mech Ageing Dev 129:11–16, 2008.

9 Cellular Mechanisms of Aging

James L. Kirkland

INTRODUCTION

Aging changes are universal within a species and are intrinsic and progressive. They are universal; each true aging change should develop in all individuals in a species if they live long enough. Aging is intrinsic because these changes occur despite environmental cues, although the environment can alter their timing. The term *progressive* refers to the time dependency of aging processes. After adulthood, aging is associated with a general decline in cellular, tissue, and systemic function, loss of reproductive capacity, decreased resilience, and the ability to adapt to environmental perturbations and respond effectively to disease. Age-related phenotypes or diseases (e.g., development of certain cancers, such as prostate cancer, or onset of atherosclerosis) are likely predisposed to by fundamental aging processes that are operative during particular stages of life. These age-related phenotypes and diseases are heterogeneous and, unlike true aging changes, are not universal, occurring segmentally in different tissues and appearing at different times among individuals.

Recent important advances have been made in our understanding of the basic biology of aging. These insights into the cellular and molecular biology of aging have led to development of a number of interventions, both lifestyle and drugs, that extend life span and health span—the period during life free of chronic disease, pain, disability, and dependency—at least in mice. If these can be translated into humans, such interventions may prove to delay, prevent, alleviate, or even reverse the age-related diseases and disabilities that are the leading drivers of morbidity, mortality, and health expenditures in developed and developing societies. These age-related conditions include atherosclerosis, most cancers, mild cognitive impairment, dementias, Parkinson and other neurodegenerative diseases, type 2 diabetes, renal dysfunction, arthritis, blindness, frailty, and sarcopenia. For each condition, chronologic aging is a major risk factor. Indeed, for most, aging is a larger risk factor than all others combined.[1-4] Importantly, the major age-related diseases share the disturbances in tissue, cellular, and molecular function that also occur with chronologic aging. These include chronic sterile inflammation, cellular senescence, macromolecular damage (DNA, proteins, carbohydrates, and lipids), and stem and progenitor cell dysfunction. Based on these points, the geroscience hypothesis has been proposed: by targeting fundamental aging processes, it may be feasible to treat the major age-related chronic diseases and geriatric syndromes as a group, instead of one at a time. This hypothesis is being actively tested in experimental animal models and human cells. If true, and if the interventions that appear to be effective in targeting fundamental aging mechanisms in mice can be translated into humans, geriatrics practice and all of medicine as we know it could be transformed.

The basic biology of aging field has moved from an era of descriptive research to hypothesis-driven research, with a focus on elucidating mechanisms and, most recently, into developing interventions that target fundamental aging processes. The next phase, which has already started, is to translate these interventions into clinical application. Modulators and interventions that delay age-related changes in experimental animals include caloric restriction, several hundred single-gene mutations across species and, most recently several drugs. The single-gene mutations that extend life span or health span involve the growth hormone (GH)–insulin-like growth factor-1 (IGF-1)–insulin signaling pathway and other pathways related to anabolism and caloric restriction, as well as inflammation, the renin-angiotensin system, and cellular senescence, among others. In general, these genetic and pharmacologic interventions are related to inflammation, cell survival, cellular senescence, macromolecular processing, fuel and metabolic sensing and processing, caloric restriction, and stem and progenitor cell function. These interlinked processes, which appear to be the most likely targets for future clinical interventions to delay age-related dysfunction and chronic diseases as a group, are considered in this chapter.

INFLAMMATION

A general decline in immunity occurs with aging, with increased susceptibility to infections, cancers, autoimmune disorders, and associated mortality. Immune cells undergo declines in function in aging organisms—for example, there is decreased macrophage function and impaired activation potential of T cells in older individuals.[5-8] Additionally, the function of antiinflammatory pathways may also decline with aging, predisposing to development of a chronic, low-grade sterile inflammatory state that leads to tissue damage. The imbalance between proinflammatory and antiinflammatory pathways with aging has been termed *inflammaging*.[9]

Chronic, low-level, nonmicrobial (or sterile) inflammation develops in multiple tissues with both aging and age-related chronic diseases.[9-12] The source of this age-related chronic inflammation has not been pinpointed precisely. Candidate mechanisms include dysregulation of the immune system, chronic antigenic stimulation (e.g., by latent viruses), oxidative stress, increases in dysfunctional macromolecules (e.g., unfolded or aggregated proteins, glycation end products, or reactive lipids), and accumulation of senescent cells (see later).[9,13,14] Chronic inflammation can drive tissue dysfunction by at least two mechanisms. First, infiltrating immune cells can degrade tissues because they release reactive or toxic moieties. Second, inflammatory cytokines can provoke phenotypic changes in nearby cells that are independent of the immune system. For example, interleukin (IL)-6 and IL-8 can stimulate angiogenesis, disrupt cell-cell communication, impede macrophage function, induce innate immune responses, and promote epithelial and endothelial cell migration and invasion.[6,15-21] Furthermore, increases in tissue inflammation under basal conditions may contribute to an increase in susceptibility to autoimmune diseases, as well as to a restricted capacity to boost the extent of inflammation further when needed. This restriction in the dynamic range of inflammatory and cellular stress responses likely constrains the capacity to respond appropriately to infection, immunization, or injury.

Increases in inflammatory mediators, including elevated IL-6, tumor necrosis factor-α (TNF-α), and immune cell chemokine levels, are associated with multiple age-related diseases, including dementias,[22] depression,[23] atherosclerosis,[24-28] cancers,[29-31] and diabetes,[32-34] as well as mortality.[22,35,36] Sterile inflammation is perhaps the most important physiologic correlate of the age-related frailty syndrome[37-40] that encompasses heightened vulnerability to stresses (e.g., surgery, infection, trauma), muscle wasting (sarcopenia), cachexia, and adipose tissue loss.[37-39,41-49] Frailty predisposes to chronic disease, loss of independence, and mortality, as well as increased health costs.[45,47]

CELLULAR SENESCENCE

Cellular senescence refers to the essentially irreversible cell cycle arrest caused by potentially oncogenic and metabolic insults that evolved as a defense against tumor formation.[13] Senescent cells adopt a characteristic enlarged shape, increased protein content, elevated tumor suppressor proteins such as $p21^{CIP1}$ and $p16^{INH4A}$, an increase in senescence-associated β-galactosidase activity, and elevated secretion of a number of growth factors, cytokines, immune cell–attracting chemokines, and matrix remodeling factors, collectively termed the *senescence-associated secretory phenotype* (SASP) or *senescence-messaging secretome*.[50-52]

A number of inducers, including oncogene activation, DNA damage, telomere erosion, oncogenic proteins, fatty acids, oxidative stress, mitogens, cytokines, and metabolites,[52-55] can act alone or in combination to push cells into the senescent cell fate through pathways involving $p16^{INK4A}$/Rb (retinoblastoma), p53/$p21^{CIP1}$, and probably others.[13] These contribute to the widespread changes in gene expression and chromatin remodeling (heterochromatin formation) that underlie senescence-associated growth arrest and changes in morphology. In these respects, cellular senescence can be viewed as a cell fate reminiscent of differentiation, replication, or apoptosis, with external and internal cues leading to activation of transcription factor cascades, gene expression changes, chromatin remodeling, and changes in function. Intracellular autocrine loops, including loops involving interleukins and reactive oxygen species (ROS), reinforce the progression to altered gene expression, irreversible replicative arrest, and heterochromatin formation over a matter of days to weeks.

Cellular senescence contributes to age-related dysfunction and frailty and is frequently operative at sites of pathology underlying chronic age-related diseases.[4,13,56] Senescence can occur at any point during life, even in blastocysts[57] and the placenta.[58] Indeed, senescence is important in remodeling during embryogenesis.[59,60] Even though senescent cells are resistant to cell death through apoptosis,[61] they are normally removed by the immune system in younger individuals.[62] However, senescent cells accumulate in multiple tissues with advancing age.[13,63,64] Senescent cell burden is, in turn, associated with life span. At 18 months of age, long-lived Ames dwarf, Snell dwarf, and GH receptor knockout mice have fewer senescent cells in their adipose tissue than age-matched control wild-type animals, whereas short-lived GH overexpressing mice have more.[65] Caloric restriction sufficient to increase life span in mice is associated with decreased expression of $p16^{INK4A}$, a senescence marker, in multiple tissues compared to animals fed ad lib.[66] Conversely, senescent cells accumulate in fat and other tissues in obese animals and humans, especially when accompanied by diabetes.[53,67] Consistent with the geroscience hypothesis, obesity and diabetes are associated with an accelerated onset of other aging- and senescence-associated conditions, including atherosclerosis, vascular dysfunction, sarcopenia, cognitive impairment, dementia, early menopause, and cancers, including non–hormone-dependent cancers.[53,68,69] Progeroid mice, such as mouse models of Werner and Hutchinson-Guilford progerias, as well as *Klotho*-deficient, $Ercc^{-/-}$, and $BubR1^{H/H}$ mice, have increased numbers of senescent cells.[13,70-72] In comparisons across longer versus shorter lived mouse cohorts, senescent cell accumulation in liver and intestinal crypts predicted mean and maximum life spans.[73]

The SASP involves the release of proinflammatory cytokines, chemokines, prothrombotic factors, and extracellular matrix proteases that cause tissue damage, as well as extracellular matrix proteins that can contribute to dysfunctional tissue architecture. In addition to removing cells from the progenitor–stem cell pool, senescence may contribute to tissue dysfunction and chronic disease predisposition through the SASP and the chronic sterile inflammation and extracellular matrix disorganization that it causes. The associations among cellular senescence, aging, and age-related pathologies prompted testing if senescent cell clearance ameliorated dysfunction. Genetically targeting senescent cells in progeroid mice that expressed a drug-activatable so-called suicide gene only in senescent cells enhanced health span.[74] Even clearing only around 30% of senescent cells from these mice led to partial reversal of age-related lipodystrophy and decreased progression of frailty, sarcopenia, and cataract formation.[13,74]

Furthermore, senescent cell removal later in life delayed progression of age-related pathology, even after it had emerged. Drugs that selectively eliminate senescent cells—senolytic drugs— have been discovered.[75] These drugs alleviate age-related cardiac and carotid vascular dysfunction in old mice, radiation-induced muscle dysfunction in younger mice, and neurologic dysfunction, osteoporosis, and frailty in progeroid mice. Cellular senescence is associated with many of the chronic diseases and disabilities that are leading drivers of morbidity, mortality, and health costs.[4,13,56] Senescent cells have been identified at sites of pathology in a number of these conditions and may have systemic effects that predispose to others (Table 9-1). These findings support a link between senescent cells and age-related dysfunction. There is now the prospect that drugs that target senescent cells and the SASP might come into clinical use to delay, prevent, ameliorate, or even reverse age- and senescence-related dysfunction and diseases in humans.

MACROMOLECULAR DYSFUNCTION

Aging is associated with the accumulation of damaged macromolecules, including DNA, proteins, carbohydrates, and lipids in and around cells. In most cases, these damaged macromolecules or the processes underlying their accumulation are related to chronic inflammation, cellular senescence, and stem and progenitor cell dysfunction, as well as to the major age-related chronic diseases. As considered later, many of the drugs that show promise for enhancing health or life span act on processes responsible for the generation or effects of these damaged macromolecules.

DNA

Genomic damage accumulates over time due to environmental exposure and effects of metabolic byproducts, requiring DNA repair mechanisms to deal with these insults. Consistent with this, DNA repair and longevity are positively correlated.[76] Premature aging phenotypes develop in mice with genetic ablation of genome repair mechanisms. Mitochondrial DNA damage, thought to be caused by ROS, may contribute to mitochondrial dysfunction with age, leading to inefficient adenosine triphosphate (ATP) production. Age-related mitochondrial dysfunction could play an important part in metabolic, cardiovascular, skeletal, and other age-related disorders.[77] Genetic regulation at other levels can also become dysfunctional with aging—for example, at the level of noncoding RNA. Dysregulation of microRNAs (miRNAs), which have widespread effects on gene expression and cell function, and potentially also of proinflammatory noncoding RNAs, appears to be related to an age-related decline in Dicer protein, which processes miRNAs and other types of RNAs.[78]

Telomeres

Telomeres are structures at the ends of chromosomes, They comprise repeated TTAGGG nucleotide sequences in chromosomal DNA and several proteins that bind to telomeric DNA and cap the ends of chromosomes. During DNA replication, as cells

TABLE 9-1 Conditions Associated with Cellular Senescence

Condition	Examples	References
Metabolic	• Diabetes • Obesity • Metabolic syndrome • Age-related lipodystrophy	53, 67
Cardiovascular disorders	• Atherosclerosis • Hypertension • Heart failure • Peripheral vascular disease	4, 126-129
Frailty	• Sarcopenia	13, 74
Loss of resilience	• Side effects shortly or many years after chemotherapy or radiation • Delayed recovery after elective surgery • After acute events such as myocardial infarction	4, 13, 130-132
Impaired vision	• Cataracts • Glaucoma • Macular degeneration	74, 133, 134
Neurodegenerative diseases	• Alzheimer disease • "Tau-opathies" • Parkinson • "Chemobrain" after, for example, *cis*-platinum • HIV dementia	4, 135-138
Bone disorders	• Osteoporosis • Osteoarthritis • Fracture nonunion	71, 139-141
Lung conditions	• Idiopathic pulmonary fibrosis • Bleomycin lung and other drug- or environmental toxin–related lung diseases • Chronic obstructive pulmonary disease	142-146
Liver disease	• Primary biliary cirrhosis	147
Renal and genitourinary dysfunction	• Age-related glomerulosclerosis • Predisposition to acute tubular necrosis • Diabetic renal disease • Prostatic hypertrophy	4, 148-151
Skin disorders	• Melanocytic nevi • Chronic skin ulcers (bedsores)	152, 153
Cancers		4, 154, 155
Drugs	• Alkylating and other chemotherapeutic agents • HIV protease inhibitors • Long-term growth hormone treatment • Toxins	65, 131, 156, 157
Radiation	• Long-term effects of therapeutic or accidental radiation	132
Genetic disorders	• Progerias	158
Infections	• Human immunodeficiency virus	156
Chronologic aging		13, 63

divide, stretches of telomeric DNA at the ends of chromosomes, often 50 to 100 base pairs (bp) long, are lost at each division. Some cells, including germline, stem, cancer, and certain immune system cells, express telomerase, an enzyme complex that can regenerate telomeric DNA during each cell division, preventing telomere erosion. Loss of telomeric DNA alters the binding of proteins to telomeres and can result in unfolding or uncapping of chromosomal ends, which initiates cellular damage responses that can lead to loss of cellular replicative potential, loss of capacity to differentiate into specialized cell types, cell death, senescence, mitochondrial dysfunction with ROS generation, and inflammation. As individuals age, and cells have undergone increasing numbers of cell divisions, telomere erosion progresses and appears to contribute to tissue dysfunction and aging phenotypes.

Accumulation of Dysfunctional Proteins

Accumulation of damaged, misfolded, abnormally glycated, oxidized, cross-linked, and aggregated proteins occurs in many tissues with aging and at sites of pathology in many age-related chronic diseases. Aggregated proteins contribute to the pathogenesis of many diseases, such as dilated cardiomyopathy, Alzheimer disease, Parkinson disease, insulin-dependent diabetes, and glomerulosclerosis.[79] Slowed protein turnover and decreased protein clearance, which is normally promoted by proteasomal degradation and autophagy, occur with aging. Damaged proteins can induce cellular stress responses that can lead to inhibition of the capacity for progenitors to differentiate into specialized cells, cell death, inflammation, and cellular senescence.

Autophagy

Degradation of damaged intracellular components by lysosomes or autophagy is part of the response to stress in many cells.[80,81] By removing defective or damaged cellular components, autophagy contributes to cellular quality control. It is involved in cellular responses to proteotoxicity, genotoxicity, metabolic stress, and immune stress. Autophagy helps return cells to homeostasis by removing damaged or malfunctioning cellular structures, eliminating exogenous cellular damaging factors, or providing alternative sources of energy to help in resolving dysfunction by facilitating the turnover and recycling of essential constituents.[82-84] It contributes to cell remodeling and differentiation by mediating the relative abundance of different proteins and eliminating damaged or excess cellular structures.[85] It also contributes to immune responses and mitigates cellular damage.[86,87] The central role for autophagy in regulating cellular function is disrupted in certain neurodegenerative disorders, leading to poor quality control of cellular components, in diabetes and obesity, resulting in altered energetic balance, and in autoimmune disorders and infections due to interference with immune responses.[80,81,88] Blocking autophagy in muscle causes an accumulation of oxidized proteins, dysfunctional mitochondria, denervation, and decreased fiber force.[89]

Three autophagy pathways have been described in mammals—macroautophagy, chaperone-mediated autophagy, and microautophagy. During macroautophagy, targeted cytoplasmic cellular structures or macromolecules are isolated from the rest of the cell within a double-membraned vesicle, an autophagosome. The autophagosome then fuses with a lysosome, where its cargo is degraded and recycled. Chaperone-mediated autophagy is a process in which chaperone proteins selectively bind to dysfunctional cellular constituents and facilitate their importation and destruction by lysosomes. Macroautophagy and chaperone-mediated autophagy gradually become dysfunctional with aging.[79,90,91] Effective autophagy has been associated with longevity and health span in genetic studies.[79,90]

Rapamycin extends life span and health span in mice.[92] One mechanism may be through enhancing autophagy. Rapamycin inhibits the mammalian target of rapamycin (mTOR) protein, a kinase that promotes protein synthesis and inhibits autophagy. The activity of mTOR is increased in response to elevated amino acid availability, IGF-1, insulin, and other growth signals, whereas mTOR inhibition recapitulates some but not all of the effects of caloric restriction. A net effect of mTOR inhibition by rapamycin is an increase in protein quality, as well as decreases in the SASP and other effects. Clinical trials of rapamycin and related compounds are currently under way for a variety of age-related conditions and diseases, including dementias and cardiovascular diseases, and to enhance influenza vaccine responses in older populations.

Carbohydrates

Glycation can affect phospholipids and nucleic acids to form what are known as advanced glycation end products (AGEs) through the Maillard reaction. Hemoglobin A_{1c} is an example of a protein with which reducing sugars have reacted to form a Maillard adduct. With aging, defenses against the formation of glycation adducts become less active. AGEs can activate proinflammatory signaling cascades through a cell surface receptor–mediated mechanism involving receptors for advanced glycation end products (RAGEs),[93] which SASP factors can also activate. AGEs accumulate in normal brain and other tissues with aging, but have also been implicated in cultured neuronal toxicity as well as β-amyloid aggregation in Alzheimer disease.[94,95] AGEs are involved in the pathogenesis of diabetes and its complications,[96] perhaps contributing to susceptibility to type 2 diabetes and diabetes complications in old age.

Lipids

Ectopic lipids are deposited in nonadipose tissues such as muscle, liver, bone marrow, and pancreatic beta cells with aging.[97] The bone marrow is often filled with yellow fat in older subjects, and age-related sarcopenia is closely associated with fatty infiltration of muscle. Ectopic lipid deposition may occur, in part, because of age-related decreases in adipose tissue capacity to store lipids effectively. This in turn is associated with failure of fat cell progenitors to differentiate into fully functioning fat cells. Ectopically deposited lipids include highly reactive, cytotoxic fatty acids and ceramides that cells other than fat cells are poorly equipped to sequester, store, or protect themselves against. Reduced autophagy with aging also contributes to intracellular cytotoxic lipid accumulation. Ectopic lipids can lead to lipotoxicity, which contributes to metabolic dysfunction and inflammation, particularly in the setting of overnutrition.[98] Aging also is related to declines in defenses against lipotoxicity at the cellular and organismal levels,[99,100] potentially amplifying the adverse effects of ectopic lipid deposition in old age.

PROGENITOR AND STEM CELL DYSFUNCTION

A general feature of aging is a decline in regenerative capacity after tissue damage. The basis for this involves cell dynamic changes in stem and progenitor cell function, including declines in capacities for replication and full differentiation into specialized cell types, as well as changes in propensities for senescence, apoptosis, and necrosis.

Adult stem cells are multipotent—that is, capable of differentiating into different types of specialized cells. Mesenchymal stem cells are an example; they can become committed to the adipocyte, bone, chondrocyte, muscle, or neuronal lineages, among others. Adult stem cells are capable of self-renewal, but unlike true stem cells, are not capable of forming an entire embryo and placenta, at least without genetic modification. Adult stem cells reside in protected niches in most, if not all tissues. Generally, they divide infrequently, unless new progenitors need to be generated during rapid tissue turnover or after injury.

Here, progenitor cells are considered to be cells capable of self-renewal that are committed to develop into a specialized type of cell on differentiation. Cells in most or perhaps all human organs turn over throughout life, including the brain and heart. The extent of turnover varies considerably among tissues, with gut epithelial cells being replaced every few days, skin every few weeks, red blood cells every few months, adipose tissue every few years, and cardiomyocytes once or twice in a lifetime. Turnover is increased after injury, with replication of committed progenitors, differentiation of progenitors into specialized cells, and recruitment and commitment of stem cells. Apoptosis, senescence, and necrosis are also accelerated as regenerating tissues are shaped and remodeled during repair.

Stem cell and progenitor pools are not unlimited, but can become depleted with age and through increased utilization for tissue repair. Autonomous and nonautonomous cell changes can occur during aging that restrict cellular replicative potential and thereby interfere with repair following injury or diseases.[101] Declines in adult stem cell recruitment are partly due to noncell autonomous changes in the stem cell niche or microenvironment. Chronic sterile inflammation associated with aging may contribute to a toxic or suppressive microenvironment that impedes proper stem cell function. Cross-talk among organ systems—for example, between adipose tissue and bone—can affect progenitor cell function and become dysregulated with aging.[102] Age-related changes in the microenvironment have been demonstrated in parabiosis experiments in which old and young mice are joined surgically so that they share circulations for several weeks or months.[103] When heart or skeletal muscle injury is sustained by the older animal, circulating factors from the young animal hasten repair by the older animal's own progenitors compared to parabiotic pairs of old with old animals. Conversely, factors from the old animals impede progenitor function and repair of tissues in cross-circulated young animals compared to parabiotic pairs of young animals with young animals. Thus, inflammation, cellular senescence, and circulating or paracrine factors appear to be important drivers of age-related dysfunction of adult stem cells. Aging progenitor cells may have at least some preservation of inherent function that is suppressed by the aging microenvironment. It appears that the provision of circulating factors from young to old animals, including growth and differentiation factor 11 (GDF-11), can restore progenitor potential and function of the brain, heart, and muscle of old mice,[104,105] suggesting that drugs based on these factors could one day be developed to enhance regeneration in older humans.

Multipotent adult stem cells can become committed to particular lineages through determination, which is mediated by external and internal signals and paracrine, metabolic, and hormonal factors. Even if adult stem cells can proliferate and produce committed progenitors that can differentiate, these cells may produce a skewed population of progenitors—for example, with a skew toward the myeloid lineage with aging in the hematopoietic system.[106]

Unlike adult stem cells, committed progenitors usually do not express telomerase and, due to this and other mechanisms, have limited replicative potential in vitro and in vivo. Over the course of a lifetime, the cumulative replicative history of progenitors is increased, and telomere length is decreased. Partly related to this, progenitors isolated from fat, marrow, skin, and other tissues of older subjects have an overall reduction in capacity for further proliferation compared to cells from younger subjects. Although colonies of cells derived from single progenitors isolated from older subjects undergo fewer divisions than clones isolated from younger subjects on average, some individual clones from older subjects can behave like those from younger individuals, and vice versa.[53,107]

The capacity of committed progenitors to differentiate into specialized cell types declines in several tissues, such as adipose tissue, with aging.[53] This is evident even in colonies derived from single progenitors isolated from older compared to younger individuals. However, as for age-related declines in replicative potential, there are some clones originating from older individuals that behave like cells isolated from younger individuals.[107] Impaired differentiation is associated with decreased signaling through the transcription factor cascades that regulate differentiation. Increases in inflammatory mediators with aging appear to contribute to declines in capacity for differentiation, at least in the case of adipose tissue. Decreased capacity of fat cell progenitors to differentiate into fat cells may contribute to age-related insulin resistance, diabetes, and lipotoxicity, which contributes to further inflammation. Consistent with this age-related decline in capacity for differentiation, undifferentiated progenitors tend to increase in a number of tissues relative to specialized cells with aging, including in adipose tissue and the intestine.

Thus, there are overall cell autonomous declines in progenitor replicative potential and capacity to differentiate with increasing age. These declines may contribute to decreased tissue repair capacity and resilience, although there remains a pool of stem cells and functional progenitors that can repair tissues, particularly if the aging tissue microenvironment can be made more favorable. Interventions to achieve this appear possible in experimental animals, and exciting opportunities to extend the power of regenerative biology to older adults may be feasible.

INTERVENTIONS

Although aging has long been recognized as the leading risk factor for chronic diseases and frailty, it has only recently become widely viewed as a potentially modifiable risk factor. Supporting this view are findings that include the following:

1. Maximum life span is extended and age-related diseases are delayed across species by a number of single gene mutations,[108] suggesting the pathways affected by these mutations could be therapeutic targets.
2. Humans who live beyond the age of 100 years, a partly heritable trait, frequently have delayed onset of age-related diseases and disabilities,[109] leading to compression of morbidity and enhanced health span.
3. Rapamycin, metformin, acarbose, 17α-estradiol, angiotensin-converting-enzyme (ACE) inhibitors, and other agents increase health span and life span in mouse models.[92,110,111] These agents may also delay age-related diseases and dysfunction. For example, rapamycin appears to delay cancers and age-related cognitive decline.[112]
4. Caloric restriction, which increases maximum life span, is associated with delayed onset of multiple chronic diseases in animal models.[113]
5. Factors produced by stem cells from young individuals ameliorate dysfunction in older individuals.[103,114]
6. Senescent cell accumulation is associated with chronic inflammation, which in turn promotes many age-related chronic diseases and frailty.[115] Importantly, senescent cell elimination enhances health span in mice.[74,75]

Because interventions that increase life span and health span in mammals now exist, it appears plausible that by targeting fundamental mechanisms of aging, clinical interventions might be developed that could delay or prevent age-related diseases and disabilities as a group, rather than one at a time. Even if a major chronic disease such as atherosclerotic heart disease were eradicated, as transformative as such an advance would be, it would only add around 3 years to life expectancy.[116,117] However, attacking the intersection between fundamental aging mechanisms and processes that lead to age-related chronic diseases could delay these diseases and enhance health span. This would have a substantially larger impact on morbidity and health costs than curing any one of the major chronic diseases, such as atherosclerosis, cancers, or dementias.

It is impractical to study the effectiveness of experimental strategies to extend health span or, especially, life span in humans. Therefore, feasible and clinically relevant clinical trials paradigms must be established to test whether agents that target fundamental aging processes can be translated into clinical use. These may include measures of frailty or resilience—for example, recovery after elective surgery, chemotherapy, therapeutic radiation, myocardial infarction, immunization, or other clinically relevant perturbations. They might also include multiple age-related chronic disease outcomes in subjects with comorbidities. Effects on symptoms and signs of progerias might also be a reasonable clinical trial paradigm. In addition, short-term studies may be appropriate for agents that are expected to reverse age-related pathology in older individuals.

Caloric restriction (CR) extends life span in yeast, worms, flies, and rodents and affects a large number of downstream metabolic and posttranscriptional pathways.[118] Studies in nonhuman primates have not definitively linked CR with life span extension, but CR enhanced health span and delayed the onset of age-related phenotypes.[119,120] Although humans practicing CR exhibit a range of improved metabolic phenotypes, such as decreased body weight and fasting glucose levels, increased insulin sensitivity, and low prevalence of metabolic syndrome, CR has also has adverse effects on the quality of life. These include irritability, lethargy, slow wound healing, decreased libido, and reduced body temperature.[121]

In addition to CR, factors that are known to affect maximum life span include several hundred single-gene mutations across species and an increasing number of pharmacologic agents. There are currently at least a half-dozen drugs reported to increase life span in various model organisms, including the following: rapamycin (see earlier),[92,122] curcumin,[123] metformin,[110] and several agents that have preferential effects on male mice; aspirin (which enhances median, but perhaps not maximum life span)[124]; and 17α-estradiol, acarbose, and nordihydroguaiaretic acid (NDGA).[111] In general, these agents alleviate inflammation, cellular senescence, and/or pathways related to CR, metabolic function, or macromolecular processing (see earlier).

Cellular senescence has been implicated in chronic sterile inflammation, age-related diseases, and the promotion of tumor spread. As previously mentioned, clearance of senescent cells in mice has beneficial effects on the amelioration of preexisting disease phenotypes and on the prevention of onset of age-related disease phenotypes. Therefore, there is interest in translating these results into the prevention and treatment of human disease.[13,125] This requires selective targeting of senescent cells, without disruption of surrounding normal cells, while preserving normal tissue architecture. Senolytic drugs that can do this have been developed.[75] Another strategy to prevent the detrimental effects of senescent cells is to target SASP components, individually or as a group.

Many theories exist to explain why we age, but the common biologic mechanisms underlying the aging process are becoming clearer through aging biology research, a field that has been moving rapidly in the past decade. By understanding the basic mechanisms of aging, including inflammation, cellular senescence, accumulation of damaging macromolecules, and stem and progenitor cell dysfunction, as well as understanding the basis for heterogeneity of longevity, it may become feasible to devise clinical strategies to reverse or prevent age-related processes. Therapeutics that target aging mechanisms have the potential to prevent or treat age-related disorders as a whole, rather than one at a time. We are at the point where it seems increasingly likely that interventions that target fundamental aging mechanisms could begin to be tested for diseases and disabilities that afflict older adults.

KEY POINTS

- Aging processes are universal within a species and are intrinsic and progressive.
- Chronologic age is the main risk factor for most of the chronic diseases that account for the bulk of morbidity, mortality, and health expenditures in modern society.
- Interventions that target fundamental aging mechanisms may one day be used to delay, prevent, alleviate, or even reverse multiple chronic diseases and age-related disabilities as a group, instead of one at a time, enhancing health span.
- Age-related dysfunction and chronic diseases are related to the following: (1) chronic, low-grade, sterile inflammation; (2) cellular senescence; (3) macromolecular dysfunction (accumulation of damaged DNA and proteins, protein aggregates, advanced glycation end products, cytotoxic lipids); and (4) stem cell–progenitor dysfunction at sites of pathology or tissue dysfunction.
- Interventions that target fundamental aging processes have been discovered that enhance health span or life span in mice. One day, these interventions could be translated into clinical application, potentially transforming geriatric medicine.

For a complete list of references, please visit www.expertconsult.com.

KEY REFERENCES

2. Goldman DP, Cutler D, Rowe JW, et al: Substantial health and economic returns from delayed aging may warrant a new focus for medical research. Health Aff (Millwood) 32:1698–1705, 2013.
3. Kirkland JL: Translating advances from the basic biology of aging into clinical application. Exp Gerontol 48:1–5, 2013.
13. Tchkonia T, Zhu Y, van Deursen J, et al: Cellular senescence and the senescent secretory phenotype: therapeutic opportunities. J Clin Invest 123:966–972, 2013.
39. Leng SX, Xue QL, Tian J, et al: Inflammation and frailty in older women. J Am Geriatr Soc 55:864–871, 2007.
48. Rockwood K, Mitnitski A: Frailty defined by deficit accumulation and geriatric medicine defined by frailty. Clin Geriatr Med 27:17–26, 2011.
65. Stout MB, Tchkonia T, Pirtskhalava T, et al: Growth hormone action predicts age-related white adipose tissue dysfunction and senescent cell burden in mice. Aging (Albany NY) 6:575–586, 2014.
73. Jurk D, Wilson C, Passos JF, et al: Chronic inflammation induces telomere dysfunction and accelerates ageing in mice. Nat Commun 2:4172, 2014.
74. Baker DJ, Wijshake T, Tchkonia T, et al: Clearance of p16Ink4a-positive senescent cells delays ageing-associated disorders. Nature 479:232–236, 2011.
75. Zhu Y, Tchkonia T, Pirtskhalava T, et al: The Achilles' heel of senescent cells: from transcriptome to senolytic drugs. Aging Cell 14:644–658, 2015.
77. Dai DF, Chiao YA, Marcinek DJ, et al: Mitochondrial oxidative stress in aging and health span. Longev Healthspan. 3:6, 2014.
78. Mori MA, Raghavan P, Thomou T, et al: Role of microRNA processing in adipose tissue in stress defense and longevity. Cell Metab 16:336–347, 2012.
81. Sridhar S, Botbol Y, Macian F, et al: Autophagy and disease: always two sides to a problem. J Pathol 226:255–273, 2012.
92. Harrison DE, Strong R, Sharp ZD, et al: Rapamycin fed late in life extends life span in genetically heterogeneous mice. Nature 460:392–395, 2009.
101. Jones DL, Rando TA: Emerging models and paradigms for stem cell ageing. Nat Cell Biol 13:506–512, 2011.
104. Sinha M, Jang YC, Oh J, et al: Restoring systemic GDF11 levels reverses age-related dysfunction in mouse skeletal muscle. Science 344:649–652, 2014.
108. Bartke A: Single-gene mutations and healthy ageing in mammals. Philos Trans R Soc Lond B Biol Sci 366:28–34, 2011.
110. Martin-Montalvo A, Mercken EM, Mitchell SJ, et al: Metformin improves health span and life span in mice. Nat Commun 4:2192, 2013.
111. Harrison DE, Strong R, Allison DB, et al: Acarbose, 17-alpha-estradiol, and nordihydroguaiaretic acid extend mouse life span preferentially in males. Aging Cell 13:273–282, 2014.
113. Anderson RM, Weindruch R: The caloric restriction paradigm: implications for healthy human aging. Am J Hum Biol 24:101–106, 2012.
125. Kirkland JL: Tchkonia T. Clinical strategies and animal models for developing senolytic agents. Exp Gerontol 28:2014.
138. Hudson MM, Ness KK, Gurney JG, et al: Clinical ascertainment of health outcomes among adults treated for childhood cancer. JAMA 309:2371–2381, 2013.

10 The Premature Aging Syndrome: Hutchinson-Gilford Progeria Syndrome—Insights Into Normal Aging

Leslie B. Gordon

Hutchinson-Gilford progeria syndrome (HGPS) is an extremely rare, uniformly fatal, segmental premature aging disease in which children exhibit phenotypes that may give us insights into the aging process at the cellular and organism levels. This chapter will compare HGPS to normal aging with respect to its genetics, biology, clinical phenotype, clinical care, and treatment. By looking carefully at one of the rarest diseases on earth, we gain novel and important insights into the most common conditions affecting quality and longevity of life—aging and cardiovascular disease (CVD).

DISEASE DESCRIPTION

Hutchinson-Gilford progeria syndrome is, in most cases, a sporadic, autosomal dominant, so-called premature aging disease in which children die primarily of heart attacks at an average age of 14.6 years (range, 1 to 26 years).[1] Incidence is estimated at 1 in 8 million live births,[2] and the prevalence is 1 in 18 million living individuals.[3] Children experience normal fetal and early postnatal development. Between several months and 1 year of age, abnormalities in growth and body composition are readily apparent (Figure 10-1).[4] Severe failure to thrive ensues, heralding generalized lipoatrophy, with apparent wasting of the limbs, circumoral cyanosis, and prominent veins around the scalp, neck, and trunk.[5] Children reach a final height of approximately 1 m (3.3 ft) and weight of approximately 14 kg (31 lb). Bone and cartilaginous changes include clavicular resorption, coxa valga, distal phalangeal resorption, facial disproportion (small slim nose and receding mandible), and short stature. Dentition is severely delayed.[6] Tooth eruption may be delayed for many months, and primary teeth may persist for the duration of life. Secondary teeth are present, but may or may not erupt. Skin looks thin, with sclerodermatous areas and almost complete hair loss.[7] Skin findings are variable in severity and include areas of discoloration, stippled pigmentation, tightened areas that can restrict movement, and areas of the dorsal trunk where small (1 to 2 cm), soft, bulging skin is present. Joint contractures, due to ligamentous and skin tightening, limit range of motion. Intellectual development is normal in HGPS. Transient ischemic attacks (TIAs) and strokes may ensue as early as 4 years of age, but more often they occur in the later years.[8] Death results primarily from sequelae of widespread arteriosclerosis. In a comprehensive retrospective study, causes of death in HGPS were cardiovascular failure (80%), head injury or trauma (10%), stroke (4%), respiratory infection superimposed on CVD (4%), and complications from anesthesia during surgery (2%).[1]

MOLECULAR GENETICS AND CELL BIOLOGY:

Lamin A

HGPS is a member of the family of genetic diseases known as the laminopathies, whose causal mutations lie along the *LMNA* gene (located at 1q21.2).[9] The *LMNA* gene codes for at least four isoforms—two major (lamin A and lamin C) and two minor (lamin AΔ10 and lamin C2).[10,11] These diverge in structure, function, expression pattern, and binding partners. Only the lamin A isoform is associated with mammalian disease. The lamin proteins are the principal proteins of the nuclear lamina, a structure located inside the inner nuclear membrane.[12] Lamin A, like all lamin molecules, contains an N-terminal head domain, coiled coil α-helical rod domain, and carboxy terminal tail domain.[13] Tail domains contain the nuclear localization sequences essential for protein targeting to the nucleus after posttranslational processing in the endoplasmic reticulum. Lamin monomers first dimerize, the dimers associate in a head to tail fashion, and then finally associate laterally. The primary RNA transcript of lamin A contains 12 exons that are spliced and then translated to produce a lamin A precursor, prelamin A. This precursor is posttranslationally processed via farnesylation, cleavage of the last three amino acid residues at its carboxy terminal, and methyl esterification (Figure 10-2). Prelamin A subsequently undergoes proteolysis of its C-terminal 18 amino acids, which includes the farnesyl group, to become mature lamin A.[14-16] The loss of the farnesyl anchor presumably releases prelamin from the nuclear membrane, rendering it free to participate in the multiprotein nuclear scaffold complex just internal to the nuclear membrane, affecting nuclear structure and function.[15] The integrity of the lamina is crucial to many cellular functions, including mitosis, creating and maintaining structural integrity of the nuclear scaffold, DNA replication, RNA transcription, organization of the nucleus, nuclear pore assembly, chromatin function, cell cycling, and apoptosis.

Mutations in *LMNA* Cause Hutchinson-Gilford Progeria Syndrome

HGPS is almost always a sporadic autosomal dominant disease. There have been two identified cases of germline mosaicism[17] (see the Progeria Research Foundation diagnostics program at www.progeriaresearch.org). Classic HGPS patients have a single C to T transition at nucleotide 1824 that does not change the translated amino acid (Gly608Gly), but activates a seldom used internal splice site, resulting in the deletion of 150 base pairs in the 3′ portion of exon 11[18,19] (see Figure 10-2). A minority of patients with atypical HGPS have progerin-producing pathogenic single-base mutations within the spliceosome recognition sequence of intron 11 of *LMNA*.[20] In these cases, instead of optimizing the internal splice site, the mutation decreases use of the intronic splice site in favor of the internal site. In classic and atypical HGPS, progerin is produced. Translation followed by posttranslational processing of this altered mRNA produces a shortened abnormal protein with a 50–amino acid deletion near its C-terminal end, termed *progerin*, or lamin AΔ50. The 50–amino acid deletion does not affect the ability of progerin to localize to the nucleus or dimerize because the necessary components for these functions are not deleted.[15] Importantly, however, it does remove the recognition site that leads to proteolytic cleavage of the terminal 18 amino acids of prelamin A (see Figure 10-2), along with the phosphorylation site(s) involved in the dissociation and reassociation of the nuclear membrane at each cell division.[14,15]

The multisystem and primarily postnatal disease manifestation in HGPS is not surprising, because lamin A is normally

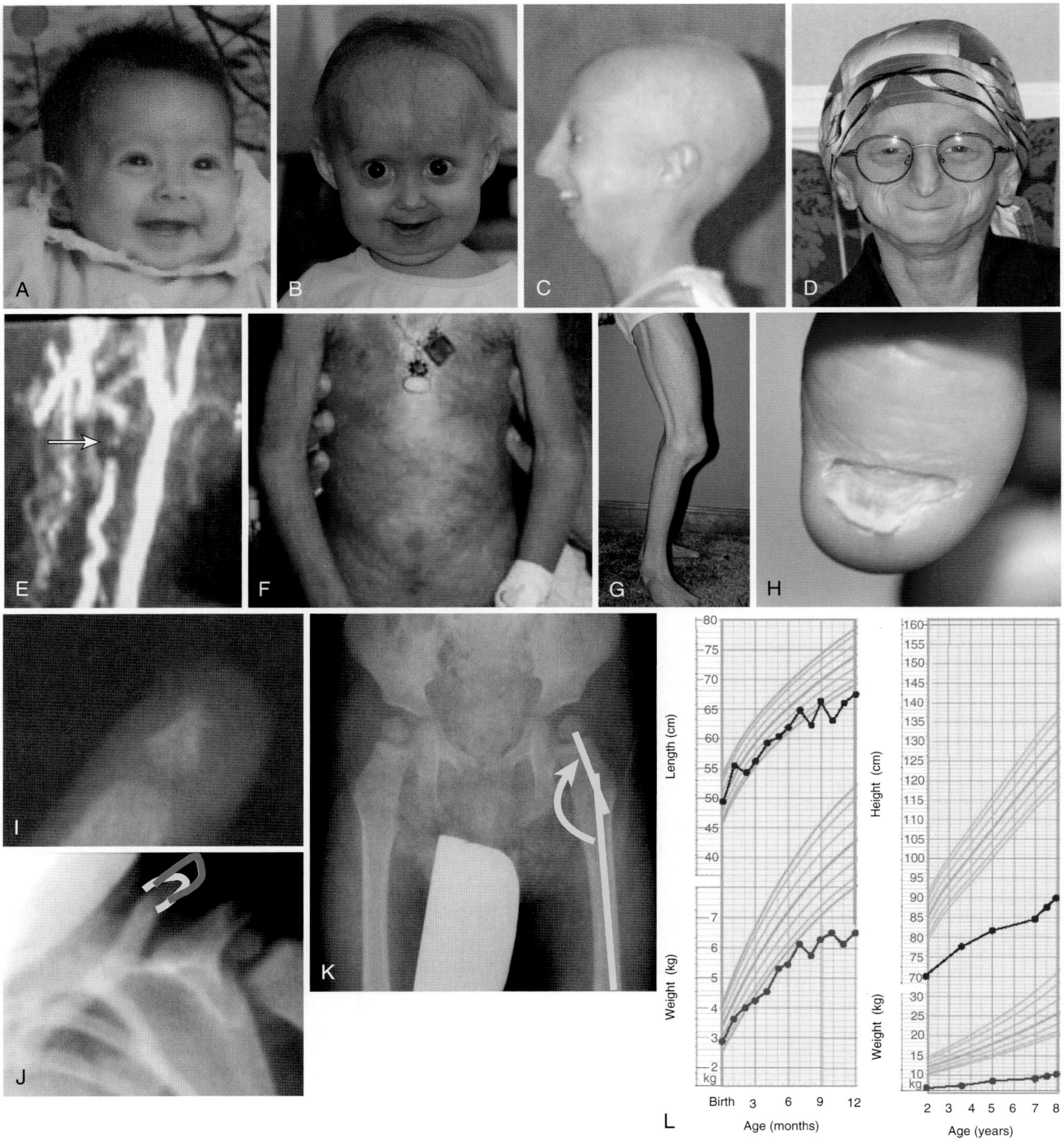

Figure 10-1. Physical characteristics of Hutchinson-Gilford Progeria syndrome. Shown are four different children at various ages: **A,** 3 months (girl); **B,** 2.2 years (girl); **C,** 8.5 years (boy); **D,**16 years (boy). **E,** Carotid artery MRI scan with contrast in a 4-year-old with HGPS demonstrates patency of right common carotid artery, and 100% occlusion of left common carotid artery (*arrow*). **F,** Truncal skin showing areas of discoloration, stippled pigmentation, tightened areas that can restrict movement, and areas of the dorsal trunk where small (1 to 2 cm), soft, bulging skin is present in a 7-year-old boy. **G,** Knee joint restriction in a 12-year-old boy. **H,** Nail dystrophy and distal phalangeal tufting in a 10-year-old boy. Typical X-ray findings: acro-osteolysis of the distal phalange (**I**); clavicular shortening (**J**); coxa valga (**K**). **L, M,** Growth characteristics showing normal birth weight and length, followed by failure to thrive. Average length (*blue*) and weight (*black*) for age for 10 girls during birth to 12 months (**K** and **I**) 2 to 8 years (**L**). Standard deviation is less than 6% for each data point. Data for boys are not significantly different from those of girls ($P < .005$; data not shown). *(Photographs courtesy Progeria Research Foundation (PRF); data courtesy PRF Medical and Research Database; growth charts adapted from Centers for Disease Control and Prevention, National Center for Health Statistics: Clinical growth charts.* http://www.cdc.gov/*growthcharts/clinical_charts.htm. Accessed January 6, 2016.)*

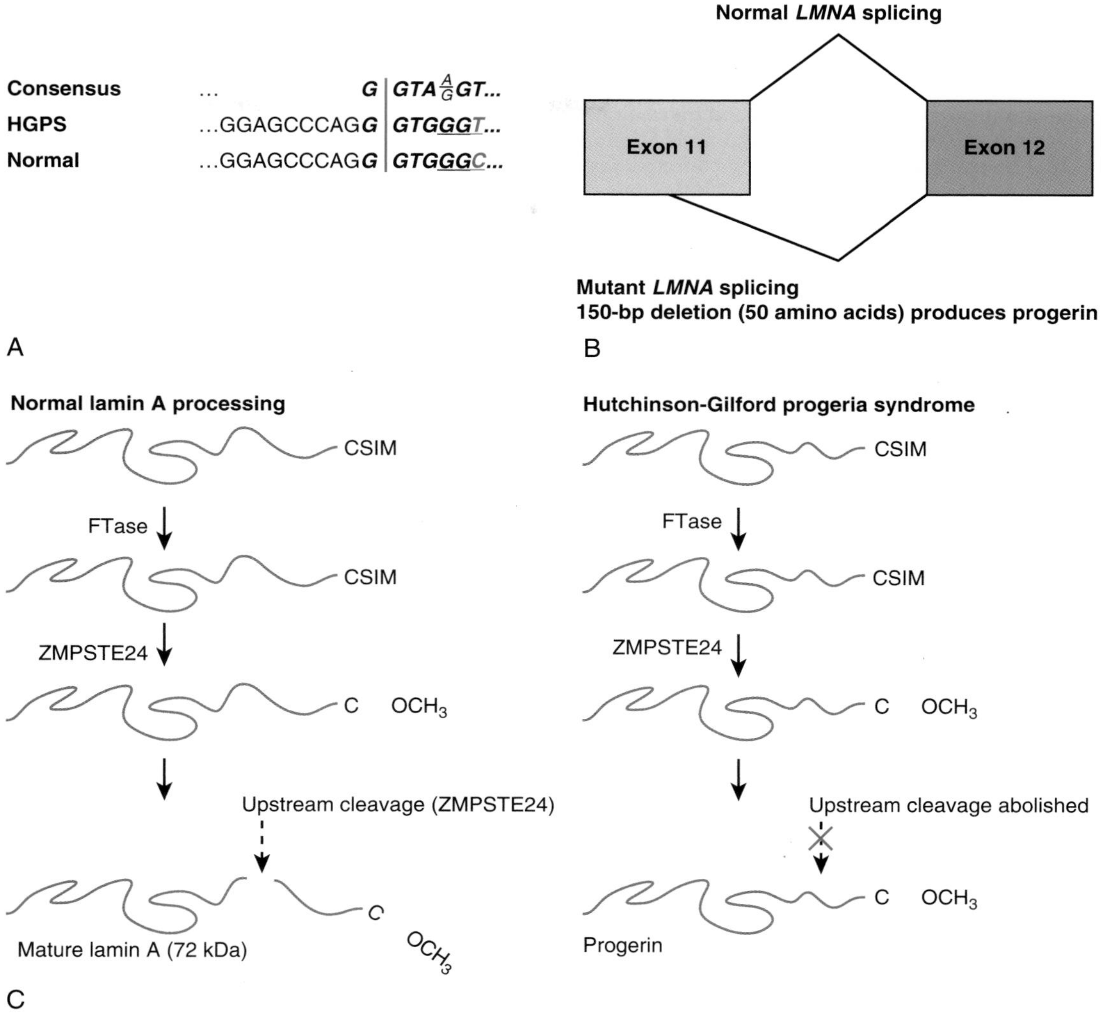

Figure 10-2. Abnormal splicing in the Hutchinson-Gilford progeria syndrome (HGPS) and normal *LMNA*. **A,** Sequences in bold and italics represent a potential splice donor sequence. Shown is a partial DNA sequence for and ideal consensus splice donor sequence (seven bases, *top line*), which shares six of seven bases with HGPS (*middle line*) and five of seven bases with normal *LMNA* (*bottom line*). Codes for glycine are underlined. Mutant transitions (C to T) are shown in *red*. The *vertical red line* represents a splice point used variably in HGPS and in normal cells (less frequently). **B,** Representation for mutant splicing that results in a 50–amino acid deletion from lamin A, thus creating progerin. **C,** Translation of the *LMNA* gene yields the prelamin A protein, which requires posttranslational processing for incorporation into the nuclear lamina. The prelamin A protein has the amino acids, CSIM, at the C terminus. This comprises a CAAX motif, where C is cysteine, A is an aliphatic amino acid, and X is any amino acid, which signals for isoprenylation—in this case, the addition of a farnesyl group to the cysteine by the enzyme farnesyltransferase (FTase). After farnesylation, the terminal three amino acids (SIM) are cleaved by the ZMPSTE24 endoprotease, and the terminal farnesylated cysteine undergoes carboxymethylation. A second cleavage step by ZMPSTE24 then removes the terminal 15 amino acids, including the farnesyl group. This final cleavage step is blocked in HGPS. *(Adapted from Capell BC: Inhibiting the farnesylation of progerin prevents the characteristic nuclear blebbing of Hutchinson–Gilford progeria syndrome. Proc Natl Acad Sci USA 102:12879–12884, Copyright 2005, National Academy of Sciences, USA.)*

expressed by most differentiated cells, preserving function in undifferentiated cells that dominate fetal development (reviewed by Gruenbaum and colleagues[21]). Lamin A expression is developmentally regulated and displays cell and tissue specificity, primarily in differentiated cells, including fibroblasts, vascular smooth muscle cells, and vascular endothelial cells.[10,22,23] The alternate splicing in HGPS leads to decreased levels of lamin A. One chromosome is not mutated and transcribes lamin A normally, whereas the other is mutated, and the splicing machinery transcribes progerin instead of lamin A for some fraction of the time (estimated to be from 40% to 80%).[24] However, decreasing lamin A levels does not seem to affect cell function significantly. A mouse model entirely lacking lamin A has shown no signs of disease.[25] HGPS is therefore a dominant negative disease; it is the action of progerin, not the diminution of lamin A, that causes the disease phenotype.

Treatment Pathways Based on Pathobiology of Disease

Preclinical evidence for effective treatment pathways has used our current understanding of the transcriptional and translational processing for progerin and its differences from normal lamin A (see Figure 10-2). The splicing defect can be ameliorated with antisense oligotherapy, both in vitro and in an HGPS mouse model.[26,27] At the protein level, one key to disease in HGPS is the persistent farnesylation of progerin, which renders it permanently intercalated into the inner nuclear membrane, where it can accumulate and exert progressively more damage to cells as they age. The hypothesis that failure to remove the farnesyl group is at least in part responsible for the phenotypes observed in HGPS has been strongly supported by studies on cell and mouse models that have been engineered to produce a nonfarnesylated progerin product or treated with a drug that inhibits farnesylation, rendering a nonfarnesylated progerin product. Drugs tested have included farnesyltransferase inhibitors, statins, and nitrogen-containing bisphosphonates, all of which work at different points along the pathway that leads to farnesylation of the abnormal lamin A proteins produced in progeria (Figure 10-3).[9] By preventing the initial attachment of the farnesyl group to newly synthesized preprogerin molecules, progerin is thought to be unable to carry out its aberrant function at the inner nuclear membrane. In many in vitro and mouse model studies, some or all of the phenotypes of HGPS were reversed toward normal.[28-30]

A human trial administering the farnesyltransferase inhibitor lonafarnib succeeded in ameliorating some aspects of disease, including cardiovascular pathology. Subgroups of patients experienced an increased rate of weight gain, decreased vascular stiffness measured via decreased carotid-femoral pulse wave velocity (PWV_{cf}) and carotid artery echodensity, increased radial bone structural rigidity, and/or improved sensorineural hearing.[31] Arterial stiffness normally increases with age and, although the HGPS cohort initially exhibited a PWV_{cf} equivalent to the age range of 60 to 69 years, the median end of therapy PWV_{cf} value was in the range of a typical 40- to 49-year-old. Based on studies of non-HGPS patients with diabetes, in whom aortic PWV_{cf} increments as small as 1 m/sec had a significant independent effect on reduced mortality,[32] the median 4.5-m/sec decrease detected in this study implies a potential for benefit to cardiovascular mortality in children with HGPS. In addition, before treatment, more than 50% of the study participants had a history of headaches, four had a history of TIA or strokes, and four had a history of prior seizure. During treatment, stroke frequency was decreased, and the prevalence and frequency of headaches were reduced.[33] These data suggest that disease-modifying treatment may also alter the progression of underlying CVD and cerebrovascular disease. Finally, after 5 years of study duration, the estimated life span was improved.[1] Dermatologic and dental problems, joint contractures, insulin resistance, lipodystrophy, and bone mineral density were unaffected by drug treatment. Other successful preclinical treatment strategies have included reducing progerin methylation by

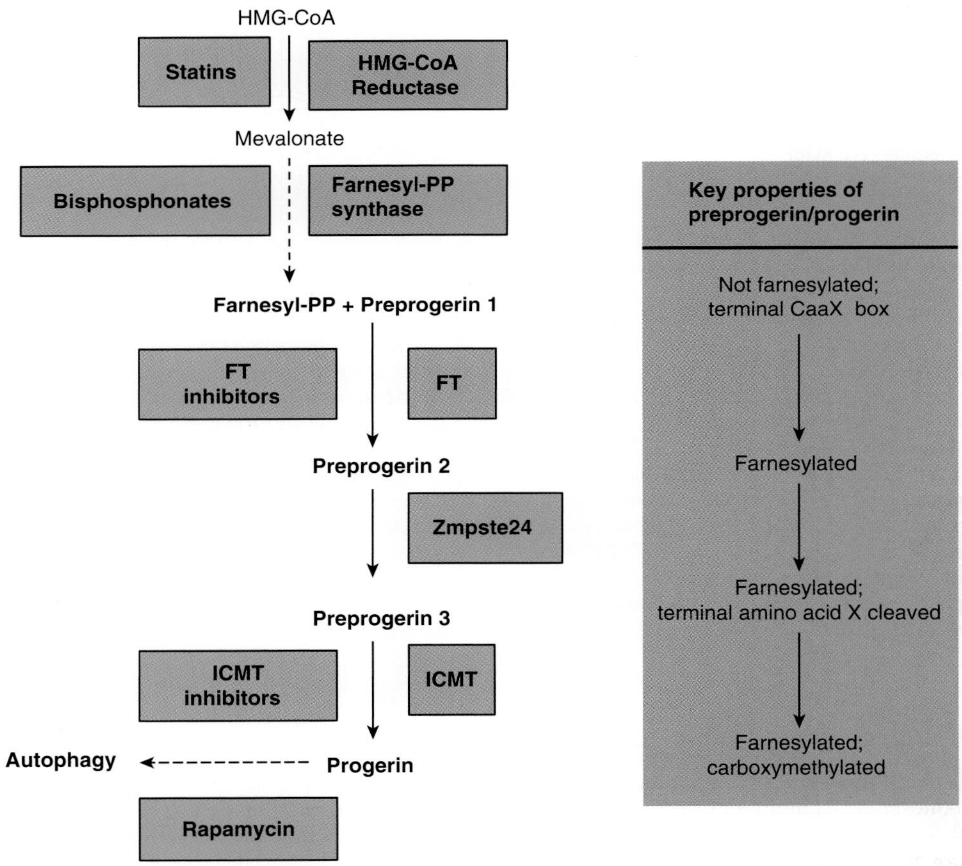

Figure 10-3. Progerin posttranslational processing pathway and potential target points for treatment. Enzymes shown in green; enzyme inhibitors shown in orange. *Solid arrow,* single step; *dashed arrow,* multiple steps; *FT,* farnesyltransferase; *ICMT,* S-isoprenylcysteine O-methyltransferase.

decreasing isoprenylcysteine carboxyl methyltransferase activity,[34] accelerating progerin autophagic cellular clearance with the mammalian target of rapamycin (mTOR) inhibitor rapamycin,[35-37] antioxidant sulforaphane[38] activation of the protein deacetylase SIRT1 by resveratrol,[39] and inhibition of the acetyltransferase protein NAT10 with remodeling (see Figure 10-3).[40]

AGING AND THE HUTCHINSON-GILFORD PROGERIA SYNDROME

HGPS is described as a segmental premature aging syndrome because it shares some phenotypes with normal aging, but not all. Cancer, Alzheimer disease, and various other sequelae of aging are not present in HGPS. Clinical characteristics common to both, but accelerated in HGPS, include progressive CVD, loss of subcutaneous fat (lipoatrophy), and hair loss. There are a number of laminopathies that have progeroid and nonprogeroid phenotypes, but HGPS has been the best studied for its commonalities with aging, senescence, and arteriosclerosis.[9]

HGPS and aging share a variety of cellular elements key to aging at the cellular level, including decreased resistance to oxidative stress, increased DNA damage, decreased ability to repair that damage, abnormal nuclear shape (blebbing; Figure 10-4),[12] and decreased resilience in response to mechanical strain, telomere function,[41,42] and a host of signaling pathways that change with senescence and age. These include the mTOR, peroxisome proliferator-activated receptor (PPAR), mitochondrial dysfunction,[43] and Notch pathways, which are important for the maintenance of stem cells (including mesenchymal stem cells), differentiation pathways, and cell death.[44] Perhaps the most exciting clue about the aging process is the presence of progerin protein at increasing concentrations as HGPS and normal cells age.[45,46]

Normal fibroblasts senesce, but HGPS fibroblasts senesce more rapidly, usually within 15 passages.[47] Oxidative stress, in the form of superoxide radicals and hydrogen peroxide, has been found to induce senescence and apoptosis and has been implicated in the cause of atherosclerosis[48] and normal aging.[49,50] Antioxidants such as superoxide dismutase, catalase, and glutathione peroxidase help eliminate superoxide radicals and hydrogen peroxide. Yan and associates[51] have demonstrated significantly decreased glutathione peroxidase, magnesium superoxide dismutase and catalase levels in HGPS fibroblast cultures compared with normal control cultures. Normal cellular senescence is also marked by increasing rates of DNA damage and a decline in the ability to repair this damage.[52] Progeria cells accumulate double-stranded DNA (dsDNA) breaks and impaired DNA repair.[53-55] An aberrant nuclear shape (called blebbing or lobulation) occurs in normal fibroblasts undergoing apoptosis as an antecedent to apoptosis and senescence[12] (see Figure 10-4). A consistent phenotype in HGPS cells is the same aberrant shape of their nuclei, which is readily detected following staining with antilamin antibodies.[12,56] The blebbing is a structural sign of cellular decline in normal and HGPS cell cultures. Another structural weakening associated with aging cells and HGPS is the response to mechanotransduction (applied force).[57,58] When strain is applied to early-passage wild-type fibroblast nuclei, they remain stiff.[59] Although progeria fibroblasts show normal rigidity during early passages (when progerin levels and nuclear blebbing are at a minimum), late-passage nuclei show dramatically increased rigidity over wild-type fibroblasts. In addition, whereas wild-type cells enter the S and G2 phases in response to mechanical stretch, HGPS cells do not proliferate in response to stretch. Microarray

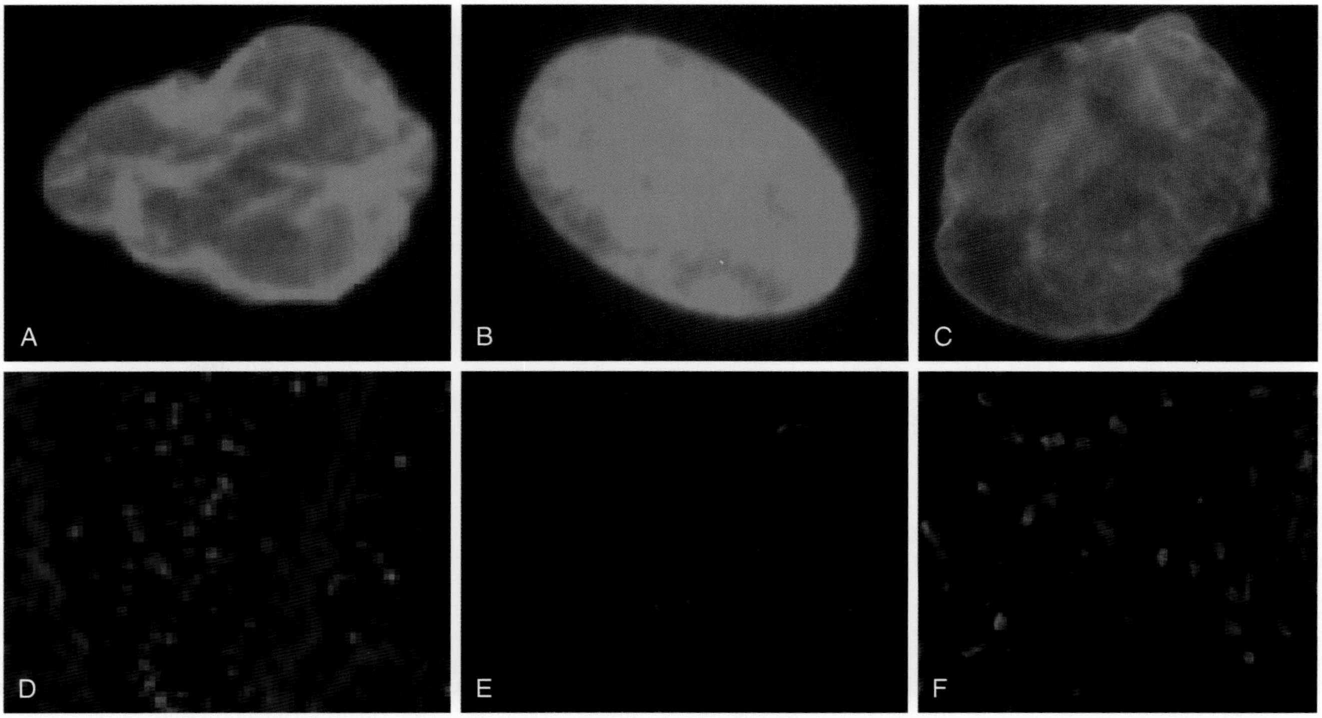

Figure 10-4. Nuclear blebbing and presence of progerin in Hutchinson-Gilford progeria syndrome (HGPS) and aging. Fibroblast nuclei were stained with antilamin antibody for **A,** passage 4 HGPS; **B,** passage 10, normal; **C,** passage 40, normal. Skin biopsies stained with antiprogerin antibody shown here at ×40 for **D,** HGPS, donor age 10 years old; **E,** normal newborn; **F,** normal, donor age 90 years old.

studies have revealed significant overlap between cell signaling in senescing cells and HGPS fibroblasts as compared to early-passage normal cells.[43]

The discovery that progeria is caused by a mutation in lamin A, which had not previously been implicated in the mechanisms of aging, has led to an entirely new question—are defects in lamin A implicated in normal aging? The first positive evidence was reported by Scaffidi and Misteli in 2006,[60] who showed that cell nuclei from normal individuals have acquired similar defects as those in progeria patients, including changes in histone modifications and increased DNA damage. Younger cells show considerably fewer of these defects. They further demonstrated that the age-related effects are the result of the production of low levels of preprogerin mRNA produced by activation of the same cryptic splice site that functions at much higher levels in progeria and is reversed by inhibition of transcription at this splice site. Cao and coworkers,[61] studying the same phenomenon, have shown that among interphase cells in fibroblast cultures, only a small fraction of the cells contains progerin. The percentage of progerin-positive cells increased with passage number, suggesting a link to normal aging. Notably, McClintock and colleagues have found progerin in skin biopsies of older donors, whereas young donors had no detectable progerin. This was the first human in vivo demonstration of a buildup of progerin with normal aging (see Figure 10-4).[46] The newly discovered relationship between HGPS and lamin A has opened the doors of scientific exploration into how lamins play a role in heart disease and aging in the general population.

A key element when considering treatment for HGPS or for arteriosclerosis and normal aging is progerin's dosage effect. In HGPS, the nonmutated *LMNA* gene splices normally producing full-length lamin A, and only rarely uses the cryptic splice site to produce progerin. The other (mutated) *LMNA* gene produces progerin in substantial amounts and a minor amount of lamin A. Different individuals may produce more or less progerin and within an individual, different cell types may produce varying amounts of progerin versus normal lamin A. In normal fibroblast cells in culture, the cryptic splice site is used about 50-fold less as compared to HGPS fibroblasts. However, because progerin protein accumulates with increasing age in skin biopsies (see Figure 10-4) and in vitro with increasing passage number,[12] the influence of progerin on health in the general population probably also increases as aging occurs. Clinical support for the dosage effect hypothesis has been found in the study of a 45-year-old man with a progeroid laminopathy, whose mutation in *T623S* produced a cryptic splice site abnormality in *LMNA*, but the splice site was used 80% less frequently than in classic HGPS.[62] His phenotype mimicked that of HGPS, but to a milder degree. Therefore, we can assume that decreasing the levels of progerin by a relatively modest percentage will significantly ameliorate disease. In addition, it is highly possible that one component of genetic predisposition to atherosclerosis lies in the amount of progerin that an individual accumulates in his or her lifetime.

Overlap between Hutchinson-Gilford Progeria Syndrome and Arteriosclerosis of Aging

Hypertension, angina, cardiomegaly, and congestive heart failure are common end-stage events in HGPS.[63-66] The underlying pathology is primarily a vascular disease, characterized by early and accelerated vascular stiffening. This is followed by small- and large-vessel occlusive disease due to atherosclerotic plaque formation and, in later years, by valvular and cardiac insufficiency.[5,67] Typical cardiac manifestations include increased afterload, angina, and late findings, such as dyspnea on exertion. Hypertension is considered a later sign of vascular disease. Gerhard-Herman and associates have found evidence of vascular dysfunction in 100% of a cohort of 26 children with HGPS as young as 3 years of age,[67] with a dramatically elevated PWV_{cf} and changes to the carotid artery wall. Death occurs by myocardial infarction or stroke, generally between the ages of 6 and 20 years, with an average life span of 14.6 years.[1]

HGPS is a unique example of atherosclerosis caused by the presence of a single toxic protein, uncluttered by factors such as smoking, exercise, and diet that contribute to the multifactorial causes of CVD in aging. Unlike CVD in the general population, the intima-media thickness of the carotid artery is normal, as are cholesterol, low-density lipoprotein (LDL), and high-sensitivity C-reactive protein levels, all factors in the chronic lipid-driven inflammation of atherosclerosis.[8] Instead, the HGPS vascular phenotype resembles an arteriosclerosis, which is characterized by hardening of the vessels (decreased compliance) in medium and large vessels and affects millions of aging individuals. HDL and adiponectin (a secretory product of adipose tissue) levels decrease with increasing age in HGPS,[68] and insulin resistance is prevalent.[67] Declines in HDL and adiponectin levels have been implicated in other lipodystrophic syndromes and lipodystrophy associated with type 2 diabetes.[69] Adiponectin has been emerging as an independent CVD risk factor that may directly regulate endothelial function and that also correlates with HDL levels in type 2 diabetes.

To date, the fewer than 20 autopsies on children with HGPS have revealed focal plaques throughout large and small arteries, including all coronary artery branches.[65,66,70-74] The plaques are markedly calcified and contain cholesterol crystals and a nearly acellular hyaline fibrosis. Vessel cross sections at autopsy of a 22-year-old woman with clinical features of HGPS revealed no indication of vasculature inflammation.[75] The vascular media no longer contained smooth muscle cells, and the elastic structure was destroyed and replaced with extracellular matrix or fibrosis, with profound adventitial thickening and a depleted media. Presumably, the primary loss of smooth muscle cells initiates vascular remodeling by secondary replacement with matrix in the large and small vasculature.

In the arteriosclerosis of aging, apoptosis occurs in vascular smooth muscle cells prior to the development of calcification[76] and may even be required for calcification to occur. Because vascular calcification is a requisite event in plaque formation,[77] apoptosis may be a key element in the development of disease in HGPS and arteriosclerosis.[47,57,78]

Autopsy studies have also revealed that HGPS is a disease involving abnormalities in the extracellular matrix, with increased collagen and elastin secretion, disorganized dermal collagen, decreased decorin, and increased aggrecan and ankyrin G compared with normal controls.[79-84] Extracellular matrix molecules have structural and cell signaling functions in skin, bone, and the cardiovascular system,[85-91] all of which are severely affected in HGPS. In pathologic and clinical studies, mesoderm-derived tissues and their extracellular matrices are targets of principal defects. Gene expression studies of HGPS fibroblasts are consistent with these findings.[92,93] Aneurysms, noted in several cases of HGPS,[71,74,94] are derived from medial necrosis, which could reflect a connective tissue problem, with concurrent death of smooth muscle cells.

In summary, the study of HGPS has provided a completely new molecule, progerin, which may play an integral role in general vascular biology and health. The progeria vasculature is characterized by global stiffness, tortuosity, and loss of smooth muscle cells in the media, with subsequent extracellular replacement. Biochemical abnormalities include progressively decreasing HDL and adiponectin levels. Smooth muscle cell dropout is unique to progeria, whereas global stiffness and tortuosity and decreased HDL and adiponectin levels are observed in arteriosclerosis and type 2 diabetes in the normal aging population.

With a potentially causal relationship to CVD with aging, progerin is found in all vascular layers, as well as plaques in HGPS,[22] and is similarly present at lower levels in non-HGPS vasculature.[45,46]

CLINICAL CARE

Diagnostics and Genetic Counseling

Initial indications for HGPS include failure to thrive, skin signs, stiffened joints, delayed dentition, gradual hair loss, and subcutaneous loss of fat, with normal developmental milestones. Average age at diagnosis is 2 years (see www.genetests.org). The Progeria Research Foundation (www.progeriaresearch.org) is the only patient advocate organization worldwide that is solely dedicated to discovering the cause, treatments, and cure for progeria. It provides services for families and children with progeria, such as patient education and communication with other progeria families. It serves as a resource for physicians and medical caregivers of these families via clinical care recommendations[95] and http://www.progeriaresearch.org/patient_care.html, a diagnostics program, clinical and research database, and funding source for basic science and clinical research in HGPS.

Cardiac and Neurovascular Care: Hydration and Low-Dose Aspirin

Children with HGPS are at high risk for heart attacks and strokes at any age. The following tests should be considered annually and more often if recommended by the family physicians— cardiology visit with cardiac auscultation and physical examination, blood pressures, electrocardiography, carotid duplex ultrasound, pulse wave velocity, and echocardiography. Once a child begins to develop signs or symptoms of vascular decline, such as hypertension, TIA, strokes, seizures, angina, dyspnea on exertion, electrocardiographic changes, echocardiographic changes, and/or heart attacks, a higher level of intervention is warranted. Antihypertensive, anticoagulant, antiseizure, and other medications usually administered to adults with similar medical issues have been given to children with HGPS.

Neurovascular morbidity is high, with up to 50% of children with HGPS experiencing silent strokes.[8] Thus, stroke remains a frequent cause of concern and morbidity in children with HGPS. If a stroke or acute neurologic symptom occurs that raises concern for TIA or stroke, management of blood pressure—specifically, maintenance of adequate blood pressure and cerebral perfusion—is imperative. In the case of a more serious stroke, monitoring in an intensive care setting is often indicated until the child's condition is stabilized. Pharmacologic treatment is often considered at that time.

Antiplatelet agents (e.g., aspirin) are often given to prevent clot formation and, ideally, to prevent future strokes from occurring. Based on evidence from adult studies, 2 to 3 mg/kg body weight per day is recommended. This dosage will inhibit platelet aggregation but will not inhibit prostacyclin activity.

Acute neurologic symptoms are often brought on by activities that involve hyperventilation, reduction in blood pressure, or dehydration. For these reasons, it is important that children remain well-hydrated at all times, especially during travel.

Intubation

Intubation is difficult in the child with progeria due to the small oral aperture with retrognathia, little flexion or extension in the cervical spine, relatively large epiglottis, and small glottic opening. A nasal fiberoptic intubation may be difficult due to the unusual glottic angle. Intubation with direct visualization is therefore recommended. For nonoral procedures, mask ventilation or laryngeal mask airway is recommended over intubation.

Physical Therapy and Occupational Therapy

Children with progeria need physical therapy (PT) and occupational therapy (OT) as often as possible (optimally, 2 or 3 times each per week) to ensure maximum range of motion and optimal daily functioning throughout their lives. Each regimen should be tailored to the child's individual needs and according to cardiac status in consultation with the child's physician. The role of PT and OT is to maintain range of motion, strength, and functional status. Proactive PT and OT are important, because all children with progeria develop restrictions in range of motion in a progressive manner (see Figure 10-1). Bony abnormalities are almost always evident on x-rays by the age of 2 years.[4,96] Range of motion may be restricted because of progressive joint contractures, primarily in the knees, ankles, and fingers due to tendinous abnormalities, hip abnormalities due primarily to progressive coxa valga, and shoulder restrictions due to clavicular resorption; tightened skin can also restrict range of motion. Skin tightening can be almost absent in some children or can be severe and restrict chest wall motion and gastric capacity in others.

Acknowledgment

I wish to gratefully acknowledge the children with progeria and their families for participation in progeria research.

KEY POINTS

- Hutchinson-Gilford progeria syndrome (HGPS) is a rare segmental premature aging syndrome in which children die primarily of heart attacks or strokes between the ages of 1 and 26 years.
- The underlying pathology in HPGS is primarily that of a vascular disease. It resembles the arteriosclerosis of aging, with hypertension, vascular stiffening, vessel wall remodeling with abnormal extracellular matrix, plaque formation in the presence of normal cholesterol levels, cardiac valve calcification, and cardiac hypertrophy with strain, culminating in cardiac failure.
- HGPS is a segmental premature aging syndrome, sharing features with normal aging, but not all. For example, there is no increased risk of cancer or Alzheimer disease.
- HGPS is an autosomal dominant disease caused by a single-base mutation in *LMNA*, leading to a silent mutation that optimizes an internal splice site.
- Lamin A is an inner nuclear membrane protein that is central to cellular structure and function, primarily in differentiated cell types.
- The abnormal lamin A protein produced in HGPS, called progerin, is not only generated in HGPS, but is also generated to a lesser extent in the normal population.
- Progerin accumulates with increased age in non-HGPS individuals and is likely associated with cellular aging and vascular disease in the general population.
- Clinical trials in HGPS using a farnesyltransferase inhibitor have demonstrated improved vascular distensibility and a small increase in estimated life span.

For a complete list of references, please visit www.expertconsult.com.

KEY REFERENCES

1. Gordon LB, et al: Impact of farnesylation inhibitors on survival in Hutchinson-Gilford progeria syndrome. Circulation 130:27–34, 2014.

3. Gordon LB: PRF by the numbers. http://www.progeriaresearch.org/prf-by-the-numbers.html. Accessed September 25, 2013.
5. Merideth MA, et al: Phenotype and course of Hutchinson-Gilford progeria syndrome. N Engl J Med 358:592–604, 2008.
9. Capell BC, Collins FS: Human laminopathies: nuclei gone genetically awry. Nat Rev Genet 7:940–952, 2006.
12. Goldman RD, et al: Accumulation of mutant lamin A causes progressive changes in nuclear architecture in Hutchinson-Gilford progeria syndrome. Proc Natl Acad Sci U S A 101:8963–8968, 2004.
13. Shumaker D, Kuczmarski E, Goldman R: The nucleoskeleton: lamins and actin are major players in essential nuclear functions. Curr Opin Cell Biol 15:358–366, 2003.
15. Sinensky M, et al: The processing pathway of prelamin A. J Cell Sci 107:61–67, 1994.
19. De Sandre-Giovannoli A, et al: Lamin A truncation in Hutchinson-Gilford progeria. Science 300:2055, 2003.
20. Gordon LB, Brown WT, Collins FS: Hutchinson-Gilford progeria syndrome. http://www.ncbi.nlm.nih.gov/books/NBK1121. Accessed January 6, 2016.
26. Osorio FG, et al: Splicing-directed therapy in a new mouse model of human accelerated aging. Sci Transl Med 3:106–107, 2011.
31. Gordon LB, et al: Clinical trial of a farnesyltransferase inhibitor in children with Hutchinson-Gilford progeria syndrome. Proc Natl Acad Sci U S A 109:16666–16671, 2012.
41. Cao K, et al: Progerin and telomere dysfunction collaborate to trigger cellular senescence in normal human fibroblasts. J Clin Invest 121:2833–2844, 2011.
45. Olive M, et al: Cardiovascular pathology in Hutchinson-Gilford progeria: correlation with the vascular pathology of aging. Arterioscler Thromb Vasc Biol 30:2301–2309, 2010.
46. McClintock D, et al: The mutant form of lamin A that causes Hutchinson-Gilford progeria is a biomarker of cellular aging in human skin. PLoS ONE 2:e1269, 2007.
52. Campisi J, d'Adda di Fagagna F: Cellular senescence: when bad things happen to good cells. Nat Rev Mol Cell Biol 8:729–740, 2007.
60. Scaffidi P, Misteli T: Lamin A-dependent nuclear defects in human aging. Science 312:1059–1063, 2006.
67. Gerhard-Herman M, et al: Mechanisms of premature vascular aging in children with Hutchinson-Gilford progeria syndrome. Hypertension 59:92–97, 2012.
73. Stehbens WE, et al: Smooth muscle cell depletion and collagen types in progeric arteries. Cardiovasc Pathol 10:133–136, 2001.
95. Progeria Research Foundation: The progeria handbook: a guide for families and caregivers of children. http://www.progeriaresearch.org/assets/files/PRFhandbook_0410.pdf. Accessed January 6, 2016.

11 The Neurobiology of Aging: Free Radical Stress and Metabolic Pathways

Tomohiro Nakamura, Louis R. Lapierre, Malene Hansen, Stuart A. Lipton

Environmental stressors and several genetic pathways play complex and crucial roles in the neurobiology and control of aging. This chapter will summarize current knowledge on these two specific research areas divided into two sections, one on free radical stressors and the other on genetic control of metabolic pathways.

I Nitrosative and Oxidative Stress in the Neurobiology of Aging

Tomohiro Nakamura, Stuart A. Lipton

Aging represents a major risk factor for neurodegenerative diseases, such as Parkinson disease (PD), Alzheimer disease (AD), amyotrophic lateral sclerosis (ALS), polyglutamine (polyQ) diseases such as Huntington disease (HD), glaucoma, human immunodeficiency virus (HIV)–associated neurocognitive disorder (HAND), multiple sclerosis, and ischemic brain injury, to name but a few.[1-5] Although many intra- and extracellular molecules may participate in neuronal injury and loss, the accumulation of nitrosative and oxidative stress, due to excessive generation of reactive nitrogen species (RNS) such as nitric oxide (NO) and of reactive oxygen species (ROS), appears to be a potential factor contributing to neuronal cell damage and death.[6,7] A well-established model for NO production entails a central role of the *N*-methyl-D-aspartate (NMDA)–type glutamate receptors in the nervous system. Excessive activation of NMDA receptors drives Ca^{2+} influx, which in turn activates neuronal NO synthase (nNOS) as well as the generation of ROS (Fig. 11-1).[8,9] Accumulating evidence suggests that NO can mediate protective and neurotoxic effects by reacting with cysteine residues of target proteins to form S-nitrosothiols (SNOs), a process termed *S-nitrosylation* because of its effects on the chemical biology of protein function. Importantly, normal mitochondrial respiration also generates free radicals, principally ROS, and one such molecule, superoxide anion (O_2^-), reacts rapidly with free radical NO under nitrosative stress conditions to form the very toxic product peroxynitrite ($ONOO^-$) (Fig. 11-2).[10,11]

An additional feature of most neurodegenerative diseases is accumulation of misfolded and/or aggregated proteins.[12-15] These protein aggregates can be cytosolic, nuclear, or extracellular. Importantly, protein aggregation can result from a mutation in the disease-related gene encoding the protein, or posttranslational changes to the protein engendered by nitrosative and oxidative stress.[16] A key theme of this chapter, therefore, is the hypothesis that age-related nitrosative or oxidative stress contributes to protein misfolding in the brains of neurodegenerative patients. In the first section of this chapter, we discuss specific examples showing that S-nitrosylation of ubiquitin E3 ligases such as parkin or endoplasmic reticulum (ER) chaperones such as protein disulfide isomerase (PDI) are critical factors for the accumulation of misfolded proteins in neurodegenerative diseases such as PD and other conditions.[17-20]

PROTEIN MISFOLDING IN NEURODEGENERATIVE DISEASES

A shared histologic feature of many neurodegenerative diseases is the accumulation of misfolded proteins that adversely affect neuronal connectivity and plasticity and trigger cell death signaling pathways.[12,15] For example, degenerating brains contain aberrant accumulations of misfolded aggregated proteins, such as α-synuclein and synphilin-1 in PD, and amyloid-β (Aβ) and tau in AD. The inclusions observed in PD are called Lewy bodies (LBs) and are mostly found in the cytoplasm. AD brains show intracellular neurofibrillary tangles, which contain tau, and extracellular plaques, which contain Aβ. Other disorders manifesting protein aggregation include HD (polyQ), ALS, and prion disease.[14] These aggregates may consist of oligomeric complexes of non-native secondary structures and demonstrate poor solubility, even in the presence of detergents.

In general, protein aggregates do not accumulate in unstressed healthy neurons due in part to the existence of cellular quality control mechanisms. For example, molecular chaperones are believed to provide a defense mechanism against the toxicity of misfolded proteins because chaperones can prevent inappropriate interactions within and between polypeptides and can promote refolding of proteins that have been misfolded because of cell stress. In addition to the quality control of proteins provided by molecular chaperones, the ubiquitin-proteasome system (UPS) and autophagy-lysosomal degradation are involved in the clearance of abnormal or aberrant proteins.[21] When chaperones cannot repair misfolded proteins, they may be tagged via the addition of polyubiquitin chains for degradation by the proteasome. In neurodegenerative conditions, intra- or extracellular protein aggregates are thought to accumulate in the brain as a result of a decrease in molecular chaperone or proteasome activities. In fact, several mutations that disturb the activity of molecular chaperones or UPS-associated enzymes can cause neurodegeneration.[15,22,23] Along these lines, postmortem samples from the substantia nigra of PD patients manifest a significant reduction in proteasome activity compared to non-PD controls.[24]

Historically, lesions that contain aggregated proteins were considered to be pathogenic. Several lines of evidence have suggested that aggregates are formed through a complex multistep

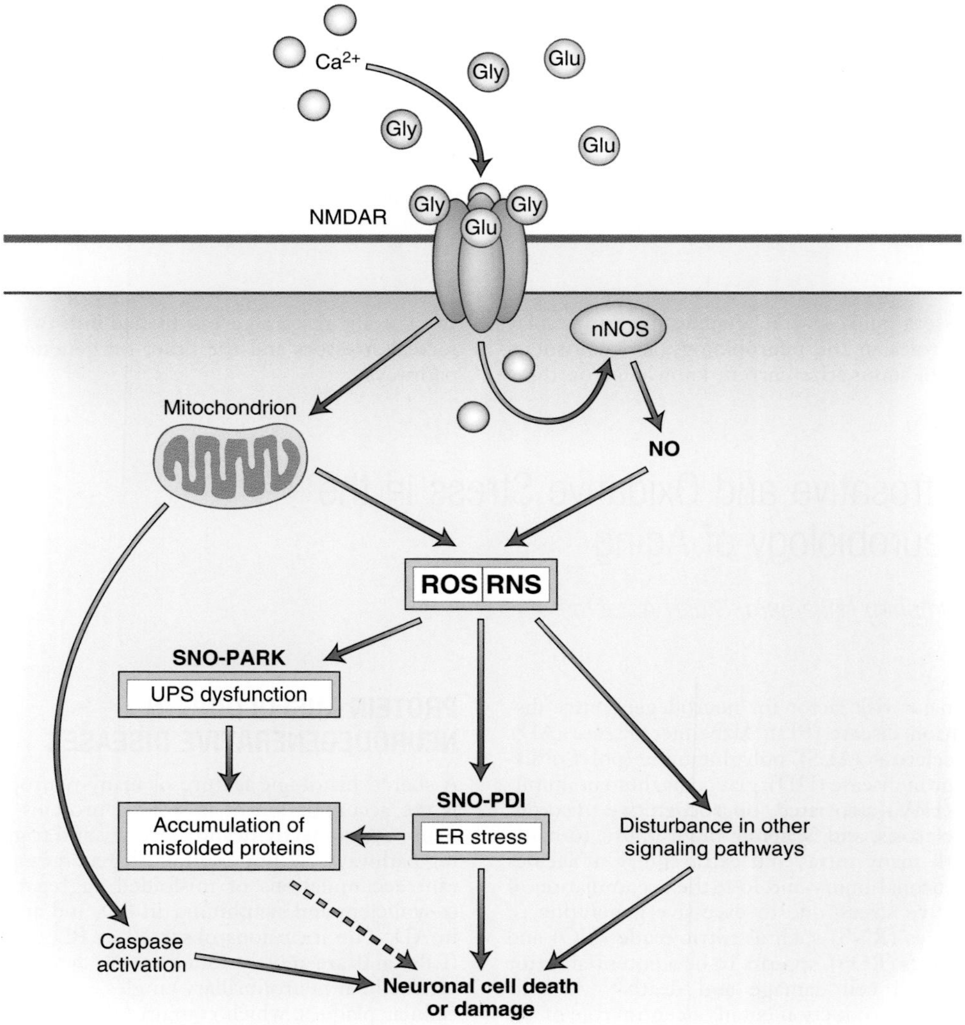

Figure 11-1. Activation of the NMDA receptor (NMDAR) by glutamate (Glu) and glycine (Gly) induces Ca^{2+} influx and consequent ROS and RNS production. NMDAR hyperactivation triggers the generation of ROS and RNS and cytochrome C release from mitochondria associated with subsequent activation of caspases, causing neuronal cell death and damage. SNO-PARK, S-nitrosylated parkin; SNO-PDI, S-nitrosylated PDI.

process whereby misfolded proteins assemble into inclusion bodies; soluble oligomers of these aberrant proteins are thought to be the most toxic forms via interference with normal cell activities, whereas large insoluble aggregates may be an attempt by the cell to wall off potentially toxic material.[25,26]

GENERATION OF REACTIVE OXYGEN AND REACTIVE NITROGEN SPECIES

Induction of Ca^{2+} Influx by NMDA Receptor–Mediated Glutamatergic Signaling Pathways

It is well known that the amino acid glutamate is the major excitatory neurotransmitter in the brain. Glutamate is present in high concentrations in the adult central nervous system and is released for milliseconds from nerve terminals in a Ca^{2+}-dependent manner. After glutamate enters the synaptic cleft, it diffuses across the cleft to interact with its corresponding receptors on the postsynaptic face of an adjacent neuron. Excitatory neurotransmission is necessary for the normal development and plasticity of synapses and for some forms of learning and memory; however, excessive activation of glutamate receptors is implicated in neuronal damage in many neurologic disorders, ranging from acute hypoxic-ischemic brain injury to chronic neurodegenerative diseases. It is currently thought that overstimulation of extrasynaptic NMDA receptors mediates this neuronal damage, whereas, in contrast, synaptic activity may activate survival pathways.[27-29] Intense hyperstimulation of excitatory receptors leads to necrotic cell death, but milder or chronic overstimulation can result in apoptotic cell death.[30-32]

NMDA receptor–coupled channels are highly permeable to Ca^{2+}, thus permitting Ca^{2+} entry after ligand binding if the cell is depolarized to relieve block of the receptor-associated ion channel

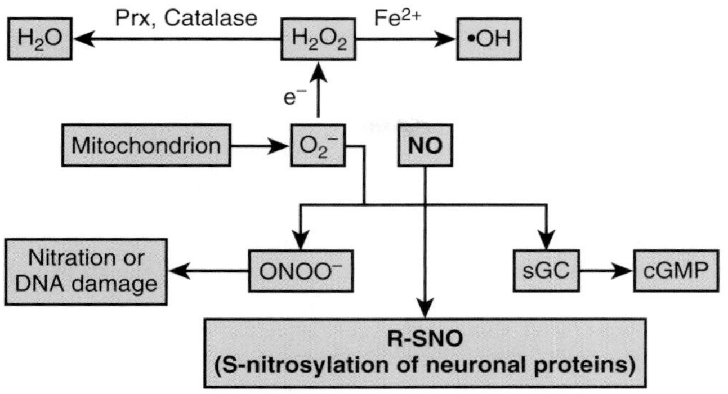

Figure 11-2. Pathways of ROSand RNS neurotoxicity. NO activates soluble guanylate cyclase (sGC) to produce cyclic guanosine monophosphate (cGMP), which in turn activates cGMP-dependent protein kinase. Excessive NMDA receptor activity, leading to the overproduction of NO, can be neurotoxic. For example, S-nitrosylation of parkin and PDI can contribute to neuronal cell damage and death, in part by triggering accumulation of misfolded proteins. Other neurotoxic effects of NO are mediated by peroxynitrite ($ONOO^-$), a reaction product of NO and superoxide anion (O_2^-). In contrast, S-nitrosylation can also mediate neuroprotective effects—for example, by inhibiting caspase activity and preventing overactivation of NMDA receptors.

by Mg^{2+}.[33,34] Subsequent binding of Ca^{2+} to various intracellular molecules can lead to many significant consequences. In particular, excessive activation of NMDA receptors leads to the production of damaging free radicals (e.g., NO and ROS) and other enzymatic processes, contributing to cell death.*

Ca^{2+} Influx and Generation of Reactive Oxygen and Reactive Nitrogen Species

Excessive activation of glutamate receptors is implicated in neuronal damage in many neurologic disorders. Olney coined the term *excitotoxicity* to describe this phenomenon.[37,38] This form of toxicity is mediated at least in part by excessive activation of NMDA-type receptors,[6,7,39] resulting in excessive Ca^{2+} influx through a receptor's associated ion channel.

Increased levels of neuronal Ca^{2+}, in conjunction with the Ca^{2+}-binding protein Ca^{2+} calmodulin (CaM), trigger the activation of nNOS and subsequent generation of NO from the amino acid L-arginine.[8,40] NO is a gaseous free radical (thus highly diffusible) and a key molecule that plays a vital role in normal signal transduction but, in excess, can lead to neuronal cell damage and death. This discrepancy in NO effects on neuronal survival can also be caused by the formation of different NO species or intermediates—NO radical (NO·), nitrosonium cation (NO^+), nitroxyl anion (NO^-, with a high-energy singlet and lower energy triplet forms).[11]

Studies have further pointed out the potential connection between ROS-RNS and mitochondrial dysfunction in neurodegenerative diseases, especially in PD.[5,41] Pesticide and other environmental toxins that inhibit mitochondrial complex I result in oxidative and nitrosative stress, with consequent aberrant protein accumulation.[17,18,20,42,43] Administration to animals of complex I inhibitors, such as 1-methyl-4-phenyl-1,2,3,6-tetrahydropyridine (MPTP), 6-hydroxydopamine, rotenone, and paraquat, which result in the overproduction of ROS-RNS, reproduces many of the features of sporadic PD, such as dopaminergic neuron degeneration, upregulation and aggregation of α-synuclein, LB-like intraneuronal inclusions, and behavioral impairment.[5,41]

*References 6, 11, 31, 32, 35, and 36.

Increased nitrosative and oxidative stress are associated with chaperone and proteasomal dysfunction, resulting in the accumulation of misfolded aggregates.[16,44] However, until recently, little was known regarding the molecular and pathogenic mechanisms underlying the contribution of NO to the formation of inclusion bodies, such as amyloid plaques in AD or LBs in PD.

PROTEIN S-NITROSYLATION AND NEURONAL CELL DEATH

Chemical Biology of S-Nitrosylation

Early investigations indicated that NO mediates cellular signaling pathways, which regulate broad aspects of brain function, including synaptic plasticity, normal development, and neuronal cell death.[35,45-47] In general, NO exerts physiologic and some pathophysiologic effects via stimulation of guanylate cyclase to form cyclic guanosine-3′,5′-monophosphate (cGMP) or through S-nitros(yl)ation of regulatory protein thiol groups (Fig. 11-2).[9,11,44,48-50] S-Nitrosylation is the covalent addition of an NO group to a critical cysteine thiol sulfhydryl (RSH or, more properly, thiolate anion, RS^-) to form an S-nitrosothiol derivative (R-SNO). Such modification modulates the function of a broad spectrum of mammalian, plant, and microbial proteins. In general, a consensus motif of amino acids comprised of nucleophilic residues (generally an acid and base) surrounds a critical cysteine, which increases the cysteine sulfhydryl's susceptibility to S-nitrosylation.[51,52] Our group first identified the physiologic relevance of S-nitrosylation by showing that NO and related RNS exert paradoxic effects via redox-based mechanisms. NO is neuroprotective via S-nitrosylation of NMDA receptors (as well as other subsequently discovered targets, including caspases) and yet can also be neurodestructive by the formation of peroxynitrite (or, as later discovered, a reaction with additional molecules such as matrix metalloproteinase-9 [MMP-9] and glyceraldehyde-3-phosphate dehydrogenase [GAPDH]).[11,53-60] Examples of SNO proteins known to be present in neurons or brains are listed in Table 11-1. Over the past decade, accumulating evidence has suggested that S-nitrosylation can regulate the biologic activity of a great variety of proteins, in some ways akin to phosphorylation.*

Chemically, NO is often a good "leaving group," facilitating further oxidation of a critical thiol to a disulfide bond between neighboring (vicinal) cysteine residue or, via reaction with ROS, to sulfenic (–SOH), sulfinic ($–SO_2H$), or sulfonic ($–SO_3H$) acid derivatization of the protein, as occurs, for example, on the enzyme MMP-9.[18,20,59,68] Alternatively, S-nitrosylation may possibly produce a nitroxyl disulfide, in which the NO group is shared by vicinal cysteine thiols.[69]

In addition, S-nitrosylation has been reported to influence other oxidative posttranslational modifications of cysteine residues. For example, S-nitrosylated as well as sulfenated cysteine residues may react with glutathione, producing S-glutathionylated proteins.[70] Moreover, S-sulfhydration (modification of a cysteine residue by hydrogen sulfide [H_2S]) generally occurs on the same cysteine residue(s) that can also undergo S-nitrosylation,[71,72] suggesting that S-nitrosylation may potentially promote the formation of S-sulfhydration.[73] Further studies are needed to reveal the chemical relationship between S-nitrosylation and other types of posttranslational modifications of thiol. Protein S-nitrosylation and other reactions with cysteine sulfhydryls should not be confused with protein nitration, in which NO is also implicated often via peroxynitrite ($ONOO^-$) reacting with a tyrosine residue to generate a nitro-tyrosine adduct.

Analyses of mice deficient in nNOS or iNOS (inducible NOS) have confirmed that NO is an important mediator of cell injury and death after excitotoxic stimulation; NO generated from

*References 11, 17, 18, 20, 52, and 59-67

TABLE 11-1 Examples of S-Nitrosylated Proteins Confirmed in Neurons or Brains

S-Nitrosothiol Targets	Effects of S-Nitrosothiol	Reference
Akt	Decreased kinase activity Increased cell death	210, 211
Caspases	Decreased activity Suppression of cell death	56, 54, 212, 55
Cdk5	Activation of kinase activity Augmentation of cell death	213-215
Dexras1	Activation of GTPase Regulation of iron homeostasis	216, 217
Drp1	Excessive mitochondrial fission Synaptic damage	218-220
NSF	Enhanced interaction with GluR2 Regulation of exocytosis	221, 222
GAPDH	Enhanced interaction with Siah1 Activation of p300 and CBP Augmentation of cell death	60, 223, 224
MAP1B	Enhanced interaction with microtubules Axon retraction	225
MMP-9	Activation Augmentation of cell death	59
NMDAR (NR1 and NR2A)	Inhibition Suppression of cell death	11, 58
Parkin	Decrease in E3 ligase activity Augmentation of cell death	17, 18
PDI	Decreased activity Accumulation of misfolded proteins Augmentation of cell death	20, 121-123
Prx2	Decreased peroxidase activity Augmentation of cell death	226
PTEN	Decrease in phosphatase activity Augmentation of cell survival	227, 228
XIAP	Decrease in E3 ligase activity Augmentation of cell death	229, 230

CBP, CREB binding protein; *GluR2*, glutamate receptor subunit 2; *GTPase*, guanosine triphosphate phosphohydrolase; *Siah1*, seven in absentia homolog 1.

nNOS or iNOS can be detrimental to neuronal survival.[74,75] In addition, inhibition of NOS activity ameliorates the progression of disease pathology in animal models of PD, AD, and ALS, suggesting that excess generation of NO plays a pivotal role in the pathogenesis of several neurodegenerative diseases.[76-79] Although the involvement of NO in neurodegeneration has been widely accepted, the chemical relationship between nitrosative stress and accumulation of misfolded proteins has remained obscure. Some studies, however, have shed light on molecular events underlying this relationship. Specifically, we recently presented physiologic and chemical evidence that S-nitrosylation modulates the ubiquitin E3 ligase activity of parkin,[17-19] and chaperone and isomerase activities of PDI,[20] contributing to protein misfolding and neurotoxicity in models of neurodegenerative disorders.

S-Nitrosylation and Parkin

Identification of errors in the genes encoding parkin (an ubiquitin E3 ligase) and ubiquitin carboxyl-terminal hydrolase L1 (UCH-L1) in rare familial forms of PD has implicated possible dysfunction of the UPS in the pathogenesis of sporadic PD as well. The UPS represents an important mechanism for proteolysis in mammalian cells. Formation of polyubiquitin chains constitutes the signal for proteasomal attack and degradation. An isopeptide bond covalently attaches the C-terminus of the first ubiquitin in a polyubiqutin chain to a lysine residue in the target protein. The cascade of activating (E1)-, conjugating (E2)-, and ubiquitin-ligating (E3)–type enzymes catalyzes the conjugation of the ubiquitin chain to proteins. In addition, individual E3 ubiquitin ligases play a key role in the recognition of specific substrates.[80]

PD is the second most prevalent neurodegenerative disease and is characterized by the progressive loss of dopamine neurons in the substantia nigra pars compacta. The appearance of LBs that contain misfolded and ubiquitinated proteins generally accompanies the loss of dopaminergic neurons in the PD brain. Such ubiquitinated inclusion bodies are the hallmark of many neurodegenerative disorders. Age-associated defects in intracellular proteolysis of misfolded or aberrant proteins might lead to the accumulation and ultimately deposition of aggregates within neurons or glial cells. Although such aberrant protein accumulation had been observed in patients with genetically encoded mutant proteins, evidence from our laboratory suggests that nitrosative and oxidative stress are potential causal factors for protein accumulation in the much more common sporadic form of PD. As illustrated later, nitrosative and oxidative stress, commonly found during normal aging, can mimic rare genetic causes of disorders, such as PD, by promoting protein misfolding in the absence of a genetic mutation.[17-19] For example, S-nitrosylation and further oxidation (e.g., sulfonation) of parkin result in dysfunction of this enzyme and thus of the UPS.[17,18,81-85] We and others have found that nitrosative stress triggers S-nitrosylation of parkin (forming SNO-parkin), not only in rodent models of PD but also in the brains of human patients with PD and the related α-synucleinopathy DLBD (diffuse LB disease). Parkin has multiple cysteine residues that can react with NO to form SNO-parkin. S-Nitrosylation of parkin initially stimulates ubiquitin E3 ligase enzymatic activity, followed by a decrease in enzyme activity, producing a futile cycle of dysfunctional E3 ligase–UPS stimulation.[18,19,86] We also found that the pesticide rotenone led to the generation of SNO-parkin and thus consequent inhibition of ubiquitin E3 ligase activity. Moreover, S-nitrosylation–induced inactivation of E3 ligase activity is also associated with a decreased neuroprotective effect of parkin.[17] Along these lines, SNO-parkin is increased in PD patients' brains, suggesting that long-term S-nitrosylation of parkin may be pathogenic.[17-19] Nitrosative and oxidative stress can also alter the solubility of parkin via post-translational modification of cysteine residues, which may concomitantly compromise its protective function.[85,87-89]

In contrast, S-sulfhydration of parkin activates its enzymatic activity and its neuroprotective effect.[72] Mass spectrometry analysis was used to identify five cysteine residues (Cys59, -95, -182, -212, and -377) as S-sulfhydration sites, among which Cys95 appeared to be the principal site of S-sulfhydration. Interestingly, Cys95 also serves as a target for S-nitrosylation.[72] Moreover, S-sulfhydration of parkin is markedly decreased in PD brains, consistent with the notion that parkin sulfhydration has beneficial effects. Thus, although further studies will be needed to reveal the relationship of S-nitrosylation and S-sulfhydration in individual proteins, at least in the case of parkin, it appears that the two gasotransmitters (i.e., NO and H_2S) may influence PD pathogenesis via cysteine modifications.

In addition to rare mutations in *parkin* causing familial PD, mutations in the gene *PINK1* are also associated with hereditary PD cases. Emerging evidence points to the possibility that parkin, together with PINK1, participates in mitophagy, whereby damaged mitochondria are removed by the cellular recycling process of autophagy (see next section).[90] In the proposed model, PINK1 is initially translocated to impaired mitochondria, which in turn recruit parkin from the cytosol to the damaged mitochondrial membrane. Recent evidence suggests that PINK1-phosphorylated mitofusin 2 may be a receptor for parkin on the mitochondrial membrane.[91] Parkin then ubiquitinates mitochondrial outer membrane proteins to enhance the autophagic removal of the unhealthy mitochondria. New evidence suggests that SNO-parkin can promote the removal of damaged mitochondria.[92] That report showed that S-nitrosylation of Cys323 transiently activates its E3 ligase activity, facilitating the mitochondrial degradation process. This finding raises the interesting hypothesis that nitrosative stress initially induces S-nitrosylation of parkin at Cys323, resulting in a short-lived increase in its E3 ligase activity. In turn, this activation of parkin mediates a neuroprotective effect of NO via promotion of mitophagy and hence disposal of unhealthy mitochondria. In contrast, pathologically prolonged generation of NO would S-nitrosylate additional cysteine residues in parkin, inhibiting its E3 ligase and neuroprotective activities. Further work will be needed, however, to elucidate more clearly these opposing effects of SNO-parkin on neuronal survival.

In addition to its E3 ligase activity, parkin also suppresses the transcription of the oncogene p53, contributing to its neuroprotective action against PD-associated apoptosis of dopaminergic neurons.[93] We recently reported that S-nitrosylation of parkin decreases its activity as a transcriptional repressor of p53, leading to the upregulation of p53 expression and thus neuronal cell death.[94] Consistent with this notion, in postmortem human PD brains, the levels of SNO-parkin and p53 are increased in a correlative manner. Hence, S-nitrosylation appears to affect both the ubiquitin E3 ligase and transcriptional repressor activities of parkin, coordinately contributing to the pathogenesis of sporadic PD.

S-Nitrosylation of Protein Disulfide Isomerase

This mediates protein misfolding and neurotoxicity in cell models of PD and AD. The ER normally participates in protein processing and folding but undergoes a stress response when immature or misfolded proteins accumulate.[95-98] ER stress stimulates two critical intracellular responses. The first represents expression of chaperones that prevent protein aggregation via the unfolded protein response (UPR), and is implicated in protein refolding, posttranslational assembly of protein complexes, and protein degradation. This response is believed to contribute to adaptation during altered environmental conditions, promoting maintenance of cellular homeostasis. The second ER stress response, termed *ER-associated degradation* (ERAD), specifically recognizes terminally misfolded proteins for retrotranslocation across the ER membrane to the cytosol, where they can be degraded by the UPS. Additionally, although severe ER stress can induce apoptosis, the ER withstands relatively mild insults via expression of stress proteins such as glucose-regulated protein (GRP) and PDI, which ameliorate the accumulation of misfolded proteins. These proteins behave as molecular chaperones that assist in the maturation, transport, and folding of secretory proteins.

During protein folding in the ER, PDI (designated PDIA1) can introduce disulfide bonds into proteins (oxidation), break disulfide bonds (reduction), and catalyze thiol-disulfide exchange (isomerization), thus facilitating disulfide bond formation, rearrangement reactions, and structural stability.[99] PDI has four domains that are homologous to thioredoxin (TRX; a, b, b′, and a′). Only two of the four TRX-like domains (a and a′) contain a characteristic redox-active CXXC motif, and these two thiol-disulfide centers function as independent active sites.[100-103] Several mammalian PDI homologues, such as ERp57 (PDIA3) and PDIp (PDIA2), also localize to the ER and may manifest similar functions.[104,105] Increased expression of PDIp in neuronal cells under conditions mimicking PD suggest the possible contribution of PDIp to neuronal survival.[104]

In many neurodegenerative disorders and cerebral ischemia, the accumulation of immature and denatured proteins results in ER dysfunction,[104,106-108] but upregulation of PDI represents an adaptive response promoting protein refolding and may offer neuronal cell protection.[104,105,109,110] In addition, it is generally accepted that excessive generation of NO can contribute to activation of the ER stress pathway, at least in some cell types[111,112] Molecular mechanisms whereby NO induces protein misfolding and ER stress, however, have remained enigmatic until recently. The ER normally manifests a relatively positive redox potential in contrast to the highly reducing environment of the cytosol and mitochondria. This redox environment can influence the stability of protein S-nitrosylation and oxidation reactions.[113] Interestingly, we previously reported that excessive NO can lead to S-nitrosylation of the active site thiol groups of PDI, and this reaction inhibits its isomerase and chaperone activities.[20] Mitochondrial complex I insult by rotenone can also result in S-nitrosylation of PDI in cell culture models. Moreover, we found that PDI is S-nitrosylated in the brains of virtually all cases examined of sporadic AD and PD. Under pathologic conditions, it is possible that both cysteine sulfhydryl groups in the TRX-like domains of PDI form S-nitrosothiols. Unlike formation of a single S-nitrosothiol, which is commonly seen after denitrosylation reactions catalyzed by PDI,[63] dual nitrosylation may be relatively more stable and prevent subsequent disulfide formation on PDI. Therefore, we speculate that these pathologic S-nitrosylation reactions on PDI are more easily detected during neurodegenerative conditions.

Additionally, it is possible that vicinal (nearby) cysteine thiols reacting with NO can form nitroxyl disulfide,[69] and such a reaction may potentially occur in the catalytic site of PDI to inhibit enzymatic activity. To determine the consequences of S-nitrosylated PDI (SNO-PDI) formation in neurons, we exposed cultured cerebrocortical neurons to neurotoxic concentrations of NMDA, thus inducing excessive Ca^{2+} influx and consequent NO production from nNOS. Under these conditions, we found that PDI was S-nitrosylated in an NOS-dependent manner. SNO-PDI formation led to the accumulation of polyubiquitinated misfolded proteins (e.g., synphilin-1 and α-synuclein) and activation of the UPR.[20,114-116] Moreover, S-nitrosylation abrogated the inhibitory effect of PDI on the aggregation of proteins observed in LB inclusions.[20,117] Other studies have also demonstrated that in AD, PDI accumulates in neurofibrillary tangles, which contain hyperphosphorylated aggregated tau protein, suggesting that SNO-PDI may also contribute to the accumulation of aggregated tau.[118,119] S-Nitrosylation of PDI also prevented its attenuation of neuronal cell death triggered by ER stress, misfolded proteins, or proteasome inhibition. Further evidence has suggested that SNO-PDI may in effect transport NO to the extracellular space, where it could conceivably exert additional adverse effects.[63] In addition, S-nitrosylation of PDI at its active cysteine sites may facilitate S-glutathionylation of this protein.[120] Thus, the potential role of S-glutathionylated PDI in neurodegeneration needs to be elucidated in future studies.

Similar to the finding that SNO-PDI contributes to the pathogenesis of AD and PD, SNO-PDI may also exacerbate pathologic conditions such as ALS, stroke, prion disease, and sleep disorders. For example, in cellular models of ALS, S-nitrosylation of PDI increases aggregation of the G93A mutant of superoxide dismutase 1 (mutSOD1), which is linked to a familial form of ALS, and increases neuronal cell death.[121-123] Also, S-nitrosylation of PDI in a stroke model contributes to the accumulation of ubiquitinated protein aggregates.[124] Moreover, S-nitrosylation of PDI mediates selective degeneration of hypothalamic orexin-containing neurons in a model of sleep disorders.[125] Finally, consistent with its pathologic role, substantial levels of SNO-PDI are present in the spinal cords of mutSOD1 mice and human patients with sporadic ALS, in brains of an animal model of prion disease, and in the hypothalamus of sleep-deprived mice.[121-123,125,126]

Next, rather than neurodegenerative disorders, we consider the normal aging brain. The quality control machinery for protein expression, composed of molecular chaperones, the UPS, and the autophagy-lysosome system, have been reported to be impaired in the aging brain.[21,127] Additionally, inclusion bodies similar to those found in neurodegenerative disorders can appear in brains of normal aged individuals as well as in those with subclinical manifestations of disease.[128] However, we have not found detectable quantities of SNO-parkin or SNO-PDI in the normal aged brain.[17,18,20] Hence, we speculate that S-nitrosylation of these proteins and others may further disrupt the quality control machinery, thus contributing to the susceptibility of the aging brain to neurodegenerative conditions.

II Metabolic Insulin Signaling in the Control of Aging and Neurodegeneration

Louis R. Lapierre, Malene Hansen

Many conserved metabolic pathways can affect organismal aging in a conserved fashion. Because of the complex regulatory systems that modulate life span, a successful approach to elucidate such longevity mechanisms has been the use of the simple invertebrate models, in particular the nematode *Caenorhabtidis elegans* and the fruit fly *Drosophila melanogaster*. Although multiple genes and processes have been linked to aging, the most well-understood example is the insulin/insulin-like growth factor 1 (IGF-1) signaling (IIS) pathway. Importantly, research has also shown a mechanistic link between IIS and neurodegenerative diseases. In this section, we discuss the mechanisms whereby IIS affects aging and neurodegeneration and briefly highlight examples of additional longevity paradigms with metabolic functions—namely, dietary restriction, target of rapamycin (TOR), and AMPK (5′-adenosine monophosphate–activated protein kinase).

INSULIN/INSULIN-LIKE GROWTH FACTOR 1 SIGNALING PATHWAY AND ORGANISMAL AGING

Evidence from multiple model organisms, ranging from worms to mice, has shown that moderately reduced activity of the IIS pathways extends life span. This discovery is particularly striking because severely impaired IIS function causes detrimental effects, including death during embryogenesis and diabetes. In addition, alterations of IIS pathway activity can have profound effects on reproduction, stress resistance, and metabolism.[129] Studies have started to unravel the underlying mechanism of IIS-mediated life span modulation.

In studies using the short-lived nematode *C. elegans*, the first long-lived IIS mutant (*age-1*) was identified through a genetic screen for genes that alter life span.[130] This mutant gene encodes the worm phosphoinositide-3-kinase (PI3K),[131,132] which supported additional findings in *C. elegans* demonstrating that mutations in the insulin/IGF-1 receptor DAF-2 increase life span and that this effect depends on the FOXO transcription factor DAF-16.[130,133-135] With the discovery that mutations in the insulin receptor (InR) or its substrate CHICO could extend the life span of *Drosophila*,[136,137] these findings collectively suggest that reduced IIS activity is an evolutionarily conserved mechanism to extend life span. This remarkable concept was further supported when rodents were shown to live longer if the insulin or the IGF-1 signaling pathways were disrupted,[138-141] indicating that the evolutionary conservation extends to mammals. This functional conservation may even extend to humans because alterations in the IIS pathway have been observed in centenarians.[142] These findings also provided a possible explanation for the long life span observed in growth hormone–deficient Ames dwarf mice and growth hormone receptor knockout (GHRKO) mice, because s growth hormone positively regulates the production of IGF-1.[143,144]

Figure 11-3 summarizes IIS interventions that have so far been shown to modulate life span in worms, flies, and mice.

Cellular Mechanisms Whereby IIS Affects Organismal Life Span

Because IIS coordinates nutritional availability and growth, it is not surprising that long-lived IIS mutants have changes in metabolic profiles (e.g., altered fat content) as well as delayed development, decreased adult body size, reduced fecundity, and increased stress resistance.[129,145] Each of these processes can make contributions to the extended longevity phenotype due to reduced IIS pathway activity.[145] Another important feature of reduced IIS function is the promotion of a longer health span as well as longer life spans in some cases. For example, experiments have demonstrated protective effects of IIS mutants that extend life span in invertebrate models against specific aging-related diseases such as cancer,[146-148] cardiac failure,[149] and AD (see later).[150,151]

Research efforts have focused on understanding when and where IIS modulates life span. To address the temporal requirements for reduction of IIS in determining life span, IIS was decreased in *C. elegans* during adulthood by administration of bacteria engineered to express double-stranded RNA for *daf-2*, and this treatment was sufficient to extend life span.[152] Consistent

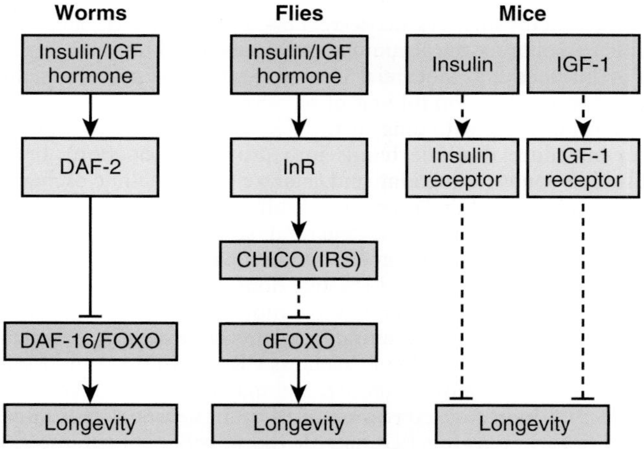

Figure 11-3. The insulin–IGF-1 pathway regulates aging in multiple organisms. Shown are the molecular components of the insulin–IGF-1 signaling pathway that have been shown to influence the life span of worms, flies and mice. See text for more details. *Dashed lines,* Plausible regulatory relationships.

with this, adult-only expression of dFOXO in the adipose tissue of flies was demonstrated to be sufficient to extend life span.[153,154] Similarly, adult-specific overexpression of dPTEN and ablation of the insulin-producing neurons in the last stage of preadult development was found to be sufficient to enhance longevity.[153,155]

The tissue-specific requirements for IIS to modulate life span have also been investigated in some detail and have pointed toward important roles for neuronal and fat tissues. For example, replacement of the insulin–IGF-1 receptor DAF-2 in neurons in *daf-2(–)* worms shorten life span back to that of wild type.[156,157] This is somewhat in contrast to the downstream effector of the *daf-2*/insulin–IGF-1 signaling pathway, the FOXO transcription factor DAF-16, which has been found to function primarily in the intestine—the worm's adipose tissue—to regulate life span downstream of the *daf-2*/insulin/IGF-1 receptor.[158] Thus, IIS in neural tissues controls signals that act in the periphery to modulate life span. Consistent with specific roles in neuronal and fat tissues, as mentioned previously, ablation of the insulin-producing neurons is sufficient to enhance longevity, whereas fat-specific overexpression of the pathway antagonists dPTEN or dFOXO can extend life span in flies via nonautonomous signaling to the insulin-producing neurons.[153,154] Finally, fat-specific knockout of the insulin receptor in mice can also extend life span.[139] Determining the nature of the signals and their cross-talk between the peripheral tissues remains a critical area of research. These results also highlight the potential autonomous and nonautonomous contributions as well as acute versus chronic consequences of altering insulin metabolic signaling in age-dependent diseases. How IIS orchestrates organ senescence, including neurodegenerative diseases and longevity, remains an important area of future studies.

Molecular Mechanisms Whereby IIS Influences Aging and Neurodegenerative Diseases

To gain deeper insight into the downstream effectors of IIS, unbiased approaches have been pursued, including gene expression profiling to understand the FOXO transcriptome in long-lived IIS mutant worms. In these studies, genes required for metabolism, stress response, and detoxification of oxidative damage have been identified.[159-164] Coordinated activation of the expression of several genes acting in these effector mechanisms is required for cellular benefits because the effect of individually altering expression of these genes results is minor.[161] Many FOXO-regulated genes are required to act additively to improve proteostasis and produce the profound life span effects seen in long-lived IIS mutants. Several studies performed in *C. elegans* and *Drosophila* proteotoxicity models have indicated that IIS links directly to the onset of toxic protein aggregation—for example, of the Aβ peptide causing AD via polyQ stretches, similar to those found in HD.[165-168] These studies have started to elucidate the mechanism whereby IIS affects neurodegeneration and suggest that IIS can protect against misfolded aggregates in AD by multiple mechanisms.[169] The primary mechanism involves disaggregation of toxic species to enable their degradation via small heat shock proteins (regulated by the heat shock factor protein-1 [HSF-1] transcription factor), whereas the secondary mechanism, regulated by DAF-16/FOXO, involves aggregation of proteins into high-molecular-weight species that are less toxic to the cell.[165] Studies in long-lived *C. elegans* IIS mutants with activated FOXO have shown that autophagy, a cellular process whereby cytoplasmic components are degraded and recycled, is a central effector mechanism in somatic maintenance.[170-172] Dysfunctional autophagy exacerbates neurodegeneration.[173] On the other hand, overexpression of at least some autophagy-related proteins can extend life span.[174,175] Interestingly, the role of FOXO in autophagy activation is conserved,[176] and maintenance of autophagy is emerging as a protective mechanism in neuromuscular junction degeneration,[177] suggesting a broad role for the FOXO-autophagy link in preventing neurologic aging.

ADDITIONAL METABOLIC LONGEVITY PATHWAYS WITH ROLES IN NEURODEGENERATION

Reduced food intake without malnutrition, referred to as dietary restriction (DR), has also been extensively studied in model organisms as a means to extend life span in a variety of species.[178] The extent of mechanistic overlap between DR and the IIS pathway is not fully understood. In *C. elegans*, the long life span of IIS mutants are completely dependent on the FOXO transcription factor DAF-16,[179] whereas some forms of DR function independently of DAF-16/FOXO, and others partially require DAF-16/FOXO.[180] In addition, a chemoattraction memory study has suggested that DR and IIS improve memory at different times during adulthood, but both require the activity of the bZIP transcription factor CREB.[181] In *Drosophila*, dFoxo null mutant flies still show life span extensions following DR.[153,182] The effects of DR on IIS in mammals are less clear, because long-lived Ames mice (see earlier) subjected to DR show a further increase in life span,[183] whereas GHRKO mice subjected to DR fail to increase life span.[184] The complexity of mammalian IIS suggests a more integrated interaction with DR, because DR leads to increased insulin sensitivity. Importantly, DR protects against neurodegeneration in mouse models,[185] and diet-restricted worms show reduced proteotoxicity mediated by the transcription factor HSF-1, similar to IIS mutants.[186]

A key player in the regulation of life span by DR is the nutrient sensor TOR. TOR exists in two distinct complexes, termed *TORC1* and *TORC2* (for review, see Wullschleger, Sarbassov, and colleagues[187,188]). Reduction of TOR function has been shown to increase life span in yeast, worms, and flies,[189-191] and pharmacologic inhibition of TOR with rapamycin extends life span in mice.[192] TOR regulates multiple processes linked to aging, including metabolism, messenger RNA (mRNA) translation, and autophagy.[148,187,188] Specifically, reduced mRNA translation extends life span in yeast, worms, flies, and mice (for review, see Kaeberlein, Selman, and associates[193,194]), and autophagy is required for multiple longevity paradigms to extend life span.[172] TOR interacts with the IIS pathway,[187] and this also seems to be the case in the context of aging, because inhibition of TOR and IIS in *C. elegans* does not extend life span further.[195,196] This functional overlap is supported by studies showing that reduced TOR activity leads to the activation of DAF-16/FOXO in *C. elegans*.[197,198] A regulatory feedback loop may exist because the TOR binding partner Raptor, called *daf-15* in worms, is a transcriptional target of DAF-16/FOXO.[190]

A new and common effector in DR, IIS, and the TOR pathway has recently been found, the transcription factor EB (TFEB). TFEB has been found to localize to the nucleus in TOR-inhibited or nutrient-restricted states and to regulate the expression of multiple lysosomal and autophagy genes, enhancing autophagic flux.[199,200] In *C. elegans*, the transcription factor HLH-30 mimics TFEB and is nuclear-localized in TOR-inhibited, dietary-restricted, and IIS mutants and is required for their life span, suggesting a common mechanism in the induction of autophagy.[201] In mammals, TFEB overexpression results in increased degradation of various types of disordered proteins involved in neurodegeneration, including mutant huntingtin (mHTT) and α-synuclein.[202,203] Therefore, activating TFEB may be beneficial to enhance lysosomal function to prevent neurodegenerative diseases. Currently, understanding how TOR regulates growth, metabolism, aging, and neurodegenerative diseases remains a critical area of research.

The energy sensor AMP-activated kinase (AMPK) has also been suggested to play an important role in longevity. Similar to TOR, AMPK plays a role in aging, stress resistance, and tumorigenesis.[204-206] AMPK also interacts with the IIS pathway, because life span extension via reduced IIS is dependent on the worm orthologue of the AMPK α subunit, *aak-2*, and the overexpression of AAK-2 and AMPK extends *C. elegans* and *Drosophila* life span, respectively.[174,206,207] Additionally, AMPK may have a neuroprotective role, because loss of AMPK causes a dramatic increase in neurodegeneration in flies.[208,209] AMPK may have additional roles in regulating neural function and may function downstream of actual chemosensory nutrient-sensing pathways, which allows the animal to detect and respond to changes in food availability. Future work will improve our understanding of how nutrient-sensing pathways are linked to neurodegeneration, aging, and life span.

Figure 11-4 summarizes the proteins and processes with metabolic functions linked to organismal aging discussed in this section.

Acknowledgment

The authors wish to thank Dr. Sean Oldham for his contributions to an earlier version of the chapter. This work was supported in part by grants from the National Institutes of Health (K99 AG042494 [LRL]; R01 AG038664 and R01 AG039756 [MH]; P30 NS076411, R01 NS086890, R01 ES017462, P01 HD029587, and R21 NS080799 [SAL]), the Brain and Behavior Research Foundation (SAL), and the Michael J. Fox Foundation (SAL and TN).

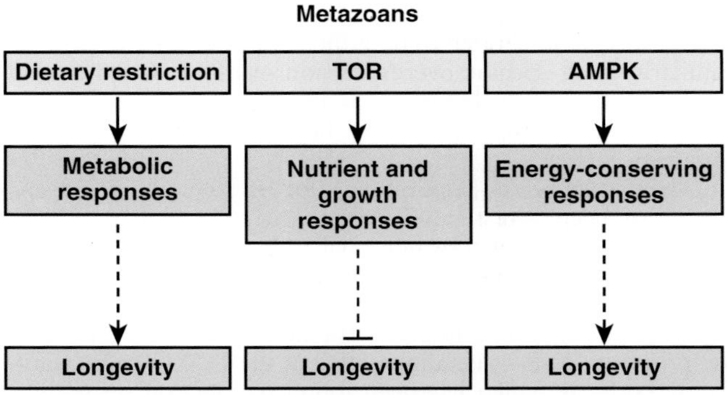

Figure 11-4. Additional processes and genes with metabolic functions that regulate aging in metazoans. Examples shown are dietary restriction, nutrient sensor target of rapamycin (TOR), and energy sensor AMP-activated kinase (AMPK). See text for more details. *Dashed lines,* Plausible regulatory relationships.

KEY POINTS: THE NEUROBIOLOGY OF AGING: FREE RADICAL STRESS AND METABOLIC PATHWAYS

- Excessive NMDA receptor activation and/or mitochondrial dysfunction trigger excessive nitrosative and oxidative stress that may result in malfunction of the UPS or molecular chaperones.
- Excessive production of ROS and RNS may contribute to abnormal protein accumulation and neuronal damage in sporadic forms of neurodegenerative diseases.
- S-Nitrosylation of specific molecules such as parkin and PDI provides a mechanistic link among free radical production, abnormal protein accumulation, and neuronal cell injury in neurodegenerative disorders such as PD and AD.
- Elucidation of these new pathways may lead to the development of additional new therapeutic approaches to prevent aberrant protein misfolding by targeted disruption or prevention of nitrosylation of specific proteins (e.g., parkin, PDI, peroxiredoxin 2).
- Single-gene mutations in the insulin and insulin-like growth factor signaling pathway can lengthen life span in worms, flies, and mice, implying evolutionary conservation of these mechanisms.
- Such mutations can keep the animals healthy and disease-free for longer periods and alleviate certain aging-related pathologies. Determination of the tissue requirements, genetic interactions, and timing of these effects remains an important area for further research, including in mammals.
- Additional conserved longevity pathways and genes can prolong life span in a conserved manner, such as dietary restriction, reduced levels of TOR, and activation of AMPK. A common factor for these paradigms, at least in simpler model organisms, is that they seem to use autophagy as an important effector mechanism.
- Autophagy is a central mechanism to rid cells of damaged organelles and macromolecules and promote survival. Uncovering autophagy enhancers in the context of neurodegenerative diseases is an emerging field of interest.

For a complete list of references, please visit www.expertconsult.com.

KEY REFERENCES

11. Lipton SA, Choi YB, Pan ZH, et al: A redox-based mechanism for the neuroprotective and neurodestructive effects of nitric oxide and related nitroso-compounds. Nature 364:626–632, 1993.
17. Chung KK, Thomas B, Li X, et al: S-Nitrosylation of parkin regulates ubiquitination and compromises parkin's protective function. Science 304:1328–1331, 2004.
18. Yao D, Gu Z, Nakamura T, et al: Nitrosative stress linked to sporadic Parkinson's disease: S-nitrosylation of parkin regulates its E3 ubiquitin ligase activity. Proc Natl Acad Sci U S A 101:10810–10814, 2004.
20. Uehara T, Nakamura T, Yao D, et al: S-Nitrosylated protein-disulphide isomerase links protein misfolding to neurodegeneration. Nature 441:513–517, 2006.
35. Dawson VL, Dawson TM, London ED, et al: Nitric oxide mediates glutamate neurotoxicity in primary cortical cultures. Proc Natl Acad Sci U S A 88:6368–6371, 1991.
51. Stamler JS, Toone EJ, Lipton SA, et al: S)NO signals: translocation, regulation, and a consensus motif. Neuron 18:691–696, 1997.
52. Hess DT, Matsumoto A, Kim SO, et al: Protein S-nitrosylation: purview and parameters. Nat Rev Mol Cell Biol 6:150–166, 2005.
58. Choi YB, Tenneti L, Le DA, et al: Molecular basis of NMDA receptor-coupled ion channel modulation by S-nitrosylation. Nat Neurosci 3:15–21, 2000.
59. Gu Z, Kaul M, Yan B, et al: S-Nitrosylation of matrix metalloproteinases: signaling pathway to neuronal cell death. Science 297:1186–1190, 2002.
60. Hara MR, Agrawal N, Kim SF, et al: S-Nitrosylated GAPDH initiates apoptotic cell death by nuclear translocation following Siah1 binding. Nat Cell Biol 7:665–674, 2005.
131. Friedman DB, Johnson TE: A mutation in the age-1 gene in Caenorhabditis elegans lengthens life and reduces hermaphrodite fertility. Genetics 118:75–86, 1988.
133. Kenyon C, Chang J, Gensch E, et al: A C. elegans mutant that lives twice as long as wild type. Nature 366:461–464, 1993.
134. Kimura KD, Tissenbaum HA, Liu Y, et al: DAF-2, an insulin receptor-like gene that regulates longevity and diapause in Caenorhabditis elegans. Science 277:942–946, 1997.
152. Dillin A, Crawford DK, Kenyon C: Timing requirements for insulin/IGF-1 signaling in C. elegans. Science 298:830–834, 2002.
156. Wolkow CA, Kimura KD, Lee MS, et al: Regulation of C. elegans life-span by insulin-like signaling in the nervous system. Science 290:147–150, 2000.
161. Murphy CT, McCarroll SA, Bargmann CI, et al: Genes that act downstream of DAF-16 to influence the lifespan of Caenorhabditis elegans. Nature 424:277–283, 2003.
163. Lee SS, Kennedy S, Tolonen AC, et al: DAF-16 target genes that control C. elegans life-span and metabolism. Science 300:644–647, 2003.
171. Melendez A, Talloczy Z, Seaman M, et al: Autophagy genes are essential for dauer development and life-span extension in C. elegans. Science 301:1387–1391, 2003.

192. Harrison DE, Strong R, Sharp ZD, et al: Rapamycin fed late in life extends lifespan in genetically heterogeneous mice. Nature 460:392–395, 2009.
196. Hansen M, Taubert S, Crawford D, et al: Lifespan extension by conditions that inhibit translation in Caenorhabditis elegans. Aging Cell 6:95–110, 2007.
197. Lapierre LR, Gelino S, Melendez A, et al: Autophagy and lipid metabolism coordinately modulate life span in germline-less C. elegans. Curr Biol 21:1507–1514, 2011.
200. Sardiello M, Palmieri M, di Ronza A, et al: A gene network regulating lysosomal biogenesis and function. Science 325:473–477, 2009.
213. Qu J, Nakamura T, Cao G, et al: S-Nitrosylation activates CDK5 and contributes to synaptic spine loss induced by beta-amyloid peptide. Proc Natl Acad Sci U S A 14330–14335, 2011.
218. Cho DH, Nakamura T, Fang J, et al: S-Nitrosylation of Drp1 mediates beta-amyloid-related mitochondrial fission and neuronal injury. Science 324:102–105, 2009.
229. Nakamura T, Wang L, Wong CC, et al: Transnitrosylation of XIAP regulates caspase-dependent neuronal cell death. Mol Cell 39:184–195, 2010.

12 Allostasis and Allostatic Overload in the Context of Aging

Bruce S. McEwen

INTRODUCTION

"Stress" is often identified as a factor in accelerated aging,[1] an important factor in disorders such as cardiovascular disease and depression, and a contributor to other disorders.[2] Being "stressed out" is a commonly used expression that generally refers to experiences that cause feelings of anxiety, anger, and frustration because they push a person beyond his or her ability to successfully cope. Besides time pressures and daily hassles at work and home, there are stressors related to economic insecurity, poor health, and interpersonal conflict. More rarely, there are situations that are life-threatening (e.g., accidents, natural disasters, violence), and these evoke the classic "fight or flight" response. In contrast to daily hassles, these stressors are acute and yet they also can lead to depression, anxiety, posttraumatic stress disorder, and other forms of chronic stress in the aftermath of the tragic event.

The most common stressors are, therefore, ones that operate chronically, often at a low level, and cause us to behave in certain ways. For example, being "stressed out" may promote anxiety or depressed mood, poor sleep, eating of comfort foods and overconsumption of calories, smoking, or drinking alcohol excessively. Being stressed out may reduce social interactions or regular physical activity. Not infrequently, anxiolytics and sleep-promoting agents are used, but, with continuation of this state, the body may increase in weight, develop metabolic dysregulation, and build up atherosclerotic plaque.

The brain is the organ that decides what is stressful and determines the behavioral and physiologic responses, whether health promoting or health damaging. The brain is a biologic organ that changes under acute and chronic stress and directs many systems of the body (metabolic, cardiovascular, immune, renal) that are involved in the short- and long-term consequences of being stressed out.

What does chronic stress do to the body and brain, particularly in relation to the aging process? This chapter summarizes some of the current information, emphasizing how the stress hormones and related mediators can play both protective and damaging roles in the brain and body, depending on how tightly their release is regulated. The chapter also discusses some of the approaches for dealing with stress in a complex world.

DEFINITION OF STRESS, ALLOSTASIS, AND ALLOSTATIC LOAD AND OVERLOAD

Stress is an ambiguous term and the actual stress response has protective, as well as potentially damaging, effects.[3] On the one hand, the body responds to almost any novel or challenging event by releasing catecholamines that increase heart rate and blood pressure and help adapt to the situation. Yet, chronically increased heart rate and blood pressure produce a chronic wear and tear on the cardiovascular system that can result, over time, in disorders such as atherosclerosis, strokes, and heart attacks. Sterling and Eyer[4] introduced the term *allostasis* to refer to the active process by which the body responds to daily events and maintains homeostasis (allostasis literally means "achieving stability through change"). Because chronically increased allostasis can lead to disease, we introduced the term *allostatic load or overload* to refer to the wear and tear that results from either too much stress or from inefficient management of allostasis (e.g., not turning off the response when it is no longer needed). Other states that lead to allostatic overload,[5] a term referring to pathophysiologic consequences, otherwise referred to as "toxic stress," are summarized in Figure 12-1 and involve not turning on an adequate response in the first place or not habituating to the recurrence of the same stressor, which then fails to dampen the allostatic response.[25]

PROTECTION AND DAMAGE AS THE TWO SIDES OF THE RESPONSE TO STRESSORS

Protection and damage are the two contrasting sides of the physiology that defend the body against the challenges of daily life, whether or not we call them "stressors." In addition to epinephrine and norepinephrine, many other mediators participate in allostasis, and they are linked together in a network of regulation that is nonlinear (Figure 12-2), meaning that each mediator has the ability to regulate the activity of the other mediators, sometimes in a biphasic manner. Glucocorticoids are the other major "stress hormones." Proinflammatory and antiinflammatory cytokines are produced by many cells in the body, and they regulate each other and are, in turn, regulated by glucocorticoids and catecholamines. Whereas catecholamines can increase proinflammatory cytokine production, glucocorticoids are known to inhibit this production.[6,7] The parasympathetic nervous system also plays an important regulatory role in this nonlinear network of allostasis, since it generally opposes the sympathetic nervous system and, for example, slows the heart and also has antiinflammatory effects.[8,9]

What this nonlinearity means is that when any one mediator is increased or decreased, there are compensatory changes in the other mediators that depend on time course and level of change of each of the mediators. Unfortunately, we cannot measure all components of this system simultaneously and must rely on measurements of only a few of them in any one study. Yet the nonlinearity must be kept in mind in interpreting the results.

MEASUREMENT OF ALLOSTATIC LOAD

Measurement of allostatic load and overload involves sampling of key mediators that may be elevated in what are called "allostatic states,"[10] as well as markers of cumulative change like abdominal fat. Allostatic states refer to the response profiles of the mediators (see Figure 12-1). On the other hand, allostatic overload focuses on the tissues and organs and other end points that show the cumulative effects of overexposure to the mediators of allostasis. These are done by collecting samples from subjects in a minimally invasive and cost-effective manner. This limits the choice to the circulating mediators such as glucocorticoids, dehydroepiandrosterone (DHEA), catecholamines, and certain cytokines. Salivary assays are particularly attractive, but the question is how to sample over time to get an adequate representation of a dynamic system, since the levels of the mediators may fluctuate

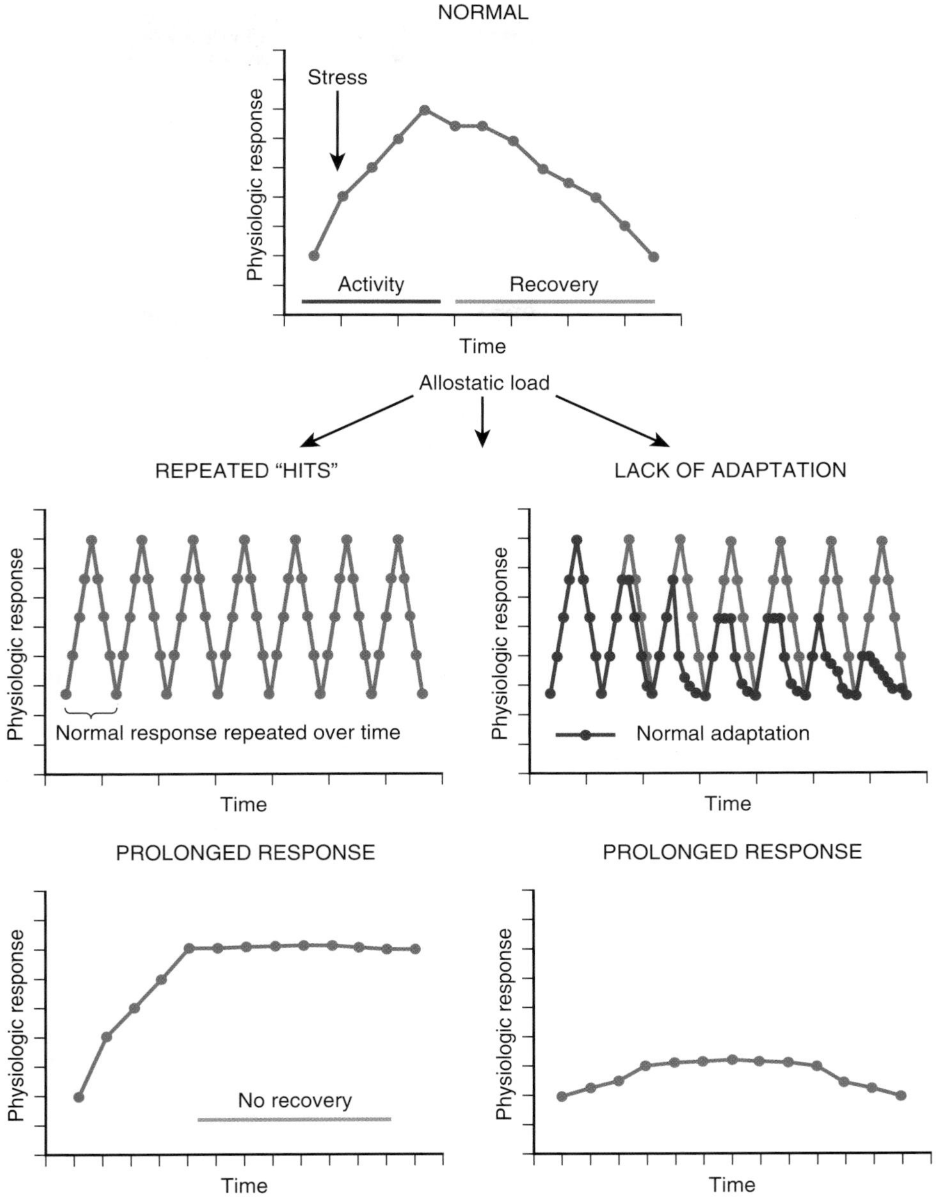

Figure 12-1. Four types of allostatic load. The top panel illustrates the normal allostatic response, in which a response is initiated by a stressor, sustained for an appropriate interval, and then turned off. The remaining panels illustrate four conditions that lead to allostatic load. *Middle, left:* repeated "hits" from multiple stressors. *Middle, right:* lack of adaptation. *Bottom, left:* prolonged response due to delayed shutdown. *Bottom, right:* inadequate response that leads to compensatory hyperactivity of other mediators (e.g., inadequate secretion of glucocorticoid, resulting in increased levels of cytokines that are normally counter-regulated by glucocorticoids). *(Modified from McEwen BS: Protective and damaging effects of stress mediators. New Engl J Med 338:171–179, 1998, by permission.)*

during the day and night. This is a topic unto itself and has been the subject of a number of methodologic studies (see website for MacArthur Research Network on Socioeconomic Status and Health: www.macses.ucsf.edu/). Box 12-1 summarizes a list of some end points that can be used for cumulative assessment of allostatic overload in different systems of the body.[11,12] These end points are currently in use in the Coronary Artery Risk Development in Young Adults (CARDIA) study and have been shown to have predictive power for a number of health outcomes.[7,13-15]

BEING "STRESSED OUT"—ESPECIALLY SLEEP DEPRIVATION AND ITS CONSEQUENCES

The common experience of being "stressed out" has as its core the elevation of some of the key systems that lead to allostatic load: these are cortisol, sympathetic activity, and proinflammatory cytokines, with a decline in parasympathetic activity. Nowhere is this better illustrated than for sleep deprivation, which is a frequent result of experiencing a lot of stress. Sleep

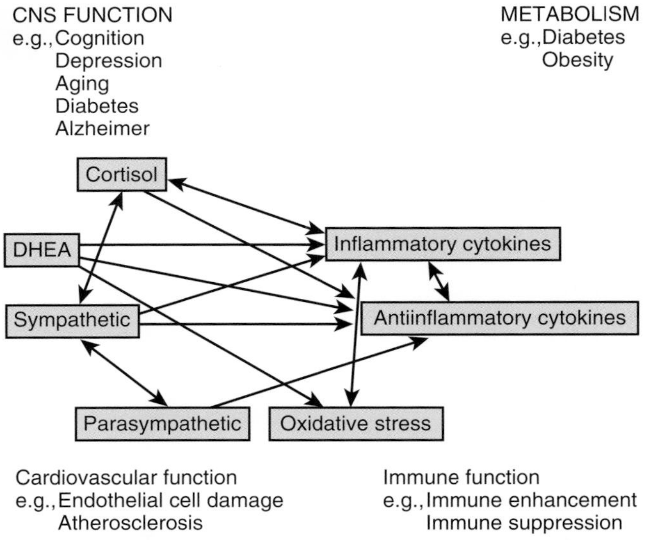

Figure 12-2. Nonlinear network of mediators of allostasis involved in the stress response. Arrows indicate that each system regulates the others in a reciprocal manner, creating a nonlinear network. Moreover, there are multiple pathways for regulation—e.g., inflammatory cytokine production is negatively regulated via antiinflammatory cytokines, as well as via parasympathetic and glucocorticoid pathways, whereas sympathetic activity increases inflammatory cytokine production. Parasympathetic activity, in turn, contains sympathetic activity. *(Modified from Dialogues in clinical neuroscience with the permission of the publisher (Les Laboratoires Servier, Suresnes, France) McEwen BS: Protective and damaging effects of stress mediators: central role of the brain. Dial in Clin Neurosci Stress 8:367-381, 2006.)*
CNS, Central nervous system; *DHEA,* dehydroepiandrosterone.

BOX 12-1 Measurements of Allostatic States and Allostatic Overload in CARDIA Study

Urine: 12-hr overnight
1. Urinary norepinephrine
2. Urinary epinephrine
3. Urinary free cortisol

Saliva: six saliva samples over 1 day assayed for cortisol

Blood
1. Total and HDL cholesterol
2. Glycosylated hemoglobin
3. IL-6
4. CRP
5. Fibrinogen

Other
1. Waist-hip ratio
2. Systolic and diastolic BP (seated/resting)
3. Heart rate variability

Modified from Seeman T, Epel E, Gruenewald T, et al: Socio-economic differentials in peripheral biology: cumulative allostatic load. Ann N Y Acad Sci 1186:223–239, 2010; Seeman T, Gruenewald T, Karlamangla A, et al: Modeling multisystem biological risk in young adults: the Coronary Artery Risk Development in Young Adults study. Am J Hum Biol 22:463–472, 2010.
BP, Blood pressure; *CARDIA,* Coronary Artery Risk Development in Young Adults (study); *CRP,* C-reactive protein; *HDL,* high-density lipoprotein; *IL-6,* interleukin-6.

deprivation produces an allostatic overload that can have deleterious consequences, which are particularly evident in aging: for example, poor sleep in aging women has been associated with elevated levels of interleukin-6 (IL-6).[16] Sleep restriction to 4 hours of sleep at night increases blood pressure, decreases parasympathetic tone, increases evening cortisol and insulin levels, and promotes increased appetite, possibly through increases in ghrelin and decreases in leptin.[17-19] Proinflammatory cytokine levels are increased, along with performance in tests of psychomotor vigilance, and this has been reported to result from a modest sleep restriction to 6 hours a night.[20] Moreover, reduced sleep duration has been reported to be associated with increased body mass and obesity in the National Health and Nutrition Survey (NHANES).[21] Sleep deprivation also causes cognitive impairment.[19]

KEY ROLE OF THE BRAIN IN RESPONSE TO STRESS

The brain is the master regulator of the neuroendocrine, autonomic, and immune systems, along with determining behaviors that contribute to unhealthy or health lifestyles, which, in turn, influence the physiologic processes of allostasis[3] (Figure 12-3). Alterations in brain function by chronic stress can, therefore, have direct and indirect effects on the cumulative allostatic overload. Allostatic overload resulting from chronic stress in animal models causes atrophy of neurons in the hippocampus and prefrontal cortex, brain regions involved in memory, selective attention, and executive function, and causes hypertrophy of neurons in the amygdala, a brain region involved in fear and anxiety, as well as aggression.[19] Thus, the ability to learn and remember and make decisions may be compromised by chronic stress and may be accompanied by increased levels of anxiety and aggression. A recent study has shown increased reactivity of the amygdala to neutral facial expressions, indicating an increase in anxiety and reactivity, resulting from a few days of sleep deprivation.[22]

TRANSLATION TO THE HUMAN BRAIN

Much of the impetus for studying the effects of aging and stress on the structure of the human brain has come from animal studies, summarized elsewhere.[19] Age-related reductions in entorhinal and hippocampal volume have been associated with mild cognitive impairment and early stages of Alzheimer disease, and a longitudinal study of aging Montreal residents revealed a smaller hippocampus and impaired hippocampal spatial and memory functions in those who showed rising cortisol levels during a yearly examination.[23] Although it is not possible to pinpoint causal factors in these age-related changes, stress and glucose regulation, along with depression and other mood and anxiety disorders, must be considered.

Regarding stress, although there is very little evidence regarding the effects of ordinary life stressors on brain structure, there are indications from functional imaging of individuals undergoing ordinary stressors (such as counting backward) that there are changes in neural activity.[24] There are also long-term effects: for example, chronic transcontinental air travel with short turnaround time, a type of chronic stress, is associated with a smaller hippocampus,[25] and a 20-year history of high perceived stress has been associated with smaller hippocampal volumes.[26]

Stress causes depressive illness in individuals with certain genetic predispositions,[19,27] and the hippocampus, amygdala, and prefrontal cortex show altered patterns of activity in positron emission tomography (PET) and functional magnetic resonance imaging (fMRI) and changes in volume, that is, decreased volume of hippocampus and prefrontal cortex and amygdala, although amygdala volume has been reported to increase in the first episode of depression, whereas hippocampal volume is not decreased.[28]

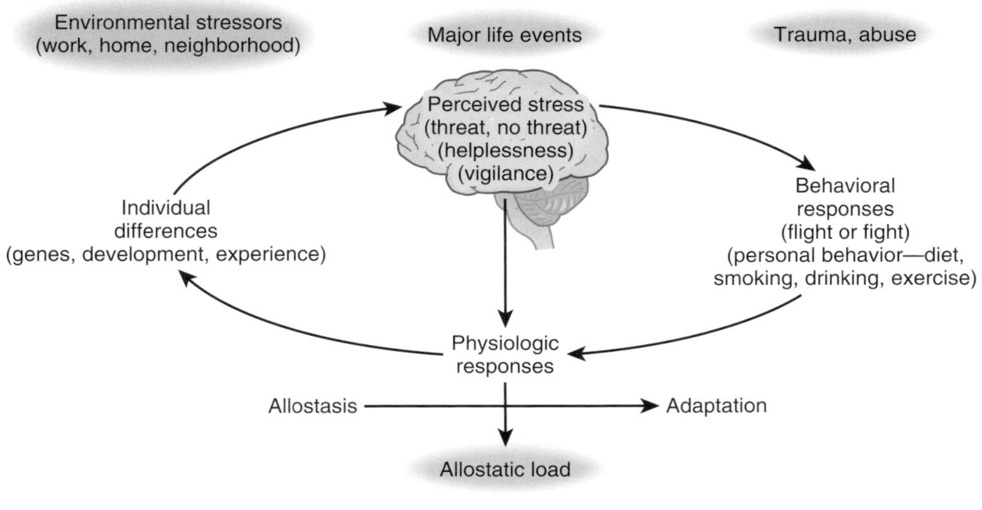

Figure 12-3. Central role of the brain in allostasis and the behavioral and physiologic response to stressors. *(Modified from McEwen BS: Protective and damaging effects of stress mediators. New Engl J Med 338:171–179, 1998, by permission.)*

There is hippocampal volume loss in individuals with Cushing disease along with cognitive impairment and depressed mood that can be relieved by surgical correction of the hypercortisolemia.[29] Moreover, there are a variety of other anxiety-related disorders, such as posttraumatic stress disorder and borderline personality disorder, in which there is atrophy of the hippocampus.[19] Another important factor in hippocampal volume and function is glucose regulation. Poor glucose regulation is associated with smaller hippocampal volume and poorer memory function in individuals in their 60s and 70s who have "mild cognitive impairment,"[30] as well as in those with frank type 2 diabetes.[31]

On a more positive note, a recent review of literature on the aging brain reveals a complex and more positive picture that leaves open the ability of positive interventions to benefit brain health:

> *Cognitive neuroscience has revealed aging of the human brain to be rich in reorganization and change. Neuroimaging results have recast our framework around cognitive aging from one of decline to one emphasizing plasticity. Current methods use neurostimulation approaches to manipulate brain function, providing a direct test of the ways that the brain differently contributes to task performance for younger and older adults. Emerging research into emotional, social, and motivational domains provides some evidence for preservation with age, suggesting potential avenues of plasticity, alongside additional evidence for reorganization. Thus, we begin to see that aging of the brain, amidst interrelated behavioral and biologic changes, is as complex and idiosyncratic as the brain itself, qualitatively changing over the life span.*[32]

POSITIVE AFFECT, SELF-ESTEEM, AND SOCIAL SUPPORT

Having a positive outlook on life and good self-esteem appears to have long-lasting health consequences,[33] and good social support is also a positive influence on the measures of allostatic load.[34] Positive affect, assessed by aggregating momentary experiences throughout a working or leisure day, was found to be associated with lower cortisol production and higher heart rate variability (showing higher parasympathetic activity), as well as a lower fibrinogen response to a mental stress test.[35]

On the other hand, poor self-esteem has been shown to cause recurrent increases in cortisol levels during a repetition of a public speaking challenge in which those individuals with good self-esteem are able to habituate (i.e., attenuate their cortisol response after the first speech).[36] Furthermore, poor self-esteem and low internal locus of control have been related to 12% to 13% smaller volume of the hippocampus in both younger and older subjects, as well as higher cortisol levels during a mental arithmetic stressor.[37]

Related to both positive affect and self-esteem is the role of friends and social interactions in maintaining a healthy outlook on life. Loneliness, often found in people with low self-esteem, has been associated with larger cortisol responses to wakening in the morning and higher fibrinogen and natural killer cell responses to a mental stress test, as well as sleep problems.[38] In contrast, having three or more regular social contacts, as opposed to zero to two such contacts, is associated with lower allostatic load scores.[34]

DELETERIOUS ROLE OF ADVERSE EARLY LIFE EXPERIENCE

The aging process begins at conception, and experiences early in life have a profound influence on the quality and length of life. Early life experiences perhaps carry an even greater weight in terms of how an individual reacts to new situations,[19] as demonstrated by the Adverse Childhood Experiences study by the Centers for Disease Control and Prevention, which shows that people who have had adverse early life experiences involving physical and sexual abuse and neglect carry with them a life-long burden of behavioral and pathophysiologic problems,[39,40] and cold and uncaring families produce long-lasting emotional problems in children.[41] These adverse experiences affect brain structure and function and carry the risk for later depression and posttraumatic stress disorder.[42-44]

INTERVENTIONS

Because environmental factors and experiences play a large role in the aging process, understanding and manipulating those factors can reduce the accumulation of allostatic overload. There are a number of approaches to deal with stress and allostatic overload as they affect the life course and affect health later in life. For the individual, these include lifestyle and personal habits, as well as pharmaceutical agents. For society, there are policies of government and the private sector.

For the individual, life-long habits may be hard to change, and it is often necessary to turn to pharmacologic interventions. Sleeping pills, anxiolytics, β-blockers, and antidepressants are all drugs that are used to counteract some of the problems associated with the accumulation of allostatic overload. Likewise, drugs that reduce oxidative stress or inflammation, block cholesterol synthesis or absorption, and treat insulin resistance or chronic pain can help deal with the metabolic and neurologic consequences of being chronically stressed out. All of these agents have value, and yet each one has side effects and limitations that are based in part on the fact that all of the systems that are dysregulated in allostatic overload are also systems that interact with each other and perform normal functions when properly regulated (as described in Figure 12-2). Because of the nonlinearity of the systems of allostasis, the consequences of any pharmaceutical treatment may be either to inhibit the beneficial effects of the systems in question or to perturb other systems in a direction that promotes an unwanted side effect. Examples of the former include the problems with cyclooxygenase-2 (COX-2) inhibitors,[45] and examples of the latter include the obesity-inducing effects of some of the atypical antipsychotics that are widely used to treat schizophrenia and bipolar disorder.[46]

The private sector has a powerful role, and businesses that encourage healthy lifestyle practices among their employees are likely to gain reduced health insurance costs and possibly a more loyal workforce.[47,48] Moreover, governmental policies are important, and the Acheson report[49] from the United Kingdom in 1998 recognized that no public policy should be enacted without considering the implications for health of all citizens. Thus basic education, housing, taxation, setting of a minimum wage, and addressing occupational health and safety and environmental pollution regulations are all likely to affect health via myriad mechanisms. At the same time, providing high-quality food and making it affordable and accessible in poor (as well as affluent) neighborhoods is necessary for people to eat better, providing they also learn what types of food to eat and can afford them. Likewise, making neighborhoods safer and more congenial and supportive[50] can improve opportunities for positive social interactions and increased recreational physical activity.

For the older adult population, community centers and activities that promote social interactions and physical activity have been demonstrated to be beneficial.[51,52] In that connection, there are programs that combine some of the key elements just described, namely, education, physical activity, and social support, along with one other ingredient that is hard to quantify: namely, finding meaning and purpose in life. One example is the Executive Volunteer Corps and another is the Experience Corps, which takes older volunteers and trains them as teachers' assistants for younger children in the neighborhood schools.[53,54] Not only does this program improve the education of the children, it also benefits the older volunteers and improves their physical and mental health[54]; it does so, in part, by providing meaning and purpose in life and a sense of psychological well-being, referred to as "eudaimonia."[55] Meaning and purpose in life is associated with reduced incidence of dementia.[56] In a study of "eudaimonic" versus "hedonic" lifestyles, those people with the "eudaimonic" lifestyle showed lower levels of inflammatory mediators than those with a purely "hedonic" lifestyle.[57] Based upon information discussed earlier, reduced inflammatory tone is consistent with a healthier physiology and an indication of lower allostatic load or overload.

CONCLUSION

There is a new way to conceptualize "stress" that emphasizes the role of the brain and its regulation of systemic physiology for the purpose of adaptation to a changing social and physical environment. It is the overuse and dysregulation of this adaptive response that leads to a cumulative burden on the body and brain, called *allostatic load* and *allostatic overload* to refer to more pathophysiologic outcomes. It is important to emphasize that the brain is a target of stress and shows allostatic load or overload resulting in remodeling of brain architecture that, in turn, alters how the brain regulates systemic physiology. Finding ways of improving the social and physical environment in which people live their lives should reduce the need for more direct medical and psychiatric interventions for everyone, particularly older adults, by allowing more physical activity, positive social interactions, and engagement in meaningful activities, among other positive outcomes.

KEY POINTS

- Events of daily life can produce the feeling of being "stressed out" and elevate and sustain activities of physiologic systems, as well as promote health-damaging behaviors and poor sleep.
- Accumulated over time, this results in wear and tear on the body, which is called "allostatic load/overload," the overload referring to pathophysiologic changes. This accumulated wear and tear reflects not only the impact of experiences but also genetic constitution, individual behaviors and lifestyle habits, and early life experiences that set life-long patterns of behavior and physiologic reactivity.
- Hormones and other mediators associated with stress and allostatic overload, including autonomic, metabolic, and immune system mediators, protect the body in the short term and promote adaptation by the process known as allostasis.
- The brain is the key organ of stress, allostasis, and allostatic overload because it determines what is threatening and, therefore, stressful, and also determines the physiologic and behavioral responses. Brain regions such as the hippocampus, amygdala, and prefrontal cortex respond to acute and chronic stress by undergoing structural remodeling, which alters behavioral and physiologic responses.
- Imaging studies of the human brain show smaller hippocampal volume in people with mild cognitive impairment resulting from aging, type 2 diabetes, and prolonged major depressive illness, as well as in individuals with low self-esteem. Structural and functional alterations in the amygdala and prefrontal cortex are also reported.
- Besides pharmaceutical agents, approaches to alleviate chronic stress and prevent diseases related to allostatic overload include changes in personal habits and lifestyle, as well as policies of government and business that would improve the ability of individuals to reduce their own chronic stress burden as they become older.
- Finally, increasing evidence shows that, along with diet, exercise, adequate sleep, and positive social support, meaning and purpose in life and "eudaimonia" (sense of well-being) are associated with healthier physiology and lower incidence of dementia, among other consequences.

For a complete list of references, please visit www.expertconsult.com.

KEY REFERENCES

1. Geronimus AT, Hicken M, Keene D, et al: "Weathering" and age patterns of allostatic load scores among blacks and whites in the United States. Am J Public Health 96:826–833, 2006.
4. Sterling P, Eyer J: Allostasis: a new paradigm to explain arousal pathology. In Fisher S, Reason J, editors: Handbook of life stress, cognition and health, New York, 1988, Wiley & Sons, pp 629–649.
6. Sapolsky RM, Romero LM, Munck AU: How do glucocorticoids influence stress responses? Integrating permissive, suppressive, stimulatory, and preparative actions. Endocr Rev 21:55–89, 2000.

8. Thayer JF, Lane RD: A model of neurovisceral integration in emotion regulation and dysregulation. J Affect Disord 61:201–216, 2000.
11. Seeman T, Epel E, Gruenewald T, et al: Socio-economic differentials in peripheral biology: cumulative allostatic load. Ann N Y Acad Sci 1186:223–239, 2010.
16. Friedman EM, Hayney MS, Love GD, et al: Social relationships, sleep quality, and interleukin-6 in aging women. Proc Natl Acad Sci U S A 102:18757–18762, 2005.
17. Spiegel K, Leproult R, Van Cauter E: Impact of sleep debt on metabolic and endocrine function. Lancet 354:1435–1439, 1999.
23. Lupien SJ, de Leon M, de Santi S, et al: Cortisol levels during human aging predict hippocampal atrophy and memory deficits. Nat Neurosci 1:69–73, 1998.
30. Convit A, Wolf OT, Tarshish C, et al: Reduced glucose tolerance is associated with poor memory performance and hippocampal atrophy among normal elderly. Proc Natl Acad Sci U S A 100:2019–2022, 2003.
34. Seeman TE, Singer BH, Ryff CD, et al: Social relationships, gender, and allostatic load across two age cohorts. Psychosom Med 64:395–406, 2002.
38. Steptoe A, Owen N, Kunz-Ebrecht SR, et al: Loneliness and neuroendocrine, cardiovascular, and inflammatory stress responses in middle-aged men and women. Psychoneuroendocrinology 29:593–611, 2004.
39. Felitti VJ, Anda RF, Nordenberg D, et al: Relationship of childhood abuse and household dysfunction to many of the leading causes of death in adults. The Adverse Childhood Experiences (ACE) study. Am J Prev Med 14:245–258, 1998.
52. Rovio S, Kareholt I, Helkala EL, et al: Leisure-time physical activity at midlife and the risk of dementia and Alzheimer's disease. Lancet Neurol 4:705–711, 2005.
56. Boyle PA, Buchman AS, Barnes LL, et al: Effect of a purpose in life on risk of incident Alzheimer disease and mild cognitive impairment in community-dwelling older persons. Arch Gen Psychiatry 67:304–310, 2010.
57. Fredrickson BL, Grewen KM, Coffey KA, et al: A functional genomic perspective on human well-being. Proc Natl Acad Sci U S A 110:13684–13689, 2013.

13 Neuroendocrinology of Aging

Roberta Diaz Brinton

Neuroendocrine aging is a multifactorial process that typically spans years and is characterized by sequential phase transitions.[1] These transitions are progressive in nature and are typified by stages of system-level changes in function, followed by compensatory adaptations. Furthermore, phase transitions are typically nonlinear processes that are more consistent with a step function from one state to another. Transition states are separated by intervening periods of apparent stability, during which the neuroendocrine system undergoes systematic dismantling and is often followed by the activation of compensatory adaptive responses. Adding to the complexity is individual variability derived from genetic, environmental, and experiential factors that alone and in concert can influence the rate of neuroendocrine aging.

Neuroendocrine aging is an illustrative example of the integrated coordination of chronologic and endocrine aging programs.[2] Both these programs of aging are modifiable by endogenous and exogenous modifiers (see Chapter 23).[3] Increasingly, the aging of neuroendocrine systems is recognized as a fundamental modifier of chronologic aging. For example, the development of insulin resistance at any age adversely modifies the trajectory of chronologic aging in women and men. This brief review focuses on two illustrative broad and interrelated aspects of neuroendocrine aging, reproductive senescence and metabolic dysfunction in women and men. Aging of both these neuroendocrine systems provides specific examples of fundamental principles of neuroendocrine aging in women and men, including phase transitions, adaptive compensatory responses, and biologic resilience.

NEUROENDOCRINE AGING IN WOMEN

Typically, the first indication of neuroendocrine aging in women is the transition to reproductive senescence, which usually begins during the mid-40s and ends in the early to mid-50s.[4,5] For some women, however, reproductive senescence can commence during the third decade of life.[4] The female reproductive axis is comprised of the hypothalamic-pituitary-ovarian-uterine axis and undergoes accelerated aging relative to other systems, which are otherwise healthy.[1,5]

Reproductive senescence in women is defined by oocyte depletion, which begins at birth and proceeds as a continuum until menopause has been undergone. A woman is endowed at birth with a finite number of oocytes that are arrested in prophase I of meiosis. Reproductive aging consists of a steady loss of oocytes through ovarian follicular atresia or ovulation, which does not necessarily occur at a constant rate.[6] The relatively wide age range for menopause in normal women (42 to 58 years) seems to indicate that women are endowed with a highly variable number of oocytes or the rate of oocyte loss varies greatly.[1] Menopause occurs at an average age of 51.4 years, with a Gaussian distribution from 40 to 58 years.[1] In the United States, approximately 1.5 million women reach menopause each year, and more than 45 million women will be older than 55 years in 2020.[7]

Perimenopause and Postmenopause

Perimenopause

Characteristics inherent to the perimenopausal transition have been extensively documented and chronicled.[4,5] The Stages of Reproductive Aging Workshop (STRAW) criteria,[4] an international collaborative effort, along with the Study of Women Across the Nation (SWAN), based on an ethnically diverse U.S. population,[8] have contributed to the classification of the perimenopausal transition while simultaneously identifying the complexity of symptoms and ethnic diversity of perimenopausal phenotypes. Normal reproductive aging in women is characterized by three distinct phases that can span years—perimenopause (also known as the menopause transition), menopause, and postmenopause.[5] According to STRAW, reproductive senescence can be subdivided into three distinct stages—perimenopause, menopause, and postmenopause.[4] Variable cycle length, variable intervals between cycles, vasomotor symptoms (hot flushes), and wide variations in steroid hormone levels characterize the menopausal transition.[4] One year of amenorrhea is considered to be the end of the perimenopause stage and onset of menopause. The end of the amenorrheic year commences the onset of the postmenopausal stage, which is also subdivided into early and late components. Early postmenopause is defined as 4 years since the last menstrual period and is followed by late-stage postmenopause, which thereafter defines the neuroendocrine state.[4,5]

Perimenopause is characterized by menstrual and endocrine changes in the hypothalamic-pituitary-ovarian-uterine axis that lead inexorably to reproductive senescence.[1] During perimenopause, ovulation occurs irregularly as a result of fluctuations in hypothalamic and pituitary hormones.[4,5] In late-phase perimenopause, nearly half of the cycles are anovulatory.[4,5] In the ovulatory cycles, follicle-stimulating hormone (FSH), luteinizing hormone (LH), and 17β-estradiol levels increase with progression of the stage of reproductive aging and, in the luteal phase, the serum progesterone level is decreased. The early-cycle (ovulatory and anovulatory) inhibin B level decreases steadily across the STRAW stages and is largely undetectable during elongated ovulatory and anovulatory cycles during the transition. The decline of inhibin B levels during early perimenopause results in an increase in follicle-stimulating hormone (FSH) levels, with no significant change in inhibin A or estradiol levels.[4] FSH levels may rise during some cycles but return to premenopausal levels in subsequent cycles.[1] Further complicating the determination of FSH concentration is the pulsatile pattern of secretion. The variability in hormone levels creates difficulties in interpreting a single laboratory test result[9] but an increase in FSH levels continues to be a clinical marker of ensuing menopause and postmenopause.[4]

In late-stage perimenopause, concentrations of 17β-estradiol are highly variable; levels can be persistently low, as might be expected, but can also be abnormally high.[1,4] A high 17β-estradiol concentration is associated with increased vulnerability to neurodegenerative insults and neuronal cell death,[10] but does not reduce the persistently high FSH and LH levels.[11,12] Remarkably, the cyclicity of progesterone appears to remain generally intact, whereas the level of progesterone can vary from a normal value to a high spike of progesterone to an undetectable level.[13] When considering relationship between steroid exposure and neurologic symptoms of menopausal transition, plasma levels of ovarian hormones are not predictive of brain concentrations of steroids.[2]

The hallmark symptom of the menopausal transition is the hot flush, also referred to as hot flashes. Although the hot flush is evidenced by vasodilation, the signal to vasodilate is neurologic.[1] The neural mechanisms underlying the signature symptom of menopause remain unclear. Hot flushes are most likely to occur during late-stage perimenopause and early-stage postmenopause.[4,14] The prevalence of hot flushes increases substantially in early perimenopause, reaches a maximum in late-stage perimenopause, remains high into the early postmenopausal stage, and returns to a low but persistent prevalence in late-stage postmenopause.[14-16] The prevalence of hot flushes can range from 30% to 80%, depending on ethnicity, with African American women experiencing the greatest frequency and longest duration.[17] Women aged 40 to 60 years who have had a hysterectomy and oophorectomy are at high risk for hot flushes.[4] In most women, hot flushes are transient. Hot flush frequency and severity abate within a few months in 30% to 50% of women and resolve in 85% to 90% of women within 4 to 5 years. However, 10% to 15% of women continue to have hot flashes into late-stage postmenopause.[17]

Although the mechanism underlying hot flushes remains unknown, the resemblance to heat dissipation responses has led to a focus on thermoregulation by the anterior hypothalamus. However, the exact role of estrogen in the pathogenesis of hot flushes remains unresolved. Increasingly, evidence has linked metabolic dysregulation to the occurrence of hot flashes.[1,18,19] Estrogen levels do not differ substantially between postmenopausal women who have hot flushes and those who do not, but the withdrawal of estrogen can induce hot flushes in women with gonadal dysgenesis who have undergone estrogen therapy that was subsequently discontinued, suggesting that estrogen withdrawal plays a role in the cause of hot flashes.[1] In SWAN, a large U.S. multicenter cohort study, higher levels of FSH were the only hormonal measure independently associated with flushing after adjustment for levels of estradiol and other hormones.[5] Women undergoing pharmacologic therapy to antagonize estrogen receptor activation by selective estrogen receptor modulators (SERMs) or inhibit estrogen synthesis using 5α-reductase inhibitors for breast cancer experience a significant increase in the frequency of hot flashes.[20]

Postmenopause

Like perimenopause, postmenopause is separated into early and late stages. Early postmenopause is defined as 4 years since the final menstrual cycle.[7] Levels of FSH continue to be high during early menopause and remain elevated throughout the late stage of postmenopause.[5,7] During the early postmenopause phase, there is a significant decline in ovarian hormones to a permanently low level, which is associated with accelerated bone loss.[5,21,22] Postmenopausal women undergo two phases of bone loss, whereas aging men undergo only one.[22] In women, menopause initiates an accelerated phase of predominantly trabecular bone (also known as cancellous and spongy bone) loss that declines over 4 to 8 years; this is followed by a slow phase that disappears after 15 to 20 years, when severe depletion of trabecular bone stimulates counterregulatory forces that limit further loss.[22] The accelerated phase results from the loss of the direct repressive effects of estrogen on bone turnover, which is mediated by estrogen receptors in osteoblasts and osteoclasts. During menopause, bone resorption increases by 90%, whereas bone formation markers increase by only 45%. In the ensuing slow phase, the rate of trabecular bone loss is reduced, but the rate of cortical bone loss can be increased.[22] Bioavailable serum estrogen and testosterone levels decline in aging men, and bioavailable estrogen is the major predictor of their bone loss. Thus, both sex steroids are important for developing peak bone mass, but estrogen deficiency is the major determinant of age-related bone loss in both genders.[22] Trabecular bone has low density and strength but a very high surface area and fills the inner cavity of long bones. The external layer of trabecular bone contains red bone marrow, in which hematopoiesis occurs and most of the arteries and veins of bone organs are found.

A wide range of pharmacologic agents are available to prevent and treat osteoporosis, including antiresorptive estrogen, SERMs, bisphosphonates, calcitonin, and anabolic therapies, including parathyroid hormone (PTH—PTH1-34 or PTH 1-84) and agents with an as yet undetermined mechanism of action, such as strontium ranelate.[23,24] Corrections in general deficiencies in calcium, vitamin D, or both are first-line therapeutic interventions.[23,24]

Therapeutic Horizons

Therapeutic intervention for endocrine aging-related symptoms continues to evolve, with increased attention to timing of intervention, dose of intervention, route of administration, and treatment regimen. Adverse outcomes of hormone therapy in late-state postmenopausal women, in particular conjugated equine estrogens plus medroxyprogesterone acetate, have led to a reevaluation of its use and delineation of factors regarding efficacy versus harm.[5] Hormone therapy for women has evolved to a greater extent than for men, for whom many of the same issues found with hormone therapy for women have been emerging in the clinical use of androgen therapy in men. As in women,[5] the efficacy of hormone therapy for men is age-sensitive, health status–sensitive and dose-dependent, with health risks associated with dosage and duration of use.[25]

Multiple pharmacologic and nonpharmacologic interventions have been used to treat hot flushes, with the most common pharmacologic intervention being estrogen or hormone therapy.[5,26-28] Multiple types of estrogen, doses, and routes of administration have been developed. Each formulation targets cessation of hot flashes and prevention of osteoporosis with near equal efficacy, depending on the dose. A position statement from the North American Menopause Society (NAMS) has supported the initiation of estrogen or hormone therapy around the time of menopause to treat menopause-related symptoms.[29] The use of hormone therapy was supported to treat or reduce the risk of certain disorders, such as osteoporosis or fractures and hot flashes in select postmenopausal women. Analysis of the risk-benefit ratio of hormone therapy for menopausal women has indicated a favorable benefit close to menopause but decreased benefit with aging and longer time since menopause in previously untreated women.[29] The attendant risks and side effects of estrogen or hormone therapy are substantial, which has led to behavioral and alternative therapies. However, there is no convincing evidence that acupuncture, yoga, Chinese herbs such as dong quai, evening primrose oil, ginseng, kava, red clover extract, or vitamin E relieve hot flushes.[30-35] Clinical trials of soy phytoestrogens have been inconsistent in showing benefit, with most randomized double-blind clinical trials indicating no significant benefit for the treatment of hot flashes.[36]

The association between hormone therapy and an increased risk of neoplasias in women's reproductive organs (see Chapter 86) has led to the development of SERMs in attempt to activate the beneficial effects of estrogen selectively while the reducing risks of therapy. In recent years, an increasing number of estrogen receptor ligands and novel SERMs have been identified from nature, and others have been designed and synthesized de novo in academia and the pharmaceutical industry.[26-28,37] The U.S. Food and Drug Administration (FDA)–approved indications for hormone therapy in women is for the treatment of hot flushes and prevention of osteoporosis, whereas SERMS have been approved for breast cancer prevention and treatment of osteoporosis. Thus, pharmaceutical industry efforts have focused on FDA-approved indications, along with antineoplastic actions in the breast and uterus. The oldest and most studied SERM is tamoxifen (TMX), a triphenylethylene derivative, nonsteroidal, first-generation SERM.[37] A minor metabolite of TMX is 4-hydroxytamoxifen (OHT), which has a shorter half-life but binds to estrogen receptors (ERs) with a binding affinity 20 to 30 times greater than that of TMX and equivalent to that of 17β-estradiol.[37] Tamoxifen functions as an ER antagonist in breast, but can act as an ER agonist activity in bone, liver, and uterus.[37]

Since 1971, TMX has been used to treat breast cancer in premenopausal and postmenopausal women and, in 1999, TMX was recommended for use in breast cancer prevention.[37] Another nonsteroidal SERM for the treatment of osteoporosis is raloxifene (RAL), a benzothiophene derivative, nonsteroidal, second-generation SERM. Similar to TMX, RAL has a mixed pharmacologic profile, acting as an ER agonist and antagonist in a tissue-specific manner. In the breast and uterus, RAL acts as a typical antiestrogen to inhibit the growth of mammary or endometrial carcinoma, whereas in nonreproductive tissues, it acts as a partial estrogen agonist to prevent bone loss and lower serum cholesterol levels, with a pharmacologic profile similar to that of 17β-estradiol in ovariectomized rats and postmenopausal women.[37,38] An increasing number of novel SERMs have now been identified and developed in academia and the pharmaceutical industry.[37,38] With enhanced efficacy, specificity, and antineoplastic action in the breast and uterus, novel SERMs have demonstrated more potential clinically therapeutic uses for the prevention or treatment of menopause-related symptoms, such as hot flushes and osteoporosis. Increasingly, combination therapy of a SERM plus estrogen therapy is being used to promote estrogenic action in nonreproductive organs while inhibiting proliferation in reproductive organs such as the breast, uterus, and ovaries.[26-28,38,39]

Unresolved Issues in Neuroendocrine Aging in Women

Currently, there has been no pharmacogenomic strategy for identifying women appropriate for hormone therapy and, if so, for determining the hormone therapy most likely to be most efficacious. Genomic strategies to date have identified ER polymorphisms associated with an increased risk of cognitive impairment in older women. However, several single-nucleotide polymorphisms (SNPs) on *ERα* (*ESR1*) and *ERβ* (*ESR2*) genes have been associated with a range of hormone-sensitive diseases, such as breast cancer and osteoporosis. ER genetic variations may also influence cognitive aging and was investigated in a cohort of 1343 women (mean age, 73.4 years) and 1184 men (mean age, 73.7 years).[40] Among women, two of the *ERα* SNPs (reference SNP cluster identification, rs—rs8179176, rs9340799)[40,41] and two of the *ERβ* SNPs (rs1256065, rs1256030) were associated with a likelihood of developing cognitive impairment.[40] In men, one of the *ERα* SNPs (rs728524) and two of the *ERβ* SNPs (rs1255998, rs1256030) were associated with cognitive impairment. These findings suggest that ER genetic variants may play a role in cognitive aging. Tailoring hormone therapy for women and men based on their ER SNP profile remains uncharted territory.

The timing of hormone therapy intervention is of critical importance, and several studies have attempted to determine the impact of timing of hormone therapy. Evidence has supported a critical window of therapeutic opportunity[42] that is related to the healthy cell bias hypothesis of estrogen action.[43,44] This hypothesis predicts that estrogen therapy, if initiated at the time of perimenopause to menopause, when neurologic health is not yet comprised, will be of benefit, manifested as reduced risk for age-associated neurodegenerative diseases such as Alzheimer and Parkinson diseases.[43,44]

Major challenges for optimal estrogen and hormone therapy remain. Beyond the timing issue,[42,43] the real and perceived risks of hormone therapy remain and were amplified by results of the Women's Health Initiative trial and Women's Health Initiative Memory Study.[45-47] It is clear that many but not all women could potentially benefit from estrogen or hormone therapy intervention.[1] Biomarkers to identify women appropriate for this type of therapy and to determine which type of hormone regimen is most appropriate remains largely undeveloped beyond the treatment of hot flashes.[1] Hormone therapy interventions that selectively target the benefits of estrogen while avoiding untoward risk factors remain an unmet need in women's health. Estrogen alternatives that activate estrogen mechanisms in the brain but not in the breast or uterus, such as NeuroSERMs and PhytoSERMs, are promising strategies for sustaining the benefits of estrogen in the brain to prevent age-associated neurodegenerative disease.[44]

NEUROENDOCRINE AGING IN MEN

Andropause

The endocrine system in the male undergoes chronologic and endocrine aging with a pattern distinct from the female.[25,48] In recent years, greater clinical and scientific focus on the endocrinology of the aging male has provided substantial evidence for andropause in the male as a medically definable condition.[25,48,49] Arguments in favor of clinical significance are the similarities between the symptomatology of aging and that of androgen deficiency in young hypogonadal men.[50] Opposing arguments cite the near-ubiquitous decline of almost all physiologic systems; thus; the decline in testosterone synthesis by the gonads is considered just one part of the complex mosaic of aging.[51] As such, the terms *partial androgen deficiency of the aging male* or *late-onset hypogonadism* have been proposed as alternatives to andropause or male climacteric because of the connotation of a generalized phenomenon and permanent infertility.

Like the female reproductive endocrine system, the male system reproductive axis is comprised of the hypothalamic-pituitary-gonadal (HPG) axis but, unlike women, the male reproductive system does not undergo accelerated aging, and fertility can be sustained throughout the life span.[50] Unlike women, for whom menopause leads to the irreversible end of reproductive life, an end of gonadal function and, as a consequence, low sex hormone levels in all postmenopausal women, fertility persists in men until very old age.[25,48] Neuroendocrine aging in men is characterized by dysregulation of the pulsatile release pattern of LH secretion, whereas the regulation of FSH secretion is essentially maintained.[50] This is therapeutically significant because the testicular residual secretory capacity could allow many older men to raise their serum testosterone levels substantially, provided there was physiologically appropriate LH activation. This change in the LH secretory pattern is due to changes in the feedback regulatory mechanisms within the hypothalamus because pituitary secretory capacity is preserved in older adults.[50]

Age-associated decline in testosterone levels is, under normal aging circumstances, slowly progressive, with 10% to 15% of men aged 65 and older experiencing low total testosterone levels of <8 nmol/L.[25] The prevalence of low testosterone is 3.2% of men aged 60 to 69 years and 5.1% of men aged 70 to 79 years.[25] A substantial proportion of men in their 80s still have bioavailable testosterone levels comparable to the normal range of young men.[48] As a rule, androgen deficiency is only partial.[50] However, the threshold level(s) of testosterone below which consequences of androgen deficiency become manifest, and the clinical symptoms, frequency, and/or severity required to establish the diagnosis of androgen deficiency, are multifaceted.[25] Men with age-associated low testosterone levels can be classified into those with primary (age-related) or secondary hypogonadism (obesity-related). Both have a serum total testosterone less than 10.5 nmol/L and LH level less than 9.4 U/L) or, with compensated hypogonadism, a serum total testosterone level more than 10.5 nmol/L and LH level more than 9.4 U/L.[25] Testosterone levels in the plasma of adult men exhibit a diurnal variation, with the highest levels in the early morning and a progressive decline to a nadir in the evening.[48] This diurnal cycle of testosterone is blunted in older men.[48]

Age-related decline in the testosterone level (primary hypogonadism) has been linked to functional decline in multiple androgen-dependent systems, including muscle (mass and strength), bone (bone mineral density, geometry, and quality), reproduction (low libido), and hematopoiesis.[25] A decline in these systems is associated with frailty, falls, fractures, limitation in mobility, diabetes mellitus, metabolic syndrome, coronary artery disease, cardiovascular events, anemia, and overall mortality.[25]

Testosterone is largely bound to plasma proteins; only 1% to 2% is free testosterone, with 40% to 50% loosely bound to albumin and 50% to 60% specifically and strongly bound to the steroid hormone-binding globulin (SHBG).[50,52] Unbound testosterone diffuses passively through the cell membranes into the target cell, where it binds to a specific androgen receptor (AR).[50] Androgen concentration in target tissues depends on the plasma concentration of bioavailable androgen, local androgen metabolism, and presence of the AR.

Androgenic actions of testosterone and its active metabolite, dihydrotestosterone (DHT), are mediated via binding to the AR. Remarkably, the level of DHT remains constant with age, despite the decline of its precursor, testosterone.[48] Although testosterone and dihydrotestosterone bind to the same receptor, the affinity of DHT for the AR is greater than that of testosterone. The expression of the AR is increased by androgens and estrogens, especially in the prostate, and decreases with aging. In the prostate, almost all androgenic effects are exerted by DHT via conversion of testosterone by 5α-reductase type 2.[50] In many tissues, DHT mediates most of the androgenic effects of testosterone. A notable exception is muscle, where testosterone is the active androgen.[50] In addition to the well-characterized nuclear AR that activates gene transcription, testosterone can also exert rapid nongenomic effects, in part via binding to a G protein–coupled membrane receptor. The AR is highly expressed in male accessory sex organs and in some areas of the brain. A lower level of AR expression occurs in skeletal muscle, heart and vascular smooth muscle, and bone.[50] Sensitivity of the AR to androgens is modulated by AR polymorphisms. The AR gene, located on the X chromosome, contains a polymorphic trinucleotide CAG repeat in exon 1, which encodes a functionally relevant polyglutamine tract of variable length. A CAG repeat length exceeding the normal range of 15 to 31 results in diminished AR transactivation function. Clinical studies have indicated that AR polymorphisms are associated with a higher prevalence of several androgen-sensitive diseases, including prostate cancer.[50]

A subset of the physiologic actions of testosterone derives from its aromatization to 17β-estradiol, which binds to ERs.[50,53,54] Documented estrogen-mediated actions of testosterone in men include a role in the feedback regulation of LH and regulation of skeletal homeostasis, as well as lipid metabolism and cardiovascular physiology, brain development, and spermatogenesis.[50] It appears that declining bioavailable estrogen levels in men can play a significant role in age-related bone loss and fracture risk, similar to what occurs women.[55,56] Consistent with a role of estrogen in bone development and remodeling, men with a homozygous deletion of the *ERα* gene or aromatase deficiency have unfused epiphyses, elevated markers of bone remodeling, and low bone mass, despite normal or elevated testosterone levels.[55]

Therapeutic Horizons

Androgen hormone therapy is available in multiple formulations; these include oral tablets, transdermal gels and patches, buccal adhesives, and long-acting intramuscular injectables.[57] As with hormone therapy in women, testosterone therapy may be associated with an increased risk of serious adverse effects in men.[58,59] Metastatic prostate cancer and breast cancer are hormone-dependent cancers that may be stimulated to grow during testosterone treatment.[60] Consequently, the use of testosterone therapy, with its potential to increase the risk and/or progression of prostate tumorigenesis, has been controversial and has led to the development of selective androgen receptor modulators (SARMs). These lack significant androgen action in the prostate but exert agonist effects in select androgen-responsive tissues of interest, including the brain, muscle, and bone.[61]

Several strategies of SARM design have been pursued.[61-63] The first has been to develop novel steroidal compounds that are not substrates for the 5α-reductase enzyme that converts testosterone to DHT. As mentioned earlier, prostate growth is largely induced by DHT, rather than testosterone, because DHT exhibits about a 10-fold greater potency for AR, which reflects a higher binding affinity for AR and slower dissociation rate from AR.[64] SARMs that are not 5α-reductase substrates, and thus do not form DHT or DHT-like derivatives, have relatively low androgen action in prostate. There are several synthetic androgens in this class that are potentially promising candidates, with varied affinity for AR and androgenic activity, including 7α-cyano-19-nortestosterone, 7α-acetylthio-19-nortestosterone, 19-nor-4-androstene-3β, 17β-diol-3β, 19-nortestosterone, and 4-estren-3α-17β-diol.[63] The most promising SARM found in this category was 7α-methyl-19-nortestosterone, commonly referred to as MENT.[65-68] MENT, developed by the Population Council, has been in clinical trials as an androgen therapy for hypogonadal men; it exhibits low androgen activity in the prostate but is more potent than testosterone in other peripheral androgen-responsive tissues, including bone.[63] Although not a substrate for 5α-reductase, MENT is a substrate for aromatase and thus, like testosterone, can be converted to estradiol. Because many cellular effects of testosterone result from aromatization to estradiol and subsequent activation of ER-dependent signaling, there is potentially a strong benefit in a SARM that exhibits androgen and estrogen functions. The effects of MENT on neural function are virtually unknown. The testosterone-based structure of MENT strongly suggests blood-brain barrier permeability.

Another promising SARM in this class is 19-nor-4-androstene-3β,17β-diol (also called estren-β). Estren-β has a high affinity for ERs and ARs. A second SARM design strategy has been the development of nonsteroidal synthetic AR ligands.[69] Of particular interest are compounds that bind AR but have altered interactions with AR binding pocket side chains that underlie tissue specificity.[63] An example of this class is BMS-564929, which has been in clinical trials to improve musculoskeletal end points in hypogonadal men.

Unresolved Issues in Reproductive Senescence in Men

Many of the issues that are unresolved for reproductive senescence in women are applicable to men. The issue of hormone therapy for androgen deficiency remains controversial.[60] Lowering testosterone concentrations in adult men by surgical orchiectomy or by administration of a gonadotropin-releasing hormone (GnRH) agonist or antagonist is associated with rapid and marked loss of bone mineral density, increase in fat mass, and loss of muscle mass and strength.[55,70] Lowering of testosterone concentrations also results in hot flashes and a decrease in overall sexual activity, thoughts, and fantasies.[70] Hot flashes are common among men treated with androgen deprivation therapy for prostate cancer.

Testosterone therapy may be associated with an increased risk of serious adverse effects in men.[25,59,60] Metastatic prostate cancer and breast cancer are hormone-dependent cancers that may be stimulated to grow during testosterone treatment.[57] Because prostate cancer is usually a function of age, the long-term consequences of surgical or pharmacologic orchiectomy, beyond the effects on bone and blood, has not been established in men, nor have biomarkers been developed to identify men appropriate for androgen or SARM therapy.

To date, no personalized medical strategy to determine which men are suitable for hormone therapy, type of hormone therapy, or dose or treatment regimen has been developed. Given the adverse health impact of hypogonadism in men and the potential benefit of hormone therapy for hypogonadal older men, the development of precision medical strategies for hormone therapy has the potential for identifying men for whom hormone therapy is appropriate and the formulation, dose, and treatment regimen to achieve benefit and reduce risk.

NEUROENDOCRINE AGING AND BRAIN METABOLISM: IMPLICATIONS FOR NEURODEGENERATIVE DISEASE

On average, the adult human brain represents approximately 2% of body weight but accounts for 20% of the oxygen and, hence, calories consumed by the body, which is 10 times that expected on the basis of its weight alone.[71] The high rate of metabolism is remarkably constant, despite widely varying mental and motor activities.[71] Ongoing metabolic activity consists largely of the oxidation of glucose to carbon dioxide and water, resulting in the production of large amounts of energy in the form of adenosine triphosphate (ATP). Most of the energy used in the brain is required for the propagation of action potentials and for restoring postsynaptic ion fluxes after receptors have been stimulated by the neurotransmitter. Thus, the greatest majority of the metabolic activity in brain is devoted to synaptic processes.[71]

The significant portion of energy metabolism in brain devoted to maintaining synaptic transmission and integrity suggests that decrements in energy production would first affect synaptic transmission and physiology. Consistent with this postulate, mounting evidence has suggested that Alzheimer disease (AD) begins with subtle alterations of hippocampal synaptic efficacy prior to frank neuronal degeneration.[72] Furthermore, hypometabolism in the brain predicts cognitive decline years in advance of the clinical diagnosis of AD.[73] The association between mitochondrial dysfunction and neurodegenerative diseases such as AD and Parkinson disease has been increasing, along with evidence that hypometabolism and a concomitant reduction and dysfunction in mitochondrial gene expression in the brain are antecedents to the cognitive deficits of AD.[73-76] The association between hypometabolism and AD is based on multiple levels of analysis and experimental paradigms, which range from genomic analyses in animal models and autopsies on the human brain postmortem to in vitro cell model systems to brain imaging in humans. Overall, each of these levels of analysis has indicated that dysfunction in glucose metabolism, bioenergetics, and mitochondrial function are consistent antecedents to the development of AD pathology in males and females.[73,76-83] The decline in brain glucose metabolism and mitochondrial function can appear decades prior to diagnosis and thus may serve as a biomarker of AD risk, as well as a therapeutic target.[73,79,83,84]

A growing body of evidence has indicated that postmenopausal women experience a decline in brain metabolism that is prevented by estrogen therapy. As part of a 9-year study in the Baltimore Longitudinal Study of Aging, Resnick and colleagues[85] conducted positron emission tomography (PET) studies to assess regional cerebral blood flow in a small cohort of women who were estrogen therapy (ET) users versus women who were not. Their results have shown that ET users and nonusers show significant differences in PET regional cerebral blood flow relative to activation patterns during memory tasks. ET users had better performance on neuropsychological tests of figural and verbal memory and on some aspects of the PET activation tests.

In a follow-up longitudinal study of the same cohort of healthy menopausal women, Maki and Resnick[86] have found that regional cerebral blood flow is increased in ET users relative to nonusers in the hippocampus, parahippocampal gyrus, and temporal lobe, regions that form a memory circuit and that are sensitive to preclinical AD. Furthermore, they found that the increase in regional cerebral blood flow was associated with higher scores on a battery of cognitive tests.[86] In a separate 2-year follow-up analysis, Rasgon and associates[87] detected a significant decrease in metabolism of the posterior cingulate cortex among postmenopausal women who did not receive ET, whereas those women who were estrogen users did not exhibit significant metabolic changes in the posterior cingulate. These findings—that estrogen use may preserve regional cerebral metabolism and protect against metabolic decline in postmenopausal women, especially in the posterior cingulate cortex—is particularly important, given that metabolism in this region of the brain declines in the earliest stages of AD.[76,87]

As might be expected from reduced energy metabolism, postmenopausal women are at greater risk for developing metabolic syndrome. A longitudinal 9-year study of 949 participants, the Study of Women's Health Across the Nation (SWAN), investigated the natural history of the menopausal transition in women of five ethnicities at seven geographic sites.[88] By the onset of menopause, 13.7% of the women had new-onset metabolic syndrome. Odds of developing the metabolic syndrome per year during perimenopause were 1.45 (95% confidence interval [CI], 1.35 to 1.56) and, after menopause, it was 1.24 (95% CI, 1.18 to 1.30). Surprisingly, an increase in bioavailable testosterone or decrease in SHBG levels increased the odds of developing metabolic syndrome in women. This longitudinal study of the largest cohort of middle-aged women undergoing the menopausal transition has indicated that the prevalence of metabolic syndrome increases significantly during perimenopause and early postmenopause, independent of aging and other known cardiovascular disease risk factors such as weight gain and smoking. Increased bioavailable testosterone emerged as an independent predictor, after controlling for aging and cardiovascular disease risk factors. These findings suggest that progression through menopause, with the associated decrease in estrogen level, results in a progressively androgen-dominated hormonal milieu, which can increase the risk of developing metabolic syndrome in women.[88]

In contrast to the association of testosterone and risk of metabolic syndrome in women, a low serum testosterone level is associated with metabolic syndrome in healthy men.[89] In a cohort study of 571 men aged 30 to 79 years, low testosterone levels predicted central obesity in men 12 years later.[50] Increased adiposity is itself partially responsible for a decrease of testosterone levels. Moreover, decreased growth hormone levels, as observed in older men, may also play a role in the age-associated changes in body composition.[50] Genetic analyses, functional imaging, and animal models of differential aerobic capacity have indicated a role of decreased mitochondrial function and the metabolic disturbances characteristic of insulin-resistant states in men.[90] In men of Northern European descent with impaired glucose tolerance (IGT) and type 2 diabetes, dysfunctional mitochondria were evidenced by decreased maximal aerobic capacity and decreased expression of mitochondrial genes involved in oxidative phosphorylation.[90] Hypogonadal men with low testosterone levels had a threefold higher prevalence of metabolic syndrome relative to men with normal testosterone levels.[90] Low serum testosterone levels were associated with an adverse metabolic profile; this has suggested that low testosterone levels and impaired mitochondrial function promote insulin resistance in men.[90]

Collectively, these findings indicate that decrements in gonadal hormones are associated with hypometabolism in the brain, increased risk of metabolic syndrome, and decreased glucose metabolism in the brain, characteristic of AD. Furthermore, early intervention with hormone therapy has been found to reverse the hypometabolism associated with hypogonadal hormone status.

Acknowledgments

Research and preparation of this review were supported by grants from the National Institute on Aging (P01-AG026572; U01-AG047222; UF1-AG046148; R01-AG033288).

KEY POINTS

- Neuroendocrine senescence is a multifactorial process with a high degree of interpersonal variability and subject to a host of beneficial or detrimental influences.
- Normal reproductive aging in women is characterized by three distinct phases that can span years: perimenopause (also known as the menopause transition), menopause that typically occurs between 49 and 51 years of age, and postmenopause.
- Increasing evidence indicates that an oophorectomy before the natural menopause transition has profound consequences for subsequent risk of neurodegenerative disease.
- In men, fertility persists until very old age and the age-associated decrease in testosterone levels is slowly progressive.
- Loss of gonadal hormones can be associated with dysfunction in glucose metabolism, bioenergetics, and mitochondrial function in the brain. Decreased brain metabolism precedes development of Alzheimer pathology, can be manifested decades before diagnosis, and may serve as a biomarker of Alzheimer disease risk and as a therapeutic target.

For a complete list of references, please visit www.expertconsult.com.

KEY REFERENCES

1. Brinton RD, et al: Perimenopause as a neurological transition state. Nat Rev Endocrinol 11:393–405, 2015.
2. Yin F, et al: The perimenopausal aging transition in the female rat brain: decline in bioenergetic systems and synaptic plasticity. Neurobiol Aging 36:2282–2295, 2015.
3. Vitale G, Salvioli S, Franceschi C: Oxidative stress and the ageing endocrine system. Nat Rev Endocrinol 9:228–240, 2013.
4. Harlow SD, et al: STRAW 10 Collaborative Group: Executive summary of the Stages of Reproductive Aging Workshop + 10: addressing the unfinished agenda of staging reproductive aging. Menopause 19:387–395, 2012.
5. Davis SR, et al: Menopause. http://www.nature.com/articles/nrdp20154. Accessed February 9, 2015.
6. Finch CE: The menopause and aging, a comparative perspective. J Steroid Biochem Mol Biol 142:132–141, 2014.
15. Cray LA, et al: Symptom clusters during the late reproductive stage through the early postmenopause: observations from the Seattle Midlife Women's Health Study. Menopause 19:864–869, 2012.
16. Greendale GA, et al: Predicting the timeline to the final menstrual period: the study of women's health across the nation. J Clin Endocrinol Metab 98:1483–1491, 2013.
17. Freeman EW, Sammel MD, Sanders RJ: Risk of long-term hot flashes after natural menopause: evidence from the Penn Ovarian Aging Study cohort. Menopause 21:924–932, 2014.
18. Thurston RC, et al: Vasomotor symptoms and insulin resistance in the study of women's health across the nation. J Clin Endocrinol Metab 97:3487–3494, 2012.
19. Thurston RC, et al: Adipokines, adiposity, and vasomotor symptoms during the menopause transition: findings from the Study of Women's Health Across the Nation. Fertil Steril 100:793–800, 2013.
25. Spitzer M, et al: Risks and benefits of testosterone therapy in older men. Nat Rev Endocrinol 9:414–424, 2013.
26. Genazzani AR, Komm BS, Pickar JH: Emerging hormonal treatments for menopausal symptoms. Expert Opin Emerg Drugs 20:31–46, 2015.
27. Pinkerton J, Thomas S: Use of SERMs for treatment in postmenopausal women. J Steroid Biochem Mol Biol 142:142–154, 2014.
28. Komm BS, Mirkin S: An overview of current and emerging SERMs. J Steroid Biochem Mol Biol 143:207–222, 2014.
30. Taylor M: Complementary and alternative approaches to menopause. Endocrinol Metab Clin North Am 44:619–648, 2015.
31. Ohn Mar S, et al: Use of alternative medications for menopause-related symptoms in three major ethnic groups of Ipoh, Perak, Malaysia. Asia Pac J Public Health 27(Suppl):19S–25S, 2015.
32. Lindh-Astrand L, et al: Hot flushes, hormone therapy and alternative treatments: 30 years of experience from Sweden. Climacteric 18:53–62, 2015.
33. Dittfeld A, et al: [Phytoestrogens—whether can they be an alternative to hormone replacement therapy for women during menopause period?]. Wiad Lek 68:163–167, 2015.
34. Carroll DG, Lisenby KM, Carter TL: Critical appraisal of paroxetine for the treatment of vasomotor symptoms. Int J Womens Health 7:615–624, 2015.
35. Alipour S, Jafari-Adli S, Eskandari A: Benefits and harms of phytoestrogen consumption in breast cancer survivors. Asian Pac J Cancer Prev 16:3091–3096, 2015.
38. Maximov PY, Lee TM, Jordan VC: The discovery and development of selective estrogen receptor modulators (SERMs) for clinical practice. Curr Clin Pharmacol 8:135–155, 2013.
39. Ellis AJ, et al: Selective estrogen receptor modulators in clinical practice: a safety overview. Expert Opin Drug Saf 14:921–934, 2015.
49. Fukui M, et al: Andropausal symptoms in men with type 2 diabetes. Diabet Med 29:1036–1042, 2012.
53. Walsh JS, Eastell R: Osteoporosis in men. Nat Rev Endocrinol 9:637–645, 2013.
54. Matsumoto AM: Reproductive endocrinology: estrogens—not just female hormones. Nat Rev Endocrinol 9:693–694, 2013.
56. Manolagas SC, O'Brien CA, Almeida M: The role of estrogen and androgen receptors in bone health and disease. Nat Rev Endocrinol 9:699–712, 2013.
59. Vigen R, et al: Association of testosterone therapy with mortality, myocardial infarction, and stroke in men with low testosterone levels. JAMA 310:1829–1836, 2013.
60. Wierman ME: Risks of different testosterone preparations: too much, too little, just right. JAMA Intern Med 175:1197–1198, 2015.
89. Rao PM, Kelly DM, Jones TH: Testosterone and insulin resistance in the metabolic syndrome and T2DM in men. Nat Rev Endocrinol 9:479–493, 2013.

14 Frailty: The Broad View

Matteo Cesari, Olga Theou

Demographic trends show that independently of geographic regions and socioeconomic background, the absolute and relative number of older persons is increasing worldwide. It has been estimated that the prevalence of persons aged 65 years and older worldwide will increase from 7.7% in 2010 to 15.6% in 2050. This trend is evident even among the subpopulation of those aged 80 years and older, which is predicted to more than double in size from 2010 to 2050 (1.6% and 4.1%, respectively).This is not exclusive to more developed countries, because similar trends have even been reported in the least developed regions of the world.[1] The reduction of mortality risk at advanced age is largely the result of scientific advancements and improvement of life conditions.[2] At the same time, as the aging population seeks care, simply extending current practices is threatening the sustainability of the health care system. In particular, current models of care do not sufficiently take into account the new (and still unmet) needs of the changing population. Not surprisingly, a recent alert by the Royal College of Physicians (London) indicated the necessity of "more consultants with skills in acute, general and geriatric medicine to be able to cope with the ageing population."[3]

One of the major challenges of health care systems is to face the severe burden imposed by disabling conditions of old age.[4] Because disability in the older person has to be considered as an almost irreversible condition, because it is largely caused by lifelong accrual of deficits,[5] attention must be focused on preventing the disabling cascade[6] and on managing people in ways that aim to mitigate, or at least not add to, their level of dependence.

During the past 2 decades, a large body of evidence has been developed to identify biomarkers and instruments capable of measuring the biologic age of the older individual. Given the increasing number of older persons requiring assistance and the high economic burdens imposed by disabling conditions, the identification of "biologically aged" (rather than "chronologically aged") subjects is today both necessary and urgent.[4,7]

The need to reshape the traditional idea of the geriatric patient is obvious. The commonly adopted criterion of chronologic age based on the number of years lived is no longer sufficiently selective for identifying the right target population requiring adapted care and special resources. It is necessary to replace the term *chronologic age* with a parameter capable of measuring the biologic status of an individual more in-depth.

The age criterion is not the only thing that needs to be redefined in the clinical and research settings to develop the optimal care of older adults. A significant and important transition from disease-oriented toward function-oriented medicine is necessary. In fact, with advancing age, the meaning of traditional diseases becomes lost, because these conditions are largely modified by the effects of the aging process. This issue is at the very basis of the so-called evidence-based medicine issue in geriatrics, largely because the social, clinical, and biologic characteristics of older adults do not reflect those on which international recommendations and guidelines are developed.[5]

The frailty concept might offer a solution in this context. Fried and coworkers have provided a perfect description of the role played by frailty. They stated that "the cornerstone, even the raison d'etre, of geriatric medicine concerns the identification, evaluation, and treatment of frail older adults and prevention of loss of independence and other outcomes for which they are at risk."[8] It is on this type of patient that the field of geriatric medicine has built up its knowledge and developed its own specific methodology—the comprehensive geriatric assessment.[9,10] This chapter focuses on the how frailty is defined and assessed, how we can treat frailty, and why it needs to be considered within our health care system.

FRAILTY

To better appreciate the heterogeneous health status of the older persons, the frailty concept was introduced in geriatric and gerontology literature about 20 years ago. Frailty is now noncontroversially understood as the concept of increased vulnerability to adverse outcomes among people of the same chronologic age. It is the term used to indicate the geriatric syndrome or state characterized by a reduction of the organism's homeostatic reserves. The lower capacity of the organism to face entropic forces (coming from endogenous and exogenous sources) exposes an individual to an increased risk of negative health-related events, including falls, hospitalizations, worsening disability, institutionalization, and mortality.[8,11-13] In a frail individual, a clinically irrelevant endogenous or exogenous stressor may become the trigger for the initiation of the burdening disabling cascade.[13]

Frailty has been defined by an international consensus of experts as "a multidimensional syndrome characterized by decreased reserve and diminished resistance to stressors."[11] A widely accepted definition of frailty was provided in Orlando, Florida, by an international consensus group in 2012. It stated that frailty is "a medical syndrome with multiple causes and contributors that is characterized by diminished strength, endurance, and reduced physiologic function that increases an individual's vulnerability for developing increased dependency and/or death."[6]

In a recent review paper, Clegg and colleagues clearly depicted frailty not as a syndrome but as a state of vulnerability that challenges the maintenance of homeostasis in older persons.[12] Similarly, the deficit accumulation approach sees frailty as a multidimensional risk state that can be measured by the quantity rather than by the nature of health problems.[14] This approach proposes that frail older adults have many things wrong with them; the more things they have wrong, the higher the likelihood that they will be frail and the greater their risk of adverse health outcomes. Based on this definition, frailty arises from a multisystem decline, which compromises the body's ability to repair damage that arises externally or as the byproduct of internal processes, (e.g., metabolic, respiratory, inflammatory), including genetically induced damage.[15]

However, frailty is not all or none; grades of frailty make a difference. Still, many studies classify people simply as frail or nonfrail. In some settings, such as comparing frailty prevalence in different samples, this can be useful; however, even in this case, important information gets lost. Many clinical decisions require greater precision than a nonfrail-frail status.[16] In addition, frailty is a dynamic process where transitions across states of frailty are common. On average, health tends to decline with age, and the population-based trajectories of frailty are consistent, showing acceleration in deficit accumulation. The frailty index increases, on average, tenfold between 20 and 90 years. Even so, individual trajectories of the frailty index are generally irregular, showing that frailty reflects a stochastic dynamic process. For an individual, most transitions are gradual, and the likelihood to change their frailty level is largely conditioned on their previous frailty level. Therefore, transitioning from a nonfrail state to a severely frail state (and vice versa) is not very common.[17] In individuals, including older adults, frailty levels increase nonmonotonically over time; however, health status can improve, which will result in a transition from a higher to a lower frailty level state.[18]

In a study conducted by Gill and associates,[19] nondisabled subjects aged 70 years and older were followed over time to monitor changes in their frailty status. Among the 754 participants, more than half (57.5%) experienced at least one transition across any of the frailty states during the 54-month follow-up period. It was also reported that 44.3% of robust participants at the baseline transitioned to a prefrailty (40.1%) or frailty (4.2%) condition during the first 18 months of follow-up. Among participants presenting as frail at baseline, most (63.9%) remained frail, whereas 23.0% improved to a healthier condition, and 13.1% died. Consistent results showing the positive and negative changes of the frailty condition over time have also been reported in data collected as part of the Survey of Health, Ageing, and Retirement in Europe (SHARE).[20] Recent studies have started exploring which conditions may be associated with improvement or worsening of the frailty condition. For example, Lee and coworkers[21] reported the significant association of specific characteristics with negative modifications (e.g., older age, history of cancer, hospitalization events, chronic obstructive pulmonary disease, cerebrovascular disease, osteoarthritis) and positive modifications (e.g., higher cognitive function, absence of diabetes, higher socioeconomic status, no history of cerebrovascular disease) across frailty states. Even though these characteristics can accelerate frailty, typically frailty develops slowly, even insidiously, and can vary in important ways among individuals.

It is well established that although they frequently coexist in the older person, frailty, comorbidity (the concurrent presence of two or more medically diagnosed diseases), and disability (the difficulty or dependency in carrying out activities of daily life) are distinct conditions.[22] For example, in the Cardiovascular Health Study, Fried and colleagues[22] reported that comorbidity, disability, and the two together coexist in 67.7%, 27.2%, and 21.5% of frail participants, respectively. On the other hand, people who meet the criteria for the frailty might do so in the absence of comorbidity and disability, as reported in 26.6% of cases in the same study.

Recently, the concept of "resilience" (the individual's ability to adapt in the face of stresses and adversities) has become increasingly used in parallel with frailty.[23] Although resilience is still is not adequately framed and defined, it is possible that it might be a field of promising research in the near future. Low versus high resilience may indeed make a difference and explain why individuals with the same frailty status follow opposite trajectories (i.e., toward disability and robustness, respectively). Although resilience is still only a briefly stated concept, its quantification may provide important insights in the assessment of the older person's risk profile. As with the frailty syndrome, resilience also results from the complex network of biologic, clinical, social, and environmental factors characterizing each individual. We also need to consider that some degree of variability in health outcomes is to be expected in relation to frailty. Some people who are severely frail can survive in highly protective environments, whereas some nonfrail people will die. This could be related to the degree of damage to which an individual is exposed or to the resources available to assist with the repair of that damage. Even in Canada, a higher income country with a universal health care system, among individuals who are considered the fittest (lowest level of frailty), 5-year mortality is doubled among those classified with high social vulnerability levels compared to those with the lowest social vulnerability levels.[24]

Prevalence of Frailty

In a recent systematic review,[25] Collard and associates provided estimates of frailty prevalence, analyzing data from 21 cohort studies (>61,500 community-dwelling older persons). The reported prevalence substantially varied across the studies examined, ranging from 4% to 59.1%, according to the adopted operational definition of frailty and the characteristics of the studied sample. Nevertheless, when analyses were restricted to studies using the most common model of operationalization (i.e., the frailty phenotype proposed by Fried and coworkers[26]), the weighted average prevalence rate was 9.9% (95% confidence interval [CI], 9.6% to 10.2%) for frailty and 44.2% (95% CI, 44.2% to 44.7%) for prefrailty, whereas in the only study included that used the frailty index, the prevalence was 22.7%.[25] Similarly, using data from SHARE, it was reported that 11% of Europeans older than 50 years were identified as frail based on the frailty phenotype approach, and 21% were frail based on the frailty index approach.[27]

Available evidence also tends consistently to report different prevalence of frailty according to age,[28-30] gender (e.g., higher estimates in women compared to men),[25,28] ethnic groups (e.g., higher prevalence in Hispanic and African Americans),[26,31] migrant groups,[32] individual socioeconomic characteristics (e.g., poor education and poverty are closely associated with frailty),[26,33,34] and macro socioeconomic factors (e.g., gross domestic product and health care expenditures of country of residence).[35]

Biology of Frailty

Frailty has been described as a phase of acceleration occurring during the aging process due to endogenous and exogenous stimuli.[36] It results from the age-related cumulative declines occurring across multiple physiologic systems.[5] The biology of frailty has its origins in the most intimate roots of the aging process. The parallelism between aging and frailty implicitly leads to the existence of a shared pathophysiologic substrate between the aging process and frailty.[5]

Such hypotheses can easily find support in the growing body of evidence showing that the same pathways indicated as crucial for the aging process (e.g., inflammation, oxidative damage, immune function, telomeres, natural selection) also represent key determinants in the development and maintenance of the frailty phenotypic syndrome.[37-41] Furthermore, it cannot be ignored that specific innate capacities (e.g., mobility[42]) characteristic of living beings across species (from *Drosophila* to humans) are strongly correlated with frailty and age-related conditions.[7]

Based on the deficit accumulation approach, frailty arises from the accumulation of microscopic damage (cellular and subcellular deficits) that are not repaired or removed and may reach macroscopic deficits—clinical detectable deficits at the organ and system levels. As organ level deficits accumulate, they may give rise to symptoms or signs, thereby presenting as clinically evident disease.[43] Also, damage in one organ system may predispose to damage in another organ system, showing that deficit accumulation and repair are intertwined. A recent study showed this association between the clinical macroscopic and subclinical microscopic deficit accumulation using a frailty index constructed by routine laboratory data.[44] This supports the notion that frailty that is macroscopically detectable represents the buildup of subcellular, tissue, and organ deficits from damage that is not removed or repaired.

Assessment of Frailty

Although the theoretical foundations of frailty are well established and largely agreed, controversies exist about its operational assessment. Multiple instruments have been developed over the years to capture in a standardized way the presence of frailty objectively. Unfortunately, the available instruments (stemming from different perspectives and purposes) are all predictive of negative health-related outcomes, but have modest agreement among them.[27,45,46] Analyses conducted by van Iersel and colleagues[47] compared the prevalence of frailty using four different defining tools—frailty phenotype, frailty index, usual gait speed, and hand grip strength. Results showed that the prevalence of frailty was different using different criteria. Moreover, there was only partial overlapping among the populations classified by these scales as frail. A study using SHARE data compared eight frailty scales and showed that among all scales, about half of participants (49.3%) were categorized as nonfrail and 2.4% as frail, and for 48.3% of participants, the eight scales did not classify them identically as frail or nonfrail.[27] In other words, every assessment tool was capturing a different risk profile, and none of them was completely exhaustive by itself. Such heterogeneity of results is in line with the nature of frailty but, at the same time, may require special caution when asked to choose one single operational definition. It is possible that the choice of the most appropriate frailty instrument should rely on the purpose of the evaluation, outcome for which the definition was originally validated, validity of the tool, population studied, and setting where the assessment will be conducted.

The most commonly used and widely diffused instruments for measuring frailty are the frailty index[14] and the frailty phenotype.[26] Building on these two models, several other frailty scales have been proposed during the past several years.[48-53] Also, performance-based measures have been used to predict adverse health outcomes in older adults, suggesting that they could also be used as frailty screening tools.

Frailty Index

The frailty index was proposed by Rockwood and associates and was initially validated in the Canadian Study of Health and Aging.[14] This instrument is designed to measure the age-related deficit accumulation using a mathematical approach. It is the ratio between the number of deficits that a person may experience (e.g., signs, symptoms, diseases, disabilities) and the total number of considered deficits (e.g., someone with 20 deficits out of 40 counted has a frailty index score of 20/40 = 0.5). In this way, the frailty index score is continuous (ranging from 0 to 1), and the higher the score of an individual, the more likely that this person is vulnerable to adverse health outcomes.

This approach proposes that in terms of understanding system behavior, knowing what exactly is wrong is less important than knowing how many things people have wrong. The index can be built up without the need of special resources, and not every frailty index needs to include the same items. In this way, the items included in a frailty index should not be included or excluded a priori as long as items are age-related, associated with adverse outcomes and, when combined, capable to cover several organ systems.[54] Given that the frailty index is not based on preset items, it is particularly useful for being applied to existing cohort data collected for different purposes a retrospective according to available data. At least 20 items should be considered to generate a frailty index; 30 or more is preferred to achieve stable estimates. Regardless of the nature and number of items included in the frailty index and whether the sample included community, institutionalized, or hospitalized older adults, it has remarkably similar measurement properties and substantive results.

As discussed earlier, one strength of the frailty index approach is that it can be developed from any existing biomedical database and even constructed solely by self-reported items. Because it requires the inclusion of at least 20 items, clinicians are often skeptical about its feasibility. However, in the era of the electronic health record, frailty indices can be constructed in clinical settings using routinely collected data, without requiring additional assessment. For example, a frailty index can be constructed based on a standard comprehensive geriatric assessment derived from a clinical examination[55] or a questionnaire that can be completed by care partners.[56] Also, recently, a frailty index was constructed using routine blood tests plus measured systolic and diastolic blood pressures.[44] Interestingly, the frailty index has been used as a model for developing frailty instruments in animal models. Following the approach of counting the accumulation of deficits for measuring the frailty condition, studies have replicated the frailty index in mice.[57-59] Such an extension of the frailty index implicitly provides the opportunity to develop frailty research in the preclinical setting and in translational research. Moreover, it provides further proof of the biologic substrate characterizing the validity of the instrument.[60]

Rockwood and coworkers also generated a screening instrument (largely based on the clinical judgement of the physician) to indicate the different stages of the patient's frailty, intended as poor health status.[6,61] The Clinical Frailty Scale is a seven- or nine-item scale that can indicate the global clinical status of the older person based on the evaluation of his or her status in the domains of mobility, energy, physical activity, and function. Future studies need to investigate how these frailty scales compare to other commonly used clinical instruments, such as the Karnofsky Performance Status[62] or Eastern Cooperative Oncology Group (ECOG) Performance Status[63] scales.

Frailty Phenotype

Comparatively, the frailty phenotype was designed by Fried and colleagues and was initially validated in the Cardiovascular Health Study.[26] It is based on the evaluation of five defining criteria—involuntary weight loss, exhaustion, slow gait speed, muscle weakness, and sedentary behavior. Each criterion was operationalized following an epidemiologic approach that took advantage of the Cardiovascular Health Study database. The phenotype distinguished three consecutive states, robustness (defined as the absence of criteria), prefrailty (presence of one or two criteria), and frailty (when three or more criteria are present).

In theory, the frailty phenotype finds its best application in nondisabled older persons. Looking at signs and symptoms, it generates a preclinical risk estimation primarily aimed at indicating the individual in need of a comprehensive geriatric assessment.[60] Therefore, its design closely resembles that of a screening tool. However, such a characteristic also represents a major limitation failing of not being informative about the potential causes of the condition of interest. For example, the involuntary weight loss criterion might be due to social isolation, unknown diseases, or unhealthy behavior, with different causes requiring completely different interventions. As is evident, the phenotype is particularly focused at exploring the physical domain of the older person to capture the overall risk profile for negative outcomes. Such an approach has been proposed in the literature, because potentially limiting to a specific function or domain is thought to be insufficient for capturing the heterogeneity, multidimensionality, and complexity of the frailty condition. For example, several groups of researchers have discussed the need for extending the frailty phenotype to other health domains, which may improve the assessment of the risk profile in the older adults (e.g., cognition, mood, social status).[64] Although the frailty phenotype is commonly referred to as the instrument most adopted for assessment of the syndrome, such a statement might be arguable. It is very rare to have the original phenotype applied without adaptations in the definition of the five criteria and/or modifications of the thresholds of risk. Such qualitative and quantitative deviations from the version proposed by Fried and associates[26] are often necessary for adapting the assessment to the available resources and data, and/or the population being studied.

Physical Performance Measures

In the context of uncertainty about the identification of a clear gold standard assessment tool for frailty, it has been proposed to restrict the focus to the inner core of frailty and the primary outcome of geriatric medicine (i.e., physical disability).[65] The domain that is usually considered as a core feature of frailty more than others is surely the physical one.[66] Given the frequent use of frailty as a predisability condition, the assessment of physical performance is also a particularly suitable indicator of this concept. Therefore, it is not surprising that consensus is mounting toward the adoption of physical performance measures (in particular, gait speed[67] and Short Physical Performance Battery [SPPB][68,69]) to estimate objectively the vulnerability of the older person to endogenous and exogenous stressors (i.e., indicators of frailty).[70]

The predictive value of physical performance measures for negative outcomes in older adults is well established.[68,69,71,72] Moreover, most of the instruments specifically looking at frailty consider physical performance as one of the key determinants of the risk profile.[26,48] The assessment of frailty using physical parameters may also facilitate the systematic clinical implementation of frailty because physical performance measures are easy to assess, clinically friendly, inexpensive, objective, standardized, repeatable, and highly reliable, even in primary care.[7,65] Interestingly, the adoption of physical performance measures as frailty screening tools may indirectly capitalize on the vast evidence coming from the widespread use of these physical performance parameters in clinical and research settings.[67-69,71,73,74]

Finally, it should not be underestimated that the use of objective tests such as physical performance measures may at least partially solve potential social, cultural, clinical, and environmental issues characterizing the administration of questionnaires. For example, the same question might be differently understood by the person being interviewed according to who is asking, how, and where. The conceptualization of the answer to a question might also be affected by the social and geographic context. Conversely, the use of a standardized performance test will reduce (although not completely eliminate[75]) such issues and render the detection of a frail individual more consistently based on her or his physiologic makeup. At the same time, a major limitation of physical performance tests needs to be mentioned—many frail individuals are unable to perform physical performance tests. Such an incapacity may introduce the risk of a potentially biased misclassification of the subject due to the floor effect caused by the nonperformance.[76,77] Mainly because of this, physical performance measures may more likely find their optimal place in the screening of frailty in nondisabled individuals.

Although the SPPB and usual gait speed were not originally designed to measure frailty (not yet conceptualized at that time), they still adequately respond to the need of predicting which older person will be vulnerable to stressors and exposed to a higher risk of negative health-related events (including disability). In other words, the theoretical concepts underlying the definition of frailty[6,11-13,26] are associated with these physical performance measures, which could themselves be used as frailty screening tools. How these tools will be incorporated into everyday care in the clinical setting and how they will benefit clinical decisions need to be the focus of translational research programs.

Short Physical Performance Battery. The SPPB was developed by Guralnik and coworkers to measure lower extremity function objectively.[68] It is composed of three subtests evaluating usual gait speed, ability to rise from a chair, and standing balance. For the gait speed subtest, the subject is asked to walk at his or her usual pace, starting from a standing still position behind a line along a 15-foot- or 4-m-long corridor. The subtest is timed and repeated twice. The faster of the two trials (in seconds) is subsequently used for the calculation of the summary score. For the chair stand subtest, the subject study participant is asked to rise from a chair and sit down five times as quickly as possible with hands folded across the chest. The performance is expressed as total time (in seconds) to complete the test. For the standing balance test, the study participant is asked to stand in three increasingly challenging positions for 10 seconds each: a side by side feet standing position, semitandem position, and full tandem position. The results of the three timed tasks are scored from 0 (worst performers) to 4 (best performers) according to predetermined cut points. The sum of scores from the three subtests then generates a summary score of physical performance ranging from 0 (worst performance) to 12 (best performance).[68,69,72]

Usual Gait Speed. It is noteworthy that usual gait speed is part of the SPPB, but has also been used as a stand-alone parameter for predicting the increased vulnerability to stressors of the older individual.[71] Guralnik and colleagues[69] have shown that the predictive value of the gait speed for major health-related outcomes (in particular, disability and mortality) is similar to the one shown by the complete SPPB.[69] The usual gait speed (measured on short track lengths) has shown to predict hospitalizations, institutionalization, disability, and mortality in older persons.[69,73,74] Studenski and associates[67] have demonstrated that it is possible to estimate life expectancy of an older person accurately by simply knowing her or his age, gender, and gait speed. Not surprisingly, the usual gait speed parameter has even been proposed as a new vital sign for older people.[7,65,78]

Interestingly, several medical specialties in addition to geriatrics have also raised interest in the role that physical performance measures may play in the field of frailty. For example, physical performance measures have already been successfully used in cardiosurgery,[79,80] cardiology,[81] respiratory medicine,[82,83] and oncology[84] for identifying older persons in need of adapted medical care.

TREATMENT OF FRAILTY

As mentioned above, frailty (or the biologic age of the individual) is a dynamic and complex condition, largely determined by endogenous and exogenous stressors experienced by individuals during their lifetime. Thus, it is also implicitly assumed that age is a continuous variable, and the manifestations of the aging process follow dynamic and continuous patterns during the entire course of the life experience.[5] Every positive or negative stressor experienced during the life course may differently affect health status and determine deviations from the reference status of successful aging. Thus, it is implied that through a careful evaluation of a person's background and history, the current health status of the person should be assessed not only cross-sectionally, but also longitudinally. This also means that preventive interventions for age-related conditions should not necessarily be applied only to older adults. Age-related conditions can be successfully prevented if the modification of risk factors (e.g., poor socioeconomic conditions, unhealthy lifestyle and behaviors, little access to health care services) also involves younger adults.

For successfully targeting frailty in the prevention of negative outcomes, it is recommended to adopt a multidimensional approach. In this context, the scientific literature about the importance of conducting a comprehensive geriatric assessment (CGA) in frail older adults is vast. The multidimensional and multidisciplinary approach to geriatric syndromes has documented beneficial effects when applied in multiple clinical settings and conditions. Several trials have demonstrated that person-tailored interventions based on results of a CGA are able to prevent major negative health-related outcomes in older persons living in community,[85] home care,[86] hospital,[87] and nursing home settings.[88] As an example, it is important to cite the meta-analysis conducted in 1993 by Stuck and associates.[10] In this study, the authors examined results of 28 randomized controlled trials (more than 9000 participants) testing the effects of CGA-based interventions versus controls. Findings clearly demonstrated that CGA-based programs linking geriatric evaluation with strong long-term management are effective for improving survival and function in older persons. A recent meta-analysis also showed how using inpatient CGA improves health outcomes.[89] In particular, a CGA of older adults admitted to a hospital increases their likelihood of returning home and reduces institutional admissions compared with usual care, and these benefits can potentially mitigate the health care costs of an aging population.

Several studies have shown that multidomain approaches simultaneously acting on different features and components of frailty may be beneficial for improving the subjective perception of health and objective functional status of the older person.[90,91] Interestingly, multidomain interventions against disability also seem to be particularly cost-effective for frail older adults.[92] Different interventions may be appropriate based on the level of frailty, and the proposed models of care should be flexible enough for modifications based on the individual needs of patients. Fairhall and coworkers[93] proposed the following principles for implementing interventions to treat frailty: (1) individualized long-term support; (2) consistent management in the presence of an acute health event; (3) interventions to improve physical, cognitive, and social function to increase independence and self-management and decrease vulnerability to adverse outcomes; (4) adherence to the intervention; and (5) involvement of caregivers.

In addition, there is strong evidence that exercise prescription is more beneficial than any other individual intervention for the health of frail people. This could be related to the impact of exercise across a variety of systems and its potential effect on intrinsic repair mechanisms. Multicomponent exercise interventions composed of aerobic, strength, and balance training seem to be the best strategy to improve health, treat frailty, and prevent disability in frail older adults.[94-96] However, the optimal design of the exercise protocol in this population is not clear. An example of the capacity to intervene successfully in the health status of frail older adults by using exercise interventions to prevent negative health-related outcomes has recently been provided by the Lifestyle Interventions and Independence for Elderly (LIFE) trial.[96] This multicenter study recruited 1635 community-dwelling sedentary older persons with physical limitations but able to walk 400 m. Participants were randomized in two groups, an intervention group undergoing a moderate intensity physical activity protocol and a control group receiving a health education program. Results showed that after 2.6 years of intervention, the physical activity protocol significantly reduced the onset of mobility disability compared to the health education program. Interestingly, the LIFE study (as well as secondary analyses conducted on its pilot trial) suggests that individuals with more comorbidities and lower physical performance at baseline are those who obtain most benefit from the physical exercise intervention.[96-98]

FRAILTY IN HEALTH CARE SYSTEMS

Based on the Web of Science database, approximately 1100 articles were published on frailty in 2014. Only half of them were published in the geriatrics and gerontology research areas; cardiology, surgery, neuroscience and neurology, and general internal medicine were the other areas with the most frailty articles. Whether frailty screening and protocol-driven care plans can yield benefits for medical teaching units is not yet known. What is known is that specialized geriatric wards that provide older adult–friendly acute medical care improve outcomes, whereas consultation teams on their own do not significantly benefit the care of patients.[89]

Probably orthopedic surgery represents the first discipline, which has successfully implemented a close collaboration with geriatricians for the assessment and management of older persons (e.g., hip fracture patients). For example, Antonelli Incalzi and colleagues[99] have demonstrated that assigning a geriatrician to assist with the medical care of older patients (hip fracture) in orthopedic wards was associated with increased rates of surgery, decreased mortality, and shortened length of stay. More recently, oncologists[100] and cardiosurgeons[80] have started looking at the CGA more frequently as a means for guaranteeing more access to standard interventions for more of their older patients. The search for such collaborations is easily explained by the common presence of geriatric patients, with all their complexities and peculiarities, in almost every hospital ward and service. Several medical specialties are today facing the effects of global aging on the patients' populations they have traditionally been targeting, with the treatment of older adults being the mainstay of their activities.

Not all older patients are frail, but many are, particularly those seen in clinical settings. Older adults who are fit become ill in ways similar to those of younger people: they show typical symptoms and signs, stable social situations, and predictable drug handling, recovery from surgery, and symptom resolution. In contrast, people who are frail have multiple interacting medical and social problems. Illnesses can present as nonspecific problems in walking, thinking, or function. Even easily identifiable symptoms, such as impaired balance, translate poorly into expected medical causes such as ataxia, arthritis, or anemia. Most importantly, standard treatments for such symptoms often make situations worse for frail patients. They require adaptations of care, personalization of interventions, and modifications of standard protocols that can be reached only through the implementation of a CGA. As such, identifying frailty early in clinical care is vital.[101]

The positive results obtained in specific clinical settings have recently encouraged geriatric researchers to try and extend the use of the multidimensional and multidisciplinary approach in primary care and as part of preventive strategies dedicated to community-dwelling older persons.[102-104] These novel health care services are mainly aimed at supporting the general practitioner in the assessment of the community-dwelling older person to promote a healthier lifestyle and facilitate the early detection of still undiagnosed medical conditions, thus increasing the possibility of success for the intervention. It is noteworthy that the assessment of frailty and the identification of its causes require a coordinated and multidisciplinary evaluation of the older person.[9,10,105]

More detailed frailty evaluation in general practice might be a place to start, where frailty assessments can lay the groundwork for preventive interventions (e.g., vaccination, fall reduction, exercise). Also, because family physicians are able to take into consideration the social context of the patient and how this affects health status, frailty assessments in this context can assist with implementing care planning centered on patient and carer goals. Nevertheless, when discussing preventive strategies for age-related conditions, the potential presence of several barriers should not be underestimated.

Multiple factors, such as comorbidities, social isolation, and poor education, may render the successful modification of (often chronic) habits and conditions that may expose the older person to negative outcomes particularly challenging. The value of prevention remains the same, regardless of age, because adherence to healthy lifestyle recommendations has been shown to be beneficial, even among the oldest and frailest individuals.[88] However, because the health profile at an advanced age largely results from the lifelong experience of the subject, the implementation of behaviors contributing to active and healthy aging should be promoted and encouraged from a very young age.[5]

SUMMARY

In conclusion, providing health care to an aging population presents important challenges and opportunities. On the frontier of these challenges and opportunities is how we understand and respond to frailty, an important issue faced by those involved in health care. The identification of frailty as a clear target for implementing preventive interventions against age-related conditions (in particular, disability) is pivotal. The frailty condition and related literature should always be considered, together with the large amount of evidence supporting the adoption of a CGA in older persons. People should be informed about the risk of the disabling cascade and should be provided with the necessary educational and therapeutic means for counteracting this detrimental phenomenon of old age. Every effort should be made by health care authorities for maximizing efforts in this field and for balancing priorities, needs, and resources.

Furthermore, prevention of frailty should not be considered a task exclusively for older adults. An effective prevention of age-related conditions starts at an early age. Thus, the promotion of a healthy lifestyle, correction of unhealthy behaviors, and improvement of health care services (actions directed toward the entire population) are crucial for implementing real prevention of age-related conditions. Such evaluations should be particularly focused on limiting the risk of overdiagnosis to ensure an ethical and cost-effective conduction of the intervention.[106] More studies are required to demonstrate that such a multidimensional and multidisciplinary approach is also beneficial when applied to community-dwelling older persons for the prevention of disability.

KEY POINTS

- Frailty is a multidimensional condition characterized by a state of vulnerability to stressors due to the individual's diminished reserves and reduced physiologic function.
- Frailty is associated with an increased risk of developing negative health-related outcomes, including disability, institutionalization, and mortality.
- The operationalization of frailty supports the discrimination between "normal" and "pathologic" aging, indirectly allowing the measurement of the individual's biologic age.
- The clinical implementation of frailty is necessary for promoting the adaptation of health care services to the needs, still largely unmet, of the aging population.

For a complete list of references, please visit www.expertconsult.com.

KEY REFERENCES

3. Royal College of Physicians: Hospital workforce: fit for the future? https://www.rcplondon.ac.uk/sites/default/files/hospital-workforce-fit-for-the-future.pdf. Accessed September 24, 2015.
5. Cesari M, Vellas B, Gambassi G: The stress of aging. Exp Gerontol 48:451–456, 2013.
6. Morley JE, Vellas B, Abellan van Kan G, et al: Frailty consensus: a call to action. J Am Med Dir Assoc 14:392–397, 2013.
8. Fried LP, Walston JD, Ferrucci L: Frailty. In Halter JB, Ouslander JG, Tinetti ME, et al, editors: Hazzard's geriatric medicine and gerontology, New York, 2009, McGraw-Hill, pp 631–645.
10. Stuck AE, Siu AL, Wieland GD, et al: Comprehensive geriatric assessment: a meta-analysis of controlled trials. Lancet 342:1032–1036, 1993.
11. Rodríguez-Mañas L, Féart C, Mann G, et al: Searching for an operational definition of frailty: a Delphi method based consensus statement: the frailty operative definition-consensus conference project. J Gerontol A Biol Sci Med Sci 68:62–67, 2012.
12. Clegg A, Young J, Iliffe S, et al: Frailty in elderly people. Lancet 381:752–762, 2013.
14. Mitnitski A, Mogilner A, Rockwood K: The accumulation of deficits as a proxy measure of aging. Scientificworldjournal 1:323–336, 2001.
15. Mitnitski A, Song X, Rockwood K: Assessing biological aging: the origin of deficit accumulation. Biogerontology 14:709–717, 2013.
19. Gill TM, Gahbauer EA, Allore HG, et al: Transitions between frailty states among community-living older persons. Arch Intern Med 166:418–423, 2006.
20. Borrat-Besson C, Ryser VA, Wernli B: Transitions between frailty states—a European comparison. In Börsch-Supan A, Brandt M, Litwin H, et al, editors: Active ageing and solidarity between generations in Europe. First results from SHARE after the economic crisis, Berlin, Germany, 2013, De Gruyter, pp 175–185.
21. Lee JS, Auyeung TW, Leung J, et al: Transitions in frailty states among community-living older adults and their associated factors. J Am Med Dir Assoc 15:281–286, 2014.
22. Fried LP, Ferrucci L, Darer J, et al: Untangling the concepts of disability, frailty, and comorbidity: implications for improved targeting and care. J Gerontol A Biol Sci Med Sci 59:255–263, 2004.
25. Collard RM, Boter H, Schoevers RA, et al: Prevalence of frailty in community-dwelling older persons: a systematic review. J Am Geriatr Soc 60:1487–1492, 2012.
26. Fried LP, Tangen CM, Walston J, et al: Frailty in older adults: evidence for a phenotype. J Gerontol A Biol Sci Med Sci 56:M146–M156, 2001.
27. Theou O, Brothers TD, Mitnitski A, et al: Operationalization of frailty using eight commonly used scales and comparison of their ability to predict all-cause mortality. J Am Geriatr Soc 61:1537–1551, 2013.
44. Howlett SE, Rockwood MR, Mitnitski A, et al: Standard laboratory tests to identify older adults at increased risk of death. BMC Med 12:171, 2014.
47. van Iersel MB, Rikkert MG: Frailty criteria give heterogeneous results when applied in clinical practice. J Am Geriatr Soc 54:728–729, 2006.
61. Rockwood K, Song X, MacKnight C, et al: A global clinical measure of fitness and frailty in elderly people. CMAJ 173:489–495, 2005.
67. Studenski S, Perera S, Patel K, et al: Gait speed and survival in older adults. JAMA 305:50–58, 2011.
68. Guralnik JM, Ferrucci L, Simonsick EM, et al: Lower-extremity function in persons over the age of 70 years as a predictor of subsequent disability. N Engl J Med 332:556–561, 1995.
69. Guralnik JM, Ferrucci L, Pieper CF, et al: Lower extremity function and subsequent disability: consistency across studies, predictive models, and value of gait speed alone compared with the short physical performance battery. J Gerontol A Biol Sci Med Sci 55:M221–M231, 2000.
93. Fairhall N, Langron C, Sherrington C, et al: Treating frailty—a practical guide. BMC Med 9:83, 2011.
96. Pahor M, Guralnik JM, Ambrosius WT, et al: Effect of structured physical activity on prevention of major mobility disability in older adults: the LIFE study randomized clinical trial. JAMA 311:2387–2396, 2014.
99. Antonelli Incalzi R, Gemma A, Capparella O: Effect of structured physical activity on prevention of major mobility disability in older adults Continuous geriatric care in orthopedic wards: a valuable alternative to orthogeriatric units. Aging (Milano) 5:207–216, 1993.

15 Aging and Deficit Accumulation: Clinical Implications

Kenneth Rockwood, Arnold Mitnitski

INTRODUCTION

Overview of Frailty

Geriatricians have an affinity for frail older people, or should. The complex care of older adults who are frail is the very stuff of geriatric medicine.[1-8] This chapter argues that the formal assessment of complexity can be used to understand the scientific basis of the analyses of frailty, with insights for the practice of geriatric medicine. It takes the view that aging can be understood as the process of deficit accumulation, from subcellular to tissue to organ levels, becoming manifest clinically along the way. Although everyone, as they grow older, has a greater risk of death, not everyone of the same age has the same risk. People at an increased risk are frail for their age; those at lower risk are fit. Although related to age, there is some level of risk that conveniently defines everyone at that level as frail; a corollary is that there is likely some age at which everyone can be considered frail.

The basis for the variable risk of adverse outcomes of people of the same age lies in the variable rates at which people accumulate deficits.[1,2,6,8] In essence, people with the greatest number of health deficits are at the greatest risk of death. The reason that the risk of death, on average, rises with age is because, on average, health deficits accumulate, and this occurs, in general because recovery times increase.[8] In short, frail older adults are at an increased risk, compared with others of the same chronologic age, as a consequence of having multiple, interacting, age-related physiologic impairments, some of which cross clinical thresholds to be recognized as diseases and others as disabilities. These impairments, diseases, and disabilities typically interact with various social vulnerability factors, which commonly travel with the frail to increase the risk of adverse health outcomes further.

The view of frailty as a multiple-determined, at-risk state is reasonably noncontroversial.[1-7] By contrast, how best to operationalize frailty consumes a lot of discussion. As outlined in Chapter 14, the "phenotypic" definition of frailty used in the Cardiovascular Health Study[9] is popular. So too is the view of frailty as deficit accumulation, the focus of this chapter.

Overview of Complex Networks

The idea of complex networks being susceptible to formal analysis, and of those analyses extending to biologic systems and in particular, medical applications, is proving to be an important conceptual advance.[10,11] Understanding how networks operate from subcellular levels on[12] appears to have transformative potential. In general, a network can be understood as a collection of items (called nodes or vertices) defined by the connectedness of the items (with connections also known as edges). For network purposes, the items are defined by their connections, such as whether they have many or few connections or the distance between one node and the next. As it turns out, a wide array of sets of items shows network properties, from how items in a physiologic system interact to how emails get answered to how scientists cite the work of others. Network properties define types of networks. For example, scale-free networks follow a power law relationship and are marked by many items (nodes), with few connections, and a few with very many connections. Airports are one such example, with a few heavily travelled international hubs, then more regional hubs, and finally a large number of local airports that might only have a few flights a day.

In contrast to heterogeneity in the distribution of connections between nodes found in a scale- free network, small world networks have a more homogenous distribution. Small world networks have many nodes that are highly connected, with short path lengths. Small world networks have been analyzed in relation to Alzheimer disease to show that it is characterized by widespread loss of connectivity, reflected in increased path lengths between functional brain areas.[13,14] Network analyses are relatively new, so that the area remains somewhat tricky. The several challenges are both in our understanding of how network connectivity arises and in technical matters, such as clustering around electroencephalographic or magnetoencephalographic sensors might give spurious connections between nodes. Advances, however, are being made swiftly, so that understanding Alzheimer disease and other brain illnesses as types of disconnections of usual cortical activity can yield insights into the normal functioning of neural networks and how they become disrupted by disease.

Even recognizing that these are initial steps, progress can be made in relation to aging. Network theories of aging are not new, and many dozens of papers have elaborated them. A few recent papers have incorporated complex network analyses. One network model of aging introduced the interdependence of fault-prone agents on one another.[15] The model showed that aging patterns do not depend on the details of the network structure. This suggests that aging is a widely distributed systemic effect, and its features do not depend on exactly which things go wrong, given the multiplicity of things that subtly go awry.[16] Our group, in a simulation study, found that deficit accumulation is responsible for the observed slowing down in the rate of repair of interconnected nodes. The model reproduced not only the major patterns of deficit accumulation observed in a wide variety of countries, but also the Gompertz law of the exponential increase in the rate of mortality with age.[17]

The translation of these ideas into tractable clinical insights remains challenging. It is evident that aging humans constitute aging systems, both as individuals and as groups. Similarly, within the human organism, different organ systems and host environment interactions can be viewed as complex networks.[11-14,17-20] Even so, the specification of complex networks in relation to organ systems—where does the vascular system end and the immunologic system begin?—often results in some arbitrariness. Such arbitrariness is best not ignored when considering a phenomenon as all-encompassing as the passage of time. Furthermore, how to specify the interconnectedness of organs in the body as people age is not clear. It is clear, however, that there is an interconnectedness of health characteristics (interdependence of variables). For now, we limit ourselves to the observation that network analysis allows a great deal of information about the state of a system (e.g. the degree of interconnectedness) to be summarized as a single number and to come from a set of numbers with characteristic distributions. This is the insight that has motivated our particular approach to understanding aging, and especially frailty, in relation to the extent to which people accumulate

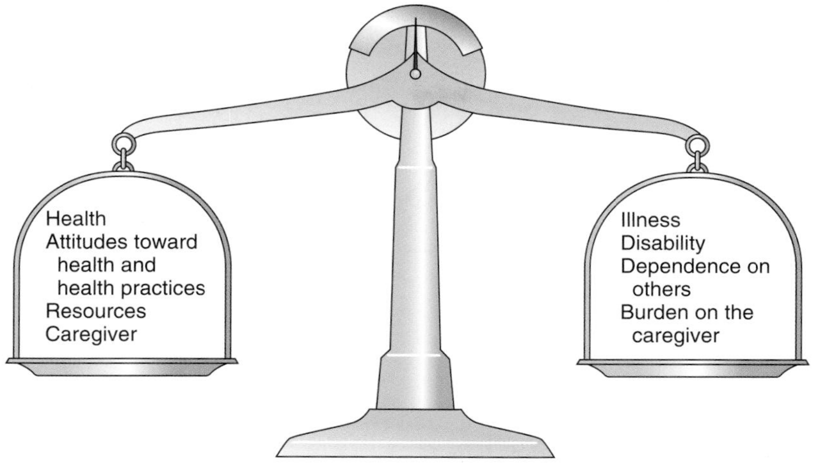

Figure 15-1. The balance beam model of changes in frailty states. The beam illustrates a multicomponent, dynamic state. *(From Rockwood K, Fox RA, Stolee P, et al: Frailty in elderly people: an evolving concept. CMAJ 150:489–495, 1994.)*

health-related deficits. Our claim is that an individual's state of health can be summarized by a single number—the frailty index—and that the properties or behavior of that number (e.g., how the frailty index changes with age) can be considered as an area of investigation in and of itself. To continue that example, we have shown that the distribution of the frailty index with age has distinctive characteristics.[21,22] These characteristics can be studied using network models, which offer an apparatus for such analyses, based on stochastic dynamics.[23] One example is the idea that heterogeneity (here, of the distribution of the frailty index with age)[21,24] arises as a consequence of the stochastic dynamics of complex systems. This approach to studying heterogeneity can be readily summarized using a network approach and has had wide applicability from cortical networks in Alzheimer disease[25] to capital markets[26] to gas furnace pressures.[27]

$$P_{nk} = \frac{\rho_n^k}{k!} \exp(-\rho_n)(1 - P_{nd})$$

Figure 15-2. Formal model of changes in frailty states, expressed as the probability of a person with n deficits at baseline surviving to have k deficits at follow-up. P_{nk} is represented by the Poisson law with a state-dependent Poisson mean, $\rho_n = a_0 + a_1 n$; P_{nd} is the probability of dying fitted by the log odds function of n, $logit(P_{nd}) = b_0 + b_1 n$. Note that a_0 and b_0 are the characteristic risks associated with no deficits. The two parameters a_1 and b_1 describe, respectively (given the current number of deficits, n), the increments of their expected change and the risk of death. Note that the model can be elaborated to include the effects of specific covariates such as age, gender, or social vulnerability.

Frailty in Relation to Deficit Accumulation

The fundamental idea of the frailty index is that the more deficits that people have (the more things people have wrong with them), the more likely they are to be frail. Deficits arise when damage goes unremoved or unrepaired. The damage is widespread and typically starts at subcellular levels. By ways that are not yet clear, the damage scales up, like aging itself, to become manifest at cellular, tissue, and organ levels. As discussed later, at some point, these changes become clinically visible health deficits.[28]

In an early attempt to characterize how frailty came about, we represented it as a state that arises from a dynamic interplay between assets and deficits (Fig. 15-1).[29] When people are fit, their assets greatly outweigh their deficits. As they accumulate deficits, the balance can shift, but because this is a dynamic state, it can also shift back. The model suggests that people with, for example, many social assets, will be harder to tip into frailty than those with fewer social assets. Most recently, we have operationalized this by considering health deficits and protective factors in modeling the risk of adverse outcomes in relation to the frailty index.[30]

Although cartoon models such as 15-1 have many uses and the advantage of readily illustrating complicated ideas, they cannot offer the precision of formal quantitative models, as depicted in Figure 15-2.[31] It demonstrates changes in frailty states, from having n deficits at baseline to k deficits at follow-up. Let P_{nk} be the probability of transitions from n deficits at baseline to k deficits at follow-up of those who did not die during the follow-up. The probability of transition from n to k deficits can be approximated by the Poisson law,[22,31] which is characterized by a single parameter, the Poisson mean, ρ{ΣB}v{/ΣB}. The Poisson mean depends on baseline state n and, in general, on covariates, such as the level of education.

The probability P_{nd} of dying during a given follow-up period for people who have n deficits at the start of that period can be approximated as a sigmoid logistic function.[22] This reflects that the probability of death increases as the number of things wrong (n) increases; because no probability can be greater than 1, the probability of dying with n saturates approaching 1. For any given n state (e.g., $n = 1$, $n = 2$), the chance of having any k deficits at follow-up proceeds in a highly ordered way, with incremental change. For example, for most baseline states, the single most likely number of deficits that an individual will have at follow-up is one more than they had at baseline. (Formally, this can be summarized as saying that the mode of k is $n + 1$.) There is a slightly smaller chance of staying the same and about the same chance of having two things wrong more than at baseline, a smaller chance again of improving, and so on. The probabilities of achieving any given k therefore arise as a function of n and follow an ordered set of changes. On average, n increases, but for virtually any value of n, there is still some chance of improvement (and likewise of stabilization or decline). Large jumps in n to k states are uncommon; when large changes in the value of n do occur, they usually go from a low n state (i.e., few deficits, good health) to a high k state. Empirically, the fit to this model is high (Fig. 15-3).

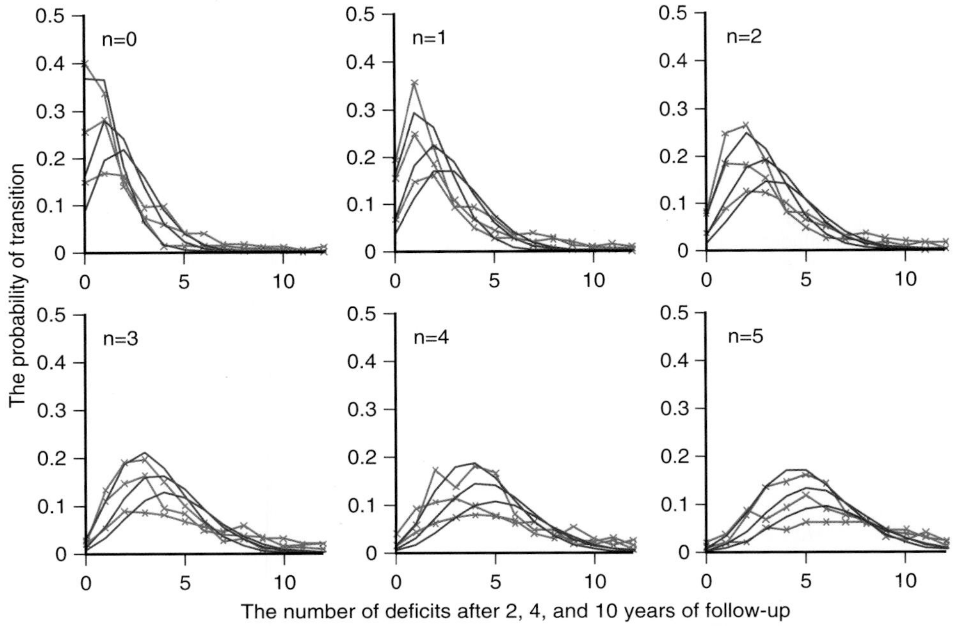

Figure 15-3. The probability of transition from *n* to *k* deficits in relation to the starting n deficits during 2 *(upper curves and crosses)*, 4 *(middle curves and crosses)*, and 10 years *(lower curves and crosses)*. *Crosses* represent observational transitional frequencies, and *lines* represent the model fit (see Fig. 15-2). In each subplot, *n* indicates the number of deficits (state) at baseline. *(From Mitnitski A, Song X, Rockwood K: Trajectories of changes over twelve years in the health status of Canadians from late middle age. Exp Gerontol 47:893–899, 2012.)*

Two other points are especially of note. One is that the chance of moving from any given n state to any k state P_{nk} depends on the present value of n and the general (ambient or background) changes in the environment. This is captured in the formula by saying that the Poisson mean increases proportionally to n, $\rho(n) = a_0 + a_1 n$, where a_0 describes the chance of accumulating deficits for people who have nothing wrong at baseline (i.e., who at baseline are in the "zero [deficit] state.") The parameter a_1 describes, given the current nonzero number of deficits, the increments of their expected change.[22] Of course, the same is true for the risk of death—that is, $logit(P_{nd}) = b_0 + b_1 n$; b_0 is the logit (log odds) of dying for people who have nothing wrong at baseline. Here, parameter b_1 describes, again given the current (nonzero) number of deficits, the associated risk of death.[22] In this way, it can be seen that the zero state appears to be informative about the environment in which a given population ages. Finally, we note that this is a simplified model, which can be adjusted to evaluate the impact of various covariates. For example, to understand the impact of high versus low level of education, we can evaluate its impact on a_0 and b_0.

The move from the operationalization of the concepts of deficits in dynamic balance in Figure 15-1 to the terms specified in Figure 15-2 has taken place over some years, but each agrees on the following essential points: frailty is a multiply determined state of risk and is formally complex—that is, its component parts, which interact in ways which cannot always be summarized at the level of the individual parts—and dynamic—the interactions produce further interactions, and change with time. In Figure 15-1, items that relate to health are envisaged as weights on the balance beam. For example, various health assets, such as a positive health attitude[32] or positive health practices such as exercise,[33] fit on the left hand side of the balance, giving positive weight to assets. Others, such as illness, the particular illness that gives rise to disabilities, and the particular disabilities that result in dependence on others are seen to weigh on the negative side. As more health deficits mount up and a person becomes more frail, the assets and deficits come into a precarious balance. In this context, an acute illness can be an important deficit, and can even tip the balance between assets and deficits. As attractive as this model is—it is easy to understand, accommodates multiple factors, and is complex and dynamic—unless and until it can be quantified, it cannot rise beyond the status of a metaphor. In its earliest operationalization, the deficits were quantified as grades of disability, cognitive impairment, and poor health attitude.[34,35]

By contrast, Figures 15-2 and 15-3 illustrate that changes in health status, changes in grades of frailty, occur as a function of the number of things that people have wrong with them. It says that the chance that people with that number of things wrong with them will change their health status in relation to a known distribution of the range of chances. These changes can be stability, worsening, or improvement. The distribution suggests that most people do not change their health status that much (i.e., a person with n things wrong with them is most likely, when followed up, to have $n + 1$ things wrong, or to show a slight worsening), but also could stay at just n things wrong, or improve to $n - 1$ things wrong. For most people, the chance of improvement to $n - 1$ is about the same as the chance of worsening to $n + 2$ things wrong. However, those discrete states (slightly better, the same, or one or two more things wrong) consist of over half of the possible outcomes. The model assigns all possible outcome states (better, same, worse, or dead) typically with high precision based on just four parameters, a staggering degree of dimensionality reduction compared with most multivariable models. As the equation shows, each of the four parameters becomes an object of investigation. Thus, the motivation to continue this line of inquiry is very strong.

Even so, most readers, especially most medical readers, for whom the mathematics is stereotypically not their strong suit, will worry that whatever apparent precision in these estimates might be obtained by the quantitative model, it comes at a very high price of comprehensibility. The balance beam is much easier to understand. For now, we will make the claim that almost everything that is in the balance beam can be included in the quantitative model; the model helps us understand how to quantify what our clinical intuition tells us is the case. An important addendum—what compels us to say "almost everything" and not "everything" is that some elements important in the balance beam need a more elaborate model to achieve full specification. For example, the balance beam posits an interaction between so-called medical and social factors. As covered in a later chapter of this text, on social vulnerability (see Chapter 30), social deficits appear to operate in a way that has much in common with frailty, but at a level that is separable from it.[36]

A useful way to understand the dynamics of deficit accumulation is to consider what Benjamin Gompertz quantified in 1825[37]; the older people are, the more likely they are to die as a precise function (± one or two error terms)[38,39] of the logarithm of their age (see Figure 15-2). However, it is not as though people suddenly drop dead as they age. Instead, before death, they accumulate deficits, and they accumulate them exponentially with age.[40] In fact, it is the deficit count, more than chronologic age that correlates most with the risk of death at any age.[40-42] The deficits that we can see accumulate clinically—the symptoms, signs, diseases, disabilities, and laboratory abnormalities that we typically count in frailty indices—begin as subcellular impairments.[28,43] Recent insights into how deficits scale from the subcellular to clinical level have come from work on a frailty index made up of 21 laboratory abnormalities and measured systolic and diastolic blood pressure (the FI-LAB).[44] Drawing on experience in developing a frailty index for use with mice has suggested that such measures could be combined to define groups at greater risk.[45] Using data from 1013 clinical examinations conducted in the first wave of the Canadian Study of Health and Aging (CSHA), the FI-LAB showed several important characteristics seen with any frailty index. These included a skewed distribution with a long right tail (Fig. 15-4), an increase in the mean value with age, and an increase in mortality with increasing FI-LAB scores (Fig. 15-5).[44]

DEVELOPMENT OF A FRAILTY INDEX BASED ON COMPREHENSIVE GERIATRIC ASSESSMENT

We began work on the frailty index by counting deficits in existing databases, chiefly epidemiologic ones. Over the years, we have collaborated with several groups to build a frailty index in epidemiologic databases. This has justifiably caused concern in some quarters about the clinical usefulness of the approach,[46,47] especially because an optimal frailty index should contain no fewer than 30 to 40 items. (The lowest practical limit seems to be about 10 to 15 although, at that point, selection of the items to be counted becomes more important.[47,48]) We have also built versions of the frailty index prospectively from standardized comprehensive geriatric assessment forms. For example, a one-page comprehensive geriatric assessment (CGA) form used routinely by our group readily can count up to 50 items (+10 items relating to social vulnerability). (The form can be downloaded at http://geriatricresearch.medicine.dal.ca.)

The frailty index derived from the CGA form is built like any other, which is to say that it counts deficits. (We have built other frailty index measures based on the CGA.[49,50]) In open access journal publications, we have described how to create a frailty index[51] and addressed its scoring.[52] A video is also available at http://geriatricresearch.medicine.dal.ca. By convention, we give any deficit a score of 1 if it is present and 0 if it is absent, although increments can be used.[52] On the CGA form, for example, under the section "Communication," we would give one point each for problems of vision, hearing, and speech. Similarly, we would give one point for impaired mobility or a recent fall. In addition, we count each of the comorbidities that an individual might have and score one point for each. We count additional deficits for

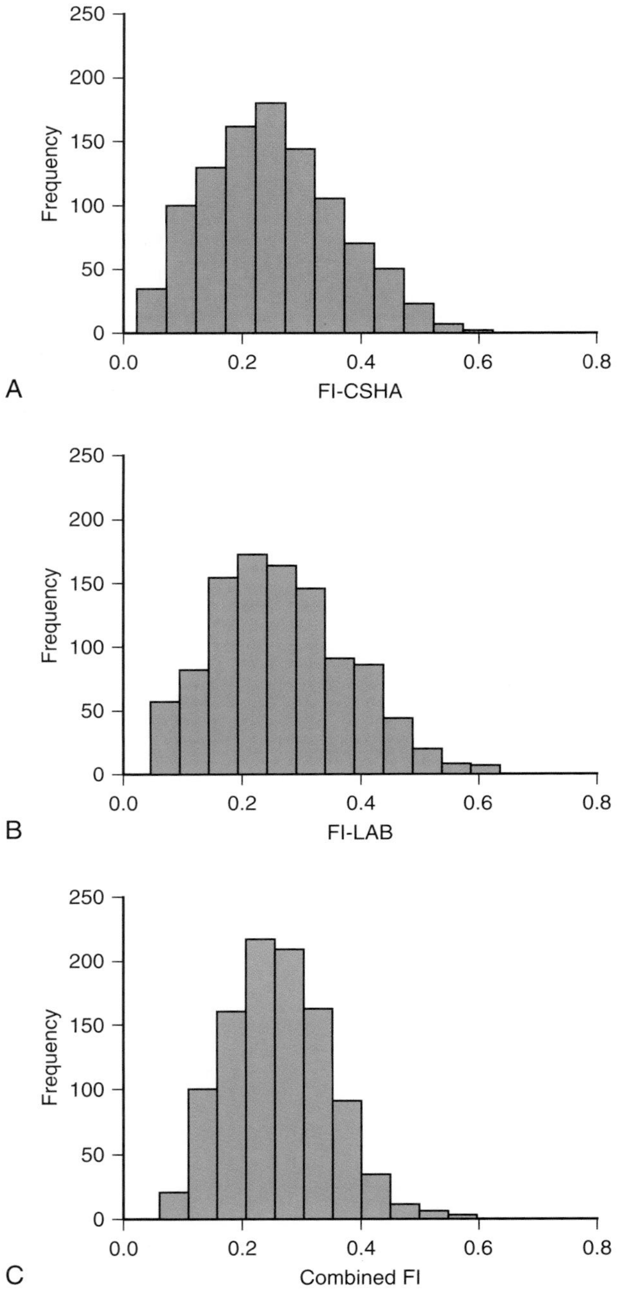

Figure 15-4. Frequency distributions for the frailty index (FI)–CSHA and FI-LAB. **A**, The frequency distribution for the FI-CSHA data was somewhat skewed to the left, with a median of 0.24 and a long right tail. The maximum FI-CSHA score was 0.72. **B,** Histogram showing the frequency distribution for the FI-LAB data collected in this study. The distribution had a median FI-LAB value of 0.27, and the maximum observed FI-LAB score was 0.63. **C,** The distribution of the combined FI scores was slightly skewed to the left, with a median value of 0.26 and a maximum of 0.59. The value of *n* was 1013 participants in each group. *FI-CSHA,* Frailty index—Canadian Study of Health and Aging; *FI-LAB,* laboratory frailty index. *(From Howlett SE, Rockwood MR, Mitnitski A, Rockwood K: Standard laboratory tests to identify older adults at increased risk of death. BMC Med 12:171, 2014.)*

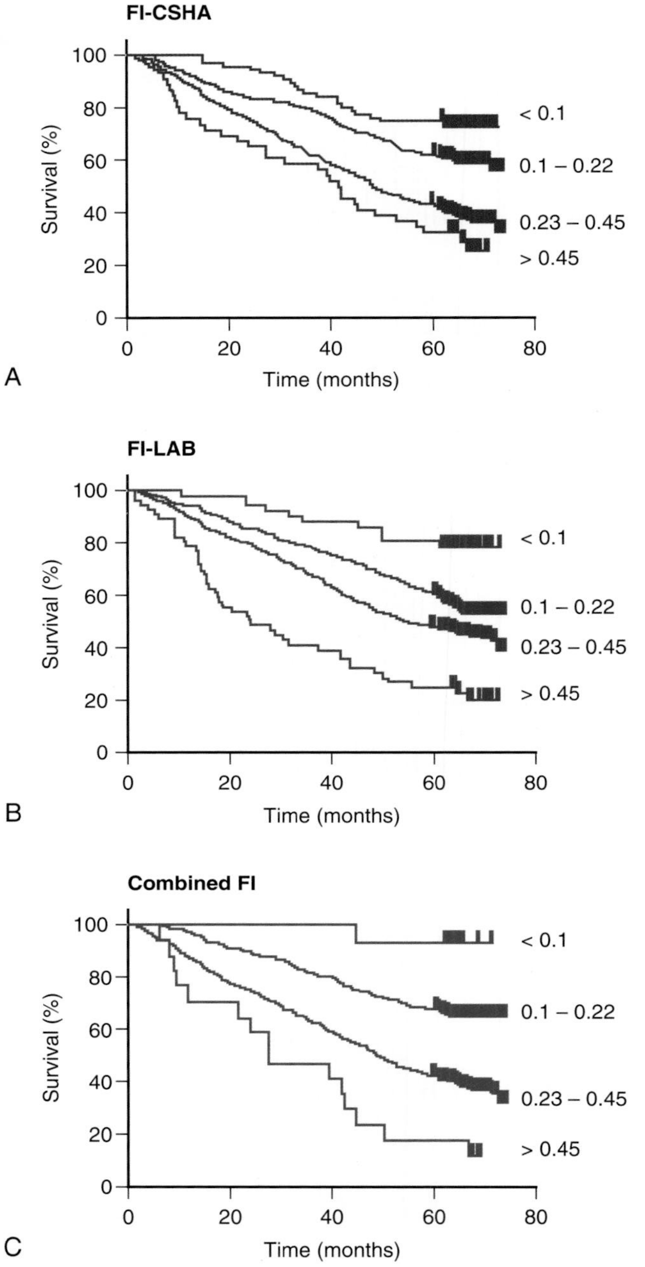

Figure 15-5. Kaplan-Meier survival curves for grades of the frailty index (FI). **A,** Survival over the course of the study plotted as a function of grades of the FI-CSHA. The least frail group (frailty score < 0.10) showed little mortality over the course of the study, whereas the most frail group (frailty score > 0.45) showed very high mortality. Differences between groups were statistically significant between all four grades of frailty when analyzed with a log-rank test ($P < .05$). **B,** Survival curves for grades of frailty assessed by the FI-LAB scores. There were significant differences in survival between subjects at all four levels when FI-LAB scores were used to grade frailty ($P < .05$; log rank test). **C,** Kaplan-Meier survival curves for "combined" FI scores obtained by merging the FI-CSHA and the FI-LAB scores. Differences in mortality between the four grades of frailty were most evident when the combination FI scores were used ($P < 0.05$; log rank test). FI-CSHA, standard frailty index; FI-LAB, laboratory frailty index. *(From Howlett SE, Rockwood MR, Mitnitski A, Rockwood K: Standard laboratory tests to identify older adults at increased risk of death. BMC Med 12:171, 2014.)*

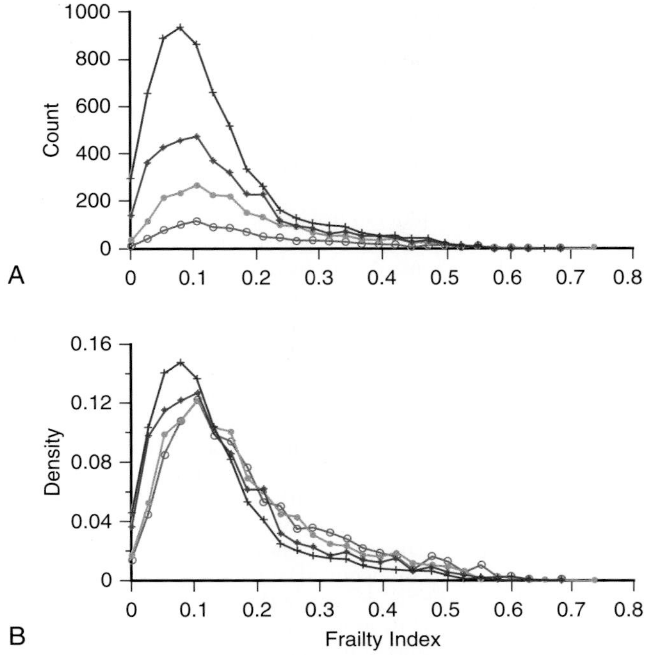

Figure 15-6. Distribution of the frailty index by the number of people at each wave shown in absolute numbers (**A**) and as a percentage (**B**). For both **A** and **B** baseline, *crosses*; 2-year follow-up, *stars*; 4-year follow-up, *dots*; 7-year follow-up, *circles*. *(From Bennett S, Song X, Mitnitski A, et al: A limit to frailty in very old, community-dwelling people: a secondary analysis of the Chinese longitudinal health and longevity study. Age Ageing 42:372–377, 2013.) Used with permission.*

every five medications prescribed beyond five (e.g., five through nine medications, one deficit point; 10 through 14 medications, two deficit points). Any asymptomatic risk factor where modification would have a mortality benefit (e.g., hypertension or antiplatelets in secondary vascular prevention) would be considered as a further deficit if left untreated.

An important point about the frailty index and CGA is that almost all deficits can be measured in every patient, so there should be few missing data, typically less than 5% for any given item. This requirement has the effect of excluding many performance-based measures from frailty index variables, at least from survey data in which they typically have considerably more than 5% missing data.[53] If they are to be included, then it seems to be useful to assign missing data to the score associated with worst performance status.[53] Several groups have now reported using frailty index CGAs. Even though each has been modified locally, they seem to yield similar results,[54-59] especially in relation to the distribution, including a submaximal limit.

The presence of a limit to frailty is one of the more intriguing characteristic behaviors of the frailty index. In a large number of datasets, both clinical (including the intensive care unit) and epidemiologic, less than 1% of people have frailty index scores higher than 0.7. Despite speculation, why this proportion exists as the limit is not clear, but its replicability is impressive. Figure 15-6 offers an example from the Chinese Health and Longevity Longitudinal Survey. There, in successive waves of the survey, the median and modal values of the frailty index stayed approximately the same, and the limit was not exceeded. In Figure 15-6*A*, the actual numbers are presented; the decreasing area under the curve corresponds to the loss to follow-up due to mortality at the advanced ages (80 to 99 years at baseline) of the sample.[60] In reports using self-report data, the limit to the frailty index

TABLE 15-1 Clinical Frailty Scale

Grade	Plain Language Descriptor	Common Characteristics	Usual Frailty Index Values
1	Very fit	Robust, active, energetic, well motivated, and fit; these people usually exercise regularly and are in the fittest group for their age and commonly describe their health as "excellent"	0.09 (0.05)
2	Well	Without active or symptomatic disease, but less fit than people in category 1	0.12 (0.05)
3	Well, with treated comorbid disease	Disease symptoms are well controlled compared with those in category 4	0.16 (0.07)
4	Apparently vulnerable	Although not frankly dependent, these people commonly complain of being "slowed up" or have disease symptoms or self-rate health as "fair," at best. If cognitively impaired, they do not meet dementia criteria	0.22 (0.08)
5	Mildly frail	Shows limited dependence on others for instrumental activities of daily living	0.27 (0.09)
6	Moderately frail	Help is needed with instrumental and some personal activities of daily living. Walking commonly is restricted	0.36 (0.09)
7	Severely frail	Completely dependent on others for personal activities of daily living	0.43 (0.08)
8	Terminally ill	Terminally ill	

seems to be higher in women than in men, but still does not exceed 0.7.[61]

Frailty Index as a Clinical State Variable

If variation in grades of the frailty index reflects variation in the risk of adverse health outcomes, it is reasonable to suppose that these grades in the frailty index represent different states of health. To this end, we have proposed that the frailty index can be considered as a clinical state variable.[2] A state variable is one that quantitatively summarizes the state of an entire system; a classic example is temperature, which can be measured as a single number on a graded scale. The number has a known meaning—as the average of the kinetic energies of the molecules that make up a given system. These individual kinetic energies are indeterminate. By contrast, temperature is more stable and can behave in ways that can be known with precision. An important trait of a state variable is that it can be described using plain language descriptions. Temperature can be meaningfully communicated as, for example, hot, warm, cool, cold, or freezing. These descriptions can also be contextualized. In a biologic context, scaling would have a precise clinical meaning. These attributes appear to be particularly worthwhile in grading frailty and allow some precision to be brought to the question of which procedures might safely be entertained in a frail patient. This grading of risk in relation to the severity or load of the intervention and the responsiveness or frailty of the individual is an active area of inquiry. For now, the interim answer seems to be to translate the frailty index into terms used. One aspect of the frailty index as a clinical state variable that has yet to be fully explored is its translation into plain language: what is the analogue to "hot" versus "tepid" with respect to frailty? Pending this answer being fully worked out, the high correlation between the frailty index and the CSHA Clinical Frailty Scale[62] makes that measure seem to be a reasonable way to grade degrees of fitness and frailty quickly (Table 15-1).

Another consequence to flow from the idea that the frailty index defines discrete health states is that how these states change might be informative. As noted, this appears to be the case (see Figs. 15-2 and 15-3). The probability for a given individual of a change in the number of deficits that he or she has depends on two factors. The first is the number of deficits that that individual has at baseline and the number of deficits that are accumulated, on average, by a person who has no deficits at baseline. Another notable feature of the reproducibility of the changes in health states represented by variable deficit counts or grades of frailty is that these estimates are very robust. The estimates noted previously do not just come from different countries, but were developed using different versions of the frailty index, which typically

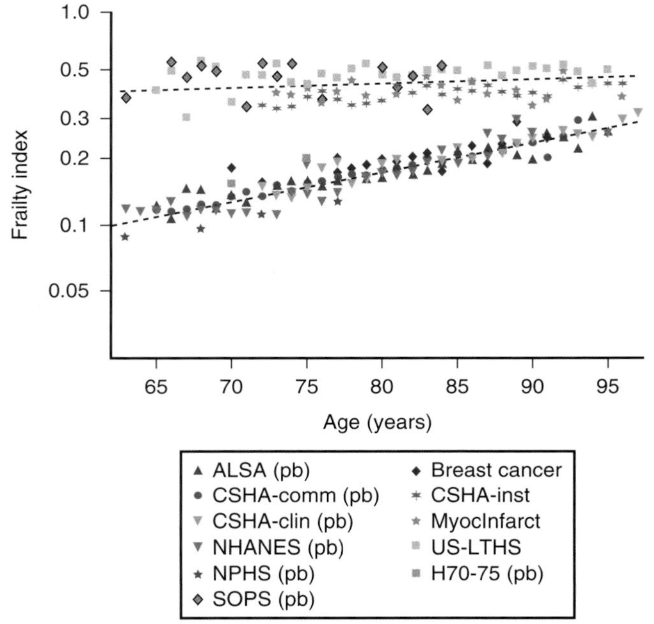

Figure 15-7. The relationship between the frailty index and age. Across a number of surveys, the frailty index accumulates in community-dwelling older adults at a rate of about 3%/year, on a log scale *(lower line)*. By contrast, in clinical samples and among institutionalized older adults, the values of the frailty index are much higher on average and show almost no accumulation with age.

has not been constructed in the same way in any two studies (Fig. 15-7).[63] The examples quoted use iterations of the frailty index that use different types of variables (e.g., self-reported in the National Population Health Survey, clinically assessed [CSHA, Gothenburg H-70 cohort study], or laboratory data [Gothenburg H-70]), and often different numbers of variables (from 39 in the National Population Health Survey to 70 in the Canadian Study of Health and Aging to 100 in the Gothenburg H-70 study).[63]

The frailty index has often been referred to as a measure of biologic age.[64-66] If we consider that biologic age derives its rationale not as time since birth, which is already well handled by chronologic age, but as the time to death, then the high correlation between the frailty index and mortality can be usefully exploited to calculate biologic age. Here is how.[64] Consider two people (A and B) of the same chronologic age—say, 80 years old

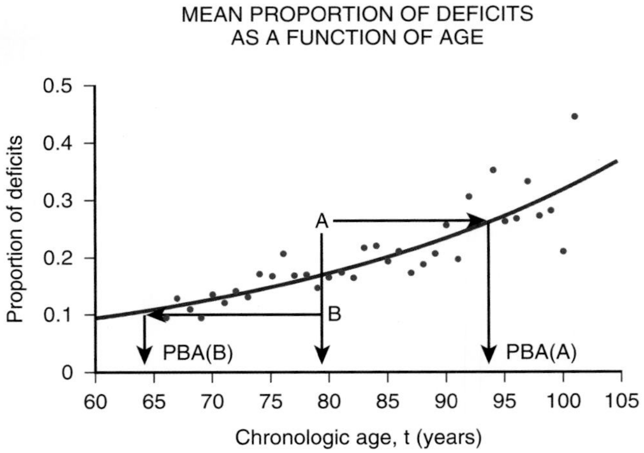

Figure 15-8. Personal biologic age. Because the mean value of the frailty index is so highly correlated with mortality (r^2 typically > 0.95), it can be used to estimate personal biologic age, understood as a measure of the proximity to death. Consider two men, each with the same (chronologic) age of 78 years. Person A has a value of the frailty index that corresponds to the mean frailty index value for 93-year-olds. In that sense, he has a personal biologic age of 93 years. By contrast, person B has a value of the frailty index that is seen, on average, at age 63 years. That person would have a mortality risk of a 63 year old.

(Fig. 15-8). One has a frailty index score of 0.11, which by interpolation we can see is the mean value, on average, of the frailty index at age 65 years. We can this say that this person has a biologic age of 65 years. The second person has a frailty index value of 0.28, which corresponds to the mean value of the frailty index at age 95 years, meaning that this person has a biologic age of 95 years. In multivariable models, which include chronologic age and the frailty index, each contributes independently, but with more information, typically coming from the frailty index.[41,42] In addition, people who accumulate deficits more quickly have a higher mortality rate.

The frailty index CGA is one example of a clinical state variable, with a single number summarizing the overall clinical state of the individual. Other candidate clinical state variables can be considered, of which mobility and balance appears to be an example, as reviewed in Chapter 102. Any clinical state variable should represent the functioning of a system, so from that standpoint must be high order. For humans, the evolutionary high order functions are upright bipedal ambulation, opposable thumbs, divided attention, and social interaction. In consequence, candidate clinical state variables logically can be sought in measures of mobility and balance, function, divided attention, and social withdrawal. Any geriatrician will recognize in this a short list of important so-called geriatric giants—impaired mobility ("taking to bed," "off legs"), falls, functional decline, social withdrawal, or caregiver distress. This text has chapters on each topic, and each is moving toward better quantification of the underlying phenomena. The disorders have also been referred to as frailty syndromes, which in this context makes sense,[1] although it must be noted that severe illness (or relevant focal disorders, such as delirium from meningitis) in a fit person can also cause similar presentations. The value of considering the overall state of an individual is well illustrated by recent work that has examined risks for common late life illnesses and their adverse outcomes. For example, the risk of dementia appears to be correlated to the degree of frailty[67]; so, too, does disease expression.[68] These associations seem to be more powerful than traditional dementia risk factors. Similarly, work on osteopororis and the risk of fragility fractures favors frailty over traditional risk factors, although all are important.[69,70] A similar case has recently been found in relation to the risk for death and hospitalization in patients with coronary heart disease.[71] These findings represent a first step in understanding how age operates as risk in late life illness.

Good geriatric medicine has always had an intuitive grasp of the nature of complexity, as manifest in the frail older patient for whom geriatricians are privileged to care. The intent in making the analysis of complexity explicit is to build on this intuition, not substitute for it. As has been argued, providing a scientific basis for the specialty of geriatric medicine, rather than its existence as a set of utilitarian values—we do these things because they seem to work—is essential to advancing the care of frail older patients with complex needs.[72]

KEY POINTS

- Frailty is an important issue for geriatricians; geriatric medicine chiefly consists of the complex care of older people who are frail.
- Frailty is a state of increased risk of adverse health outcomes.
- Frailty can be operationalized in relation to a deficit count; the more things people have wrong, the more likely they will be frail. This is captured by a frailty index, which is the ratio of the number of health deficits that an individual has to the number of health deficits counted (e.g., in a geriatric assessment or health questionnaire).
- The frailty index can be considered as a clinical state variable, a single number that allows the overall clinical state to be summarized. The frailty index, a deficit count, is one example of the chronic health state. Mobility and balance, appropriately measured, appears to be another clinical state variable, more applicable for acute changes in health.
- A comprehensive geriatric assessment and the evaluation of delirium, falls, and immobility are intrinsic to geriatric medicine. Each is a response to the analysis of complex systems at high risk for failure.

For a complete list of references, please visit www.expertconsult.com.

KEY REFERENCES

1. Clegg A, Young J, Iliffe S, et al: Frailty in elderly people. Lancet 381:752–762, 2013.
2. Rockwood K, Mitnitski A: Frailty defined by deficit accumulation and geriatric medicine defined by frailty. Clin Geriatr Med 27:17–26, 2011.
7. Cesari M, Gambassi G, van Kan GA, et al: The frailty phenotype and the frailty index: different instruments for different purposes. Age Ageing 43:10–12, 2014.
8. Mitnitski A, Song X, Rockwood K: Assessing biological aging: the origin of deficit accumulation. Biogerontology 14:709–717, 2013.
9. Fried LP, Tangen CM, Walston J, et al: Frailty in older adults: evidence for a phenotype. J Gerontol A Biol Sci Med Sci 56:M146–M156, 2001.
16. López-Otín C, Blasco MA, Partridge L, et al: The hallmarks of aging. Cell 153:1194–1217, 2013.
22. Mitnitski A, Song X, Rockwood K: Trajectories of changes over twelve years in the health status of Canadians from late middle age. Exp Gerontol 47:893–899, 2012.
30. Wang C, Song X, Mitnitski A, et al: Effect of health protective factors on health deficit accumulation and mortality risk in older adults in the Beijing Longitudinal Study of Aging. J Am Geriatr Soc 62:821–828, 2014.
38. Vaupel JW, Manton KG, Stallard E: The impact of heterogeneity in individual frailty on the dynamics of mortality. Demography 9:439–454, 1979.
41. Kulminski AM, Ukraintseva SV, Kulminskaya IV, et al: Cumulative deficits better characterize susceptibility to death in elderly people

than phenotypic frailty: lessons from the cardiovascular health study. J Am Geriatr Soc 56:898–903, 2008.
44. Howlett SE, Rockwood MR, Mitnitski A, et al: Standard laboratory tests to identify older adults at increased risk of death. BMC Med 12:171, 2014.
46. Martin FC, Brighton P: Frailty: different tools for different purposes? Age Ageing 37:129–131, 2008.
67. Song X, Mitnitski A, Rockwood K: Age-related deficit accumulation and the risk of late-life dementia. Alzheimers Res Ther 6:54, 2014.
58. Dent E, Chapman I, Howell S, et al: Frailty and functional decline indices predict poor outcomes in hospitalised older people. Age Ageing 43:477–484, 2014.
60. Bennett S, Song X, Mitnitski A, et al: A limit to frailty in very old, community-dwelling people: a secondary analysis of the Chinese longitudinal health and longevity study. Age Ageing 42:372–377, 2013.
65. Goggins WB, Woo J, Sham A, et al: Frailty index as a measure of biological age in a Chinese population. J Gerontol A Biol Sci Med Sci 60:1046–1051, 2005.
69. Kennedy CC, Ioannidis G, Rockwood K, et al: A frailty index predicts 10-year fracture risk in adults age 25 years and older: results from the Canadian Multicentre Osteoporosis Study (CaMos). Osteoporos Int 25:2825–2832, 2014.

16 Effects of Aging on the Cardiovascular System

Susan E. Howlett

Advanced age is a major risk factor for the development of cardiovascular disease. Why age increases the risk of cardiovascular disease is debatable. The increased risk might arise simply because there is more time to be exposed to risk factors such as hypertension, smoking, and dyslipidemia. In other words, the aging process itself has little impact on the cardiovascular system. However, an emerging view is that the accumulation of cellular and subcellular deficits in the aging heart and blood vessels renders the cardiovascular system susceptible to the effects of cardiovascular diseases. Although increased exposure to risk factors likely contributes to the development of cardiovascular disease in aging, there is considerable evidence that the structure and function of the human heart and vasculature change importantly as a function of the normal aging process. These changes occur in the absence of risk factors other than age and in the absence of overt clinical signs of cardiovascular disease.

AGING-ASSOCIATED CHANGES IN VASCULAR STRUCTURE

Studies in blood vessels from apparently healthy humans have shown that the vasculature changes with age, a process known as remodeling. The centrally located large elastic arteries dilate, something that is evident to the naked eye, and that is well seen in arterial radiographic studies. Structural changes due to remodeling are apparent even in early adulthood and increase with age.[1-3] Aging-related arterial remodeling is important, because it is thought to provide an ideal setting in which vascular diseases can thrive. Structural changes that occur in the arteries of normotensive aging humans are observed in hypertensive patients at much younger ages.[3]

These readily visible changes arise from microscopic changes in the wall structure of these large elastic arteries.[1-3] The arterial wall is composed of three different layers, or tunics. The outermost layer, tunica adventitia, is composed of collagen fibers and elastic tissue. The thicker middle layer, the tunica media, is composed of connective tissue, smooth muscle cells, and elastic tissue. The contractile properties of the arterial wall are determined primarily by variations in the composition of the media. The innermost layer of the arterial wall, tunica intima, consists of a connective tissue layer and an inner layer of endothelial cells. Endothelial cells are squamous epithelial cells that play an important role in the regulation of normal vascular function, and endothelial dysfunction contributes to vascular disease.[4] Age-associated changes in these different layers have a profound effect on the structure and function of the vasculature in older adults.

One of the most prominent age-related changes in the structure of the vasculature in humans is dilation of large elastic arteries, which leads to an increase in lumen size.[2,5] In addition, the walls of large elastic arteries thicken with age. Studies of carotid wall intima plus media (IM) thickness in adult human arteries have shown that IM thickness increases almost threefold by 90 years of age.[2,5] Increased IM thickness is an important risk factor for atherosclerosis independent of age.[6] Thickening of the arterial wall in aging is due mainly to an increase in the thickness of the intima.[1] Whether thickening of the media occurs in aging is controversial. However, studies have shown that the number of vascular smooth muscle cells in the media declines with age, whereas the remaining cells increase in size.[1] Whether these hypertrophied smooth muscle cells are fully functional or whether this is one way in which aging is deleterious to vascular function is not yet clear. The major structural changes in the vasculature with age are illustrated in Figure 16-1.

Age-associated thickening of the intima is due, in part, to an increase in infiltrating vascular smooth muscle cells.[3] In addition, the collagen content of the intima and collagen cross-linking increase markedly with age in human arteries.[3,7,8] However, the elastin content of the intima declines, and elastin fraying and fragmentation occur.[7,8] It has been proposed that repeated cycles of distention followed by elastic recoil may promote the loss of elastin and deposition of collagen in aging arteries.[8] These changes in collagen and elastin content are believed to have important effects on the distensibility or stiffness of aging arteries, as discussed in more detail later (see "Arterial Stiffness in Aging Arteries").

In addition to alterations in intimal connective tissues in aging, studies in human arteries have shown that the aging process modifies the structure of endothelial cells themselves. Endothelial cells increase in size with age or hypertrophy. In addition, endothelial cell shape becomes irregular.[3] The permeability of endothelial cells increases with age, and vascular smooth muscle cells may infiltrate the subendothelial space.[1,3,8] There also is considerable evidence that the substances released by the endothelium are modified by age.[9,3] The impact of these changes on vascular function is discussed in more detail in the next section.

ENDOTHELIAL FUNCTION IN AGING

Once regarded as an almost inert lining of the blood vessels, the vascular endothelium is now recognized to be a metabolically active tissue involved in the maintenance and regulation of blood flow. In younger adults, the vascular endothelium synthesizes and releases a variety of regulatory substances in response to chemical and mechanical stimuli. For example, endothelial cells release substances such as nitric oxide, prostacyclin, endothelins, interleukins, endothelial growth factors, adhesion molecules, plasminogen inhibitors, and von Willebrand factor.[4,10] These substances are involved in the regulation of key functions, including vascular tone, angiogenesis, thrombosis, and thrombolysis. There is growing evidence that the aging process may disrupt many of these normal functions of the vascular endothelium.[2,3]

Endothelial dysfunction is usually measured as a disruption in endothelium-dependent relaxation. Endothelium-dependent relaxation is mediated by nitric oxide, which is released from the endothelium by mechanical stimuli, such as increased blood flow (shear stress), and by chemical stimuli (e.g., acetylcholine, bradykinin, adenosine triphosphate [ATP]).[4] When nitric oxide is released from the endothelium, it causes vascular smooth muscle relaxation by increasing intracellular levels of cyclic guanosine monophosphate (cGMP). The increased cGMP prevents the interaction of the contractile filaments actin and myosin.[11] The increase in vascular stiffness in aging arteries is partly explained by a decrease in the production of nitric oxide by the vascular endothelium.[9] This leads to impairment in blood vessel relaxation as people age.

The mechanism whereby nitric oxide activity is reduced in aging remains controversial. Nitric oxide is synthesized in endothelial cells by a constitutive enzyme called endothelial nitric oxide synthase (eNOS or NOS III).[11] There is evidence that the levels of eNOS are reduced in aging, which could account for the decrease in nitric oxide activity in aging vasculature.[2,3] Other studies have suggested that factors such as the production of oxygen free radicals in aging endothelial cells may impair nitric oxide production.[3] Further studies will be needed to understand fully the mechanism or mechanisms responsible for endothelial dysfunction in aging vasculature.

There is good evidence that endothelial dysfunction is an important cause of cardiovascular disease, independent of age.[2,11] Therefore, age-related endothelial dysfunction is likely to make a major contribution to the increased risk of cardiovascular disease in older adults.

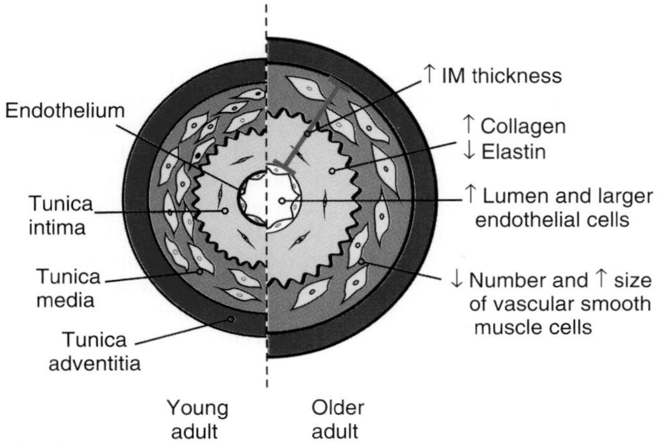

Figure 16-1. Remodeling of the central elastic arteries with age. The layers of the arterial wall are labeled as shown. There are marked changes in central elastic arteries as a consequence of the aging process. The diameter of the lumen increases with age. Intima plus media (IM) thickness also increases, primarily as a consequence of an increase in the thickness of the tunica intima. An increase in collagen deposition and decrease in elastin are responsible for intimal remodeling in aging arteries. The number of vascular smooth muscle cells in the tunica media decreases, whereas the remaining cells hypertrophy. Endothelial cell hypertrophy also occurs in aging arteries.

ARTERIAL STIFFNESS IN AGING ARTERIES

Aging-related remodeling of the large central elastic arteries has a major impact on the function of the cardiovascular system. One of the best-characterized functional changes in aging arteries is a decrease in the compliance or distensibility of aging arteries.[2,12] This resistance of arteries to deflection by blood flow is known as stiffness. Increased arterial stiffness in aging impairs the ability of the aorta and its major branches to expand and contract with changes in blood pressure. The lack of deflection of the blood flow increases the velocity at which the pulse wave travels within large arteries in older adults.[12-14] Increased pulse wave velocity is related to hypertension, but pulse wave velocity can be measured separately from blood pressure. An increase in pulse wave velocity in aging is an important risk factor for future adverse cardiovascular events.[12-14]

The structural changes in the arterial wall described are implicated in the increase in arterial stiffness observed in central elastic arteries in the aging heart. The increased collagen content and increased collagen cross-linking that occur in aging arteries are believed to increase arterial stiffness.[3,8,15] Other factors such as reduced elastin content, elastin fragmentation, and increased elastase activity also are thought to increase stiffness in aging arteries.[3,15] Alterations in the endothelial regulation of vascular smooth muscle tone and changes in other aspects of the arterial wall and vascular function may also contribute to the age-associated increase in arterial stiffness.[8,15]

Arterial stiffness is thought to be responsible for some of the changes in blood pressure that are reported in older adults.[15,16] In younger adults, recoil in the elastic central arteries transmits a portion of each stroke volume in systole and a portion of each stroke volume in diastole, as illustrated in Figure 16-2, *A*. However, with aging, the increase in stiffness of large arterial walls contributes to the increase in systolic pressure and decrease in diastolic pressure that are characteristically observed in aging.[14-16] In this way, stiff central arteries can lead to an increase in pulse pressure in aging.[14-16] These changes occur because increased stiffness abolishes elastic recoil in central elastic arteries. This means that blood flow is transmitted during systole, which leads to a high systolic pressure.[15,16] As blood flow is transmitted in systole, the elastic recoil does not dissipate in diastole and diastolic pressure declines with age, as shown diagrammatically in Figure 16-2, *B*. This increase in systolic pressure with no

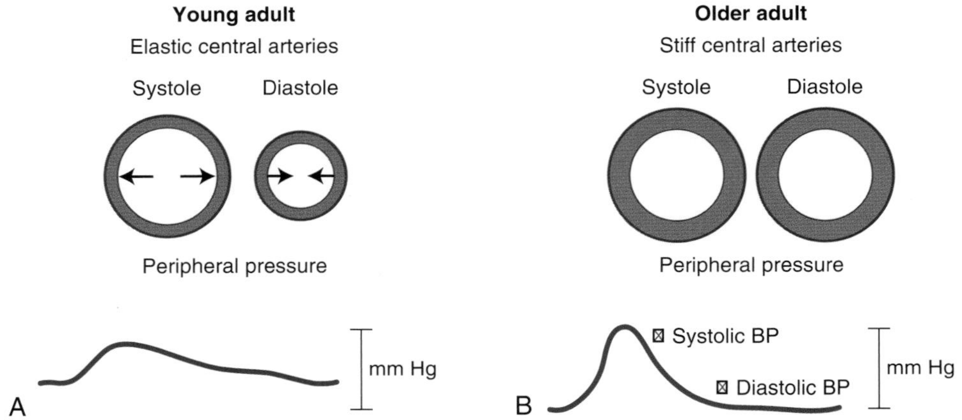

Figure 16-2. The age-associated increase in central artery stiffness has important effects on peripheral pressure. **A,** In young adults, the elastic central arteries expand with each cardiac contraction, so that part of the stroke volume is transmitted peripherally in systole and the remainder is transmitted in diastole. **B,** In older adults, stiff central arteries do not expand with each contraction, so stroke volume is transmitted in systole. This leads to an increase in systolic blood pressure and a decrease in diastolic blood pressure in older adults. *(Adapted from Izzo JL Jr: Arterial stiffness and the systolic hypertension syndrome. Curr Opin Cardiol 19:341–352, 2004.)*

TABLE 16-1 Age-Related Changes in the Vasculature

Age-Associated Changes in Vasculature	Clinical Consequences
↑ Intimal thickness	Promotes atherosclerosis
↑ Collagen, reduced elastin, ↑ vascular stiffness	Systolic hypertension
Endothelial cell dysfunction	↑ Risk of vascular disease

change or a reduction in diastolic pressure leads to isolated systolic hypertension, which is the most common form of hypertension in older adults.[17] Studies have shown that isolated systolic hypertension increases the risk of cardiovascular disease.[18] Therefore, aging-related changes in the stiffness of large elastic arteries can explain many of the changes in blood pressure observed in aging and help increase the risk of cardiovascular disease in older adults. This increase in central artery stiffness is also thought to play a role in some of the age-associated changes in the heart, both by increasing the work of the heart and decreasing coronary artery flow, as discussed in the next section.

Age-related changes in blood vessels may vary among different vascular beds. The structural changes that lead to increased arterial stiffness are much more pronounced in large elastic arteries, such as the carotid artery, than in smaller muscular arteries, such as the brachial artery.[8] However, progressive stiffening of the central arteries in aging can lead to high pulsations in the microvasculature and cause damage in vital organs such as the brain and kidney.[13] There is also evidence for age-related changes in vascular reactivity in vessels other than the central elastic arteries. For example, the responsiveness of arterioles to drugs that stimulate α_1-adrenergic receptors declines with aging.[19] Vascular responsiveness to endothelin or angiotensin receptor agonists may also decline with age, although this has not been extensively investigated, and there is no evidence for such changes in humans.[19] Few studies have investigated the impact of age on vascular responsiveness in veins, but most studies have reported that age has little effect on the responsiveness of veins to a variety of pharmacologic agents.[19] Investigation of age-dependent alterations in vascular reactivity is an important area of inquiry; such changes would affect the responsiveness of the aging vasculature to drugs that target blood vessels in humans. Table 16-1 summarizes the major age-associated changes in the vasculature, along with the clinical consequences of these alterations.

EFFECT OF THE AGING PROCESS ON THE STRUCTURE OF THE HEART

The aging process has obvious effects on the structure of the heart at the macroscopic and microscopic levels. At the macroscopic level, there is a noted increase in the deposition of fat on the outer epicardial surface of the aging heart.[20] Calcium deposition in specific regions of the heart, known as calcification, is commonly observed.[5] The gross morphologic structure of individual heart chambers also is modified by age. There is an age-dependent increase in the size of the atria.[21] Furthermore, the atria dilate, and their volume increases with age.[21] Although some studies have reported that the mass of the left ventricle increases with age, more recent work has shown that left ventricular mass does not change in women and actually declines with age in men if those with underlying heart disease are excluded.[2,5] There is general agreement that left ventricular wall thickness increases progressively with age, whereas left ventricular volume declines in both systole and diastole.[5]

Age-related changes in heart structure are apparent not just macroscopically but at the level of individual heart cells, known as cardiomyocytes. Beginning at age 60 years, there is a noticeable reduction in specialized pacemaker cells in the sinoatrial node, which is the normal pacemaker of the heart.[5,22] The total number of ventricular muscle cells also declines, and this decrease is greater in males than in females.[20] Cell loss is thought to occur through apoptotic and necrotic cell death, although autophagy may also be implicated.[23-25] The loss of cardiomyocytes in the aging heart leads to an increase in size (hypertrophy) of the remaining cells, something that is more pronounced in men than women.[20] Interestingly, this parallels the age-dependent decrease in left ventricular mass seen in men but not women, as noted earlier.[2,5] Cardiomyocyte hypertrophy may compensate, at least in part, for the loss of contractile cells in the aging heart. However, unlike cardiac hypertrophy that occurs as a result of exercise, hypertrophy of cells in the aging heart results from the loss of myocytes, which may increase the mechanical burden on the remaining cells.[26] Interestingly, recent evidence from animal studies has shown that cardiomyocyte hypertrophy may more closely reflect biologic age (known as frailty) rather than chronologic age.[27] These findings suggest that age-dependent cardiac remodeling may be more closely linked to frailty than chronologic age, although further studies are required.

In addition to cardiomyocytes, the heart contains large numbers of fibroblasts, which are the cells that produce connective tissues such as collagen and elastin. Collagen is a fibrous protein that holds heart cells together, and elastin is a connective tissue protein responsible for the elasticity of body tissues. Because the number of myocytes progressively declines with age, there is a relative increase in the number of fibroblasts.[28] The amount of collagen increases with age, and there is an increase in collagen cross-linking between adjacent fibers.[5,28,29] Increased collagen leads to interstitial fibrosis in the atria and ventricles.[5,28,29] There also are structural alterations in elastin, and these changes may reduce elastic recoil in the aging heart.[30] Together with changes in the myocytes, these structural modifications in connective tissues increase myocardial stiffness, decrease ventricular compliance, and thereby impair passive left ventricular filling.[28] The idea that these age- and frailty-dependent cellular deficits scale up to affect function at the organ and system levels has been recently proposed.[31] The impact of these cellular changes on myocardial function is considered in more detail next.

MYOCARDIAL FUNCTION IN THE AGING HEART AT REST

The changes in the heart outlined above are maladaptive and lead to abnormalities in systolic and especially diastolic function in older adults. Functional abnormalities are most apparent during exercise, although some changes are evident even at rest. When individuals are reclining at rest, the heart rate is similar in younger and older subjects. However, when older individuals move from a supine to seated position, the heart rate increases less in older adults than in younger adults.[21] This impaired ability to augment heart rate in response to a positional change may be linked to the age-related reduction in responsiveness to the sympathetic nervous system discussed later (see "Response of the Aging Heart to Exercise"). In contrast, left ventricular systolic function, which is a measure of the ability of the heart to contract, is well preserved at rest in older adults.[2,5,21] Other measures of cardiac contractile function at rest also are unchanged with age. The volume of blood ejected from the ventricle per beat (stroke volume) is generally comparable or slightly elevated in older adults when compared with their younger counterparts.[21] Similarly, the left ventricular ejection fraction, which is the ratio of the stroke volume to the volume of blood left in the ventricle at the end of diastole, is unchanged in aging.[2,5,21] Thus, systolic function is relatively well preserved in healthy older adults at rest.

Unlike systolic function, diastolic function is profoundly altered in the hearts of older adults at rest. The rate of left ventricular filling in early diastole declines by up to 50% between

20 and 80 years of age.[2,21] Several mechanisms have been implicated in the reduction of left ventricular filling rate aging. There is evidence that age-associated structural changes in the left ventricle impair early diastolic filling. Specifically, the increase in collagen and modifications in elastin combine to increase left ventricular stiffness.[32] This increased ventricular stiffness reduces the compliance of the ventricle and impairs passive filling.[32] An additional mechanism involves changes at the level of the cardiomyocyte. The uptake of intracellular calcium into internal stores is disrupted in myocytes from the aging heart.[33] As a result, residual calcium from the previous contraction may cause persistent activation of contractile filaments and delay cardiomyocyte relaxation in the aging heart.[32,33] It also has been suggested that diastolic dysfunction reflects, at least in part, an adaptation to the age-related changes in the vasculature. Increased vascular stiffness leads to increased mechanical load and subsequent prolongation of contraction time.[2]

The age-associated increase in stiffness of the aorta has other effects on the heart. Stiffness in the aorta increases the load that the heart must work against (afterload), which is thought to promote the increase in left ventricular wall thickness observed in the aging heart.[2,5] Together, these adaptive changes may serve to preserve systolic function at the expense of diastolic function. This age-dependent slowing of relaxation in diastole may predispose the aging heart toward heart failure with preserved ejection fraction (HFpEF), which is common in older adults.[32-34]

In the hearts of young adults, left ventricular filling occurs early and very rapidly due primarily to ventricular relaxation. Only a small amount of filling occurs as a result of atrial contraction later in diastole in the young adult heart.[2,21] In contrast, early left ventricular filling is disrupted in the aging heart. This increased diastolic filling pressure results in left atrial dilation and atrial hypertrophy in the aging heart.[2] The more forceful atrial contraction observed in the aging heart promotes late diastolic filling and compensates for the reduced filling in early diastole.[2,21] Because the atria make such an important contribution to ventricular filling in older adults, loss of this atrial contraction due to conditions such as atrial fibrillation can lead to a marked reduction in diastolic volume and can predispose the aging heart to diastolic heart failure.[2] Atrial dilation and fibrosis can promote the development of atrial fibrillation and other arrhythmias in the aging heart.[2,21,22] Despite this evidence for diastolic dysfunction, left ventricular end-diastolic pressure does not decline with age in older healthy adults at rest. Aging is actually associated with a small increase in left ventricular end-diastolic pressure, in particular in older men.[21] Thus, although the filling pattern in diastole is altered in aging, this does not lead to notable changes in end-diastolic pressure in older hearts at rest.

RESPONSE OF THE AGING HEART TO EXERCISE

Although many aspects of cardiovascular performance are well preserved at rest in older adults, aging has important effects on cardiovascular performance during exercise. The decline in aerobic capacity with age in individuals with no evidence of cardiovascular disease is attributable in part to peripheral factors, such as increased body fat, reduced muscle mass, and a decline in O_2 extraction with age.[35,36] However, there is strong evidence that age-associated changes in the cardiovascular system also help reduce exercise capacity in older individuals. Studies have shown that the VO_{2max}, which is the maximum amount of oxygen that a person can use during exercise, declines progressively with age, starting in early adulthood.[2,35,36] Age-related changes in maximum heart rate, cardiac output, and stroke volume described below compromise delivery of blood to the muscles during exercise and contribute to this decline in VO_{2max} in aging.

The maximum heart rate attained during exercise declines gradually with age in humans, a fact well known by widely distributed posters commonly seen in exercise facilities.[2,37] Several mechanisms have been implicated in the reduction in maximum heart rate during exercise in aging. One mechanism involves a decrease in the sensitivity of the aging myocardium to sympathetic stimulation. Normally, the sympathetic nervous system becomes activated during exercise and releases catecholamines (noradrenaline and adrenaline) to act on β-adrenergic receptors in the heart. This β-adrenergic stimulation leads to an increase in heart rate and augments the force of contraction of the heart. However, it is well established that the responsiveness of the heart to β-adrenergic stimulation declines with age.[21,37] This is thought to be due to the high circulating levels of noradrenaline present in older adults.[37] These high levels of catecholamines in older adults arise from a decrease in plasma clearance of noradrenaline and an increase in the spillover of catecholamines from various organ systems, including the heart, into the circulation.[2,37] Chronic exposure to high levels of catecholamines is thought to desensitize elements of the β-adrenergic receptor signaling cascade in the aging heart and limit the rise in heart rate during exercise.[21,37] These age-dependent changes are thought to impair the response of the heart to sympathetic stimulation during exercise.

The lower maximal heart rates during exercise have a major impact on the response of the aging cardiovascular system to exercise. Both heart rate and stroke volume are important determinants of cardiac output. Therefore, a lower maximum heart rate during exercise would be expected to have an impact on cardiac output during exercise in older adults. Although this has not been extensively investigated, there is evidence that cardiac output during exercise is lower in older adults compared with their younger counterparts.[2] This lower cardiac output during exercise is not attributable to age-associated alterations in stroke volume.[2] However, reduced responsiveness to β-adrenergic receptor stimulation in the heart may limit the increase in myocardial contractility in response to exercise in older adults.[2,37] These changes in cardiovascular function in aging are thought to be mitigated by an increase in left ventricular end-diastolic volume during exercise in older adults.[2] This increases the amount of blood in the ventricle at the end of diastole and increases the stretch on the heart. It is well established that an increase in the amount of blood in the ventricle at the end of diastole results in an increase in the strength of contraction of the heart, a property known as the Frank-Starling mechanism. Thus, an increase in reliance on the Frank-Starling mechanism may at least partially compensate for the decrease in heart rate and contractility during exercise in aging.[2]

Although a decrease in cardiovascular performance and an increase in susceptibility to cardiovascular diseases are inevitable consequences of aging, there is evidence that regular exercise has numerous beneficial effects on the aging cardiovascular system. Endurance exercise blunts the decline in VO_{2max} that occurs as a consequence of the aging process.[35] Also, the age-associated decline in cardiac output can be partially overcome by regular aerobic training.[35] However, endurance training does not modify the age-related decline in maximal heart rate during exercise.[35] This might occur because exercise increases the levels of circulating catecholamines, which have been implicated in the decline in maximal heart rate in older adults, as discussed earlier.[2,35] Regular endurance exercise also attenuates the increased arterial stiffness that is observed in central elastic arteries from sedentary older adults and protects the heart from the age-dependent increase in fibrosis and apoptosis.[38-40] Finally, habitual aerobic exercise can protect the aging heart from detrimental effects of cardiovascular diseases such as myocardial ischemia.[41] Therefore, there is good evidence that exercise can mitigate at least some of the detrimental effects of age on the cardiovascular system. The major age-related changes in the heart and the clinical consequences of these changes are summarized in Table 16-2.

TABLE 16-2 Age-Related Changes in the Heart

Age-Associated Changes in the Heart	Clinical Consequences
↑ Collagen, changes in elastin, ↑ left ventricular wall thickness	Impairs passive left ventricle filling
↑ Left ventricular stiffness, prolonged availability of intracellular calcium	Promotes diastolic dysfunction, predisposes towards HFpEF
Left atrial fibrosis and hypertrophy	↑ Susceptibility to atrial arrhythmias
↓ Sensitivity to β-adrenergic receptor stimulation	Impaired ability to ↑ heart rate and contractility in exercise

SUMMARY

There are prominent changes in the structure and function of the vasculature and myocardium in older adults when compared to younger adults. These changes are apparent, even in the absence of risk factors other than age and in the absence of overt cardiovascular disease. Nevertheless, age-dependent remodeling of the vasculature and the heart may render the cardiovascular system more susceptible to the detrimental effects of cardiovascular disease.

KEY POINTS: EFFECTS OF AGING ON THE CARDIOVASCULAR SYSTEM

- The structure and function of the human heart and vasculature change as a function of the normal aging process.
- The age-associated increase in stiffness of central elastic arteries promotes systolic hypertension in older adults.
- Diastolic dysfunction in the aging heart arises from impaired left ventricular filling, increased afterload, and prolonged availability of intracellular calcium and can promote HFpEF.
- Decreased responsiveness to β-adrenergic receptor stimulation limits the increase in heart rate and contractility in response to exercise in older adults.
- Despite limits on the ability of the aging cardiovascular system to respond to exercise, regular exercise attenuates the adverse effects of aging on the heart and vasculature and protects against the development of cardiovascular disease in older adults.

For a complete list of references, please visit www.expertconsult.com.

KEY REFERENCES

1. Collins JA, Munoz JV, Patel TR, et al: The anatomy of the ageing aorta. Clin Anat 27:463–466, 2014.
2. Fleg JL, Strait J: Age-associated changes in cardiovascular structure and function: a fertile milieu for future disease. Heart Fail Rev 17:545–554, 2012.
3. Lakatta EG, Wang M, Najjar SS: Arterial ageing and subclinical arterial disease are fundamentally intertwined at macroscopic and molecular levels. Med Clin North Am 93:583–604, 2009.
5. Strait JB, Lakatta EG: Ageing-associated cardiovascular changes and their relationship to heart failure. Heart Fail Clin 8:143–164, 2012.
8. Najjar SS, Scuteri A, Lakatta EG: Arterial ageing: is it an immutable cardiovascular risk factor? Hypertension 46:454–462, 2005.
12. Sethi S, Rivera O, Oliveros R, et al: Aortic stiffness: pathophysiology, clinical implications, and approach to treatment. Integr Blood Press Control 7:29–34, 2014.
14. Lee HY, Oh BH: Ageing and arterial stiffness. Circ J 74:2257–2262, 2010.
15. Lim MA, Townsend RR: Arterial compliance in the elderly: its effect on blood pressure measurement and cardiovascular outcomes. Clin Geriatr Med 25:191–205, 2009.
16. Izzo JL, Jr: Arterial stiffness and the systolic hypertension syndrome. Curr Opin Cardiol 19:341–352, 2004.
21. Lakatta EG, Levy D: Arterial and cardiac ageing: major shareholders in cardiovascular disease enterprises: part II: the ageing heart in health: links to heart disease. Circulation 107:346–354, 2003.
27. Parks RJ, Fares E, Macdonald JK, et al: A procedure for creating a frailty index based on deficit accumulation in ageing mice. J Gerontol A Biol Sci Med Sci 67:217–227, 2012.
28. Chen W, Frangogiannis NG: The role of inflammatory and fibrogenic pathways in heart failure associated with ageing. Heart Fail Rev 15:415–422, 2010.
29. Dun W, Boyden PA: Aged atria: electrical remodeling conducive to atrial fibrillation. J Interv Card Electrophysiol 25:9–18, 2009.
31. Howlett SE, Rockwood K: New horizons in frailty: ageing and the deficit-scaling problem. Age Ageing 42:416–423, 2013.
32. Loffredo FS, Nikolova AP, Pancoast JR, et al: Heart failure with preserved ejection fraction: molecular pathways of the aging myocardium. Circ Res 115:97–107, 2014.
33. Feridooni HA, Dibb KM, Howlett SE: How cardiomyocyte excitation, calcium release and contraction become altered with age. J Mol Cell Cardiol 83:62–72, 2015.
34. Kaila K, Haykowsky MJ, Thompson RB, et al: Heart failure with preserved ejection fraction in the elderly: scope of the problem. Heart Fail Rev 17:555–562, 2012.
35. Goldspink DF: Ageing and activity: their effects on the functional reserve capacities of the heart and vascular smooth and skeletal muscles. Ergonomics 48:1334–1351, 2005.
36. Tanaka H, Seals DR: Endurance exercise performance in Masters athletes: age-associated changes and underlying physiological mechanisms. J Physiol 586:55–63, 2008.
37. Ferrara N, Komici K, Corbi G, et al: β-Adrenergic receptor responsiveness in aging heart and clinical implications. Front Physiol 4:396, 2014.

17 Age-Related Changes in the Respiratory System

Gwyneth A. Davies, Charlotte E. Bolton

RESPIRATORY FUNCTION TESTS

The commonly used respiratory function tests are presented in this chapter. In addition, patterns of lung function abnormality seen in some of the common types of condition are also presented. Breathing parameters include the following:

- Forced expiratory volume (L) in 1 second, FEV_1. This is the volume of air expired during the first second of a forced expiratory maneuver from vital capacity (maximal inspiration); it is measured by spirometry.
- Forced vital capacity (L), FVC. This is the total volume of air expired during forced expiration from the end of maximum inspiration. A slow vital capacity (SVC) is the volume of air expired, but this time through an unforced maneuver. In the young, these are similar, but in emphysema, where there is loss of elastic recoil, FVC may fall disproportionately more than SVC. These are also measured by spirometry.
- Peak expiratory flow rate (L/min), PEFR. This is the maximal expiratory flow rate measured using a peak flow meter, a more portable method; therefore, serial home measurements may be performed by patients.

The following parameters require more detailed lung physiology testing:

- Total lung capacity (L), TLC. This is the volume of air contained in the lung at the end of maximal inspiration; it is measured by helium dilution or body plethysmography together with the next two tests.
- Functional residual capacity (L), FRC. This is the amount of air left in the lungs after a tidal breath out and indicates the amount of air that stays in the lungs during normal breathing.
- Residual volume (L), RV. This is the amount of air left in the lungs after a maximal exhalation. Not all the air in the lungs can ever be expired.
- Transfer factor (mmol/min), TL_{CO}. This is a measure of the ability of the lung to oxygenate hemoglobin. It is usually measured with a single breath hold technique using low-concentration carbon monoxide.
- Transfer coefficient (mmol/min/k/Pa/L_{BTPS}), K_{CO}. This is the TL_{CO} corrected for the lung volume.

In addition, blood gas measurements are often performed to assess acid-base balance and oxygenation. The most important measures for respiratory disease are the partial pressure of oxygen (PaO_2), partial pressure of carbon dioxide ($PaCO_2$), and the pH. A low PaO_2 (hypoxemia) with a normal $PaCO_2$ indicates type I respiratory failure. An increased $PaCO_2$ with hypoxemia indicates type II respiratory failure. A rapidly rising $PaCO_2$ will result in a fall in the pH—for example, that seen in an acute exacerbation of chronic obstructive pulmonary disease (COPD). Renal compensation occurs in response to a chronically high $PaCO_2$, with correction of the pH to normal or near-normal levels, but this renal compensation takes several days to occur. Hyperventilation, associated with excess expiration of CO_2, as seen in anxiety attacks but also in altered respiratory control such as Cheyne-Stokes respiration, will result in an increase in pH as a result of a drop in $PaCO_2$. Pure anxiety-related hyperventilation will not cause hypoxemia but other causes for this altered respiratory control may cause hypoxemia.

There are two main characteristic patterns of respiratory disease based on spirometric evaluation, the obstructive and restrictive patterns.

An obstructive pattern is seen in several situations including in patients with asthma and COPD. It is characterized by the following:

- Reduced FEV_1 and PEFR
- Normal or reduced FVC (if FVC is reduced, it is disproportionately less reduced than FEV_1)
- Reduced FEV_1/FVC ratio

A restrictive pattern is characterized by the following:

- Reduced FEV_1
- Reduced FVC
- Normal or high FEV_1/FVC ratio

Conditions relating to both these spirometric patterns, with more detail about lung function patterns and the use of other lung physiology parameters to characterize and diagnose conditions, will be discussed elsewhere in this text.

AGE-RELATED CHANGES IN THE RESPIRATORY SYSTEM

Lungs age over a lifetime but there is, in addition, an accumulation of environmental insults to which an individual has been exposed, given that the lungs have direct contact with the atmosphere. The key exposure is smoking in the form of direct smoke but also second-hand passive smoking, the impact of which has been increasingly recognized.[1,2] A quantitative evaluation of a person's smoking habit is usually classed in relation to the number of pack-years (e.g., 20 cigarettes/day =1 pack/day; for 10 years, this equates to a 10-pack-year history).

Oxidative stress is an important mechanism of lung function decline, with oxidants both from cigarette smoke and other causes of airway inflammation.[3,4] Oxidants and the subsequent release of reactive oxygen species (ROS) lead to the reduction and inactivation of proteinase inhibitors, epithelial permeability, and enhanced nuclear factor κB (NF-κB), which promotes cytokine production and, in a cyclic fashion, is capable of recruiting more neutrophils. There is also plasma leakage, bronchoconstriction through elevated isoprostanes levels, and increased mucus secretion. The lung has its own defensive enzymatic antioxidants, such as superoxide dismutase (SOD), which degrades superoxide anion and catalase, and glutathione (GSH), which inactivates hydrogen peroxide and hydroperoxidases. Both are found intracellularly and extracellularly. In addition there are nonenzymatic factors that act as antioxidants, such as vitamins C and E, β-carotene, uric acid, bilirubin, and flavonoids.[5]

There has been a renewed interest in the effect of critical early life periods determining peak lung function and the subsequent "knock-on" effect on the adult and older adult's lungs. If peak lung function reserve is not attained, then even the natural trajectory of decline may lead to symptomatic lung impairment in midlife or later life. Such factors in early life would include premature birth, asthma, environmental exposure, nutrition, and respiratory infection.[6,7] In addition, the effects of environmental pollution, nutrition, respiratory infections, and physical inactivity on lung function decline have been reported.[8,9] The mechanisms affecting respiratory function are likely to be multiple and cumulative. Interestingly, in the Inuit community, where their lifestyle has gradually become more westernized—and with a reduction in fishing and hunting activities and the community developing a more sedentary lifestyle—there has been acceleration in age-related lung function decline.[10]

In the aging lung, there are structural and functional changes within the respiratory system and, in addition, immune-mediated and extrapulmonary alterations. These are discussed in detail in this chapter.

Structural Changes

There are three main structural changes in the aging lung—altered lung parenchyma and subsequent loss of elastic recoil, stiffening of the lung (reduced chest wall compliance), and the respiratory muscles.

The main change is the loss in the alveolar surface area as the alveoli and alveolar ducts enlarge. There is little alteration to the bronchi. The small airways suffer qualitative changes far more than quantitative changes in the supporting elastin and collagen, with disruption to fibers and loss of elasticity leading to the subsequent dilation of alveolar ducts and air spaces, known as senile emphysema. The alveolar surface area may drop by as much as 20%. This leads to an increased tendency for small airways to collapse during expiration because of the loss of surface tension forces.[11] In a healthy older individual, this is probably of little or no significance, but reduction in their reserve may unearth difficulties during an infection or superadded respiratory complication. Amyloid deposition in the lung vasculature and alveolar septae occurs in older adults, although its relevance is unclear. Within the large airways, with aging, there is a reduction in the number of glandular epithelial cells, resulting in a reduced production of mucus and thus impairing the respiratory defense against infection.

Chest wall compliance is decreased in older adults. Contributing to this increasing stiffness of the lungs are loss of intervertebral disc space, ossification of the costal cartilages, and calcification of the rib articulatory surfaces, which combine with muscle changes to produce impaired mobility of the thoracic cage. In addition to these, additional insults from osteoporosis leading to vertebral collapse have been shown to result in a 10% reduction in FVC,[12] probably through developing kyphosis and increased anterior-posterior diameter—the barrel chest. Such vertebral collapse is frequently found in older adults, increasing with age, if determined through appropriate imaging. These structural alterations lead to suboptimal force mechanics of the diaphragm and increasing chest wall stiffness. Rib fractures, again common in older adults, may further limit respiratory movements.

The predominant respiratory muscle is the diaphragm, making up about 85% of respiratory muscle activity, with the intercostal, anterior abdominal, and accessory muscles also contributing. The accessory muscles are used by splinting of the arms, a feature commonly associated with the emphysematous COPD patient. Inspiration leading to chest expansion is brought about by these muscles contracting, whereas expiration is a passive phenomenon. The accessory muscles are used when there is increased ventilatory demand, such as in the COPD patient. The respiratory muscles are made up of type I (slow), type IIa (fast fatigue-resistant), and type IIx (fast fatigable) fibers. The difference in the muscle fibers is based on the aerobic capacity and adenosine triphosphate (ATP) activity of the myofibrils and confers differing physiologic properties. The major age-related change in the respiratory muscles is a reduction in the proportion of type IIa fibers, which thus impairs strength and endurance.[13] An increasing reliance on the diaphragm due to loss of intercostal muscle strength and the less advantageous diaphragmatic position to generate force add to breathlessness. Globally, there is reduced muscle myosin production, and this is likely to confer a disadvantage to the respiratory muscles also. Comorbid conditions, such as COPD and congestive heart failure, are associated with altered muscle structure and function, as is poor nutrition.[14-16] Physical deconditioning and sarcopenia, hormone imbalance, and vitamin D deficiency will exacerbate the age-related lung structural changes; the body becomes less adaptive to the respiratory limitations. Medications, especially oral corticosteroids, may cause problems, particularly with regard to respiratory and peripheral muscle strength. Acute infection puts added demands on the respiratory system and may expose the limited respiratory reserve.

Age-Related Functional Changes

Both FEV_1 and FVC decrease with age. Flow within the airways also falls. The ratio of FEV_1 to FVC decreases annually as a result of a greater reduction in the FEV_1 parameter relative to FVC with time. For this reason, it has been proposed to consider an abnormal ratio as being less than the lower limit of normal (lower than the fifth percentile of healthy subjects, determined by using equations that take into account age, height, gender, and ethnicity) as opposed to a fixed ratio of a less than 0.7 ratio.[17] A fixed ratio will overdiagnose airflow obstruction in older adults.

The TLC does not change significantly with age because the loss of elastic recoil and increased elastic load of the chest wall counteract each other. The RV and FRC increase due to reduced elastic recoil, causing the premature closure of the airways and stiffness of the chest wall. The older adult thus breathes at a higher lung volume, placing additional burden on the respiratory muscles, and has a higher energy expenditure of up to 120% that of a young adult. The closing volume is the lung volume at which the dependent airways begin to close during expiration. This is increased in older adults because of a lack of support and tethering of the terminal airways by collagen and elastin and may lead to closure during normal tidal breathing,[18] leading to a ventilation-perfusion (V/Q) mismatch that may be responsible for lower resting arterial oxygen tensions.[17] Although arterial oxygen tensions tend to be lower in older adults, unless there is coexistent respiratory disease, the PaO_2 is sufficient for adequate hemoglobin saturation. There is reduced gas transfer (TL_{CO}) because of the structural changes and V/Q mismatch. In addition, there is a reduction in pulmonary capillary blood volume and density of the capillaries.

The impaired respiratory muscle strength and endurance may be of little or no functional significance in the healthy older adult, but may lead to impaired reserve to combat respiratory challenges consequent to acute respiratory disease. Measures of respiratory muscle strength, such as the maximal inspiratory pressure (MIP), maximal expiratory pressure (MEP), and sniff nasal inspiratory pressure (SNIP), fall with age.[14]

In older adults, there are alterations in the regulation and control of breathing. Older adults breathe with a similar minute ventilation as younger subjects but at a smaller tidal volume and higher respiratory frequency. A blunted response to hypoxia and hypercapnia has been reported,[19-21] with Poulin[22] demonstrating impaired response to hypoxia during sustained hypercapnia. Older adults show an increased ventilatory response to exercise,[20] which may be more pronounced in men.[23] Maximal oxygen uptake (VO_{2max}) declines with age, with a parallel decline in exercise capacity, having reached a peak as a young adult. This is due to a combination of cardiovascular (such as reduced cardiac output) and respiratory causes, including V/Q mismatch. The decline in maximal oxygen uptake with age can be attenuated to some degree by maintaining regular exercise.[24,25]

Older adults are less able to perceive acute bronchoconstriction objectively.[26,27] Moreover, airway β_2-adrenoceptor responsiveness is reduced in old age, as evidenced by impaired responses to β-agonists in healthy older adults.[28] Altered chemoreceptor sensitivity to hypoxia, reduced ability to perceive elastic loads on inspiration or expiration, impaired perception of tactile sensation and joint movement, or age-associated central processing abnormalities may all be contributing factors.[29,30] Subsequently, this is likely to mask deteriorating respiratory symptoms and may delay presentation to health care services.

Sleep-disordered breathing is more common in healthy older adults,[31] yet older subjects appear less likely to seek medical review or have the sleep disorder diagnosed due to a high prevalence of tiredness, fatigue, and snoring in this age group, generally along with concurrent other medical illness and the use of sedating medications, including benzodiazepines. Cerebrovascular disease is associated with sleep-disordered breathing,[32] and obstructive sleep apnea in stroke patients is a predictor of death.[33] There is increased upper airway resistance in older adults, with a reduced respiratory effort to try and overcome this obstruction. There is a high prevalence of sleep-disordered breathing in patients with congestive heart failure,[34] and it is said to be greater in patients with Alzheimer disease,[35] both of which have become increasingly prevalent in older adults. In addition, and conversely, sleep-disordered breathing can contribute to cardiovascular disease and impaired cognitive function.[36,37]

Effects of Aging on Pulmonary Host Defense and Immune Response

The immune system is described as comprising two separate but interacting components. Innate immunity is the rapid nonspecific system that functions as the first line of defense against invading microorganisms. Adaptive (or acquired) immunity, mediated by B and T lymphocytes, is antigen-specific and involves the development of memory cells, allowing a future antigen-specific response. There is impaired immune function in older adults, both of the innate and adaptive components.

Aging leads to breakdown of the mucosal barrier of the lung and reduced mucociliary clearance enabling invasion by pathogenic organisms. In the aged lung, the innate immune system is increasingly challenged by greater contact with pathogens and cumulative exposure to environmental insults, such as smoking. Aging-related changes in human lung innate immunity have a similar pattern to those seen in COPD.[38] There is impaired chemotaxis and phagocytosis, reduced superoxide generation, and reduced bactericidal activity of neutrophils.[39] Dendritic cells are less efficient at antigen presentation. In addition, although the number of natural killer (NK) cells increases with advanced age, there is a reduction in NK cytotoxicity.[40] In vitro evidence has suggested that macrophage function is impaired with age, with a reduced capacity to generate ROS and proinflammatory cytokines, and reduced expression of certain pattern recognition receptors, such as Toll-like receptors.[41,42]

Healthy older adults have been shown to demonstrate a hyperinflammatory state, so-called inflamm-aging.[43] This is associated with increased circulating proinflammatory cytokines, such as interleukin-6 (IL-6), tumor necrosis factor (TNF), IL-1β, prostaglandin E_2, and antiinflammatory mediators, including soluble TNF receptors, IL-1 receptor antagonists, and acute phase proteins (e.g., C-reactive protein, serum amyloid A). This progressive proinflammatory state affects the phenotype and function of cells in the aged lung and contributes to a poorer outcome when host defenses are challenged. Alterations in cell-mediated adaptive immunity include atrophy of the thymus together with aging in the T cell pool, including altered memory T cell function and a shift from a TH1 to TH2 profile.[41] There is a reduction in naïve T lymphocyte production and absolute numbers of $CD3^+$, $CD4^+$, and $CD8^+$ T cells. Other changes include a smaller T cell receptor repertoire and reduced proliferative responses to antigens, which has implications with respect to reduced efficacy of vaccinations in older immune systems. A decrease in B cell numbers, impaired production of memory B cells, and reduced antibody responses affect humoral immunity in older adults.

Immunosenescence explains a large part of the increased susceptibility to lower respiratory tract infection in older adults, with impaired neutrophil migration likely to play a role. However, causes that contribute to pneumonia risk in this population are multifactorial. Bacterial colonization of the upper respiratory tract is not uncommon in older adults.[43] This may be associated with colonization of the stomach, which itself is more common in old age and may be preceded by antacids or H_2 blockers.[44,45] The older person with swallowing difficulties, particularly in association with cerebrovascular disease and other neurologic diseases with associated cognitive impairment, is more prone to aspiration. Similarly, tracheal intubation or the presence of nasogastric tubes increases aspiration risk. Malnutrition and the presence of chronic disease such as diabetes or renal failure will also contribute to pneumonia susceptibility. An age-related decline in immune function leads to a reduced response to vaccination, including influenza vaccination and increased susceptibility to respiratory infection and pneumonia.

In conclusion, there are structural and functional changes in the lungs, together with alterations in the control of breathing and more general immunologic alterations, in older adults. The changes are not just a direct consequence of age but are also affected by environmental exposures and coexistent comorbidities.

KEY POINTS: AGE-RELATED CHANGES IN THE RESPIRATORY SYSTEM

- There are both age-related changes and true aging changes in the respiratory system.
- Most of the available information comes from cross-sectional studies rather than longitudinal studies.
- There are structural and functional changes to the lung in the elderly. In addition, there are alterations to respiratory control and immunologic alterations that can all contribute to age-related changes of the respiratory system. Such alterations may be synergistic.
- The proinflammatory state of "inflamm-aging" affects the phenotype and function of cells in the aged lung and contributes to a poorer outcome when host defenses are challenged.
- Exercise exerts additional demands on the respiratory system that may reveal respiratory limitation. Further, although alterations in the respiratory system may not be apparent in the healthy elderly person, acute illness may unearth the diminished respiratory reserve.
- Elderly people are less able to perceive bronchoconstriction and other symptoms. In parallel, there is thus relative underreporting of symptoms.

For a complete list of references, please visit www.expertconsult.com

KEY REFERENCES

1. Griffith KA, Sherrill DL, Siegel EM, et al: Predictors of loss of lung function in the elderly: the cardiovascular health study. Am J Respir Crit Care Med 163:61–68, 2001.
8. Pelkonen M, Notkola I, Lakka T, et al: Delaying decline in pulmonary function with physical activity: a 25-year follow-up. Am J Respir Crit Care Med 168:494–499, 2003.
10. Rode A, Shepherd RJ: The ageing of lung function: cross-sectional and longitudinal studies of an Inuit community. Eur Respir J 9:1653–1659, 1994.
11. Verbeken EK, Cauberghs M, Mertens I, et al: The senile lung: comparison with normal and emphysematous lungs. 1: structural aspects. Chest 101:793–799, 1992.

12. Leech JA, Dullberg C, Kellie S, et al: Relationship of lung function to severity of osteoporosis in women. Am Rev Respir Dis 141:68–71, 1990.
19. Kronenberg RS, Drage CW: Attenuation of the ventilatory and heart responses to hypoxia and hypercapnia with ageing in normal men. J Clin Invest 52:1812–1819, 1973.
21. García-Río F, Villamor A, Gómez-Mendieta A, et al: The progressive effects of ageing on chemosensitivity in healthy subjects. Respir Med 101:2192–2198, 2007.
27. Killian KJ, Watson R, Otis J, et al: Symptom perception during acute bronchoconstriction. Am J Respir Crit Care Med 162:490–496, 2000.
36. Dealberto M, Pajot N, Courbon D, et al: Breathing disorders during sleep and cognitive performance in an older community sample: the EVA study. J Am Geriatr Soc 44:1287–1294, 1996.
37. Golbin JM, Somers VK, Caples SM: Obstructive sleep apnea, cardiovascular disease, and pulmonary hypertension. Proc Am Thorac Soc 5:200–206, 2008.
38. Shaykhiev R, Crystal RG: Innate immunity and chronic obstructive pulmonary disease: a mini-review. Gerontology 59:481–489, 2013.
39. Gomez CR, Boehmer ED, Kovacs EJ: The aging innate immune system. Curr Opin Immunol 17:457–462, 2005.
42. Meyer KC: The role of immunity and inflammation in lung senescence and susceptibility to infection in the elderly. Semin Respir Crit Care Med 31:561–4374, 2010.
43. Franceschi C, Bonafe M, Valensin S, et al: Inflamm-aging. An evolutionary perspective on immunosenescence. Ann N Y Acad Sci 908:244–254, 2000.

18 Neurologic Signs in Older Adults

James E. Galvin

Neurologic disorders are a common cause of morbidity, mortality, institutionalization, and increased health care costs in the older adult population.[1] Not only does advancing age increase the frequency and severity of neurologic disease, but it may also play an important role in modifying disease presentation. Although physical difficulties can occur independently of cognitive decline, physical difficulties coexist with cognitive impairment in many seniors.[2] Data from the Behavioral Risk Factor Surveillance System have suggested that cognitive impairment is present in 12.7% of individuals aged 60 years and older.[3] Of these, 35.2% also report physical functional difficulties. Having cognitive and physical functional impairment may be particularly taxing on the affected individuals and their caregivers. Thus, the geriatric neurologic examination is a critical part of any encounter with older adults but can be challenging, even for the most experienced clinicians. Normal aging may be associated with the loss of normal neurologic signs or the exaggeration of others. It may be associated with the appearance of findings considered abnormal in younger patients or the reappearance of physical signs usually seen in infancy and early stages of development.

The geriatric neurologic examination is also frequently influenced by the involvement of other systems (e.g., endocrinologic or rheumatologic disease), the co-occurrence of multiple chronic conditions in a single patient, and the presentation of nonneurologic disorders (e.g., myocardial infarction, urinary tract infection, fecal impaction) as neurologic signs (e.g., gait difficulty, confusion). When establishing a neurologic diagnosis, the clinical history—history of the present illness, past medical history, social habits, occupational experience, family history, and review of systems and medications—assists the clinician in generating a differential diagnosis that can be further explored and refined by pertinent observations documented on the mental status and neurologic examinations. Therefore, it is important to appreciate the multitude of age-related changes in the central and peripheral nervous systems (Box 18-1).

MENTAL STATUS

Because the frequency of cognitive disorders increases dramatically with advancing age, examination of mental status is one of the most important components of the neurologic examination. Unfortunately, it is often one of the more time-consuming parts of the examination and can be difficult to interpret, particularly in new patients for whom no baseline performance data exist. In general, the fund of knowledge and vocabulary continues to expand throughout life, and learning ability does not appreciably decline in older adults without a neurocognitive disorder. Cognitive changes associated with normal aging include decreases in processing speed, cognitive flexibility, visuospatial perception (often in conjunction with decreased visual acuity), working memory, and sustained attention.[4] Other cognitive abilities such as access to remotely learned information and retention of encoded new information appear to be spared in aging, allowing their use as sensitive indicators for disease processes.[3]

Crystallized intelligence characterized by practical problem solving, knowledge gained from experience, and vocabulary tends to be cumulative and does not generally decline with aging.[5] On the other hand, fluid intelligence characterized by the ability to acquire and use new information, as measured by solutions to abstract problems and speeded performance (e.g., performance on the Raven's Progressive Matrices and Digit Symbol of the Wechsler Adult Intelligence Scale) has been shown to decline gradually with aging.[6]

Longitudinal studies of memory and aging demonstrate considerable variability of cognitive abilities between different individuals (interindividual variability) as well as of different cognitive domains within the same individual (intraindividual variability).[7] At least part of this variability may be attributed to different study designs; however, it is very important to take the intraindividual and interindividual variability into consideration when defining neuropsychological norms for older adults to ensure that clinical samples are not contaminated by individuals with mild forms of cognitive impairment. Some authors have suggested that age-weighted rather than age-corrected norms for cognition should be used, whereas other investigators have stressed the influence of other factors such as culture, experience, educational background, and motor speed on cognitive performance. For example, whereas older adults generally perform less well on the verbal and performance subtests of the Wechsler Adult Intelligence Scale compared with young adults, these differences are minimized when corrected for motor slowing and educational level. Other situational factors that may affect individual performance on cognitive tasks include fatigue, emotional status, medications, and stress. Moreover, it may be very difficult to attribute impaired cognition to aging in the presence of underlying conditions such as depression, dementia, and delirium, all of which are common, and often unrecognized, in the older adult population.[8]

The elements of a comprehensive mental status examination include the assessment of cognitive, functional, and behavioral domains. The initial contact with the patient affords the opportunity to assess whether a cognitive, attention, affective, or language disorder is present. If available, questioning of an informant may reveal changes in cognition, function, and behavior of which the patient is not aware or denies.

Screening for cognitive disorders in the older adult may include performance and informant measures. Examples of brief tests of mental status include the Mini-Mental State Examination,[9] Mini-Cog,[10] and Montreal Cognitive Assessment.[11] Decrements in cognitive ability are compared to published norms, often adjusted for age and education. Examples of brief informant assessments include the AD8[12] and Informant Questionnaire on Cognitive Decline in the Elderly.[13] These scales detect intraindividual decline by comparing current performance on cognitive and functional tasks to prior levels of performance, although patients may perform differently, depending on the level of impairment.[14] Combining performance and informant measures may increase the likelihood of detecting cognitive disorders.[15]

CRANIAL NERVE FUNCTION

Smell and Taste

Normal aging is associated with decrements in olfaction at threshold and suprathreshold concentrations. Older adults also have a reduced capacity to discriminate the degree of differences between odors of different qualities and have impaired performance on tasks that require odor identification.[16] Impaired olfaction with aging may be due to structural and functional changes

BOX 18-1 Neurologic Changes Associated With Normal Aging

- Psychomotor slowing
- Decreased visual acuity
- Smaller pupil size
- Decreased ability to look upward
- Decreased auditory acuity, especially for spoken language
- Decreased muscle bulk
- Mild motor slowing
- Decreased vibratory sensation
- Mild swaying on Romberg test
- Mild lordosis and restriction of movement in neck and back
- Depression of Achilles tendon reflex

in the upper airway, olfactory epithelium, olfactory bulb, or olfactory nerves.[17] It is important to recognize that although impaired smell can be associated with aging, it can also be the result of medications, viral infections, and head trauma. Moreover, there appears to be early involvement of olfactory pathways in neurodegenerative diseases such as Alzheimer disease (neurofibrillary tangles)[18] and Parkinson disease (Lewy bodies).[19] Taste, which in turn is greatly dependent on olfaction, also decreases with advanced age, with a reduced sensitivity for a broad range of tastes compared to young adults.[20,21] Although the number of taste buds does not seem to be significantly decreased in older adults, some studies have suggested decreased responses in electrophysiologic recordings from taste buds. A number of other factors, such as medications, smoking, alcohol, head injuries, and dentures, may contribute to decreased taste and smell.

Vision

Age-related changes have been documented in visual acuity, visual fields, depth perception, contrast sensitivity, motion perception, and perception of self-motion in relation to external space (optical flow). Visual acuity declines due to a number of ophthalmologic (e.g., cataracts, glaucoma) and neurologic (e.g., macular degeneration) causes. Pupillary size is typically smaller with age, and pupils are less reactive to light and accommodation, forcing many older adults to use glasses for reading.[4] There is also a restriction in eye movement in upward gaze. Anatomic and physiologic studies have demonstrated a gradual decline in photoreceptors after the age of 20 years, resulting in decreased visual acuity in older adults.[22,23] This is especially apparent in conditions with low contrast and luminance. There is also age-related impairment in accommodation, which leads to farsightedness (presbyopia) and a decrease in accommodation due to rigidity of the lens.[24] Relaxation and accommodation times increase progressively and peak around the age of 50 years. Therefore, many older adults are forced to use glasses for reading. Moreover, ophthalmologic conditions such as cataracts, glaucoma, and macular degeneration occur commonly with advancing age and contribute significantly to the decreased visual acuity seen with aging.

Pupillary abnormalities can also been seen with normal aging. These include smaller pupils (senile miosis), which may be due to decreased preganglionic sympathetic tone, sluggish reaction to light, and decrease or even loss of the near or accommodation response.

Age-associated changes in extraocular motility include decreased velocity of saccades, prolonged latency, decreased accuracy, and prolonged duration and reaction time.[25] There is also an age-related limitation of upgaze, but not downgaze, slowing of smooth pursuits. and impaired visual tracking.[26] Vertical gaze changes begin in middle age and decline in the upward plane from 40 degrees between the ages of 5 and 14 years to 16 degrees between the ages of 75 and 84 years.[27,28] Vertical gaze palsy is an important consideration in the evaluation of driving abilities in older adults (street signs, traffic lights). Other changes of eye movements with aging include loss of the Bell phenomenon—upward and outward deviation of the eyes in response to attempted forced closure of the eyelids.

Hearing and Vestibular Function

Gradual loss of cochlear hair cells, atrophy of the stria vascularis, and thickening of the basement membrane may account for the impaired hearing commonly seen with aging. This is often referred to as presbycusis and predominantly affects higher frequencies.[29,30] Other changes include impaired speech discrimination, increase in pure tone threshold averages (approximately 2 dB/year), and decreased discrimination scores.[31] Vestibular function may also be affected with age.[32] There is a decrease in vestibulospinal reflexes and in the ability to detect head position and motion in space. These may be secondary to loss of hair cells and nerve fibers, as well as neuronal loss in the medial, lateral, and inferior vestibular nucleus in the brainstem.[26]

MOTOR FUNCTION

There is a progressive decline in muscle bulk associated with aging, sometimes referred to as sarcopenia. This is most obvious in the intrinsic muscles in the hands and feet, particularly the dorsal interossei and thenar muscles, as well as around the shoulder cap (deltoid and rotator cuff muscles).[4] Atrophy of the thenar muscles, without weakness or fasciculations, may be present in over 50% of older adult patients.[33] Results of different longitudinal studies have been inconsistent regarding the predominant fiber type affected by aging, with reports of loss of type IIb (fast twitch) fibers, reduction in the percentage of type 1 fibers, with no change in type I or II mean fiber area, decrease in the capillary-to-fiber ratio, and increase in the percentage of type I fibers.[34] The decrease in muscle mass is associated with electrophysiologic evidence of denervation and muscle fiber atrophy.[35] However, the consistent presence of fasciculations is not a normal sign of aging and, if present, should warrant a search for pathologic causes (e.g., motor neuron disease, compressive cervical myelopathy, multifocal motor neuropathy). A decrease in muscle strength often accompanies the decrease in muscle bulk,[36] with up to a 50% decrease in maximal voluntary contraction force and twitch tension in the quadriceps. Hand grip strength decreases significantly after the age of 50 years, but strength in the arms and shoulders does not change until after the age of 60. Weakening of abdominal muscles may accentuate lumbar lordosis and contribute to low back pain.[4]

In addition to motor bulk and strength, there also appears to be loss of speed and coordination of movement with aging.[37] Speed of hand and foot tapping was reduced by 20% in one study, and a mild terminal tremor, mild bradykinesia, rigidity, and mild dysmetria on finger-nose and heel-shin testing can also be found in isolation in up to 40% of older adults. In one study of 467 patients, the prevalence of parkinsonian signs defined as the presence of signs of two or more categories (rigidity, bradykinesia, tremor, gait disturbance) increased gradually from 14.9% for those aged 65 to 74 years to 52.4% for those 85 years and older.[38] These may interfere with activities of daily living, such as dressing, eating, and getting out of a chair, and may be an important source of disability. Another finding in that study was that the presence of parkinsonism was associated with a twofold increase in mortality, mostly due to gait instability.

Paratonia

Paratonia (gegenhalten) represents increased motor tone with rapid passive movements of the limbs (flexion and extension), often suggestive of deliberate resistance.[39] Unlike the rigidity of Parkinson disease, it is not constant and tends to disappear with slow movements of the limbs. Paratonia can be detected when the patient's arms, suspended 15 cm above the lap, remain elevated after being released, despite instructions to the patient to relax. The prevalence of paratonia increases with advancing age, with a prevalence of 4% to 21%.[4] It is considered by some to be a postural reflex or a cortical release sign. Similar to other primitive release signs, its prevalence is higher in patients with Alzheimer disease and other forms of dementia and correlates with the severity of cognitive impairment. Paratonia may also represent a sign of age-related changes in the basal ganglia.

Tremor

Physiologic tremor may occur at any age. There are different types of physiologic tremor—rest tremor (with a frequency of 8 to 12 Hz), postural tremor when the patient holds out the arms during isometric contractions of the muscles against gravity (with a frequency of 8 to 12 Hz), and action or volitional tremor during isotonic contraction (with a frequency of 7 to 12 Hz). The prevalence of physiologic tremor in healthy older adults is controversial.[40] Postural tremor is more likely secondary to other causes such as medications, alcohol, disease states such as hyperthyroidism, hyperadrenergic states, or dystonia. When no obvious secondary factors are evident, essential tremor should be considered in the diagnosis. Its prevalence has been reported to range from 1.7% to 23% of healthy older adults aged 65 years or older. In the absence of secondary causes for tremor, and when the tremor does not fit the criteria for essential tremor, it is often referred to as senile tremor. Senile tremor is very common, affecting 98% of older patients in one community-based case-control study. It is often a mild asymptomatic tremor and frequently does not require treatment. It is unclear if it represents an exaggerated physiologic tremor or a mild form of essential tremor. A rhythmic, usually asymmetric, rest tremor is often indicative of Parkinson disease and is rarely seen in healthy older adults.[26,39]

Changes in Gait and Station

There is a tendency to develop a flexed posture with advanced age. This may be due to decreased muscle strength, weakening of abdominal muscles, arthritis and degenerative joint disease, diminished vibration and position sense, and/or impairment in motor speed and coordination.[4] Increased postural sway is a normal phenomenon in older adults and is seen in two different frequencies. Fast oscillations are dependent on proprioceptive input from the lower extremities, and slow oscillations are dependent, at least partially, on vestibular input. Looking at the feet exaggerates this normal sway by interfering with visual compensation. Postural righting reflexes may be slowed and have reduced amplitude in older adults. Control of stance, as judged by the amplitude of sway, is poor in childhood, peaks in adulthood, and decreases with age. In one study, almost one third of patients older than 60 years were unable to minimize their sway with visual endeavors and therefore had a significant risk for falls.[41]

Examination of gait in older adults is an essential part of the neurologic examination, given the high risk of falls in this population. Gait is composed of equilibrium (maintaining an upright posture) and locomotion (gait ignition and steppage), both of which appear to be decreased with aging. Healthy older adults have difficulty maintaining balance on one foot with the eyes closed. Quantitative studies have also shown that older people have greater body sway and exhibit significant reduction in the velocity of gait and length of stride. Therefore, older adults may have difficulty with tandem gait or heel to toe walking for extended periods of time.

When assessing gait in the older adult, it is important to recognize gait abnormalities that may be secondary to joint pain and arthritic conditions. Gait is assessed by having the patient walk straight for at least 10 yards, making a turn, and maneuvering in a tight corridor while noting stride length, arm swing, and posture. The patient should also be asked to tandem-walk, walk on his or her toes and heels and, if possible, walk up a few steps. Postural stability is assessed by asking the patient to stand with their legs shoulder width apart. A forceful pull is given to their shoulders, and the righting response is assessed; the clinician should be prepared to catch the patient if she or he stumbles. One or two steps of retropulsion is considered normal. Despite multiple factors, age alone does not generally affect postural righting reflexes or cause recurrent falls. If present, these should be investigated to rule out underlying disorders, such as Parkinson disease.

Sensory Examination

The most common and evident abnormality in the sensory examination associated with aging is decreased vibration and, to a lesser extent, proprioception.[42] Both of these sensory modalities are carried by the dorsal column; their impairment with age may be due to proliferation of connective tissue, arteriosclerotic changes in the arterioles, degeneration in nerve fibers, or loss of axons in the dorsal column.[43,44] The sensory examination is subjective, and it is important to consider the consistency of responses and how sensory complaints relate to other signs and symptoms. Peripheral causes of sensory loss typically present bilaterally and are largely symmetric. Unilateral sensory loss occurs with lesions of primary sensory cortex or its projections.

Vibration sense is impaired in 12% to 68% of older adults between the ages of 65 and 85 years and becomes more impaired with advanced age.[4,42] The loss of vibration affects upper and lower extremities and often begins distally. This can be demonstrated with a 128-Hz tuning fork at the metatarsals or medial malleolus of the ankle. Using quantitative measurements, it has been shown that the sensitivity of vibration decreases with age in the high-frequency range but does not change in the low-frequency range (25 to 40 Hz).[43]

Proprioception is also affected to a lesser extent, with a prevalence ranging from 2% to 44% in different studies.[45] This often manifests as a mild sway on the Romberg test.There is a paucity of data regarding the involvement of tactile sensation in older adults. Some reports have suggested that age is associated with increased thresholds for light touch, but it is unclear whether these age-related changes are clinically meaningful.[44,46]

Reflexes

Deep Tendon Reflexes

The ability to detect reflexes can be limited by conditions such as apprehension or joint disease in older adults. Hyporeflexia or areflexia of the ankle jerks has been reported in older adults aged 60 years or older.[4] Asymmetry of reflexes was reported in 3% of older adults in one study. Electrophysiologic studies have suggested that the afferent and efferent limbs of the reflex are decreased with age, and mild asymmetry may be detected. The ankle jerk is usually the first reflex to decrease or disappear with aging, although there have been reports of loss of patella tendon reflexes as well.[42] Lateralized hyperactive reflexes in conjunction with spasticity and the Babinski sign are indicative of a contralateral lesion of the pyramidal system.

Superficial reflexes (abdominal, cremasteric, and plantar responses) may become sluggish or disappear with advanced age. Corticospinal lesions above T6 may lead to the loss of all superficial abdominal reflexes, but all are spared in lesions below T12.

Lesions between T10 and T12 may lead to selective loss of the lower reflexes only, with a positive Beevor sign (upward movement of the umbilicus in a supine patient attempting to flex the head). Extension or dorsiflexion of the big toe, with fanning of the toes induced by stroking the lateral aspect of the sole, is called the Babinski sign. It is considered to be a primitive reflex that when present beyond the first 2 years of life, is a reliable sign of upper motor neuron pathology. No consistent changes have been documented with normal aging, and there is often some degree of interobserver variability in eliciting this reflex.

Primitive Reflexes

Primitive reflexes, or so-called archaic or developmental reflexes, represent the loss of cortical inhibition on reflex associations present at early stages of development and later suppressed with brain maturation.[47] Their reappearance in adult life has been associated with atrophic changes predominantly involving the frontal lobes (e.g., dementia syndromes, demyelinating disease, cerebrovascular disease) and are sometimes referred to as cortical release signs. However, these reflexes are sometimes seen in otherwise healthy older adults, and some (e.g., the palmomental reflex) can be elicited at all ages. The exact pathophysiologic mechanisms underlying these reflexes are not completely understood. In isolation, they are neither sensitive nor specific for any neurologic disease. Although some can be seen in normal aging, their occurrence in combination should necessitate investigation for underlying disease (e.g., neurodegenerative disease, dementia) and should not be attributed to normal aging alone.

Grasp Reflex. There are three different types of grasp reflex that reflect three different levels of severity of cortical disinhibition.[48] The first, called tactile grasp, is elicited by applying firm pressure across the palm from the ulnar to the radial side while distracting the patient (e.g., asking the patient to count backward from 20). It is considered positive if the patient grasps the examiner's fingers or flexes the fingers with adduction of the thumb in response to stroking the palm. Traction grasp is described as the patient counter pulling when the examiner attempts to pull away from the patient's grip. Magnetic grasp is when the patient follows or reaches for the examiner's hand to grasp it. It is generally considered a pathologic sign and often occurs as a result of contralateral or bilateral damage to medial frontal or basal ganglia structures. However, tactile grasp responses can be seen in many healthy older adults and generally increases with advanced age. It is also more frequent in Alzheimer disease and correlates with the degree of cognitive impairment. Analogous to the grasp reflex in the hand is flexion and adduction of the toes, with inversion and incurving of the foot in response to tactile stimulation or pressure on the sole. This reflex is seen invariably in neonates; it may reappear in older adults and contribute to gait difficulty and interference with activities of daily living.[48]

Glabellar Tap Reflex. Other names for this reflex include the glabella tap sign, orbicularis oculi sign, blinking reflex, and Myerson sign.[49] It is elicited by tapping between the eyebrows with the finger at a rate of 2 per second and avoiding a visual threat response. A normal response consists of blinking in response to the first three to nine taps, followed by cessation of the response with further tapping. It is considered positive or abnormal if blinking continues with further tapping. An abnormal glabellar tap was first described in Parkinson disease patients and was considered to be diagnostic for that disease. However, it can occur with normal aging, as well as other neurodegenerative disorders. It is found in over 50% of normal older adults, and it is debatable whether it becomes more prevalent with older age. It is different from the other primitive reflexes in that it mainly results from basal ganglia lesions, rather than cortical disinhibition.[49]

Palmomental Reflex. Contraction of the mentalis muscle in the lower jaw is elicited by stroking the ipsilateral thenar eminence. It is a polysynaptic and nociceptive reflex, with the afferent arm traveling through the median and ulnar nerves and the efferent arm in the facial nerve. The threshold for eliciting the palmomental reflex varies greatly among individuals. The palmomental reflex is seen in up to 27% of individuals younger than 50 years and in over 35% of individuals older than 85% years. The appearance of the palmomental reflex may reflect frontal lobe dysfunction.[49]

Snout or Pout Reflex. This is elicited by pressing or gently tapping over the philtrum of the upper lip in the midline, which results in pouting or pursing of the lips.[47] It is a nociceptive reflex of the perioral muscles carried by the trigeminal and facial nerves for the afferent and efferent limbs. Unlike the palmomental reflex, it is generally not seen before the age of 40 to 50 years; however, the incidence increases with age, with a prevalence of 73% by 85 years of age.[50] The occurrence of this reflex correlates well with impaired performance on psychometric testing and corresponds to the loss of large pyramidal neurons in the anterior cingulate gyrus.

Suck Reflex. This is elicited by stroking the lips with the index finger or a reflex hammer. The response could be incomplete, with the lips closing around the finger or object, or complete, resulting in sucking movements in the lips, tongue, and jaw. If the stimulus is applied to the lateral margins of the lips, the head turns toward the side of the stimulus. Although it can be seen in 6% of normal older adults, it is more common in the presence of dementia and correlates with the severity of cognitive impairment.[50] The snout and suck reflexed appear to be more common with prolonged use of antipsychotic medications.

CONCLUDING COMMENTS

A variety of neurologic disorders (e.g., stroke, Parkinson disease, Alzheimer disease) preferentially affect older adults. To document normal findings and detect abnormal signs, a comprehensive mental status and neurologic examination should be performed in every older adult.

Altered cognitive function in the setting of a clear sensorium is consistent with dementia secondary to a neurodegenerative process (Alzheimer disease, Parkinson disease, Pick disease) or medical illness (cerebrovascular disease, vitamin B_{12} deficiency, hypothyroidism). Delirium, on the other hand, causes alterations in the sensorium and level of consciousness and may be due to medications, infection, head injury, or metabolic derangement. Associated features include disruption of the sleep-wake cycle, intermittent drowsiness and agitation, restlessness, emotional lability, and frank psychosis (e.g., hallucination, illusions, delusions). Predisposing factors include advanced age, dementia, impaired physical or mental health, sensory deprivation (poor vision or hearing), and placement in an intensive care unit.

A functional decline in some aspects of cranial nerve function (e.g., vision, hearing, vestibular function, taste, smell) can be readily detected on examination. In the absence of other findings, this may be considered part of the normal aging process. However, a constellation of abnormalities usually represents a pathologic condition afflicting the nervous system. Similarly, older individuals experience decreased mobility, coordination, sensation, and strength as they age. However, more profound changes that significantly alter mobility or present as focal neurologic signs should alert the clinician to a neuropathologic disorder and warrants diagnostic testing.

In conclusion, neurologic findings of normal aging include subtle declines in cognitive function, mildly impaired motor function, and altered sensory perceptions. However, exaggerated impairments in cognitive, behavioral, motor, and sensory function suggest the onset of neurologic diseases that commonly afflict the older adult. A comprehensive mental status and neurologic examination, in addition to a detailed general physical examination, is the foundation for identifying neuropathologic conditions that necessitate further investigation.

Acknowledgments

This chapter was supported by a grants from the National Institute on Aging (P30 AG008051, R01 AG040211) and the New York State Department of Health (DOH-2011-1004010353).

KEY POINTS

- Neurologic disorders are a common cause of morbidity, mortality, institutionalization, and increased health care costs in older adults.
- Normal aging may be associated with the loss of normal neurologic signs or the exaggeration of others.
- Cognitive changes associated with normal aging include decrease in processing speed, cognitive flexibility, and visuospatial perception; other domains, such as new learning and language, are resistant to age effects, allowing the use of list learning, paragraph recall, and category fluency as sensitive markers of cognitive decline.
- Aging is associated with changes in taste, smell, sight, hearing, proprioception, and balance. Other neurologic findings warrant further investigation.
- There is a progressive decline in muscle bulk associated with aging (sarcopenia), which tends to be symmetric, and involves the intrinsic muscles of the hands and feet. Focal loss of strength is not a feature of normal aging.
- A comprehensive mental status and neurologic examination, in addition to a detailed general physical examination, is the foundation for identifying neuropathologic conditions that necessitate further investigation.

For a complete list of references, please visit www.expertconsult.com.

KEY REFERENCES

1. Olesen J, Gustavsson A, Svensson M, et al: CDBE2010 study group; European Brain Council. The economic cost of brain disorders in Europe. Eur J Neurol 19:155–162, 2012.
2. Tolea MI, Galvin JE: Sarcopenia and impairment in cognitive and physical performance. Clin Interv Aging 10:663–671, 2015.
5. Harada CN, Natelson Love MC, Triebel KL: Normal cognitive aging. Clin Geriatr Med 29:737–752, 2013.
7. Galvin JE, Powlishta KK, Wilkins K, et al: Predictors of preclinical Alzheimer disease and dementia: a clinicopathologic study. Arch Neurol 62:758–765, 2005.
8. Karantzoulis S, Galvin JE: Distinguishing Alzheimer's disease from other major forms of dementia. Expert Rev Neurother 11:1579–1591, 2011.
11. Nasreddine ZS, Phillips NA, Bedirian V, et al: The Montreal cognitive assessment, MoCA: a brief screening tool for mild cognitive impairment. J Am Geriatr Soc 53:695–699, 2005.
12. Galvin JE, Roe CM, Powlishta KK, et al: The AD8: a brief informant interview to detect dementia. Neurology 65:559–564, 2005.
17. Doty RL, Kamath V: The influences of age on olfaction: a review. Front Psychol 5:20, 2014.
18. Braak H, Braak E: Neuropathological staging of Alzheimer-related changes. Acta Neuropathol 82:239–259, 1991.
19. Braak H, Del Tredici K, Rub U, et al: Staging of brain pathology related to sporadic Parkinson's disease. Neurobiol Aging 24:197–211, 2003.
21. Imoscopi A, Inelmen EM, Sergi G, et al: Taste loss in the elderly: epidemiology, causes and consequences. Aging Clin Exp Res 24:570–579, 2012.
22. Klein R, Klein BE: The prevalence of age-related eye diseases and visual impairment in aging: current estimates. Invest Ophthalmol Vis Sci 54:ORSF5–ORSF13, 2013.
35. Rudolf R, Khan MM, Labeit S, et al: Degeneration of neuromuscular junction in age and dystrophy. Front Aging Neurosci 6:99, 2014.

18

19 Connective Tissues and Aging

Nicholas A. Kefalides, Zahra Ziaie, Edward J. Macarak*

Aging is a continuous process that constitutes a cycle studded with events that affect all systems in the body, including the connective tissues. The interrelationship between the aging process and connective tissues is complex, involving a variety of factors and interactions acting in a reciprocal fashion. One could inquire into the effects of aging on connective tissues and, conversely, one may ask how the components of connective tissue contribute to the aging process. To answer these questions, it is important to have some understanding of the structural biochemistry of connective tissues, knowledge of the processes involved in their biosynthesis, modification, extracellular organization, molecular genetics, and of the factors affecting the properties of connective tissue cells and the extracellular matrix (ECM). Since the last edition, new data have become available that highlight the progress made regarding the mechanisms responsible for the alterations in connective tissue components in diseases associated with aging. Armed with this knowledge, it becomes apparent that there can be a huge number of events in the development of connective tissues that may be associated, directly or indirectly, with the processes or effects of aging. These have been and continue to be areas of intensive research.

This chapter presents an abbreviated discussion of the various components of the ECM and their structure, molecular organization, biosynthesis, modification, turnover, and molecular genetics. It discusses some concepts on the effects of aging on the ECM and effects of aging on the properties of various connective tissues, as well as the involvement of connective tissue physiology on diseases associated with aging.

PROPERTIES OF CONNECTIVE TISSUES

The properties of connective tissues are derived primarily from the properties of the components of the ECM surrounding, and secreted by, the cells of those tissues. Some connective tissues, such as cartilage or tendons, are products primarily of a single cell type (e.g., chondrocytes, fibroblasts) whose synthesis and secretion of ECM and other factors largely determine the properties of the tissue. Some structures, such as bone, blood vessels, and skin contain a number of different connective tissue cell types, such as osteoblasts and osteoclasts in bone, endothelial, and smooth muscle cells, fibroblasts in blood vessels, and fibroblasts, epithelial cells, and adipocytes cells in skin, which contribute to their structural and functional properties. Other tissues and organs, such as cardiac muscle and kidney, may have properties dependent on connective tissue components whose biologic roles are separate from the major physiologic function of the tissue and that may influence the properties of that tissue during the process of aging. Different cell types will exhibit different phenotypic patterns of ECM production that in turn will influence the structural properties of a given connective tissue.

The major components of the ECM fall into three general classes of molecules: (1) the structural proteins, which include the collagens (of which there are now 28 recognized types) and elastin; (2) the proteoglycans, which contain several structurally distinct molecular classes, such as heparan sulfate and dermatan sulfate; and (3) the structural glycoproteins, exemplified by fibronectin (FN) and laminin (LM), whose contributions to the properties of connective tissues have been recognized only within the past 35 to 40 years. The interactions among these materials determine the development and properties of the connective tissues.

Collagens

Structure

The collagens are a family of connective tissue proteins characterized by the presence of three polypeptides called alpha chains, which contain molecular domains that are wound together in a ropelike super helix. Collagens are rich in the amino acids proline and glycine, which play roles in the formation and stability of the triple-stranded super helix. The reader is referred to two reviews on collagen biochemistry.[1,2]

The genes of at least 28 distinct collagen types have been characterized.[3] The interstitial collagens, types I, II, III, and V, exist as large extended molecules that tend to organize into fibrils that may be heterotypic[1]—that is, there may be more than one collagen type within these fibrils.[4] Type IV collagen, also termed *basement membrane* (BM) *collagen*, does not exist in fibrillar form but is in a complex network of collagen molecules linked by disulfide and other cross-linkages and associated with noncollagenous molecules, such as LM, entactin, and proteoglycans, to form an amorphous matrix.[5,6] Although at least 28 collagen types are recognized, the protein of only the first 11 collagens has been isolated from tissues.

Table 19-1 presents a summary of the collagen family (a modification of the one reported by Canty and Kadler[3]). There are 46 genes corresponding to the alpha chains of 28 collagen types. Collagen type I is the most abundant collagen and protein in the body. The basic unit of the type I collagen fibril is a triple helical heterotrimer, tropocollagen, consisting of two identical chains, alpha 1(I), and a third chain, alpha 2(I).[1] The other collagen types have been given similar designations; however, some of the types are homotrimers containing three identical chains and some contain three genetically distinct chains.

The collagen alpha chain has a unique amino acid composition, with glycine occupying every third position in the sequence. Thus, the collagenous domains consist of a repeating peptide triplet, -Gly-X-Y-, in which X and Y are amino acids other than glycine. A large percentage of amino acids in the Y position is occupied by proline. In addition, collagen contains two unique amino acids derived from posttranslational modifications of the protein, 4- and 3-hydroxyproline and hydroxylysine. The presence of 4-hydroxyproline provides additional sites along the alpha chain capable of forming hydrogen bonds with adjacent alpha chains, which are important in stabilizing the triple helix so that it maintains its structure at body temperatures. If hydroxyproline formation is inhibited, the triple helix dissociates into its component alpha chains at 37° C, making it structurally unstable.

The presence of glycine in every third position, along with the extensive hydrogen bonding, provides the triple helix with a compact protected structure resistant to the action of most proteases. The alpha chains of the collagen superfamily are encoded

*Dr. Nicholas A. Kefalides died on December 6, 2013. This manuscript is dedicated to his memory and his many notable contributions to the field of connective tissue research.

TABLE 19-1 Collagen Types

Type	Genes	Tissue Distribution
I	*COL1A1, COL1A2*	Skin, tendon, bone, cornea, blood vessels
II	*COL2A1*	Cartilage, intervertebral discs, vitreous body
III	*COL3A1*	Skin, blood vessels
IV	*COL4A1, COL4A2, COL4A3* *COL4A4, COL4A5, COL4A6*	Basement membranes (BMs)
V	*COL5A, COL5A2, COL5A3*	Placenta, skin, cardiovascular system
VI	*COL6A1, COL6A2, COL6A3* *COL6A4, COL6A5, COL6A6*	Cornea, blood vessels, lung, testis, colon, kidney, liver, spleen, thymus, heart, skeletal muscle, articular cartilage
VII	*COL7A1*	Skin, cornea, gastrointestinal tract
VIII	*COL8A1, COL8A2*	Cardiovascular system, placenta, cornea
IX	*COL9A1, COL9A2, COL9A3*	Cartilage, cornea
X	*COL10A1*	Cartilage
XI	*COL11A1, COL11A2, COL2A1*	Cartilage
XII	*COL12A1*	Tendons, periosteum
XIII	*COL13A1*	Many tissues
XIV	*COL14A1*	Skin, bone, cornea, blood vessels
XV	*COL15A1*	Placenta, heart, colon
XVI	*COL16A1*	Placenta, heart, colon
XVII	*COL17A1*	Skin hemidesmosomes
XVIII	*COL18A1*	Several tissues, particularly kidney and liver
XIX	*COL19A1*	Rhabdomyosarcoma cells
XX	*COL20A1*	Corneal epithelium, embryonic skin, sternal cartilage, tendon
XXI	*COL21A1*	Heart, stomach, kidney, skeletal muscle, placenta, blood vessel
XXII	*COL22A1*	Articular cartilage, skin, tissue junctions—cartilage synovial fluid, myotendinous junctions in skeletal and heart muscle
XXIII	*COL23A1*	Lung, cornea, tendon, brain, skin, kidney
XXIV	*COL24A1*	Bone and cornea
XXV	*COL25A1*	Amyloid plaques in the brain
XXVI	*COL26A1*	Testis, ovary
XXVII	*COL27A1*	Cartilage, tendon, stomach, lung, gonad, skin, cochlea, tooth
XXVIII	*COL28A1*	Kidney, skin, calvaria, nerves, BM of certain Schwann cells

with information that specifies self-assembly into fibrils, microfibrils, and networks that have diverse functions in the ECM.[6] The structures of collagens can be stabilized further through the formation of covalent cross-linkages derived from modification and condensation of certain lysine and hydroxylysine residues on adjacent alpha chains.[2] Cross-linkage formation is important in stabilizing collagen fibrils and contributes to their high tensile strength, equivalent to that of fine steel wire.

Biosynthesis

Type I collagen alpha chains are synthesized as a larger precursor, procollagen, containing noncollagenous sequences at their C and N termini.[7] As each pro–alpha chain is synthesized, intracellular prolyl and lysyl hydroxylases act to form hydroxyproline and hydroxylysine. The triple helix is formed intracellularly and stabilized by the formation of interchain disulfide bonds near the carboxyl termini of the component pro–alpha chains. After secretion of the triple helical collagen, procollagen peptidases remove most of the noncollagenous portions at each end of the procollagen. Extracellular lysine and hydroxylysine oxidases oxidize the epsilon amino groups of lysine or hydroxylysine to form aldehyde derivatives, which can go on to form Schiff base adducts, the first cross-linkages. These can rearrange and become reduced to form the various other cross-linkages. Increased number of collagen cross-linkages have been reported in a pathologic state known as scleroderma.

Degradation of Connective Tissue Components

The role played by matrix metalloproteinases (MMPs) in connective tissue turnover has gained prominence in the past 40 years as information on the mechanisms whereby MMPs mediated synovial joint inflammation, as well as ECM turnover, in arthritides became available.[8] Extracellular degradation of collagen is accomplished by enzymes known as tissue collagenases. These enzymes cleave triple helical collagen at a site three quarters from the amino terminus, resulting in the formation of two triple helical fragments that become denatured at temperatures above 32° C to form nonhelical peptides, which can be degraded by tissue proteinases. Cleavage by tissue collagenase is considered to be the rate-limiting step in the collagenolysis of triple helical collagen. Collagenolysis is the subject of reviews by Kleiner and Stetler-Stevenson[9] and Tayebjee and colleagues.[10]

Collagenolysis is an important physiologic process responsible to a large extent for the repair of wounds and processes of tissue remodeling in which undesired accumulations are removed as new connective tissue is laid down. However, in conditions such as rheumatoid arthritis and osteoporosis (OS), as well as aging, the production of collagenases may be stimulated, resulting in an elevated degradation of synovial tissue or bone. Degradation of elastin by elastases, belonging to a family of serine, metallo, or cysteine proteinases, gives rise to the generation of elastin fragments, designated as elastokines.[11]

Tissue collagenases are secreted by connective tissue cells as a precursor procollagenase, which must be activated to become enzymatically functional. This can be achieved in vitro by the action of trypsin on the latent enzyme. Other proteinases, including lysosomal cathepsin B, plasmin, mast cell proteinase, and plasma kallikrein, also can activate latent collagenases. Thus, inflammatory cells can secrete factors that lead to collagenase activation, accounting for the inflammatory sequelae of the arthritides. Collagenases are also under the influence of plasma inhibitors, of which α_2-macroglobulin accounts for most of the inhibitory process. In addition, inhibitors of plasminogen activation can indirectly prevent the activation of procollagenases by plasmin. Fibroblasts and other connective tissue cells also secrete inhibitors of collagenases, suggesting a complex system of extracellular control of collagenolysis.[9,10]

Elastin

The biochemistry and molecular biology of elastin have been subjects of excellent reviews.[12,13] As in interstitial collagens, glycine makes up about one third of the amino acid content of elastin. Unlike collagen, however, glycine is not present in every third position. In addition, elastin is an exceedingly hydrophobic protein, with a large content of valine, leucine, and isoleucine.

Elastin is synthesized as a precursor molecule, tropoelastin, with a molecular weight of about 70 kDa. However, in tissues, elastin is found as an amorphous macromolecular network. This is because of the condensation of tropoelastin molecules through the formation of covalent cross-linkages unique to elastin. These cross-linkages arise through the condensation of four lysine residues on different tropoelastin molecules to form the cross-linking amino acids, desmosine and isodesmosine, that are characteristic of tissue elastin. The reader is referred to reviews by Bailey and associates[2] and Wagenseil and Mecham[12] for a more detailed discussion of collagen and elastin cross-linking.

The hydrophobicity, together with the formation of cross-linkages, endow elastin with its elastic properties as well as its extreme insolubility and amorphous structure. Elastin accounts for most of the elastic properties of skin, arteries, ligaments, and the lungs. The presence of elastin has been demonstrated in other organs, such as the eye and kidney. In most tissues, elastin is found in association with microfibrils, which contain several glycoproteins, including fibrillin. Microfibrils have been identified in many tissues and organs, and the importance of their assembly as determinants of connective tissue architecture has been brought into focus by the identification of mutations in fibrillin in the heritable connective tissue disorder, Marfan syndrome.[13]

An elegant review has summarized knowledge of the structure of the elastin gene, including consideration of the heterogeneity observed in immature mRNA due to alternative splicing in the primary transcript.[14] Analyses of the bovine and human elastin genes have revealed the separation of those exons coding for distinct hydrophobic and cross-linking domains. Comparison of the cDNA and genomic sequences, as well as S1 analyses, have demonstrated that the primary transcript of both species is subject to considerable alternative splicing. It is likely that this accounts for the presence of multiple tropoelastins found in several species. It has been suggested that the differences in alternative splicing may be correlated with aging.[14]

Proteoglycans

Proteoglycans are characterized by the presence of highly negatively charged, polymeric chains (glycosaminoglycans [GAGs]) of repeating disaccharide units covalently attached to a core protein. The disaccharide units comprise an N-conjugated amino sugar, either glucosamine or galactosamine, and a uronic acid, usually D-glucuronic acid or, in the case of dermatan sulfate, heparan sulfate, and heparin, L-iduronic acid. In cartilage and in the cornea, another GAG, keratan sulfate, containing D-glucose instead of a uronic acid, has been demonstrated. The amino group of the hexosamine component is generally acetylated, and the GAGs are usually O-sulfated in hexosamine residues with some N-sulfation, instead of acetylation, in the case of heparan sulfate and heparin. Depending on the source and type of proteoglycan, the number of GAGs attached to the core protein can vary from three or four to more than 20, with each GAG having a molecular size in the tens of thousands of daltons. In addition, as in the case of the cartilage proteoglycans, there may be more than one type of GAG attached to the core protein. In cartilage, several proteoglycan molecules may be associated with another very large GAG, hyaluronic acid, consisting of disaccharide units of glucuronyl N-acetylglucosamine. The compositional structure of the GAGs is summarized in Table 19-2.

TABLE 19-2 Properties and Tissue Distribution of Glycosaminoglycans (GAGs)

GAGs	Composition	Tissue Distribution
Hyaluronic acid	*N*-Acetylglucosamine D-Glucuronic acid	Blood vessels, heart, synovial fluid, umbilical cord, vitreous
Chondroitin sulfate	*N*-Acetylgalactosamine D-Glucuronic acid 4- or 6-O-sulfate	Cartilage, cornea, tendon, heart valves, skin
Dermatan sulfate	*N*-Acetygalactosamine L-Iduronic acid 4- or 6-O-sulfate	Skin, lungs, cartilage
Keratan sulfate	*N*-Acetyglucosamine D-Galactose O-Sulfate	Cornea, cartilage, nucleus pulposus
Heparan sulfate	*N*-Acetylglucosamine	Blood vessels, basement membranes, lung, spleen, kidney
Heparin	*N*-Sulfaminoglucosamine D-Glucuronic acid L-Iduronic acid O-Sulfates	Mast cells, lung, Glisson membranes

The overall effect of these structures is the creation of huge, negatively charged highly hydrophobic complexes. The hydration and charge properties of these complexes cause them to become highly extended, occupying a hydrodynamic volume in the tissue much larger than that which would be predicted from their chemical composition. In the case of synovial cartilage, it is suggested that the hydration endows the tissue with shock-absorbing properties in which applied pressure to the joint is counteracted by the extrusion of water from the complex, forcing a compression of the negative charges within the molecule. On the release of pressure, the electronegative repulsive forces drive the charges apart, with a concomitant influx of water to restore the initial hydrated state. The metachromatic staining properties of connective tissues are mainly because of their proteoglycan content. There have been several excellent reviews of proteoglycan biochemistry.[15-17]

In recent years, several proteoglycans have been identified in the pericellular environment, associated with cell surfaces or interacting with ECM components, such as interstitial collagens, FN, and transforming growth factor-β (TGF-β). Reviews by Groffen and coworkers[15] and Schaefer and Iozzo[16,17] have described the structures of the protein cores and their gene organization, functional characteristics, and tissue distribution. Table 19-3 (a modification of that published by Schaefer and Iozzo[16]) lists the biologic characteristics of pericellular proteoglycans. Several of the proteoglycans on the list constitute a group of small, leucine-rich proteoglycans (SLRPs). Notable among them are decorin[17] and perlecan.[18] They are multidomain assemblies of protein motifs with relatively elongated and highly glycosylated structures and have several protein domains shared with other proteins. In their review, Groffen and colleagues[15] discussed the role of perlecan as a crucial determinant of glomerular BM permselectivity and suggested that the additional presence of agrin, another heparan sulfate proteoglycan species, makes the latter important contributors to glomerular function.

Lumican, one of the leucine-rich proteoglycans, is found in relative abundance in articular cartilage,[17] which, along with its size, varies with age. In adult cartilage extracts, it exhibits a molecular size in the range of 55 to 80 kDa. Extracts from juvenile cartilage have a more restricted size variation corresponding to the higher molecular size range present in the adult. In the neonate, the sizes are in the range of 70 to 80 kDa.

The biosynthesis of proteoglycans begins with the synthesis of the core protein. The sugars of the GAG chain, in most cases, are sequentially added to serine residues of the protein using uridine diphosphate conjugates of the component sugars, with sulfation following as the chain elongates. Most of the chain elongation and sulfation is associated with the Golgi apparatus. The degradation of proteoglycans is mediated through the action of lysosomal glycosidases and sulfatases specific for the hydrolysis of the various structural sites within the GAG chain. Genetic abnormalities in the production or synthesis of these enzymes have been shown to be the main causes of the mucopolysaccharidoses, whose victims may exhibit severe tissue abnormalities and a high incidence of mental retardation.

Structural Glycoproteins

In addition to the collagen and elastin components of connective tissues, there are groups of glycoproteins, the structural glycoproteins, that have important roles in the physiology and

TABLE 19-3 Properties of Secreted Pericellular Proteoglycans

Designation (Gene Product)	Protein Core Size (kDa)	Chromosomal Location (human)	Tissue Distribution
Decorin	36	12q21.3–q23	Ubiquitous; collagenous matrices, bone, teeth, mesothelia, floor plate, sclera, lung
Biglycan	38	Xq28	Sclera, teeth, bone, articular cartilage
Fibromodulin	42	1q32	Collagenous matrices, sclera
Lumican	38	12q21.3–q22	Cornea, intestine, liver, muscle, cartilage, sclera
Epiphycan	36	12q21	Epiphyseal cartilage, ligament, placenta
Versican	265-370	5q14.2	Blood vessels, brain, skin, cartilage
Aggrecan	220	15q26.1	Cartilage, brain, blood vessels
Neurocan	136	19p12	Brain, cartilage,
Brevican	100	1q31	Brain
Perlecan	400-467	1p36.33	Basement membranes (BMs), cell surfaces, sinusoidal spaces, cartilage
Agrin	200	1p32-pter 1p36.33	Synaptic sites of neuromuscular junctions, renal basement membranes, colon
Testican	44	5q31.2	Seminal fluid
Asporin	39	9q21.3-q22	Articular cartilage, heart skeleton, specialized connective tissues, liver meniscus, aorta, uterus
Chondroadherin	36	17q21.33	Cartilage
ECM2	79.8	9q22.31	Adipose tissue, female-specific organs—mammary gland, ovary, uterus
Keratocan	37	12q21.3-q22	Cornea, trachea, intestine, ovary , lung, skeletal muscle
Opticin	35	1q31	Retina, ligament, skin
Osteoadherin (Osteomodulin)	49	9q22.31	Primary bone spongiosa, odontoblasts, bone, dentin, bone trabeculae, mature odontoblasts, human pulpal fibroblasts
PRELP	45	1q32	BM, connective tissue extracellular matrix, sclera, articular cartilage
Nyctalopin	52	Xp11.4	Kidney, retina, brain, testis, muscle
Podocan	68.98	1p32.3	Kidney, heart, brain, pancreas, vascular smooth muscle
Osteoglycin	33.9	9q22	Bone
Tsukushu	37.8	11q13.5	Uterus, placenta, colon (protein evidence at transcript level)

structural properties of connective and other types of tissues. These proteins, which include FN, LM, entactin-nidogen, thrombospondin (TSP), and others, are involved during development, in cell attachment and spreading, and in tissue growth and turnover.

Fibronectin

One of the best characterized of the structural glycoproteins is fibronectin. It was originally isolated from serum, where it was referred to as cold-insoluble globulin (CIG). As it became recognized that FN was an important secretory product of fibroblasts and other types of cells, and was involved in cell adhesion, the term *fibronectin* replaced CIG. Comprehensive reviews on the structure and function of FN have been published by Haranuga and Yamada[20] and Schwarzbauer and DeSimone.[21]

FN exists as a disulfide-linked dimer with a molecular weight of about 450 kDa, with each monomer having a molecular size of 250 kDa. FN exists in at least two forms, a cell-associated form and a plasma form. Plasma FN is synthesized by hepatocytes and secreted into the circulation. It is somewhat smaller and more soluble at a physiologic pH than the cellular form. Spectrophotometric and ultracentrifugal studies have indicated that both forms are elongated molecules composed of structured domains separated by flexible, extensible regions. Limited proteolytic digestion studies have revealed the presence of specific binding sites for a number of ligands, including collagen, fibrin, cell surfaces, heparin (heparan sulfate proteoglycan), factor XIIIa, and actin.

FN plays a role in blood clotting by becoming cross-linked to fibrin through the action of factor XIIIa transamidase, which catalyzes the final step in the clotting cascade.[22] Fibroblasts and other cell types involved in the repair of injury adhere to the clot by interacting with the cell-binding domain of FN. FN contains a unique peptide sequence, arginyl-glycyl-aspartyl-serine (RGDS, RGD), which binds to specific cell surface proteins (integrins) that span the plasma membrane.[21] Purified RGD can inhibit FN from binding the cells and can even displace bound FN. The integrins have a complex molecular organization and appear to interact with certain intracellular proteins, thereby providing a mechanism for the control of a number of events by components of the extracellular environment.

FN is encoded by a single gene, and its complete primary structure has been determined by the DNA sequencing of overlapping complementary DNA (cDNA) clones.[23] From such studies, it became recognized that there are peptide segments derived from alternative splicing of FN mRNA at three distinct regions, termed *extradomain A* (ED-A), ED-B, and connecting segment (CS) III. A middle region of FN containing homologous repeating segments of about 90 amino acids, called type III homologies, has been identified.[24,25] Using immunologic techniques with monoclonal antibodies, it was shown that the ED-A exon is omitted during splicing of the FN mRNA precursor in arterial medial cells; the expression of FN containing ED-A, however, is characteristic of multiple cell types involved in wound healing and tissue and organ fibrotic diseases characterized by the overproduction of connective tissue proteins. In such disorders, EDA-FN synthesis precedes that of collagens and is a requirement for the TGF-β–induced differentiation of fibroblasts into myofibroblasts. The contributions of myofibroblast differentiation and expression of the EDA-FN isoform to the aging process are problematic because of their close association with the early stages of fibrotic diseases.[26] Genetic studies have shown that ED-A is not required for normal development, but significant abnormalities were noted in adult mice that lacked the ED-A gene.[27] Increased ED-A FN has been demonstrated in the skin of patients with scleroderma.[28] ED-A FN also is found during embryonic development where it plays a role in cell migration. In addition, recent evidence has shown the presence of EDA-FN in keloid scars.[29]

This could be the source of differences between the plasma and cellular forms of FN. This phenomenon of alternative splicing may also be involved in the synthesis of collagens and elastin and may well be implicated in the processes of aging.

TABLE 19-4 Isoforms of Laminin (LM)*

Laminin	Chain Composition	Abbreviated New Nomenclature	Tissue Distribution
1	α1β1γ1	LM-111	All basement membranes (BM) except skeletal muscle
2	α2β1γ1	LM-211	Striated muscle, peripheral nerve, placenta
3	α1β2γ1	LM-121	Synapse, glomerulus, arterial blood, vessel walls
4	α2β2γ1	LM-221	Myotendinous junction, trophoblast
5 or 5A	α3Aβ3γ2	LM-332 or LM-3A32	Dermal-epidermal junction, stromal-epidermal junction
5B	α3Bβ3γ2	LM-3B32	Dermal-epidermal junction, stromal-epidermal junction
6 or 6A	α3β1γ1	LM-311 or LM-3A11	Dermal-epidermal junction, stromal-epidermal junction
7 or 7A	α3Aβ2γ1	LM-321 or LM-3A21	Amnion, fetal skin
8	α4β1γ1	LM-411	Lung, heart, blood vessels, smooth muscle, endothelial cells, placenta
9	α4β2γ1	LM-421	Heart, blood vessels, placenta, lung
10	α5β1γ1	LM-511	Heart, blood vessels, placenta, lung, kidney
11	α5β2γ1	LM-521	Corpus luteum, breast, glomerular BM, neuromuscular system, stroma and capillaries of placenta, lung, synaptic cleft, trophoblastic BM
12	α2β1γ3	LM-213	BM, kidney, testis
14	α4β2γ3	LM-423	Central nervous system (CNS), retinal matrix, malignant fibrous histiocytomas
†	α5β2γ2	LM-522	Skeletal muscle, kidney, prostate, lung
15	α5β2γ3	LM-523	CNS, retinal matrix

*Based on a new nomenclature,[33] new laminins should not be given a new two-digit number, but should be referred to by their constituent chains.
†No LM has been designated number 13.

Laminin

LM is the major structural glycoprotein of BMs. In addition to its association with the molecular components of BMs (e.g., type IV collagen, entactin-nidogen, heparan sulfate proteoglycan), it plays an important role in cell attachment and neurite growth.[30-32] LM is difficult to isolate from whole tissues or from BMs owing to its poor solubility, so most of our knowledge of it is derived from extracts of tumor matrices.

LM is a very large complex composed of at least three protein chains associated by disulfide linkages. The largest of these, the alpha 1 chain, has a molecular weight of about 440 kDa, whereas the smaller units, beta 1 and gamma 1 chains, have molecular weights of about 200 to 250 kDa, respectively. Several LM isoforms have been described in recent years,[32] necessitating a new nomenclature of its component chains.[33] The first new chain (alpha 2) has been found in preparations from normal tissues but is absent in those from neoplastic tissues.[34,35] Table 19-4 lists the various LM isoforms and their tissue distribution. LM has been shown to have a twisted cruciform shape consisting of three short arms and a single long arm, with globular domains at the extremities of each arm. In several of the newer isoforms of LM, the alpha 1 chain has a smaller molecular size and lacks a portion of its amino terminus.

LM can influence processes of differentiation, cell growth, migration, morphology, adhesion, and agglutination. It plays a major role in the structural organization of BMs and exhibits a preferential binding to type IV collagen compared with other collagen types.[36] LM contains domains similar to those of FN that bind to different proteins and cell surface components containing an RGD sequence on the alpha 1 chain and a YlGSR sequence on the beta 1 chain, both of which bind to different integrins on the cell surface and are involved in cellular attachment and migratory behaviors.

Entactin-Nidogen

Entactin-nidogen, a sulfated glycoprotein, is an intrinsic component of BMs. Entactin was first identified in the ECM synthesized by mouse endodermal cells in culture.[37] Subsequently, a degraded form, termed *nidogen*, was isolated from the Engelbreth-Holm-Swarm sarcoma and mistakenly identified as a new BM component, although both terms are used interchangeably in the modern literature.[38] Entactin-1–nidogen-1 and entactin-2–nidogen-2 are differentially expressed in myogenic differentiation.[39]

Entactin-nidogen forms a tight stoichiometric complex with LM. Rotary shadowing electron microscopy has revealed its association with the gamma 1 chain of LM. Entactin-nidogen has been shown to promote cell attachment via an RGD sequence, and calcium ions have been implicated in its properties.[40] Its role along with LN in BM assembly and epithelial morphogenesis was noted earlier. It has been shown that entactin-1–nidogen-1 regulates LM-1–dependent mammary gland specific gene expression.

Thrombospondin

Thrombospondins (TSPs) are a family of extracellular, adhesive proteins that are widely expressed in vertebrates. Five distinct gene products, designated TSP 1-4 and cartilage oligomeric matrix protein (COMP), have been identified. TSP-1 and TSP-2 have similar primary structures. The molecule (450 kDa) is composed of three identical disulfide-linked protein chains. It is one of the major peptide products secreted during platelet activation, and it is also secreted by a diversity of growing cells. TSP has 12 binding sites for calcium ion, required for its conformational stability. It binds to heparin, heparan sulfate proteoglycan, and cell surfaces, and appears to modulate a number of cell functions, including platelet aggregation, progression through the cell cycle, and cell adhesion and migration.[41,42] Genetic studies have shown associations of single-nucleotide polymorphisms in three of the five TSPs with cardiovascular disease.[41] Both TSP-1 and TSP-2 are best known for their antiangiogenic properties and their ability to modulate cell-matrix interactions.[42]

Integrins and Cell Attachment Proteins

As indicated earlier, cell surfaces contain groups of proteins, integrins, that mediate cell-matrix interactions. The integrins behave as receptors for components of the ECM and also interact with components of the cytoskeleton.[43] This provides a mechanism for the mediation of intracellular processes by components of the ECM, including control of cell shape and metabolic activity. The integrins exist as paired molecules containing alpha and beta subunits. They appear to have a significant degree of specificity for ECM proteins, which apparently is conferred by a combination of different alpha and beta subunits.

In addition to the integrins, cell attachment proteins (CAMs) are present on the cell surface. These confer specific cell-cell recognition properties. For reviews on integrins and CAMs, see Albelda and Buck,[43] Danen and Yamada,[44] Takagi,[45] and Lock and associates.[46]

AGING AND THE PROPERTIES OF CONNECTIVE TISSUES

From the foregoing discussion, it becomes apparent that there can be a multitude of possible loci in the development, structural organization, metabolism, and molecular biology of connective tissues for the introduction of alterations in the properties of these tissues. For a given tissue, changes in the composition of the ECM or changes in the factors that control the production of ECM can feed back through complex mechanisms to induce changes in tissue properties. The process of aging may well involve some of these factors. It is probable that during the aging process, the phenotypical expression of ECM—that is, the patterns of ECM composition—will change. It is also probable that many of the components of the ECM may evolve with time as a function of their long biologic half-lives and the enzymatic and nonenzymatic modifications that take place. These can include processes of maintenance and repair, responses to inflammation, nonenzymatic glycosylation (glycation), and cross-linkage formation.

In a sense, it may be important to differentiate between those processes of senescence that are genetically programmed (innate senescence) and the contributions to aging induced by environmental factors. However, it becomes difficult to distinguish whether a given alteration is an effect or a cause of aging.

In this section, we will discuss some of the factors and conditions involving connective tissues that may be associated with the aging process. These include aspects of cellular senescence, inflammatory and growth factors, photoaging of the skin, diabetes mellitus, nonenzymatic glycosylation, the cause of OS, osteoarthritis (OA), atherosclerosis, Werner syndrome (WS), and Alzheimer disease (AD).

Cellular Senescence

A large body of research has established conclusively that normal diploid cells have a limited replicative life span and that cells from older animals have shorter life spans than those from younger animals. Thus, the process of aging could be attributed to cellular senescence. A number of observations have suggested that connective tissue proteins may be affected during cellular senescence. In an extensive study on the properties of murine skin fibroblasts, van Gansen and van Lerberghe[47] concluded that among the main effects of cellular mitotic age were a depression of chromatin plasticity, changes in the organization of cytoplasmic filaments, and changes in the organization of the ECM. They implicated an involvement of collagen fibers in the intracellular events in vivo and in vitro. Although senescent fibroblasts may not be dividing, they are biosynthetically active, showing an increased synthesis of FN and increased levels of FN mRNA. However, both senescent and progeroid cells demonstrated a decreased chemotactic response to FN and developed a much thicker extracellular FN network than young fibroblasts.[48] There is some indication that with increasing age, cells become less able to respond to mitogens, which may have a bearing on age-related differences in wound healing.[49] It was also shown that the presence of senescent chondrocytes increases the risk of articular cartilage degeneration, which is associated with fibrillation of the articular surface and increased collagen cross-linking.[50] Thus, it would appear that there is some correlation between cellular senescence and changes in the regulation of connective tissue metabolism and cellular interactions.

Inflammatory and Growth Factors

An active area of contemporary connective tissue biology is the study of the influence of inflammatory and growth factors on the properties of connective tissues. It is well recognized that inflammatory cells accumulate in damaged and infected tissues as part of the inflammatory response. These cells secrete lymphokines such as the interleukins and other factors that may influence connective tissue metabolism. In addition, a number of growth factors, including epidermal growth factor (EGF), platelet-derived growth factor (PDGF), fibroblast growth factors (FGFs), and transforming growth factors (TGFs), can have extensive control over connective tissue metabolism. As indicated above, senescent cells may not respond to these factors as young cells. In addition, it is possible that stimulation of cell replication by certain of these factors may accelerate the progression of cells toward senescence. To add to the complexity are the findings that many cells can synthesize some of these factors, including interleukin-1, PDGF, FGFs, and TGFs, endowing the cellular components of tissues with autocrine and paracrine properties.

In studies reported by Furuyama and colleagues,[51] alveolar type II epithelial cells cultured on collagen fibrils in a medium supplemented with TGF-β1 synthesized a thin continuous BM. Immunohistochemical studies revealed the presence of type IV collagen, LM, perlecan and entactin-nidogen. Similar stimulatory effects of TGF-β1 on BM protein synthesis in rat liver sinusoids were reported by Neubauer and associates.[52] The role of a variety of growth factors and cytokines in the development of inflammatory synovitis accompanied by the destruction of joint cartilage was demonstrated in studies by Gravallese.[53] Studies by Takehara[54] have suggested that the growth of skin fibroblasts is regulated by a variety of cytokines and growth factors, with a resultant increase in ECM protein production. The extent of involvement of these interacting factors in the aging process is not clear, but it is probable that they contribute to the process.

Mechanisms of Cutaneous Aging

Cutaneous aging is a complex biologic activity consisting of two distinct components: (1) intrinsic, genetically determined degeneration; and (2) extrinsic aging due to exposure to the environment, also known as photoaging. These two processes are superimposed in the sun-exposed areas of skin, with their profound effects on the biology of cellular and structural elements of the skin.[55,56] The symptoms of photoaging are different from those of intrinsic aging, and evidence suggests that these two processes have different mechanisms.

A variety of theories have been advanced to explain aging phenomena, and some of them may be applicable to innate skin aging as well. It was postulated that diploid cells, such as dermal fibroblasts, have a finite life span in culture.[54] This observation, when extrapolated to the tissue level, could be expected to result in cellular senescence and degenerative changes in the dermis. Others have suggested that free radicals may damage collagen in the dermis,[57] and a third theory implicates nonenzymatic glycosylation of proteins, such as collagen, leading to increased cross-linking of collagen fibrils. It has been postulated that this process is the major cause of dysfunction of collagenous tissues in old age.[58] Finally, cutaneous aging may be attributed to differential gene expression of the ECM of connective tissue. It has been demonstrated that the rate of collagen biosynthesis is markedly reduced in the skin of older people.[59] Collectively, the observations on dermal connective tissue components in innate aging suggest an imbalance between biosynthesis and degradation, with less repair capacity in the presence of ongoing degradation.

Additional changes in the aged dermis concern the architecture of the collagen and elastin networks. The spaces between fibrous components are more compact owing to a loss of noncollagenous components. Collagen bundles appear to unravel, and there are signs of elastolysis. Scanning electron microscopic studies of the three-dimensional arrangement of rat skin from animals ranging in age from 2 weeks to 24 months showed that during postnatal growth, there was a dynamic rearrangement of the collagen and elastic fibers, with an ordered arrangement of mature collagen bundles being attained by producing distortions of relatively straight elastic fibers. During adulthood, there is a tortuosity of these elastic fibers, coupled with an incomplete restructuring of the elastic network that was deposited to interlock with the collagen bundles.

The effects of photodamage on dermal connective tissue are exemplified in the histopathologic pictures of photoaging. The hallmark of photoaging is the massive accumulation of the so-called elastotic material in the upper and mid-dermis. This phenomenon, known as solar elastosis, has been attributed to changes in elastin.[60] Solar elastotic material is composed of elastin, fibrillin, versican, a large proteoglycan, and hyaluronic acid. Even though the elastotic material contains the normal constituents of elastic fibers, the supramolecular organization of solar elastotic material and its functionality are severely perturbed. It was also found that elastin gene expression is markedly activated in cells within the sun-damaged dermis. In addition, it has been shown that the accumulation of elastotic material is accompanied by degeneration of the surrounding collagen meshwork. Parallel studies provide evidence implicating MMPs as mediators of collagen damage in photoaging.[59]

It would appear that the main culprit in photoaging appears to be the ultraviolet B (UVB) portion of the UV spectrum, although UVA and infrared radiation also contribute to the damage. In UVA-irradiated hairless mice, there appears to be alteration in the ratio of type III to type I collagen in addition to the elastosis. It has been shown that UV irradiation of fibroblasts in culture enhances expression of MMPs.[59] There is also an increase in the levels of the components of the ground substance in photoaged skin (predominantly dermatan sulfate, heparan sulfate, and hyaluronic acid). In human aged skin, mast cells are numerous and appear to be degranulated. These cells are known to produce a variety of inflammatory mediators, so that photoaged skin is chronically inflamed. In innate aging, the skin tends to be hypocellular. The microcirculation of the skin is also affected, becoming sparse, with the horizontal superficial plexus almost destroyed. Although atrophy may be present in end-stage photoaging in older adults, ongoing photoaging is characterized by more, not less elastotic components.

The effects of photoaging could be totally prevented by the use of broad-spectrum sunscreens. Although severe photoaging in humans is considered to be irreversible, in hairless mice it was found that repair could take place after the cessation of irradiation, with the newly deposited collagen appearing totally normal. A similar repair was observed in biopsies of severely photodamaged human skin after several years of avoidance of exposure to the sun.

Diabetes Mellitus

Currently, two types of diabetes mellitus are recognized clinically, type 1 diabetes (DM 1), which is insulin-dependent and is caused by beta cell destruction, and type 2 diabetes (DM 2), formerly known as non–insulin-dependent diabetes. Diabetics often show signs of accelerated aging, primarily as a result of the complications of vascular disease and impaired wound healing so common in this disease. It is well-documented that diabetics will exhibit a thickening of vascular BMs.[5] The biologic basis for this thickening is as yet obscure but could well be related to abnormalities in cell attachment or the response to factors affecting BM formation, to excessive nonenzymatic glycosylation of proteins, or to an abnormal turnover of BM components. Fibroblasts from diabetic individuals exhibit a premature senescence in culture.[61]

The role of inhibitors of aldose reductase was investigated by Sibbitt and colleagues.[62] They showed that in normal human fibroblasts, the mean population doubling times, population doublings to senescence, saturation density at confluence, tritiated thymidine incorporation, and response to PDGF were inhibited with increasing glucose concentrations in the media. They found that inhibitors of aldose reductase, sorbinil and tolrestat, completely prevented these inhibitions. Myoinositol had similar effects, but no data were presented to indicate that aldose reductase inhibitors would reverse the premature senescence in fibroblasts from diabetic individuals. Thus, it is unclear whether prevention of the formation of reduced sugars can have a therapeutic effect, nor is it clear that all the aging effects of diabetes are mediated by reduced sugars.

One of the lesser known complications of DM 1 and DM 2 is bone loss. This complication has been receiving increased attention because DM 1 diabetics are living longer owing to better therapeutic measures; however, they are faced with additional complications associated with aging, such as OS.[63] Both DM 1 and DM 2 diabetic patients are at high risk of cardiovascular disease. Uncontrolled hyperglycemia may give rise to nonenzymatic glycosylation of proteins, which may lead to the generation of reactive oxygen species, increased intermolecular and intramolecular cross-linking, with subsequent vessel damage, and atherogenesis.[64,65]

Nonenzymatic Glycosylation (Glycation) and Collagen Cross-Linking

When enzymes attach sugars to proteins, they usually do so at sites on the protein molecule dictated by the specificity of the enzyme for the regional sequence to be glycosylated. On the other hand, glycation, a process long known to cause food discoloration and toughness, proceeds nonspecifically at any site that is sterically available.[65] The longer a protein is in contact with a reducing sugar, the greater the chance for glycation to occur. In uncontrolled diabetics, elevated circulating levels of glycosylated hemoglobin and albumin are found. Because erythrocytes turn over every 120 days, the levels of hemoglobin A_{1c} are an index of the degree of control of hyperglycemia over a 120-day period. The same is true for glycosylated albumin over a shorter period. Proteins such as collagen, which is extremely long-lived, have also been shown to undergo glycation. Paul and Bailey[66] have demonstrated that the glycation of collagen forms the basis of its central role in the complications of aging and diabetes mellitus.

The glycation reactions between glucose and proteins are collectively known as the Maillard or Browning reaction. The initial reaction is the formation of a Schiff base between glucose and an amino group of the protein. This is an unstable structure, and it can spontaneously undergo an Amadori rearrangement, in which a new ketone group is generated on the adduct. This can condense with a similar product on another peptide sequence to produce a covalent cross-linkage.[64] Initially, glycation affects the interaction of collagen with cells and other matrix components, but the most damaging effects are caused by the formation of glucose-mediated, intermolecular cross-linkages. These cross-linkages decrease the critical flexibility and permeability of the tissues and reduce turnover. Another fibrous protein that is similarly modified by glycation is elastin.[66] Verzijl and associates[67] have shown that during aging, nonenzymatic glycation results in the accumulation of the advanced glycation end product pentosidine in an articular cartilage aggrecan.

The Arthritides

Osteoarthritis

The development of rheumatoid diseases, particularly OA, is a common event in aging individuals. The cause of OA and OP is based on a variety of factors, ranging from genetic susceptibility and endocrine and metabolic status to mechanical and traumatic injury events.[68] With aging, the bone loss in OA is lower compared to OP. The lower degree of bone loss with aging is explained by the lower bone turnover, as measured by bone resorption-formation parameters.[69] In the initial stages of OA, there is increased cell proliferation and synthesis of matrix proteins, proteinases, growth factors, and cytokines synthesized by adult articular chondrocytes. Other types of cells and tissues of the joint, including the synovium and subchondral bone, contribute to the pathogenesis.[70]

In inflammatory arthritis, degradative enzymes, including tissue collagenases and MMPs, are present in the rheumatoid lesion, leading to degradation of cartilage and bone. It is believed that inflammatory factors stimulate abnormal levels of these enzymes.[71] Studies by Iannone and Lapadula[72] have demonstrated that interleukin-1 (IL-1) is produced by synovial cells. IL-1, TNF-β, and other cytokines are also mitogenic for synovial cells and can stimulate the production of collagenases, proteoglycanases, plasminogen activator, and prostaglandins. It has been suggested that IL-1 plays an important role in the pathogenesis of rheumatoid arthritis.

Osteoporosis

OP is a systemic skeletal disease comprised of rarefaction of bone structure and loss of bone mass, leading to increased fracture risk. The frequency of this disorder increases with aging. Twin and family studies have demonstrated a genetic component of OP regarding parameters of bone properties, such as bone mineral density, with a heredity component of 60% to 80%.[73] OP affects most women older than 80 years; at the age of 50 years, the lifetime risk of suffering an OP-related fracture approaches 50% in women and 20% in men. Studies have indicated that genetic variations explain as much as 70% of the variance for bone mineral density in the population.[74] The National Organization of Osteoporosis recommends bone density testing for all women older than 65 years and earlier (around the time of menopause) for women who have risk factors.

Viguet-Carrin and coworkers[75] have demonstrated that different determinants of bone quality are interrelated, especially mineral content and modifications in collagen. Different processes of maturation of collagen occur in bone involving enzymatic and nonenzymatic reactions. The latter type of collagen modification is age-related and may impair the mechanical properties of bone. In a study of human trabecular bone taken at autopsy, Oxlund and colleagues[76] examined collagen and reducible and nonreducible collagen cross-linkages in relation to age and OP. The extractability of collagen from vertebral bone of control individuals increased with age. Bone collagen of those with OP showed increased extractability and a marked decrease in the concentration of the divalent reducible collagen cross-linkages compared with gender- and age-matched controls. No alterations were observed in the concentration of trivalent pyridinium cross-linkages. These changes would be expected to reduce the strength of the bone trabeculae and could explain why those with OP had bone fractures, although the collagen density did not differ from that of the gender- and age-matched controls.

Croucher and associates[77] have quantitatively assessed cancellous structure in 35 patients with primary OP. Their data demonstrated that for a given cancellous area, structural changes in primary OP are similar to those observed during age-related bone loss in normal subjects. These findings strongly implicate an abnormal increase in the activity (or activities) of osteoclast-derived resorption enzymes, acting on the degradation of the ECM, in the cause of OP.

Arterial Aging

In young healthy individuals, the resiliency function of elastic arteries, principally the aorta, results in optimal interaction with the heart and optimal steady flow through peripheral resistance vessels. As the arteries age, changes in their composition and structure lead to an increase in the stiffness of their walls, resulting in increased pulse pressure, hypertension, and greater risk of cardiovascular disease. Another effect of aortic stiffening is transmission of flow pulsations downstream into vasodilated organs, principally the brain and kidney, where pulsatile energy is dissipated and fragile microvessels are damaged. This accounts for microinfarcts and microhemorrhages, with specialized cell damage, cognitive decline, and renal failure.[78]

The arterial media responsible for arterial stiffness and resilience is composed of elastin, collagen, vascular smooth muscle cells, and noncollagenous proteins. Elastin comprises 90% of arterial elastic fibers. The generalized age-related stiffening (arteriosclerosis) is confined primarily to the media of arteries. Elastin content in the aorta has been shown to be relatively constant with aging; however, because collagen content increases with aging, the absolute amount of elastin actually decreases. These changes likely affect the mechanical properties of the aorta.[79] Although the absolute amounts of collagen and elastin in arteries fall with age, the ratio of collagen to elastin increases.

In addition, with age, elastic lamellae undergo fragmentation and thinning, leading to ectasia and a gradual transfer of mechanical load to collagen, which is 100 to 1000 times stiffer than elastin. Possible causes of this fragmentation are mechanically (fatigue failure) or enzymatically driven by MMP activity.[79] MMPs navigate the behavior of vascular wall cells in different atherosclerosis stages, adaptive remodeling, normal aging and nonatherosclerotic vessel disease.[80] In arteries, accumulation of advanced glycation end products over time leads to cross-linking of collagen and consequent increases in its material stiffness. Furthermore, the remaining elastin itself becomes stiffer because of calcification and the formation of cross-links resulting from the increased presence of advanced glycation end products, a process that affects collagen even more strongly.[79] These changes are accelerated in the presence of disease, such as hypertension, diabetes, and uremia. Most studies have shown that arterial stiffening occurs across all age groups in DM 1 and DM 2. Arterial stiffening in DM-2 results, in part, from the clustering of hyperglycemia, dyslipidemia, and hypertension, all of which may promote insulin resistance, oxidative stress, endothelial dysfunction, and the formation of proinflammatory cytokines and advanced glycosylation end products.[81]

Although there is ample evidence for the link between arteriosclerosis and the degradation and remodeling of collagen and elastin, much remains unknown about the detailed mechanisms.

Werner Syndrome

WS is a rare autosomal recessive premature aging disease manifested by age-related phenotypes, such as atherosclerosis, cataracts, OP, soft tissue calcification, premature graying, and loss of hair, as well as a high incidence of some types of cancer.[82] The gene product, *WRN*, which is defective in WS, is a member of the RecQ family of DNA helicases.[83] Clinical and biologic manifestations in four major body tissues and/or systems—nervous, immune, connective, and endocrine systems—similar to normal aging, appear at an early stage of the patient's life. WS may cause abnormalities in the cardiovascular system that are manifested as restrictive cardiomyopathy.[84,85] Ostler and coworkers[86] have reported that WS fibroblasts show a mutator phenotype, abbreviated replicative life, and accelerated cellular senescence. They also demonstrated that T cells derived from WS patients have the mutator phenotype. Increased collagen synthesis in fibroblasts from two WS patients has been reported. This was accompanied by a near doubling of the levels of procollagen mRNA over normal controls. Similarly, studies by Hatamochi and colleagues[87] have demonstrated that a WS fibroblast-conditioned medium activated normal fibroblast proliferation but failed to alter the relative rates of collagen and noncollagenous protein synthesis by these fibroblasts.

Alzheimer Disease

AD is a disease of old age. The characteristic pathophysiologic changes at autopsy include neurofibrillary tangles, neuritis plaques, neuronal loss, and amyloid angiopathy. Mutations in chromosomes 1, 12, and 21 cause familial AD. Susceptibility genes do not cause the disease by themselves but, in combination with other genes, modulate the age of onset and increase the probability of AD.[87] Significant progress has been made in identifying the mutations in the tau protein and dissecting the crosstalk between tau and the second hallmark lesion of AD, the Aβ peptide-containing amyloid plaque.[88]

Studies of familial AD have demonstrated reduction or loss of smooth muscle actin in the media of cerebral arterioles. Intracerebral arterioles and numerous capillaries were laden with amyloid deposits. There was marked expression of collagen type III and BM collagen type IV. Fibers of both amyloid and collagen were found within the BM.[89]

Clinical and experimental studies have shown that cerebral perfusion is progressively decreased as aging progresses, and this decrease in brain blood flow is significantly greater in AD.[90] Studies by Carare and associates[91] have shown that capillary and arteriole BMs seem to act as lymphatics of the brain for drainage of fluid and solutes. Amyloid beta is deposited in BM drainage pathways in cerebral amyloid angiopathy and may impede the elimination of amyloid beta and interstitial fluid from the brain in AD.

The localization of BM components such as LM, entactin-nidogen and collagen type IV to the amyloid plaques has suggested that these components may play a role in the pathogenesis of AD.[91] The work of Kiuchi and coworkers[92,93] has shown that entactin-nidogen, collagen type IV, and LM had the most pronounced effect on preformed Aβ 42 fibrils, causing disassembly of Aβ protein fibrils. Circular dichroism studies have indicated that high concentrations of BM components induce structural transition in Aβ 42 beta sheets to random structures.

It has been suggested that the vascular BM may serve as a nidus for senile plaque, playing a role in the development of amyloid and neuritic elements in AD.

SUMMARY

This chapter has reviewed some aspects of biochemistry and molecular biology, as well as the involvement of connective tissue in the process of aging. There is a complexity inherent in the control of connective tissue structure, metabolism, and molecular biology, and aging might contribute to alterations in these, and vice versa. Among the phenomena that may prove central to the aging process are the processes of collagen cross-linking and glycation. Advanced glycation end products and their receptors induce inflammation, which can be destructive; however, there are also protective effects on tissues. Alternative gene splicing of many interacting connective tissue proteins leads to altered interactions and reciprocal changes in the communication between cells and their surrounding connective tissues. Also involved in the aging process are the effects of solar radiation, interplay of cytokines, growth factors, and hormones on the control of connective tissue and muscle phenotype,[94] production and action of degradative enzymes, factors that affect cell replication, connective tissue diseases, and intracellular factors that control senescence. The causes and effects of aging are an active area of contemporary research in which the involvement of connective tissue is an important element.

KEY POINTS: CONNECTIVE TISSUES AND AGING

- Changes in the structural integrity and production of connective tissue macromolecules are associated with the process of aging.
- Loss of tissue function in aging is associated with increased cross-linking of collagen and elastin fibrils and subsequent decrease in their turnover.
- Alternative splicing in the mRNA of the connective tissue macromolecules has been implicated in the process of aging.
- There is a correlation between cellular senescence and changes in the regulation of connective tissue metabolism.
- Glycation of collagen and elastin is accelerated with aging and may be associated with changes in diabetes.
- In age-related osteoporosis, a decrease in divalent reducible collagen cross-linkages may lead to reduced bone strength and may explain increased bone fractures.
- In aging and in senile dementia of the Alzheimer type, there is co-localization of type IV collagen, laminin, heparan sulfate proteoglycan and amyloid plaques in the brain vasculature.

For a complete list of references, please visit www.expertconsult.com.

KEY REFERENCES

1. Brodsky B, Persikov AV: Molecular structure of the collagen triple helix. Adv Protein Chem 70:301–339, 2005.
2. Bailey AJ, Paul RG, Knott L: Mechanisms of maturation and aging of collagen. Mech Ageing Dev 106:1–56, 1998.
5. Kefalides NA, Borel JP: Basement membranes: cell and molecular biology, San Diego, 2005, Academic Press.
10. Tayebjee MH, Lip GY, MacFadyen RJ: Metalloproteinases in coronary artery disease: clinical and therapeutic implications and pathological significance. Curr Med Chem 12:917–925, 2005.
18. Iozzo RV, Shaefer L: Proteoglycans in health and disease: novel regulatory signaling mechanisms evoked by the small leucine-rich proteoglycans. FEBS J 277:3864–3875, 2010.
21. Schwarzbauer JE, DeSimone DW: Fibronectins, their fibrillogenesis, and in vivo functions. Cold Spring Harb Perspect Biol 3:a005041, 2011.
26. Hinz B, Phan SH, Thannickal VJ, et al: Recent developments in myofibroblast biology: paradigms for connective tissue remodeling. Am J Pathol 180:1340–1355, 2012.
27. Muro AF, Chauhan AK, Gajovic S, et al: Regulated splicing of the fibronectin EDA exon is essential for proper skin wound healing and normal lifespan. J Cell Biol 162:149–160, 2003.
28. Bhattacharyya S, Tamaki Z, Wang W, et al: Fibronection EDA promotes chronic cutaneous fibosis through Toll-like receptor signaling. Sci Transl Med 6:232ra50, 2014.
29. Andrews JP, Marttala J, Macarak E, et al: Keloid pathogenesis: potential role of cellular fibronectin with the EDA domain. J Invest Dermatol 135:1921–1924, 2015.
30. Domogatskaya A, Rodin S, Tryggvason K: Functional diversity of laminins. Annu Rev Cell Dev Biol 28:523–553, 2012.
42. Bornstein P, Agah A, Kyriakides TR: The role of thrombospondins 1 and 2 in the regulation of cell-matrix interactions, collagen fibril formation, and the response to injury. Int J Biochem Cell Biol 36:1115–1125, 2004.

59. Uitto J, Bernstein EF: Molecular mechanisms of cutaneous aging: connective tissue alteration in the dermis. J Investig Dermatol Symp Proc 3:41–44, 1998.
66. Paul RG, Bailey AJ: Glycation of collagen: the basis of its central role in the late complications of ageing and diabetes. Int J Biochem Cell Biol 28:1297–1310, 1996.
78. O'Rourke MF: Arterial aging: pathophysiological principles. Vasc Med 12:329–341, 2007.
79. Tsamis A, Krawiec JT, Vorp DA: Elastin and collagen fibre microstructure of the human aorta in ageing and disease: a review. J R Soc Interface 10:20121004, 2013.
80. Greenwald SE: Ageing of the conduit arteries. J Pathol 211:157–172, 2007.
83. Ozgenc A, Loeb LA: Current advances in unraveling the function of the Werner syndrome protein. Mutat Res 577:237–251, 2005.
88. Cummings JL, Vinters HV, Cole GM, et al: Alzheimer's disease: etiologies, pathophysiology, cognitive reserve, and treatment opportunities. Neurology 51:S2–S17, 1998.
94. Tarantino U, Baldi J, Celi M, et al: Osteoporosis and sarcopenia: the connections. Aging Clin Exp Res 25(Suppl 1):S93–S95, 2013.

20 Bone and Joint Aging

Celia L. Gregson

The musculoskeletal system serves three primary functions: (1) it enables an efficient means of limb movement; (2) it acts as an endoskeleton, providing overall mechanical support and protection to soft tissues; and (3) it serves as a mineral reservoir for calcium homeostasis. In older adults, the first two of these functions frequently become compromised; musculoskeletal problems are a major cause of pain and physical disability in older adults and represent a significant contributor to the global burden of disease.[1] Furthermore, fracture incidence rises steeply with age[2] (Figure 20-1). Several factors contribute to the age-related decline in musculoskeletal function:

1. Effects of aging on components of the musculoskeletal system (e.g., articular cartilage, skeleton, soft tissues), contributing to the development of osteoporosis and osteoarthritis as well as a reduced range of joint movement, stiffness, and difficulty in initiating movement
2. Age-related rise in the prevalence of common musculoskeletal disorders beginning in young adulthood or middle age and causing increasing pain and disability without shortening life span (e.g., seronegative spondyloarthritis, musculoskeletal trauma)
3. High incidence of certain musculoskeletal disorders in older adults (e.g., polymyalgia rheumatica, Paget disease of bone, crystal-related arthropathies)

A number of interrelated hypotheses have been proposed to explain the high prevalence of bone, muscle and joint problems in older adults[3-6]:

1. Our long life span results in increasing accumulation of mechanical damage to the musculoskeletal system, potentially exacerbated by rising levels of obesity.
2. There is a lack of genetic investment in the repair of age-related tissue damage developing in the postreproductive phase of life.
3. The musculoskeletal system in humans has not fully adapted to the upright posture and prehensile grip because of lack of evolutionary pressure. Hence, many of our bones and joints are inappropriately shaped and underdesigned to cope with the stresses endured.
4. Our modern sedentary lifestyle mean that people today tend to be exposed to less mechanical stress than our ancestors. Because musculoskeletal strength is governed by the mechanical strains to which it is exposed, our weaker musculoskeletal systems may not be so well adapted for episodes of sudden major stress.

Several different mechanisms are involved in musculoskeletal tissue aging, including the following[7-10]:

- Reduced synthetic capacity of differentiated cells such as osteoblasts and chondrocytes, with a consequent loss of ability to maintain matrix integrity
- Accumulation of degraded molecules, such as proteoglycan fragments, in musculoskeletal tissue matrices
- Decline in mesenchymal stem cell (MSC) populations
- Changes in posttranslational modification of structural proteins such as collagen and elastin
- Aberrant epigenetic modification altering cell regulation
- Induction of inflammatory mediators with accumulation of proinflammatory cytokines
- Increased production of reactive oxygen species and mitochondrial dysfunction, leading to oxidative stress, which contributes to stress-induced senescence
- Decreased levels of trophic hormones and growth factors such as insulin-like growth factor 1 (IGF-1) or altered cellular responsiveness to these factors
- Alterations in the loading patterns of tissue or the tissue's response to loading
- Decreased capacity for wound healing and tissue repair, which may be the result of some or all of the mechanisms described above

The major tissues pivotal to the integrity of the musculoskeletal system are articular cartilage, skeleton, and soft tissues. Age-related changes in these structures will now be described in more detail.

ARTICULAR CARTILAGE

The structure of a mammalian synovial joint is summarized in Figure 20-2. Much of its function derives from the properties of articular cartilage, which cushions the subchondral bone beneath and provides a low-friction surface necessary for free movement. Articular cartilage contains very few cells, is aneural and avascular, and yet in health its integrity is maintained throughout a lifetime of biomechanical stress. A certain amount of mechanical loading is known to be necessary for cartilage homeostasis, because joint damage develops following immobilization.[11] The chief cells in cartilage are chondrocytes; the extracellular matrix is composed principally of type II collagen and aggrecan (aggregating proteoglycans). Collagen molecules consist of a triple helix of three polypeptide chains, cross-linked to form collagen fibrils, which are bound to hyaluronic acid and aggrecan and form a network of collagen fibrils.[12,13] Aggrecan has many glycosaminoglycan side chains, which help retain water molecules within the matrix.[13] Over two thirds of the articular cartilage weight is water, and this high water content is vital to maintain the tissue's viscoelastic properties.[12] The collagen fibrillar network confers tensile strength to the articular cartilage, whereas aggrecan produces stiffness under compression.[12,13]

With age, articular cartilage thins and changes color from a glistening white to a dull yellow, and its mechanical properties deteriorate. There is a decrease in tensile stiffness, fatigue resistance, and strength, but no significant change in its compressive properties; these changes are partly caused by a decrease in water content. The morphology and function of the chondrocytes and nature of aggrecan and type II collagen also change with age. Osteoarthritis (OA) is the name given to a number of characteristic pathologic changes occurring in synovial joints and adversely affecting joint function. OA is thought to arise when there is an imbalance between the mechanical forces acting on or within a joint and the ability of the articular cartilage and other joint tissues to withstand these forces. Damage can be caused by abnormal mechanical forces acting on normal joint tissues or by normal forces acting on already damaged or abnormal tissues.[14] Although OA is not an inevitable consequence of aging, aging

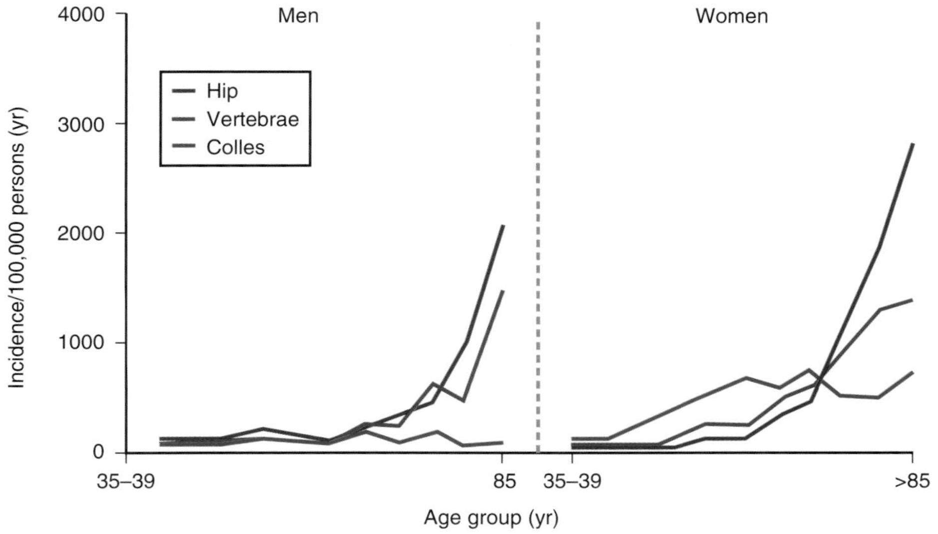

Figure 20-1. Age-specific incidence rates for hip, vertebral, and distal forearm (Colles) fractures in Rochester, Minnesota, men and women. *(Adapted from Cooper C, Melton LJ III: Epidemiology of osteoporosis. Trends Endocrinol Metab 3:224–229, 1992; with permission.)*

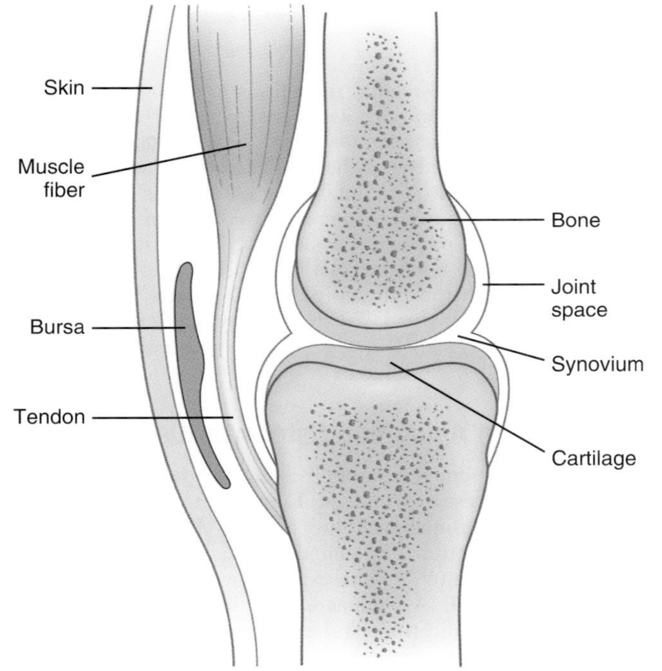

Figure 20-2. The synovial joint. The histologic appearances of the main tissues are highlighted. *(Courtesy Dr. J.H. Klippel and Dr. P.A. Dieppe.)*

adds to the risk of developing OA because it is associated with a number of joint changes affecting all the different joint tissues (Figure 20-3).

The chondrocyte's principal function is to maintain cartilage homeostasis. However, with age, chondrocytes develop a senescent phenotype with impaired synthetic activity such that the proteoglycans they produce become small and irregular. The response by chondrocytes to changes in anabolic and catabolic stimuli (e.g., IGF-1, osteogenic protein-1, transforming growth factor-β [TGF-β], interleukins [ILs]) tips the balance toward catabolism, which increases OA susceptibility.[7] In OA, excess catabolic activity disrupts cartilage homeostasis, causing cartilage matrix breakdown, principally orchestrated by proinflammatory cytokines and catabolic mediators (e.g., MMPs [matrix metalloproteinases]) and ADAMTS (***a d****isintegrin* ***a****nd* ***m****etalloproteinase with* ***t****hrombo****s****pondin motifs*). Replicative senescence, due to telomere shortening with consequent telomere dysfunction, may contribute to chondrocyte aging. However, slow chondrocyte turnover rates reduce susceptibility. Instead, stress-induced senescence, due to telomere damage from oxidative stress, activated oncogenes, mitochondrial dysfunction, and inflammation, is thought to play a greater role. The senescent chondrocytes produce ILs and MMPs, mediating cartilage matrix damage. Autophagy, a homeostatic mechanism of cell recycling that removes damaged and/or redundant organelles and proteins, becomes deregulated in aging cartilage. Excess activation of the protein kinase mammalian target of rapamycin (mTOR), which suppresses autophagy, has been associated with aging. Interestingly, senescent cells, enlarged from accumulated proteins, can be rescued by rapamycin, an mTOR inhibitor.[15] Chondrocyte loss can also occur through increased apoptosis, a normal physiologic process involved in the removal of potential carcinogenic and damaged cells. High-mobility group box protein (HMGB2), whose levels decline with age, has emerged as an important regulator of chondrocyte survival.[16]

Proteoglycan depletion is one of the earliest signs of articular cartilage loss in OA. Proteoglycans consist of a protein core and two major glycosaminoglycan (GAG) side chains, chondroitin sulfate (CS) and keratin sulfate (KS). CS, the predominant GAG chain in human articular cartilage, is made up of oligosaccharide (sugar) chains containing a basic disaccharide repeat of two sugar molecules (*N*-acetylgalactosamine and glucuronic acid), which carry a sulfate group on the sixth (C6) or fourth (C4) carbon atom. Changes in the C6/C4 sulfation ratio show marked changes with aging and in OA, potentially making the cartilage more susceptible to cytokine-mediated damage.[17,18] The main proteoglycan, aggrecan, binds with hyaluronan to form massive hydrophilic aggregates that expand the collagen framework, providing compressive and tensile strength. With age, proteoglycan aggregation reduces, with the synthesis of smaller proteoglycans with increased KS and reduced CS content and increased aggrecanase production, leading to aggrecan degradation.

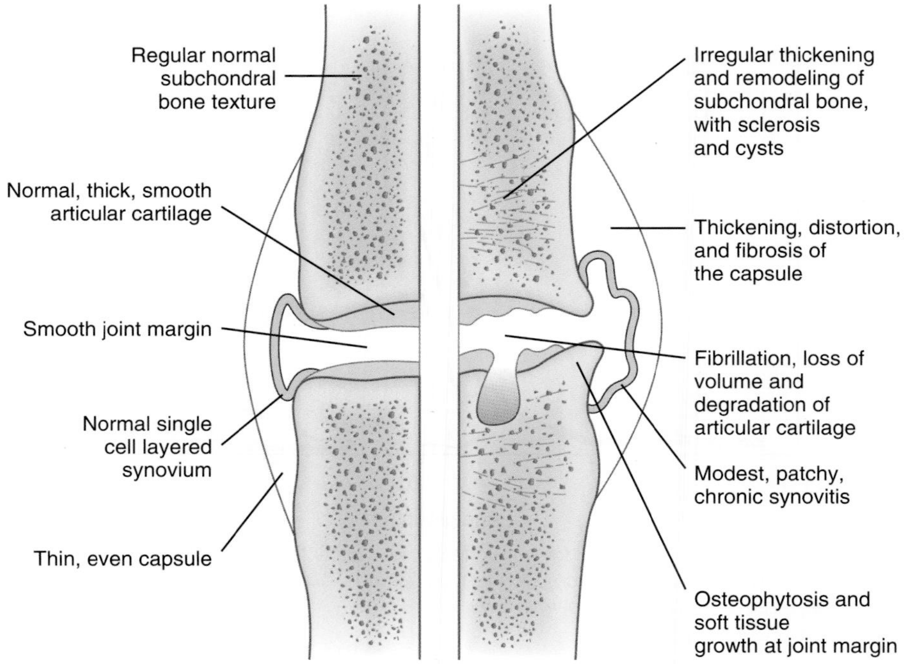

Figure 20-3. Normal versus whole synovial joint osteoarthritis. *(Courtesy Dr. J.H. Klippel and Dr. P.A. Dieppe.)*

Collagen also changes with age, with increases in fiber diameter and cross-linking. Fiber cross-linking may be enzymic or nonenzymic; the former process involves the enzyme lysyl hydroxylase. In young growing bone, collagen turnover is high, and enzymic divalent and trivalent cross-links stabilize the collagen fibers, with almost complete hydroxylation of telopeptide lysines. With age, lysyl hydroxylase activity wanes, causing incomplete hydroxylation of telopeptide lysines. However, further increases in collagen fiber cross-linking occur with age due to nonenzymatic reactions between glucose and lysine, forming glucosyl lysine and related molecules. Subsequent oxidative and nonoxidative reactions produce stable end products, known as advanced glycation end products (AGEs), some of which can act as collagen cross-links and produce fibers too stiff for optimal function, making cartilage more vulnerable to mechanical failure.[19,20] In chondrocytes, AGEs can suppress type II collagen production, simulate MMP and ADAMTS expression, and increase inflammation through the production of TNF-α (tumor necrosis factor-α), prostaglandin E2, and nitric oxide.[21,22] Hyperglycemia and oxidative stress increase AGE production, and dietary AGE intake may also be an important factor.[23,24] Elastin, which conveys extensibility and elastic recoil in some ligaments, is also stabilized by cross-linking, and AGE production can also prompt age-related stiffening.[25] Accumulation of reactive oxygen species (ROS) in the chondrocyte with aging, due in part to mitochondrial dysfunction, increases oxidative stress, which has a series of consequences, including DNA damage, telomere shortening, loss of anabolic activity, increased production of inflammatory cytokines and MMPs, chondrocyte senescence, and apoptosis.[8]

As well as changes to the articular cartilage, aging also adversely affects other tissues of the joint. Below the basal layer of articular cartilage (calcified cartilage) lies subchondral bone; an emerging body of evidence has now suggested that the metabolism of cartilage and bone is tightly coupled within joints and that this is important in the pathogenesis of OA.[26] Certainly, distinct bone changes are seen as OA progresses—increased subchondral bone turnover, hypomineralization of the underlying trabecular bone, subchondral sclerosis, and the formation of osteophytes and bone marrow lesions. The latter is predictive of the pain of OA.[27] Age-related reductions in estrogen, as seen in postmenopausal women, are associated with increases in bone turnover and cartilage degradation.[28] Correspondingly, use of estrogen replacement therapy has been associated with a reduced prevalence of OA.[29] Studies linking increased rates of bone turnover to OA progression have suggested a role for increased osteoclast activity in the pathogenesis of OA.[30] Thus, there is current interest in targeting bone and cartilage with antiresorptive medications,[26] although the efficacy of this approach has yet to be demonstrated in humans.[31] Further age-related changes within periarticular soft tissue structures that may also adversely affect joint health are discussed later.

Epigenetics in Aging and Osteoarthritis

The role of epigenetic regulation in aging and the cause of OA has been of growing research interest. Epigenetics may explain some of the so-called missing heritability of OA, a disease that can have a strong familial pattern. Epigenetic mechanisms are stable and inherited determinants of gene expression involving no changes in the underlying DNA sequence. They include DNA methylation; histone; modification; and small, noncoding microRNAs (miRNAs). Generally, methylation levels are reduced with age. Hypomethylation of a number of MMP promoters has been seen in cartilage affected by OA.[32] Furthermore, histone methylation has been shown to regulate the nuclear factor of activated T cells (NFAT); transcription factors in articular chondrocytes, as an age-dependent mechanism controlling chondrocyte homeostasis that when perturbed, manifests an OA-like phenotype.[33] Already a wide variety of miRNAs has been identified, with a range of roles in cartilage and the development of OA.[9] Research into the epigenetic mechanisms underlying aging and OA has been gaining momentum, offering the potential for novel insights into the mechanisms of disease, aging, and future therapies.

THE SKELETON

Weight-bearing bones consist of an outer shell of cortical bone, designed for maximum strength. In addition, certain sites, such

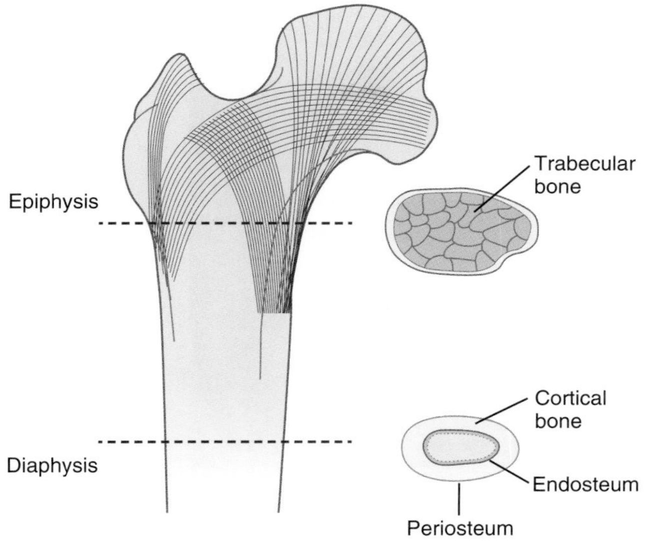

Figure 20-4. The macroscopic organization of bone. *(Courtesy Dr. J.H. Klippel and Dr. P.A. Dieppe.)*

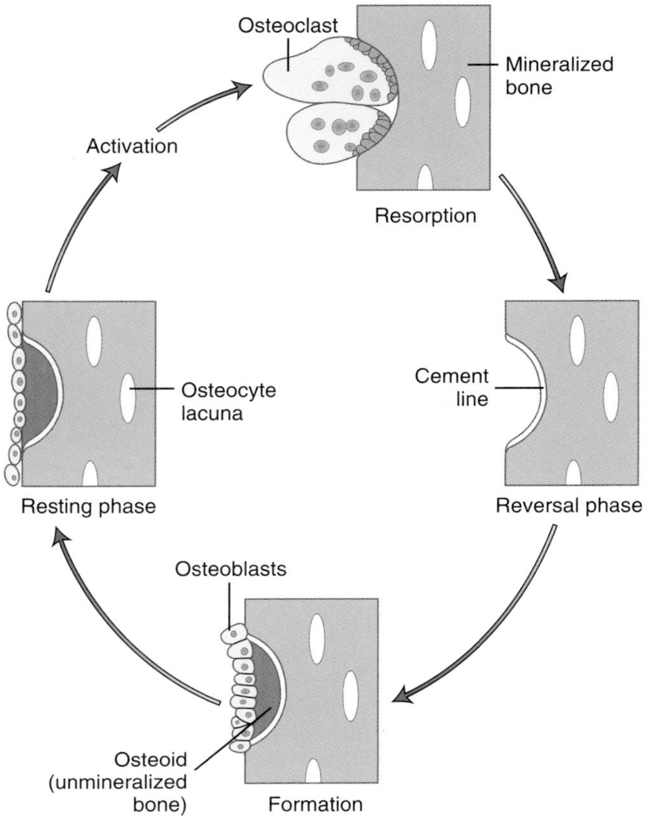

Figure 20-5. The bone remodeling sequence. This commences with osteoclastic bone resorption, after which a cement line is laid down (reversal phase). Osteoblasts then fill up the resorption cavity with osteoid, which subsequently mineralizes, and the bone surface is finally covered by lining cells and a thin layer of osteoid.

as vertebrae and metaphyses, contain an inner meshwork of trabecular bone, which acts as an internal scaffold (Figure 20-4). Microscopically, the skeleton is made up of interconnecting fibrils of type I collagen, which provide tensile strength. Hydroxyapatite crystals, comprised of calcium and phosphate, are deposited among the collagen fibrils, giving bone its rigidity. Adult bone continuously undergoes self-renewal. This process, known as bone remodeling, occurs at discrete sites throughout the skeleton, called bone remodeling units. Bone remodeling involves the coordinated activity of cells responsible for bone formation and resorption (osteoblasts and osteoclasts, respectively) in a continuous cycle aimed at repairing microdamage and adapting bone density and shape to the patterns of forces it endures (Figure 20-5). Osteoclasts differentiate from hematopoietic precursors shared with macrophages, whereas osteoblasts, which produce osteoid and promote mineralization, arise from MSCs, which also give rise to fibroblasts, stromal cells, and adipocytes. Osteocytes, the most numerous and long-lived of the bone cells, reside within the bone canaliculi. They are increasingly appreciated as important regulators of bone homeostasis; for example, osteocytes are the key mechanosensory cell in bone. Both osteoblasts and osteocytes produce membrane-bound receptor activator of nuclear factor-kappa B ligand (RANKL), which binds to the osteoclast's RANK receptor and stimulates osteoclast differentiation, averting cell death.[34] This process is regulated by osteoblasts, which also produce osteoprotegerin, a decoy receptor.[35] Multiple factors influence the RANK–RANKL–OPG system, including parathyroid hormone (PTH), vitamin D, cytokines, ILs, prostaglandins, thiazolidines, estrogen, mechanical forces, and TGF-β. Monoclonal antibodies to RANKL are now used to treat osteoporosis, reducing osteoclastic bone resorption.

Structural Changes in the Skeleton

Once middle age is reached, the total amount of calcium in the skeleton (bone mass) starts to decline, a process that accelerates during the first few years following menopause in women.[36] This is associated with changes in skeletal structure, whereby the skeleton becomes weaker and more prone to fracture. Trabecular bone is affected; individual trabeculae undergo thinning followed by perforation and ultimately removal, leading to deterioration of the trabecular network (Figure 20-6). The bony cortex also becomes considerably weaker during aging through a combination of thinning as a result of expansion of the inner medullary cavity and an increase in the size, number, and clustering of haversian canals. In addition to deterioration in skeletal architecture, the material strength of bone may also decline significantly with age; microfractures are thought to build up within bone tissue with increasing age, representing the accumulation of fatigue damage.[37] In addition, adverse biochemical changes may occur, such as a decline in cross-linking efficiency, required for stabilizing collagen fibrils.[38]

Changes in Skeletal Metabolism

Bone loss in older adults is largely a result of excess osteoclast activity, which causes an expansion in the total number of remodeling sites and an increase in the amount of bone resorbed per individual site, resulting in a bone remodeling imbalance. The rise in osteoclast activity in older women partly reflects the decline in ovarian hormone production following menopause because estrogens exert an important restraining influence on bone resorption by reducing RANKL production and promoting osteoclast apoptosis, also exerting antiapoptotic effects on osteoblasts.[39] Originally, the age-related declines in bone density were thought to be due to falling estrogen levels in women and testosterone levels in men. However, estrogens have also emerged as the dominant sex steroid in males, regulating bone loss later in

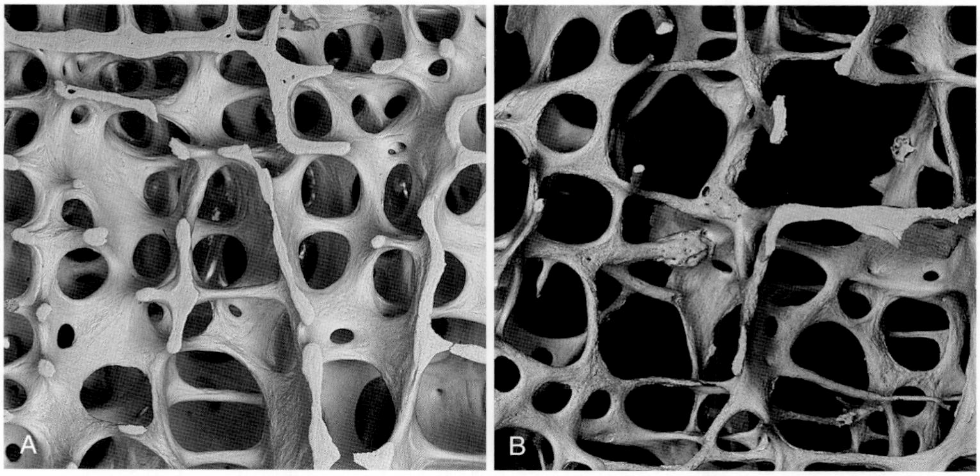

Figure 20-6. Changes in trabecular structure associated with osteoporosis. Shown are scanning electron micrographs of lumbar vertebrae (×20) obtained from a 31-year-old man **(A)** and an 89-year-old woman **(B)**. Note the loss of bone tissue, associated with thinning and removal of trabecular plates. *(Courtesy Professor A. Boyde, Department of Anatomy and Developmental Biology, University College, London.)*

life, as well as acquisition of peak bone mass in early life in combination with testosterone.[40] Serum estradiol and bioavailable estradiol levels are strongly correlated with bone mass density (BMD), which is not the case for testosterone. Progesterone, androgen, and inhibin levels also decline around the time of menopause, although their precise roles in bone remain to be determined.[41] Aging also alters the MSC population within bone marrow, slowing proliferation, reducing osteoblast differentiation, and leading to age-related impairment of bone formation. Oxidative stress, telomere shortening, local inflammation, and DNA damage are all thought to contribute to this osteoblast senescence.[42] Furthermore, aging leads to a gradual decline in circulating growth hormone (GH) and IGF-1, with consequent declines in bone density, lean body mass, and skin thickness, the so-called somatopause.[43] Reductions in these trophic factors encourage local expression of molecules (e.g., TNF-α, ILs), which increase osteoclasts, decrease osteoblast activity, and downgrade the differentiation potential of bone marrow MSCs.[44]

Osteoclast activity can be elevated in older adults as a consequence of vitamin D deficiency, which is widespread.[45] Low dietary vitamin D intake, combined with reduced sunlight exposure and a reduced capacity to synthesize vitamin D in aging skin, leads to mild secondary hyperparathyroidism.[46-48] These effects of vitamin D deficiency on bone metabolism are aggravated by age-related declines in the efficiency of gastrointestinal calcium absorption and of renal 1α-hydroxylation of vitamin D. Low vitamin D levels influence MSC differentiation toward greater adipogenesis at the expense of osteoblastogenesis.[49] Despite subclinical evidence of osteomalacia, many patients present in the same way as those with osteoporosis (e.g., with fractures of the femoral neck). Immobilization is recognized to cause bone loss, whereas physical activity can help attenuate rates of age-related bone loss. Reductions in physical activity often accompany aging, thereby reducing the quality and quantity of mechanical skeletal stimulation. A reduced mechanical load is sensed by osteocytes, which increases the expression of sclerostin, an inhibitor of canonical Wnt signaling and a potent inhibitor of osteoblastic bone formation. Sclerostin levels rise with age and immobility.[41,50] However, to what extent sclerostin explains age-related declines in osteoblastic bone formation has yet to be determined. Interestingly, sclerostin antibodies are currently in a phase 3 trial as a future anabolic osteoporosis treatment.[51]

SOFT TISSUES

Age-related changes occur in other bone and joint-related tissues, largely due to reduced synthesis and posttranslational modification of collagen, leading to reduced ligament elasticity. For example, the tensile strength of tendons and ligament-bone complexes declines with age, and the integrity of joint capsules may be lost. This may result in disorders such as rotator cuff dysfunction in the shoulder, in which communication between the shoulder joint and subachromial bursa may be seen. In addition, there is a gradual loss of connective tissue resistance to calcium crystal formation with age, leading to an increase in the incidence of crystal-related arthropathies. Functional impairment within soft tissues may also adversely affect joint biomechanics, which may represent an important initiating factor in OA development. For example, age-specific differences in the response of the meniscus to injury have been described, such that catabolic activity may predict progression of OA.[52]

Back and neck pain and stiffness are common complaints among older adults and can reflect age-related changes in intervertebral discs. The latter consist of an outer fibrous ring, the annulus fibrosus, and an internal gelatinous (semifluid) structure, the nucleus pulposus. As people get older, the diameter of the nucleus pulposus and hydrostatic pressure in this region decrease, resulting in increased compressive stress within the annulus.[53] Thus, with age, the intervertebral discs become compressed, reducing intervertebral spaces and leading to overall height loss. The extracellular matrix of the disc contains a network of collagen fibers (types I and II) responsible for tensile strength and aggregating proteoglycans that help the disc resist compressive forces. Changes in the distribution and concentrations of these macromolecules in later life can also significantly alter the mechanical properties of the disc. In many ways, these age-related changes in extracellular matrix metabolism in intervertebral discs are rather similar to those taking place in articular cartilage. For example, there is increased degradation and reduced synthesis of type II collagen and reduced glycosaminoglycan and collagen levels.[54]

Sarcopenia is the slow and progressive age-related loss of skeletal muscle, resulting in reduced muscle power and function. The consequences of increased falls, and hence increased fracture risk with associated loss of independence, can be devastating.

Sarcopenia involves reductions in muscle fiber number and size (atrophy), with type II fibers being particularly vulnerable. Sarcopenia has complex causes and is an area of ongoing research. Declining levels of anabolic factors are thought to be important, such as estrogen and vitamin D levels in women, testosterone and physical performance in men, in addition to waning GH and IGF-1 levels. Loss of central and peripheral innervations with reductions in motor units, and nutritional changes with altered protein synthesis also contribute. Increased levels of catabolic inflammatory cytokines and adipokines have also been implicated—IL-6, particularly in older women, and TNF-α, particularly affecting muscle mass in men.[55-57] Interestingly, activin pathway and myostatin inhibitors are now on the horizon; targeting such myokine pathways offers promise of future anabolic treatments for sarcopenia.[58]

CONSEQUENCES OF BONE AND JOINT AGING

Musculoskeletal problems cause a huge burden of pain and physical disability for older adults. The most important functional impairments include marked loss of muscle strength, reduced range of movement of the spine and peripheral joints, and loss of joint proprioception, contributing to impaired balance. In addition, spinal osteoporosis causes progressive kyphotic deformity and height loss, which in some individuals may be relatively asymptomatic, but in others is a major cause of pain and reduced function. The key symptoms are pain and stiffness. Although pain thresholds may increase, there is still a very high prevalence of musculoskeletal pain. For example, some 25% of individuals older than 55 years complain of current knee pain. Stiffness and difficulty in initiating movement are almost universal in those older than 70 years.

Bone and soft tissues changes make the whole musculoskeletal system more susceptible to trauma. Periarticular pain syndromes and spinal disorders related to minor trauma are common, but the most important consequence is the high incidence of fractures. These partly reflect the age-related increase in skeletal fragility that characterizes osteoporosis and partly the age-related increase in falls. Osteoporosis predisposes to an increased risk of fracture at all skeletal sites other than flat bones such as the skull, although fractures of the vertebrae, distal radius, and hip are the most common (see Figure 20-1). The relative rise in hip fractures in very old individuals may also be related to changes in the pattern of falling, because older adults, with slower motor function, may be less likely to fall onto an outstretched arm.

The magnitude of disability related to musculoskeletal changes has been well described in community-based epidemiologic studies. Problems with reaching and locomotion are particularly frequent, with the latter contributing extensively to the isolation of older adults. Importantly, among those who sustain a hip fracture, most will fail to regain their prefracture level of function. There is also an appreciable excess mortality, with 8% dying within the first month and approximately 30% dying within 1 year of sustaining a hip fracture.[59,60]

THE FUTURE

With our population aging, the burden of musculoskeletal disease will rise. Fragility fractures are expensive, in terms of direct medical costs and also through the costs of their social sequelae. Furthermore, globally, the prevalence of obesity is rising at an alarming rate. The cumulative physical consequences of a life of repetitive excessive skeletal loading is likely to manifest in substantially greater morbidity in the years to come. Current treatments for osteoporosis mostly focus on suppressing bone resorption, but in the future we are likely to see greater use of anabolic therapies, which stimulate osteoblastic bone formation. Although current treatments for osteoarthritis focus on symptom control, we will hopefully see the emergence of drugs that modify the structure of joints, potentially targeting cartilage and subchondral bone.

KEY POINTS

- Musculoskeletal problems are a huge burden for older adults due to a combination of pain and functional impairment.
- These problems result partly from the increased incidence of common musculoskeletal disorders in older adults, such as rheumatoid arthritis and polymyalgia rheumatica.
- The high burden of musculoskeletal disease in older adults also reflects the impact of the aging process on the musculoskeletal tissue, articular cartilage, muscle, and bone.
- There have been considerable advances in recent years in the understanding of the cellular and molecular mechanisms that underlie these age-related changes.

For a complete list of references, please visit www.expertconsult.com.

KEY REFERENCES

3. Hutton CW: Generalised osteoarthritis: an evolutionary problem? Lancet 1:1463–1465, 1987.
7. Lotz M, Loeser RF: Effects of aging on articular cartilage homeostasis. Bone 51:241–248, 2012.
9. Barter MJ, Bui C, Young DA: Epigenetic mechanisms in cartilage and osteoarthritis: DNA methylation, histone modifications and microRNAs. Osteoarthritis Cartilage 20:339–349, 2012.
16. Taniguchi N, et al: Aging-related loss of the chromatin protein HMGB2 in articular cartilage is linked to reduced cellularity and osteoarthritis. Proc Natl Acad Sci U S A 106:1181–1186, 2009.
19. Avery NC, Bailey AJ: Enzymic and non-enzymic cross-linking mechanisms in relation to turnover of collagen: relevance to aging and exercise. Scand J Med Sci Sports 15:231–240, 2005.
21. Nah S-S, et al: Effects of advanced glycation end products on the expression of COX-2, PGE2 and NO in human osteoarthritic chondrocytes. Rheumatology 47:425–431, 2008.
23. Peppa M, Uribarri J, Vlassara H: Aging and glycoxidant stress. Hormones (Athens) 7:123–132, 2008.
26. Karsdal MA, et al: The coupling of bone and cartilage turnover in osteoarthritis: opportunities for bone antiresorptives and anabolics as potential treatments? Ann Rheum Dis 73:336–348, 2014.
29. Szoeke CE, et al: Factors affecting the prevalence of osteoarthritis in healthy middle-aged women: data from the longitudinal Melbourne Women's Midlife Health Project. Bone 39:1149–1155, 2006.
31. Davis AJ, et al: Are bisphosphonates effective in the treatment of osteoarthritis pain? A meta-analysis and systematic review. PLoS One 8:e72714, 2013.
34. Nakashima T, et al: Evidence for osteocyte regulation of bone homeostasis through RANKL expression. Nat Med 17:1231–1234, 2011.
43. Sattler FR: Growth hormone in the aging male. Best Pract Res Clin Endocrinol Metab 27:541–555, 2013.
44. Troen BR: The regulation of cathepsin K gene expression. Ann N Y Acad Sci 1068:165–172, 2006.
45. Lips P: Vitamin D status and nutrition in Europe and Asia. J Steroid Biochem Mol Biol 103:620–625, 2007.
50. Gaudio A, et al: Increased sclerostin serum levels associated with bone formation and resorption markers in patients with immobilization-induced bone loss. J Clin Endocrinol Metab 95: 2248–2253, 2010.
55. Payette H, et al: Insulin-like growth factor-1 and interleukin 6 predict sarcopenia in very old community-living men and women:

the Framingham Heart Study. J Am Geriatr Soc 51:1237–1243, 2003.
58. Girgis C, Mokbel N, DiGirolamo D: Therapies for musculoskeletal disease: can we treat two birds with one stone? Curr Osteoporos Rep 12:142–153, 2014.
59. Roche JJW, et al: Effect of comorbidities and postoperative complications on mortality after hip fracture in elderly people: prospective observational cohort study. BMJ 331:1374, 2005.
60. Royal College of Physicians, Falls and Fragility Fracture Audit Programme (FFFAP): National Hip Fracture Database (NHFD) extended report. http://www.nhfd.co.uk/20/hipfractureR.nsf/vwcontent/2014reportPDFs/$file/NHFD2014ExtendedReport.pdf?OpenElement. Accessed November 16, 2015.
61. Cooper C, Melton LJ, III: Epidemiology of osteoporosis. Trends Endocrinol Metab 3:224–229, 1992.

21 Aging and the Gastrointestinal System

Richard Feldstein, David J. Beyda, Seymour Katz

More than 20% of our population is expected to exceed 65 years of age by 2030,[1] with the most rapidly growing segment older than 85 years.[2] In 2050, the population aged 65 years and older is projected to be over 83 million, almost double its estimated population of 43 million in 2012. The baby boomers are largely responsible for this increase in the older population because they began turning 65 in 2011. By 2050, the surviving baby boomers will be older than 85 years, which is the group most likely to require health care services.[3] Of necessity, gastroenterologists will be increasingly confronted with digestive diseases in older adult patients. Gastrointestinal disease is the second most common indication for hospital admission of older adult patients,[4] who account for four times as many hospitalizations as younger patients.[1] In the outpatient setting, patients 75 years and older visit internists six times more frequently than younger adults.[4]

NORMAL PHYSIOLOGY OF AGING

With a few notable exceptions, the digestive system maintains normal functioning in older adults. To distinguish between the expected age-related alterations of the gut and symptoms attributable to pathologic conditions, the clinician must have an understanding of the normal physiology of aging. One must also appreciate the interactions between the gastrointestinal (GI) tract and long-standing exposures to environmental agents (e.g., medications, tobacco, alcohol) and chronic non-GI disease states (e.g., congestive heart failure, diabetes mellitus, chronic obstructive pulmonary disease [COPD], dementia, depression).[5] With this knowledge, it will become apparent that most new GI complaints in otherwise healthy older adults are due to disease rather than to aging alone and therefore merit appropriate investigation and treatment.

Aging is not associated with a difference in the desire to eat or the hunger response prior to meal intake, but postprandial hunger and desire to eat are reduced.[6,7] One explanation may be that fasting and intraduodenal lipid-stimulated plasma concentrations of cholecystokinin (CCK), a physiologic satiety factor; leptin, a hormone that functions mainly as a signal of adiposity eliciting long-term satiety; and GLP-2, an incretin hormone mainly released by the L cells of the distal small intestine in response to nutrient ingestion, have been found to be higher in older than in younger men.[8-13] In addition, ghrelin, a growth hormone–releasing peptide from the stomach that functions as a potent stimulator of energy intake, is one-third lower in older adults.[13] However, anorexia in older adults should not be attributed to advanced age alone. This symptom warrants evaluation to exclude a medical or psychological cause or a medication-induced adverse effect.[6]

Up to 40% of healthy older adults subjectively complain of dry mouth. Although baseline salivary flow probably decreases with aging, as noted with decreased salivary bicarbonate (involved in neutralization of refluxed acid), stimulated salivation is unchanged in healthy and edentulous geriatric patients.[14-18] Chewing power is diminished, probably because of decreased bulk of the muscles of mastication,[19,20] although perhaps attributable in part to preclinical manifestations of neurologic disease rather than to the normal aging process.[18] Although many older patients are edentulous to some degree, better dental care has now enabled more of them to have intact teeth than in the past.[6,21,22]

Gustatory and olfactory sensation tend to decrease with aging.[12,23] The ability to detect and discriminate among sweet, sour, salty, and bitter tastes deteriorates as one gets older.[6,12,23,24] Thresholds for salt and bitter taste show age-related elevations, whereas that for sweet taste appears stable.[6,25] Olfaction decreases dramatically following the fifth decade of life, frequently resulting in anosmia after the age of 90 years, when the olfactory threshold increases by about 50%, contributing to poor smell recognition.[6,12,26] Increasingly, chronic diseases observed during aging (Alzheimer or Parkinson diseases) may be responsible for such a decline, and recent studies have focused on the sensation of smell as a predictor of disease presentation.

Despite early data to the contrary, the physiologic function of the esophagus in otherwise healthy individuals is well preserved with increasing age, with the exception of very old patients.[27,28] Studies from the early 1960s introduced the concept of the term *presbyesophagus*, based on cineradiographic and manometric data,[29,30] but the term has been abandoned.[31] Other studies study that excluded patients with diabetes or neuropathy found no increase in dysmotility in older men.[32] Investigators have also found that minor alterations may occur in some octogenarians, including decreased pressure and delayed relaxation of the upper esophageal sphincter and reduction in the amplitude of esophageal contraction.[33,34] Furthermore, one study has shown that age-related changes of increased stiffness and reduced primary and secondary peristalsis in the human esophagus is associated with a deterioration of esophageal function beginning after the age of 40 years.[30] In addition, in a study comparing esophageal manometry and scintigraphic examinations of gastroesophageal reflux in groups of healthy volunteers ranging from 20 to 80 years of age, it was determined that although the number of reflux episodes per volunteer was similar in the various age groups, the duration of reflux episodes was longer in older volunteers. The older participants had impaired clearance of refluxed materials due to a high incidence of defective esophageal peristalsis.[35] Similarly, in another study, age was shown to correlate inversely with lower esophageal sphincter (LES) pressure and length, upper esophageal sphincter (UES) pressure and length, and peristaltic wave amplitude and velocity, suggesting that normal esophageal motility deteriorates with advancing age.[36] It was also noted that hiatal hernias are more common with increasing age and are found in up to 60% of patients older than 60 years.[37] Together, these findings may help explain the high prevalence of reflux symptoms in older adults.

Most studies on gastric histology have found evidence of an increased prevalence of atrophic gastritis in people older than 60 years.[38,39] Consequently, it has been suggested that aging results in an overall decline in gastric acid output.[27,40,41] However, more recent data have demonstrated that gastric atrophy and hypochlorhydria are not normal processes of aging. Rather, *Helicobacter pylori* infestation, which is more common in older adults, not advancing age itself, appears to be the more likely cause of these histologic and acid secretory changes.[38,42-47] The literature remains conflicted over the issue of whether aging alone, rather than factors such as increased *H. pylori* infestation and decreased smoking, leads to altered pepsin secretion.[7,44,46] However, given recent trends, many older adult patients also retain their acid secretion ability in old age as a result of increased *H. pylori* treatment and cure. This can in turn raise the risk for reflux symptoms, given the peristaltic dysfunction associated with aging.[48] Data are scarce in relation to gastric motility, emptying, and gastroduodenal reflux and their relationship to gastric function and acid production. Intrinsic factor secretion is usually maintained into advanced age and is retained longer in the setting of gastric atrophy than acid or pepsin secretion.[49,50] Gastric prostaglandin synthesis, bicarbonate, and nonparietal fluid secretion may diminish, making older adults more prone to nonsteroidal inflammatory drug (NSAID)–induced mucosal damage.[6,7,12] Finally, most (but not all) studies have shown that gastric emptying of solids remains intact in older adults, although liquid emptying is prolonged.[51-56]

Small bowel histology[57-59] and transit time[12,55,60-62] do not appear to change with age in humans, although increased epithelial proliferation in response to cellular injury has been found in a rodent model.[63] Splanchnic blood flow is reduced in older adults.[7] Small bowel absorptive capacity for most nutrients remains intact, but there are some exceptions, especially those due to effects of disease (e.g., chronic gastritis, bacterial overgrowth) and medications on micronutrient absorption.[12] However, the increase in small bowel bacterial overgrowth seen in older adults may be attributed to medications (slow gut transit), diseases such as diabetes, and mobility impairment, which lead to malnutrition and changes in gut immune function, and not to advancing age.[64] No change with aging was found in duodenal brush border membrane enzyme activity of glucose transport.[65] D-Xylose absorption testing remains normal after correction for renal impairment, except perhaps in octogenarians.[66,67] Jejunal lactase activity decreases with age, whereas that of other disaccharides remains relatively stable, declining only during the seventh decade.[68] Protein digestion and assimilation[27,69] and fat absorption remain normal with aging, although the latter has a more limited adaptive reserve capacity.[70-73] Absorption of fat-soluble vitamin A is increased in the older adult population,[12,49,74] whereas vitamin D absorption may be impaired,[49,75-77] and a reduction in vitamin D receptor concentration and responsiveness occurs.[6,21,75] Absorption of the water-soluble vitamins B_1 (thiamine),[78] B_{12} (cyanocobalamin),[70,72,79] and C (ascorbic acid)[80] remains normal, whereas disparate data exist on folate absorption with aging.[81,82] Iron absorption is maintained in healthy older adults who are not hypochlorhydric,[83,84] but absorption of zinc[49,85] and calcium[49,86-88] declines with age.

Several histologic changes have been demonstrated in the colon, including increased collagen deposition,[7] atrophy of the muscularis propria, with an increase in the amount of fibrosis and elastin[27,89] and an increase in proliferating cells, especially at the superficial portions of the crypts.[63,90] Some studies have found that colonic transit time increases with aging to varying degrees,[73,91,92] perhaps due to the increase with age in the number of abnormally appearing myenteric ganglia in the human colon,[93] resulting in myenteric dysfunction, whereas others have not shown any change.[94,95] Prolonged transit time in older adults with constipation is due to factors associated with aging (e.g., comorbidity, immobilization, drugs) rather than to aging per se.[96] It is currently believed that colonic motility and the colon's response to feeding are largely unaffected by healthy aging; however, conditions such as pelvic floor dysfunction and impaired rectal sensation and poor distention all contribute to impaired colonic function and altered bowel habits.

Anorectal physiologic changes have been well documented. Aging is associated with decreased resting anal sphincter pressure in men and women and decreased maximal sphincter pressure in women.[97-100] This may be due in part to age-related changes in muscle mass and contractility and in part to pudendal nerve damage associated with perineal descent in older women.[100-102] The closing pressure—that is, the difference between the maximum resting anal pressure and rectal pressure—also falls in older women.[102] Maximum squeeze pressure declines with age, particularly in postmenopausal women,[10] as does rectal wall elasticity.[103,104] An age-dependent increase in rectal pressure threshold producing an initial sensation of rectal filling has also been demonstrated.[105] The combined effects of reduced rectal compliance, sensation and perineal laxity may be the predisposing factors to fecal incontinence in older women.[99] Defecation dynamic studies in older women have shown a significant failure of rectal evacuation because of insufficient opening of the recto-anal angle and an increased degree of perineal descent compared with younger women.[96,106] Histologic[107] and endosonographic[108] studies on anorectal structure have revealed that the internal anal sphincter develops fibrofatty degeneration and increased thickness, respectively, with aging.

The pancreas undergoes minor histologic changes with aging.[27,109,110] There also appears to be a steady increase in the caliber of the main pancreatic duct, with other branches showing areas of focal dilation or stenosis, without any apparent disease or functional age-related changes[111,109] In fact, 69% of patients older than 70 years without pancreatic pathology have a so-called dilated duct when criteria developed for younger patients are applied.[112] However, any duct larger than 3 mm should be regarded as pathologic.[113] High echogenicity of the pancreas is a normal finding on ultrasonography.[113,114] Aging reduces exocrine pancreatic flow rate and secretion of bicarbonate and enzymes, and the rate falls significantly with repeated stimulation.[11,109,110,115,116] However, other studies have shown a lack of reduced pancreatic secretions with age, independent of disease and the effect of drugs.[116] Given that a variable degree in functional reserve of different organ systems occurs in the aging process, it is not clearly known whether pancreatic insufficiency occurs as a sole consequence of aging.[117]

Anatomic studies on the liver reveal an age-related decrease in weight, both absolute and relative to body weight, as well as the number and size of hepatocytes.[118,119] Pseudocapillarization of the hepatic sinusoid (morphologic changes such as defenestration and thickening of the liver sinusoidal endothelial cell, increased numbers of fat-engorged, nonactivated stellate cells), lipofuscin accumulation, bile duct proliferation, fibrosis, and nonspecific reactive hepatitis are histologic changes more common in older adults.[119-121] The major functional changes in older adult patients are reduction in hepatic blood flow,[116,121] altered clearance of certain drugs, and delayed hepatic regeneration after injury.[121-124] The altered drug clearance is due to age-related reductions in phase I reactions (e.g., oxidation, hydrolysis, reduction), first-pass hepatic metabolism, and serum albumin–binding capacity. Phase II reactions (e.g., glucuronidation, sulfation), however, remain unaffected by aging.[118,119,122,123] There are no age-specific alterations in conventional liver blood test results.[124]

Although a cholecystographic study found that gallbladder emptying remained stable with increasing age, other studies have shown that gallbladder contraction in older adults may be less responsive to CCK.[125-127] Increases in the proportions of the phospholipid and cholesterol components of bile raise the lithogenicity index,[128,129] leading to an increased occurrence of gallstones in older adults.[27] Furthermore, the decline in bile salt synthesis, deconjugation of bile salt pigments, and increase in bactobilia are all speculated as being factors in the increased incidence of gallstone disease.[130] Choledocolithiasis is particularly common; in older adult patients who have undergone an emergency cholecystectomy, the incidence of bile duct stones approached 50%.[131] Even in the absence of bile duct stones or other pathology, older adult patients generally have larger common bile duct diameters than younger patients.[132]

ALTERED MANIFESTATION OF ADULT GASTROINTESTINAL DISEASES

Although there are certain disorders that occur almost exclusively in older adults, most diseases afflicting older adults are those that affect younger adults as well. However, these illnesses may have typical features that must be recognized by clinicians and represent a formidable challenge. In older adults with an acute abdomen, the initial diagnostic impression has been found to be incorrect in up to two thirds of patients[133]; the mortality in octogenarians is 70 times that in young adults.[134]

Acute abdominal pain appears mute with age.[50,135] Theories explaining this phenomenon include increased endogenous opiate secretion, a decline in nerve conduction, and mental depression.[136] Pain localization is often atypical in older adult patients. Furthermore, age-dependent decline in immune function, along with a well-documented delay in pain perception, can give rise to an atypical or even absence of a febrile response, leukocytosis, and pain severity.[137] For example, in a study of acute appendicitis, 21% of patients older than 60 years presented with atypical pain distribution, whereas this occurred in only 3% of patients younger than 50 years.[138] Following appendectomy, morbidity and mortality in older adults carry a higher risk, up to 70% as compared to 1% in the general population.[139,140]

The causes of acute abdominal pain differ as well. Acute cholecystitis, rather than nonspecific abdominal pain or acute appendicitis, was found to be the most common cause in one large survey.[134,135] In this series, 10% of patients older than 70 years were found to have a vascular cause for their pain, such as mesenteric ischemia, embolus, or infarction. Furthermore, retrospective studies have shown that in older adult patients with acute cholecystitis, over 60% of them did not present with the typical back or flank pain, and 5% had no pain at all. In addition, 40% denied nausea, over 50% were afebrile, and 41% had a normal white cell count. Overall, 13% of older adult patients had no fever, leukocytosis, or abnormal liver function test results.[135] A multicenter review has found that 25% of emergency patients older than 70 years had cancer (usually colorectal in Europe and North America, and hepatocellular in tropical regions)[134] as the cause of pain, whereas patients younger than 50 years had malignancy as the explanation in fewer than 1% of cases.[141]

Acute appendicitis may have few overt abdominal signs[142,143,135] and may therefore progress more frequently to gangrene and perforation.[143] Perforation rates range from 20% to 30% in the general population but increase to 50% to 70% in older adults.[135] Older adults account for 50% of all deaths from appendicitis.[144] Other intraabdominal inflammatory conditions, such as diverticulitis, may have rather nonspecific symptoms, including anorexia, altered mental status, low-grade or absence of fever, relatively little tenderness, and late-stage complications (e.g., hepatic abscess). Even biochemical abnormalities such as leukocytosis may be absent in a large number of cases.[144] Furthermore, perforation of a viscus may lack the typical dramatic manifestations.[48,136] Possible explanations for the paucity of tenderness in some cases include altered sensory perception, use of psychotropic drugs, and absence of chemical peritonitis if the patient is hypochlorhydric.[50] The site of perforation also differs with age. Colonic perforation is more common than perforated peptic ulcer disease or appendicitis, the two most common causes for generalized peritonitis in younger patients.[134]

Studies vary regarding whether there is a higher prevalence of gastroesophageal reflux disease (GERD) in older adults,[145-148] but several studies have suggested that the frequency of GERD complications is significantly higher in older adults.[145,146,149,150] Older adult patients have more intense abnormal acid contact time and advanced erosive disease.[150] Severe esophagitis is much more common in patients older than 65 years than in younger people.[149-151] Esophageal sensitivity seems to decrease with age,[152] so very severe esophagitis may be associated with a relative paucity of symptoms. In fact, one study has shown that more than 75% do not experience acid regurgitation as an initial symptom.[145] Therefore, manifestations of GERD are more likely to be late-stage complications, such as bleeding from hemorrhagic esophagitis,[151] dysphasia from a peptic stricture, or adenocarcinoma in the setting of a Barrett esophagus. Esophagitis accounts for a higher incidence of GI bleeding in persons older than 80 years.[150] GERD-induced chest pain may mimic or occur concomitantly with cardiac disease; thus, reflux must be excluded in any older adult patient with all but very typical angina.[28] Aspiration from occult GERD should be considered in older adult patients with recurrent pneumonia or exacerbations of underlying COPD.[28] Early endoscopy is indicated in all older adult patients with GERD, regardless of symptom severity.[145,146] The medical and surgical treatment of GERD in older adult patients follows the same principles as for young patients.[146] Proton pump inhibitors (PPIs) as a class are considered first-line treatment for GERD and erosive esophagitis in older adults,[145,153] although they may require a greater degree of acid suppression than younger patients to heal their esophagitis.[148] Also, with the advent of newer PPIs (e.g., pantoprazole), studies have shown good tolerability, even for long-term therapy due to minimal interactions with other drugs because of a lower affinity for cytochrome P450.[154] This is especially important in patients on clopidogrel, a prodrug that is metabolized to its active form by the same cytochrome p450 as most other PPIs and is used to prevent vascular events. Initial concern involved the potential to decrease efficacy; however, recent guidelines for the treatment of GERD have lessened any association.[150]

Gastroduodenal ulcer disease has a several-fold greater incidence, hospitalization rate, and mortality in older adults,[155-157] with up to 90% of ulcer-related mortality in the United States occurring in patients older than 65 years.[157] This is due to an increase in injurious agents (e.g., *H. pylori* and NSAIDS, two factors that do not seem to act synergistically)[158,159] and to impaired defense mechanisms (e.g., lower levels of mucosal prostaglandins).[12,160] In fact, from 53% to 73% of older peptic ulcer patients are *H. pylori*–positive, yet eradication of the infection remains very low.[161] There may be a paucity or distortion of classic burning epigastric pain, temporal features related to food intake, and typical patterns of radiation.[50] Pain was absent in one third of older hospitalized patients with peptic ulcer disease.[162] As a result, older adult patients more frequently develop complications, such as bleeding or perforation. Giant benign ulcers of older adults can mimic malignancy by presenting with weight loss, anorexia, hypoalbuminemia, and anemia. Despite the increased morbidity and mortality of upper GI bleeding in older adults, endoscopic and clinical criteria have been reported that would allow for successful outpatient management.[159,163-165]

The manifestation of celiac sprue differ considerably in older adults because features are generally more subtle than in young patients.[50,166] Only 25% of newly diagnosed older adult patients with celiac disease present primarily with diarrhea and weight loss.[167] Vague symptoms, including dyspepsia or an isolated folate or iron deficiency, may be the patient's sole manifestation.[166,168,169] In one study, the mean delay to diagnosis in those aged 65 years and older was 17 years.[170] Irritable bowel syndrome was the most erroneous diagnosis made in older adult patients with presenting symptomatology.[169] Severe osteopenia and osteomalacia[166] and a bleeding diathesis due to hypoprothrombinemia are more common in older adults than in younger individuals.[50] Not uncommonly, the initial presentation in older adults may be a perforated viscus, given the multifocal and ulcerative lesions seen in the enteropathy-associated T cell lymphomas associated with celiac disease.[169] Small bowel lymphoma may be particularly common when celiac disease occurs in older adults,[170,171] specifically in patients who were diagnosed between 50 and 80 years of age.[169] Therefore, older adult patients with persistent symptoms, including weight loss, pain, and bleeding, despite strict adherence to a gluten-free diet, require careful evaluation to exclude GI malignancy.[172]

Constipation is perceived by older adult patients to be straining during defecation rather than decreased bowel frequency,[173-175] and it may be manifested in unusual ways. Many older adult patients with constipation may meet diagnostic criteria for functional defecation disorders, such as rectal outlet delay. Excessive defecatory straining in older adult patients with underlying cerebrovascular disease or impaired baroreceptor reflexes can present as syncope or a transient ischemic attack. When unrelieved constipation progresses to fecal impaction, an overflow paradoxic diarrhea may occur, even in patients with relatively normal anal sphincter pressure. If the clinician does not recognize this and prescribes standard antidiarrheal therapy, the underlying impaction will only worsen and potentially lead to other serious complications, such as stercoral ulcers, volvulus, and bleeding.[174,175]

New-onset Crohn disease in older adults is thought to account for almost one third of new cases.[176] Patients older than 60 years account for 10% to 30% of the total irritable bowel disease (IBD) population, with an equal male-to-female ratio. The incidence of IBD in older adults decreases with age, with a 65% occurrence between the ages of 60 to 70 years but only 10% in patients older than 80 years.[176] Misdiagnosis on initial presentation is more common in older adults, with an average delay of up to 6 years.[176,177] Crohn disease has been commonly reported to be limited to the colon more often than is in younger patients.[178] The colitis is more often left-sided in older adults, whereas proximal colonic involvement is more common in younger individuals.[179,180] However, the severity of disease is less severe in older adults, as exhibited by a lower incidence of fistula or stricture formation.[178] Older adult patients are less likely to have close relatives affected by Crohn disease and to have abdominal pain, weight loss, or anemia as a presenting symptom.[177] Crohn disease in older adults develops more rapidly, may be more severe on initial presentation, and is characterized by a shorter time interval between onset of symptoms and first resection.[177] Older adult patients with Crohn disease may suffer fewer relapses,[50] and their postoperative recurrence rate is lower than or equal to that of younger people.[178] However, in older adult patients who do have postoperative recurrence, it occurs more rapidly than in younger patients.[177] Whereas those few young Crohn disease patients who die do so because of their disease, death in older adult patients is usually due to unrelated causes.[178] Older adult patients are more prone to steroid-induced osteoporosis,[172] but bisphosphonates prevent and effectively treat bone loss in these patients,[181] and their use must be strongly considered in this setting. Extraintestinal manifestations were found to be similar in younger and older adults.

The manifestations of ulcerative colitis are generally the same in the young and the old, including extraintestinal manifestations.[180] In older adults, proctosigmoiditis is more common, with a lower incidence of proximal extension over time; pancolitis and the need for surgery are less common. Colectomy rates are lower in older adults with ulcerative colitis when compared to younger patients.[176]

Therapy for inflammatory bowel disease in older adults can follow the same stepwise regimen as in the younger population. However, a clear distinction must be made between the fit older adult and the frail older adult. Studies have shown that the fit older adult can tolerate therapeutic modalities similar to those of the younger generation, with minimal additional risk or morbidity.[182] However, it is imperative to take into account comorbidities, potential drug-drug interactions, and malignancy potential when considering therapy. Furthermore, a stepwise progression and "go slow" approach may be prudent in treatment of the older IBD patient.

The most common manifestation of gallstone disease in older adults are acute cholecystitis and cholangitis.[50] Biliary tract disease is the most common indication for surgical intervention in patients presenting with acute abdominal pain older than 55 years.[135] Cholecystitis in older adults may have nonspecific symptoms, including vague mental and physical disability.[135,183,184] Pain may be muted[135] or absent, even in the presence of gallbladder empyema, leading to a delay in hospitalization.[185] Typical features of cholangitis may be absent. Therefore, blood cultures are critical to exclude bacteremia as the sole evidence of an infected biliary tract, which can result in greater mortality in older adults.[186,187] Older adult patients who require an emergency cholecystectomy have a higher mortality rate than younger patients, but can do well with elective operations, aside from longer operative time and postoperative hospital stay.[188] Thus, surgery should not be denied to the healthy older adult patient with recurrent biliary colic based on age alone.[131,189] Minimally invasive procedures, such as endoscopic retrograde cholangiopancreatography and laparoscopic cholecystectomy, should be used whenever possible.[131]

The clinical course of liver disease in older adults is usually similar to that in younger adults, although complications are less well tolerated.[50,190] Chronic hepatitis C, along with alcoholic liver disease, has been emerging as the most common cause of chronic parenchymal liver disease in older adultsopulation.[124,191] The Centers for Disease Control and Prevention has recommended screening for hepatitis C virus (HCV) for all subjects born between 1945 and 1965, many of whom will be older than 60 years. This group represents 75% of all those infected with HCV in the United States.[192] Viral hepatitis more commonly has a prolonged and cholestatic picture in older adults, although data are equivocal on whether they are more or less likely to suffer severe or fulminant hepatitis.[119] Although the risk of death from fulminant liver failure from acute hepatitis A infection appears to increase with age,[191] acute hepatitis B in older adult patients is usually a mild subclinical disease, and the risk of fulminant disease is not increased.[193] However, a higher risk for progressing to chronic infection exists for those who acquire the disease after 65 years of age.[191] Advanced age at the onset of infection with HCV is associated with an increased mortality rate.[193] This is related to a more rapid rate of fibrosis, whose cause is unknown but is presumed to be related to the decline in immune function with age.[191] When fulminant hepatic failure develops from any cause, advanced age is an adverse prognostic variable.[124] Certain conditions, including alcoholic liver disease, hemochromatosis, primary biliary cirrhosis, and hepatocellular carcinoma, are often seen in more advanced stages when they first present in older adult patients.[119]

Nonalcoholic fatty liver disease (NAFLD) is the most common liver disorder in the United States and worldwide[194] and is seen with increasing prevalence in older adults.[195] However, studies have shown a lack of association with the metabolic syndrome, a clear distinction from the disease in adulthood.[195] In addition, the natural progression of NAFLD with associated liver complications is typically noted between the sixth and eight decades of life,[196] with progression to advanced fibrosis, cirrhosis, and mortality in older adult patients. Patient with NAFLD are at increased risk for hepatocellular carcinoma but this is likely limited to those with advanced fibrosis and cirrhosis.[197] Therefore, the diagnosis of cryptogenic cirrhosis in older adults may be directly related to the ever-rising epidemic of fatty liver in adulthood.

GASTROINTESTINAL PROBLEMS UNIQUE TO OLDER ADULTS

Certain gastrointestinal symptoms and diseases occur primarily, or even exclusively, in the older adult population. In the esophagus, a posterior hypopharyngeal (Zenker) diverticulum may form as a result of reduced muscle compliance of the UES.[198,199] The most common presentation is dysphagia, but serious complications include aspiration and malnutrition. Neurologic disorders, particularly cerebrovascular insult (e.g., small basal ganglia infarcts)[12] and Parkinson disease, account for 80% of cases of oropharyngeal dysphasia in older adults.[200] It has been postulated that dysphagia in older adults can also be caused, in part, by subtle changes in LES function that are noted on motility studies when compared to younger controls.[201] Dysphasia aortica is a syndrome in which symptoms are caused by extrinsic compression of the esophagus by a large thoracic aneurysm or a rigid atherosclerotic aorta.[34] Although cervical osteophytes are common in the older adult population, they are thought to be a very rare cause of dysphasia.[34]

Stomach disorders generally confined to older adults include atrophic gastritis, with or without pernicious anemia. As mentioned previously, prolonged *H. pylori* infection rather than aging alone may be responsible for this condition. A Dieulafoy lesion, resulting from a nontapering ectatic submucosal artery, may be an obscure cause of upper GI bleeding in patients of all ages but is particular frequent in older adults.[202,203]

The prevalence of small bowel diverticulosis increases greatly in older people.[204] The condition may be limited to a single large duodenal diverticulum or may be characterized by numerous diverticula throughout the jejunum. Although most cases are completely asymptomatic, some lead to perforation, hemorrhage, or bacterial overgrowth–induced malabsorption.[50,204,205] Additionally, there is moderate villous atrophy that occurs with aging in the small bowel. A notable outcome of this includes a decrease in the efficiency of calcium absorption secondary to a decrease in vitamin D receptors.[35,206]

Chronic mesenteric ischemia, manifested by intestinal angina, is a very rare form of mesenteric vascular disease seen in older adult patients with atherosclerosis.[207,208] Mesenteric artery stenosis is found in 17.5% of patients older than 70 years.[207] Colonic ischemia may be found in all age groups but studies have shown an increase in those older than 49 years, with a noted female predominance, especially after the age of 69 years.[209] Aortoenteric fistula, an uncommon cause of life-threatening GI hemorrhage, occurs in older adult patients with prior graft placement for an abdominal aortic aneurysm (AAA) or, rarely, with an untreated AAA. It can also occur in patients who have undergone aortoiliac bypass surgery (0.5%) and in patients with native anatomy and after enteral stent placement.[210]

NSAID-induced enteropathy, characterized by ulceration, leading to acute or occult bleeding, ileal stenosis, strictures, protein loss, or iron deficiency, has been increasingly recognized.[172]

Age is a strong risk factor for colon polyps and cancer. Guidelines that advise colorectal screening examinations beginning at age 50 years in average-risk patients and at age 40 years for certain high-risk patients do not provide upper age constraints for colorectal screening. Some experts have suggested an age cutoff at 80 years for screening[211] and 85 years for surveillance for patients who have had only small tubular adenomas.[212] A more recent study has shown that in unscreened older adults with no comorbid conditions that colorectal cancer screening was cost-effective in those up to to the age of 83 years and in those 80 years of age with moderated comorbid conditions.[213] Others, however, disagree with this. Most notably, a recent retrospective cohort study advocating for an age cutoff of 75 years old found that some 24.9% of colonoscopies in Texas were potentially inappropriate based on this cutoff age.[214] Because these age cutoffs are somewhat arbitrary, colorectal screening and surveillance in older adults must be individualized based on comorbidity and life expectancy.[215,216] Colonoscopic polypectomy, rather than surgery, has been advocated for the treatment of large polyps in healthy older patients up to 90 years old for whom life expectancy is at least 5 years.[211]

Several other colonic disorders are seen far more commonly in older adult patients than in younger patients. These include colonic diverticulosis, a condition found on postmortem examination in more than 50% of people older than 70 years.[217] A recent study has estimated its prevalence to be 65% in elderly patient's greater than 65 years of age.[218] Also common are segmental colitis associated with sigmoid diverticulosis,[219,220] sigmoid volvulus; vascular ectasia in the cecum,[221] stercoral ulcer in the setting of fecal impaction, fecal incontinence[173,222-224] (the second leading cause of institutionalization of older adults[100,224]), and *Clostridium difficile* infection, a frequent cause of diarrhea in older adults[220,225] and the most common cause of nosocomial infectious diarrhea in the nursing home setting.[226] In recent studies, the incidence has been shown to be as high 57% in residents in long-term care facilities,[227] where transmission is predominately nosocomial, from surface contamination and hand carriage from staff and infected patients.

Most older adult patients with jaundice have biliary tract obstruction as the cause, rather than hepatocellular disease. Malignancy is more common than choledocholithiasis as a cause of obstruction. Because an older adult with malignant obstructive jaundice rarely survives more than 4 months, endoscopic rather than surgical biliary decompression is appropriate.[131] In this setting, endoscopic biliary stenting for palliation of the jaundice has been advocated to restore a sense of well-being, avoid early liver failure and encephalopathy, and improve the patient's nutritional and immunologic status.[131,228] However, with the advent of improved surgical techniques and decreased postoperative mortality, surgery has expanded to a greater number of patients during the past decade and has found increased use in patients older than 70 years.[228] When acute hepatitis occurs, one third of cases are commonly drug-induced and not viral, as in young people.[119,191] Pyogenic liver abscesses primarily affect older adult patients and should be considered in the differential diagnosis of fever or bacteremia of unclear cause.[193]

SUMMARY

The GI tract generally maintains normal physiologic functioning in older adults. Most new GI symptoms in otherwise healthy older patients are due to pathology rather than to the aging process alone. These patients merit attentive and expeditious evaluation and management because their ability to tolerate illness is lower than that of younger patients.

KEY POINTS: EVALUATION AND TREATMENT OF GASTROINTESTINAL DISORDERS

- Normal physiologic changes in the older adult GI tract are few, so clinicians must seek out and actively treat GI disorders (e.g., oropharyngeal dysphasia, malabsorption, abnormal liver enzyme levels) and not ascribe these signs and symptoms to the aging process.
- Older adult patients have diminished reserve capacity to accommodate illness and should be thoughtfully evaluated and treated early in the course of disease to prevent irreversible deterioration.
- Goals of treatment must be realistic and individualized, with an emphasis on returning the patient to a functional lifestyle.
- Comorbid conditions and concomitant medications have a dramatic effect on the presentation and prognosis of GI disease in older adults.
- To improve compliance, clinicians must avoid prescribing medications that are expensive and/or are taken frequently throughout the day if alternatives are available because older adult patients may be on a fixed income, subject to polypharmacy, or have memory impairment.

Continued

- Clinicians should avoid prescribing drugs more likely to cause adverse effects (e.g., isoniazid, corticosteroids, opiates, mineral oil, NSAIDs, anticholinergics) if reasonable alternatives are available and should avoid overprescribing tranquilizers and antidepressants for symptoms thought to be due to somatization.
- Although irritable bowel syndrome of new onset may occur in older adults, 90% of cases first appear before the age of 50 years. Therefore, this diagnosis should be rendered only after thorough evaluation to exclude other diseases, including malignancies or ischemia.
- Endoscopy and abdominal surgery can be performed safely in older adults. Morbidity and mortality are related to the degree of concomitant disease and the emergent or elective nature of the procedure. An unnecessary delay in surgery is often lethal.
- Chronologic age need not be an absolute contraindication to aggressive therapeutic measures, such as chemotherapy or organ transplantation, because the tolerance of these interventions correlates more with the overall physiologic condition.

For a complete list of references, please visit www.expertconsult.com.

KEY REFERENCES

3. Ortman JM, Velkoff V, Hogan H: An aging nation: the older population in the United States. Current Population Reports. http://www.census.gov/prod/2014pubs/p25-1140.pdf. Accessed October 25, 2015.
7. Blechman MB, Gelb AM: Aging and gastrointestinal physiology. Clin Geriatr Med 15:429–438, 1999.
9. Ahmed T, Haboubi N: Assessment and management of nutrition in older people and its importance to health. Clin Interv Aging 5:207–216, 2010.
13. Deniz A, Nerys MA: Anorexia of aging and gut hormones. Aging Dis 4:264–275, 2013.
23. Boyce JM, Shone GR: Effects of ageing on smell and taste. Postgrad Med J 82:239–241, 2006.
35. Gregersen H, Pedersen J, Drewes AM: Deterioration of muscle function in the human esophagus with age. Dig Dis Sci 53:3065–3070, 2008.
55. Madsen JL, Graff J: Effects of ageing on gastrointestinal motor function. Age Ageing 33:154–159, 2004.
97. Orozco-Gallegos JF, Orenstein-Foxx AE, Sterler SM, et al: Chronic constipation in the elderly. Am J Gastroenterol 107:18–26, 2012.
99. Fox JC, Fletcher JG, Zinsmeister AR, et al: Effect of aging on anorectal and pelvic floor functions in females. Dis Colon Rectum 49:1726–1735, 2006.
117. Bhavesh BS, Farah KF, Goldwasser B, et al: Pancreatic diseases in the elderly. http://www.practicalgastro.com/pdf/October08/Oct08_ShahArticle.pdf. Accessed October 25, 2015.
130. Shah BB, Agrawal RM, Goldwasser B, et al: Biliary diseases in the elderly. http://www.practicalgastro.com/pdf/September08/ShahArticle.pdf. Accessed October 25, 2015.
140. Bhullar JS, Chaudhary S, Cozacov Y, et al: Appendicitis in the elderly: diagnosis and management still a challenge. Am Surg 80:295–297, 2014.
150. Achem SR, DeVault KR: Gastroesophageal reflux disease and the elderly. Gastroenterol Clin North Am 43:147–160, 2014.
155. Zullo A, Hassan C, Campo SM: Bleeding peptic ulcer in the elderly: risk factors and prevention strategies. Drugs Aging 24:815–828, 2007.
161. Pilotto A: Aging and upper gastrointestinal disorders. Best Pract Res Clin Gastroenterol 18(Suppl):73–81, 2004.
169. Rashtak S, Murray JA: Celiac disease in the elderly. Gastroenterol Clin North Am 38:433–446, 2009.
223. Crane SJ, Talley NJ: Chronic gastrointestinal symptoms in the elderly. Clin Geriatr Med 23:721–734, 2007.
191. Junaidi O, Di Bisceglie AM: Aging liver and hepatitis. Clin Geriatr Med 23:889–903, 2007.
208. Sreenarasimhaiah J: Chronic mesenteric ischemia. Curr Treat Options Gastroenterol 10:3–9, 2007.
216. Lin OS, Kozarek RA, Schembre DB, et al: Screening colonoscopy in very elderly patients: prevalence of neoplasia and estimated impact on life expectancy. JAMA 295:2357–2365, 2006.
218. Comparato G, Pilotto A, Franzè A, et al: Diverticular disease in the elderly. Dig Dis 25:151–159, 2007.
206. Salles N: Basic mechanisms of the aging gastrointestinal tract. Dig Dis 25:112, 2007.
213. van Hees F, Habbema JD, Meester RG, et al: Should colorectal cancer screening be considered in elderly persons without previous screening? A cost-effectiveness analysis. Ann Intern Med 160:750–759, 2014.
214. Sheffield K, Han Y, Kuo Y, et al: Potentially inappropriate screening colonoscopy in Medicare patients. JAMA Intern Med 173:542–550, 2013.
227. Surawicz CM, Brandt LJ, Binion DG: Guidelines for diagnosis, treatment, and prevention of *Clostridium difficile* infections. Am J Gastroenterol 108:478–498, 2013.
197. Chalasani N, Younossi Z, Lavine JE: The diagnosis and management of non-alcoholic fatty liver disease: practice guideline by the American Association for the Study of Liver Diseases, American College of Gastroenterology, and the American Gastroenterological Association. Am J Gastroenterol 107:811–826, 2012.

22 Aging of the Urinary Tract

Philip P. Smith, George A. Kuchel

INTRODUCTION

Although traditional classification considers the upper and lower urinary tracts as part of one system, each serves a distinct function. In this edition, upper and lower urinary tract components will be considered, emphasizing the known effects of aging on each system. Nevertheless, a number of potentially pertinent topics will not be discussed in this chapter. For example, age-related changes in the renal handling of water and electrolytes are addressed in Chapter 82, and diseases that commonly affect the aged kidney, prostate, and gynecologic structures are discussed in Chapters 81, 83, and 85, respectively. Given the multifactorial systemic complexity inherent to aging and common geriatric syndromes (Chapter 15),[1] the discussion will need to cross traditional organ-based boundaries. Therefore, we will also discuss the ability of age-related declines in renal function to influence key geriatric measures, such as cognitive function and mobility performance. Conversely, given growing evidence that oxidative stress, inflammation, and nutrition can influence aging- and disease-related processes across many different organs, the ability of these systemic factors to modify urinary tract aging will also be considered. Finally, the contribution of lower and upper urinary tract dysfunction to urinary incontinence, a major geriatric syndrome, is discussed in Chapter 106.

UPPER URINARY TRACT: KIDNEYS AND URETERS

Overview

Declines in renal function represent one of the best documented and most dramatic physiologic alterations in human aging. In spite of great progress, important issues remain. For example, it has been difficult to explain why renal aging can be so variable between seemingly "normal" individuals and to establish which of these changes may potentially be reversible. Nevertheless, developments and continuing research in this area offer unique opportunities for improving the lives of older adults.[2-5]

Glomerular Filtration Rate

Age-related declines in glomerular filtration rate (GFR) are well-established, yet contrary to general belief, GFR does not inevitably decrease with age. Among Baltimore Longitudinal Study of Aging participants, mean GFR declined approximately 8.0 mL/min per 1.73 m^2 per decade from the middle of the fourth decade of life.[6] However, these decrements were not universal, with approximately one third of these subjects showing no significant decrease in GFR over time.[6] This high degree of interindividual variability among relatively healthy older adults has raised the hope that age-related declines in GFR may not be inevitable and could ultimately be preventable, even in the absence of an overt disease process. At the same time, clinicians wishing to prescribe renally excreted medications to healthy older adults clearly require reliable tools to estimate GFR accurately.

The decrease in GFR with age is generally not accompanied by elevations in serum creatinine levels[6] because age-related declines in muscle mass tend to parallel those observed for GFR, causing overall creatinine production also to fall with age. Thus, serum creatinine levels generally overestimate GFR with age, and in women and underweight individuals, the serum creatinine level is most insensitive to impaired kidney function.[7] Although many formulas have been devised for estimating creatinine clearance based on normative data,[8,9] their reliability in predicting individual renal function is poor.[10,11] In frail and severely ill patients on multiple medications, where the need for accurate estimation is greatest, the reliability of such estimates may be the most questionable. In consequence, timed short-duration urine collections for creatinine clearance measurement are generally recommended.[10,12] In contrast to the poor predictive ability of low creatinine levels, elevations in serum creatinine levels above 132 mmol/L (1.5 mg/dL) reflect declines in GFR greater than what would be typically expected with normal aging, representing likely underlying pathology. Ultimately, even creatinine clearance has limitations and may underestimate GFR.[13] Cystatin C, a measure of kidney function that is independent of muscle mass, has been advocated as an improved marker of reduced GFR in older adults with creatinine levels within the normal range.[14] Although U.S. Food and Drug Administration (FDA)–approved kits for its measurement have been available since 2001, and in spite of its potential attraction in the management of frail older adults, the precise role of cystatin C measurements in clinical decision making remains to be clearly defined.

Renal Blood Flow

On average, aging is associated with a progressive decrease in renal plasma flow.[15,16] Losses of 10% per decade have been described, with typical values declining from 600 mL/min in a young adult to 300 mL/min at 80 years of age.[15,16] Perfusion of the renal medulla is maintained in the presence of lower blood flow to the cortex, which can be observed as patchy cortical defects on renal scans obtained in healthy older adults. Regional renal flow and GRF are determined by a balance between the vascular tone involving the afferent and efferent renal blood supply. Generally, renal vasoconstriction increases in old age, whereas the capacity of the vascular bed to dilate is decreased. Responsiveness to vasodilators (e.g., nitric oxide, prostacyclin) appears to be attenuated, whereas responsiveness to vasoconstrictors (e.g., angiotensin II) is enhanced.[5] Basal renin and angiotensin II levels are significantly lower in older adults, and the ability of various different stimuli to activate the renin-angiotensin-aldosterone system (RAAS) is blunted.

Tubular Function

The ability of the tubules to excrete and reabsorb specific solutes plays a crucial role in maintaining normal fluid and electrolyte balance. The impact of aging and specific disease processes on the ability of tubules to handle specific solutes is discussed elsewhere (Chapter 82). Nevertheless, some overarching principles, are worthy of note[2,5,17]:

1. Overall tubular function appears to decline with aging.
2. The ability to handle water, sodium, potassium and other electrolytes is generally impaired with aging.
3. Such physiologic declines do not generally affect the ability of older adults to maintain normal fluid and electrolyte balance under basal conditions.

4. Older adults are less capable of maintaining normal homeostasis when exposed to specific fluid and electrolyte challenges.

For example, the ability to conserve and excrete sodium is impaired, with reduced salt resorption in the ascending loop of Henle, reduced serum aldosterone secretion, and a relative resistance to aldosterone and angiotensin II.[2,5] As a result, older adults take longer to reduce their sodium excretion in response to a salt-restricted diet; conversely, older adults take longer to excrete a sodium load. Qualitatively similar changes have been described in regard to the tubular capacity to adjust to changes in water.

Structural Changes

The aged kidney is granular in appearance, with modest declines in parenchymal mass.[2,5] The most impressive changes involve a reduction in the number and size of nephrons in the renal cortex, with a relative sparing of the medullary regions. Loss of parenchymal mass leads to a widening of interstitial spaces between the tubules and an increase in interstitial connective tissue. The numbers of visible glomeruli in aged kidneys decline in parallel with change in weight, with an increasing percentage of sclerotic glomeruli. Sclerosis is associated with lost lobulation of the glomerular tuft, increased mesangial cells, and decreased epithelial cells, resulting in decreased effective filtering surface. In response, remaining nonsclerotic glomeruli compensate by enlarging and hyperfiltering.

Even in the absence of hypertension and other relevant diseases, important changes of the intrarenal vasculature can be observed in old age.[2,5] Larger renal vessels may show sclerotic changes, whereas smaller vessels generally are spared. Nevertheless, arteriolar-glomerular units demonstrate distinctive changes in old age.[2,5,18] Cortical changes are more profound, with hyalinization and collapse of glomerular tufts, luminal obliteration within preglomerular arterioles, and decreased blood flow. Structural changes within the medulla are less pronounced, and juxtamedullary regions demonstrate evidence of anatomic continuity and functional shunting between afferent and efferent arterioles.

Mechanistic Considerations

The hyperfiltration theory suggests that a loss of glomeruli results in increased capillary blood flow through the remaining glomeruli and a correspondingly high intracapillary pressure.[2,5] Such age-related increases in intracapillary pressure (or shear stress) can also result in local endothelial cell damage and glomerular injury, contributing to the progressive glomerulosclerosis.[2,5,19] Cytokines and other vasoactive humoral factors have been implicated in this type of pressure-mediated renal damage.[2,5,20] Also in support of the hyperfiltration theory, restricted protein intake[21] and antihypertensives that reduce single-nephron GFR (e.g., angiotensin-converting-enzyme [ACE] inhibitors and angiotensin II blockers)[21] reduce glomerular capillary pressure and glomerular injury and prevent measurable declines in renal function.

Other factors and mechanisms contribute to age-related declines in renal function. For example, individuals born with a reduced nephron mass could be more vulnerable to all categories of renal injury, including those associated with aging. A growing body of research has linked renal aging to the damaging effects of normal metabolism through the accumulation of toxins, such as reactive oxygen species (ROS), advanced glycosylation end products (AGEs), and advanced lipoxidation end products (ALEs).[2,3,5,22,23] This toxin-mediated theory has many attractions:

1. These toxins accumulate with aging and can induce structural and functional changes.
2. They provide vital linkages between efforts to understand aging at the level of a single organ and traditional gerontologic research into longevity (see Chapter 5).
3. Nutritional and potentially pharmacologic interventions may allow individuals to decrease exposure to such toxins and ultimately prevent or delay renal aging.
4. Such research has permitted the development of a pathophysiologic framework within which different risk factors (e.g., underlying genetic predisposition, renal progenitor cell behavior,[24] gonadal hormone levels,[25] diet,[22] smoking,[26] subclinical processes) can all influence how renal aging manifests in individuals.[2,5,23]

System-Based Perspective

Renal aging cannot be viewed in isolation from aging at the systemic level. Not only are most patients with chronic kidney disease (CKD) older adults, but these patients are frail and at high risk of being disabled.[4] Individuals with advanced CKD have an especially high risk of developing cardiovascular disease,[27] cognitive declines,[25-30] sarcopenia,[31-33] and poor physical performance.[27,34] It remains to be seen to what extent milder declines in renal function, more consistent with normal aging, may contribute to altered body composition and physiologic performance seen in generally healthy older adults. As discussed, creatinine-based estimates of GFR depend on skeletal muscle mass and tend to overestimate GFR in older adults. Thus, it is interesting that even mild declines in GFR, as measured using cystatin C, were associated with poorer physical function, whereas creatinine-based GFR estimates demonstrated a relationship only when less than 60 mL/min/1.73 m^2.[35] Ultimately, the development of an approach that places renal aging in a systems-based context, in which key functional issues are considered, may offer most exciting opportunities for developing interventions that will help maintain function and independence in late life.

LOWER URINARY TRACT: BLADDER AND OUTLET

Overview

By storing and periodically releasing urine on a volitional basis, the lower urinary tract (LUT) serves to isolate the kidneys from the exterior environment while providing controlled elimination of metabolic byproducts. The anatomic arrangement of the nonrefluxing ureterovesical junction, fluid-tight urethral sphincteric mechanism, and interposed chamber—the bladder—create an effective barrier to the retrograde passage of infectious agents into the kidneys and from there into the bloodstream. Presumably, as the result of evolutionary pressures, the bladder and its outlet normally function as a urine storage structure sufficiently capacious to accept several hours' volume of renal output while an efficient evacuation mechanism under voluntary permissive control can be quickly and voluntarily activated and then returned to storage status. Under normal circumstances, this process is under socially appropriate voluntary control in response to nonnoxious perceptions related to bladder volume and voiding flow.

The requirements for proper function of this system include normal sensory transduction of normal physiologic bladder filling, central transmission and subconscious processing, appropriate conscious recognition and processing, coordination of sphincteric relaxation and bladder pressurization via detrusor contraction, and normal biomechanical function of the bladder and its outflow, as well as intact urethral and bladder guarding and voiding reflexes. The individual experiences the perception of these processes. Biomechanical and functional changes as a result of the aging process per se involving the LUT and nervous system may alter an individual's storage and evacuation capabilities. Bidirectional convergence of peripheral and central signaling pathways, including from the gut and skin,[36] provide a physiologic basis for urinary symptoms arising from nonurinary sources. The association between mobility and cognition of urinary symptoms and dysfunction[37-41] points to the centrality of integrative processes to effective urinary performance. In a broader perspective especially relevant to aging, the complexity of control and perception suggests that functional disturbances and urinary symptoms represent thresholds of failure of an integrative homeostatic system. Symptoms and objective dysfunctions thus should be regarded as syndromic, involving diverse nongenitourinary systems such as fluid balance and mobility, as well as sensory and decision making processes rather than as being reflective of merely isolated LUT pathology.[42]

Despite the nominal implications of current terminology, the relationships of LUT mechanistic capabilities, descriptive LUT physiology, and perceptions of urinary status (including the voluntary control of storage vs. voiding) are not reliable and are likely not fixed over the life span. Clinically measurable LUT function (e.g., flow rates, urodynamics, postvoid residual volumes) is the result of brain control over end-organ structures as controlled by cognitive (including perceptual) processes. The poor correlation between symptoms and objective function has long been recognized.[43] A urodynamic study of continent older adults found that 63% were symptom-free, and 52% were both symptom-free and free of any potential confounding disease or medication use.[44] Nevertheless, only 18% of these individuals were also free of any urodynamic abnormality.[44] Moreover, nonvoiding bladder contractions during filling (so-called detrusor overactivity [DO]) unrelated to identifiable disease were observed in 53% of these individuals, with no correlation to gender or age.[45] Variability in postvoid residual volumes also increases with aging, resulting in asymptomatic, elevated, postvoid residual volumes in some people.[46,47] The perception of voiding difficulties (underactive bladder [UAB]) may relate more to abnormal bladder sensations than to a weak detrusor muscle contraction during voiding.[48]

Patient-perceived symptoms are clearly clinically important, especially when bothersome. Nevertheless, as a result of the complex syndromic nature of symptoms and dysfunction in older adults, and the related unreliable correlation of symptoms, dysfunction, and cause, the physiologic meaning of urinary symptoms and objective dysfunction in the older adult must be approached with caution. Relatively simplistic algorithmic care derived from studies of younger adults may represent a special case of a broader pathophysiologic model and therefore may not always be applicable in older adults.

Mechanistic Considerations

The mechanical interaction of the detrusor smooth muscle with nonmuscular components of the bladder wall gives the bladder its ability to distend compliantly (i.e., hold urine under low pressure) during storage and create expulsive force during voiding. The expression of bladder wall forces during voiding as a measurable detrusor pressure and/or urinary flow rate is dependent on the degree of urethral dispensability, which is itself the mechanical consequence of the interaction of urethral musculature and nonmuscular components. Furthermore, these wall forces relate to the sensitivity of afferent activity generated in response to volume and flow[49,50] and thus to the LUT sensory information provided to brain control and perceptual processes. Finally, the smooth muscle of the detrusor and urethra are under autonomic control, potentially providing adjustability to this sensitivity in addition to the accepted importance of autonomic input in mediating urine storage and voiding. Although all these elements are subject to age-associated changes, the complex and centrifugal nature of urinary control by an integrative brain means that the functional impact of any individually changed parameter cannot always be reliably predicted. Even though the prevalence of LUT symptoms and dysfunction increases with aging, many older adults remain free of LUT problems despite harboring many age-related physiologic changes involving the LUT and associated structures.

Much of the mechanistic research literature addressing LUT disorders in later life is based on animal modeling. This literature must be interpreted with caution for two reasons. First, unless at least three age groups are compared (young, mature, old), the biologic effects of maturation cannot be distinguished from those of aging. And, unless a fourth oldest-old group is included, effects observed in old animals may be more reflective of robust aging rather than late life frailty, thus limiting the translation of findings to the most problematic human clinical conditions. Second, animal model systems lack the human perceptual overlay and associated high-level cortical brain functions. Studies have suggested that cognitive processes related to perception have an active role in measurable function during filling and voiding, so the impact of mechanistic change on function should not be overinterpreted. Furthermore, animal models cannot provide direct information about symptom complexes such as overactive and underactive bladder because these symptoms are by definition perceptual.

Aspects of cellular and structural contributors to detrusor muscular force creation demonstrate changes with aging, resulting in altered responsiveness of the detrusor muscle to neuropharmacologic stimulation. Structurally, aging is classically associated with a decrease in detrusor muscle–to–collagen ratio[51] and nerve density in the bladder and urethra,[52-54] but sensory neurons may be relatively spared.[55] Quantitative assessment in a rat model demonstrated no diminution in nerve density at the bladder neck in aged compared to mature rats[56,57] nor in the content of contractile proteins.[58] Smooth and striated muscle thickness and fiber density in the bladder neck and urethra have been found to be diminished in older women relative to young women.[59-62] Striated muscle changes are circumferentially uniform, although the decrease in smooth muscle is most pronounced on the dorsal-vaginal aspect of the urethra.

The detrusor normally contracts in response to M3 muscarinic receptor activation via pelvic nerve efferent release of acetylcholine—M2 receptors are also present, but their precise role is not known.[36] M3 receptor numbers decrease with age,[63] and M3-stimulated activity is diminished, although the clinical importance of decreased contractile sensitivity is unclear.[64] Against the decline in M3 responsiveness, other factors appear to become more important, including purinergic transmission,[65-68] non-neuronal urothelial acetylcholine release,[67]and an increased contractile response to norepinephrine.[60] Agonist-invoked mobilization of intracellular calcium is less in old mice, suggesting a reduced size of releasable calcium stores important for contraction.[69] Rho kinase–mediated responses to carbachol correlate with age, whereas myosin light chain kinase–mediated contractions do not, indicating changes in the intracellular responses to stimulation.[70] A 50% reduction in caveolae, specialized cell membrane regions important to detrusor muscle contraction, has been reported in a rat model.[71]

Diminished coordination and reactivity of autonomic discharge could contribute to inefficient use of available resources.[72] Advances in functional neuroimaging have resulted in improved understanding of LUT control and the impact of aging and disease.[73,74] Diminished activation in brain areas related to bladder sensory function and coordination are associated with aging.[75] Some of these same regions are key to the ability to focus attention selectively on sensory input in preparation for conscious perception and action (attentional biasing).[76-79] Frontal cortical areas monitor continuously increasing LUT afferent outflow during bladder filling, anticipating the threshold of afferent activity that requires action.[80] Cognitive declines with aging and age-associated brain degenerative disorders such as white matter hyperintensities may interfere with the subconscious registration and transmission of LUT sensory information, precluding normal homeostatic control. Impaired sensory registration might also result in ill-prepared motor areas (bladder-sphincter and somatic-mobility centers), slowing responses and thus contributing to symptom severity and collateral dysfunctions. In view of all these considerations, geriatric incontinence may result from diminished capability of these individuals to sense, process, make decisions, and then execute decisions in the face of an unexpected bladder contraction, as opposed to being the result of the sensation of urgency developing in the first place.

Functional Considerations

Available studies on functional changes with aging must also be approached with care. The physiology of bladder function in animal models frequently differs significantly from humans. For example, rodents do not void with the synergic detrusor-sphincter coordination characteristic of the pontine-organized human void, complicating voiding studies and research into sphincteric incontinence using rodent models. Furthermore, it is much easier to obtain human research data from symptomatic individuals because invasive urodynamic studies and research requiring tissue biopsies are difficult to carry out in healthy asymptomatic individuals. Aging is characterized by a decline in the ability to adapt to physiologic challenges, thus implying a level of biologic adaptability to control on measurable function. It would therefore be unlikely that normal function in the older adult—especially in well-adapted later life—can be characterized by the same normative values on clinical testing as in younger adults. However, it is exactly these data that are frequently missing in human clinical research. How then can accurate statements about pathologic function be made? Great caution is advised when interpreting the scientific literature on LUT function and aging.

Urinary symptoms are the perception, on the part of the patient and/or caregiver, of lower urinary tract dysfunction. Symptoms can be broadly categorized into irritability (e.g., overactive bladder; frequency, urgency, nocturia), obstructive-retentive (e.g., underactive bladder; hesitancy, abnormal stream, incomplete emptying), and incontinence. The prevalence of all such symptoms increases with age in women and men, with moderate to severe symptoms roughly doubling between 40 to 49 years of age and after 80 years.[44] Overactive bladder symptoms, including incontinence, were experienced more commonly and earlier in life in women than in men, with 19% of women and 8% to 10% of men older than 65 years reporting some degree of urinary incontinence. The NOBLE study reported data on 5204 randomly selected participants. Overactive bladder symptoms were experienced by 5% to 10% of people younger than 35 years, increasing to 30% to 35% in those older than age 75 years, with no gender differences.[81] Especially in the older adult, symptomatology often extends beyond the patient in the examination room. Urinary incontinence in older adults significantly burdens their caregivers,[82,83] increasing the risk of nursing home placement.[84]

Urodynamically, aging is associated with sensory and motor changes. Older asymptomatic women demonstrate diminished sensitivity to bladder volume, although bladder capacity remains unchanged.[85,86] Loss of bladder volume sensitivity can lead to diminished warning time between the first urge to urinate and urgency with leakage[37] and impaired bladder emptying. The resultant decreased functional capacity may then aggravate symptoms of urinary frequency, urgency, or urge incontinence by perpetuation of bladder volumes in the narrow functional zone between the first desire to urinate and leakage. The impact of aging on detrusor strength remains controversial. A significant contributor to this controversy is the difficulty in assessing detrusor strength. Any measurement of detrusor strength must account for the expression of contractile force as pressure (a static measure) and flow (a work function), as well as consideration of the thermodynamics of muscular contraction. The available literature is complicated by a frequent lack of pressure and flow assessment and population selection,[87,88] and there are no reports evaluating the impact of age on detrusor muscular energetics. The use of the common stop test to assess isovolumetric detrusor contractility has been inconclusive,[89,90] possibly due to variable effects of methodologic perturbations of bladder outlet function. Urodynamic calculations such as the Watts factor and bladder contractility index make a number of assumptions (including thermodynamic) that limit their applicability in aging studies.

In animal models, aging is associated with less frequent but higher volume voiding, with increased pressure thresholds for voiding and no difference in maximal pressure,[91,92] indicating that the functional impact of aging may be more on sensory than motor functions. Enhanced afferent activity with increased intraluminal release of the relevant neurotransmitters ATP and acetylcholine has been reported in old versus young (immature) mice,[93] suggesting that the decreased sensitivity observed in other studies may be a loss of central sensitivity to afferent activity. Diminished detrusor muscle shortening velocity, perhaps an early marker of impending detrusor underactivity,[94] does not diminish with age in vitro.[58] In contrast, another study has reported that total detrusor effort does not change with age; however, aging was associated with failure of contraction initiation and slowed contraction velocities.[95] Maximum detrusor pressures associated with detrusor overactivity decrease with age,[85] suggesting larger absolute but decreased functional bladder capacity and diminished voiding efficiency. The finding of greater contractility (by the stop test) in older patients with detrusor overactivity at lower bladder volumes as compared to patients without detrusor overactivity[90] suggests that maximal contractility is preserved and that functional deficits (evidenced as detrusor underactivity) are due to an inability to maintain a contractile state.

Urethral function is also affected by aging; findings in women probably are more representative of intrinsic urethral function per se due to the confounding influence of the prostate in men. Urodynamic evaluation has demonstrated lower detrusor pressures at opening and closing of the urethra in older women,[56,96] along with maximum closure pressures and a short functional length.[97] These findings all suggest a lack of sphincteric action inherent to the urethra. In addition to potentially contributing directly to incontinence, loss of urethral resistance to flow could reduce urethral afferent activity during flow, compounding an age-associated loss of urethral sensitivity.[98] Diminishing the reinforcing urethral-detrusor reflex during voiding[99,100] can contribute to symptoms associated with voiding dysfunction. Maximum detrusor pressure and detrusor pressure at maximum flow are not a function of age in symptomatic unobstructed, unoperated men and women older than 40 years, although unadjusted flow rates decrease with age.[101] In contrast to younger patients, in whom DO during bladder filling is often accompanied by sphincteric relaxation and some consequent leakage, DO in older adults is more likely to result in bladder emptying but is accompanied by a steady sphincter.[102] This implies a different mechanism underlying detrusor overactivity as well as more disastrous results for the older patient in the event of DO.

Other Considerations

It is certainly true for LUT symptoms and function that the relative contributions of aging per se are difficult to disentangle from those of the common coconditions of menopause, pelvic organ prolapse, and benign prostatic hyperplasia (BPH) and the more classic disease model comorbidities (e.g., obesity, cardiovascular insufficiency, dementia, diabetic and other neuropathies).

The impact of prostatic hypertrophy (BPH) in men on lower urinary tract function is discussed elsewhere (see Chapter 86). In women, pelvic organ prolapse may have direct and indirect relationships to lower urinary tract dysfunction.[103] About 40% of women with LUT symptoms have vaginal prolapse, and vice versa. Lower urinary tract symptoms correlate moderately well with the severity of vaginal prolapse.[104] Anterior and posterior vaginal prolapse to levels above the introitus may be associated with irritative and incontinence symptoms, and anterior and apical vaginal prolapse beyond the introitus may produce bladder outlet obstruction. Significantly, sphincteric incompetence may be masked by significant anterior prolapse; we await reliable methods to assess sphincteric competence in these patients.

The impact of estrogen loss with menopause and aging on lower urinary tract function has not been well characterized. In mature rodents, oophorectomy results in decreases in detrusor smooth muscle, axonal degeneration, and electron microscopic findings of sarcolemmal dense band patterns with diminished caveolar numbers, suggesting impaired contractile properties as a result of de-estrogenization.[105,106] In a study of symptomatic premenopausal and postmenopausal women, a lower mean maximum detrusor pressure was observed during voiding in postmenopausal women, suggesting that menopause may influence LUT function by impaired detrusor function or reduced outlet resistance.[107] Additive effects of intravaginal estrogens and pelvic floor rehabilitation on symptoms and urodynamic parameters have suggested a dynamic influence of hormonal status rather than fixed tissue–based relationships.[108] The clinical impact of estrogen replacement on symptoms of bladder overactivity and incontinence are contradictory and incomplete.

System-Based Perspective

Aging is associated with an increased prevalence of bothersome lower urinary tract symptoms, as well as demonstrable alterations of function. The determinants of urine storage and voiding functions include renal output, LUT biomechanical and sensorimotor function, and central processing abilities integrating urinary control with multiple other physiologic demands, including mobility. Age-associated changes in end-organ functional capabilities place increased adaptive demands on diminishing cognitive functions. Relevant normal function involves not only baseline performance, but also what is necessary to provide system (including perceptual) homeostasis in the face of specific challenges, and this may not align with published norms. Perceptual processes critical to control and the distinction of sensations versus symptoms may diminish with cognitive decline. Degradation of the ability to store and appropriately evacuate urine normally thus has many contributors, both external and inherent to the lower urinary tract. These alterations are complicated by other age-related physiologic changes and comorbidities.

KEY POINTS

- Although a decline in the glomerular filtration rate is common with age, it is not inevitable.
- Although older adults are able to preserve renal function under normal basal conditions, the ability to respond to stressors is commonly reduced, giving rise to common problems such as water and electrolyte disorders.
- Aspects of renal aging reflect exposure to toxins over the life course. Structural changes in adaptation to loss that can accelerate other effects of aging, such as increased capillary blood flow, with higher intracapillary pressures, in response to the loss of glomeruli.
- Urinary symptoms and functional disturbances commonly go beyond the urinary system because they represent thresholds of failure of an integrative homeostatic system.

For a complete list of references, please visit www.expertconsult.com.

KEY REFERENCES

1. Inouye SK, Studenski S, Tinetti ME, et al: Geriatric syndromes: clinical, research, and policy implications of a core geriatric concept. J Am Geriatr Soc 55:780–791, 2007.
2. Zhou XJ, Rakheja D, Yu X, et al: The aging kidney. Kidney Int 74:710–720, 2008.
20. Schmitt R, Cantley LG: The impact of aging on kidney repair. Am J Physiol Renal Physiol 294:F1265–F1272, 2008.
22. Vlassara H, Uribarri J, Cai W, et al: Advanced glycation end product homeostasis: exogenous oxidants and innate defenses. Ann N Y Acad Sci 1126:46–52, 2008.
27. Lin CY, Lin LY, Kuo HK, et al: Chronic kidney disease, atherosclerosis, and cognitive and physical function in the geriatric group of the National Health and Nutrition Survey 1999-2002. Atherosclerosis 202:312–319, 2009.
29. Kurella TM, Wadley V, Yaffe K, et al: Kidney function and cognitive impairment in US adults: the Reasons for Geographic and Racial Differences in Stroke (REGARDS) Study. Am J Kidney Dis 52:227–234, 2008.
39. Ouslander JG, Palmer MH, Rovner BW, et al: Urinary incontinence in nursing homes: incidence, remission and associated factors. J Am Geriatr Soc 41:1083–1089, 1993.
41. Wakefield DB, Moscufo N, Guttmann CR, et al: White matter hyperintensities predict functional decline in voiding, mobility, and cognition in older adults. J Am Geriatr Soc 58:275–281, 2010.
44. Araki I, Zakoji H, Komuro M, et al: Lower urinary tract symptoms in men and women without underlying disease causing micturition disorder: a cross-sectional study assessing the natural history of bladder function. J Urol 170:1901–1904, 2003.
52. Gilpin SA, Gilpin CJ, Dixon JS, et al: The effect of age on the autonomic innervation of the urinary bladder. Br J Urol 58:378–381, 1986.
53. Elbadawi A, Yalla SV, Resnick NM: Structural basis of geriatric voiding dysfunction. II. Aging detrusor: normal versus impaired contractility. J Urol 150:1657–1667, 1993.
72. Hotta H, Uchida S: Aging of the autonomic nervous system and possible improvements in autonomic activity using somatic afferent stimulation. Geriatr Gerontol Int 10(Suppl 1):S127–S136, 2010.
73. Griffiths D, Tadic SD: Bladder control, urgency, and urge incontinence: evidence from functional brain imaging. Neurourol Urodyn 27:466–474, 2008.
85. Pfisterer MH, Griffiths DJ, Rosenberg L, et al: Parameters of bladder function in pre-, peri-, and postmenopausal continent women without detrusor overactivity. Neurourol Urodyn 26:356–361, 2007.
86. Pfisterer MH, Griffiths DJ, Schaefer W, et al: The effect of age on lower urinary tract function: a study in women. J Am Geriatr Soc 54:405–412, 2006.
101. Madersbacher S, Pycha A, Schatzl G, et al: The aging lower urinary tract: a comparative urodynamic study of men and women. Urology 51:206–212, 1998.

23 Endocrinology of Aging

John E. Morley, Alexis McKee

HISTORICAL OVERVIEW

The concept that hormones play a role in the aging process originated in the nineteenth century.[1] Based on monkey studies, Hanley stated that myxedema resembled old age (senility), and this included "imbecility." Brown-Sequard's experiments found that testicular extracts rejuvenated rodents and, through experiments on himself, reported that these extracts allowed him "to approximate the strength of a younger person." By the start of the twentieth century, the concept that the decline of hormones was a major cause of aging was well accepted, as chronicled by Lorand, who coined the term *geriatrics* in his book, *Old Age Deferred* (1910):

> *We can produce experimentally typical symptoms of old age in young animals by extirpation of the ductless glands....The memory shows the same typical deficiency, events of long ago being more easily remembered than those of a quite recent date. There often is great fatigue, slow speech and an apathetic condition in both these states.*
>
> **Arnold Lorand**

Throughout the first part of the twentieth century, the concept of a hormonal fountain of youth was spurred on by so-called monkey gland transplants pioneered by Serge Voronoff in Europe and goat gland transplants in the United States. During World War II, the precursor of adrenal cortical hormones, pregnenolone, was shown to enhance visuospatial functioning. In 1957, dehydroepiandrosterone (DHEA) was shown to decline with aging.[2] The antiaging effects of estrogen were chronicled in Wilson's book in 1966, entitled *Feminine Forever*.[3] In 1964, Wesson wrote an article on the "Value of testosterone to men past middle age."[4] This heralded the era of the andropause.[5] Then, in 1990, Rudman and colleagues[6] published their seminal article on growth hormone and aging in men older than 60 years.

This historical overview helps explain how, in the early twenty-first century, there is a raging battle among academics of whether or not a hormonal fountain of youth exists, allowing a great opportunity for antiaging quackery to be used to seduce older adults. A balanced view suggests that although some of these claims may have validity, they need to be balanced against many that are clearly wrong—for example, the growth hormone saga—and that when hormones are given to older persons, they can also produce a number of adverse effects.[7]

This chapter will attempt to provide perspective on how hormones change with aging and how the clinician should interpret these changes. Table 23-1 lists the changes seen in hormones with aging. Most hormone levels decline with aging, with the decline beginning at about 30 years of age and the rate of decline being slightly under 1%/year. In addition, there is a decline in the circadian rhythm seen in most hormones during the aging process. When hormones increase with aging, this is mostly due to a failure of its receptor or postreceptor mechanisms. Overall, these changes lead to an increase in hormonal deficiencies with aging (Fig. 23-1). In addition, older persons are more likely to have autoimmune hormonal deficiency diseases. Box 23-1 summarizes the effects of aging on endocrine disorders.

HORMONAL CHANGES

Thyroid

With aging, there is an increase in nodularity of the thyroid gland and an increase in thyroid neoplasms. Papillary thyroid cancer is the most common cancer in older persons. Aging is associated with an increased likelihood of a mutated *BRAF* gene, with a poorer prognosis.[8] Rapidly growing thyroid nodules in older persons are usually anaplastic carcinomas or lymphomas. Follicular thyroid cancer is much less aggressive, but can metastasize to remote sites. When medullary thyroid cancer occurs in older persons, it is usually the sporadic form.

The decline in the production of thyroxine is balanced by a decreased clearance rate and thus results in no change in circulating thyroxine levels. With the extremes of age, there tends to be a decrease in triiodothyronine (T_3) and an increase in reverse T_3. Because of the decline in the thyroxine clearance rate, most older persons require lower replacement doses of L-thyroxine (~75 μg/day). When older adults are taking higher doses, the physician should check that they are not taking it with calcium or iron supplements, which block absorption. Overreplacement of thyroid hormone leads to osteoporosis and hip fracture. In general, trials treating subclinical hypothyroidism have failed to show clinical benefit.[9]

In rodents, low levels of thyroxine are associated with a longer life span. Similarly, centenarians and their close relatives have a decrease in T_3 levels.[10] There is evidence that mild increases in thyroid-stimulating hormone (TSH) are associated with increased longevity.[11,12] This has been associated with a decrease in TSH receptor function.

Hypothyroidism occurs in 2% to 4% of older persons, with it being more common in men than women.[13] Subclinical hypothyroidism (a raised TSH level with a normal thyroxine level) occurs in 3% to 16% in those older than 60 years. A common cause of an increased TSH level is thyroiditis. Persons with autoimmune hypothyroidism can be identified by measuring antithyroid peroxidase (microsomal) antibodies. The classic symptoms of hypothyroidism, such as fatigue, hoarse voice, dry skin, muscle cramps, puffy eyes, cold sensitivity, cognitive dysfunction, and constipation are commonly seen in older persons, making a clinical diagnosis very difficult. A delayed return of tendon reflexes is a typical finding but requires expertise to detect. Thus, it is important to do biochemical testing for hypothyroidism in those older than 60 years with one or more nonspecific complaints.

The prevalence of hyperthyroidism is substantially lower than hypothyroidism in older persons (≤0.7%).[14] The symptoms of hyperthyroidism are much less common in older compared to younger persons. In older adults, only tachycardia occurs in over 50% of persons with hyperthyroidism. Tremor and nervousness occur in 30% to 40%, and heat intolerance occurs in just over 10%. Appetite increase is rare in older persons. Atrial fibrillation is a relatively common presentation, as is depression. This apathetic presentation has suggested that older adults have a degree of thyroid hormone resistance at the receptor or postreceptor level. In older adults, radioactive iodine appears to be the best option with the least side effects for treating hyperthyroidism. There is evidence that thyroidectomy can be safely carried out in older adults.

Subclinical hyperthyroidism (low TSH level with normal thyroxine level) occurs in about 8% of persons 65 years of age and older. Subclinical hyperthyroidism has been associated with atrial fibrillation, coronary heart disease, and fractures. However, others have failed to confirm these findings, and the progression of subclinical hyperthyroidism to clinical disease is rare.[15] This controversy may be due to the fact that older adults may have physiologically suppressed TSH levels, especially when associated with physical and psychological disorders. In addition, acute thyroiditis can cause TSH suppression. High doses of β-blockers increase circulating thyroxine levels, leading to a decrease in TSH levels. In general, the evidence for treating subclinical hyperthyroidism is controversial.

TABLE 23-1 Hormonal Alterations Associated With Aging

Decreased	Increased	Unchanged
Growth hormone	ACTH	LH (men)
Insulin growth factor-1	Cortisol	Thyroxine
Pregnenolone	Insulin	Epinephrine
Dehydroepiandrosterone sulfate	Amylin	Prolactin
	FSH	
Aldosterone	LH (women)	
Estrogen (women)	Parathyroid hormone	
Testosterone	Norepinephrine	
Triiodothyronine (T_3)	Arginine vasopressin (daytime)	
Arginine vasopressin (nocturnal rise)	TSH	
Vitamin D	Reverse T_3	

Growth Hormone

Growth hormone (GH) release from the somatotropes in the pituitary is under positive regulation of growth hormone-releasing hormone (GHRH) and negative regulation of somatostatin. With aging, there is a decrease in the amount of growth hormone produced per pulsatile burst.[16] This is in part due to the decline in estradiol that occurs at menopause in women and in

BOX 23-1 Effects of Aging on Endocrine Disorders

- Age-related biochemical decline in hormones produces diagnostic difficulty.
- Illnesses can produce declines in hormone levels.
- Decreased functional reserve increases the propensity to endocrine deficiency.
- Decline in plasma clearance leads to lower hormonal replacement doses.
- A decrease in T suppressor lymphocytes and increase in autoantibodies result in increased autoimmune endocrine disease and polyglandular failure.
- Cancer produces ectopic hormones such as AVP and ACTH.
- Decreased receptor and postreceptor responsiveness lead to atypical presentations that often mimic aging changes.
- Polypharmacy results in the following:
    - Abnormal biochemical measurements
    - Decreased absorption of hormone replacement (e.g., iron, calcium)
    - Altered circulating hormone levels (e.g., phenytoin, thyroxine)
    - Drug-hormone interactions
    - Metabolic abnormalities (e.g., vitamin A, hypercalcemia)
- Cognitive dysfunction leads to poor compliance with hormonal replacement.

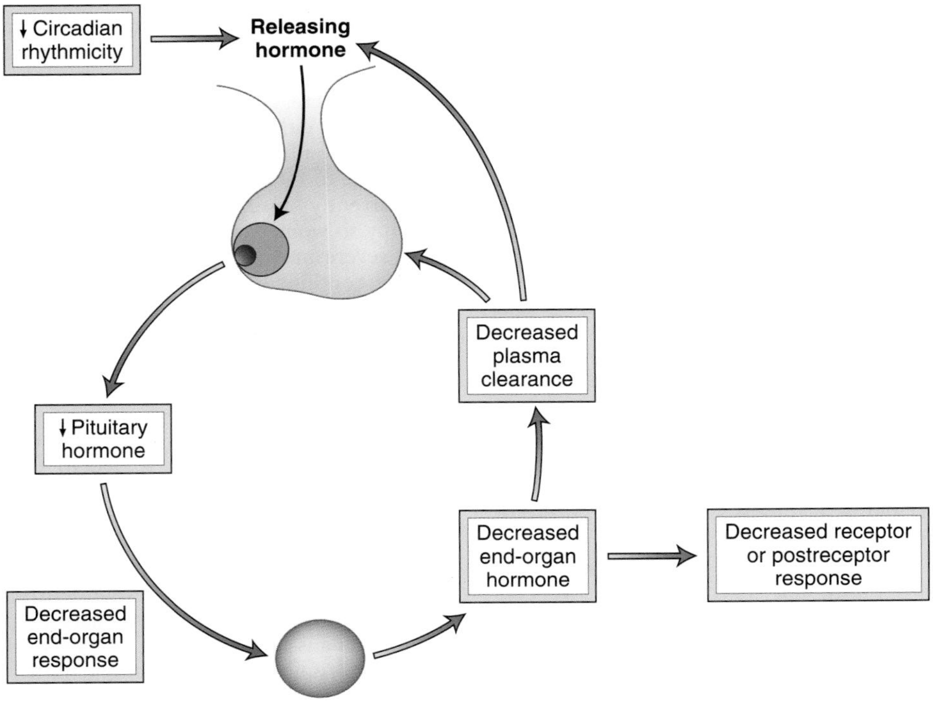

Figure 23-1. Hormonal changes with aging.

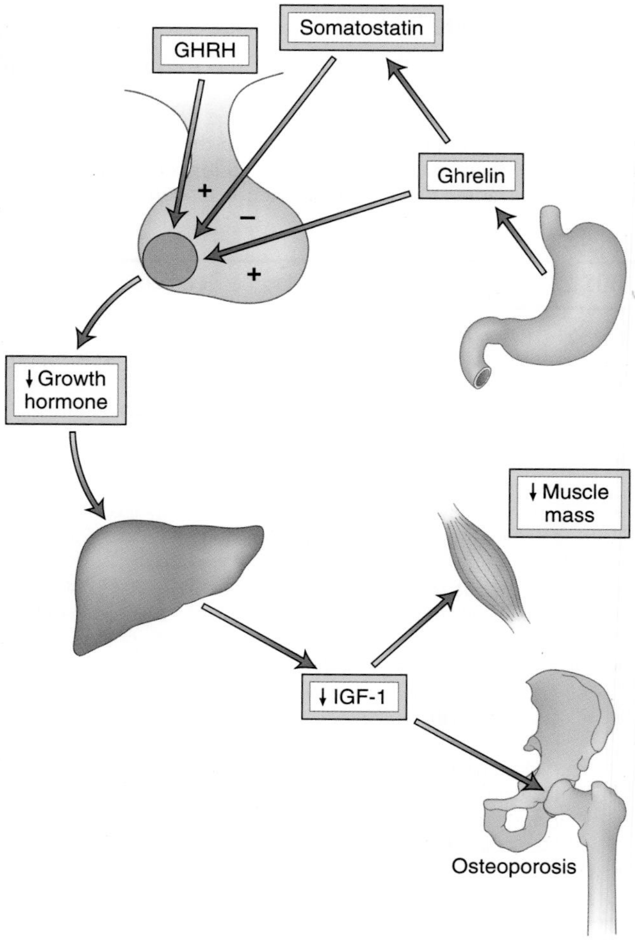

Figure 23-2. Changes in growth hormone with aging.

men by the decline in testosterone. GH release is also under the control of ghrelin, a hormone produced from the fundus of the stomach. The decline in GH production leads to a decrease in insulin-like growth factor 1 (IGF-1) from the liver (Fig. 23-2).

In animals, the Ames dwarf mouse lives longer than controls, suggesting that GH leads to a reduction in survival.[7] A GHRH antagonist in an older mouse model of Alzheimer disease (SAMP8) resulted in increased survival, enhanced memory and telomerase activity, and decreased oxidative damage.[17] Similarly, in the Paris prospective study, persons whose GH level was in the upper range of normal had a higher cardiovascular and total mortality.[18]

In studies in which older adults received GH, GH increased nitrogen retention, weight gain, and muscle mass.[7] It did not increase muscle strength. The lack of increase in muscle strength was because GH increases protein synthesis but not satellite cell formation. In older adults, GH causes arthralgias, carpal tunnel syndrome, soft tissue edema, and insulin resistance.[19] Increased IGF-1 levels are associated with tumors of the breast, prostate, and colon in older adults.

When given as a transgene, IGF-1, which is under GH control, produces hypertrophy and regeneration in senescent muscle.[20] However, IGF-2 (mechano growth factor), which is not under GH control and is produced in muscle, increases satellite cell proliferation. This may explain the failure of GH alone to produce strength. An IGF-1 receptor abnormality has been associated with longevity.

Ghrelin enhances food intake, improves memory, and increases GH levels.[21] Studies with ghrelin agonists in older adults have suggested that it can produce a mild degree of functional improvement.[22]

Dehydroepiandrosterone

DHEA and its sulfate levels decline dramatically with aging. This has led to numerous epidemiologic studies, which found a positive association between the decline in DHEA and DHEA sulfate levels and a higher degree of physical disability.[23] However, high-quality intervention studies such as the DHEAge study found only a small effect on libido in older women and no effect on muscle strength or volume.[24] Similarly, despite the fact that pregnenolone (the DHEA precursor) and DHEA are potent enhancers of memory in mice, no effects have been seen in humans.[7] Furthermore, many of the DHEA products on the market have been found to have no DHEA in them. Overall, the replacement of DHEA in older adults has been shown to be ineffectual and of no benefit.

Estrogen

Menopause in women occurs around the age of 52 years. Women who have a later menopause tend to live longer. Estrogen given at the time of the menopause decreases hip fractures and improves quality of life, predominantly by reducing hot flashes, night sweats, vaginal dryness, and sexual function. Preliminary data from the KEEPS Kronas study have suggested that giving estrogen in lower doses than in the Women's Health Initiative (WHI) trial[25] produced these effects when given for 48 months without increasing cardiovascular events, venous thromboembolism, and breast or endometrial cancer.

The WHI trial studied women aged 50 to 79 years who received placebo, premarin alone in hysterectomized women, or premarin plus progesterone. The trial was stopped early (average, 5.2-year follow-up) because of side effects.[25] Overall, in the combination therapy, there was an increase in coronary heart disease, stroke, pulmonary embolism, venous thromboembolism, breast cancer, gallbladder disease, incontinence, and dementia. Improvements were noted in hip fractures, total fractures, diabetes, and colorectal cancer. In the estrogen-alone group, there was no increase in coronary heart disease. Although embolism and dementia increased, it was not significant. Total mortality was not increased in either treatment group (Table 23-2). Overall, estrogen alone had a small number of statistically negative effects compared to the combination therapy.

Currently available data would support giving hormone therapy to women with premature menopause and women who have severe menopausal symptoms. This should most probably not be continued for more than 5 years beyond the age of 52 years. There is no evidence to support hormone therapy in women older than 60 years.

Testosterone

Total testosterone declines at the rate of 1%/year in older men. About half of this decline is due to the increase in body fat that occurs with aging. Sex hormone-binding globulin (SHBG) increases with age, so there is a greater decline in free or bioavailable (free and albumin-bound) testosterone. The decline in testosterone level is due to a decrease in Leydig cell function, as demonstrated by a decreased response to human chorionic gonadotropin, and to a decrease in hypothalamic-pituitary function (Fig. 23-3). Aging is associated with a decrease in the circadian rhythm of gonadotropin-releasing hormone (GnRH) release. In addition, there is a decrease in pulsatility and pulse magnitude with aging. This leads to a decrease in luteinizing hormone (LH) pulse

TABLE 23-2 Effects of Estrogen (E) and Progesterone (P) and Estrogen Alone on Outcomes*

	Positive Effects		No Effect		Negative Effects	
Outcome	*E + P*	*E Alone*	*E + P*	*E Alone*	*E + P*	*E Alone*
Total mortality	—	—	0.98	1.04	—	—
Coronary heart disease	—	—	—	0.95	1.24	—
Stroke	—	—	—	—	1.31	1.37
Pulmonary embolism	—	—	—	1.37	2.13	—
Venous embolism	—	—	—	1.32	2.06	—
Breast cancer	—	—	—	0.80	1.24	—
Colorectal cancer	0.56	—	—	1.08	—	—
Endometrial cancer	—	—	0.81	—	—	—
Hip fractures	0.67	0.65	—	—	—	—
Total fractures	0.76	0.71	—	—	—	—
Diabetes	0.79	—	—	1.01	—	—
Gallbladder disease	—	—	—	—	1.59	1.67
Stress incontinence	—	—	—	—	1.87	2.15
Dementia	—	—	—	1.49	2.05	—

*Numbers represent the odds ratio.

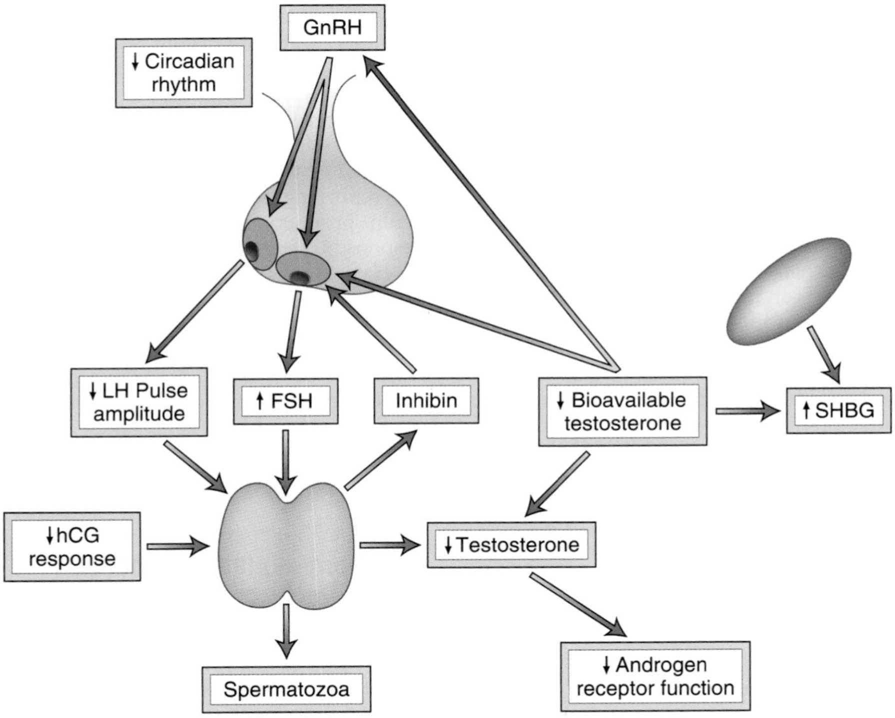

Figure 23-3. Effects of aging on the hypothalamic-pituitary-testicular axis. hCG, Human chorionic gonadotropin.

amplitude. In addition, it appears that there may be a decrease in androgen receptor function, with a decline in intracellular β-catenin activity.[26]

Epidemiologic studies have shown a clear relationship of testosterone and muscle mass with strength, frailty, hematocrit, bone mineral density, hip fractures, sexual function, and cognition.[7,27,28] Persons with mild cognitive impairment who have low bioavailable testosterone levels have a rapid transition to Alzheimer disease.[29] Testosterone also has been shown to improve lower urinary tract syndrome (LUTS).[30]

The relationship of testosterone to mortality is less clear. Although most studies have shown that low testosterone is related to mortality, some studies have failed to show this relationship.[31] A variety of diseases are associated with low testosterone levels. The studies that failed to show a relationship of mortality to testosterone examined very healthy or very sick persons. This suggests that the increased mortality in other studies could be due to ill persons in the cohort having lower testosterone levels.

Controlled studies have shown that testosterone replacement increases hematocrit, muscle mass and strength, quality of life, memory, and bone mineral density.[7,32] A number of studies have shown that testosterone increases strength and function in frail older persons and also in those with end-stage heart failure.[33,34] The testosterone dose required to increase strength is higher than the dose needed to increase muscle mass.

The side effects of testosterone are not absolutely clear. Although two large epidemiologic studies have suggested that persons receiving testosterone have an increase in myocardial infarction, both studies had a number of flaws.[35,36] A meta-analysis of controlled studies found no increase in myocardial infarction.[37]

Because testosterone increases hematocrit, it is possible that in patients not followed appropriately, the hematocrit can be allowed to increase above 55%, resulting in an increased propensity to form thrombi. In addition, it needs to be recognized that testosterone causes water retention, which in frail older persons produces edema, and this could be inaccurately attributed to heart failure.

Similar controversy exists on the role of testosterone in prostate cancer. Overall, little evidence indicates that testosterone is responsible for prostate cancer, but it can clearly accelerate it when present. It is now acceptable to give testosterone to persons who have had prostate cancer treated by surgery or radiation and have a low prostate-specific antigen (PSA) level.[38]

Testosterone seems to make sleep apnea worse in the first 3 months with this disorder. However, by 6 months, this is no longer true.[39]

The approach to the diagnosis of male hypogonadism requires the presence of symptoms, predominantly decreased libido or soft erections. Questionnaires such as the Aging Male Survey or the St. Louis University ADAM questionnaire can be used.[40,41] If the person has symptoms, depression needs to be ruled out. Testosterone and bioavailable testosterone testing should then be performed; if either is low, a trial of testosterone for 3 months is warranted. If the symptoms do not improve, treatment should be stopped (Fig. 23-4).

A variety of measures to deliver testosterone are available. These include oral skin patches, gels, buccal patch, nasal, pellets, and injections. Overall, testosterone injections are the least expensive and probably the easiest to manage.

There are a number of selective androgen receptor molecules (SARMs) available to treat frailty and/or disability. Nandrolone, an intramuscular SARM, was shown to have small effects on function. Similarly, enobosarm is an investigational oral drug that has been shown to have effects on muscle mass and power.[42]

Testosterone levels decline in females rapidly from 30 years of age to menopause and then more gradually thereafter.[43] In postmenopausal women, testosterone has been shown to improve libido, general well-being, mastalgia, headaches, bone mineral density, and muscle mass. At present, there are no recommendations to use testosterone for these purposes in women.

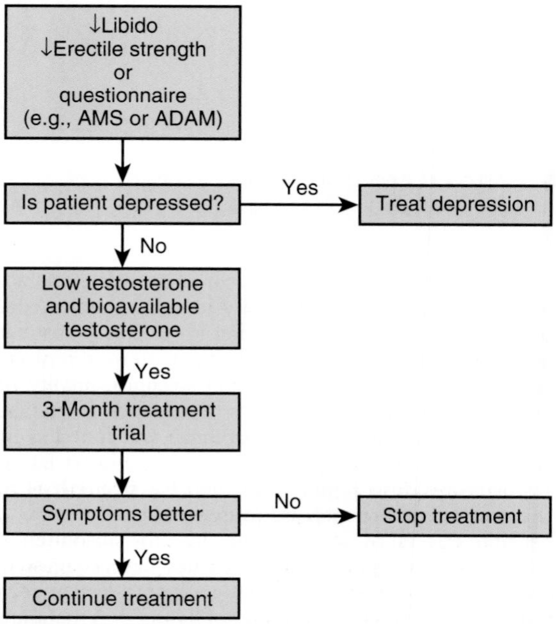

Figure 23-4. Algorithm for the diagnosis of male hypogonadism in an older male.

Hypothalamic-Pituitary-Adrenal Axis

Corticotropin-releasing hormone (CRH) from the hypothalamus causes the release of adrenocorticotropic hormone (ACTH) from the pituitary, which regulates the release of cortisol and, to a lesser extent, aldosterone, from the adrenal cortex. In general, it is believed that the hypothalamic-pituitary-adrenal axis is overactive with aging, with an increase in 24-hour total and free plasma and salivary cortisol.[44] This is associated with phase advancement of morning cortisol and increased fragmentation of cortisol secretion. There is a decreased rate of plasma cortisol clearance. The response to CRH is unchanged, but dexamethasone fails to inhibit the cortisol response to the same extent as in younger persons. There is a decreased adrenal production of cortisol when ACTH is administered exogenously. It has been postulated that the increased circulating cortisol levels are due to an increase in conversion of corticosterone to cortisol in adipose tissue.

With aging, increased cortisol can have many detrimental effects, including acceleration of neuronal damage, leading to cognitive decline, as well as increasing the risk of osteopenia and subsequent hip fractures. Excess cortisol also leads to muscle wasting, causing sarcopenia, frailty, and disability. Accelerated visceral obesity and insulin resistance and consequent atherosclerosis and an increased risk of infection due to decreased immune function are also results of elevated cortisol levels [45,46]

Aldosterone is produced by the zona glomerulosa of the adrenal. With aging, there is a small decrease in aldosterone production to ACTH.[47] The major controller of aldosterone is the renin-angiotensin-aldosterone system. There is a decline in renin production and decrease in aldosterone production in response to angiotensin II with aging.[48]

Hyperaldosteronism occurs in about 10% of older adults. This is due, in most cases, to bilateral adrenal hyperplasia. Some of these cases have multiple microadenomas due to a KLNJ5 gain in function mutation.[49] In older adults with hypokalemia and hypertension, hyporeninemic hyperaldosteronism should be suspected and is treatable with spironolactone.

Finally, in older adults under stress or who are depressed, it needs to be recognized that increases in hypothalamic corticotropin-releasing hormone can lead to anorexia and weight loss.

Adrenomedullary Hormones

With aging, there is an increase in sympathetic (norepinephrenic) tone.[50] On the other hand, the adrenomedullary release of epinephrine is decreased in older compared to younger persons.[51] Plasma levels, however, are only mildly decreased because there is also a decrease in plasma clearance activity with aging. Finally, with aging, there is a decrease in sympathetic receptor activity due to receptor desensitization.[52] The increase in orthostatic hypotension with aging is predominantly due to catecholamine receptor or postreceptor defects.

Arginine Vasopressin

In 1949, Findley suggested that there were alterations in the neurohypophyseal-renal axis with aging.[53] This was confirmed by the studies of Miller and associates,[54,55] who reported that hyponatremia was present in 115 of ambulatory older persons over a 2-year period and in 53% of nursing home residents over 1 year. These studies suggested that most of them had a syndrome similar to the syndrome of inappropriate antidiuretic hormone secretion (SIADH).

Hyponatremia in older adults is associated with an increase in inpatient and outpatient mortality.[56] Asymptomatic hyponatremia is associated with an unstable gait, increased falls, and an increase in hip fractures. Much of this hyponatremia is also related to

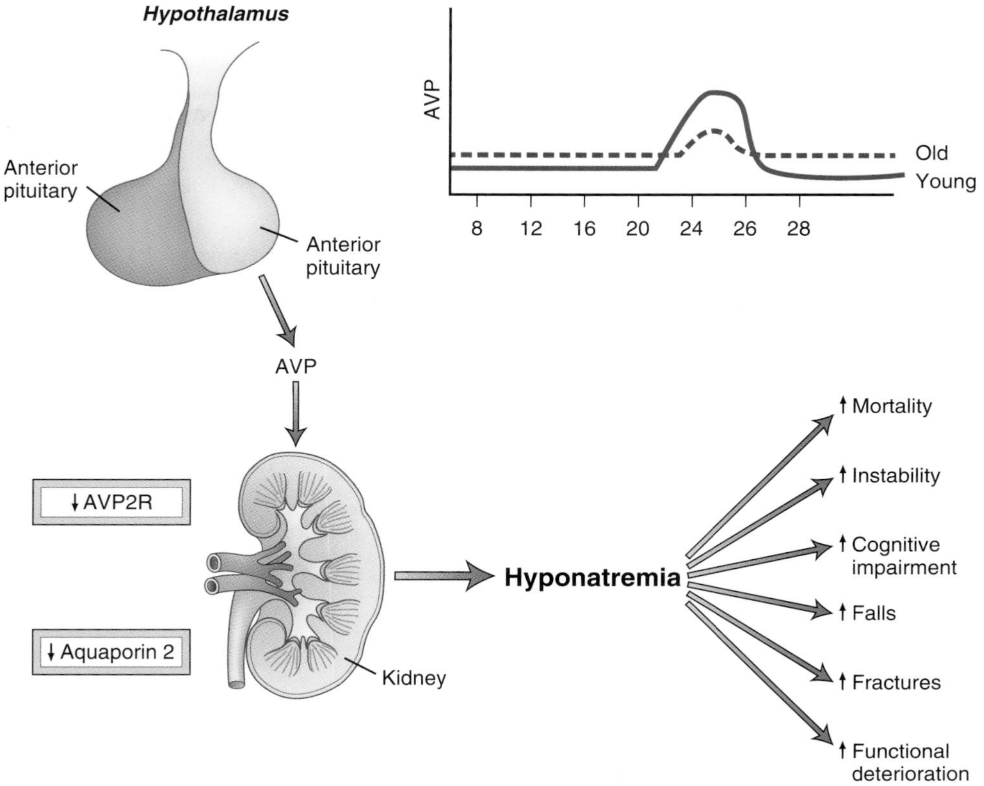

Figure 23-5. Changes in arginine vasopressin (AVP) and its effects on aging.

attention deficits and a mild delirium. Hyponatremia has also been related to functional decline.

Circulating arginine vasopressin (AVP) levels are increased during the daytime in older adults.[57] However, this is offset by a blunting of the nocturnal rise in AVP levels. This blunting is responsible for the increase in nocturia in older adults. With aging, there is a blunted kidney response to AVP, despite the elevated daytime circulating levels. Animal studies have suggested that aging is associated with a decrease in AVP V2 receptors with aging. The V2 receptor controls the shuttling of the aquaporin 2 water channels from intracellular water channels to the apical membrane to form channels that allow water absorption from the collecting ducts of the kidney. There is some evidence that there is a decline in aquaporin 2 activity with aging.

Figure 23-5 depicts an overview of the changes in AVP with aging and its effects.

Melatonin

Melatonin is produced from tryptophan in the pineal gland. This is under the regulation of the suprachiasmatic nucleus. Melatonin levels decline gradually throughout the life span. Low levels of melatonin at night have been associated with disturbances in the sleep-wake rhythm in older adults,[58] and this is particularly true in persons with Alzheimer disease. Melatonin and ramelteon (a melatonin 1 and 2 receptor agonist) have both been shown to produce small improvements in sleep. There is increasing evidence that melatonin and ramelteon may be useful for delirium and sundown syndrome.[59,60]

Melatonin also has a number of effects on the immune system. It stimulates a number of immune cells, especially natural killer cells and CD4 T helper lymphocytes.[61] Melatonin is also an antioxidant. Melatonin increases GH hormone and IGF-1 levels.[62] Melatonin also has been shown to have effects on DNA methylation and histone production, suggesting a role in epigenetic modulation. Low levels of melatonin are associated with an increased risk of prostate cancer.[63]

CONCLUSION

Numerous hormonal changes occur with aging. Most of these begin around 30 years of age and gradually decline. The role of these hormonal changes in aging, whether they accelerate the aging process or are perhaps protective, is uncertain. Future studies using physiologic replacement doses over prolonged periods will be necessary to determine whether a so-called hormonal fountain of youth is mythology or has some scientific validity.

KEY POINTS

- Hypothyroidism occurs in 2% to 4% of older adults.
- The decrease in thyroxine clearance in older adults means that they need lower L-thyroxine replacement doses than younger persons
- Studies do not support the replacement of growth hormone in older adults.
- Testosterone levels decline at the rate of 1%/year in men.
- Although testosterone replacement in older adults is controversial, it does increase strength in frail older adults.
- Hyporeninemic hyperaldosteronism is not uncommon in older adults with hypertension.
- The syndrome of inappropriate antidiuretic hormone is common in older adults.
- Testosterone, growth hormone, DHEA, and IGF-1 all play a role in the pathophysiology of sarcopenia.

For a complete list of references, please visit www.expertconsult.com.

KEY REFERENCES

7. Morley JE: Scientific overview of hormone treatment used for rejuvenation. Fertil Steril 99:1807–1813, 2013.
9. Bensenor IM, Olmos RD, Lotufo PA: Hypothyroidism in the elderly: diagnosis and management. Clin Interv Aging 7:97–111, 2012.
10. Tabatabaie V, Surks MI: The aging thyroid. Curr Opin Endocrinol Diabetes Obes 20:455–459, 2013.
13. Gesing A, Lewinski A, Karbownik-Lewinska M: The thyroid gland and the process of aging; what is new? Thyroid Res 5:16–20, 2012.
19. Nass R: Growth hormone axis and aging. Endocrinol Metab Clin North Am 42:187–199, 2013.
22. Morley JE, von Haehling S, Anker SD: Are we closer to having drugs to treat muscle wasting disease? J Cachexia Sarcopenia Muscle 5:83–87, 2014.
32. Matsumoto AM: Testosterone administration in older men. Endocrinol Metab Clin North Am 42:271–286, 2013.
33. Morley JE: Sarcopenia in the elderly. Fam Pract 29(Suppl 1):i44–i48, 2012.
37. Corona G, Maseroli E, Rastrelli G, et al: Cardiovascular risk associated with testosterone-boosting medications: A systematic review and meta-analysis. Expert Opin Drug Saf 13:1327–1351, 2014.
38. Balbontin FG, Moreno SA, Bley E, et al: Long-acting testosterone injections for treatment of testosterone deficiency after brachytherapy for prostate cancer. BJU Int 114:125–130, 2014.
39. Wittert G: The relationship between sleep disorders and testosterone. Curr Opin Endocrinol Diabetes Obes 21:239–243, 2014.
40. Morley JE, Perry HM 3rd, Kevorkian RT, et al: Comparison of screening questionnaires for the diagnosis of hypyodonadism. Maturitas 53:424–429, 2006.
44. Veldhuis JD, Sharma A, Roelfsema F: Age-dependent and gender-dependent regulation of hypothalamic-adrenocorticotropic-adrenal axis. Endocrinol Metab Clin North Am 42:201–225, 2013.
55. Miller M, Morley JE, Rubenstein LZ: Hyponatremia in a nursing home population. J Am Geriatr Soc 43:1410–1413, 1995.
56. Cowen LE, Hodak SP, Verbalis JG: Age-associated abnormalities of water homeostasis. Endocrinol Metab Clin North Am 42:349–370, 2013.
57. Moon DG, Jin MH, Lee JG, et al: Antidiuretic hormone in elderly male patients with severe nocturia: a circadian study. BJU Int 94:571–575, 2004.
59. Tsuda A, Nishimura K, Naganawa E, et al: Ramelteon for the treatment of delirium in elderly patients: a consecutive case series study. Int J Psychiatry Med 47:97–104, 2014.
60. Lammers M, Ahmed AI: Melatonin for sundown syndrome and delirium in dementia: is it effective? J Am Geriatr Soc 61:1045–1046, 2013.
62. Jenwitheesuk A, Nopparat C, Mukda S, et al: Melatonin regulates aging and neurodegeneration through energy metabolism, epigenetics, autophagy and circadian rhythm pathways. Int J Mol Sci 15:16848–16884, 2014.

24 Aging and the Blood

Michael A. McDevitt

INTRODUCTION

Age-related changes to normal blood cell development and function remain poorly understood but measurably evident. In 1961, Hayflick and Moorhead described experiments that established the concept that normal somatic cells have a finite number of cell divisions.[1] After completing this limiting number of cell divisions, a resting cellular phase, or senescence, is irreversibly entered. These postmitotic cells do not immediately die, however. They may survive for several years with normal function but with biochemical changes that ultimately affect themselves and potentially neighboring cells. Cellular senescence has long been used as a cellular model for understanding the mechanisms underlying the aging process, and this may be particularly important for age-related blood cell changes. Extensive observations have suggested that DNA damage accumulates with age and may be due to an increase in the production of reactive oxygen species (ROS) and a decline in DNA repair capacity with age. Mutation or disrupted expression of genes that increase DNA damage often result in premature aging. In contrast, interventions that enhance resistance to oxidative stress and attenuate DNA damage contribute toward longevity.

In this chapter, we will update observations that characterize aging blood cells with the hope that these findings will help provide insight into underlying mechanisms associated with aging, particularly those that can be altered by interventions. Overlap with and potential significance for aging of recently discovered genetic and epigenetic changes identified in several hematologic conditions will be explored. Finally, highlights in the area of blood cell immunosenescence will be discussed. In that blood, bone marrow, and lymphoid tissues are among the most accessible of tissues for human experimental study, advances in this area continue to provide insights into our general understanding of the normal and pathologic physiology of aging. Age-related cytopenias, myelodysplastic and myeloproliferative disorders, chronic lymphocytic leukemia, and other clonal lymphoid disorders are increasingly being recognized as ideal model systems to study the intersection of tissue aging, molecular changes, and physiologic effects.

SITES OF BLOOD CELL DEVELOPMENT: BONE MARROW AND STROMA

Healthy individuals produce billions of red and white blood cells every day under normal conditions. With infection, bleeding, or other stresses, production is increased in response to complex physiologic mechanisms. The process of hematopoiesis begins with a limited number of hematopoietic stem cells (HSCs), which serve as the reservoir for the progenitors that generate mature blood cell production while maintaining the stem cell compartment.[2] The sites of hematopoiesis change during mammalian development.[3] During the first 6 to 8 weeks of human embryonic life, the yolk sac is the site of hematopoiesis, followed by a fetal liver stage. With further development, the bone marrow becomes the major site of hematopoiesis, other than pathologic disorders such as myeloproliferative neoplasms (MPN) and thalassemia, in which extramedullary hematopoiesis in the spleen, liver, and other sites outside of the bone marrow may occur. Elegant murine studies have tracked the migration of HSCs through these various tissues and identified the earliest site of definitive hematopoiesis in the embryo as the aorta-gonad-mesonephros (AGM) region.[4]

The bone marrow is a complex specialized environment. At birth, the bone marrow is a fully hematopoietically active tissue but, with aging, there is replacement with hematopoietically inactive adipose tissue. A transition of approximately 1%/year in the bone marrow is a rough standard when assessing clinical bone marrow sample cellularity in individuals of different ages.[5] Bone marrow is a diverse cellular mix, minimally including fibroblasts, macrophages, mast cells, reticular cells, endothelial cells, osteoid cells, and adipocytes. Conventional histologic and immunohistologic analysis has identified a generally orderly arrangement of developing cells in the bone marrow, including localization of early granulocytic cells along the bony trabecular margins and erythroid islands, megakaryocytes, and occasional lymphoid nodules positioned in the intertrabecular spaces. Examples of special cellular niche relationships include megakaryocyte localization near draining venules to facilitate platelet release into the bloodstream[6] and juxtaposition of central macrophages and surrounding developing erythroid clusters.[7,8] Age-related histologic findings include marrow necrosis and fibrosis, loss of bone substance, increase in bone marrow iron stores, expansion of adipose tissue, and accumulation of benign lymphoid aggregates.[9] Although analysis of individual cytokines, cellular compositions, and supportive stromal functions can be measured to decrease with aging, underlying mechanisms have been elusive.

Recent advances have identified a specialized component of the bone marrow microenvironment termed the *niche*. This three-dimensional functional hematopoietic unit has specialized anatomic relationships among bone, blood vessels, and differentiating hematopoietic cells. The HSC niche functions as an anatomically confined regulatory environment governing HSC numbers and fate.[10-13] Niche cellular relationships include vascular endothelial and perivascular cells and sympathetic innervation and osteoclasts. Several spatially and likely functionally distinct bone marrow microenvironments and niches have been proposed.[14,15] The endosteal HSC niche contains osteoblasts as the main supportive cell type. The vascular niche has HSCs associated with the sinusoidal endothelium in the bone marrow and spleen.[16,17] These environments serve as sites for local cytokine production. Factors implicated in HSC function include the Notch ligands Delta and Jagged, involved in the generation, antidifferentiation, and expansion of HSCs.[18,19] Wnt signaling is involved in HSC generation and expansion and the maintenance of HSCs in a quiescent state.[20,21] Bone morphogenic proteins (BMPs) and transforming growth factor-β (TGF-β) regulate HSC activity,[22] and BMP appears to regulate the size of the endosteal niche.[23] Many other soluble factors are also under investigation.[24,25]

Many of these niche components and relationships have been identified so recently that their potential roles in age-related bone marrow functional changes have not yet been investigated. Based on the importance to normal steady-state hematopoiesis, the niche has been investigated in disease pathogenesis, however. The human myeloproliferative neoplasm primary myelofibrosis (PMF), long known as a disorder of abnormal marrow fibrosis leading to so-called wandering stem cells,[26] has been proposed to be a clonal disorder of the stem cell niche deregulation and abnormal stroma.[27] Myelofibrosis is one of the classic myeloproliferative neoplasms (MPNs) that also include essential thrombocytosis (ET) and polycythemia vera (PV). These and many other myeloid and lymphoid malignancies have been diagnosed at increasing frequency in aging individuals. Niche perturbations have also been observed in a myeloproliferative disorder that develops in retinoic acid gamma receptor microenvironment murine knockouts.[28] Lyer and colleagues[29] have found that the HSC compartment expands significantly when aged in a niche that contains SHIP1 (Src homology 2-domain-containing inositol 5′-phosphatase 1)-deficient mesenchymal stem cells and also provides potential insight into the development of MPN in older adults.

The bone marrow microenvironment and niche abnormalities have been increasingly implicated in other hematopoietic malignancies frequently found in older adults as well.[30] The myelodysplastic syndromes (MDSs), for example, are a diverse group of clonal hematopoietic malignancies characterized by ineffective hematopoiesis, progressive bone marrow failure, cytogenetic and molecular abnormalities, and risk of progression to acute myelogenous leukemia. Using a retroviral model of induced acute myeloid leukemia (AML), Lane and associates[31] have identified a leukemia stem cell (LSC) niche that is physically distinct and independent of the constraints of Wnt signaling that apply to normal HSCs. Donor cell leukemia (DCL), a rare complication of bone marrow transplantation, has been linked to niche damage from inflammation triggered by the primary underlying malignancy, active chemotherapeutic and radiation conditioning, or transplantation-related immune modulatory treatment, all leading to extrinsic leukemic influences on donor HSCs.[32]

To summarize, the discovery of the niche and stromal contributions to hematopoiesis represent major new areas for the investigation of normal physiology and aging. In addition to serving as a primary site of hematopoiesis, the bone marrow has also been identified as a tissue source of cells for nonhematopoietic wound healing or regeneration. Examples of potential bone marrow-derived tissue contributors include mesenchymal stem cells[33-35] and fibrocytes.[36] Mesenchymal stem cells (MSCs) are multipotent stem cells. Although originally identified in bone marrow and described as marrow stromal cells, they have since been identified in many other anatomic locations. MSCs can be isolated from bone marrow, adipose tissue, umbilical cord, and other tissues but the richest tissue source of MSCs is fat.[35] Because they are adherent to plastic, they may be expanded in vitro. MSCs have a distinct morphology and express a specific set of cell surface molecules. Under appropriate conditions, MSCs can proliferate and give rise to other cell types and are under evaluation as tissue sources for the treatment of systemic inflammatory and autoimmune conditions and as a replacement for injured tissue following injury or trauma. The heart,[37] cornea,[38] and liver[39] are among many other tissues that are being examined as potential target organs for bone marrow–derived regenerating tissue grafts.

HEMATOPOIETIC STEM CELLS

The stem cell model of hematopoiesis starts with the totipotent HSC that has the capacity for self-renewal to prevent exhaustion of the HSC compartment. The asymmetric proliferation and differentiation produce large numbers of lineage-restricted hematopoietic cells daily and the ability to reconstitute hematopoiesis in a lethally irradiated host.[2] Although intrinsic and extrinsic control of the early developmental steps from self-renewing HSCs and cells committed to differentiation are poorly understood, these represent an excellent general model system to define basic mechanisms of mammalian cell development and differentiation. The ability of transferred HSCs to reconstitute hematopoiesis provides the clinical basis for bone marrow transplantation. The earliest description of stem cell transplantation (SCT) was based on studies showing murine bone marrow transplanted into lethally irradiated mice, rescuing the recipient by reconstituting donor hematopoiesis.[40] Remarkably, intravenous injection is possible because the HSCs are able to home to the bone marrow and identify and interact with the niche. The biology and physiology of the HSC is enormously complex and has been the subject of many reviews that include descriptions of the characterization and developmental origins of HSCs, enumeration of cellular sources, regulation of cell fate decisions, and clinical implications for bone marrow transplantation.[2,3,41] Detailed studies of aging hematopoietic stem cells have provided unique insights into the aging process.

Telomeres and telomerase have been specifically investigated as potential components of age-related bone marrow failure, including hematopoietic stem cell dysfunction. Short telomeres have been linked to the cause of degenerative diseases, including idiopathic pulmonary fibrosis, cryptogenic liver cirrhosis, and bone marrow failure.[42] Natural mutations to the core complex were first discovered in the rare bone marrow failure syndrome dyskeratosis congenita (DC).[43] Heterozygous mutations of these genes have been described for patients with DC, bone marrow failure, and idiopathic pulmonary fibrosis.[42] Mutations in the telomerase RNA (*TERC*) or telomerase reverse transcriptase component (*TERT*) apparatus associated with telomerase dysfunction have been identified in sporadic and familial MDS and AML.[44] The spectrum of mutations in *TERT* and *TERC* varies for these diseases and appear, at least in part, to explain the clinical differences observed, including bone marrow failure. Environmental insults and genetic modifiers that accelerate telomere shortening and increase cell turnover may exaggerate the effects of telomerase haploinsufficiency, contributing to the variability of age of onset and tissue-specific organ pathology.

Telomere dysfunction in mouse models has been associated with alveolar stem cell failure.[45] Warren and Rossi, in 2008, reviewed the general lack of direct evidence for progressive depletion of the hematopoietic stem cell pool based on telomere shortening with aging.[46] Serial bone marrow transplantation experiments in mice have suggested that that although the replicative potential of HSCs is finite, there is little evidence that replicative senescence causes depletion of the stem cell pool during the normal life span of mice or humans. Evidence has suggested that HSC numbers substantially increase with advancing age in mice.[47] The expansion of the HSC pool is a cell-autonomous property—HSCs from older donors exhibit a greater capacity than younger controls on transplantation into younger recipients.[48] Although there is an increase in the number of HSCs with age, they have functional deficiencies, including altered homing and mobilization properties[49,50] and decreased competitive repopulation abilities.[47] Remarkably, a skewing of lineage potential from lymphopoiesis to myelopoiesis has been observed with advancing age.[41] There are reduced lymphoid progenitors in older mice and are maintained to increased myeloid progenitors. These HSC cell-autonomous transplantable property findings may explain age-related immune cell senescence and an increase in myelogenous hematologic malignancy with age.

The reproducible finding of altered lymphoid-to-myeloid blood cell ratios with age has been a focus of intensive molecular investigations. Analysis of a single HSC in long-term transplantation assays and genetic differences in HSC behavior in different strains of inbred mice have demonstrated that many HSC behaviors are fixed intrinsically through genetic or epigenetic mechanisms.[41,51] A striking example of epigenetically fixed heterogeneity among HSCs is found in myeloid-biased HSCs. These HSCs make typical levels of myeloid cells but generate too few lymphocytes. The diminished lymphoid progeny have impaired responses to interleukin-1 (IL-7).[52] Using highly purified HSCs from young and aged mice, Chambers and colleagues have identified functional deficits as well as an increase in stem cell numbers with advancing age.[53] Gene expression analysis has identified approximately 1,500 of more than 14,000 genes that were age-induced and 1,600 that were age-repressed. Genes associated with the stress response, inflammation, and protein aggregation dominated the upregulated profile, whereas the genes involved in chromatin remodeling and preservation of genomic integrity were downregulated. Many chromosomal regions showed a coordinate loss of transcriptional regulation and an overall increase in transcriptional activity with age, and an inappropriate expression of genes normally regulated by epigenetic mechanisms was observed.

Sun and colleagues have recently extended the observations described earlier. They performed an intensive analysis of highly purified HSC populations comparing genomic properties of young and old murine HSCs with coordinate analyses of global changes in the transcriptome, histone modifications, and DNA methylation.[54] Their group reported a significant link between aging-associated changes in the deposition of histone marks with changes in RNA expression, coding, and noncoding. Pathway analysis revealed a high percentage of aging-associated changes in gene expression related to ultimately decreased TGF-β signaling, as well as upregulation of genes encoding ribosomal proteins. The study by Sun and associates[54] has strongly supported emerging evidence that deregulated epigenetic status represents one of the driving forces behind age-related alterations in the functionality of stem cells. Further work is needed to connect the alterations in DNA methylation and histone modifications and associated changes in gene expression related to increased self-renewal and myeloid-skewed differentiation of aging HSCs.

Epigenetic alterations are pharmacologically targetable. Epigenetic chromatin-modifying drugs have been applied to normal HSC cultures with cytokines with the goal of preserving marrow-repopulating activity.[55] Activation of several genes and their products implicated in HSC self-renewal were observed compared with cells exposed to cytokines alone, which lost their marrow-repopulating activity. Previous attempts to expand HSCs resulted in HSC differentiation and stem cell exhaustion or, at best, asymmetric cell division and maintenance of the same numbers of HSCs. These observations suggest that chromatin-modifying agents may allow for the symmetric division of HSCs and expansion of potential therapeutic grafts, with preservation of stem cell function. Molecular analysis of patients with an informative clonal marker and neutrophil response has indicated that restoration of normal nonclonal hematopoiesis may be a significant component of the epigenetic agent 5-aza-2′-deoxycytidine (decitabine, DAC) used in the treatment of MDS and AML.[56]

Additional support for age-related biologic differences in HSCs and how detailed investigations of malignant hematopoietic disorders provide insight into the aging of blood has been illustrated by recent studies comparing the clinical outcomes of stem cell transplantations using younger or older stem cell donors. Kroger and coworkers[57] have investigated whether a young human leukocyte antigen (HLA)–matched unrelated donor (MUD) should be preferred as the donor to an HLA-identical sibling (matched related donor, MRD) for older patients with MDS who underwent allogeneic stem cell transplantation. Transplantation from younger MUDs had a significantly improved 5-year overall survival in comparison with MRDs and older MUDs. In a multivariate analysis, transplantation from young MUDs remained a significant factor for improved survival in comparison with MRDs. These are not definitive results but illustrate one of the clinical issues related to understanding the age-associated function of the HSCs.[57]

Alternative sources of HSCs for stem cell therapy and regenerative medicine have been sought through the use of embryonic stem cell (ESC) and induced pluripotent stem cell (iPSC) technologies.[58,59] These strategies have yet to yield fully functional cells. More recent approaches have also investigated transcription factor (TF) overexpression to reprogram PSCs and various somatic cells.[60] The induction of pluripotency with just four TFs[61] provides the rationale for an approach to convert cell fates and demonstrates the feasibility of using terminally differentiated cells to generate cells with multilineage potential.

Progenitor Compartment

Lineage-restricted progenitor cells derived from HSCs allow amplification of numbers and differentiation into separate lineage effector cells. Ultimately, more than 10 different mature cell types are derived from the HSC through these progenitors. Within a pathway, there are early and late progenitors, which differ in the number of potential proliferative cell divisions. Early models proposed a linear development from primitive HSCs to late HSCs through a simple bifurcation of common myeloid progenitors (CMPs) and common lymphoid progenitors (CLPs) to generate the full set of blood cell lineages,[62] with additional downstream binary pathways. These proposals correlate nicely with transcriptional regulatory mechanisms, with positive and negative feedback loops.[3,63-67] Additional technical advances in single-cell isolation and molecular studies continue to add to our knowledge and challenge recognized models.[68] Paul and coworkers have found that myeloid progenitors appear to commit very early to differentiation toward distinct blood lineages.[69] Contrary to previous beliefs,[67] very few progenitors express multiple transcription factors regulating different fates. Studies by Perié and colleagues[70] and Notta and associates[71] have all been consistent with finding that most myeloid progenitors from adult humans are committed to a single lineage. Interestingly, most of the myeloid blood cell output appears to be driven by a transient clonal succession of lineage-restricted cells, in which a pool of progenitors is committed to lineages upstream of the common myeloid progenitor.[72] These and other findings have significant implications for our understanding of normal hematopoiesis and leukemogenesis.[68]

The identification and study of progenitors has been greatly facilitated through the development of in vitro culture systems, including the identification of growth factors necessary to prevent apoptosis, an important default regulatory pathway in many, if not all, hematopoietic lineages. Transcription factors represent intrinsic determinants of cellular phenotype and differentiation. Particularly informative has been the study of transcription factor knockout and transgenic mice in elucidating hematopoietic regulatory roles.[3,63] One set of observations has demonstrated how alterations in transcriptional regulators may connect age-associated alterations in blood cell development. Quéré and coworkers have observed that young mice deleted for transcription intermediary factor 1γ (Tif1γ) in HSCs developed an accelerated aging phenotype.[73] Supporting this, they found that Tif1γ is downregulated in HSCs during aging in wild-type mice and that Tif1γ controls TGF-β signaling. Their data provide connections between transcriptional regulators (Tif1γ) and downstream signaling (TGF-β) in regulating the balance between lymphoid- and myeloid-derived HSCs, with implications for HSC aging. Analysis of transcription factor knockout or knockdown at aging time points for other transcription factors is an important step in identifying potential phenotypes.[74,75]

Based on the importance of transcriptional control mechanisms on the regulation of hematopoiesis and the hypothesis that aging is the outcome of accelerated accumulation of somatic DNA mutations,[76] accumulation of mutations in key regulatory transcription factors has been proposed as an explanation for age-associated deficits in hematopoiesis, a hypothesis termed *transcriptional instability*. Early studies did not support this genetic hypothesis,[77] however, although analysis of the nematode *Caenorhabditis elegans* has identified an association between alterations in three GATA transcription factors—ELT-3, ELT-5, and ELT-6—and global aging of the worm.[78]

Two recent advanced exome sequencing studies have identified age-dependent clonal expansion of somatic mutations in the human hematopoietic system associated with an increased risk of future hematopoietic malignancies and other illnesses. Jaiswal and colleagues[79] and Genovese and associates[80] carried out whole-exome sequencing on blood samples from 17,182 and 12,380 people, respectively, who had no clinically apparent hematologic pathologies. Somatically acquired driver mutations were identified. Both groups found that the most frequent mutations were in three chromatin-related genes—DNA methyltransferase 3A (*DNMT3A*), TET methylcytosine dioxygenase 2 (*TET2*, involved in DNA demethylation), and the Polycomb group gene *ASXL1*, which maintains repressive chromatin. Remarkably, the mutation frequencies increased with age; mutations in any of these genes were found in = 1% of people younger than 50 years of age but in = 10% of people older than 65 years. There was a greater than 10-fold increased risk for subsequent hematologic malignancies in those with a mutation present. Somatic variants also increased the risks of noncancerous adverse events and death; for example, Jaiswal and coworkers have identified an increased risk of coronary heart disease and stroke through unknown mechanisms.[79]

Further studies have indicated that the mutant cells detected in healthy individuals appear to be genuine premalignant cells that can progress to cancer through further mutagenesis. The presence of mutations in a given individual has only limited predictive power, however. Conversion to a hematologic malignancy was rare, regardless of mutation status (even for mutation carriers, only ~1% progressed to malignancy per year). These results are consistent with early observations of recurrent somatic *TET2* mutations in normal older adults with clonal hematopoiesis[81] and with findings by Laurie and colleagues[82] and Jacobs and associates[83] that detected acquired clonal mosaicism in older adults. Wahlestedt and coworkers tested the hypothesis that HSC aging is driven by the acquisition of genetic mutations in a series of functional experiments.[84] Their data have demonstrated remarkably similar functional properties of iPS-derived and endogenous blastocyst-derived HSCs, despite the extensive chronologic and proliferative age of the former; this favors a model in which an underlying but reversible epigenetic component is a hallmark of HSC aging rather than a permanent genetic mutation.

In summary, mutations in transcriptional and other pathways and epigenetic chromatin alterations represent potential mechanisms of age-related changes in blood cell production and function. MicroRNAs (mRNAs; short noncoding sequences that regulate gene expression, as in FOXO3, later) are critical alternate pathway posttranscriptional regulators of hematopoietic cell fate decisions.[85] Several have been implicated in age-associated blood cell changes—for example, the mRNA-212/132 cluster.[86] These mRNAs are enriched in HSCs and are upregulated during aging. Both overexpression and deletion of mRNAs in this cluster (Mirc19) lead to inappropriate hematopoiesis with age. The miR-132 may exert its effect on aging HSCs by targeting the transcription factor FOXO3, a known aging-associated gene. The application of large-scale, multilevel analyses, such as those by Sun and colleagues,[54] will be needed for the optimal definitions of critical pathways and molecular targets associated with the regulation of age-related changes in blood cell production and function.

Circulating Blood Cells

Circulating blood cells derived from HSCs and downstream progenitors represent the third class of hematopoietic cells in Metcalf's original classification of hematopoiesis.[87] The cellular components of circulating blood include granulocytes, monocytes, eosinophils, basophils, erythroid cells, and lymphocytes. As critical physiologic cellular effectors, age-related changes in number and/or function of these cells have been proposed to contribute to the fragility that develops in older adults.

Granulocytes

Granulocytes, including neutrophils, eosinophils, and basophils, are components of the innate immune response to bacterial, fungal, and protozoal infections. As one of the most important cellular components of the innate immune response, polymorphonuclear neutrophils (PMNs) are the first cells to be recruited to the site of inflammation. They have a short life span and die by apoptosis. However, their life span and functional activities can be extended in vitro by a number of proinflammatory cytokines, including the granulocyte-macrophage colony-stimulating factor (GM-CSF). It has been shown that the functions and rescue from apoptosis of PMNs tend to diminish with aging. With aging, there is also an alteration of other receptor-driven functions of human neutrophils, such as superoxide anion production and chemotaxis. Observations of molecular defects in neutrophil receptor–mediated signaling,[88-90] taken together, describe an acquired defect in innate immunity with aging that at least in part might partially explain the higher incidence of sepsis-related deaths in older adults, and may affect frailty. Clinical studies investigating whether hematopoietic growth factors at pharmacologic doses (including granulocyte colony-stimulating factor [G-CSF] and GM-CSF) improve outcomes in older adults with cancer have demonstrated some success, but have significant financial, disease, and treatment-specific implications.[91,92]

Recent studies have suggested that environment and microbiota can significantly influence neutrophil function and provide additional parameters to investigate as we seek to understand potential mechanisms of blood cell senescence. Although neutrophils are generally considered to be a relatively homogeneous population, evidence for heterogeneity has been emerging. Aged neutrophils upregulate CXCR4, a receptor allowing their clearance in the bone marrow, with feedback inhibition of neutrophil production via the IL-17/G-CSF axis and rhythmic modulation of the hematopoietic stem cell niche.[93] Neutrophil aging is driven by the microbiota via Toll-like receptor and myeloid differentiation factor 88–mediated signaling pathways. Depletion of the microbiota significantly reduces the number of circulating aged neutrophils and dramatically improves the pathogenesis and inflammation-related organ damage in mouse models. Other innate immunity mechanisms have been identified to be impaired in neutrophils from older adults,[94] as well as cross-talk interactions with other components of the inflammatory response, with implications for age-related diseases.[95] Following is a discussion of the potential role of neutrophil senescence in cancer surveillance.

Eosinophils, Basophils, and Mast Cells. Eosinophils function in host defense, allergic reactions, other inflammatory responses, tissue injury, and fibrosis. Age-related changes in eosinophil function have been identified by Mathur and associates.[96] Basophils are the least common of the human granulocytes and are implicated in immediate hypersensitivity reactions, urticaria, asthma, and allergic rhinitis. Basophils and mast cells are effectors of immediate allergic reaction via their high-affinity receptors for immunoglobulin E (IgE). The role of abnormal peripheral blood eosinophil and bone marrow–derived mast cell effector functions in the pathophysiology of inflammatory conditions such as asthma have been evolving.[97] Specific innate changes that might affect the severity of asthma in older patients include changes in airway neutrophil, eosinophil, and mast cell numbers and function and impaired mucociliary clearance. Age-related altered antigen presentation and decreased specific antibody responses might increase the risk of respiratory tract infections. Nguyen and coworkers[98] have identified age-induced reprogramming of mast cell degranulation, and Sparrow and colleagues have identified inflammatory airway mechanisms involving basophils in older men, which may participate in asthmatic inflammatory responses in older patients.[99]

Mast cells and basophils also contribute to innate immunity against pathogens and venoms.[100] Mast cells appear to be capable of releasing a variety of molecules that may participate in many physiologic and pathologic processes, including immunomodulatory and antimicrobial functions.[101-103] Mast cells are derived from progenitors through a developmental transcriptional program that includes Pu.1 and the mast cell regulators Mitf and c-fos.[104,105]

Monocytes and Macrophages

Monocytes and macrophages are closely related to neutrophils developmentally, generated from progenitors through complex molecular mechanisms.[106,107] Monocytes originate in the bone marrow from a common myeloid progenitor that is shared with the neutrophils and are released into the peripheral blood, where they circulate for several days before entering the tissues and replenishing tissue macrophage populations. Circulating monocytes give rise to a variety of tissue-resident macrophages and specialized cells throughout the body, such as osteoclasts and dendritic cells (DCs).[108,109] Circulating monocytes represent 5% to 10% of human peripheral blood leukocytes in nonpathologic situations. The many functional roles of monocyte, macrophage, dendritic, and osteoclast cells in the maintenance of tissue homeostasis through the clearance of senescent cells, remodeling and repair of tissues after inflammation, antigen presentation, and other immune functions through the production of inflammatory cytokines are only partially understood.[110,111] Some tumors even recruit infiltrating monocytes as part of their immune escape mechanisms.[112,113] Similar to the age-related immune response changes in neutrophil signaling pathways described earlier, monocyte-macrophage signaling, including through Toll-like receptors, has also been reported to be altered.[114]

In addition to being a major source of regulatory cytokine production, monocytes and macrophages are particularly metabolically active. Differences in lipid metabolism have been associated with age-related disease development and life span. Inflammation is a common link between metabolic dysregulation and aging. Saturated fatty acids (FAs) initiate proinflammatory signaling from many cells, including monocytes.

Pararasa and associates[115] have investigated age-associated changes in individual FAs in relation to inflammatory phenotype. Plasma-saturated, poly-unsaturated, and mono-unsaturated FAs were found to increase with age. Circulating tumor necrosis factor-α (TNF-α) and IL-6 concentrations increased with age, whereas IL-10 and transforming growth factor-β1 (TGF-β1) concentrations decreased. Plasma oxidized glutathione concentrations were higher, and ceramide-dependent peroxisome proliferator-activated receptor γ (PPARγ) pathways were investigated. These data provide an example of how the monocytes and macrophages may be central to age-associated proinflammatory and metabolic reprogramming.

The macrophage is also central to the normal physiologic clearing of senescent red cells through signaling pathways that continue to be elucidated, including CD47–signal regulatory protein α (SIRPα),[116] which may be involved in tissue aging as well. For example, efficient engulfment of apoptotic cells is critical for maintaining tissue homoeostasis. When phagocytes recognize so-called eat me signals presented on the surface of apoptotic cells, this subsequently induces cytoskeletal rearrangement of phagocytes for the engulfment.[117] The role of CD47 and other molecular interactions as “do not eat me” or “eat me” signals also may be a tumor avoidance mechanism and is being tested as a therapeutic target in clinical trials.[118,119]

Red Cells

Erythrocytes transport hemoglobin, the major oxygen carrier, and thus facilitate tissue gas exchange. Gender, hormones that change with age, hypoxia, and other factors influence red cell numbers in mammals. Age-related changes in red cell number is not infrequent in older adults. Anemia for all adult ranges is one of the most frequent hospital diagnoses.[120] Potential mechanisms that have been investigated include overexpression of inflammatory cytokines such as IL-6,[121] which may negatively influence hematopoiesis through multiple mechanisms, including antagonizing function and impairing erythropoietin production.[122] Mouse models also support the role of inflammatory cytokines as inhibitors of hematopoiesis.[123,124]

Artz and coworkers have tested the hypothesis that unexplained anemia in the elderly (UAE) shares features of anemia of inflammation through the analysis of serum or plasma samples from control subjects participating in the Baltimore Longitudinal Study of Aging or from older adults with UAE evaluated in the University of Chicago anemia referral clinic.[125] This analysis demonstrated that a small but well-characterized cohort of older adults, with no known cause for anemia, have features of anemia associated with inflammation. Supporting an inflammatory mechanism, significantly higher hepcidin levels were found in participants with anemia of inflammation, anemia of kidney disease, and with unexplained anemia relative to participants without anemia in the Leiden Plus 85 study.[126] Hepcidin is an important regulator of iron homeostasis and has been suggested to be causally related to the anemia of inflammation.[127] Identifying the cause, finding diagnostic tests, and developing effective treatments for UAE remain a significant unmet medical need.[120]

LYMPHOID DEVELOPMENT

Like myelopoiesis, lymphoid development has intrinsic and extrinsic controls and requires specific environmental interactions and gene regulatory networks.[128-131] Understanding these developmental stages is critical to understanding normal and abnormal immunity and lymphogenesis. The peripheral immune system develops from stem cells originating in the bone marrow. Lymphoid progenitors, including B and T cells, migrate from the bone marrow to specialized peripheral sites, including the thymus, spleen, Peyer patches, Waldeyer ring, and lymph nodes to undergo further maturation, differentiation, and acquisition of self- and nonself-training. On identification of a danger signal or foreign invader, innate immune cells (natural killer [NK] cells) respond by destroying infected cells and releasing cytokines and chemokines to recruit additional immune cells to fight the invader or infection and alter the host environment (inflammation). This innate immune response is often followed by an adaptive (antigen-specific) immune response with the recruitment of effector B and T lymphocytes. Following effective clearance of the invading pathogen, the host immune response must return to the quiescent state to prevent damage from an excessive immune response. A specialized subset of T cells, called regulatory T cells (Tregs), participate in this process and are discussed below.[132]

AGING AND BLOOD CELLS

T Cells

T cells become specialized in the thymus to provide adaptive cellular immunity via CD8$^+$ cytotoxic T cells and play important roles in B cell–mediated humoral immunity through helper functions. T cells have been identified as highly susceptible to age-related changes. A number of factors have been linked to the decline in T cell function with age and age-induced thymic atrophy, and decreased output of naïve T cells has been implicated as a critical factor.[133] Changes in the composition of the bone marrow stroma with age and decreased nurturing of hematopoietic precursors contribute to decreased T cell production with aging. Cytokine profiles can be modified with aging—for example, changes in T helper cells (Th cells; e.g., Th1 vs. Th2 cytokine expression balance). Secretion of IL-7, an essential T-lineage survival cytokine, is decreased in the aged bone marrow.[134]

The precise nature and identity of the bone marrow–derived, earliest committed T cells remains controversial, which complicates quantitation with age. Early T-lineage progenitors (ETPs), which give rise to T cells, are generated in the bone marrow. Thymocyte progenitor cells then enter the thymus and begin their differentiation and education process with changes in surface marker expression, rearrangement of their T cell receptor, and positive and negative cellular selection. The overall process of T cell maturation and education is modulated by cytokines, hormones, epithelial cells, macrophages, dendritic cells, and fibroblasts in the thymic stroma. Increasing understanding of the thymic epithelial-hematopoietic cell interactions include identification of Notch pathway receptors and ligands required for T cell development.[135] As an individual ages, the thymus involutes, and the output of T cells falls significantly.[136,137] By 70 years of age, the thymic epithelial space shrinks to less than 10% of the total tissue. New techniques to monitor newly produced (naïve) recent thymic emigrants (RTEs) have provided powerful molecular tools to evaluate the attenuation of thymopoiesis with aging.[138] $CD4^+$-$CD8^+$ recent thymic emigrant numbers diminish with age, and RTE maturation and activation are suboptimal in aged mice. These and other observations[139] have provided promise that therapeutic regeneration of the functional thymic epithelial space in older adults could potentially reverse some of the age-related T cell deficits. This remains a very active area of research.[140-143]

With aging, the decrease in naïve T cells is accompanied by an increase in memory T cells in the periphery. Impaired T cell contributions to humoral immunity are numerous, including IL-2 production, germinal center defects, reduced activation, differentiation, and cytokine production.[144-146] Impaired $CD8^+$ cytotoxic effector T cell function is also diminished when influenza responses in murine models or humans are analyzed.[147] These and other studies[148-150] have provided some of the mechanisms that might explain the disease-related immune system senescence effects associated with aging. Studies have focused on Tregs; $CD4^+$/$CD25^+$/$Foxp3^+$ regulatory T cells play a key role in controlling the host immune response to prevent excessive immune response and damage.[132,151,152] Quantitation and functional evaluation of these cells in disease and aging have been under active investigation.[153-155]

B Cells

B lymphocyte development begins in the fetal liver and bone marrow in defined stages characterized by the status of immunoglobulin gene rearrangement in cells expressing combinations of specific cell surface antigens.[129] The production of B lymphocytes begins to decline steadily in adulthood and is severely compromised in older adults.[156-158] There may be differences among lymphocyte subsets and steady-state levels, however.[159]

In addition to reduced production of B-lineage cells in aged mice and older adults, studies have shown that the numbers of all B cell progenitors, including elastin-like-peptide (ELP), collagen-like peptide (CLP), pre-/pro-B, and pro-B cells, are reduced in old bone marrow.[160] The decline in B cell production is not restricted to very old mice.[161] Gene profiling of young and old HSCs[41] has suggested that age-related defects in the hematopoietic system appear to be different between lymphoid and myeloid lineages. The expression of lymphoid-specific gene sets were significantly decreased in old HSCs, whereas genes directing myeloid development were upregulated. Numerous biochemical and differentiation defects have been identified at multiple levels of B cell development and aging.[156,160,162] Cell culture and murine transplant studies have also provided evidence for additional stromal contributions to B cell age-related senescence.[163,164]

The plasma cell proliferative disorders—monoclonal gammopathy of undetermined significance (MGUS) and multiple myeloma (MM)—are characterized by an accumulation of transformed clonal B cells in the bone marrow and production of a monoclonal immunoglobulin. They typically affect an older population, with median age of diagnosis of approximately 70 years.[165] In both disorders, there is an increased risk of infection due to the immunosuppressive effects of the underlying disease, as well as the concomitant therapy in MM. Response to vaccination to counter infection is compromised.[166] Also, confounding the weakened immune response in MGUS and MM is the contribution of normal aging, which quantitatively and qualitatively hampers humoral immunity to affect responses to infection and vaccination. Like the recently described clonal hematopoiesis of indeterminate potential (CHIP) relative to myelodysplastic syndrome, and monoclonal B cell lymphocytosis (MBL) relative to chronic lymphocytic leukemia (CLL),[167-170] the relationship between MGUS and MM remains incompletely characterized. MGUS and MM have variable rates of disease progression, and genetic and epigenetic underpinnings have been under intense study.[171,172]

IMMUNOSENESCENCE AND CANCER

Hanahan and Weinberg have summarized six biologic capabilities acquired during the multistep development of human tumors as an organizing principle for rationalizing the complexities of neoplastic disease.[173] They include sustaining proliferative signaling, evading growth suppressors, resisting cell death, enabling replicative immortality, inducing angiogenesis, and activating invasion and metastasis. It has become increasingly clear that mutated cells that progress to a tumor also have to learn how to thrive in a chronically inflamed microenvironment, evade immune recognition, and suppress immune reactivity. These three immune hallmarks of cancer are now also considered as critical to carcinogenesis models and represent therapeutic targets.[174-177]

Among the most promising approaches to activating therapeutic antitumor immunity is the blockade of immune checkpoints. It is now clear that tumors co-opt certain natural regulatory immune checkpoint pathways as a major mechanism of immune resistance, particularly against T cells that are specific for tumor antigens.[177] Because many of the immune checkpoints are initiated by ligand-receptor interactions, they can be readily blocked by antibodies or modulated by recombinant forms of ligands or receptors. Cytotoxic T-lymphocyte–associated antigen 4 (CTLA4) antibodies were the first of this class of immunotherapeutics to receive U.S. Food and Drug Administration (FDA) approval.[175] Targeting additional immune checkpoint proteins, such as programmed cell death protein 1 (PD1) and programmed cell death ligand 1 (PD-L1), represent additional clinical opportunities.[175,176]

These anticancer therapies may bypass the toxic and often only modestly effective approaches using conventional chemotherapy, but rely on an intact immune system. The potential role of decreased immunosurveillance against cancer both contributing to the increase of cancer in older adults and affecting response to immune checkpoint and other immunotherapy treatments, such as tumor vaccination, remain to be determined.

KEY POINTS: AGING AND THE BLOOD

- Intensive investigation of aging hematopoietic stem cells are providing general insights into age-related genetic, epigenetic, biochemical, and cellular alterations. This includes identifying gene regulatory networks that direct hematopoietic and stromal cell fate in normal and aging blood cell producing tissues. Translation of this information will likely lead to effective cellular therapies.
- Continued study of acquired abnormalities in signaling and other mechanisms of effector cell dysfunction with aging, particularly inflammation, will likely provide significant new insights and approaches to hematopoietic aspects of frailty.
- Pathways and molecules linked to the cellular aging process in other tissues and model systems are often reproducibly altered in aging hematopoietic cells as well, warranting further intensive investigation; examples include TGF-β, WNT, Notch, FoxO3, and p16.
- The bone marrow and related hematopoietic tissues continue to be evaluated as a source of alternative cellular regenerative therapies. Better understanding of stem cell biology, lineage plasticity, and stroma–hematopoietic cell interactions are critical to advancing this field.
- There is an evolving convergence of clinical characterization of age-related clonal disorders such as clonal cytopenia of unknown significance, MGUS, MDS, MPN, CLL, and related hematologic malignancies, with genetic and epigenetic pathway investigations, including characterization of acquired mutations in epigenetic regulators.
- Increased understanding of innate and acquired immunity and immunosenescence mechanisms offer potential for the following:
  - Better understanding and prevention of age-related, increased susceptibility to infections
  - More effective vaccinations of older adults
  - Increasing understanding of immune escape as a fundamental cancer development pathway
  - More effective application of new checkpoint inhibitors and immunostimulatory factors for optimal responses to novel cancer therapies

For a complete list of references, please visit www.expertconsult.com.

KEY REFERENCES

2. Eaves CJ: Hematopoietic stem cells: concepts, definitions, and the new reality. Blood 3;125:2605–2613, 2015.
3. Orkin SH, Zon LI: Hematopoiesis: an evolving paradigm for stem cell biology. Cell 132:631–644, 2008.
12. Boulais PE, Frenette PS: Making sense of hematopoietic stem cell niches. Blood 125:2621–2629, 2015.
13. Reagan MR, Rosen CJ: Navigating the bone marrow niche: translational insights and cancer-driven dysfunction. Nat Rev Rheumatol 2015.
30. Balderman SR, Calvi LM: Biology of BM failure syndromes: role of microenvironment and niches. Hematology Am Soc Hematol Educ Program 2014:71–76, 2014.
41. Rossi DJ, Jamieson CH, Weissman IL: Stem cells and the pathways to aging and cancer. Cell 132:681–696, 2008.
42. Armanios M: Telomeres and age-related disease: how telomere biology informs clinical paradigms. J Clin Invest 123:996–1002, 2013.
44. Townsley DM, Dumitriu B, Young NS: Bone marrow failure and the telomeropathies. Blood 124:2775–2783, 2014.
54. Sun D, Luo M, Jeong M, et al: Epigenomic profiling of young and aged HSCs reveals concerted changes during aging that reinforce self-renewal. Cell Stem Cell 14:673–688, 2014.
62. Akashi K, Traver D, Miyamoto T, et al: A clonogenic common myeloid progenitor that gives rise to all myeloid lineages. Nature 404:193–197, 2000.
69. Paul F, Arkin Y, Giladi A, et al: Transcriptional heterogeneity and lineage commitment in myeloid progenitors. Cell 163:1663–1677, 2015.
72. Busch K, Klapproth K, Barile M, et al: Fundamental properties of unperturbed haematopoiesis from stem cells in vivo. Nature 518: 542–546, 2015.
79. Jaiswal S, Fontanillas P, Flannick J, et al: Age-related clonal hematopoiesis associated with adverse outcomes. N Engl J Med 371:2488–2498, 2014.
80. Genovese G, Kähler AK, Handsaker RE, et al: Clonal hematopoiesis and blood-cancer risk inferred from blood DNA sequence. N Engl J Med 371:2477–2487, 2014.
81. Busque L, Patel JP, Figueroa ME, et al: Recurrent somatic TET2 mutations in normal elderly individuals with clonal hematopoiesis. Nat Genet 44:1179–1181, 2012.
93. Zhang D, Chen G, Manwani D, et al: Neutrophil ageing is regulated by the microbiome. Nature 525:528–532, 2015.
127. Weiss G: Anemia of chronic disorders: new diagnostic tools and new treatment strategies. Semin Hematol 52:313–320, 2015.
130. Singh H, Khan AA, Dinner AR: Gene regulatory networks in the immune system. Trends Immunol 35:211–218, 2014.
143. Al-Chami E, Tormo A, Pasquin S, et al: Interleukin-21 administration to aged mice rejuvenates their peripheral T-cell pool by triggering de novo thymopoiesis. Aging Cell 2016.
167. Steensma DP, Bejar R, Jaiswal S, et al: Clonal hematopoiesis of indeterminate potential and its distinction from myelodysplastic syndromes. Blood 126:9–16, 2015.
174. Hanahan D, Weinberg RA: Hallmarks of cancer: the next generation. Cell 144:646–674, 2011.
175. Sharma P, Allison JP: The future of immune checkpoint therapy. Science 348:56–61, 2015.
176. Pardoll D: Cancer and the immune system: basic concepts and targets for intervention. Semin Oncol 42:523–538, 2015.

25 Aging and the Skin

Desmond J. Tobin, Emma C. Veysey, Andrew Y. Finlay

INTRODUCTION

The last 25 years has seen enormous growth in our knowledge of skin function, with new subspecialties of cutaneous biology emerging during that time, not least of which is cutaneous neuroendocrinology. The position of the skin, our largest organ by weight (≈12% of total body weight) and extent, and as a sensor of the periphery has prompted some researchers to describe skin as our "brain on the outside."[1] Although now over a decade old, we think that the best single discussion on the function of skin can be found in the multiauthor discussion review, "What is the 'true' function of skin?"[2] From an anatomic and physiologic perspectives alone, it is clear that skin is truly a biologic universe in that it incorporates all the body's major support systems—blood, muscle, and innervation, and including immunocompetence, psychoemotional reactivity, ultraviolet radiation sensing, and endocrine function. These functions participate in the homeostasis not just of skin and its appendages but also of the entire mammalian body. Although this view was initially polemic to some, particularly many in the endocrinology community, it now appears self-evident given that the skin occupies such a strategic location between the noxious external and biochemically active internal environments. Thus, skin can rightfully be expected to be critical in preserving the constancy of our body's internal environment. Despite exquisite adaptations driven from a raft of key evolutionary selective pressures for life on an ultraviolet radiation (UVR)–drenched terrestrial planet, still skin conditions still rank as the fourth leading cause of nonfatal disease burden,[3] with this burden rising still further as we age.[4]

It may be impossible to describe the true function of skin, but rather we should ask "Is there anything that the skin can't contribute to?" Research on the skin's remarkable stress sensing, much of which is transduced via its equivalent of the hypothalamic-pituitary-adrenal and thyroid axes, provides us with an opportunity to assess how age may affect these key axes in terms of skin physiology. Well-nourished and UVR-protected skin and associated integumental adnexa exhibit truly remarkable resilience to chronologic (or intrinsic) aging. In this chapter, we will examine the structural changes to the skin as a consequence not only of this type of aging, but will also examine the contributors to so-called extrinsic aging (e.g., UVR, trauma, chemical) and how both types of aging present challenges to skin integrity.

The two main global giveaways of our lost youth are most readily detected by changes to our skin, including so-called wrinkling and changes to the skin's principal appendage, the hair follicle, especially canities or common graying and hair thinning and baldness. Increasingly, we appear to be less and less keen to sport this universally recognized aging phenotype. Our expectations for the extension of optimal functioning continue to grow well into our 70s and beyond. This is not unreasonable because life expectancy in the West is expected to be 100 years of age in the next decade,[5] with further extensions to 120 years in the decades beyond 2025. The implications of this demographic change for skin aging, which has no precedent in human history, has even more significant implications for women because they will spend up to half of their lives postmenopause, during which falling estrogen levels adversely affect skin integrity and function. Aspirations for healthy and functional aging continue to drive a rapidly expanding skin and hair care market that brings increasingly sophisticated cosmetics and cosmeceuticals, pharmaceuticals, and surgeries to the palette of options to assuage our vanities, but also to aid our increasingly dry and itchy,[6] infection-prone,[7] immune-unstable[8] skin, with its vascular complications and increasing risk of cutaneous malignancy.

Given its strategic interface position on the body, the skin is uniquely subject to a wide range of aging drivers, not only to intrinsic (chronologic) aging, which are generally under genetic and hormonal influences, but also to extrinsic aging caused by environmental factors, principally including UVR, smoking, diet, chemicals, and trauma. UVR-induced aging is so powerful that it has been designated separately by the term *photoaging*. The sheer differential impact of the latter can be seen when comparing sun-protected buttocks skin with sun-exposed hand or facial skin in an older, but active, white adult. Both types of aging have their distinct morphologic and histologic features, with only some overlapping biologic, biochemical, and molecular mechanisms.[9] Interestingly, analyses of composite facial images created from women who were considered to look young or old for their age have reported that changes to the structure of subcutaneous tissue were also partly responsible for this perceived effect. Moreover, when the heritability of these appearance traits (e.g., perceived age, pigmented age spots, skin wrinkles, sun damage) was analyzed, it was reported that these features were more or less equally influenced by genetic and environmental factors.[10]

Finally, we will focus here on reevaluating some older accepted data of skin aging, including its "yin-yang" relationship to the sun, but also will see how cell, molecular biologic, and other discoveries may help develop approaches to maintain this evolutionarily, highly selected for organ at optimum function during our ever-increasing longevity.[11]

INTRINSIC AGING

The very slow process of intrinsic aging varies among populations, between individuals of the same ethnicity, and between different sites on the same individual. This type of aging is essentially only visible at old age and is characterized by unblemished, smooth, pale(r), drier, less elastic skin, with fine wrinkles and somewhat exaggerated expression lines (reflecting additional subcutaneous changes).[12,13] The process of intrinsic aging falls into two categories—one engendered within the tissue itself, including reductions in dermal mast cells, fibroblasts, and collagen production, flattening of the dermal-epidermal junction, and loss of rete ridges, and one caused by the influence of aging in other organs (e.g., age-related hormonal changes). Flattening of the epidermis is perhaps the most striking feature of intrinsically aged skin. This is caused by a loss of reciprocal interdigitation of capillary-rich dermal papillae, a likely consequence of reduced nutrient support by the vascularized dermis to the avascular epidermis. Together these are thought to contribute to the increase fragility of intrinsically aged skin in the very old. Intrinsically aged epidermis is also controlled by progressive telomere shortening, compounded by low-grade oxidative damage to telomeres and other cellular constituents.[14] A study of normal human epidermis has established that progressive telomere shortening associated with aging is characterized by tissue-specific loss rates.[15]

EXTRINSIC AGING

Given that the regulation of intrinsic aging is largely beyond our influence (e.g., short of hormone supplementation, albeit with associated health implications), significant consideration is being directed toward the prevention and treatment of extrinsic aging-associated changes to skin structure and appearance. The greatest source of extrinsic aging comes from accumulated sun (unprotected) exposure called photoaging and so is largely confined to the face, neck, and hands and less so to the lower arms and legs. It has been estimated that over 80% of aging of the face is due to chronic UVR exposure, whereas acute UVR exposure of the skin will cause sunburn, tanning, inflammation, immunosuppression, and damage to the connective tissue of the dermis.[16,17] It should be noted that the impact of environmental factors on so-called extrinsic aging cannot be completely separated from how the skin will respond to chronologic aging, given the significant impact of exogenous factors on how skin physiology is regulated (e.g., pro-oxidant and antioxidant influences on cell turnover via neuroendocrine and immune biologic response modifiers). The characteristics of extrinsically aged skin include coarse wrinkling, rough texture, sallow complexion with mottled pigmentation, and loss of skin elasticity. Much of this change can be ascribed to the effects of UVR-induced photoaging.

Photoaging

Photoaging is caused by solar irradiation. At the earth's surface, sunlight consists mostly of infrared light, with 44% visible light and only 3% UVR (when it is cloudless and the sun is directly overhead). The earth's atmosphere blocks the vast majority of the sun's UVR (100 to 400 nm). UVR reaching our planet's surface (and so potentially our skin and eyes) consists of more than 95% UVA (315 to 400 nm) and about 5% UVB (280 to 315 nm). Germicidal UVC (100- to 280-nm) radiation is extremely hazardous to skin but is completely absorbed by the ozone layer and atmosphere, fortunately. Another important consideration is the ratio of UVA to UVB reaching our skin, which depends on the latitude (and thus the height of the sun), season, and time of day. More UVB is present is midday sun during summer than at other times of the day or year. Most studies in the literature have used solar-simulated radiation with a spectrum (UVA/UVB ratio < 18, and often much lower) as a proxy for the noon summer sun on a clear day, although a more representative real-world UVA/UVB ratio is 25.[18]

Although researchers believe that the deeply penetrating UVA damages connective tissue in the dermis and also increases risk for skin cancer, UVB only penetrates as far as the epidermis, where it can cause sunburn, tanning, and photocarcinogenesis.[19] UVB is the major cause for direct DNA damage and induces inflammation and immunosuppression.[20] UVA is thought to play a greater role in skin photoaging given its greater abundance in sunlight and the greater average depth of penetration into the skin's dermis and epidermis.[20] In pale-skinned whites, the first signs of extrinsic aging on exposed sites are already apparent by 15 years of age,[21] whereas on nonexposed sites, they are not apparent until age 30 years.[22] Worryingly, the pursuit of a tan remains a high priority in Western culture, associated as it is with ever-rising rates of skin cancer and prematurely aged skin. Moreover, the increasing use of sun protection, such as topical sunscreen cream with so-called sun protection factor (SPF) ratings, has not come without problems. For example, stated protection levels can require the topical application of an unrealistic (i.e., cosmetically unacceptable) amount of cream, and users are often misguided in thinking that a single suboptimal application of a nonwaterproof sunscreen permits them to increase their time in the sun significantly, including with intervening swims. It has recently been proposed that even when applied correctly, sunscreen use will result in suberythemal exposure,[23] and we have still to learn more about the ideal ratio of UVB/UVA protection needed to improve long-term photoprotection outcomes.

In addition to the negative effects of exposure to UVA and UVB (e.g., induction of melanoma and nonmelanoma skin cancers, cataract formation, systemic immunosuppression that may reactivate latent viral infection, skin aging), it should be remembered that exposure to UVB radiation also has positive effects. These include suppression of autoimmune reactivity, mood enhancement via endorphin production, and vitamin D synthesis to aid calcium homeostasis. There is increasing concern about the rising incidence of vitamin D deficiency or at least its insufficiency.

Clinically, photoaged skin is characterized by deep wrinkles, laxity, roughness, a sallow or yellow color, increased fragility, purpura formation, mottled pigmentary changes, telangiectasia, impaired wound healing, and benign and malignant growths. The degree of accumulated sun exposure determines the magnitude of the associated skin changes. The mechanisms through which UVR induces accelerated aging are discussed later in this chapter. The second most powerful inducer of extrinsic aging is cigarette smoking.

Smoking

Smoking is an independent risk factor for premature facial wrinkling after controlling for sun exposure, age, gender, and skin pigmentation.[14,24] The relative risk of moderate to severe wrinkling for current smokers was found to be 2.3 for men and 3.1 for women.[15,25] There is a clear dose-response relationship, with facial wrinkling increasing in individuals who smoke longer and with increasing numbers of cigarettes daily.[24] When smoking and excessive sun exposure combine, the effect on wrinkling multiplies in that the risk of developing wrinkles increases to 11.4 times that in a normal age-controlled population.[26] The exact mechanism for the aging effects of smoking is poorly understood. The effects may be topical, due to the drying or irritating effect of smoke on the skin; systemic, with induction of matrixmetalloproteinase-1 (MMP-1)[27]; or by negatively affecting cutaneous microvasculature. Specifically, the dermal microvasculature is constricted by acute and long-term smoking, the severity of which is independently related to duration and intensity of exposure to smoking.[28]

Skin Type

Pigmentation of the skin is protective against the cumulative effects of photoaging. When populations with Fitzpatrick classification types I to VI (ranging from always burn never tan to always tan and never burns) were compared, it was found that those with skin type VI (black) show little difference between exposed and unexposed sites.[29] Moreover, the much higher rates of skin cancer rates among whites compared with African Americans reflects the significant protection from UVR damage that pigmentation provides (up to 500-fold).[30] The appearance of photodamaged skin differs for those with skin types I and II (red hair, freckles, burns easily) and those with skin types III and IV (darker skin, tans easily). The former tend to show atrophic skin changes, but with fewer wrinkles, and focal depigmentation (guttate hypomelanosis) and dysplastic changes, such as actinic keratoses and epidermal malignancies. In contrast, those with types III and IV skin develop hypertrophic responses, such as deep wrinkling, coarseness, a leather-like appearance, and lentigines.[20] Basal cell carcinoma and squamous cell carcinoma occur almost exclusively on sun-exposed skin of light-skinned people. A large and statistically robust study evaluated skin thickness in chronologic aging and photoaging conditions; it was reported that although increases and decreases in skin thickness can be seen in different body sites, there was no general relationship between skin thickness and age.[30,31]

Thus, it appears that the epidermis thins with age at some body sites, such as the upper inner arm[32,33] and back of the upper arm,[34] but remains constant at others, such as the buttocks, dorsal forearm, and shoulder.[35] This variation is clearly not accounted for by sun or environmental exposure alone.[30] Differences in study method, population, and body site likely account for different results reported in different studies. Although epidermal thickness appears to remain largely constant with advancing age, there is some variability in keratinocyte shape and size with age, specifically that these cells become shorter and flatter in contrast to an increase in corneocyte size, potentially as a result of decreased epidermal cell turnover with age.[13] Wrinkling in Asian skin has been documented to occur later and with less severity than in white skin.[22]

EPIDERMIS

The epidermis is composed of an outer nonviable layer called the stratum corneum, and the bulk of the viable epidermis consists primarily of keratinocytes (90% to 95% of cells), with smaller populations of Langerhans cells (2%, or 1 for every 53 keratinocytes), melanocytes (3%, or 1 for every 36 with viable keratinocytes, the so-called epidermal melanin unit), and Merkel cells (0.5%).[1]

The stratum corneum is the body's principal barrier to the environment and also plays a major role in determining the level of cutaneous hydration. Its structure is often described by the bricks and mortar model, consisting of protein-rich corneocytes, which are embedded in a matrix of ceramides, cholesterol, and fatty acids.[30] These lipids form multilamellar sheets amid the intercellular spaces of the stratum corneum and are critical to its mechanical and cohesive properties, enabling it to function as an effective water barrier.[36] There is general agreement that the thickness of the stratum corneum does not change with age,[37] and that barrier function does not alter significantly. However, certain features of aging skin do indicate an abnormal skin barrier—namely, the extreme skin dryness (xerosis) and increased susceptibility to irritant dermatitis that accompanies old age. Furthermore, there is evidence of altered permeability to chemical substances[38] and reduced transepidermal water flux in aged skin.[30] It seems that baseline skin barrier function is relatively unaffected by age.[37] This is perhaps counterintuitive, but substances recoverable from the skin surface (e.g., sebum, sweat, components of natural moisturizing factor, corneocyte debris) were not significantly affected by age or ethnicity and gender.[39]

If the skin is subjected to sequential tape stripping, the barrier function in aged skin (>80 years) is much more readily disrupted than in young skin (20 to 30 years).[37] In addition, the same study found that after tape stripping, barrier recovery was greatly disturbed in the older age group. The reason for this abnormality is not entirely understood; however, it appears that there is a global reduction in stratum corneum lipids, which affects what binds the corneocytes. Studies have confirmed that in moderately aged individuals (50 to 80 years), abnormal stratum corneum acidification results in delayed lipid processing, delayed permeability barrier recovery, and abnormal stratum corneum integrity.[40] Not only does the rise in stratum corneum pH interfere with lipid production, it also accelerates the degradation of intercorneocyte connections, the corneodesmosomes.[41] The abnormal acidification is linked to decreased membrane Na^+/H^+ transport protein.[40] In addition, with age, stratum corneum turnover time lengthens with protracted replacement.[42]

In a recent study of adult female skin, skin surface pH on the forehead, temple, and volar forearm were reported to increase only slightly with age.[43] This information is crucial for the development of medical and cosmetic skin care products.

The most consistent change found in aged skin is flattening of the dermoepidermal junction at sites that were highly corrugated in youth (Fig. 25-1, *A* and *B*).[44] The flattening creates a thinner looking epidermis primarily because of retraction of the rete ridges.[30] With this reduced interdigitation between layers, there is less resistance to shearing forces.[13,22] There is also a reduced surface area over which the epidermis communicates with the dermis, accompanied by a reduced supply of nutrients and oxygen.[8] It is likely that much of this effect is influenced from so-called solar elastosis changes in the papillary dermis (see below)—that is, changes in the elastic fiber network, including tropoelastin and fibrillin-1.[45] Even with minimal photoaging, one can appreciate the loss of fibrillin-rich microfibrils in the dermal-epidermal junction, so this can be viewed as an early marker of photoaging.[46-48] There is general agreement that epidermal cell turnover is 50% lower between the third and seventh decades of life.[49,50] This is consistent with the observation that wound-healing capacity deteriorates in old age.[51]

Keratinocytes

With age, there is increasing atypia of the basal layer keratinocytes.[33] Involucrin, a differentiation marker normally expressed by irreversibly differentiated keratinocytes in the stratum corneum, has been found to have increased expression in sun-damaged skin.[52] This is consistent with the fact that keratinocyte differentiation is impaired by UVR. In addition, in basal epidermal cells, there is downregulation of certain β_1-integrins,[52] which are markers of keratinocyte differentiation and adhesion to the extracellular matrix, suggesting that proliferation and adhesion of keratinocytes in photodamaged aged skin are abnormal.

Melanocytes

With age, there is a reported reduction in the number of functional (tyrosinase-positive and tyrosinase-active) melanocytes in the basal layer of the human epidermis, from 8% to 20% per decade.[53] Paradoxically, there may be an increase in the number of melanocytes in photodamaged skin, although these cells tend to be smaller than normal and often exhibit cellular activation with marked nuclear heterogeneity, large intracytoplasmic vacuoles, and more frequent contact with Langerhans cells.[54] This overall reduction in melanocyte number and/or function in aging skin is also reflected by a reduction in melanocytic nevi in older patients.[55] With reducing melanocyte numbers, there is an associated loss of melanin in the skin, which means less protection against the harmful effects of UV radiation. Consequently, older adults are more susceptible to skin cancers, and sun protection remains very important for this group, despite the fact that most of an individual's harmful sun exposure occurs in the first 2 decades of life.[56]

There are also dramatic changes to pigment cell function in the graying hair follicle that are directly linked to the cyclic activity of the hair growth cycle (see later).[57] One of the most striking changes in aged skin in those of most ethnicities is the dramatic increase in so-called age spots, or solar lentigo lesions. For those of Asian ethnicity, these pigmentary changes contribute more to perceived age than wrinkling. Age spots are usually up to 1 cm in diameter, with major histologic changes to the basal layer of the epidermis, especially the elongation of epidermal rete ridges (in contrast with the epidermal flattening seen with general skin aging). Although it first appears that these areas of hyperpigmentation are due to an increase of melanocytes, this finding has not been confirmed in several reports. In a report by Kadono and associates, the numbers of tyrosinase-positive melanocytes per length of the dermal-epidermal interface appeared to be increased twofold in the solar lentigo versus the unaffected skin.[58] Other studies have reported increased melanocyte size, dendrite

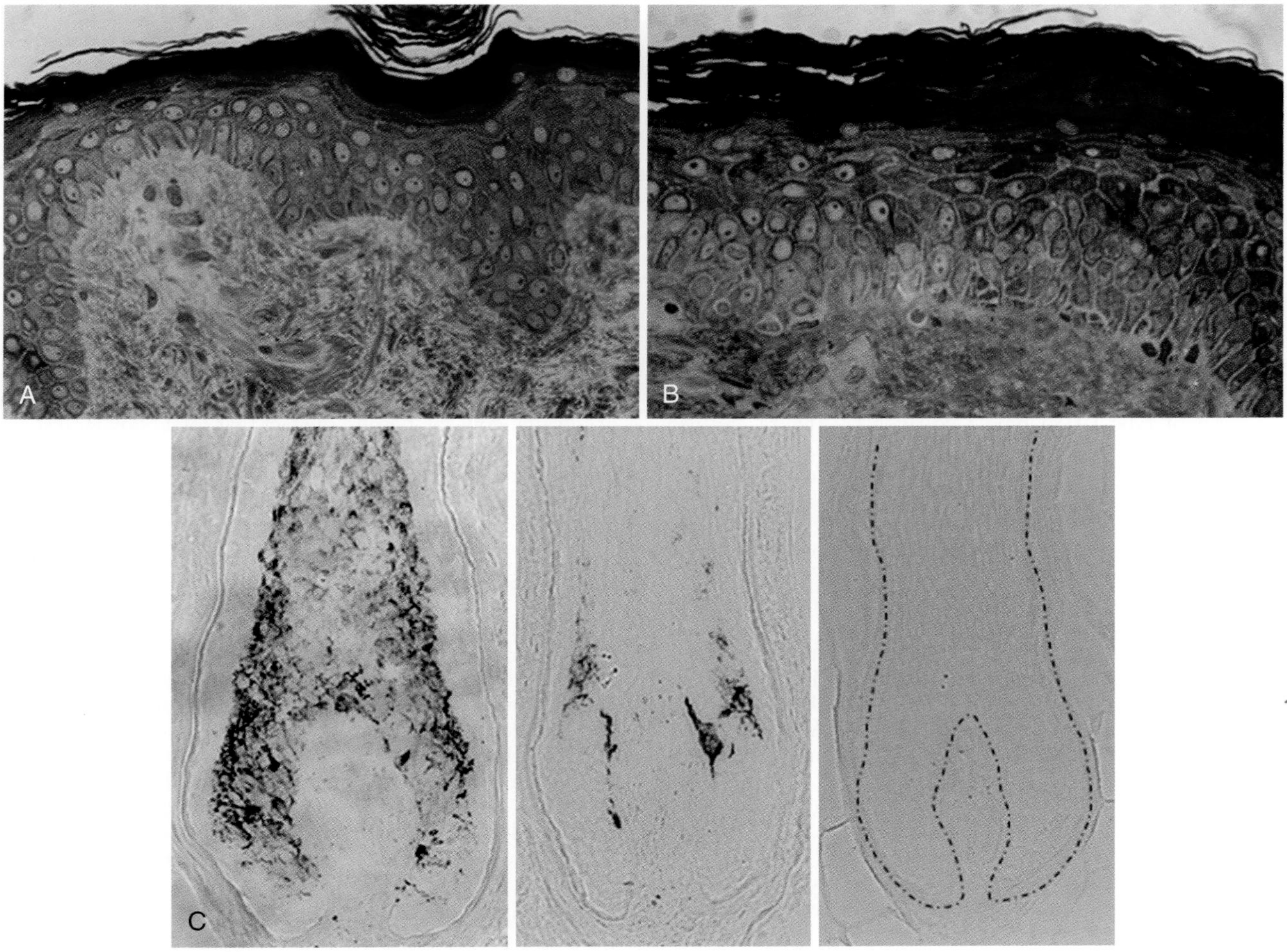

Figure 25-1. Human skin and hair follicle changes with age. **A,** Toluidine blue–stained vertical section of male forearm skin (32-year-old man; ×1200). **B,** Toludine blue-stained vertical section of male forearm skin (67-year-old man; ×1200). **C,** Unstained vertical sections (×1000) of lower anagen scalp hair follicles of 23-year-old man (pigmented, *left*), 66-year-old woman (graying, *middle*), and 55-year-old woman (white, *right*).

elongation, and alterations in melanosomes and their organization, but not increased cell numbers. Endothelin-1 and the stem cell factor appear to be key regulators in the development of hyperpigmentation in solar lentigo lesions, with alterations in the epidermal-dermal melanin axis, including dermal melanin incontinence and factor XIIIa–positive melanophages in senile lentigo and aging skin.[59]

DERMIS

The dermis consists predominantly of connective tissue and contains blood vessels, nerves, and the adnexal structures, including sweat glands and pilosebaceous units. Its main role is to provide a tough and flexible layer that supports the epidermis and binds to the subcutis, the fatty layer deep to the dermis. Dermal connective tissue contains collagen and elastin. Collagen fibers collectively contribute the largest volume of the skin and give this organ its tensile strength, whereas elastin fibers contribute to elasticity and resilience.[60] As with studies of the aging human skin epidermis, analysis of studies on dermal changes with age also yield conflicting results; some show thinning with age and others no change.[30] It has been suggested that the initial effect of photodamage at a young age is skin thickening due to solar elastosis. This is in contrast to aging changes in the dermis of older adults that exhibit severe damage where there appears to be notable thinning.[61] However, despite extensive data, it is extremely difficult to define the effects of aging on skin thickness, partly because of interindividual and interbody site variations and differences in methodology among different studies.[30] This is a rather unsatisfactory situation, given that it is generally accepted that changes in the dermis are responsible for wrinkling, a key change perceived with skin aging. Although the mechanism of wrinkle formation is not entirely understood,[44] there is general atrophy of the extracellular matrix accompanied by a decrease in cellularity, especially of the fibroblasts, with associated reduction in their synthesizing ability.[62,63] Photoaged skin has been reported to exhibit histologic features of chronic inflammation without significant evidence of clinical or molecular abnormalities, suggesting that UVR induces infiltration but not necessarily activation of innate immune cells in areas of elastolysis.[64] There are more abnormalities of collagen and elastic fibers in sun-exposed sites versus those in sun-protected skin.[65,66]

Collagen

Collagen is the most abundant protein found in humans and, as the primary structural component of the dermis, it is responsible for conferring strength and support to human skin. Alterations in collagen play an integral role in the aging process.[56] In the dermis of young adults, collagen bundles are well organized; they are arranged in such a way that allows for extension, with return to their resting state facilitated by the interwoven elastic fibers.[44] With aging, there is an increase in the density of collagen bundles[67] and they may lose their extensible configuration and become fragmented, disorganized, and less soluble.[65,68]

Both UVR and the intrinsic aging process, mainly through the production of reactive oxygen species (ROS), result in upregulation of the collagen-degrading enzymes MMPs.[69] In addition, there is a decrease in collagen synthesis,[70] and thus a shift in the balance between synthesis and degradation occurs.[8,13] Different collagens in the skin have different functions, all affected differently by the aging process. In young skin, collagen I comprises 80% of dermal collagen and type III makes up 15%; however, with age, there is a decrease in collagen I, with a resultant increase in the ratio of type III to type I collagen.[68,71] There are also changes in the levels of collagens IV and VII. Collagen IV, an integral part of the dermoepidermal junction, provides a structural framework for other molecules and plays a key role in maintaining mechanical stability.[59] Collagen VII is critical for basement membrane binding to the underlying papillary dermis.[59] There are significantly lower levels of collagens IV and VII at the base of wrinkles, and it is speculated that loss of these collagens contributes to wrinkle formation.[72] MMPs can act independently or together to degrade elements of collagenous and elastic scaffolds. These enzymes are expressed at a low level in normal skin, but even lifestyle changes such as smoking have been shown to increase the expression of some (e.g., MMP-1). MMPs are also upregulated by UVR, and MMP-9 is a most potent lytic enzyme for elastic fibers and fibrillin.

Elastin

Human skin is uniquely rich in elastic fibers, where they are entwined with collagen bundles, especially in the reticular dermis. There is also significant regional variation in the density of elastic fiber meshes. Elastin exhibits numerous age-related changes, and remodeling of elastic fibers in response to UVR is mostly regulated by activation of MMPs. These include slow elastin degradation,[73,74] accumulation of damage in existing elastin with intrinsic aging,[73] increased synthesis of apparently abnormal elastin in photoexposed areas,[75] and abnormal localization of elastin in the upper dermis of photodamaged skin.[30]

Histologically, one of the most striking features of photodamaged skin is the change in elastotic material. On hematoxylin and eosin staining, there is an area of amorphous blue staining in the superficial to mid-dermis referred to as solar elastosis. This represents a tangled mass of degraded elastic fibers accompanied by amorphous material composed of disorganized tropoelastin and fibrillin in the upper dermis, including adjacent to the key anatomic feature of the dermis-epidermis junction.[20] Even in sun-protected sites, most elastin fibers appear abnormal after the age of 70 years and exhibit increased calcification.[66,76] This abnormal elastotic material provides neither elasticity nor resilience to the skin. Although recovery from mechanical depression takes only minutes in young skin, this can be as long as more than 24 hours in older adults.

Glycosaminoglycans, Water Content, and Dermal Adipose

Glycosaminoglycans (GAGs), along with collagen and elastin, are major constituents of the skin and include hyaluronic acid, dermatan sulfate, and chondroitin sulfate.[56] The key role of these molecules is to bind water, and their presence enables the skin to remain plump, soft, and hydrated.[56] In photoaged skin, the level of GAGs increases[77,78]; however, these molecules are unable to exert their hydrating effect because they are deposited on elastotic material rather than scattered diffusely in the dermis, as in young or photoprotected skin.[78] Young skin is well hydrated because most of the water is bound to proteins.[79] Water molecules that are not bound to proteins bind to each other and form what is known as tetrahedron or bulk water.[79] In intrinsically aged skin, water structure and binding do not appear to be altered significantly.[77] In photoaged skin, there is an increase in total water content.[77] However, because proteins are more hydrophobic[80] and folded[77,79] than those in sun-protected skin, and GAGs are deposited on elastotic material, water binds to itself rather than to these molecules and so is present mostly in the tetrahedron form.[77] In addition, tetrahedron water does not offer the same level of hydration and turgor as the bound form of water, thus contributing to the dry xerotic appearance of photoaged skin.[30]

Aging is also associated with an overall reduction in the volume of subcutaneous fat, despite the fact that total body fat (especially in the thighs, waist, and abdomen) typically continues to increase until approximately 70 years of age, especially in those living in the West. There is also a change in the regional distribution in fat, with greatest loss detected in the face, feet, and hands.[55,80]

Nerves and Sensation

It has been reported that skin enervation is little affected by aging and, although end-organs such as Meissner corpuscles are little changed, they may appear enlarged and distorted. Some studies have reported a decrease in sensory perception and an increase in pain threshold with age.[81] It has been demonstrated that there is loss of Meissner corpuscle density in the little finger from over 30/mm^2 in young adults to approximately 12/mm^2 by the age of 70 years.[82] Some loss of nerve support can be seen in bald versus haired scalp but, again, these changes are more likely driven by hair follicle miniaturization than by skin aging per se.[82]

Dermal Vasculature

Although not all studies are in agreement, it appears that increased age may be associated with decreased cutaneous perfusion, especially in photoexposed areas.[30] One study has demonstrated a 35% reduction in venous cross-sectional area in aged skin as opposed to young skin.[83] This reduction in vascularity is particularly noticeable in the papillary dermis (superficial dermis), where there is loss of the vertical capillary loops from the now absent rete ridges. Reduced vascularity results in skin pallor, depleted nutrient exchange, and disturbed thermoregulation.[56] There is some evidence that the vasoconstrictive or vasodilatory responses to cold and heat, respectively, are delayed in older adults, further diminishing thermoregulatory reponses.[30] In addition, dermal vasculature in mildly photodamaged skin displays venule wall thickening. However, in severely photodamaged skin, the walls are thinned and become dilated, manifesting clinically as telangiectasia.[20] Some studies have compared the vasculature of bald versus nonbald scalp and found a significant reduction in superficial capillary loops and tufts in the papillary dermis in the former. However, the miniaturization of hair follicles in balding scalp is likely to have caused some of this change (see later), because balding can already be advanced, even at a young age.

SKIN APPENDAGES

Sweat Glands

Eccrine Sweat Glands

There is a reduction in the number of eccrine sweat glands[84] and output per gland[85] in skin with increasing age, which also affects whole body thermoregulation, although without apparent significant reduction in neural support. There is an equally reduced response to the effects of epinephrine in older adults; however, there is a far greater decrease in response to acetylcholine in older men than in older women. This suggests that the effects of cholinergic sweating are indirectly affected by hormones.[85] Further evidence for this has been provided by the observation that the maximum rate of cholinergic sweating is far greater in adult males than in adult females or juveniles and is probably therefore androgen dependent.[86]

Apocrine Sweat Glands

Apocrine gland activity is diminished in old age, probably as a consequence of declining testosterone levels, leading to a reduction in pheromone secretion and consequent body odor.[87]

Nails

Nail growth increases until about the age of 25 years; thereafter, it starts to decrease.[44] Until the age of 70 years, nail growth is greater in men than women, after which the situation appears to be reversed.[88] Nails become more brittle in older adults and develop beaded ridging. This brittleness may be caused by a reduction in lipophilic sterols and free fatty acids.[89]

Pilosebaceous Unit

The pilosebaceous unit, including the hair follicle and its associated sebaceous glands, exhibits perhaps the most profound age-associated changes. These can be readily seen with enlargement changes during puberty. For example, during puberty, there is a striking transformation of low sebum–secreting fine and nearly invisible hair fibers produced by vellus hair follicle units to high sebum–secreting pigmented, coarse, terminal hair-producing follicles on the male chin. Paradoxically, there is miniaturization of hair follicles during age-related male pattern alopecia (common baldness). These anatomic changes in the hair follicle, i.e., enlargement and miniaturization, result in a significant remodeling of the dermis in the adjacent interfollicular skin, as highlighted by the significant reduction in the subcutaneous fat layer of the bald scalp, which increases the likelihood of cuts and bruising in this area.[90] Although age does not significantly alter the absolute number of pilosebaceous units per unit area on the scalp (until perhaps very late in life), the sebaceous glands themselves may become hyperplastic and larger,[91] including those in photoaged skin, and may present as giant comedones. Despite this increase in size, there is a 50% reduction in sebum production,[92] suggesting reduction in holocrine sebocyte turnover, which contributes to the xerosis of aged skin. Some investigators believe that this is due to decreased levels of testosterone,[93] although this does not explain the hyperplasia. Sebum secretion is also significantly reduced in postmenopausal women, suggesting that these glands are also estrogen sensitive. In addition, the constituency of sebum is altered in aging skin in that it contains less free cholesterol and more squalene.[94]

Hair

The hair follicle is a very complex multicellular tissue system (a veritable miniorgan) and is susceptible to similar underlying processes that control the functional longevity of organs and tissues. The hair follicle is somewhat unusual among mammalian tissues, however, in that it is a veritable histologic mélange of multiple cell types (e.g., epithelial, mesenchymal, neuroectodermal) that function concomitantly in all stages of their life histories (e.g., stem cells, transient amplifying cells, terminally differentiating cells). It is notable that some of these interactive cell systems are nonessential for overall hair follicle survival (e.g., melanocytes). Perhapse surprisingly, graying or white hair follicles may grow even more vigorously than their pigmented predecessors. Powerful evolutionary selection ensures that the hair follicle is generally hard-wired against significant aging-related loss of function, even after as much as 12 decades or more decades of life, although some would argue with this view, if only on purely hair aesthetics grounds.[90] Processes underlying aging in general (e.g., oxidative damage, telomere shortening, age-associated deficiencies related to nuclear and mitochondrial DNA damage and repair, age-related reductions in the cells' energy supply) will all affect whether some follicular cell subpopulations will enter cellular senescence.

Chest, axillary, and pubic hair all decrease in density with age; however, in men, there is often increased hair growth vigor in other body sites such as the eyebrows, around the external auditory meatus, and in the nostrils, and this may reflect the maintenance of high testosterone levels in men into their 70s.[44] In older women, there is a similar conversion of vellus to coarse terminal hairs on the chin and mustache areas, which is thought to reflect an unmasking of testosterone's influence in the context of now-diminished estrogen balance.

Aside from intrinsic aging, a principal influence on the characteristics of hair growth with age is the condition androgenetic alopecia. This is a distinct entity from the more aging-related hair thinning recently described as senescent alopecia,[95] because androgenetic alopecia (or common male pattern baldness) can manifest very early, even in the late teenage years. Moreover microarray analysis has now shown that androgenetic and senescent alopecia differ significantly in their respective gene expression profiles. The former is the result of dihydrotestosterone action on so-called androgen-sensitive hair follicles,[96] whereas senescent alopecia may more accurately represent true aging effects on the hair follicle. By contrast, so-called female-patterned alopecia may be truly androgenetic for only a small number of women with thinning hair. Thus the majority of age-associated alopecias in women are likely to have other causes.[97] Regardless of cause, age-related alopecia affects at least 50% of men by the age of 50 years and 50% of women by the age of 60 years.[98] Hairs in the affected area become finer and less pigmented until they resemble vellus hairs.[98]

Hair color in children tends to darken in about their first decade, and it is not unusual for a blond child to be dark-haired, even before the onset of puberty. Similarly, the phenomenon of heterochromia is much more apparent after puberty; color differences between scalp and beard are not uncommon.[90] The fine scalp hair of the growing child and adolescent exhibits striking changes with increasing age to mature adulthood, not only in color but also by showing a coarsening of the hair fibers themselves. Also, there is a tendency for miniaturizing hairs in the aging scalp (especially in older men) to be less medullated than terminal scalp hairs. By contrast, the loss of melanocytes from hair follicles that produce hair fibers of normal caliber (during hair graying or canities) may result in a concomitant change in the structure of these hair fibers. This is perhaps not surprising, given the close interaction between melanin granule–transferring melanocytes and hair shaft–forming and melanin-accepting precortical keratinocytes.[99]

Briefly, there is evidence that gray and white hair fibers exhibit different mechanical properties compared to adjacent pigmented hairs. Pigment-free hairs are not only coarser but also can be wavier than pigmented hairs, and some have reported that the average diameter of white hair fibers is significantly greater than that of pigmented hairs.[99] White hair was thicker on average, showed more central medulla component, and grew faster than pigmented hair. Interestingly, these researchers also described an age-related reduction in hair growth rate, but noted that this was broadly limited to pigmented hairs. Thus, the implication is that, counterintuitively, the apparently more aged white hairs may be partially spared these aging changes. The tensile strength of hair also decreases with age, having increased from birth to the second decade. However, the unpigmented hair of menopausal women grew at the same rate when compared with similar hair from much younger women. The biology underlying these events requires further investigation, particularly in terms of observed regional variability and the potential influence of androgens or other hormonal factors involved.

Changes in hair color and density are very visible indicators of age and are the target of endless manipulation to maintain a youthful appearance. An oft-quoted rule of thumb is that by the age of 50 years, approximately 50% of people are 50% gray, irrespective of hair color and gender.[100] However, a recent reevaluation of this concept suggests that this is exaggerated; it is more likely to be 6% to 23% of people, depending on ethnic and geographic origin and original natural hair color.[101] Hair graying appears to be a consequence of an overall and specific depletion of hair bulb melanocytes, less so in the outer root sheath and sebaceous gland basal layer.[102,103] The mechanism for this steady depletion remains uncertain, but appears to involve the stability and survival of melanocyte stem cells and bulbar melanocytes (see Fig. 25-1, *C*), especially in the context of their relative sensitivity to an increasingly friable oxidant and antioxidant protection status.[104,105]

Immune Function

The skin, apart from the immune-privileged transient portion of the growing hair follicle, is a potent immunocompetent tissue. It is so powerful that some have even been tempted to elevate skin to near-secondary lymphoid organ status. Indeed many of the tenets of modern immunology were deduced from graft-host responses using transplanted skin in mice. The density of Langerhans cells in the skin decreases greatly in older adults, even in sun-protected sites.[106,107] Not only is there a reduction in the number, but these cells have a reduced ability to migrate from the epidermis in response to cytokines (e.g., tumor necrosis factor-α).[108] Similarly, T lymphocytes are reduced in number and become less responsive to specific antigens.[42,109] Aging skin also appears to have a reduced ability to produce certain cytokines (e.g., interleukin-2[110]), whereas the production of others (e.g., interleukin-4) is increased.[110] The consequence of these changes is a reduced intensity to delayed hypersensitivity reactions[8] and increased susceptibility to photocarcinogenesis and chronic skin infections.[49]

Women

Reduced estrogen levels in postmenopausal women contributes to wrinkling, dryness, atrophy and laxity, in addition to poor wound healing, and vulvar atrophy.[111] Studies have suggested that the loss of collagen is more closely related to postmenopausal age than chronologic age, and thus reflects hormonal effects.[112,113] Estrogen therapy (hormone replacement therapy [HRT]) appears to prevent collagen loss in women with higher baseline levels of collagen and stimulates synthesis of collagen in those that have lower initial collagen levels.[114,115] Studies have also supported a relationship between estrogen deprivation and degenerative changes of dermal elastic tissue.[116] However, it remains uncertain whether there are beneficial effects of estrogen therapy on skin elasticity.[117] There is some evidence that HRT improves skin dryness[118] and wound healing[119] and increases skin surface lipids.[120,121] The role of estrogens in skin aging has recently been reviewed.[122]

MECHANISMS OF AGING

Previously cited literature reports make reference to several proposed modes of aging in terms of their cellular and molecular biologic mechanisms. However, like several aging theories, it is not at all clear whether they adequately address the primary cause(s) of aging. For example, a failing melanocyte could be expected to exhibit free radical–associated anomalies, although these may not have originated the degenerative changes. Nevertheless, the production of ROS or free radicals, through UVR exposure, smoking, pollution, and normal endogenous metabolic processes, is thought to contribute to the process of aging in the skin. ROS induce gene expression pathways that result in increased degradation of collagen and accumulation of elastin.[123] ROS not only directly destroy interstitial collagen, but also inactivate tissue inhibitors of MMPs and induce the synthesis and activation of matrix-degrading MMPs.[123] Hormones have also been shown to play a role. Postmenopausal hormone changes are responsible for a rapid worsening of skin structure and function, which can be at least partially repaired by HRT or local estrogen treatment.[113,124]

Mitochondrial DNA (mtDNA), due to repeated constitutional oxidative stress, incurs regular DNA damage and, in particular, deletion of a specific length of DNA, which is known as the common deletion. This deletion is 10 times more common in photodamaged than in sun-protected skin. It results in decreased mitochondrial function and resultant further accumulation of ROS, with additional damage to the cell's ability to generate energy. The extent of mtDNA damage in photodamaged skin does not correlate with the chronologic age of the person, but rather with photodamage severity.[20] Interestingly, this common deletion was also detected more frequently in graying hair follicles than in their pigmented counterparts.[125]

UVR can accelerate telomere shortening, which occurs ordinarily with every cell division. This results in the activation of DNA damage response proteins such as p53, a tumor suppressor protein, thereby inducing proliferative senescence or apoptosis, depending on the cell type.[14,126]

TREATMENT AND PREVENTION

Sun avoidance and adequate sunscreen use are central to preventing age-related skin changes. Aside from these, there are a number of products of proven and/or still controversial efficacy. Topical retinoids can significantly improve skin surface roughness, fine and coarse wrinkling, mottled pigmentation, and sallowness.[127] Histologically, there is reduction and redistribution of epidermal melanin, increased papillary dermal collagen deposition, and increased vascularity of the papillary dermis. Tretinoin treatment not only improves photodamage but also reverses the histologic changes associated with intrinsic aging.[128,129] These effects are thought to be mediated via the nuclear retinoic acid receptors. Retinoids not only improve the cosmetic appearance of aging, but also help prevent skin cancer.[20]

There are also many novel therapies undergoing investigation, including the treatment of dyspigmentation (e.g., solar lentigo). These include the delivery of enzymes that assist in DNA repair, antioxidants such as the polyphenols, flavonoids, alpha-hydroxy acids, and melanin synthesis and melanin transfer inhibitors. Reconstitution of lost extracellular matrix components is another potentially exciting avenue and antiaging strategy to bolster dermis function and structure.[130] Dietary lipids appear to play a role in skin aging.[131] There is evidence that a low-fat diet provides some protection against the development of actinic keratoses,[132] and certain dietary fats appear to be protective against UV-induced damage.[20] Future treatments include inducing/boosting cutaneous pigmentation, thus protecting the skin from UVR damage and various approaches to this are in development.[20] Nonmedical therapies include laser treatment, injectable fillers, botulinum toxin, and surgery.

CONCLUSION

Skin is subject to a complex blend of intrinsic and extrinsic aging processes, and given its strategic location as an interface organ, is particularly vulnerable to environmental insults—principally, UVR. Although there are numerous defense mechanisms to protect the skin from damage, the efficacy of these diminishes over time, resulting in the clinical features associated with aging and development of skin cancers. Sun protection is the key to prevention, and novel and more practical therapies continue to be developed.

KEY POINTS: AGING AND THE SKIN

- Aging of the skin is affected by intrinsic and extrinsic factors.
- UV radiation is responsible for most of the visible signs of aging and is known as photoaging.
- Photoaging is seen on sun-exposed sites, such as the face and forearms.
- Photoaging results in increased degradation of collagen and increased deposition of abnormal elastin in the dermis.
- Intrinsic aging is associated with fine wrinkling, xerosis (dryness), and skin laxity. Extrinsic aging is associated with coarse wrinkles, xerosis, mottled dyspigmentation, skin laxity, roughness, and the development of malignant neoplasms.
- The mechanisms for aging skin include the actions of ROS, mtDNA mutations, and telomere shortening.
- Hormonal changes, particularly in women, are important for skin aging.
- The key to treatment is prevention through sun protection, and novel therapies have been developed.

For a complete list of references, please visit www.expertconsult.com.

KEY REFERENCES

1. Tobin DJ: Biochemistry of human skin—our brain on the outside. Chem Soc Rev 35:52–67, 2006.
10. Gunn DA, Rexbye H, Griffiths CE, et al: Why some women look young for their age. PLoS ONE 1(4):e8021, 2009.
15. Nakamura KI, Izumiyama-Shimomura N, Sawabe M, et al: Comparative analysis of telomere lengths and erosion with age in human epidermis and lingual epithelium. J Invest Dermatol 119:1014–1019, 2002.
20. Yaar M, Gilchrest BA: Photoageing: mechanism, prevention and therapy. Br J Dermatol 157:874–887, 2007.
22. Grove GL: Physiologic changes in older skin. Clin Geriatr Med 5:115–125, 1989.
30. Waller JM, Maibach HI: Age and skin structure and function, a quantitative approach (I): blood flow, pH, thickness, and ultrasound echogenicity. Skin Res Technol 11:221–235, 2005.
36. Escoffier C, de Rigal J, Rochefort A, et al: Age-related mechanical properties of human skin: an in vivo study. J Invest Dermatol 93:353–357, 1989.
44. Graham-Brown RAC: Old age. In Burns T, Breathnach S, Cox N, et al, editors: Rook's textbook of dermatology, vol 6, Oxford, England, 2004, Blackwell Science.
46. Watson RE, Griffiths CE, Craven NM, et al: Fibrillin-rich microfibrils are reduced in photoaged skin. Distribution at the dermal-epidermal junction. J Invest Dermatol 112:782–787, 1999.
49. Cerimele D, Celleno L, Serri F: Physiological changes in ageing skin. Br J Dermatol 122(Suppl 35):13–20, 1990.
57. Tobin DJ: Gerontobiology of the hair follicle. In Trueb RM, Tobin DJ, editors: Aging hair, Berlin-Heidelberg, 2010, Springer-Verlag, pp 1–8.
60. Farage MA, Miller KW, Elsner P, et al: Structural characteristics of the aging skin: a review. Cutan Ocul Toxicol 26:343–357, 2007.
65. Uitto J: Connective tissue biochemistry of the aging dermis. Age-related alterations in collagen and elastin. Dermatol Clin 4:433–446, 1986.
80. Farage MA, Miller KW, Maibach HI: Degenerative changes in aging skin. In Farage MA, Miller KW, Maibach HI, editors: Textbook of aging skin, Berlin-Heidelberg, 2010, Springer-Verlag, pp 25–35.
95. Karnik P, Shah S, Dvorkin-Wininger Y, et al: Microarray analysis of androgenetic and senescent alopecia: comparison of gene expression shows two distinct profiles. J Dermatol Sci 72:183–186, 2013.
99. Trueb RM, Tobin DJ, editors: Aging hair, Berlin-Heidelberg, 2010, Springer-Verlag.
103. Tobin DJ, Paus R: Graying: gerontobiology of the hair follicle pigmentary unit. Exp Gerontol 36:29–54, 2001.
111. Hall G, Phillips TJ: Estrogen and skin: the effects of estrogen, menopause, and hormone replacement therapy on the skin. J Am Acad Dermatol 53:555–568, 2005.
122. Thornton MJ: Estrogens and aging skin. Dermatoendocrinol 5:264–270, 2013.
127. Gilchrest BA: A review of skin ageing and its medical therapy. Br J Dermatol 135:867–875, 1996.

26 The Pharmacology of Aging

Patricia W. Slattum, Kelechi C. Ogbonna, Emily P. Peron

Each day, worldwide, older adults consume millions of doses of medications. This remarkable amount of medication use benefits many older people by preventing and treating disease, preserving functional status, prolonging life, and improving or maintaining good quality of life. However, this level of medication exposure may harm older people via adverse drug reactions and is associated with other problems, such as drug interactions. The responses of older individuals to drugs, both beneficial and harmful, are partially dependent on age-related physiologic changes that influence how the body handles a given drug (pharmacokinetics) and what a drug does to the body (pharmacodynamics). To obtain the desired therapeutic response and prevent drug-related problems, it is also useful to have an understanding of drug use patterns in the geriatric population. Therefore, this chapter first examines the epidemiology of drug use in older adults around the world, followed by age-related alterations in drug pharmacokinetics and pharmacodynamics, and finally drug interactions.

EPIDEMIOLOGY OF DRUG USE

In general, the number of medications (prescription and nonprescription) used by older adults is greater than the number used by younger persons.[1-3] In the United States, older adults account for 13% of the population but for 34% of all prescription drugs dispensed.[4] The number and type of medications used by older adults are based in part on their living situation and access to medications.

Living Situation

Community-Living Adults

Of adults aged 57 to 85 years in the United States, 81% have reported taking at least one prescription medication.[5] Although the prevalence of medication users has not changed over time, the prevalence of polypharmacy (the use of multiple medications) has increased in recent years.[6] On average, community-dwelling older adults take from two to nine medications.[7] In the United States, race has been associated with differences in medication use among older adults, with older African Americans and Hispanic Americans demonstrating less use than older whites and Native Americans.[1] Older women also take more medication overall than older men.[8-10]

Rates of polypharmacy also vary by country. In one international survey of adults 55 years and older, 53% of older adults in the United States reported taking four or more prescription medications.[11] Approximately 40% of older adults in eight other countries—Australia, Canada, Germany, the Netherlands, New Zealand, Norway, Sweden, and the United Kingdom—reported the same medication-taking behavior, and those least likely to report this rate of medication use were from France (29%) and Switzerland (29%).

Also, the use of dietary supplements has been on the rise in the United States, with estimates of use in older adults rising from 14% in 1998[10] to 49% in 2006.[5] Although dietary supplement use appears to be more common among women than men, rates of nonprescription use overall are similar, with 42% of men and women aged 57 to 85 years in the United States using nonprescription medication.[5] Cardiovascular drugs were found to be the most commonly used medications among all prescription and nonprescription medications in the population studied.

Hospitalized Older Adults

Medication use by hospitalized older adults tends to be slightly higher than that of community-dwelling older adults. However, there is a paucity of information with regard to the types of medications used by older adults in this setting. Reported rates of prescription medication use among hospitalized older adults have ranged from a mean of 5 per patient in Italy[12] and Ireland[13] to 7.5/patient in the United States[14] and Austria.[15] One study, using pharmacy records from the University of Pittsburgh Medical Center, a tertiary academic medical center in southwestern Pennsylvania, identified the top 50 oral drugs prescribed for older hospitalized patients.[16] Warfarin, potassium, and pantoprazole were the most commonly prescribed oral drugs.

Older Adults in Long-Term Care Facilities

The level of medication use by older adults in long-term care facilities (LTCFs) is generally higher than that of older adults living at home in the community. There is a notable disparity worldwide in the percentages of LTCF residents taking large numbers of medications. In the United States and Iceland, 33% of LTCF residents take 7 to 10 medications, whereas only 5% of residents exhibit this degree of use in Denmark, Italy, Japan, and Sweden.[17] In one survey of United States LTCFs, 40% of residents (and 45% of those ≥85 years) received nine or more medications.[18] Gastrointestinal agents, central nervous system agents, and pain relievers were the most commonly used agents among patients receiving polypharmacy in that study.

Although the use of multiple medications may be necessary in some patients, the potential for inappropriate prescribing and drug-related problems are of concern. Overuse of certain centrally active medications—namely, antipsychotics—can be a particular problem in the LTCF setting.[19] In 1987, federal legislation was enacted in the United States that defined clear indications for appropriate prescribing of these agents and mandated close monitoring of them (Omnibus Budget Reconciliation Act [OBRA], 1987).[20] In 2005, the U.S. Food and Drug Administration (FDA) added a black box warning to the labeling of second-generation antipsychotics regarding the increased mortality risk associated with their use in older adults with dementia. This labeling change was then expanded to include all antipsychotics (first and second generation) in 2008. There have been decreases in antipsychotic prescribing in LTCFs since then,[21,22] but additional efforts are needed to continue to reduce antipsychotic use, particularly among patients at risk of significant harm, such as older adults with dementia.

Access to Medications

Universal public health insurance programs for older adults in Australia, Sweden, Canada, France, Germany, Japan, New Zealand, and the United Kingdom provide some level of drug benefit coverage, with the drug benefits differing in the amount of cost sharing, maximum amount of coverage, and specific pharmaceuticals covered.[23] The U.S. health insurance program for

TABLE 26-1 Age-Related Changes in Drug Pharmacokinetics

Pharmacokinetic Phase	Pharmacokinetic Parameters
Gastrointestinal absorption	Unchanged passive diffusion and no change in bioavailability for most drugs ↓ Active transport and ↓ bioavailability for some drugs ↓ First-pass effect and ↑ bioavailability for some drugs
Distribution	↓ Volume of distribution and ↑ plasma concentrations of water-soluble drugs ↑ Volume of distribution and ↑ terminal disposition half-life ($t_{1/2}$) for fat-soluble drugs ↑ or ↓ free fraction of highly plasma protein-bound drugs
Hepatic metabolism	↓ Clearance and ↑ $t_{1/2}$ for some oxidatively metabolized drugs ↓ Clearance and ↑ $t_{1/2}$ of drugs with high hepatic extraction ratio
Renal excretion	↓ Clearance and ↑ $t_{1/2}$ of renally eliminated drugs

↑, Increased; ↓, decreased.

older adults, Medicare, began coverage of outpatient drugs in 2006 via Medicare Part D. Although characterized by substantial copayments and an absence of coverage over a small but fixed drug cost range (the so-called doughnut hole), older adults in the United States are now protected from catastrophic out of pocket costs for outpatient drugs. This, in turn, has improved adherence and reduced the need for older adults to forgo necessities to purchase medications.[24-26] Notably, in many developing countries, medicines are the largest household health expenditure. Moreover, the supply of medications in developing countries may be inadequate or too expensive for older adults to purchase.[27,28]

ALTERED PHARMACOKINETICS

Table 26-1 presents an overview of age-related changes in drug pharmacokinetics.[29,30] This chapter details these changes in drug absorption, distribution, metabolism, and elimination. Frailty, a syndrome characterized by weight loss, fatigue, weakness, slowed walking speed, and low physical activity that is associated with advanced age and increased risk of adverse drug events, is probably more important than chronologic age as a risk factor for altered pharmacokinetics in older adults.[31]

Absorption

Numerous changes occur in the physiology of the gastrointestinal (GI) tract as a function of advancing age that might be expected to affect the absorption of drugs administered orally.[29,32] Gastric pH rises because of the development of atrophic gastritis, as well as the use of acid-suppressive medications to treat age-related GI disorders, such as peptic ulcer and gastroesophageal reflux. Gastric emptying is somewhat delayed and decreases are seen in intestinal blood flow (30% to 40% from age 20 to 70 years), intestinal motility, and number of functional absorptive cells.

Most drugs administered orally are absorbed via the process of passive diffusion, a process minimally affected by aging. A few agents require active transport for GI absorption, and their bioavailability may be reduced as a function of aging (e.g., calcium in the setting of hypochlorhydria). Of more significance is the decrease in first-pass hepatic extraction that occurs with aging, resulting in an enhancement in systemic bioavailability for drugs such as propranolol and labetalol and reduced bioavailability of some prodrugs such as enalapril and codeine after oral administration.[29,32] The bioavailability of drugs that are cytochrome P450 (CYP450), isoenzyme 3A4, and/or P-glycoprotein substrates (e.g., midazolam, verapamil) may be increased in older women, but no dosage adjustment recommendations have as yet been made.[33] The effects of aging on modified-release dosage forms are not known, although absorption might be affected by changes in GI motility or pH for some dosage forms in some patients. The effects of aging on drug absorption from other sites of administration such as the rectum, muscle, and skin are poorly understood.

Distribution

A number of changes in physiology occur with aging that may affect drug distribution. Body fat as a proportion of body weight rises from 18% to 36% in men and from 33% to 45% in women from age 20 to 70 years, whereas lean body mass decreases by 19% in men and by 12% in women, and plasma volume decreases by 8% from age 20 to 80 years. Total body water decreases by 17% from age 20 to 80 years and extracellular fluid volume decreases by 40% from 20 to 65 years of age. In addition, cardiac output declines approximately 1%/year from age 30 years, and brain and cardiac vessel blood flow rates decline 0.35% to 0.5% and 0.5%/year, respectively, beyond age 25 years. Additionally, frailty and concurrent disease may result in substantial changes in the serum concentrations of the two major drug-binding plasma proteins—albumin, which binds acidic drugs, decreases, whereas α_1-acid glycoprotein, which binds basic drugs, remains the same or rises.[34]

As a result of these factors, the volume of distribution of water-soluble (hydrophilic) drugs is generally decreased and that of fat-soluble (lipophilic) drugs is increased. Moreover, changes in volume of distribution can directly affect the loading doses of medications. For many drugs, loading doses will be lower in older versus younger patients and lowest in older white and Asian women (and thus use weight-based regimens routinely).[33] Decreases in serum albumin concentration can lead to a reduction in the degree of plasma protein binding of acidic drugs, such as naproxen, phenytoin, tolbutamide, and warfarin, therefore increasing the unbound fraction of the drug. Increases in α_1-acid glycoprotein because of inflammatory disease, burns, or cancer can lead to enhancement in the degree of plasma protein binding of basic drugs such as lidocaine, β-blockers, quinidine, and tricyclic antidepressants, thus reducing the unbound fraction of the drug. Provided there is no compromise in excretory pathways, these potential changes are unlikely to be clinically significant. However, plasma protein binding changes can alter the relationship of unbound (free) and total (unbound plus bound) plasma drug concentrations, making drug concentration interpretation more difficult. In these cases, the measurement of free plasma drug concentrations may be preferable to the usual use of total plasma drug concentrations.

Permeability across the blood-brain barrier may also be altered in older adults, affecting distribution of drugs into the central nervous system (CNS). Cerebrovascular P-glycoprotein is responsible in part for the transport of drugs across the blood-brain barrier. Studies using verapamil labeled with carbon-11 (a positron emitter) and positron emission tomography have demonstrated reduced P-glycoprotein activity in the blood-brain barrier with aging. As a result, the brain of older adults may be exposed to higher levels of drugs.[35]

Metabolism

Although drug metabolism can occur in numerous organs, most of the available data concern the effects of aging on the liver. Variations in drug metabolism and those resulting in altered drug clearance are a major source of variability in the response to medications in older adults.[36,37] Hepatic metabolism of drugs depends on perfusion, liver size, activity of drug-metabolizing enzymes, transporter activity, and protein binding, all of which may be altered by aging. Drugs are metabolized by two types of reactions—phase I (oxidative reactions) and phase II (conjugative or synthetic reactions, wherein an acetyl group or sugar is conjugated to the drug to enhance its polarity, water solubility, and hence excretion via the kidneys). Generally, drugs that undergo phase I metabolism demonstrate reduced clearance, whereas drugs undergoing phase II metabolism are preserved with aging.[36] For drugs with high intrinsic clearance (high hepatic extraction ratio), drug clearance is dependent on hepatic blood flow, is termed *flow-limited metabolism*. For drugs with low intrinsic clearance (low hepatic extraction ratio), clearance depends on hepatic enzyme activity, termed *capacity-limited metabolism*.

Age-associated reductions in hepatic blood flow can reduce the clearance of high hepatic extraction ratio drugs such as amitriptyline, lidocaine, morphine, diltiazem, and propranolol.[29,36] Hepatic blood flow may decline by 20% to 50%, resulting in reduced clearance of drugs such as propranolol by 40% or more in older adults.[31] Understanding the effect of age on the metabolism of drugs undergoing capacity-limited metabolism is more complex. For these drugs, total clearance depends on the fraction unbound in blood and intrinsic hepatic clearance. Many but not all studies report reduced size of the liver and reduced enzyme content in older adults.[36] Total hepatic clearance for drugs with capacity-limited metabolism many be increased (e.g., ibuprofen, naproxen), reduced (e.g., lorazepam, warfarin), or unchanged (e.g., temazepam, valproic acid) with aging.[36] Hepatic clearance of unbound drug rather than total hepatic clearance, which includes bound and unbound drugs, may be more relevant for understanding the effect of age on hepatic clearance.[36] Numerous confounders such as race, gender, frailty, smoking, diet, and drug interactions can significantly enhance or inhibit hepatic drug metabolism in older adults.[37] Frail older adults, for example, may experience reduced phase II metabolism. Although frailty remains challenging to define, it is characterized by reduced lean body mass, muscle loss, malnourishment, reduced functional status, and reduced endurance.[36] Frailty is associated with inflammation, which may downregulate drug metabolism and transport.[38] The interplay between drug transporters and drug-metabolizing enzymes may also play a role in the hepatic clearance of drugs with aging, but these relationships have remained largely unexplored.[29]

Elimination

Renal excretion is a primary route of elimination for many drugs and their metabolites. Aging is associated with a significant reduction in renal mass and number and size of nephrons. In addition, the glomerular filtration rate (GFR), tubular secretion, and renal blood flow decrease approximately 0.5%, 0.7%, and 1%/year, respectively, in those older than 20 years. At all ages, these three parameters are lower in women than in men.[33] However, older adults are a heterogeneous group, with up to one third of healthy older adults having no decrement in renal function as measured by creatinine clearance, a surrogate for glomerular filtration. In addition, tubular secretion and glomerular filtration may not decline in parallel.[39] Changes in kidney function with aging may be associated with hypertension or heart disease rather than with aging itself.[29] The estimation of creatinine clearance (CrCl), using any of a number of equations, serves as a useful screen for renal impairment in lieu of the use of serum creatinine (SCr), which is an imperfect marker of renal function in older adults because of the reduction of muscle mass with advancing age (i.e., a normal serum creatinine level does not equate with normal renal function in older adults).[40] One commonly used estimation equation for creatinine clearance used for dosage adjustment in older adults is the Cockcroft and Gault equation[41]:

$$\text{Creatinine clearance} = \frac{(140 - \text{age}) \times (\text{actual body weight})}{72 \times \text{SCr}}$$

where age is in years, actual body weight in kilograms, and serum creatinine concentration in milligrams per deciliter. For females, multiply the result by 0.85.

The Modified Diet in Renal Disease[42] equation and the Chronic Kidney Disease Epidemiology Collaboration[43] equation have been used more recently for the estimation of glomerular filtration rate based on SCr. The validity of each of these equations for estimating GFR in older adults has been advocated and challenged.[44-46] Dosing guidelines for primarily renally cleared medications are still based on estimated CrCl determined using the Cockcroft and Gault equation, and current consensus is to continue to use the Cockcroft and Gault equation for renal drug dosing in older adults. Frailty is associated with renal impairment, and the Cockcroft and Gault equation for renal dosing is not reliable in frail older adults. Research continues to identify improved methods to estimate CrCl in frail older adults for the purpose of drug dosing.[31]

Numerous medications are primarily renally excreted and/or have renally excreted active metabolites. There is evidence of age-related reductions in the total body clearances of drugs that are primarily cleared renally. The risk of adverse clinical consequences is likely increased for drugs with a narrow therapeutic index (e.g., digoxin, aminoglycosides, chemotherapeutics). Consensus guidelines for oral dosing of primarily renally cleared drugs in older adults have been developed.[47] Medications to avoid in older adults with CrCl lower than 30 mL/min include chlorpropamide, colchicine, cotrimoxazole, glyburide, meperidine, nitrofurantoin, probenecid, spironolactone, and triamterene. Oral medications with recommended dosage adjustments for reduced renal function in older adults include acyclovir, amantadine, ciprofloxacin, gabapentin, memantine, metformin, ranitidine, rimantadine, and valacyclovir. Dosage adjustment for renal impairment is easily accomplished once CrCl has been estimated using information provided in the package insert or other drug-dosing reference sources.

ALTERED PHARMACODYNAMICS

In contrast to the relationship of aging to altered pharmacokinetics, fewer data are available investigating the effect of aging on pharmacodynamics (drug response). Most studies documenting age-related differences in pharmacodynamics have focused on medications acting on the CNS and cardiovascular system. Theoretically, altered pharmacodynamics could be due to two basic mechanisms: (1) altered sensitivity because of changes in receptor number or affinity or changes in postreceptor response; and (2) age-related impairment of physiologic and homeostatic mechanisms.[48,49] This section reviews altered responses of older adults to medications mediated by these two mechanisms.

ALTERED SENSITIVITY

Table 26-2 lists medications for which there is reasonable documentation of altered drug sensitivity in older adults. There is

TABLE 26-2 Drugs Whose Sensitivity Is Altered With Advancing Age

β-Agonists (↓)	H_1-antihistamines (↑)
β-Blockers (↓)	Metoclopramide (↑)
Benzodiazepines (↑)	Neuroleptics (↑)
Calcium antagonists (↓↑)	Opioids (↑)
Dopaminergic agents (↑)	Warfarin (↑)
Furosemide (↓)	Vaccines (↓)

↑, Increased; ↓, decreased.

evidence that older adults are less responsive to β-blockers and β-agonists.[50,51] There is also good evidence that older adults are more sensitive to the effects of benzodiazepines. Using psychomotor testing, this has been established for diazepam, flurazepam, loprazolam, midazolam, nitrazepam, and triazolam.[48,49] Enhanced sensitivity has also been demonstrated for opioids, metoclopramide, dopamine agonists, levodopa, and antipsychotics.[48,49] Age-related changes in pharmacodynamics have been reported for calcium channel blockers (increased hypotensive and bradycardic effects), β-blockers (reduced blood pressure response), diuretics (reduced effectiveness), and warfarin (increased risk of bleeding), but not with angiotensin-converting enzyme inhibitors or angiotensin receptor blockers.[48,49]

Alterations in Physiologic and Homeostatic Mechanisms

Physiologic and homeostatic changes in older adults may affect drug responses, altering baseline performance and the ability to compensate for the effects of medications. Examples of homeostatic mechanisms that may become impaired with advanced age include postural or gait stability, orthostatic blood pressure responses, thermoregulation, cognitive reserve, and bowel and bladder function.[52-54] The loss of efficiency of homeostatic mechanisms puts older adults at risk of symptomatic orthostasis and falls (with antihypertensives, antipsychotics, and tricyclic antidepressants), urinary retention and constipation (with drugs with anticholinergic properties), falls and delirium (with virtually every sedating drug), and accidental hypothermia or heat stroke (with neuroleptics).[52,53] Medications are a common contributor to geriatric syndromes such as falls, delirium, functional decline, and constipation.[55]

DRUG INTERACTIONS

Drug-drug interactions can be defined as the resulting effect or consequence that one drug has on another when co-administered.[56] The two major types of drug-drug interactions include pharmacokinetic interactions, wherein drug absorption, distribution, metabolism, and excretion are affected, and pharmacodynamic interactions, wherein pharmacologic effects are altered. Drugs may also interact with food, nutritional status, herbal products, alcohol, and preexisting disease.[57-60]

Pharmacokinetic Interactions

Increased drug bioavailability may be seen with the concurrent ingestion of grapefruit juice owing to its inhibitory effect on CYP450 isoenzyme 3A4–mediated first-pass metabolism in the gut wall and liver. This may result in exaggerated pharmacologic effects.[61] Decreased bioavailability can be seen when phenytoin is administered with enteral feedings.[62] Multivalent cations (e.g., antacids, sucralfate, iron, calcium supplements) can reduce the bioavailability of tetracycline and quinolone antimicrobials.[63]

Drug interactions involving drug distribution are primarily related to altered plasma protein binding. Although a number of drugs may displace other drugs from plasma protein–binding sites, especially acids such as salicylate, valproic acid, and phenytoin, this type of drug interaction is rarely clinically significant.

Drug interactions most likely to be clinically significant are those that involve the inhibition or induction of metabolism of narrow therapeutic margin drugs.[64] Table 26-3 illustrates selected CYP450 enzyme inducers and inhibitors. It does not appear that younger and older individuals differ in the magnitude of hepatic enzyme inhibition after exposure to drugs such as cimetidine, macrolide antimicrobials (e.g., erythromycin, clarithromycin), quinidine, and ciprofloxacin.[63,65] However, there is controversy regarding the effect of hepatic enzyme inducers in younger versus older individuals, with some studies demonstrating no difference between the age groups and others suggesting that older adults do not respond as well to enzyme induction.[36,66-68] It may be that these effects are substrate- and/or inducer-specific.

TABLE 26-3 Selected Cytochrome P450 Inducers and Inhibitors by Isoenzyme

CYP1A2	CYP2C	CYP2D6	CYP3A4
INDUCERS			
Char-broiled beef	Rifampin	None known	Carbamazepine
Cruciferous vegetables			Phenytoin
Omeprazole			Rifampin
Smoking			St John's wort
INHIBITORS			
Cimetidine	Amiodarone	Fluoxetine	Erythromycin
Ciprofloxacin	Fluconazole	Paroxetine	Ketoconazole
Fluvoxamine	Fluvastatin	Quinidine	Nefazodone
		Ritonavir	

Inhibition of renal clearance of one drug by another drug can also result in clinically significant effects.[69] Many of these drug-drug interactions involve competitive inhibition of tubular secretion of anionic or cationic drugs. Cationic agents include amiodarone, cimetidine, digoxin, procainamide, quinidine, ranitidine, trimethoprim, and verapamil. Anionic agents include cephalosporins, indomethacin, methotrexate, penicillins, probenecid, salicylates, and thiazides.

Drug interactions with herbal and over-the-counter (OTC) products are frequently overlooked. In one series, 52% of all moderate- or high-risk interactions occurred between prescription drugs and herbal and/or OTC products.[70] The interaction potential of herbal products is enhanced because of frequent contamination with heavy metals and adulteration with prescription drugs (e.g., nonsteroidal anti-inflammatory drugs [NSAIDs], corticosteroids, psychotherapeutics, and phosphodiesterase-5 inhibitors, such as sildenafil).[71] Table 26-4 illustrates the most common herbal-drug interactions.[71,72]

Pharmacodynamic Interactions

Some drugs may alter the response of another drug and produce adverse effects. A good example of this is the synergistic effect of taking more than one anticholinergic agent concurrently, which can result in delirium, urinary retention, constipation, and other problems.[56] Other examples include additive bradycardia when β-blockers are administered concurrently with verapamil or diltiazem, additive hypotension when several antihypertensives are administered concurrently, and sedation or falls when several CNS depressants (e.g., benzodiazepines, sedative-hypnotics, antidepressants, neuroleptics) are administered concurrently.

Drug-Disease Interactions

Drug interactions can also be considered in a broader sense when they involve medications that can affect and can be affected by disease states. Older adults are at higher risk for adverse outcomes with drug–disease state interactions because of alterations in homeostatic mechanisms, diminished physiologic reserve, and multiple comorbidities. Avoiding inappropriate medications, and identifying medication-related adverse events and drug interactions, coupled with patient participation, can have favorable effects on patient outcomes.[73] Expert panels in Canada and the United States have developed guidelines to identify potentially clinically important drug–disease state interactions (Table 26-5).[74,75] Unfortunately, explicit quality indicators (e.g., the Beers list[75]) cannot be easily transferred from one country to another,

TABLE 26-4 Most Common Herbal-Drug Interactions

Interacting Drug	Herb (Vernacular Name)	Description of the Effect of Herbs on Drug Kinetics and Activity
Warfarin	St John's wort, ginseng	↓ INR
	Garlic, danshen, gingko, devil's claw, dong quai, papaya, glucosamine	↑ INR
	Garlic, ginseng, gingko, ginger, feverfew	↑ Bleeding time
ASA, NSAIDs, dipyridamole, clopidogrel-ticlopidine	Gingko	↑ Bleeding time
Amitriptyline	St John's wort	↓ Drug concentration
Warfarin		
Theophylline		
Simvastatin		
Alprazolam		
Verapamil		
Digoxin		
Iron		
Ethanol	Ginseng	
Phenytoin	Shankhapushpi	
Phenytoin	Gingko	
Valproate		
Iron	Feverfew	
	Camomile	
Metformin	Guar gum	
Glibenclamide		
Digoxin		
Lithium	Psyllium	
ASA	Tamarind	↑ Drug concentration
Nifedipine	Gingko	
Sertraline	St John's wort	Serotonin syndrome (mild)
Paroxetine		
Trazodone		
Nefazodone		
Chlorpropamide	Garlic	↓ Glucose concentration
Antidiabetic drugs	Fenugreek	
MAOIs	Ginseng	Manic-like symptoms, headache, tremors
Thiazides	Gingko	↓ Drug effect
	Dandelion	
	Uva-ursi	
Thyroxine	Horseradish	
	Kelp	
Phenytoin	Shankhapushpi	
Warfarin	Gingko	↑ Drug effect
ASA		
NSAIDs		
Dipyridamole		
Clopidogrel/ticlopidine		
Benzodiazepines	Kava	
Barbiturates		
Opioids		
Ethanol		
Barbiturates	Valerian	
Other CNS depressants		
Digoxin	Hawthorn	
Thiazides	Gossypol	
Levodopa	Gingko	↑ "Off" periods in Parkinson disease
Anabolic steroids	Echinacea	↑ Hepatotoxicity risk
Amiodarone		
Methotrexate		
Ketoconazole		
Caffeine	Ma huang	Hypertension, insomnia, tachycardia, nervousness, tremor, headache, seizures; ↑ MI, stroke risk
Stimulants		
Decongestants		
Tricylic antidepressants	Yohimbine	Hypertension
Heparin	Fenugreek	↑ Bleeding risk
Clopidogrel-ticlopidine		
Warfarin		

Adapted from Skalli S, Zaid A, Soulaymani R: Drug interactions with herbal medicines. Ther Drug Monit 29:679–686, 2007.
↑, Increased; ↓, decreased; *ASA,* aspirin; *CNS,* central nervous system; *INR,* international normalized ratio (of prothrombin time); *MAOI,* nonselective monoamine oxidase inhibitor; *MI,* myocardial infarction; *NSAID,* nonsteroidal anti-inflammatory drug.

TABLE 26-5 Drug-Disease Interactions to Avoid in Older Adults*

Disease or Condition	Drug or Drug Class
Heart failure	NSAIDs and COX-2 inhibitors; nondihydropyridine CCBs (avoid only for systolic heart failure); pioglitazone, rosiglitazone; cilostazol; dronedarone
Syncope	AChEIs; peripheral α-blockers (e.g., doxazosin prazosin, terazosin); tertiary TCAs (e.g., amitriptyline, clomipramine, doxepin, imipramine, trimipramine); chlorpromazine; thioridazine; olanzapine
Chronic seizures or epilepsy	Bupropion; chlorpromazine; clozapine; maprotiline; olanzapine; thioridazine; thiothixene; tramadol
Delirium	Anticholinergics; benzodiazepines; chlorpromazine; corticosteroids; H_2 receptor antagonists; meperidine sedative-hypnotics; antipsychotics
Dementia and cognitive impairment	Anticholinergics; benzodiazepines; H_2 receptor antagonists; nonbenzopdiazepine hypnotics (eszopiclone, zolpidem, zaleplon); antipsychotics
History of falls or fractures	Anticonvulsants; antipsychotics; benzodiazepines; nonbenzodiazepine hypnotics (eszopiclone, zaleplon, zolpidem); TCAs; SSRIs; opioids
Insomnia	Oral decongestants (e.g., pseudoephedrine and phenylephrine); stimulants (e.g., amphetamine, methylphenidate, armodafinil, modafinil); theobromines (e.g., theophylline and caffeine)
Parkinson disease	All antipsychotics (except for aripiprazole, quetiapine and clozapine); antiemetics (metoclopramide, prochlorperazine, promethazine)
History of gastric or duodenal ulcers	Aspirin (>325 mg/day); non–COX-2 selective NSAIDs
Chronic kidney disease stages IV and V	NSAIDs
Urinary incontinence in women	Estrogen (oral and transdermal), peripheral alpha-1 blockers (doxazosin, prazosin, terazosin)
Lower urinary tract symptoms, benign prostatic hyperplasia	Strongly anticholinergic drugs, except antimuscarinics for urinary incontinence

AChEI, Acetylcholinesterase inhibitor; *CCB,* calcium channel blocker; *COX,* cyclooxygenase; *NSAID,* nonsteroidal anti-inflammatory drug; *SSRI,* selective serotonin reuptake inhibitor; *TCA,* tricyclic antidepressant.

*As defined by explicit criteria (see reference 73 for detailed description of rationale and level of evidence).

or even from one setting to another, without being modified and revalidated because of contextual differences.[73] Implicit criteria, such as the Screening Tool of Older Person's Prescriptions (STOPP), may be more advantageous when applying patient specific characteristics.[76] However, none of these tools provide an exhaustive list of scenarios encountered in geriatric practice.

SUMMARY

Older adults consume a disproportionate share of medications. Factors enhancing medication use include the concurrent presence of multiple diseases, female gender, increasing level of care, and increasing age. Other factors that probably influence drug use in older adults include provider prescribing behaviors, cultural milieu, psychosocial issues (e.g., living alone, anxiety, depression), and direct to consumer advertising by the pharmaceutical industry.

The most common classes of medications used by older adults include cardiovascular, GI, CNS, and analgesic agents. Many studies have documented that the aging process alters drug disposition and response. Phase I hepatic metabolism is often reduced in older adult patients, resulting in reduced clearance and increased terminal disposition half-life for many commonly used drugs. Age-related decline in renal function decreases clearance and increases the terminal disposition half-life of renally eliminated drugs and metabolites. Pharmacodynamic studies have indicated that older adults tend to be more sensitive to the effects of benzodiazepines, opioids, dopamine receptor antagonists, and warfarin. Drug-drug and drug-disease interactions may also affect the well-being of older adults.

Comorbidities, concurrent medications, social factors, and functional and cognitive status, along with physiologic changes associated with aging, must be considered when selecting appropriate drug therapies and doses to achieve maximal benefits of medications for older adults while minimizing or preventing drug-related problems.

KEY POINTS: PHARMACOLOGY OF AGING

- Older adults are avid consumers of medications.
- Age-related alterations in drug pharmacokinetics are most pronounced in terms of the decline in the hepatic metabolism and renal elimination of certain drugs.
- Age-related alterations in drug pharmacodynamics have not been studied extensively, but older adults appear to be more sensitive to the effects of benzodiazepines, opioids, dopamine receptor antagonists, and warfarin.
- Drug-drug and drug-disease interactions are common in older adults and may have a negative impact on health-related quality of life.

For a complete list of references, please visit www.expertconsult.com.

KEY REFERENCES

5. Qato DM, Alexander GC, Conti RM, et al: Use of prescription and over-the-counter medications and dietary supplements among older adults in the United States. JAMA 300:2867–2878, 2008.
29. Shi S, Klotz U: Age-related changes in pharmacokinetics. Curr Drug Metab 12:601–610, 2011.
30. Corsonello A, Pedone C, Incalzi RA: Age-related pharmacokinetic and pharmacodynamic changes and related risk of adverse drug reactions. Curr Med Chem 17:571–584, 2010.
31. Hubbard R, O'Mahoney M, Woodhouse K: Medication prescribing in frail older people. Eur J Clin Pharmacol 69:319–326, 2013.
36. McLachlan AJ, Pont LG: Drug metabolism in older people-A key consideration in achieving optimal outcomes with medicines. J Gerontol A Biol Sci Med Sci 67A:175–180, 2012.
47. Hanlon JT, Aspinall SL, Semla TP, et al: Consensus guidelines for oral dosing of primarily renally cleared medications in older adults. J Am Geriatr Soc 57:335–340, 2009.
48. Bowie MW, Slattum PW: Pharmacodynamics in older adults: a review. Am J Geriatr Pharmacother 5:263–303, 2007.
49. Trifior G, Spina E: Age-related changes in pharmacodynamics: focus on drugs acting on central nervous and cardiovascular systems. Curr Drug Metab 12:611–620, 2011.
57. Mallet L, Spinewine A, Huang A: The challenge of managing drug interactions in elderly people. Lancet 370:185–191, 2007.
59. Mason P: Important drug-nutrient interactions. Proc Nutr Soc 69:551–557, 2010.
75. American Geriatrics Society 2012 Beers Criteria Update Expert Panel: American Geriatrics Society updated Beers Criteria for potentially inappropriate medication use in older adults. J Am Geriatr Soc 60:616–631, 2012.
76. Gallagher P, Ryan C, Byrne S, et al: STOPP (Screening Tool of Older Person's Prescriptions) and START (Screening Tool to Alert doctors to Right Treatment). Consensus validation. Int J Clin Pharmacol Ther 46:72–83, 2008.

27 Antiaging Medicine

Ligia J. Dominguez, John E. Morley, Mario Barbagallo

Attempts to reverse the aging process stretch back to the time when Adam and Eve were expelled from the Garden of Eden. Since then, wise sages and charlatans have made numerous pronouncements on what the populace should do to extend their life span. In most cases, this has required that those who wish to benefit pay exorbitant sums of money to those who have developed the magical elixir of longevity. This has led to the concept that antiaging medicine is a scam.

On the other hand, we have seen a remarkable extension in longevity over the last century. In the United States, at the start of the twentieth century, half of the population was dead by 50 years of age, whereas by the dawn of the twenty-first century, half of women lived to older than 80 years. These dramatic changes were brought about by public health measures such as improved sanitation, greatly improved and available food supply, introduction of antibiotics, vaccinations, improved care of pregnant women and the birthing process, enhanced surgical techniques and, to a lesser extent, a variety of new medications introduced in the second half of the twentieth century. One needs also to give credit to the improved work environment and decrease in excessive manual labor.

The secret to longevity appears often to follow a healthy lifestyle and avoiding excesses. In the thirteenth century, Friar Roger Bacon in England wrote a best-selling antiaging book.[1] His secrets to longevity were as follows:

- A controlled diet
- Proper rest
- Exercise
- Moderation in lifestyle
- Good hygiene
- Inhaling the breath of a young virgin

George Valiant, a Harvard psychiatrist, studied inner city individuals and Harvard graduates from their mid-50s.[2] His studies suggested that aging successfully occurred in those individuals who did the following:

- Got some exercise
- Did not smoke
- Managed crises well
- Did not abuse alcohol
- Enjoyed a stable marriage
- Were not obese (although this applied only to those in the inner city)

The Norfolk-EPIC study found that persons who followed four simple lifestyle habits were physiologically 14 years younger than those who did none of them.[3] The four magical ingredients that produced this greatly improved outcome were as follows:

- Not smoking
- Getting some exercise
- Eating five helpings of fruit and vegetables each day
- Drinking 1 to 14 glasses of alcohol per week

A higher score of adherence to the modifiable lifestyle factors described in the Northfolk-EPIC study was significantly associated with a higher quality of life.[4]

Because long-lived populations tend to come from places such as Japan, Macau, and Hong Kong, where there is a high preponderance of fish in the diet, it is probably reasonable to suggest that fatty fish intake, rich in eicosahexanoic and docosahexaenoic acids, should be included in a diet of a person who wishes to live for a long time.[5]

BRIEF HISTORY OF ANTIAGING MEDICINE

In ancient Egypt, the olive leaf was used to improve beauty and extend life.[6] This is paralleled in the twenty-first century by the recognition that the Mediterranean diet is associated with longer and healthier lives. Ayurvedic medicine in India developed specific diets, lifestyle practices, and herbs that would extend life.

The search for the Fountain of Youth was first made famous by Ponce de Leon, the Governor of Puerto Rico, who went searching for Bimini, where it was believed that there was a fountain of youth. Instead, he discovered Florida, a modern day haven for retirees in the United States. In 1933, in the novel *Lost Horizon*, James Hilton created a paradise where no one got older, called Shangri-La. So riveting was this concept for the public that a number of expeditions set out to try and find this paradise in the Himalayan Mountains. Nobel Prize winner (for physiology or medicine) Elie Metchnikoff mistakenly believed that Bulgarians lived extremely long lives, and this was due to yogurt. This created an antiaging cult based on eating yogurt.

The modern quasiscientific approach to antiaging medicine was expressed in the book *Life Extension* by Durk Pearson and Sandy Shaw, published in 1982.[7] In an 858-page volume, they provided detailed accounts of animal experiments that increased longevity, claiming that their book was "for anyone, regardless of age, who seeks greater youthfulness-*starting right now*." This book opened the door to multiple others where snippets of animal science were fed to the public, suggesting that these findings should be used by humans who wished to live a long life.

The American Academy of Anti-Aging Medicine (A4M) was founded in 1992 by Dr. Ronald Klatz and Dr. Robert Goldman. Its avowed purpose is to advance "technology to detect, prevent and treat aging related disease and promote research into methods to retard and optimize the human aging process." It provides a number of certifications for physicians in antiaging medicine. It claims to have more than 26,000 members from more than 120 countries (www.worldhealth.net). It produces the *International Journal of Anti-Aging Medicine*.

The Life Extension Foundation, founded by Saul Kent in 1980, is based in Florida and produces the monthly magazine, *Life Extension*. Its readership is thought to be around 350,000. It also sells dietary supplements by mail order. Two more mainstream physicians whose books have promoted antiaging philosophies are Andrew Weil and Deepak Chopra.

Aubrey De Grey, a Cambridge-educated scientist, has developed a theory called "Strategies for Engineered Negligible Senescence (SENS)." He has been extraordinarily successful at promoting his theories to the lay public. He suggested that there are seven types of aging damage, which are readily open to treatment:

- Cancer mutations
- Mitochondrial mutations
- Intracellular junk

- Extracellular junk
- Cell loss
- Cell senescence
- Extracellular cross-links

The De Grey SENS proposal has been widely criticized by gerontologists: "Each one of the specific proposals that comprise the SENS agenda is, at our present stage of ignorance, exceptionally optimistic," and it "will take decades of hard work, if [these proposals] ever prove to be useful."[8] His approach is a classic example of the quasiscientific methods that have been used to create antiaging literature.

The most extensive criticism of the modern antiaging medicine came in 2002 from Olshansky and colleagues.[9] The article stated that:

> *...no currently marketed intervention has yet been proved to slow, stop or reverse human aging.... The entrepreneurs, physicians and other health care practitioners who make these claims are taking advantage of consumers who cannot easily distinguish between the hype and reality of interventions designed to influence the aging process and age-related diseases.*

Caloric Restriction

In 1934, Mary Crowell and Clive McKay at Cornell University published a series of experiments showing that limiting the food intake of laboratory rats (dietary restriction) resulted in prolongation of their lives.[10] Subsequently, studies in some species have shown that caloric restriction (CR) results in a prolongation of lives. Some studies have suggested that caloric restriction needs to be started in younger animals, and it fails to prolong life in older animals.[11]

Studies in monkeys have suggested that dietary restriction improves the metabolic profile (glucose, cholesterol) in these animals[12] and may attenuate Alzheimer-like amyloid changes in their brains.[13] However, these animals also showed a loss of bone and an increased propensity to develop hip fractures. Two studies addressing the effect of CR on nonhuman primates have reported contrasting results. The University of Wisconsin-Madison (UWM) study showed prolonged life span under CR,[14] but a National Institute of Aging (NIA) study did not.[15] A possible explanation may lie in the diet composition—the high sugar concentration in the ad lib diet of the control group in the UWM study[14] may have led to a shortened life span compared to the group under CR. Conversely, the ad lib healthier diet in the NIA study[15] led to longer life span in the control group without conferring additional benefit for those under CR.

Numerous theories exist about why CR may enhance longevity. The hormesis theory suggests that CR represents a low level of stress, which allows the animal to develop enhanced defenses that slow the aging process. It has also been suggested that CR reduces oxidative damage, enhances insulin sensitivity, and decreases tissue glycation. CR reduces the release of growth factors such as growth hormone, insulin, and insulin-like growth factor 1 (IGF-1), which have been associated to accelerated aging and increased mortality in diverse organisms.[16] The silent information regulator (*Sir*) gene is upregulated by CR in yeast and in mammals. However, the role of *Sir* genes in longevity is controversial. For example, the polyphenol resveratrol found in grapes and in red wine has been shown to prolong the life span of mice fed a high-fat diet, flies, and worms, mimicking CR by a suggested interaction with sirtuins.[17] However, recent data have indicated that the degree of life span extension in worms and flies on resveratrol supplementation may be shorter than previously reported.[18]

The Caloric Restriction Society was founded in 1984 by Roy and Lisa Walford and Brian Delaney. Members of this society practice CR to varying degrees. Studies of members of this society have suggested that they have lower blood pressure, glucose, and cholesterol values.[19] The National Institutes of Health has funded a number of short-term studies to determine the utility of CR in middle-aged persons. The enthusiasm for CR in older persons has been tempered by multiple studies in persons older than 60 years showing that weight loss is associated with increased institutionalization, increased mortality, and increased hip fracture.[20] In younger populations, prolonged CR may decrease fertility and libido, lead to wound-healing problems, amenorrhea, osteoporosis, and decreased potential to combat infections and be harmful in lean humans.[16]

At present, there are a number of CR diets that are advertised to the public as a method for life prolongation. The CRON diet (***c****aloric* ***r****estriction with* ***o****ptimal* ***n****utrition*) was developed by Walford and Delaney. It was based on the research conducted in the Biosphere. In general, this diet recommends a 20% CR based on determining one's basal metabolic rate. The Okinawa diet is a low-calorie, nutrient-rich diet based on the original diet of people living on the Japanese island of Okinawa (Ryukyu Islands). Its popularity is based on the large number of centenarians who used to live in the Ogimi Village on Okinawa. The diet is calorie-restricted compared with the Japanese diet. It predominantly consists of vegetables (especially sweet potatoes), a half-serving of fish per day, legumes, and soy. It is low in meat, eggs, and dairy products. The New Longevity Diet of Henry Mallek represents a popularization of other longevity diets. It needs to be recognized that none of these diets has been proven to extend longevity. It is interesting to note that Roy Walford, a major proponent of dietary restriction, died at 79 years of age of amyotrophic lateral sclerosis (ALS). Animal studies have suggested that CR is especially bad for animals with ALS.

Exercise

Exercise in moderation appears to be a cornerstone of longevity. Mice with an excess of phosphoenolpyruvate carboxykinase (PEPCK-C) in their skeletal muscle are more active than their controls and can run for 5 km at a speed of 20 m/min compared with 0.2 km for control mice.[21] These mice live longer than controls, and females remain reproductively active until 35 months of age.

Observational studies in humans have strongly suggested that those who are physically active live longer. In a study of 70- to 80-year-olds, those with a higher total energy expenditure lived longer than those with less energy expenditure.[22] A major factor in enhancing energy expenditure was stair climbing. Interestingly, long-lived Okinawan people usually combine an above-average amount of daily exercise with a below-average food intake.[23]

Fries found that older runners compared with sedentary older adults tended to become disabled 13 years later.[24] The LIFE pilot study has shown that a structured physical activity program significantly improves functional performance.[25] Walking speed is associated with decreased disability. Physical activity is associated with decreased dysphoria. Persons aged 50 years of age who exercise regularly are less liable to develop Alzheimer disease as they age.[26] Regular physical activity reduces the rate of deterioration in persons with dementia.[27] CR and exercise seem to stimulate diverse molecular pathways, but both induce autophagy[28] (from the Greek *auto-*, "self," and *phagein*, "to eat"), a catabolic process that degrades defective cellular components for recycling.

THE HORMONAL FOUNTAIN OF YOUTH

Since the publication of Wilson's *Feminine Forever* in the 1950s, touting the role of estrogen to maintain youth, there has been

TABLE 27-1 Does Low Testosterone Predict Death?

Author, Year	Population	Predicts Death?
Morley et al, 1996[33]	Healthy men in New Mexico,14-yr follow-up	No
Shores et al, 2006[34]	Veteran population, 8-yr follow-up	Yes
Araujo et al, 2007[35]	Massachusetts Male Aging Study	No
Khaw et al, 2007[37]	Europe	Yes
Laughlin et al, 2008[36]	Rancho Bernardo, CA, 11.8-yr follow-up	Yes

increasing interest in the antiaging effects of hormones.[5] Previously, toward the end of the nineteenth century, Brown-Séquard had suggested that a testicular extract produces remarkable antiaging effects. It is unlikely that this extract had any testosterone, demonstrating the powerful effect of the placebo. This led to a large number of wealthy men in Europe and the United States receiving monkey testicular implants, which were claimed to rejuvenate them. Brinkley, in the United States, pioneered a series of goat gland extracts, which were equally ineffective but made him a rich man. Subsequently, almost every hormone has been touted to produce antiaging effects. In general, it can be said that the more enthusiasm that the lay public has expressed in these hormones, the less likely they are to be effective.

Vitamin D (25[OH] vitamin D) levels decline with aging.[29] Low levels of vitamin D have been associated with increased mortality.[30] In persons with 25(OH) vitamin D levels below 30 ng/mL, replacement has been demonstrated to enhance function, decrease falls, and decrease hip fracture.[31] Vitamin D replacement of more than 625 IU/day in a meta-analysis led to decreased mortality.[32] It is now generally accepted that older adults should get regular skin exposure (15 to 30 min/day) without sun block or should take 800 to 1000 IU of vitamin D/day. All persons older than 70 years should have their 25(OH) vitamin D levels measured at least annually (preferably in winter) because they may need higher doses of vitamin D to raise their level above 30 ng/mL.

Studies on men with low testosterone levels have shown conflicting results concerning whether low testosterone is associated with an increased mortality rate (Table 27-1).[33-37] Overall, testosterone should be considered a quality of life drug and not a life extension drug. The major effects of testosterone are to enhance libido and sexual function.[38] Testosterone also increases muscle and bone mass and muscle strength in hypogonadal males.[39] No studies have evaluated its effect on hip fracture. Testosterone also increases visuospatial cognition.[40] Studies have suggested that testosterone may be cardioprotective.[41] Despite multiple potential positive effects of testosterone, recommendations for its use in older men, from the International Society for the Study of the Aging Male, are that it should only be given to men who have symptoms and are biochemically hypogonadal.[42] Either the Aging Male Survey or the St. Louis University Androgen Deficiency in the Aging Male (ADAM) questionnaire[43,44] can be used to screen for symptoms (Table 27-2).

Testosterone levels decline rapidly in women between 20 to 45 years of age.[45] The reason for this rapid decline is uncertain. Studies have suggested that testosterone replacement in women may improve libido to a small extent.[46]

The role of estrogen replacement in females following the menopause was muddied by the Women's Health Initiative.[47,48] It appears clear that in women older than 60 years, estrogen replacement will increase cardiovascular disease and mortality. This is similar to the finding of the HERS study.[49] It remains unclear whether there is a place for estrogen at the time of menopause. In women with premature menopause, estrogen replacement

TABLE 27-2 Androgen Deficiency in the Aging Male (ADAM) Questionnaire

Question	Answer (Circle One)*	
1. Do you have a decrease in libido (sex drive)?	Yes	No
2. Do you have a lack of energy?	Yes	No
3. Do you have a decrease in strength and/or endurance?	Yes	No
4. Have you lost height?	Yes	No
5. Have you noticed a decreased enjoyment of life?	Yes	No
6. Are you sad and/or grumpy?	Yes	No
7. Are your erections less strong?	Yes	No
8. Have you noticed a recent deterioration in your ability to play sports?	Yes	No
9. Are you falling asleep after dinner?	Yes	No
10. Has there been a recent deterioration in your work performance?	Yes	No

*A positive answer represents yes to question 1 or 7 or any three other questions.

appears to be reasonable until the age of 52 years. Women with menopause who are between the ages of 45 to 55 years may benefit from estrogen replacement in low doses, both to treat symptoms and delay the loss of bone. At this time, its effect on cardiovascular disease is uncertain, but some authorities believe that it may be cardioprotective at this time period (the critical period hypothesis). In women with normal menopause, estrogen should most probably not be used for more than 5 years. Similar caveats exist for the use of progesterone and, when necessary to use, one should consider a progestogen with aldosterone antagonistic properties.

Rudman and associates[50] created a craze for growth hormone replacement as a "fountain of youth" based on their article in the *New England Journal of Medicine*. Their paper, citing the negative effects of growth hormone in older men, was published later in *Clinical Endocrinology* and has been generally ignored by antiaging pundits.[51] However, a meta-analysis published in 2007 could find no positive effects of growth hormone in older adults.[52] Studies with ghrelin agonists in older adults have been equally disappointing. Ghrelin is a peptide hormone released from the fundus of the stomach that increases appetite, releases growth hormone, and enhances memory.[53] A Google search for "growth hormone and aging" resulted in 1,360,000 citations. These included a large number of sponsored links selling growth hormone or physicians who prescribe it. These advertisements included statements such as "Using growth hormone combats the ravages of aging," "Can aging be reversed," and "Growth hormone releaser: fight the aging process effectively." Dehydroepiandrosterone (DHEA) and its sulfate levels fall dramatically with increasing age.[54] This has resulted in multiple claims that DHEA can rejuvenate older adults. However, large well-controlled studies have failed to show any effects of DHEA on aging.[55] A Google search for "DHEA and aging" yielded 758,000 citations. A quotation from one of these sites says that "DHEA stands out as a multitalented star with amazing ways...."

On the Internet, pregnenolone has been called "the feel-good hormone" or "the mother hormone." Our studies in mice have shown that pregnenolone is a potent memory enhancer.[56] However, the ability to demonstrate similar effects in humans has been largely negative; at present, there is no evidence that pregnenolone in humans is a memory enhancer or antiaging hormone.[57]

Levels of melatonin, a hormone produced by the pineal gland, also decline with aging. It has antioxidant properties and, as such, has been touted as an antiaging hormone and soporific. Overall, it appears to have minimal effects.

Marcus Tullius Cicero (106-43 BC) said that "Old age must be resisted and its deficiencies restored." With the exception of vitamin D, there is little evidence that hormone replacement should be used in an attempt to reverse the aging process. Despite this, it would appear that unscrupulous charlatans will continue to prescribe and supply them inappropriately, and the aging populace will hungrily devour them with the hope of staying young forever.

ANTIOXIDANTS AND AGING

Multiple animal studies have shown a role for oxidative stress in aging.[58] Oxidative damage has also been implicated in the pathogenesis of age-related diseases, such as atherosclerosis and Alzheimer disease. It is clear that consumption of fruits and vegetables that are rich in antioxidants appears to prevent disease. However, there is no evidence that persons taking vitamin supplements have a longer life than those who do not take supplements. Studies of vitamin E and cardiovascular disease in humans have found that supplementation has no effect or is harmful.[59] Similarly, effects of vitamin E on cancer have suggested mixed results. Vitamin E had minimal effects on people with Alzheimer disease.

β-Carotene in the ATBC trial resulted in an increase in lung, prostate, and stomach cancers.[60] The CARET study also resulted in an increase in lung cancer deaths in people previously exposed to asbestos.[61] No positive effects of β-carotene on cardiovascular disease have been found in a number of studies.[62] Similarly, vitamin C has been shown to have minimal beneficial effects.

α-Lipoic acid is a powerful antioxidant. It has been shown to be useful in the treatment of diabetic neuropathy.[63] It has reversed memory disturbances in SAMP8 mice, a partial model of Alzheimer disease.[64] However, our unpublished studies in mice have shown that it increased mortality rates.

Overall, human studies do not support the use of antioxidant vitamin supplementation. The one exception may be the use of high-dose multivitamins in age-related macular degeneration. Based on the available data, high-dose vitamin supplementation cannot be considered to be benign.

PHOTOAGING

Skin aging occurs because of environmental damage, which interacts with chronologic aging.[65] Photoaging occurs as a result of ultraviolet light exposure. With the aging of the population, there has been an explosion of medications, cosmetics, and dermatologic procedures that attempt to reverse the aging process (Table 27-3). These modalities are used to remove or prevent wrinkles, rough skin, telangiectasia, actinic keratosis, brown spots, and benign neoplasia. In 2002, more than $13 billion was spent on 5 million cosmetic procedures and more than 1 million plastic surgery procedures. Relatively common antiaging plastic surgery procedures include rhytidectomy (face lift), blepharoplasty, abdominoplasty (tummy tuck), and lipectomy or liposuction. These procedures are costly and pander to the vanity of our new aging population.

OTHER CONSIDERATIONS

Today's science fiction may well represent tomorrow's antiaging technology. The rapid advances in robotic prosthesis and exoskeletons will further enhance the ability of older adults to function well in late life.

Antiaging medicine raises a number of ethical issues, such as the following:

- In a society of limited resources, is extending the life of older adults appropriate?
- Is extending life without improved quality appropriate?
- What if life extension were associated with cognitive impairment?
- How long is it appropriate to extend life—5, 10, 20, 50, or even 100 years?

There are no simple answers to any of these questions, and the answers depend not only on scientific and philosophical studies, but also on religious views and fiscal realities.

Every year, changes in medical knowledge are leading to increased longevity and improved quality of life. It needs to be recognized that not all advances in mainstream medicine have positive effects but, overall, medical advances are at present the strongest antiaging medicine. In contrast, the aging public continues to spend billions of dollars on antiaging potions of little proven value. Geriatricians will continue to be at the forefront of educators on how to age successfully.

TABLE 27-3 Cosmetic Antiaging Products

Product	Action	Side Effects
Sunscreen with a sun protection factor (SPF) > 15	Decrease actinic keratosis and squamous cell carcinoma	Allergic reactions occur in one in five persons
α- and β-Hydroxyl acids	Exfoliants—decrease roughness and some pigmentation	Irritation of skin
Retinoids (tretinoin and tazarotene)	Decrease pigmentation, wrinkling, and roughness	Irritation of skin
Fluorouracil cream	Actinic keratosis	Irritation of skin
Laser therapy	Wrinkles, pigmentation, telangiectasia	Scarring, hypopigmentation, bruising
Dermabrasion	Wrinkles, actinic keratoses	Scarring, pain, infection
Skin fillers (collagen and hyaluronic acid)	Wrinkles	Pain, allergic reactions
Botox	Wrinkles	Bruising, ptosis, headaches

CONCLUSION

Amazing breakthroughs in the understanding of the aging process are occurring almost daily in cellular and animal models. Gerontologists, like Tantalus (a Greek mythologic figure), are consistently being tempted to apply these findings instantly in humans before appropriate controlled trials are carried out. As history has shown, this is a dangerous precedent. Treatments that are highly effective in animals can be highly toxic in humans. The geriatrician plays an important role in being able to educate older adults regarding the positives and negatives of antiaging medicines.

Two areas that have the potential to change the antiaging field are stem cells and computers. Studies with stem cells carrying muscle IGF-1 in rodents have shown that they can reverse muscle loss in old animals.[66] The potential for stem cells to rejuvenate a variety of tissues is enormous but its application to humans is in its infancy. Also, we are beginning to see computer-enhanced technology used to reverse age-related deficits. Examples are cochlear implants and retinal computer chips. As computer technology advances, Kurzweil has suggested that hippocampal computer chips could be used to treat Alzheimer disease.

KEY POINTS: ANTIAGING MEDICINE

- The factors best demonstrated to delay aging are fruit and vegetables, exercise, not smoking, drinking one or two glasses of alcohol daily, and fish consumption.
- Vitamin D replacement in persons with low 25(OH) vitamin D levels decreases hip fractures, improves muscle strength, enhances function, and decreases mortality.
- Antiaging medicine has been hijacked by charlatans who promote unproven or dangerous remedies to a naïve aging public.
- Too often, animal studies that produce longevity are directly applied to humans before appropriate clinical trials have been carried out.
- There is no evidence that hormones or megadoses of vitamins prolong life.
- Numerous products of varying quality are available to slow photoaging and remove skin blemishes.

For a complete list of references, please visit www.expertconsult.com.

KEY REFERENCES

5. Morley JE, Colberg ST: The science of staying young, New York, 2007, McGraw-Hill.
6. Morley JE: A brief history of geriatrics. J Gerontol A Biol Sci Med Sci 59:1132–1152, 2004.
15. Mattison JA, Roth GS, Beasley TM, et al: Impact of calorie restriction on health and survival in rhesus monkeys from the NIA study. Nature 489:318–321, 2012.
17. Bauer JA, Sinclair OA: Therapeutic potential of resveratrol: the in vivo evidence. Nat Rev Drug Discov 5:493–506, 2006.
23. Willcox BJ, Willcox DC: Calorie restriction, calorie restriction mimetics, and healthy aging in Okinawa: controversies and clinical implications. Curr Opin Clin Nutr Metab Care 17:51–58, 2014.
31. Morley JE: Should all long-term care residents receive vitamin D? J Am Med Dir Assoc 8:69–70, 2007.
65. Stern RS: Clinical practice. Treatment of photoaging. N Engl J Med 350:1526–1534, 2004.
66. Musaro A, Giacinti C, Borsellino G, et al: Stem cell–mediated muscle regeneration is enhanced by local isoform of insulin-like growth factor 1. Proc Natl Acad Sci U S A 101:1206–1210, 2004.

28 Normal Cognitive Aging*

Jane Martin, Clara Li

This chapter provides an overview of the principal features of cognitive functioning in normal aging adults. The first part of this chapter considers intelligence and the importance of estimating premorbid intellectual ability to detect discrepancies in functioning, followed by the concept of cognitive reserve being protective as we age. The cognitive functions of attention and processing speed, memory, verbal abilities, and executive functions are discussed before a final section regarding the lifestyle factors associated with cognitive functioning. "Normal" in the present context refers to older adults with no discernible mental illness and whose physical health is typical of their age group.

INTELLIGENCE AND AGING

The U.S. Bureau of the Census[1] projected that between 2010 and 2050, the United States is expected to experience rapid growth in its older population and, in 2050, the number of Americans aged 65 years and older is estimated to be 88.5 million. According to the Alzheimer's Association,[2] an estimated 5.2 million Americans would have had Alzheimer disease in 2014, including approximately 200,000 individuals younger than age 65 years who have younger onset Alzheimer's. Thus, cognitive studies of older adults are an important area of research. There is a need to understand what is normal or typical aging in contrast to the development of a disease process and to understand what factors contribute to improved cognitive status with increasing age.

Literature on cognitive aging is based on studies of performance on standardized intelligence and neuropsychological tests. "IQ" refers to a derived score used in many test batteries designed to measure a hypothesized general ability, intelligence. The accepted definition is that general intelligence, or *g*, is a measure of overall ability on all types of intellectual tasks. General intelligence can be more specifically divided into the concepts of fluid intelligence and crystallized intelligence.[3] Fluid intelligence is the primary factor of most intelligence tests, measuring the degree to which an individual can solve novel problems without any previous training. On the other hand, crystallized intelligence is the amount of knowledge and information from the world that one brings to the testing situation. It has been established that fluid intelligence declines in older adults, and crystallized intelligence is well preserved. The general theory is that fluid intelligence increases throughout childhood into young adulthood, but then plateaus and eventually declines; crystallized intelligence increases from childhood into late adulthood.[3]

Because a multitude of cognitive functions are assessed in an intelligence battery, and IQ scores represent a composite of performances on different kinds of items, the meaningfulness of IQ is often questioned.[4] The only widely agreed on value of IQ tests is that IQ scores are good predictors of educational achievement and, consequently, occupational outcome. The argument about the usefulness of IQ scores is that a composite score does not highlight important information that is only obtainable by examining discrete scores. Consequently, most widely used tests, such as the Wechsler Adult Intelligence Scale (WAIS-IV),[5] now include measures of more discrete factors and domains. Even with limitations, IQ scores help provide a baseline of overall intellectual functioning from which to assess performance on cognitive tests as we age.

Premorbid Ability

Lezak and colleagues have cautioned that an estimate of premorbid ability should never be based on a single test score, but should take into account as much information about the individual as possible.[4] Thus, a good premorbid estimation of intelligence in adults uses current performance on tasks thought to be fairly resistant to neurologic change and demographics, such as educational and occupational attainment. This approach uses test scores obtained in the formal testing session of "hold" tests—that is, tests that tap abilities considered resistant to the effects of cerebral insult.[6] Aspects of cognitive functioning that involve overlearned activities change very little in the course of aging, whereas functions that involve processing speed, processing unfamiliar information, complex problem solving, and delayed recall of information typically decline with age.[7] On the WAIS-IV,[5] tests such as vocabulary and information are considered relatively resistant to the effects of aging and thus are useful hold tests to help estimate overall premorbid levels of cognitive functioning. However, there are limitations that must be considered. For example, the information subtest reflects an individual's general fund of information, and the score may be misleading, because this test is strongly affected by level of education. Scores on word reading tests, such as the National Adult Reading Test (NART),[8] developed in Britain, and the subsequent American National Adult Reading Test (AMNART),[9] for use in the United States, correlate highly with IQ and have been found to be relatively resistant to cerebral insult.[6] However, the AMNART is not useful for an aphasic individual or someone with visual or articulatory problems. Again, the practice of using many sources of information to estimate an individual's premorbid level of cognitive functioning is essential.

Premorbid estimation of overall intellectual functioning is important to establish to compare current performance against some standard measure. However, comparing an individual's performance to a general population average score is misleading because it is only useful if the individual matches the population in terms of demographic measures, such as IQ and education. For example, average performance may be considered functioning at a normal level for one individual and may represent a significant decline for another individual. Thus, a more useful approach is to compare an individual's current performance against an individualized standard. Only in this way can deficits or a diagnosis be discerned. Because premorbid neuropsychological test data are rarely available, it becomes necessary to estimate an individual's premorbid level of intellectual functioning against which present test scores can be compared to determine a change in cognitive functioning. Assessing a deficit involves comparing an individual's present performance on cognitive tests to an estimate of the

*Material in this chapter contains contributions from the previous edition, and we are grateful to the previous authors for the work done.

individual's original ability level (premorbid level) and evaluating the discrepancies.[4]

Cognitive Reserve

The concept of cognitive reserve[10-12] proposes that there are differences in how individuals are able to compensate once pathology disrupts the brain networks that normally underlie performance. Thus, variability exists across individuals in their ability to compensate for cognitive changes as they age. The cognitive reserve model evolved in response to the fact that often there is no direct relationship between the degree of brain pathology that disrupts performance and the degree of disruption in actual performance across individuals. In other words, individuals with a similar degree of brain pathology often differ in their clinical presentation of functional ability. Reserve may represent naturally occurring individual differences in the ability to perform a task or deal with increases in task difficulty. These differences may be due to innate intellectual ability, such as IQ, and/or they may be altered by experiences of education, occupation, or leisure activities.[11,12] Stern and associates[11,12] have suggested that higher neural reserve might mean that brain networks that are more efficient or more flexible in the presence of increased demand may be less susceptible to disruption. This model suggests that the brain actively attempts to compensate for the challenge represented by brain disease and hypothesizes that adults with higher initial cognitive ability are better able to compensate for the effects of aging and dementia.[10,12] However, the cognitive or neural mechanism that underlies cognitive reserve remains unknown. Research in the area of cognitive reserve has recently focused on using functional brain imaging (fMRI) to identify networks that might mediate cognitive reserve.[12] Stern and coworkers have proposed two forms of neural mechanisms that underlie cognitive reserve, neural reserve and neural compensation. Neural reserve refers to the idea that reserve may be associated with individual differences in the utility of preexisting cognitive networks. Neural compensation refers to the idea that some individuals may be better able to use compensatory resources than others.[12] Recent neuroimaging studies have supported the view that older cognitively normal adults, with higher cognitive reserve, have neural networks that operate more efficiently when task demands increase.[12,13]

According to the cognitive reserve model, impairments in cognition become apparent after a reserve is depleted. Individuals with less reserve are likely to exhibit clinical impairments because they have relatively fewer resources to maintain them in the course of normal aging and disease-related changes, whereas individuals with more initial reserve can function longer without obvious clinical impairments because their supply of resources is greater.[14] The initial level of cognitive reserve may be determined by numerous factors, such as innate intellectual ability and differences in cognitive activity as the brain matures throughout the life span. It has been found that early education and higher levels of intellectual ability and activity are associated with slower cognitive decline as individuals age.[12,14-17] Fritsch and associates[14] found that IQ and education had direct effects on global cognitive functioning, episodic memory, and processing speed, but that other midlife factors, such as occupational demands, were not significant predictors of late life cognition. Studies of the relationship between childhood intelligence and cognitive decline in later life have found that individuals with lower childhood mental ability experience greater cognitive decline than those with higher childhood mental ability, suggesting that higher premorbid cognitive ability is protective of decline in later life.[15] Kliegel and coworkers[16] found that early education and lifelong intellectual activities seem to be important to cognitive performance in old age; higher early education and the greater number of intellectual activities continued throughout life served as a buffer against becoming cognitively impaired. Cognitive reserve research suggests that an active engaged lifestyle, emphasizing mental activity and educational pursuits in early life, has a positive impact on cognitive functioning in later life. Thus, individuals whose baseline cognitive functioning is at higher levels and who have an engaged lifestyle, which typically includes interpersonal relationships and productive activities, will likely show less cognitive decline with age. Cognitive reserve is not a fixed entity but can change across the life span, depending on exposure and behavior, which suggests that changes in lifestyle, even later in life, can provide cognitive reserve against age- or disease-related pathology.[12]

Attention and Processing Speed

Attention relates to one's ability to focus and concentrate on a given stimuli for a sustained period of time. Attention is a complex process that allows one to filter stimuli from the environment, hold and manipulate information, and respond appropriately.[6] Models of attention typically divide attention into various processes, such as alertness and arousal, selective attention, divided attention, and sustained attention. There is a limited amount of information that the brain can process at a given time. Attention allows one to function effectively by selecting the specific information to be processed and filtering out the unnecessary information.

It is difficult to assess pure attention because many tests of attention overlap with tests of executive function, verbal and visual skills, motor speed, information processing speed, and memory. Traditional methods of assessing attention involve timed tasks and tests of working memory. The Wechsler subtest, digit span,[5] is a common method for assessing attention span for immediate verbal recall of numbers. Digit span involves the examiner reading progressively longer strings of digits for the individual to repeat forward, backward, and in sequence. Thus, repeating and manipulating the digits requires auditory attention and is dependent on short-term memory retention. Another commonly used test to assess attention is the Continuous Performance Test of Attention (CPTA).[18] The CPTA is administered on a computer and consists of the individual seeing and listening to a series of letters and tap with a finger each time the target letter is presented.

Attentional processes, like other cognitive functioning, change over the course of the life span, but attention is particularly vulnerable to the process of aging. Moreover, the effects of aging on attention are related to the complexity of the task. Attention on simple tasks, such as the digit span task, is relatively well preserved into the 80s. On the other hand, on tasks that require divided attention, older adults respond more slowly and make more errors. In normal aging, there is typically a decline in sustained and selective attention and an increase in distractibility.[19]

With regard to aging and cognition, attention is a prerequisite for healthy memory functioning. Attention is necessary in the process of encoding information for future retrieval from memory and, as we age, the complex processes of encoding and retrieving information require greater attentional resources. Intact attention is also required for the processing of information; processing speed is the rate at which one can process information. Cognitive processing speed refers to how fast a person can execute the mental operations needed to complete the task at hand.[20] It is widely believed that the age-related slowing in processing speed underlies declines in other cognitive areas, including memory and executive functioning.[21] It is often difficult to assess pure processing speed because many tasks also reflect a visual and/or motor component. Timed tests can measure processing speed and also help the examiner to gain a better understanding of attentional deficits.[22] Slowed processing speed is demonstrated in slower reaction times and in a longer than average performance time.[6]

One test frequently used to assess processing speed is the Trail Making Test, Part A.[6] This is a timed sequencing test that requires individuals to draw a line from one number to the next in numeric order. Timed visual scanning tasks, requiring a target letter, number, or symbol to be identified, are also used to assess processing speed.

The processing speed theory proposes that the decline seen in memory and other cognitive processes with normal aging is due, in part, to slow processing speed. It has been estimated that older adults' response time is approximately 1.5 times slower than that of younger adults.[23] It is hypothesized that slower processing speed affects cognition in two ways, the limited time mechanism and the simultaneity mechanism.[24] The limited time mechanism occurs when relevant cognitive processes are performed too slowly and therefore cannot be accomplished in the expected time. The simultaneity mechanism occurs when slower processing reduces the amount of information available for later processing to be completed. In other words, relevant information may not be accessible when it is needed because it was not encoded. However, slower processing speed associated with normal aging does not affect an individual's performance across all tasks. Processing speed has a stronger relationship to tasks of fluid intelligence than crystallized intelligence. Slower processing speed in older adults accounts for the decline in fluid ability (e.g., memory, spatial ability) with aging, but not crystallized ability (e.g., verbal ability).[25] Longitudinal data on cognitive performance across the life span have suggested that the decline in processing speed performance begins at an earlier age and progresses at a steeper rate compared to memory functioning, which declines later in life.[26]

Memory

Memory is commonly thought of as the ability to recall past events and learned information. However, aside from remembering information from the past, memory includes memory for future events (remembering an appointment), autobiographical information, and keeping track of information in the present (e.g., a conversation or reading prose). Memory can be discussed in terms of the complex processes whereby the individual encodes, stores, and retrieves information. Memory can also be divided into the length of time the items have been mentally stored—thus, the distinction between short-term memory and long-term memory. In addition, memory can be organized by the type of material being stored, such as visual or verbal or autobiographical information. Similar to other areas of cognitive functioning, different aspects of memory differ in how they change with aging.

Working Memory (Short-Term Memory)

Working memory or short-term memory is seen as a limited capacity store for retaining information over the short term (seconds to 1 to 2 minutes) and for performing mental operations on the contents.[6] Immediate memory, the first stage of short-term memory, temporarily holds information and may also be thought of as one's immediate attention span. The recognized limited capacity store of approximately seven bits of information[27] requires that information is transferred from short-term memory to a more permanent store for later recall. Baddeley and Hitch have proposed a model that divides short-term or working memory into two systems—one phonologic, for processing language (verbal) information, and one visual-spatial, for processing visual information.[28-30] This model holds that short-term memory is controlled by a limited capacity attentional system and thus is organized by a so-called central executive. The central executive assigns information to be remembered to the visuospatial sketch pad (for memory of visual and spatial information) or the phonologic loop (for verbal materials). The overall concept is that more specialized storage systems exist in the limited short-term store that distinguish between verbal and visual information to be stored. Through rehearsal in working memory (e.g., repetition), copies of the information are sent for long-term storage. Regardless of the particular memory model, the overall idea is that short-term memory is a temporary holding ground for information that can be processed or encoded into long-term memory.

Working memory is typically assessed by asking an individual to recall or repeat back words, letters, or numbers, often with sequences of varying length. Using this method, short-term memory span shows only a slight age effect.[4] However, short-term memory becomes vulnerable to aging when the task becomes more complex and requires mental manipulation. For example, on Wechsler's subtest, digit span, individuals are presented with progressively longer strings of numbers verbally and are asked to recall immediately digits in a forward order, reverse order, and in sequence from lowest to highest. It is when the task requires more than attention span and individuals have to recall the numbers backward and in sequence, thus manipulating the material, that older adults perform disproportionately weaker than younger adults.[4]

The issue of how aging affects short-term or working memory is associated with the level of complexity of the particular task and presence of a distracting task. Older adults have been found to have difficulty suppressing irrelevant information from the recent past.[31] Difficulties in processing due to changes in inhibitory control result in increased difficulty for selecting relevant information on which to focus in working memory, as well as difficulty in shifting focus while ignoring distracting information.[32] Although working memory capacity is an important facet in the process of learning new information, attention and processing speed are inextricably linked to one's ability to learn. In daily life, older adults perform cognitively best when they focus on one task at a time because attention and processing speed are not divided. Simple memory strategies, such as writing down information or rehearsing information aloud, can help compensate for memory changes as we age. Such mental techniques aid older adults' ability to move information from short-term to long-term memory. It is important to note that short-term memory decline is part of normal aging, and generally these age-related changes do not affect daily functioning in the disruptive way that the presence of dementia affects daily functioning.

Long-Term Memory

Long-term memory refers to the acquisition of new information that is available for access at a later point in time and involves the processes of encoding, storage, and retrieval of information. Although long-term memory typically means memory for information from the past, it also involves memory for future events or what is termed *prospective memory*. An example of prospective memory is remembering a future physician's appointment or remembering to take medication; it requires that a memory be maintained about what must be done before the action takes place. Despite numerous theories about the stages of memory or processing levels, the dual system conceptualization of two long-term memory systems (explicit and implicit) provides a useful model for clinical use to understand patterns of functioning and deficits.[4,6,30,33] Explicit memory refers to the intentional recollection of previous experiences; an individual consciously attempts to recall information and events. To assess explicit memory, verbal or visual information (e.g., words or pictures) is presented and, after a delay, the individual is asked to recall the material through simple recall or a recognition task. Implicit memory, on the other hand, relates to knowledge that is observable in performance, but without the awareness that one holds this information. For example, the ability to ride a bicycle does not depend on the conscious awareness of the particular skills involved in the activity.

Explicit Memory. Explicit memory, often referred to as declarative memory, can further be divided into episodic memory and semantic memory. Episodic memory refers to the ability to recollect everyday experiences.[34] More specifically, episodic memory is the conscious recollection of personal events, along with the specific time and place (context) that they occurred. Episodic material includes autobiographical information, such as the birth of a child or graduation from high school, and includes personal information, such as a meal from the previous day or a recent golf game. These are memories that relate to an individual's own unique experience and include the details of "when and where" an event occurred. Most memory tests assess episodic memory and usually involve a free recall (retrieval), cued recall, and recognition trial and rely on an individual's ability to recollect the material to which he or she was previously exposed.[6] Compared to younger adults, older adults typically perform better on recognition tasks as opposed to recall tasks. Recognition requires less cognitive effort because a target or cue is provided as a prompt to aid recall, as opposed to a recall task, which requires an individual to recall the material to which she or he was previously exposed, without any prompt. Overall, older adults are most disadvantaged when tests use explicit memory, in particular episodic memory, compared to younger adults.[35,36]

Semantic memory is an individual's knowledge about the world and includes memory of the meanings of words (vocabulary), facts, and concepts and, contrary to episodic memory, is not context-dependent. Knowledge is remembered regardless of when and where it was learned, such as word definitions or knowing the years when WWII occurred. Tests that assess semantic memory include vocabulary and word identification tests (e.g., AMNART),[9] category fluency tasks (e.g., Animal Naming Test),[37] and confrontational or object naming tests (e.g., Boston Naming Test).[38] When most older adults report memory complaints, they are often referring to their difficulty in remembering words and names of objects and people.[39]

Tests that require recall of semantically unrelated material, such as the Rey Auditory-Verbal Learning Test (RAVLT)[40] word lists, are seen as more difficult because they require more effortful strategies for encoding and retrieval than story recall tests, such as Wechsler's Logical Memory (WMS-IV, Logical Memory)[41] or semantically related word lists, such as the California Verbal Learning Test (CVLT-II).[42] When information is presented in a context, or words on a list belong to a category and are semantically related, the material presented is already organized in a meaningful way, which aids the recall processes. These memory tests include delayed recall and recognition trials to discern whether a deficit relates to the storage rather than retrieval of information.[4]

Implicit Memory (Procedural Memory). Implicit memory, often referred to as nondeclarative memory, does not require the conscious or explicit recollection of past events or information, and the individual is unaware that remembering has occurred. Implicit memory is usually thought of in terms of procedural memory, but also involves the process of priming. Priming is a type of cued recall in that an individual is exposed to material without his or her awareness, and this prior exposure aids a future response. For example, having been shown the word *green*, individuals will be more likely to respond "green" when later asked to complete the word fragment g_e_ _, even though *great* is a more common word.[43] Similarly, the prior brief presentation of a word increases the likelihood of identifying it correctly when presented with a choice of words at a later time.[44] Advertising is based on the concept of priming because the exposure to a product may lead to selecting that product for future purchase.

Procedural memory relates to skill learning and includes motor and cognitive skill learning, as well as perceptual or "how to" learning.[4] Riding a bicycle, driving a car, and playing tennis are examples of procedural memory. It is generally accepted that implicit memory processes are relatively unimpaired in older adults; on simple tasks, there is little or no difference between older and younger adults, although greater age deficits emerge when the implicit learning task is more complex.[35] A good example of how implicit (procedural) memory is preserved with aging is the observation of patients with amnesia who lack the ability to learn new information, but still remember how to walk, dress, and perform other skill-dependent activities.[45] Most research on implicit memory has focused on the finding that the repetition of information aids performance, even when conscious memory of the prior experience is not needed.[44] The overall conclusion from research on implicit memory is that there is relatively little age-related change in this area compared to explicit memory tasks, which involve active recall or recognition of information.

Overall Age-Related Changes in Memory

Retrieval of information is an important part of daily functioning. With normal aging, memory deficits are associated primarily with the storage of long-term episodic memories. Information that places little demand on attention, such as implicit memory tasks, results in very little age-related changes in performance. The advantage that older adults experience on recognition tasks indicates that their memory storage and retrieval may be much less efficient than that of younger adults. A processing speed perspective illustrates that normal aging is accompanied by a slowing in overall cognitive processing, and it is accepted that older adults process information at a slower rate compared to younger adults. Salthouse[24] found that after statistically controlling for processing speed, age was only weakly related to memory. Memory functioning in normal aging is thus mediated by processing speed. The reduced attentional resources concept[23,46] suggests that a limited amount of cognitive resources are available for a given task and, consequently, a more complex task requires more attentional capacity than a simpler task. It follows that because the amount of attentional resources is reduced with aging, the processes of encoding and retrieval of information use a larger proportion of available resources for older adults than for younger adults. Thus, research suggests that overall cognitive slowing and changes in attentional ability account for much of the change in memory functioning as we age.

Verbal Abilities

Most verbal abilities remain intact with normal aging.[47] Therefore, vocabulary and verbal reasoning scores remain relatively constant in normal aging and may even show minor improvements. The two main areas of verbal abilities that are frequently discussed in terms of aging are verbal fluency (semantic and phonemic) and confrontation naming. Verbal fluency is the ability to retrieve words based on their meaning or their sounds. Confrontation naming describes the ability to identify an object by its name.

Two common tests used to assess verbal fluency are the Controlled Oral Word Association Test (COWAT)[48] and the Semantic Fluency Test.[37] COWAT is perhaps the most widely used test of phonemic fluency. The COWAT task requires individuals to generate as many words as quickly as they can that begin with a specific letter. The semantic fluency task is a timed test that requires the individual to generate examples in a specific category (e.g., Animal Naming Test).

The Boston Naming Test[35] is a commonly used test to measure confrontation naming ability because individuals are required to name the object in the presented picture. Confrontation naming is comprised of several different processes—an individual must perceive the object in the picture correctly, identify the semantic concept of the picture, and retrieve and express the appropriate name for the object.[49] Confrontation naming ability is associated with the tip-of-the-tongue phenomenon (TOT). TOT occurs when an individual knows the name of a person or object and is able to retrieve the semantic information about the object, but cannot retrieve the name of the object.[50] Although an individual is unable to retrieve the target word, he or she will often try to describe the term using other words.[51] Throughout all of adulthood, proper nouns comprise most of the TOT experiences. However, the increase in TOT among older adults is due to their greater difficulty in retrieving proper nouns.[50] There is no significant age difference in the frequency of TOT episodes for simple words. However, older adults have significantly more TOT experiences than younger adults for difficult words.[51] Thus, word-finding difficulty and TOT moments are the most common cognitive complaints of older adults.

Most cross-sectional studies have found that older adults have lower scores on the Boston Naming Test compared to younger individuals. It should be noted that although subjective complaints of word-finding difficulties increase with age, significantly lower performance on tasks of confrontation naming only emerges after age 70.[50] Zec and colleagues[52] found that confrontation naming ability, as measured by the Boston Naming Test, improves when individuals are in their 50s, remain the same in their 60s, and decline in the 70s and 80s; it should be noted that the magnitude of these age-related changes is relatively small. It was found that there was an approximate one-word improvement in the 50s age group and a 1.3-word decline in the 70s age group. There is some indication that there is an accelerated rate of decline in confrontation naming ability with age.[50]

Normal aging is associated with a decline in verbal fluency. It is important to note that the normal age-related decline seen in verbal fluency performance may be partially mediated by reduced psychomotor speed rather than by true deficits in verbal ability. Slower handwriting and reading speed in older adults was predictive of poorer performance on verbal fluency tests.[53] Rodriguez-Aranda and Martinussen[54] found a decline in verbal fluency, as measured by the COWAT, after age 60. The ability to generate words beginning with a particular letter improves until the third decade of life and remains constant through the 40s. Subsequently, a significant decline occurs in phonemic naming ability and continues to worsen gradually until the late 60s. Phonemic verbal fluency ability continues to decline rapidly through the late 80s. Gender and education may affect a person's phonemic verbal fluency across the life span. Women may slightly outperform men on tasks of phonemic verbal fluency. Individuals with higher levels of education (beyond high school) show greater verbal fluency ability, as measured by the COWAT, compared to individuals with lower levels of education (≤12 years).[55]

Executive Functions

Executive functions describe a wide range of abilities that relate to the capacity to respond to a novel situation.[19] Executive functions include abilities such as mental flexibility, response inhibition, planning, organization, abstraction, and decision making.[56,57] Executive function can be thought of as having four distinct components—volition, planning, purposive action, and effective performance.[4] Volition is a complex process that refers to the ability to act intentionally. Planning is the process and steps involved in achieving the goal. Purposive action refers to the productive activity required to execute a plan. Effective performance is the ability to self-correct and monitor one's behavior while working. All of the components of executive functioning are necessary for problem solving and appropriate social behavior.

Another term for executive functions is *frontal lobe functions*, because these abilities are localized in the prefrontal cortex.[58] The Frontal Aging Hypothesis refers to the idea that the frontal lobes, a late myelinating region, are most vulnerable to age-related deterioration.[59] Thus, normal aging, which is associated with a loss of volume in the prefrontal cortex, is associated with cognitive deficits. Prefrontal deterioration plays a key role in many of the age-related changes in cognitive processes, such as memory, attention, and executive function.[60]

Like many cognitive processes, it is difficult to assess pure executive function because many of the measures used in its assessment rely on other cognitive processes, such as working memory, processing speed, attention, and visual spatial abilities. The Wisconsin Card Sorting Task (WCST)[61] is a popular test used to measure executive function. The WCST requires an individual to sort a set of cards based on different categories. Individuals are not informed about how to sort the cards and must deduce the correct sorting strategies through the limited feedback that is provided. After a particular category is achieved (e.g., a set number of correct responses), based on a particular characteristic (e.g., color or shape), the sorting strategy changes, and the individual must shift strategies accordingly. Once the test is completed, the examiner is provided with several measures related to executive function—for example, categories and perseverative errors. A category is achieved when a specific number of cards have been sorted correctly based on the particular criterion, such as, color. Perseverative errors occur when an individual continues to give the wrong response when provided with feedback that the strategy is not or is no longer correct, thus demonstrating a lack of cognitive flexibility.

On the WCST, older adults achieve significantly fewer categories than younger adults.[58] The most significant decline in performance on this test is seen in adults age 75 years and older. Individuals in this age group achieve significantly fewer categories and more perseverative errors compared to younger individuals. However, changes in executive functioning, as measured by neuropsychological assessment such as the WCST, can be seen in adults aged 53 to 64 years, but these adults do not show deficits on more real-world executive tasks.[62] Thus, although individuals in midadulthood may show a decline in executive functioning on structured neuropsychological tests, their real-world executive skills remain intact.

Other measures used in the assessment of executive functioning included the Trail Making Test, Part B,[6] and the WAIS-IV subtests,[5] matrix reasoning and similarities. Trail Making, Part B, is a timed visual-spatial sequencing task requiring an individual to draw connecting lines alternating between numbers and letters in numeric and alphabetic order. Matrix reasoning is an untimed task that measures one's nonverbal analytic thinking abilities. The matrix reasoning task requires an individual to identify the missing element of an abstract pattern from a variety of choices. The WAIS-IV similarities subtest measures an individual's verbal abstract reasoning skills by asking an individual to describe how two different objects or concepts are alike.

Normal aging is generally associated with a decline in executive functioning.[63] When reasoning and problem solving involve material that is novel or complex, or requires the ability to distinguish relevant from irrelevant information, older adults' performance suffers because they tend to think in more concrete terms, and there is a decline in the mental flexibility required to form new abstractions and concepts.[4] Compared to younger adults, older adults also show a decreased capacity to form conceptual links as mental flexibility diminishes.[4] Executive functions serve as the overseer of brain processing and are essential for purposeful, goal-directed behavior. Deficits in executive functioning can be seen in difficulties with planning and organizing, difficulties implementing strategies, and inappropriate social behavior or poor judgment.

LIFESTYLE FACTORS ASSOCIATED WITH COGNITIVE FUNCTIONING

Leisure Activities

The mental exercise hypothesis refers to the idea that keeping mentally active will help maintain an individual's cognitive functioning and prevent cognitive decline. Many activities such as playing bridge, doing crossword puzzles, studying a foreign language, and learning to play an instrument have been suggested to help prevent cognitive decline.[64,65] There is a growing interest in computer-based training games and video games as an effective way of improving aspects of cognition and increasing neural plasticity in older adults.[66] However, the research regarding the mental exercise hypothesis has been varied, and there is currently no definitive answer regarding the role of leisure activities in preventing cognitive decline.

It is suggested that engaging in leisure activities, especially ones that are cognitively demanding, maintains or improves cognitive functioning.[67] However, there is also evidence that individuals with high levels of intellectual functioning engage in more cognitively demanding activities, making it difficult to discern the exact role of mental activities in preventing cognitive decline. This line of research suggests that it is not the activity per se that is responsible for maintaining cognitive functioning, but rather specific lifestyles and living conditions.[67]

Although there is no conclusive evidence regarding the protective factors of leisure activities, several research studies have shown that leisure activities reduce the risk of dementia in older adults.[65-70] Reading, playing board games, learning a musical instrument, visiting friends or relatives, going out (e.g., movies or restaurant), walking for pleasure, and dancing are associated with a reduced risk of dementia.[68,69] Such leisure activities have been shown to protect against memory decline even after controlling for age, gender, education, ethnicity, baseline cognitive status, and medical illness. Participation in an activity for one day per week was found to reduce the risk of dementia by 7%.[68] Individuals who participated in many leisure activities (i.e., six or more activities a month) had a 38% lower risk of developing dementia.[69]

It has been also hypothesized that leisure activities reduce the risk of cognitive decline by enhancing cognitive reserve. A decrease in activity results in reduced cognitive abilities.[71] Engaging in leisure activities may also provide structural changes in the brain that protect against cognitive decline, given that certain areas of the adult brain are able to generate new neurons (plasticity). Stimulation, such as engaging in social, intellectual, and physical activities, is suggested to promote increased synaptic density.[66] Enhanced neuronal activation has been proposed to hinder the development of disease processes, such as dementia.[65,69] However, research has also shown that changes in cognitive reserve are more likely to occur early in life; it is primarily the early experiences of education and intellectual activity that increases cognitive reserve the most.[14] Despite the varied findings, the following should be noted[64]:

> *People should continue to engage in mentally stimulating activities because even if there is not yet evidence that it has beneficial effects in slowing the rate of age-related decline in cognitive functioning, there is no evidence that it has any harmful effects, the activities are often enjoyable and thus may contribute to a higher quality of life, and engagement in cognitively demanding activities serves as an existence proof—if you can still do it, then you know that you have not yet lost it.*
>
> **T.A. Salthouse**

Physical Activities

In 1995, the Centers for Disease Control and Prevention (CDC) and the American College of Sports Medicine (ACSM) published national guidelines on physical activity and public health that recommended 30 minutes or more of moderate-intensity physical activity on most days of the week.[70] It has been hypothesized that engaging in physical activities may enhance cognition and prevent decline in late life because physical activities enhance blood flow to the brain and oxygenation, processes known to slow biologic aging.[14,72] Physical activities reduce cardiovascular and cerebrovascular risk factors that may reduce the risk of vascular dementia and Alzheimer disease.[73] There is also evidence that physical activity may directly affect the brain by preserving neurons and increasing synapses.[74]

Moderate and strenuous physical activity is associated with a decreased risk of cognitive decline. Moderate activity includes playing golf on a weekly basis, playing tennis twice a week, and walking 1.6 m/day. Research has found that long-term regular physical activity, such as walking, is associated with less cognitive decline in women.[75] The benefits of walking at least 1.5 hours/week at a 21- to 30-minute-mile pace are similar to being about 3 years younger and are associated with a 20% reduced risk of significant cognitive decline. In addition, aerobic exercise has been found to have an overall benefit on episodic memory, attention, processing speed, and executive function in nondemented older adults.[76] It has been shown that short-term aerobic training (e.g., 4 to 6 months) increases whole brain and hippocampal volume and regional gray and white matter volumes in the prefrontal cortex.[72] Thus, numerous studies have suggested that exercise can enhance brain structure and function in healthy older adults.

Social Activities

Social support has also been suggested to serve as a protective factor in cognitive decline. Social support may serve as a buffer against stress and may lead to decreased cortisol production in the brain. Lower levels of cortisol result in better performance on tests of episodic memory.[77] Interacting with others may also prevent cognitive decline by providing an individual with increased mental stimulation[78] and may also protect an individual from depression, which has been shown to affect cognition negatively.[79] Depression and mood disorders are associated with an accelerated cognitive decline as people age.[80] Processing speed, attention, and consequently memory may all be affected by depression. In addition, a lack of social interaction also affects older adults' well-being. It has been found that individuals who live alone or have no intimate relationships are at an increased risk of developing dementia; those who are classified as having a poor social network are 60% more likely to develop dementia.[81] Individuals in their 70s who report having limited social support at baseline show greater cognitive decline at follow-up assessments.[79] On the other hand, individuals with greater emotional supports have better performance on cognitive tests.[79] Rowe and Kahn[82] have proposed a model of successful aging as being composed of three main components—avoidance of disease-related disability, maintenance of physical and cognitive functioning, and active engagement in life. Active engagement with life involves maintaining interpersonal relationships, and it has been found that social environment and emotional supports may be protective against cognitive decline and result in a slower decline in functional status.

HEALTH FACTORS

Several medical conditions are associated with cognitive decline. Hypertension is the most prevalent vascular risk factor in older adults.[83] Chronic hypertension has been shown to result in deficits in brain structure, including the reduction of white and gray matter in the prefrontal lobes, atrophy of the hippocampus, and increased white matter hypertensities.[84] Research has found that uncontrolled hypertension can lead to cognitive decline that is independent of normal aging, aside from posing a risk for stroke.[83,85,86] Older adults with hypertension have mild but specific cognitive deficits in the areas of executive function, processing speed, episodic memory, and working memory.[85]

Diabetes mellitus has also been associated with cognitive decline.[87,88] Lipids and other metabolic markers may play a role in the relationship between diabetes and cognition.[89] Diabetes may also affect cognition through confounding factors such as hypertension, heart disease, depression, and decreased physical activity.[89] Diabetes and hypertension are conditions that are typically associated with ischemic lesions in the brain, and there is evidence that these conditions are associated with Alzheimer disease pathology and brain atrophy.[86] Individuals with type 1 diabetes display a slower processing speed and a decline in mental flexibility.[88] Type 2 diabetes is also associated with cognitive decline; longer duration of type 2 diabetes results in greater cognitive decline.[90] Older women with type 2 diabetes have a 30% greater risk of cognitive decline compared to those without diabetes, with a 50% greater risk for individuals with a 15-year or longer history of diabetes.

Dietary factors and vitamin deficiencies have also been associated with cognitive decline in older adults. Individuals with cognitive decline associated with normal aging should be investigated for vitamin B_{12} deficiency. Research has demonstrated that vitamin B_{12} injections may improve executive and language functions in patients with cognitive decline, but will rarely reverse dementia.[91] Low vitamin B levels may be associated with impaired cognitive performance through several possible mechanisms, including multiple central nervous system functions, reactions involving DNA, and the overproduction of homocysteine, which could potentially damage neurons and blood vessels.[92] Low levels of vitamin B_{12} and folic acid result in poorer performance on tasks of free recall, attention, processing speed, and verbal fluency.[93] Overall, research studies have suggested that the effects of vitamin deficiency are most likely seen on complex cognitive tasks that demand greater executive functions.

CONCLUSION

Cognitive decline is a natural part of aging throughout the life span. However, the extent of decline varies across individuals and across the specific cognitive domain being assessed. The cognitive reserve perspective maintains that individual differences with regard to cognitive aging are related to an individual's reserve, which is built on early life factors (educational and intellectual experiences).[10] Although cognitive reserve can be increased in later life, it is more amenable to change in early life. Cognitive decline is inevitable, but all areas of functioning do not change equally. It is well established that older adults process, store, and encode information less efficiently than younger adults. The cognitive functions related to fluid intelligence, such as the ability to solve novel or complex problems, tend to decline with aging, whereas cognitive functions related to crystallized intelligence, such as school-based knowledge, vocabulary, and reading, generally remain stable throughout the life span. Processing speed and attentional capacity are particularly vulnerable to aging, especially on more challenging tasks, and mediate multiple areas of cognitive functioning. For example, a memory problem is often, more accurately, a problem with poor attention and/or slower speed of processing information.

Although research has found cognitive decline in the areas of attention, processing speed, episodic memory, and executive function, research has also shown that older adults have cognitive (or brain) plasticity and may benefit from cognitive training and physical activities.[66,70,72,94] However, the results of cognitive training with normal aging adults has been varied; although improved performance on a specific task can be seen, there is a lack of generalizability to daily functioning in the long term.[95] Nevertheless, maintaining an engaged and healthy lifestyle (social, physical, and intellectual) improve one's quality of life and may contribute to successful aging. One problem is the assumption that successful aging means that there is no discernible change in memory and overall cognitive functioning from the previous level of functioning. Changes in cognition are a normal part of aging and not necessarily a cause for concern or precursor to dementia. It is important that older adults develop a realistic idea of normal aging, focus on reducing risk factors of cognitive decline, and remain active mentally, socially, and physically.

KEY POINTS: NORMAL COGNITIVE AGING

- Variability exists across individuals in their ability to compensate for cognitive changes as they age.
- An active engaged lifestyle, emphasizing mental activity and educational pursuits in early life, has a positive impact on cognitive functioning in later life.
- Participation in physical activity, particularly aerobic exercise, is associated with a lower risk of cognitive decline.
- In normal aging, there is typically a decline in sustained attention, selective attention, and processing speed and an increase in distractibility.
- Older adults' response time is approximately 1.5 times slower than younger adults.
- Most verbal abilities remain intact with normal aging.
- Normal aging is generally associated with a decline in executive functioning.
- Memory deficits associated with normal aging are primarily related to episodic memory.
- Implicit (procedural) memory tasks result in few age-related changes in performance.

For a complete list of references, please visit www.expertconsult.com.

KEY REFERENCES

4. Lezak MD, Howieson DB, Bigler ED, et al: Neuropsychological assessment, ed 5, New York, 2012, Oxford University Press.
6. Strauss E, Sherman EMS, Spreen O: A compendium of neuropsychological tests: administration, norms, and commentary, New York, 2006, Oxford University Press.
10. Stern Y: The concept of cognitive reserve: a catalyst for research. J Clin Exp Neuropsychol 25:589–593, 2003.
12. Stern Y: Cognitive reserve in ageing and Alzheimer's disease. Lancet Neurol 11:1006–1012, 2012.
43. Balota DA, Dolan PO, Duchek JM: Memory changes in healthy older adults. In Tulving E, Craik FIM, editors: The Oxford handbook of memory, New York, 2000, Oxford University Press, pp 395–409.
47. Hannay HJ, Howieson DB, Loring DW, et al: Neuropathology for neuropsychologist. In Lezak MD, Howieson DB, Loring DW, editors: Neuropsychological assessment, ed 4, New York, 2004, Oxford University Press, pp 286–336.
59. Lu PH, Lee GJ, Raven EP, et al: Age-related slowing in cognitive processing speed is associated with myelin integrity in a very healthy elderly sample. J Clin Exp Neuropsychol 33:1059–1068, 2011.
64. Salthouse TA: Mental exercise and mental aging: evaluating the validity of the "use it or lose it" hypothesis. Perspect Psychol Sci 1:68–87, 2006.
68. Verghese J, Lipton RB, Katz MJ, et al: Leisure activities and the risk of dementia in the elderly. N Engl J Med 348:2508–2516, 2003.

76. Smith PJ, Blumenthal JA, Hoffman BM, et al: Aerobic exercise and neurocognitive performance: a meta-analytic review of randomized controlled trials. Psychosom Med 72:239–252, 2010.
89. Kumari M, Marmot M: Diabetes and cognitive function in a middle-aged cohort: Findings from the Whitehall II study. Neurology 65:1597–1603, 2005.
93. Bäckman L, Wahlin A, Small BJ, et al: Cognitive functioning in aging and dementia: the Kungsholmen project. Aging Neuropsychol Cognition 11:212–244, 2004.
94. Ball K, Berch DB, Helmers KF, et al: Effects of cognitive training interventions with older adults: a randomized control trial. JAMA 288:2271–2281, 2002.

29 Social Gerontology

Paul Higgs, James Nazroo

INTRODUCTION

Social gerontology, as the term suggests, is concerned with the study of the social aspects of aging and old age. These include a large range of topics, disciplines, and methods requiring a good understanding of the clinical and economic dimensions of aging. This chapter includes the following discussions: individual experiences of aging (e.g., age identities, social networks and supports, life events, coping, and resilience); the social institutions that provide health and social care services to older adults; how old age is socially constructed and the age-related inequalities that flow from this; the factors that drive social and health inequalities in older age, such as class, gender, ethnicity, and race; and the broad social impact of our aging populations. Central to these studies, however, has been a concern to understand the factors that promote or undermine the well-being, or quality of life, of older adults.

Conclusions from research on older adults' quality of life and their clinical implications were well summarized in Hepburn's chapter in a previous edition of this volume, which focused on factors that contribute to social functioning—social status, social connections, occupations, activities, personal resources, and life events.[1] Here we take a broader view of the social context of aging, describing the development of approaches in social gerontology that seek to theorize and understand the aging experience. We illustrate how these ideas have developed in ways that reflect changes in the experience of aging and show how the drivers of these changes relate to social inequalities at older ages. We begin by describing the tendency in social gerontology to problematize the circumstances of later life through accounts of adjustment, disengagement, dependency, and poverty and through a conceptualization of increasing life expectancy in terms of the potential difficulties that are brought about as populations age. We argue that as later life becomes more of a potentially positive experience for greater numbers of people, such an approach is not the most useful way to view old age. We suggest that we are seeing dramatic changes in the experience of aging that need to be understood in terms of changes to the health and wealth of older adults and in terms of the cultural context of cohorts, such as the baby boomer generation, now entering retirement. These "new" older people challenge much of the thinking about old age and how it relates to gerontology, as well as the reordering of later life into what can be referred to as the third and fourth ages. We conclude by returning to the theme of inequality by exploring the heterogeneity of aging experiences and how these relate to class, gender, ethnicity, and race.

THE "PROBLEM" OF OLD AGE

As Cole, Achenbaum and Katz have observed, current academic concerns with aging have tended to focus on the problem of old age.[2-4] The perception of older adults as a social problem has a long history in social and health research, and this preoccupation with the problems of senescence characterizes the development of gerontology, including social gerontology. Katz[4] has quoted the first article in the first issue of the newly established *Journal of Gerontology* in 1946, which stated that "Gerontology reflects the recognition of a new kind of problem that will increasingly command the interest and devotion of a variety of scientists, scholars, and professional workers."[5] How this influenced the development of specifically social approaches to later life can be seen with the establishment of a Committee on Social Adjustment in Old Age by the U.S. Social Science Research Council in 1944 and a Research Unit into the Problems of Aging by the Nuffield Foundation (England) in 1946. In this immediate postwar period, Sauvy suggested that Britain's economic difficulties were largely the result of an aging population. Furthermore, he claimed that "The danger of a collapse of western civilization owing to a lack of replacement of its human stock cannot be questioned. Perhaps we ought to regard this organic disease, this lack of vitality of the cells, as a symptom of senility of the body politic itself and thus compare social biology with animal biology."[6]

This sense of foreboding had been a strong theme driving earlier developments in social policy. The introduction of old age pensions in Britain in 1908 was not only intended to eliminate extreme poverty in old age, but also to lower "poor law" expenditure on older people.[7] By the mid-1920s, the effects of economic turbulence had moved the terms of debate in the direction of the capacity of retirement to alleviate unemployment. In this formulation, removal from active participation in the workforce was the main motivation for retirement, which in time led to a lowering of the retirement age to 65 years.

In the United States, there were similar concerns to take older workers out of the workforce, with the economic depression of the 1930s creating an impetus for change. However, several factors complicated matters, including the fact that most older people in the United States were still employed. In addition, legislators had to deal with the federal structure of the government, the confusing pattern of Civil War pension entitlements for which many were eligible, and the wide array of pension schemes operating across companies and occupations.[8,9] In this context, the Townsendite movement of the 1930s, named after Dr. Francis E. Townsend, argued for a tax-funded state pension rather than one based on a contributory principle. Furthermore, in advocating the reflationary potential of creating a large number of state-funded consumers, the movement reconceptualized retirement with the slogan "Youth for work, age for leisure."[9] However, the New Deal and its Social Security pension, when it was established in 1935, was much more conventional in its conception, acting as a poverty alleviation program and as a way of dealing with unemployment by using retirement to release jobs to younger workers.

The identification of the old as a problem that needed to be resolved continued along these lines for much of the second half of the twentieth century, although with different national emphases. In Britain, the tradition that included Rowntree's studies of poverty[10,11] continued in the work of Townsend[12] and has been a continuing theme of social gerontologists into the twenty-first century.[13] Conversely, in the United States, the successful selling of retirement after World War II led to research initiatives and programs on successful and productive aging, concerned with investigating adaption to the circumstances of retirement. Whatever the national differences, the collection of data to answer questions posed as the problem of aging has continued to the present day, although more recently within the context of population aging and the economic consequences that accompany it. Paradoxically, this has meant that research is now directed at the problems posed by "a rapidly growing population of rather healthy and self-sufficient persons whose collective dependence is now straining the economies of western nations."[4] We will return to this theme shortly but first will describe the early theoretical perspectives that have underpinned social gerontology.

THEORETICAL APPROACHES: FROM FUNCTIONALISM TO STRUCTURED DEPENDENCY

Much of the reason for social gerontology's focus on the problems associated with later life lies in the emergence of retirement, in the 1940s in the United States[9] and the 1960s in Britain,[14] as a distinct part of the life course. This led sociologists working within the functionalist tradition such as Parsons and Burgess[15,16] (an approach concerned with how elements of society operate in complementary ways) to worry about the "roleless role" of the retired person, a population defined by its permanent exit from the labor market rather than indigence. Obviously, this referred mainly to men, for whom their social role and employment were seen as largely interchangeable, whereas a consistent domesticated role was assumed for women. Criticism of this view, and the corresponding assumption that retirement was therefore relatively nonproblematic for women, came from Beeson,[17] who noted that it was not based on any empirical evidence and ignored the existence of working women.

Some approached this roleless state through the prism of disengagement theory,[18] focusing on the social and psychological adjustment of the older person to after work and after married life. Theorizing the wider processes that accompanied retirement, this theory hypothesized that older adults in industrial societies disengaged themselves from the roles they occupied so that younger generations would have opportunities to develop and take on their socially necessary roles. Consequently, disengagement was assumed not only to occur in relation to work roles, but also in relation to families, when retired generations became much less central to the lives of their children. Focusing on a psychological approach, disengagement theory saw itself as influenced by the work of Erikson and the notions of life review.[19] A considerable amount of research was undertaken in the United States during the 1960s to provide evidence for this theory. A longitudinal study in Kansas City showed that older adults did indeed disengage, although women were observed to start this process at widowhood and men began on retirement.[20] This approach, which for a long time was one of the dominant paradigms in social gerontology, saw the way in which old age occurred in modern societies as an inevitable and natural process. Questions about whether older adults wanted to disengage, or were forced to do so by society, were not asked. The emphasis on psychological adjustment also avoided looking at the very real social processes that structured old age.

Although disengagement theory centered on the perspective of the individual older person, the analysis put forward by the predominantly British structured dependency approach stressed the importance of social policy.[21] For writers in this school and those who described themselves as adopting the political economy approach to aging, the problem of old age was not one of individual social and psychological adjustment but of a dependency structured by the circumstances of retirement, something that was set by government social policy.[22-24] Townsend noted that retirement not only marks a withdrawal from the formal labor market, but also indicates a shift from making a living through earning a wage to being dependent on a replacement income.[21] The fact that this income was often funded by the state demonstrated the role of social policy in structuring the dependency that many older people experienced after retirement. In Britain, for example, the relatively low levels at which the state pension was paid out indicated the low priority that older adults had in decisions about state welfare. As Walker[22] and others have noted, the continuing impact of social class into later life was also indicated in the relative imbalance among the levels of state retirement pensions that funded most working class retirees' old age and the amounts paid out by the better funded occupational pensions enjoyed by the middle class. Those reliant on state retirement pensions, consequently, were seen as a residual category of the population drawing resources from public funds, a problem that led to considerable interest in researching poverty in later life.

It is also argued that structured dependency is not just limited to the economic sphere, but pervades social processes more generally. Townsend suggested that the association of age with infirmity and dependency not only represents the position of older adults, but also justifies the inferior status of older adults and their exclusion from various forms of social participation.[25] Ageism also emerges out of the cultural valorization of youthfulness, which not only defines aging in negative terms, but also clears the way to make it acceptable to discriminate against older people. This can manifest itself in policies seeking to limit medical or health care resources to older people, in discriminatory employment practices, and in the treatment of physically frail or mentally confused older adults.[25] For writers such as Townsend and Walker, with a focus on well-being and social inequality, the disengaged position of later life is not only a social construct, but also something that should be challenged by campaigns for the restoration of full citizenship rights to older adults.[26]

INCREASING LIFE EXPECTANCY AND COMPRESSION OF MORBIDITY: A GOLDEN AGE

As described elsewhere in this text, there are many who argue that the human life span is malleable, with mortality only occurring as a result of an accumulation of damage in cells and tissues and limitations in investments in somatic maintenance.[27] And, more controversially, writers such as de Grey have argued that longevity can be extended upward once the basic biologic processes have been understood.[28] Although these views have been heavily criticized, there is now recognition at a population level that life expectancy is increasing rapidly, perhaps at an accelerating rate. For example, Rau and colleagues[29] have shown that for men aged 80 to 89 years, mortality rates dropped by 0.81% in the 1950s and 1960s but by 1.88% in the 1980s and 1990s, whereas for women of the same age group the figures were 0.91% and 2.45%, respectively. The rate of acceleration in decline in mortality rates is greatest for older adults. Given a focus on the problem of age, it is not surprising that concerns have been expressed that increased longevity might lead to higher rates of morbidity and/or disability, a failure of success in which industrial societies have passed through an epidemiologic transition that has shifted the burden of disease onto chronic conditions in later life.[30] However, this conclusion has been challenged by evidence that suggests that increased life expectancy does not come at the cost of an expansion of morbidity.[31] Researchers such as Fries have proposed a thesis built around a compression of morbidity, in which even under the conditions of increased life expectancy, the proportion of life spent in ill health is concentrated into an ever-shorter period prior to death.[32,33]

Although this view challenged many of the assumptions made about the connection between aging and chronic illness, there has been considerable support for the claim that chronologic age in itself is not a factor in increasing levels of disability and chronic illness.[34] Although analyses based on subjective measures of health have suggested an increasing disease burden in later life,[35] more objective indicators of disability suggest a more positive view of healthy life expectancy.[36,37] Analyses of disability rates in the United States have suggested that not only are disability rates falling, they are falling at an accelerating rate, much in the same way as mortality rates are falling at an accelerating rate. For

30 Social Vulnerability in Old Age

Melissa K. Andrew

People's lives are embedded in rich social contexts; many social factors affect each of our lives every day. This is perhaps more noticeable for older adults because declines in health and functional status may increase reliance on social supports and diminish opportunities for social engagement, even in the face of social circles dwindling due to declining health and function among peers.

This chapter will provide an overview of how social factors affect health in old age, through a discussion of the concept of social vulnerability. Association with health outcomes relevant to geriatric medicine, including function, mobility, cognition, mental health, self-assessed health, frailty, institutionalization, and death, will be the focus, with particular emphasis on the relationship between social vulnerability and frailty. Detailed discussion of social gerontology and of standardized instruments and measurement scales used in the social assessment of older people is beyond the scope of this chapter; interested readers are referred to Chapters 29 and 36 on these topics.[1,2]

BACKGROUND AND DEFINITIONS

Many social factors influence health, including socioeconomic status, social support, social networks, social engagement, social capital, and social cohesion.[3-10] As such, the social context is key to a broad understanding of health and illness. Perhaps due in part to the numerous disciplines in which this line of inquiry has been investigated, including epidemiology, sociology, geography, political science, and international development, terminology and methods of approach have differed. In some cases, the same terminology has been used to refer to different ideas, whereas in others, divergent terminology obscures underlying commonalities. There has also been debate surrounding the level, from individual to communal, at which some elements of the social context are relevant and, as such, how they can be measured.[3,11,12] In the following section, various terms and concepts will be defined and discussed, and each will be placed in context on the continuum from individual to group influence (Fig. 30-1).

Socioeconomic Status

Socioeconomic status (SES) is a broad concept that includes factors such as educational attainment, occupation, income, wealth, and deprivation. There are three broad theories of how socioeconomic status might relate to health.[13] The materialist theory states that gradients in income and wealth are associated with varying levels of deprivation, which in turn affects health status because those with fewer means have inferior access to health care and the necessities of life. Another view is that education influences health through lifestyle and health-related behaviors such as diet, substance use, and smoking. A third theory sees social status (often measured by occupation) and personal autonomy as key influences on health, particularly through the stresses that accompany low social status and low autonomy.[13] Measurement of each of these elements of SES may present difficulties in the older adult population. Older adults are likely to be retired, and some older women may never have worked outside the home, making occupational assessments problematic. Income is associated with employment status, and many income supplements and benefits are available to those with disability and poor health, raising problems of reverse causation.[13] Educational opportunities available to older cohorts may have been limited, creating a "floor effect," in which it is difficult to differentiate among the majority whose educational attainment is low.[13] Additionally, information may be missing when a proxy respondent has been used, depending on how well the proxy knows the subject. Socioeconomic status is a property of individuals; however, aggregates of such measures can be used to describe the social context in which people live. For example, average income, employment rates, or educational attainment may be useful descriptors when applied to groups of people living in relevant geographic areas such as housing complexes or neighborhoods and may allow for a study of contextual effects on health.[14-20]

Social Support

Social support refers to the various sources of help and resources obtained through social relationships with family, friends, and other caregivers. Types of social support include emotional (including the presence of a close confidante), instrumental (help with activities of daily living, provided through labor or financial support), appraisal (help with decision making), and informational (provision of information or advice).[21] Various measures of social support have been studied, with some tending to be more objective (based on reports of actual use of services and tangible help received in the various domains) and others being more subjective, based on the individual's perception of the adequacy and richness of the supports to which he or she has access. Social support can also, importantly, be seen as a two-way transaction, with older adults receiving supports in some areas while providing support in others. For example, within spousal relationships, each spouse may have complementary strengths and weaknesses; between generations, older adults may provide care for grandchildren and financial support for adult children while receiving instrumental support.[22]

Social Networks and Social Engagement

Social networks are the ties that link individuals and groups in social relationships. Various characteristics can be measured, including size, density, relationship quality, and composition.[3] Social networks and social support are generally seen as individual-level resources and are measured at an individual level.[5,21,23] Through social networks, individuals can access social support, material resources, and various other forms of capital (e.g., cultural, economic, social).[24]

Social engagement represents an individual's participation in social, occupational, or group activities, which may include formal organized activities such as religious meetings, service groups, and clubs. More informal activities such as card groups, trips to the bingo hall, and cultural outings to see concerts or visit art galleries can also be considered as social engagement. Volunteerism is often considered separately,[3] but can also be seen as an important measure of social engagement.

Social Capital

Social capital is a broad term that has been used inconsistently in the literature, and there is ongoing debate about its nature and

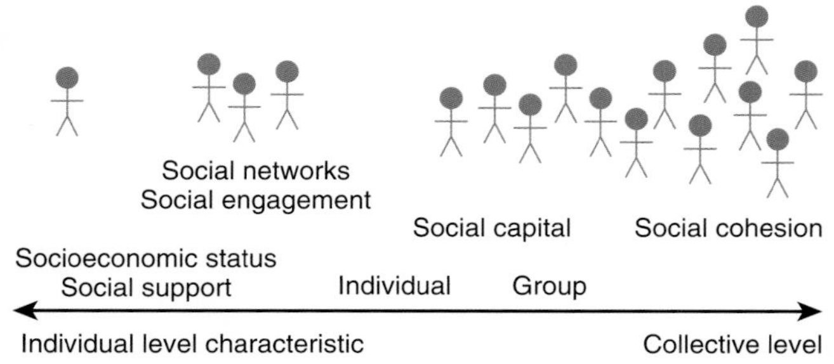

Figure 30-1. Continuum of social factors that influence health, acting from individual to group levels.

measurement. For example, Bourdieu has defined social capital as "the aggregate of the actual or potential resources which are linked to possession of a durable network of more or less institutionalized relationships."[24] This definition is consistent with the idea that social capital is a resource that can be accessed and measured at an individual level, stating that "the volume of social capital possessed by a given agent thus depends on the size of the network of connections he [or she] can effectively mobilize and the volume of the capital … possessed by each of those to whom he [or she] is connected."[24] However, this definition is also consistent with the view that social capital is a property of the relationships within the network; if there are no connections between individuals, there would be no social capital. Coleman has made a similar argument, stating that "Unlike other forms of capital, social capital inheres in the structure of relations between actors and among actors. It is not lodged either in the actors themselves or in the physical implements of production."[25] Coleman also sees social capital as a resource accessible by individuals: "social capital constitutes a particular kind of resource available to an actor."[25]

Putnam has defined social capital as "the features in our community life that make us more productive—a high level of engagement, trust, and reciprocity"[26]—and sees it as "simultaneously a 'private good' and a 'public good'" with both individual and collective aspects.[27] To access the private good benefits of social capital, an individual would need to be integrated into a network and have direct connections with other members. However, the public good effects of social capital would accrue to everyone in the community, regardless of their personal connections to others. The public good conception of social capital is shared by others, including Kawachi and colleagues, who see social capital as an ecologic level characteristic that can only properly be measured at a collective level; they noted that "social capital inheres in the structure of social relationships; in other words, it is an ecological characteristic," which "should be properly considered a feature of the collective (neighborhood, community, society) to which an individual belongs."[5,16,23,28]

Measures of social capital are as varied as its definitions and include structural elements (e.g., social networks, relationships, group participation) and cognitive ones (e.g., trust in others, voting behavior, newspaper subscription, feelings of obligation, reciprocity, and cooperation, and perceptions of neighborhood security).[3,12,25]

Social Cohesion

The concept of social cohesion implies collectivity of definition and measurement. Again, definitions vary, but generally relate to ideas of cooperation and ties that unite communities and societies. For example, Stansfeld has defined social cohesion as "the existence of mutual trust and respect between different sections of society."[29] For Kawachi and Berkman, social cohesion relies on two key features of a society, the absence of social conflict and presence of social bonds.[5]

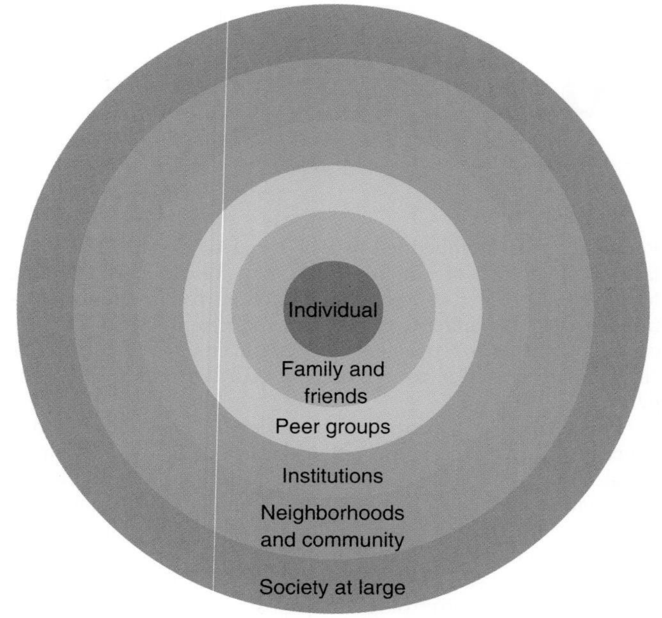

Figure 30-2. Social ecology framework of social vulnerability. *(Adapted from Andrew M, Keefe J: Social vulnerability among older adults: a social ecology perspective from the National Population Health Survey of Canada. BMC Geriatr 14:90, 2014.)*

Social Isolation

Social isolation is another term encountered in the literature relating social circumstances and health. It is related to ideas of loneliness, reduced social and religious engagement, and reduced access to social supports. It may also incorporate properties of the older adult's environment, such as difficulty with transportation. As with many other social factors, social isolation can be subjective, as perceived by older adults themselves, such as loneliness, or objective, based on outside measures or assessments by others.

Social Vulnerability

The concept of social vulnerability addresses the understanding that the reason we are interested in the social environment is not merely as a descriptor, but as an attempt to quantify an individual's relative vulnerability (or resilience or invulnerability) to perturbations in his or her environment, social circumstances, health, or functional status. Older adults' social circumstances are complex, with multiple factors that may interact in potentially unforeseen ways. A global measure of social vulnerability would thus account for this complexity while providing descriptive and predictive value. A measure of social vulnerability should be broad enough to capture a rich description of the social deficits (or problems) that an individual has, readily and practically measurable in population and clinical settings, responsive to meaningful changes, and predictive of important health outcomes. Ideally, a measure of social vulnerability would incorporate factors that come into play across the continuum, from an individual to a group level. A social ecology framework (Fig. 30-2) is a useful tool for considering social vulnerability as a broad construct, seeing individuals nested within expanding spheres of social influence. This approach considers how social factors at each of these levels—from the individual to family and friends, peer groups, institutions, neighborhoods, and communities, and society at large—contribute to overall social vulnerability.[30]

HOW CAN WE STUDY SOCIAL INFLUENCES ON HEALTH?

A study of how social factors influence health requires careful consideration of analytic design in relation to the specific questions being asked (Table 30-1). Possible approaches include traditional "one thing at a time" analyses, in which a single social factor (e.g., the social network) is related to the outcome of interest, ideally adjusting for possible confounders in a multivariable model. This approach has certain benefits, chief among them simplicity and clarity in execution and interpretation. For example, it allows for clear statements of important findings such as "An extensive social network seems to protect against dementia."[31] This approach can be carried out using single variables considered individually, a combination of variables relating to different aspects of the same theme (e.g., several variables that relate to the size and quality of the social network), or set instruments that have been previously validated to measure the social factor of interest (e.g., the Berkman and Syme Social Network Index and Lubben Social Network Scale).[32] The standardized psychometric properties of such scales add to the reliability and validity of studies that use them, but their use does have drawbacks, including relative rigidity and longer administration time. Their use may also be limited or impossible with existing data sets due to challenges encountered in their faithful reconstruction. Also, considering single variables one at a time may lead to oversimplification of older adults' complex social circumstances. For example, two older women who live alone may be classified as vulnerable in a study on "living alone." If one woman is well integrated into the community, with strong social networks and family ties, and the other woman is truly isolated, with no one to count on for help, we understand that they have very different profiles of social vulnerability. Considering single variables one at a time, even with attempts to adjust for other variables in statistical models, risks misclassification of true vulnerability.[30,33]

Deficit accumulation offers another potential approach to the study of social influences on health. Akin to the frailty index, which readers will find described elsewhere in this volume (see Chapter 15),[34] a social vulnerability index, operationalized as a count of deficits relating to many social factors, offers a means of considering an individual's broad social circumstance and the potential vulnerability of her or his health and functional status. The index has a number of benefits, including the following: (1) the potential to include many different categories of social factors (e.g., SES, social support, social engagement, social capital); (2) the commonly encountered difficulty of embodying social and socioeconomic characteristics using single variables in studies of older adults is alleviated by including consideration of different factors; (3) related factors are not arbitrarily separated into distinct categories for separate analysis; and (4) representation of gradations in social vulnerability is improved compared with consideration of one or a few binary or ordinal social variables. This last point is particularly important, given that studies using the social vulnerability index in two cohorts of older adults have found that no one was completely free of social vulnerability (i.e.,

TABLE 30-1 Analytic Approaches for Studying Social Influences on Health

Analytic Approach	Example(s)	Benefits	Drawbacks
"One Thing at a Time"			
Single variables considered individually	Size of the social network	Simple and clear execution and interpretation	May result in overly simplistic understanding of associations
Combination of variables relating to the same theme	Several variables describing the social network	Allows simultaneous investigation of several variables, adjusting for one another and for relevant confounders	• Validity considerations—must be addressed • Models may become too complex with technical challenges (e.g., collinearity)
Validated measurement instrument	Lubben's Social Network Scale	Use of standardized and validated instruments—enhances reliability and validity	• Lengthy administration time • Rigidity • Use may be limited with existing data sets if difficult to reconstruct faithfully
"Many Things at Once"			
Index approach—deficit accumulation	Social vulnerability index, frailty index	• Takes many aspects of social circumstances into account simultaneously • Does not rely on use of single variables, which may present measurement challenges in some older adults • Related factors not arbitrarily separated • Allows representation of gradations in exposure • Potential applicability to most data sets and clinical situations	• Represents risk relating to composite social circumstances rather than single identifiable factors in isolation • Complex modeling based on novel techniques
Options for Studying the Social Context			
"Horizontal" analyses	Multivariable regression modeling	Simple and clear execution and interpretation	• May not provide a full understanding of the social context • Technical problems for models; observations not really independent
"Vertical" analyses	Multilevel modeling, hierarchical linear modeling	• Yields more detailed understanding of contextual effects • Preserves independence of observations • Avoids loss of meaning due to data aggregation	• Complex models • Not all data sets lend themselves to these models; need sufficient numbers in groups with shared characteristics

no individual had a zero score on the index).[33] Use of a deficit accumulation approach to social vulnerability also presents a fifth great benefit, that of scaling. As readers will note elsewhere in this text (Chapters 5, 14, 15, and 16), deficit accumulation can be seen in cells, tissues, animals, and people. Considering the bigger picture of social circumstances, here we can scale this measure of vulnerability up to the societal level.[35]

In addition to these analytic considerations of how the social factor(s) of interest is (are) measured, incorporating the social context into the analyses can be done in different ways. More traditional horizontal approaches might add a summary variable that describes the individual's social context (e.g., mean neighborhood income or educational attainment) as a variable or confounder attached to the individual in the multivariable model.[18,19] This approach can yield useful findings and has the advantage of simplicity, but some might argue that it does not provide a full understanding of the importance of the contextual variable(s) and that it presents statistical problems in terms of independence of observations—individuals are no longer truly independent if they share these important characteristics of the groups to which they belong. Multilevel (vertical) modeling (e.g., hierarchical linear modeling) is another option; here, the individual is nested within layers of group influence, with collective characteristics treated as attributes of the group rather than of the individual.[36] This approach offers the advantage of allowing for a more detailed understanding of the contextual effects, preserving the independence of observations, and not losing information, as occurs when data are aggregated.[36]

The consideration of contextual or group-level variables such as neighborhood and community characteristics is particularly relevant to the study of how social factors affect health because many social factors are properties of the groups or communities in which individuals live and may be best measured on a group level. As we have seen, there is active debate about whether social capital is a property of individuals or of groups.[3,11] Most theories of social capital are consistent with the idea that it is a property of relationships between individuals and within societies, rather than residing within individuals per se. The heart of the issue, which continues to divide theorists, is whether social capital is a resource that an individual can be said to draw on and thus, in practical research terms, whether it can legitimately be measured at an individual level.

This debate has clear implications for the design and interpretation of research studies that aim to investigate how social factors influence health; valid and useful findings can rest only on sound theoretical foundations. In this regard, a second distinction may be helpful; the answer may depend on whether the question applies to where social capital exists (is it a property of individuals or of relationships?) or to how it is measured and accessed.[11] Practically speaking, measurement issues and data availability may strongly influence analytic design. The issue of how social factors should be studied in relation to older adults' health is therefore ideally guided by a balance of theoretical considerations and analytic pragmatism.

SUCCESSFUL AGING

This concept has been the subject of numerous enquiries in the academic literature and popular press.[37-39] Definitions of successful aging vary and generally fall into psychosocial and biomedical camps, with contributory factors that include physical functioning, social engagement, well-being, and access to resources.[38] Psychosocial conceptualizations emphasize compensation and contentedness, in which biomedical definitions are based on the absence of disease and disability.[40] The concept of successful aging recognizes that the aging process is variable, and that how older adults adapt to later life changes associated with aging influences how successfully they will age. Ideally, research into this area would identify potentially modifiable factors are at play that help some age better and more successfully than others.

There is a potential downside to the idea of successful aging: if successful aging is applied as a value judgment, it may be at the cost of blaming and further marginalizing the so-called unsuccessful agers, those who are not so fortunate as to have the good health and functional status that might allow them to be doing aerobics at the age of 102 years or volunteering with "the old people" at 99 years of age.[37] Such stereotypes, based on rare aging successes and on the undercurrent of ageism that is common in our society, also influence the portrayal of older adults in the popular media. Positive and negative stereotypes run the risk of perpetuating the marginalization of the most vulnerable older adults, regardless of whether their unsuccessful aging is implied or emphasized.[37]

Another way to think about successful aging is to consider individuals who overcome their expected trajectory in the natural history of decline for a given level of frailty. Work with the frailty index has shown that trajectories of decline are established early, and that such declines are well predicted using mathematical models.[41,42] However, there are some older adults who improve or transition to lower levels of frailty—who are able to "jump the curve" from their own predicted course and outcomes to attain the outcomes that would be expected for people with a lower baseline level of frailty. This might be a useful subgroup in which to study predictors and correlates of this successful aging.

ASSOCIATIONS WITH HEALTH

The various social factors discussed here have been associated with health outcomes that are important for older adults. Readers interested in broad-based discussions of how social circumstances relate to health, as well as to other attributes of societies, are referred to the studies of Marmot, Wilkinson, Putnam and their associates, who have each made strong and comprehensive cases that weak social cohesion and declines in social capital contribute to poor health[27] and may explain associations between poor health and income inequalities[43] and social status inequalities.[8] As in many areas of geriatric medicine, studies pertaining specifically to older adults are limited in number. These will be discussed here, along with important findings from general population studies in relation to health outcomes that are important in geriatric medicine.

Survival

Numerous studies have found associations between social factors and survival. Perceived social support and social interaction were associated with lower 30-month mortality in a cohort of 331 community-dwelling adults aged 65 years and older in Durham County, North Carolina.[44] In the Alameda County 1965 Human Population Laboratory study, those with a richer social network, more contact with friends and family, and church or other group membership (used to generate a social network index), including older adults, had lower mortality over 9 years of follow-up.[45] Using 17-year follow-up data from the same study, social connectedness predicted better survival at all ages, including those aged 70 years and older.[7] Older individuals with few social ties also had reduced survival in a cohort study conducted in Evans County, Georgia.[4] In another study, increased social ties predicted 5-year survival in two of three community-based cohorts.[46] The Whitehall studies of men employed in the British civil service identified an impressive gradient in survival across levels in the occupational hierarchy; in middle age, office workers in the lowest ranking jobs had four times the mortality of those in the highest ranking "administers" category. This gradient persisted after retirement, although it decreased to twice the risk of mortality, in the oldest age group studied, aged 70 to 89 years.[8,9]

High social vulnerability, as measured using a social vulnerability index, increased the risk of mortality over 5- and 8-year follow-up in two separate longitudinal studies of older Canadians, the Canadian Study of Health and Aging (CSHA) and the National Population Health Survey.[33] Even among the fittest older Canadians, those with no health deficits, there was an absolute mortality difference of 20% between those with low versus high social vulnerability.[47] In keeping with the social ecology perspective on social vulnerability, social context is important; in a cross-national comparison in the Survey of Health and Retirement in Europe (SHARE), high social vulnerability predicted mortality in countries with continental and Mediterranean social welfare models, but not in Nordic countries.[48] Ecologic (collective-level) analyses using multilevel modeling have also linked high social capital, defined by high trust and membership in voluntary associations, with reduced mortality at state[20] and neighbourhood[16] levels in the United States. In a Chinese study, factors commonly included in a social vulnerability index—being married; having a good spousal relationship, good financial status, high education, access to television or radio; reading newspapers, books, or magazines; and playing cards, chess, or mahjong—were included in a so-called protection index. In a multivariable model, they mitigated some of the risk conferred by a frailty index.[49]

Cognitive Decline and Dementia

In a study of 2812 older adults living in New Haven, Connecticut, social disengagement was associated with 3-, 6-, and 12-year incident cognitive decline, defined as a transition to a lower category of performance on the 10-item Short Portable Mental Status Questionnaire.[50] Greater emotional social support predicted better cognitive function measured by a battery of tests assessing language, abstraction, spatial ability, and recall over 7.5 years in the MacArthur Studies of Successful Aging.[51] Among 2468 CSHA participants aged 70 years and older, high social vulnerability was associated with a 35% increase in the odds of clinically meaningful cognitive decline (a decline $\geq$ 5 points[52] on the Modified Mini Mental State Examination [3MS]) over 5 years.[53] In a cohort of 1203 older adults in Kungsholmen, Sweden, those with a limited social network (including consideration of marital status, living arrangement, and contacts with friends and relatives) had a 60% increased risk of dementia over an average of 3 years of follow-up, whereas the incidence of dementia decreased in a stepwise fashion with increasing social contectedness.[31]

The association of strong social networks and participation in mental and physical leisure activities with reduced incidence of dementia was also supported by a systematic review.[54] A U.S. study of 9704 older women found that a richer social network (defined as the top two tertiles on the Lubben Social Network Scale) was associated with maintenance of optimal cognitive function (i.e., not experiencing age-related declines in cognition) over 15 years of follow-up.[55] Loneliness has also been associated with lower levels of baseline cognition in older adults, more rapid cognitive decline, and twice the risk of pathologically diagnosed Alzheimer dementia.[56] Interestingly, feeling lonely, more than being alone, was associated with dementia when the two were examined separately.[57] Social interaction and engagement reduced the probability of declines in orientation and memory in a 4-year study of community-dwelling Spanish older adults,[58] and greater social resources (networks and engagement) were similarly associated with reductions in cognitive decline in older adults.[59]

SES status has also been studied in relation to cognition and cognitive declines in late life. Low SES (as measured by education, income, and assets) was associated with cognitive decline ($\geq$5-point decline in the 3MS over 4 years) independent of biomedical comorbidity in a cohort of 2574 older participants aged 70 to 79 years in the Health, Aging, and Body Composition study.[60] In a study that measured performance on complex memory tasks and electroencephalographic recordings of event-related potentials, older women ($\geq$65 years) of high SES performed similarly to younger women in complex source memory tasks and appeared to make use of neural compensation strategies not used by their lower SES counterparts and not required by the younger subjects.[61] In the Chicago Health and Aging project study of 6158 older adults aged 65 years and older, early life SES (both of the individual's family and birth county) was associated with late life cognitive performance but not with subsequent rate of decline.[62] A report from the English Longitudinal Study of Ageing (ELSA) found that neighborhood-level SES was associated with cognitive function independent of individual SES.[18] Using hierarchic linear modeling, neighborhood-level educational attainment was associated with cognitive function of Americans aged 70 years and older participating in the Study of Assets and Health Dynamics Among the Oldest Old (AHEAD). This was independent of individual factors, including educational attainment and neighborhood measures of income, leading the authors to conclude that promoting educational attainment in the general population may help older residents maintain cognitive function.[63]

Functional Decline and Dependence

Low levels of social engagement among older adults have been associated with increased disability, measured as impairment in activities of daily living (ADLs), mobility, and upper and lower extremity function, over 9 years of follow-up.[6] Older adults ($\geq$72 years) with dense social networks showed delayed onset of self-perceived disability over 8 years of follow-up in a panel study of 1000 residents of three retirement communities in Florida.[64] Social engagement through group participation, social support, and trust and reciprocity were each associated with reduced functional impairment in community dwellers in a cross-sectional analysis of the Health Survey for England. The association between group participation and functional impairment was also statistically significant among residents of institutional care homes.[65] Social conditions across countries also influence the association between social circumstances and disability. In the SHARE study, the relationship between social vulnerability and function in basic ADLs varied by social welfare model; social vulnerability predicted incident disability in countries with continental and Mediterranean social welfare models, but not in Nordic countries.[48]

Mobility

Various social factors have been associated with risk of falls and subsequent injury. For example, one Australian population-based study found that older adults with lower SES, those living alone, and those needing repairs to their home were more likely to have fallen.[66] Another study identified protective factors for fall-related hip fractures that included being currently married, living in the same place for more than 5 years, having private health insurance, and engaging in social activities.[67] These associations in older adults parallel what is seen in the population in general, in which lower SES is linked to a variety of unintentional injuries and death.[68] Neighborhood-level deprivation has been associated with incident self-reported mobility difficulties and measured impairment in gait speed, independent of individual SES and health status, in ELSA.[19]

Institutionalization

Because most studies in this field have been done using surveys or cohorts with community-based sampling frames, there has been a paucity of research that included residents of long-term care facilities. However, severe lack of social support was associated with higher odds of care home residence[65] and is a risk factor for care home placement.[69,70] The issue of how social factors and social vulnerability affect the health of older residents of institutions requires further study. In a cross-sectional analysis of the Health Survey for England, in which associations between social capital and health were found among care home residents, these associations were generally weaker than in the community setting, suggesting that the importance of social capital may vary according to living situation.[65]

Mental Health

Low perceived neighborhood social capital and high social disorganization were associated with psychiatric and physical morbidity in a study of British adults.[71] Mental health has also been found to be associated with the strength and nature of social ties, although protective effects do not appear to be uniform across all population groups.[72] For example, a study of 1714 older Cubans found that social networks (particularly those centered on children and extended family) were associated with reduced depressive symptoms in women, whereas being married and not living alone were more important for men.[73] Among community-dwelling older adults, social support, group participation, and trust and reciprocity were each associated with better mental health, as measured by the General Health Questionnaire, an instrument that has been validated to detect mild psychiatric morbidity. Social support was also associated with reduced psychiatric morbidity among older adults who resided in care homes.[65] Lower neighborhood SES and higher population density were associated with depression and anxiety among people aged 75 years and older in Britain, but in this study the effect of neighborhood SES was explained by individual SES and health factors.[74]

Self-Assessed Health

SES (income adequacy and education) is strongly associated with better self-rated health in older adults.[75] Individual-level social capital, as defined by religious participation, trust, and having a helpful friend, was associated with better self-assessed health among Swedish-speaking adults in a bilingual region of Finland.[76] High community-level social trust and membership in voluntary associations were also associated with better self-assessed health among community-dwelling adults in multilevel analyses adjusting for individual-level influences on health in two large U.S. studies (N = 167,259 and 21,456).[15,17] Among 1677 community-dwelling older adult participants in the Health Survey for England, higher levels of social support, group participation, and trust *and* reciprocity were associated with better self-assessed health.[65] At a neighborhood level, low SES (including poverty, unemployment, low education, and reliance on public assistance) was associated with poor self-assessed health of Americans aged 70 years and older in the AHEAD study, independent of individual-level health and SES factors. This association with self-assessed health held, even though the neighborhood-level attributes were not independently associated with cardiovascular disease and functional status.[77]

Frailty

Social position (educational and income) was strongly associated with frailty in a gradient (rather than a threshold) fashion in a Canadian study of older adults.[78] In two other cohorts of older Canadians, social vulnerability was moderately correlated with frailty, but was distinct from it. Both frailty and social vulnerability contributed independently to the risk of mortality.[33] Several social determinants of frailty were identified in a Chinese population aged 70 years and older; these included low SES (occupational category and inadequate income), having few or little contact with relatives and neighbors, low participation in community and religious activities, and reporting low social support.[79] Low perceived social support was found to be an independent predictor of frailty development following myocardial infarction[80] and predicted attenuated increases of frailty in a prospective cohort of older Mexican American adults.[81] Increased social support and resilience were associated with lower frailty among homeless middle-aged and older adults.[82] On an international level, average levels of frailty across Europe are correlated with national economic indicators, such as gross domestic product (GDP).[83]

MECHANISMS OF HOW SOCIAL FACTORS AFFECT HEALTH

Various mechanisms have been proposed to explain how social factors might affect health. Broadly speaking, these can be broken down into four groups—biologic and physiologic, behavioral, material, and psychological. The study of neurophysiology and neuroanatomy may also contribute to understanding the relationship between social factors and health.

Physiologic Factors

Chronic and sustained stress responses exert powerful effects on health through complex hormonal regulatory systems, with myriad downstream effects on tissues and organs. Various animal studies have found effects on the hypothalamic-pituitary-adrenal axis. Chronically elevated levels of glucocorticoids in socially isolated rats accelerated aging processes, including hippocampal cell loss and cognitive impairment.[21] Social support has also been linked to immune function in humans and animals, with social isolation and loneliness compromising immunocompetence, even among otherwise healthy medical students.[21]

Behavioral Factors

Socioeconomic inequalities (including employment and educational opportunities) and the norms and influences exerted through social networks and communities may affect health-related behaviors, such as diet, smoking, substance use, and exercise. This may partially explain social influences on health; however, many studies in which these behaviors were taken into account found that social circumstances exert additional independent effects on health.[15,21,44,45]

Material Factors

SES and social support networks clearly affect access to goods and services. This access accrues in three broad ways—through financial resources (what you have), social status (who you are), and social contacts (who you know). Those with financial means and high social status can afford to make healthy lifestyle choices (e.g., balanced diet, opportunities for exercise, avoiding smoking and substance abuse) and have access to health care services, which may be difficult to obtain without such resources. There are also strong systemic and societal factors that serve to maintain the social exclusion of marginalized individuals and groups. Those with strong social support resources can access financial and instrumental assistance in time of need.

Psychological Factors

Self-efficacy and adaptive coping strategies are important for health and are some of the potential psychological mechanisms through which social factors may influence health.[21] Low self-efficacy (having low confidence in one's abilities) is associated with fear of falling, with important functional and mobility ramifications for older adults.[84] Low self-efficacy has also been found to predict functional decline in older adults with impaired physical performance.[6] Social supports and engagement may bolster feelings of self-efficacy and self-confidence.

Neurophysiology and Neuroanatomy

Studies of patients with neurologic conditions have historically been a rich source of insight into the function of the brain and nervous system. Whereas the potential mechanisms discussed in the last few paragraphs have attempted to explain how social circumstances themselves might influence health, here we consider the reverse. By studying people with neurologic conditions, including dementia, we may be able to learn more about how the brain influences social factors such as engagement, participation in social networks, and perceptions of others, such as trust and reciprocity, which are important to the idea of social capital. For example, some individuals with dementia become socially withdrawn and apathetic, suspicious, and less trusting or have other personality changes that influence their social function. Study of the localization and function of such problems (e.g., with functional imaging techniques and more traditional neuropathologic measures) may help elucidate the links between social function and social circumstances and health. This field is in its early stages but, as an example, "agreeableness" in frontotemporal dementia (which is often characterized by personality changes and problems with social function) has been shown to be positively correlated with the volume of the right orbitofrontal cortex and negatively correlated with left-sided orbitofrontal volume.[85] In addition to the role of the frontal lobes in social behavior, other brain structures are likely to be implicated, especially in the face of complex inter-connections. For example, the hippocampus appears to have an important social influence through flexible cognition. This will have particular relevance to the study of social behavior in dementia given the well-known role of the hippocampus in memory.[85a] Animal studies may also contribute to this area of inquiry. For example, a study of hyenas has shown that the four distinct species of hyenas can be placed on a continuum of increasing social complexity. Interestingly, the volume of the frontal cortex (as determined by internal measurements of their skulls) is directly proportional, with the hyenas that have the most complex social relationships having the greatest frontal lobe volumes.[86]

FRAILTY, EXCLUSION, AND "SILENCE BY PROXY"

Older adults who are frail and/or cognitively impaired present a unique challenge for research in this field for many reasons. These include exclusion from research, reliance on proxy informants, problematic assessment of social situation and SES, and controversy regarding informed consent.

Many frail older adults may be excluded from population-based research if the sampling frame excludes nursing homes (as is commonly the case) or if persons unable to answer for themselves are not included in surveys. Even if efforts are made to include these groups by using proxy respondents, subjective reports and personal historical details may be missing or unreliable.[11,65]

This so-called silence by proxy presents great challenges in research involving frail older adults because it is often hardest to gather information from those who are the most frail, particularly in institutions where family may be unavailable to fill in historical details. One might imagine that social support and social interactions could be more relevant to health in frail older adults because they might be most reliant on family and friends for care and encouragement, and benefits of social engagement could be greater in terms of mobility and optimizing function appropriate to their level of ability. As such, the associations found in studies from which they are excluded could be underestimates.

POLICY RAMIFICATIONS AND POTENTIAL FOR INTERVENTIONS

Although there are not many intervention studies in which social vulnerability is reduced and health outcomes studied, some studies have suggested hope in this regard. For example, there is evidence that participation in some type of volunteer group may help buffer the negative psychological effects of functional decline.[87] Intervention trials with so-called befriending services, in which social support is offered by a volunteer visitor, have had mixed results, possibly due in part to limited uptake.[88] There is a large literature and clinical experience with structured peer support groups—for example, those provided through various disease-specific community organizations. However, a discussion of these is beyond the scope of this chapter.

One area in which social interventions have the potential to improve health is in the design of senior housing. Given the mounting evidence that social engagement and interaction with neighbors improves health, these principles could considered as housing developments and facilities for older people are designed, built, and renovated. Cannuscio and coworkers have described such senior housing strategies as a "promising mode of delivery of social capital to the aging population."[28] Long-term care facilities could be designed to encourage interaction by residents among themselves and within the wider community. Residents' rooms spread out along long hallways, inaccessible to those with mobility impairment, might be replaced by rooms organized into pods around shared common areas.[29] Planned care environments, in which a continuum of living arrangements from independent apartments through to full nursing care within a single complex might foster neighborhood cohesion and reduce residential mobility, which has been shown to affect the formation of social ties negatively.[14,28] Community planning on a larger scale may also help address many of the challenges to mobility and community interaction faced by older adults. Sidewalks and crosswalks wide enough and in good enough repair to allow the use of mobility aids, traffic lights with cycles long enough to allow safe crossing, accessible public transportation, and availability of services in local residential neighborhoods are strategies that benefit the health of people of all ages. For example, these issues, which take such policy considerations to national and international levels, are at the core of the World Health Organization's Age-Friendly World project.[89]

One specific policy use of understanding social vulnerability is that of how to respond to disasters. Frail and socially vulnerable older adults are overrepresented among those most harmed by a range of disasters, so there is considerable interest in understanding the degree of risk. Even so, little work has specifically targeted older adults in this regard.[90]

CONCLUSIONS

Although further research is required to clarify and contextualize the relationships between social circumstances and health in older adults, it has become increasingly clear that social factors exert great influence. In this chapter, the various social factors that have been studied in relation to health have been reviewed, along with their relationship to the concept of overall social vulnerability. Specific associations with health outcomes that are important in geriatric medicine, including frailty, have been discussed.

The deficit accumulation approach to social vulnerability has numerous advantages, including theoretical grounding in understanding the continuum of social influences on health and in relation to work on frailty, consideration of numerous different domains of social factors at once, sensible positioning within a social ecology framework, and great potential for clinical applicability. For example, a social ecology framework of social vulnerability provides a useful basis for a structured approach to the challenge of social admission to acute care hospitals.[91] From the point of view of clinical services providing care in geriatric medicine, the issue is not only which deficits an individual has, but how they add up to contribute to that person's vulnerability perturbations in their social environment, personal health, or functional state in ways that might predispose them to adverse outcomes. As such, a composite measure of social vulnerability may be a useful and potentially clinically relevant starting point to conceptualize the social circumstance of older adults encountered in the course of clinical care. This points to the need for clinical operationalization and testing of such measures of social circumstances.

KEY POINTS

- Social factors are important for older adults' health, particularly in the context of frailty.
- Social circumstances are complex; a deficit accumulation approach to social vulnerability embraces this complexity by considering multiple social factors at once and expressing vulnerability as a gradient.
- A social ecology framework is useful for considering contributions of social factors at various levels from the individual to family and friends, peer groups, institutions, neighborhoods, communities, and society at large.
- Understanding older older adults' social circumstances is important as a predictor of health outcomes and for practical purposes, such as planning care and community support.

For a complete list of references, please visit www.expertconsult.com.

KEY REFERENCES

3. Baum FE, Ziersch AM: Social capital. J Epidemiol Community Health 57:320–323, 2003.
5. Kawachi I, Berkman LF: Social cohesion, social capital, and health. In Berkman LF, Kawachi I, editors: Social Epidemiology, Oxford, England, 2000, Oxford University Press, pp 174–190.
9. Marmot MG, Shipley MJ: Do socioeconomic differences in mortality persist after retirement? 25-year follow-up of civil servants from the first Whitehall study. BMJ 313:1177–1180, 1996.
13. Grundy E, Holt G: The socioeconomic status of older adults: how should we measure it in studies of health inequalities? J Epidemiol Community Health 55:895–904, 2001.
18. Lang IA, Llewellyn DJ, Langa KM, et al: Neighborhood deprivation, individual socioeconomic status, and cognitive function in older people: analyses from the English Longitudinal Study of Ageing. J Am Geriatr Soc 56:191–198, 2008.
27. Putnam RD: Bowling alone: The collapse and revival of American community, New York, 2000, Simon & Schuster.
30. Andrew M, Keefe J: Social vulnerability among older adults: a social ecology perspective from the National Population Health Survey of Canada. BMC Geriatr 14:90, 2014.
31. Fratiglioni L, Wang HX, Ericsson K, et al: Influence of social network on occurrence of dementia: a community-based longitudinal study. Lancet 355:1315–1319, 2000.
38. Cosco TD, Prina AM, Perales J, et al: Operational definitions of successful aging: a systematic review. Int Psychogeriatr 26:373–381, 2014.
42. Mitnitski A, Song X, Rockwood K: Improvement and decline in health status from late middle age: modeling age-related changes in deficit accumulation. Exp Gerontol 42:1109–1115, 2007.
47. Andrew M, Mitnitski A, Kirkland SA, et al: The impact of social vulnerability on the survival of the fittest older adults. Age Ageing 41:161–165, 2012.
48. Wallace L, Theou O, Pena F, et al: Social vulnerability as a predictor of mortality and disability: Cross-country differences in the Survey of Health, Aging, and Retirement in Europe (SHARE). Aging Clin Exp Res 27:365–372, 2015.
49. Wang C, Song X, Mitnitski A, et al: Effect of health protective factors on health deficit accumulation and mortality risk in older adults in the Beijing Longitudinal Study of Aging. J Am Geriatr Soc 62:821–828, 2014.
50. Bassuk SS, Glass TA, Berkman LF: Social disengagement and incident cognitive decline in community-dwelling elderly persons. Ann Intern Med 131:165–173, 1999.
54. Fratiglioni L, Paillard-Borg S, Winblad B: An active and socially integrated lifestyle in late life might protect against dementia. Lancet Neurol 3:343–353, 2004.
78. St John PD, Montgomery PR, Tyas SL: Social position and frailty. Can J Aging 32:250–259, 2013.
79. Woo J, Goggins W, Sham A, et al: Social determinants of frailty. Gerontology 51:402–408, 2005.
82. Salem BE, Nyamathi AM, Brecht ML, et al: Correlates of frailty among homeless adults. West J Nurs Res 35:1128–1152, 2013.
83. Theou O, Brothers TD, Rockwood MR, et al: Exploring the relationship between national economic indicators and relative fitness and frailty in middle-aged and older Europeans. Age Ageing 42:614–619, 2013.
89. World Health Organization: Age-friendly world. http://agefriendlyworld.org/en. Accessed February 3, 2015.

31 The Aging Personality and Self: Diversity and Health Issues

Julie Blaskewicz Boron, K. Warner Schaie, Sherry L. Willis

Personality may be defined as the pattern of thoughts, feelings, and behaviors that shape an individual's interface with the world, distinguish one person from another, and manifest across time and situation.[1-3] Personality is impacted by biologic, cognitive, and environmental determinants, including the impact of culture and cohort. Theoretical approaches to personality are as varied as the breadth of the construct they attempt to describe and explain yet each approach, to varying degrees, emphasizes stability and change within individuals across time and situation.

The impact of personality across the adult life span touches every domain—personal, professional, spiritual, and physical. Certainly, personality characteristics have direct and indirect influences on health status, health behaviors, and behavioral interactions with health care professionals. Although no single chapter can adequately condense such rich empirical and theoretical research, we will attempt to provide a concise overview of stage models, trait theory, and social-cognitive approaches to personality. As such, we will focus on aspects of personality development among cognitively intact older adults, not personality changes that may ensue as the result of dementia.

Each section of this chapter contains four subsections. For each of the three major approaches—stage, trait, social-cognitive—we first provide an overview of classic along with the most current research on stability and maturational and environmental changes in the adult personality. Our focus will be on findings from longitudinal data. Second, we include cross-cultural comparisons of adult personality, where available. This focus provides a unique contribution to reviews of adult personality and aging.[4,5] Third, we examine the health correlates of adult personality, focusing on morbidity and mortality, well-being, life satisfaction, positive and negative affect, anxiety, and depression. Finally, we discuss measurement issues and provide examples of current assessment instruments.

PERSONALITY STAGES AND EGO DEVELOPMENT

Freudian Theory

The psychoanalytic approach to adult personality development has its roots in the theories of Sigmund Freud. His theories encompassed four domains—level of consciousness, personality structure, defense mechanisms, and stages of psychosexual development.[6,7] Freudian theory postulates that adult personality is made up of three aspects: (1) the id, operating on the pleasure principle generally within the unconscious; (2) the ego, operating on the reality principle within the conscious realm; and (3) the superego, operating on the morality principle at all levels of consciousness. The interplay of these personality structures generates anxiety that must be reduced through various defense mechanisms. These mechanisms act to obscure the true, anxiety-laden reasons for one's behavior.

Although seminal in the expansion of our understanding of the human psyche, Freud's specific theories receive little attention in the scientific study of personality today.[6] His theories are not easily amenable to scientific inquiry in that they frequently lead to nonspecific hypotheses, wherein failure to find expected effects may simply be a result of unknown defense mechanisms. Additionally, having postulated that personality development associated with his stages of psychosexual development essentially ends in adolescence, Freud's theories have limited applicability to the fields of gerontology and geriatric medicine.

Post-Freudian Theorists

In contrast, some post-Freudian theorists have conceptualized personality development as a continuing process focused on current interpersonal and/or family of origin issues as the source of individual distress and coping patterns. Carl Jung proposed that as individuals age, they achieve a balance between the expression of their masculine characteristics (animus) and feminine characteristics (anima).[8,9] Findings regarding increased balance of gender roles with age have emerged in different cultures, lending some support to Jung's hypothesis.[2]

Erik Erikson's stages of psychosocial development are perhaps the best known of the stage theories of adult personality. The sequence of Erikson's eight stages of development is based on the epigenetic principle, which means that personality moves through these stages in an ordered fashion at an appropriate rate.[3,10] Two of the eight stages describe personality change during the adult years. Although the identity crisis is placed in adolescence, deciding "who you are" is a continual process that is reflected throughout adulthood, even in old age.[11] In the midlife stage of generativity versus stagnation, individuals seek ways to give their talents and experiences to the next generation, moving beyond the self-concerns of identity and interpersonal concerns of intimacy.[5] Successful resolution of this stage results in the development of a sense of trust and care for the next generation and assurance that society will continue. Unsuccessful resolution of this stage results in self-absorption.

Ego integrity versus despair is Erikson's final stage of ego development, beginning around the age of 65 years and continuing until death. In this stage, individuals become increasingly internally focused and more aware of the nearness of death. Successful resolution of this stage results in being able to look back on one's life and find meaning, developing a sense of wisdom before death. Alternatively, meaninglessness and despair can ensue if this process of life review results in focus on primarily negative outcomes.

Difficulties arising from attempts to investigate Erikson's theory empirically include the assertion that stages must be encountered in order and there is lack of specification regarding how developmental crises are resolved, so that an individual may move from one stage to the next. However, the environmental influences of culture and cohort on adult personality have been minimized. One 22-year investigation found significant age changes supportive of Erikson's theory.[12] Middle-aged adults expressed emotions and cognitions consistent with successful completion of more psychosocial developmental crises than younger adults. In addition, Ackerman and colleagues found a stronger association between generativity in midlife compared with that in young adulthood.[13] Some theorists have postulated that the ego integrity versus despair period initiates a process of life review.[14]

Life Review

The concept of life review is the exception to this lack of empirical investigation regarding stage theories of adult personality.[14,15] Life review can be thought of as a systematic cognitive-emotional process occurring late in life in which an individual thinks back across his or her life experiences and integrates disparate events into general themes. The portion of life review focusing on recall of primarily positive life experiences is reminiscence. Reminiscence has been linked to successful aging[16] by contributing to sustained identity formation and self-continuity, a sense of mastery, meaning, and coherence in life, and acceptance and reconciliation of one's life.[17] Although this approach to adult personality development can be conceptualized as a cognitive process in which identity emerges from the story of one's life, we have chosen to include it with stage models because it is most frequently described as occurring near the completion of one's life. Nevertheless, it should be acknowledged that individuals likely undergo a process of life review periodically throughout the adult years, including young adulthood[18] and midlife.[19,20]

Stage Theory

Stage Theories and Diversity

Few studies investigating stage theories of personality have focused on diverse cultural or racial and ethnic groups. Most of the stage models, such as Freud's original theories, were based on highly select samples. Only a few investigations of life review have succeeded in recruiting participants reflecting the general population of interest.[21-23] Cross-cultural evidence has indicated that life review programs have improved self-esteem and life satisfaction in Taiwanese older adults,[24] depressive symptoms in community-dwelling Chinese older adults,[25] and depression and anxiety symptoms in Dutch older adults.[26] Data reflecting the broader diversity of the population are needed for examining the universality of life review and generalizability of the basic assumptions.

Stage Theories and Health

There has been limited investigation of the relation between stage approaches to adult personality and health. One study on generativity found that those perceiving more generativity in their lives had fewer activity of daily living impairments and decreased risk of mortality 10 years later.[27] However, most research has focused on life review processes. Several intervention studies have supported the contention that life review, in comparison with nonspecific but supportive interventions, has a positive impact on health, life satisfaction, well-being, and depression.

A meta-analysis on reminiscence and well-being in older adulthood has demonstrated that although reminiscence was moderately (effect size, 0.54) associated with life-satisfaction and well-being in older adulthood, engaging in life review had a stronger effect.[17] This suggests that consideration of all major life events, positive and negative, as is typical for life review, has a greater impact on well-being in older adulthood. Furthermore, another meta-analysis by Bohlmeijer and associates have investigated the effects of life review on late-life depression.[28] Results suggested that life review and reminiscence may be an effective treatment for depressive symptoms in older adults. Additional research has supported the utility of life review interventions to decrease depressive symptoms and improve life satisfaction in older adults.[29-33] Recent research has considered the effects of psychological resources and found that mastery and meaning in life mediated the relationship between negative reminiscence and psychologically distressing symptoms consistent with depression and anxiety.[34] Finally, participants in life review programs have demonstrated wider psychological benefits, including increased autonomy, environmental mastery, personal growth, positive relations with others, purpose in life, and self-acceptance in comparison to control groups.[35]

Measurement Issues

The primary methodologic problem plaguing empirical research involving stage theory approaches to adult personality development has been the lack of specification of change mechanisms and limitations in psychometrically reliable and valid measures. Personality stability is assumed with these stage theories. This is not necessarily problematic; however, measuring how people progress through the proposed stages, including the order of progression, and whether non-normative life events can lead to changes in personality, is not captured through current measures, nor is the consideration of age changes versus cohort differences.[36] The most current stage approach to adult personality in our organizational scheme involves the concept of life review near the end of life. Bohlmeijer and coworkers have noted the lack of standardized protocols to life review as a therapeutic technique in the delivery of interventions.[17]

A common methodologic limitation in much of this research is the problem of making causal inferences of age-related personality change from cross-sectional studies. In these studies, age-related differences could be observed because of the impact of aging or due to cohort differences. Without cohort sequential data, it is impossible to tease apart these influences. Thus, although stage theories of adult personality have intuitive appeal, their contribution is limited by vague delineation of constructs and methodology.

Personality Traits

In contrast to stage approaches to adult personality development, empirical research regarding trait approaches has experienced a significant boom in recent years. The Big Five Factor Model of Personality provides a broad framework for organizing the hundreds of traits, or individual differences, that characterize people.[37] These five core dimensions have been demonstrated at most life stages through extensive factor analyses of personality descriptors.[38,39] A description of the most commonly identified five factors can be found in Box 31-1.

Early studies suggested that maturational changes in personality occur in young adulthood until approximately the age of 30 years, with relative intraindividual stability in traits thereafter.[40-44]

BOX 31-1 The Big Five Personality Traits

1. **Emotional stability versus neuroticism—**anxiety, depression, emotional instability, self-consciousness, hostility, and impulsiveness vs. relaxation, poise, and steadiness
2. **Extraversion or surgency—**gregariousness, assertiveness, activity level, and positive emotions versus silence, passivity, and reserve
3. **Culture and intellect or openness to experience—**imagination, curiosity, and creativity versus shallowness, imperceptiveness, and stupidity
4. **Agreeableness or pleasantness**—attributes such as kindness, trust, and warmth that are considered pleasant and attractive to others versus hostility, selfishness, and distrust
5. **Conscientiousness or dependability**—encompasses organization, responsibility, ambition, perseverance, and hard work versus carelessness, negligence, and unreliability

Adapted from Goldberg LR: The structure of phenotypic personality traits. Am Psychol 48:26–34, 1993.

However, stability of personality across adulthood lacks consensus. The debate as to whether personality remains stable or changes in adulthood may be based on different criteria for determining change. Roberts and Mroczek have described various forms of change, including mean-level change, rank-order consistency, structural consistency, and individual differences in change.[45] Usually, research supporting stability refers to rank-order consistency, whereas research emphasizing change focuses on individual differences in change. Consistent with cross-sectional results,[41] longitudinal assessments and meta-analyses[46] have shown small age-related declines in neuroticism, extraversion, and openness to experience, with age-related increases in agreeableness and conscientiousness in adults up to the age of 70 years (declines in neuroticism persisted until age 80). However, this research is often cited as supporting stability of personality in adulthood. Although mean-level changes are shown, individuals maintain their rank-order on the personality domains.[47] Findings from other research teams have contributed support for stability.[48-52]

Studies of variability in individual rates of change have provided support for the notion that personality may change, even in adulthood.[53-57] Together these studies suggest that some individuals change more or less than other individuals in terms of personality traits. Thus, studies have attempted to investigate factors that may contribute to these varying rates of individual change. In a 12-year longitudinal study of middle-aged to older men, Mroczek and Spiro found cohort, incidence of marriage or remarriage, spousal death, and memory complaints to be associated with differential rates of change in personality.[55] Individual differences in life circumstances or other environmental sources were also found to be associated with differential rates of change in personality, affecting overall well-being.[58] Social support, unmet needs, health, and psychosocial needs are examples of various life circumstances found to be significant predictors of differential rates of change in older women.[59] Thus, specific life experiences may have an impact on personality. Consideration of the various definitions of change and the factors accounting for change is important when reviewing research on personality stability or change.

Trait Theories and Diversity

Cross-cultural studies have most frequently compared non-Hispanic whites in the United States with individuals living in other countries.[60-62] These studies seek to estimate the effects of environment on different age cohorts by comparing adults in cultures with different recent histories. Using the NEO Personality Inventory-R, McCrae and colleagues studied parallels in adult personality traits across cultures in five countries—Germany, Italy, Portugal, Croatia, and South Korea.[61] Once again, different patterns of age changes would result if environmental factors play a major role in adult personality development. In contrast, intrinsic maturational perspectives would suggest that even widely different cultures should show similar age trends. Results have shown that across cultures, midlife adults scored higher on measures of agreeableness and conscientiousness and lower on neuroticism, extraversion, and openness than 18- to 21-year-olds. Congruence was strongest for openness and weakest for neuroticism, for which only two cultures (Germany and South Korea) replicated the American pattern.

Using the California Psychological Inventory (CPI), factor structures similar to the Big Five were compared among adults in the United States and the People's Republic of China; comparisons revealed very similar patterns of age correlations.[60,62] In a study by Yang and associates,[62] the Chinese sample was an average of 25 years younger than the U.S. sample, and age effects were smaller in the U.S. sample. Likewise, Labouvie-Vief and associates found high congruence on all four personality factors derived from the CPI—extraversion, control-norm orientation, flexibility, and femininity-masculinity.[60] Older cohorts across cultures had lower scores on extraversion and flexibility and higher scores on control-norm orientation. Once again, age differences were more pronounced among Chinese than U.S. adults. Smaller cultural differences were found among the youngest age groups than among the oldest groups.

In general, the results of these cross-cultural studies are consistent with the hypothesis that there are universally intrinsic maturational changes in personality.[60-62] Yang and coworkers reported, however, that across the span from 18 to 65 years, age never accounted for more than 20% of the variance in CPI scale scores.[62] Gender did not influence the pattern of results in these cross-cultural studies. The authors differed in their interpretation of the influence of environmental factors. In the Yang and McCrae studies,[61,62] the authors maintained that the results offered little support for historical cohort effects being major determinants of cross-sectional age differences in adult personality traits. Although noting the high degree of similarity in personality traits across cultures, Labouvie-Vief and colleagues also noted that cultural climate and cultural change do affect the relationship between age and personality.[60]

Trait Theories and Health

There is extensive literature on the association of adult personality and health. Neuroticism is one of the traits most frequently studied in relation to health. Neuroticism has been associated with greater reactivity to stress,[63] whereas high levels of personal control or mastery serve as a protective factor in regard to the impact of stress on health.[64,65] In a recent review of the literature, Hill and Roberts documented several physiologic markers of aging associated with personality traits. In particular, lower interleukin-6 levels, affecting inflammation and C-reactive protein, also influential for acute injuries, have been associated with higher conscientiousness and lower neuroticism.[66] Siegman and associates found the dominance factor derived from the Minnesota Multiphasic Personality Inventory (2-MMPI) to be an independent risk factor for incidence of fatal coronary heart disease and nonfatal myocardial infarction among older men, with an average age of 61 years.[67] Niaura and coworkers found that among older men, greater hostility may be associated with a pattern of obesity, central adiposity, and insulin resistance, which can exert effects on blood pressure and serum lipid levels.[68] A study of Japanese older adults found extraversion, conscientiousness, and openness to be negatively associated with 5-year mortality rates.[69] Overall, several studies have documented an association between personality and mortality, indicating that higher levels of neuroticism and lower levels of conscientiousness serve as risk factors of mortality.[70-73]

Measurement Issues

There are multiple instruments of personality traits that measure the Big Five.[74-76] Regardless of the specific measurement instrument used, however, these measures demonstrate remarkable consistency in the derivation of five dimensions of personality via factor analysis.[37] However, multiple methodologic issues remain. One major complication of stability estimates in adult personality research involves the type of stability that is under consideration. The impact of cohort and time of measurement on trait consistency within the longitudinal studies conducted to date has not been fully considered.[51] Studies of gender role differences have shown that age is not as good a predictor as the life experiences of different cohorts on personality traits of men and women across time.[77-79] Thus, it may be that earlier born cohorts developed more consistent personality traits earlier in life as the result of numerous social, historical, and life span–related influences.

More extensive consideration of the relative impact of biologic and environmental variables on stability and change in adult personality is essential. Although the influence of genetic factors has been investigated in the development of personality among monozygotic and dizygotic twins over a 10-year period, no such investigations have addressed the contribution of genetics to the maintenance of personality across the adult age range. Regarding the impact of environmental influences, with time and age individuals may encounter fewer novel experiences.[52] Thus, the stability of personality factors may be causally related to the decreasing novelty of the environment in which individuals live rather than genetic factors. Finally, prior research on traits has been primarily descriptive and would profit from a theory-driven approach.

SOCIAL-COGNITIVE APPROACHES TO PERSONALITY

The social-cognitive approach to the study of adult personality and the self focuses on the processes underlying stability and change in one's perception of the self and emphasizes the impact of necessary, adaptive adjustments in one's personality. An individual's sense of self is proposed to develop through the interaction of internal and environmental factors, influencing maturational changes and cohort differences. Although the content of the developing self may change, this model proposes that the mechanisms whereby changes are integrated into the concept of self are stable. Thus, the development of the self as a dynamic construct reflects one's identity, perception of possible selves, sense of control or personal mastery, and perception of the remaining life span.

Identity and Personal Control

Whitbourne and Connolly have described a life span approach to one's core identity development. The term *identity* is defined as an individual's developing sense of self, an organizing schema through which internal and external life experiences are interpreted.[80] Identity includes physical functioning, cognition, social relationships, and environmental experiences.[81,82] The identity process theory posits that changes in identity with age occur through assimilation, accommodation, and balance.[70] Successful aging consists of integrating information about the self and achieving equilibrium between assimilation and accommodation. Similar to the identity process with age, a sense of control or personal mastery, the degree to which people believes that they can affect and influence outcomes in their life, also requires aging individuals to adapt their beliefs as age-related changes in physical functioning, cognition, social relationships, and environmental experiences occur.

Whitbourne and Collins have examined the self-reports of adults aged 40 to 95 years regarding the relation between identity and changes in physical functioning.[83] Older adults who focused more on perceived changes in competence were more likely to use identity assimilation (i.e., reinterpretation of experiences to coincide with the self) in the area of cognitive functioning than were other age groups. In a clinical trial on cognitive training, personal control in regard to cognitive functioning was found to increase in older adults as a function of cognitive training on inductive reasoning or speed of processing[84]; thus, this facet of personality may vary as a result of experience and can experience positive effects from intervention. Another study by Sneed and Whitbourne has highlighted the importance of assimilation over accommodation, because those who engaged in identity assimilation and identity balance were associated with increased self-esteem, whereas accommodation resulted in decreased self-esteem.[85] Finally, in a study of identity and self- consciousness, identity accommodation was positively associated with self-reflection and public self-consciousness.[86]

Researchers interested in understanding the self from a life span perspective often use the theoretical framework provided by the "possible selves" model.[87] The construct of possible selves postulates that individuals are guided in their actions by aspects of the self that represent what the individual could become, would like to become, and is afraid of becoming. Possible selves serve as psychological resources that may motivate an individual and direct future behavior.

Ryff's research has provided empirical support for the concept of possible selves.[88] Young, middle-aged, and older adults were asked to judge their past, present, future, and ideal selves on dimensions related to self-acceptance, positive relations with others, autonomy, environmental mastery, purpose in life, and personal growth. Older adults were more likely than younger adults to adjust their ideal self downwardly and to view their past more positively.[88] Over a 5-year period in old age, hoped and feared possible selves were found to remain stable.[89] Goal orientation shifted with age; specifically, older adults focused on maintenance and loss prevention, and this orientation was associated with well-being.[90] A shift in goal orientation in regard to possible selves may contribute to perceived control and stability of possible selves. Furthermore, this reflects the shift with age from focusing on primary control, efforts directed at changing the environment, to secondary control, attempts to manage emotions or internal processes rather than external processes.[91] Recent research has suggested that although both types of control increase as a function of age, with secondary control increasing to a greater extent, primary control was more predictive of life satisfaction.[92] However, in older adults, perceived secondary control influenced perceived primary control, thus indirectly influencing life satisfaction. Perceived control over development is associated with subjective well-being across adulthood.[93]

Socioemotional Selectivity Theory

Carstensen's socioemotional selectivity theory (SST) focuses on the agentic choices made by adults in their social world for the purpose of regulating knowledge-oriented and emotional goals.[94-96] The purposeful selective reduction in social interaction begins in early adulthood, and emotional closeness remains stable or increases within selected relationships as one ages.[94-96] When time is perceived as open-ended, acquisition of knowledge is prioritized. When time is perceived as limited, however, emotional goals assume primacy. Older adults select social relationships in which they want to invest their resources and in which they expect reciprocity and positive affect, thereby optimizing their social networks. Furthermore, those maintained in older adults' social networks were reported to elicit more positive and fewer negative emotions, which in turn positively affected daily emotional experiences.[97] Thus, older adults' social networks are reduced by choice as individuals decrease contact with acquaintances but seek to maintain contact with relatives and friends as a function of increased saliency of emotional attachment to one's life goals.[94-96]

The perception of time left in life (future time perspective) is postulated to be fundamental to motivation, and age is correlated with time perspective.[98] Perceiving an ending plays an important role in identity processes, such that endings promote greater self-acceptance and less striving toward an abstract ideal.[88,99] Thus, due to changes in the perceived time left to live, older adults have been shown to be more present-oriented than concerned about the past and less concerned than young adults about the future.[100] This has also been associated with an increased focus on positive emotions, compared to negative. Rather than age being the causal factor in shifts in self-perception and social goals, it is the inverse association of chronologic age with number of years left to live that produces observed relations. Experimental research has demonstrated the malleability of this shift based on age perspective. When adopting a younger adult perspective, younger and older adults showed a negativity effect, whereas a positivity effect was observed in both age groups when taking an older adult perspective.[101]

Social-Cognitive Theories and Diversity

There have been few empirical investigations of cultural or racial and ethnic diversity in the study of social-cognitive approaches to adult personality development. Cross-cultural research on SST mostly supports similarities in age differences across cultures, rather than cultural differences. The experience of increased positive and decreased negative affect was found in both U.S. and Chinese older adults; however, although U.S. older adults reported higher self-life satisfaction overall, perceived family life satisfaction was found to be more influential to self-life satisfaction for Chinese older adults.[102]

Waid and Frazier have compared older Spanish-speaking natives and white non-Hispanic, English-speaking natives.[103] Cultural differences in hoped and feared possible selves were present, primarily reflecting traditional differences in individualistic (English speakers) and collectivist (Spanish speakers) cultures, with physical concerns and loss of loved ones endorsed most for these two groups, respectively. Frequently cited hoped-for selves included family-oriented domains for Spanish-speaking natives and advances in the abilities and education domain for English-speaking natives. Thus, the cultural differences evident for possible selves and control revolve around differences attributed to individualistic and collectivist cultures. In a Taiwanese sample, possible selves who focused on the physical self were associated with engagement in physical activity.[104]

Gross and colleagues found consistent age differences in the subjective report of emotional experience and control across diverse cultures—Norwegians, Chinese Americans, African Americans, European Americans, and Catholic nuns.[105] Across all groups, older adults reported fewer negative emotional experiences and greater emotional control. Likewise, Fung and associates found support for the notion that socioemotional selectivity is due to perceived limitations in time among adults in the United States and Hong Kong[106] and among adults in Taiwan and Mainland China.[107]

An investigation exemplifying the importance of perceived time left to live was conducted following the terrorist attacks of September 11, 2001, in the United States and the severe acute respiratory syndrome (SARS) epidemic in Hong Kong. By investigating social goals before and after these events, Fung and Carstensen found increased motivation to focus on emotional goals, regardless of age.[108]

Social-Cognitive Theories and Health

In general, empirical research regarding identity and the self has explored relationships with physical health outcomes, whereas research regarding socioemotional selectivity theory has focused on relationships with emotional outcomes. As one advances in age, people define themselves increasingly in terms of health and physical functioning.[21] In a study of older adults aged 60 to 96 years, leisure was an important domain for the young-old, whereas health was the most important self-domain for the oldest-old.[109] It appears that adults cognitively manage their expectations and social comparison processes so that they are, in general, no less satisfied with their health status, despite increasing physical limitations. Zhang and colleagues found that older adults were more likely to engage in positive health behavior change if the information presented to them included emotional compared to nonemotional goals.[110] Given the increase in chronic disease management in older adulthood, framing health-relevant goals in a way that appeals to emotional goals is an important way to positively affect quality of life in later life.

The content of possible selves and perceived control have been examined in relation to subjective well-being, health, and health behaviors. Hooker and Kaus have found that having a possible self in the realm of health was more strongly related to reported health behaviors than was a global measure of health values.[111] Furthermore, those focusing on health and reporting more health-related fears in regard to their possible selves endorsed fewer depressive symptoms, suggesting a benefit to prioritizing health in older adulthood.[112] Stability in perceived control provides a protective benefit to health. Older adults exhibiting variability in perceived control had poorer health, functional status, more physician visits and hospital admissions.[113,114] Individuals higher on personal mastery were less likely to rate themselves as in fair or poor health, whereas those endorsing more perceived constraints were more likely to rate their health as poor.[115] Finally, individuals with higher self-efficacy, the belief that people have the ability to exert control over themselves and their environment, interpret and manage stressors in ways that promote health.[116]

With regard to SST, negative exchanges with one's social network have a detrimental impact on daily mood and, if encountered frequently, can increase the incidence of depression, whereas positive exchanges can serve to buffer the impact of negative exchanges.[117]

Measurement Issues

Comparisons of findings from studies focusing on possible selves, compared with socioemotional selectivity, are limited by the different measurement approaches used. The possible selves construct is measured using a questionnaire inventory.[99] SST, in contrast, has relied on self-report, observation of marital interactions, and card sorting of potential social partners on the basis of similarity judgments, with the resulting categories submitted to multidimensional scaling analysis.[98]

A strength of social-cognitive approaches is the positing of explanatory processes for personality development. The identification of specific testable processes such as identity assimilation, identity accommodation, possible selves, or socioemotional selectivity promotes theoretical advances via empirical hypothesis testing.

Social cognitive researchers interested in personality and self in later life investigate domains emphasizing growth and development in old age. This contributes to an individual's perception of possible selves, need for affiliation, and content of life review.

SYNTHESIS AND FUTURE DIRECTIONS

In this chapter, we have reviewed the psychological literature concerning personality development across the adult life span. We have considered stage, trait, and social-cognitive approaches to the study of adult personality. Within each section, we reviewed literature on diversity and health outcomes, where available. We also included a measurement section highlighting particular assessment instruments and providing an overview of methodologic strengths and weaknesses for each approach.

We have reviewed several issues central to the conceptualization of adult personality. The issue of stability versus maturational change or cohort differences in personality development is dependent on the theory and measurement approach used. For example, the relative stability found in the trait approaches (e.g., the Big Five) may be in part a result of the aggregation of multiple personality facets. Examination of stability at the facet and aggregate levels is needed to investigate whether personality may be dependent on genetic or biologic factors. In contrast, measurement of more precise traits (e.g., facets) may be influenced more by cognitive and environmental (i.e., cohort) influences. Thus, specific individual traits would be expected to be less stable across time than the Big Five personality aggregates. As stated in the section on trait theory, clarity in the definition of stability (i.e., intraindividual, mean-level, or ordinal) is critical to ensure that conclusions drawn from differing research methodologies are interpreted uniformly.

In the effort to tease apart the influence of environmental and biologic influences on stability and change, cross-cultural comparisons of adult personality have been particularly useful. Comparisons of adults of the same age who have experienced different environments across their life span provide evidence regarding the extent of environmental influence on personality. More research is needed, however, to address the personality development of very old individuals in diverse cultures. Additionally, investigation of health effects of adult personality in diverse cultures provides invaluable information for health service provision and the development of preventive interventions.

Finally, it would be useful to apply the wealth of accumulated information regarding personality across adulthood to the provision of services designed to enhance quality of life. Identification of personality processes that drive specific behaviors and choices (e.g., medical treatment) is needed. There is powerful evidence that personality characteristics can affect health status and health behaviors. For example, interventions such as life review have successfully enhanced quality of life. Using social-cognitive approaches to adult personality development and the processes of identity assimilation, identity accommodation, and socioemotional selectivity could inform interventions designed to improve the process of advance care planning for the implementation of life-sustaining or palliative treatments at the end of life.

Furthermore, applied intervention research will not only enhance service provision, but will also drive theoretical advances in the concept of the self in old age. For example, palliative care and/or hospice interventions designed to provide services targeting personal, physical, and spiritual needs can inform aspects of SST involving present-time orientation and time remaining to live. Incorporating aspects of life review could also provide advances in theories driving therapeutic approaches for depression. Interventions for bereaved personal and professional caregivers and interventions for the terminally or chronically ill older adult are desperately needed. It is our contention that the time to apply our knowledge of adult personality across the life span is now, thereby deriving benefit from our accumulated knowledge and driving advances in theory.

KEY POINTS: THE AGING PERSONALITY AND SELF

- Personality is the pattern of thoughts, feelings, and behaviors that shape an individual's interface with the world, distinguish one person from another, and manifest across time and situations. It is affected by biologic, cognitive, and environmental determinants.
- Stage theorists include Freud, Jung, and Erikson. The psychoanalytic approach to adult personality encompasses four domains—level of consciousness, personality structure, defense mechanisms, and stages of psychosexual development. Erikson's eight stages of development are based on the idea that the growing personality moves through stages in an ordered fashion. Few studies investigating stage theories of personality have focused on diverse cultures, racial and ethnic groups, or health.
- Trait approaches are currently the standard method of personality assessment, with multiple instruments available. The Big Five personality traits are neuroticism. extraversion, openness to experience, agreeableness, and conscientiousness. In general, the results of cross-cultural studies are consistent with the hypothesis that there are universal intrinsic maturational changes in personality. Neuroticism, in particular, has been associated with several health outcomes, including stress, chronic conditions, and mortality.
- The social-cognitive approach focuses on the individual's sense of self, developing through the interaction of internal and environmental factors. Social-cognitive theories have incorporated physical health and emotional outcomes.
- The socioemotional selectivity theory (SST) focuses on the agentic choices made by adults in their social world for the purpose of regulating knowledge-oriented emotion goals. In SST, individuals alter their environmental interactions such that optimization of emotional experience is prioritized later in life. There have been few empirical investigations incorporating diverse cultural or racial and ethnic groups in the study of social-cognitive approaches to adult personality development; existing evidence suggests similar age differences across cultures.

For a complete list of references, please visit www.expertconsult.com.

KEY REFERENCES

1. Allport GW: Personality, New York, 1937, Holt, Rinehart, and Winston.
7. Freud S: Three essays on the theory of sexuality. In Freud S, editor: The standard edition, vol VII, London, 1953, Hogarth.
8. Jung CG: Analytical psychology: its theory and practice, New York, 1968, Vintage Books.
10. Erikson E: Childhood and society, ed 2, New York, 1963, Norton.
17. Bohlmeijer E, Roemer M, Cuijpers P, et al: The effects of reminiscence on psychological well-being in older adults: a meta-analysis. Aging Ment Health 11:291–300, 2007.
25. Chan M, Ng S, Tien A, et al: A randomised controlled study to explore the effect of life story review on depression in older Chinese in Singapore. Health Soc Care Community 21:545–553, 2013.
27. Gruenewald T, Liao D, Seeman T: Contributing to others, contributing to oneself: perceptions of generativity and health in later life. J Gerontol B Psychol Sci Soc Sci 67B:660–665, 2012.
32. Chippendale T, Bear-Lehman J: Effect of life review writing on depressive symptoms in older adults: A randomized controlled trial. Am J Occup Ther 66:438–446, 2012.
34. Korte J, Cappeliez P, Bohlmeijer E, et al: Meaning in life and mastery mediate the relationship of negative reminiscence with psychological distress among older adults with mild to moderate depressive symptoms. Eur J Ageing 9:343–351, 2012.
42. Costa PT, McCrae RR: Longitudinal stability of adult personality. In Hogan R, Johnson J, Briggs S, editors: Handbook of Personality Psychology, San Diego, CA, 1997, Academic Press.
46. Debast I, van Alphen S, Rosowsky E, et al: Personality traits and personality disorders in late middle and old age: do they remain stable? A literature review. Clin Gerontol 37:253–271, 2014.
57. Specht J, Egloff B, Schmukle S: Stability and change of personality across the life course: The impact of age and major life events on mean-level and rank-order stability of the Big Five. J Pers Soc Psychol 101:862–882, 2011.
58. Kandler C, Kornadt A, Hagemeyer B, et al: Patterns and sources of personality development in old age. J Pers Soc Psychol 109:1751–1791, 2015.
66. Hill PL, Roberts BW: Personality and health: reviewing recent research and setting a directive for the future. In Schaie KW, Willis SL, editors: Handbook of the psychology of aging, ed 8, San Diego, CA, 2016, Academic Press, pp 206–219.
69. Iwasa H, Masui Y, Gondo Y, et al: Personality and all-cause mortality among older adults dwelling in a Japanese community: a five-year population-based prospective cohort study. Am J Geriatr Psychiatry 16:399–405, 2008.
77. Schmitt DP, Realo A, Voracek M, et al: Why can't a man be more like a woman? Sex differences in big five personality traits across 55 cultures. J Pers Soc Psychol 94:168–182, 2008.

84. Wolinsky F, Vander Weg M, Tennstedt S, et al: Does cognitive training improve internal locus of control among older adults? J Gerontol B Psychol Sci Soc Sci 65:591–598, 2010.
92. de Quadros-Wander S, McGillivray J, Broadbent J: The influence of perceived control on subjective wellbeing in later life. Soc Indic Res 115:999–1010, 2014.
97. English T, Carstensen L: Selective narrowing of social networks across adulthood is associated with improved emotional experience in daily life. Int J Behav Dev 38:195–202, 2014.
101. Lynchard N, Radvansky G: Age-related perspectives and emotion processing. Psychol Aging 27:934–939, 2012.
102. Pethtel O, Chen Y: Cross-cultural aging in cognitive and affective components of subjective well-being. Psychol Aging 25:725–729, 2010.
104. Hsu Y, Lu F, Lin L: Physical self-concept, possible selves, and well-being among older adults in Taiwan. Educ Gerontol 40:666–675, 2014.
110. Zhang X, Fung H, Ching B: Age differences in goals: Implications for health promotion. Aging Ment Health 13:336–348, 2009.
112. Bolkan C, Hooker K, Coehlo D: Possible selves and depressive symptoms in later life. Res Aging 37:41–62, 2015.
115. Ward M: Sense of control and self-reported health in a population-based sample of older Americans: Assessment of potential confounding by affect, personality, and social support. Int J Behav Med 20:140–147, 2013.

32 Productive Aging

Jan E. Mutchler, Sae Hwang Han, Jeffrey A. Burr

INTRODUCTION

Far from being years of leisure and inactivity, later life is increasingly recognized as being characterized by high levels of productivity. The concept of productive aging captures both paid and unpaid activities that have social value and are performed by adults during the later years of the life course. Late life engagement in activities such as paid work, volunteering, informal helping, caregiving, and taking on the role of a grandparent caregiver are widely accepted as markers of productive aging. Estimates from the Health and Retirement Study (HRS) suggest that well over half of U.S. adults age 65 and older engage in at least one of these productive activities, with participation in volunteering and informal helping being especially common.

Productive aging has consequences for society as well as for the participant. The productive engagements of older adults are widely acknowledged to contribute substantially to society as a whole, and especially to the social groups, communities, and networks that directly benefit from the contributions. Older adults contribute millions of hours in unpaid productive activity, and many of these valued services would need to be paid for if they were not contributed by older adults. For example, Johnson and Schaner[1] place a dollar value on these activities and estimate that in 2002, Americans age 55 and older generated $162 billion in unpaid activity through volunteering and caregiving alone.

As well, participation in productive activities often directly benefits the older adult who participates in them. Some research finds participating in productive activities is linked to avoiding disease and even prolonging survival.[2,3] In this respect, a clear pathway is evident between "productive aging" (participation in activities that have intrinsic value and contribute to the well-being of others) and "successful aging," that is, aging with good health, high functioning, and active involvement.[4]

The focus of this chapter is on factors that shape engagement in productive activities in later life, referred to here as *antecedents* of productive aging, and on the *consequences* of productive aging. In considering antecedents, we review both individual-level factors that promote or inhibit participation and societal and cultural factors that shape the opportunities for older adults to participate. In addition, in reviewing consequences of productive activity, we offer a brief summary of the societal-level consequences, and we focus especially on the scientific literature suggesting that participation in productive activities contributes to health and well-being in later life.

Previous editions of this volume included a chapter on productive aging authored by Robert N. Butler, MD, widely regarded as the founder of the concept. Butler traced the creation of the concept of productive aging to the recognition that older adults had much to contribute well into later life, yet they encountered societal barriers to participation in the form of ageism and prejudice. Indeed, early in the development of this concept, Butler[5] suggested that ageism should be treated as a disease, with productive aging pursued as a remedy. Butler's insights, and his advocacy on behalf of older adults, established a framework for re-envisioning later life and promoting activity as a means of preserving health and well-being. The following discussion highlights the enduring usefulness of these insights.

A PORTRAIT OF PRODUCTIVE AGING IN THE UNITED STATES

The research literature on productive aging places emphasis on five forms of productive activities frequently performed by older adults: paid work, volunteering, caregiving, informal helping, and grandparenting. In this section, we describe these activities and offer recent evidence on how participation in each is related to age and gender. The data used here to describe productive activity among middle-aged and older adults are taken from the 2010 version of the HRS. The HRS contains a nationally representative sample of adults in the United States age 51 and older. The HRS is one of only a handful of data files that contain national-level information on all five of these forms of productive activity. Other sources of information describing some of these specific activities are available, and the statistics generated from the HRS may not match those generated from these other sources, largely because of differences in research design. Readers should keep this in mind when comparing our numbers to those generated from other sources.

Paid Work

The capacity of the older population to serve in the paid labor force was, and sometimes still is, considered as the standard indicator of productivity by some observers. Typical indicators of economic performance, such as the gross domestic product, omit estimated monetary values of voluntary activities and informal contributions made by older adults.[6] Despite the distinctive age curve in labor force participation, which peaks during late middle age and declines thereafter,[7] a considerable number of older workers remain in the labor force well into the later stages of the life course. We estimate that about 18 million adults ages 51 to 64, and 7.5 million age 65 and older, were working for pay in 2010 (see Table 32-1). Moreover, older adults are expected to comprise a larger share of the workforce in coming years. Estimates suggest that the share of the labor force composed of workers age 55 years and older will increase to 26% in 2022, up from 12% in 2012.[8] As demonstrated with HRS data (Table 32-1), there is a considerable difference in labor force participation between older males and females, with males being more likely than females to be in the labor market in later life. However, recent data suggest a narrowing of the gender differences, as a result of declining participation among men and rising participation among women contributing to the trend.

Older workers do not show much difference in the type of work they do and what they do when compared with their younger counterparts, as they can be found in most industries and occupations, broadly classified. However, older workers are more likely than younger workers to be self-employed or to work part-time.[9] For some older adults, these forms of employment may be pursued as part of a phased retirement strategy, working fewer hours for the same employer, or working in a bridge job

TABLE 32-1 Productive Activity Participation Rates by Age Group and Sex (Estimated from the 2010 Health and Retirement Study*)

	Paid Work†		Volunteering†		Informal Help†		Grandparenting†		Caregiving†	
	Percentage of Population	*Number‡*	*Percentage of Population*	*Number‡*	*Percentage of Population*	*Number‡*	*Percentage of Population*	*Number‡*	*Percentage of Population*	*Number‡*
Total										
51-64	62.8%	17,734	41.6%	11,751	66.0%	18,643	13.7%	3,874	21.0%	5,933
65+	**19.8%**	**7,488**	**35.7%**	**13,517**	**49.0%**	**18,562**	**9.3%**	**3,528**	**15.2%**	**5,743**
Male										
51-64	66.5%	8,281	39.74%	4,949	71.67%	8,926	10.4%	1,292	17.9%	2,219
65+	**25.1%**	**4,119**	**34.64%**	**5,693**	**55.86%**	**9,180**	**10.3%**	**1,689**	**14.0%**	**2,365**
Female										
51-64	59.9%	9,453	43.12%	6,801	61.60%	9,717	16.4%	2,582	23.5%	3,713
65+	**15.7%**	**3,369**	**36.45%**	**7,824**	**43.71%**	**9,382**	**8.6%**	**1,839**	**16.1%**	**3,379**

Based on data from the 2010 Health and Retirement Study.

*Health and Retirement Study (HRS) is a panel survey based on a national probability sample of adults age 51 and older. For more information, refer to http://hrsonline.isr.umich.edu/.

†The following questionnaire items from the HRS were used to assess productive activity participation among older adults. **Paid Work**: *Are you doing any work for pay at the present time?* **Volunteering:** *Have you spent any time in the past 12 months doing volunteer work for religious, educational, health-related, or other charitable organizations?* **Informal Help:** *Have you spent any time in the past 12 months helping friends, neighbors, or relatives who did not live with you and did not pay you for the help?* **Grandparenting:** *Did you spend 100 or more hours in total in the last two years taking care of grandchildren?* **Caregiving:** *How often do you care for a sick or disabled adult? (Respondents were counted as a caregiver if they provide care at least once a month.)*

‡Numbers in thousands; respondent weights were used to produce estimates that are representative of the U.S. population.

with a different employer, each serving as a stepping-stone from full-time work to full retirement.

Volunteering

Volunteer work includes unpaid work performed through an organization with the intent of benefitting others. Volunteering can be distinguished from other forms of productive activities, such as informal helping or caregiving, not only by the context of a formal organizational structure within which the activity is performed but also with reference to those who receive the help. Typically, volunteers have no contractual, familial, or friendship relationships with the persons or groups who are helped.[10] Historically, volunteer work has been regarded as an important form of productive activity in old age, as volunteering was one of the few formal roles available to older adults in their postretirement years.[11]

Similar to paid work, volunteering shows a distinct life-course pattern, where the rate of volunteering peaks during middle age and diminishes somewhat in later life.[12] In 2010, about 36% of respondents in the HRS who were age 65 and older reported participating in formal volunteer activities, showing a slightly lower level of participation in this activity as compared with middle-aged adults (42%, see Table 32-1). Yet the number of hours committed per volunteer is higher among older volunteers as compared to middle-aged volunteers.[12] Gender differences in rates of volunteer are minimal, as shown in Table 32-1.

Informal Helping

Although volunteering is defined as unpaid work provided through formal organizations, observers agree that focusing only on help provided in these contexts excludes important *informal* help provided by older adults.[13] Accordingly, many scholars have acknowledged informal helping behavior as an alternative type of volunteerism that occurs out of public view and in support of neighbors, friends, and others who live outside of one's own household.[13,14] Informal helping is relatively understudied compared to other forms of productive activities. Evidence from the HRS shows that a substantial fraction of the population of middle-aged and older adults are engaged in informal helping (66% and 49%, respectively), with informal helping surpassing formal volunteering in number of participants (see Table 32-1).[15]

Grandparenting

The term *grandparenting* encompasses a wide range of care-providing activities. These include occasional babysitting for grandchildren, taking on supplemental or co-parenting responsibilities in multigenerational households, and taking primary responsibility for raising one or more grandchildren.[16] Recent reports indicate that a growing number of older adults may be involved in grandparenting in a co-parenting situation: in 2011, about 7 million grandparents were co-residing with their grandchildren, which marks a 22% increase from 2000. More than 2.7 million grandparents are also found to be the primary caregiver for a grandchild.[17] Moreover, a substantial portion of older adults are also engaged in occasional grandparenting. As shown in Table 32-1, approximately 7 million grandparents age 51 and older are providing more than occasional grandchild care (e.g., at least 50 hours annually). Although the research literature makes clear that grandmothers are more likely than grandfathers to serve as substitute parents for their grandchildren, data from the HRS (see Table 32-1) suggest that men age 65 and older may be involved in at least some forms of grandparenting at a greater rate than women.

Caregiving

Caregiving is another form of intrafamily productive activity that is gaining more attention in light of the growing need for informal, unpaid care work. A sizable portion of the adult population provides care to a parent, spouse, sibling, or adult child who is ill or disabled. Approximately 21% of middle-aged and 15% of older adult respondents report providing care for another adult at least once a month (see Table 32-1). Women are somewhat more likely than men to participate in caregiving. In caregiving, as with other forms of productive activity, gender comparisons are highly sensitive to measures used, with the result that different studies report different levels of gender disparity.

A recent study suggests that what sets older caregivers apart from their younger counterparts is their level of involvement in caregiving: caregivers aged 65 and older provided 31 hours in an average week of caregiving, whereas those in the younger age group provided 17 hours. As well, older (65 years and older) and middle-aged (age 50 to 64) caregivers occupy the caregiving role for a longer period of time (7.2 and 4.9 years, respectively) compared to caregivers aged 49 and younger (3.7 years). The care recipient's relationship to the caregiver is also age-graded. Whereas caregivers 65 and older are more likely than younger caregivers to care for a spouse or a sibling, younger caregivers are more likely than older caregivers to care for family members of an older generation, such as their parent or parent-in-law.[18]

ANTECEDENTS OF PRODUCTIVE ACTIVITY IN LATER LIFE

Participation in productive activities is shaped by both individual-level characteristics of the older adult and features of the society that shape perceived opportunities and obligations. Taking paid work as an example, we note that the age at which one leaves the labor force is structured by a combination of individual factors shaping capacity and preference for working, as well as societal factors that create obstacles and disincentives, including private and public pension provisions. Personal characteristics and resources can diminish the feasibility or capacity for continued work. For example, older adults face a higher exposure to risk of a physically disabling condition that may make continued paid employment more challenging. Older adults are also at greater risk of a decline in cognitive ability, which in turn diminishes the feasibility of continued work in later life. As well, training and skills accumulated decades ago by an older worker may have reduced value in the labor market, lessening their employability. Many older adults prefer to work part-time; yet opportunities to work part-time in occupations consistent with their experience, and at a fair level of compensation, are often limited.[9]

Ageism in the workplace negatively impacts the ability of older adults to find appropriate employment and may discourage some from seeking work at all.[19] As noted by Butler,[6] many employers fail to take advantage of older adults' maturity and prior work experience, due to their misperceptions that older workers are inflexible and lack the ability to learn new skills. In the United States, age-graded access to Social Security benefits shape older adults' decisions about working. In recent history, sizable drops in the labor force participation rate at age 62 (designated as early retirement with respect to Social Security benefits) and age 65 (the age at which full retirement benefits may be received, for persons born prior to 1938) demonstrate the extent to which policies shaping access to non-earned income condition work behavior. In an effort to safeguard the solvency of the Social Security system, the U.S. Congress implemented a set of increases in the age at which full Social Security benefits may be obtained. The age of eligibility is dependent on year of birth, where, for example, persons who were born in 1960 or later will not be eligible to receive full benefits until age 67.[20]

Reversing a long-term trend, age at retirement has been rising in the United States, from age 59 in 2002 to age 62 in 2014, according to a recent Gallup poll.[21] Increases in late-life labor force participation are likely to continue as the baby boom generation reaches retirement age. The expected shortage of younger workers as a result of demographic shifts, the declining rates of disability among older adults, the rising inadequacy of public and private pension levels in the context of cost of living, and strengthened interest among employers in creating flexible work arrangements may support higher levels of productive engagement in paid work by older adults in the future.[9] Indeed, evidence collected by AARP shows that a majority of nonretired baby boomers in the United States expect to work at least part-time after they retire.[22]

Other forms of productive activity are also age-graded, as described in the previous section. Rates of volunteering; informally helping relatives, friends, and neighbors; caregiving for persons who are ill or disabled; and caring for grandchildren are lower among older adults than among their middle-aged counterparts (see Table 32-1), although for some of these activities the differences are not large. Some research evidence suggests relinquishing the responsibilities of paid work and completing the obligations of building young families provide an opportunity for older adults to contribute to their community and the larger society.[23] Additional factors known to shape the likelihood of involvement in nonpaid forms of productive activity include human capital (education, work experience), as well as health and functional capacity. Those with more education and higher income and wealth are more likely to participate in formal volunteering. Poor health conditions can be a barrier to unpaid activity just as it is for paid work; for example, older adults with significant physical disability or cognitive impairment are less likely to be engaged in unpaid productive activities.[24] However, the impact of health and disability is less pronounced for some unpaid involvements, especially where the tasks are not overly demanding and hours are flexible.

Another important factor shaping the level of involvement in unpaid productive activity among older adults is the size and composition of their social networks. Adults are often drawn into participating in unpaid productive activity through their involvement in social networks; conversely, participating in these activities can serve to strengthen and expand an older adult's social support. Involvement in productive activity serves as a basis for building *social capital*, defined as a reserve of potential support developed through social relationships. In the case of formal volunteering, for example, two key predictors of volunteering include being married (especially if one's spouse is a volunteer) and simply being asked by a friend, family member, or other acquaintance to participate. Informal helping typically involves contributing time to helping family members who do not live with the older adult, including adult children, siblings, friends, or neighbors. And adults are nearly always drawn into caregiving by their close attachments to a parent, spouse, or other relative. Thus being embedded in a social network helps older adults become aware of opportunities to be engaged productively; in addition, their participation can strengthen existing relationships and create new ones resulting from that involvement.

Additional factors beyond the older adult's characteristics shape participation in productive activities. Broader environmental features, including social and political factors, influence the set of activity choices. Thus the likelihood of engaging in productive activities later in life is not simply a reflection of intrinsic motivations and preferences on the part of individuals. Rather, institutional and social influences shape expected roles for older adults; in turn, institutional features may either serve as opportunities or challenges to participation.

International comparisons of productive aging shed light on the types and impact of environmental features on the behavior of older adults. A recent analysis of productive activity, including volunteering, informal helping, and caregiving, across 11 European countries found considerable variability in participation rates.[25] For example, rates of volunteering were as low as 3% in Spain but more than 20% in the Netherlands. Informal helping was also low in Spain (at about 5%) but near 40% in Sweden. Spain and Italy had relatively low rates of caregiving (about 3%), compared to between 8% and 9% in Belgium, Switzerland, and Sweden. In these countries, the association between participation and individual-level characteristics (age, gender, education, and health) was similar to that documented in the United States. Features of a society shaping predispositions to engage in productive activities, as well as variation in opportunity structures that shape the extent to which caring activities are available, account for differences across countries. A positive association between government social spending and probability of volunteering, informal helping, and caregiving is evident, suggesting that "the private initiative of individuals seems to require public support."[25] Based on these findings, the report concludes that "culturally blind 'one-size-fits-all' strategies to foster social participation and productive aging are … unlikely to be successful."[25]

Scientific research on the antecedents of engagement in productive activity in later life highlights the importance of both individual-level factors and societal-level features that may promote or discourage participation. At the individual level, preferences for involvements (e.g., a preference for working part-time) and capacity for involvement (e.g., presence and level of disability) play a role. At the societal level, opportunities for and barriers to meaningful engagement shape participation levels not only in paid work but also in unpaid activities such as caregiving and grandparenting. The importance of social networks as a mechanism by which older adults become aware of opportunities for involvement and become drawn into participation is also highlighted. Successful strategies for increasing the level of productive aging would include building opportunities that align with older adults' preferences and capacities and proactively reaching out to older adults as a significant societal resource.

CONSEQUENCES OF PRODUCTIVE ACTIVITY IN LATER LIFE

Remaining productive in later life is a component of the more general conceptual framework of successful aging.[26] A focus on productive aging and well-being is directly embedded in a paradigm shift from the medical model of aging, with its attendant focus on physical deterioration, frailty, and death, to a vision of later life as characterized by active engagement with sweeping consequences for positive and negative outcomes, defined broadly. Paid work has consequences for older persons in at least two ways. If older adults wish to work and can find meaningful work, then psychological and social benefits may accrue. If older adults find that their retirement savings and pensions are insufficient with respect to their desired lifestyle, continuing a relationship with the labor market past the normative retirement age benefits them economically. Yet working when one prefers to be retired, or when one has health conditions that make it difficult to work, may yield negative consequences for overall well-being. We focus the remainder of this discussion on the unpaid forms of productive activity, which in essence reflect different types of helping behaviors (volunteering, informal help, grandparenting, caregiving), distinguished in part by where the activity occurs, what the relationship is between the helper and helped, and where the activity lies on a continuum of the discretionary-obligatory nature of the activity.

A number of scholarly disciplines have contributed to our understanding of the implications of volunteering for formal organizations and providing care to family members for overall well-being. In both cross-sectional and longitudinal research in the United States, volunteering has been related to lower levels of depression, greater life satisfaction, and higher self-rated health. Cross-national work on the consequences of volunteering for well-being typically shows similar results in Europe, Asia, and Canada. The relative consistency in the cross-cultural patterns linking volunteering and health demonstrate the generalizability of these results. Volunteers are less likely than non-volunteers to report physical functioning deficits and disability. Volunteers are also less likely to be obese (except with respect to volunteering for religious institutions[27]), have lower risk of hypertension,[2] and have lower risk of inflammation, as measured by C-reactive protein levels.[28] Several reviews of current research show that volunteering is also related to a lower risk of death.[29,30]

In contrast, some caregiving roles are associated with increased risk of health decline and mortality among older adults largely as a result of the emotional, physical, and social burdens related to caring intensively for a loved one.[31] The burden and subsequent insults to health are especially pernicious when caring for a person with dementia. However, many caregivers are not excessively burdened by the demands of this form of productive activity and may take satisfaction from being able to provide care. A relatively small fraction of caregivers experience sufficient levels of burden that their health is impaired, and recent research shows that some caregivers have a lower risk of mortality than their non-caregiving counterparts.[32] Although this finding may be due to a selection process, whereby healthier persons are drawn into caregiving, research regarding the issue of reciprocal causation and selectivity bias is ongoing.

Comparatively, we have much less research evidence on the potential health effects of the two remaining forms of productive activity, that is, grandparenting and informal helping. What evidence is available shows that grandparenting is positively associated with well-being when the grandparent's caregiving activity is less demanding and does not involve full-time caretaking. When the older adult does not live in the same household as grandchildren, has access to adequate economic resources, and has a good relationship with the parent(s) of the grandchild, then grandparenting is a positive experience, promoting the well-being of the grandparent. When engagement in grandparenting is coupled with other stressors (poverty, crowded households, conflicts with the parent, single grandparenting), health status may deteriorate (for a review of health and grandparenting, see Grinstead and colleagues[33]).

The small amount of published research on the implications of informal helping for well-being is inconclusive. Generally, when alternative explanations for health decline are considered, the role of informal helping in models of well-being is not statistically significant. However, some recent research shows informal helping is related to better mental health.[34,35] Additional research is needed to better understand how this form of productive activity is related to morbidity and mortality, as well as for the other forms of well-being (social integration and social capital, financial health), in part because this is a very common mode of productive activity in later life.

Although a linkage between productive involvement and health benefits is established in the scientific literature, the causal relationship between productive engagements and health is uncertain. Our review has emphasized evidence suggesting that productive involvement leads to positive health outcomes; yet some research demonstrates that health also predicts the capacity to participate in paid work, volunteering, informal helping, grandparenting, and caregiving.[36] Undoubtedly, both causal processes are evident. Although most of the research linking productive aging and health is based on observational data, two recent studies of volunteering and well-being using randomized controlled trial (RCT) designs provide evidence that volunteering is a predictor of better health among older adults[37] and adolescents.[38] Thus studies based on experimental designs provide results consistent with the much larger body of research based on surveys. Prospects may be limited for evaluating the health consequences of other forms of productive activity using RCT designs. Because participation in caregiving, grandparenting, and other forms of helping often occurs based on perceived obligations to close family members, testing the health consequences of these engagements using RCT designs may not be possible.

Gerontologists and other observers recognize that engagement in activities defined as "productive" may not unambiguously yield benefits for participants. Some scholars have argued that promoting the idea that productive engagement is necessary in order to age "successfully" has negative consequences for those who are unable to be productive or for those for whom such engagements are simply not desirable.[39,40] Older adults who reach the "third age" may not have the physical wherewithal to work in the paid labor force. Some older adults lack the executive function skills or physical and mental capacity requisite for continuing to work, volunteer, or act as effective caregivers. Providing intensive caregiving or informal help to others may not be based on choice or free will but rather may be seen as compulsory, yielding intrapersonal and interpersonal conflict. Grandparenting may be seen as a positive experience for those who do not live with their grandchildren, but those who are compelled to raise their grandchildren in their homes and cannot leave these responsibilities behind are not necessarily benefiting from the experience. The potential consequences of being labeled "unproductive" in later life include social ostracism, status reduction, insults to self-esteem, and economic stress.

Despite limitations of the current evidence on individual-level health consequences of productive activities, and the criticisms of the concept of productive aging more generally, our interpretation of the scientific evidence is that the benefits of productive aging are clear, and immense, for those who are helped and supported by older adults and for the macro-economic and social systems that rely on their contributions. The benefits of productive activities are more often than not unmeasured and possibly unmeasurable, but analysts who have estimated the economic values of unpaid activities provide a sense of the magnitude of older adults' contributions. For example, the economic value of services provided by older volunteers was estimated to be $64 billion[41] and the value of grandparent-provided care was estimated to be $39 billion.[42] As well, older adults are responsible for a substantial portion of the caregiver services provided by family caregivers (up to 80% of all care provided), which were valued at $450 billion per year in 2009.[18]

SUMMARY

The productive contributions of older adults are considerable. A perhaps surprising number of older adults participate in the paid workforce, and researchers speculate that the proportion doing so will continue to rise in coming years. Even among those who do not work for pay, many contribute time and effort to important unpaid activities that benefit members of their personal networks as well as the communities within which they live. Formal volunteering, helping neighbors and friends, caring for disabled and frail loved ones, and helping to care for grandchildren are common activities in later life that yield enormous benefits. By documenting the contributions of older adults through productive activity more completely, it may be possible to correct misperceptions that limit the opportunities available to older adults. Ideally, this effort will proceed without stigmatizing the older adults who are unable to or uninterested in participating in activities conventionally defined as productive.

Evidence is plentiful suggesting that, at least under some circumstances, engaging in productive activity is healthful for the older participant. Participating in unpaid helping activity (volunteering, providing informal help, grandparenting, caregiving) and paid work are related positively to a myriad of indicators of well-being, including social integration and social capital, mental and physical health, and longevity. However, excessive amounts of productive activity, and engagement in productive activities that are perceived as burdensome, show negative relationships with several forms of well-being.

More research is needed on the pathways between productive aging and health. Understanding how much participation yields maximum benefit and how much is instead burdensome to the participant is a challenging but valued goal. Which groups benefit the most in terms of health outcomes? Which activities yield the most benefit, and in what "dose"? What are the mechanisms by which productive activity generates healthfulness? Such mechanisms may include the alleviation of stress; improvements in "under the skin" biologic systems (immune system, metabolic system); and improved health behaviors, such as adherence to health care provider recommendations, reductions in smoking, better nutrition, and moderate alcohol consumption. Continued support by the National Institutes of Health and other funding agencies for research across the globe will help us to better understand productive aging and its implications for well-being across cultures, across political settings, and in different types of economies.

Robert Butler, founder of the concept of productive aging, believed that productive engagements in later life were the key to eliminating ageism in society. Indeed, previous models of age and aging are gradually being replaced by new images focusing on vitality, productivity, and purpose. Yet, despite high levels of productive aging and numerous models of productive older adults such as Dr. Butler,[43] ageism is alive and well, creating and reinforcing barriers encountered by older adults as they age. Continued efforts to document the consequences of productive aging for individuals, organizations, and societies will need to be pursued for Dr. Butler's vision to be realized.

KEY POINTS

- The concept of productive aging captures both paid and unpaid activities that have social value and are performed by adults during the later years of the life course. Late life engagement in activities such as paid work, volunteering, informal helping, caregiving, and taking on the role of a grandparent caregiver are widely accepted as markers of productive aging.
- The productive engagements of older adults are widely acknowledged to contribute substantially to society as a whole, and especially to the social groups, communities, and networks that directly benefit from the contributions. As well, participation in productive activities often directly benefits the older adult who participates in them.
- Scientific research on the antecedents of engagement in productive activity in later life highlights the importance of both individual-level factors and societal-level features. Individual factors such as human capital, health and disability, and characteristics of one's social network can shape the likelihood of involvement in different forms of productive activity. At the societal level, opportunities for and barriers to meaningful engagement shape participation levels not only in paid work but also in unpaid activities.
- Research to date indicates that there is a linkage between productive involvement and health benefits. Evidence is plentiful suggesting that at least under some circumstances, engaging in productive activity is related positively to a myriad of indicators of well-being. However, gerontologists also recognize that engagement in activities defined as "productive" may not unambiguously yield benefits for participants.

For a complete list of references, please visit www.expertconsult.com.

KEY REFERENCES

1. Johnson RW, Schaner SG: Value of unpaid activities by older Americans tops $160 billion per year, Washington, DC, 2005, Urban Institute.
2. Burr JA, Tavares J, Mutchler JE: Volunteering and hypertension risk in later life. J Aging Health 23:24–51, 2011.
3. Glass TA, de Leon CM, Marottoli RA, et al: Population based study of social and productive activities as predictors of survival among elderly Americans. BMJ 319:478–483, 1999.
4. Johnson KJ, Mutchler JE: The emergence of a positive gerontology: from disengagement to social involvement. Gerontologist 54:93–100, 2014.
6. Butler RN: Productive aging. In Fillit HM, Rockwood K, Woodhouse K, editors: Brocklehurst's textbook of geriatrics and clinical gerontology, ed 7, Philadelphia, 2010, Elsevier, pp 193–197.
9. Rix SE: Employment and aging. In Binstock RH, George LK, editors: Handbook of aging and the social sciences, ed 7, Amsterdam, 2011, Academic Press, pp 193–206.

11. O'Neill G, Morrow-Howell N, Wilson SF: Volunteering in later life: from disengagement to civic engagement. In Settersten RA, Angel JL, editors: Handbook of sociology of aging, New York, 2011, Springer, pp 333–350.
12. Cutler SJ, Hendricks J, O'Neill G: Civic engagement and aging. In Binstock RH, George LK, editors: Handbook of aging and the social sciences, ed 7, Amsterdam, 2011, Academic Press.
14. Burr JA, Mutchler JE, Caro FG: Productive activity clusters among middle-aged and older adults: intersecting forms and time commitments. J Gerontol B Psychol Sci Soc Sci 62:S267–S275, 2007.
15. Zedlewski SR, Schaner SG: Older adults engaged as volunteers perspectives on productive aging, Washington, DC, 2006, Urban Institute.
18. National Alliance for Caregiving, AARP: Caregiving in the U.S. 2009. http://www.caregiving.org/data/Caregiving_in_the_US_2009_full_report.pdf. Accessed January 16, 2016.
23. Mutchler JE, Burr JA, Caro FG: From paid worker to volunteer: leaving the paid workforce and volunteering in later life. Soc Forces 81:1267–1293, 2003.
28. Kim S, Ferraro KF: Do productive activities reduce inflammation in later life? Multiple roles, frequency of activities, and C-reactive protein. Gerontologist 54:830–839, 2014.
29. Anderson ND, Damianakis T, Kröger E, et al: The benefits associated with volunteering among seniors: a critical review and recommendations for future research. Psychol Bull 140:1505–1533, 2014.
30. Jenkinson C, Dickens A, Jones K, et al: Is volunteering a public health intervention? A systematic review and meta-analysis of the health and survival of volunteers. BMC Public Health 13:1–10, 2013.
35. Kahana E, Bhatta T, Lovegreen LD, et al: Altruism, helping, and volunteering: pathways to well-being in late life. J Aging Health 25:159–187, 2013.
37. Fried LP, Carlson MC, McGill S, et al: Experience Corps: a dual trial to promote the health of older adults and children's academic success. Contemp Clin Trials 36:1–13, 2013.
39. Estes CL, Mahakian JL, Weitz TA: A political economic critique of "productive aging.". In Estes CL, editor: Social policy and aging: a critical perspective, Thousand Oaks, CA, 2001, SAGE Publications.
41. Martin J: (2011). Senior volunteers: serving their communities and their country. http://blog.aarp.org/2011/09/20/senior-volunteers-serving-their-communities-and-their-country/. Accessed November 1, 2014.
43. Achenbaum WA: Robert N. Butler, MD: visionary of health aging, New York, 2013, Columbia University Press.

33 Presentation of Disease in Old Age

Maristela B. Garcia, Sonja Rosen, Brandon Koretz, David B. Reuben

Although diseases occur more commonly as people get older, many become more challenging to diagnose accurately in older adults. Classic presenting symptoms may be absent, or nonspecific symptoms such as altered mental status, weight loss, fatigue, falls, dizziness, or functional decline may be the earliest or only manifestations in this age group. For example, common infections (e.g., pneumonia, urinary tract infection) may present with a change in mental status such as lethargy or confusion but with few or no symptoms related to the source of the infection. Similarly, older adults who experience myocardial infarction may not report having chest pain.

A number of possible explanations may account for such atypical presentations. Comorbid conditions may alter the presentation of disease, and age-related physiologic changes may alter the perception of stimulus. For example, because of age-related changes in immunity, the febrile response may be absent in infected older adults.[1] Furthermore, cognitive impairment may prevent the patient from providing an accurate history. As a result, these atypical presentations may be more common than classic presentations. Atypical presentations may predict poor outcomes for hospitalized older patients,[2] perhaps as a result of delays in diagnosis and initiation of appropriate therapy. Moreover, nonspecific symptoms may result in overutilization of diagnostic tests and procedures.[3,4]

Because older patients may often have nonspecific symptoms and/or atypical symptoms for disease, we have chosen to present this material in two different sections. First, this chapter examines six nonspecific presentations of disease—altered mental status, weight loss, fatigue, dizziness, and falls and fever. Next, we review some common diseases, discussed by organ system, to explore the differences in disease presentation between younger and older patients.

NONSPECIFIC CLINICAL PRESENTATIONS OF DISEASE IN THE OLDER POPULATION

As noted in Table 33-1, six nonspecific presentations may be caused by diverse disorders. We review the major diseases responsible for these presentations and provide approaches to determining the causes. Although these often occur independently, they may also occur in clusters. For example, weight loss and fatigue are two of the criteria for the frailty syndrome (see later), which may be a nonspecific presentation for diseases listed in Table 33-1 or an outcome of some of these diseases (e.g., heart failure, chronic obstructive pulmonary disease [COPD]).

Altered Mental Status

Altered mental status (AMS) may often be the only indicator of a serious underlying disease.[5] Presenting symptoms can include disorientation, decreased or nonsensical verbalization, and somnolence or hyperactivity or a mixture of both. When AMS is of rapid onset, accompanied by disturbed consciousness (especially decreased attention) and is due to a medical condition, it meets the criteria for delirium. Delirium can also be associated with sleep disturbances and hallucinations. Delirium is a common presentation of disease in older adult patients and is the most common complication associated with inpatient hospital admission among older adults.[6] The symptoms of delirium may persist for months and are associated with adverse outcomes.[7]

The differential diagnosis of AMS in older adult patients is very broad and encompasses many systems. The presence of preceding clinical symptoms (e.g., change in urine frequency, color, cloudiness, cough, skin tears or sores), low-grade fever, or leukocytosis may suggest an infectious cause. As noted, because of age-related changes in immunity, older adults may not necessarily exhibit a fever or leukocytosis.[1] The most common infectious causes of delirium include respiratory, urine, and skin infections. Another cause may be iatrogenic secondary to medications.

Estimates have suggested that up to 39% of delirium in older adults is attributable to medications owing to the altered pharmacokinetics and pharmacodynamics, as well as the presence of comorbidities and polypharmacy in this population.[8] Medications with a narrow therapeutic index and/or those that cross the blood-brain barrier are the most common culprits, including anticholinergics and benzodiazepines. A systematic review of prospective studies investigating the association between medications and delirium among patients older than 65 years has suggested a higher risk of delirium with the use of opioids, benzodiazepines, and H1 antihistamines such as diphenhydramine. The association is less with corticosteroids, tricyclic antidepressants (TCAs), and digoxin.[8,9] It is important to note that although opioid use increases the risk of delirium, untreated pain itself can cause delirium. Another cause of drug-related delirium that is frequently underrecognized is serotonin syndrome, a serious adverse reaction that is a predictable result of serotonin excess. The constellation of signs and symptoms of serotonin syndrome that may include delirium often occurs in temporal association with the recent addition of a serotonergic agent or an increase in the dose of drugs known to have serotonergic activity by blocking serotonin reuptake (e.g., selective serotonin reuptake inhibitors [SSRIs], tramadol, trazodone, chlorpheniramine, dextromethorphan), augmentation of serotonin release (e.g., codeine, levodopa, monoamine oxidase [MAO] inhibitors), or inhibition of serotonin metabolism (e.g., linezolid).[10] Alcohol intoxication or withdrawal should also be considered. Metabolic disorders include electrolyte imbalances, especially sodium disorders, dehydration, hypoglycemia, and hypoxia. Cardiovascular causes of altered mental status include heart failure and myocardial infarction.[11] CNS causes such as infections (e.g., meningitis, encephalitis),[12] stroke,

TABLE 33-1 Nonspecific Presentations of Various Disorders

		Nonspecific Presentation					
Category	**Disease Examples**	*Altered Mental Status*	*Weight Loss*	*Fatigue*	*Dizziness*	*Falls*	*Fever*
Infection	Urosepsis	X		X	X	X	X
	Pneumonia	X		X	X	X	X
	Subacute endocarditis	X		X	X	X	X
	Cellulitis	X		X		X	X
	Meningoencephalitis	X				X	X
Metabolic	Hypoxia	X	X	X	X	X	
	Dehydration	X		X	X	X	
	Hyponatremia	X		X	X	X	
	Hypoglycemia	X		X		X	
Cardiopulmonary	Heart failure		X	X			
	COPD		X	X			
Cancer			X	X			X
Psychiatric		X	X	X	X		
Cerebrovascular		X			X	X	
Rheumatologic	Pseudogout (CPPD)	X	X	X			X
	Rheumatoid arthritis	X		X			X
	Temporal arteritis	X		X			X
	Adult-onset Still disease			X			X
Endocrine	Hyperthyroidism	X	X	X			X
	Hypothyroidism	X		X			

CPPD, Calcium pyrophosphate deposition disease.

seizures, and subdural hematomas are less common. Finally, miscellaneous causes of altered mental status in older adults include urinary retention and fecal impaction.[13]

Acute abnormal mental status may also occur in the absence of delirium. For example, psychiatric causes, such as dementia with psychosis, psychotic depression, and bipolar disorder, may present with changes in mental status. Psychosis may be accompanied by delusions and hallucinations and is one of the most common noncognitive symptoms associated with Alzheimer dementia.[14] The second most common cause of psychosis in older adults is depression.[15] Mania, although less common in older adults, is characterized by hyperactivity, but patients generally remain oriented.

When patients' mental status is too altered for them to give a reliable history, clinicians must obtain additional information about the history of present illness from family members, friends, caregivers, or health care workers for patients who live in institutional settings. It is also important to review medications with a focus on recent changes and over-the-counter (OTC) medications that may have anticholinergic properties (e.g., those containing diphenhydramine). For the most part, infection and other major medical causes can be identified with a set of simple laboratory studies, including a complete blood cell count with differential, comprehensive metabolic panel, urinalysis, chest x-ray, electrocardiography and, depending the on patient's clinical status, cardiac enzyme levels.

If an infectious cause is suspected but no clear source can be found, a lumbar puncture may be warranted,[16] although a retrospective analysis of 232 hospitalized patients with fever and altered mental status demonstrated that lumbar punctures for suspected nosocomial meningitis in nonsurgical patients have a low yield.[17] Although AMS is unusual in meningitis, it may be a sign of other CNS infection, particularly meningoencephalitis. Furthermore, older patients may not mount the typical immune response associated with these infections, such as fever or leukocytosis. Brain imaging is of value in ruling out stroke or subdural hematoma if there is clinical suspicion of either diagnosis or if the evaluation of AMS is otherwise unrevealing. Recent studies have shown that the routine use of head imaging in the evaluation of older patients with AMS following cardiac surgery and total hip arthroplasty is rarely useful in the absence of focal neurologic deficits.[3,4] Finally, electroencephalography (EEG) is helpful in diagnosing occult seizures and sometime to distinguish delirium from psychosis.

Weight Loss

Undernutrition is indicated by unintentional weight loss of more than 5% within a year.[18] Unintentional weight loss occurs in up to 15% of community-dwelling older persons, between 20% to 65% of hospitalized patients, and 5% to 85% of institutionalized older persons.[19] Unintentional weight loss is often a marker of severity of comorbidities or undiagnosed disease and may be divided into three causes—social, psychological, and medical.[19]

Social reasons include poverty, functional impairment, social isolation, poor nutritional knowledge, and elder abuse. Most surveys have shown that poverty is the single most important social cause of weight loss.[20] Dependence in activities of daily living (ADLs) and instrumental activities of daily living (IADLs), such as needing assistance with feeding, shopping, or food preparation, are also important factors.

Psychological reasons include psychiatric problems such as depression, paranoia, and bereavement. Depression has been shown to be the major cause of weight loss in the outpatient setting.[21] Of older adults with depression, 90% have weight loss compared to 60% of younger adults with that diagnosis.[22] Depression is also an important cause of weight loss in institutionalized patients.

Medical reasons include dementia, pulmonary and cardiac diseases, malignancy, medications, alcoholism, infectious diseases, poor dentition, endocrine abnormalities, especially hyperthyroidism and diabetes, malabsorption, and dysphagia.

The first step in determining the cause is to assess whether patients have adequate dietary intake.[23] If they have inadequate nutrition, medical and psychosocial factors should be investigated. Medical factors include nausea, constipation, poor oral health, and/or health problems that lead to functional dependence. Medication side effects may also be contributory factors. For example, opioids and anticholinergics may cause constipation, which in turn may cause bloating and poor appetite. Psychosocial factors, including poverty, dementia, depression, and social isolation, should be investigated. The use of geriatric assessment tools such as the Mini-Cog,[24] Mini Mental State Examination (MMSE),[25] or Montreal Cognitive Assessment (MOCA)[26] to screen for cognitive impairment, and the Patient Health Questionnaire-9 (PHQ-9)[27] to screen for depression can help elucidate the cause.

On the other hand, if patients have adequate dietary intake, a search must be undertaken for underlying disease by careful history and physical examination, with special attention paid to symptoms that may suggest malignancy (e.g., cough, constipation, gastrointestinal bleeding), or cardiac, pulmonary, inflammatory bowel, or rheumatic disease. The physical examination should evaluate for lymphadenopathy, palpable masses, and breast or thyroid abnormalities. Initial laboratory testing should include complete blood cell count with differential, comprehensive metabolic panel, determination of levels of prealbumin, albumin, thyroid-stimulating hormone (TSH), and lactate dehydrogenase (LDH), urinalysis, erythrocyte sedimentation rate (ESR), and chest x-ray.[28] Because of its shorter half-life compared to albumin, the prealbumin level is a better indicator of the more acute changes in nutritional state that occur in the inpatient setting. Depending on the patient's clinical findings and preliminary laboratory results, further evaluation may be necessary to determine the cause of the weight loss. However, when investigating potential causes, it is important to keep in mind that weight loss in older adults may not have a disease-based cause but may occur as a consequence of aging and frailty from the so-called physiologic anorexia of the aging[29] and age-related sarcopenia.[30] However, this is often a diagnosis of exclusion.

Fatigue

Fatigue can be defined as tiredness or decreased energy, but excessive daytime fatigue is not a normal process of aging.[31] As the body protects its functional reserve, fatigue may be associated with generalized weakness.[32] Fatigue may be acute or chronic, the latter of which is the result of physical and/or psychological factors. Physiologic causes of fatigue by body systems include hematologic and oncologic (e.g., anemia, cancer, cancer-related therapy), cardiac (e.g., congestive heart failure), renal or liver disease, endocrine (thyroid disease, diabetes), and pulmonary (sleep-related breathing disorders, severe obstructive or restrictive lung diseases).

Fatigue is one of the most common side effects of cancer treatment, with 70% of cancer patients receiving radiation and chemotherapy experiencing this symptom, and that may also persist for years after treatment.[33] Fatigue is also the most common symptom of congestive heart failure (CHF) and is the initial presenting complaint in 10% to 20% of new CHF diagnoses.[34] Obstructive sleep apnea (OSA) is common in patients older than 60 years, with a reported prevalence of 37.5% to 62%; daytime sleepiness is a prominent symptom.[35] Other sleep disorders, such as insomnia or disturbances in sleep-wake cycles that may occur with dementia, can also lead to daytime fatigue. Some chronic infections, such as subacute endocarditis, may also present with fatigue as a chief complaint. Medications are also a common culprit of fatigue in older adults (Table 33-2), particularly antihistamines, anticholinergic medications, sedatives or nonsedating hypnotics, and antihypertensive medications (especially β-blockers at high doses). Finally, psychiatric illnesses, most commonly depression, can cause excessive fatigue.

The evaluation of fatigue begins with a history, with a focus on any symptoms of concern for malignancy (e.g., weight loss) or other body system diseases that may suggest a cause (e.g., dyspnea suggesting anemia, CHF, ischemia, or pulmonary disease, recent bereavement suggesting depression). Geriatric assessment tools such as the PHQ-9[26] or Geriatric Depression Scale (GDS)[36] can be performed to screen for depression. The Mini-Cog,[24] MOCA,[26] or MMSE[25] can be used to screen for cognitive impairment. Similarly, the physical examination should focus on any red flags (e.g., weight loss suggesting malignancy, edema suggesting CHF).

TABLE 33-2 Common Groups of Medications That Cause Fatigue

Drug Class	Examples
Benzodiazepines	Diazepam, temazepam
Antihistamines, first generation	Diphenhydramine, hydroxyzine
Centrally acting α-adrenergic agonists	Clonidine
β-Adrenergic antagonists and other antihypertensives	Propranolol
Antiepileptic drugs	Carbamazepine, valproic acid
Muscle relaxants	Baclofen
Opioids	Morphine, hydrocodone,
Diuretics	Furosemide

Fatigue is a frequent side effect of many medications that older adults commonly use. A careful review of medications, including OTC drugs and a temporal association between the onset of fatigue and the addition or dose increase of a medication known to cause fatigue may be simple and helpful step in identifying the cause of the symptom. The list of pharmacologic agents that can cause fatigue is long. Drugs cause fatigue by various mechanisms, most of which are through CNS depression by decreasing excitatory CNS activity or increasing inhibitory CNS activity.[37] A number of drugs used by older adults (e.g., anticonvulsants, antipsychotics, antimicrobials, chemotherapeutic agents, medications used to treat rheumatoid arthritis) cause hematologic toxicity resulting in symptomatic anemia. Other drugs cause fatigue by unknown mechanisms.

Laboratory and diagnostic testing in the evaluation of fatigue must be tailored toward identifying potential causes after obtaining a thorough history and physical examination. Basic laboratory tests (e.g., complete blood cell count, comprehensive metabolic panel, TSH, urinalysis) may be helpful; additional diagnostic tests may be carried out based on history and physical findings (e.g., electrocardiography, echocardiography, brain natriuretic peptide [BNP] level) may be ordered in someone suspected of having CHF; an overnight sleep study might be ordered if obstructed sleep apnea is suspected.

Dizziness

Dizziness is prevalent among older adults in the community and is the presenting complaint of up to 7% of older patients in the primary care setting.[38] Although common, dizziness is not a normal process of aging and can be a vexing clinical problem to diagnose and treat. Dizziness in most older adults has a benign cause but dizziness may also be indicative of a more serious underlying medical condition. One study of patients older than 60 years having dizziness found that 28% had a cardiovascular diagnosis and 14% had a central neurologic disorder. Of note, 22% had no attributable cause of the symptoms identified.[39] Psychological disorders are rare as the primary cause of dizziness, but may be contributing or modulating factors in older adults with dizziness.[40] Furthermore, patients with dizziness may develop a fear of falling, falls,[41] and subsequent disability in daily activities secondary to their symptoms.[42]

To determine the cause of dizziness, it is important first to determine the nature of the presenting symptoms. Dizziness can be classified into four symptom categories—vertigo, presyncope, dysequilibrium, and nonspecific dizziness[43]:

1. Vertigo is defined as a feeling that one's surroundings are moving and can be episodic or continuous. Causes of vertigo

include benign paroxysmal positional vertigo, acute labyrinthitis, Menière disease, vertebrobasilar insufficiency, brain stem stroke, tumors, and cervical vertigo.
2. Presyncope is defined as a lightheaded feeling or impending faint. It is commonly due to orthostatic hypotension, vasovagal attacks, and decreased cardiac output, such as significant valvular lesions or arrhythmias.
3. Dysequilibrium is defined as a sense of unsteadiness or imbalance where a person feels as if he or she is going to fall and is usually constant, occurring primarily while standing. It is generally the result of vestibular loss (e.g., acoustic neuroma), proprioceptive (e.g., spinal stenosis) or somatosensory loss (e.g., peripheral neuropathy), a cerebellar or motor lesion (e.g., subcortical or cerebellar infarct, tumor), or multiple neurosensory impairments, such as those occurring in Parkinson disease.
4. Finally, some nonspecific dizziness symptoms do not fit into any of these categories. They may be described as mild lightheadedness but also may be difficult for patients to describe. Infections (e.g., urinary tract infections), anxiety, or hyperventilation are commonly responsible for nonspecific dizziness.

The evaluation of the differential diagnosis begins with a history and physical examination, with a focus on the nature of the patient's symptomatology. A dizziness simulation battery can be performed to delineate further the type of dizziness from which the patient suffers.[44] For example, reproduction of symptoms with nystagmus in response to the Barany or Dix-Hallpike maneuver is diagnostic for vertigo. Further vestibular concerns can be evaluated with audiometry, brain magnetic resonance imaging (MRI), and/or referral to an otolaryngologist. Presyncope should be evaluated with screening laboratory tests, including a complete blood cell count, comprehensive metabolic panel, urinalysis and thyroid function, electrocardiography, and possible further cardiac studies (e.g., event monitoring, echocardiography) or neurologic testing (e.g., carotid ultrasound, brain MRI), depending on clinical presentation and history. In addition, dysequilibrium may require a neurology evaluation and further neurologic testing.

Falls

Over one third of community-dwelling persons older than 65 years fall each year, and more than 50% of these patients have recurrent falls.[45] Falls are responsible for two thirds of accidental deaths, which are the fifth leading cause of death in older adults.[46] In addition, 20% to 30% of those who fall suffer moderate to severe injuries such as lacerations, hip fractures, or head trauma.[47,48] Falls are also independently associated with functional and mobility decline. All patients older than 65 years should be screened for a history of falling in the last year because patients who have fallen in the last year are at higher risk for falling again.[49]

Although the cause of most falls is multifactorial in nature, it is useful to understand the separate entities that may be contributing factors or may independently cause falls. These include the following physiologic contributors: cardiac disease (e.g., orthostatic hypotension, arrhythmia, valvular lesions, ischemia); neurologic disease (e.g., stroke, Parkinson disease, subdural hematomas in recurrent fallers, peripheral neuropathy; cognitive impairment); musculoskeletal disorders (e.g., osteoarthritis, leg asymmetry, muscle weakness); sensory impairment (visual and hearing impairment); iatrogenic factors (e.g., medications, physical restraints in institutionalized settings); and primary gait and balance impairments. There are also several other nonphysiologic factors that may cause or contribute to falls, including incorrect use of walking aids, environmental hazards (e.g., loose carpets), performing several activities simultaneously, inappropriate footwear, and hazardous behavior.[50]

If a patient has fallen in the last year, a multifactorial evaluation of the cause(s) should be undertaken. This begins with a history to determine the circumstances surrounding the falls (e.g., loss of balance, tripping secondary to poor vision, presyncopal symptoms). A review should be performed of prescription and nonprescription medications that may be contributing to falls (e.g., sedatives, anticholinergics, nonsedating hypnotics). The physical examination should include orthostatic vital signs, visual acuity testing, and a gait and balance evaluation. The physician can most efficiently observe a patient's gait while the patient is entering and leaving the examination room. Simple tests of balance include observing the patient's ability to stand side by side, semitandem, and full tandem for 10 seconds each and stability during a 360-degree turn.[51] The neurologic examination should evaluate for any focal or generalized weakness, impaired cognition, signs of parkinsonism (e.g., rigidity, tremor), and/or poor proprioception. For patients who are found to have cognitive impairment or focal weakness, further evaluation may include brain imaging to assess for vascular disease. In addition, patients with focal weakness may require musculoskeletal imaging (e.g., to evaluate for osteoarthritis, spinal stenosis, mass lesions) and electromyographic studies to evaluate for possible peripheral neuropathy. The cardiovascular examination should include evaluation for valvular lesions, arrhythmias, and carotid lesions. An electrocardiogram should be obtained, with further cardiac testing if patients have presyncopal or syncopal symptoms (see earlier, "Dizziness"). The musculoskeletal examination should focus on any muscle weakness or atrophy, joint abnormalities, foot deformities, or leg asymmetry.

Fever

Fever is the prototypical sign of many infections (most commonly—urinary tract, infections, pneumonias, skin, and intraabdominal infections; less commonly—endocarditis and osteomyelitis), and some malignancies (e.g., lymphoma, renal cell carcinoma, hepatic cell carcinoma) and rheumatologic diseases (e.g., calcium pyrophosphate dihydrate deposition disease, rheumatoid arthritis, temporal arteritis, adult-onset Still disease). Other less common causes include drug reactions, hematomas, and thyroid storm.

The presence of fever serves as a warning sign for potentially life-threatening diseases.[52] However, as noted, the febrile response may be absent in infected older patients. Although errors in measurement may account for some of this variability,[53] older patients, on average, have a lower basal temperature than younger persons.[54] To compensate for this, some have suggested that the use of change from basal temperature might be more sensitive for the presence of infection than absolute temperature.[53] In older adults, an oral temperature higher than 99° F should be considered elevated.[1] One study examined the importance of fever in 470 consecutive older patients who were seen in an emergency room with a temperature of 100.0° F or higher.[55] Three quarters of these patients were classified by the authors as seriously ill.

The fever workup should begin with a history focusing on evaluation for infection, malignancy, or rheumatologic disease. The physical examination should pay attention to the cardiac (e.g., murmurs suspicious for endocarditis) and pulmonary examination (e.g., rales or rhonchi indicating possible pneumonia), lymphadenopathy, skin findings, joint abnormalities, and gastrointestinal examination (e.g., pain, organomegaly or other masses). The laboratory evaluation should begin with a complete blood cell count with differential, urinalysis, urine culture, chest x-ray, and ESR or C-reactive protein (CRP). The last two tests should be done if there is clinical suspicion for osteomyelitis, endocarditis, temporal arteritis/polymyalgia rheumatica, or lymphoma. Further imaging may be warranted if there is clinical suspicion for occult disease, such as intraabdominal abscesses or neoplasm.

TABLE 33-3 Common Diseases and Their Atypical Presentations in Older Adults

Disease	Typical Presentation in Younger Persons	Atypical Presentation in Older Persons
GERD	Postprandial burning with reclining	Regurgitation, dysphagia, chronic cough, hoarseness
PUD	Epigastric abdominal pain	Bleeding, nausea and vomiting, anorexia, abdominal pain not relieved by eating or drinking
Appendicitis	Peritoneal signs localizing to right lower quadrant, nausea and vomiting, leukocytosis	Abdominal rigidity, abdominal pain—generalized, decreased bowel sounds, nausea and vomiting, leukocytosis
Cholecystitis	Right upper quadrant pain, Murphy sign, fever, nausea and vomiting, leukocytosis	Generalized abdominal pain, fever, nausea and vomiting
Myocardial infarction	Substernal chest pain radiating to left arm or jaw	Chest pain, dyspnea, vertigo, altered mental status, heart failure, weakness
Pneumonia	Fever, cough, chills, pleuritic chest pain	Tachypnea, altered mental status, decreased oral intake, fever, cough, chest pain
Gout	Male predominance, monoarticular	Indolent course, polyarticular
Rheumatoid arthritis	Indolent course	Acute onset, fever, weight loss, fatigue
Urinary tract infection	Dysuria, fever	Altered mental status, dizziness, nausea

ATYPICAL PRESENTATIONS OF COMMON DISEASES IN OLDER ADULTS

As noted in Table 33-3, common diseases may often have atypical presentations in older adults. In this section, we review some of these common diseases and discuss the differences in disease presentation between younger and older patients.

Gastrointestinal Diseases

Gastroesophageal Reflux Disease

Gastroesophageal reflux disease (GERD) is common among older adults; however, the classic symptom of heartburn found in younger patients may occur less frequently in older adults. A study involving 195 older adults (mean age, 74 years) who underwent upper endoscopy to evaluate abdominal symptoms and anemia found that of the 18% of patients diagnosed with esophagitis, the main symptoms reported were regurgitation, dysphagia, respiratory symptoms such as chronic cough, wheezing, hoarseness, and vomiting.[56] A post hoc analysis of pooled baseline data from five prospective, randomized, double-blind multicenter trials in the United States found that patients older than 70 years with severe esophageal erosions on endoscopy had less frequent symptoms of severe heartburn compared to the younger age group with similar findings.[57] Thus, in older patients with erosive esophagitis, the reported degree of heartburn symptoms does not reliably correlate with the severity of the esophageal disease.

Peptic Ulcer Disease

Among patients with endoscopically diagnosed ulcers, older adults are less likely to present with abdominal pain.[58,59] One study found that 65% of patients older than 80 years who presented with peptic ulcer disease (PUD)–related gastrointestinal bleed did not have pain symptoms.[60] Older adults with PUD are more likely to have bleeding, a shorter duration of symptoms, and other symptoms not typically considered to be associated with peptic ulcer disease (e.g., nausea, vomiting, anorexia, abdominal pain not relieved by eating or drinking).[61] Complications may not also present typically; only about 20% of older patients with perforated PUD manifest abdominal rigidity on physical examination.[62]

Appendicitis

Although appendicitis is more common in younger patients, its mortality is substantially higher among older adults.[63] The classic pattern of periumbilical pain that eventually localizes to the right lower abdominal quadrant occurs in only about one third of older patients with acute appendicitis.[62] Although the typical presentation may not be as common compared to younger patients, most older adults will develop right lower quadrant tenderness at some time during the illness. However, although most older patients exhibited right lower quadrant pain, anorexia, and leukocytosis, less than 50% of patients presented with fever. Overall, less than one third of older patients present with all four classic findings of fever, anorexia, right lower quadrant pain, and leukocytosis.[64] Misdiagnosis of acute appendicitis in older persons on admission occurs in up to 54% of cases[64]; awareness of its variation from the typical presentation, along with better imaging techniques, may improve diagnostic accuracy.

Cholecystitis

The typical presentation of cholecystitis in the younger patient is right upper quadrant pain, fever, nausea, and vomiting. In one retrospective cross-sectional study of 168 patients older than 65 years, 84% had neither epigastric nor right upper quadrant pain, and 5% had no pain whatsoever, on presentation to the emergency room. More than 50% the patients were afebrile; 57 % had nausea, 38% had vomiting, and 36% had back or flank pain radiation.[65] The white blood cell (WBC) count may be normal in 30% to 40% of patients, and liver function tests may not show any abnormality.[66]

Cardiovascular Diseases

Myocardial Infarction

Older adults with acute myocardial infarction may present with altered mental status, neurologic symptoms, weakness, and worsening heart failure; however, chest pain remains the most common chief complaint.[67] A retrospective multicenter study in France of 255 patients aged 75 years and older admitted to the emergency room with ST-segment elevation myocardial infarction (STEMI), 41% presented with chest pain, 16% with faintness and/or fall, 16% with dyspnea, 10% with digestive symptoms, 7% with impaired general condition, and 6% with delirium, and the remainder presented with other unspecified symptoms.[68] Those who present with atypical symptoms tend to belong to the more vulnerable category of older adults (i.e., those who reside in the nursing homes, have dementia, are functionally dependent, and have communication difficulties).[68]

Pulmonary Diseases

Pneumonia

Pneumonia is the fifth leading cause of death among older adults. Unlike the typical presentation of pneumonia consisting of fever, cough, chills, and pleuritic chest pain, atypical presentations occur more frequently in older adults.[69] Atypical presentations include decreased oral intake, falling, confusion, or an abrupt worsening of an underlying chronic medical condition (e.g., hemiplegia from a prior stroke). Tachypnea is common; 75% or more of older patients with pneumonia may present with respiratory rates greater than 20 breaths/min[70,71] and may be one of the earliest signs of pneumonia, often occurring 24 to 48 hours before the clinical diagnosis.[72] Fever has been reported in 27% to 80% of older patients with pneumonia.[71,73,74,75] A cough has been noted in 54% to 82% of older patients admitted to the hospital with community-acquired pneumonia.[76,77] Chills or rigors are noted in about 25% of patients, and a similar percentage have had falls.[65] Chest pain is present in one third.[69] Although most older adults still present with symptoms suggestive of pneumonia, delirium is the most likely presentation among the nonspecific symptoms associated with advancing age.[78]

Rheumatologic Diseases

Gout

The presentation of gout in the older person may follow a more indolent course and is more likely to be polyarticular.[79] The male predominance noted in younger patients does not seem to be present among older adults.[80] There is a strong association with long-term diuretic use, in part because of inhibited renal excretion of uric acid due to volume contraction.[81,82] For the same reason, tophaceous deposits are more likely to be present in older adults.

Rheumatoid Arthritis

Compared with younger persons, older patients who develop rheumatoid arthritis (RA) tend to have more constitutional symptoms (e.g., fever, weight loss, fatigue), have more shoulder involvement, and are more likely to have an acute onset of arthritis and a negative assay for rheumatoid factor (RF).[83-86] However, there have been some concerns about the methodologic rigor of the studies on which these conclusions are based.[87] The timely diagnosis of older-onset RA may be challenging because of the occurrence of other painful joint conditions in older adults that may present similarly, such as polymyalgia rheumatica (PMR), pseudogout, gout, and osteoarthritis.[88] Radiologic evaluation may only reveal nonspecific findings of joint swelling and osteopenia, and thus may not be always helpful as a diagnostic tool, especially early in the disease process.[88] Furthermore, the higher prevalence of autoantibodies in the healthy older adult population affects the usefulness of the RF assay in the diagnosis of RA. Because of its better specificity, anti–cyclic citrullinated peptide antibody (anti-CCP) may be more helpful in the diagnosis of RA.[89,90]

Systemic Lupus Erythematosus

Characteristically a disease of reproductive age women, systemic lupus erythematosus (SLE) has been increasing in incidence among older adults, with an estimated 4% to 18% of cases occurring after 50 years of age. Late-onset SLE has a lower female predominance.[91,92] The clinical manifestation of late-onset SLE appears to be modified with the aging process, with older adults presenting with a more subtle course, less major organ involvement, and lesser degree of disease severity.[92] Pooled data analyses from the literature have suggested that in late-onset SLE, serositis, pulmonary involvement, and RF positivity occur more frequently, whereas the classic malar rash, photosensitivity, lymphadenopathy, arthritis, nephropathy, and neuropsychiatric manifestations appear less commonly.[93] Because of its often insidious presentation and the frequent presence of comorbidities that may explain some symptoms, the diagnosis of late-onset SLE is often delayed in many patients and is often only confirmed after an extensive investigation.[92] It is important to remember that because this disorder afflicts older patients who are also likely getting treatment for other chronic conditions, it is valuable to perform a thorough review of the medication history and recognize the possibility of a drug-induced lupus (e.g., due to procainamide, hydralazine, diltiazem, isoniazid).[91]

Genitourinary Disorders

Urinary Tract Infection and Urosepsis

Bacteriuria becomes increasingly common with advancing age. In the absence of symptoms, its association with increased mortality is controversial.[94] It is clear, however, that the urinary tract is the most common source for bacteremia in older patients admitted to a hospital.[71] The typical symptoms associated with lower tract infections—dysuria, urgency, and suprapubic pain—are commonly absent in older patients with bacteriuria.[95] Similarly, the flank pain, fevers, and chills that typically accompany upper urinary tract infections may be absent. The clinical picture of urinary tract infections in older patients is variable. In one series of older patients with bacteremia from urinary sources, 30% had confusion, 29% had a cough, and 27% had dyspnea.[95,96] Other studies have suggested that the febrile response to urinary tract infection remains intact, but also that confusion is a common presenting sign.[97]

Neuromuscular Disorders

Myasthenia Gravis

The incidence of myasthenia gravis (MG) among those older than 65 years has significantly increased in the past 2 decades.[98,99] In contrast to early-onset disease, males are more commonly affected in late-onset myasthenia gravis (LOMG).[100,101] Immunologic features in LOMG include lower titers of acetylcholine receptor antibodies (AchRAbs)[102] and the more frequent presence of striational antibodies.[103] Although the characteristic clinical features may not vary considerably from early-onset MG, literature reports have indicated that in some parts of the world, such as Japan, LOMG presents more commonly with ocular manifestations[104]; however, a U.S. study suggested that bulbar symptoms manifest more likely at onset in patients aged 50 years and older.[105] Prompt diagnosis of MG in older adults can be difficult. Symptoms during the initial presentation may lead to a workup for more familiar disorders, such as brain stem strokes. In the presence of multiple comorbidities, the presenting symptom of weakness in older adult patients may initially be attributed to other disease states.

CONCLUSION

Many studies support the notion that common diseases present differently in the older adult population. What is less clear is whether it is appropriate to call these presentations atypical. In fact, when the atypical presentation is more common than the classic presentation described for younger persons, perhaps it should be termed the *typical presentation* in the older age group. Rather than using the 25-year-old as the reference standard for all age groups, practitioners should remain aware that diseases have different clinical features, depending on the age of the affected patient. Physicians should also be aware of common nonspecific presentations of illness, their differential diagnosis, and appropriate evaluation to help lead them to the right diagnosis.

KEY POINTS: PRESENTATION OF DISEASE

- Nonspecific presentations of disease maybe the earliest or only manifestations of disease in older adults.
- Six common nonspecific presentations of disease are altered mental status, weight loss, fatigue, falls, dizziness, and fever.
- Practitioners should remember that many common diseases may present differently in younger and older patients.
- Cognitive impairment may prevent the ability of the patient to provide an accurate history; whenever possible, obtain collateral information from sources who are knowledgeable about the patient.

For a complete list of references, please visit www.expertconsult.com.

KEY REFERENCES

2. Jarrett PG, Rockwood K, Carver D, et al: Illness presentation in elderly patients. Arch Intern Med 155:1060–1064, 1995.
5. Inouye SK, Westendorp RG, Saczynski JS: Delirium in elderly people. Lancet 383:911–922, 2014.
23. Alibhai SM, Greenwood C, Payette H: An approach to the management of unintentional weight loss in elderly people. Can Med Assoc J 172:773–780, 2005.
26. Nasreddine ZS, Phillips NA, Bédirian V, et al: The Montreal Cognitive Assessment, MoCA: a brief screening tool for mild cognitive impairment. J Am Geriatr Soc 53:695–699, 2005.
30. Fried LP, Tangen CM, Walston J, et al: Frailty in older adults: evidence for a phenotype. J Gerontol A Biol Sci Med Sci 56:M146–M156, 2001.
35. Norman D, Loredo JS: Obstructive sleep apnea in older adults. Clin Geriatr Med 24:151–165, 2008.
43. Eaton DA, Roland PS: Dizziness in the older adult, part 2. Treatments for causes of the four most common symptoms. Geriatrics 58:46–52, 2003.
44. Eaton DA, Roland PS: Dizziness in the older adult, part 1. Evaluation and general treatment strategies. Geriatrics 58:28–30, 33–36, 2003.
45. Tinetti ME: Clinical practice: preventing falls in elderly persons. N Engl J Med 348:42–49, 2003.
49. Ganz DA, Bao Y, Shekelle PG, et al: Will my patient fall? JAMA 297:77–86, 2007.
66. Martinez JP, Mattu A: Abdominal pain in the elderly. Emerg Med Clin North Am 24:371–388, 2006.
68. Grosmaitre P, Le Vavasseur O, Yachouh E, et al: Significance of atypical symptoms for the diagnosis and management of myocardial infarction in elderly patients admitted to emergency departments. Arch Cardiovasc Dis 106:586–592, 2013.
78. Johnson JC, Jayadevappa R, Baccash PD, et al: Nonspecific presentation of pneumonia in hospitalized older people: age effect or dementia? J Am Geriatr Soc 48:1316–1320, 2000.
81. Michet CJJ, Evans JM, Fleming KC, et al: Common rheumatologic diseases in elderly patients. Mayo Clin Proc 70:1205–1214, 1995.
90. Soubrier M, Mathieu S, Payet S, et al: Elderly-onset rheumatoid arthritis. Joint Bone Spine 77:290–296, 2010.
93. Boddaert J, Huong DL, Amoura Z, et al: Late-onset systemic lupus erythematosus: a personal series of 47 patients and pooled analysis of 714 cases in the literature. Medicine (Baltimore) 83:348–359, 2004.

34 Multidimensional Geriatric Assessment

Laurence Z. Rubenstein, Lisa V. Rubenstein

Geriatric assessment is a multidimensional, usually interdisciplinary, diagnostic process intended to determine a frail older person's medical, psychosocial, and functional capabilities and problems, with the objective of developing an overall plan for treatment and long-term follow-up. It differs from the standard medical evaluation in its concentration on frail older adults, with their complex problems, emphasis on functional status and quality of life, and frequent use of interdisciplinary teams and quantitative assessment scales.

The process of geriatric assessment can range in intensity from a limited assessment by primary care physicians or community health workers focused on identifying an older person's functional problems and disabilities (screening assessment) to a more thorough evaluation of these problems by a geriatrician or multidisciplinary team (comprehensive geriatric assessment [CGA]), often coupled with initiation of a therapeutic plan. This chapter discusses limited geriatric assessment, such as that which can be performed by a single practitioner in an office setting, and CGA, usually requiring a specialized geriatric setting.

Because the ultimate goal of geriatric assessment is to improve the quality of life for older adults, readers may find Figure 34-1 helpful.[1] As diagrammed, quality of life includes health status and socioeconomic and environmental factors. Health status can be quantified by measures of disease, such as signs, symptoms, and laboratory tests, and by measures of functional status. By functional status, we mean the individual's ability to participate fully in the physical, mental, and social activities of daily life. The ability to function fully in these areas is strongly affected by an individual's physiologic health and can often be used as a measure of the seriousness of a patient's multiple diseases. A CGA should be able to evaluate and plan care for all these areas.

BRIEF HISTORY OF GERIATRIC ASSESSMENT

The basic concepts of geriatric assessment have evolved over the past 80 years by combining elements of the traditional medical history and physical examination, social worker assessment, functional evaluation, treatment methods derived from rehabilitation medicine, and psychometric methods derived from the social sciences. By incorporating the perspectives of many disciplines, geriatricians have created a practical means of viewing the whole patient.

The first published reports of geriatric assessment programs came from the British geriatrician Marjory Warren, who initiated the concept of specialized geriatric assessment units during the late 1930s while in charge of a large London infirmary. This infirmary was filled primarily with chronically ill, bedridden, and largely neglected older patients who had not received proper medical diagnosis or rehabilitation and who were thought to be in need of lifelong institutionalization. Good nursing care kept the patients alive, but the lack of diagnostic assessment and rehabilitation kept them disabled. Through evaluation, mobilization, and rehabilitation, Warren was able to get most of the long bedridden patients out of bed and often discharged home. As a result of her experiences, Warren advocated that every older adult patient receive comprehensive assessment and an attempt at rehabilitation before being admitted to a long-term care hospital or nursing home.[2]

Since Warren's work, geriatric assessment has evolved. As geriatric care systems have been developed throughout the world, geriatric assessment programs have been assigned central roles, usually as focal points for entry into the care systems.[3] Geared to differing local needs and populations, geriatric assessment programs vary in intensity, structure, and function. They can be located in different settings, including acute hospital inpatient units and consultation teams, chronic and rehabilitation hospital units, outpatient and office-based programs, and home visit outreach programs. Despite diversity, they share many characteristics. Virtually all programs provide multidimensional assessment using specific measurement instruments to quantify functional, psychological, and social parameters. Most use interdisciplinary teams to pool expertise and enthusiasm in working toward common goals. Additionally, most programs attempt to couple their assessments with an intervention, such as rehabilitation, counseling, or placement.

Today, geriatric assessment continues to evolve in response to increased pressures for cost containment, avoidance of institutional stays, and consumer demands for better care. Geriatric assessment can help achieve improved quality of care and plan cost-effective care. This has generally meant more emphasis on noninstitutional programs and shorter hospital stays. Geriatric assessment teams are well positioned to deliver effective care for older adults with limited resources. Geriatricians have long emphasized the judicious use of technology, systematic preventive medicine activities, and less institutionalization and hospitalization.

STRUCTURE AND PROCESS OF GERIATRIC ASSESSMENT

Geriatric assessment begins with the identification of deteriorations in health status or the presence of risk factors for deterioration. These deteriorations include worsening of disease and worsening of functional status. If disease alone has worsened, without affecting function, the patient should be able to be cared for in the usual primary care settings. In addition, when functional status problems are mild and are not rapidly progressive, it is appropriate for a primary care practitioner to proceed with the assessment. However, because families and patients identify functional status problems early, and because internists and family practitioners often are unfamiliar with the concept of "treating" functional status impairment as a problem in its own right, patients often self-refer to geriatric care settings for these functional status problems, when such settings are available. Patients who have new severe or progressive deficits should ideally receive comprehensive multidisciplinary geriatric assessment. Figure 34-2 outlines an approach for evaluating older outpatients with health status deterioration and deciding who should be referred to multidimensional geriatric assessment settings.

Using this approach, an older patient with a deteriorating health status of any type, whether it is a markedly elevated blood glucose level, vertebral collapse, or new inability to perform errands, should be evaluated briefly to determine the full extent of functional disabilities. Many experts believe that frail older adults, defined generally as people older than 75 years or older than 65 years with chronic disease, should also be screened for

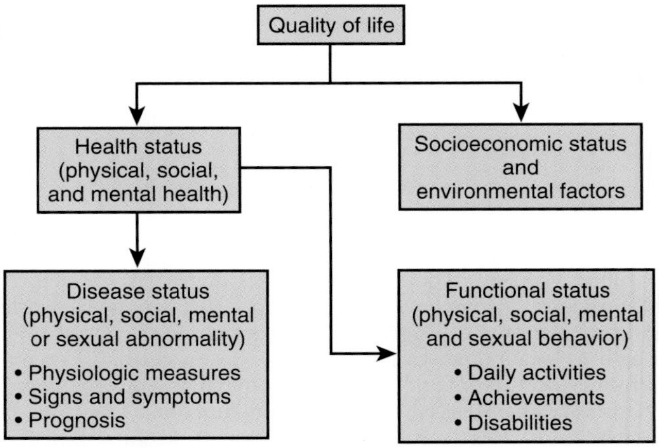

Figure 34-1. Conceptual components of quality of life-relationship to health and functional status. *(Adapted from Rubenstein LV, Calkins DR, Greenfield S, et al: Health status assessment for elderly patients. Report of the Society of General Internal Medicine Task Force on Health Assessment. J Am Geriatr Soc. 37:562-569, 1989.)*

functional disability or risk factors at regular intervals, such as once a year, even when no known acute health insults have occurred.[1,4-7] When a new disability or high-risk state is detected through screening, such patients may also be appropriate for a full geriatric assessment.

A typical geriatric assessment begins with a functional status review of systems that inventories the major domains of functioning. The major elements of this review of systems are captured in two commonly used functional status measures—basic activities of daily living (ADLs) and instrumental activities of daily living (IADLs). Several reliable and valid versions of these measures have been developed,[8-12] perhaps the most widely used being those by Katz and colleagues,[13] Lawton and Brody,[14] and Wade and Colin.[15] These scales are used by clinicians to detect whether the patient has problems performing activities that people must be able to accomplish to survive without help in the community. Basic ADLs include self-care activities, such as eating, dressing, bathing, transferring, and toileting. Patients unable to perform these activities will generally require 12- to 24-hour support by caregivers. IADLs include heavier housework, going on errands, managing finances, and making phone calls, activities that are required if the individual is to remain independent in a house or apartment.

To interpret the results of impairments in ADLs and IADLs, physicians will usually need additional information about the patient's environment and social situation. For example, the amount and type of caregiver support available, strength of the patient's social network, and level of social activities in which the patient participates will all influence the clinical approach taken in managing deficits detected. This information could be obtained by an experienced nurse or social worker. A screen for mobility and fall risk is also extremely helpful in quantifying function and disability, and several observational scales are available.[16,17] An assessment of nutritional status and risk for undernutrition is also important in understanding the extent of impairment and for planning care.[18] Likewise, a screening assessment of vision and hearing will often detect crucial deficits that need to be treated or compensated for.

Two other key pieces of information must always be gathered in the face of functional disability in an older adult. These are a screen for mental status (cognitive) impairment and a screen for depression. Of the many validated screening tests for cognitive function, the Folstein Mini-Mental State Examination and the Kokmen Short Test of Mental Function are among the best because they efficiently test the major aspects of cognitive functioning and have been available for many years.[19,20] Of the various screening tests for geriatric depression, the Yesavage Geriatric Depression Scale[21] and PHQ-9 (depression screen of the Patient Health Questionnaire)[22] are in wide use, and even shorter screening versions are available without significant loss of accuracy.[23]

The major measurable dimensions of geriatric assessment, together with examples of commonly used health status screening scales, are listed in Table 34-1.[7-36] The instruments listed are short, have been carefully tested for reliability and validity, and can be easily administered by virtually any staffperson involved with the assessment process. Both observational instruments (e.g., physical examination) and self-report (completed by patient or proxy) are available. Their components of them, such as watching a patient walk, turn around, and sit down, are routine parts of the geriatric physical examination. Many other types of assessment measures exist and can be useful in certain situations. For example, there are several disease-specific measures for stages and levels of dysfunction for patients with specific diseases such as arthritis,[30] dementia,[31] and parkinsonism.[32] There are also several brief global assessment instruments that attempt to quantify all dimensions of the assessment in a single form.[33-36] These latter instruments can be useful in community surveys and some research settings but are not detailed enough to be useful in most clinical settings. More comprehensive lists of available instruments can be found by consulting published reviews of health status assessment.[7-12,37]

A number of factors must be taken into account in deciding where an assessment should take place, outlined in Table 34-2. Mental and physical impairment make it difficult for patients to comply with recommendations and navigate multiple appointments in multiple locations. Functionally impaired older adults must depend on families and friends, who risk losing their jobs because of chronic and relentless demands on time and energy in their roles as caregivers, and who may be older adults themselves. Each separate medical appointment or intervention has a high time cost to these caregivers. Patient fatigue during periods of increased illness may require the availability of a bed during the assessment process. Finally, enough physician time and expertise must be available to complete the assessment within the constraints of the setting.

Most geriatric assessments do not require the full range of technology nor the intense monitoring found in the acute-care inpatient setting. However, hospitalization becomes unavoidable if no outpatient setting provides sufficient resources to accomplish the assessment fast enough. A specialized geriatric setting outside an acute hospital ward, such as a day hospital or subacute inpatient geriatric evaluation unit, will provide the easy availability of an interdisciplinary team with the time and expertise to provide needed services efficiently, an adequate level of monitoring, and beds for patients unable to sit or stand for prolonged periods. Inpatient and day hospital assessment programs have the advantages of intensity, rapidity, and ability to care for particularly frail or acutely ill patients. Outpatient and in-home programs are generally cheaper and avoid the necessity of an inpatient stay.

Assessment in the Office Practice Setting

A streamlined approach is usually necessary in the office setting. An important first step is setting priorities among problems for initial evaluation and treatment. The best problem to work on first might be the problem that most bothers a patient or, alternatively, the problem on which resolution of other problems depends—alcoholism or depression often fall into this category.

The second step in performing a geriatric assessment is to understand the exact nature of the disability through performing a task or symptom analysis. In a nonspecialized setting, or when

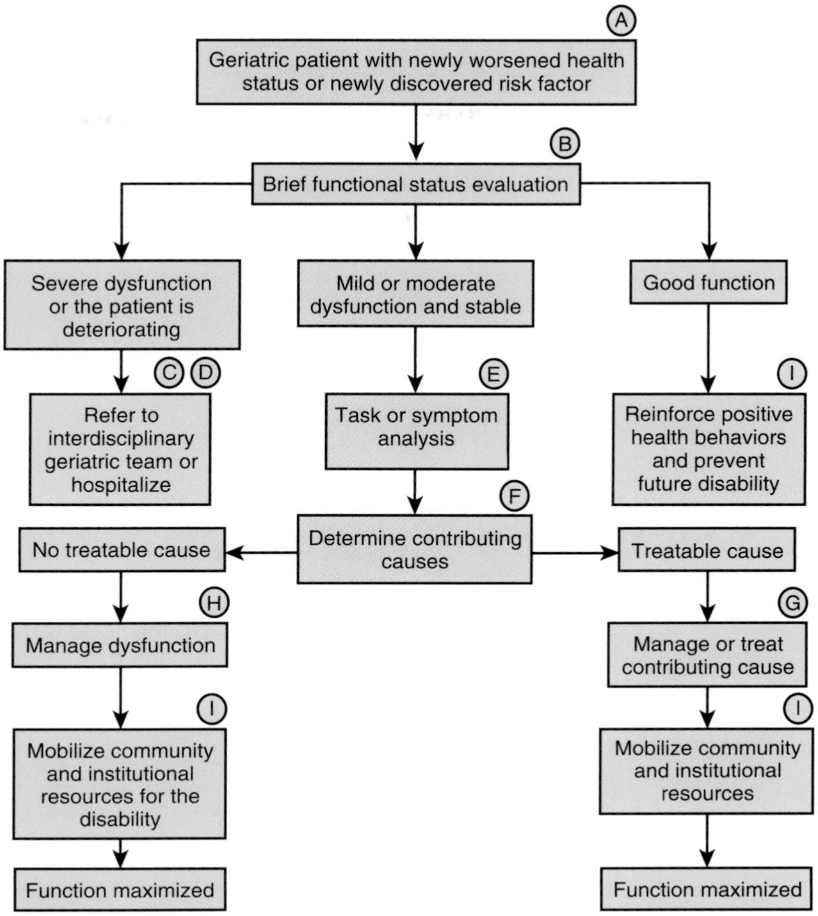

Figure 34-2. Evaluating and treating health status deterioration among geriatric outpatients. **A,** Older adults with a new deterioration in health status or newly discovered risk factor(s) may need geriatric assessment. Examples of patients needing assessment include the following: (1) frail older adults with a new functional disability or risk factor for deterioration detected on routine screening; (2) older adults with a new or worsened medical complaint or laboratory finding (e.g., "I fell last week" or x-ray that revealed a new vertebral compression fracture); (3) older adults with a new or worsened functional disability complaint ("I can't go to church because of my health"). **B,** Brief functional status evaluation should include the following: (1) activities of daily living (ADLs)[13-15,24]; (2) instrumental activities of daily living (IADLs)[14,24]; (3) mental status (e.g., Folstein Mini-Mental State Examination)[19]; (4) affective status (e.g., Yesavage Geriatric Depression Scale)[21-23]; **C,** Full multidimensional geriatric assessment and/or hospitalization is necessary for older patients with new severe or progressive functional disability. **D,** Targeted assessment for patients in office practice is appropriate for the following: (1) patients whose functional disabilities or medical problems are mild enough to make multiple appointments feasible; (2) patients whose disability is stable enough to permit assessment over weeks to months. **E,** To perform task or symptom analysis, select the patient's major symptom or disability or chief complaint (the one that bothers him or her the most, the disability on which resolution of other health problems depends, or the one that is the most treatable). Then determine the exact maneuvers necessary to complete the task or the exact components of the symptom (e.g., difficulty getting dressed due to difficulty putting on shoes because of inability to bend or difficulty with housework because of failure to complete tasks despite adequate physical ability to perform them). **F,** To determine contributing causes, the following should be carried out: (1) perform a targeted history, guided by the functional disabilities detected and by the known common occult causes of disability in older adults (see text); (2) perform a targeted physical examination, always including postural blood pressure changes, vision and hearing screening, observations of gait (at least, get up, walk 25 feet, turn around, sit down). Determine all specific physical disabilities, such as hip flexor weakness or poor hand mobility, that explain the observed functional disability. **G,** Manage or treat contributing cause(s). Begin appropriate medical treatments and evaluations. Mobilize community and institutional resources as appropriate (e.g., low-vision resources for blindness, Alcoholics Anonymous for alcoholics). Identify key members of the multidisciplinary team and refer as needed (e.g., social worker for social isolation, physical therapist for gait disorder, psychiatrist for depression). **H,** When the disability cannot be reversed, maximize function using available services and behavioral or physical adaptation. For example, rearranging schedule to maximize activity, providing adaptive devices, or arranging for home support services might be indicated. **I,** Always reinforce positive health behaviors.

TABLE 34-1 Measurable Dimensions of Geriatric Assessment

Dimension	Basic Context	Examples
Basic ADLs[24]	Strengths and limitations in self-care, basic mobility, and incontinence	Katz (ADLs)[13]; Lawton Personal Self-Maintenance Scale[14]; Barthel index[15]
IADLs[24]	Strengths and limitations in shopping, cooking, household activities, and finances	Lawton (IADLs)[14]; Older Americans Resources and Services, IADL section[28]
Social activities and supports[25]	Strengths and limitations in social network and community activities	Lubben Social Network Scale[29]; Older Americans Resources and Services, social resources section[28]
Mental health, affective[27]	The degree to which the person feels anxious, depressed, or generally happy	Yesavage Geriatric Depression Scale[21,23]; PHQ-9[22]
Mental health, cognitive[27]	The degree to which the person is alert, oriented, and able to concentrate and perform complex mental tasks	Folstein Mini-Mental State[19]; Kokmen Short Test of Mental Function[20]
Mobility, gait, and balance[9,11]	Quantitative scale of gait, balance, and risk of falls	Tinetti Performance-Oriented Mobility Assessment[16]; Get Up and Go Test[17]
Nutritional adequacy[18]	Current nutritional status and risk of malnutrition	Nutrition Screening Initiative Checklist[18]; Mini-Nutritional Assessment[26]

ADLs, Activities of daily living; *IADLs,* instrumental activities of daily living.

TABLE 34-2 Determining Intensity and Location of the Geriatric Assessment

Parameter	Office Setting	Outpatient or Home Care Team	Inpatient Unit or Team
Level of disability	Low	Intermediate	High
Cognitive dysfunction	Mild	Mild to severe	Moderate to severe
Family support	Good	Good to fair	Good to poor
Acuity of illness	Mild	Mild to moderate	Moderate to severe
Complexity	Low	Intermediate	High
Transportation access	Good	Good	Good to poor

the disability is mild or clear-cut, this may involve only taking a careful history. When the disability is more severe, more detailed assessments by a multidisciplinary or interdisciplinary team may be necessary. For example, a patient may have difficulty dressing. There are multiple tasks associated with dressing, any one of which might be the stumbling block (e.g., buying clothes, choosing appropriate clothes to put on, remembering to complete the task, buttoning, stretching to put on a shirt, reaching downward to put on shoes). By identifying the exact areas of difficulty, further evaluation can be targeted toward solving the problem.

Once the history has revealed the nature of the disability, a systematic physical examination and ancillary laboratory tests are needed to clarify the cause of the problem. For example, difficulty dressing could be caused by mental status impairment, poor finger mobility, or dysfunction of shoulders, back, or hips. Evaluation by a physical or occupational therapist may be necessary to pinpoint the problem adequately, and evaluation by a social worker may be required to determine the extent of family dysfunction engendered by or contributing to the dependency. Radiologic and other laboratory testing may be necessary.

Each abnormality that could cause difficulty dressing suggests different treatments. By understanding the abnormalities that contribute most to the functional disability, the best treatment strategy can be undertaken. Often, one disability leads to another. Impaired gait may lead to depression or decreased social functioning, and immobility of any cause, even after the cause has been removed, can lead to secondary impairments in performance of daily activities because of deconditioning and loss of musculoskeletal flexibility.

Almost any acute or chronic disease can reduce functioning. Common but easily overlooked causes of dysfunction in older adults include impaired cognition, impaired special senses (e.g., vision, hearing, balance), unstable gait and mobility, poor health habits (e.g., alcohol, smoking, lack of exercise), poor nutrition, polypharmacy, incontinence, psychosocial stress, and depression. To identify contributing causes of the disability, the physician must look for worsening of the patient's chronic diseases, occurrence of a new acute disease, or appearance of one of the common occult diseases listed earlier. The physician does this through a refocused history guided by the functional disabilities detected, their differential diagnoses, and a focused physical examination. In addition to usual evaluations of the heart, lungs, extremities, and neurologic function, the physical examination always includes postural blood pressure, vision and hearing screening, and careful observation of the patient's gait. A cognitive assessment screen, already recommended as part of the initial functional status screen, may also determine which parts of the physical examination require particular attention as part of the evaluation of dementia or acute confusion. Finally, basic laboratory testing, including a complete blood count, blood chemistry panel, and tests indicated on the basis of specific findings from the history and physical examination, will generally be necessary.

Once the disability and its causes are understood, the best treatments or management strategies for it are often clear. When a reversible cause for the impairment is found, a simple treatment may eliminate or ameliorate the functional disability. When the disability is complex, the physician may need the support of a variety of community or hospital-based resources. In most cases, a strategy for long-term follow-up and, often, formal case management should be developed to ensure that needs and services are appropriately matched up and followed through.

Comprehensive Geriatric Assessment

If referral to a specialized geriatric setting has been chosen, the process of assessment will probably be similar to that described, except that the greater intensity of resources and special training of all members of the interdisciplinary team in dealing with geriatric patients and their problems will facilitate carrying out the proposed assessment and plan more quickly and in greater breadth and detail. In the usual geriatric assessment setting, key disciplines involved include, at a minimum, physicians, social workers, nurses, and physical and occupational therapists, optimally, may include those in other disciplines such as dieticians, pharmacists, ethicists, psychologists, and home care specialists. Special geriatric expertise among the interdisciplinary team members is crucial.

The interdisciplinary team conference, which takes place after most team members have completed their individual assessments, is critical. Most successful trials of geriatric assessment have included such a team conference. By bringing the perspectives of all disciplines together, the team conference generates new ideas, sets priorities, disseminates the full results of the assessment to all those involved in treating the patient, and avoids duplication or incongruity. Development of fully effective teams requires commitment, skill, and time as the interdisciplinary team evolves through the so-called forming, storming, and norming phases to reach the fully developed performing stage.[38] Involvement of the patient (and caregiver, if appropriate) at some stage is important in maintaining the principle of choice.[38,39]

EFFECTIVENESS OF GERIATRIC ASSESSMENT PROGRAMS

A large and still growing literature supports the effectiveness of geriatric assessment programs (GAPs) in a variety of settings. Early descriptive studies indicated a number of benefits from GAPs, such as improved diagnostic accuracy, reduced discharges to nursing homes, increased functional status, and more appropriate medication prescribing. Because they were descriptive studies, without concurrent control patients, they were not able to distinguish the effects of the programs from simple improvement over time, nor did these studies look at long-term or many short-term outcome benefits. Nonetheless, many of these early studies provided promising results.[40-44]

Improved diagnostic accuracy was the most widely described effect of geriatric assessment, most often indicated by substantial numbers of important problems uncovered. Frequencies of new diagnoses found ranged from almost one to more than four per patient. Factors contributing to the improvement of diagnosis in GAPs include the validity of the assessment itself (the capability of a structured search for geriatric problems to find them), the extra measure of time and care taken in the evaluation of the patient (independent of the formal elements of the assessment), and a probable lack of diagnostic attention on the part of referring professionals.

Improved living location on discharge from a health care setting has been demonstrated in several early studies, beginning with Williams and associates' classic descriptive study of an outpatient assessment program in New York, before and after assessment.[45] Of patients referred for nursing home placement in the county, the assessment program found that only 38% actually needed skilled nursing care, whereas 23% could return home, and 39% were appropriate for board and care or retirement facilities. Numerous subsequent studies have shown similar improvements in living location.[46-59] Several studies that examined mental or physical functional status of patients before and after CGA, coupled with treatment and rehabilitation, showed patient improvement on measures of function.[46-50,52,56]

Beginning in the 1980s, controlled studies appeared that corroborated some of the earlier studies and documented additional benefits, such as improved survival, reduced hospital and nursing home use and, in some cases, reduced costs.[46-67] These studies were by no means uniform in their results. Some showed a whole series of dramatic positive effects on function, survival, living location, and costs, whereas others showed relatively few, if any, benefits. However, the GAPs being studied were also very different from each other in terms of process of care offered and patient populations accepted. To this day, controlled trials of GAPs continue and, as results accumulate, we are able to understand which aspects have contributed to their effectiveness and which have not.

One striking effect confirmed for many GAPs has been a positive impact on survival. Several controlled studies of different basic GAP models have demonstrated significantly increased survival, reported in different ways and with varying periods of follow-up. Mortality was reduced for Sepulveda geriatric evaluation unit patients by 50% at 1 year, and the survival curves of the experimental and control groups still significantly favored the assessed group at 2 years.[46,60,61] Survival was improved by 21% at 1 year in a Scottish trial of geriatric rehabilitation consultation.[56] Two Canadian consultation trials demonstrated significantly improved 6-month survival.[52,53] Two Danish community-based trials of in-home geriatric assessment and follow-up demonstrated reduction in mortality,[47,58] and two Welsh studies of in-home GAPs had beneficial survival effects among patients assessed at home and followed for 2 years.[49,50] On the other hand, several other studies of geriatric assessment found no statistically significant survival benefits.[51,55,56]

Multiple studies have followed patients longitudinally after the initial assessment and thus were able to examine the longer term utilization and cost impacts of assessment and treatment. Some studies found an overall reduction in nursing home days.[46,56,62] Hospital use was examined in several reports. For hospital-based GAPs, the length of hospitalization was obviously affected by the length of the assessment itself. Thus, some programs appeared to prolong the initial length of stay,[44,63,64] whereas others reduced initial stay.[58,65] However, studies following patients for at least 1 year have usually shown reduction in use of acute-care hospital services, even in those programs with initially prolonged hospital stays.[46,47,54]

Compensatory increases in use of community-based services or home care agencies might be expected with declines in nursing home placements and use of other institutional services. These increases have been detected in several studies[47,49,52,66] but not in others.[46,54,59] Although increased use of formal community services may not always be indicated, it usually is a desirable goal. The fact that several studies did not detect increases in the use of home and community services probably reflects the unavailability of community service or referral networks, rather than that more of such services were not needed.

The effects of these programs on costs and utilization parameters have seldom been examined comprehensively owing to methodologic difficulties in gathering comprehensive utilization and cost data and statistical limitations in comparing highly skewed distributions. The Sepulveda study found that total first-year direct health care costs had been reduced owing to overall reductions in nursing home and rehospitalization days, despite significantly longer initial hospital stays in the geriatric unit.[46] These savings continued through 3 years of follow-up.[60] Hendriksen and coworkers' program[47] reduced the costs of medical care, apparently through successful early case finding and referral for preventive intervention. Williams and colleagues' outpatient GAP[54] detected reductions in medical care costs owing primarily to reductions in hospitalization. Although it would be reasonable to worry that prolonged survival of frail older patients would lead to increased service use and charges—or, of perhaps greater concern, to worry about the quality of the prolonged life—these concerns may be without substance. Indeed, the Sepulveda study demonstrated that a GAP could improve not only survival but prolong high-function survival,[46,60] while at the same time reducing the use of institutional services and costs.

A 1993 meta-analysis attempted to resolve some of the discrepancies among study results and tried to identify whether particular program elements were associated with particular benefits.[68,69] This meta-analysis included published data from the 28 controlled trials completed as of that date, involving nearly 10,000 patients, and was also able to include substantial amounts of unpublished data systematically retrieved from many of the studies. The meta-analysis identified five GAP types—hospital units (six studies), hospital consultation teams (eight studies), in-home assessment services (seven studies), outpatient assessment services (four studies), and hospital-home assessment services (three studies), the latter of which performed in-home assessments on patients recently discharged from hospitals. The meta-analysis confirmed many of the major reported benefits for many of the individual program types. These statistically and clinically significant benefits included reduced risk of mortality (by 22% for hospital-based programs at 12 months and by 14% for all programs combined at 12 months), improved likelihood of living at home (by 47% for hospital-based programs and by 26% for all programs combined at 12 months), reduced risk of hospital (re)admissions (by 12% for all programs at the study's end), greater chance of cognitive improvement (by 47% for all programs at the study's end), and greater chance of physical function improvement for patients on hospital units (by 72% for hospital units).

Clearly, not all studies have shown equivalent effects, and the meta-analysis was able to indicate a number of variables at the program and patient levels that tended to distinguish trials with large effects from those with more limited ones. When examined on the program level, hospital units and home visit assessment teams produced the most dramatic benefits, whereas no major significant benefits in office-based programs could be confirmed. Programs that provided hands-on clinical care and/or long-term follow-up were generally able to produce greater positive effects than purely consultative programs or ones that lacked follow-up. Another factor associated with greater demonstrated benefits, at least in hospital-based programs, was patient targeting; programs that selected patients who were at high risk for deterioration yet still had rehabilitation potential generally had stronger results than less selective programs.

The meta-analysis confirmed the importance of targeting criteria in producing beneficial outcomes. In particular, when use of explicit targeting criteria for patient selection was included as a covariate, increases in some program benefits were often found. For example, among the hospital-based GAP studies, positive effects on physical function and likelihood of living at home at 12 months were associated with studies that excluded patients who were relatively "too healthy." A similar effect on physical function was seen in the institutional studies that excluded persons with relatively poor prognoses. The reason for this effect of targeting on effect size no doubt lies in the ability of careful targeting to concentrate the intervention on patients who could benefit, without diluting the effect with persons too ill or too well to show a measurable improvement.

Studies performed after the 1993 meta-analysis have been largely corroborative. A 2005 meta-analysis confirmed that inpatient GAPs for hospital older patients may reduce mortality, increase the chances of living at home in 1 year, and improve physical and cognitive function,[70] and a 2011 meta-analysis that included 22 randomized trials of inpatient GAPs confirmed that patients undergoing in-hospital CGA were more likely to be alive and living in their homes at follow-up and less likely to be living in residential care homes.[71] However, with principles of geriatric medicine becoming more diffused into usual care, particularly at places where controlled trials are being undertaken, differences between GAPs and control groups seem to be narrowing.[72-76] For example, a 2002 study of inpatient and outpatient GAPs failed to demonstrate substantial benefits.[77] Other studies have continued to reveal major benefits of inpatient programs.[78,79] Effects of outpatient GAPs have been less impressive, with a 2004 meta-analysis showing no favorable effects on mortality outcome.[80] For cost reasons, the growth of inpatient units has been slow, despite their proven effectiveness, whereas outpatient programs have increased, despite their less impressive effect size in controlled trials. However, other trials of outpatient programs have shown significant benefits in areas not found in earlier outpatient studies, such as functional status, psychological parameters, and well-being, which may indicate improvement in the outpatient care models being tested.[72-76,79]

A 2002 meta-analysis of preventive home visits revealed that home visitation programs are consistently effective if they are based on multidimensional geriatric assessments, use multiple follow-up visits, and are offered to older adults with relatively good function at baseline.[81] The NNV (number needed to visit) to prevent one hospital admission in programs with frequent follow-up was shown to be about 40. An expanded 2008 meta-analysis of preventive home visits largely confirmed the earlier findings on the importance of multidimensional assessment and higher function, but not on multiple follow-up visits.[82] It has also been confirmed that a key component of successful programs is a systematic approach for teaching primary care professionals. These results have important policy implications. In countries with existing national programs of preventive home visits, the process and organization of these visits should be reconsidered on the basis of the criteria identified in this meta-analysis. In addition, there are a variety of chronic disease management programs specifically addressing the care needs of older adults.[83] Engrafting the key concepts of home-based preventive care programs into these programs should be feasible and cost-effective as they continue to evolve. Identifying risks and dealing with them as an essential component of the care of older adults is central to reducing the emerging burden of disability and improving the quality of life for older adults.

A continuing challenge has been obtaining adequate financing to support adding geriatric assessment services to existing medical care. Despite GAPs' many proven benefits, and their ability to reduce costs documented in controlled trials, health care financiers have been reluctant to fund geriatric assessment programs, presumably out of concern that the programs might be expanded too fast and that costs for extra diagnostic and therapeutic services might increase out of control. Many practitioners have found ways to unbundle the geriatric assessment process into component services and receive adequate support to fund the entire process. In this continuing time of fiscal restraint, geriatric practitioners must remain constantly creative to reach the goal of optimal patient care.

CONCLUSION

Published studies of multidimensional geriatric assessment have confirmed its efficacy in many settings. Although there is no single optimal blueprint for geriatric assessment, the participation of the interdisciplinary team and optimization of functional status and quality of life as major clinical goals are common to all settings. Although the greatest benefits have been found in programs targeted to the frail subgroup of older adults, a strong case can be made for a continuum of GAP screening assessments performed periodically for all older adults and comprehensive assessment targeted to frail and high-risk older patients. Clinicians interested in developing these services would do well to heed the experiences of the programs reviewed here in adapting the principles of geriatric assessment to local resources. Future research is still needed to determine the most effective and efficient methods for performing geriatric assessment and develop strategies for best matching needs with services.

KEY POINTS

- Geriatric assessment is a systematic multidimensional approach to improving diagnostic accuracy and planning care for frail older adults.
- Controlled trials have documented many benefits from geriatric assessment, including improved functional status and survival and reduced hospital and nursing home admissions.

For a complete list of references, please visit www.expertconsult.com.

KEY REFERENCES

1. Rubenstein LV, Calkins DR, Greenfield S, et al: Health status assessment for elderly patients: reports of the society of general internal medicine task force on health assessment. J Am Geriatr Soc 37:562–569, 1989.
2. Matthews DA: Dr. Marjory Warren and the origin of British geriatrics. J Am Geriatr Soc 32:253–258, 1984.
5. Rubenstein LZ, Josephson KR, Nichol-Seamons M, et al: Comprehensive health screening of well elderly adults. J Gerontol 41:343–352, 1986.
9. Rubenstein LZ, Wieland D, Bernabei R: Geriatric assessment technology: the state of the art, Milan, Italy, 1995, Kurtis.
10. Kane RL, Kane RA: Assessing older persons, New York, 2000, Oxford University Press.
11. Osterweil D, Brummel-Smith K, Beck JC: Comprehensive geriatric assessment, New York, 2000, McGraw-Hill.
42. Brocklehurst JC, Carty MH, Leeming JT, et al: Medical screening of old people accepted for residential care. Lancet 2:141–143, 1978.
46. Rubenstein LZ, Josephson KR, Wieland GD, et al: Effectiveness of a geriatric evaluation unit: a randomized clinical trial. N Engl J Med 311:1664–1670, 1984.
47. Hendriksen C, Lund E, Stromgard E: Consequences of assessment and intervention among elderly people: three-year randomized controlled trial. BMJ 289:1522–1524, 1984.
68. Stuck AE, Siu AL, Wieland GD, et al: Comprehensive geriatric assessment: a meta-analysis of controlled trials. Lancet 342:1032–1036, 1993.
71. Ellis G, Whitehead MA, Robinson D, et al: Comprehensive geriatric assessment for older adults admitted to hospital: meta-analysis of randomized controlled trials. BMJ 343:d6553, 2011.
82. Huss A, Stuck AE, Rubenstein LZ, et al: Multidimensional preventive home visit program for community-dwelling older adults: a systematic review and meta-analysis of randomized controlled trials. J Gerontol A Biol Sci Med Sci 63:298–307, 2008.

35 Laboratory Diagnosis and Geriatrics: More Than Just Reference Intervals for Older Adults

Alexander Lapin, Elisabeth Mueller

INTRODUCTION

Radical improvements in health care and general lifestyle have brought about longer life expectancy and, with it, a demographic phenomenon that has never been observed before. The steady growth of the proportion of older adults in the general population, especially in industrialized countries, has resulted in what is called an inverse demographic pyramid.

Concurrently, the subject of geriatric medicine has also gained in popularity, both among the members of the professional community and in the general public, but not so in laboratory medicine. Here, except for an occasional call to adjust the reference intervals for specific tests, there has been no fundamental discussion of the consequences of the current demographic trend in the population—that is, until now. This chapter should provide some insights into this problem.

Objectivity as a Basic Principle of In Vitro Diagnosis

Since antiquity, the in vitro diagnosis has followed the same principle. A biologic sample such as blood or urine collected from the patient would be analyzed for its physical and/or chemical properties, and the result would then be interpreted in terms of clinical information indicating the health status of the patient.

If the procedure is properly calibrated, the results can be expressed quantitatively and described not in words, as is the case for other diagnostic disciplines, such as pathology or radiology, but as an exact numeric value. Thus, the result of a laboratory analysis is not a descriptive observation derived from a subjective experience of the operator, but is an objective measurement, which always is related to a deductive postulated standard. Because most of the results provided by laboratory investigations can be considered as data that are generally reproducible and comparable, laboratory analysis represents a valid instrument of modern, evidence-based medicine.

To keep the clinical interpretation of these data objective, as much as possible, every numeric test result is usually completed by a reference interval, which is listed on the same line next to the test result value. The reference intervals have been derived from the standard statistical distribution of test results obtained from a demographic sample drawn from the normal adult population; normal is understood to be synonymous with healthy.[1]

However, because the statistical reference interval is based on the 95th percentile of Gaussian normal distribution (the bell curve), 5% of results obtained from healthy individuals will always be outside the reference range yet have no pathologic correlation. It follows that even in the case of a healthy individual, the probability that a random test result value would fall outside the reference interval proportionally increases with the number of the same laboratory tests performed on that same healthy individual.

Thus, ironically, the larger the number of tests undertaken, the higher the probability of a patient not being found normal,[1] which shows that the statistically based reference concept[2] has its limits. Every person is not just an anonymous member of a collective, but a unique unrepeatable individual.

Geriatric Individuality

You cannot step twice into the same rivers.

Attributed to Heraclitus

From the point of view of the sociology, the answer to the question whether an older adult is healthy or sick can neither be based on actual performance at work nor reduced to the fact of whether he or she has secured a physician's note from the employer. By contrast, in older adults, more than in younger adults, the difference between being healthy or sick is based on a very subjective feeling reflecting the quality of one's life.

However, there is yet another aspect to be considered in geriatric laboratory medicine. It is the continuous progressive decline of physiologic functions in an aging human body. Age-dependent impairment of renal and pulmonic functions, progression of osteoporosis, decrease of various endocrine functions, and general weakening of immunity at an older age are typical examples.[3-6]

Attempts to establish age-related reference intervals, similar to those used in pediatrics, have proven to be unsuccessful. Such intentions failed because the approach did not and could not address the individuality and variability of the senescent process from the clinical and biologic point of view for each patient (Figure 35-1).

In pediatrics, as well as in the adult medicine, most of the population is healthy, and those who are sick usually have only one cause (rarely more than one) for their illness. The primary aim of pediatric and adult medicine is to detect and cure the disease as efficiently as possible to protect the future life chances of the patients. Adult medicine strives to return adult patients to their normal productive (working) life as quickly as possible.

Geriatrics is different. Here, the clinical histories of older adults who have reached the last part of their lives are much more complex than those in the previous stages of their life.

Past crises and emergency situations, but also periods of prosperity and affluence—perceived as the good times—all have influenced the actual health state of an older adult. Diseases and trauma, which randomly occur in the course of life and have left more or less relevant after effects and physical and emotional scars in all of us, contribute to the specificity of the clinical status of each older adult. Moreover, with advancing age, the probability of manifestation of genetically or secondarily predisposed diseases increases progressively. To describe all these inputs, clinical geriatrics uses the term *multimorbidity*. It is a very important term because it characterizes the occurrence of several diseases and/or pathologic processes to which an older patient is subjected, often in oligosymptomatic and atypical ways.

Many different involute processes can be considered as typical physiologic processes of older age. They all can occur with individual accentuation and can be triggered by different random events at different moments of the life. In this context, it becomes more and more difficult to define unequivocally the meaning of the term *biologic age*.[7] Finally, one has to accept that death itself is often a result of one or more diseases breaking out during the ultimate period of life (Figure 35-2).

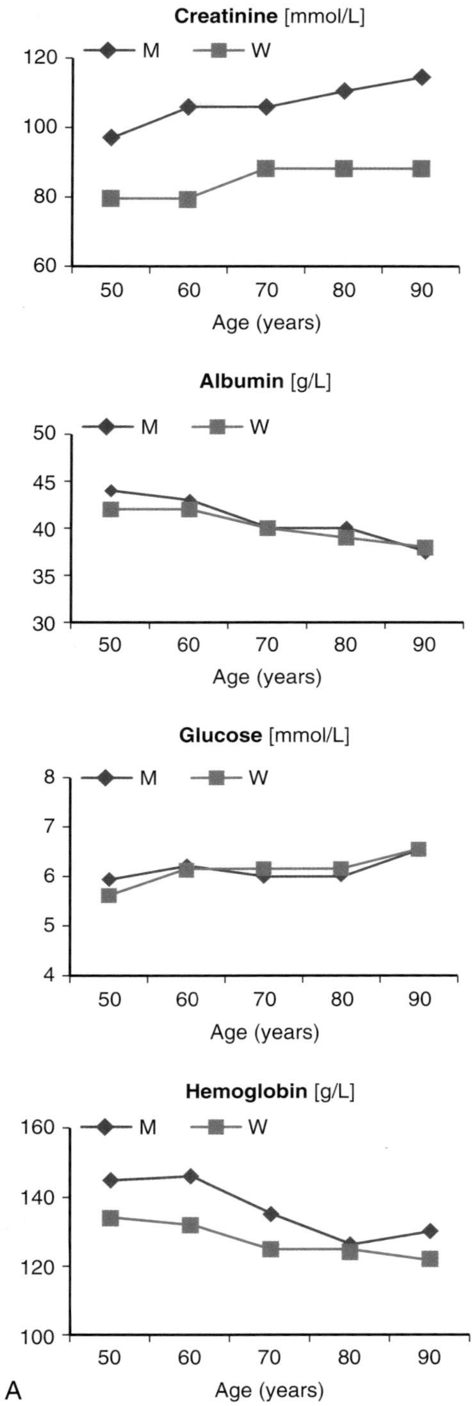

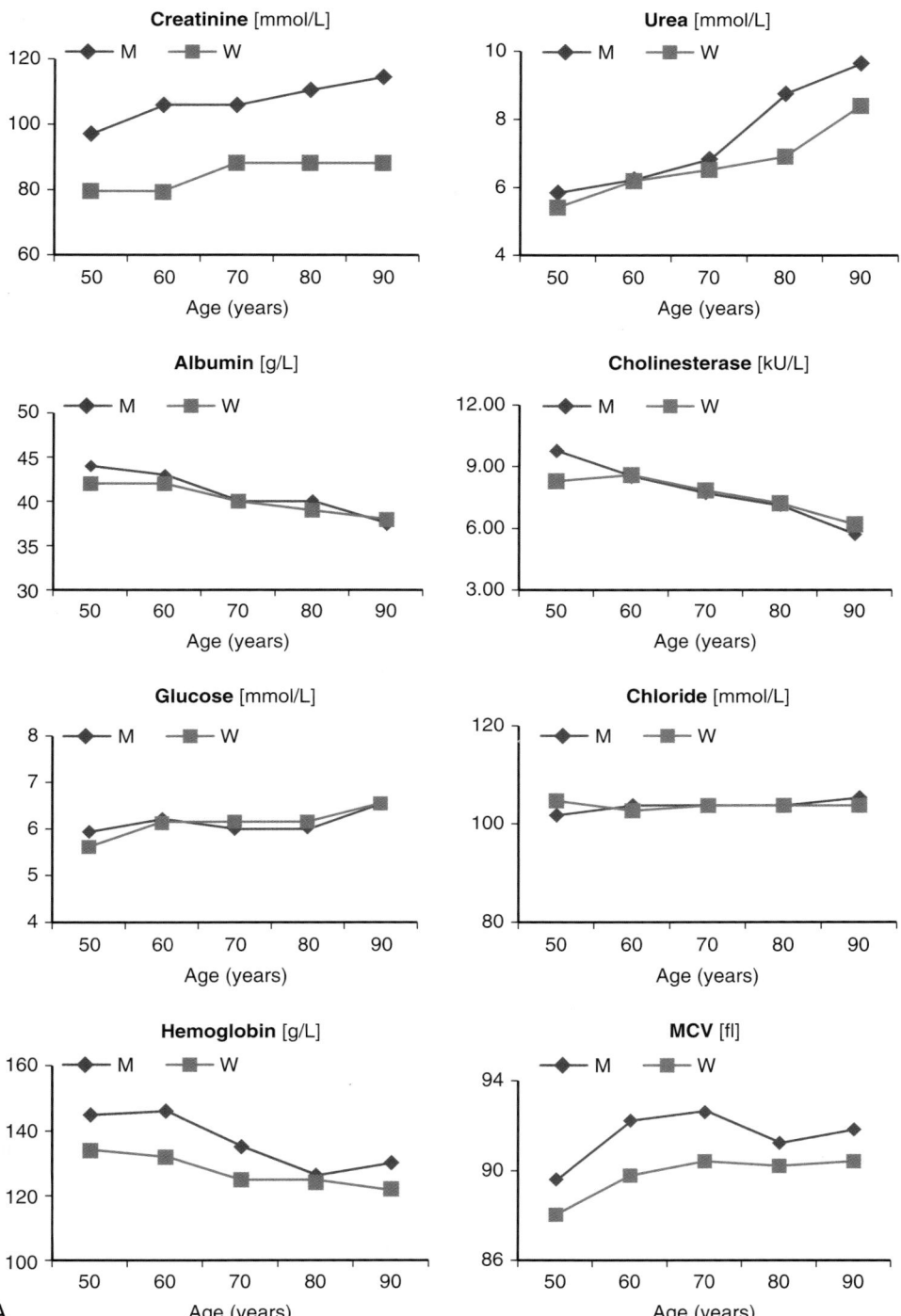

Figure 35-1. A, Correlation of different laboratory parameters with age. The best correlation shows albumin (r < 0.5).

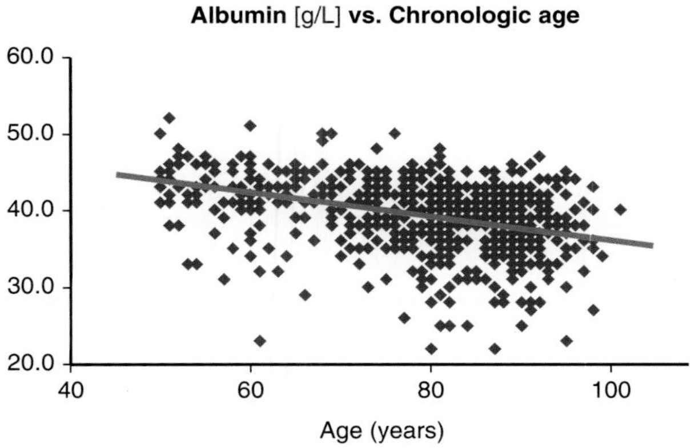

Figure 35-1, cont'd. B, Correlation of different laboratory parameters with age. The best correlation shows albumin (r < 0.5). MCV,

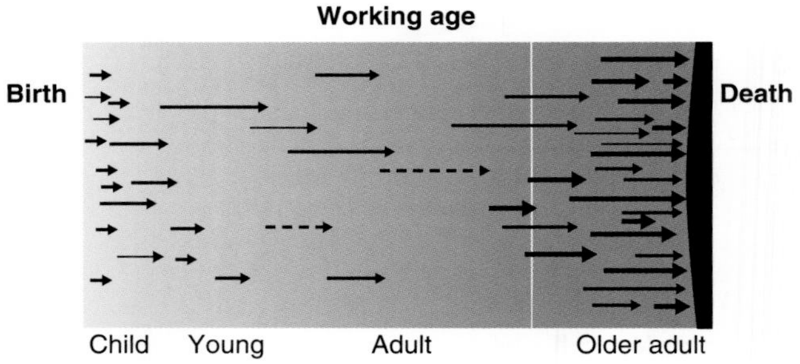

Figure 35-2. The course of life *(horizontal axis)* and randomly occurring diseases and traumas (→), and their after effects (—): At the end of life, they are contributing in an additive way to the final clinical status. *(From Lapin A, Böhmar F: Laboratory diagnosis and geriatrics: more than just reference intervals for the elderly. ... Wien Med Wochenschr 155:30–35, 2005.)*

To sum up, when speaking about the normality of patients in geriatrics, it has to be kept in mind that an older, perfectly healthy individual is a biologic rarity, rather than the normal case.[8]

From Screening to Monitoring

The opinion that geriatric reference intervals can be estimated by large-scale studies seems to be spurious, even from a theoretical point of view. According to Harris,[9] the width of the reference interval is determined by three types of variation, which can be characterized by appropriate coefficients of variation, C_V:

- C_{VA}—analytic variation, due to the imprecision of an analytic method
- C_{VB}—biologic variation, accounting for variations within one individual
- C_{VC}—interindividual variation, due to differences among several individuals

The total variation (C_{VTOT}) results from the geometric sum of these three variations:

$$C_{VTOT} = SQRT[(C_{VA})^2 + (C_{VB})^2 + (C_{VC})^2]$$

In practice, it can be assumed that the analytic variation (C_{VA}) is almost negligible due to the high technical standards of the analytic method. Hence, the total reference interval (C_{VTOT}) is determined by the biologic (C_{VB}) and the interindividual (C_{VC}) variations alone. There are two extreme cases to be considered (Figure 35-3):

1. In the first case, the reference interval of a parameter is almost identical with the biologic variation (C_{VB}) that is nearly the same in all healthy individuals—that is, $C_{VC} \rightarrow 0$ (e.g., glucose).
   Should a particular individual disease break out, the probability that the corresponding value will be shifted out of the reference range increases. In such conditions, the pathology would be detected early, and the probability to obtain a result outside the reference interval would be increased by repeating the test (see Figure 35-3).
2. By contrast, in another situation the parameter would show a very narrow biologic variation ($C_{VB} \rightarrow 0$), but the mean values (medians) of this variation would differ from individual to individual (as with the uric acid).

In this case, the reference interval relies preferentially on the distribution of the mean values (medians) of such individual variations (C_{VC}). Strictly speaking, such a test is less suitable for diagnostic use, especially for early detection of a disease. A minor pathologic change, which occurs in one individual, would merely cause a shift out of that individual's interval of the biologic variation, but not necessarily outside the reference interval that was determined for all the considered individuals in the sample or collective (C_{VTOT}). Evidently, such pathologic change could remain undetected, despite repeated measurements. To increase the diagnostic significance of such tests, it is necessary to perform the stratification of the reference collective—that is, to determine the reference intervals in different subpopulations separately, which in turn should be defined according to more specific criteria such as gender, age, and other demographic parameters.

This is not the case in geriatrics. In geriatrics, such an approach would not suffice unless the proposed stratification also considers other criteria, such as physical constitution, nutritional status, mobility, cognitive activity, and predominant disease. By pushing stratification to the extreme, it becomes more and more difficult to find and establish a statistically relevant reference group of individuals with the same characteristics. The lack of such reliable groups creates a major problem in establishing an age-dependent reference interval in geriatrics.[10,11]

On the other hand, the ultimate stratification could be achieved when the actual result (the present measured value) is compared to the previous results obtained for the same person. And here, parameters of narrow biologic variation but of wide interindividual differences are not useful for screening (e.g., to detect a new disease) but are well suited for monitoring dynamic changes in the individual's clinical status. However, a basic condition for the realization of such long-term monitoring is the assessment of the long-time stability and the quality of the laboratory tests applied, which may occasionally deliver somewhat questionable results, especially in older adults.

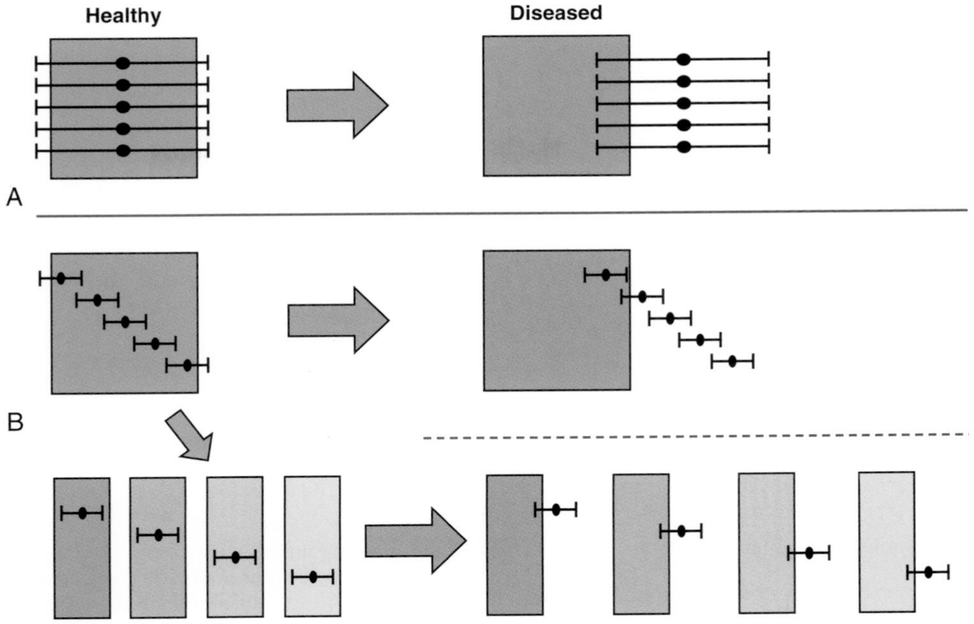

Figure 35-3. Influence of illness on two types of laboratory investigations. **A,** The width of the reference interval is determined by biologic factors (e.g., intraindividual variation, C_{VB}). Due to an illness, all values are shifted out from the reference interval. **B,** The width of the reference interval is determined by intraindividual variation (C_{VC}), whereas interindividual variation is negligible ($C_{VB} \rightarrow 0$). An illness would shift the values only in a segment of individuals of the considered collective. To improve the diagnostic relevance of this test, stratification (e.g., redefinition of the subreference intervals) has to be performed. *(Adapted from Harris EK. Effects of intra- and interindividual variation on the appropriate use of normal ranges. Clin Chem 20:1535–1542, 1974.)*

Monitoring in Geriatrics

One of the actual trends of today's laboratory medicine is the consolidation of laboratories, which has been imposed on the existing laboratory community by the markedly improved efficiency of laboratory testing as a whole. Usually, this means the concentration of medical laboratories in large, semi-industrial diagnostic institutions,[12] a hub to which the work is outsourced. The separation of laboratory medicine from clinical institutions has brought about the depersonalization of the communication between clinicians and laboratory specialists.[13,14] Consequently, certain aspects, which have theoretically been known to affect the diagnostic significance of laboratory testing, have gained an unexpected actuality. One of these concerns the preanalytic studies.

Such preanalytic conditions include orthostatic effects (especially in patients with edema), effects related to impaired mobility and/or nutritional status, and seasonal influences.[15] Because of impairment of the functionality of different organs (e.g., liver, kidney, lung, immune system) in older adults, minor pathologic influences will be compensated for with less elasticity. This, in turn, is reflected by the higher variability of laboratory results.

Moreover, the poor venous status of some older patients can cause difficulties in regard to phlebotomy and blood collection, which are then responsible for hemolytic sera and inadequate sample volumes that might be too small for an optimal analytic process.

The fact that the sheer number of samples sent to the laboratory by geriatric practitioners can be far less than those that originate, for example, in the intensive care unit, can lead to negligence and sloppiness. This can result in geriatric samples being treated with less interest and therefore given the lowest priority. Well known are situations when, in a nursing home, the collected samples are ignored by the courier and left behind on the counter for a later batch in the day or even for the next day's collection. The increased turnaround time is always disadvantageous, whether because of the stability of the analyte (substance, enzymatic activity, or other subject of chemical analysis[15]) or the actual diagnostic information to be submitted for review by the attending physician.

The consolidation of laboratory medicine has brought about another trend, known as point of care testing (POCT). Using modern testing devices, which are usually based on dry chemistry principles, analyses can now be performed in situ and the results obtained faster and much more effectively than before, when a distant laboratory was used.[16] The POCT is also of particular interest in geriatrics because of the growing scope of available tests.

Although the use of POCT has become a generally accepted procedure, some disadvantages such as calibration, documentation, and especially uncontrolled performance by untrained personnel are still being discussed in the laboratory medicine community. A serious problem can arise when laboratory data, provided by different sources (e.g., by diagnostic institutions and/or by different POCT devices) are clinically evaluated and included in the patient's history.[17] Older adult patients are the most prone to such variations because they are often being treated by several health care providers—in a physician's office, in a nursing home as a resident, and in a hospital as an emergency patient.

Medical Significance of Laboratory Results in Older Adults

Finally, there is the issue of the medical significance of laboratory analyses in the context of clinical geriatrics. This can be different from adult medicine, not only in physiologic parameters, but also in demographic changes, life expectancy, and clinical consequences (Table 35-1).

TABLE 35-1 Possible Clinically Significant Alterations of Laboratory Parameters Used for Older Adults

Parameter	Usual Significance in Adults	Possible Alternative Significance in Older Adults
Blood urea nitrogen	Renal insufficiency	Acute catabolism (often reversible)
Albumin	Renal or hepatic insufficiency	Biologic age, malnutrition, frailty
Cholesterol	Risk of atherosclerosis (high cholesterol)	Malnutrition, marker of fatal prognosis (low cholesterol)
γ-Glutamyl transpeptidase	Alcoholism, cholestasis, hepatitis	Liver congestion (due to heart insufficiency)
Amylase	Pancreatitis	Parotitis (often during summer season); macroamylase
Lactate dehydrogenase	Parenchymal damages, hemolysis	Phlebotomy problem
Total protein	Chronic inflammation	Exsiccation, myeloma
C-reactive protein	Inflammation, acute phase	Infection, necrosis (sometimes unique conclusive marker)
Erythrocyte sedimentation rate	Chronic inflammation	Occult neoplasm
Partial thromboplastin time	Heparin, hemophilia	Lupus inhibitor
Hemoglobin	Bleeding	Anemia of older adults, myelodysplastic syndrome
Mean corpuscular volume	Alcohol abuse	Deficiency of vitamin B_{12} or folic acid

Adapted from Campion EW, deLabry LO, Glynn RJ: The effect of age on serum albumin in healthy males: report from the normative aging study. J Gerontol 433:M18–M20, 1988; Goichot B, Schlienger JL, Grunenberger F, et al: Low cholesterol concentrations in free-living elderly subjects: relations with dietary intake and nutritional status. Am J Clin Nutr 1995;62:547–553, 1995; and Rudman D, Mattson DE, Nagraj HS, et al: Prognostic significance of serum cholesterol in nursing home men. JPEN J Parenter Enteral Nutr 12:155–158, 1998.

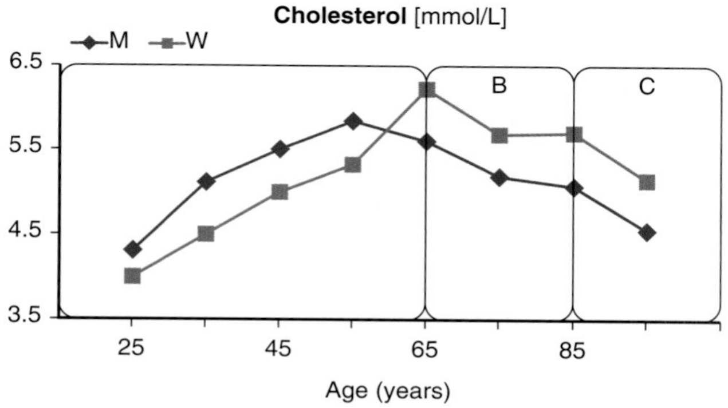

Figure 35-4. Age-dependent course of cholesterol. *(From Lapin A, Böhmer F. Laboratory diagnosis and geriatrics: more than just reference intervals for elderly. … Wien Med Wochenschr 155:30–35, 2005.)*

A good example of a change in diagnostic significance during the life course can be seen in the case of cholesterol (Figure 35-4). Usually, the mean level of cholesterol in serum correlates with the cardiovascular risk, which increases with age. However, starting from the sixth decade of life, this increase stops, and cholesterol levels begin to decrease. Such behavior can be explained by the successive demographic change of the cohort. Individuals, who as younger adults maintained a high level of cholesterol, slowly became victims of their own increased risk and now are simply being excluded from the higher age cohort as a result of their increased mortality.[18] At the same time, cholesterol has also became a marker for nutritional status because its decrease correlates with malnutrition.[19] Finally, at the end of this age-dependent correlation, the sudden decrease of the cholesterol level may indicate a worsening life expectancy prognosis.[20]

Due to symptomatic, supportive, and palliative therapy, which is more important in geriatrics than in adult medicine, the geriatrician is sometimes forced to undergo therapeutic compromises—for example, using corticosteroids in patients with diabetes mellitus. In this situation, to optimize the individual therapeutic strategy, it is not enough to monitor clinical status. It is more important is to estimate the still remaining functional capacity of different organs and systems. For example, it is useful to monitor renal function by measuring the serum creatinine level, but it would be more conclusive to determine creatinine clearance to learn the proportion of renal functional reserve that remains intact. In other words, parameters that enable the estimation of still remaining functional capacity and/or parameters that provide prognostic information are of particular importance in older adults. A good example of such an important parameter is the amount of brain natriuretic peptide (BNP) in the patient's blood because it provides quantitative information about the degree of cardiac insufficiency as it relates to congestive heart failure.

Another important feature of geriatrics is the frequent presence of multimorbidity. In this context, Fairweather and Campbell have demonstrated that in older adults, "failing to make diagnosis when the disease is present or making a diagnosis when a disease is not present is likely to occur twice as often as in younger patients."[21] In the same way, an autopsy study has shown that the accuracy rate of the clinical diagnosis of the immediate cause of death is no higher than roughly 50%.[22]

In this sense, it is meaningful to differentiate between multipathology and multicausality. Because multipathology can be seen as a complex of several impairments of the organism, the term *multicausality* is a more complicated one. It characterizes several dynamic pathologic processes, often convoluted in each other.

Often, pathologic conditions such as infections, cardiovascular diseases, acute abdomen, hyperthyroidism, and depression occur in older adults in an atypical and nonspecific way and with correspondingly atypical symptoms, physical findings, and laboratory results.[23] However, the adequate estimation of multiple causative factors that are contributing to the current status of the patient can be more difficult. Frequently, due to the propensity to think in terms of a single disease, it can be difficult for the clinician to decide which of the actual factors are important and will benefit the patient if treated. At the same time, the underestimation of multicausality, together with the progressive decline of the cognitive and physical status of the patient, can aggravate the problem of degradation of the diagnostic information.[21] However, especially in view of the prognosis of the patient, there can be a discrepancy between the necessity of a diagnostic and therapeutic intervention on one side and the need for caring for a patient with appropriated dignity on the other side. In this case, even laboratory medicine faces ethical limits.

CONCLUSION

With the growing proportion of older adults in industrialized countries, the role of geriatric medicine will grow accordingly. The trend will, in turn, create corresponding requirements for better efficiency in laboratory diagnoses. It is imperative to distinguish between geriatric medicine, which deals with the wide variety of individuals rather than samples, collectives, or groups of people, common in classic medicine.

It is to be expected that soon geriatric laboratory medicine will be subjected to a radical change of paradigms. Not only the statistically revealed evidence, as obtained from studies of a large number of individuals, but also consideration of the individual patient, with his or her clinical individuality, status, predispositions, physiologic reserves, and prognosis, will need a thorough, in-depth review.

It will not be sufficient to consider health solely from the deterministic point of view, observing differences between physiology and pathology of the laboratory findings. Similarly, it will be important to consider clinical individuality as a relative risk in the dimension of time for the rest of the patient's life.[24]

From the practical point of view, it would be necessary to pay more attention to limits of the diagnostic significance of laboratory testing of older adults. This should be considered especially for education programs for specialists in geriatric medicine. Research in geriatrics should concentrate on new diagnostic parameters that would enable a better estimation of the clinical risk to the patients.

KEY POINTS

- **Normality in geriatrics.** The perfectly healthy individual is a biologic rarity rather than the normal case. In geriatrics, it is a problem to postulate generally applicable references.*
- **Multimorbidity.** When approaching the end of life, the sum of after effects of previous diseases and the probability of manifestation of predisposed diseases increase. The individuality of a person increases by his or her life itinerary.
- To keep the best possible quality of life requires monitoring of individual clinical status, rather than screening for potentially occurring diseases, with the aim of a complete cure.
- Laboratory parameters that provide information about the still available physiologic reserves are especially valuable. Clinical interpretation of some laboratory tests may be modified by life expectancy of the patient.
- Laboratory medicine in geriatrics should be performed with long-time quality assessment, professional logistics, and with special consideration of the preanalytics.

*Other terms used more or less correctly for the same purpose are the reference range and normal values.

For a complete list of references, please visit www.expertconsult.com.

KEY REFERENCES

2. Solberg HE: International Federation of Clinical Chemistry (IFCC), Scientific Committee, Clinical Section, Expert Panel on Theory of Reference Values, International Committee for Standardization in Haematology (ICSH), Standing Committee on Reference Values: Approved recommendation on the theory of reference values. Part 1. The concept of reference values. J Clin Chem Clin Biochem 25:337–342, 1987.
3. Rowe JW, Andres R, Tobin JD, et al: The effect of age on creatinine clearance in men: a cross-sectional and longitudinal study. J Gerontol 31:155–163, 1976.
7. Martin H, Huth M, Kratzsch J, et al: Age dependence of laboratory parameters in a health study—attempt at calculating a laboratory index for assessing biological aging. Z Gerontol Geriatr 35:2–12, 2002.
9. Harris EK: Effects of intra- and interindividual variation on the appropriate use of normal ranges. Clin Chem 20:1535–1542, 1974.
11. Kallner A, Gustavsson E, Hendig E: Can age- and sex-related reference intervals be derived for non-healthy and non-diseased individuals from results of measurements in primary health care? Clin Chem Lab Med 38:633–654, 2000.
15. Young DS: Conveying the importance of the preanalytical phase. Clin Chem Lab Med 41(7):884–887, 2003.
18. Bush TL, Linkenns R, Maggi S, et al: Blood pressure changes with aging: evidence for a cohort effect. Aging (Milano) 1:39–45, 1989.
20. Brescianini S, Maggi S, Frachi G, et al: Low total cholesterol and increased risk of dying: are low levels clinical warning signs in the elderly? Results from the Italian longitudinal study on ageing. J Am Geriatr Soc 51:991–996, 2003.
21. Fairweather DS, Campbell AJ: Diagnostic accuracy. The effects of multiple aetiology and the degradation of information in old age. J R Coll Physicians Lond 25:105–110, 1991.
22. Attems J, Arbes S, Böhm G, et al: The clinical diagnostic accuracy rate regarding the immediate cause of death in a hospitalized geriatric population; an autopsy study of 1594 patients. Wien Med Wochenschr 154:159–162, 2004.
23. Kim R, Emmett MD: Nonspecific and atypical presentation of disease in the older patient. Geriatrics 53:50–60, 1998.

36 Social Assessment of Older Patients

Sadhna Diwan, Megan Rose Perdue

Social assessment is an integral part of a comprehensive multidimensional assessment of older adult patients. Many studies on the effectiveness of comprehensive geriatric assessment include a social worker on the assessment team, whose mandate typically includes identifying and addressing social and community living needs.[1] Social assessment is a broad construct, encompassing many aspects of an older individual's life. It includes assessment of functional ability, as measured by the ability to perform the basic activities of daily living (ADLs) and instrumental activities of daily living (IADLs), social functioning (the older adult's social network and support system), the need for supportive services, screening for cognitive function, and an assessment of psychological well-being (e.g. mood, quality of life, life satisfaction). Regardless of whether an older person lives in the community or in an institution, supportive activities provided by social networks are key to ensuring adequate care and maintaining well-being. Social functioning encompasses many aspects of a person's relationships and activities, and a social assessment provides a snapshot of the resources and risks related to health and wellness experienced by an older patient.

The objectives of this chapter are as follows: (1) provide an overview of the relevance of social assessment in comprehensive geriatric assessments and to care provided by physicians; (2) describe various aspects of social functioning, their relationship to health and wellness, and key screening tools relevant for social assessment; (3) describe the impact of chronic illnesses and dementia on social functioning as related to the concept of caregiver burden; (4) discuss cultural considerations in social assessment.

RELEVANCE OF SOCIAL ASSESSMENT IN COMPREHENSIVE GERIATRIC ASSESSMENT

A great deal of attention has been given by researchers to social issues and their impact on health and wellness of older adults. Recalling that frail older adults are at increased risk compared with others their own age, there is discussion about how to conceptualize where the risk comes from. A common formulation, typified in this book, is to distinguish between intrinsic risk and extrinsic risk. Intrinsic risk is reflected in ill health and factors of known, uncertain, or variable modifiability (e.g., exercise, epigenetics, genome, microbiome, smoking) and extrinsic risk. In this conceptualization, social vulnerability becomes an extrinsic risk. Clearly, protective and mitigating factors are also present, and these too can be seen as largely intrinsic or extrinsic.

Extrinsic social factors have been studied in different ways. One line of work on social issues, which is covered in Chapter 30 of this text, looks at social vulnerability, focuses on concepts such as social determinants of health,[2] and typically refers to the impact of macrosocial issues such as poverty, education, neighborhood conditions, and the built environment[3] on the health status of individuals. Another line of research, which this chapter will address, focuses on the health impact of microsocial issues or social functioning and examines the role of formal and informal social networks, social support, social isolation, loneliness, and caregiver burden on individual health and functioning.

Impact of Social Functioning on Health and Well-Being

A large body of research exists on the impact of social functioning on the health and well-being of older adults. Research on older adults in several countries (Denmark, Holland, Japan, Britain, and the United States) has found that social isolation and loneliness are associated with increased mortality.[4] Multiple studies have found greater level of social support to be related to better self-management of diabetes and dietary and exercise behaviors.[5] Furthermore, social relationships such as marital status and friendship networks influence the practice of healthy behaviors such as smoking, alcohol use, physical activity, and dental visits, where dissolution of marriage or weaker social networks are associated with lower levels of healthy behaviors.[6] In a meta-analysis of available studies, Barth and colleagues[7] noted that good evidence exists for the positive relationship between lower perceived social support and a poorer prognosis for coronary heart disease (CHD). They suggested that an important step in increasing the survival of patients after a cardiac event might be a more thorough monitoring of patients with low social support to improve compliance with medication and adherence to healthy behaviors.

Finally, most older patients receive some level of care and support from family and friends, and for many this constitutes their sole source of support.[8] Many caregivers of older persons are themselves older (typically a spouse or adult child). Caregiving for older persons with limitations in ADLs, chronic illnesses, or dementia is physically and emotionally challenging and has been documented to have serious adverse physical and mental health consequences, such as declining health and increased mortality among older caregivers.[8] The experience of caregiver burden can result in impaired ability to provide adequate care to the older patient and may lead to medication errors, elder mistreatment or neglect, and family conflict.[8,9] Caregiver strain or burden is also associated with increased likelihood of institutionalization for the older patient.[10] Therefore, including an assessment of an older adult's ADL and IADL functioning, social functioning, including met and unmet need for services, and status of the caregiver(s) are critical components of a social assessment.

FUNCTIONAL ABILITY TO PERFORM ACTIVITIES OF DAILY LIVING

Since the development of the landmark Katz Index of Activities of Daily Living in 1963,[11] many scales have been developed to assess a person's ability to perform the tasks involved in basic and instrumental activities of daily living. Activities categorized as basic ADLs include personal care (e.g., dressing, bathing, eating, grooming, toileting, getting in and out of bed or a chair, urinary and bowel continence) and mobility, which includes walking and climbing stairs. IADLs, on the other hand, include activities necessary for living in a community setting (e.g., cooking, cleaning, shopping, money management, use of transportation, telephone, medication administration). The measurement of the ability to perform these activities varies in terms of observation by professionals or self-reports by the older adult. The performance of these activities is usually assessed in terms of being independent, needing assistance (help from another person or mechanical device), or completely dependent on help from another person to perform the various activities. Increasing levels of difficulty in performing ADLs and IADLs are associated with an older adult's progression along the continuum of care from independent to assisted living to nursing home care. See Chapter 36 for more details.

Limitations in the performance of ADL and IADL tasks are a prerequisite for eligibility for services in all publicly funded home and community-based services programs. Many factors influence the performance of ADL and IADL tasks. These include an individual's physical condition (frailty), emotional status (depression, anxiety, fear of falling), social issues (availability of social support), and external environment (type of dwelling, neighborhood conditions, climate), all of which can impede task performance and call for changes in a person's living conditions.[12] A thorough social work assessment of functional ability as well as other factors influencing the performance of ADL and IADL tasks can be instrumental in developing a care plan that includes adequate service provision for the older adult and their caregiver, if applicable.

ASPECTS OF SOCIAL FUNCTIONING AND ASSESSMENT TOOLS

Social functioning is a multidimensional term used broadly to describe the social contexts through which individuals live out their lives. It includes concepts such as interpersonal relationships, social adjustment, and spirituality, which have been operationalized in the literature.[13,14] The assessment of social functioning may be complicated by personal biases and values (e.g., ageism, stereotypes, culture) that can influence the practitioner's and older adult's assessment.[15] These issues may also influence a practitioner's perception of how much social support or how large a social network is needed to protect an older adult from social isolation. Similarly, satisfaction with one's level of social support may be influenced by one's life experiences, personal values, group membership, and self-concept. Even so, physicians only need to identify older adults whom they have determined to be at risk for social isolation. In the following section, we present the most relevant aspects of social functioning to consider when providing geriatric care, which include the following concepts: social networks, social support, social roles, and social integration.

Social Networks

A social network is an aspect of social functioning that describes a person's web of social relationships.[16-18] It is an objective concept that quantitatively describes a person's combined social relationships instead of focusing on more subjective considerations, such as a person's feelings about the quality of these relationships. Aspects of a person's social network include the following: size (number of people considered to be part of the network); density (connectedness of the members); boundedness (traditional boundaries that define group members, such as family, neighbors, and church); homogeneity (similarities of members); frequency of contacts (regularity of member transactions); multiplexity (single or multiple transactions between members); duration (how long members have known one another); and reciprocity (the extent to which transactions of the members are reciprocal).[16,17]

A person's social network can be further understood as social relationships that exist along a continuum of proximity, often referred to as primary and secondary social relationships. A primary relationships consists of individuals with whom a person has the most frequent interactions, such as family members, spouses or partners, and good friends, whereas a secondary relationship refers to people with whom a person interacts less frequently, such as the mail carrier, grocery clerk, and members of a faith-based congregation.[17] Within a social network, a person's relationships can also be classified by degree of formality.[18] Informal social networks are those made up of naturally forming social relationships, such as that of a friend, child, and spouse or partner. Semiformal networks are made up of social relationships formed as a result of joining a preexisting social structure, such as a neighborhood, church, club, or senior center. Finally, formal social networks are those social relationships or interactions with professional service staff, such as case managers, social workers, physicians, and nurses found in a formal organization, such as a medical clinic, hospital, or social welfare agency.

Although there are many aspects included in the concept of social network, it is not necessary for a physician to obtain such detailed information about a patient's social relationships during a social assessment. Instead, a physician can condense his or her knowledge of social networks into several questions that can identify patients who are risk for social isolation. One way for physicians to accomplish this is to ask patients about the number and frequency of their social contacts (daily, weekly, monthly), as well as asking them to identify the nature of these contacts (in person, by telephone, by mail).[15] Another more structured way to accomplish this is for the physician to administer a short evidenced-based screening tool, such as the Berkman-Syme Social Network Index,[19] Social Network List,[20] or Lubben Social Network Scale-6 (LSNS-6).[21] The LSNS-6, presented in Box 36-1, has been recommended for use in health care settings to help physicians identify patients who may be at risk for social isolation and in need of a more thorough social assessment by a social worker.[17,21] The LSNS-6 contains six questions that ask patients about the size of their social network and the tangible and emotional support received through their identified networks. Each of the six questions has a possible score of 0 to 5; a score of 0 indicates a lack of social network, and 5 indicates an above adequate social network, with the lowest total score being 0 and the highest score being 30. It is recommended that any

BOX 36-1 Lubben Social Network Scale-6 (LSNS-6)

Use the following response categories for each question below (0 = none; 1 = one; 2 = two; 3 = three or four; 4 = five through eight; 5 = nine or more):

FAMILY: Consider the people to whom you are related (e.g., by birth, marriage, adoption).

1. How many relatives do you see or hear from at least once a month?
2. How many relatives do you feel at ease with that you can talk to about private matters?
3. How many relatives do you feel close to so that you could call on them for help?

FRIENDSHIPS: Consider all your friends, including those who live in your neighborhood.

4. How many of your friends do you see or hear from at least once a month?
5. How many friends do you feel at ease with that you can talk to about private matters?
6. How many friends do you feel close to so that you could call on them for help?

The LSNS-6 total score is an equally weighted sum of these six items. Scores range from 0 to 30.

Modified from Lubben J, Blozik E, Gillmann G, et al: Performance of an abbreviated version of the Lubben social network scale among three European community-dwelling older adult populations. Gerontologist 46:503–513, 2006.

older adult who scores at or below 12 on the LSNS-6 be referred to a social worker for a more in-depth social assessment.[21]

Social Support

Although an understanding of a person's social network may help the geriatric care team identify persons at risk for social isolation, this basic understanding does not allow the care team to understand how well their patients are supported by members within their social networks. For this reason, an assessment of social support is more important than an assessment of a social network because social support is more closely related to an older adult's ability to remain independent in the community.[22-24] In spite of a large social network, without adequate social supports in place an older adult who experiences significant functional decline will be unable to safely remain living outside of an institutional setting.[22-24] In addition, studies have shown that without a robust social support system, older adults are less likely to follow medical advice[17] and are at greater risk for significant negative health outcomes[22] such as increased comorbidities,[25] cognitive decline,[26] depression,[27,28] poorer self-rated health,[29] and mortality.[16] The convoy model of social relations can also help the geriatric care team understand the concept of social support within the context of their patients' lives. According to this model, older adults surround themselves with social supports that move with them throughout their life course and largely contribute to their well-being. This theory maintains that the quality of social support is more important than the quantity. The longer the supports have been in place, the more significance they hold for older adults, and the more likely they will contribute to their satisfaction with social supports and, as a result, their overall well-being.[30]

For the purposes of geriatric assessment, social support is defined as the tangible and intangible assistance derived from an older adults' social network and the older person's satisfaction with that help.[15,17,22,31] Social support may be given in the form of the following: (1) emotional support (love and caring most often provided by a family member, spouse, or close friend); (2) instrumental support (tangible help with ADLs and IADLs); and (3) appraisal or informational support (providing information or advice to help someone make a decision about something that concerns them).[16,17,31] Each of these types of social support is delivered through the informal, semiformal, or formal networks described earlier and is subjective, meaning that an older adult's perception of that help is just as important as the actual help received. In fact, there is evidence that suggests that a person's satisfaction with her or his level of social support is more closely correlated with psychological well-being than the actual help received.[22,31]

Similar to the concept of a social network, a physician does not need to master all the concepts included in the description of social support. Instead, a physician could condense this knowledge to identify patients who may be at risk of adverse health outcomes or premature institutionalization due to inadequate social support. One approach would be to ask patients to identify the types of help they need in ADLs and IADLs, find out who is available to offer the appropriate assistance for these things, and determine who would be able to step in if this person became unavailable.[15] If the patient is independent in all ADLs and IADLs, the most appropriate approach would be to pose these questions hypothetically. Another approach is for physicians to use an evidence-based screening tool to screen for patients who may need additional interventions from the geriatric team. There are many screening tools that may be appropriate for this purpose, such as the Social Support Questionnaire,[32,33] Interpersonal Support Evaluation List,[34] MOS (Medical Outcomes Study) Social Support Survey,[35] and Enhancing Recovery in Coronary Heart Disease Patients (ENRICHD) Social Support Instrument (ESSI).[36] A short instrument developed for use in a medical setting is the ESSI (Box 36-2), which is a seven-item self-report questionnaire. The ESSI was developed to examine the relationship between social support and cardiovascular disease outcomes because lower levels of perceived functional support and network support have been found to be associated with increased mortality and morbidity among patients with cardiovascular disease.[37] The ESSI measures a patient's perception of his or her emotional, instrumental, informational, and appraisal social support systems. Possible scores range from 7 to 35, with a score at or below 18 indicating poor social support.[36,38] Thus, it is recommended that patients with a score at or below 18 on the ESSI be referred to a social worker for additional follow-up.

BOX 36-2 Enriched Social Support Instrument (ESSI)

Use the following response categories for each of the questions below (1 = none of the time; 2 = a little of the time; 3 = some of the time; 4 = most of the time; 5 = all the time).

Please read the following questions and circle the response that most closely describes your current situation.

1. Is there someone available to you whom you can count on to listen to you when you need to talk?
2. Is there someone available to you to give you good advice about a problem?
3. Is there someone available to you who shows you love and affection?
4. Is there someone available to help you with daily chores?
5. Can you count on anyone to provide you with emotional support (talk over problems or help you make a difficult decision)?
6. Do you have as much contact as you would like with someone you feel close to, someone in whom you can trust and confide?
7. Are you currently married or living with a partner?

Modified from Vaglio J, Conard M, et al: Testing the performance of the ENRICHD social support instrument in cardiac patients. Health Qual Life Outcomes, 2:1–5, 2004.

Social Support and Elder Mistreatment

When assessing an older adult's social support system, it is also important to screen for elder mistreatment, because research studies have shown that elder abuse is often perpetrated by members of an older adult's support system. According to researchers for the World Health Organization,[39] older adults may be at risk for elder mistreatment in the form of physical abuse, emotional abuse, and neglect when they are cared for by someone who is stressed by caregiving responsibilities, lives with a caregiver, is socially isolated, and/or has functional impairments. Although different definitions and reporting requirements make it difficult to measure the extent of the problem across national lines, combined studies from five developed countries have revealed that 4% to 6% of older adults in domestic settings and 4% to 7% in institutional settings, such as nursing homes, reported being abused.[39] Based on the risk for and incidence of elder mistreatment across developed counties, it is important for geriatric providers to screen every older adult for possible mistreatment during the social assessment process. One elder mistreatment screening tool recommended for physician use is the Health and Safety Screen (Box 36-3), which is a short six-question survey that can be given to patients prior to their appointment or can be administered by the physician. If the patient answers yes to any of the questions asked, it is recommended that the physician make a social work referral for a more in-depth assessment.[40]

BOX 36-3 Elder Abuse Screening Protocol for Physicians

- Has anyone close to you called you names or put you down recently?
- Are you afraid of anyone in your life?
- Are you able to use the telephone anytime you want to?
- Has anyone forced you to do things you didn't want to do?
- Has anyone taken things or money that belong to you without your OK?
- Has anyone close to you tried to hurt you or harm you recently?

Modified from University of Maine Center on Aging: Elder abuse screening protocol for physicians: lessons learned from the Maine Partners for Elder Protection Pilot Project (2007). http://umcoa.siteturbine.com/uploaded_files/mainecenteronaging.umaine.edu/files/elderabusescreeningmanual.pdf. Accessed October 14, 2015.

Social Role and Social Integration

Within the context of an older adult's social networks and social support systems, it is also useful for the geriatric care team to understand their patients' social roles and assess their level of integration within their social setting based on these roles. Social roles, or the social identities that an older adult holds within her or his social relationships, such as partner, parent, grandparent, friend, church member, and volunteer, are important in shaping older adults' self-concept and indicative of their integration in society. As compared to someone with few social roles, an older adult who holds more social roles may feel a stronger degree of social belonging and connectedness, which is related to positive emotional well-being in later life.[41-43] In addition, a strong sense of social integration has been linked to better health outcomes, not the least of which is decreased mortality.[25] However, as older adults age and their functional abilities decline, they may begin to experience role loss and become at risk for social isolation. Thus, it is important for the geriatric team to ask older adults about their social roles and feelings of social connectedness so as to identify older adults who may be appropriate for a targeted intervention to reduce or limit negative health outcomes associated with social isolation. Zunzunegui and associates[28] have used three simple questions with yes or no responses to assess social integration:

1. Are you a member of any community organizations?
2. Do you attend any religious services at least once a month?
3. Do you visit any community center for social or recreational activities?

In addition to these questions, a physician might also ask the following two basic questions:

1. How do you spend your time every day?
2. How satisfied are you with your daily activities or routine?

Socially isolated individuals will likely have very few activities and roles that occupy their time and may report some dissatisfaction with their daily routine.

Consequences of Social Isolation and Loneliness

By assessing older adults' social functioning through the concepts explained earlier, it is hoped that the geriatric care team will be able to identify and intervene with older adults for whom there is risk for or the existence of social isolation. Decline in physical functioning, chronic conditions, and terminal diseases are some of the most recognized causes of social isolation.[27] In addition, poor health outcomes are not only a cause of social isolation, but they are also a consequence. Social isolation can have devastating effects on an older adult's physical, emotional, and cognitive well-being and has been linked to increased comorbidities, chronic illness, poor self-rated health, substance abuse, depression, suicidal ideation, and suicide completion.[27,44,45] This makes the assessment of risk for social isolation even more relevant for health care facilities that treat frail older adults. By conducting routine social assessments and/or screenings at medical appointments, physicians can help prevent these negative health outcomes by identifying patients at risk and referring them to a social worker for additional intervention.

SOCIAL SUPPORT AND CAREGIVER BURDEN

Informal caregivers, defined as family or friends within an older adult's social support system who provide unpaid assistance with ADLs and IADLs, play an important role in helping older adults avoid hospital readmissions and premature institutionalization.[10] In the United States, 78% of all caregiving services are provided by informal caregivers, making up more than 43.5 million adults who provide consistent unpaid caregiving services to older adults, 14.9 million of whom care for someone with a diagnosis of Alzheimer disease or dementia.[46,47] The economic value of this unpaid care has been calculated to be nearly $450 billion in the United States alone.[48]

Research has shown that informal caregivers provide care to older adults at great cost to their own physical and mental health. Although there is evidence that caregiving does have positive effects on the caregiver, such as feeling fulfilled and satisfied with providing a quality of life to a loved one,[49] an overwhelming amount of research highlights the detrimental effects of caregiving for patients who are dependent in one or more ADLs, have a chronic illness, or have a diagnosis of dementia with behavioral disturbances.[50] Studies have suggested that the unpredictability of caregiving and the prolonged strain on all aspects of the caregiver's life sets up caregivers to have a chronic stress experience.[50] A nonexhaustive list of the many negative health effects of informal caregiving on the caregiver include the following: premature death,[51] increased health risk behaviors,[52] poorer sleep practices and fatigue,[53] higher risk for cardiovascular disease and coronary heart disease,[54] higher rates of depression and anxiety,[55] feelings of loneliness and isolation,[56] and higher emergency room utilization.[57] Caregiver burden and its impact on caregiver health is particularly acute with patients diagnosed with dementia or Alzheimer disease.[58] These health consequences affect both the caregiver and care recipient because the caregiver may not be able to sustain the caregiver role as a result of her or his own failing health.[59,60]

To assess the sustainability of the informal care received by an older adult and to provide interventions and supportive services to the informal caregiver, it is important to assess caregiver burden during a comprehensive geriatric assessment. Reinhard and coworkers[8] have even gone as far as suggesting that informal caregivers be treated as secondary patients during an assessment so as to identify and meet caregiver needs, which can directly affect the primary patient's health and social situation. An important consideration when assessing the caregiver is the relationship of the caregiver to the care recipient and any additional care responsibilities that the caregiver may have for other members of the family, such as older patients' children who find themselves in the sandwich generation or caregivers who continue to work outside the home while still providing primary care for an older family member.[15] Beyond these initial considerations, many tools have been developed to assess three areas of the caregiving experiencing, including caregiver burden, caregiver needs, and quality of life for the caregiver. A meta-analysis[61] of these assessment domains has found that tools designed to measure caregiver burden and quality of life may be most appropriate for clinicians trying to understand the overall mental and physical health of a caregiver, whereas a needs assessment may be more appropriate when trying to understand the effects of an intervention on caregiver health. For the purposes of comprehensive geriatric assessments and physician screening, evidence-based screening tools that measure caregiver burden are recommended. Given and colleagues'[62] caregiver reaction assessment is an in-depth screening tool that covers caregiver esteem, lack of family support, finances, schedule, and health in a 24-item, five-point Likert scale that can be used for a more comprehensive screening purposes. Another widely used tool, the Zarit Burden Interview, originally a 21-item scale used to assess caregiver burden, is now available in other versions—a short 12-item version and four-item screening version.[63] The screening version, which can be used for most caregivers of community dwelling older adults consists of the following four questions:

1. Do you feel that because of the time you spend with your relative that you don't have enough time for yourself?
2. Do you feel stressed between caring for your relative and trying to meet other responsibilities (work, family)?
3. Do you feel strained when you are around your relative?
4. Do you feel uncertain about what to do about your relative?

The following Likert-type responses are used for each question: never (0), rarely, sometimes, quite frequently, or nearly always. A score of 8 or more may indicate higher caregiver burden and referral for social work assessment.

CULTRAL CONSIDERATIONS IN SOCIAL ASSESSMENT

The growing ethnic and cultural diversity among older populations in developed countries has led to an increased focus on providing culturally competent care that acknowledges the influence of older persons' values, preferences, and cultural background on maintaining health and well-being. Studies have indicated the prevalence of health disparities in health care and health access among people of color,[64] especially among those with limited English proficiency[65] and lower health literacy.[66] Thus, ethnogeriatrics, which is a synthesis of aging, health, and cultural concerns related to health and social services, has become an important area of investigation in research and clinical practice.[67]

Older adults from diverse ethnic backgrounds may have culturally grounded belief systems regarding illness and health that can be in conflict with the biomedical model of health care used in Western countries.[68] For example, older adults with ethnically traditional beliefs may use concepts such as balance or nature or supernatural forces such as spirits to understand their health conditions and consequently focus on traditionally prescribed remedies to address these conditions.[22] Differences also exist in cultural expectations of the involvement of family members in health care decision making.[67] Thus, in addition to asking about the older person's preferences for care, it is useful to examine the values of the client and family regarding expectations of family members in decision making and invite family participation in the assessment, if indicated.[69,70]

Ethnogeriatric assessment in the context of social functioning can include an assessment of an individual's culturally defined health beliefs and the role of the family and other social support systems in the cultural context.[22] Because there are no clinical tools available for assessing care preferences arising from cultural values, several conceptual frameworks have been developed to help elicit patients' health-related beliefs and values that may be influenced by culture. These frameworks include the modified ABCDE model (***a***ttitudes, ***b***eliefs, ***c***ontext, ***d***ecision making, ***e***nvironment),[71] LEARN model (***l***isten, ***e***xplain, ***a***cknowledge, ***r***ecommend, ***n***egotiate),[72] explanatory model,[73] and Culturagram.[74]

Social Work Intervention in Social Assessment

When a social worker receives a referral from a physician or other member of the geriatric care team based on a preliminary social screening, he or she can meet with the patient to complete a more thorough assessment and develop an appropriate care plan, with meaningful interventions. As part of the assessment process, the social worker will spend time with the patient and caregiver to provide emotional support and active listening and learn more about the patient's social resources. Within the assessment process, the social worker may use a combination of evidence-based screening tools and carefully planned out questions to obtain information about an older adults' socioeconomic, disability, insurance, retirement and veteran status, as well as to learn more about her or his social contexts, including access to transportation, adequate housing, and food. Depending on the social welfare system in the state, province, or country in which the older adult resides, answers to these questions will help the social worker to identify and connect the older adult to resources that will help him or her improve social functioning. Social workers will also assess the older adults' past and current coping strategies to determine appropriate interventions, such as individual or group therapy, support groups, or peer counseling, which may help them overcome feelings of loneliness or lack of social connections.

KEY POINTS

- Social functioning is a multidimensional concept referring to the social context of an individual's life and influences the health outcomes experienced by older adults.
- Social assessment of older adults should include an assessment of their social networks, social support systems, social roles, and social integration.
- It is important to obtain objective and subjective evaluations of social functioning.
- Physicians can use short evidence-based screening tools to identify older adults with poor social functioning who may be at risk for social isolation or loneliness.
- When at-risk patients are identified, physicians can refer these patients to social workers for further assessment and intervention.
- Informal caregivers, especially those who care for individuals diagnosed with dementia or Alzheimer disease, can experience many negative health outcomes due to the chronic stress experience that caregiving can create.
- Screening tools that assess the degree of caregiver burden are useful in helping clinicians understand the overall mental and physical health of a caregiver.
- Caregivers identified as at risk should be referred to social workers for further assessment and support.
- Culturally competent care should include an ethnogeriatric assessment of an older adult's social functioning. Aspects of social functioning to consider in such an assessment include an individual's culturally defined health beliefs and the role of the family or other social support systems within the individual's cultural context.

For a complete list of references, please visit www.expertconsult.com.

KEY REFERENCES

4. Hawkley LC, Cacioppo JT: Loneliness matters: a theoretical and empirical review of consequences and mechanisms. Ann Behav Med 40:218–227, 2010.
5. Gallant MP: The influence of social support on chronic illness self-management: a review and directions for research. Health Educ Behav 30:170–195, 2003.

6. Watt RG, Heilmann A, Sabbah W, et al: Social relationships and health related behaviors among older US adults. BMC Public Health 14:1–11, 2014.
7. Barth J, Schneider S, von Känel R: Lack of social support in the etiology and the prognosis of coronary heart disease: a systematic review and meta-analysis. Psychosom Med 72:229–238, 2010.
8. Reinhard SC, Given BG, Petlick NH, et al: Supporting family caregivers in providing care. In Hughes RG, editor: Patient safety and quality: an evidence-based handbook for nurses, Rockville, MD, 2008, Agency for Healthcare Research and Quality, pp 1–64.
13. Kane RL, Kane RA, editors: Assessing older persons: measures, meaning, and practical applications, New York, 2000, Oxford University Press.
17. Lubben J, Girondo M: Centrality of social ties to the health and well-being of older adults. In Berkman B, Harootyan L, editors: Social work and health care in an aging society, New York, 2006, Springer, pp 319–350.
18. Morano C, Morano B: Social assessment. In Gallo JJ, Bogner HR, Fulmer T, et al, editors: Handbook of geriatric assessment, ed 4, Sudbury MA, 2006, Jones and Bartlett.
22. Diwan S, Balaswamy S, Lee S: Social work with older adults in healthcare settings. In Gehlert S, Browne T, editors: Handbook of health social work, ed 2, Hoboken, NJ, 2012, John Wiley.
39. Wolf R, Daichman L, Bennett G: Elder abuse. In Krug EG, Dahlberg LL, Mercy JA, editors: World report on violence and health, Geneva, 2002, World Health Organization.
50. Schulz R, Sherwood PR: Physical and mental health effects of family caregiving. Am J Nurs 108:23–27, 2008.
53. Willette-Murphy M, Todero C, Yeaworth R: Mental health and sleep of older wife caregivers for spouses with Alzheimer's disease and related disorders. Issues Ment Health Nurs 27:837–852, 2006.
58. Sansoni J, Anderson KH, Varona LM, et al: Caregivers of Alzheimer's patients and factors influencing institutionalization of loved ones: some considerations on existing literature. Ann Ig 25:235–246, 2013.
68. Yeo G: How will the U.S. healthcare system meet the challenge of the ethnographic imperative? J Am Geriatr Soc 57:1278–1285, 2009.
69. Andrulis DP, Brach C: Integrating literacy, culture, and language to improve health care quality for diverse populations. Am J Health Behav 31(Suppl 1):S122–S133, 2007.
72. Berlin EA, Fowkes WC: A teaching framework for cross-cultural health care: application in family practice. West J Med 139:934–938, 1983.

37 Surgery and Anesthesia in the Frail Older Patient

Jugdeep Kaur Dhesi, Judith Partridge

INTRODUCTION

In recent years, there has been a growing recognition of the role for geriatric medicine specialists in the care of older surgical patients.[1-4] This has been fueled in part by the increasing numbers of older people undergoing elective and emergency surgery and in part by the increasing medical complexity of older surgical patients. The increase in numbers is due to changing global demographics, resulting in an age-related increase in the prevalence of degenerative and neoplastic pathology, for which surgery is often the best treatment option, and to advances in surgical and anesthetic technique. Furthermore, patient expectations and health care professional attitudes and behaviors have evolved, with impetus provided by legislation against age discrimination. The overall impact is that rates of surgical procedures in older adults are now significantly higher than in any other age group.[5,6]

Although rates of surgery in the older population have increased, they have not kept pace with the observed prevalence of conditions requiring surgery. It appears that surgery may still not be offered to older patients where it would be offered to younger patients, either for symptomatic or curative benefit. For example, the rates of hip arthroplasty decline steadily beyond the age of 70 years, as do resection rates for curable cancer across a range of tumor sites.[1] This is despite the fact that older adults have much to gain from surgery for symptomatic control (as in joint replacement surgery) and improved survival (as in colorectal cancer). The apparently limited access to surgery seen in some older adults may occur for a number of different reasons, but a likely contributor is the complex analysis of risk or harm versus benefit of surgery in older adults. It requires an understanding of not only the surgical and anesthetic issues, but also of life expectancy with and without surgery, alternative treatment options, modifiable risk factors, and management of predictable and unpredictable postoperative complications. Such analysis needs to be presented in a manner appropriate to the patient to facilitate shared decision making.

The complexity of the older surgical population, which makes the assessment of the risk-to-benefit ratio difficult, relates to the association of aging with physiologic decline, multimorbidity, and frailty, all of which are independent predictors of adverse postoperative outcome.[7] With such a profile, it is no surprise that in comparison to the younger population, older patients suffer from higher rates of postoperative morbidity and mortality when undergoing emergency and elective surgery across various surgical subspecialties.[8,9] Furthermore, in older adults, a surgical procedure with associated hospitalization is more likely to result in impaired functional recovery, with a consequent need for rehabilitation, complicated hospital discharge, and increased home care or new institutionalization.[10,11] This complexity in older surgical patients presents challenges throughout the surgical pathway, from the preoperative decision making phase to medical management in the postoperative period.

It is increasingly apparent from recent reports and research that to achieve quality care for the older patient throughout the surgical pathway, collaboration among surgeons, anesthetists, and geriatricians is necessary.[1,2,12] For these reasons, the geriatrician should be equipped with a basic understanding of the issues presented in this chapter.

THE FRAIL OLDER SURGICAL PATIENT

When considering the older surgical patient known to be at risk of an adverse postoperative outcome, the following issues are relevant.

Physiologic Reserve

Surgery results in a stress response and increased metabolic requirements, often compounded by a catabolic state secondary to the malignancy or inflammation that necessitated the surgery. Withstanding this surgical insult requires adequate physiologic or functional reserve (capacity).[13,14] Unsurprisingly, poor cardiorespiratory reserve is an established predictor of postoperative morbidity and mortality.[15] Because aging, even in the absence of pathology, is associated with a decline in the physiologic reserve of all major organs, particularly cardiorespiratory reserve, evaluation and, where possible, optimization of reserve are essential.

The principal purpose of assessing preoperative exercise capacity is to anticipate whether the patient will be able to increase oxygen delivery during the perioperative period. Traditionally, cardiorespiratory reserve has been described by asking patients about their exercise tolerance. An attempt has been made to formalize this assessment by considering metabolic equivalents (METs). The MET is a unit used to estimate the amount of oxygen used by the body during physical activity. One MET is the basal metabolic rate of a 40-year-old, 70-kg man at rest, which equates to 3.5 mL/kg/min. METs can be measured objectively using exercise testing but are more often described subjectively by estimating the ability to perform activities of daily living (ADLs). Poor physiologic reserve is defined as a MET less than 4 (unable to climb one flight of stairs). Limitations of such an approach include the lack of reliability in self-reporting ADLs, lack of additional value (when combined with age and ASA) in predicting outcome, and limited evidence of validity in specialties other than cardiothoracic surgery. Furthermore, METs may lack discriminatory power in older adults with other noncardiorespiratory reasons for the inability to complete ADLs, such as osteoarthritis.[16]

More recently, objective testing of reserve has been used in clinical practice using techniques such as the 6-minute shuttle walk, gait speed, or cardiopulmonary exercise testing (CPET). As with estimation of METS, the shuttle walk and gait speed can equally be affected by noncardiorespiratory pathology or general deconditioning. In contrast, CPET provides information on cardiorespiratory fitness. It allows measurement of oxygen uptake and carbon dioxide production while the patient exercises (using feet or hands) on a cycle ergometer attached to 12-lead electrocardiography. Various parameters can be measured, but the most frequently described is the anaerobic threshold (AT), the threshold at which aerobic metabolism switches to anaerobic. Evidence suggests that measurement of the AT can help triage patients as high or intermediate perioperative risk. Studies have used this description of risk to allocate postoperative level 2 and 3 care beds with the aim of reducing postoperative morbidity and mortality.[17] Concerns regarding the use CPET include the inability of older adults to complete the test due to noncardiorespiratory issues (e.g., fatigue, motivation, joint disease), need for skilled interpretation of data, extrapolation of evidence from colorectal and vascular surgery to other surgical populations, and potential exclusion of older adults from surgical intervention on the basis of a CPET test result.[18]

Multimorbidity

The presence of coexisting disease—in particular anemia, diabetes, and cardiac, respiratory, and renal disease—increases the risk of adverse postoperative outcome. Although each individual condition increases this risk, a combination of more than three coexisting conditions (multimorbidity) is highly predictive of postoperative complications, poor functional outcome, and mortality.[19] Because increasing age is associated with multimorbidity, with more than 40% of community-dwelling people older than 70 years living with multimorbidity,[7] older adults presenting for surgery are a vulnerable population. Various scores are available to describe and measure comorbidities (e.g., the Charlson Comorbidity Index). These are useful for comparison between patient groups and stratification of risk and thus for coding and research, but their clinical utility in the surgical population is limited.

Furthermore, the severity of the coexisting condition and its related complications is more important in affecting outcome than merely its presence. For example, poorly controlled diabetes associated with untreated diastolic heart failure is of more significance than well-controlled diabetes and mild optimized chronic obstructive pulmonary disease (COPD), despite the fact that the comorbidity count would be the same. Recognition of the impact of comorbidity on postoperative outcome has led to the publication of resources to guide perioperative assessment and optimization of specific comorbidities. These resources include guidelines covering cardiac disease (e.g., coronary artery disease, valve disease, cardiac failure), anemia, and diabetes (Table 37-1). Interestingly, although it is intuitive that optimization of such comorbidities should reduce the risk of poor outcome, there are little data to support such hypotheses (e.g., there are no reliable studies to date demonstrating that preoperatively reducing hemoglobin A1c [HbA1c] levels in patients with diabetes results in improved postoperative outcomes).

Frailty

In recent years, there has been a surge of interest in frailty in the medical, surgical, and anesthetic literature. In various surgical populations, frailty has been described as an independent risk factor for postoperative morbidity, mortality, prolonged hospitalization, and institutional discharge. Combining a measure of frailty (based on Fried criteria) with other preoperative risk assessment tools (e.g., American Society of Anesthesiologists [ASA] class, Lee index) increases the predictive power relating to postoperative morbidity, length of stay, and institutionalization.[20,21] Furthermore, frailty is common in older surgical patients, with a quoted prevalence of between 40% and 50% in those undergoing elective surgery.[21-25] This is in comparison to the cited prevalence of frailty in less than 10% of older community-dwelling individuals (aged 65 to 74 years [26]), suggesting the relative vulnerability of the older surgical population. The cause of frailty is incompletely understood, but is thought to be related to the dysregulation of inflammatory pathways, with several inflammatory cytokines independently associated with frailty, including interleukin-6, tumor necrosis factor-α and chemokine ligand-10.[27] Many conditions that are treated surgically (e.g., neoplastic conditions, degenerative or inflammatory arthropathies, arterial pathology) also result in the dysregulation of inflammatory processes. Thus, frail older adults may be more susceptible to developing such diseases or, alternatively, patients with such inflammatory, neoplastic, or vascular-type pathology may be more likely to be frail.

Interpreting the literature examining frailty in surgical patients is hampered by inconsistent definitions of frailty and the use of different tools for measuring frailty. The measurement of frailty will depend on the intention (e.g., screening, case finding, assessment, prognostication), setting (e.g., research, clinical, community, inpatient, outpatient), and clinician (e.g., researcher, allied health care professional, geriatrician). At present, two approaches are generally used—scoring systems based on assessment across multiple domains, which include comorbidity, cognition, function, and psychosocial status (e.g., Edmonton Frail Scale, Canadian Study of Health and Aging [CSHA] Clinical Frailty Scale, Groningen Index) or surrogate single measures, such as grip strength, gait speed, or timed get-up-and-go (TGUG) test. The anesthetic literature tends to focus on the use of surrogate markers. This approach has two potential drawbacks. First the sensitivity and specificity of these surrogate markers in identifying frailty are not yet well established and second, identifying frailty to use it simply as a predictor of outcome may limit the potential to modify the perioperative risk related to frailty. The more detailed multidomain scoring systems may be more useful in this situation to identify individual components of frailty that can be modified using targeted interventions. For example, patients could be assessed using a tool such as the Edmonton Frail Scale to screen for frailty-associated perioperative risk, prompting optimization in the high-risk group using comprehensive geriatric assessment. Such an approach has yet to be evaluated.[28]

TABLE 37-1 Some Resources to Facilitate Assessment and Optimization of Comorbidity

Comorbidity	Resource
Anemia	NATA guidelines—www.nataonline.com[48]
Diabetes	http://www.asgbi.org.uk/en/searchresult/index.cfm/str/diabetes/category/webpage
Cardiac disease	www.escardio.org/GUIDELINES-SURVEYS/ESCGUIDELINES/Pages/perioperative-cardiac-care.aspx http://circ.ahajournals.org/content/130/24/e278[16]
Respiratory disease	http://annals.org/article.aspx?articleid=722320&resultClick=3 http://annals.org/article.aspx?articleid=722395&resultClick=3.[49,50]
Kidney	http://bja.oxfordjournals.org/content/101/3/296.full.pdf+html?sid=b3c9565d-2a77-4441-a101-3562a7d513e6[51]

Cognitive Syndromes

Cognitive syndromes are commonly encountered in older adult patient undergoing surgical procedures. To date, the literature has lacked clarity regarding the causation, overlap, or relationship among postoperative delirium, postoperative cognitive dysfunction, and longer term cognitive impairment. Furthermore, and possibly incorrectly, these terms are sometimes used interchangeably. Postoperative delirium (POD), similar to delirium attributable to a medical cause, is well defined by the DSM-5 (*Diagnostic and Statistical Manual of Mental Disorders*, fifth edition) criteria. It is known to be common, occurring in about one third of patients following hip fracture fixation[29] and open abdominal aortic aneurysm repair.[30] Regardless of the surgical subspecialty, POD is consistently shown to be an independent predictor of postoperative morbidity, mortality at up to 1 year after surgery,[31] and new institutionalization at hospital discharge.[32] Furthermore, it has emotional and psychological sequelae beyond the index period, not only for the patient, but also for caregivers and staff,[33] and can worsen the trajectory of underlying cognitive impairment. Reliable and valid tools for the assessment of delirium risk are still lacking, but a pragmatic interpretation of the robust literature on delirium predictors can be interpreted into preoperative clinical practice.[3]

In contrast, another entity, described as postoperative cognitive dysfunction (POCD), is less clearly defined, although it is often described as neurobehavioral change occurring in the postoperative period. Its natural history has not been clearly delineated, and longer term consequences are not yet described. Interpretation of the literature is hampered by the use of various neurocognitive assessment tools, the use of different cutoff values for what constitutes change, and the differing time points at which cognition is assessed.[34] The main limitation in the published research examining POCD is the lack of systematic identification of POD, which makes it difficult to conclude that POD and POCD are distinct entities. This picture is further confounded by the high prevalence of underlying cognitive impairment or dementia in the older surgical population, which is often unrecognized at preoperative assessment and not fully accounted for in the literature examining POCD.[35-37]

Cognitive impairment or dementia is relevant during the perioperative pathway of care for several reasons—it raises the likelihood that the patient may not have the capacity to consent to surgery, it influences the shared decision making process, and it is associated with adverse in-hospital outcomes, including increased falls, delirium, and longer length of hospital stay. Furthermore, there are specific considerations, such as the patient taking cholinesterase inhibitors as a treatment for dementia, because these agents can potentiate the actions of muscle relaxants used in general anesthesia. Although the preoperative assessment clinic may not be the most appropriate setting for the formal diagnosis of dementia, it remains important to include cognition as part of the holistic assessment, given that there are such clear implications on outcome. Assessment should include screening for undiagnosed cognitive impairment and a description of severity in known dementia using tools and measures such as the Montreal Cognitive Assessment validated across geriatric populations.[12]

SURGICAL AND ANESTHETIC CONSIDERATIONS FOR THE GERIATRICIAN

Timing of Surgery

Surgery can be defined as elective (performed at a time that suits the patient and surgeon), urgent (performed within 24 hours of admission), or emergency (carried out within 2 hours of admission or in conjunction with resuscitation).[2] Within the elective group, the timing will depend on the pathology; for example, surgery for neoplastic pathology is more urgent than joint replacement for degenerative disease. Emergency and urgent surgery remain higher risk than elective surgery in terms of morbidity and mortality. This relates to the physiologic insult of an acute illness, with the associated so-called cytokine storm that it induces. It is therefore preferable, where possible, to perform elective surgery rather than postponing surgery until presentation as an emergency. For example, the outcome for a patient with a known abdominal aortic aneurysm measuring more than 6.5 cm in diameter will be much improved if the surgery is performed electively rather than as an emergency at the time of rupture.

Surgical Techniques

Surgery has evolved dramatically over the past 20 years, now using new techniques such as minimally invasive and robotic surgery. Such approaches can reduce surgical insult, thereby reducing duration of hospital stay and improving outcomes. Examples include the use of endovascular aortic aneurysm repair, which allows early mobilization, functional recovery, and reduced length of stay and, although there is no longer term mortality benefit over open repair, the rapid recovery has clear advantages for a frail older patient.[38] Another example is holmium enucleation of the prostate (HoLEP), which reduces the risk of postoperative hyponatremia in comparison to transurethral resection of the prostate, which may be particularly relevant in a patient with an underlying electrolyte disturbance. However, the geriatrician should be aware of some of the practicalities of such approaches, which may have adverse implications for the frail older patient. For example, minimally invasive or keyhole procedures often require a longer period of general anesthesia (than open surgery) and often require a patient to be head down throughout the operation. This may not be appropriate for certain patients—for example, for those with underlying autonomic dysfunction secondary to diabetes. Overall, however, the significant advantages of newer techniques should not be underestimated.

Anesthetic Techniques

The major advances in anesthesia that are relevant to the frail older adult patient include the evolution of regional anesthetic techniques, technologic advances in intraoperative monitoring, and new modalities for the delivery of analgesia. There is a perception that regional anesthesia may pose less of a physiologic insult than general anesthesia, but the evidence does not suggest a significant difference in postoperative outcome between the two. This may be because primary outcomes studied do not directly relate to anesthesia (e.g., length of hospital stay and 30-day mortality) or because studies are confounded by the frequent concomitant administration of intravenous sedation with regional anesthesia.[39] Advances in monitoring may reduce the incidence and severity of postoperative complications. For example, monitoring of intraarterial blood pressure is now routine to prevent, diagnose, and treat hypotension, thus reducing the risk of vital organ perfusion problems, including cardiac and cerebral ischemia. Bispectral index monitoring (BIS) can be used to guide the depth of anesthesia and sedation, with possible reduction in hypotensive episodes and postoperative cognitive dysfunction,[40] and neuromuscular function monitoring could avoid prolonged neuromuscular blockade. Although goal-directed fluid therapy using technology such as esophageal Doppler monitoring has been widely advocated,[41] the evidence in older adult patients is limited. This may be because aging can affect the compliance of the aorta so that cardiac output may be overestimated and lead the clinician to deliver insufficient fluid resuscitation.

Poorly controlled preoperative pain can increase analgesic requirements postoperatively[42] and, as such, requirements for preoperative analgesia should be actively reviewed and adjusted. Although it is widely acknowledged that inadequate control of postoperative pain results in a poor outcome (e.g., increased risk of delirium, immobility), it is often poorly assessed and treated, particularly in patients with cognitive impairment. This is despite the availability of guidance and protocols outlining the indications for and use of multimodal analgesia (including pharmacologic and nonpharmacologic approaches), which have been demonstrated to improve the patient experience.[43] Although evidence is limited showing that frail older patients can use modalities such as patient-controlled analgesia, expert consensus advocates the use of such modalities, even in those with cognitive impairment. The benefits of early mobilization with neuroaxial blockade are particularly important in frail older patients for reducing the risk of respiratory complications and functional decline.

SURGICAL OUTCOMES

The measurement of outcomes in the surgical and anesthetic literature has traditionally focused on clinician-reported outcomes and process measures. There has been an emphasis on

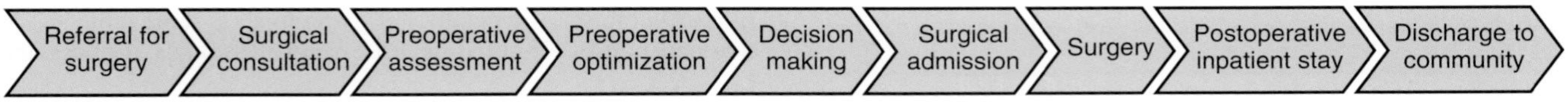
Referral for surgery
Surgical consultation
Preoperative assessment
Preoperative optimization
Decision making
Surgical admission
Surgery
Postoperative inpatient stay
Discharge to community

Figure 37-1. The surgical pathway.

describing postoperative surgical and medical morbidity and 30-day mortality. Surgical morbidity is often described as individual complications (e.g., reoperation rates, wound complications), whereas composite measures of medical morbidity (e.g., cardiovascular, respiratory, and renal complications) are frequently reported using measures such as postoperative morbidity survey (POMS), or major adverse cardiac events (MACE). Thirty-day postoperative mortality is now widely reported and, in most settings, will include adjustment for baseline characteristics of the patient population. Process measures such as length of hospital stay and readmission rates can provide useful measures of quality and efficiency of care, but may be affected by local medical, rehabilitation, and care services, resulting in the potential for misinterpretation.

These clinician-reported outcomes and process measures are important, are relatively easy to measure, and provide a measure of safety, but they have limitations in the evaluation of effectiveness, efficiency, and quality of perioperative care. This is particularly the case for frail older surgical patients; if the baseline descriptors fail to capture their medical and functional complexity accurately, the frequency and severity of observed adverse outcomes may appear exaggerated. There is concern that publication of 30-day mortality may, on the one hand, deter surgery in high-risk patients and surgery for palliation and, on the other hand, may paradoxically influence postoperative decision making. For example, once a patient has had surgery, even with palliative intent, there may be a misplaced or futile emphasis on preserving or extending life at any cost simply because the patient has undergone a surgical procedure.

To deliver patient-centered efficacious care, it is imperative to measure patient-reported outcomes (PROMs) along with clinician-reported outcomes. The tools currently available include generic measures of PROMs, such as the EuroQol Quality of Life Scale (EQ-5D), Short Form-36 (SF36), or more disease-specific measures, such as the Oxford Hip and Knee Score. However, to inform clinical practice, patient-reported outcomes should also include measurement against the goals of surgery. For example, these could include the impact of peripheral arterial bypass surgery on postoperative exercise tolerance at 3 months or the effect of palliative surgery for an obstructing colonic cancer on nausea and vomiting. Furthermore, outcome reporting should include information on the unintentional effect of surgery on functional and cognitive status. Many older patients and their caregivers request such information, but to date there are limited data and, where it does exist, suggests that functional and cognitive recovery to preoperative baseline may take 6 to 12 months.[10,44] Most of the existing evidence regarding postoperative functional recovery comes from the hip fracture population. This may relate to the now long-established involvement of geriatric medicine in the care of hip fracture patients, resulting in more of a focus on traditional geriatric syndromes.

The advent of PROMs has prompted the need for clear communication and documentation of the intended benefit of surgery between the health care team and the patient and caregivers. This can provide an opportunity to discuss alternative treatment options, postoperative management, including the use of life-supporting treatments, and resuscitation status, thus informing advance care directives. The effectiveness of patient engagement can be measured in terms of patient experience, thus helping formulate measures for patient-reported experiences (PREMs).

TABLE 37-2 Components of Preoperative Assessment of Older Surgical Patients

Assessment	Physiologic reserve; morbidity (existing and previously undiagnosed); frailty; cognition; capacity to consent; patient and caregiver expectations of surgery
Optimization	Physiologic reserve; multimorbidity; frailty; psychosocial issues; social setting
Prediction	Organ-specific postoperative risk; risk of functional postoperative decline; perioperative mortality
Management of medications	To do the following: preoperatively rationalize drug regimen pharmacologically optimize comorbidity; plan for necessary preoperative cessation of medications (e.g., anticoagulants); ensure accurate postoperative prescription (e.g., of Parkinson disease medications)
Communication to promote shared decision making regarding	Risk-to-benefit ratio of surgery; decide whether surgery is the best option or whether alternative treatments should be used
Collaboration	Via interspecialty team (surgeons, anesthetists, geriatricians); interdisciplinary team (medical and allied health professionals); integrated work between hospital and community
Planning of postoperative care	Planned use of levels 2 and 3 care; standardized management of predictable postoperative complications; proactive rehabilitation and discharge planning
Improvement	In the following: clinician-reported outcomes; process measures; patient-reported outcome measures; patient-related experience measures; cost

THE OLDER PATIENT AND THE SURGICAL PATHWAY

The surgical pathway (Fig. 37-1) provides many opportunities to improve patient outcomes and experiences for older surgical patients. As in many settings, the key is standardization of processes and pathways while individualizing care for the frail older patient.

Preoperative Considerations

Preoperative Assessment

Traditionally, the preoperative assessment process estimates anesthetic or on-table risk and aims to prevent late cancellation of surgery. However, the scope in frail older patients is much broader. It provides an opportunity to assess risk versus benefit of surgery, identify and optimize modifiable factors, and improve patient experience and outcome (Table 37-2).

The depth and focus of preoperative history, examination, and investigation are dictated by the time that is available and perceived risk of surgery in an individual patient. For example, in a hip fracture patient, the impetus is on improving physiologic status and proceeding with surgery within 24 hours, whereas a longer period may be available for assessment and optimization

TABLE 37-3 Identification of Geriatric Issues in the Preoperative Setting

Domain	Suggested Screening Tool
Cognition	Montreal Cognitive Assessment, Mini-Cog, CLOX
Frailty	Edmonton Frailty Scale
Depression	Patient Health Questionnaire-2, Geriatric Depression Scale, Hospital Anxiety and Depression Scale
Anxiety	Hospital Anxiety and Depression Scale
Alcohol	CAGE questionnaire
Nutrition	Malnutrition universal screening tool, body mass index
Functional status	Activities of daily living, instrumental activities of daily living, Nottingham Extended Activities of Daily Living, timed get-up-and-go, gait velocity, Barthel index
Functional capacity	6-minute walk test
Polypharmacy	STOPP; START—***s****creening* ***t****ool of* ***o****lder adults'* ***p****otentially inappropriate* ***p****rescriptions;* ***s****creening* ***t****ool to* ***a****lert physicians to* ***r****ight (appropriately indicated)* ***t****reatment*

in a patient with a malignancy and an even longer period in a patient awaiting a joint replacement. A minor procedure, even in a relatively frail older patient, may not require a detailed assessment (e.g., a cataract operation), but a complex procedure likely to cause physiologic insult necessitates a full preoperative assessment in all older adult patients, regardless of frailty.

Comprehensive evaluation of the frail older patient is likely to require additional resources and time in the preoperative period, but may be offset by the benefits of identifying high-risk patients, reducing postoperative complications, and improving the patient experience. Ensuring a comprehensive baseline assessment is key and requires a thorough history, examination, and targeted investigations to identify recognized and unrecognized conditions, which may affect the perioperative period. This may be facilitated by using screening tools and comprehensive geriatric assessment (CGA) methodology (Table 37-3).[45] Note should be made of the possible masking of typical symptoms by the underlying condition requiring surgery. For example, a patient awaiting surgery for peripheral arterial disease, with a typical vascular risk profile, may have underlying, undiagnosed, ischemic heart disease but may not complain of symptoms of angina because activity is reduced to a level at which exertional symptoms do not occur. Furthermore, the opportunity to assess and optimize the older adult patient comprehensively should include the shorter term preoperative optimization and also involve longer term management plans, which are made collaboratively with patients and primary care teams to maximize potential benefits on morbidity and mortality.

In terms of investigations, all older adult patients undergoing intermediate or high-risk surgery should have a preoperative complete blood count, renal function tests, and electrocardiography to identify modifiable risk factors (e.g., anemia, electrolyte disturbance, asymptomatic cardiac disease), assess the presence and severity of coexisting disease, and inform perioperative management of medications, including anesthetic agents. The need for further investigations will be informed by the preoperative clinical assessment and by disease-specific guidelines for perioperative assessment and management (see Table 37-1)

Preoperative Optimization

Preoperative assessment should lead to optimization aiming to modify risk factors and improve postoperative outcomes. This is likely to require a multidisciplinary approach involving physiotherapists, occupational therapists, dieticians, social workers, and other allied health care professionals, if necessary.

Optimization of Physiologic Reserve. Physiologic function can be optimized through preoperative exercise interventions (prehabilitation). Although prehabilitation using continuous or interval training improves fitness, even in older patients, the impact on surgical outcomes has been less well described.[46,47] Evidence supports the use of preoperative inspiratory muscle training to reduce postoperative pulmonary complications in cardiac and abdominal surgical patients. As these data on exercise emerge, clinicians will face challenges in translating the likely benefits seen in research studies into clinical practice. Potential barriers to effective translation include practicalities and cost of attending exercise programs for patients, incorporating exercise interventions into the already time-pressured timeline to surgery, and the potential reluctance to participate in an exercise program observed in older patients.

Optimization of Multimorbidity. Preoperative optimization of multimorbidity should be undertaken according to published guidance on organ-specific conditions, regardless of patient age. Examples of such resources are provided in Table 37-1. The role of the geriatric medicine specialist in this process is to use these guidelines to tailor a patient-specific optimization plan. Formulating this plan can require deviation from guidance for clinical reasons, patient choice, or clinical pragmatism. For example, a patient with anemia, Parkinson disease, and ischemic heart disease may need more cautious uptitration of β-blockers and angiotensin-converting-enzyme (ACE) inhibitors, given their risk of postural hypotension. Furthermore, assessment and optimization of the anemia should be undertaken while being aware of the potential impact on ischemic heart disease and the patient's experience of attending multiple appointments. Similarly, the geriatrician will need to rationalize medications and advise on drugs to be omitted or drugs to be continued—for example, weighing the advantages of continuing antiplatelet agents throughout the surgical period to prevent cardiac ischemia against the potential risks of bleeding.

Optimization of Frailty. No single modifier of frailty exists, although literature is evolving. The geriatrician will need to draw on evidence from nonsurgical groups and apply it to the surgical setting. As with exercise interventions targeting physiologic reserve, progressive resistance training is positively linked to improved muscle strength and function, but the impact on modifying frailty or sarcopenia over the longer term is less clear. There is similarly no current evidence for this in surgical populations. Although nutritional compromise is an aspect of the frailty syndrome and should be treated, there is little evidence at present that preoperative nutritional supplementation affects postoperative outcomes, except for the use of carbohydrate loading prior to colorectal surgery to improve gut function.

However, there is emerging evidence for the use of multimodal interventions. In an elective orthopedic population, preoperative comprehensive geriatric assessment and optimization with follow-through on the surgical pathway reduced postoperative medical and geriatric complications and length of stay.[52] Similarly, in an older colorectal surgical population, a trimodal prehabilitation program (nutritional support, anxiety reduction, exercise) resulted in 80% of patients in the intervention group returning to baseline function at 8 weeks compared to 40% in the control arm.[53] A systematic review of the use of CGA methodology in the preoperative setting has concluded that it is likely to have a positive impact on postoperative outcomes in older patients undergoing elective surgery, but further definitive research is required.[45] Although the results of this research is awaited, based on the available evidence at present, clinical services providing preoperative comprehensive geriatric assessment for older surgical patients should be considered.

Optimization of Cognitive Syndromes. The mainstay of preoperative intervention for POD is prevention of the condition rather than treatment once it has developed. There have been one or two studies reporting that the prophylactic use of medications (haloperidol, melatonin) in at-risk medical inpatients and preoperative older surgical patients may reduce delirium incidence, but this has not yet been conclusively established, and the preoperative use of drugs to prevent delirium is not currently part of routine clinical care.[3] In contrast, multicomponent nonpharmacologic interventions are evidence-based methods of delirium prevention and are now widely incorporated into routine practice. These multicomponent interventions have been shown to be effective in preventing postoperative delirium in those with hip fracture who are known to be at high risk for delirium.[54] Interventions target the likely precipitants of postoperative delirium, using support or treatment to mitigate against them. For example, pain and constipation are actively sought and managed, dehydration is prevented through regular provision of oral fluids, day-night reversal is avoided by promotion of exercise during the day and good sleep hygiene at night, and drugs known to precipitate delirium are avoided, if possible. Although the literature regarding multicomponent interventions is robust, the practical translation of this into the clinical setting can be problematic and often requires local adaption of guidelines based on available resources.[3]

Preoperative Decision Making

The decision to operate in a frail older patient is difficult and requires an analysis of the risk related to surgery compared to the intended benefits of surgery, taking into account the individual patient and his or her specific treatment goals. Furthermore, the risk-to-benefit ratio of surgery may be modified by optimizing the patient and so will need to be reviewed at different points in the surgical pathway. Regardless of the complexity, the first step in this process must always be to assess the capability of the patient to make a decision regarding the treatment options for a specific pathology. This needs to be conducted in the context of legislation (e.g., the U.K. Mental Capacity Act). If the patient has the capacity, available algorithms can be followed.[55] If the patient does not have the capacity, surrogates can be involved in a best interest decision making process. This process should be conducted within the legal framework provided by national legislation.

Use of Surgical Risk Stratification Tools

With the advent of routine reporting of surgical outcomes and the recognition that most complications occur in a relatively small proportion of the surgical population, there is an impetus to identify the high-risk surgical patient and quantify perioperative risk. Such an assessment is essential in informing clinical decision making (e.g., whether or not to operate, whether level 2 or 3 care will be required) and facilitating the consent process, as well as providing the denominator for clinical audit and comparison between units.

Risk stratification tools can take the form of risk scores or of risk prediction models. Risk scores use weighting of independent predictors of outcome to provide a score on a scale whereby patients may be compared to others, but this approach does not provide an individualized prediction of perioperative risk. The ASA physical status score is the most widely known of the risk scores and is commonly used, often with the misunderstanding that it provides an individual risk score. Other recognized deficiencies of the ASA include interobserver variability and lack of discriminatory power in older adult patients, for whom the majority are classified as ASA class 2 or 3.

In contrast, risk prediction models can provide estimates of individualized perioperative risk. However, they are less frequently used in the clinical setting, probably due to the complexity of such tools, often requiring more than 15 variables to provide an accurate estimate of risk. The Portsmouth modification of the Physiological and Operative Severity Score for the enUmeration of Mortality and Morbidity (PPOSSUM) is the most validated model, but requires preoperative and intraoperative variables and tends to overestimate risk, particularly in low-risk patients. In comparison to PPOSSUM, the surgical risk scale (SRS) consists only of preoperative variables, but contains the ASA (subject to its own limitations) and requires coding of surgical severity (using the British United Provident Association system). As age, comorbidities, and abnormal blood results (e.g., estimated glomerular filtration rate [eGFR], sodium and hemoglobin levels) are usual inclusions in many of the available risk prediction tools, their utility in the frail older surgical patient is limited due to floor effect—that is, most older patients are deemed to be high risk. Although decisions to operate should not be made on the basis of such tools alone, they can be useful for initiating a discussion within the team and with the patient regarding the risk-to-benefit ratio of surgery.[56]

INTRAOPERATIVE AND POSTOPERATIVE CONSIDERATIONS

Intraoperative Period

The discussion of intraoperative anesthesia in the frail older surgical patient is beyond the scope of this chapter.

Postoperative Period

Organ-Specific Complications

The rate of surgical complications (e.g., anastomotic leak following bowel resection) remains much the same across age cohorts, whereas postoperative medical complications occur more frequently in older surgical patients than in younger.[57] The most commonly affected systems are the cardiac, pulmonary, and renal systems. Medical complications affecting these organs have significant implications in terms of short- and long-term mortality and functional outcome[58] and can be difficult to manage in the context of multimorbidity and frailty.

In older surgical patients, the most frequently encountered cardiac complications are acute coronary syndromes, arrhythmias, and heart failure. Such complications are not only more common in older compared with younger patients but also more significant, as demonstrated by the higher mortality rate associated with perioperative myocardial infarction.[59,60] In frail older patients, the underlying causes and contributing factors for such complications are different from those of younger patients, hemodynamic shifts are less likely to be well tolerated in an older patient with underlying anemia and small-vessel cardiac disease secondary to diabetes, fast atrial fibrillation is more likely to occur in a patient with structural heart disease and underlying thyroid disease, and heart failure is likely to be more difficult to manage in a patient with malnutrition, low serum albumin level, and poor oncotic pressure.

Pulmonary complications (e.g., atelectasis, lower respiratory tract infection, respiratory failure) occur as frequently as cardiac complications and contribute similarly to morbidity, mortality, and length of stay.[61] In fact, in older patients, respiratory complications may be stronger predictors of long-term mortality than cardiac complications.[62] Simple measures to reduce the incidence and severity of such complications include early mobilization, continuation of usual inhaled drugs, and lung expansion physiotherapy techniques.[49,50]

The impact of acute kidney injury on short-term outcomes and the trajectory of chronic kidney disease has now been recognized. Baseline assessment of renal function is critical in informing perioperative drug prescribing and fluid balance management. Postoperative management of acute kidney injury should be undertaken using strict adherence to "bundles of care," with close liaison with renal physicians, when required.

Geriatric Syndromes

Postoperative Cognitive Disorders. Despite preoperative efforts to prevent postoperative delirium, it remains a common postoperative complication and requires prompt diagnosis, standardized management and, where appropriate, follow-up after resolution. Several tools are discussed here to aid in the detection and diagnosis of delirium. These can be used interchangeably between delirium attributed to a medical cause or postoperative delirium. They include the Confusion Assessment Method (CAM), a version validated for use in intensive care unit (ICU) patients (CAM–ICU); the 4AT or more detailed scales are suited to the research setting, such as the delirium rating scale (DRS) and memorial delirium assessment scale (MDAS). Following the accurate identification of delirium, it should be managed according to published guidelines (e.g., from the National Institute for Health and Clinical Excellence [NICE])[63] or the American Geriatrics Society (AGS).[3] Such guidance focuses initially on nonpharmacologic management, including identification and treatment of underlying precipitants (e.g., infection, pain, constipation), ensuring a safe environment for the patient (e.g. appropriate hospital bed to reduce risk of pressure ulcers, minimizing risk of falls) and, where necessary, using de-escalation techniques and one-to-one special nursing support if patients are presenting a danger to themselves or others. The use of medications to treat delirium is reserved for those whose behavior makes it difficult to provide treatment safely—for example, the cautious use of drugs in patients who require intravenous antibiotics but are refusing cannulation or those who cannot lie still for essential imaging. With the expert advice of a geriatrician or old age psychiatrist, patients with protracted postoperative delirium or that thought to be significantly hampering functional recovery may also be treated with medications. Most guidelines recommend the first-line use of dopamine antagonists (e.g., haloperidol), with benzodiazepines reserved for patients with coexistent Parkinson disease or a long QT interval. Medications should be started at the lowest dose possible, using the least invasive route of delivery (i.e., PO rather than IM or IV) and discontinued as early as possible. Furthermore, whenever treatments are administered to noncapacitous patients, a full assessment of best interests should be used and accurately documented. Such management should occur within the relevant legal framework (e.g., U.K. Mental Capacity Act).

Given the emotional and psychological sequelae reported during and after delirium,[33] the perioperative geriatrician and surgical nursing staff should also ensure that patients and family are fully informed about the condition, its precipitants and expected course, and any treatment to be used. In select patients, it may also be necessary to provide follow-up once delirium has resolved. This should be done to ensure that cognition is formally assessed (in case there is underlying dementia) and also to provide support to those who have significant psychological sequelae related to recall of the postoperative delirium.

Functional Decline. Despite the regular requests for information from older adult patients regarding functional recovery following surgery, there is a paucity of evidence for this, with most work having been done in hip fracture surgery. Hospitalization for any reason, including surgery, is known to increase disuse atrophy of muscle and decline in functional status, especially in frail patients. Furthermore, frail older surgical patients are at higher risk of discharge to a facility other than their usual place of residence following surgery.[11,20] However, it remains unclear whether there is a relationship between preoperative functional status and rate of functional decline.[64,65] This lack of clarity may relate to the use of measures such as the Barthel index, which is limited by floor effects in the older surgical population. Regardless of baseline function, it is increasingly apparent that full functional recovery in terms of a return to normal ADLs can take up to 3 to 6 months.[10]

To improve rates of recovery, it is essential that baseline information regarding functional status is used to involve the multidisciplinary team preoperatively, not only to optimize physical and psychosocial aspects but also to ensure a proactive approach to rehabilitation in the postoperative period. Maintaining existing function and maximizing rehabilitation should be undertaken holistically, ensuring that issues known to hamper this process are also addressed. For example, if pain is inadequately managed, patients will be reluctant to participate in therapy; similarly, nutrition should be proactively managed to attain the best functional outcomes. Furthermore, in the postoperative period, the clinician must distinguish between whether there is still rehabilitation potential or whether maximal recovery has been attained. This will directly influence the discharge destination—a rehabilitation program at home or in a rehabilitation facility or appropriate services at home or in a care home to meet functional needs.

MODELS OF CARE

Traditional Model

In many centers, the traditional model of preoperative assessment involves a physician in training or nurse-led medical history and examination, focusing predominantly on anesthetic risk. Although this may be appropriate for younger patients with single-organ pathology, can be relatively inexpensive to run, and can reduce same-day cancellation, it is less well suited to older, multimorbid frail patients. It fails to assess preoperative risk factors comprehensively for full medical, cognitive, and functional recovery (see Table 37-2) and lacks the optimization component, which often relies on referral back to primary care. Furthermore, there is fragmentation of care, with no further involvement of the health professional undertaking the preoperative assessment during the remainder of the surgical pathway. Postoperative care in this model is provided by the surgical team, often with limited knowledge or skills in the specific management of frail older patients and subsequent reliance on various organ specialists for advice regarding the management of postoperative medical complications. Geriatricians are frequently involved in a reactive manner (once the geriatric complications have become established) and often late in the pathway, when functional recovery may be less achievable. In recent years, there has been an emphasis on moving the traditional model of care toward enhanced recovery programs with the aim of improving pre-, intra-, and postoperative delivery of care. These programs have demonstrated improvements in surgical and process-related outcomes, but the evidence is less robust in older patients, possibly due the relatively young age of the study participants.[66]

Anesthetist-Led Model of Care

With the recognition that preoperative risk assessment is key to improving outcomes in high-risk patients, other centers have developed anesthetist-led models of care. In such settings, the anesthetist preoperatively assesses high-risk patients, often defined by the surgical procedure (e.g., major and complex surgery) or by patient-related factors (screening using functional status and morbidity). The focus of such a review is to quantify risk using objective measurement (e.g., using cardiorespiratory exercise testing and risk stratification tools), identify the need for intervention (often referral back to primary care or organ specialist), and inform postoperative management (particularly in the setting of level 2 or 3 care). Often, in these models, preoperative optimization and postoperative management of complications are again deferred to other specialties.

Hospitalist Model of Care

As anesthetist-led models of care have evolved, so have hospitalist models of care, particularly in the United States. Their focus has been on providing medical expertise throughout the surgical pathway. In some centers, these models have incorporated the anesthetist delivering the preoperative risk assessment component and the generalist or hospitalist delivering the postoperative component. In others, the hospitalist has taken on the delivery of preoperative assessment and postoperative management, working as a team with surgeons and anesthetists. Before and after studies have suggested that collaborative working between generalists and surgical teams can reduce length of stay and improve outcome, but are yet to be translated into health care systems other than those in the United States.[67]

Geriatrician-Led Model of Care

Another approach is for the patient to be preoperatively assessed and optimized is by a geriatrician-led multidisciplinary team, with hands-on follow-through from the surgical admission to manage postoperative medical and geriatric complications. This model allows the application of the knowledge and skills of a multidisciplinary team in the following: the assessment and optimization of frail, multimorbid, older surgical patients (in a one-stop service); communication of risks and benefits of intervention (often with patients who may have sensory and cognitive disorders); management of postoperative medical complications in the context of multimorbidity and frailty; and rehabilitation and discharge planning. Comprehensive geriatric assessment methodology is the mainstay of such an approach. A number of before and after studies have demonstrated promising results, with the proactive care of older patients undergoing surgery service (POPS) demonstrating reductions in postoperative medical- and discharge-related complications, with improvements in length of hospital stay.[52,68] However, these services have not yet become widespread, which may relate to the need for a better evidence base, cultural change required to develop cross-specialty work, workforce, and resource issues, and the need for education and training for geriatricians in a new subspecialty of perioperative medicine

EDUCATION AND TRAINING

It is increasingly apparent that frail older surgical patients pose a challenge to medical and allied health care professions. Cross-specialty education and training are required to ensure the development of a workforce that has the knowledge and skills necessary for the optimal management of the older patient throughout the surgical pathway. Recent studies have suggested that current undergraduate and postgraduate surgical, anesthetic, and physician training programs do not provide this.[69] With the increase in the number and complexity of older adults undergoing surgery, all health care professionals should be educated and trained in the provision of basic care for older surgical patients. For example, they all should understand the concept of capacity to consent, have knowledge regarding screening for common geriatric syndromes (e.g., cognitive impairment, frailty) and have skills in communication with the older patient. However, there is a role for specialists in perioperative medicine optimally to manage and advise on the care of the frail, multimorbid older surgical patient.

FUTURE AREAS FOR RESEARCH

In reading this chapter, the reader will appreciate that there are numerous unanswered questions regarding the optimal management of the frail older surgical patient. These questions range from unexplained basic science to the translation of research findings into the clinical setting. Some of these areas of interest will be the same as in the younger population—for example, optimal management of anemia in the perioperative period. However, the translation of evidence may require a different approach (e.g., in a multimorbid older patient scheduled for colorectal cancer surgery who has anemia in the context of chronic kidney disease). Similarly, many areas of interest will overlap with research questions in the general geriatric population but will require answers specific to the surgical population, such as the identification of a valid and feasible tool for screening for frailty in the surgical population as compared to a community-dwelling population. In response to such questions, a number of research collaborations have been established by international geriatric medicine associations, working collaboratively with surgical and anesthetic colleagues. The rapid expansion in the field of perioperative medicine for older adult patients makes it an exciting field for geriatricians in regard to practice and research, with the aim of standardizing and improving outcomes from and access to surgery for the growing aging population.

KEY POINTS

- Increasing numbers of older adults are undergoing elective and emergency surgery.
- Older adult patients are less likely than younger patients to have access to curative and symptomatic surgery.
- With increasing age, there are increased rates of postoperative morbidity, mortality, and functional deterioration, likely related to physiologic changes with age, multimorbidity (including cognitive impairment), and frailty.
- Older surgical patients require specialist preoperative assessment, multidisciplinary optimization, and collaborative decision making which can be delivered using different models of care but should ideally include the involvement of geriatricians.
- All health care professionals involved in the care of older surgical patients should receive education and training in geriatric medicine.
- Research in perioperative medicine for older adult patients should focus on addressing unanswered questions, from basic science to the translation of research findings into the clinical setting.

For a complete list of references, please visit www.expertconsult.com.

KEY REFERENCES

2. Wilkinson K: An age-old problem: a review of the care received by elderly patients undergoing surgery: a report by the National Confidential Enquiry into Patient Outcome and Death, London, 2010, National Confidential Enquiry into Patient Outcome and Death.
4. Chow WB, et al: Optimal preoperative assessment of the geriatric surgical patient: a best practices guideline from the American College of Surgeons National Surgical Quality Improvement Program and the American Geriatrics Society. J Am Coll Surg 215:453–466, 2012.
8. Hamel MB, et al: Surgical outcomes for patients aged 80 and older: morbidity and mortality from major noncardiac surgery. J Am Geriatr Soc 53:424–429, 2005.

10. Lawrence VA, et al: Functional independence after major abdominal surgery in the elderly. J Am Coll Surg 199:762–772, 2004.
11. Makary MA, et al: Frailty as a predictor of surgical outcomes in older patients. J Am Coll Surg 210:901–908, 2010.
16. Fleisher LA, et al; American College of Cardiology; American Heart Association: 2014 ACC/AHA guideline on perioperative cardiovascular evaluation and management of patients undergoing noncardiac surgery: a report of the American College of Cardiology/American Heart Association Task Force on Practice Guidelines. J Am Coll Cardiol 64:e77–e137, 2014.
27. Clegg A, et al: Frailty in elderly people. Lancet 381:752–762, 2013.
34. Nadelson MR, Sanders RD, Avidan MS: Perioperative cognitive trajectory in adults. Br J Anaesth 112:440–451, 2014.
45. Partridge JS, et al: The impact of pre-operative comprehensive geriatric assessment on postoperative outcomes in older patients undergoing scheduled surgery: a systematic review. Anaesthesia 69(Suppl 1):8–16, 2014.
48. Goodnough LT, et al: Detection, evaluation, and management of preoperative anaemia in the elective orthopaedic surgical patient: NATA guidelines. Br J Anaesth 106:13–22, 2011.
49. Smetana GW, et al: Preoperative pulmonary risk stratification for noncardiothoracic surgery: systematic review for the American College of Physicians. Ann Intern Med 144:581–595, 2006.
51. Craig RG, Hunter JM: Recent developments in the perioperative management of adult patients with chronic kidney disease. Br J Anaesth 101:296–310, 2008.
52. Harari D, et al: Proactive care of older adults undergoing surgery ('POPS'): designing, embedding, evaluating and funding a comprehensive geriatric assessment service for older elective surgical patients. Age Ageing 36:190–196, 2007.
54. Marcantonio ER, et al: Reducing delirium after hip fracture: a randomized trial. J Am Geriatr Soc 49:516–522, 2001.

38 Measuring Outcomes of Multidimensional Geriatric Assessment Programs

Paul Stolee

Although frailty in older adults may be associated with an underlying loss of complexity in many physiologic systems,[1] the clinical conditions and geriatric syndromes[2,3] that are commonly present in frail older adults are often highly complex. This clinical complexity, including the presence of multiple interacting medical and social concerns, is the challenge and also the joy of geriatrics.[4,5]

Geriatric services respond to this complexity with comprehensive approaches to assessment, multidisciplinary teams, and multidimensional interventions. Although there may be widespread agreement on the need for comprehensive, multidisciplinary, and multicomponent approaches, there is less agreement on the specific elements of these approaches. It is also not always clear which specific interventions or aspects of care (or combinations thereof) make a difference for an individual patient or for groups of patients—hence, the references to the black box of geriatrics.[6,7] Clinical complexity and comorbidity have often meant that frail older adults are excluded from many clinical trials,[8] although there have been recent efforts to rectify this.[9-11] This exclusion is problematic in terms of the interventions being tested and results of the studies, which are not relevant or generalizable to many frail older adult patients.[12,13] Multicomponent interventions have been found to be more effective than single-component interventions for frail older patients[14] but these types of programs are much more difficult to evaluate in the context of clinical trials.[12] Allore and colleagues[15] have made a distinction between statistical and analytic considerations and clinical considerations in the design of such trials. Statistical or analytic considerations would suggest that one specific intervention should target a single outcome or risk factor, the basis on which power calculations are generally undertaken.[8] Clinically, however, it makes sense for interventions to target more than one outcome or risk factor, and many interventions are likely to have overlapping effects.[15] For studies of interventions for frail older patients, clinical and analytic considerations are particularly at odds.

Given the heterogeneity of the patient population and the heterogeneity of clinical interventions, it is not surprising that evidence for the effectiveness of geriatric interventions has been hard to establish. Rubenstein and Rubenstein[16] have closely observed this literature over the years and have pointed out a number of factors associated with an increased likelihood of demonstrating their effectiveness. These include appropriate targeting, more intensive interventions, control over longer term management, and a usual care control group. To this list, it is suggested here that an additional consideration be added, the selection of meaningful and responsive outcome measures. The selection of appropriate outcome measures for geriatric interventions is not straightforward and has been identified as a priority for research.[17,18] In the early 1990s, a working group of the American Geriatrics Society achieved a consensus on measures appropriate for measuring outcomes of geriatric evaluation and management units.[19] The consensus statement recommended 12 physical outcomes, three psychological and social functioning outcomes, and 17 outcomes related to health care utilization and cost, reflecting concerns about future implementation and funding. The number and variety of these measures reflect the multidimensional nature of geriatric care as well as its potential system impact. Although all these measures may have relevance to specialized geriatric interventions, few, if any, of these measures would be relevant for all patients. The question therefore becomes how to achieve nonarbitrary dimensionality reduction from multidimensional interventions with multidimensional outcomes.

A more recent attempt to achieve a consensus on outcome measurement for older patients was undertaken by a U.S. National Institute on Aging (NIA) expert panel in 2001.[20] This working group was charged to "recommend the content of a core set of well-validated universal patient-centered outcome measures that could be routinely measured and recorded widely in health care delivery"[20] for older persons with multiple chronic conditions. This group recommended an initial composite measure, such as the SF-36[21] or the Patient-Reported Outcomes Measurement Information System 29-item Health Profile (PROMIS-29)[22] be used, with these results forming a basis for targeting additional follow-up measures. This approach has the potential to be more feasible in routine clinical practice, but still may require a fairly large array of outcome measures. The working group was unable to achieve consensus on appropriate follow-up measures in several important assessment domains, including disease burden, cognitive function, and caregiver burden. Also, despite an intention to recommend patient-centered measures, patients were not included in the consensus process nor were measures proposed to elicit patient preferences and values, which would be fundamental to a patient-centered approach.[23]

Some of the challenges associated with measuring outcomes of multidimensional geriatric interventions can be gauged by reviewing the outcome measures used in randomized controlled trials (RCTs) of these interventions. Relevant studies were identified from selected major systematic reviews and meta-analyses, beginning with the seminal meta-analysis of comprehensive geriatric assessment services published by Stuck and associates in 1993.[24] Other reviews included a review of studies specifically focused on outpatient geriatric assessment,[25] two reviews of studies focused on preventive home visits,[26,27] and one review that specifically targeted multicomponent interventions.[15] Collectively, these reviews reported results from 56 RCTs (see Appendix Table 38-1). Outcome measures were categorized into mortality, self-rated health, health care utilization, three assessment domains (physical function, cognitive function, and psychosocial outcomes), and an "other" category. These 56 studies are summarized as follows (see Appendix Table 38-1):

- Physical function was measured in 54 studies, using 77 different measures, of which 23 were statistically significant.
- Cognitive function was measured in 32 studies, using 12 different measures, of which six were statistically significant.
- Psychosocial function was measured in 39 studies, using 43 different measures, of which 13 were statistically significant.
- Self-rated health was measured in 18 studies, using nine different approaches, of which five were statistically significant.
- Health care utilization outcomes were measured in 46 studies, using 27 different measures, of which 26 were statistically significant.

- Other outcomes were measured in 32 studies, using 31 different measures, producing statistically significant results in 14 studies.

This review illustrates several points. Geriatric services were associated with statistically significant benefits in each category of outcome measure in at least some studies, but no category of outcome was significantly improved in all studies. None of the studies reported significant improvement in all the outcomes measured. The review also highlights the range of outcomes considered meaningful and plausible for geriatric services. Mortality is a clear end point and amenable to summation and comparison in meta-analyses, but is not necessarily the most meaningful outcome for programs serving a frail clientele for whom life expectancy is limited.[8] Indicators related to health care utilization are of great relevance to the health care system and, although they may relate to an older person's quality of life (e.g., for some older adults their quality of life may be higher in a community setting than in a long-term care home), these are at best indirect measures of quality of life from a patient's perspective. Within each of the other domains, there is further evidence of heterogeneity; each domain has multiple aspects, and a large variety of instruments and approaches have been used to measure these. Even within the "other" category, an outcome such as falls is itself a multifactorial syndrome.[15]

GERIATRIC ASSESSMENT OUTCOMES AND QUALITY OF LIFE MEASURES

The assessment domains commonly measured in geriatric intervention studies can be seen as major components of quality of life. If outcomes commonly targeted by multidimensional geriatric interventions can be considered, collectively, as a reflection of quality of life as the overarching domain of importance, a sufficiently comprehensive quality of life measure could be a good choice as an outcome measure for common use in geriatric intervention studies. A candidate measure is the SF-36,[21] or one of its variants with subsets of items, which has been very widely used as a health-related measure of quality of life.[28] Unfortunately, testing of its use with older adults has not been extensive,[8] and results of these studies have suggested that the utility of this measure with older patients may be limited.[29-32] A promising measure is the EQ-5D,[33] which quantifies an individual's health-related quality of life into a single index value and provides a descriptive profile. It has proven to be a valid, reliable, and easy to use measure.[34-41] However, it has also been shown to have limitations—predominantly, ceiling effects and poor sensitivity at the top of the scale.[36,37,39,42-44] A revised five-level version (EQ-5D-5L) has shown promise in addressing these limitations.[45-47] A few studies have tested the EQ-5D in populations that include older subjects[40,41,48,49]; further work in this area would be welcome.

Despite some promising work in quality of life measurement, the development of any measure that could achieve wide acceptance has been hindered by the lack of a common conceptual or theoretical understanding of the meaning of quality of life and by lack of agreement on its constituent elements.[50] Spitzer has argued that the development of a gold standard measure is possible, even for a subjective construct such as quality of life: "We fail to have a Gold Standard…because no one has made it his or her primary objective to develop a Gold Standard either for measures of health status or for measures of quality of life…I believe Marilyn Bergner and her co-workers have a sufficiently long head start that they deserve support from all the rest of us."[51] Although Spitzer pointed to the work of Bergner on the Sickness Impact Profile[52] as the best candidate for further development as a gold standard quality of life measure, Bergner turned out not to share this view: "The bitter truth is that there is no gold standard, there is unlikely ever to be one, and it is unlikely to be desirable to have one."[53]

STANDARDIZED ASSESSMENT SYSTEMS

Another approach that aims at providing a comprehensive assessment of health and social functioning is the use of a standardized assessment system, of which the interRAI minimum data set (RAI or MDS) assessment systems are the most prominent. The interRAI instruments are a comprehensive assessment and problem identification system developed by an international consortium of researchers.[54] The original interRAI assessment was developed for long-term care homes (MDS 2.0) in response to U.S. government regulations (Omnibus Budget Reconciliation Act of 1987) aimed at improving nursing home quality.[55] The interRAI home care assessment instrument (RAI-HC or MDS-HC)[56] has been developed for home care settings. Other versions have been developed for use in mental health, acute care, palliative care, and other settings.[57-59] RAI assessment items include personal items, referral information, cognition, communication and hearing, vision, mood, behavior, physical functioning, continence, disease diagnoses, preventive health measures, nutrition status, oral health, skin condition, environmental assessment, and formal and informal service use. Specific scales have been derived from RAI assessment items, including measures of activities of daily living (ADLs), cognitive impairment, depression, and pain.[60-63] Application of the RAI system has been linked with reduced institutionalization and functional decline.[64] The approach to data collection is one of best available information, which may be done by an interview or observation of the older adult via an interview of their caregiver (paid or unpaid) or through chart review. Although this approach may suggest the possibility of inconsistent data collection, it should be noted that there has been growing support for outcome measurement that incorporates a variety of perspectives, including self-report, proxy, and objective measures.[8,65] Briefer screening tools have been developed as part of the RAI system, including the RAI contact assessment.[66] When articulated with the more comprehensive RAI assessments such as the MDS 2.0 and the RAI-HC, the RAI system could thus be seen as an alternative strategy to achieve the aims of the NIA working group mentioned earlier[20] (i.e., a screening tool followed by more in-depth assessment).

An important advantage of the interRAI system is that it allows for consistency in data collection across sites and across types of care settings; the various versions of the RAI instruments use similar questions and data collection approaches. This advantage is particularly strong when contrasted to the alternative practice of trying to achieve consensus on the battery of measures that should be used in clinical practice and outcome evaluation. Even if a particular group achieves consensus on a set of tools (e.g., as noted by Dickinson[67]), another group is likely to agree on a different set (e.g., as noted by Pepersack[68]), and it is unlikely that all members of either group will be consistent in their use of the prescribed measures.

A limitation of the interRAI assessment systems is the same as for other approaches aiming to achieve a comprehensive, multidimensional assessment; not all the assessment areas will point to relevant clinical outcomes for all patients, and it would still be necessary to identify the specific outcomes of interest for a specific intervention or for a specific patient. In the interRAI system, this is addressed to some extent through the use of triggers used to identify issues warranting further investigation, referred to as resident assessment protocols (RAPs)[69] or clinical assessment protocols (CAPs).[70]

INDIVIDUALIZED OUTCOME ASSESSMENT AND PATIENT-CENTERED CARE

The inadequacies of outcome measures have often been suggested as a possible explanation for negative or ambiguous results of intervention trials. This is illustrated in the following comments from several studies:

- "The fact that we observed no significant differences in the prevention of decline in activities of daily living or cognitive function in our study may be explained in several ways … (including) … insensitivity of our outcome measures to improvements that did occur."[71]
- "There might, however, have been positive effects which we could not detect. Our measurements on the health state may not have been sensitive enough to show relevant effects."[72]
- "The outcome variables may have been wrongly chosen to measure the effects of this kind of program."[73]
- "Common measures of disability may be insensitive to change in the outpatient setting of the day hospital."[74]
- "For most of the published programs, efficacy was tested on questionable indicators (e.g., mortality, health services use), on a crude proxy for functional decline (e.g., admission to a nursing home) or using a global unresponsive measure of functional autonomy."[75]
- "It is possible that the measures we used to evaluate health-related quality of life lacked sufficient sensitivity."[76]

A point made clear in Appendix Table 38-1 is the lack of consensus and consistency in the selection of outcome measures for geriatric interventions. The heterogeneous and individualized nature of geriatric programs and their patients makes such a consensus unlikely. Williams[77] has argued strongly for the individualized nature of geriatric care:

> *It is clear, first, that there are immense individual differences among older people, more than at any earlier age, in virtually all types of characteristics—physical, mental, health, socioeconomic. Thus when we consider what quality of life means to an older person and what features of quality of care may contribute to that quality of life, we must arrive at highly individualized conclusions. This principle is of course recommended for all ages, but it may not be so essential in some aspects of earlier life as it is in the lives of older people.*

One attempt to reflect the individualized nature of older adults in outcome measurement is the use of clinical judgment, with such measures as the Clinical Global Impression[78] or Clinician Interview-Based Impression.[79] These approaches allow a clinically experienced rater to reflect individual characteristics and health concerns in an overall assessment of improvement. They provide a role for informed clinical judgment in outcome assessment, but do not provide details on the specific aspects of a patient's health or quality of life that may have been improved as the result of an intervention.

The individualized nature of geriatric care can also be addressed through individualized outcome measures. These could also be used to reflect individual patient preference, goals, and values in a manner consistent with a patient-centered care approach.[80] Individualized outcome measures allow for specific measurement domains to be selected that are most relevant for individual patients. Individualized measures can be used to generate clinical insights into the nature of the effects of geriatric interventions, and particularly into understanding the effects of Alzheimer disease treatment[81]:

> *To the extent that standard measures do not record ways in which important improvements or deteriorations occur, they miss an opportunity to enhance our understanding of what Alzheimer's disease looks like when it gets better, and to provide clinical correlates of supposed pharmacologic changes. In this regard, I believe that the developments of individualized outcome measures may provide some useful insights into patterns of clinically important changes and heterogeneous disease conditions.*[82]

A number of fully or semi-individualized measures have been developed for use in a variety of settings.[83] The most widely known of these is likely Goal Attainment Scaling (GAS), which was proposed by Kiresuk and Sherman in the 1960s as a tool for evaluating human service and mental health programs.[84] GAS is an individualized goal setting and measurement approach that enables users to individualize goals to the needs, concerns, and wishes of a specific patient and to individualize the scale on which attainment of these goals is measured. GAS accommodates multiple individualized goals and also permits calculation of an overall score that enables comparisons among individuals or groups of patients. GAS differs from other individualized measures in two important respects. First, GAS allows for the individualization of the scales on which goals are measured, as well as the goals. Second, GAS requires a judgment to be made at the beginning of treatment on the level of goal attainment that will be considered to be a successful outcome—rather than, for example, subjectively rating achievement of outcome on 10-point scales, as in the Canadian Occupational Performance Measure.[85]

Individual goals are scaled on a five-point rating scale of expected outcomes: −2, much less than expected; −1, somewhat less than expected; 0, expected level (program goal); +1, somewhat better than expected; and +2, much better than expected. The steps to construct a GAS follow-up guide are detailed in Box 38-1. An example follow-up guide is provided in Table 38-1. Goals can be weighted in terms of their relative importance, although equally weighted goals are generally recommended.[86] A summary goal attainment score (T score) allows comparison of outcomes for different patients or for groups of patients. GAS scores for a

BOX 38-1 Developing a Goal Attainment Scaling (GAS) Follow-up Guide

1. Identify the issues that will be the focus of treatment.
   - Focus on problems that are important to the patient and that the intervention is expected to change.
2. Translate the selected problems into goals—aim for at least three.
   - It must be possible to observe or elicit the patient's level of attainment on these goals at the time of follow-up.
3. Choose a brief title for each goal.
4. Select an indicator for each goal.
   - The indicator is the behavior or state that clearly represents the goal and can be used to indicate progress in meeting the goal.
5. Specify the expected level of outcome for the goal.
   - Predict the status of the patient on the selected goal at the end of treatment or at a prespecified follow-up time.
6. Describe the patient's current status in relation to the goal indicator.
   - Typically this is at the "somewhat less" or "much less" level.
   - This is usually designated with a check mark on the guide.
7. Specify the remaining "somewhat better" and "somewhat less" than expected levels of outcome for the goal.
   - These are more or less likely but still realistically attainable outcomes.
8. Specify the remaining "much better" and "much less" than expected levels of outcome.
   - These are achievable, still realistic limits of the indicator.
   - These represent outcomes that might be expected 5% to 10% of the time.
9. Repeat scaling steps for each of the goals.
   - Try not to skip any of the five levels for each goal.
10. Although GAS is an individualized approach, descriptors, items, or scores from standardized measures may be useful in scaling some GAS goals.
11. On follow-up, rate the level for each goal that best reflects the patient's current state. This is usually designated with an asterisk on the guide.
12. Determine the GAS follow-up score (see Table 38-1).

TABLE 38-1 Goal Attainment Scaling Follow-Up Guide

Attainment Level	Score	Mobility	Activities of Daily Living (ADLs)	Future Care Arrangements
Much better than expected	+2	>200 yards with walker, or independent with cane	Independent in ADLs and instrumental ADLs	Home with no need for home support
Somewhat better than expected	+1	Independent with walker (100-200 yards)*	Independent in ADLs and instrumental ADLs, except outside activities	Home with weekly home support
Expected level (program goal)	0	Independent with walker, limited distance (<100 yards)	Independent with ADLs, needs help with meal preparation, housework, and transportation*	Home with home support 2-3 times/wk*
Somewhat less than expected	−1	Walker with assistance✓	Dependent in ADLs, except dressing✓	Discharged to nursing home
Much less than expected	−2	Bedfast	Dependent in ADLs, including dressing	On rehabilitation unit > 7 wk✓
Comment				Patient does not wish nursing home placement

*Asterisks designate the level for each goal that best reflects the patient's current state. The patient's current status is designated with a check mark (✓).

large group of patients are expected to have a mean of 50 and a standard deviation of 10. The GAS score can be calculated using a formula[84] or looked up in a table (e.g., see Zaza and coworkers' study[87]) if goals are unweighted. A standardized menu approach has been proposed as a means to facilitate goal setting.[88]

The first published use of GAS in geriatrics was in 1992.[89] Since then, the measurement properties of GAS in geriatric settings have been tested in a number of studies.[90] GAS has been found to have good interrater reliability (intraclass correlation coefficients of 0.87 to 0.93[89,91,92]) and to correlate with standardized measures such as the Barthel index and with global ratings.[92] Of particular significance for outcome measurement in geriatrics is that GAS has consistently been found to be very responsive to change. This has been demonstrated in before and after studies, including a multisite study and in the context of a randomized controlled trial.[91-96] GAS has been used as an outcome measure in randomized trials of a geriatric assessment team and an antidementia medication.[97-99] In both cases, GAS measured statistically significant benefits of the intervention. The clinical utility of GAS in geriatrics has been assessed using qualitative methods.[100]

GAS is a measure that seems to be a particularly strong fit for the measurement needs and constraints of multidimensional geriatric interventions. It has potential as a research measure and a clinical tool. Although goal priorities may differ among patients, caregivers, and clinicians,[101,102] involving diverse perspectives can generate rich insights into the interventions that will most benefit older patients and into the effects of these interventions.

Reuben and Tinetti have recently recommended that a goal-oriented approach, such as GAS, be used for patient-centered outcome measurement.[80] They argued that such an approach facilitates decision making for patients with multiple conditions and aligns decision making with individual goals rather than universally desired health outcomes. This position can be contrasted with the aim of the NIA working group to achieve a set of universally applied measures.[20]

In addition to the measurement of individual health outcomes, patient-centered care approaches are increasingly concerned with active engagement of patients in their care and with the measurement and understanding of patients' experiences of care.[103-105] Measurement of patient experience can yield insights that are valuable in identifying priorities for quality improvement.[106] Older patients and their families often feel disengaged in their care, and greater understanding and measurement of their experiences may lead to improved quality and outcomes of geriatric services.[107-109]

CONCLUSION

Measuring the outcomes of multidimensional geriatric interventions presents significant challenges. These challenges have resulted in frail older patients often being excluded from studies of interventions from which they might benefit and in potential benefits of geriatric interventions not being detected by the measures used. After 30 years of controlled trials in geriatrics, it seems unlikely or perhaps even inappropriate that consensus will be achieved on a set of standardized measures that will have wide applicability. Application of a universal set of outcome measures may also compromise efforts to achieve patient-centered care approaches that reflect individual patient preferences and needs. For multidimensional geriatric interventions, goal setting and outcome measurement thus need to balance the values of patient-centered care with the benefits of consistent data collection.

For consistency of data collection and to provide comprehensive assessment information, there is a strong rationale to move toward standardized health information systems, such as the interRAI. In measuring outcomes, GAS is an effective, clinically useful, and patient-centered approach to addressing the challenges of outcome measures for heterogeneous, frail older adults.

Acknowledgments

I am grateful to Sarah Meyer and Miranda McDermott for assistance in reviewing background literature for the development of this paper.

KEY POINTS

- Geriatric services respond to the clinical complexity of frail older adults with comprehensive approaches to assessment, multidisciplinary teams, and multidimensional interventions. This complexity presents challenges for evaluation and outcome measurement.
- A review of randomized controlled trials of multidimensional geriatric interventions has revealed a wide range of targeted outcomes and a lack of consensus on appropriate measures.
- Efforts to obtain consensus on appropriate outcome measures for geriatric interventions have resulted in recommendations for a wide range of measures, but have not achieved consensus on some important domains and have arguably not reflected a patient-centered approach.
- Identification or development of a widely accepted quality of life measure has been hindered by the lack of a common conceptual understanding of the meaning of quality of life and its constituent elements.
- Standardized assessment systems, such as those developed by interRAI, have shown promise in allowing consistent collection of comprehensive health information across care settings.
- The individualized nature of geriatric care of a heterogeneous population of older patients suggests a role for individualized and patient-centered measures, such as Goal Attainment Scaling.

For a complete list of references, please visit www.expertconsult.com.

Appendix

APPENDIX TABLE 38-1 Randomized Controlled Trials of Geriatric Interventions and Associated Outcome Measures

			Outcome Measures						
Study	**Setting**	**Study Description (Duration, No. of Subjects)**	*Physical Function*	*Cognitive Function*	*Psychosocial*	*Self-Rated Health*	*Mortality*	*Health Care Utilization*	*Other*
Allen et al, 1986[1]	IGCS (United States)	1 yr, *N* = 185; evaluated whether a geriatric consultation service (GCS) can provide additional input into patient care and strategies that improve compliance to this input	Katz Index of activities of daily living,[2] Older American's Resources and Services (OARS), instrumental activities of daily living (IADLs) scale[3]	Pfeiffer short portable mental status questionnaire[4]	Center for Epidemiologic Studies Depression Scale (CES-D)[5]			Admitting service used, number of days in institution	Veterans Alcoholism Screening Test,[6] time of yr of consultation, number of medical problems/patient, compliance rates of recommendation; direct discussion with house staff led to increased compliance in intervention group (P = .0030)
Alessi et al, 1997[7]	HAS (United States)	3 yr, *N* = 202; measured the process of comprehensive geriatric assessment (CGA) and determined: (1) major findings in CGA; (2) emergence of annual clinical yield of CGA; and (3) factors that affect patient adherence with recommendations	Oral health assessment,[8] vision and hearing test,[9] gait and balance assessment,[10] functional status assessment,[11] hematocrit and glucose testing, urinalysis, fecal occult blood testing	Kahn-Goldfarb mental status questionnaire[12]	Social assessment, Geriatric Depression Scale (GDS)[13]				Percentage of ideal body weight,[14] medication review,[15] environmental assessment, adherence to recommendations; subjects more likely to adhere to recommendations involving referral to a physician than a nonphysician professional, for community service, or for recommendations involving self-care activities (P < .001)
Applegate et al, 1990[16]	GEMU (United States)	1 yr, *N* = 155; evaluated whether care for older patients in a geriatric assessment unit would affect their function, rate of institutionalization, and mortality	Self-reported ability to perform physical activities,[17] performance on timed physical tests,[18] self-reported ADLs showed significant improvement in study group than control in first 6 mo (P < .05)	Folstein Mini-Mental State examination (MMSE)[19]	CES-D[5]	Acute Physiology and Chronic Health Evaluation (APACHE) II score[20]	Control group patients at lower risk of immediate nursing home placement had significantly higher mortality at 6 mo (95% CI, 1.2 to 15.2; P < .05); was no significance in higher risk stratum	After 6 wk, significantly fewer study patients living in an institution (P < .01); no significance at 6 mo; significantly fewer study patients institutionalized at 1 yr (P < .05), risk of nursing home admission 3.3 times higher in control group (95% CI, 2.6 to 3.8; P < .001), study group spent more days in rehabilitation than control group (P < .0001)	

Continued

APPENDIX TABLE 38-1 Randomized Controlled Trials of Geriatric Interventions and Associated Outcome Measures—cont'd

			Outcome Measures						
Study	**Setting**	**Study Description (Duration, No. of Subjects)**	*Physical Function*	*Cognitive Function*	*Psychosocial*	*Self-Rated Health*	*Mortality*	*Health Care Utilization*	*Other*
Beyth et al, 2000[21]	GEMU (United States)	6 mo; *N* = 325; studied the effectiveness of multicomponent management program of warfarin therapy and warfarin-related major bleeding in older patients	Recurrent venous thromboembolism, therapeutic control of anticoagulant therapy measured by patient-time approach[22] and INR[23]; intervention group within therapeutic range at each time period significantly more often than controls (*P* < .001)				No significant difference between groups		Bleeding Severity Index[24] showed significantly more incidence of bleeding in control group at 1, 3, and 6 mo (*P* = .0498)
Boult et al, 2001[25]	OAS (United States)	18 mo, *N* = 568; studied the effectiveness and costs of geriatric evaluation management (GEM) in preventing disability	Bed disability days (BDDs), restricted activity days (RASs),[26] sickness impact profile (SIP): physical functioning dimension[27]; treatment group lost less function after 12 and 18 mo (aOR = .67; 95% CI, 0.47-0.99), had fewer health-related restrictions in ADLs (aOR = .60; 95% CI = .37-.96)		GDS[28]; treatment group less depressed at 12 mo (*P* < .01) and 18 mo (*P* < .01)	Individual questions on general health[29]	No significant difference	Costs, Medicare expenditure, individual questions on use of nursing home and home health services; treatment group used less home health services (aOR = .60; 95% CI, 0.37-0.92)	
Burns et al, 2000[30]	OAS (United States)	2 yr; *N* = 98; aimed at comparing the effectiveness of long-term primary care management by interdisciplinary geriatric team	Katz Index,[2] instrumental ADL (IADL) deficits [31] significantly better in GEM group at 1 yr (*P* = .006),[11] study subjects showed improvement in Rand general well-being inventory[32] (*P* = .001)	Study group showed increase in MMSE[19] at 2 yr (*P* = .025)	Study group showed improvement on perceived global social activity (GSA)[33-35] (*P* = .001), on CES-D[5] (*P* = .003), and on perceived global life satisfaction (GLS) scale[33-35] (*P* < .001) at 2 yr	Study subjects showed improvement on global health perception[33-35] (*P* = *.001*) at 2 yr	No significant difference	Number of days in institution, study subjects had smaller increases in number of clinical visits (*P* = .019) at 2 yr	
Carpenter et al, 1990[36]	HAS (United Kingdom)	3 yr, *N* = 539; tested benefits of regular surveillance on older adults living at home	Winchester Disability Rating Scale[36]				No significant difference	Geriatric and psychogeriatric community support services, primary health care team contacts, use of community support services, control group spent 33% more days in an institution than study group (*P* = .03)	Falls doubled in control group but remained unchanged in study group (*P* < 0.05)

Clarke et al, 1992[37]	HAS (United Kingdom)	3 yr, N = 523; tested the effect of social intervention in terms of mortality and morbidity on older adults living alone	ADLs[38]	Measure of cognitive impairment and simple screening tool for dementia[39]	Wenger scale (measure of support networks),[40] Wenger modification of the Philadelphia Geriatric Morale Scale,[40,41] social contact score[42]	Perceived health status significantly greater in treatment group[†]	No significant difference		
Cohen et al, 2002[43]	GEMU/OAS (United States)	3 yr, N = 1388; assessed the effects of inpatient units and outpatient clinics on survival and functional status	Survival and quality of life with Medical Outcomes Study 36-Item Short-Form General Health Survey (MOS SF-36),[44,45] Katz ADLs,[2,46] physical performance test,[47] positive effects on bodily pain at 12 mo in GEMU treatment group (P = .01)*				No significant difference	Use of health services, costs, GEMU treatment group experienced more days in hospital (P < .001)	
Counsell et al, 2000[48]	GEMU (United States)	3 yr, N = 1531; tested whether multicomponent intervention, called Acute Care for Elders, improved functional outcomes and the process of care in hospitalized older patients	Mobility index,[49] physical performance and mobility examination (PPME),[50] Charlson comorbidity score,[51] IADLs,[31] Katz Index[2] decline at 12 mo favored intervention group (P = .037); fewer intervention patients experienced composite outcome of ADL decline from baseline or nursing home placement at discharge (P = .027), persisted at 1-yr follow-up (P = .022)	Pfeiffer short portable mental status questionnaire[4]	CES-D (short form),[52] physicians more often recognized depression in intervention group than in controls (P = .02), patient satisfaction with hospitalization[53] higher in intervention group (P = .001), along with caregiver satisfaction (P < .05)	Overall health status, APACHE II[20]		Reason for hospitalization, time from admission to initiation of discharge planning, social work consultations, orders for bed rest, physical therapy consults, application of physical restraints, length of stay, costs, intervention; physicians significantly reported no difficulty getting treatment plans carried out (P = .010) and that they were often informed of useful information on discharge plans (P = .015); intervention nurses reported higher satisfaction with extent of care (P = .001) and extent to which issues were discussed (P = .001)	Medications
Epstein et al, 1990[54]	HAS (United States)	1 yr, N = 600; studied effectiveness of consultative geriatric assessment and follow-up for ambulatory patients	Physical examination,[55] new diagnoses, functional impact of patient diagnosis, Katz Index,[2] OARS (IADLs),[56] SIP[57]	MMSE[19] showed significantly better cognitive function at 3 mo than controls (P < .05); those > 80 yr improved more than those who were younger (P < .05)	Social support, social activities,[58] coping style, emotional health adapted from RAND Health Insurance Study,[59] satisfaction[60] showed significant benefits for those in lowest quintile of functional health at 1 yr (P < .05)	Changes in health status, overall perceived health with adapted RAND[61]	No significant difference	Nursing home placement, incidence of hospitalization, costs, length of stay, office visits, use of diagnostic tests	Medications, nutrition, economic issues, environmental issues

Continued

APPENDIX TABLE 38-1 Randomized Controlled Trials of Geriatric Interventions and Associated Outcome Measures—cont'd

			Outcome Measures						
Study	**Setting**	**Study Description (Duration, No. of Subjects)**	*Physical Function*	*Cognitive Function*	*Psychosocial*	*Self-Rated Health*	*Mortality*	*Health Care Utilization*	*Other*
Fabacher et al, 1994[62]	HAS (United States)	1 yr, $N = 254$; examined the effectiveness of preventive home visits in improving health and function in older adults	Physical examination, health behavior inventory, gait and balance assessment,[63] Katz Index,[64] IADLs[31] significantly higher in intervention group at 1 yr ($P < .05$)	MMSE[19]	GDS[28]			Intervention group had significantly increased likelihood of having primary care physician at 1 yr ($P < .05$)	Environmental hazards, falls, immunization rates significantly improved in intervention group at 1 yr ($P < .05$); nonprescription drug use increased significantly for control group at 1 yr ($P < .05$)
Fretwell et al, 1990[65]	IGCS (United States)	6 mo, $N = 436$; assessed whether early interdisciplinary geriatric assessment could prevent mental, physical, and emotional decline without increasing hospital stay or costs	Katz Index[66]	MMSE[67]	Zung Self-Rating Depression Scale (SDS),[68] treatment groups emotional function improved ($P = .045$) at 6 wk		No significant difference	Costs, number of days in institution	
Gayton et al, 1987[69]	IGCS (Canada)	6 mo, $N = 222$; evaluated effects of interdisciplinary geriatric consultation team in an acute care hospital	Barthel Index,[70] level of rehabilitation scale (LORS)[71]	Pfeiffer short portable mental status questionnaire[4]			No significant difference	Health care use, number of days in institution, place of residence at discharge	
Gilchrist et al, 1988[72]	GEMU (United Kingdom)	22 mo, $N = 222$; tested efficacy of an orthopedic geriatric unit in managing older women with proximal femoral fractures	General medical assessment, hip and chest X-ray; more patients in study group found to have new medical disorders than those in control (95% CI, 3.4 to 28.5; $P < .025$)	Mental function[73,74]			No significant difference	Placement of patients, length of hospital stay	
Gunner-Svensson et al, 1984[75]	ICGS (Denmark)	11 yr, $N = 343$; assessed whether social medical intervention would help avoid relocation in nursing homes	Unspecified questions on somatic symptoms, functions, activities	Unspecified questions on mental condition, with emphasis on dementia	Unspecified questions on communication		No significant difference	Housing, medical contact, help in illness, relocations significantly differed in favor of intervention group for women > 80 yr, old ($P < .05$)	Diet, demographic information (age, gender, marital status)
Hall et al, 1992[76]	HAS (Canada)	3 yr, $N = 167$; evaluated a local health program (LTC program of the British Columbia Ministry of Health) to assist frail older adults living at home	ADLs, chronic disease		Memorial University Happiness Scale,[77] UCLA Loneliness Scale,[78] Social Readjustment Rating Scale,[79] social support	MacMillan Health Opinion Survey,[80] health locus of control (HLC)[81]	Significantly higher survival rates for those in treatment group at 3 yr ($P = .054$)	At 2 yr, significantly more of treatment group remained at home ($P = .02$), and at 3 yr ($P = .04$)	Smoking, alcohol consumption, nutrition, number of prescription medications

Hansen et al, 1992[82]	HHAS (Denmark)	1 yr, N = 344; evaluated nurse- and physician-led follow-up model of home visits to older patients after discharge from hospital	General medical data		Unspecified social data		No significant difference	Number of days in institutions, number of readmissions to hospital, intervention patients were admitted to nursing home significantly less than controls (P < .05) at 1-yr follow-up	
Harris et al, 1991[83]	GEMU (Australia)	1 yr, N = 267; aimed at testing differences in medical management and clinical outcome between a designated geriatric assessment unit and two general medical units	ADLs,[84] radiology and pathology tests, discharge diagnosis	MMSE[19]			No significant difference	Accommodation prior to hospitalization, length of admission, accommodations following discharge	Procedures performed, medications on admission and discharge showed that patients in the GAU discharged on fewer drugs (P < .04)
Hebert et al, 2001[85]	HAS (Canada)	1 yr, N = 503; tested efficacy of multidimensional program aimed at functional decline of older adults	Functional Autonomy Measurement System (SMAF),[86] hearing		General well-being schedule,[87,88] Social Provisions Scale[89]		No significant difference	Admissions, use of health services	Medications, risk of falls
Hendrikson et al, 1984[90]	HAS (Denmark)	3 yr, N = 572; measured the effects of preventative community measures for older adults living at home			Social services, intervention group received more home help (P < .05)		Significantly more deaths in control group than intervention group (P < .05)	Contact with GPs, admissions into nursing home, significantly more medical calls registered to control group (P < .05), significant reduction in hospital admissions in intervention group (P < .01)	
Sorensen and Sivertsen, 1988[91]	HAS (Denmark)	3 yr, N = 585; tested effectiveness of sociomedical intervention aimed at relieving unmet medical and social needs of older adults	ADLs and IADLS[92]		Quality of life	Self-rated health	No significant difference	Practical help received, need for more help, number of institutionalizations	
Hogan and Fox, 1990[93]	IGCS (Canada)	1 yr, N = 132; conducted trial of geriatric consultation team in acute care setting	Improved Barthel Index[94] at 1 yr in intervention group (P < .01)	Mental status scale[95]			Intervention group had improved 6-mo survival (P < .02) at 4 mo	Number of days in institution, living arrangements post discharge, referrals to hospital services	

Continued

APPENDIX TABLE 38-1 Randomized Controlled Trials of Geriatric Interventions and Associated Outcome Measures—cont'd

Study	Setting	Study Description (Duration, No. of Subjects)	Outcome Measures						
			Physical Function	*Cognitive Function*	*Psychosocial*	*Self-Rated Health*	*Mortality*	*Health Care Utilization*	*Other*
Hogan et al, 1987[96]	IGCS (Canada)	1 yr, *N* = 113; assessed effectiveness of GCS on outcomes related to hospital stay	Barthel Index[94]	Improvement in metal status score[95] in intervention group (*P* < .01)			Lower short-term death rates in intervention group (*P* < .05)	Costs, number of days in institution, number of referrals to community services at discharge higher in intervention group (*P* < .005), referrals to hospital services, intervention group more likely to receive in-hospital physiotherapy and occupational therapy (*P* < .025, *P* < .005, respectively)	Falls, treatment group received fewer medications at discharge (*P* < .05)
Inouye et al, 1999[97]	GEMU (United States)	2 yr, *N* = 852; evaluated a multicomponent strategy for prevention of delirium in hospitalized older patients	IADLs,[31] Katz Index,[2] Jaeger vision test, Whisper test,[98] APACHE II[20]	Confusion assessment method,[99] MMSE,[19] digit span test,[100] modified Blessed dementia rating scale[101,102] showed significantly less incidence of delirium (*P* = .02), total number of days of delirium (*P* = .02) and total number of episodes (*P* = .03) in intervention group					Adherence to intervention
Jensen et al, 2003[103]	ICGS (Sweden)	45 wk, *N* = 362; assessed effectiveness of a multifactorial program for prevention of falls and injury on older adults with high and low levels of cognition	Hearing and vision, Barthel ADL Index,[70,104] mobility interaction fall chart,[105] DiffTUG (measures ability to walk and carry a glass of water)[106]	MMSE,[19] concentration					Environmental hazards, medications, falls [number of residents sustaining falls, number of falls, and time to occurrence of first fall significantly longer in high MMSE intervention group (*P* < .001)], fall-related injuries using Abbreviated Injury Scale[107] showed increased injuries in low MMSE control group (*P* = .006)

Kennie et al, 1988[108]	IGCS (United Kingdom)	18 mo, $N = 144$; assessed whether collaborative care between orthopedic surgeons and geriatric physicians could reduce various outcome measures in women with femoral fractures	Katz Index,[2] ADLs significantly better in treatment group ($P = .005$)	Pfeiffer short portable mental state questionnaire[4]	Social prognosis[109]			Significantly fewer discharges of patients in treatment group to NHS or private nursing care ($P = .03$), length of stay in hospital shorter in control group[†]	
McEwen et al, 1990[110]	HAS (United Kingdom)	20 mo, $N = 296$; tested effectiveness of nurse-run screening program	ADLs, McMaster health index,[111] functional and problem evaluation interview[112]		Nottingham health profile,[113] Philadelphia Morale Scale,[114] significantly better in test group with respect to attitude in own ageing ($P < .01$) and loneliness ($P < .05$) at 20-mo follow-up, emotional reaction ($P < .05$) and isolation ($P < .01$) perceived to be worse in control group at 20-mo follow-up		No significant difference	Contact with health and social services	Compliance with medication
Melin and Bygren, 1992[115]	HHAS (Sweden)	17 mo, $N = 249$; assessed impact of primary home care intervention program on patient outcomes after discharge from a short-stay hospital	Modified Katz Index,[66] IADLs[116,117] increased at follow-up in study group ($P = .04$), medical disorders declined in study group at 6-mo follow-up ($P < .001$); indoor walking,[118] outdoor walking[118] significantly improved in study group ($P = .03$)	MMSE[19,119]	Social function ratings on activities attended, contacts made during preceding week significantly higher in study group ($P = .01$) at 6-mo follow-up			Number of admissions to short- term care and rehabilitative care hospitals, number of inpatient care days and outpatient care days showed that study group spent more days in home care than controls ($P < .001$) but fewer days in long-term hospital care than controls ($P < .001$)	Number of medications increased in control group at 6 month follow-up ($P = .02$)
Newbury et al, 2001[120]	HAS (Australia)	2 yr, $N = 100$; measured effectiveness of nurse-led health assessment of older adults living independently at home	Hearing and vision, physical condition, Barthel Index,[70] mobility	MMSE[19]	Unspecified social factors, SF-36 Quality of Life Questionnaire[121] and GDS-15[13] showed significant improvement in intervention group at 1 yr ($P = .032$, .05, respectively)	Self-rated health	No significant difference	Housing, admission to institutions	Medication, compliance, vaccinations, alcohol and tobacco use, nutrition, number of problems in each group, number of participants with problems, number of self-reported falls showed significant improvement in intervention group ($P = .033$)

Continued

38

APPENDIX TABLE 38-1 Randomized Controlled Trials of Geriatric Interventions and Associated Outcome Measures—cont'd

			Outcome Measures						
Study	**Setting**	**Study Description (Duration, No. of Subjects)**	*Physical Function*	*Cognitive Function*	*Psychosocial*	*Self-Rated Health*	*Mortality*	*Health Care Utilization*	*Other*
Pathy et al, 1992[122]	HAS (United Kingdom)	3 yr, *N* = 725; evaluation of case- finding and surveillance program of older patients at home	Townsend score[123]		Nottingham Health Profile,[112] Life Satisfaction Index[124]	Self-rated overall health significantly higher in intervention group ($P <$ .05)	Significantly lower in intervention group ($P =$ .05)	Use of services [domiciliary visits less frequent in intervention group ($P < .01$), contact with GP, podiatrist, and attendance allowance], questions about meals on wheels and home help, hospital admissions did not differ but duration of stay shorter in younger intervention group ($P < .01$)	
Powell and Montgomery, 1990[125]	GEMU (Canada)	3 mo, *N* = 203; studied effectiveness of inpatient geriatric unit at a hospital	Functional activity	Cognitive function improved between discharge and home visit in intervention group[†]	Depression, life satisfaction		Fewer patients died in intervention group[†]	Length of stay higher in intervention group but overall admissions lower[†]	
Reuben et al, 1999[126]	OAS (United States)	15 mo, *N* = 363; tested effectiveness of outpatient CGA coupled with an adherence intervention	NIA lower extremity battery,[127] functional status questionnaire,[128] MOS SF-36[129,130] showed change scores for treatment group in physical functioning ($P =$ .021); RAS, and BDD[131] significantly lower in treatment group ($P = .006$); physical performance test[47] showed treatment effect ($P =$ .019)	MMSE,[19] mental health summaries showed significant treatment effect ($P = .006$)	Patient satisfaction questionnaire,[132] Perceived Efficacy in Patient-Physician Interaction scale,[133] treatment group benefited on social functioning scale ($P = .01$), and emotional well-being ($P =$ .016) at 15 mo	Treatment group reported less pain[129] than control group ($P = .043$)	No significant difference		Falls

Rubenstein et al, 1984[134]	GEMU (United States)	2 yr, N = 123; assessed effectiveness of geriatric evaluation unit at improving patient outcomes	IADLs,[31] personal self-maintenance scale[31] showed significant improvement in study patients (P < .01); almost five times as many new diagnoses were made in study group than in controls (P < .001)	Kahn-Goldfarb Mental Status Questionnaire[12]	Philadelphia Geriatric Morale Scale[114] showed significant improvement at 1-yr follow-up for study patients (P < .05)		Mortality significantly higher in control group at 1-yr follow-up (P < .005)	Utilization costs, initial placement at discharge, significantly more study patients discharged to their home than controls (P < .05), more than twice as many controls discharged to nursing home (P < .05), study patients underwent more specialized screening examinations and consultations than controls (P < .001), at 1-yr follow-up, controls averaged more than twice as many nursing home days (P < .05)	Medications
Rubin et al, 1992[135]	HHAS (United States)	1 yr, N = 200; studied effectiveness of GEM program of health care charges and Medicare	Medical history, Katz Index,[66] IADLs	Sensory and communication abilities,[136] MMSE[56]	Social history, affective, and behavioral status[136]			Experimental group significantly more likely to receive home health care than control (P < .01), control group had significantly greater inpatient charges (P < .03) and Medicare reimbursement (P < .005)	Medications
Rubin et al, 1993[137]	OAS (United States)	1 yr, N = 200; assessed effectiveness of outpatient GEM on physical function, mental status, and well-being	Katz Index,[66] IADLs[46] showed greater improvement and less decline in treatment group at 1 yr (P = .038)		Life Satisfaction Index-Z (LSI-Z)[138]	Self-perception of health status (OARS)[56] significantly higher for treatment group (P = .006); perceived less decline in health (P = .007) and less activity limitations (P = .024)	No significant difference	No significant differences between groups on long-term nursing placements	
Shaw et al, 2003[139]	IGCS (United Kingdom)	1 yr, N = 274; determined effectiveness of multifactorial intervention after falls in older patients with cognitive impairments and dementia	General medical examination, mobility assessment,[140] assessment of walking aids, feet, and footwear[141]				No significant difference	Fall-related attendance at accident and emergency department, fall-related hospital admissions	Number of falls, time to first fall, injury rates, medications, environmental hazards[142]

Continued

APPENDIX TABLE 38-1 Randomized Controlled Trials of Geriatric Interventions and Associated Outcome Measures—cont'd

Study	Setting	Study Description (Duration, No. of Subjects)	Outcome Measures						
			Physical Function	*Cognitive Function*	*Psychosocial*	*Self-Rated Health*	*Mortality*	*Health Care Utilization*	*Other*
Silverman et al, 1995[143]	OAS (United States)	1 yr, *N* = 442; studied process and outcomes of outpatient CGAs	ADLs,[3,144] Barthel Index,[94] urinary and bowel incontinence identified significantly more in study group ($P < .0001$)	MMSE,[19] Clinical Dementia Rating (CDR) scale,[145] cognitive impairment identified significantly more in study group ($P < .0001$)	Measures of social support, patient satisfaction with care,[146] clinical depression and anxiety sections of diagnostic interview schedule (DIS)[147,148] showed significantly lessened anxiety in study group at 1 yr ($P = .036$); depression identified significantly more in study group ($P = .0004$)	Self-perceived health status		Nursing home institutionalizations	Changes in participants status, caregiver stress[149] significantly less at 1 yr in study group ($P = .002$)
Strandberg et al, 2001[150]	OAS (Finland)	5 yr, *N* = 400; determined effectiveness of multifactorial prevention program for composite major cardiovascular events in older adults with atherosclerotic disease	General medical examination, cardiovascular tests (blood pressure, heart rate, and 12-lead resting ECG), blood tests, physical function,[151] clinical events	Consortium to Establish a Registry for Alzheimer disease tool (CERAD)[152]	Health-related quality of life using the 15D,[153,154] Zung questionnaire		No significant difference	Health care resource use, hospitalizations, permanent institutionalization	
Stuck et al, 1995[155]	HAS (United States)	3 yr, *N* = 414; evaluated effect of in-home CGA and follow-up of older adults	Geriatric Oral Health Assessment Index,[8] balance and gait,[156] vision and hearing,[9] treatment group required less assistance in basic ADLs[11] ($P = .02$) at 3 yr; IADLs,[11] combined basic and instrumental activities[117,157]	Kahn-Goldfarb mental status questionnaire[12]	GDS,[13] extent of social network and quality of social support[158]			Costs, admissions to acute care hospital, short-term nursing home admissions, significantly more visits to GP among intervention group ($P = .007$), permanent nursing home admission higher among control group ($P = .02$)	Medications, environmental hazards, percentage of ideal body weight[159]

Stuck et al, 2000[160]	OAS (Switzer-land)	3 yr, N = 791; examined effects of preventive home visits with annual multidimensional assessments on functional status and institutionalization between high- and low-risk older persons	Gait and balance performance,[63] ADLs and IADLs[11]; intervention group at low baseline less dependent in IADLs (95% CI, 0.3 to 1.0; P = .04)	MMSE[19]	GDS[13]	Self-perceived general health,[161] self-reported chronic conditions		Costs, permanent nursing home admission higher in high-risk intervention group (P = .02)	Medication use[15]
Teasdale et al, 1983[162]	GEMU (United States)	1 yr, N = 124; assessed whether a geriatric assessment unit using multidisciplinary team approach affected patient placement outcomes					No significant difference	Source of admission, placement at discharge, location 6 mo postadmission, location of patient after discharge, mean length of stay significantly higher in intervention group (P < .001)	
Thomas et al, 1993[163]	IGCS (United States)	1 yr, N = 120; tested effectiveness of inpatient geriatric consultation team	Functional Assessment Inventory (FAI),[164] physical and activities scales, Katz scale[2]		FAI, psychological and social scale[164]		Significantly more patients died in control group at 6 mo (P = .01)	Referrals to community service, number of postdischarge GP visits, discharge destination, number of days in institution, control group had significantly more readmissions (P = .02)	FAI—economic scale[164]
Timonen et al, 2002[165]	OAS (Finland)	9 mo, N = 68; studied effects of multicomponent training program focused on strength training after hospitalization	Strength and physical performance (walking speed and Berg Balance scores) significantly improved after the intervention in the study group at 3 mo (P < 0.05). Isometric hip abduction and walking speed significantly improved after the intervention in the study group at 9 mo (P < 0.05).					Community services use	Medication

Continued

APPENDIX TABLE 38-1 Randomized Controlled Trials of Geriatric Interventions and Associated Outcome Measures—cont'd

			Outcome Measures						
Study	**Setting**	**Study Description (Duration, No. of Subjects)**	*Physical Function*	*Cognitive Function*	*Psychosocial*	*Self-Rated Health*	*Mortality*	*Health Care Utilization*	*Other*
Tinetti et al, 1994[167]	HAS (United States)	1 yr, $N = 301$; evaluated effect of multiple risk factor reduction on incidence of falls	Presence of chronic disease, ADLs,[31] vision[168] and hearing,[169] Sickness Impact Profile (ambulation and mobility subscales),[27] risk factor for balance impairment reduced in intervention group at 1 yr ($P = .003$), impairment in balance and bed to chair transfers reduced ($P = .001$), impairment in toilet transfers reduced ($P = .05$)		Depressive symptoms[170]		No significant difference	Costs, hospitalizations, number of hospital days, intervention group received more home visits ($P < .001$)	Room by room number of hazards for falling, falls efficacy scale[171]; at 1 yr, control group fell significantly more ($P = .04$), intervention group significantly reduced number of medications ($P = .009$)
Toseland et al, 1997[172]	OAS (United States)	2 yr, $N = 160$; investigated effectiveness of an outpatient GEM team by examining changes in health status, health care utilization, and costs	SF-20,[173] (FIM)[174-176]				No significant difference	Outpatient utilization (visitation of UPC/GEM clinic, medicine clinic, surgery clinic, emergency room, and total clinic visits), inpatient utilization (number of hospital admissions, hospital days of care, nursing home admissions and nursing home days of care); GEM patients used significantly fewer emergency room services ($P \leq .05$), GEM patients used significantly more total outpatient clinic services ($P \leq .01$), costs (total inpatient costs, total outpatient costs, nursing home costs, institutional costs, total health care costs); significantly more outpatient cost in GEM patients over 2 yr ($P \leq .05$)	

Tucker et al, 1984[177]	OAS (New Zealand)	5 mo, N = 120; assessed effectiveness of day hospital in geriatric service	Significant increase in Northwick Park ADL index[178] at 6 wk for intervention group (P = .002)	Cognitive function[179]	Zung index,[68] intervention group showed improved mood at 5 mo (P =.011)			Domiciliary services, day hospital costs one third more than alternative	
Tulloch and Moore, 1979[180]	OAS (United Kingdom)	2 yr, N = 295; evaluated effects of geriatric screening and surveillance program on older adults	Screening for medical disorders found significantly greater incidence in study group compared to controls (P < .01); greater proportion of medical problems unrecognized in control group (P < .001)					Rate of hospital admission, outpatient referrals significantly higher in study group (P < .01), time spent in hospital less for the study group than controls (P < .01)	Socioeconomic problems
van Haastregt et al, 2000[181]	HAS (Netherlands)	18 mo, N = 316; assessed whether multifactorial program of home visits reduces falls and mobility impairments in older adults	Physical health, control scale, and mobility range scale of SIP 68,[182,183] number of physical complaints, Frenchay daily activities[184,185]	Mental health section of RAND-36[186,187]	Social functioning,[188] psychosocial functioning	Perceived health by RAND-36,[186,187] perceived gait problems			Falls efficacy scale,[171,189] falls, medications, environmental hazards[190]
van Rossum et al, 1993[191]	HAS (Netherlands)	3 yr, N = 580; tested effectiveness of preventive home visits to older adults	Self-rated functional state, hearing and vision problems	Memory disturbances[179]	Self-rated well-being,[192] loneliness,[193] modified Zung index[68]	Self-rated health	No significant difference	Costs, use of community and institutional care	
Vetter et al, 1984[194]	HAS (United Kingdom)	2 yr, N = 1286; evaluated effectiveness of health visitors on older population of urban (Gwent) and rural (Powys) towns	Townsend score[123]		Mental disability,[195,196] use of social contacts, self-rated quality of life		Significantly more deaths in Powys (P < .01)	Use of medical and social services, Gwent intervention group used podiatrists significantly more than Powys group (P = .02), significantly more home visits for Gwent intervention group (P = .005)	Availability of caregiver, composition of household, type and quality of housing, participants in Gwent attended more lunch clubs than Powys (P < .05)
Vetter et al, 1992[197]	HAS (United Kingdom)	4 yr, N = 674; assessed whether health visitors reduced incidence of fractures in older adults	Townsend score,[123] medical condition, assessment and improvement of general muscle tone						Falls and fractures, nutrition, medications, environmental hazards

Continued

APPENDIX TABLE 38-1 Randomized Controlled Trials of Geriatric Interventions and Associated Outcome Measures—cont'd

			Outcome Measures						
Study	**Setting**	**Study Description (Duration, No. of Subjects)**	*Physical Function*	*Cognitive Function*	*Psychosocial*	*Self-Rated Health*	*Mortality*	*Health Care Utilization*	*Other*
Wagner et al, 1994[198]	HAS (United States)	2 yr, *N* = 1559; tested multicomponent program to prevent disability and falls in older adults	Fitness test, hearing and vision, control group worsened in RAS[199] (*P* < .05), BDD[131] (*P* < .01) and MOS[200,201] (*P* = .05) at 1-yr follow-up			Self-rated health and practices questionnaire			Environmental hazards, alcohol consumption, medications; significantly fewer members of intervention group reported falling than control (difference = 9.3%; CI, 4.1%-14.5%) at 1-yr follow-up
Williams et al, 1987[202]	OAS (United States)	1 yr, *N* = 117; evaluated whether team-oriented assessment can improve traditional health care approaches	Functional status and medical diagnoses[203,204]		Social supports[203,204]			Health care use, degree of client satisfaction with evaluation, health service use behaviors	
Winograd et al, 1991[205]	IGCS (United States)	1 yr, *N* = 197; studied effect of inpatient multidisciplinary geriatric consultation service on health care utilization and functional and mental status	Physical Self-Maintenance Scale, ADLs, IADLs*	MMSE[19]	Philadelphia Geriatric Morale Scale[114]			Health care use	
Yeo et al, 1987[206]	OAS (United States)	18 mo, *N* = 205; compared effects of two models of outpatient care on functional health and subjective well-being	SIP[57] showed significantly less functional decline in intervention patients (*P* = .029) and its physical dimension (*P* = .011)		Zung Self-Rating Depression Scale (SDS),[68,207] Life Satisfaction Index-A (LSI-A)[208] Affect Balance Scale (ABS),[209] psychosocial dimension of SIP[57]	Self-rated health measure[210,211]	No significant difference		

aOR, Adjusted odds ratio; *BDD,* bed disability day; *CI,* confidence interval; *ECG,* electrocardiogram; *FAI,* Functional Assessment Inventory; *GEMU,* Geriatric and Evaluation Management Unit; GP, general practitioner; *HAS,* Home Assessment Service; *HHAS,* Hospital Home Assessment Service; *IGCS,* Inpatient Geriatric Consultation Service; *INR,* international normalized ratio; *MMSE,* Folstein Mini-Mental State Examination; *NHS,* National Health Service; *NIA,* National Institute on Aging; *OAS,* Outpatient Assessment Service; RAS, restricted activity day; *SIP,* Sickness Impact Profile; *UPC/GEM,* usual outpatient primary care/geriatric evaluation and management.

*Variation in significance at other follow-up times.

†No *P* value given.

APPENDIX TABLE 38-2 Summary of Outcome Measures Used in Randomized Controlled Trials of Geriatric Interventions

	Outcome Measures						
	Physical Function	*Cognitive Function*	*Psychosocial*	*Self-Rated Health*	*Mortality*	*Health Care Utilization*	*Other*
Tests Used	Acute Physiology and Chronic Health Evaluation APACHE[†] II[20] **(1)*** Barthel Index[70,94] **(6)** Berg Balance Scale[166] **(1)** Bed disability days and restricted activity days[26,131,199] **(3)** DiffTUG[106] **(1)** Frenchay daily activities[184,185] **(1)** Functional Autonomy Assessment System (SMAF)[86] **(1)** Functional Independence Measure (FIM)[174-176] **(1)** Functional and problem evaluation interview[112] **(1)** Functional Status Questionnaire[128] **(1)** General functional assessment[11,17,151,203,204] **(10)** General gait and balance assessment[10,63,156] **(4)** Hearing and vision tests[9,168,169] **(9)** Katz Index of Activities of Daily Living[2,46,64,66,92] **(14)** Level of Rehabilitation Scale (LORS)[71] **(1)** McMaster health index[111] **(1)** Mobility Index[49,140] **(3)** Mobility Interaction Fall Chart[105] **(1)** NIA lower extremity battery[127] **(1)** Northwick Park ADL Index[178] Older American's Resources and Services Inventory (OARS)[3,56]/ Functional Assessment Inventory (FAI)[164] **(4)** Oral health assessment[8] **(2)** Other **(43)** Personal self-maintenance scale[31] **(1)** Physical Assessment[17,18,47,55] **(10)** Physical Performance and Mobility Examination (PPME)[50] **(1)** Physical Self-Maintenance Scale **(1)** RAND Medical Outcomes Study Short Form General Health Survey (MOS SF-36)[32,44,45,129,130,200,201] **(4)** SF-20[173] **(1)** Sickness Impact Profile (SIP): Physical Functioning Dimension[27,57,182,183] **(5)** Townsend score[123] **(3)** Unspecified ADLs[11,31,38,84,92] **(13)** Unspecified IADLs[11,31,46,92,116,117] **(12)** Winchester Disability Rating Scale[36] **(1)**	Blessed Dementia Rating Scale[101,102] **(1)** Consortium to Establish a Registry for Alzheimer's Disease tool (CERAD)[152] **(1)** Clinical Dementia Rating Scale (CDR)[145] **(1)** Confusion Assessment Method[98] **(1)** Digit Span Test[100] **(1)** Folstein Mini-Mental State Examination (MMSE)[19,56,67,119] **(15)** General mental function[39,73,74,95,179] **(10)** Kahn-Goldfarb Mental Status Questionnaire[12] **(3)** Pfeiffer Short Portable Mental Status Questionnaire[4] **(4)** RAND MOS SF-36, mental health section[186,187] **(1)** Sensory and communication abilities[136] **(1)** Unspecified dementia screening tool[39] **(1)**	Affect Balance Scale (ABS)[209] **(1)** Center for Epidemiological Studies' Depression Scale (CES-D)[5,52,170] **(5)** Diagnostic Interview Schedule (DIS), depression and anxiety sections[147,148] **(1)** General depression **(1)** General well-being schedule[87,88] **(1)** General social functioning[188] **(3)** General social support[158,203,204] **(6)** Geriatric Depression Scale (GDS)[13,28] **(6)** Global life satisfaction scale (GLS)[33-35] **(1)** Global social activity (GSA)[33-35] **(1)** Life Satisfaction Index-Z (LSI-Z)[124,138,208] **(3)** Memorial University Happiness Scale[77] **(1)** Nottingham Health Profile[113] **(2)** OARS/FAI: Psychological and social scale[164] **(1)** Other **(16)** Patient-Physician Interaction scale[133] **(1)** Patient Satisfaction Questionnaire[132] **(1)** Philadelphia Geriatric Morale Scale[40,41,114] **(4)** Quality of life **(2)** RAND MOS SF-36 emotional health questions[59] **(1)**, Quality of life questions[121] **(1)** SIP: psychological dimension[57] **(1)** Social contact score[42] **(1)** Social Provisions Scale[89] **(1)** Social Readjustment Rating Scale[79] **(1)** UCLA Loneliness Scale[78] **(1)** Wenger Scale[40] (measure of support networks) **(1)** Zung Questionnaire[68,207] **(5)** 15D (Health-Related Quality of Life)[153,154] **(1)**	APACHE II[20] **(2)** Global health perception[33-35] **(1)** Health Locus of Control (HLC)[81] **(1)** MacMillan Health Opinion Index[80] **(1)** OARS/FAI[56] **(1)** Other **(2)** RAND MOS SF-36[61,129,186,187] **(3)** Unspecified measure of perceived health[29,161,210,211] **(12)**		Admitting service used **(2)** Application for physical restraints **(1)** Client satisfaction **(1)** Costs **(13)** General health and support services utilization **(24)** Housing **(2)** Institutionalization **(22)** Number of days in institution **(23)** Number of days in rehabilitation **(1)** Number of readmissions **(2)** Number of referrals **(4)** Other **(9)** Place of residence at admission **(1)** Place of residence at discharge **(7)** Practical help received **(1)** Primary health care team contacts **(1)** Reason for hospitalization **(1)** Relocations **(1)** Use of diagnostic tests **(1)**	Abbreviated Injury Scale[107] **(1)** Alcohol consumption **(3)** Bleeding severity index[24] **(1)** Compliance rates **(5)** Environmental assessment **(10)** FAI—economic scale[164] **(1)** Falls efficacy scale[171,189] **(2)** Immunization rates **(2)** Medication review[15] **(2)** Nutrition **(5)** Other **(16)** Percentage of ideal body weight[14,159] **(2)** Tobacco use **(2)** Veterans Alcohol Screening Test[6] **(1)** Unspecified measure of falls **(10)** Unspecified measure of medications **(18)**
Conclusions	Out of 56 studies described, 54 measured physical function, using 77 different measures, of which 23 studies reported statistical significance.	Out of 56 studies described, 32 measured cognitive function, using 12 different measures, of which 6 studies reported statistical significance.	Out of 56 studies described, 39 measured psychosocial function, using 43 different measures, of which 13 studies reported statistical significance.	Out of 56 studies described, 18 measured self-rated health, using 9 different measures, of which 5 studies reported statistical significance.	Out of 56 studies described, 36 measured mortality, of which 9 studies reported statistical significance.	Out of 56 studies described, 46 measured health care utilization, using 27 different measures, of which 26 studies reported statistical significance.	Out of 56 studies described, 32 measured "other" outcomes, using 31 different measures, of which 14 studies reported statistical significance.

*Numbers in bold denote the frequency of instruments used within the collective studies.
[†]Instruments categorized in terms of reported use within each study (e.g., SF-36 may be used as a measure of physical function, self-rated health, or quality of life).

APPENDIX TABLE REFERENCES

1. Allen CM, Becker PM, McVey LJ, et al: A randomized, controlled clinical trial of a geriatric consultation team: compliance with recommendations. JAMA 255:2617–2621, 1986.
2. Katz S, Ford AB, Moskowitz RW, et al: Studies of illness in the aged: the index of ADL: a standardized measure of biological and psychosocial function. JAMA 185:914–919, 1963.
3. Pfeiffer E: Multidimensional functional assessment: the OARS methodology, Durham NC, 1975, Duke University, Center for the Study of Aging and Human Development.
4. Pfeiffer E: A short portable mental status questionnaire for the assessment of organic brain deficit in elderly patients. J Am Geriatr Soc 23:433–441, 1975.
5. Radloff LS: The CES-D scale: a self-report depression scale for research in the general population. Appl Psychol Meas 1:385–401, 1977.
6. Magruder-Habib K: Validation of the Veterans Alcoholism Screening Test. J Stud Alcohol 43:910–926, 1982.
7. Alessi CA, Stuck AE, Aronow HU, et al: The process of care in preventive in-home comprehensive geriatric assessment. J Am Geriatr Soc 45:1044–1050, 1997.
8. Atchinson KA, Dolan TA: Development of a geriatric oral health assessment index. J Dent Ed 54:680–687, 1990.
9. Lachs MS, Feinstein AR, Cooney LM, et al: A simple procedure for general screening for functional disability in elderly patients. Ann Intern Med 112:699–706, 1990.
10. Tenetti ME: Performance-oriented assessment of mobility problems in elderly patients. J Am Geriatr Soc 34:119–126, 1986.
11. Lawton MP, Moss M, Fulcomer M, et al: A research and service oriented multilevel assessment instrument. J Gerontol 37:91–99, 1982.
12. Kahn RL, Goldfarb AI, Pollack M, et al: A brief objective measures for the determination of mental status in the aged. Am J Psychiatry 117:326–328, 1960.
13. Sheikh JI, Yesavage JA: Geriatric Depression Scale (GDS): recent evidence and development of a shorter version. Clin Gerontol 5:122–125, 1986.
14. Master AM, Lasser RP, Beckman G: Tables of average weight and height of Americans aged 65 to 94 years. JAMA 172:658–663, 1960.
15. Stuck AE, Beers MH, Steiner A, et al: Inappropriate medication use in community-residing older persons. Arch Intern Med 154:2195–2200, 1994.
16. Applegate WB, Miller ST, Graney MJ, et al: A randomized controlled trial of a geriatric assessment unit in a community rehabilitation hospital. N Engl J Med 322:1572–1578, 1990.
17. Jette AM, Branch LG: The Framingham disability study. II. Physical disability among the aging. Am J Public Health 71:1211–1216, 1981.
18. Williams ME, Hadler NM, Earp JAL: Manual ability as a marker of dependency in geriatric women. J Chronic Dis 35:115–122, 1981.
19. Folstein M, Folstein S, McHugh PR: Mini-Mental State: A practical method for grading the cognitive state of patients for the clinician. J Psychiatr Res 12:189–198, 1975.
20. Knaus WA, Draper EA, Wagner DP, et al: APACHE II: A severity of disease classification system. Crit Care Med 13:818–829, 1985.
21. Beyth RJ, Quinn L, Landefeld CS: A multicomponent intervention to prevent major bleeding complications in older patients receiving warfarin: a randomized controlled trail. Ann Intern Med 133:687–695, 2000.
22. Rosendaal FR, Cannegieter SC, van der Meer FJM, et al: A method to determine the optimal intensity of oral anticoagulant therapy. J Thromb Haemost 69:236–239, 1993.
23. Hirch J, Dalen JE, Deykin D, et al: Oral anticoagulants. Mechanism of action, clinical effectiveness, and optimal therapeutic range. Chest 108(Suppl):231S–246S, 1995.
24. Landefeld CS, Anderson PA, Goodnough LT, et al: The bleeding severity index: validation and comparison to other methods for classifying bleeding complications of medical therapy. J Clin Epidemiol 42:711–718, 1989.
25. Boult C, Boult LB, Morishita L, et al: A randomized clinical trial of outpatient geriatric evaluation and management. J Am Geriatr Soc 49:351–359, 2001.
26. The design (1973-84) and procedures (1975-83) of the National Health Interview Survey. Vital Health Stat 1:1–127, 1985.
27. Bergner M, Bobbitt RA, Carter WB, et al: The Sickness Impact Profile: development and final revision of a health status measure. Med Care 19:787–805, 1981.
28. Yesavage JA, Brink TL: Development and validation of a geriatric depression screening scale: a preliminary report. J Psychiatr Res 17:37–49, 1982.
29. Kovar MG, Fitti JE, Chyba MM: The longitudinal study of aging. Vital Health Stat 1:1–248, 1992.
30. Burns R, Nicols LO, Martindale-Adams J, et al: Interdisciplinary geriatric primary care evaluation and management: two-year outcomes. J Am Geriatr Soc 48:8–13, 2000.
31. Lawton MP, Brody EM: Assessment of older people: self-maintaining and instrumental activities of daily living. Gerontologist 9:179–186, 1969.
32. Brook RH, Ware JE, Davies-Avery A, et al: Overview of adult health status measures fielded in Rand's health insurance study. Med Care 17(Suppl 17):1–131, 1979.
33. Applegate WB, Phillips HL, Schnaper H, et al: A randomized controlled trial of the effects of three antihypertensive agents on blood pressure control and quality of life in older women. Arch Intern Med 151:1817–1823, 1991.
34. Engle VF, Graney MJ: Self-assessed and functional health of older women. Int J Aging Hum Dev 22:301–313, 1986.
35. Cantril H: The pattern of human concerns, New Brunswick, NJ, 1965, Rutgers University Press.
36. Carpenter GI, Demopoulos GR: Screening the elderly in the community. BMJ 300:1253–1256, 1990.
37. Clarke M, Clarke SJ, Jagger C: Social intervention and the elderly. Am J Epidemiol 136:1517–1523, 1992.
38. Jagger C, Clarke M, Davies RA: The elderly at home: indices of disability. J Epidemiol Community Health 40:139–142, 1984.
39. Clarke M, Jagger C, Anderson J, et al: The prevalence of dementia in a total population: A comparison of two screening instruments. Age Ageing 20:396–403, 1991.
40. Wegner GC: The supportive network, London, 1984, Allen & Unwin.
41. Morris JN, Sherwood S: A retesting and modification of the Philadelphia Geriatric Center Morale Scale. J Gerontol 30:77–84, 1975.
42. Tunstall J: Old and alone: a sociological study of old people, London, 1966, Routledge & Kegan Paul.
43. Cohen HJ, Feussner JR, Weinberger M, et al: A controlled trial of inpatient and outpatient geriatric evaluation and management. N Engl J Med 346:905–912, 2002.
44. Tarlow AR, Ware JE, Greenfield S, et al: The Medical Outcomes Study: an application of methods for monitoring the results of medical care. JAMA 262:925–930, 1989.
45. Weinberger M, Oddone EZ, Henderson WG: Does increased access to primary care reduce hospital readmission? N Engl J Med 334:1441–1447, 1996.
46. Fillenbaum G: Screening the elderly: a brief instrumental activities of daily living measure. J Am Geriatr Soc 33:698–706, 1985.
47. Rueben DB, Siu AL: An objective measure of physical function of elderly outpatients: the Physical Performance Test. J Am Geriatr Soc 38:1105–1112, 1990.
48. Counsell SR, Holder CM, Liebnauer LL, et al: Effects of a mulitcomponent intervention on functional outcomes and process of care in hospitalized older patients: A randomized controlled trial of acute care for elders (ACE) in a community hospital. J Am Geriatr Soc 48:1572–1581, 2000.
49. Stewart AL, Ware JE, Brook RH: Advances in the measurement of functional status: construction of aggregate indexes. Med Care 19:473–488, 1981.
50. Winograd CH, Lemsky CM, Nevitt MC, et al: Development of a physical performance and mobility examination. J Am Geriatr Soc 42:743–749, 1994.
51. Charlson ME, Pompei P, Ales KL, et al: A new method of classifying prognostic comorbidity in longitudinal studies: Development and validation. J Chronic Dis 40:373–383, 1987.
52. Kohout FJ, Berkman L, Evans DA, et al: Two shorter forms of the CES-D depression symptoms index. J Aging Health 5:179–193, 1993.
53. Ware JE, Hays RD: Methods for measuring patient satisfaction with specific medical encounters. Med Care 26:393–402, 1988.

54. Epstein AM, Hall JA, Fretwell M, et al: Consultative geriatric assessment for ambulatory patients. A randomized trial in a health maintenance organization. JAMA 263:538–544, 1990.
55. National Institute of Health Consensus Development Conference statement: geriatric assessment methods for clinical decision making. J Am Geriatr Soc 36:342–347, 1988.
56. Duke University Center for the Study of Aging and Human Development: Multidimensional functional assessment: the OARS methodology, Durham, NC, 1978, Duke University, Center for the Study of Aging and Human Development.
57. Bergner M, Bobbitt RA, Pollard WE, et al: The sickness impact profile: reliability of a health measure. Med Care 14:57–67, 1976.
58. Wan TTH: Stressful life events, social-support networks, and gerontological health: a prospective study, Lexington, MA, 1982, Lexington Books.
59. Ware JE, Johnston SA, Ross Davies A, et al: Conceptualization and measurement of health for adults in the health insurance study, vol III, mental health, Santa Monica, CA, 1979, RAND Corporation.
60. DiMatteo MR, Hays R: The significance of patients' perceptions of physician conduct: a study of patient satisfaction in a family practice center. J Community Health 6:18–34, 1980.
61. Ware JE, Davis-Avery A, Donald CA: Conceptualization and measurement of health insurance study, vol V, general health perceptions, Santa Monica, CA, 1978, RAND Corporation.
62. Fabacher D, Josephson K, Pietruszka F, et al: An in-home preventive assessment program for independent older adults. J Am Geriatr Soc 42:630–638, 1994.
63. Tinetti ME, Williams TF, Mayewski R: Fall index for elderly patients based on number of chronic disabilities. Am J Med 80:429–434, 1986.
64. Katz S, Downs TD, Cash HR, et al: Progress in the development of the index of ADL. Gerontologist 10:20–30, 1970.
65. Fretwell MD, Raymond PM, McGarvey ST, et al: The senior care study. A controlled trial of a consultative/unit-based geriatric assessment program in acute care. J Am Geriatr Soc 38:1073–1081, 1990.
66. Katz S, Akpom CA: A measure of primary sociobiological functions. Int J Health Servs 6:493–508, 1976.
67. Klein LE, Roca RP, McArthur J, et al: Diagnosing dementia: univariate and multivariate analyses of the mental status examination. J Am Geriatr Soc 33:483–488, 1985.
68. Zung WWK: A self-rating depression scale. Arch Gen Psychiatry 12:63–70, 1965.
69. Gayton D, Wood-Dauphinee S, de Lorimer M, et al: Trial of a geriatric consultation team in an acute care hospital. J Am Geriatr Soc 35:726–736, 1987.
70. Mahoney FI, Barthel DW: Functional evaluation: the Barthel index. Md State Med J 14:61–65, 1965.
71. Carey GC, Posavac EH: Program evaluation of a physical medicine and rehabilitation unit. Arch Phys Med Rehabil 59:330–337, 1978.
72. Gilchrist WJ, Newman RJ, Hamblen DL, et al: Prospective randomized study of an orthopaedic geriatric inpatient service. BMJ 297:1116–1118, 1988.
73. Still CN, Goldschmidt TJ, Mallin R: Mini object test: a new brief clinical assessment for aphasia-apraxia-agnosia. South Med J 76:52–54, 1983.
74. Hughes AM, Gray RF, Downie DIV: Brief cognitive assessments of the elderly—the mini object test and the Clifton assessment procedures for the elderly. Br J Clin Psychol 3:81–83, 1985.
75. Gunner-Svensson F, Ipsen J, Olsen J, et al: Prevention of relocation of the aged in nursing homes. Scand J Prime Health Care 2:49–56, 1984.
76. Hall N, De Beck P, Johnson D, et al: Randomized trial of a health promotion program for frail elders. Cana J Aging 11:72–91, 1992.
77. Kozma A, Stones MS: The measurement of happiness: development of the Memorial University of Newfoundland Scale of Happiness (MUNSH). J Gerontol 35:906–912, 1980.
78. Russell D, Peplau LA, Cutrona CE: The revised UCLA Loneliness Scale: concurrent and discriminant validity evidence. J Personality Social Psychol 39:472–480, 1980.
79. Masuda M, Holmes TH: Magnitude estimations of social readjustments. J Psychosom Res 11:219–225, 1967.
80. MacMillan AM: The Health Opinion Survey: technique for estimating prevalence of psychoneurotic and related types of disorders in communities. Psychol Rep 3:325–339, 1957.
81. Wallston BS, Wallston KA, Kaplan GD, et al: Development and validation of the Health Locus of Control (HLC) scale. J Consult Clin Psychol 44:580–585, 1976.
82. Hansen FR, Spedtsperg K, Schroll M: Geriatric follow-up by home visits after discharge from hospital: a randomized controlled trial. Age Aging 21:445–450, 1992.
83. Harris RD, Henschke PJ, Popplewell PY, et al: A randomised study of outcomes in a defined group of acutely ill elderly patients managed in a geriatric assessment unit or a general medical unit. Aust N Z J Med 21:230–234, 1991.
84. Sheikh K, Smith DS, Meade TW, et al: Repeatability and validity of modified activities of daily living (ADL) index in studies of chronic disability. Int Rehabil Med 1:51–58, 1979.
85. Hébert R, Robichaud L, Roy PM, et al: Efficacy of a nurse-led multidimensional preventive programme for older people at risk of functional decline: a randomized control trial. Age Ageing 30:147–153, 2001.
86. Hébert R, Carrier R, Bilodeau A: The functional autonomy measurement system (SMAF): description and validation of an instrument for the measurement of handicaps. Age Ageing 17:293–302, 1988.
87. Dupuy HJ: Self-representation of general psychological well-being of American adults. Presented at the American Public Health Association Meeting, Los Angeles, CA, October 17, 1978.
88. Bravo G, Gaulin P, Dubois MF: Validation d'une échelle de bien-être général auprès d'une population francophone âgée de 50 à 75 ans. Can J Aging 15:112–118, 1996.
89. Cutrona C, Russell DW: The provisions of social support and adaptation to stress. Adv Personal Relationships 1:37–67, 1987.
90. Hendriksen C, Lund E, Stromgard E: Consequences of assessment and intervention among elderly people: a three-year randomised controlled trial. BMJ 289:1522–1524, 1984.
91. Sorensen K, Sivertsen J: Follow-up three years after intervention to relieve unmet medical and social needs of old people. Compr Gerontol [B] 2:85–91, 1988.
92. Katz S: Assessing self-maintenance. J Am Geriatr Soc 31:721–727, 1983.
93. Hogan DB, Fox RA: A prospective controlled trial of a geriatric consultation team in an acute-care hospital. Age Ageing 19:107–113, 1990.
94. Granger CV, Albrecht GL, Hamilton BB: Outcome of comprehensive medical rehabilitation: Measurement by PULSES profile and the Barthel Index. Arch Phys Med Rehabil 60:145–154, 1979.
95. Hodkinson HM: Evaluation of a mental test score for assessment of mental impairment in the elderly. Age Ageing 1:233–238, 1972.
96. Hogan DB, Fox RA, Badley BWD, et al: Effect of a geriatric consultation service on management of patients in an acute care hospital. CMAJ 136:713–717, 1987.
97. Inouye SK, Bogardus ST, Charpentier PA, et al: A multicomponent intervention to prevent delirium in hospitalized older patients. N Engl J Med 340:669–676, 1999.
98. MacPhee GJ, Cowther JA, McAlpine CH: A simple screening test for hearing impairment in elderly patients. Age Ageing 17:347–351, 1988.
99. Inouye SK, van Dyck CH, Alessi CA, et al: Clarifying confusion: the Confusion Assessment Method: a new method for detection of delirium. Ann Intern Med 113:941–948, 1990.
100. Cummings J: Clinical neuropsychiatry, Orlando, FL, 1985, Grune & Stratton.
101. Blessed G, Tomlinson BE, Roth M: The association between quantitative measures of dementia and of senile change in the cerebral grey matter of elderly subjects. Br J Psychiatry 114:797–811, 1968.
102. Ulhmann RF, Larson EB, Buchner DM: Correlations of Mini-Mental State and modified Dementia Rating Scale to measures of transitional health status in dementia. J Gerontol 42:33–36, 1987.
103. Jensen J, Nyberg L, Gustafson Y, et al: Fall and injury prevention in residential care—effects in residents with higher and lower levels of cognition. J Am Geriatr Soc 51:627–635, 2003.
104. Wade DT, Collin C: The Barthel ADL index. A standard measure of physical disability? Int Disabil Stud 10:64–67, 1988.
105. Lundin-Olsson L, Nyberg L, Gustafson Y: The mobility interaction fall chart. Physiother Res Int 5:190–201, 2000.
106. Lundin-Olsson L, Nyberg L, Gustafson Y: Attention, frailty, and falls: the effect of a manual task on basic mobility. J Am Geriatr Soc 46:758–761, 1988.

107. Committee on Injury Scaling: The abbreviated injury scale, Morton Grove, IL, 1990, American Association for Automotive Medicine.
108. Kennie DC, Reid J, Richardson IR, et al: Effectiveness of geriatric rehabilitative care after fractures of the proximal femur in elderly women: a randomised clinical trial. BMJ 297:1083–1086, 1988.
109. Jensen JS, Bagger J: Long-term social prognosis after hip fractures. Acta Orthop Scand 53:97–101, 1982.
110. McEwen RT, Davison N, Forster DP, et al: Screening elderly people in primary care: a randomized controlled trial. Br J Gen Pract 40:94–97, 1990.
111. Chambers LW, MacDonald LA, Tugwell P, et al: The McMaster health index questionnaire as a measure of the quality of life. J Rheumatol 9:780–784, 1982.
112. Weed LA: Medical records, medical education and patient care, Cleveland, 1971, The Press of Case Western Reserve University.
113. Hunt SM, McEwan J, McKenna P: Measuring health status, London, 1986, Croom Helm.
114. Lawton MP: The Philadelphia Geriatric Center morale scale: a revision. J Gerontol 30:85–89, 1975.
115. Melin AL, Bygren LO: Efficacy of the rehabilitation of elderly primary health care patients after short-stay hospital treatment. Med Care 30:1004–1015, 1992.
116. Spector WD, Katz S, Murphy JB, et al: The hierarchical relationship between activities of daily living and instrumental activities of daily living. J Chronic Dis 40:481–489, 1987.
117. Kane RA, Kane RL: Assessing the elderly. A practical guide to measurement, Lexington, MA, 1986, Lexington Books.
118. Katz S, Ford AB, Heiple KG, et al: Studies of illness in the aged: recovery after fracture of the hip. J Gerontol 19:285, 1964.
119. Galasko D, Klauber MR, Hofstetter R, et al: The Mini-Mental State Examination in the early diagnosis of Alzheimer's disease. Arch Neurol 47:49–52, 1990.
120. Newbury JW, Marley JE, Beilby JJ: A randomized controlled trial of the outcome of health assessment of people aged 75 years and over. Med J Aust 175:104–107, 2001.
121. Medical Outcomes Trust: SF-36 health survey. Scoring manual for English language adaptations: Australia/New Zealand, Canada, United Kingdom, Boston, MA, 1994, Medical Outcomes Trust.
122. Pathy MSJ, Bayer A, Harding K, et al: Randomised trial of case finding and surveillance of elderly people at home. Lancet 340:890–893, 1992.
123. Townsend P: Poverty in the United Kingdom, Harmondsworth, England, 1979, Penguin Books.
124. Neugarten BL, Navighurst RJ, Tobin SS: The measurement of life satisfaction. J Gerontol 16:134–143, 1961.
125. Powell C, Montgomery P: The age study: the admission of geriatric patients through emergency. J Am Geriatr Soc 38:A35, 1990.
126. Reuben DB, Frank JC, Hirsch SH, et al: A randomized clinical trial of outpatient comprehensive geriatric assessment coupled with an intervention to increase adherence to recommendations. J Am Geriatr Soc 47:269–276, 1999.
127. Guralnik JM, Simonsick EM, Ferrucci L, et al: A short performance battery assessing lower extremity function: association with self-reported disability and prediction of mortality and nursing home admission. J Gerontol 49:M85–M94, 1994.
128. Jette AM, Davies AR, Cleary PD, et al: The functional status questionnaire: Reliability and validity when used in primary care. J Gen Intern Med 1:143–149, 1986.
129. Ware JE, Sherbourne CD: The MOS 36-item Short-Form Health Survey (SF-36): 1. Conceptual framework and item selection. Med Care 30:473–483, 1992.
130. Hays RD, Sherbourne CD, Mazel RM: The RAND 36-item health survey 1.0. Health Econ 2:217–227, 1993.
131. Current estimates from the National Health Interview Survey: United States 1985. Vital Health Stat 10:160, 1986.
132. Ware JE, Snyder MK, Wright WR, et al: Defining and measuring patient satisfaction with medical care. Eval Prog Planning 6:247–263, 1982.
133. Maly RC, Frank JC, Marshall GN: Perceived efficacy in patient-physician interactions (PEPPI): validation of an instrument in older persons. J Am Geriatr Soc 46:889–899, 1998.
134. Rubenstein LZ, Josephson KR, Wieland GD, et al: Effectiveness of a geriatric evaluation unit: a randomized clinical trial. N Engl J Med 311:1664–1670, 1984.
135. Rubin CD, Sizemore MT, Loftis PA, et al: The effect of geriatric evaluation and management on medicate reimbursement in a large public hospital: a randomized clinical trial. J Am Geriatr Soc 40:989–995, 1992.
136. National Center for Health Statistics: Long-term health care: minimum data set, Washington, DC, 1978, U.S. Government Printing Office.
137. Rubin CD, Sizemore MT, Loftis PA, et al: A randomized, controlled trial of outpatient geriatric evaluation and management in a large public hospital. J Am Geriatr Soc 41:1023–1028, 1993.
138. Wood V, Wylie ML, Sheafor B: An analysis of a short self-report measure of life satisfaction: correlation with rater judgements. J Gerontol 24:465–469, 1969.
139. Shaw FE, Bond J, Richard DA, et al: Multifactorial intervention after a fall in older people with cognitive impairment and dementia presenting to the accident and emergency department: Randomised controlled trail. BMJ 326:73–78, 2003.
140. Tinetti ME: Performance-oriented assessment of mobility problems in elderly patients. J Am Geriatr Soc 34:119–126, 1986.
141. Koch M, Gottschalk M, Baker DI, et al: An impairment and disability assessment and treatment protocol for community living elderly persons. Phys Ther 74:286–298, 1994.
142. Tideiksaar R: Preventing falls: home hazard checklists to help older people protect themselves. Geriatrics 41:26–28, 1986.
143. Silverman M, Musa D, Martin DC, et al: Evaluation of outpatient geriatric: a randomized multi-site trial. J Am Geriatr Soc 43:733–740, 1995.
144. George LK, Fillenbaum GG: OARS methodology. A decade of experience in geriatric assessment. J Am Geriatr Soc 33:607–615, 1985.
145. Berg L, Hughes CP, Coben LA: Mild senile dementia of the Alzheimer's type: research diagnostic criteria, recruitment, and description of a study population. J Neurol Neurosurg Psychiatry 45:962–968, 1982.
146. McCusker J: Development of scales to measure satisfaction and preferences regarding long-term and terminal care. Med Care 22:476–493, 1984.
147. Helzer JE, Robins LN: The diagnostic interview schedule: its development, evolution, and use. Soc Psychiatry Psychiatr Epidemiol 23:6–16, 1988.
148. Robins LN, Helzer JE, Croughan J, et al: National Institute of Mental Health diagnostic interview schedule: its history, characteristics, and validity. Arch Gen Psychiatry 38:381–389, 1981.
149. Morycz RK: Caregiving strain and the desire to institutionalize family members with Alzheimer's disease. Res Aging 7:329–361, 1985.
150. Strandberg TE, Pitkala K, Berglind S, et al: Multifactorial cardiovascular disease prevention in patients aged 75 years and older. A randomized controlled trial. Am Heart J 142:945–951, 2001.
151. Ettinger WH, Fried LP, Harris T, et al: Self-reported causes of physical disability in older people: the Cardiovascular Health Study. CHS Collaborative Research Group. J Am Geriatr Soc 42:1035–1044, 1994.
152. Clark CM, Ewbank D, Lerner A, et al: The relationship between extrapyramidal signs and cognitive performance in patients with Alzheimer's disease enrolled in the CERAD Study. Consortium to Establish a Registry for Alzheimer's Disease. Neurology 49(Suppl):70–75, 1997.
153. Hirvonen J, Blom M, Tuominen U, et al: Health-related quality of life in patients waiting for major joint replacement. A comparison between patients and population controls. Health Qual Life Outcomes 4:3, 2006.
154. Rissan P, Sogaard J, Sintonen H, et al: Do QOL instruments agree? A comparison of the 15D (health-related quality of life) and NHP (Nottingham Health Profile) in hip and knee replacements. Int J Technol Assessment Health Care 16:696–705, 2000.
155. Stuck AE, Aronow HU, Steiner A, et al: A trial of annual in-home comprehensive geriatric assessments for elderly people living in the community. N Engl J Med 333:1184–1189, 1995.
156. Tinetti ME, Baker DI, McAvay G, et al: A multifactorial intervention to reduce the risk of falling among elderly people living in the community. N Engl J Med 331:821–827, 1994.
157. Kempen GI, Suurmeijer TP: The development of a hierarchical polychotomous ADL-IADL scale for noninstitutionalized elders. Gerontologist 30:497–502, 1990.
158. Rubenstein LZ, Aronow HU, Schloe M, et al: A home-based geriatric assessment, follow-up and health promotion program: design,

methods and baseline findings from a 3-year randomised clinical trial. Aging Clin Exp Res 6:105–120, 1994.
159. Master AM, Lasser RP, Beckman G: Tables on average weight and height of Americans aged 65 to 94 years. JAMA 172:658–663, 1960.
160. Stuck AE, Minder CE, Peter-Wuest I, et al: A randomized trial of in-home visits for disability prevention in community-dwelling older people at low and at high risk for nursing home admission. Arch Intern Med 160:977–986, 2000.
161. Nelson EC, Landgraf JM, Hays RD, et al: The functional status of patients: how can it be measured in physicians' offices? Med Care 28:1111–1116, 1990.
162. Teasdale TA, Shuman L, Snow E, et al: A comparison of outcomes of geriatric cohorts receiving care in a geriatric assessment unit and on general medicine floors. J Am Geriatr Soc 31:529–534, 1983.
163. Thomas DR, Brahan MD, Haywood BP: Inpatient community-based geriatric assessment reduces subsequent mortality. J Am Geriatr Soc 41:101–104, 1993.
164. Pfeiffer E, Johnson T, Chiofolo R: Functional assessment of elderly subjects in four service settings. J Am Geriatr Soc 29:433–437, 1981.
165. Timonen L, Rantanen T, Ryynänen OP, et al: A randomized controlled trial of rehabilitation after hospitalization in frail older women: effects on strength, balance, and mobility. Scand J Med Sports 12:186–192, 2002.
166. Berg KO, Wood-Dauphinee SL, Williams JI, et al: Measuring balance in the elderly. Validation of an instrument. Can J Public Health 83(Suppl 2):S7–S11, 1992.
167. Tinetti ME, Baker DI, McAvay G, et al: A multifactorial intervention to reduce the risk of falling among elderly people living in the community. N Engl J Med 331:821–827, 1994.
168. Spaeth EB, Fralick FB, Hughes WF: Estimation of loss of visual efficiency. Arch Ophthalmol 54:462–468, 1955.
169. Macphee GJA, Crowther JA, McAlpine CH: A simple screening test for hearing impairment in elderly patients. Age Ageing 17:347–351, 1988.
170. Radloff LS: The CES-D scale: a self-report depression scale for research in the general population. Appl Psychol Meas 1:385–401, 1977.
171. Buchner DM, Hornbrook MC, Kutner NG, et al: Development of the common data base for the FICSIT trials. J Am Geriatr Soc 41:297–308, 1993.
172. Toseland RW, O'Donnell JC, Engelhardt JB, et al: Outpatient geriatric evaluation and management: is there an investment effect? Gerontologist 37:324–332, 1997.
173. Stewart AL, Hays RD, Ware JE: The MOS short-form General Health Survey: reliability and validity in a patient population. Med Care 26:724–735, 1988.
174. Granger CV, Hamilton BB: UDS report: The uniform data system for medical rehabilitation report of first admissions for 1990. Am J Phys Med Rehabil 71:108–113, 1992.
175. Granger CV, Hamilton BB, Keith RA, et al: Advances in functional assessment for medical rehabilitation. Top Geriatr Rehabil 1:59–74, 1986.
176. Linacre JM, Heinemann AW, Wright BD, et al: The structure and stability of the functional independence measure. Arch Psychol Med Rehabil 75:127–132, 1994.
177. Tucker MA, Davison JG, Ogle SJ: Day hospital rehabilitation—effectiveness and cost in the elderly: a randomised controlled trial. BMJ 289:1209–1212, 1984.
178. Benjamin J: The Northwick Park ADL index. Br J Occup Ther 12:301–306, 1976.
179. Qureshi KM, Hodkinson HM: Evaluation of a 10-question mental test in the institutionalised elderly. Age Ageing 3:152–157, 1974.
180. Tulloch AJ, Moore V: A randomized controlled trial of geriatric screening and surveillance in general practice. J R Coll Gen Pract 29:733–742, 1979.
181. van Haastregt JCM, Diederiks JPM, van Rossum E, et al: Effects of a programme of multifactorial home visits on falls and mobility impairments in elderly people at risk: randomized controlled trial. BMJ 321:994–998, 2000.
182. De Bruin AF, Diederiks JPM, de Witte LP, et al: The development of a short generic version of the sickness impact profile. J Clin Epidemiol 47:407–418, 1994.
183. De Bruin AF, Buys M, de Witte LP, et al: The sickness impact profile: SIP68, a short generic version; first evaluation of the reliability and the reproducibility. J Clin Epidemiol 47:863–871, 1994.
184. Holbrook M, Skilbeck CE: An activities index for use with stroke patients. Age Ageing 12:166–170, 1983.
185. Schuling J, de Haan R, Limburg M, et al: The Frenchay activities index: assessment of functional status in stroke patients. Stroke 24:1173–1177, 1993.
186. RAND Health: Rand 36-item health survey from the RAND Medical Outcomes Study. http://www.rand.org/health/surveys_tools/mos/mos_core_36item.html. Accessed November 17, 2015.
187. Van der Zee I, Sanderman R: Het meten van de algemene gezondheidstoestand met de RAND-36: een handleiding, Groningen, Netherlands, 1993, Noordelijk Centrum voor Gezondheidsvraagstukken.
188. Ware JE, Johnston SA, Ross Davies A, et al: Conceptualization and measurement of health for adults in the health insurance study, vol III, mental health, Santa Monica, CA, 1979, RAND Corporation.
189. Tinetti ME, Richman D, Powell L: Falls efficacy as a measure of fear of falling. J Gerontol 45:239P–243P, 1990.
190. Stalenhoef P, Diederiks J, Knottnerus A, et al: How predictive is a home safety checklist of indoor fall risk for the elderly living in the community? Eur J Gen Pract 4:114–120, 1998.
191. van Rossum E, Frederiks CMA, Philipsen H, et al: Effects of preventative home visits to elderly people. BMJ 307:27–32, 1993.
192. Templeman CJJ: Welbevinden bij ouderen. Konstruktie van een meetinstrument, Groningen, Netherlands, 1987, University of Groningen, pp 56–82. PhD thesis.
193. De Jong-Gierveld J, Kamphius FH The development of a Rasch-type loneliness scale. http://conservancy.umn.edu/bitstream/handle/11299/102185/v09n3p289.pdf?sequence=1&isAllowed=y>. Accessed November 17, 2015.
194. Vetter NJ, Jones DA, Victor CR: Effect of health visitors working with elderly patients in general practice: a randomised control trial. BMJ 288:369–372, 1984.
195. Foulds GA, Bedford A: Manual of the delusions-symptoms-states inventory, Windsor, England, 1979, NFER Publishing.
196. McNab A, Philip AE: Screening an elderly population for psychological well-being. Health Bull (Edinb) 38:160–162, 1980.
197. Vetter NJ, Lewis PA, Ford D: Can health visitors prevent fractures in elderly people? BMJ 304:888–890, 1992.
198. Wagner EH, LaCroix AZ, Grothaus L, et al: Preventing disability and falls in older adults: a population-based randomized trial. Am J Public Health 84:1800–1806, 1994.
199. Scholes D, LaCroix AZ, Wagner EH, et al: Tracking progress toward national health objectives in the elderly: what do restricted activity days signify? Am J Public Health 8:485–488, 1991.
200. Ware JE: Reliability and validity of general health measures, Santa Monica, CA, 1976, RAND Corporation.
201. Ware JE, Sherbourne CD, Davis A, et al: The MOS short-form general health survey: development and test in a general population, Santa Monica, CA, 1988, RAND Corporation.
202. Williams ME, Williams TF, Zimmer JG, et al: How does the team approach to outpatient geriatric compare with traditional care: a report of a randomized control trial. J Am Geriatr Soc 35:1071–1078, 1987.
203. Eggert GM, Brodows BS: The ACCESS program: assuring quality in long-term care. QRB 9–15, 1982.
204. Eggert GM, Bowlyow JE, Nichols CW: Gaining control of the long-term care system: first returns from the ACCESS experiment. Gerontologist 20:356–363, 1980.
205. Winograd CH, Gerety M, Lai N: Another negative trial of geriatric consultation: is it time to say it doesn't work? J Am Geriatr Soc 39:A13, 1991.
206. Yeo G, Ingram L, Skurnick J, et al: Effects of a geriatric clinic on functional health and well-being of elders. J Gerontol 42:252–258, 1987.
207. Zung WW: Depression in the normal aged. Psychosomatics 8:287–292, 1967.
208. Carp FM, Carp A: Structural stability of well-being factors across age and gender, and development of well-being unbiased for age and gender. J Gerontol 38:572–581, 1983.
209. Bradburn NM: The structure of psychological well-being, Chicago, 1969, Aldine.
210. Blazer D, Houpt J: Perception of poor health in the healthy older adult. J Am Geriatr Soc 27:330–334, 1979.
211. Mossey JM, Shapiro E: Self-rated health: a predictor of mortality among the elderly. Am J Public Health 72:800–806, 1982.

KEY REFERENCES

8. Ferrucci L, Guralnik JM, Studenski S, et al; The Interventions on Frailty Working Group: Designing randomized, controlled trials aimed at preventing or delaying functional decline and disability in frail, older persons: a consensus report. J Am Geriatr Soc 52:625–634, 2004.
12. Working Group on Functional Outcome Measures for Clinical Trials: Functional outcomes for clinical trials in frail older persons: time to be moving. J Gerontol A Biol Sci Med Sci 63:160–164, 2008.
19. Hedrick SC, Barrand N, Deyo R, et al: Working group recommendations: measuring outcomes of care in geriatric evaluation and management units. J Am Geriatr Soc 39:48S–52S, 1991.
20. Working Group on Health Outcomes for Older Persons with Multiple Chronic Conditions: Universal health outcomes measures for older persons with multiple chronic conditions. J Am Geriatr Soc 60:2333–2341, 2012.
24. Stuck AE, Siu AL, Wieland GD, et al: Comprehensive geriatric assessment: a meta-analysis of controlled trials. Lancet 342:1032–1036, 1993.
25. Kuo H, Scandrett KG, Dave J, et al: The influence of outpatient comprehensive geriatric assessment on survival: a meta-analysis. Arch Gerontol Geriatr 39:245–254, 2004.
26. van Haastregt JCM, Diederiks JPM, van Rossum E, et al: Effects of preventive home visits to elder people living in the community: systematic review. BMJ 320:754–758, 2000.
27. Stuck AE, Egger M, Hammer A, et al: Home visits to preventnursing home admission and functional decline in elderly people. Systematic review and meta-regression analysis. JAMA 287:1022–1028, 2002.
50. Mor V, Guadagnoli E: Quality of life measurement: a psychometric tower of Babel. J Clin Epidemiol 41:1055–1058, 1988.
53. Bergner M: Quality of life, health status, and clinical research. Med Care 27:S148–S156, 1989.
54. Hirdes JP, Fries BE, Morris J, et al: Integrated health information systems based on the RAI/MDS series of instruments. Healthc Manage Forum 12:30–40, 1999.
77. Williams TF: Geriatrics: A perspective on quality of life and care for older people. In Spilker B, editor: Quality of life assessment in clinical trials, New York, NY, 1990, Raven Press, pp 217–223.
80. Reuben DB, Tinetti ME: Goal-oriented patient care—an alternative health outcomes paradigm. N Engl J Med 366:777–779, 2012.
82. Rockwood K: Use of global assessment measures in dementia drug trials. J Clin Epidemiol 47:101–103, 1994.
86. Kiresuk TJ, Smith A, Cardillo JE, editors: Goal attainment scaling: applications, theory, and measurement, Hillsdale, NJ, 1994, Lawrence Erlbaum.
87. Zaza C, Stolee P, Prkachin K: The application of goal attainment scaling in chronic pain settings. J Pain Symptom Manage 17:55–64, 1999.
89. Stolee P, Rockwood K, Fox RA, et al: The use of goal attainment scaling in a geriatric care setting. J Am Geriatr Soc 40:574–578, 1992.
92. Stolee P, Stadnyk K, Myers AM, et al: An individualized approach to outcome measurement in geriatric rehabilitation. J Gerontol A Biol Sci Med Sci 54:M641–M647, 1999.
95. Stolee P, Awad M, Byrne K, et al; Regional Geriatric Programs of Ontario Day Hospital Research Group: A multi-site study of the feasibility and clinical utility of Goal Attainment Scaling in geriatric day hospitals. Disabil Rehabil 34:1716–1726, 2012.
96. Rockwood K, Howlett S, Stadnyk K, et al: Responsiveness of goal attainment scaling in a randomized trial of comprehensive geriatric assessment. J Clin Epidemiol 56:732–743, 2003.
97. Rockwood K, Stadnyk K, Carver D, et al: A clinimetric evaluation of specialized geriatric carefor rural dwelling, frail older people. J Am Geriatr Soc 48:1080–1085, 2000.
103. Berwick DM: What "patient-centered" should mean: confessions of an extremist. Health Aff (Millwood) 28:w555–w565, 2009.

39 Chronic Cardiac Failure

Neil D. Gillespie, Miles D. Witham, Allan D. Struthers

Cardiac failure increases in prevalence and incidence with age. It is a disease of middle and old age, although the underlying causes differ considerably with age. In younger patients with cardiac failure, the cause is frequently coronary artery disease or a cardiomyopathy of uncertain cause, whereas in the older patient, valvular disease and hypertension are more often implicated. Heart failure remains a severely debilitating condition for many older adults, but advances continue to be made in diagnosis, treatment, and organization of care. The challenge is to ensure that these advances can be translated to older adults with multiple comorbid diseases and to understand how best to deliver high-quality heart failure care to the frailest older adults.

The pool of patients at risk of heart failure continues to rise as more patients survive myocardial infarction as a result of percutaneous coronary intervention, thrombolytic therapy, and adjunctive drug treatment. In addition, patients with hypertension are surviving longer as a result of continued improvements in treatment, which includes the prevention of strokes. Fortunately, it appears that the effective treatment of hypertension may in fact prevent the onset of heart failure, even in the very old.[1] However, as more older adults live to extremes of age, it is almost inevitable that if they survive long enough, they will develop some degree of heart failure, even if it is not diagnosed until they are very frail.[2]

When considering the epidemiology of heart failure, it is important to note that it is defined as the presence of symptoms and signs of cardiac decompensation, together with objective evidence of underlying structural heart disease. These are the definitions used by the European Society of Cardiology[3] and the American Heart Association,[4] who have similar consensus statements on the diagnosis and management of heart failure. These agreements are important because they have resulted in a more focused approach when considering precisely which disease entity is being treated in individual patients. In the United Kingdom, the National Institute for Healthcare Excellence (NICE) guidelines give additional advice about treatment and, in Scotland, the Scottish Intercollegiate Guideline Network (SIGN) provides evidence-based advice. In this chapter, however, we will also consider issues particularly relevant to older adults and consider some of the very real challenges faced when managing older adults who are frail and often have many additional medical problems, as well as heart failure.

Heart failure is of major economic significance; in the United Kingdom, it accounts for up to 5% of hospital admissions, and across the world hospitalization for heart failure is a significant financial burden.[5] Many older adults with heart failure also have multiple pathologies and coexistent diseases, including cognitive impairment, which can make the diagnosis more difficult.[6]

EPIDEMIOLOGY

The prevalence of heart failure rises with age, with this phenomenon seen in multiple cohorts, including the Framingham cohort,[7] Scandinavian cohorts,[8,9] and community-based screening cohorts.[10] In the Framingham study, the prevalence of heart failure reached 10% in those older than 80 years; similar prevalence figures have been obtained from other cohorts.[11] Echocardiographic screening studies suggest that as many of the population have asymptomatic left ventricular systolic dysfunction as have clinically overt heart failure.[11] Many but not all cohort studies have suggested that the age-adjusted incidence of new heart failure diagnoses is rising over time[12,13]; this may reflect improved survival from ischemic heart disease and stroke, leading to a larger pool of at-risk individuals who then go on to develop clinically overt heart failure.

The proportion of heart failure patients with heart failure with reduced ejection fraction (HFREF) compared with those suffering from heart failure with reduced ejection fraction (HFPEF) changes with age.[14] Younger patients (i.e., those < 65 years) suffer predominantly from HFREF and are predominantly men. In those older than 80 years, however, the number of women affected is similar to the number of men affected, driven in part by their greater longevity in most populations. In parallel, numbers with HFPEF are similar to numbers with HFREF in those older than 80 years.

Because frailty is linked to age, it can be expected that frailty and heart failure will often coexist, and this appears to be the case. In addition, frailty has been demonstrated to be a risk factor for heart failure[15]; it also seems likely, given elements of shared pathophysiology, that heart failure will make frailty worse.[16]

DISEASE COURSE AND PROGNOSIS

Heart failure has a variable prognosis, but despite improvements in survival with pharmacologic and device therapy, the prognosis remains worse than that of many major cancers.[17] Key determinants of prognosis that are useful in clinical practice include ejection fraction, exercise capacity (as measured by maximal oxygen uptake or simpler tests such as the 6-minute walk test), symptoms (e.g., New York Heart Association [NYHA] class), renal impairment, and high natriuretic peptide levels.[4] Patients admitted to hospital with acute decompensation of heart failure have a particularly poor prognosis, with high death rates in the 3 to 6 months after admission. Among older adults hospitalized with heart failure, mean survival is about 2.5 years.[9] However, there is considerable heterogeneity in survival. The degree to which heart failure itself contributes to poor prognosis, rather than frailty or comorbid disease, can be difficult to discern, but the presence of chronic heart failure in older adults may result in an approximately 50% reduction in life expectancy.

Heart failure is a leading cause of hospitalization for older adults. Although there are data suggesting that heart failure as a primary cause of hospitalization is static or declining (possibly due to improved therapy), all-cause hospitalization for patients with heart failure continues to rise.[12] Data from North America suggest that there is a high rate of readmission in heart failure patients, and it is noteworthy that readmissions are often not due to heart failure exacerbation.[18] Evidence suggests that a multidisciplinary approach to the treatment of heart failure may reduce the need for hospitalization in older adult patients with the condition.[19]

TABLE 39-1 New York Heart Association Classification of Heart Failure (HF)

Class	Features
I	No symptoms
II	Symptoms with ordinary activity
III	Symptoms with less than ordinary activity
IV	Symptoms at rest

BOX 39-1 Factors That May Precipitate Heart Failure in Older Adults

Anemia
Alcohol
Intercurrent infection, including pneumonia, endocarditis
Fluid overload (often postoperatively)
Thyrotoxicosis
Drugs (e.g., nonsteroidal antiinflammatory drugs [NSAIDs], thiazolidinediones)
Atrial fibrillation
Myocardial ischemia
Altered drug adherence
Pulmonary emboli
Obstructive sleep apnea

Assessing factors that go beyond heart function is therefore critical in older adult patients, suggesting that elements of frailty assessment should inform heart failure management.[20,21] Such an approach is crucial in the older adult patient for whom issues such as adherence to treatment plans, cognition, and continence figure prominently in the clinical decision making process.

The prognosis for heart failure, although improved in recent years by drug treatment, is nevertheless still poor. Most patients with NYHA Class IV disease (Table 39-1) will be unlikely to survive 1 year.

A study of older men admitted as inpatients with heart failure revealed that the 1-year mortality was about 50%,[22] although the mortality rate is reduced in those who survive for the first few months after hospitalization. Given this poor prognosis, alleviation of symptoms and improving daily function are as important as any potential mortality benefits for many older adult patients.[23]

CAUSES OF HEART FAILURE

Heart failure has been described as a syndrome rather than a diagnosis or disease, and the underlying cause must always be sought in patients having the syndrome. HFREF is most frequently caused by ischemic heart disease, particularly previous myocardial infarction, although hypertension and diabetes also contribute to the cause. However, in older adult patients, valvular heart disease may cause left ventricular (LV) systolic dysfunction or exacerbate HFREF caused primarily by ischemic heart disease. Less frequently, HFREF in the older adult patient may be caused by one of the cardiomyopathies (e.g., viral or idiopathic), amyloidosis, storage diseases (e.g., hemochromatosis), secondary to chemotherapy (e.g., doxorubicin, trastuzumab [Herceptin]), or vitamin B deficiencies.

Furthermore, many patients have symptoms associated with heart failure in the presence of normal systolic function and no evident valvular disease. HFPEF may be responsible for as much as 50% of heart failure in the older adult population. Hypertension is a key driver of HFPEF, often through the development of left ventricular hypertrophy, which leads to stiffening of the ventricle, but other factors, including microvascular endothelial dysfunction,[24] mild degrees of valvular dysfunction, and atrial fibrillation, with the loss of atrial kick to assist with filling a stiff ventricle, may also contribute. Recent data have suggested that obesity is also an important causative factor in HFPEF, in part by alteration of hemodynamics and respiratory function, but also via the effects or, or resistance to, adipocytokine secretion (e.g., adiponectin, leptin).[25] Not infrequently, heart failure will be precipitated by anemia, alcohol, and a number of other factors.[26] Obstructive sleep apnea is frequently underdiagnosed, often coexists with obesity, and is itself a risk factor for cardiovascular disease, as well as a precipitant for heart failure (Box 39-1).

PATHOPHYSIOLOGY

It is now clear than heart failure is a systemic disease, affecting not just the heart and vasculature, but involving most organ systems, including lung, skeletal muscle, brain, kidneys, gut, and adipose tissue. The relationships among these involved organs are mediated by derangements of inflammation and immunologic signaling, neurohormonal axes, and other circulating factors, several of which are also implicated in relation to frailty.[16] As previously noted, heart failure may occur with reduced ejection fraction (HFREF) or preserved ejection fraction (HFPEF); these entities share some common risk factors but have important differences in pathophysiology.

The pathophysiology of heart failure is multifactorial, especially in older adult patients in whom hypertensive heart disease and valvular heart disease are more common. There may be structural abnormalities within the heart, together with overcompensatory mechanisms in the renin-angiotensin-aldosterone system (RAAS), sympathetic nervous system, and peripheral vasculature. Although there are specific changes in the cardiovascular system with age (see Chapter 14) such as increased calcification, increased myocardial fibrosis, and reduced ventricular compliance, most older adult patients with heart failure have additional pathology to explain their symptoms. In patients with heart failure due to ischemia, remodeling can result in alterations in the shape and morphology of the left ventricle,[27] ultimately with left ventricular dilation and a large end-diastolic volume. In addition to changes in the structure of the left ventricle, many older adult patients have associated calcific degeneration of the aortic and mitral valves, with functional and hemodynamically significant consequences. The cardiomyopathies are also a small but significant cause of heart failure in older adult patients, although the widely seen asymmetric septal hypertrophy itself is not of great significance.[28] In hypertensive patients with left ventricular hypertrophy, the increase in collagen content of the ventricular wall and associated myocardial fibrosis may lead to diastolic filling abnormalities, which may contribute to the symptoms of heart failure, and represent a pathophysiologic substrate for HFPEF. In addition, loss of atrial contraction can result in significant hemodynamic deteriorations because atrial systole has an increased importance in older adult patients when left ventricular wall stiffness is increased.[29,30]

In a healthy person, cardiac output is influenced directly by stroke volume and heart rate. In the failing heart, stroke volume is maintained by increasing the left ventricular end-diastolic pressure and volume, which is the basis of the Starling law of the heart. However, eventually, at very high left ventricular end-diastolic volumes, there will be no subsequent compensatory increase in cardiac output. One of the aims of heart failure treatment is to minimize increases in left ventricular end-diastolic pressure so that cardiac output can be maintained and subsequent tissue oxygenation will be adequate for perfusion of the vital organs.

In older adults, heart failure with preserved systolic function (HFPEF) becomes increasingly more common. Although this entity shares risk factors (e.g., hypertension, diabetes) with HFREF, it appears to be pathophysiologically distinct. A history of myocardial infarction is less common, obesity is more common, and derangements of adipokine levels and function appear to play a role. Although subtle derangements of systolic function are seen in HFPEF, impaired relaxation and ventricular filling are important. Left ventricular dilation is not a feature, and cardiac output remains well matched to the degree of peripheral vasodilation.[31] Similar systemic derangements, including those of neurohormonal systems, cytokines, and skeletal muscle function, are seen in HFPEF and HFREF, but the reasons why some patients develop HFPEF and some develop HFREF are poorly understood.

The autonomic nervous and neuroendocrine systems initially support the failing heart, but ultimately the compensatory mechanisms may themselves prove harmful. Activation of the RAAS can result in increased levels of angiotensin and aldosterone in the heart, kidney, brain, and vascular system, with undesirable consequences.[32] Furthermore, the associated high levels of plasma adrenaline and noradrenaline (epinephrine and norepinephrine) are associated with a poor prognosis due to deleterious effects on myocardial function, autonomic balance, and peripheral vascular function.

In both HFREF and HFPEF, changes in the morphology of skeletal muscle may explain the fatigability seen in heart failure patients over and above that expected with reduced tissue blood supply.[33,34] Disruption of the microvasculature is also seen with impaired endothelial function. These changes are usually consequences of the disease process and not merely related to age, although in extremely old patients with mild symptoms of cardiac failure, true pathologic processes and age-related processes may be difficult to differentiate. Such age-related changes include a reduction of cardiac output on exercise, increase in end-systolic volume, decrease in ejection fraction with exercise, and reduced heart rate with exercise. It is important to note, however, that heart failure is a disease with systemic effects—derangements of immune function cause a proinflammatory response[35] that may in itself be cardiotoxic and contributes to the development of anemia; circulating cytokines may also help drive the prominent skeletal myopathy that accompanies heart failure and is the major cause of tiredness and breathlessness in heart failure patients. This skeletal myopathy in turn causes abnormalities of ergoreceptor function[36] that drive further sympathetic nervous system activation. Disturbance of lung architecture and gas exchange are seen in the lungs of heart failure patients, even in the absence of overt fluid overload, a further contributor to the symptoms of heart failure.

DIAGNOSIS OF HEART FAILURE

It is often straightforward to recognize heart failure when the patient has pronounced symptoms and signs accompanied by echocardiographic evidence of left ventricular dysfunction. The diagnosis is often more difficult when symptoms are mild; signs may be absent in the early stages of the disease and, even later, might chiefly be due to frailty syndrome or functional decline without overt dyspnea. Differentiating HFPEF from other causes of exercise intolerance and breathlessness may be particularly difficult.

The European Society of Cardiology (ESC) has developed guidelines for the diagnosis of heart failure[3] (Table 39-2). The American College of Cardiology (ACC) and American Heart Association (AHA) guidelines[4] approach diagnosis in a similar way. For the clinician who is faced with an older adult patient with suspected heart failure, two questions should be considered before further assessment:

1. Are the patient's symptoms at least partly cardiac in origin?
2. If so, what type of cardiac disease is producing these symptoms?

TABLE 39-2 Diagnosis of Heart Failure (HF)

HFREF: All Three Present	HFPEF All Four Present
Symptoms typical of HF	Symptoms typical of HF
Signs typical of HF	Signs typical of HF
Reduced LVEF	Normal or only mildly reduced LVEF; left ventricle not dilated
	Relevant structural heart disease (LVH, enlarged left atrium, diastolic dysfunction)

Modified from McMurray JJ, Adamopoulos S, Anker SD, et al: ESC guidelines for the diagnosis and treatment of acute and chronic heart failure 2012: the Task Force for the Diagnosis and Treatment of Acute and Chronic Heart Failure 2012 of the European Society of Cardiology. Developed in collaboration with the Heart Failure Association (HFA) of the ESC. Eur Heart J 33:1787–1847, 2012.

HFREF, Heart failure with reduced ejection fraction; *HFPEF,* heart failure with preserved ejection fraction; *LVEF,* left ventricular ejection fraction; *LVH,* left ventricular hypertrophy.

TABLE 39-3 Symptoms and Differential Diagnoses of Heart Failure in Older Patients

Classic Symptoms	Atypical Features	Differential Diagnoses
Dyspnea	Lethargy	Anemia
Orthopnea	Confusion	Chronic obstructive pulmonary disease
Peripheral edema	Falls	Depression or anxiety
	Dizziness	Hypothyroidism
	Syncope	Hypoalbuminemia
	Immobility	Malnutrition
		Renal disease
		Neoplasia
		Lymphedema

Table 39-3 lists the typical and atypical symptoms in the older adult patient with suspected heart failure and potential differential diagnoses.

The diagnosis of heart failure is especially difficult because it is not defined by an absolute level of any one parameter, as is the case with a number of other diseases. Consequently the diagnosis is a judgment based on a careful history and examination, chest radiology, electrocardiography, echocardiography, and other routine baseline investigations, such as complete blood count, serum biochemistry, and thyroid function.

Clinical History

The most classic symptom of heart failure is exertional breathlessness. However, this is a common symptom and is often a result of chronic obstructive pulmonary disease (COPD), deconditioning, obesity, or interstitial lung disease. Most people will experience some breathlessness with moderate exertion and, during exercise, the stage at which breathlessness is experienced depends on the overall level of fitness.

Anemia and obesity are confounding factors that make exertional dyspnea a very nonspecific symptom. Orthopnea is a more specific symptom that does not occur in normal patients and is not usually a feature in respiratory disease. However, the disease process has to be relatively advanced before orthopnea occurs and, even if it is present, diuretics have often been instituted by the patient's general practitioner to relieve this symptom. Likewise, paroxysmal dyspnea (PND) is a more extreme version of dyspnea and is a result of fluid redistribution, which increases the left ventricular end-diastolic pressure. Again, PND is specific but is an insensitive symptom because it signifies significant fluid overload, which should have been noted and previously treated.

Fatigue and lethargy are other common problems in heart failure, but they are even harder to define and assess than dyspnea, particularly in older adult patients. Fatigue is common in people who are ill and more common still in older adults who are frail; indeed, it forms one of the components of Fried and colleagues' phenotypic definition of frailty.[38]

Ankle edema is a common presenting feature but, again, there are many alternative causes, such as cor pulmonale, deep venous thrombosis, dependent edema, or hypoalbuminemia.

Risk factors for heart failure may also assist the diagnosis. In particular, myocardial infarction is a key risk factor for future HFREF.[39] Although hypertension is an important risk factor for both HFREF and HFPEF, the prevalence of hypertension is so high in older adults that it becomes less useful as a diagnostic discriminator. Additional features that may suggest the diagnosis of heart failure include excessive alcohol intake, history of rheumatic fever, or presence of atrial fibrillation. Note too, however, that heart failure is associated with cognitive impairment, including memory impairment and frontal lobe dysfunction, which often manifests with slowness and decreased initiative.[6] In consequence, it is easy in a busy clinical practice to be misled by incomplete or seemingly vague answers; both false-positive and false-negative responses can put the history off track.

Physical Signs

Many of the physical signs of heart failure are nonspecific and of relatively low predictive value. These include tachycardia, pulmonary crepitations, and peripheral edema. Equally, many of the physical signs that are specific to heart failure are insensitive because they occur only once the heart failure has become severe. These include elevation of the jugular venous pressure, a gallop rhythm, and displacement of the cardiac apex beat. The situation is further compounded by the variable ability of physicians to detect these clinical signs.[40] As a result, diagnosis may be difficult, especially in older adults who may be less likely to present with typical signs. Signs are less likely to manifest in mild heart failure, and diuretic therapy often leads to rapid resolution of signs of fluid overload. Such a response to diuretic therapy can be used to assist with the diagnosis. The probability of the diagnosis of heart failure thus requires signs and symptoms to be considered by the individual clinician, making full use of clinical judgment.

Investigations

Investigations in patients with suspected heart failure are aimed at the following: (1) confirming the diagnosis; (2) searching for other diseases likely to contribute to the symptom complex (such diseases often coexist with heart failure); and (3) defining the cause and subtype of heart failure.

Chest X-Ray

Chest x-ray should be performed routinely. Cardiac enlargement (cardiothoracic ratio > 50%) implies cardiomegaly and, if present, suggests a higher probability of HFREF.[41] However, many heart failure patients do not exhibit cardiomegaly, so it is a specific but insensitive test. Other helpful chest x-ray findings are pulmonary edema, upper lobe diversion, fluid in the horizontal fissure, and Kerly B lines in the costophrenic angles. In severe cases, pleural effusions may be present, although there may be alternative explanations for them, such as bronchial carcinoma, pneumonia, or pulmonary emboli.

A chest x-ray can reveal other clues about noncardiac disease that might be causing breathlessness. A lung tumor might be obvious, and evidence of COPD or pulmonary fibrosis may also be present. Nevertheless, the chest x-ray should be seen as a whole. For example, the finding of cardiomegaly plus bilateral pleural effusions, with no other parenchymal lung disease, makes heart failure likely—although the presence of structural heart disease should still be confirmed by echocardiography.

Electrocardiography

The 12-lead electrocardiogram (ECG) should be obtained routinely. Left ventricular systolic dysfunction is rare in the presence of a completely normal 12-lead ECG, making it a useful rule-out test. For HFREF, an abnormal resting ECG is sensitive (94%), with excellent negative predictive value (98%), but is much less specific (61%) and has a poor positive predictive value (35%).[42] Most studies suggest that this is the case; where there is doubt, an echocardiogram should be obtained.

Other abnormalities on the ECG may be useful in the assessment of patients. For example, the presence of atrial fibrillation may be useful in concluding whether the patient should receive additional anticoagulation.

Echocardiography

The optimum investigation in the older adult patient with suspected heart failure is echocardiography. Measurement of the left ventricular ejection fraction is the preferred index of systolic function[43] because it is simple and less prone to error from regional wall motion abnormalities than alternatives. Regional wall motion indices are an alternative approach, but these are less widely used in practice. Echocardiography can clearly distinguish whether the left ventricle is dilated; this approach for assessing left ventricular dimensions is superior to chest x-ray.

Echocardiography can also identify patients with mitral valve disease or aortic stenosis, which may both contribute to the syndrome of heart failure and indicate who may benefit from surgery. It can also assess left ventricular wall thickness, and hence hypertrophy, and left atrial size, both important for making a diagnosis of HFPEF. Finally, echocardiography can be used to assess diastolic dysfunction. Debate continues about the optimum way to assess this, and an array of indices should be measured and reported. Key measurements include the mitral inflow pattern and tissue Doppler measures of longitudinal shortening of the ventricle.

When echocardiography proves to be technically difficult, objective assessments of left ventricular function may be made by radionuclide ventriculography or by cardiac magnetic resonance (MRI) scanning. Figure 39-1 suggests an approach for diagnosing heart failure in practice.

Natriuretic Peptides

The natriuretic peptides (NPs) released from the atrium and ventricles have a variety of cellular effects, act as vasodilators, and cause a natriuresis. They have been shown to reflect left ventricular wall stress. Natriuretic peptide levels (usually B-type natriuretic peptide [BNP] or its cleavage product, N-terminal [NT] pro-BNP) are useful in excluding heart failure in acute and chronic situations. Low levels (<35 pg/mL of BNP or <125 pg/mL of NT pro-BNP) are thresholds recommended by the ESC[3] in the chronic situation to rule out heart failure and should prompt a search for alternative diagnoses, especially if the ECG is also normal. Higher levels do not make the diagnosis of heart failure, because any cardiac abnormality (e.g., myocardial ischemia, atrial fibrillation, left ventricular hypertrophy) can lead to elevated BNP levels. However, elevated levels should prompt further investigations, including echocardiography.

In summary, the diagnosis of heart failure is a sequential one that relies on a clear clinical history and examination followed by electrocardiography, chest radiology, or echocardiography. Echocardiography is desirable in all cases, although it may not be

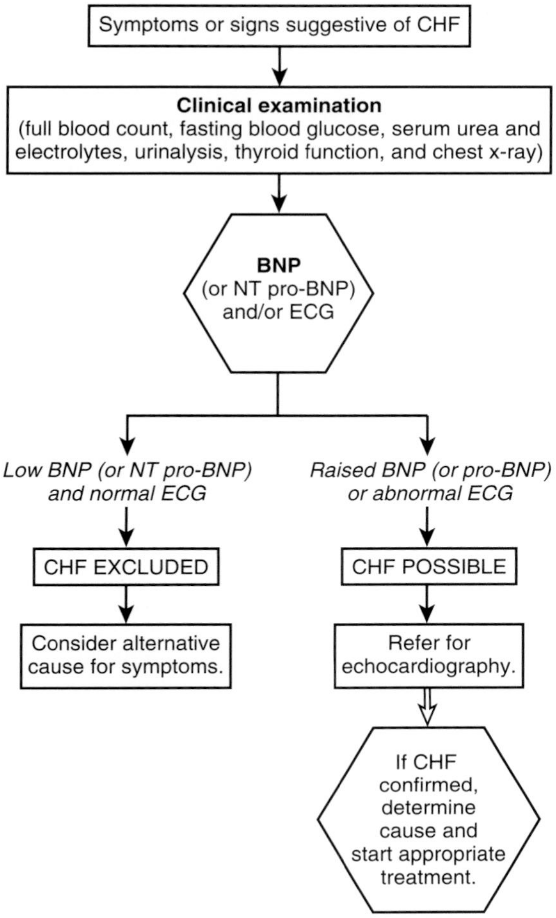

Figure 39-1. Diagnostic algorithm for patients with suspected chronic heart failure (CHF). BNP, B-type natriuretic peptide; ECG, electrocardiogram; NT pro-BNP, N-terminal pro-BNP.

readily available in the community or in small hospitals. Nevertheless, it is probably more important to obtain an echocardiogram for the older adult patient before initiating treatment because structural abnormalities are more common, and optimum treatment requires as accurate a diagnosis as possible so that adverse effects may be kept to a minimum.

TREATMENT OF HEART FAILURE

General Issues

Since the 1960s, when loop diuretics were introduced, treatments for heart failure have diversified. As the pathophysiology of heart failure has become clearer, treatment options have broadened and a number of agents, including angiotensin-converting enzyme (ACE) inhibitors, β-blockers, and aldosterone antagonists, have now been shown to improve prognosis. It is now known that the impairments in left ventricular function and the peripheral circulation can be treated, with consequent hemodynamic improvement. Neurohumoral activation can be blocked and left ventricular remodeling reduced. These adverse consequences of heart failure are the targets of drug treatment. As a result, patients may require multidrug treatment, and priorities need to be established. It is important that patients and their caregivers understand the implications of their treatment.

TABLE 39-4 Summary of Treatment Options for Heart Failure in Older People

	HFREF	HFPEF
Recommended	Diuretics; ACE inhibitor or ARB β-blocker, aldosterone antagonist	Diuretics
Adjunctive therapy	Nitrates or hydralazine (if ACE inhibitor– or ARB-intolerant), digoxin, biventricular pacing (if dyssynchrony), intravenous iron	Intravenous iron
Possible benefit	Exercise training	ACE inhibitor or ARB, exercise training

ACE, Angiotensin-converting enzyme; *ARB,* angiotensin receptor blocker; *HFREF,* heart failure with reduced ejection fraction; *HFPEF,* heart failure with preserved ejection fraction.

In the frail older adult patient, quality of life and alleviation of symptoms are especially important. The major clinical trials of heart failure have generally excluded older patients, so that most patients enrolled in studies are in the age range of 50 to 70 years, favoring single-system and single-cause disease. Although the mean age of patients enrolled in heart failure trials is rising, it still lags behind the age of most heart failure patients.[44] Typical heart failure patients are not only old but are often frail, with many active comorbid illnesses that may require management.

Such complex patients require multidimensional evaluation and management in the hospital and in the community. This ensures that a full picture of the patient's abilities, needs, and wishes is obtained, so that the goals of treatment are fully aligned with what the patient requires. It is clearly of little use to treat heart failure with all the recommended therapies but to impair function and quality of life further through the development of intolerable side effects.

As with all medication use in older adults, a drug should be started at a low dose and titrated in relation to the response, especially because patients may be taking over-the-counter preparations, and the potential for drug interactions is considerable.[45] Each of the aforementioned drug classes will be considered in more detail but, in addition to the main therapeutic options, drugs that have less proven efficacy will be discussed (Table 39-4).

Pharmacologic Agents

Diuretics

Diuretics are fundamental to the treatment of chronic heart failure. The loop diuretics introduced in the 1960s were shown to be very effective in reducing symptoms associated with fluid retention, and they had a clear hemodynamic benefit. Studies have shown deterioration in symptomatic heart failure when diuretics are withdrawn,[46] and diuretics have been shown to reduce mortality and hospitalization in chronic heart failure.[47]

The loop diuretics, which include furosemide and bumetanide, block the sodium-potassium-chloride transport exchange in the ascending limb of the loop of Henle. Thiazides have a different site of action and work in the distal convoluted tubule. Spironolactone has a different mode of action, antagonizing the aldosterone-mediated sodium exchange with potassium and hydrogen in the collecting ducts. In older adult patients with heart failure, the rate of absorption of loop diuretics and time to peak plasma concentration are reduced because renal function is often impaired. High doses of diuretics may need to be used to produce a diuresis because the coexisting relative acidosis results in increased competition for the organic acid transport pathway at the proximal tubule. The bioavailability of furosemide can be vary considerably, from 20% to 80%, but is more consistent with bumetanide.[48] Most of the loop diuretics have a fairly short half-life, about 1 to 2 hours. In contrast, the thiazide and potassium-sparing diuretics have longer half-lives, which allow once-daily doses to be given. Tolerance can occur to diuretics, and this has clinical relevance. The natriuretic response diminishes after the first dose, but this can be reversed by restoring intravascular volume. Long-term administration of a loop diuretic can also result in tolerance, which can be addressed by combining loop and thiazide diuretics together.

When furosemide is given to patients with severe acutely decompensating heart failure, high doses should be used until symptoms and signs of fluid overload have been controlled. An intravenous dose of 40 to 50 mg is often sufficient to control the symptoms; but when resistance to loop diuretics occurs, up to 250 to 500 mg/day may be required. In resistant cases, furosemide can be given by a continuous infusion, up to 4 g/day.

Thiazides (e.g., metolazone, high-dose bendroflumethiazide) can be used for resistant edema and heart failure. They block sodium reabsorption in the proximal convoluted tubule, along with having effects on the distal convoluted tubule. They can result in a profound diuresis, and postural hypotension may be significant if intravascular volume depletion is too extreme. Close monitoring of electrolytes is essential.

When patients with heart failure are being treated with a diuretic, it is essential to monitor plasma biochemistry regularly. Particular electrolyte disturbances include the following: hypokalemia, which may precipitate cardiac arrhythmias; hyponatremia, which may cause drowsiness and fits; and hypomagnesemia, which may cause a number of cellular effects, including muscle weakness and arrhythmias. Hypokalemia may be alleviated by the concomitant use of potassium-sparing diuretics such as spironolactone or by using an ACE inhibitor (see later discussion). Diuretic treatment can also result in disturbances of lipid metabolism, glucose intolerance, and hyperuricemia.

In addition to these diuretic side effects, older adult patients are prone to difficulties with urinary incontinence, immobility, postural hypotension, dehydration, and confusion. These problems should be prominent in the prescriber's mind when initiating treatment in an individual patient. It is also important not to administer intravenous furosemide rapidly because this may precipitate an irreversible hearing loss.

A study of older adults[49] assessed the impact of discontinuing diuretic therapy for those with relatively mild symptoms of heart failure; patients with severe symptoms and acute heart failure and those requiring intravenous diuretics were excluded. In the follow-up period, diuretic therapy had to be reintroduced in half of the patients in whom it had been withdrawn because of symptomatic deterioration. Even though the patients in whom diuretic therapy had to be restarted were relatively well, this study highlights the likelihood of a recurrence of symptoms if diuretics are discontinued in an older adult population.

Angiotensin-Converting Enzyme Inhibitors

ACE inhibitors block overactivity of the RAAS and sympathetic nervous system. In addition to these effects, ACE inhibitors enhance the bradykinin–nitric oxide system in the vascular endothelium.[50] They may also have an influence outside the circulation in various tissues, including skeletal muscle.[51] ACE inhibitors are now known to reduce morbidity and mortality in patients with left ventricular systolic dysfunction, regardless of symptom severity,[52-54] and are also effective at improving exercise capacity and symptoms, even in very old heart failure patients.[55,56] Mechanistically, ACE inhibitors are vasodilators with subsequent reduction in cardiac preload and afterload, resulting in hemodynamic and symptomatic improvement for patients with heart failure. In addition to reducing the pathologic overactivity of the RAAS, ACE inhibitors have beneficial effects on the endothelium and may also have antiischemic effects.[57] ACE inhibitors inhibit adverse remodeling of the myocardium after infarction and lead to reductions in ventricle size and improvements in ejection fraction in patients with LV systolic dysfunction.

The main contraindications to treatment with ACE inhibitors are severe aortic stenosis and renal impairment. Patients who are volume-depleted are more likely to experience hypotension with the initial dose, so ACE inhibitors should be introduced when patients are euvolemic or fluid-overloaded. Treatment should be started at a low dose and gradually uptitrated until the maximum achievable dose is obtained. In general terms, the optimal benefit is obtained at the top end of the dosage range. The ATLAS study[58] compared low and high doses of lisinopril in heart failure, and patients with higher dosages fared better. However, a low dose of ACE inhibitor is likely to be of more benefit than none. Renal function and electrolytes should be monitored at regular intervals, initially every few days or weekly and then every 3 to 6 months. It may be possible to reduce the dose of maintenance diuretic therapy once the patient has been established on ACE inhibition. Although aortic stenosis has traditionally been thought of as a contraindication to ACE inhibitor therapy, patients with mild to moderate aortic stenosis started on an ACE inhibitor appear to have a lower mortality than controls in observational studies.[59] Severe aortic stenosis, however, remains a contraindication to ACE inhibitor therapy.

The effects of ACE inhibitors on heart failure appear to be a class effect, and there is little to choose among the once-daily ACE inhibitors in current use. The main side effects of ACE inhibitors include cough, hypotension, hyperkalemia and, rarely, angioneurotic edema. The occurrence of a cough with ACE inhibitors should prompt a switch to an angiotensin receptor blocker (ARB). Although orthostatic hypotension can occur in patients treated with an ACE inhibitor, this is much less common with once-daily agents and is often precipitated by hypovolemia due to overdiuresis or by underlying vascular disease, rather than the treatment itself. Rather than stopping the ACE inhibitor, the first response should be to reduce the diuretic dose.

The clear benefit of ACE inhibitors in HFREF is not mirrored in patients with HFPEF. The PEP-CHF study[60] compared perindopril with a placebo in older adult patients with preserved systolic function heart failure. There was no significant reduction in mortality, but symptoms and hospitalization were improved in the perindopril group. A recent meta-analysis has confirmed the lack of benefit of ACE inhibitors on mortality in HFPEF[61] and also does not suggest benefit in hospitalization or symptoms. In practice, however, many older adults with HFPEF will require an ACE inhibitor for another indication, such as myocardial infarction, hypertension, or stroke disease.

β-Blockers

Overstimulation of the sympathetic nervous system is an important component of the pathophysiology underlying heart failure, and β-blockers are now well established as a key component of therapy for HFREF. An improved understanding of the pathophysiology of heart failure has highlighted the role for β-blockers in reducing the effects of vasoconstriction and fluid retention associated with heart failure. Blockade of the sympathetic nervous system by β-blockers complements the beneficial effects of ACE inhibitors on the RAAS. β-Blockers also have an antiarrhythmic effect and also facilitate coronary blood flow by prolonging diastole. Blockade of the adrenergic system may reduce adrenaline (epinephrine)-mediated myocyte cell loss and myocyte dysfunction, thus reducing associated left ventricular systolic dysfunction.[62] Furthermore, the promotion of cellular growth and ventricular remodeling, which is mediated by noradrenaline (norepinephrine), is blocked by β-blockers. It also appears that β-blockade may reduce some of the uncoupling of the β-receptors from their G protein at a cellular level, preventing further deterioration in systolic function.[63]

A meta-analysis of several very large trials has confirmed that β-blockers reduce overall mortality, overall hospitalization and heart failure specific death, and hospitalization. The most recent estimate of effect size suggests a 27% reduction in mortality.[64] Older adults (≥75 years) appear to benefit, although the benefit appears much less than in those with atrial fibrillation. Although the major trials of β-blockade used bisoprolol, metoprolol, or carvedilol, network meta-analysis has suggested no significant differences in efficacy across a range of different β-blockers, suggesting that the benefit is a class effect.[65]

It is important that the dose be carefully titrated, with a close evaluation following each uptitration to detect worsening heart failure or associated hypotension. Uptitration of the dose should occur only when the patient is stable, but β-blockers should not be discontinued during admissions for decompensated heart failure unless cardiogenic shock supervenes. Although most patients will show some improvement in their clinical condition, and the progression of heart failure is reduced, exercise capacity may be only marginally improved by treatment. However, hospital admissions for decompensated heart failure are less frequent overall.

Contraindications include bradycardia, atrioventricular block beyond the first degree, hypotension, asthma, or COPD with significant reversibility. It is worth noting that many patients with COPD can tolerate β-blockade, and such patients were successfully enrolled in the CIBIS II trial of bisoprolol in heart failure.[66] Problems with tolerability may be accentuated if the patient is taking other cardioactive medications. Patients with peripheral vascular disease may also find β-blockers difficult to tolerate.

Until recently, data on the tolerability of β-blockade in older heart failure patients were lacking. Some studies have suggested that β-blockers are tolerated by most older heart failure patients,[67] and the SENIORS trial[68] specifically evaluated a cohort of older patients with heart failure (mean age, 76 years). In this study, nebivolol had a significant effect on reducing hospital admissions, although the impact on all-cause mortality did not reach significance, and the effects in patients older than 75 years appeared less than in the younger old.

β-Blockers are not specifically indicated for treatment of HFPEF; current evidence suggests no benefit on hospitalization or mortality.[69] However, the high prevalence of comorbid cardiovascular disease (especially atrial fibrillation, angina, and hypertension) in this group of patients means that many will have other indications for β-blockade.

Aldosterone Antagonists

Aldosterone is another key hormone with a wide range of deleterious effects, including worsening of endothelial function, myocyte hypertrophy, increased afterload, and myocardial fibrosis. In HFREF, aldosterone antagonists have been shown to reduce mortality and hospitalization in NYHA classes II, III, and IV heart failure.[70,71] Small doses of spironolactone (25 to 50 mg/day) were well tolerated in the RALES trial and reduced total mortality by 30% in the treatment group. Deaths from progressive heart failure and sudden deaths were reduced equally, and the incidence of severe hyperkalemia was low in both arms of the study. Similar, albeit small, benefits were seen in patients with LV systolic dysfunction after myocardial infarction who were taking the aldosterone antagonist eplerenone.[72] In both cases, aldosterone antagonists were used in addition to ACE inhibitors or ARBs. The evidence that spironolactone improves exercise capacity in heart failure is less strong, and trial data are limited in the very old.

Clinical experience of spironolactone in older adults with heart failure suggests the need for caution. The incidence of renal dysfunction and hyperkalemia in older adults in clinical practice is up to 10 times that seen in the RALES trial, and inappropriate use of spironolactone outside the indications used in the RALES trial may lead to a high incidence of side effects, possibly negating the beneficial effects seen in the trials.[73,74] Dehydration due to intercurrent illness (e.g., diarrhea, vomiting) commonly precipitates acute kidney injury in older adult patients taking aldosterone antagonists; this situation requires very close monitoring of renal function and possibly withdrawal of aldosterone antagonists for a few days until the intercurrent illness has resolved.

Spironolactone is not currently indicated for patients with HFPEF; the recent TOPCAT trial[75] failed to reduce a composite outcome of death or hospitalization in this patient group, although heart failure–specific hospitalization was reduced by 17%.

Digoxin

Digoxin has been used in the treatment of heart failure for over 200 years. It is a positive inotrope, and the effects of digoxin are mediated by inhibition of Na^+,K^+-ATPase, which influences intracellular sodium, with resultant influences on sodium-calcium exchange across the sarcolemmal membrane. It has a relatively narrow therapeutic window, with the result that side effects are common, particularly in older adults with renal impairment and hypokalemia.

In addition to its effects on the myocardium, digoxin is a weak diuretic, can cause gastric irritation, and has a mild estrogenic effect. It also has anticholinergic effects,[76] which may increase the risk of falls and delirium. In HFREF, digoxin improves the cardiac output and stroke volume index, with a resultant improvement in hemodynamic status in heart failure patients. The side effects of digoxin are more pronounced in patients with hypokalemia because potassium competes for the binding site at the site of action.

Evidence from the DIG trial,[77] which examined the effect of digoxin in HFREF patients in sinus rhythm, showed that total mortality was no different between the digoxin and placebo groups. Heart failure deaths were reduced in the digoxin group, but there was a trend toward an increase in deaths because of arrhythmias or myocardial infarction. Hospital admissions were significantly reduced. The trial was, however, performed before current triple-therapy regimens were in widespread use. Thus, digoxin may have a role in HFREF patients who are intolerant of standard therapy or remain symptomatic, despite standard therapy. Digoxin has multiple side effect, however, and, even for HF patients in atrial fibrillation, it is a less effective therapeutic choice than β-blockers for rate control. β-Blockers not only control rate better, especially during exertion, but have proven benefits on mortality, hospitalizations, and symptoms.

In older adult patients, close monitoring of digoxin therapy is essential. With impaired renal function and reduced clearance of the drug, symptomatic nausea and fatigue are probably the most frequent complication, together with bradycardia. A number of therapeutically important drug interactions also exist with digoxin, particularly with quinidine and amiodarone. It is also sometimes difficult to distinguish between digoxin toxicity and the underlying symptoms of cardiac failure; digoxin is also capable of precipitating delirium in older adults. Digoxin is the third most commonly implicated drug in admissions precipitated by medication side effects; the balance between potential benefits for patients with refractory heart failure must always be carefully weighed against this side effect profile.

The maintenance dosage of digoxin in heart failure should not usually exceed 125 μg/day in older adults because side effects are more common if the dosage is higher. In addition, patients in the intervention arm of the DIG trial with plasma levels of digoxin above 1.2 ng/mL had a higher risk of death than those in the placebo arm.[78] Clinical response, not digoxin level, should guide dosing; the digoxin level is a poor guide to tissue levels or effects of digoxin.

Angiotensin Antagonists

Blockade of the angiotensin receptor provides an alternative method for attenuating the deleterious effects of angiotensin II without the side effects of increasing bradykinin levels that are caused by ACE inhibition. A meta-analysis have suggested that similar benefits accrue from ARB therapy as for ACE inhibitor therapy in HFREF, with a more favorable side effect profile.[79] Studies comparing ARBs with placebo are less common; meta-analysis of these studies has suggested a borderline significant reduction in mortality of 13%. In a recent meta-analysis examining the effect of ARB therapy in patients with HFPEF, no benefit was seen in all-cause mortality or cardiovascular mortality,[61] although a trend to reduced hospitalization with ARB use was seen, driven by the results from the CHARM Preserved Trial of candesartan.[80]

These agents are generally well tolerated and should be used as an alternative therapy in patients who are intolerant of ACE inhibition because of cough. Concern exists, however, that multiple blockade of the RAAS may lead to an increased incidence of side effects, particularly renal impairment, which may limit the usefulness of this approach. Older adults, who are more likely to suffer from renal impairment, falls, or intercurrent illness, are likely to be particularly at risk from dual blockade, and this should be avoided. A meta-analysis of trials in HFREF, in which ARBs were added to baseline ACE inhibitor therapy, has confirmed that such an approach does not reduce mortality or hospitalization, but does increase the risk of adverse events.[79] The effect of ARBs on exercise capacity in older adults people are not well studied, but ARBs may improve exercise time.[81]

Ivabradine

Reduction in heart rate has physiologic benefits in the failing myocardium, independently of the mechanism by which this is achieved—diastolic filling is improved, coronary blood flow is enhanced, and myocardial ischemia is ameliorated. Ivabradine acts to block the I_f channel in the sinoatrial node, thus reducing heart rate. The large SHIFT trial[82] compared ivabradine with placebo in 6552 patients with HFREF, who were in sinus rhythm with a heart rate higher than 70 beats/min. Patients could be taking β-blockers but have inadequate rate control or could be intolerant of β-blockers. Although only marginal, nonsignificant reductions were seen for all-cause and cardiovascular mortality; there were significantly fewer hospitalizations for heart failure or for all causes in the ivabradine group.

Ivabradine may thus have a role as adjunctive therapy in older adults who are unable to tolerate β-blockers at sufficient dose to bring their heart rate below 70 beats/min. Ivabradine is also effective as an antianginal agent, so it provides an additional treatment option for patients with a combination of heart failure and angina. The rate of symptomatic bradycardia is higher in patients treated with ivabradine, which may be of particular importance for those at risk of falls. It is also important to note that ivabradine is ineffective in patients with atrial fibrillation due to its selective action on the sinoatrial node. Caution is warranted, however; few older adult patients were enrolled in SHIFT, and the benefits appeared markedly attenuated in those older than 65 years. In small trials in younger patients, ivabradine improved exercise capacity and health-related quality of life[83-85]; the improvements seen with ivabradine were considerably greater than those seen with β-blockers. There is, however, no information about whether these findings hold true in older HFREF patients. One trial showed improvements in exercise capacity in patients with HFPEF,[86] but no large-scale trials of ivabradine in HFPEF have been reported to date.

Other Pharmacologic Agents

Nitrates and Hydralazine. In the first Veterans Administration Cooperative Heart Failure trial (V-HeFT 1), isosorbide dinitrate and hydralazine[87] were compared with prazosin and placebo in patients with NYHA class II or III heart failure. There was a mild improvement in mortality in the nitrate and hydralazine group, and ejection fraction and exercise performance also improved. The most notable effect was seen in patients of African ethnicity, and these findings were confirmed in patients with severe heart failure in the more recent A-HeFT study.[88] This highlights the potential value of nitrates and hydralazine as an intervention for patients unable to tolerate ACE inhibition who remain severely symptomatic.

Inotropes. Chronic use of positive inotropes has been largely unhelpful, with most trials showing no effect or increased mortality.[89-91] Short-term use of intravenous positive inotropes may be useful in select patients—for example, as a bridge to ventricular assist device placement—but their overall benefit is limited.

Iron Therapy. Anemia commonly accompanies heart failure. As a chronic inflammatory state, heart failure may induce anemia of chronic disease, and coexisting renal dysfunction may further exacerbate anemia. Iron deficiency from other pathologies may also coexist, thus worsening symptoms. For clear iron deficiency, investigation of the cause, with oral iron replacement, may suffice. For anemia of chronic disease, oral iron is unlikely to provide benefit, and intravenous iron is preferred; in select patients with renal impairment, erythropoietin may be required as well. Intravenous iron improves symptoms and exercise capacity and reduces hospitalization in patients with heart failure and low serum ferritin levels, and this benefit is not restricted to those with anemia at baseline.[92]

Arrhythmia Management. Cardiac arrhythmias are common in patients with heart failure. Patients with atrial fibrillation should be managed with anticoagulation and rate control where possible; β-blockers are more effective and less toxic than digoxin. Conversion to sinus rhythm can prove difficult because the atrial fibrillation is often long-standing, and rhythm control has little benefit in most patients.[93] Ventricular arrhythmias are also relatively common in patients with heart failure. These ventricular arrhythmias may cause considerable hypotension and may even be fatal. Implantable cardioverter-defibrillators (ICDs) are now first-line therapy for malignant ventricular arrhythmias in patients with reduced ejection fraction, although amiodarone may be required to reduce the frequency of shocks. Amiodarone may also be used as an alternative therapy in patients with frequent arrhythmias and significant frailty or comorbid disease, for whom the survival benefit offered by ICD implantation is unlikely to be realized.

Antianginal Therapy. Patients with heart failure who have associated angina and myocardial ischemia should be treated for their ischemic heart disease by conventional means. Patients may require treatment with aspirin, β-blockade, statins, oral nitrates, non–rate-reducing calcium antagonists, or other nonpharmacologic measures. In patients with symptomatic ischemic heart disease and LV systolic impairment, LV performance may be improved by coronary bypass surgery. Such patients may have a hibernating area of myocardium, which could potentially be salvaged following bypass surgery. The large Surgical Treatment for Ischaemic Heart Failure (STICH) trial,[94] however, did not find a reduction in overall mortality with revascularization, although cardiovascular deaths were lower in the surgical arm compared to medical therapy alone.

Combined Inhibitors. Results from combining inhibitors of neprilysin (an enzyme that breaks down natriuretic peptides) with ACE inhibitors have been disappointing, with high rates of angioedema as a side effect.[95] However, a recent large trial of HFREF patients receiving joint inhibition of neprilysin with angiotensin receptor blockade suggested a significant reduction in death, heart failure, hospitalization, and symptoms with joint inhibition compared to enalapril therapy.[96] Questions remain, however, about whether the comparison group were adequately treated, and experience of these new agents in a wider population of older adults is required before firm conclusions about their place in the therapeutic armamentarium can be reached.

Multidisciplinary Team Interventions

There is evidence to support multidisciplinary intervention and involvement in older heart failure patients. The combination of nurse specialist intervention, pharmacist medication review, and education, plus physician intervention, led to reduced hospitalization and improved symptom control and quality of life in a U.S. trial.[19]

Both clinic-based and home-based multidisciplinary team (MDT) models have been used successfully. The addition of telemonitoring—for example, of weight and symptoms—or using more sophisticated invasive measures of hemodynamic function may be a useful adjunct to standard approaches. Systematic reviews have suggested a reduction in mortality and hospitalization with telemonitoring and structured telephone follow-up,[97] but care is required because the mean age for most trial participants was younger than 75 years, and the benefits of telemonitoring in older frail populations with multiple comorbidities are less apparent.[98] Given the burden of symptoms and need for regular health care input, the general support provided by members of the MDT can have considerable impact on the well-being and general care provided to the older adult patient with heart failure. Traditional medicine for older adult outpatients is also an area in which coordinated care with several health care professionals can improve patient experiences when more assistance is required than with outpatient clinic consultation.

Role of the Heart Failure Nurse

Heart failure nurses have a critical role to play in coordinating heart failure care, monitoring patients' symptoms, educating patients and caregivers, and uptitrating medications. They are therefore a pivotal member of the MDT. Older heart failure patients, with their complex care needs, are particularly well placed to benefit from the skills of the heart failure nurse. Studies have confirmed that case management led by a heart failure nurse leads to lower levels of mortality and readmission in heart failure patients.[99]

When quality of life is a major consideration, coordination of care from heart failure nurses, often in conjunction with a palliative care team, can result in better control of symptoms and ensure that patients remain in community-based settings rather than in larger hospitals, where they would be more prone to develop iatrogenic problems, including delirium.

Other Considerations

Exercise in Congestive Heart Failure. There is good evidence that at least for younger heart failure patients, regular submaximal aerobic or resistance exercise training leads to important improvements in symptoms, quality of life, reduction in hospitalizations, and reduction in mortality.[100,101] However, there are few studies in older heart failure patients to guide the type, duration, and intensity of exercise intervention best suited to older heart failure patients.

In younger old patients, group circuit exercise in cardiac rehabilitation classes[102] appears successful, but in older frailer patients, neither gentle seated exercise[103] nor more vigorous exercise[104] appear to be efficacious. Alternative exercise regimens, perhaps based more around resistance training, may be needed.[105]

Patients with uncontrolled atrial fibrillation, active sepsis, decompensated fluid overload, severe aortic stenosis, or malignant ventricular arrhythmias (unless an ICD is placed) should probably not participate in exercise but, for other patients, exercise appears remarkably safe. An exercise intensity of up to 70% to 80% of maximal should be the aim; in practical terms, this is a level at which patients can still talk. The optimal session frequency and length have yet to be determined, but will depend on symptoms and practicalities such as a suitable venue and transportation. It is important to note that exercise training needs to be continued for sustained benefit; improvements in exercise capacity are lost rapidly on cessation of exercise. Exercise programs should therefore be capable of being continued at home, unsupervised, rather than being confined to supervised sessions in a hospital or outpatient setting. As with any exercise intervention program, the challenge is to ensure that the specific regimen can be maintained long enough for the older adult patient to derive benefit from the intervention.

Smoking Cessation. Smoking increases the chance of further myocardial ischemic events and directly worsens tissue oxygenation. Smoking should always be actively discouraged in patients with heart failure, however old they are. Counseling remains the cornerstone of intervention for those prepared to cease smoking. Nicotine replacement may be used with care in patients with stable coronary artery disease and no history of malignant ventricular arrhythmias, and bupropion may be useful in carefully selected patients without other contraindications.

Alcohol. Alcohol has depressant effects on the myocardium and also interacts with common comorbid diseases, particularly urinary incontinence, in which the excess of fluid and decreased sensation caused by alcohol may worsen incontinence. Consumption in older people should therefore be limited to one or two units daily, in line, with current population-level guidance. Patients with alcoholic cardiomyopathy should be strongly encouraged to abstain totally.

Diet. Surprisingly little data exist to guide practice regarding diet in heart failure. Many older adults with heart failure are overweight and, although obesity may reduce exercise tolerance still further, cohort studies have suggested that overweight heart failure patients survive longer than patients of normal weight. The value of calorie restriction in heart failure has not been subjected to randomized controlled trials, and caution thus seems appropriate in recommending this, even in obese patients.

Cardiac cachexia is associated with advanced disease and a particularly poor prognosis. Dietary approaches to reversing cardiac cachexia have not been subjected to randomized trials but may not be successful, given that cachexia is a syndrome of catabolism resistant to protein supplementation. Nevertheless, a pragmatic approach to dietary intervention in underweight heart failure patients is probably merited, given the overlap with other chronic causes of frailty and undernutrition seen in older adults.

Although salt and fluid restriction has long been promoted as beneficial in controlling heart failure symptoms, practical issues limit the applicability of this advice. Efforts should be made to avoid excessive fluid consumption, but salt restriction below the recommended 6 g/day limit is often difficult in older adult patients who may have deeply ingrained cooking habits and a reliance on preprepared foods, and for whom the flavor-enhancing properties of salt are important in stimulating appetite and food intake.

FRAILTY, SARCOPENIA, AND HEART FAILURE

Frailty is common in patients with heart failure; this is perhaps not surprising because several of the cardinal features of heart failure, such as low activity levels and exhaustion, are also components of the phenotype of frailty. Between 15% and 45% of heart failure patients fulfil the criteria for frailty,[21] with an additional 30% in the prefrail category. Frail heart failure patients are more likely to be hospitalized and more likely to die than nonfrail patients; interestingly, frail patients without heart failure are also more likely to develop incident heart failure, perhaps because of the relationship between underlying vascular disease and skeletal muscle dysfunction.

Frailty is closely related to sarcopenia, the loss of muscle mass that commonly accompanies ageing. However, the sarcopenia of age is typified by the loss of type II muscle fibers and loss of maximum muscle strength, whereas the myopathy commonly seen in heart failure is characterized by a loss of endurance and selective loss of type I muscle fibers.[106] Overlap syndromes may well occur in older adults, and this area requires further research. Heart failure and sarcopenia share a number of pathophysiologic features, including elevated proinflammatory cytokine profiles and deleterious effects of RAAS system activation.

Evaluating frailty is important for prognostication in older heart failure patients and may also be a useful tool for selecting patients for therapies such as ventricular assist devices; further research is needed in this area. Frail adult patients are those most likely to benefit from comprehensive geriatric assessment; therefore, screening for frailty, especially by nongeriatricians, can provide a way to determine those patients for whom collaborative management between cardiology and geriatric medicine teams is of particular value.[21]

OTHER PROBLEMATIC DISEASE INTERACTIONS

Heart failure in older adults never exists in isolation, and the essence of good care of older adults with heart failure is to balance the management of their heart failure with management of their comorbid diseases, taking into account their physical and psychologic state, quality of life, and treatment preferences. Comorbidity in heart failure patients may cause specific problems, including delayed diagnosis, because of confusion about the relevance of particular symptoms. Treatment options may be limited because of contraindications or cautions with particular drug treatments, and patients may be hospitalized for other treatment, including surgical problems (e.g., fracture of the femoral neck). Some comorbidities are so common in heart failure (e.g., cardiovascular disease, diabetes, hypertension, renal dysfunction) to merit being considered as part of the heart failure syndrome; management of these conditions in heart failure is well covered elsewhere and will not be discussed here.[107] The following comorbid conditions often lead to particular problems in patients with heart failure and are of particular importance in older heart failure patients.

Chronic Obstructive Pulmonary Disease

Because s smoking is a risk factor for heart failure and COPD, the syndromes often coexist. This may make diagnosis more challenging; in older adults experiencing breathlessness, it is often necessary to investigate for both syndromes. Severe COPD may also lead to right heart dysfunction as the underlying cause of the heart failure syndrome.

Management of heart failure in the presence of COPD still involves ACE inhibitors and diuretics; however, overdiuresis may cause a precipitous drop in cardiac output and blood pressure if the right ventricle is impaired because the impaired ventricle requires high filling pressures. β-Blockers can be used in many patients with COPD unless significant reversible airway obstruction is present. There are theoretical advantages to using β_1-selective agents. In many patients, only an empirical trial of β-blockers will show if they are tolerated.

Patients with COPD often have pulmonary hypertension. The more severe the pulmonary hypertension, the worse the prognosis and, in patients with severe pulmonary hypertension, pulmonary artery pressure is a stronger predictor of prognosis than other cardiac parameters.

Exercise in the form of pulmonary rehabilitation is an important component of therapy for COPD, and exercise training should thus be encouraged when both conditions exist. Smoking, needless to say, should be firmly discouraged.

Urinary Incontinence

Incontinence, always a prevalent problem in older adults, is a particular problem in older patients with heart failure. Reduced mobility and exercise capacity mean that reaching a toilet in time may be difficult, and the use of diuretics may lead to large urine volumes accumulating, with little warning. This in turn leads to activity restriction because patients are worried about leaving the house after taking diuretics or, worse, patients deliberately miss diuretics, leading to decompensation of heart failure. Nocturia may also be a problem in patients with heart failure; lying flat causes excess fluid to redistribute from the lower extremities, increasing renal blood flow and urine excretion.

Careful adjustment of the dose and timing of diuretics is needed to circumvent these problems. Dividing doses, avoiding diuretics late in the day, or using diuretics with a slower onset of action such as torasemide[108] may all help. Use of interventions such as ACE inhibitors and exercise may help improve exercise capacity, thus allowing patients to reach the toilet more easily.

Cognitive Impairment

Cognitive impairment is common in older patients with heart failure, almost certainly a result of the two major causes of cognitive impairment that share vascular risk factors with heart failure.[6] Several cognitive impairment syndromes are more likely in those with heart failure, including delirium, cognitive impairment from vascular causes that might not meet dementia criteria, and dementia itself—for example, Alzheimer disease, vascular dementia, and mixed syndromes.[109] Any degree of cognitive impairment may cause problems with adherence to medication, the ability to undertake self-monitoring (e.g., weight), and the ability to understand and retain information about the illness, medications, and prognosis.

Such problems should be anticipated, and strategies to manage issues such as medication (e.g., dosette boxes), close involvement of caregivers in education, fluid management, meal preparation, and medication administration are vital. Heart failure itself is not necessarily a contraindication to anticholinesterase inhibitor therapies, but care is needed to ensure that there is no evidence of underlying atrioventricular (AV) or sinoatrial (SA) node disease or that other rate-limiting drugs do not cause heart block.

It is worth noting that the risk of progression to dementia in patients with heart failure is up to twice that of healthy older people.[110,111] Although cognitive impairment is associated with hypotension, anemia, and hyperglycemia, there is no robust evidence that addressing these issues can prevent or modify the problem of cognitive impairment, although improvements may occur in some individual patients, particularly after treatment of very low-output states in those with advanced heart failure.[112]

Depression

Depression is common in heart failure patients, as is the case for many older adults with chronic disease. Debate continues as to whether depression is truly an independent risk factor for death in heart failure, although some evidence has suggested that this may be the case, but there is no doubt that it exacerbates symptoms and worsens an already poor quality of life.

As with all unwell older adults, depression should be sought whenever a comprehensive assessment is performed, preferably using a screening tool such as the Geriatric Depression Scale or the Hospital Anxiety and Depression Scale. Psychological interventions (particularly cognitive behavioral therapy) remain the cornerstone of treatment for mild to moderate depression in the general older adult population; more severe depression may require drug treatment. Existing data on the treatment of heart failure (specifically in heart failure) are mixed. Cognitive behavioral therapy has not shown benefit in heart failure patients with depression, and selective serotonin reuptake inhibitors (SSRIs) have shown mixed results.[113] The known cardiotoxic side effects of tricyclic antidepressants mean that this class should be avoided. Other evidence has suggested that SSRIs and related classes are relatively safe for use in those with heart failure. Despite the evidence base suggesting benefits of treatment, many older adults remain reluctant to undergo treatment for their depression.

Other Considerations

Rationalizing the Drug Burden

Heart failure as a disease entity often entails a large number of extra medications. Added to the medications that patients often need to take for their comorbid diseases, this presents a substantial burden (including financial) to patients, increases the chances of drug-drug interactions, and makes adherence to therapy less likely.[114]

It is possible to use heart failure treatments for multiple indications, especially for multiple vascular diseases, which may help reduce the burden of therapy. ACE inhibitors will help treat hypertension and reduce the risk of myocardial infarction; β-blockers can be used for rate control in atrial fibrillation (AF), reducing blood pressure and treating angina. If further antianginals are needed, nitrates can have further beneficial effects on blood pressure and heart failure. Such approaches may provide a way of reducing the number of vascularly active medications taken by a patient. In some patients, sodium restriction and the use of ACE inhibitors may even allow diuretics to be withdrawn, with consequent improvement in urinary continence and urge symptoms. Such an approach may then allow other medications aimed at the urinary tract to be reduced or stopped. Patients generally are compliant in taking their heart failure medication because they often have experienced disabling symptoms that they do not want to recur. Caution is particularly required when treating coexisting conditions. In this regard, a clinical pharmacist can often provide timely advice regarding potential adverse effects.

Device Therapy

Two major advances in device therapy for heart failure have become commonplace rather recently—ICDs and cardiac resynchronization therapy (CRT), also known as biventricular pacing. The two devices can also be combined into a single unit (ICD-CRT).

In patients with a significantly impaired ejection fraction, ICDs are known to reduce mortality rates by providing timely treatment of ventricular arrhythmias.[115] However, considerable discussion is required before using such devices in older heart failure patients with multiple comorbid diseases; these devices do not improve physical function or quality of life, may cause significant psychological distress (not to mention physical discomfort from defibrillation shocks), and will not prolong life in the presence of the multiple system failures that are the hallmark of frailty.

Cardiac resynchronization on the other hand may dramatically improve cardiac function, exercise capacity, symptoms, and quality of life in carefully selected patients with HFREF and significant dyssynchrony between the left ventricular septum and free wall—in particular those with left bundle branch block. Patients with relatively mild disease (NYHA classes I and II) can benefit, as well as those with severe symptoms.[60,116] Such devices may also allow sufficient hemodynamic improvement for other medications to be tolerated, such as ACE inhibitors and β-blockers.

Advanced Therapies

Few very old patients with heart failure are likely to be eligible for cardiac transplantation; in many countries, age is still an explicit contraindication to transplantation listing. Recent advances in left ventricular assist devices (LVADs) have brought the possibility of using such devices as destination therapy, rather than merely as a bridge to transplantation and, in carefully selected older adults with otherwise end-stage heart failure, such devices can avoid certain death. Experience is beginning to accrue with implantation in those 70 years of age and older,[117] but careful selection is likely to be needed to ensure that the benefits of such devices are not cancelled by the high complication rates and considerable burden of therapy.[118]

Palliative Care for Congestive Heart Failure

For patients with end-stage heart failure, there is good evidence to suggest that control of symptoms can be effectively managed by palliative care teams. The emphasis of most medical treatment approaches in heart failure is extending the duration of life but, sadly, there are many heart failure patients who do not have the opportunity to die a good death. However, involvement of palliative medicine specialists in the care of heart failure patients is now becoming more widespread, in part via clinical networks. Palliative care specialists, general practitioners, community nursing teams, heart failure specialist nurses, geriatricians, and physicians working in managed clinical networks provide opportunities for relevant health care professionals to access expert symptom control and end of life care planning and execution. It is important to ensure that palliative expertise is deployed well before the end of life; such approaches can and should be used along with conventional life-prolonging therapies. As heart failure becomes more advanced, the emphasis shifts more toward the relief of symptoms and away from simply prolonging life. Sometimes difficulties occur when trying to predict an individual patient's prognosis accurately; the disease trajectory in heart failure is often one of relapses and remissions, often making identification of the terminal phase of the illness difficult. This is particularly the case in older heart failure patients, in whom frailty and other comorbid diseases, each with their own effects on symptoms, function, and prognosis, will interact with heart failure. Close teamwork can facilitate decisions to optimize palliative care in this setting, without prematurely withdrawing treatment.

Communication is key; ideally, patients should appreciate the prognosis in heart failure, which is worse than for breast and colorectal cancers. As the illness advances, sensitive discussions should take place to explore whether patients would like life-prolonging therapy, including hospital admission, intubation, and inotropic support during exacerbations, and whether they would like to undergo cardiopulmonary resuscitation in the event of cardiac arrest. Involvement of caregivers, as desired by patients, together with meticulous documentation of such discussions, can go a long way toward preparing the patients and their friends and family for the day when further efforts to prolong life become futile. Perhaps, in older adult patients, it is easier to have these discussions when the person has lived a full life, but even when this is the case, discussions have to be very sensitive because patient's families often find the discussions more painful than the patients themselves.

Near the end of life, some medications may be withdrawn if they are not contributing to symptom management. Similarly, some devices, particularly ICDs, may be deactivated to prevent inappropriate shocks when such therapy will no longer prolong an acceptable quality of life. Intractable breathlessness may be alleviated by small doses of opiates; older adult patients with end-stage heart failure commonly also have pain, which is underreported.[119] Good palliative care involves the provision of support for all the patient's needs, including psychosocial and spiritual. Thus, the narrow medical model used to manage heart failure or other chronic disease early in the course of the disease becomes less and less relevant as the illness progresses. In the final stages of heart failure, the environment of the patient may be just as important as any other factor. Purpose-built palliative care facilities (hospices) can help provide a more calm environment, but patients would more often prefer to be in their own homes at the end of life.

CONCLUSIONS

Chronic heart failure is a major cause of morbidity and mortality in older adult patients. Optimum treatment requires an accurate diagnosis. Clinical and examination findings should be confirmed by objective assessments, including chest radiology, electrocardiography, and particularly echocardiography.

Once an accurate diagnosis has been established, treatment should follow the recent guidelines of the ESC and the AHA, where possible, with consideration of the specific requirements of the individual patient. ACE inhibitors and β-blockers should be tried in all patients with HFREF, with the addition of aldosterone blockers in select cases, where they are tolerated. The prognosis for chronic heart failure is poor and, when treating the older adult patient, emphasis should always be on improving the patient's quality of life and symptom control, rather than merely delaying death.

Other agents should be chosen in the light of contraindications to these major treatments. Digoxin, nitrates, hydralazine, and device therapy, especially biventricular pacing, are potentially useful adjunctive therapies. Multidisciplinary care is crucial, as with all older patients, and staff skilled in the care of older adults should be closely involved in teams caring for heart failure patients. Exercise training, smoking cessation, and avoidance of excessive fluid and salt are important adjuncts to pharmacologic therapy.

KEY POINTS

- Heart failure is common in older adults and frequently coexists with frailty syndromes.
- Half of older heart failure patients have heart failure with preserved ejection fraction (HFPEF).
- Echocardiography remains essential to guide therapy, even in the oldest frailest patients. B-type natriuretic peptide can also help diagnose or exclude heart failure.
- Therapy for heart failure with reduced ejection should be based on β-blockers and RAAS inhibitors, but with the caveat that few trials have included very old people.
- There is still little evidence to guide therapy for heart failure with preserved ejection fraction.
- Biventricular pacing and exercise training may have significant benefits in select patients.
- Therapy must be adapted to the large burden of comorbid disease that typically accompanies heart failure in older adults.
- A multidisciplinary approach to care can improve heart failure management; good palliative care and planning for the end of life are essential in managing heart failure in older adults.

For a complete list of references, please visit www.expertconsult.com.

KEY REFERENCES

2. Yousaf F, Collerton J, Kingston A, et al: Prevalence of left ventricular dysfunction in a UK community sample of very old people: the Newcastle 85+ study. Heart 98:1418–1423, 2012.
3. McMurray JJ, Adamopoulos S, Anker SD, et al: ESC guidelines for the diagnosis and treatment of acute and chronic heart failure 2012: the Task Force for the Diagnosis and Treatment of Acute and Chronic Heart Failure 2012 of the European Society of Cardiology. Developed in collaboration with the Heart Failure Association (HFA) of the ESC. Eur Heart J 33:1787–1847, 2012.
4. Yancy CW, Jessup M, Bozkurt B, et al: 2013 ACCF/AHA guideline for the management of heart failure: a report of the American College of Cardiology Foundation/American Heart Association Task Force on Practice Guidelines. J Am Coll Cardiol 62:e147–e239, 2013.
11. McDonagh TA, Morrison CE, Lawrence A, et al: Symptomatic and asymptomatic left-ventricular systolic dysfunction in an urban population. Lancet 350:829–833, 1997.
13. Owan TE, Hodge DO, Herges RM, et al: Trends in prevalence and outcome of heart failure with preserved ejection fraction. N Engl J Med 355:251–259, 2006.
19. Rich MW, Beckham V, Wittenberg C, et al: A multidisciplinary intervention to prevent the readmission of elderly patients with congestive heart failure. N Engl J Med 333:1190–1195, 1995.
30. Fleg JL: Alterations in cardiovascular structure and function with advancing age. Am J Cardiol 57:33C–44C, 1986.
44. Masoudi FA, Havranek EP, Wolfe P, et al: Most hospitalized older persons do not meet the enrollment criteria for clinical trials in heart failure. Am Heart J 146:250–257, 2003.
56. Abdulla J, Abildstrom SZ, Christensen E, et al: A meta-analysis of the effect of angiotensin-converting enzyme inhibitors on functional capacity in patients with symptomatic left ventricular systolic dysfunction. Eur J Heart Fail 6:927–935, 2004.

68. Flather MD, Shibata MC, Coats AJ, et al: Randomized trial to determine the effect of nebivolol on mortality and cardiovascular hospital admission in elderly patients with heart failure (SENIORS). Eur Heart J 26:215–225, 2005.
70. Pitt B, Zannad F, Remme WJ, et al: The effect of spironolactone on morbidity and mortality in patients with severe heart failure. Randomized Aldactone Evaluation Study Investigators. N Engl J Med 341:709–717, 1999.
77. The effect of digoxin on mortality and morbidity in patients with heart failure. N Engl J Med 336:525–533, 1997.
80. Yusuf S, Pfeffer MA, Swedberg K, et al: Effects of candesartan in patients with chronic heart failure and preserved left-ventricular ejection fraction: the CHARM-Preserved Trial. Lancet 362:777–781, 2003.
82. Swedberg K, Komajda M, Bohm M, et al: Ivabradine and outcomes in chronic heart failure (SHIFT): a randomised placebo-controlled study. Lancet 376:875–885, 2010.
93. Roy D, Talajic M, Nattel S, et al: Rhythm control versus rate control for atrial fibrillation and heart failure. N Engl J Med 358:2667–2677, 2008.
97. Pandor A, Thokala P, Gomersall T, et al: Home telemonitoring or structured telephone support programmes after recent discharge in patients with heart failure: systematic review and economic evaluation. Health Technol Assess 17:1–207, 2013.
101. O'Connor CM, Whellan DJ, Lee KL, et al: Efficacy and safety of exercise training in patients with chronic heart failure: HF-ACTION randomized controlled trial. JAMA 301:1439–1450, 2009.
102. Austin J, Williams R, Ross L, et al: Randomised controlled trial of cardiac rehabilitation in elderly patients with heart failure. Eur J Heart Fail 7:411–417, 2005.
111. Vogels RL, Scheltens P, Schroeder-Tanka JM, et al: Cognitive impairment in heart failure: a systematic review of the literature. Eur J Heart Fail 9:440–449, 2007.
113. Woltz PC, Chapa DW, Friedmann E, et al: Effects of interventions on depression in heart failure: a systematic review. Heart Lung 41:469–483, 2012.
116. Cleland JG, Daubert JC, Erdmann E, et al: The effect of cardiac resynchronization on morbidity and mortality in heart failure. N Engl J Med 352:1539–1549, 2005.

40 Diagnosis and Management of Coronary Artery Disease

Wilbert S. Aronow

The most common cause of death in older adults is coronary artery disease (CAD). Coronary atherosclerosis is very common in older adults, with autopsy studies demonstrating a prevalence of at least 70% in persons older than 70 years. The prevalence of CAD is similar in older women and men.[1] In one study, clinical CAD was present in 502 of 1160 men (43%), mean age 80 years, and in 1019 of 2464 women (41%), mean age 81 years.[1] At 46-month follow-up, the incidence of new coronary events (myocardial infarction, sudden cardiac death) was 46% in the older men and 44% in the older women.[1]

CAD is diagnosed in older adults if they have coronary angiographic evidence of significant CAD, documented myocardial infarction (MI), typical history of angina pectoris with myocardial ischemia diagnosed by stress testing, or sudden cardiac death. The incidence of sudden cardiac death as the first clinical manifestation of CAD increases with age.

CLINICAL MANIFESTATIONS

Dyspnea on exertion is a more common clinical manifestation of CAD in older adults than the typical chest pain of angina pectoris. The dyspnea is usually exertional and is related to a transient rise in left ventricular (LV) end-diastolic pressure caused by ischemia superimposed on reduced LV compliance. Because older adults are more limited in their activities, angina pectoris is less often associated with exertion. Older adults with angina pectoris are less likely to have substernal chest pain, and they describe their anginal pain as less severe and of shorter duration than younger persons. Angina pectoris in older adults may occur as a burning postprandial epigastric pain or as pain in the back or shoulders. Acute pulmonary edema unassociated with an acute MI may be a clinical manifestation of unstable angina pectoris due to extensive CAD in older adults.[2]

Myocardial ischemia, appearing as shoulder or back pain in older adults , may be misdiagnosed as degenerative joint disease. Myocardial ischemia, appearing as epigastric pain, may be misdiagnosed as peptic ulcer disease. Nocturnal or postprandial epigastric discomfort that is burning in quality may be misdiagnosed as hiatus hernia or esophageal reflux instead of myocardial ischemia because of CAD. The presence of comorbid conditions in older adults may also lead to misdiagnosis of symptoms as a result of myocardial ischemia.

Older adults with CAD may have silent or asymptomatic myocardial ischemia.[3-5] In a prospective study of older adults with CAD, 133 of 195 men (68%), mean age 80 years, and 256 of 771 women (33%), mean age 81 years, had silent myocardial ischemia detected by 24-hour ambulatory electrocardiograms (ECGs).[5] At 45-month follow-up, the incidence of new coronary events in older men with CAD was 90% in those with silent myocardial ischemia versus 44% in older men without silent ischemia.[5] At 47-month follow-up, the incidence of new coronary events in older women with CAD was 88% in those with silent ischemia versus 43% in older women without silent ischemia.[5]

The reason for the frequent absence of chest pain in older patients with CAD is unclear.

RECOGNIZED AND UNRECOGNIZED MYOCARDIAL INFARCTION

Pathy[6] reported that in 387 older patients with acute MI, 19% had chest pain, 56% had dyspnea or neurologic or gastrointestinal symptoms, 8% had sudden death, and 17% had other symptoms. Another study showed that in 110 older patients with acute MI, 21% had no symptoms, 22% had chest pain, 35% had dyspnea, 18% had neurologic symptoms, and 4% had gastrointestinal symptoms (Box 40-1).[7] Other studies have also shown a high prevalence of dyspnea and neurologic symptoms in older patients with acute MI.[8-10] In these studies, dyspnea was present in 22% of 87 patients,[8] in 42% of 777 patients,[9] and in 57% of 96 patients.[10] Neurologic symptoms were present in 16% of 87 patients,[8] 30% of 777 patients,[9] and 34% of 96 patients.[10]

As with myocardial ischemia, some patients with acute MI may be completely asymptomatic or the symptoms may be so vague that they are unrecognized by the patient or physician as an acute MI. Studies have reported that 21% to 68% of MIs in older patients are unrecognized or silent.[7,11-17] These studies also found that the incidence of new coronary events, including recurrent myocardial infarction, ventricular fibrillation, and sudden death in patients with unrecognized MI is similar to[11,14-16,18] or higher[19] than in patients with recognized MI.

Older patients with acute MI have a higher prevalence of non–ST-segment elevation MI (NSTEMI) with absence of pathologic Q waves than ST-segment elevation MI (STEMI) with pathologic Q -waves.[20-22] Of 91 consecutive patients with acute MI aged 70 years and older, mean age 78 years, 61 (75%) had NSTEMI.[21] Of 4,017,367 patients aged 65 years and older with acute MI during 2001to 2010, 64.3% had NSTEMI.[22] During this period, STEMI decreased 16.4% in patients with acute MI aged 65 to 79 years and by 19% in patients with acute MI aged 80 years and older.[22]

DIAGNOSTIC TECHNIQUES

Resting Electrocardiography

In addition to diagnosing recent or prior MI, the resting ECG may show ischemic ST-segment depression, arrhythmias, conduction defects, and LV hypertrophy related to subsequent coronary events. At 37-month mean follow-up, older patients with ischemic ST-segment depression 1 mm or greater on the resting ECG were 3.1 times more likely to develop new coronary events than were older patients with no significant ST-segment depression.[23] Older patients with ischemic ST-segment depression of 0.5 to 0.9 mm on the resting ECG were 1.9 times more likely to develop new coronary events during 37-month follow-up than older patients with no significant ST-segment depression.[23] At 45-month mean follow-up, pacemaker rhythm, atrial fibrillation, premature ventricular complexes, left bundle branch block, intraventricular conduction defect, and type II second-degree atrioventricular block were associated with a higher incidence of new coronary events in older patients.[24] Numerous studies

BOX 40-1 Presenting Symptoms in 110 Older Patients With Acute Myocardial Infarction

- Dyspnea was present in 35% of patients.
- Chest pain was present in 22% of patients.
- Neurologic symptoms were present in 18% of patients.
- Gastrointestinal symptoms were present in 4% of patients.
- No symptoms were present in 21% of patients.

Modified from Aronow WS: Prevalence of presenting symptoms of recognized acute myocardial infarction and of unrecognized healed myocardial infarction in elderly patients. Am J Cardiol 60:1182, 1987.

have also demonstrated that older patients with LV hypertrophy on the ECG have an increased incidence of new coronary events.[25-27]

Many studies have found that complex ventricular arrhythmias in older adults with CAD are associated with an increased incidence of new coronary events, including sudden cardiac death.[28-31] The incidence of new coronary events is especially increased in older adults with complex ventricular arrhythmias and abnormal LV ejection fraction (LVEF)[28] or LV hypertrophy.[29] At 45-month follow-up of 395 men with CAD, mean age 80 years, complex ventricular arrhythmias detected by 24-hour ambulatory ECGs significantly increased the incidence of new coronary events by 2.4-fold.[30] At 47-month follow-up of 771 women with CAD, mean age 81 years, complex ventricular arrhythmias detected by 24-hour ambulatory ECGs significantly increased the incidence of new coronary events by 2.5-fold.[30] Over an 8-year follow-up of 2192 ambulatory volunteers aged 70 to 79 years without CAD, major baseline ECG abnormalities (Q waves, bundle branch block, atrial fibrillation or flutter, or major ST-T wave changes) were associated with a 50% increased risk of coronary events independent of conventional risk factors.[32] Minor ST-T changes were associated with a 35% increased risk of coronary events independent of conventional risk factors.[32]

Stress Testing

Exercise Stress Testing

Hlatky and colleagues[33] found the exercise ECG to have a sensitivity of 84% and specificity of 70% for the diagnosis of CAD in persons older than 60 years. Newman and Phillips[34] found a sensitivity of 85%, specificity of 56%, and positive predictive value of 86% for the exercise ECG in diagnosing CAD. The increased sensitivity of the exercise ECG with increasing age found in these two treadmill exercise studies was probably due to the increased prevalence and severity of CAD in older adults.

Exercise stress testing also has prognostic value in older patients with CAD.[35-37] Deckers and associates[37] demonstrated that the 1-year mortality was 4% for 48 patients 65 years of age or older who were able to do an exercise stress test after acute MI and 37% for the 63 older patients unable to do the exercise stress test after acute MI.

Exercise stress testing using thallium perfusion scintigraphy, radionuclide ventriculography, and echocardiography is also useful for the diagnosis and prognosis of CAD.[38-40] Iskandrian and coworkers[38] showed that exercise thallium-201 imaging can be used for risk stratification of older patients with CAD. The risk for cardiac death or nonfatal MI at 25-month follow-up in 449 patients 60 years of age or older was less than 1% in patients with normal images, 5% in patients with a single-vessel thallium-201 abnormality, and 13% in patients with multivessel thallium-201 abnormality.

Pharmacologic Stress Testing

Intravenous (IV) dipyridamole thallium imaging may be used to determine the presence of CAD in older patients who are unable to undergo treadmill or bicycle exercise stress testing.[41] In patients 70 years of age or older, the sensitivity of IV dipyridamolethallium imaging for diagnosing significant CAD was 86% and the specificity was 75%.[41] In 120 patients older than 70 years, adenosine echocardiography had a 66% sensitivity and 90% specificity in diagnosing CAD.[42] An abnormal adenosine echocardiogram predicted a threefold risk of future coronary events, independent of coronary risk factors.[42] In 120 patients older than 70 years, dobutamine echocardiography had a 87% sensitivity and 84% specificity in diagnosing CAD.[42] An abnormal dobutamine echocardiogram predicted a 7.3-fold risk of future coronary events.[42] In 101 patients older than 70 years, the sensitivity and specificity of dipyridamole thallium imaging for CAD were 86% and 75%, respectively, compared with 83% and 70%, respectively, in younger patients.[43] Dobutamine stress echocardiography predicted at 3-year follow-up in 227 octogenarians a 2.7-fold increase in all-cause mortality and a 3.2-fold increase in major cardiovascular events.[44]

Electrocardiography

Ambulatory Electrocardiography

Ambulatory electrocardiography performed for 24 hours is also useful for detecting myocardial ischemia in older adults with suspected CAD who cannot perform treadmill or bicycle exercise stress testing because of advanced age, intermittent claudication, musculoskeletal disorders, heart failure, or pulmonary disease. Ischemic ST-segment changes demonstrated on 24-hour ambulatory ECGs correlate with transient abnormalities in myocardial perfusion and LV systolic dysfunction. The changes may be associated with symptoms, or symptoms may be completely absent, which is referred to as silent myocardial ischemia. Silent myocardial ischemia is predictive of future coronary events, including cardiovascular mortality in older adults with CAD.[3-5,31,45-47] The incidence of new coronary events is especially increased in older adults with silent myocardial ischemia plus complex ventricular arrhythmias,[31] abnormal LVEF,[45] or echocardiographic LV hypertrophy.[47]

Signal-Averaged Electrocardiography

Signal-averaged electrocardiography (SAECG) was performed in 121 older postinfarction patients with asymptomatic complex ventricular arrhythmias detected by 24-hour ambulatory ECGs and an LVEF of 40% or higher.[48] At 29-month follow-up, the sensitivity, specificity, positive predictive value, and negative predictive value for predicting sudden cardiac death were 52%, 68%, 32%, and 83%, respectively, for a positive SAECG; 63%, 70%, 38%, and 87%, respectively, for nonsustained ventricular tachycardia; and 26%, 89%, 41%, and 81%, respectively, for a positive SAECG plus nonsustained ventricular tachycardia.[48]

Multislice Computed Tomography and Magnetic Resonance Imaging

A direct comparison of multislice computed tomography angiography (MSCTA) with magnetic resonance imaging (MRI) for noninvasive coronary arteriography was performed in 129 patients, mean age 64 years, with suspected CAD.[49] Sensitivity for coronary stenoses larger than 50% of luminal diameter was 82% for MSCTA versus 54% for MRI; the respective specificities were 90% and 87%. The negative predictive value was slightly higher for MSCTA (95% vs. 90%). In this study, 74% of patients preferred MSCTA over MRI. The greater diagnostic accuracy of MSCTA over MRI in this study is consistent with meta-analyses of both tests.[50,51]

64-MSCTA and coronary angiography were performed in 145 patients, mean age 67 years, and stress testing was done in 47 of these patients to determine the sensitivity, specificity, positive predictive value, and negative predictive value of these tests in diagnosing obstructive CAD in patients with suspected CAD.[52] Of 145 patients, 64-MSCTA had a 98% sensitivity, 74% specificity, 90% positive predictive value, and 94% negative predictive value in diagnosing obstructive CAD. Of 47 patients, stress testing had a 69% sensitivity, 36% specificity, 78% positive predictive value, and 27% negative predictive value for diagnosing obstructive CAD, whereas 64-MSCTA had a 100% sensitivity, 73% specificity, 92% positive predictive value, and 100% negative predictive value for diagnosing obstructive CAD. 64-MSCTA has a better sensitivity, specificity, positive predictive value, and negative predictive value than stress testing in diagnosing obstructive CAD.[52] The ability to estimate myocardial blood flow and fractional flow reserve with MSCTA may allow more accurate assessment of hemodynamically significant coronary lesions without the need for invasive coronary angiography.[53] Unrecognized MI can be detected by resting electrocardiography, echocardiography, nuclear imaging, or cardiovascular MRI.[54]

CORONARY RISK FACTORS

Cigarette Smoking

The Cardiovascular Health Study of 5201 men and women 65 years of age or older demonstrated that more than 50 pack-years of smoking increased 5-year mortality 1.6-fold.[55] The Systolic Hypertension in the Elderly Program pilot project showed that smoking was a predictor of first cardiovascular event and MI and sudden death.[56] At 5-year follow-up of 7178 persons 65 years of age or older in three communities, the relative risk for cardiovascular disease mortality was 2.0 for male smokers and 1.6 for female smokers.[57] The incidence of cardiovascular disease mortality in former smokers was similar to that in those who had never smoked.[57] At 40-month follow-up of 664 men, mean age 80 years, and at 48-month follow-up of 1488 women, mean age 82 years, current cigarette smoking increased the relative risk of new coronary events 2.2-fold in men and 2.0-fold in women.[58] At 6-year follow-up of older men and women in the Coronary Artery Surgery Study registry, the relative risk of MI or death was 1.5 for persons 65 to 69 years of age and 2.9 for persons 70 years and older who continued smoking compared with those who quit during the year before study enrollment.[59]

Older men and women who smoke cigarettes should be strongly encouraged to stop smoking to reduce the development of CAD and other cardiovascular diseases. Smoking cessation will decrease mortality from CAD, other cardiovascular diseases, and all-cause mortality in older men and women. A smoking cessation program should be instituted.[60]

Hypertension

Systolic hypertension in older adults is diagnosed if the systolic blood pressure is 140 mm Hg or higher from two or more readings on two or more visits.[61] Diastolic hypertension in older adults is similarly diagnosed if the diastolic blood pressure is 90 mm Hg or higher.[61] In a study of 1819 persons, mean age 80 years, living in the community, the prevalence of hypertension was 71% in older African Americans, 64% in elderly Asians, 62% in older Hispanics, and 52% in older whites.[62]

Isolated systolic hypertension in older adults is diagnosed if the systolic blood pressure is 140 mm Hg or higher, with a diastolic blood pressure less than 90 mm Hg.[61] Approximately two thirds of older adults with hypertension have isolated systolic hypertension.[62]

Isolated systolic hypertension and diastolic hypertension are both associated with increased CAD morbidity and mortality in older adults.[63] Increased systolic blood pressure is a greater risk factor for CAD morbidity and mortality than increased diastolic blood pressure.[63] The higher the systolic or diastolic blood pressure, the greater the morbidity and mortality from CAD in older women and men. The Cardiovascular Health Study demonstrated in 5202 older men and women that a brachial systolic blood pressure greater than 169 mm Hg was associated with a 2.4-fold greater 5-year mortality.[55]

At 30-year follow-up of persons 65 years and older in the Framingham Heart Study, systolic hypertension was related to a greater incidence of CAD in older men and women.[64] Diastolic hypertension correlated with the incidence of CAD in older men but not in older women.[64] At 40-month follow-up of 664 older men and 48-month follow-up of 1488 older women, systolic or diastolic hypertension was associated with a relative risk of new coronary events of 2.0 in men and 1.6 in women.[58] Data from the Framingham study have also suggested the importance of increased pulse pressure, a measure of large artery stiffness. Among 1924 men and women aged 50 to 79 years, at any given level of systolic blood pressure of 120 mm Hg or higher, the risk of CAD over 20 years rose with lower diastolic blood pressure, suggesting that higher pulse pressure was an important component of risk.[65] Among 1061 men and women aged 60 to 79 years in the Framingham Heart Study, the strongest predictor of CAD risk was pulse pressure (hazard ratio, 1.24).[66]

Older adults with hypertension should be treated with salt restriction, weight reduction if necessary, cessation of drugs that increase blood pressure, avoidance of alcohol and tobacco, increase in physical activity, decrease of dietary saturated fat and cholesterol, and maintenance of adequate dietary potassium, calcium, and magnesium intake. In addition, antihypertensive drugs have been shown to reduce CAD events in older men and women with hypertension.[67-75]

The Hypertension in the Very Elderly Trial (HYVET) randomized 3845 patients aged 80 years and older, mean age 84 years, with a sitting mean blood pressure of 173/90 mm Hg, to indapamide plus perindopril if needed versus a double-blind placebo.[75] The study was prematurely stopped at 2 years (median follow-up, 1.8 years) because antihypertensive drug therapy reduced fatal or nonfatal stroke by 30%, fatal stroke by 39%, all-cause mortality by 21%, death from cardiovascular causes by 23%, and heart failure by 64%.[75]

Older adults with CAD should have their blood pressure reduced to less than 140/90 mm Hg and to less than 140/90 mm Hg if diabetes mellitus or chronic renal disease is present.[61] Most older patients with hypertension will require two or more antihypertensive drugs to achieve this blood pressure goal.[61] The drugs of choice for treating CAD with hypertension are β-blockers and angiotensin-converting enzyme (ACE) inhibitors.[61,76] If a third antihypertensive drug is needed, a thiazide diuretic should be administered.[61]

Left Ventricular Hypertrophy

Elderly men and women with ECG LV hypertrophy and echocardiographic LV have an increased risk of developing new coronary events hypertrophy.[25-27,29,77] At 4-year follow-up of 406 older men and 735 older women in the Framingham study, echocardiographic LV hypertrophy was 15.3 times more sensitive in predicting new coronary events in older men and 4.3 times more sensitive in predicting new coronary events in older women than electrocardiographic LV hypertrophy.[77] At 37-month follow-up of 360 men and women with hypertension or CAD, mean age 82 years, echocardiographic LV hypertrophy was 4.3 times more sensitive in predicting new coronary events than electrocardiographic LV hypertrophy.[26]

Physicians should try to prevent LV hypertrophy from developing or progressing in older men and women with CAD. A meta-analysis of 109 treatment studies found that ACE inhibitors were more effective than other antihypertensive drugs in decreasing LV mass.[78]

Dyslipidemia

Numerous studies have demonstrated that a high serum total cholesterol level is a risk factor for new or recurrent coronary events in older men and women.[58,79-81] At 40-month follow-up of 664 older men and at 48-month follow-up of 1488 older women, an increment of 10 mg/dL of serum total cholesterol was associated with an increase in the relative risk of 1.12 for new coronary events in men and women.[58]

A low-serum, high-density lipoprotein (HDL) cholesterol level is a risk factor for new coronary events in older men and women.[58,79,82-84] In the Framingham study,[79] Established Populations for Epidemiologic Studies of the Elderly study,[81] and a large cohort of nursing home patients,[58] a low serum HDL cholesterol level was a more powerful predictor of new coronary events than total serum cholesterol. At 40-month follow-up of 664 older men and 48-month follow-up of 1488 older women, a decrement of 10 mg/dL of serum HDL cholesterol increased the relative risk of new coronary events 1.70 times in men and 1.95 times in women.[58]

Hypertriglyceridemia is a risk factor for new coronary events in older women but not in older men.[58,79] At 40-month follow-up of older men and 48-month follow-up of older women, the level of serum triglycerides was not a risk factor for new coronary events in men and was a very weak risk factor for new coronary events in women.[58]

Numerous studies have demonstrated that statins reduce new coronary events in older men and women with CAD.[85-98] The absolute reduction in new coronary events in these studies is greater for older adults than for younger persons. In an observational prospective study of 488 men and 922 women, mean age 81 years, with prior MI and a serum low-density lipoprotein (LDL) cholesterol level of 125 mg/dL or higher, 48% of persons were treated with statins.[89] At 3-year follow-up, statins reduced new coronary events by 50%.[89] The lower the LDL cholesterol level achieved in this study, the greater the reduction in new coronary events.[89]

In the 1263 persons aged 75 to 80 years at study entry and 80 to 85 years at follow-up in the Heart Protection Study, any major vascular event was significantly reduced 28% by simvastatin. Lowering the serum LDL cholesterol level from less than 116 mg/dL to less than 77 mg/dL by simvastatin caused a 25% significant reduction in vascular events.[88]

In the Heart Protection Study, 3500 persons had initial serum LDL cholesterol levels less than 100 mg/dL.[88] A decrease of the serum LDL cholesterol level from 97 to 65 mg/dL by simvastatin in these persons caused a similar decrease in risk, as did treating patients with higher serum LDL cholesterol levels. The Heart Protection Study investigators recommended treating those at high risk for cardiovascular events with statins, regardless of the initial levels of serum lipids, age, or gender.[88]

On the basis of these and other data,[89,95-98] the American College of Cardiology (ACC)/American Heart Association (AHA) guidelines[60] and updated National Cholesterol Education Program III guidelines[99] stated that in very high-risk persons, working toward a serum LDL cholesterol level of less than 70 mg/dL is a reasonable clinical strategy.

A meta-analysis was performed in nine randomized trials of statins for secondary prevention in 19,569 patients aged 65 to 82 years.[100] Over 5 years, statins reduced all-cause mortality by 22%, CAD mortality by 30%, nonfatal by MI 26%, need for revascularization by 30%, and by stroke 25%. The estimated number needed to treat to save one life was 28.[100]

The 2013 ACC/AHA lipid guidelines recommend the use of high-dose statins (20 to 40 mg daily of rosuvastatin or 40 to 80 mg daily of atorvastatin) to adults aged 75 years and younger with arteriosclerotic cardiovascular disease (ASCVD) unless contraindicated with a class I indication.[101] Moderate-dose or high-dose statins are reasonable to administer to persons with ASCVD older than 75 years with a class IIa indication. Persons aged 21 years and older with a serum LDL cholesterol level of 190 mg/dL or higher should be treated with high-dose statins with a class I indication. For primary prevention in diabetics aged 40 to 75 years and a serum LDL cholesterol level between 70 to 189 mg/dL moderate-dose statins should be administered with a class I indication. For primary prevention in diabetics aged 40 to 75 years, a serum LDL cholesterol level between 70 to 189 mg/dL and a 10-year risk of ASCVD of 7.5% or higher calculated from the pooled cohort equation, high-dose statins should be administered with a class IIa indication. For primary prevention in diabetics aged 21 to 39 years or older than 75 years and a serum LDL cholesterol level between 70 to 189 mg/dL, moderate-dose statins or high-dose statins should be administered with a class IIa indication. Adults aged 40 to 75 years without diabetes mellitus or ASCVD with a serum LDL cholesterol level between 70 to 189 mg/dL and a 10-year risk of ASCVD of 7.5% or higher calculated from the pooled cohort equation should be treated with high-dose statins or moderate-dose statins with a class I indication. Adults aged 40 to 75 years of age without diabetes mellitus or ASCVD with a serum LDL cholesterol level between 70 to 189 mg/dL and a 10-year risk of ASCVD of 5% to 7.4%, calculated from the pooled cohort equation, should be treated with moderate-dose statins with a class IIa indication.[101]

Diabetes Mellitus

Diabetes mellitus is a risk factor for new coronary events in older men and women.[58,79,102] In the Cardiovascular Health Study, an elevated fasting glucose level (>130 mg/dL) increased 5-year mortality by 1.9-fold.[55] At 40-month follow-up of 664 older men and 48-month follow-up of 1488 older women, diabetes mellitus increased the relative risk of new coronary events by 1.9-fold in men and 1.8-fold in women.[58] Older diabetics without CAD have a higher incidence of new coronary events than older nondiabetics with CAD.[103]

Persons with diabetes mellitus are more often obese and have higher serum LDL cholesterol and triglyceride levels and lower serum HDL cholesterol levels than nondiabetics. Diabetics also have a higher prevalence of hypertension and LV hypertrophy than nondiabetics. These risk factors contribute to the increased incidence of new CAD events in diabetics compared to nondiabetics. Increased age can further amplify these risk factor differences and contribute to greater CAD risk.

Diabetics with microalbuminuria have more severe angiographic CAD than diabetics without microalbuminuria.[104] Diabetics also have a significant increasing trend of HbA1c levels over the increasing number of vessels with CAD.[105]

Older adults with diabetes mellitus should be treated with dietary therapy, weight reduction if necessary, and appropriate drugs if necessary to control hyperglycemia. The HbA1c level should be maintained at less than 7%.[60,106,107] Other risk factors such as smoking, hypertension, dyslipidemia, obesity, and physical inactivity should be controlled. Diabetics should be treated with statins, as recommended by the 2013 ACC/AHA lipid guidelines.[101] The blood pressure should be reduced to less than 140/90 mm Hg.[61] Metformin is the drug of choice.[107] Sulfonylureas should be avoided in persons with CAD.[108,109]

Obesity

Obesity was an independent risk factor for new CAD events in older men and women in the Framingham Heart Study.[110] Disproportionate distribution of fat to the abdomen assessed by the waist-to-hip circumference ratio has also been shown to be a risk factor for cardiovascular disease, mortality from CAD, and total mortality in older men and women.[111,112]

Obese men and women with CAD must undergo weight reduction. Weight reduction is also a first approach to controlling mild hypertension, hyperglycemia, and dyslipidemia. Regular aerobic exercise should be used in addition to diet to treat obesity. The body mass index should be reduced to 18.5 to 24.9 kg/m^2.[54]

Physical Inactivity

Physical inactivity is associated with obesity, hypertension, hyperglycemia, and dyslipidemia. At 12-year follow-up in the Honolulu Heart Program, physically active men 65 years of age or older had a relative risk of 0.43 for CAD compared with inactive men.[113] Lack of moderate or vigorous exercise increased 5-year mortality in older men and women in the Cardiovascular Heart Study.[55]

Moderate exercise programs suitable for older adults include walking, climbing stairs, swimming, and bicycling. However, care must be taken in prescribing any exercise program because of the high risk of injury in this age group. Group or supervised sessions, including aerobic classes, offered by senior health care plans are especially appealing. Exercise training programs are not only beneficial in preventing coronary heart disease (CHD) but have also been found to improve endurance and functional capacity in older adults after MI.[114,115]

THERAPY OF STABLE ANGINA

Nitroglycerin is used for relief of the acute anginal attack. It is given as a sublingual tablet or as a sublingual spray.[116] Long-acting nitrates prevent recurrent anginal attacks, improve exercise time until the onset of angina, and reduce exercise-induced ischemic ST-segment depression.[117,118] To prevent nitrate tolerance, it is recommended that a 12- to 14-hour nitrate-free interval be established when using long-acting nitrate preparations. During the nitrate-free interval, the use of another antianginal drug will be necessary.

β-Blockers prevent recurrent anginal attacks and are the drug of choice to prevent new coronary events.[119] β-Blockers also improve exercise time until the onset of angina and reduce exercise-induced ischemic ST-segment depression.[119] β-Blockers should be administered along with long-acting nitrates to all patients with angina unless there are contraindications to the use of these drugs. Antiplatelet drugs such as aspirin or clopidogrel should also be administered to all patients with angina to reduce the incidence of new coronary events.[120-122]

There are no class I indications for the use of calcium channel blockers in the treatment of patients with CAD.[60] However, if angina pectoris persists despite the use of β-blockers and nitrates, long-acting calcium channel blockers such as diltiazem or verapamil should be used in older patients with CAD and normal LV systolic function and amlodipine or felodipine should be used in patients with CAD and abnormal LV systolic function as antianginal agents.[116]

Ranolazine reduces the frequency of angina episodes and nitroglycerin consumption and improves exercise duration and time to anginal attacks without clinically significant effects on heart rate or blood pressure.[123,124] Ranolazine should be used as combination therapy when angina is not adequately controlled with other antianginal drugs.[116,125,126] The recommended dose of sustained-release ranolazine is 750 or 1000 mg twice daily.

If angina persists despite intensive medical management, coronary revascularization with coronary angioplasty or coronary artery bypass surgery (CABS) should be considered.[127,128] Addition of percutaneous coronary intervention (PCI) to optimal medical therapy in older adult patients with stable CAD did not improve or worsen the 5-year incidence of all-cause mortality or MI.[129] The use of other approaches to manage stable angina pectoris, which persists despite antianginal drugs and coronary revascularization, is discussed elsewhere.[116]

ACUTE CORONARY SYNDROMES

Unstable angina pectoris is a transitory syndrome that results from disruption of a coronary atherosclerotic plaque, which critically decreases coronary blood flow and causes new-onset angina pectoris or exacerbation of angina pectoris.[130] Transient episodes of coronary artery occlusion or near-occlusion by thrombus at the site of plaque injury may occur and cause angina pectoris at rest. The thrombus may be labile and cause temporary obstruction to flow. Release of vasoconstrictive substances by platelets and vasoconstriction due to endothelial vasodilator dysfunction contribute to a further reduction in coronary blood flow and, in some patients, myocardial necrosis with NSTEMI occurs. Elevation of serum cardiospecific troponin I or T or creatine kinase-MB levels occur in patients with NSTEMI but not in patients with unstable angina.

Older patients with unstable angina pectoris should be hospitalized and, depending on their risk stratification, may need monitoring in an intensive care unit.[131] In a prospective study of 177 consecutive unselected patients hospitalized for an acute coronary syndrome (91 women and 86 men) aged 70 to 94 years, unstable angina was diagnosed in 54%, NSTEMI in 34%, and STEMI in 12%.[132-134] Obstructive CAD was diagnosed by coronary angiography in 94% of older men and in 80% of older women.[131]

Treatment of Unstable Angina Pectoris and Non–ST-Segment Elevation Myocardial Infarction

Treatment of patients with unstable angina pectoris and NSTEMI should be initiated in the emergency department. Reversible factors precipitating unstable angina pectoris should be identified and corrected. Oxygen should be administered to patients who have cyanosis, respiratory distress, congestive heart failure, or high-risk features. Oxygen therapy should be guided by arterial oxygen saturation and should not be given if the arterial oxygen saturation is more than 94%. Morphine sulfate should be administered IV when anginal chest pain is not immediately relieved with nitroglycerin or when acute pulmonary congestion and/or severe agitation is present.

Aspirin should be administered to all patients with unstable angina pectoris and NSTEMI unless contraindicated and continued indefinitely.[134,135] The first dose of aspirin should be chewed rather than swallowed to ensure rapid absorption.

The ACC/AHA 2011 guidelines have updated conditions for which clopidogrel should be administered in addition to indefinite use of aspirin in hospitalized patients with unstable angina pectoris and NSTEMI for whom an early noninterventional approach or PCI is planned. Clopidogrel should be withheld for 5 to 7 days in patients for whom elective coronary artery surgery is planned.[135] Prasugrel may be considered instead of clopidogrel if PCI is planned if there is a low bleeding risk, no history of stroke or ischemic attack, age younger than 75 years, body weight more than 60 kg, and the need for CABS considered unlikely.[136] Ticagrelor may also be used instead of clopidogrel if PCI is planned, but the aspirin dose must not be more than 100 mg daily.[137,138] When possible, ticagrelor should be stopped at least 5 days prior to any surgery. On the basis of data from the

Clopidogrel in Unstable Angina to Prevent Recurrent Events (CURE) trial[139,140] and Clopidogrel for the Reduction of Events During Observation (CREDO) trial,[141] 81 mg of aspirin daily plus 75 mg of clopidogrel daily should be administered to patients with unstable angina and NSTEMI for at least 1 year.

Nitrates should be administered immediately in the emergency department to patients with unstable angina and NSTEMI.[135,142] Patients whose symptoms are not fully relieved with three 0.4-mg sublingual nitroglycerin tablets or a spray taken 5 minutes apart and initiation of an IV β-blocker should be treated with continuous IV nitroglycerin.[135,142] Topical or oral nitrates are alternatives for patients without ongoing refractory symptoms.[135,142]

β-Blockers should be administered IV in the emergency department unless there are contraindications to their use, followed by oral administration and continued indefinitely.[135,142] Metoprolol may be given in 5-mg IV increments over 1 to 2 minutes and repeated every 5 minutes until 15 mg has been given, followed by oral metoprolol 100 mg twice daily. The target resting heart rate is 50 to 60 beats/min.

An oral ACE inhibitor should also be given unless there are contraindications to its use and continued indefinitely.[135,142] In patients with continuing or frequently recurring myocardial ischemia despite nitrates and β-blockers, verapamil or diltiazem should be added to their therapeutic regimen in the absence of LV systolic dysfunction (class IIa indication).[135,142] The benefit of calcium channel blockers in the treatment of unstable angina pectoris is limited to symptom control.[135,142] Intraaortic balloon pump counterpulsation should be used for severe myocardial ischemia that is continuing or occurs frequently, despite intensive medical therapy, or for hemodynamic instability in patients before or after coronary angiography.[135,142]

A platelet glycoprotein IIb/IIIa inhibitor should also be administered in addition to aspirin and clopidogrel and heparin in patients in whom coronary angioplasty is planned.[135,142] Abciximab can be used for 12 to 24 hours in patients with unstable angina/NSTEMI in whom coronary angioplasty is planned within the next 24 hours.[135,142] Eptifibatide or tirofiban should be administered in addition to aspirin and low-molecular-weight heparin or unfractionated heparin to patients with continuing myocardial ischemia, an elevated cardiospecific troponin I or T, or with other high-risk features in whom an invasive management is not planned.[135,142]

IV thrombolytic therapy is not recommended for the treatment of unstable angina and NSTEMI.[135,142] Prompt coronary angiography should be performed without noninvasive risk stratification in patients who fail to stabilize with intensive medical treatment.[142] Coronary revascularization should be performed in patients with high-risk features to reduce coronary events and mortality.[135,142-144]

On the basis of the available data, the ACC/AHA 2013 guidelines have recommended the use of statins in all patients with acute coronary syndromes without contraindications.[101] Statins should be continued indefinitely after hospital discharge.[95,99,101,142,145]

Patients should be discharged on aspirin plus clopidogrel, β-blockers, and ACE inhibitors in the absence of contraindications. Nitrates should be given for ischemic symptoms. A long-acting nondihydropyridine calcium channel blocker may be given for ischemic symptoms that occur, despite treatment with nitrates plus β-blockers. Hormone therapy should not be administered to postmenopausal women.[146,147]

Treatment of ST-Segment Elevation Myocardial Infarction

Chest pain due to acute MI should be treated with morphine, nitroglycerin, and β-blockers.[148,149] If arterial saturation is lower than 94%, oxygen should be administered. Aspirin should be given on day 1 of an acute MI and continued indefinitely to reduce coronary events and mortality.*

The first dose of aspirin should be chewed rather than swallowed. The addition of clopidogrel to aspirin is also beneficial in reducing coronary events and mortality.[152,153] Early intravenous β-blockade should be used during acute MI and oral β-blockers continued indefinitely to reduce coronary events and mortality (Table 40-1).[76,145,149,154-161] ACE inhibitors should be given within 24 hours of acute MI and continued indefinitely to reduce coronary events and mortality (Table 40-2).[76,149,161-167] Statins should be given to all patients with acute MI and no contraindications and continued indefinitely.[101,149] Statins should be continued indefinitely after hospital discharge to reduce coronary events and mortality.[99,101,145]

The ACC/AHA guidelines have stated that there are no class I indications for the use of calcium channel blockers during or after acute MI.[76] However, if older adults have persistent angina after MI, despite treatment with β-blockers and nitrates and are not suitable candidates for coronary revascularization, or if they have hypertension inadequately controlled by other drugs, a nondihydropyridine calcium channel blocker such as verapamil or diltiazem should be added to the therapeutic regimen if the LVEF is normal. If the LVEF is abnormal, amlodipine or felodipine should be added to the therapeutic regimen.

The ACC/AHA guidelines recommend using IV heparin in persons with acute MI undergoing primary coronary angioplasty or surgical coronary revascularization and in those with acute MI at high risk for systemic embolization (e.g., persons with a large or anterior MI, atrial fibrillation, history of pulmonary or systemic embolus, LV thrombus).[76,149] In persons with acute MI not receiving IV heparin, the ACC/AHA guidelines recommend

*References 76, 121, 122, 143-145, and 149-151.

TABLE 40-1 Effect of β-Blockers on Mortality in Older Patients after Myocardial Infarction

Study (Reference)	Follow-Up	Results
Goteborg Trial[154]	90 day	Compared with placebo, metoprolol caused a 45% significant decrease in mortality in patients aged 65-74 yr.
Norwegian Multicenter Study[155]	17 mo (up to 33 mo)	Compared with placebo, timolol caused a 43% significant reduction in mortality in patients aged 65-74 yr.
Norwegian Multicenter Study[156]	61 mo (up to 72 mo)	Compared with placebo, timolol caused a 19% significant decrease in mortality in patients aged 65-74 years.
Beta Blocker Heart Attack Trial[157]	25 mo (up to 36 mo)	Compared with placebo, propranolol caused a 33% significant decrease in mortality in patients aged 60-69 yr.
Carvedilol Post-Infarct Survival Control in Left Ventricular Dysfunction Trial[158]	1.3 yr	Compared with placebo, carvedilol caused a 23% significant reduction in mortality, 24% significant reduction in cardiovascular mortality, 40% significant reduction in nonfatal myocardial infarction, and 30% significant decrease in all-cause mortality or nonfatal myocardial infarction in patients, mean age 63 yr.

TABLE 40-2 Effect of Angiotensin-Converting Enzyme Inhibitors on Mortality in Older Patients after Myocardial Infarction

Study (Reference)	Follow-Up	Results
Survival and Ventricular Enlargement Trial[165]	42 mo (up to 60 mo)	In patients with MI and LVEF ≤ 40%, compared with placebo, captopril reduced mortality 25% in patients ≥ 65 yr.
Acute Infarction Ramipril Efficacy Study[166]	15 mo	In patients with MI and clinical evidence of heart failure, compared with placebo, ramipril decreased mortality 36% in patients ≥ 65 yr.
Survival of Myocardial Infarction Long-Term Evaluation Trial[167]	1 yr	In patients with anterior MI, compared with placebo, zofenopril reduced mortality or severe heart failure 39% in patients ≥ 65 yr.
Trandolapril Cardiac Evaluation Study[183]	24 to 50 mo	In patients with LVEF ≤ 35%, mean age 68 years, compared with placebo, trandolapril reduced mortality 33% in patients with anterior MI and 14% in patients without anterior MI.
Heart Outcomes Prevention Evaluation Study[184]	4.5 yr (up to 6 yr)	In patients ≥ 55 years with MI (53%), cardiovascular disease (88%), or diabetes (38%) but no heart failure or abnormal LVEF, ramipril reduced MI, stroke, and cardiovascular death by 22%.
European trial on reduction of cardiac events with perindopril in patients with stable coronary artery disease[185]	4.2 yr	In patients, mean age 60 years, with coronary artery disease and no heart failure, compared with placebo, perindopril reduced cardiovascular death, MI, or cardiac arrest by 20%.

LVEF, Left ventricular ejection fraction; *MI,* myocardial infarction.

using subcutaneous heparin 7500 U twice daily for 24 to 48 hours to decrease the incidence of deep vein thrombosis.[76,149]

Thrombolytic therapy is beneficial in the treatment of STEMI for patients younger than 75 years.[76,149,150,168-171] From the available data, one cannot conclude whether thrombolytic therapy is beneficial or harmful in patients with acute MI older than 75 years.[171] However, evidence favors the use of primary coronary angioplasty in eligible patients with acute MI younger and older than 75 years to reduce coronary events and mortality.[171-178] In patients 85 years and older, aggressive treatment of STEMI was associated with reasonable long-term survival and excellent quality of life, except in patients presenting with cardiogenic shock.[179] Administration of IV erythropoietin to older patients with STEMI was associated with increased cardiovascular events.[180]

Treatment after Myocardial Infarction

Older adults who have experienced MI should have their modifiable coronary risk factors intensively treated, as discussed previously in this chapter. Aspirin or clopidogrel should be given indefinitely to reduce new coronary events and mortality.[76,120-122,145,181,182] ACC/AHA guidelines recommend the following as class I indications for long-term oral anticoagulant therapy after MI: (1) secondary prevention of MI in post-MI patients unable to tolerate daily aspirin or clopidogrel; (2) post-MI patients with persistent atrial fibrillation; and (3) post-MI patients with LV thrombus.[76] Long-term warfarin should be given in a dose to achieve an international normalized ratio (INR) between 2.0 and 3.0.[76]

β-Blockers (see Table 40-1) and ACE inhibitors (see Table 40-2) should be given indefinitely unless there are contraindications to the use of these drugs to reduce new coronary events and mortality.[76,145,154-168,183-185] Long-acting nitrates are effective antianginal and antiischemic drugs.[116-118] There are no class I indications for the use of calcium channel blockers after MI.[76,145]

Teo and colleagues[186] have analyzed randomized controlled trials comprising 20,342 persons that investigated the use of calcium channel blockers after MI. Mortality was 4% insignificantly higher in persons treated with calcium channel blockers.[186] In this study, β-blockers significantly reduced mortality by 19% in 53,268 persons.[186] In another study, older adults treated with β-blockers after MI had a 43% decrease in 2-year mortality and a 22% decrease in 2-year cardiac hospital readmissions than older adults who were not treated with β-blockers.[187] Use of a calcium channel blocker instead of a β-blocker after MI doubled the risk of mortality.[187]

Aldosterone Antagonists

At 16-month follow-up of 6632 patients after MI, with an LVEF of 40% or less and heart failure or diabetes mellitus treated with ACE inhibitors or angiotensin receptor blockers. and 75% treated with β-blockers compared with the placebo, patients randomized to 50 mg of eplerenone daily had a significant 15% reduction in mortality and 13% significant reduction in death from cardiovascular causes or hospitalization for cardiovascular events.[188] The ACC/AHA guidelines have recommended an aldosterone antagonist in patients treated with ACE inhibitors plus β-blockers after MI if they have an LVEF of 40% or less with heart failure or diabetes mellitus if they have no significant renal dysfunction or hyperkalemia.[60,145]

Antiarrhythmic Therapy

A meta-analysis of 59 randomized controlled trials comprising 23,229 persons that investigated the use of class I antiarrhythmic drugs after MI showed that mortality was 14% significantly higher in persons receiving class I antiarrhythmic drugs than in persons receiving no antiarrhythmic drugs.[186] None of the 59 studies showed a reduction in mortality by class I antiarrhythmic drugs.[186]

In the Cardiac Arrhythmia Suppression Trials I and II, older age also increased the likelihood of adverse effects, including death, in persons after MI receiving encainide, flecainide, or moricizine.[189] Compared with no antiarrhythmic drug, quinidine or procainamide did not reduce mortality in older adults with CAD, normal or abnormal LVEF, and presence versus absence of ventricular tachycardia.[190]

Compared with placebo, D,L-sotalol did not reduce mortality in post-MI persons followed for 1 year.[191] Mortality was also significantly higher at 148-day follow-up in persons treated with D-sotalol (5.0%) than in those treated with a placebo.[192] On the basis of available data, persons who have suffered a MI should not receive class I antiarrhythmic drugs or sotalol.

In the European Myocardial Infarction Amiodarone Trial, 1486 survivors of MI with an LVEF of 40% or less were randomized to amiodarone (743 patients) or placebo (743 patients).[193] At 2-year follow-up, 103 patients treated with amiodarone and 102 patients treated with a placebo had died.[193] In the Canadian Amiodarone Myocardial Infarction Arrhythmia Trial, 1202 survivors of MI with nonsustained ventricular tachycardia or complex ventricular arrhythmias were randomized to amiodarone or placebo.[194] Amiodarone was very effective in suppressing ventricular tachycardia and complex ventricular arrhythmias.

However, the mortality rate at 1.8-year follow-up was not significantly different in those treated with amiodarone or placebo.[194] In addition, early permanent discontinuation of drug for reasons other than outcome events occurred in 36% of persons taking amiodarone.

In the Sudden Cardiac Death in Heart Failure Trial (SCD-HEFT), 2,521 patients with class II or III congestive heart failure (CHF), LVEF of 35%, and mean QRS duration of 120 msec on the resting ECG were randomized to placebo, amiodarone, or automatic implantable cardioverter-defibrillator (AICD).[195] At 46-month median follow-up, compared with placebo, amiodarone insignificantly increased mortality by 6%.[195] At 46-month median follow-up compared with placebo, ICD therapy significantly reduced all-cause mortality by 23%.[195] Of 14,700 patients with acute MI with CHF and/or LV dysfunction, 825 of them, mean age 70 years, were treated with amiodarone.[196] Amiodarone use was associated with excess early and late all-cause mortality and cardiovascular mortality.[196]

In the Cardiac Arrest in Seattle: Conventional Versus Amiodarone Drug Evaluation Study, the incidence of pulmonary toxicity was 10% at 2 years in persons receiving amiodarone at a mean dose of 158 mg daily.[197] The incidence of adverse effects for amiodarone also approached 90% after 5 years of treatment.[198] On the basis of the available data, amiodarone should not be used in the treatment of persons after MI.

However, β-blockers have been shown to reduce mortality in patients with nonsustained ventricular tachycardia or complex ventricular arrhythmias after MI in patients with a normal or abnormal LVEF.[199-202] On the basis of the available data, β-blockers should be used in the treatment of older adult patients after MI, especially if nonsustained ventricular tachycardia or complex ventricular arrhythmias are present, unless there are specific contraindications to their use.

In the Antiarrhythmics Versus Implantable Defibrillators (AVID) trial, 1016 persons, mean age 65 years, with a history of ventricular fibrillation or serious sustained ventricular tachycardia, were randomized to an AICD or drug therapy with amiodarone or D,L-sotalol.[179] Persons treated with an AICD had a 39% reduction in mortality at 1 year, 27% reduction in mortality at 2 years, and 31% reduction in mortality at 3 years.[203] If those who have suffered MI have life-threatening ventricular tachycardia or ventricular fibrillation, an AICD should be inserted.

The Multicenter Automatic Defibrillator Implantation Trial (MADIT) II randomized 1232 persons, mean age 64 years, with a prior MI and LVEF of 30% or less to an AICD or conventional medical therapy.[204] At 20-month follow-up, compared with conventional medical therapy, those with an AICD had a significantly decreased all-cause mortality of 31%, from 19.8% to 14.2%.[204] The effect of AICD therapy in improving survival was similar in persons stratified according to age, gender, LVEF, New York Heart Association class, and QRS interval.[204]

In MADIT II, the reduction in sudden cardiac death in patients treated with an AICD was significantly reduced by 68% in 574 patients younger than 65 years, by 65% in 455 patients 65 to 74 years, and by 68% in 204 patients 75 years.[205] The median survival in 348 octogenarians treated with AICD therapy was longer than 4 years.[206] These data favor considering the prophylactic implantation of an AICD in older postinfarction patients with an LVEF of 30% or lower.

Hormone Replacement Therapy

The Heart Estrogen/Progestin Replacement Study (HERS) investigated the effect of hormone therapy versus a double-blind placebo on coronary events in 2763 women with documented CAD.[207] At 4.1-year follow-up, there were no significant differences between hormone therapy and placebo in the primary outcome (nonfatal MI or CAD death) or in any of the secondary cardiovascular outcomes. However, there was a 52% significantly higher incidence of nonfatal MI or death from CAD in the first year in persons treated with hormone therapy than in those treated with the placebo.[207] Women on hormone therapy had a 289% significantly higher incidence of venous thromboembolic events and a 38% significantly higher incidence of gallbladder disease requiring surgery than women in the placebo group.

At 6.8-year follow-up in the HERS trial, hormone therapy did not reduce the risk of cardiovascular events in women with CAD.[208] The investigators concluded that hormone therapy should not be used to decrease the risk of coronary events in women with ischemic heart disease (IHD).[208] At 6.8-year follow-up in the HERS trial, all-cause mortality was insignificantly increased by 10% with hormone therapy.[208] The overall incidence of venous thromboembolism at 6.8-year follow-up was significantly increased by 208% with hormone therapy.[208] At 6.8-year follow-up, the overall incidence of biliary tract surgery was significantly increased (48%), for any cancer was insignificantly increased (19%), and for any fracture was insignificantly increased (4%).[208]

Influenza Vaccination

Evidence from cohort studies and a randomized clinical trial have indicated that annual vaccination against seasonal influenza prevents cardiovascular morbidity and mortality in patients with cardiovascular disease.[209] The ACC/AHA guidelines have recommended influenza immunization with inactivated vaccine administered intramuscularly as part of secondary prevention in patients with CAD or other atherosclerotic vascular disease with a class I indication.[145,209]

Coronary Revascularization

Medical therapy alone is the preferred treatment in older adults after MI (Box 40-2). The two indications for revascularization in

BOX 40-2 Medical Approach to Older Patients after Myocardial Infarction (MI)

1. Initiate programs to discontinue cigarette smoking.
2. Treat hypertension with β-blockers and angiotensin-converting enzyme (ACE) inhibitors; the blood pressure should be reduced to <140/90 mm Hg.
3. Treat with high-dose statins (rosuvastatin, 20-40 mg daily, or atorvastatin 40-80 mg daily)
4. Diabetes mellitus, obesity, and physical inactivity should be treated.
5. Aspirin or clopidogrel, β-blockers, and ACE inhibitors should be given indefinitely unless there are contraindications to the use of these drugs.
6. Long-acting nitrates are effective antianginal and antiischemic drugs.
7. There are no class I indications for the use of calcium channel blockers after MI.
8. Administer annual vaccination against seasonal influenza
9. Postinfarction patients should not receive class I antiarrhythmic drugs, sotalol, or amiodarone.
10. An automatic implantable cardioverter-defibrillator should be implanted in postinfarction patients at very high risk for sudden cardiac death.
11. Hormone replacement therapy should not be administered to postmenopausal women after MI.
12. The two indications for coronary revascularization in older patients after MI are prolongation of life and relief of unacceptable symptoms, despite optimal medical management.

older adults after MI are prolongation of life and relief of unacceptable symptoms, despite optimal medical management. In a prospective study of 305 patients aged 75 years and older with chest pain refractory to at least two antianginal drugs, 150 patients were randomized to optimal medical therapy and 155 patients to invasive therapy.[127,128] In the invasive group, 74% had coronary revascularization (54% coronary angioplasty and 20% CABS). During the 6-month follow-up, one third of those in the medically treated group needed coronary revascularization for uncontrollable symptoms. At 6-month follow-up, death, nonfatal MI, or hospital admission for an acute coronary syndrome was significantly higher in the medically treated group (49%) than in the invasive group (19%).[127] Revascularization by coronary angioplasty[210] or CABS[211,212] in older adults is extensively discussed elsewhere. A Medicare observational study of 262,700 patients, mean age 73 years, showed a lower incidence of mortality (25%) and of MI (23%) treated with drug-eluting stents than with bare metal stents, but randomized trial data are needed to confirm these data.[213] The ACC and AHA have established guidelines for PCI and for CABS.[214] If coronary revascularization is performed, aggressive medical therapy must be continued.

KEY POINTS

- Coronary risk factors
  - Age
  - Smoking
  - Hypertension
  - Left ventricular hypertrophy
  - Dyslipidemia
  - Diabetes mellitus
  - Obesity
  - Physical inactivity
- Therapy of stable angina pectoris
  - β-Blockers
  - Nitrates
  - Addition of calcium channel blocker as third drug if angina persists
  - Addition of ranolazine as fourth drug if angina persists
- Therapy after myocardial infarction
  - Treatment of modifiable risk factors
  - Aspirin
  - β-Blocker
  - Angiotensin-converting enzyme inhibitor
  - High-dose statin
  - Exercise training program
  - Influenza vaccination annually
  - Cardioverter-defibrillator if clinically indicated
  - Coronary revascularization if clinically indicated

For a complete list of references, please visit www.expertconsult.com.

KEY REFERENCES

1. Aronow WS, Ahn C, Gutstein H: Prevalence and incidence of cardiovascular disease in 1160 older men and 2464 older women a long-term health care facility. J Gerontol A Biol Sci Med Sci 57A:M45–M46, 2002.
7. Aronow WS: Prevalence of presenting symptoms of recognized acute myocardial infarction and of unrecognized healed myocardial infarction in elderly patients. Am J Cardiol 60:1182, 1987.
21. Woodworth S, Nayak D, Aronow WS, et al: Comparison of acute coronary syndromes in men versus women > or = 70 years of age. Am J Cardiol 90:1145–1147, 2002.
23. Aronow WS: Correlation of ischemic ST-segment depression on the resting electrocardiogram with new cardiac events in 1,106 patients over 62 years of age. Am J Cardiol 64:232–233, 1989.
27. Aronow WS, Ahn C, Kronzon I, et al: Congestive heart failure, coronary events, and atherothrombotic brain infarction in elderly blacks and whites with systemic hypertension and with and without echocardiographic and electrocardiographic evidence of left ventricular hypertrophy. Am J Cardiol 67:295–299, 1991.
28. Aronow WS, Epstein S, Koenigsberg M, et al: Usefulness of echocardiographic abnormal left ventricular ejection fraction, paroxysmal ventricular tachycardia, and complex ventricular arrhythmias in predicting new coronary events in patients over 62 years of age. Am J Cardiol 61:1349–1351, 1988.
29. Aronow WS, Epstein S, Koenigsberg M, et al: Usefulness of echocardiographic left ventricular hypertrophy, ventricular tachycardia and complex ventricular arrhythmias in predicting ventricular fibrillation or sudden cardiac death in elderly patients. Am J Cardiol 62:1124–1125, 1988.
30. Aronow WS, Ahn C, Mercando A, et al: Prevalence and association of ventricular tachycardia and complex ventricular arrhythmias with new coronary events in older men and women with and without cardiovascular disease. J Gerontol A Biol Sci Med Sci 57A:M178–M180, 2002.
52. Ravipati G, Aronow WS, Lai H, et al: Comparison of sensitivity, specificity, positive predictive value, and negative predictive value of stress testing versus 64-multislice coronary computed tomography angiography in predicting obstructive coronary artery disease diagnosed by coronary angiography. Am J Cardiol 101:774–775, 2008.
60. Smith SC Jr, Allen J, Blair SN, et al: ACC/AHA guidelines for secondary prevention for patients with coronary and other atherosclerotic vascular disease: 2006 update: endorsed by the National Heart, Lung, and Blood Institute. Circulation 113:2363–2372, 2006.
61. Aronow WS, Fleg JL, Pepine CJ, et al: ACCF/AHA 2011 expert consensus document on hypertension in the elderly: a report of the American College of Cardiology Foundation Task Force on Clinical Expert Consensus Documents developed in collaboration with the American Academy of Neurology, American Geriatrics Society, American Society for Preventive Cardiology, American Society of Hypertension, American Society of Nephrology, Association of Black Cardiologists, and European Society of Hypertension. J Am Coll Cardiol 57:2037–2114, 2011.
75. Beckett NS, Peters R, Fletcher AE, et al: Treatment of hypertension in patients 80 years of age or older. N Engl J Med 358:1887–1898, 2008.
88. Heart Protection Study Collaborative Group: MRC/BHF heart protection study of cholesterol lowering with simvastatin in 20,536 high-risk individuals: a randomised placebo-controlled trial. Lancet 360:7–22, 2002.
89. Aronow WS, Ahn C: Incidence of new coronary events in older persons with prior myocardial infarction and serum low-density lipoprotein cholesterol = 125 mg/dL treated with statins versus no lipid-lowering drug. Am J Cardiol 89:67–69, 2002.
90. Aronow WS, Ahn C, Gutstein H: Reduction of new coronary events and of new atherothrombotic brain infarction in older persons with diabetes mellitus, prior myocardial infarction, and serum low-density lipoprotein cholesterol = 125 mg/dL treated with statins. J Gerontol A Biol Sci Med Sci 57:M747–M750, 2002.
91. Aronow WS, Ahn C: Frequency of new coronary events in older persons with peripheral arterial disease and serum low-density lipoprotein cholesterol = 125 mg/dL treated with statins versus no lipid-lowering drug. Am J Cardiol 90:789–791, 2002.
94. Deedwania P, Stone PH, Merz CNB, et al: Effects of intensive versus moderate lipid-lowering therapy on myocardial ischemia in older patients with coronary heart disease: results of the Study Assessing goals in the Elderly (SAGE). Circulation 115:700–707, 2007.
101. Stone NJ, Robinson J, Lichtenstein AH, et al: 2013 ACC/AHA guideline on the treatment of blood cholesterol to reduce atherosclerotic cardiovascular risk in adults: a report of the American College of Cardiology/American Heart Association Task Force on Practice Guidelines. J Am Coll Cardiol 63:2889–2934, 2014.
116. Aronow WS, Frishman WH: Angina in the elderly. In Aronow WS, Fleg JL, Rich MW, editors: Cardiovascular disease in the elderly, ed 5, Boca Raton, FL, 2013, CRC Press, pp 215–237.
125. Fihn SD, Gardin JM, Abrams J, et al: 2012 ACCF/AHA /ACP/AATS/PCNA/SCAI/STS guideline for the diagnosis and management of patients with stable ischemic heart disease: a report of the American College of Cardiology Foundation/American Heart Association Task Force on Practice Guidelines and the American College of Physicians, American Association for Thoracic Surgery,

Preventive Cardiovascular Nurses Association, Society for Cardiovascular Angiography and Interventions, and Society of Thoracic Surgeons. J Am Coll Cardiol 60:e44–e164, 2012.
146. Hulley S, Grady D, Bush T, et al: Randomized trial of estrogen plus progestin for secondary prevention of coronary heart disease in postmenopausal women. JAMA 280:605–613, 1998.
149. O'Gara PT, Kushner FG, Ascheim DD, et al: 2013 ACCF/AHA guideline for the management of ST-elevation myocardial infarction: executive summary: a report of the American College of Cardiology Foundation/American Heart Association Task Force on Practice Guidelines developed in collaboration with the American College of Emergency Physicians and Society for Cardiovascular Angiography and Interventions. Circulation 127:529–555, 2013.
161. Aronow WS, Ahn C, Kronzon I: Reduction of incidences of new coronary events and of congestive heart failure by beta blockers alone, by angiotensin-converting enzyme inhibitors alone, and by beta blockers plus angiotensin-converting enzyme inhibitors with prior myocardial infarction and asymptomatic left ventricular systolic dysfunction. Am J Cardiol 88:1298–1300, 2001.
201. Aronow WS, Ahn C, Mercando AD, et al: Effect of propranolol versus no antiarrhythmic drug on sudden cardiac death, total cardiac death, and total death in patients > or = 62 years of age with heart disease, complex ventricular arrhythmias, and left ventricular ejection fraction > or = 40%. Am J Cardiol 74:267–270, 1994.

41 Practical Issues in the Care of Frail Older Cardiac Patients

George A. Heckman, Kenneth Rockwood

INTRODUCTION

Despite a decline in recent decades in overall cardiovascular mortality in developed countries, the overall burden of cardiovascular disease remains substantial.[1] The incidence of coronary artery disease (CAD), acquired valvular heart disease (VHD), and heart failure (HF) increases with age, resulting in significant growth in the prevalence of these conditions in the context of population aging.[2] The lifetime risk for symptomatic CAD after the age of 40 years is 49% in men and 32% in women, and the average age of patients suffering a first myocardial infarction is 64.9 years in men and 72.3 years in women.[2] Of those who die from CAD, over 80% are aged 80 years and older. The prevalence of acquired VHD also rises with age, from less than 2% below the age of 65 years to 13% over the age of 75 years.[3] From a population perspective, mitral regurgitation (MR) is the most common form of VHD, followed by aortic stenosis (AS).[3] However, among persons referred to hospital with VHD, AS is more common than MR, with a prevalence of 43% and 32%, respectively, in one large European study.[3] Finally, the prevalence of HF also rises with age, and octogenarians face a 20% lifetime risk of developing HF.[2]

Although the burden of heart disease is greatest among older patients, therapeutic recommendations are usually extrapolated from clinical trials conducted on relatively younger, generally healthier, and highly selected patients. Historically, a significant majority of potential candidates for these trials has been excluded because of multiple medical and age-associated comorbidities, a trend that persists today.[4,5] Furthermore, clinical trials generally measure "hard outcomes," such as rates of death or of other cardiovascular events, outcomes that may not be as important to some older patients as quality of life, preserving cognition, or maintaining functional independence in the community. The publication of the Hypertension in the Very Elderly Trial (HYVET) study illustrated some progress made in this regard, as well as the significant gaps that remain.[6] In this multicenter randomized controlled trial of 3845 patients aged 80 years and older, treatment of hypertension with indapamide, with or without perindopril for 2 years, was well-tolerated and reduced the risk of stroke, death, and HF; there were no differences in the number of trial participants who experienced cognitive decline.[7] In contrast to most prior cardiovascular trials, HYVET specifically targeted older patients, with the average age of participants being almost 84 years, thus filling an important gap in hypertension management literature. However, compared to the general population, HYVET participants had fewer comorbid conditions, were not demented, and outcomes such as functional decline, caregiver burden, or institutionalization have not been reported.

Clinicians are thus left with the difficult task of determining how best to apply the results of clinical trials to real-life older patients. The purpose of this chapter is to provide a framework to assist clinicians in the process of determining the most appropriate courses of action for frail older cardiac patients.

MAKING TREATMENT DECISIONS IN OLDER ADULTS: SHOULD AGE MATTER?

In patients with cardiovascular disease, older age is often associated with a reduced likelihood of receiving recommended therapies, despite evidence of equivalent, and in some cases, greater benefit than in younger persons with similar conditions.[8-12] Underlying these findings appears to be the assumption that aging is a homogenous phenomenon and that all older cardiac patients require the same, often nihilistic, approach. Clearly, people age with variable degrees of success; consider the prominent roles played by Queen Elizabeth and Nelson Mandela well into their 80s. Some octogenarians require caregiver support to remain in their own homes, whereas others require institutional care. When it comes to health, aging is a heterogeneous process, making chronologic age alone an inadequate criterion on which to base treatment decisions.

Some of the heterogeneity seen in aging can be accounted for by the development of chronic illnesses. According to the Canadian National Population Health Survey, the proportion of persons with no chronic illness declines with increasing age, from 44% of those aged 40 to 59 years to 12% of those 80 or older.[13] In contrast, the proportion of persons with three or more chronic conditions in the same age brackets rises from 12% to 41%, respectively. However, the difference between successful and unsuccessful aging reflects more than just the burden of chronic disease and is a manifestation of underlying frailty (see Chapter 14). Although consensus on an operational definition of frailty has yet to be achieved, frailty can be understood as a state of increased vulnerability to health stressors due to reduced physiologic reserve that is usually, but not exclusively, found in older persons.[14] Frailty is not exclusive to chronic disease; whereas some older patients with chronic illness are frail, many are not, and a small minority of frail older persons have no history of chronic disease.[15] However, a systematic review has confirmed the strong association between frailty and a wide range of chronic cardiovascular conditions, both clinical and subclinical.[16] Furthermore, this association may be, as in the case of HF, bidirectional—frail persons may be more likely to develop HF with time, and patients with HF are more likely to become frail.[16] This review also confirms that the presence of frailty in a person with cardiovascular disease is associated with an increased risk of adverse outcomes, including mortality, morbidity, health service utilization, and impaired quality of life.[16]

Assessing frailty can be considered akin to estimating a person's biologic age. A frailty index was developed using data collected from the inception cohort of the Canadian Study of Health and Aging (CSHA).[17] This 20-item index, which considers not only the presence of chronic vascular disease but other symptoms and signs elicited during a structured clinical examination, permits the determination of a person's biologic age as a reflection of underlying frailty and was shown to be a more important predictor of mortality than chronologic age.[17] This approach was recently replicated in a population-based study comparing traditional cardiac risk factors to a frailty index in predicting incident CAD hospitalization and death.[18] The frailty index, which consisted of 25 items, including traditional cardiovascular risk factors and conditions usually considered unrelated to CAD, was more predictive of CAD outcomes (adjusted hazard ratio [aHR], 1.61; 95% confidence index [CI], 1.40 to 1.85) than traditional risk factors (aHR, 1.31; 95% CI, 1.14 to 1.51). These data suggest that chronologic age per se is not an adequate factor on which to base treatment decisions for older persons, but rather that a comprehensive assessment of frailty, reflecting biologic age, provides more useful information on which to base treatment recommendations. Note, also, that patients who have many age-related illnesses also have more deficits. These include subclinical age-related problems, such as motor slowing, abnormal laboratory test results, and less initiative. It is this whole package of health deficits, not just diseases or disabilities, that makes people frail.[19,20] This is a triple whammy, in that frail older adults are more likely to become ill and be less likely to respond to and more likely to be harmed by usual care.[21]

INCORPORATING FRAILTY ASSESSMENT INTO CLINICAL DECISION MAKING

Frailty, as a state of heightened vulnerability, leads to an increased risk of poor outcomes when an affected person is challenged by a health stressor. Conceptually, the degree of risk can be understood as being proportional to the interaction between the degree of frailty and severity of the stressor, which can be expressed mathematically by the following equation:

$$\text{Risk} \propto C \times \text{frailty} \times \text{stressor}$$

where C is a constant specific to an outcome of interest. Risk, therefore, depends on the particular outcome under consideration, or it can be modified by interventions that focus on frailty itself that mitigate or reduce the impact of a stressor on the individual, or both. This conceptualization of risk has a number of implications:

1. Assessing frailty can identify persons at lower risk despite their advanced age and others at high risk despite their relative youth.
2. All outcomes of interest must be identified.

Different outcomes will entail different and potentially competing degrees of risk. Frail individuals may have far more to gain from the success of an intervention than nonfrail individuals; similarly, they may also have far more to lose from adverse events. It is essential to consider patient values and preferences when discussing competing risks. For example, although a patient might benefit from a successful surgical procedure, the risk of an adverse event that could lead to permanent disability—for example, a stroke—might inform their ultimate decision.[22]

3. Risk can be modified by intervening on the frail state itself, usually through multicomponent procedures such as the comprehensive geriatric assessment (see Chapter 34) or by targeting components of the frail state through focused physical therapy or nutritional interventions.[23]
4. Risk can also be modified by intervening on the stressor and mitigating, if not avoiding altogether, its impact on the frail person.

Examples of such interventions include senior-friendly hospital strategies (see Chapter 118), modified anesthetic techniques, or minimally invasive surgical techniques.[24,25]

5. The degree of frailty may be so great that any potential benefits of a proposed intervention are outweighed by the risks related to their severity as a stressor. However, risk and frailty are never so great as to preclude sound palliative care.

CASE STUDY 41-1

Ludwig is a bright, relatively healthy, 85-year-old retired engineer with a history of hypertension controlled with indapamide. He is fully independent in performing his basic and instrumental activities of daily living (BADLs and IADLs) and passed a driving test the year before. He stopped playing golf last year to look after his 75-year-old wife, who has moderately severe Alzheimer disease. He experiences a 1-hour episode of retrosternal chest pressure radiating to his left shoulder, but does not seek medical attention because he has to look after his wife. When he finally sees his family physician 1 week later, an ECG demonstrates new inferior Q waves, and an echocardiogram demonstrates an ejection fraction of 55% with hypokinesis of the inferior wall of the left ventricle, consistent with a recent myocardial infarction (MI). An incidental note is made of mild to moderate aortic stenosis. His family physician prescribes enteric-coated acetylsalicylic acid, an ACE enzyme inhibitor, and a β-blocker, all of which are well tolerated. Ludwig declines further investigations because he now feels well and wants to resume looking after his wife. A cholesterol profile demonstrates a low-density lipoprotein (LDL) cholesterol level of 145 mg/dL and a high-density lipoprotein (HDL) cholesterol level of 35 mg/dL. Should Ludwig be prescribed a statin for secondary prevention of cardiovascular events?

TABLE 41-1 Canadian Study of Health and Aging Frailty Scale

Frailty Level	Description
1. Very fit	Robust, active, energetic, well-motivated and fit; these people commonly exercise regularly and are in the most fit group for their age
2. Well	Without active disease, but less fit than people in category 1
3. Well, with treated comorbid disease	Disease symptoms well controlled compared with those in category 4
4. Apparently vulnerable	Although not frankly dependent, commonly complain of being "slowed up" or have disease symptoms
5. Mildly frail	With limited dependence on others for instrumental activities of daily living
6. Moderately frail	Help is needed with instrumental and noninstrumental activities of daily living
7. Severely frail	Completely dependent on others for the activities of daily living or terminally ill

Modified from Mitnitski AB, Graham JE, Mogilner AJ, Rockwood K: Frailty, fitness and late-life mortality in relation to chronological and biological age. BMC Geriatrics 2:1, 2002.

The case studies discussed in this chapter illustrate how to incorporate these considerations into clinical decision making for older patients with cardiovascular disease. The first is illustrated in Case Study 41-1.

Clinical trials have demonstrated that statins reduce the risk of subsequent coronary events and mortality in patients who have suffered a myocardial infarction (MI). However, clinical trials have only included patients up to the age of 82 years.[26,27] The family physician must consider whether the results of these trials are applicable to Ludwig, who is 85 years old. Using the CSHA frailty scale (Table 41-1), the family physician determines that Ludwig falls into category 3 (well, with treated comorbid disease), which is associated with a relatively good prognosis and thus corresponds to a biologic age of younger than 85 years.[28] In that case, the potential for benefits likely offsets the risk of adverse events.[29] The arguments for and against treating Ludwig with a

TABLE 41-2 Arguments for and Against Treating Ludwig With a Statin

Arguments Favoring Statin Therapy	Arguments Against Statin Therapy
• Ludwig is not very frail: he is old chronologically, but less old biologically. • There is no compelling evidence that atherosclerosis is substantially different in an 85-year-old adult than in an 80-year-old adult. • Ludwig is otherwise healthy, has no other competing comorbidities, and therefore has a remaining life expectancy of approximately 5 years. • In the PROSPER trial, benefits of statin therapy became apparent after 1 year. • Ludwig is at high risk for a recurrent cardiac event, which might leave him unable to care for his wife.	• Ludwig's age exceeds clinical trial inclusion criteria and he is therefore too old. • Potential risk for adverse events

CASE STUDY 41-2

Ludwig's 75-year-old wife Thelma has moderately severe Alzheimer disease. She requires assistance for all IADLs, as well as with washing, grooming, and dressing. She has episodes of urinary incontinence because she cannot always find her way to the bathroom. She has had falls, requires a walker, and cannot leave the house unattended. Otherwise, she has no cardiovascular risk factors or other comorbid conditions and has never sustained a cardiovascular event. Routine cholesterol profile reveals an LDL of 145 mg/dL and HDL of 35 mg/dL. Should Thelma be prescribed a statin for the primary prevention of cardiovascular events?

statin are presented in Table 41-2. In this situation, the balance of arguments weighs in favor of offering Ludwig a statin.

The next study involves Ludwig's wife, Thelma (Case Study 41-2). Statins are often recommended for the primary prevention of cardiovascular events, although the benefits may be attenuated in older patients with no other concomitant cardiovascular risk factors.[30,31] The family physician determines that Thelma falls within category 6 (moderately frail) of the CSHA frailty scale, which is associated with a poor prognosis over the medium term.[28] Furthermore, the family physician considers the results of the NHANES I (the first National Health and Nutrition Examination Survey) study, which found that high cholesterol was associated with CAD only in active individuals aged 65 to 74 years.[32] Her frailty puts her at increased risk of side effects from the statin, which are not worth the minimal benefits of treatment.[29,31] The arguments for and against treating Thelma with a statin are presented in Table 41-3. In this situation, the balance of arguments weighs against offering Thelma a statin.

In both these cases, considering frailty (biologic age) rather than chronologic age facilitated individualized clinical decision making in the absence of directly applicable evidence from clinical trials. These examples also illustrate the importance of considering patient and caregiver needs and preferences.

Case Study 41-3 illustrates the importance of identifying all relevant outcomes and competing risks. In this situation, a successful procedure will allow Ludwig to fulfil his goals; an adverse event might affect his ability to look after his wife, causing her to be institutionalized. However, most clinical trials in cardiology focus on mortality, hospitalization, coronary interventions, and other objective assessments of cardiovascular events. Very few trials have examined outcomes of interest to older adults, such as preventing functional and cognitive decline, caregiver stress, and

TABLE 41-3 Arguments for and Against Treating Thelma With a Statin

Arguments Favoring Statin Therapy	Arguments Against Statin Therapy
• Even a remotely small reduction in the risk of a cardiovascular event might permit Ludwig to look after his wife at home as long as possible.	• Thelma is frail. Her biologic age is greater than her chronologic age. • Thelma is inactive according to the NHANES I definition and therefore her cholesterol level is unlikely to be a risk factor for a coronary event. • Marginal benefit of statins in persons at low cardiovascular risk • Increased polypharmacy • Potential risk for adverse events

CASE STUDY 41-3

Following his MI, Ludwig continues to look after his wife at home. He remains independent in his IADLs and ADLs. Six months after his MI, he develops angina. Despite optimal medical therapy with an ACE inhibitor, acetylsalicylic acid, statin, β-blocker, nitrates, and calcium channel blocker, his chest pain continues to be brought on by climbing six steps and occasionally when he helps his wife dress. Clinical evaluation and investigations reveal no new changes in the ECG or evidence of HF. An echocardiogram demonstrates no change in left ventricular function and minimal worsening of his aortic stenosis. Ludwig states that his priority is to continue looking after his wife, Thelma, who has remained relatively stable, at home and for as long as possible. Should he undergo revascularization?

institutionalization. However, emerging evidence in the treatment of cardiovascular disease has underlined the importance of these domains.

Evidence from smaller trials and observational data suggest that the benefits of cardiovascular therapies in older adult patients may include the preservation of function and cognition.[33] In a randomized placebo-controlled trial of 60 New York Heart Association (NYHA) class II and III patients with HF from left ventricular (LV) systolic dysfunction aged 81 ± 6 years, perindopril over 10 weeks was associated with a 37-m increase in 6-minute walking distance compared to baseline versus no significant change in the control group ($P < .001$).[34] A supervised exercise program over 18 weeks in 20 NYHA class III HF patients aged 63 ± 13 years and left ventricular ejection fraction (LVEF) of 35% or less resulted in improvements in psychomotor speed and attention.[35] Numerous observational studies have suggested that angiotensin-converting enzyme (ACE) inhibitors prescribed to older HF patients may result in improved cognition, less depression, slower functional decline, and less institutionalization.[33] ACE inhibitors may also preserve cognitive function in hypertensive persons with Alzheimer's disease, as well as physical function in older persons without HF.[36-38] Although these data require confirmation by larger clinical trials, they do support the notion that standard cardiovascular therapies have the potential to address outcomes of importance to frail older adults.

Among older adult patients with CAD, increasing numbers of revascularization procedures are being performed. The Trial of Invasive versus Medical therapy in Elderly patients (TIME) trial, one of a few trials to focus exclusively on older adults, randomized 305 patients aged 75 years and older, 78% of whom had chronic Canadian Cardiovascular Society (CCS) class III or IV angina despite at least two antianginal drugs, to optimal medical therapy (148 patients) or early invasive therapy (153 patients).[39] In the early invasive therapy group, 72% of patients underwent revascularization (28% had coronary artery bypass grafting [CABG]), which was associated with an early mortality hazard, but there were no significant mortality differences at 1 and 4 years.[40] Early invasive therapy led to greater and more rapid improvements in quality of life and functional capacity than medical therapy, although differences disappeared after 1 year, likely because almost half of the medical therapy patients eventually underwent revascularization. Subsequent health service use was also lower among early intervention patients. The results of this trial suggest that older patients with intolerable angina who proceed with an early invasive approach to treatment face an early mortality hazard that is offset by earlier improvements in quality of life and functional capacity. Patients who tolerate their angina may choose to undergo revascularization at a later date, at the expense of greater health care utilization, but with no overall mortality penalty.

The rising number of cardiac surgeries being performed in older adults has been facilitated by improvements in surgical and anesthetic methods over time. As a result, CABG and valve replacement surgeries are being routinely conducted in appropriately selected octogenarians and increasingly among nonagenarians and even centenarians.[41-44] Studies of these practices have been primarily observational and have shown significant variability with respect to periprocedural outcomes, with mortality rates in octogenarians ranging from 4% to 14% and rates of stroke ranging from 0.5% to almost 8%.[41-44] CABG in older adult patients can lead to significant deconditioning and functional decline, with discharge rates to skilled nursing facilities ranging from 16% to almost 70% and functional recovery taking as long as 2 years.[45-53] Postoperative cognitive dysfunction may occur in over 50% of patients following cardiac surgery, and although most recuperate or even improve from baseline, recovery may take up to 1 year.[54,55]

Clearly, appropriate selection of surgical candidates is often in the eye of the beholder. Although older studies linked adverse outcomes to comorbidities and urgent or repeat revascularization, more recent studies have indicated frailty as an important determinant.[56] Combining frailty measures with surgical, physiologic, and functional assessments improves the accuracy of risk stratification in older adults undergoing cardiac surgery.[57,58] Following cardiac surgery, frailty has been associated with an increased risk of periprocedural mortality and complications, including delirium, pneumonia, prolonged ventilation, increased length of stay, stroke, renal failure, reoperation, and deep sternal infection.[59,60] Frailty is also associated with poor late outcomes. In a cohort of 629 patients age 74.3 ± 6.4 years undergoing percutaneous revascularization, frailty, as measured by the Fried phenotype, was associated with an increased risk of myocardial infarction and death.[61] In a retrospective cohort study of 3826 patients undergoing cardiac surgery, frailty, as determined by the presence of functional, cognitive, or gait difficulties, was associated with a greater likelihood of requiring prolonged institutional care after discharge (48.5% vs. 9%; odds ratio, 6.3; 95% CI, 4.2 to 9.4).[60]

Arguments for and against Ludwig undergoing a coronary intervention are summarized in Table 41-4. Details are described in Case Study 41-4.

Treatment modalities for cardiovascular disease can have an important impact on outcomes of relevance to older adults, including functional independence and cognition. Furthermore, evidence has suggested that frailty is an important mediator in determining the potential benefits and risks associated with cardiac interventions in the short-term and in the medium to long term. Eliciting patient preferences, values, and goals, and discussing how these may be affected by the short-term and longer term impact of proposed treatments, is central to optimal care planning.

Case Study 41-5 illustrates a common scenario, whereby an older adult with underlying cardiovascular disease becomes frail and also develops HF, often concurrently. This study illustrates how the manifestations of heart disease in frail or functionally impaired older adults are often at variance with the classical syndromes of HF or angina pectoris and include geriatric syndromes such as falls, delirium, functional decline, and incontinence.[33,62] Although such manifestations are often referred to as atypical disease presentations, they are in reality common among frail seniors and should be more properly referred to as nonclassical rather than atypical.

Nonclassical and nonspecific presentations in older adult patients with HF are common.[33] Patients who are sedentary from other comorbidities may not experience exertional symptoms. In bedridden patients, edema may accumulate over the sacrum rather than in the legs and may reflect venous insufficiency, treatment with calcium channel blockers, reduced oncotic pressure, or pulmonary disease rather than HF.[63] Nonspecific sleep disturbances may be manifestations of orthopnea, paroxysmal nocturnal dyspnea, or nocturia due to the mobilization of peripheral

TABLE 41-4 Arguments for and Against Ludwig Undergoing a Coronary Intervention

Arguments Favoring Intervention	Arguments Against Intervention
• He is not frail and therefore is likely to avoid periprocedural and postprocedural complications. • Successful intervention would allow him to continue caring for his wife. • Delaying the intervention will result in ongoing angina and an increased likelihood of a coronary event in the near future, which would interfere with his ability to care for his wife. • He may as well undergo the procedure now, because there is a high likelihood that he will require one in the near future.	• There is a risk of complications such as stroke or death that would preclude him from looking after his wife. • He can always undergo the procedure at a later date.

CASE STUDY 41-4

Ludwig undergoes a coronary angiogram. He has an 80% stenosis of the mid–left anterior descending (LAD) artery; mild, nonhemodynamically significant coronary stenosis in his circumflex; and a distal obstruction of the right coronary artery. He undergoes percutaneous revascularization to the LAD lesion, with resolution of his angina. The procedure is complicated by a false aneurysm of the right femoral artery, treated conservatively. He also experiences a transient ischemic attack affecting his speech, but with no permanent sequelae. His acetylsalicylic acid is replaced by clopidogrel. His is able to continue caring for his wife, who eventually dies at home from pneumonia 6 months later.

CASE STUDY 41-5

Ludwig is now 91 years old. He has not experienced any angina since his coronary procedure. However, over the last 2 years, his children have noticed that he has slowed down. He has had two falls in the last months, requires a walker, and needs help to bathe. His children assist with meals, medication, and finances, because Ludwig is at times forgetful. He has been hospitalized three times, presenting once with resting dyspnea, once with a fall, and once with delirium. In all cases, he was diagnosed with heart failure, and was eventually referred to a heart failure clinic.

edema in the recumbent position.[33] Urinary incontinence may develop due to ACE inhibitor–associated cough, persistent volume overload, elevated natriuretic peptide levels, or underlying sleep apnea.[33] Neuropsychiatric symptoms, including delirium, anxiety or depressive symptoms, may be associated with symptomatic or undertreated HF in frail older adults.[33,63]

Nonclassical symptoms also occur in frail older adults with CAD. In a cross-sectional cohort of 1939 persons aged 67 ± 11 years and hospitalized with an acute coronary syndrome, presenting symptoms included weakness and fatigue in over 50%, anxiety in 34%, and vertigo or presyncope in 26%.[64] In a cross-sectional analysis of 247 older adult patients aged 76 ± 6 years hospitalized after an acute myocardial infarction (MI), only 22% presented with classical chest pain.[65] Almost 30% presented with symptoms of fatigue, sleep disturbance, psychological distress, dyspnea, and moderate pain, and almost 50% presented with multiple mild respiratory and gastrointestinal symptoms, fatigue, sleep disturbances, and pain. Delirium is one of the most common complications of MI in persons 90 years and older.[66]

The consequences of delayed or missed diagnoses as a result of nonclassical presentations can be significant. Hospitalized patients presenting with nonclassical symptoms are more likely to be suffer adverse consequences, such as being restrained or institutionalized.[62] Data from the Cardiovascular Health Study have demonstrated that unrecognized MI in older adults presenting without classical angina or clinical evidence of HF are very common and are associated with a prognosis similar to that of recognized MI.[67] It is therefore imperative that clinicians assessing acutely ill older adults with nonspecific symptoms, particularly those with cardiovascular risk factors or who are frail or functionally impaired, must maintain a high index of suspicion for an acute cardiac event. Furthermore, such patients are often frail and may benefit from a comprehensive geriatric assessment.

Persons with advanced cardiovascular conditions such as HF are best cared for in disease management programs (see Chapter 39). For example, HF management programs, designed for patients with frequent HF exacerbations, improve outcomes by considering concomitant comorbidities, including cognitive impairment, and providing individualized and intensive support to individuals and their caregivers. HF management programs are more likely to succeed when patient goals are taken into account.[68] Furthermore, frail seniors with HF are most likely to benefit from HF management programs. A randomized trial of an HF management intervention stratified participants using a frailty index that considered advanced age, cognition, physical function, incontinence, and mobility.[12] All-cause and HF hospitalizations were reduced among patients with mild to moderate frailty, and HF hospitalizations were reduced for those with any degree of frailty, whereas nonfrail patients derived no additional benefits compared to usual care. The intervention was cost-effective among patients with mild to moderate frailty.

Ludwig has developed symptomatic severe aortic stenosis (AS; Case Study 41-6), which, if left untreated, is associated with a 2-year mortality rate of 50% to 80%.[25] The definitive treatment for AS is surgical aortic valve replacement (SAVR), which is associated with an overall periprocedural mortality rate of 3% (within 30 days of surgery).[69] A seminal study of 299 patients who were offered SAVR showed that the 3-year survival rate of those who underwent surgery was 87% compared to 21% among the 49 operative candidates who turned down surgery.[70] A recent meta-analysis of 48 studies of 13,216 octogenarians undergoing isolated SAVR found a perioperative mortality of 5.8% from 2000 to 2006, compared to 7.5% from 1982 to 1999; the stroke rate was 2.6%.[71] This review found that pooled survival rates at 1, 3, 5, and 10 years were 87.6%, 78.7%, 65.4%, and 29.7%, respectively.[71] Outcomes among octogenarians who undergo combined SAVR and CABG are somewhat worse, with periprocedural mortality and stroke rates of 8.2% and 3.7%, respectively, and survival rates at 1, 3, 5 and 10 years of 83.2%, 72.9%, 60.8%, and 25.7%, respectively.[72]

CASE STUDY 41-6

As part of his evaluation in the heart failure clinic, an echocardiogram is performed. This shows that his left ventricular ejection fraction is now 40%, and he now has severe aortic stenosis. Should Ludwig undergo aortic valve replacement?

Despite the effectiveness of SAVR, between 30% and 40% of patients with severe AS are not offered surgery because of an increased risk of poor outcomes related to technical (e.g., porcelain aorta) or clinical (e.g., frailty) considerations. Therapeutic options for such patients have been hitherto limited to valvuloplasty or medical therapy, with the former demonstrating short-term quality of life benefits over the latter, but no survival advantage.[25] The advent of minimally invasive transaortic valve implantation (TAVI) has been touted as a potentially effective option for nonoperative patients, particularly those who are frail. However, identifying those who are too frail for SAVR but who would benefit from TAVI, and those who are too frail to benefit meaningfully from either intervention (i.e., who are more likely to die with AS than from AS) remains challenging.[73,74] This challenge is best framed by referring back to the equation on the degree of risk (see earlier) and considering different potential outcomes and severity of the stressors that represent SAVR and TAVI.

Outcomes are best considered in relation to their timing, distinguishing periprocedural outcomes from longer term outcomes measured in months to years. The importance of this distinction is underlined by the results of a small but highly informative single-center study of 84 octogenarians (83.7 ± 3.3. years; range, 80 to 94 years) who underwent SAVR (35% also underwent simultaneous CABG) and who were followed for up to 3 years.[75] In this group, periprocedural mortality was 16.7%; survival among those remaining was 86% and 69% at 1 and 3 years, respectively. Of these survivors, 32% described poor to very poor self-rated health, 23% described poor to very poor self-rated quality of life, and almost 40% would elect not to repeat SAVR due to the resulting loss of autonomy, depression, and ongoing cardiac symptoms. In all, 86% of survivors suffered from at least one geriatric syndrome—mood, falls, gait abnormality and loss of autonomy. In another series of octogenarians undergoing combined aortic and mitral valve replacement, frailty, as measured using Karnofsky performance status, was also associated with periprocedural and 1-year mortality.[76] These data emphasize the importance of not only considering periprocedural outcomes, but also of longer term outcomes, such as quality of life and functional status, in patients with severe AS.

From a stressor perspective, TAVI is less invasive than SAVR, suggesting that in appropriately selected patients, procedure-related complications should be minimized. In the PARTNER A trial comparing SAVR to TAVI in high surgical risk patients, periprocedural mortality was higher in the SAVR group (6.5% vs. 3.4%; $P = .07$).[77] However, the risk of periprocedural stroke was higher in the TAVI group (5.5% vs. 2.4%; $P = .04$). There were no significant mortality differences at 1 and 2 years (33.9% vs. 35.0%), although TAVI remained associated with an almost twofold risk of stroke throughout the follow-up period.[77,78] Quality of life and function improved more rapidly in patients undergoing TAVI, although no differences in these outcomes remained after 1 year.[79] Significantly, 40% of patients in either group experienced no improvements in quality of life. In the PARTNER B trial, TAVI was compared to medical therapy in patients considered inoperable due to frailty, as determined by a clinical team consensus using prespecified criteria, or to technical

CASE STUDY 41-7

Ludwig is referred to a heart team and geriatrician to be assessed. His CSHA frailty score is 6 (moderately frail). He is considered too frail for SAVR, but a potential candidate for TAVI. However, Ludwig, who always took pride in his intellect, is worried that a stroke might adversely affect his cognition. Ultimately, Ludwig, his family, and his care team arrive at a mutually agreeable decision to provide Ludwig with palliative care in his own home. Ludwig lives another 2 months and passes away quietly at home from heart failure, surrounded by his family.

reasons.[80,81] TAVI was associated with a greater risk of periprocedural stroke (5% vs. 1.1%; $P = 0.06$) and, at 1 and 2 years, greater functional status and lower mortality overall. However, mortality rates in the TAVI group remained high (30.7% and 43.3% at 1 and 2 years), and patients with a Society of Thoracic Surgeons (STS) score higher than 15% derived no survival advantage from the procedure compared to patients treated medically.[82] Among surviving patients in PARTNER B, 23% of those in the TAVI group and 66% of those in the medical therapy group reported, at most, minimal gains in quality of life at 1 year.[82] After 3 years, PARTNER B patients who underwent TAVI had a survival rate of 45.9% and a stroke rate of 15.7% versus 19.1% and 5.5% in the medical therapy group.[83]

Several conclusions can be drawn from these data. First, regardless of which treatment is received, these patients all have a high mortality rate, consistent with the severity of their cardiovascular illness, but also reflecting underlying frailty. Second, compared to SAVR, TAVI is less of a stressor from the perspective of mortality and earlier return of function, although it appears to be associated with a significantly higher risk of stroke.[84] This risk may be of particular concern among patients with preexisting cognitive impairment, in whom a stroke could lead to significantly worse function.[85] This risk may not be as significant as TAVI technology continues to evolve.[86] Third, a substantial proportion of survivors benefit minimally from either procedure, suggesting that there exists a threshold beyond which TAVI is unhelpful. Data from several TAVI registries, which used a variety of frailty measures, have shown that frailty is associated with an increased risk of not only periprocedural complications, but also of later functional decline, reduced quality of life, residual HF symptoms, and mortality.[87-90] Furthermore, causes of mortality shift over time: cardiovascular events predominate in the first year, whereas organ failure, cancer, and so-called senescence are most common beyond 2 years.[91,92] Subgroup analyses of the PARTNER trials have suggested that from a surgical risk perspective, patients with STS scores over 15% do not derive a survival benefit; a similar frailty threshold, determined using a standardized frailty instrument, remains to be established.[25]

Ludwig has been referred to a heart team (Case Study 41-7).

CONCLUSION

Assessing frailty and considering patient goals are fundamental to the appropriate management of heart disease in older persons. Although many standard cardiac therapies may be beneficial for outcomes and goals of importance to frail older cardiac patients, clinicians must weigh these potential benefits against their potential risks, which include not only the possibility of periprocedural complications but also of subsequently reduced functional capacity and quality of life. Interprofessional collaboration is essential in the care of these patients. Research priorities include the development of standardized strategies to assess frailty-related risk and guide clinical trials of cardiovascular therapies in representative populations of older cardiac patients for whom all relevant outcomes are considered.

KEY POINTS

- Evidence for the management of cardiovascular disease is drawn from clinical trials that are unrepresentative of many older adults, particularly those with complex multimorbidity and frailty.
- Frailty is intimately associated with cardiovascular disease.
- The risks associated with frailty depend on the degree of frailty, severity of a potential health stressor, and the outcome that is being considered.
- Frail older adults may have more to gain from a treatment and more to lose from an adverse event. Risk can be attenuated by comprehensive geriatric assessment, enrollment into disease management programs, use of less invasive therapies, and adoption of senior-friendly care strategies.
- Eliciting and understanding patient preferences and developing a shared understanding of the pros and cons of proposed interventions, are essential for optimal shared decision making for frail older adults with cardiovascular disease.

For a complete list of references, please visit www.expertconsult.com.

KEY REFERENCES

12. Pulignano G, Del Sindaco D, Di Lenarda A, et al: Usefulness of frailty profile for targeting older heart failure patients in disease management programs: a cost-effectiveness, pilot study. J Cardiovasc Med (Hagerstown) 11:739–747, 2010.
14. Bergman H, Ferrucci L, Guralnik J, et al: Frailty: an emerging research and clinical paradigm—issues and controversies. J Gerontol A Biol Sci Med Sci 62:731–737, 2007.
16. Afilalo J, Alexander KP, Mack MJ, et al: Frailty assessment in the cardiovascular care of older adults. J Am Coll Cardiol 63:747–762, 2014.
18. Wallace LMK, Theou O, Kirkland SA, et al: Accumulation of non-traditional risk factors for coronary artery disease is associated with incident coronary heart disease hospitalization and death. PLoS One 9:e90475, 2014.
19. Clegg A, Young J, Iliffe S, et al: Frailty in elderly people. Lancet 381:752–762, 2013.
21. Rockwood K, Mitnitski A: Frailty defined by deficit accumulation and geriatric medicine defined by frailty. Clin Geriatr Med 27:17–26, 2011.
33. Heckman GH, Tannenbaum C, Costa AP, et al: The journey of the frail older adult with heart failure: implications for management and health care systems. Rev Clin Gerontol 24:269–289, 2014.
40. Pfisterer M, Trial of Invasive versus Medical therapy in Elderly patients Investigators: Long-term outcome in elderly patients with chronic angina managed invasively versus by optimized medical therapy: four-year follow-up of the randomized Trial of Invasive versus Medical therapy in Elderly patients (TIME). Circulation 110:1213–1218, 2004.
58. Afilalo J, Mottillo S, Eisenberg MJ, et al: Addition of frailty and disability to cardiac surgery risk scores identifies elderly patients at high risk of mortality or major morbidity. Circ Cardiovasc Qual Outcomes 5:222–228, 2012.
68. Riegel B, Moser DK, Anker SD, et al: State of the science: promoting self-care in persons with heart failure: a scientific statement from the American Heart Association. Circulation 120:1141–1163, 2009.
75. Maillet J-M, Somme D, Hennel E, et al: Frailty after aortic valve replacement (AVR) in octogenarians. Arch Gerontol Geriatr 48:391–396, 2009.
77. Smith CR, Leon MB, Mack MJ, et al: Transcatheter versus surgical aortic-valve replacement in high-risk patients. N Engl J Med 364: 2187–2198, 2011.
78. Kodali SK, Williams MR, Smith CR, et al: Two-year outcomes after transcatheter or surgical aortic-valve replacement. N Engl J Med 366:1686–1695, 2012.
79. Reynolds MR, Magnuson EA, Wang K, et al: Health-related quality of life after transcatheter or surgical aortic valve replacement in high-risk patients with severe aortic stenosis: results from the PARTNER

(Placement of AoRTic TraNscathetER Valve) Trial (Cohort A). J Am Coll Cardiol 60:548–558, 2012.
80. Leon MB, Smith CR, Mack M, et al: Transcatheter aortic-valve implantation for aortic stenosis in patients who cannot undergo surgery. N Engl J Med 363:1597–1607, 2010.
81. Svensson LG, Tuzcu M, Moses JW, et al: Transcatheter aortic-valve replacement for inoperable severe aortic stenosis. N Engl J Med 366:1696–1704, 2012.
87. Stortecky S, Schoenenberger AW, Moser A, et al: Evaluation of multidimensional geriatric assessment as a predictor of mortality and cardiovascular events after transcatheter aortic valve implantation. JACC Cardiovasc Interv 5:489–496, 2012.
88. Green P, Woglom AE, Genereux P, et al: The impact of frailty status on survival after transcatheter aortic valve replacement in older adults with severe aortic stenosis: a single-center experience. J Am Coll Cardiol Intv 5:974–981, 2012.
90. Schoenenberger AW, Stortecky S, Neumann S, et al: Predictors of functional decline in elderly patients undergoing transcatheter aortic valve implantation (TAVI). Eur Heart J 34:684–692, 2013.
92. Saia F, Latib A, Ciuca C, et al: Causes and timing of death during long-term follow-up after transcatheter aortic valve replacement. Am Heart J 168:798–806, 2014.

42 Hypertension

John Potter, Phyo Myint

INTRODUCTION

Demographic changes in most Westernized societies have highlighted the increasing number of older and very old (80+ years) adults in the global population, of whom over two thirds will have raised blood pressure (BP) levels. These elevated BP levels cannot be regarded as benign, only reflecting the effects of the natural aging process on the cardiovascular system, because they are associated with significant rates of cardiovascular disease, which remains the single biggest causes of death in this age group. Intervention trials have shown the benefits of BP reduction even in those aged 90+ years in terms of reducing cardiovascular events; this evidence has perhaps swung the pendulum from reluctance to treat hypertension in older adults to active lowering of BP, even in the very old, in more recent years. Following the publication of the Hypertension in the Very Elderly Trial,[1] and other important studies involving older adults, many new and relevant guidelines have been published centered on the optimal treatment of the older hypertensive patient. This chapter deals with the epidemiologic and pathophysiologic changes associated with hypertension in older adults, as well as some of the therapeutic changes that have resulted from the more recent studies involving older hypertensive patients, to give a practical guide to diagnosis and management.

EPIDEMIOLOGY

Cross-sectional and longitudinal studies in industrialized cultures have shown an age-related rise in BP, with increases in systolic BP (SBP) being almost linear up to age 80 years, plateauing thereafter, whereas diastolic BP (DBP) levels plateau earlier, at 50 to 60 years, and then fall.[2] These changes herald the important age-related changes that occur in pulse pressure (PP), which rises steeply after the age of 60 years irrespective of SBP levels when young, whereas mean arterial pressure (MAP) shows a much greater increase with age in those with high values in their 30s and 40s and reaches a plateau after the age of 50 to 60 years.

Many factors govern these changes, genetic and environmental. For example, Afro-Caribbeans tend to have a greater age-related BP rise than whites, especially in women, and a higher prevalence of hypertension up to the age of 75 years, although this ethnic difference is significantly attenuated after this age.[3] Important gender differences in the BP changes with age are also found when comparing the results from cross-sectional and longitudinal studies, with the former showing women to have higher SBP and DBP values than men after 50 years of age. Cohort studies show a different pattern, with SBP increasing to the same degree in both genders, with little difference in age-related values, whereas DBP levels for women are consistently lower than for men, about 5 mm Hg. It is possible that some of these differences in cross-sectional studies are due to selective mortality differences (e.g., death rates being higher in those with higher BP levels), resulting in an underrepresentation of those with initially high BP levels in the older age groups. Lifestyle differences probably influence some of these age-related alterations, little change in BP being seen with advancing years in some non-Western cultures.

Prevalence and Incidence

Hypertension may be defined as the BP threshold at which the benefits of treatment outweigh those of nontreatment, but the actual BP levels and how they are measured for defining hypertension have changed considerably recently (see later). In the United Kingdom, using a threshold of 140/90 mm Hg for hypertension, the Health Survey for England found that 60% of men and 53% of women aged 60 to 69 years were hypertensive, with prevalence rates rising to 72% for men and 86% for women aged 80+ years.[4] Despite these high prevalence rates, awareness, treatment, and control rates have significantly improved over the past 2 decades, with control rates increasing from 33% in 1994 to 63% in 2011. There are, however, marked differences in prevalence rates between countries (e.g., in rural India rates ≅ 46% compared to 80% in Venezuela for those aged 65+ years).[5] In most studies, these rates are based on just two or three recordings at a single visit and, given the increased BP variability in older adults, the estimates are probably too high; rates based on repeated measurements may be up to 30% less than those quoted.[6]

SBP tends to increase to a greater extent than the DBP with advancing years, so isolated systolic hypertension (ISH) is the most common form of hypertension in older adults. Prevalence rates for ISH in the BIRNH Study were 9.9% in men and 11.7% in women aged 65 to 74 years, compared with rates for diastolic hypertension (DBP = 95 mm Hg) of 15.8% and 10.6%.[7] For those aged 75 to 89 years, ISH rates increased to 15.3% and 17.4% in men and women, whereas diastolic hypertension (DH) fell to 7.7% in men but increased slightly to 11.2% in women. Interestingly, 84% of all female hypertensives in this study were aware of their diagnosis, compared with less than 70% of men, highlighting the need for BP screening in this age group. Other studies using multiple BP recordings made on several visits have found prevalence rates for ISH of 4.2%, combined hypertension (CH) in 3.9%, and isolated DH of 1% in those aged 65 to 84 years.[6]

Increasing hypertension prevalence rates have been reported in several countries; for example, in the U.S. National Health and Nutrition Examination Survey (NHANES), rates of hypertension in men aged 70+ years increased from 56.6% in 1988 to 1994 to 63.3% in 1999 to 2004 and for women increased from 68.7% to 78.8% over the same time periods.[8] However, the Health Survey for England has shown that hypertension prevalence rates between 1994 and 2011were basically unchanged, remaining at around 30% for all age groups combined.[4] Reliable hypertension incidence data are relatively scarce, particularly in the very old population. Recent U.S. studies have shown that incidence rates vary markedly with ethnicity, with crude incidence rates/1000 person-years being 118 in blacks aged 65 to 74 years compared to 74 in whites, although no such ethnic differences are seen in older age groups.[3] However blacks had a greater awareness and were more likely to be treated for their raised BP levels than whites, although not necessarily with better BP control.

Blood Pressure and Risk

Hypertension in older adults is associated with a twofold to fourfold greater risk of a cardiovascular (CV)–related death than for age- and gender-matched normotensives. There has been much discussion as to whether the link between BP and CV morbidity and mortality is linear, U-shaped, or J-shaped, although many of the intervention studies suggesting an increased risk with lower BP levels were of relatively short duration and did not control for potentially confounding variables. The largest meta-analysis of prospective observational studies to date, involving nearly 1 million adults with no previous history of CV disease, has clearly shown a log linear relationship between increasing BP levels and CV mortality, at least up to the age of 89 years. There was no evidence of a J- or U-shaped effect down to SBP levels of 115 mm Hg and DBP values of 75 mm Hg.[9] A reduction in SBP of 20 mm Hg would potentially reduce stroke mortality by 74% in those aged 40 to 49 years but only by 33% in those aged 80 to 89 years. However, because the absolute risk of stroke and coronary heart disease (CHD) events is much greater in older adults, a 20-mm Hg lower SBP or 10-mm Hg lower DBP would result in an annual difference in absolute risk that is almost 10 times greater in those aged 80 to 89 years compared with the 50- to 59-year-old group. For the very old, some prospective observational studies have suggested that high BP is not a risk factor for mortality, and low values are more closely associated with excess deaths.[10] Little is known about the pattern and factors associated with long-term change (either rise or fall) in BP at a population level, and its impact on important outcomes, including CV incidence, mortality, and cognition, has been less well researched.

Systolic Blood Pressure, Diastolic Blood Pressure, Pulse Pressure, and Risk

Cardiovascular events are more closely related to SBP than DBP levels in older adults. In the Copenhagen Heart Study,[11] the risk ratio (RR) for stroke due to ISH (SBP = 160 mm Hg; DBP < 90 mm Hg) in men was 2.7, but for diastolic hypertension (DBP = 90 mm Hg, irrespective of SBP) it was 1.7 compared with normotensives. For myocardial infarction, no such difference was seen in the relative risk between ISH and diastolic hypertension. More importantly, borderline ISH (SBP = 140 to 159; DBP < 90 mm Hg) in the Physicians Health Study[12] was associated with a 32% increase in CV events and a 56% increase in CV deaths compared to normotensives. If future studies show that treatment of borderline ISH reduces CV risk, this will have enormous implications, because over 20% of those older than 70 years fall into this BP category.

The difference between SBP and DBP values (PP) increases greatly after the age of 50 years as a result of arterial wall stiffening with the associated increase in SBP and fall in DBP. In older age groups in the Framingham study,[13] coronary heart disease was found to be inversely related to DBP at any given level of SBP, suggesting that higher PP is as important, if not more so, than any other component of BP in predicting CHD risk. Pulse pressure was also a better predictor than SBP, independent of DBP levels, for congestive heart failure (CHF); for each 10-mm Hg increase in pulse pressure, there was a 14% increased risk of CHF compared with a 9% increase for the same change in SBP. However, for stroke, mean arterial pressure has been found, in some studies at least, to be a better predictor than SBP or PP. In the Systolic Hypertension in the Elderly Programme,[14] a 10-mm Hg increase in PP was associated with an RR of stroke of 1.11 (1.01 to 1.22) compared with 1.20 (1.02 to 1.42) for a similar MAP rise, suggesting that in older adults, CHD events are more closely related to pulsatile load than steady-state components of BP.

Blood Pressure Variability, Masked Hypertension, White Coat Hypertension, and Risk

Although much attention has previously focused on actual BP levels and CV risk, new data have highlighted the potential role of BP variability as an additional risk factor. Studies have shown that increasing visit to visit SBP variability (a feature of increasing age), as well as maximum SBP values at each visit, are associated with a greater CV risk, in particular for stroke and cognitive decline, compared to average BP values; however, this has not been found in all studies in older adults, particularly for mortality.[15,16] It has also been suggested that the reason some antihypertensive agents (e.g., calcium channels blockers) appear to reduce CV events more effectively in older adults than other agents (e.g., β-blockers) for a similar reduction in BP levels is that they reduce BP variability and/or or central aortic BP more, although this remains to be proven.

Masked hypertension (MHT—normal office BP but elevated home and ambulatory BP levels) has also been identified as another element of the BP spectrum that is important in predicting CV events. It is common (up to 40% of normotensive older adults have MHT) and is particularly common in older men, the 80+ age group, and those with diabetes, but is difficult to recognize because it is impossible to perform self-ambulatory BP measurement in all older adults. Studies have shown that it is not a benign condition, increasing the risk of CV events compared to normotensives, with a hazard ratio of 1.55 compared to 2.1 for those with sustained hypertension.[17] White coat hypertension (WCH—high clinical but normal home and ambulatory BP levels) is also common. In the HYVET trial, 50% of participants had WCH[18] but it appears to be a more benign condition, having a similar or only marginally raised CV risk compared to normotensives. As yet, however, there is no clear evidence that treating WCH or MHT is of benefit at any age.

PATHOGENESIS

MAP is determined by cardiac output and peripheral vascular resistance (PVR) and is the steady-state component of blood pressure. The dynamic component, PP, is the variation around the mean state and is influenced by large artery stiffness, early pulse wave reflection, left ventricular ejection, and heart rate. A rise in PVR and large artery stiffness will increase the systolic BP component, whereas a decrease in PVR or increase in large artery stiffness will result in a fall in diastolic BP, with the latter being the dominant change in older hypertensives.

The main cardiovascular pathophysiologic changes associated with aging are arterial dilation and a decrease in large artery compliance and increased arterial stiffness, especially in the aorta, because of the loss of elastic fibers in the vessel wall and a concomitant increase in collagen. Arterial stiffening leads to enhanced pulse wave velocity (PWV) and early reflected waves augmenting the late systolic aortic pressure wave, resulting in an SBP increase and DBP fall (the underlying findings in isolated systolic hypertension), although the BP changes with age do not generally parallel those of PWV. The rise in mean aortic pressure is augmented by the rise in PVR, seen particularly in older women, and enhanced by impaired endothelial release of nitric oxide, especially in older hypertensives. The increase in systolic load puts excess mechanical strain on the left ventricle, leading to concentric wall thickening. Because coronary artery perfusion is primarily dependent on the diastolic pressure, any reduction in DBP can have adverse effects on coronary artery perfusion, especially because left ventricular myocardial demands are increased in hypertension.

The other main features associated with hypertension in older adults are a reduction in heart rate, cardiac output, intravascular volume, glomerular filtration rate, and cardiac baroreceptor sensitivity (BRS), although cerebral autoregulation is unimpaired with normal aging and hypertension.[19,20] This decrease in cardiac BRS accounts for the increased BP variability found in older hypertensives and plays a role in the increased susceptibility to postural hypotension. Both renal plasma flow and plasma renin activity (PRA) levels decrease with age, with the fall in PRA being more marked in older adult hypertensives than in normotensives. Plasma noradrenaline (norepinephrine) levels increase with age and are associated with a decrease in β-adrenoreceptor sensitivity.

Other Cardiovascular Risk Factors

Primary prevention of CV events is based on the assessment and treatment of classical risk factors, and hypertension should not be considered in isolation, irrespective of patient age. However, it is increasingly clear that the predictive value of the usual risk factors alters with age and therefore standard risk charts, as used in many guidelines, cannot be used in the very old who, because of their age, are already at high risk.

Lipid Abnormalities

The management of dyslipidemia in older adults, especially in those 75 years and older, has been poorly studied but is important, especially because increases in lipid levels and BP are often closely related. Serum total cholesterol (TC) levels increase with age and remain a significant independent predictor for CHD in men. The effect in women is less clear because the numbers of women studied have been too small to draw firm conclusions. The SHEP study[14] found that TC and low-density lipoprotein (LDL) cholesterol levels remained significant indicators of risk in both genders, such that a 1-mmol/L increase in TC was associated with a 30% to 35% higher CHD event rate. The Prospective Studies Collaboration meta-analysis of prospective observational studies of more than 900,000 adults has shown increasing TC levels to be a risk factor for CV mortality, even in the very old. However, although the risk is attenuated with age, such that a 1-mmol/L lower TC was linked to a significant reduction in the hazard ratio (HR) for CHD in those aged 50 to 59 years to 0.57, compared with 0.85 in the 80- to 89-year-old group.[21] This effect was greater in men than women in the older age groups, but was present in both up to 90 years of age. However, for stroke, the link with TC was not as strong as for CHD. For a similar TC reduction, there was a significant lowering of the HR for stroke by 9% in 50- to 59-year-olds compared with a nonsignificant 5% increase in the HR in those aged 80 to 89 years. For CHD, but not stroke, the ratio of TC to high-density lipoprotein (HDL) cholesterol was a better predictor than TC alone, but the predictive power fell with age. A 1.33 lower ratio was related to a 31% decrease in CHD mortality in the 70- to 89-year-old group compared with a 44% reduction in 40- to 59-year-olds. For stroke in those aged 70 to 89 years, and with an SBP higher than 145 mm Hg, TC was negatively correlated with hemorrhagic and total stroke mortality.

Diabetes Mellitus

Up to 10% of older adults with hypertension will have impaired glucose tolerance, and diabetes doubles the risk of developing CHD and stroke in those aged 65 to 94 years. Like total cholesterol, however, its impact on CV events decreases with age: women remain slightly more at risk than men, although the absolute risk from diabetes is greater in older adults than in younger adults.

Body Mass Index

Increasing body mass index (BMI) is associated with a BP increase, but the risk of obesity-related hypertension declines with age compared to those of normal weight; the risk of hypertension is increased threefold in obese 20- to 45-year-olds compared to a 1.5 increase in 65- to 94-year-olds. For each unit of BMI increase (kg/m^2), SBP can be expected to increase by 1.2 mm Hg and DBP by 0.7 mm Hg. Interestingly, for older hypertensive men, the CV relative risk increases from 1.8 to 2.9 between the lowest and highest tertiles of BMI, whereas the reverse is true for women. Even so, hypertension still more than doubles the risk of developing CV disease in both genders. In the European Working Party on Hypertension in the Elderly (EWPHE) study,[22] those with the lowest total mortality and CV terminating events were found in the moderately obese group with a BMI of 28 to 29 kg/m^2, whereas those with a BMI of 26 to 27 kg/m^2 had the lowest cardiovascular mortality. Truncal obesity (reflected in an increased waist- to-hip ratio) is more strongly related to hypertension and is a better predictor for coronary heart disease and stroke than BMI alone. Adiposity tends to decrease in those 75 years and older, and the CV risk associated with increasing BMI, waist circumference, or waist-to-hip ratio is three to four times less in those 70 years and older compared to 40- to 59-year-olds.[23]

Smoking

Although the number of smokers decreases with age, smoking remains a significant risk factor for CV mortality in older adults (RR for men is 2.0 and 1.6 for women). The stroke risk among older hypertensive smokers is five times that of normotensives but 20 times that of normotensive nonsmokers. The benefits of stopping smoking in terms of reducing CHD and stroke mortality are still present, even in those 70 years and older, with the excess risk of mortality declining within 1 to 5 years of quitting. Older smokers should therefore be encouraged to stop. Encouragingly, hypertensive ex-smokers of less than 20 cigarettes/day have, after only a few years of quitting, a similar CV risk to that of hypertensive nonsmokers.

Atrial Fibrillation and Left Ventricular Hypertrophy

In patients with atrial fibrillation, hypertension doubles the stroke risk compared with normotensives. Electrocardiographically diagnosed left ventricular hypertrophy (LVH) increases with age, with reported prevalence rates of 6% in men and 5% in women aged 65 to 74 years, compared with 9.4% and 10.8%, respectively, in those older than 85 years. LVH has a significant effect on CV risk. Its presence in those aged 65 to 94 years nearly triples the risk for men and quadruples that in women, but this effect is less than that seen in younger age groups with a similar BP.

Alcohol

Increasing alcohol consumption is associated with a rise in BP, although the relationship is not linear in most epidemiologic studies, with the lowest incidence of hypertension being seen in those consuming about five to ten units of alcohol per week. Large falls in BP (19/10 mm Hg) have been recorded with abstention in those aged 70 to 74 years who had a long history of heavy alcohol intake. Excessive alcohol intake has been directly related to stroke risk; whether this is due to its direct pressor effect or to some other mechanisms, such as increased risk of atrial fibrillation, is unclear. Because there appears to be a mild protective effect of a small amount of alcohol in older adults, there is no reason to advise strict abstinence.

Diet and Physical Exercise

The relationship between dietary sodium intake and hypertension strengthens with age. For a 100-mmol/day increase, mean BP rises by 5 mm Hg in those aged 20 years but this more than doubles in those 60 to 69 years. Conversely, increasing potassium intake by 60 mmol/day reduces BP in older adults by as much as

10/6 mm Hg. Increasing potassium dietary intake may also reduce stroke risk independently of its hypotensive effect. The average daily potassium intake in older adults in the United Kingdom is about 60 to 70 mmol. This could be raised to over 100 mmol simply by increasing the consumption of vegetables and fruit.

Even mild to moderate physical exercise, such as walking for 30 minutes three to four times a week, has a hypotensive effect and reduces stroke risk, even in older age groups, and has other beneficial effects (e.g., reducing the risk of falls). Whether these effects are mediated solely through BP lowering or are a result of other mechanisms, such as exercise-induced decreases in fibrinogen levels or an increase in HDL cholesterol levels, is unknown.

COMPLICATIONS OF HYPERTENSION

Stroke

Hypertension remains the major treatable risk factor for stroke, although the attributable risk for increasing BP levels decreases with age. For a 10-mm Hg increase in usual DBP, the risk of stroke is almost doubled. A reduction of 9/5 mm Hg can be expected to produce about a 30% decrease in stroke incidence, whereas a fall of 18/10 mm Hg halves the risk; these expectations are irrespective of baseline BP levels. The relative risk of cerebral infarction varies, depending on the hypertension type in older age groups.[24] ISH is a bigger risk factor (RR, 2.3) than combined systolic and diastolic hypertension (RR, 1.5) compared to normotensives. The population-attributable risk for stroke in those aged 70 to 79 years with ISH is about 21% for women and 17% for men, whereas for those aged 50 to 59 years, the figures are 5% for women and 4% for men. Although the relative risk of stroke from raised BP decreases with age, this is not because hypertension per se loses its effect as a risk factor, but that more strokes occur in those with normal blood pressure. Intracerebral hemorrhage is also closely related to hypertension; the relative risk varies from 2.0 to 9.0 in different studies, being greater for combined hypertension than ISH, particularly in younger patients.

Blood Pressure and Asymptomatic Cerebrovascular Disease

Deep white matter lesions (leukoaraiosis) in asymptomatic hypertensive older adult patients are frequently found on magnetic resonance scanning. Whether these lesions account for the age-related cognitive impairment seen with hypertension that has been reported in many studies is unknown. It is also uncertain whether they increase the risk of subsequent cerebral infarction or hemorrhage. ISH, in particular, is associated with subcortical lesions, and good BP control appears to have a protective effect. Large diurnal falls in BP are associated with silent subcortical white matter lesions and lacunar infarcts, but these are also found in those who have marked nocturnal rises in BP.

Cognitive Impairment

The influence of blood pressure on cognitive decline and psychomotor function, over and above its association with vascular dementia, has been widely debated. Some studies have shown no such relationship, whereas others have reported a strong positive correlation with vascular and Alzheimer-type dementia. Studies have suggested that increasing BP levels in midlife are a risk factor for cognitive impairment and dementia in old age, but that there is an inverse correlation between BP measured in old age and dementia in cross-sectional studies. The results of longitudinal studies of BP and cognition in later life are inconsistent, as are those for BP and dementia, although most suggest that a low BP is common in those with severe cognitive impairment.[25] Treating hypertension, even with small decreases in BP, is associated with improvements in MMSE scores and immediate and delayed memory scores, as well as significantly reducing the risk of dementia in some but not all studies.[26,27] In a recent systematic review of placebo-controlled trials of BP reduction in older adults with dementia, Beishon and colleagues[28] showed that there was no clear evidence for benefit (or harm) on cognition or other CV outcomes from antihypertensive use. The pathogenesis of hypertension-related cognitive impairment is unclear but could be linked to a decrease in cerebral blood flow with increasing BP levels and alterations in cerebral metabolism, beyond the changes associated with leukoaraiosis. The Scottish Birth Cohorts data have suggested that the negative relationship between white matter hyperintensities and late-life intelligence is linear and increases with age and hypertension.[29]

Cardiac Disease

The relationship between CHD and hypertension is discussed in a later chapter. Hypertension accelerates the development of coronary artery atheroma via many mechanisms, particularly in association with metabolic abnormalities, as in the insulin resistance syndrome. Increased blood glucose and insulin levels, changes in total cholesterol, HDL, and LDL levels, and endothelial dysfunction result in impaired endothelial-dependent relaxation and increased leukocyte adherence, smooth muscle proliferation, intimal macrophage accumulation, fibrosis, and arterial medial wall thickening. These changes, along with increased vascular oxidative stress and free radical production, result in inflammatory changes in the arterial wall, monocyte migration into the intima, and plaque formation.

DIAGNOSIS AND EVALUATION

General Issues

Accurate measurement of BP levels in older adults is of paramount importance and, despite posing particular problems, it is essential if patients are not to receive unnecessary or inadequate treatment. Minute to minute BP variations occur with respiratory and vasomotor changes, whereas during the 24-hour period, fluctuations are related to mental and physical activity, sleep, and postprandial changes. Seasonal variations are also seen, with BP levels being higher during the winter months. Clinically important differences in BP are frequently found between individual readings at a single visit and between visits. Large falls in BP with repeated measurements in older adult hypertensives have been demonstrated in nearly every placebo-controlled interventional trial, with the effect increasing with age and amounting to as much as a 10/5 mm Hg decrease. The tendency for BP levels to decrease with time is related in part to regression to the mean and familiarity with the procedure of BP measurement.

Measuring Blood Pressure

Guidelines recommend that in uncomplicated cases, an average of two readings (although more will be required in certain cases in which variability is high, as in atrial fibrillation [AF]) be taken with the patient sitting in a quiet relaxed atmosphere on at least two separate occasions, usually during the initial assessment period. It is particularly important to measure BP levels after standing to assess postural BP change in view of the frequency of orthostatic hypotension in this age group and to use standing values if a significant postural BP is found (e.g., >20/10 mm Hg, or the patient is symptomatic).

Mercury sphygmomanometers are being phased out and replaced by semiautomatic devices, but it is important to check the accuracy of any device used and ensure that it has been properly validated in older adults. A list of validated BP measuring devices for use in younger persons and older adults is constantly updated on the British Hypertension Society website (www.bhsoc.org). Cuff size is important, because undercuffing gives falsely high BP values. The cuff width should equal two thirds of the distance between the axilla and antecubital fossa and, when the bladder is placed over the brachial artery, it should cover at least 80% of the arm's circumference, which should be kept supported at heart level. Clinicians should have standard and large cuffs available and ensure that they are used appropriately.

Measurement should be taken in both arms initially because more than 10% of older adults have at least a 10-mm Hg difference between arms. The arm with the highest reading should be used for subsequent measurements. Patients should sit quietly, legs not crossed, and be relaxed, and all measurements should be taken at least 2 hours after a meal to ensure that a falsely low level is not recorded due to postprandial decrease. All older adults should have their BP measured every 5 years if untreated, up to age 80 years at least, and in those with high-normal BP (135 to 139 mm Hg and 85 to 89 mm Hg), it should be reassessed annually.

Cuff measurements tend to underestimate intraarterial levels of SBP by up to 5 to 10 mm Hg and to overestimate DBP by about 5 to 15 mm Hg. The term *pseudohypertension* refers to falsely high noninvasive recordings caused by arterial rigidity. The prevalence of this condition in an unselected older adult population is probably very low, about 1% to 2%, but unfortunately there is no accurate clinical method of easily predicting the condition.

Ambulatory and Self-Monitoring Blood Pressure

NICE guidelines[30] have highlighted the role of ambulatory BP monitoring (ABPM) or self-BP monitoring (SBPM) in the assessment and management of older adults with hypertension; in the United Kingdom, at least routine use of ABPM or SBPM is needed to confirm the diagnosis of hypertension in those with repeatedly raised clinical values with mild hypertension (140 to 159 mm Hg; 90 to 99 mm Hg). Both forms of monitoring reduce the variability and alerting response to measurement, so that 75% of older adult hypertensives will have lower ABPM and SBPM values than clinical values. For daytime ABPM, this is about 10 to 15/5 mm Hg, with the difference increasing with age. It is suggested that for ABPM, three readings/hour are taken during the daytime (minimum, 14 readings) and hourly readings at night (11 PM to 7 AM). The value of other information that the 24-hour ABPM profile can provide, such as day-night differences, is unknown. For SBPM, there should be two readings in the morning before medication and two readings in the evening for 7 days, and the mean of all 28 readings calculated, although some authorities remove the first day's values. Both ABPM and SBPM can be used to diagnose WCH, MHT, postural and postprandial hypotension and truly resistant hypertension in older adults. SBPM, rather than ABPM, has also been used to assess BP control on treatment, although the measuring period is reduced to 3 to 4 days.

Clinical Assessment and Investigations

One common feature of hypertension in younger and older adults alike is that it is very often asymptomatic. Complaints often attributed to increased BP levels, such as headache, are unrelated in most cases. The history and examination should include assessment for the presence of important CV risk factors (e.g., diabetes) and for symptoms and signs of secondary causes of hypertension. Other important factors to be considered are the presence of confusion, urinary incontinence, decreased mobility, and other medication use (for possible drug interactions, which will affect the need for and type of antihypertensive agent), all of which will influence treatment decisions. The examination should focus on evidence of target organ damage, including peripheral pulses and bruits (renal or carotid) and cardiac murmurs. Ophthalmoscopy is used for possible malignant phase hypertension (a condition seen in older adults) and diabetic changes, and a neurologic examination is used for signs of cerebrovascular disease and vascular dementia.

Initial investigations should include height, weight, blood samples for renal function, lipid profile, glucose and HbA1c level estimations, 12-lead electrocardiogram (to exclude ischemic change, dysrhythmias, and LVH), and urine dipstick test for protein and blood. A chest x-ray is of doubtful benefit, except for those who may have heart failure or pulmonary disease, and echocardiography is rarely needed.

Renal artery stenosis is the only major secondary cause of hypertension in this age group and should be considered if there is a sudden onset or rapid progression of hypertension and BP control suddenly becomes difficult, particularly in those at greater risk of atherosclerotic renal artery stenosis (e.g., diabetics, smokers, and those with peripheral vascular disease). It should also be suspected in those who develop malignant phase hypertension and there is rapid deterioration of renal function, particularly after starting angiotensin-converting enzyme (ACE) inhibitors, and in those who develop sudden onset pulmonary edema for no other obvious cause.

Cardiovascular Risk Estimation

The contribution of high BP and hypertension to future CV risk in older adults is usually attenuated due to the accumulation of other competing risk factors associated with aging. Age itself becomes the strongest risk factor associated with CV incidence in the very old, although hypertension remains the biggest treatable risk factor. Although established risk calculators (e.g., those based on Framingham data[31] or QRISK data[32]) have been shown to be of value in the young old (up to 75 years of age), they have limited accuracy in the old old. The original Framingham risk calculator concentrated on factors such as age, gender, BP, lipid levels, diabetes, smoking, BMI, and LVH, but was not found to be accurate in some populations. The QRISK calculator based on UK data included additional factors, such as ethnicity, presence of angina, rheumatoid arthritis, renal dysfunction, AF, and Townsend deprivation score to predict risk more accurately, especially in those up to 84 years of age. More recently, the poor predictive value of using these established CV risk factors and Framingham scoring systems in very old adults has been noted, and other factors, such as homocysteine levels, may be better indicators of those at very high CV risk in the 80 years and older age group.[33] It is worthwhile noting that these risk calculators used different definitions to define CV risk, and there is a tendency for all the risk scores to overestimate the actual risk.

Hypertension Management Guidelines

Several important guidelines relating to the diagnosis and management of hypertension in older people have been published in the last 5 years from the United States,[34] United Kingdom, and Europe[30,35] and, although most offer similar advice, important differences do exist. The most recent guidelines from NICE in 2011,[30] and those subsequently from the Joint British Societies (JBS3),[36] recommended ambulatory BP monitoring (although self-monitoring was an alternative) to confirm the diagnosis of hypertension prior to treatment in those 80 years or younger with a clinical BP of 140 to 159/90 to 99 mm Hg and evidence of target organ damage, established CV disease, renal disease or diabetes, or a 10-year CV risk of 20%. For the 80 years and older

TABLE 42-1 Compelling and Potential Indications for the Main Classes of Antihypertensives in Older Adults*

Class of Drug	Compelling Indications	Possible Indications	Compelling Contraindications	Possible Contraindications
ACE inhibitors, angiotensin receptor blockers	Heart failure	Chronic renal disease, left ventricular dysfunction, diabetes with proteinurea, ARB for those with ACEI-related cough	Renal artery stenosis (particularly if bilateral)	Renal impairment
β-Blockers	Myocardial infarction, angina, atrial fibrillation	Heart failure	Asthma, COPD Heart block	Heart failure, dyslipidemia, PVD, diabetes
Calcium antagonists (dihydropyridine)	ISH, angina	Angina	—	—
Thiazide-like or thiazide diuretics	Heart failure, ISH	Osteoporosis	Gout	Dyslipidemia, renal impairment
α-Blockers	Prostatism	Dyslipidemia	Postural hypotension	Urinary incontinence
Calcium antagonists with (rate-limiting)	Angina	Myocardial infarction	Heart block, heart failure	Combination with β-blocker

ACE, Angiotensin-converting enzyme; *ISH,* isolated systolic hypertension; *COPD,* chronic obstructive pulmonary disease; *PVD,* peripheral vascular disease.
*According to the presence of comorbidities, contraindications, and cautions for their use in older adults.

age group, clinical BP values were set at 150 to 159/90 to 99 mm Hg with ABPM to confirm the diagnosis. All guidelines recommend treatment for those older than 80 years, with certain caveats, especially for the very frail older adults for whom treatment should be individualized. In those with raised BP levels but not at high enough risk for pharmacologic treatment, NICE has recommended that they receive lifestyle advice and an annual checkup. However, for older adults, because their CV risk is high due to age alone, most will be eligible for drug treatment. Other guidelines do not require ABPM and SBPM for diagnosis in those with raised clinical BP levels but propose similar clinical values to consider starting treatment, along with comparable treatment regimens and targets, as shown in Table 42-1.

PHARMACOLOGIC MANAGEMENT OF HYPERTENSION

Several large intervention studies have assessed the effects of antihypertensive drug treatment on outcome in older adults in combined and isolated hypertension, all of which have shown a positive benefit for active treatment. This is perhaps surprising, given the heterogeneity of the patients included in the trials—those with combined hypertension, combined hypertension and ISH, or ISH alone, presence or absence of target organ damage, varying CV risk factors—differences in age at entry, antihypertensive drugs used, and varying length of follow-up.

Hypertension Trials in Older Adults

The first large trial solely in older adult patients was the European Working Party Hypertension in the Elderly (EWPHE) trial, published in 1985,[22] which showed that for every 1000 older adult patients treated for 1 year, initially with a diuretic, 11 fatal cardiac events, 6 fatal and 11 nonfatal strokes, and 8 cases of congestive cardiac failure would be prevented. Subsequently, several important randomized controlled trials enrolled hypertensive patients over 75 years, including the following: Kuramoto and colleagues,[37] using thiazide diuretics as first-line therapy; Hypertension in Elderly People trial,[38] using β-blockers; MRC older adult study,[39] using thiazides or β-blockers; STOP-Hypertension trial,[40] again using thiazides or β-blockers as first-line agents; SHEP,[41] using chlorthalidone, with Syst-Eur[42] and Syst-China[43] being unique in using calcium channel blockers (CCBs) as first-line antihypertensive treatment; and, more recently, the pivotal HYVET trial, which was the first to concentrate on the old old by only enrolling those aged 80 years and older and used the nonthiazide diuretic indapamide as initial therapy.[1]

Fatal and Nonfatal Events

Of the 10 large trials that included people aged 75 years and older, only the HYVET trial reported a significant reduction in all-cause mortality following treatment (HR, 0.79; range, 0.65 to 0.95). A meta-analysis of these trials[44] has shown an overall significant reduction in mortality and morbidity from CHD (RR, 0.73; range, 0.55 to 0.96) and from cardiovascular disease (RR, 0.75; range, 0.65 to 0.86). A general picture of treatment effects on nonfatal events is difficult to formulate because different trials used different criteria for defining nonfatal events. In the nine studies for which data are available in the 75 years and older age group, nonfatal strokes were significantly reduced (RR, 0.78; range, 0.63 to 0.97), as was congestive heart failure (RR, 0.49; range, 0.37 to 0.67), but with considerable variation among trials. In HYVET, there was a significant reduction in fatal stroke of 39% but not nonfatal stroke; for all cardiovascular events there was a significant reduction of 27%, with the benefits being seen within 1 year of starting treatment. The benefits of treatment in terms of RR reduction varied markedly among studies (e.g., for nonfatal stroke it was 0.21 in the SHEP pilot but 1.16 in STOP), and the absolute benefit was seen as being related to underlying patient risk. Withdrawals due to adverse effects were increased with treatment (RR, 1.71; range, 1.45 to 2.00), but overall treatment benefited those with mild to severe systolic and/or diastolic hypertension.

A Cochrane systematic review[45] included 15 trials of over 24,000 moderately to severe hypertensive older adults aged 60 years and older (the young old and old old) who were treated in most trials with a thiazide-like diuretic as first-line therapy, for a mean duration of treatment of 4.5 years. Again, treatment significantly reduced total mortality (RR, 0.90; range, 0.84 to 0.97), total cardiovascular morbidity and mortality (RR 0.72; range, 0.68 to 0.77), and cerebrovascular morbidity and mortality (RR 0.66; range, 0.58 to 0.74). In the three trials restricted to those with ISH, similar benefits were seen.

There is thus convincing evidence that treating raised BP levels in selected older adult patients, at least up to 90 years of age (HYVET had too few patients aged 90 years and older to be conclusive), will significantly reduce CV events without causing intolerable side effects.

There is no substantial evidence that one antihypertensive drug class is significantly better than another in older adult patients but most older hypertensives will require two or three different classes. In keeping with most guidelines, for the 65 years and older age group, recommended initial therapy is a dihydropyridine CCB or thiazide-like diuretic, especially if heart failure is present, to which an ACE inhibitor (ACEI) or angiotensin receptor blocker (ARB) is added if control is not achieved. The ACCOMPLISH trial[46] has shown that the combination of an ACEI and CCB is better at reducing CV events than an ACEI and diuretic, despite similar on treatment BP levels. For those requiring triple therapy, the combination of a thiazide-like diuretic plus an ACEI and CCB is a logical regimen. The availability of low-dose combination tablets (e.g., ACEI and thiazide-like diuretic) may be easier for older adult patients who are already on multiple drug therapies. Current NICE treatment guidelines are as follows:

- Where possible, recommend treatment with drugs taken only once a day.
- Offer people aged 80 years and older the same antihypertensive drug treatment as people aged 55 to 80 years, taking into account any comorbidities.
- Offer people with isolated systolic hypertension (SBP ≥ 160 mm Hg) the same treatment as people with both raised SBP and DBP.
  - **Step 1.** Offer antihypertensive treatment with a CCB to those older than 55 years and to black people of African or Caribbean origin of any age. If a CCB is not suitable—for example, because of edema or intolerance—or if there is evidence of heart failure or high risk of heart failure, offer a thiazide-like diuretic.
  - **Step 2.** If blood pressure is not controlled by step 1, offer treatment with a CCB in combination with an ACEI or ARB. If a CCB is not suitable for step 2 treatment—for example, because of edema or intolerance—or if there is evidence of heart failure or a high risk of heart failure, offer a thiazide-like diuretic.
  - **Step 3.** If treatment with three drugs is required, the combination of an ACEI or angiotensin II receptor blocker, CCB, and thiazide-like diuretic should be used. Consider that clinical BP that remains higher than 140/90 mm Hg after treatment with the optimal or best tolerated doses of an ACEI or ARB plus CCB plus diuretic as resistant hypertension, and consider adding a fourth antihypertensive drug and/or seeking expert advice.
  - **Step 4.** For treatment of resistant hypertension, consider further diuretic therapy with low-dose spironolactone (25 mg, once daily) if the blood potassium level is 4.5 mmol/L or lower. Use particular caution in those with a reduced estimated glomerular filtration rate because they have an increased risk of hyperkalemia. Consider higher dose of thiazide-like diuretic treatment if the blood potassium level is higher than 4.5 mmol/L.
- If a diuretic treatment is to be initiated or changed, offer a thiazide-like diuretic, such as indapamide (1.5 mg modified-release or 2.5 mg once daily) in preference to a conventional thiazide diuretic, such as bendroflumethiazide.
- For people who are already being treated with a thiazide diuretic and whose blood pressure is stable and well controlled, continue current therapy.

Target Blood Pressure Levels for Treatment

Target BP levels in trials have varied considerably and have also fallen considerably over time; for example, target levels in the HEP study[38] were 170/105 mm Hg compared to lower than 140 mm Hg for SBP in SHEP.[41] The fact that the degree of CV risk reduction was so similar between studies is remarkable. However, with the concern still present about a potential U- or J-shaped relationship between BP levels on treatment and outcome, it is still unclear how far BP should be reduced and what target BP should be set. The EWPHE trial[22] suggested that all-cause mortality was lower in those with an SBP with treatment of 150 mm Hg compared with those who achieved an SBP of 130 mm Hg.

The HOT study[47] was specifically designed to determine the optimal target BP level, recruiting 18,790 patients aged 50 to 80 years (mean, 61.5 years) with a diastolic BP of 100 to 115 mm Hg and randomizing them to three target DBP groups: ≤80, ≤85, or ≤90 mm Hg. All patients received initial therapy with the dihydropyridine CCB felodipine. In addition, patients were randomized to low-dose aspirin (75 mg daily) or no aspirin. Unfortunately it proved difficult to reach target BP, particularly in the two lowest groups of DBP, despite triple therapy for most patients. No differences were seen in outcome measures between the three target BP group apart from a borderline significant reduction in myocardial infarctions in 80 mm Hg or less group compared with the 90 mm Hg or less group. However, combining all patient groups showed that the lowest risk point for major cardiovascular events was a mean achieved SBP of 138.5 mm Hg and DBP of 82.6 mm Hg; CV mortality was lowest with a BP of 138.8/86.5 mm Hg (taken as <140/90 mm Hg for guideline purposes). For stroke, the lowest estimated incidence was with an SBP of 142 mm Hg, with no definite minimum DBP level. The Valsartan in Isolated Systolic Hypertension (VALISH) trial[48] aimed to examine whether strict BP control (<140 mm Hg) was superior to moderate BP control (≥140 to <150 mm Hg) in reducing cardiovascular mortality and morbidity in older adult patients aged 70 to 84 years. The study was underpowered to answer the question but showed that BP targets of less than 140 mm Hg are safely achievable in relatively healthy patients =70 years of age with ISH. More relevant to the very old in the HYVET trial, BP was reduced by 15/6 mm Hg by 2 years compared to placebo in those with a baseline BP of 173/90 mm Hg (minimum SBP at entry > 160 mm Hg; target < 150/80 mm Hg). As noted, this brought significant levels of benefit in terms of CV event reduction without resulting in side-effects, but target BP was only achieved in just over 40% of the actively treated group. Threshold and target BP for clinical measurements, as advised by various guideline bodies, are similar (Table 42-2), although the corresponding ABPM and SBPM values vary among studies.

There are many factors that need to be taken into account when considering the need for treatment in older adults. These include the presence of conditions such as postural hypotension, atrial fibrillation, renal impairment, cognitive problems, and contraindications to certain antihypertensive medications. Compliance with medications and quality of life of the patient also need to be taken into account, as well as the overall potential benefit to the patient. It is important to bear in mind that introducing antihypertensive treatment is only part of the risk reduction process. It is the level of blood pressure while on treatment that is a much better predictor of subsequent events than baseline values—hence, the need to try and achieve these target levels. This will mean the requirement for three or more different antihypertensive agents in 20% to 30% of older adult hypertensives. BP medication should be reviewed regularly and appropriate blood tests performed (e.g., electrolyte and lipid levels, renal function). Antihypertensive treatment takes time for the full BP lowering effect to be attained, so a review 3 to 6 weeks after starting or altering therapy should be done. In some cases, SBPM has been used successfully to monitor control; recordings been obtained over 3 to 4 days rather than for 1 week, as for diagnosis. Target BP values are given in the Table 42-2. It is also important that other CV risk factors be addressed simultaneously, such as raised lipid levels and smoking.

Hypertension Treatment in Special Situations

Poststroke Patients

The management of hypertension in the acute stroke period has been the focus of much rather recent work. The SCAST study[49] enrolled patients with ischemic strokes (85%) or primary

TABLE 42-2 Treatment Target Blood Pressures for Clinical Measurements

BP Measurement	NICE/JBS3 Threshold (mm Hg)	NICE/JBS3 Treatment Target (mm Hg)	ESH/ESC Threshold (mm Hg)	ESH/ESC Treatment Target (mm Hg)	ACCF/AHA Threshold (mm Hg)	ACCF/AHA Treatment Target (mm Hg)
OFFICE						
<80 years	≥140/90	<140/90	≥140/90	<140/90	≥140/90	<140/90
≥80 years	≥160/100	<150/90	≥160/100	140-150/<90	≥140/90 (?)	<140-145/90
ABPM DAYTIME						
<80 years	≥135/85	<135/85	≥135/85	Not given	Not given	Not given
≥80years	≥150/95	<140/85	<145/85			
SBPM DAYTIME						
<80 years	≥135/85	<135/85	≥135/85	Not given	Not given	Not given
≥80years	≥150/95	<140/85	<145/85			

Modified from references 30, 34, 35, and 36.
ABPM, Ambulatory blood pressure monitoring; *SBPM,* self–blood pressure monitoring.

intracerebral hemorrhage (PICH) and an SBP more than 140 mm Hg who were randomized to candesartan or placebo within 30 hours of symptom onset. There was a very small BP reduction with active treatment (SBP decrease, 2 mm Hg at 24 hours), but no overall treatment benefit at 6 months and a suggestion of a detrimental effect in terms of functional outcome. The CHHIPS trial[50] compared the hypotensive effect of lisinopril or labetalol with placebo in hypertensive (SBP > 160 mm Hg), mild to moderate severity stroke patients (84% cerebral infarct) within 36 hours of stroke onset. At 24 hours postrandomization, the SBP difference between active and placebo arms was 10 mm Hg but no positive or negative outcomes were seen at 2 weeks; however, 6-month mortality was reduced in the actively treated group. The effect of continuing or stopping current antihypertensive immediately poststroke was assessed in the COSSACS study[51] but again, at 2 weeks and 6 months, there were no differences in death or disability between groups. A meta-analysis of BP reduction trials early poststroke showed no benefit of early treatment. However, these studies, comprised mainly of patients with cerebral infarction, suggested that PICH patients may benefit to a greater extent with acute BP lowering. This was addressed in INTERACT2,[52] a trial of rapid BP reduction within 6 hours of intracerebral hemorrhage to a target of less than 180 mm Hg or less than 140 mm Hg within 1 hour of randomization. Although the primary outcome of death and disability was not significantly reduced by intensive BP reduction, other measures of functional outcome were significantly improved in the lower target BP group.

In regard to the poststroke period, some key questions remain unanswered, in particular the timing of when to start antihypertensive treatment poststroke and target levels to be achieved. One of the key questions that remains unanswered is the optimal timing of BP lowering poststroke, although early intervention aiming to reduce BP levels seems safe. The PROGRESS trial[53] emphasized the benefit of a regimen based on a thiazide-like diuretic, with or without an ACEI, for reducing stroke recurrence in normotensive and hypertensive patients. Several important trials of BP reduction in secondary stroke prevention were subsequently published. The PRoFESS study[54] included over 20,000 patients with a history of ischemic stroke who were randomized to telmisartan or placebo, of whom nearly 75% had a history of hypertension. Surprisingly, over the 30-month follow-up period, and despite a difference of 4/2 mm Hg between the telmisartan and placebo groups, no benefit was found in terms of reducing stroke recurrence or major CV event rates. A subsequent analysis showed a J-shaped relation between achieved BP levels and stroke recurrence, with the lowest risk in those who maintained an SBP between 120 and 139 mm Hg, similar to findings in the PROGRESS trial. A meta-analysis of 10 poststroke secondary prevention studies, which included these trials, showed a significant treatment effect of BP lowering in reducing stroke recurrence (odds ratio [OR], 0.71; 95% confidence interval [CI], 0.59 to 0.86) and cardiovascular events (OR, 0.69; CI, 0.57 to 0.85), but could not provide evidence that any specific antihypertensive agent was better or stated the optimal target BP levels.

Subsequently, the SPS3 study, which aimed to assess the optimal BP levels to prevent stroke recurrence in those who had had a lacunar infarct, randomized patients to an SBP target of 130 to 149 mm Hg or less than 130 mm Hg, with no specific antihypertensive regimen being used to achieve these targets. Patients in the intensive BP reduction group at 1 year achieved a mean SBP of 127 mm Hg, compared to 138 mm Hg in the higher target group, which was associated with a 19% (nonsignificant) reduction in all stroke events and a 63% (significant) reduction in PIHC, without producing any significant adverse effects. The fact that recurrence rates were not statistically reduced was probably, at least in part, related to the fact that the stroke recurrence rate in the trial was lower than predicted and the study was therefore underpowered.

Further evidence that lower BP levels offer a better prognostic outcome has been demonstrated in the observational studies, which have shown that cerebral infarct patients receiving antithrombotic agents poststroke were less likely to develop an ICH with lower BP levels, with optimum values being less than 130/80 mm Hg. Most stroke secondary prevention trials have excluded patients with a previous intracerebral hemorrhage but, in those in which they have been enrolled, and despite the small patient numbers, the benefit of BP lowering has been as much or greater than that seen with cerebral infarction. Similarly, there are few data on BP management in those with significant carotid or vertebral artery stenosis, although some clinical expert opinion has suggested maintaining higher target BP levels (e.g., 140 to 150/85 to 90 mm Hg) so that patients remain asymptomatic, with cerebral perfusion being compromised in some of these patients due to associated impaired cerebral autoregulation. Despite limited data, there is no evidence that target BP levels following a transient ischemic attack (TIA) should be set at a different value than those following stroke.

Thus, currently, there is good evidence that antihypertensive treatment should be considered for secondary prevention in all stroke and TIA patients. For most of them, this should be started after the first week postictus if BP is sustained at 140/90 mm Hg, with the aim of a target BP of 130 to 140/80 to 85 mm Hg (although optimal target BP levels have yet to be clearly defined).

Most evidence to date suggests that treatment should be with a thiazide-like diuretic, with or without an ACEI.

Falls and Frailty

The relationship between antihypertensive treatment and falls is complex. Older adult patients with hypertension frequently have orthostatic hypotension (OH), which may be due to the effects of hypertension in reducing cardiac baroreceptor sensitivity. However, many older hypertensive patients experience postural symptoms without an obvious fall on standing in systemic BP levels, suggesting an abnormality in cerebral blood flow control. Although antihypertensive medications are known to be associated with an increased risk of OH and hence falls, and falls with injury, others causes, such as drug-related drowsiness, cognitive impairment, bradycardia, or comorbidities, should be considered as a potential fall risk. BP-lowering therapy per se may increase risk of falls by nearly 25%, although the risk of serious falls does not seem to be related to the intensity of treatment or type of antihypertensive drug group, despite the well-known link between certain drug types—for example, α-blockers, and OH.[55] Those with elevated BP levels and determined as frail (being unable to complete a 6-m walk test) had a better prognosis than those with normal BP levels in terms of reduced mortality.[56] The walking test may therefore be one way of identifying those who may not benefit from antihypertensive treatment. Fracture rates tend to be lower in those older hypertensives who are prescribed thiazide diuretics and ARBS than those on CCBs, with the highest rates occurring in those on loop diuretics.[56]

As noted, nearly all trials of antihypertensive therapy in older adults have excluded those who are physically or mentally frail. Some have suggested that a high BP in this group may be a good prognostic indicator because BP often falls in older adults in the months to years before death. The benefits and the risks of antihypertensives in those who faller and those who are frail should always be considered before prescribing; clinical judgement is paramount in decision making.

Resistant Hypertension

Resistant hypertension (RHT) is defined as a BP that remains above goal (see Table 42-2) in spite of the concurrent use of three antihypertensive agents of different classes at optimal or best tolerated doses. The prevalence of RHT is estimated at 10% to 20% among those with treated hypertension, depending on the population studied.[57] Older adults, especially those older than 75 years, with high baseline BP, presence of target organ damage (e.g., LVH, chronic kidney disease), diabetes, obesity, atherosclerotic vascular disease, female gender, black ethnicity, and excessive dietary sodium are typically present in resistant hypertension. It is important to exclude WCH prior to making a diagnosis of resistant hypertension, because up to 40% of patients defined as having RHT according to clinical BP recordings may have WCT.[58]

There is as yet no clear evidence about the best agent to add to the standard triple therapy in RHT. Possibilities for older adults include spironolactone or amiloride (while watching serum potassium levels and renal function), and/or an α- or β-blocker, but seeking specialist help is also advisable.

Type 2 Diabetes

Hypertension is common in older type 2 diabetics. Nearly two thirds will have raised BP levels that require treatment. Older diabetics should be treated aggressively in terms of BP reduction. The UK Prospective Diabetes Study[59] showed that strict BP control reduces strokes by 44% (11% to 65%) and death related to diabetes by 32% (6% to 51%). A subgroup of older diabetics in the SHEP study[41] also did well, with a 5-year reduction of major CV events of 34% (6% to 54%) compared with placebo and a reduction of nonfatal and fatal coronary heart disease (CHD) events by 54% (12% to 76%). Diabetics in the STOP-2 study[60] showed no difference in outcome between those on conventional therapy (low-dose thiazide diuretic or β-blocker) and those on the newer agents (ACEIs, CCBs). This again highlights how the degree of BP reduction and not the agent used that predicts CV risk; diabetics require lower target BP levels, as evidenced by the HOT study. Hence, in type 2 diabetics, BP levels for the introduction of therapy should be 140/90 mm Hg (with target control levels set at 130/80 mm Hg in those up to 80 years of age). Despite the high CV risk with type 2 diabetes, the ACCORD trial showed no evidence that lower BP target levels (SBP < 120 mm Hg) further reduced CV events, although more stroke events were prevented.[61] Recommended first-line agents are ACEIs; if control levels are not reached, then follow the steps outlined earlier in the chapter with a CCB as second-line agent, rather than a diuretic.

Cognitive Function, Dementia, and Quality of Life

The Medical Research Council study in older adults found no difference in the changes in cognitive function between β-blocker- or diuretic-treated patients compared with the placebo group over a 54-month follow-up.[62] Because hypertension is associated with vascular dementia and Alzheimer disease, it might be hoped that treatment could slow down or prevent cognitive decline. The Syst-Eur study,[42] encouragingly for a relatively short follow-up period of 2 years, found that active treatment reduced the incidence of dementia by 50% (although the numbers actually involved were very small) and improved the Mini-Mental State score slightly, whereas in the placebo group, scores deteriorated significantly. However, the SHEP study[41] failed to find a decrease in the incidence of dementia with active treatment. The cognitive arm of the HYVET study[27] also failed to show that BP lowering in the very old reduced dementia, but the follow-up period was probably too short to see any benefit; this might have been because the trial was too short to see an effect. Combining all trials that assessed the effects of BP lowering on dementia in older adult hypertensives found a 13% reduction with active treatment.[27]

Although there are relatively limited numbers of studies assessing the long-term effects of antihypertensives on quality of life measures, most have shown a long-term benefit. Quality of life should be an essential part of the overall patient assessment, but it does not necessarily require a lengthy or complex questionnaire. A simple clinical assessment of possible changes in physical function (e.g., mobility and balance, ability for self-care), sexual function, energy levels and mood, cognitive function, life satisfaction, and social interaction is sufficient. Of particular importance are the effects of treatment on cognitive function, mood, and mobility. Thiazide diuretics appear to be the cleanest in terms of effects on quality of life factors, but there are at present too few data on the newer agents to assess whether some of the positive qualities of these agents (e.g., improved mood with ACEI use) are borne out in large clinical trials. For those who are particularly frail, stopping antihypertensive treatment should always be considered, particularly if it might be causing symptoms.

METHODS OF BLOOD PRESSURE REDUCTION

Lifestyle and Nonpharmacologic Methods

There has been a general lack of enthusiasm for nondrug measures to reduce BP in older adult patients, despite the evidence of their efficacy (see later). Various guidelines have emphasized the importance of lifestyle modification as first-line treatment in trying to achieve normotension in those with only mild hypertension and in reducing other CV risk factors, as well as assisting the effects of antihypertensive treatment.

Weight Loss

A 2-kg weight loss in those who are overweight over a 6-month period will reduce BP by about 4/5 mm Hg in older hypertensive subjects.[63] However, constant encouragement is needed to maintain this weight loss if the long-term benefit is to be seen. A body weight within 10% of ideal (or a BMI < 26 kg/m^2) should be encouraged, not just for its hypotensive effects, but also to improve glycemic control, lipid profiles, mobility, and respiratory and cardiac function.

Dietary Mineral Intake

The hypotensive effect of reducing sodium intake increases with age. In older hypertensives, an 80-mmol/day decrease in sodium intake (roughly halving dietary intake) will result in an 8-mm Hg decrease in SBP.[43,64] This level of sodium reduction can be achieved simply by avoiding salty foods and not adding salt while cooking or at the table. Reducing salt added to processed food would make even greater reductions possible. Increasing potassium intake by 40 mmol/day will have a significant hypotensive action, reducing clinical BP by 10/6 mm Hg and 24-hour BP levels by 6/2 mm Hg.[65] The average intake of potassium in the United Kingdom is about 60 to 70 mmol/day, and an intake of 100 to 110 mmol/day can be achieved by encouraging greater consumption of fresh fruits and vegetables. Changing magnesium and calcium intake has not been found to have a significant effect on BP in older adults, although increasing vitamin C intake does have a mild hypotensive action and a positive effect on the lipid profile in older hypertensives.

Other Measures

Inquiring about, and if necessary reducing, alcohol intake is an important but often neglected method of reducing BP. Caffeine may have an acute pressor effect in caffeine-naïve persons, but regular caffeine intake does not have a pressor effect, although some studies have shown that increasing consumption is associated with an increased CHD risk. Mild aerobic exercise—walking 30 minutes/day, three to four times a week—results in important BP reductions (≈20/10 mm Hg) in older hypertensives. It also decreases stroke risk independently of its hypotensive action and improves glucose profiles, reduces weight, and benefits general well-being.

Combined Effects

The combined effect of dietary interventions has been investigated in two important studies. The Dietary Approaches to Stop Hypertension (DASH) trial[66] studied the effects of a special diet rich in vegetables and fruit and low in dairy products and compared this to a standard diet while varying levels of sodium intake in persons with and without hypertension. The DASH diet, with a low sodium intake, resulted in a BP fall of 7 mm Hg in normotensives and 11.5 mm Hg in hypertensives, effects similar to those that might be seen with a thiazide diuretic (see later).

The Trial of Non-pharmacologic intervention in the Elderly (TONE) study[63] randomized older hypertensives who were normotensive on monotherapy to drug treatment withdrawal and sodium reduction (and, if obese, sodium reduction, weight loss, or both) or usual care, with a 30-month follow-up. End points of restarting hypotensive drug treatment or developing a CV disorder were significantly reduced by all the interventions, with a 53% risk reduction in the obese on the combined sodium restriction and weight loss diet. The study was underpowered to find a significant decrease in CV events alone, but the nutritional interventions were well tolerated.

Approximately 25% of older adults with mild hypertension could remain off drug treatment for 12 months or more using nonpharmacologic measures. Predictors of those who will remain normotensive include the absence of LVH on the electrocardiogram, being nonobese, and with well-controlled SBP levels prior to withdrawal of treatment. In general, nonpharmacologic methods should be tried initially in all patients and given time to work, although constant encouragement will be needed and, in most patients, drug therapy will also be needed. Important synergistic effects between nonpharmacologic and drug treatments have been found, such as with sodium restriction of patients treated with ACEIs.

Drug Treatment

Thiazide and Thiazide-Like Diuretics

Despite low-dose thiazide-like diuretics (e.g., indapamide) being of proven benefit in the older hypertensive, with little evidence for the efficacy of true thiazide diuretics (e.g., bendroflumethiazide), the latter are often prescribed as first-line therapy for combined or isolated systolic hypertension.[24] Their mode of action has not been fully resolved, but is in part due to a reduction in peripheral vascular resistance. Although there are concerns that thiazides may induce postural hypotension, this is not a significant side effect. Mild hypokalemia, hyponatremia, hyperuricemia, dyslipidemia, and increased blood glucose levels can occur but are not normally clinically significant if low doses are used. Impotence can still be a problem with these agents in all age groups. Serum electrolyte levels should be checked a few weeks after starting treatment to assess the need for additional potassium supplementation.

Calcium Channel Blockers

Intervention studies (e.g., Syst-Eur,[42] Syst-China,[43] and HOT[47] studies) have used members of the dihydropyridine CCB group as first-line therapy and shown significant benefits, particularly in terms of stroke and CV risk reduction, and trial evidence has indicated that these agents are generally well tolerated. They are useful in those with concomitant diseases such as angina and their adverse effects (e.g., ankle swelling) are usually well tolerated if low doses are used initially and gradually increased. Short-acting CCBs have no role in the treatment of hypertension.

Angiotensin-Converting Enzyme Inhibitors and Angiotensin Receptor Blockers

In spite of the theoretical argument that ACEIs or ARBs may not be effective antihypertensives in older adults because of their low renin status, numerous trials have shown that both drug groups are effective antihypertensive agents in younger individuals and older adults, both in terms of BP reduction and prevention of CV disease. First-dose hypotension may occur, especially in patients who are on high-dose diuretics, so it is usually recommended that these agents be reduced or stopped for a few days before initiating ACEI therapy. Hyperkalemia can be a problem, so potassium-sparing diuretics should be stopped with the introduction of these drugs. Problems with renal impairment have been reported in older adult patients especially those taking nonsteroidal antiinflammatory drugs (NSAIDs) and those with preexisting renal impairment. Renal failure may be precipitated in those with occult renal artery stenosis, so it is recommended that urea and electrolyte levels be checked before and 1 to 2 weeks after starting treatment. Cough can be a problem in about 10% of

43 Valvular Heart Disease

Wilbert S. Aronow

AORTIC STENOSIS

Causes and Prevalence

Valvular aortic stenosis (AS) in older adults is usually due to stiffening, scarring, and calcification of the aortic valve leaflets. The commissures are not fused, as in rheumatic AS. Calcific deposits in the aortic valve are common in older adults and may lead to valvular AS. Aortic cuspal calcium was present in 295 of 752 men (36%), mean age 80 years, and in 672 of 1663 women (40%), mean age 82 years.[1] Of 2358 persons, mean age 81 years, 378 (16%) had valvular AS, 981 (42%) had valvular aortic sclerosis (thickening of or calcific deposits on the aortic valve cusps, with a peak flow velocity across the aortic valve = 1.5 m/sec), and 999 (42%) had no valvular AS or aortic sclerosis.[2] Calcific deposits in the aortic valve were present in 22 of 40 necropsy patients (55%) aged 90 to 103 years.[3] Calcium of the aortic valve and mitral annulus may coexist.[4-7]

In the Helsinki Aging Study, calcification of the aortic valve was diagnosed by Doppler echocardiography in 28% of 76 persons aged 55 to 71 years, in 48% of 197 persons aged 75 to 76 years, in 55% of 155 persons aged 80 to 81 years, and in 75% of 124 persons aged 85 to 86 years.[8] Aortic valve calcification, aortic sclerosis, and mitral annular calcium (MAC) are degenerative processes,[4,3,9-11] accounting for their high prevalence in older adults.

Otto and colleagues[10] have shown that the early lesion of degenerative AS is an active inflammatory process, with some similarities to atherosclerosis, including lipid deposition, macrophage and T cell infiltration, and basement membrane disruption. In a study of 571 persons, mean age 82 years, 292 (51%) had calcified or thickened aortic cusps or root.[12] A serum total cholesterol of 200 mg/dL, a history of hypertension, diabetes mellitus, and a serum high-density lipoprotein cholesterol level less than 35 mg/dL were more prevalent in older adults with calcified or thickened aortic cusps or root than in older adults with normal aortic cusps and root.[12]

In the Helsinki Aging Study, age, hypertension, and a low body mass index were independent predictors of aortic valve calcification.[13] In 5201 persons older than 65 years in the Cardiovascular Health Study, independent clinical factors associated with degenerative aortic valve disease included age, male gender, smoking, history of hypertension, height, and high lipoprotein(a) and low-density lipoprotein (LDL) cholesterol levels.[11] In 1275 older adults, mean age 81 years, AS was present in 52 of 202 (26%) with 40% to 100% extracranial carotid arterial disease (ECAD) and in 162 of 1073 (15%) with 0% to 39% ECAD.[14] In 2987 older adults, mean age 81 years, symptomatic peripheral arterial disease occurred in 193 of 462 (42%) with AS and in 639 of 2525 (25%) without AS.[15]

In 290 persons, mean age 79 years, with valvular AS, who had follow-up Doppler echocardiography, older adults with MAC had a greater reduction in aortic valve area per year than older adults without MAC.[16] Significant independent risk factors for the progression of valvular AS in 102 older adults, mean age 76 years, who had follow-up Doppler echocardiography were cigarette smoking and hypercholesterolemia.[17] Palta and associates[18] have also shown that cigarette smoking and hypercholesterolemia accelerate the progression of AS. These and other data suggest that aortic valve calcium, MAC, and coronary atherosclerosis in older adults have similar predisposing factors.[10-20]

A retrospective analysis of 180 older adult patients with mild AS who had follow-up Doppler echocardiography at 2 or more years showed that significant independent predictors of the progression of AS were male gender, cigarette smoking, hypertension, diabetes mellitus, serum LDL cholesterol level equal to 125 mg/dL at follow-up, serum high-density lipoprotein (HDL) cholesterol level less than 35 mg/dL at follow-up, and use of statins (inverse association).[21] A retrospective analysis of 174 older adult patients, mean age 68 years, with mild to moderate AS showed that statin therapy reduced the progression of AS.[22] In a retrospective study of 156 older adult AS patients, mean age 77 years, statin therapy decreased the progression of AS by 54% at 3.7-year follow-up.[23]

In a prospective open-label study of 121 patients with an aortic valve area between 1.0 and 1.5 cm^2, 61 patients with a serum LDL cholesterol level greater than 130 mg/dL were treated with rosuvastatin and 60 patients with a serum LDL cholesterol level less than 130 mg/dL did not receive statins.[24] At 73-week follow-up, patients treated with rosuvastatin had significantly less progression of AS. These data differ from the results reported in 155 patients in the Scottish Aortic Stenosis and Lipid Lowering Trial, Impact on Regression Study, which included patients with extensive aortic valve calcification.[25] Two trials are in progress investigating the effect of statins on AS.

The frequency of AS increases with age. Valvular AS, as diagnosed by Doppler echocardiography, was present in 141 of 924 older men (15%), mean age 80 years, and in 322 of 1881 older women (17%), mean age 81 years.[26] Severe valvular AS (peak gradient across aortic valve = 50 mm Hg, or aortic valve area < 0.75 cm^2) was diagnosed in 62 of 2805 older adults (2%).[26] Moderate valvular AS (peak gradient across aortic valve = 26 to 49 mm Hg, or aortic valve area = 0.75 to 1.49 cm^2) was present in 149 of 2805 older adults (5%).[26] Mild valvular AS (peak gradient across aortic valve =10 to 25 mm Hg, or aortic valve area = 1.50 cm^2) occurred in 250 of 2805 older adults (9%).[26] In 501 unselected older adults aged 75 to 86 years in the Helsinki Aging Study, critical AS was present in 3% and moderate to severe AS was present in 5% of the 501 older adults.[8]

Pathophysiology

In valvular AS, there is resistance to ejection of blood from the left ventricle into the aorta, with a pressure gradient across the aortic valve during systole and an increase in left ventricular (LV) systolic pressure. The pressure overload on the left ventricle leads to concentric LV hypertrophy, with an increase in LV wall thickness and mass, normalizing systolic wall stress, and maintenance of normal LVEF (LVEF) and cardiac output.[27,28] A compensated hyperdynamic response is common in older women.[29] Older adults with a comparable degree of AS have more impairment of LV diastolic function than younger persons.[30] Coronary vasodilator reserve is more severely impaired in the subendocardium in patients with LV hypertrophy caused by severe AS.[31]

The compensatory concentric LV hypertrophy leads to abnormal LV compliance, LV diastolic dysfunction with decreased LV diastolic filling, and increased LV end-diastolic pressure, further increased by left atrial systole. Left atrial enlargement develops. Atrial systole plays an important role in diastolic filling of the left ventricle in those with AS.[32] Loss of effective atrial contraction may cause immediate clinical deterioration in those with severe AS.

Sustained LV hypertrophy eventually leads to LV chamber dilation, with reduced LVEF and ultimately congestive heart failure (CHF). The stroke volume and cardiac output decrease, mean left atrial and pulmonary capillary pressures increase, and pulmonary hypertension occurs. Older adults with both obstructive and nonobstructive coronary artery disease have an increased incidence of LV enlargement and LV systolic dysfunction.[33] In a percentage of older adults with AS, the LVEF will remain normal, and LV diastolic dysfunction will be the main problem.

In 48 older adults with CHF associated with unoperated severe valvular AS, the LVEF was normal in 30 of them (63%).[34] The prognosis of those with AS and LV diastolic dysfunction is usually better than that of those with AS and LV systolic dysfunction, but is worse than that of those without LV diastolic dysfunction.[34,35]

Symptoms

Angina pectoris, syncope or near-syncope, and CHF are the three classic manifestations of severe AS. Angina pectoris is the most common symptom associated with AS in older adults. Coexistent coronary artery disease (CAD) is frequently present in them. However, angina pectoris may occur in the absence of CAD as a result of an increase in myocardial oxygen demand, with a decrease in myocardial oxygen supply at the subendocardial level. Myocardial ischemia in those with severe AS and normal coronary arteries is due to inadequate LV hypertrophy, with increased LV systolic and diastolic wall stresses causing reduced coronary flow reserve.[36]

Syncope in persons with AS may be caused by decreased cerebral perfusion following exertion when arterial pressure falls because of systemic vasodilation in the presence of a fixed cardiac output. LV failure with a reduction in cardiac output may also cause syncope. In addition, syncope at rest may be caused by a marked decrease in cardiac output secondary to transient ventricular or atrial fibrillation or transient atrioventricular block related to extension of the valve calcification into the conduction system. Coexistent cerebrovascular disease with transient cerebral ischemia may contribute to syncope in older adults with AS.

Exertional dyspnea, paroxysmal nocturnal dyspnea, orthopnea, and pulmonary edema may be caused by pulmonary venous hypertension associated with AS. Coexistent CAD and hypertension may contribute to CHF in older adults with AS. Atrial fibrillation may also precipitate CHF in these persons.

CHF, syncope, or angina pectoris was present in 36 of 40 older adults (90%) with severe AS, in 66 of 96 older adults (69%) with moderate valvular AS, and in 45 of 165 older adults (27%) with mild valvular AS.[37]

Sudden death occurs mainly in symptomatic AS older adults.[34,37-40] It may also occur in 3% to 5% of asymptomatic older adults with AS.[38,41] Marked fatigue and peripheral cyanosis in those with AS may be caused by a low cardiac output. Cerebral emboli causing stroke or transient cerebral ischemic attack, bacterial endocarditis, and gastrointestinal bleeding may also occur in older adults with AS.

Signs

A systolic ejection murmur heard in the second right intercostal space, down the left sternal border toward the apex, or at the apex is classified as an aortic systolic ejection murmur (ASEM).[5,41-43] An ASEM is commonly heard in older adults,[4,5,41] occurring in 265 of 565 unselected older adults (47%).[5] Of 220 older adults with an ASEM and technically adequate M-mode and two-dimensional echocardiograms of the aortic valve, 207 (94%) had aortic cuspal or root calcification or thickening.[5] Of 75 older adults with an ASEM, valvular AS was diagnosed by continuous-wave Doppler echocardiography in 42 of them (56%).[43]

TABLE 43-1 Correlation of Physical Signs of Aortic Stenosis With Severity of Aortic Stenosis in Older Adults

	Severity of Aortic Stenosis (%)		
Sign	*Mild (n = 74)*	*Moderate (n = 49)*	*Severe (n = 19)*
Aortic systolic ejection murmur	95	100	100
Prolonged duration aortic systolic ejection murmur	3	63	84
Late-peaking aortic systolic ejection murmur	3	63	84
Prolonged carotid upstroke time	3	33	53
A_2 absent	0	10	16
A_2 reduced or absent	5	49	74

Modified from Aronow WS, Kronzon I. Prevalence and severity of valvular aortic stenosis determined by Doppler echocardiography and its association with echocardiographic and electrocardiographic left ventricular hypertrophy and physical signs of aortic stenosis in elderly patients. Am J Cardiol 67:776–777, 1991.

Table 43-1 shows that an ASEM was heard in 100% of 19 older adults with severe AS, in 100% of 49 older adults with moderate AS, and in 95% of 74 older adults with mild AS.[42] However, the ASEM may become softer or absent in persons with CHF associated with severe AS because of a low cardiac output. The intensity and maximal location of the ASEM and transmission of the ASEM to the right carotid artery do not differentiate among mild, moderate, and severe AS.[5,42,43] The ASEM may be heard only at the apex in some older adults with AS. The apical systolic ejection murmur may also be louder and more musical than the basal systolic ejection murmur in some older adults with AS. The intensity of the ASEM in valvular AS increases with squatting and by inhalation of amyl nitrite and decreases during the Valsalva maneuver.

Prolonged duration of the ASEM and late peaking of the ASEM best differentiate severe AS from mild AS.[5,42,43] However, the physical signs do not distinguish between severe and moderate AS (see Table 43-1).[42,43]

A prolonged carotid upstroke time does not differentiate between severe and moderate AS in older adults.[42,43] A prolonged carotid upstroke time was palpable in 3% of older adults with mild AS, in 33% of older adults with moderate AS, and in 53% of older adults with severe AS (see Table 43-1).[42] Stiff noncompliant arteries may mask a prolonged carotid upstroke time in older adults with severe AS. The pulse pressure may also be normal or wide rather than narrow in older adults with severe AS because of loss of vascular elasticity. An aortic ejection click is rare in older adults with severe AS because of loss of vascular elasticity and because the valve cusps are immobile.[42,43]

An absent or reduced A_2 occurs more frequently in older adults with severe or moderate AS than in persons with mild AS (see Table 43-1). However, an absent or decreased A_2 does not differentiate between severe and moderate AS.[42,43] The presence of atrial fibrillation, reversed splitting of S_2, or an audible fourth heart sound at the apex also does not differentiate between severe and moderate AS in older adults.[43] The presence of a third heart sound in older adults with AS usually indicates the presence of LV systolic dysfunction and elevated LV filling pressure.[44]

Diagnosis

Electrocardiography and Chest Roentgenography

Echocardiography is more sensitive than electrocardiography in diagnosing LV hypertrophy in an older person with AS.[42] In 19 older adults with severe valvular AS, LV hypertrophy was diagnosed by electrocardiography in 58% of older adults and by echocardiography in 100% of older adults.[42] In 49 older adults with moderate AS, LV hypertrophy was diagnosed by electrocardiography in 31% and by echocardiography in 96%. In 74 older adults with mild valvular AS, LV hypertrophy was diagnosed by electrocardiography in 11% and by echocardiography in 74%.[42] Rounding of the LV border and apex may occur as a result of concentric LV hypertrophy. Poststenotic dilation of the ascending aorta is commonly seen. Calcification of the aortic valve is best seen by echocardiography or fluoroscopy.

Involvement of the conduction system by calcific deposits may occur in older adults with AS. In a study of 51 older adults with AS who underwent aortic valve replacement, conduction defects occurred in 58% of 31 older adults with MAC and in 25% of 20 older adults without MAC.[7] In another study of 77 older adults with AS, first-degree atrioventricular block occurred in 18%, left bundle branch block in 10%, intraventricular conduction defect in 6%, right bundle branch block in 4%, and left axis deviation in 17%.[45]

Complex ventricular arrhythmias may be detected by 24-hour ambulatory electrocardiography in those with AS. Older adults with complex ventricular arrhythmias associated with AS have a higher incidence of new coronary events than older adults with AS and no complex ventricular arrhythmias.[46]

Echocardiography and Doppler Echocardiography

M-mode and two-dimensional echocardiography and Doppler echocardiography are very useful in the diagnosis of AS. Of 83 persons with CHF or angina pectoris and a systolic precordial murmur in whom severe AS was diagnosed by Doppler echocardiography, AS was not clinically diagnosed in 28 of them (34%).[47] Echocardiography can detect thickening, calcification, and reduced excursion of aortic valve leaflets.[5] LV hypertrophy is best diagnosed by echocardiography.[42] Chamber dimensions and measurements of LV end-systolic and end-diastolic volumes, LVEF, and assessment of global and regional LV wall motion provide important information on LV systolic function.

Doppler echocardiography is used to measure peak and mean transvalvular gradients across the aortic valve and to identify associated valve lesions. Aortic valve area can be calculated by the continuity equation using pulsed Doppler echocardiography to measure LV outflow tract velocity, continuous-wave Doppler echocardiography to measure transvalvular flow velocity, and a two-dimensional long-axis view to measure LV outflow tract area.[48,49] Aortic valve area can be detected reliably by the continuity equation in older adults with AS.[49]

Shah and Graham[50] have reported that the agreement in quantitation of the severity of AS between Doppler echocardiography and cardiac catheterization was greater than 95%. Those with a peak jet velocity greater than 4.5 m/sec had critical AS, and those with a peak jet velocity less than 3.0 m/sec had noncritical AS. Slater and coworkers[51] demonstrated a concordance between Doppler echocardiography and cardiac catheterization in the decision to operate or not to operate in 61 of 73 older adults (84%) with valvular AS. In 75 older adults, mean age 76 years, with valvular AS, the Bland-Altman plot showed that 4 of the 75 older adults (5%) had disagreement between cardiac catheterization and Doppler echocardiography that was outside the 95% confidence limit.[52]

Cardiac catheterization was performed in 105 older adults in whom Doppler echocardiography demonstrated an aortic valve area of 0.75 cm^2 or a peak jet velocity of 4.5 m/sec, consistent with critical AS.[53] Doppler echocardiography was 97% accurate in this subgroup. Cardiac catheterization was performed in this study in 133 older adults with noncritical AS. Doppler echocardiography was 95% accurate in this subgroup. Although most older adults do not require cardiac catheterization before aortic valve surgery, they require selective coronary arteriography before aortic valve surgery. Those in whom Doppler echocardiography shows a peak jet velocity between 3.6 and 4.4 m/sec and an aortic valve area greater than 0.8 cm^2 should undergo cardiac catheterization if they have cardiac symptoms attributable to AS.[49] Those with a peak jet velocity between 3.0 and 3.5 m/sec and an LVEF less than 50% may have severe AS, requiring aortic valve replacement, and should undergo cardiac catheterization.[50] Those with a peak jet velocity between 3.0 and 3.5 m/sec and an LVEF greater than 50% probably do not need aortic valve replacement (AVR) but should undergo cardiac catheterization if they have symptoms of severe AS.[50]

Natural History

Ross and Braunwald[38] have demonstrated that the average survival rate was 3 years after the onset of angina pectoris in those with severe AS. They reported that their average survival rate after the onset of syncope was 3 years and that the average survival rate after the onset of CHF in those with severe AS was 1.5 to 2 years.

Persons with symptomatic severe valvular AS have a poor prognosis.[37-40,54] At the National Institutes of Health, 52% of those with symptomatic severe valvular AS not operated on were dead at 5 years.[39,40] At 10-year follow-up, 90% of them were dead.

At 4-year follow-up of older adult patients aged 75 to 86 years in the Helsinki Aging Study, the incidence of cardiovascular mortality was 62% in those with severe AS and 35% in those with moderate AS.[55] At 4-year follow-up, the incidence of total mortality was 76% in those with severe AS and 50% in those with moderate AS.[55]

In a prospective study, at 19-month follow-up (range, 2 to 36 months), 90% of 30 older adult patients with CHF associated with unoperated severe AS and a normal LVEF were dead.[34] At 13-month follow-up (range, 2 to 24 months), 100% of 18 older adult patients with CHF associated with unoperated severe AS and an abnormal LVEF had died.[34]

Table 43-2 shows the incidence of new coronary events in older adults with no, mild, moderate, and severe AS. Independent

TABLE 43-2 Incidence of New Coronary Events in Older Adults With Aortic Stenosis (AS)

	Severity of AS			
Parameter	*No AS (n = 1496)*	*Mild AS (n = 165)*	*Moderate AS (n = 96)*	*Severe AS (n = 40)*
Age (yr)	81	84	85	85
Follow-up (mo)	49	52	32	20
New coronary events (%)	41	62	80	93

Modified from Aronow WS, Ahn C, Shirani J, et al: Comparison of frequency of new coronary events in older adults with mild, moderate, and severe valvular aortic stenosis with those without aortic stenosis. Am J Cardiol 81:647–649, 1998.

risk factors for new coronary events in this study were prior myocardial infarction, AS, male gender, and increasing age.[37] In this prospective study, at 20-month follow-up of 40 older adults with severe AS, CHF, syncope, or angina pectoris was present in 36 of 37 (97%) who developed new coronary events and in 0 of 3 (0%) without new coronary events.[37] At 32-month follow-up of 96 older adults with moderate valvular AS, CHF, syncope, or angina pectoris was present in 65 of 77 (84%) who developed new coronary events and in 1 of 19 (5%) without new coronary events.[37] At 52-month follow-up of 165 older adults with mild AS, CHF, syncope, or angina pectoris was present in 40 of 103 older adult patients (39%) who developed new coronary events and in 5 of 62 older adult patients (8%) without new coronary events.[37]

In a prospective study of 981 older adults, mean age 82 years, with aortic sclerosis and of 999 older adults, mean age 80 years, without valvular aortic sclerosis, older adults with aortic sclerosis at 46-month follow-up had a 1.8 times higher chance of developing a new coronary event than those without valvular aortic sclerosis.[2] Otto and colleagues[56] also reported that AS and aortic sclerosis increased cardiovascular morbidity and mortality in 5621 men and women aged 65 years.

Kennedy and associates[57] followed 66 older adults with moderate AS diagnosed by cardiac catheterization (aortic valve area, 0.7 to 1.2 cm^2). In 38 older adults with symptomatic moderate AS and 28 older adults with minimally symptomatic moderate AS, the probabilities of avoiding death from AS were 0.86 and 1.0 for those with minimally symptomatic moderate AS at 1-year follow-up, 0.77 for those with symptomatic AS and 1.0 for those with minimally symptomatic AS at 2 years, 0.77 for those with symptomatic AS and 0.96 for those with minimally symptomatic AS at 3 years, and 0.70 for those with symptomatic AS and 0.90 for those with minimally symptomatic AS at 4 years.[57] During the 35-month mean follow-up in this study, 21 older adults underwent aortic valve replacement.

The Veterans Administration Cooperative Study on Valvular Heart Disease followed 106 older adults with unoperated AS for 5 years.[58] During follow-up, 60 of 106 older adults (57%) died. Multivariate analysis has demonstrated that measures of the severity of the AS, presence of CAD, and presence of CHF were the important predictors of survival in unoperated older adults.

Studies have shown that patients with asymptomatic severe AS are at low risk for death and can be followed until symptoms develop.[59-62] Turina and colleagues[59] followed 17 older adults with asymptomatic or mildly symptomatic AS. During the first 2 years, none died or had aortic valve surgery. At 5-year follow-up, 94% were alive and 75% were free of cardiac events. Kelly and associates[60] followed 51 asymptomatic older adults with severe AS. During 17-month follow-up, 21 (41%) of them became symptomatic. Only 2 of 51 (4%) died of cardiac causes. In both of them, death was preceded by the development of angina pectoris or CHF. Pellikka and coworkers[61] showed that 113 of 143 older adults (79%), mean age 72 years, with asymptomatic severe AS were not initially referred for AVR or percutaneous aortic balloon valvuloplasty. During 20-month follow-up, 37 of 113 of them (33%) became symptomatic. The actuarial probability of remaining free of cardiac events associated with AS, including cardiac death and aortic valve surgery, was 95% at 6 months, 93% at 1 year, and 74% at 2 years. No asymptomatic older adult with severe AS developed sudden death while asymptomatic.

Rosenhek and colleagues[62] followed 126 older adults with asymptomatic severe AS for 22 months. Eight of them died and 59 of them developed symptoms necessitating aortic valve replacement. Event-free survival was 67% at 1 year, 56% at 2 years, and 33% at 4 years. Five of the six deaths from cardiac disease were preceded by symptoms. Of those with moderately or severely calcified aortic valves whose aortic jet velocity increased by 0.3 m/sec or more within 1 year, 79% underwent AVR or died within 2 years of the observed increase.

However, other studies have demonstrated that those with asymptomatic severe AS should be considered for AVR (AVR).[63,64] Of 338 older adult patients with severe asymptomatic AS, mean age 71 years, 99 (29%) had AVR during a mean follow-up of 3.5 years.[63] Survival at 1, 2, and 5 years in the nonoperated patients was 67%, 56%, and 38%, respectively, compared with 94%, 93%, and 90%, respectively, in those who underwent AVR ($P < .0001$).[63] In this study, unoperated patients had a 48% significant reduction in mortality if they were treated with statins and a significant 48% reduction in mortality if they were treated with β-blockers.[63]

Data were analyzed for 622 older adult patients, mean age 72 years, with asymptomatic severe AS at the Mayo Clinic.[64] After the initial diagnosis, 166 (27%) developed chest pain, shortness of breath, or syncope and had AVR. Another 97 older adult patients (16%) had AVR in the absence of symptoms. The operative mortality was 2% for the symptomatic patients and 1% for the asymptomatic patients. The survival of the 263 older adult patients who had AVR was not significantly different from an age- and gender-matched population. The 10-year survival was 64% for symptomatic patients and 64% for asymptomatic patients who had AVR.[64] At 3 years after the diagnosis of severe AS, 52% of the 622 older adult patients had had symptoms develop, had undergone AVR, or had died.[64] Absence of AVR was an independent risk factor for mortality, with a hazard ratio of 3.53.

Treatment

Medical Management

Prophylactic antibiotics should not be used to prevent bacterial endocarditis in those with AS regardless of severity, according to current American Heart Association (AHA) guidelines.[65] Persons with CHF, exertional syncope, or angina pectoris associated with moderate or severe AS should undergo AVR promptly. Valvular surgery is the only definitive therapy in these older adults.[66] Medical therapy does not relieve the mechanical obstruction to LV outflow and does not relieve symptoms or progression of the disorder. Older adults with asymptomatic AS should report the development of symptoms possibly related to AS immediately to their physician. If significant AS is present in asymptomatic older adults, clinical examination and electrocardiography and Doppler echocardiography should be performed at 6-month intervals if AVR is not being considered. Nitrates should be used with caution in those with angina pectoris and AS to prevent the occurrence of orthostatic hypotension and syncope. Diuretics should be used with caution in those with CHF to prevent a decrease in cardiac output and hypotension. Vasodilators should be avoided. Digitalis should not be used for those with CHF and a normal LVEF unless needed to control a rapid ventricular rate associated with atrial fibrillation.

Surgical Treatment

Aortic Valve Replacement. Box 43-1 lists four class I indications and one class IIa indication for performing AVR in older adult patients with AS.[67] AVR is the procedure of choice for symptomatic older adult patients with severe AS. Other class I indications for AVR in older adult patients with severe AS include patients undergoing coronary artery bypass surgery (CABS), those undergoing surgery on the aorta or other heart valves, and those with an LVEF less than 50%.[67] Older adult patients with moderate AS undergoing CABS or surgery on the aorta or other heart valves have a class IIa indication for AVR.[67]

Although the American College of Cardiology (ACC)/AHA guidelines do not recommend AVR in older adult patients with asymptomatic severe AS and normal LVEF, other studies have suggested otherwise.[63,64] The data from these two studies favor

BOX 43-1 American College of Cardiology/American Heart Association Indications for Aortic Valve Replacement in Older Adults With Severe Aortic Stenosis (AS)

1. Older patient with symptomatic severe AS (class I indication)
2. Older patient with severe AS undergoing coronary artery bypass surgery (class I indication)
3. Older patient with severe AS undergoing surgery on the aorta or other heart valves (class I indication)
4. Older patient with severe AS and a left ventricular ejection fraction < 50% (class I indication)
5. Older patient with moderate AS undergoing coronary artery bypass surgery or surgery on the aorta or other heart valves (class IIa indication)

Modified from Bonow RO, Carabello BA, Chatterjee K, et al: ACC/AHA 2006 practice guidelines for the management of patients with valvular heart disease: executive summary. A report of the American College of Cardiology/American Heart Association task force on practice guidelines (writing committee to revise the 1998 guidelines for the management of patients with valvular heart disease). Developed in collaboration with the Society of Cardiovascular Anesthesiologists. Endorsed by the Society for Cardiovascular Angiography and Interventions and the Society of Thoracic Surgeons. J Am Coll Cardiol 48:598–675, 2006.

AVR in older adult patients with a diagnosis of asymptomatic severe AS when there is a low institutional perioperative mortality. In addition, of 197 consecutive older adult patients with asymptomatic severe AS, early AVR was performed in 102 of them (52%).[68] The estimated actuarial 6-year all-cause mortality rates were 2% for AVR and 32% for the conventional treatment group. Despite being asymptomatic, older adult patients with very severe AS have a poor prognosis.[69] Early elective AVR should be considered in these patients. Of 73 older adult patients with severe AS who did not undergo AVR, 15 (14%) died at 15-month follow-up.[70] Of these 73, symptoms were thought to be unrelated to the AS in 31 patients. Exercise stress tests for symptoms were performed in only 4% of the 42 asymptomatic older adult patients.[70]

Asymptomatic patients with low-gradient severe AS and normal LVEF with reduced stroke volume index had aortic valve events similar to those with a normal stroke volume index at 46-month follow-up.[71] Of 248 older adult patients with severe AS and normal LVEF, 94 had a low gradient (<30 mm Hg mean gradient; group 1), 87 had a moderate gradient (30 to 40 mm Hg mean gradient; group 2), and 67 had a severe gradient (>40 mm Hg mean gradient; group 3).[72] Symptoms were present in 49% of group 1 patients, in 55% of group 2 patients, and in 60% of group 3 patients (*P* not significant). At 45- to 60-month follow-up, the incidence of AVR or death was 71% for group 1, 77% for group 2, and 76% for group 3 (*P* not significant). Kaplan-Meier survival curves for time to death in all three groups were significantly better for patients with AVR versus no AVR

Echocardiography is recommended in asymptomatic patients with AS every year for severe AS, every 1 to 2 years for moderate AS, and every 3 to 5 years for mild AS.[64] AVR is the procedure of choice for symptomatic older adults with severe AS. The bioprosthesis has less structural failure in older adults than in younger persons and may be preferable to the mechanical prosthetic valve for AS replacement in older adults due to the anticoagulation issue.[73-76] Persons with mechanical prostheses need anticoagulant therapy indefinitely. Those with porcine bioprostheses may be treated with aspirin, 75 to 100 mg daily, unless he or she has atrial fibrillation, abnormal LVEF, previous thromboembolism, or a hypercoagulable condition.[67,76] Box 43-2 lists four

BOX 43-2 Indications for Antithrombotic Therapy in Older Adult Patients With Aortic Valve Replacement (AVR)

1. After AVR with bileaflet mechanical or Medtronic Hall prosthesis. If no risk factors, administer warfarin to maintain INR between 2.0 and 3.0; if risk factors are present, the INR should be maintained between 2.5 and 3.5 (class I indication).
2. After AVR with Starr-Edwards valves or mechanical disc valves (other than Medtronic Hall prostheses), in patients with no risk factors, warfarin should be administered to maintain INR between 2.5 and 3.5 (class I indication).
3. After AVR with a bioprosthesis and no risk factors, administer aspirin in a dose of 75 to 100 mg daily (class I indication).
4. After AVR with a bioprosthesis and risk factors, administer warfarin to maintain an INR between 2.0 and 3.0 (class I indication).
5. During the first 3 months after AVR with a mechanical prosthesis, it is reasonable to give warfarin to maintain an INR between 2.5 and 3.5 (class IIa indication).
6. During the first 3 months after AVR with a bioprosthesis in patients with no risk factors, it is reasonable to give warfarin to maintain an INR between 2.0 and 3.0 (class IIa indication).

Modified from Bonow RO, Carabello BA, Chatterjee K, et al: ACC/AHA 2006 practice guidelines for the management of patients with valvular heart disease: executive summary. A report of the American College of Cardiology/American Heart Association task force on practice guidelines (writing committee to revise the 1998 guidelines for the management of patients with valvular heart disease). Developed in collaboration with the Society of Cardiovascular Anesthesiologists. Endorsed by the Society for Cardiovascular Angiography and Interventions and the Society of Thoracic Surgeons. J Am Coll Cardiol 48:598–675, 2006.

class I indications and two class IIa indications for antithrombotic therapy in older adult patients with AVR.[67]

Arom and associates[77] performed AVR in 273 older adults aged 70 to 89 years (mean age, 75 years), 162 with AVR alone, and 111 with AVR plus CABS. Operative mortality was 5%. Late mortality at 33-month follow-up was 18%. At 5-year follow-up, actuarial analysis showed that overall survival was 66% for those with AVR alone, 76% for those with AVR plus CABS, and 74% for a similar age group in the general population.

Culliford and coworkers[75] performed AVR in 71 older adults aged 80 years, in 35 with AVR alone, and in 36 with AVR plus CABS. Hospital mortality was 6% in older adults s with AVR alone and 19% in older adults with both AVR plus CABS. At 1-year follow-up, survival from late cardiac death was 100% for older adults who had AVR alone and 96% for older adults who had AVR plus CABS. At 3-year follow-up, survival from late cardiac death was 100% for older adults who had AVR alone and 91% for older adults who had AVR plus CABS. Freedom from all valve-related complications (e.g., thromboembolism, anticoagulant-related complications, endocarditis, reoperation, prosthetic failure) was 93% at 1-year follow-up and 80% at 3-year follow-up. At follow-up, 65% of survivors were in New York Heart Association (NYHA) functional class I or II, 31% in NYHA functional class III, and 4% in NYHA functional class IV.

Levinson and colleagues[78] performed AVR in 71 octogenarians, mean age 82 years. The operative mortality was 9% in these older adults . At 28-month follow-up, 100% of the survivors were in NYHA functional class I or II. Actuarial 1-, 5-, and 10-year survival rates were 83%, 67%, and 49%, respectively. A U.K. heart valve registry has indicated that 30-day mortality was 6.6% in 1100 older adults aged 80 years (56% women) who underwent AVR.[79] The actuarial survival was 89% at 1 year, 79% at 3 years, 69% at 5 years, and 46% at 8 years.

AVR is associated with a reduction in LV mass and in improvement of LV diastolic filling.[80,81] Hoffman and Burckhardt[82] performed a prospective study in 100 older adults who had AVR. At 41-month follow-up, the yearly cardiac mortality rate was 8% in those with electrocardiographic LV hypertrophy and repetitive ventricular premature complexes (two couplets/24 hr during 24-hour ambulatory monitoring) and 0.6% in older adults without either of these findings.

If LV systolic dysfunction in those with severe AS is associated with critical narrowing of the aortic valve rather than myocardial fibrosis, it often improves after successful AVR.[83] In 154 older adult patients, mean age 73 years, with AS and LVEF of 35% who underwent AVR, the 30-day mortality was 9%. The 5-year survival was 69% in those without significant CAD and 39% in those with significant CAD. NYHA functional class III or IV was present in 58% of them before surgery versus 7% of them after surgery. Postoperative LVEF was measured in 76% of survivors at a mean of 14 months after surgery; improvement in LVEF was found in 76%.[83]

Balloon Aortic Valvuloplasty. AVR was a procedure for symptomatic older adults with severe AS. In a Mayo Clinic study, the actuarial survival of 50 older adults, mean age 77 years, with symptomatic severe AS in whom AVR was refused (45 persons) or deferred (5 persons) was 57% at 1 year, 37% at 2 years, and 25% at 3 years.[84] Because of the poor survival rate in this group, balloon aortic valvuloplasty should be considered when operative intervention is refused or deferred.

Balloon aortic valvuloplasty is effective palliative therapy for some older adults with symptomatic AS, although restenosis with recurrence of symptoms is common.[85-94] Rodriguez and associates[91] found that in 42 older adults undergoing aortic valvuloplasty, mean age 78 years, the 2-year survival was 36% in those with an LVEF less than 40% and 80% in those with an LVEF greater than 40%. The 2-year event-free survival (freedom from aortic valve surgery or severe CHF) was 0% in persons with an LVEF less than 40% and 34% in persons with an LVEF greater than 40%.[91] Block and Palacios[86] found recurrence of symptoms, death, or hemodynamic evidence of restenosis in 56% of 90 older adults, mean age 79 years, an average of 5.5 months after aortic valvuloplasty. Kuntz and coworkers[92] found immediate clinical improvement after successful aortic valvuloplasty in most of 205 older adults, mean age 78 years, but restenosis in more than 50% of the persons within 1 to 2 years. On the basis of the available data, balloon aortic valvuloplasty should be considered for older adults with symptomatic severe AS who are not candidates for aortic valve surgery and possibly for persons with severe LV dysfunction as a bridge to subsequent valve surgery.[92-94]

The European Society of Cardiology/European Association for Cardio-Thoracic Surgery 2012 guidelines stated that class I indications for AVR include the following: (1) symptomatic severe AS; (2) asymptomatic patients with severe AS undergoing CABS, surgery of the ascending aorta, or surgery of another valve; (3) asymptomatic severe AS with an LVEF less than 50%; and (4) asymptomatic severe AS with an abnormal exercise test showing symptoms on exercise clearly related to AS.[95] Class IIa indications for AVR include the following: (1) high-risk patients with severe symptomatic AS suitable for transapical AVR but in whom AVR is favored by a heart team based on the risk profile and anatomic suitability; (2) asymptomatic severe AS and an abnormal exercise test showing a fall in blood pressure below baseline; (3) moderate AS in patients undergoing CABS, surgery of the ascending aorta, or surgery of another valve; (4) symptomatic patients with severe AS, normal LVEF, and a low gradient (<40 mm Hg); (5) symptomatic patients with severe AS, reduced LVEF, low gradient, and evidence of flow reserve; and (6) asymptomatic severe AS with none of the above if the surgical risk is low, and the peak transvalvular velocity is greater than 5.5 m/sec (very severe AS) or there is severe aortic valve calcification and a rate of peak transvalvular velocity progression of 0.3 m/sec/year. Transapical AVR should be considered in patients with severe symptomatic AS who are considered unsuitable for surgical AVR because of severe comorbidities.[95]

Follow-up was performed at a mean of 12.6 years in older adult patients aged 65 to 80 years undergoing AVR with a biologic (24,410 patients) or mechanical (14,789 patients) prosthesis.[96] Long-term mortality rates were similar for both types of prostheses. Bioprostheses were associated with a higher risk of reoperation (255%) and endocarditis (60%) but a lower risk of stroke (13%) and hemorrhage (34%).[96]

Transcatheter Aortic Valve Implantation. Transcatheter aortic valve implantation (TAVI) may be performed in nonsurgical older adult patients with end-stage calcific AS.[97,98] Eighteen high-risk older adult patients, mean age 76 years, with severe AS and moderate CAD amenable to percutaneous coronary intervention (PCI) had combined PCI followed by minimally invasive AVR.[99] One of 18 of them (6%) died postoperatively, with no late mortality, after a mean follow-up of 19 months.[99] Of 442 older adult patients with severe AS at increased surgical risk, mean age 82 years, 78 were treated with medical management, 107 with AVR, and 257 with TAVI.[100] At 30-month follow-up, adjusted mortality was 49% significantly lower for AVR compared with medical treatment and 62% significantly lower for TAVI compared with medical treatment. At 1-year, 92.3% of AVR patients, 93.2% of TAVI patients, and 70.8% of medically treated patients were NYHA functional class I or II.[100]

In the Placement of Aortic Transcatheter Valves (PARTNER) trial, 699 high-risk older adult patients with severe AS, mean age 84 years, were randomized to AVR or TAVI.[101] All-cause mortality was 3.4% for the TAVI group versus 6.5% for the AVR group at 30 days (*P* not significant) and 24.2% for the TAVI group versus 26.8% for the AVR group at 1 year (*P* not significant). Major stroke was 3.8% for the TAVI group versus 2.1% for the AVR group at 30 days (*P* not significant) and 5.1% for the TAVI group versus 2.4% for the AVR group at 1 year (*P* not significant). Major vascular complications at 30 days were 11.0% for the TAVI group versus 3.2% for the AVR group. New-onset atrial fibrillation was 16.0% after AVR and 8.6% after TAVI. Major bleeding was found in 19.5% after AVR and 9.3% after TAVI. At 1-year follow-up, there were similar improvements in cardiac symptoms for both groups.[101] In the PARTNER trial, among inoperable patients with severe AS, TAVI caused significant improvements in health-related quality of life maintained for at least 1 year compared with standard care.[102] At 2-year follow-up of 699 high-risk patients with severe AS in the PARTNER trial, all-cause mortality was 33.9% for TAVI and 35.0% for AVR (*P* not significant).[103] The incidence of stroke was 7.7% for TAVI and 4.9% for AVR (*P* not significant). Moderate or severe paravalvular aortic regurgitation was 6.9% for TAVI and 0.9% for AVR and was associated with increased late mortality.[103]

At 2-year follow-up of 358 older adult patients, mean age 83 years, with inoperable severe AS in the PARTNER trial randomized to transcatheter AVR (TAVR) or to standard therapy with balloon aortic valvuloplasty performed in 82% of this group, 43% of the TAVR patients and 68% of the standard therapy patients were dead.[104] The rates of cardiac death at 2 years were 31% for the TAVR group versus 62% for the standard therapy group. The rates of stroke at 2 years were 14% for the TAVR group versus 6% for the standard therapy group. The rates of rehospitalization at 2 years were 35% for the TAVR group versus 73% for the standard therapy group. Echocardiographic data showed a sustained increase in aortic valve area and a reduction in aortic valve gradient, with no worsening of paravalvular aortic regurgitation.[104] These data suggest that the mortality benefit in patients with TAVR may be limited to older adult patients without extensive comorbidities.

Low flow in patients with severe AS independently predicts mortality.[105] At 2-year follow-up of 180 older adult patients, mean age 84 years, with low-flow inoperable severe AS in the PARTNER trial, the mortality was 76% in the standard therapy group versus 46% in the TAVR group.[105] At 2-year follow-up of 350 older adult patients, mean age 84 years, with low-flow severe AS in the PARTNER trial, the mortality was 40% in the AVR group versus 38% in the TAVR group (*P* not significant).[105] In the inoperable group in the PARTNER trial, at 2-year follow-up, all-cause mortality in older adult patients with a normal stroke volume index was 38% with TAVR versus 53% in those who had undergone medical management.[105]

One third of 270 patients undergoing a CoreValve TAVI needed a permanent pacemaker implanted within 30 days.[106] Periprocedural atrioventricular block, balloon predilation, use of the larger CoreValve prosthesis, increased interventricular septum diameter, and prolonged QRS duration were independently associated with the need for implantation of a permanent pacemaker.[106]

At 42-month follow-up of 339 older adult patients, mean age 81 years, who had TAVI because they were considered to be inoperable or at very high surgical risk, 188 (56%) had died.[107] The causes of late death in 152 patients were noncardiac comorbidities in 59%, cardiac death in 23%, and unknown in 18%.[107] TAVI results in similar hemodynamic and long-term clinical outcomes for high-risk surgical patients with low-gradient severe AS as for those with typical severe AS.[108]

In the United States, the Society of Thoracic Surgeons (STS)/American College of Cardiology Transcatheter Valve Therapy Registry showed that 7,710 older adult patients underwent TAVR (20% who were inoperable and 80% who were high risk but operable).[109] The median age was 84 years, 49% were women, and the median STS predicted risk of mortality was 7%. A transfemoral approach was used in 64%, a transapical approach in 29%, and other alternative approaches in 7%. In-hospital mortality was 5.5% and major vascular injury was 6.4%. At 30- day follow-up, the incidence of mortality was 7.6% (52% due to a noncardiovascular cause), of stroke was 2.8%, of dialysis-dependent renal failure was 2.8%, and of re-intervention was 0.5%.[109]

The 2012 ACCF/American Association for Thoracic Surgery/Society for Cardiovascular Angiography and Interventions/STS expert consensus document on TAVR recommended TAVR for patients with severe symptomatic calcific stenosis of a trileaflet aortic valve who have aortic and vascular anatomy suitable for TAVR and a predicted survival longer than 1 year and who have a prohibitive surgical risk. This was defined by an estimated 50% or greater risk of mortality or irreversible morbidity at 30 days or other factors such as frailty, prior radiation therapy, porcelain aorta, and severe hepatic or pulmonary disease.[110] These guidelines also stated that TAVR is a reasonable alternative to AVR in patients at high surgical risk (PARTNER trial criteria: STS = 8%). These guidelines stated that major complications from TAVR are mortality (3% to 5%), stroke (6% to 7%), access complications (17%), pacemaker insertion (2% to 9% for Sapien and 19% to 43% for CoreValve), bleeding, prosthetic dysfunction, paravalvular aortic regurgitation, acute kidney injury, coronary occlusion, valve embolization, and aortic rupture.[110]

The European Society of Cardiology/European Association for Cardio-Thoracic Surgery guidelines have stated that TAVR is indicated for patients with severe symptomatic AS who are considered unsuitable for AVR as assessed by a heart team and who are likely to gain improvement in their quality of life and have a life expectancy of more than 1 year after consideration of their comorbidities (class I indication).[95] TAVR should be considered for high-risk older adult patients with severe symptomatic AS who may still be suitable for AVR but for whom TAVR is favored by a heart team based on their individual risk profile and anatomic suitability (class IIa indication).[95] Clinical absolute contraindications to TAVR include absence of a heart team and no cardiac surgery on site, estimated life expectancy less than 1 year, improvement of quality of life by TAVR unlikely because of comorbidities, severe primary associated disease of other valves with major contribution to symptoms that can be treated only by surgery, and anatomic contraindications (e.g., inadequate annulus size, thrombus in left ventricle, active endocarditis, increased risk of coronary ostium obstruction, plaques with mobile thrombi in the ascending aorta or arch, inadequate vascular access).[95] Relative contraindications include bicuspid or noncalcified valves, untreated coronary artery disease requiring revascularization, hemodynamic instability, LVEF less than 20% and, for the transapical approach, severe pulmonary disease or the LV apex is not accessible.[95] After TAVI, treatment with clopidogrel for 3 months in addition to aspirin is widely practiced.

AORTIC REGURGITATION

Causes and Prevalence

Acute aortic regurgitation (AR) in older adults may be due to infective endocarditis, rheumatic fever, aortic dissection, trauma following prosthetic valve surgery, or rupture of the sinus of Valsalva and causes sudden severe LV failure. Chronic AR in older adults may be caused by valve leaflet disease (secondary to any cause of AS, infective endocarditis, rheumatic fever, congenital heart disease, rheumatoid arthritis, ankylosing spondylitis, following prosthetic valve surgery, or myxomatous degeneration of the valve) or by aortic root disease. The cause of aortic root disease causing chronic AR in older adults includes association with systemic hypertension, syphilitic aortitis, cystic medial necrosis of the aorta, ankylosing spondylitis, rheumatoid arthritis, Reiter disease, systemic lupus erythematosus, Ehler-Danlos syndrome, and pseudoxanthoma elasticum. Mild or moderate AR was also diagnosed by Doppler echocardiography in 9 of 29 persons (31%) with hypertrophic cardiomyopathy.

The prevalence of AR increases with age.[111-113] Margonato and colleagues[112] linked the increased prevalence of AR with age to aortic valve thickening. In a prospective study of 450 unselected older adults, mean age 82 years, AR was diagnosed by pulsed Doppler echocardiography in 39 of 114 men (34%) and in 92 of 336 women (27%).[114] Severe or moderate AR was diagnosed in 74 of 450 older adults (16%). Mild AR was diagnosed in 57 of 450 older adults (13%). In a prospective study of 924 men, mean age 80 years, and 1881 women, mean age 82 years, valvular AR was diagnosed by pulsed Doppler recordings of the aortic valve in 282 of 924 men (31%) and in 542 of 1881 women (29%).[26]

Pathophysiology

The primary determinants of AR volume are the regurgitant orifice area, transvalvular pressure gradient, and duration of diastole.[115] Chronic AR increases LV ventricular end-diastolic volume. The largest LV end-diastolic volumes are seen in those with chronic severe AR. LV stroke volume increases to maintain the forward stroke volume. The increased preload causes an increase in LV diastolic stress and the addition of sarcomeres in series, which results in an increase in the ratio of the LV chamber size to wall thickness. This pattern of LV hypertrophy is termed *eccentric left ventricular hypertrophy*.

Primary myocardial abnormalities or ischemia due to coexistent CAD decrease the contractile state. LV diastolic compliance decreases, LV end-systolic volume increases, LV end-diastolic pressure rises, left atrial pressure increases, and pulmonary venous hypertension result. When the LV end-diastolic radius-to-wall thickness ratio rises, LV systolic wall stress increases abnormally because of the preload and afterload mismatch.[28,116] Additional stress then decreases the LVEF response to exercise.[117] Eventually, the LVEF, forward stroke volume, and effective cardiac output are decreased at rest. My colleagues and I have demonstrated that an abnormal resting LVEF occurs in 8 of 25 older adults (32%) with CHF associated with chronic severe AR.[118]

In those with acute severe AR, the left ventricle cannot adapt to the increased volume overload. Forward stroke volume falls, LV end-diastolic pressure increases rapidly to high levels,[119] and pulmonary hypertension and pulmonary edema result. The rapid rise of the LV end-diastolic pressure to exceed the left atrial pressure in early diastole causes premature closure of the mitral valve.[120] This prevents backward transmission of the elevated LV end-diastolic pressure to the pulmonary venous bed.

Symptoms

Persons with acute AR develop symptoms due to the sudden onset of CHF, with marked dyspnea and weakness. Persons with chronic AR may remain asymptomatic for many years. Mild dyspnea on exertion and palpitations, especially on lying down, may occur. Exertional dyspnea, orthopnea, paroxysmal nocturnal dyspnea, fatigue, and edema are common clinical symptoms when LV failure occurs. Syncope is rare. Angina pectoris occurs less often in older adult patients with AR than in older adult patients with AS and may be due to coexistent CAD. However, nocturnal angina pectoris, often accompanied by flushing, diaphoresis, and palpitations, may develop when the heart rate slows and arterial diastolic pressure falls to very low levels. Most of those with severe AR who do not have surgery die within 2 years after CHD develops.[121]

Signs

The AR murmur is typically a high-pitched, blowing diastolic murmur that begins immediately after A_2. The diastolic murmur is best heard along the left sternal border in the third and fourth intercostal spaces when AR is due to valvular disease. The murmur is best heard along the right sternal border when AR is due to dilation of the ascending aorta. The diastolic murmur is best heard with the diaphragm of the stethoscope with the person sitting up, leaning forward, and holding the breath in deep expiration. The severity of AR correlates with the duration of the diastolic murmur, not with the intensity of the murmur.

Grayburn and associates[122] heard an AR murmur in 73% of 82 older adults with AR and in 8% of 24 older adults without AR. Saal and coworkers[123] heard an AR murmur in 80% of 35 older adults with AR and in 10% of 10 older adults without AR. Meyers and colleagues[124] heard an AR murmur in 73% of 66 older adults with AR and in 22% of 9 older adults without AR. An AR murmur was heard in 95% of 74 older adults with severe or moderate AR diagnosed by pulsed Doppler echocardiography, in 61% of 57 older adults with mild AR, and in 3% of 319 older adults with no AR.[114]

In those with chronic severe AR, the LV apical impulse is diffuse, hyperdynamic, and displaced laterally and inferiorly. A rumbling diastolic murmur (Austin Flint) may be heard at the apex, with its intensity reduced by inhalation of amyl nitrite. A short basal systolic ejection murmur is heard. A palpable LV rapid filling wave and an audible S_3 at the apex are usually found. Physical findings due to a large LV stroke volume and a rapid diastolic runoff in those with severe AR include a wide pulse pressure with increased systolic arterial pressure and abnormally low diastolic arterial pressure, arterial pulse that abruptly rises and collapses, bisferiens pulse, bobbing of the head with each heartbeat, booming systolic and diastolic sounds heard over the femoral artery, capillary pulsations, and systolic and diastolic murmurs heard over the femoral artery when it is compressed proximally and distally.

Diagnosis

Electrocardiography and Chest Roentgenography

The electrocardiogram (ECG) may initially be normal in persons with acute severe AR. In 30 necropsy findings of older adults with chronic severe AR, Roberts and Day[125] have demonstrated that the ECG did not accurately predict the severity of AR or cardiac weight. Using various electrocardiographic criteria, the prevalence of LV hypertrophy varied from 30% ($RV_6 > RV_5$) to 90% (total 12-lead QRS voltage > 175 mm). The P-R interval was prolonged in 28% and the QRS duration was 0.12 second in 20% of them.[125]

The chest x-ray in persons with acute severe AR may show a normal heart size and pulmonary edema. The chest x-ray in older adults with chronic severe AR usually shows a dilated LV, with elongation of the apex inferiorly and posteriorly and a dilated aorta. Aneurysmal dilation of the aorta suggests that aortic root disease is causing the AR. Linear calcifications in the wall of the ascending aorta are seen in syphilitic AR and in those with degenerative disease.

Echocardiography and Doppler Echocardiography

M-mode and two-dimensional echocardiography and Doppler echocardiography are very useful in the diagnosis of AR. Two-dimensional echocardiography can provide information showing the cause of the AR and measurements of LV function. Eccentric LV hypertrophy is diagnosed by echocardiography if the LV mass index is increased with a relative wall thickness less than 0.45.[126-128] Echocardiographic measurements reported to predict an unfavorable response to AVR in older adults with chronic AR include an LV end-systolic dimension greater than 55 mm,[129] LV shortening fraction less than 25%,[129] LV diastolic radius-to-wall thickness ratio greater than 3.8,[130] LV end-diastolic dimension index greater than 38 mm/m^2,[130] and LV ventricular end-systolic dimension index greater than 26 mm/m^2.[130]

Grayburn and associates[122] have found that pulsed Doppler echocardiography correctly identifies the presence of AR in 57 of 57 older adults (100%) with 2+ AR and in 22 of 25 older adults (88%) with 1+ AR. Saal and coworkers[123] have shown that pulsed Doppler echocardiography identified the presence of AR in 34 of 35 older adults (97%) with documented AR. Continuous-wave Doppler echocardiography has also been demonstrated to be very useful in diagnosing and quantitating AR.[131,132] AR is best assessed by color flow Doppler imaging.[133]

Natural History

The natural history of chronic AR is significantly different than the natural history of acute AR. Older adults with acute AR should have immediate AVR because death may occur within hours to days. In one study of older adults with hemodynamically significant chronic AR treated medically, 75% were alive at 5 years after diagnosis.[54,134] In older adults with moderate to severe chronic AR, 50% were alive at 10 years after diagnosis.[54,134] The 10-year survival rate for older adults with mild to moderate chronic AR was 85% to 95%.[54,135]

In another study of 14 older adults with chronic severe AR who did not have surgery, 13 (93%) died within 2 years of developing CHF.[121] The mean survival time after the onset of angina pectoris is 5 years.[134]

During 8-year follow-up of 104 asymptomatic older adults with chronic severe AR and normal LVEF, 2 of them (2%) died suddenly, and 23 of them (22%) had AVR.[136] Of the 104 older adults, 19 of them (18%) had AVR because of cardiac symptoms and 4 of them (4%) had AVR because of the development of LV systolic dysfunction in the absence of cardiac symptoms.

Multivariate analysis has shown that age, initial end-systolic dimension, and rate of change in end-systolic dimension and resting LVEF during serial studies can predict the outcome.

In a prospective study, at 24-month follow-up (range, 7 to 55 months) of 17 older adults, mean age 83 years, with CHF associated with unoperated severe chronic AR and normal LVEF, 15 of them (88%) had died.[118] At 15-month follow-up (range, 8 to 21 months) of 8 older adults, mean age 85 years, with CHF associated with unoperated severe chronic AR and abnormal LVEF, 8 of them (100%) had died.[118]

Medical and Surgical Management

Asymptomatic older adults with mild or moderate AR do not require therapy. Prophylactic antibiotics should not be used to prevent bacterial endocarditis in those with AR, according to current AHA guidelines.[65] Echocardiographic evaluation of the LV end-systolic dimension should be performed yearly if less than 50 mm but every 3 to 6 months if the LV end-systolic dimension is 50 to 54 mm. AVR should also be considered when the LVEF approaches 50% before the decompensated state.[130]

Older adults with asymptomatic, chronic severe AR should be treated with hydralazine,[137] nifedipine[138] or, preferably, angiotensin-converting enzyme therapy[139] to decrease the LV volume overload. Infections should be treated promptly. Systemic hypertension increases the regurgitant flow and should be treated. Drugs that reduce LV function should not be used. Arrhythmias should be treated. Older adults with AR due to syphilitic aortitis should receive a course of penicillin therapy. Prophylactic resection should be considered in persons with Marfan syndrome when the aortic root diameter exceeds 55 mm.[140]

Bacterial endocarditis should be treated with intravenous antibiotics. Indications for AVR in older adults with AR due to bacterial endocarditis are CHF, uncontrolled infection, myocardial or valvular ring abscess, prosthetic valve dysfunction or dehiscence, and multiple embolic episodes.[141-143]

CHF should be treated with sodium restriction, diuretics, digoxin if the LVEF is abnormal, vasodilator therapy, and AVR. Angina pectoris should be treated with nitrates.

Older adults with acute severe AR should undergo AVR immediately. Those with chronic severe AR should have aortic valve repair if they develop symptoms of CHF, angina pectoris, or syncope.[67,136] AVR should also be performed in asymptomatic older adults with chronic severe AR if they develop LV systolic dysfunction.[67,136] ACC/AHA indications for performing AVR in older adult patients with severe chronic AR are listed in Box 43-3.

The European Society of Cardiology/European Association for Cardio-Thoracic Surgery 2012 guidelines have stated that class I indications for AVR in older adult patients with chronic severe AR include the following: (1) symptomatic patients; (2) asymptomatic patients with a resting LVEF of 50%; and (3) patients undergoing CABS or surgery of the ascending aorta or on another valve.[95] AVR should be considered with a class IIa indication in asymptomatic older adult patients with a resting LVEF greater than 50% with severe LV dilation—LV end-diastolic dimension more than 70 mm, LV end-systolic dimension more than 50 mm, or LV end-systolic dimension more than 25 mm/m^2 of body surface area.[95] Surgery is indicated with a class I indication in patients with Marfan syndrome with aortic root disease (whatever the severity of AR) with a maximal ascending aorta diameter of 50 mm.[95] Surgery should be considered with a class IIa indication in older adult patients with Marfan syndrome with a maximal ascending aorta diameter of 45 mm, older adult patients with a bicuspid aortic valve with risk factors with a maximal ascending aorta diameter of 50 mm, and other older adult patients with a maximal ascending aorta diameter of 55 mm.[95]

BOX 43-3 American College of Cardiology/American Heart Association Indications for Aortic Valve Replacement in Older Adults With Chronic Severe Aortic Regurgitation (AR)

1. Symptomatic older patient with severe AR and normal or abnormal left ventricular ejection fraction (LVEF; class I indication)
2. Asymptomatic older patient with severe AR and LVEF ≤ 50% at rest (class I indication)
3. Older patient with severe AR undergoing coronary artery bypass surgery or surgery on the aorta or other heart valves (class I indication)
4. Asymptomatic older patient with severe AR with LVEF > 50% but LV end-diastolic dimension > 75 mm or LV end-systolic dimension > 55 mm (class IIa indication)

Modified from Bonow RO, Carabello BA, Chatterjee K, et al: ACC/AHA 2006 practice guidelines for the management of patients with valvular heart disease: executive summary. A report of the American College of Cardiology/American Heart Association task force on practice guidelines (writing committee to revise the 1998 guidelines for the management of patients with valvular heart disease). Developed in collaboration with the Society of Cardiovascular Anesthesiologists. Endorsed by the Society for Cardiovascular Angiography and Interventions and the Society of Thoracic Surgeons. J Am Coll Cardiol 48:598–675, 2006.

Older adults undergoing AVR for severe AR have an excellent postoperative survival if the preoperative LVEF is normal.[144-146] If LV systolic dysfunction has been present for less than 1 year, persons also do well postoperatively. However, if the older adult with severe AR has an abnormal LVEF, impaired exercise tolerance, and/or the presence of LV systolic dysfunction for longer than 1 year, the postoperative survival is poor.[144-146] After AVR, women exhibit an excess late mortality rate, suggesting that surgical correction of severe chronic AR should be considered at an earlier stage in women.[147]

The operative mortality for AVR in older adults with severe AR is similar to that in older adults with AVR for valvular AS. The mortality rate is slightly increased in those with infective endocarditis and in those needing replacement of the ascending aorta plus AVR. The bioprosthesis is preferable to the mechanical prosthetic valve for AVR in older adults, as in older adults with valvular AS.[73-76] Older adults with porcine bioprostheses may be treated with antiplatelet therapy alone unless they have atrial fibrillation, abnormal LVEF, previous thromboembolism, or a hypercoagulable state.[67]

Of 450 older adult patients with severe AR, 273 (61%) had an LVEF equal to 50%, 134 (30%) had an LVEF of 35% to 50%, and 43 patients (10%) had an LVEF less than 35%.[148] The operative mortality was 3.7% for patients with a normal LVEF, 6.7% for patients with an LVEF of 35% to 50%, and 14% for patients with an LVEF less than 35%.[148] At 10-year follow-up, survival rates were 70% for those with a normal LVEF, 56% for those with an LVEF of 35% to 50%, and 41% for those with an LVEF less than 35%.

In a prospective study, the AVR procedure in 38 older adults with severe AR normalized LV chamber size and mass in two thirds of those undergoing surgery.[149] At 9-month follow-up after AVR, 58% of them had a normal LV end-diastolic dimension and 50% of them had a normal LV mass. During further follow-up (18 to 56 months postoperatively), 66% had a normal LV end-diastolic dimension and 68% had a normal LV mass. The LV end-diastolic dimension normalized in 86% of those with a preoperative LV end-systolic dimension of 55 mm. A preoperative

LV end-systolic dimension greater than 55 mm was present in 81% of those with postoperative persistent LV dilation.

Moderate or severe AR was present in 11.7% after TAVR in 12,926 older adult patients (16.0% with the CoreValve and 9.1% with the Edwards valve).[150] Moderate or severe AR after TAVR increased mortality 2.95 times at 30 days and 2.27 times at 1 year follow-up, respectively.[150] Aortic valve repair is currently considered an option to treat the regurgitant AR after TAVR.[151] Data and experience with transcatheter aortic valve implantation in the treatment of severe native AR are limited.[152]

MITRAL ANNULAR CALCIUM

MAC is a chronic degenerative process that is common in older adults, especially women. The amount of calcium may vary from a few spicules to a large mass behind the posterior cusp, often extending to form a ridge or ring encircling the mitral leaflets, occasionally lifting the leaflets toward the left atrium. Sphincter function loss of the mitral annulus and mechanical stretching of the mitral leaflets can cause improper coaptation of the leaflets during systole, resulting in mitral regurgitation (MR).[6]

Although the calcific mass may immobilize the mitral valve, actual calcification of the leaflets is rare. In older adults with severe MAC, the calcification may extend inward to involve the underside of the leaflets. Mitral stenosis (MS) may result from severe calcific deposits within the mitral annulus protruding into the orifice.[153,154] Calcific deposits may extend from the mitral annulus into the membranous portions of the ventricular septum, involving the conduction system and causing rhythm and conduction disturbances.[7,155,156] Although the annular calcium is covered with a layer of endothelium, ulceration of this lining can expose the underlying calcific deposits, which may serve as a nidus for platelet-fibrin aggregation and subsequent thromboembolic (TE) episodes.[157-159] In persons with endocarditis associated with MAC, the avascular nature of the mitral annulus predisposes to periannular and myocardial abscesses.[160-163]

Prevalence

MAC is a degenerative process that increases with age and occurs more frequently in women than in men.*

MAC was present in 298 of 924 men (36%), mean age 80 years, and in 985 of 1881 women (52%), mean age 81 years.[26]

Predisposing Factors

Because calcific deposits in the mitral annulus, aortic valve cusps, and epicardial coronary arteries are commonly associated in older adults and have similar predisposing factors, Roberts[19] has suggested that MAC and aortic cuspal calcium are a form of atherosclerosis. MAC and aortic cuspal calcium may coexist.[19]

The prevalence of CAD is higher in men and women with aortic valve calcium and with MAC[1,172-174] than in men and women without aortic valve calcium and MAC.

The breakdown of lipid deposits on the ventricular surface of the posterior mitral leaflet at or below the mitral annulus and on the aortic surfaces of the aortic valve cusps is probably responsible for the calcification.[8] Increased LV systolic pressure due to AS increases stress on the mitral apparatus and may accelerate the development of MAC.[3,5,6,157,171] Tricuspid annular calcium and MAC may also coexist and have similar predisposing factors.[175]

Systemic hypertension increases with age and predisposes to MAC.†

*References 3, 5, 9, 19, 26, 157, and 164-171.

†References 3, 6, 19, 20, 157, 166, 170, 171, and 176.

Those with diabetes mellitus also have a higher prevalence of MAC than nondiabetics.[3,6,20,170] MAC occurs in the teenage years in those with serum total cholesterol levels greater than 500 mg/dL.[177] Waller and Roberts[3] have suggested that hypercholesterolemia predisposes to MAC. The prevalence of hypercholesterolemia with a serum total cholesterol level of 200 mg/dL was higher in older adults with MAC than in older adults without MAC.[20]

Roberts and Waller[178] have found that chronic hypercalcemia predisposes to MAC. Older adults with chronic renal insufficiency have a higher prevalence of MAC and aortic valve calcium than older adults with normal renal function.[179,180] Older adults undergoing dialysis for chronic renal insufficiency have an increased prevalence of MAC.[178-186] MAC has also been found to be a marker of LV dilation and reduced LV systolic function in those with end-stage renal disease on peritoneal dialysis.[186] Cardiac calcium in those with chronic renal failure has been attributed to secondary hyperparathyroidism[183,186] Nair and colleagues[170] found a similar mean serum calcium level, higher mean serum phosphorus level, and higher mean product of serum calcium and phosphorus levels in those younger than 60 years with MAC than in a control group. However, Aronow and associates[20] have demonstrated no significant difference in mean serum calcium, serum phosphorus, or product of serum calcium and phosphorus levels between older adults with and without MAC.

By accelerating LV systolic pressure, hypertrophic cardiomyopathy predisposes to MAC.[6] Kronzon and Glassman[187] diagnosed MAC in 12 of 18 persons (67%) older than 55 years with hypertrophic cardiomyopathy and in 4 of 28 persons (14%) younger than 55 years with hypertrophic cardiomyopathy. Nair and coworkers[188] observed MAC in 12 of 42 older adults (27%) with hypertrophic cardiomyopathy. Those with both MAC and hypertrophic cardiomyopathy were older than those with hypertrophic cardiomyopathy and no MAC. Motamed and Roberts[189] have demonstrated MAC in 30 of 100 necropsy studies (30%) in those with hypertrophic cardiomyopathy older than 40 years and in none of 100 necropsy studies (0%) in those younger than 40 years with hypertrophic cardiomyopathy. Aronow and Kronzon[190] have diagnosed MAC in13 of 17 older adults (76%) with hypertrophic cardiomyopathy and in 176 of 362 older adults (49%) without hypertrophic cardiomyopathy.

Diagnostic Considerations

Calcific deposits in the mitral annulus are J-, C-, U-, or O-shaped and are seen in the posterior third of the heart shadow.[157,165,181,191-197] MAC may be diagnosed by chest x-ray or fluoroscopy.[197] However, the procedures of choice for diagnosing MAC are M-mode and two-dimensional echocardiography.

Posterior MAC is diagnosed by M-mode echocardiography when a band of dense echoes is recorded anterior to the LV posterior wall and moving parallel with it.[198] These echoes end at the atrioventricular junction and merge with the LV posterior wall on echocardiographic sweep from the aortic root to the LV apex. Anterior MAC is diagnosed by M-mode echocardiography when a continuous band of dense echoes is observed at the level of the anterior mitral leaflet in systole and diastole.[198] These echoes are contiguous with the posterior wall of the aortic root. Calcification may extend from the mitral annulus throughout the base of the heart and into the mitral and aortic valves.

Using multiple echocardiographic views, MAC may be classified as mild, moderate, or severe.[195,199] The echo densities in mild MAC involve less than one third of the annular circumference (<3 mm in width) and are usually restricted to the angle between the posterior leaflet of the mitral valve and LV posterior wall. The echo densities in moderate MAC involve less than two thirds of the annular circumference (3 to 5 mm in width). The echo densities in severe MAC involve more than two thirds of the annular circumference (>5 mm in width), usually extending beneath the entire posterior mitral leaflet, with or without making a complete circle.

MAC was diagnosed in the original chest x-ray report in 3 of 8 older adults (38%) with MAC diagnosed at autopsy.[165] Schott and colleagues[181] have diagnosed MAC by chest x-ray in 2 of 41 older adults (5%) with MAC diagnosed by echocardiography. Dashkoff and associates[200] have detected MAC by chest x-ray in 5 of 8 older adults (63%) with MAC diagnosed by echocardiography.

In a blinded prospective study, MAC was diagnosed by M-mode and two-dimensional echocardiography in 55% of 604 older adults.[197] The diagnosis of MAC by chest x-ray using a lateral chest x-ray in addition to the posterior-anterior or anterior-posterior chest x-ray had a sensitivity of 12%, specificity of 99%, positive predictive value of 95%, and negative predictive value of 47%. Older adults with radiographic MAC were more likely than older adults without radiographic MAC to have a more severe form of the disease, with significant MR, functional MS, or conduction defects. However, older adults with echocardiographically severe MAC and significant MR, functional MS, or conduction defects may have no evidence of MAC on chest x-ray films.

Chamber Size

Those with MAC have a higher prevalence of left atrial enlargement and LV enlargement than those without MAC.*

In a prospective study of 976 older adults (526 with MAC and 450 without MAC), left atrial enlargement was 2.4 times more prevalent in those with MAC than in the group without MAC.[202]

Atrial Fibrillation

Those with MAC also have a higher prevalence of atrial fibrillation than those without MAC.[157,165-167,169,199,201-203] The prevalence of atrial fibrillation was increased 12-fold,[166] 5-fold,[199] and 2.8-fold[203] in those with MAC than in those without MAC.

Conduction Defects

Because of the close proximity of the mitral annulus to the atrioventricular node and bundle of His, persons with MAC have a higher prevalence of conduction defects, such as sinoatrial disease, atrioventricular block, bundle branch block, left anterior fascicular block, and intraventricular conduction defect, than persons without MAC.[7,155-157,171,199] The calcific deposits may also extend into the membranous portions of the interventricular septum involving the conduction system or may even extend to the left atrium, interrupting interatrial and intraatrial conduction. In addition, MAC may be associated with a sclerodegenerative process in the conduction system. Nair and coworkers[199] have shown in their study that those with MAC had a higher incidence of permanent pacemaker implantation because of atrioventricular block and sinoatrial disease than those without MAC.

Mitral Regurgitation

MAC is thought to generate systolic murmurs by the sphincter action loss of the annulus and mechanical stretching of the mitral leaflets causing MR and by vibration of the calcified ring or vortex formation around the annulus. Table 43-3 shows that the prevalence of apical systolic murmurs of MR in persons with MAC ranged from 12% to 100% in different studies.†

*References 157, 165-167, 169, 170, 199, and 201.

†References 153, 157, 165, 166, 168, 181, 198, and 200.

TABLE 43-3 Prevalence of Apical Systolic Murmurs of Mitral Regurgitation (MR) and Mitral Stenosis (MS) in Older Adults With Mitral Annular Calcium

Prevalence of MR Murmur		Prevalence of MS Murmur	
No.	*%*	*No.*	*%*
14/14[165]	100	3/14[165]	21
10/14[181]	71	2/14[181]	14
2/4[153]	50	1/4[153]	25
72/80[157]	90	5/59[157]	8
26/132[166]	20	2/132[166]	2
17/104[198]	12	7/104[198]	7
129/283[168]	44	28/293[168]	10
43/100[204]	43	6/100[204]	6

TABLE 43-4 Prevalence of Mitral Regurgitation (MR) and Mitral Stenosis (MS) Diagnosed by Doppler Echocardiography in Older Adults With Mitral Annular Calcium

Prevalence of MR		Prevalence of MS	
No.	*%*	*No.*	*%*
28/51[205]	55	4/51[205]	8
54/100[204]	54	6/100[204]	6
28/29[201]	97	83/1028[203]	8

Table 43-4 states the prevalence of MR diagnosed by Doppler echocardiography in persons with MAC.[201,204,205] The prevalence of mitral regurgitation associated with MAC ranged from 54% to 97% in the Doppler echocardiographic studies.[201,204,205]

The greater the severity of MAC, the greater the severity of MR associated with MAC. Moderate to severe MR was diagnosed by Doppler echocardiography in 33%with MAC by Labovitz and colleagues[205] and in 22% of 1028 older adults with MAC by Aronow and associates.[203] Kaul and coworkers[201] diagnosed severe MR in 7% of their 29 persons with MAC. Kaul and colleagues[201] also concluded from their study that MR in persons with MAC is caused by a decreased sphincteric action of the mitral annulus, with MAC preventing the posterior annulus from contracting and assuming a flatter shape during systole.

Mitral Stenosis

An apical diastolic murmur may be heard in persons with MAC as a result of turbulent flow across the calcified and narrowed annulus (annular stenosis). Table 43-3 shows that the prevalence of apical diastolic murmurs of MS in persons with MAC ranged from 0% to 25% in different studies.*

Table 43-4 indicates that MS associated with MAC was diagnosed by Doppler echocardiography in 8% of 51 older adults by Labovitz and associates,[205] in 6% of 100 older adults by Aronow and Kronzon,[204] and in 8% of 1028 older adults by Aronow and coworkers.[203]

The decrease of the mitral valve orifice in persons with MAC is due to the annular calcium and decreased mitral excursion and mobility secondary to calcium at the base of the leaflets.[204] The commissures are fused in rheumatic MS but are not fused in MS associated with MAC. The mitral leaflet margins in MAC may be thin and mobile, and the posterior mitral leaflet may move normally during diastole. However, Doppler echocardiographic recordings show increased transvalvular flow velocity and prolonged pressure half time and, therefore, a smaller mitral valve orifice in older adults with MS, regardless of the cause.

*References 157, 165-167, 169, 170, 199, and 201.

Bacterial Endocarditis

Bacterial endocarditis, with a high incidence of *Staphylococcus aureus* endocarditis, may complicate MAC.[157,160-163,169] Older adults with MAC associated with chronic renal failure are especially at increased risk for developing bacterial endocarditis.[178] The calcific mass erodes the endothelium under the mitral valve, which is exposed to transient bacteremia. The avascular nature of the mitral annulus interferes with antibiotics reaching a nidus of bacteria, predisposing to periannular and myocardial abscesses and, consequently, to a poor prognosis.[160-163] Therefore, Burnside and DeSanctis[160] have recommended prophylactic antibiotics to prevent bacterial endocarditis in persons with MAC.

Nair and colleagues[199] observed no significant difference in the incidence of bacterial endocarditis in 99 persons younger than 61 years with MAC compared with a control group of 101 persons at 4.4-year follow-up. However, Aronow and associates[169] found a 3% incidence of bacterial endocarditis in 526 older adults with MAC and a 1% incidence of bacterial endocarditis in 450 older adults without MAC at 39-month follow-up. On the basis of these data, we recommend using prophylactic antibiotics to prevent bacterial endocarditis in older adults with MAC.

Cardiac Events

In a prospective study of 107 persons (8 lost to follow-up) younger than 61 years of age with MAC and 107 age- and gender-matched control subjects (6 lost to follow-up), Nair and coworkers[199] observed that persons with MAC had a higher incidence of new cardiac events than control subjects at 4.4-year follow-up (Table 43-5). In a prospective study of 526 older adults with MAC and 450 older adults without MAC, Aronow and colleagues[169] found that the incidence of new cardiac events (myocardial infarction, primary ventricular fibrillation, or sudden cardiac death) was also higher in older adults with MAC than in older adults without MAC at 39-month follow-up.

Mitral Valve Replacement

Nair and associates[206] reported that mitral valve replacement can be accomplished in older adults with MAC with morbidity and mortality similar to those in persons without MAC. Following mitral valve replacement, subsequent morbidity and mortality were also similar in older adults with and without MAC during 4.4-year follow-up.

TABLE 43-5 Incidence of New Cardiac Events in Older Adults With and Without Mitral Annular Calcium (MAC)

	Cardiac Events		
Study	*MAC (%)*	*No MAC (%)*	*Relative Risk*
NAIR ET AL[10,99] (99 WITH MAC, 101 WITHOUT MAC)			
Total cardiac death	31	2	15.5
Sudden cardiac death	12	1	12.0
Congestive heart failure	41	6	6.8
Mitral or aortic valve replacement	9	0	—
ARONOW ET AL[169]			
Cardiac events, if atrial fibrillation (90 with MAC, 41 without MAC)*	69	54	1.3
Sinus rhythm (436 with MAC, 409 without MAC)	36	26	1.4
All persons (526 with MAC, 450 without MAC)	42	28	1.5

*Myocardial infarction, primary ventricular fibrillation, or sudden cardiac death.

Cerebrovascular Events

Although the increased prevalence of atrial fibrillation, MS, MR, left atrial enlargement, and CHF predisposes older adults with MAC to TE stroke, some investigators have considered MAC to be a marker of other vascular disease causing stroke rather than the primary embolic source.[207] However, the prevalence of prior stroke was higher in 280 African American, Hispanic, and white men with MAC (40%) than in 484 African American, Hispanic, and white men without MAC (27%) and in 876 African American, Hispanic, and white women with MAC (36%) than in 799 African American, Hispanic, and white women without MAC (22%).[208] In addition, six prospective studies have demonstrated an increased incidence of new cerebrovascular events in those with MAC than in those without MAC.[173,199,203,209-211]

Nair and coworkers[199] showed at 4.4-year follow-up in 107 individuals younger than 61 years with MAC (8 lost to follow-up) and 107 age- and gender-matched control subjects (6 lost to follow-up) that those with MAC had a five times higher incidence of new TE cerebrovascular events than those without MAC. The Framingham Heart Study observed in 160 persons with MAC and 999 persons without MAC that the incidence of stroke was increased 2.7-fold more in those with MAC than in those without MAC at 8-year follow-up.[209] At 39-month follow-up of 526 older adults with MAC and 450 older adults without MAC, Aronow and colleagues[169] observed a 1.5-fold higher incidence of new TE stroke in older adults with MAC than in older adults without MAC if atrial fibrillation were present, a 1.6-fold higher incidence of new TE stroke in older adults with MAC than in older adults without MAC if sinus rhythm were present, and a 1.7-fold higher incidence of new TE stroke in all older adults with MAC than in all older adults without MAC. At 2.2-year follow-up, the Boston Area Anticoagulation Trial for Atrial Fibrillation study demonstrated in 129 older adults with atrial fibrillation and MAC and in 291 older adults with atrial fibrillation without MAC a fourfold higher incidence of ischemic stroke in those with MAC than in those without MAC.[210] At 45-month follow-up, Aronow and associates[211] showed that the incidence of TE stroke was 1.5-fold higher in 101 older adults with 40% to 100% ECAD and MAC than in 49 older adults with 40% to 100% ECAD and no MAC and 2.2-fold higher in 365 older adults with MAC and 0% to 39% ECAD than in 413 older adults without MAC and 0% to 39% ECAD.

Table 43-6 shows the incidence of new TE stroke at 44-month follow-up in 310 older adults with chronic atrial fibrillation and in 1838 older adults with sinus rhythm, mean age 81 years.[203] MS and the severity of MR were diagnosed by Doppler echocardiography in this study. In older adults with chronic atrial fibrillation, MAC increased the incidence of new TE 2.1-fold if MS was associated with MAC, 1.7-fold if 2 to 4+ MR was associated with MAC, and 1.4-fold if 0 to 1+ MR was present.[203] In older adults with sinus rhythm, MAC increased the incidence of new TE stroke 3.6-fold if MS was associated with MAC, 3.1-fold if 2 to 4+ MR was associated with MAC, and 2.7-fold if 0 to 1 MR was present.[203]

There was a higher prevalence of MAC in older adults with 40% to 100% ECAD (67% of 150 persons) than in older adults with 0% to 39% ECAD (47% of 778 persons).[211] The increased prevalence of significant ECAD contributes to a higher incidence of TE stroke in older adults with MAC. Thrombi of the mitral annulus also contribute to TE stroke in older adults with MAC.[212-214] In addition, MAC is associated with complex intraaortic debris, which could contribute to TE stroke.[215]

Because older adults with MAC and atrial fibrillation or sinus rhythm have a higher incidence of TE stroke than older

TABLE 43-6 Incidence of New Thromboembolic (TE) Stroke at 44 Months

Study Population	TE Stroke (%)
Atrial fibrillation, no MAC (*n* = 85)	35
Atrial fibrillation with MS due to MAC (*n* = 42)	74
Atrial fibrillation with MAC and 2 to 4+ MR (*n* = 90)	59
Atrial fibrillation with MAC and 0 to 1+ MR (*n* = 93)	48
Sinus rhythm, no MAC (*n* = 1035)	9
Sinus rhythm with MS due to MAC (*n* = 41)	32
Sinus rhythm with MAC and 2 to 4+ MR (*n* = 134)	28
Sinus rhythm with MAC and 0 to 1+ MR (*n* = 625)	24

Modified from Aronow WS, Ahn C, Kronzon I, et al: Association of mitral annular calcium with new thromboembolic stroke at 44-month follow-up of 2,148 persons, mean age 81 years. Am J Cardiol 81:105–106, 1998.

MAC, Mitral annular calcium; *MR*, mitral regurgitation; *MS*, mitral stenosis.

adults without MAC, antithrombotic therapy should be considered in older adults with MAC and no contraindications to antithrombotic therapy. In the Boston Area Anticoagulation Trial for Atrial Fibrillation study, warfarin significantly reduced the incidence of TE stroke in older adults with MAC by about 90%.[216,217]

Until data from prospective randomized studies evaluating the efficacy and risk of antithrombotic therapy in older adults with MAC are available, we recommend treating older adults with MAC associated with atrial fibrillation, MS, or moderate to severe MR with warfarin treatment if they have no contraindications to anticoagulant therapy. The INR should be maintained between 2.0 and 3.0. The efficacy of antiplatelet treatment in older adults with MAC is unknown.

MITRAL STENOSIS

Prevalence and Cause

MS due to rheumatic heart disease was diagnosed by Doppler echocardiography in 3 of 924 older men (0.3%), mean age 80 years, and in 34 of 1881 older women (2%), mean age 81 years.[26] The most common cause of MS in older adults is MAC. The differentiation of MS due to rheumatic heart disease from MS caused by MAC via echocardiography was discussed earlier (see "Mitral Annular Calcium"). In a study of 1699 older adults, mean age 81 years, the prevalence of rheumatic MS was 6% in those with atrial fibrillation versus 0.4% in those with sinus rhythm.[203]

Pathophysiology

MS leads to an increase in left atrial pressure, pulmonary capillary pressure, and right ventricular and pulmonary artery systolic pressures, causing pulmonary hypertension. Atrial fibrillation predisposes older adults with MS to develop stroke, peripheral arterial embolism, and CHF.

Symptoms and Signs

If MS is moderate or severe (especially if atrial fibrillation is present), exertional dyspnea, orthopnea, paroxysmal nocturnal dyspnea, and pulmonary edema may develop. Pulmonary hypertension leads to right-sided CHF. Hemoptysis may result from ruptured bronchial veins. The loud first heart sound and opening snap heard in older adults with MS may become softer or disappear if valvular calcification is present. An apical, low-frequency, diastolic murmur with presystolic accentuation is heard as a rumble at the point of maximum apical impulse. The low-frequency diastolic murmur begins after the opening snap, is prolonged with increasing severity of the MS, and increases in intensity after inhalation of amyl nitrite. The closer the opening snap is heard to A_2, the more severe the MS. If atrial fibrillation develops, the presystolic accentuation usually disappears.

Diagnostic Tests

The ECG and chest x-ray will often show left atrial enlargement in older adults with MS. Electrocardiographic right ventricular hypertrophy (RVH) is usually present with severe MS. Documentation of MS and its severity is made by Doppler echocardiography. Echocardiography will also rule out left atrial myxoma, which can mimic mitral stenosis.

Management

A rapid ventricular rate associated with atrial fibrillation is controlled by digoxin and/or β-blockers, verapamil, or diltiazem. Diuretics should be used to control congestive symptoms. Unloading therapy with vasodilators is not beneficial and may cause a significant reduction in cardiac output. Long-term anticoagulation with oral warfarin is indicated in persons with MS and atrial fibrillation (especially) or sinus rhythm to prevent systemic embolization. The INR should be maintained between 2.0 and 3.0. Prophylactic antibiotics should not be used to prevent bacterial endocarditis in persons with MS, according to AHA guidelines.[65]

Interventional therapy is indicated for symptomatic persons with severe MS. A mitral valve area of 1.0 cm^2 or smaller is considered severe MS. Mitral valve replacement is usually performed because the calcified mitral valve is usually not amenable to open mitral commissurotomy. For the few older adults who have an uncalcified mitral valve or mild calcific deposits, flexible mitral valve leaflets, and no or mild MR, percutaneous balloon valvuloplasty is the procedure of choice.[218]

ACUTE MITRAL REGURGITATION

Acute severe MR in older adults may be caused by ruptured chordae tendineae or the development of a flail mitral valve secondary to acute myocardial infarction, infective endocarditis, papillary muscle rupture, or mucoid degeneration of the mitral valve cusps. Acute severe MR usually results in severe CHF with pulmonary edema and right-sided CHF.

Signs

The MR murmur associated with acute severe MR is characteristically a harsh systolic murmur heard at the apex, with an associated palpable thrill, which begins with the first heart sound but ends early when the noncompliant left atrium can no longer accept the large regurgitant volume. The first heart sound is soft, and the pulmonic component of the second heart sound is increased. A left ventricular third heart sound gallop and an atrial fourth heart sound gallop are heard at the apex.

Diagnosis and Management

Doppler echocardiography confirms the diagnosis of severe MR. Transesophageal echocardiography provides a highly accurate anatomic assessment of the cause of the acute MR and assists in determining whether the mitral valve can be repaired or must be replaced.[219] CHF needs to be managed medically. Infective endocarditis should be treated with appropriate antibiotics. Mitral valve surgery should be performed urgently.

CHRONIC MITRAL REGURGITATION

Prevalence and Causes

Chronic MR was present in 298 of 924 older men (32%), mean age 80 years, and in 630 of 1881 older women (33%), mean age 81 years.[26] MR 2 to 4+ was present in 10% of 2148 older adults, mean age 81 years.[203] The most common cause of MR in older adults is MAC.[168] Other causes of chronic MR in older adults include papillary muscle dysfunction after myocardial infarction, rheumatic heart disease, myxomatous degeneration of the mitral valve leaflets and chordae tendineae with mitral valve prolapse (MVP), ruptured chordae tendineae, and endocarditis. MR may also result from alteration in the geometry of the mitral annulus that occurs with dilation of the LV and CHF.

Pathophysiology

The regurgitant volume gradually increases in chronic MR, increasing the left atrial volume during systole and LV volume during diastole. Eccentric LV hypertrophy occurs. Atrial fibrillation develops, and the LV cannot maintain an effective forward stroke volume because of depressed LV contractility. Left-sided CHF develops, resulting in increased pulmonary artery and right ventricular systolic pressures and eventually right-sided CHF. Decreased LV systolic and diastolic function in older adults with chronic MR contribute to the clinical manifestations of CHF.[220] Unrecognized MR may contribute to acute pulmonary edema in older adults with normal or abnormal LV systolic function.[221]

Symptoms and Signs

Older adults with chronic MR may be asymptomatic or have a reduction in exercise tolerance, with easy fatigability. Dyspnea on exertion will develop with significant MR and progress to orthopnea, paroxysmal nocturnal dyspnea, and dyspnea at rest caused by left-sided CHF. Right-sided CHF will cause ankle swelling, anorexia, and right upper abdominal tenderness from hepatic congestion. Symptoms may also result from the development of atrial fibrillation. Atypical chest pain, palpitations, or syncope due to arrhythmias may be associated with MVP. In some older adults, acute pulmonary edema may be the initial manifestation of severe MR from MVP.[222]

The heart murmur associated with chronic MR is heard as an apical holosystolic, late systolic, or early systolic murmur beginning with the first heart sound but ending in midsystole. The holosystolic murmur may radiate to the left axilla, to the back, and over the entire precordium. A nonejection systolic click may precede the mid to late systolic apical murmur associated with MVP. With severe MR, the first heart sound becomes decreased, and a LV third heart sound is heard at the apex.

Diagnosis

Doppler echocardiography can quantitate the severity of MR and assess LV size and function. Doppler echocardiography and especially transesophageal echocardiography can also determine the cause of the MR. Vegetations are seen with infective endocarditis. MVP and thickening of the mitral valve leaflets suggest myxomatous degeneration. MAC can be diagnosed. Thickened retracted leaflets and chordal fusion suggest rheumatic heart disease as the cause of MR. A flail mitral valve and ruptured chordae tendineae can be diagnosed. The sensitivity of transesophageal echocardiography in diagnosing specific causes of MR was 82% for vegetations, 99% for MVP, 100% for a flail mitral valve, and 84% for ruptured chordae tendineae.[219] In older adults with severe chronic MR, the ECG may show atrial fibrillation or left atrial enlargement, LV hypertrophy in about 50% of older adults, and RVH in approximately 15% of older adults.

Management

Older adults with chronic MR should have Doppler echocardiography performed every 6 to 12 months. There are no long-term studies supporting the use of vasodilator therapy in asymptomatic persons with chronic MR. Angiotensin-converting enzyme inhibitors should be used in treating older adults with symptomatic chronic MR.[223] Older adults with atrial fibrillation should be treated with long-term oral warfarin therapy to maintain the INR between 2.0 and 3.0. CHF should be treated with standard medical therapy. Prophylactic antibiotics should not be used to prevent bacterial endocarditis in persons with MR, according to current AHA guidelines.[65]

Timing of Surgery

Of 478 older adults with nonischemic chronic severe MR undergoing surgery, the cause of MR was MVP in 79%, rheumatic in 8%, endocarditis in 8%, and miscellaneous in 4%.[224] Surgical repair of the mitral valve was performed in 68% and mitral valve replacement in 32% of older adults. CABS was performed in 27% of older adults in association with mitral valve surgery.[224]

The operative mortality was 0% for those younger than 75 years. In older adults 75 years of age and older, the operative mortality was 3.6% in those with NYHA class I or II symptoms and 12.7% in those with severe symptoms.[224] In older adults with an LVEF of 60%, the 10-year survival was 79% in those with class I or II symptoms versus 49% in those with class III or IV symptoms.[224] In older adults with an LVEF less than 60%, the 10-year survival was 75% in those with class I or II symptoms versus 41% in those with class III or IV symptoms.[224]

Box 43-4 lists the ACC/AHA class indications for performing mitral valve surgery in those with nonischemic severe MR.[67] Older adults with chronic nonischemic MR who have NYHA class I symptoms and normal LV function should be followed at 3- to 6-month intervals.[67] If LV dysfunction, atrial fibrillation, or pulmonary hypertension develops, the older adult should be considered for cardiac catheterization and possible mitral valve surgery, especially if it is thought that the mitral valve can be repaired.[67]

The prognosis for older adults with ischemic MR is worse than that for MR from other causes. CABS may improve LV function and decrease ischemic MR.[67] The best surgical procedure for ischemic MR is controversial.[67]

Mitral valve repair is the preferred technique when it is expected to be durable.[95] The European Society of Cardiology/European Association for Cardio-Thoracic Surgery 2012 guidelines state that class I indications for mitral valve surgery in those with chronic severe primary MR include the following: (1) symptomatic patients with an LVEF more than 30% and a LV end-systolic dimension less than 55 mm; and (2) asymptomatic patients with an LV end-systolic dimension of 45 mm and/or LVEF of 60%.[95] Surgery should be considered with a class IIa indication in the following: (1) asymptomatic patients with a normal LVEF and new onset of atrial fibrillation or a resting systolic pulmonary artery pressure higher than 50 mm Hg; (2) asymptomatic patients with a normal LVEF, high likelihood of durable repair, low surgical risk and flail leaflet, and LV end-systolic dimension of 40 mm; and (3) in patients with a LVEF less than 30% and/or a LV end-systolic dimension higher than 55 mm refractory to medical therapy, with a high likelihood of durable repair and a low comorbidity.[95] Indications for mitral valve surgery in older adults with severe chronic secondary MR are the following: (1) older patients undergoing CABS with a LVEF higher than 30% (class I indication); (2) symptomatic older

BOX 43-4 Indications for Mitral Valve Surgery in Older Adults With Nonischemic Severe Mitral Regurgitation

1. Acute symptomatic MR (class I indication)
2. Older adult with NYHA class II, III, or IV symptoms in the absence of severe LV dysfunction defined as LVEF < 30% and/or LV end-systolic dimension > 55 mm (class I indication)
3. Asymptomatic persons with mild to moderate LV dysfunction defined as LVEF of 30% to 60% and/or a LV end-systolic dimension of 40 to 55 mm (class I indication)
4. Mitral valve repair recommended over mitral valve replacement in most older patients with severe chronic MR who require surgery (class I indication)
5. Mitral valve repair reasonable for asymptomatic patients if the likelihood of successful repair without residual MR is >90% (class IIa indication)
6. Mitral valve surgery reasonable for asymptomatic patients, normal LV function, and new onset of atrial fibrillation (class IIa indication)
7. Mitral valve surgery reasonable for asymptomatic patients, normal LV function, and pulmonary artery pressure > 50 mm Hg at rest or > 60 mm Hg with exercise (class IIa indication)
8. Mitral valve surgery is reasonable in patients with a primary abnormality of the mitral apparatus, NYHA class III or IV symptoms, and severe LV dysfunction in whom mitral valve repair is highly likely (class IIa indication)

Modified from Bonow RO, Carabello BA, Chatterjee K, et al: ACC/AHA 2006 practice guidelines for the management of patients with valvular heart disease: executive summary. A report of the American College of Cardiology/American Heart Association task force on practice guidelines (writing committee to revise the 1998 guidelines for the management of patients with valvular heart disease). Developed in collaboration with the Society of Cardiovascular Anesthesiologists. Endorsed by the Society for Cardiovascular Angiography and Interventions and the Society of Thoracic Surgeons. J Am Coll Cardiol 48:598–675, 2006.

patients with an LVEF less than 30%, option for revascularization, and evidence of viability (class IIa indication); and (3) older patients with an LVEF higher than 30% who remain symptomatic despite optimal medical therapy and low comorbidity when revascularization is not indicated (class IIa indication).[95]

At 1-year follow-up of 251 older adult patients, mean age 69 years, with severe ischemic MR randomized to mitral valve repair versus replacement, there was no significant difference in LV reverse remodeling or survival but a lower rate of moderate or severe recurrent MR with mitral valve replacement (2.3%) than with mitral valve repair (32.6%).[225] At 4-year follow-up of 279 older adult patients, mean age 67 years, with severe MR randomized to percutaneous repair versus surgery, percutaneous repair was associated with similar mortality and symptomatic improvement but a higher incidence of MR needing repeat procedures and less improvement in LV dimensions than surgery.[226]

TRICUSPID REGURGITATION

In older adults, tricuspid regurgitation (TR) is usually caused by dilation of the right ventricle and tricuspid annulus associated with right-sided heart failure resulting from left-sided heart failure or pulmonary hypertension associated with pulmonary vascular disease. The murmur of TR is usually high-pitched and holosystolic, is heard in the third or fourth intercostal space at the left sternal border and occasionally in the subxiphoid area, and increases with inspiration in 50% of older adults. When TR is mild, the systolic murmur may be a short ejection murmur or an absent. P_2 is increased with pulmonary hypertension. If TR is severe, a prominent large V wave is seen in the jugular venous pulse. Systolic pulsation of an enlarged tender liver is commonly present. Ascites and peripheral edema occur frequently. Diagnosis of TR is confirmed by Doppler echocardiography. Medical treatment of CHF is indicated. Surgery is rarely necessary.

TRICUSPID STENOSIS

Tricuspid stenosis (TS) in older adults is rare and due to multivalvular rheumatic heart disease or the carcinoid syndrome. Symptoms of right-sided heart failure occur. A low-frequency diastolic rumble is heard in the third or fourth intercostal space at the left sternal border, which increases with intensity with inspiration. A prominent A wave with poor or absent Y descent is seen in the jugular venous pulse. The ECG shows tall right atrial P waves and no RVH. The chest x-ray shows a dilated right atrium without an enlarged pulmonary artery segment. Diagnosis of TS is confirmed by Doppler echocardiography.

Medical therapy is indicated for mild TS. Balloon valvotomy is recommended for older adults with TS with signs of right-sided heart failure or with a marked reduction in exercise tolerance due to an inability to increase cardiac output. If the tricuspid valve is calcified (rarely), tricuspid valve replacement is indicated. A porcine bioprosthetic heart valve is recommended in the tricuspid position.

PULMONIC REGURGITATION

In older adults, pulmonic regurgitation (PR) is almost always due to pulmonary hypertension resulting from left-sided heart failure or pulmonary vascular disease. A high-pitched, blowing decrescendo murmur beginning immediately after P_2 is heard in the second and third intercostal space to the left of the sternum. Diagnosis of PR is confined by Doppler echocardiography. Management of PR is directed at treatment of the underlying disorder and attempts to reduce pulmonary artery pressure.

KEY POINTS

- Class I indications for aortic valve replacement in older patients with aortic stenosis (AS)
  - Symptomatic severe AS
  - Older patients with severe AS undergoing coronary artery surgery
  - Older patients with severe AS undergoing surgery on aorta or other heart valves
  - Older patients with severe AS and ejection fraction 50%
- Class I indication for transcatheter aortic valve replacement in older patients with severe AS
  - Older patients with severe symptomatic AS considered unsuitable for surgical aortic valve replacement by a heart team and who are likely to have improvement of quality of life and a life expectancy longer than 1 year after consideration of their comorbidities
- Class I indications for aortic valve replacement in patients with aortic regurgitation (AR)
  - Symptomatic severe AR
  - Older patients with severe AR undergoing coronary artery surgery
  - Older patients with severe AR undergoing surgery on aorta or other heart valves
  - Older patients with severe AR and ejection fraction 50%

For a complete list of references, please visit www.expertconsult.com.

KEY REFERENCES

2. Aronow WS, Ahn C, Shirani J, et al: Comparison of frequency of new coronary events in older subjects with and without valvular aortic sclerosis. Am J Cardiol 83:599–600, 1999.
26. Aronow WS, Ahn C, Kronzon I: Prevalence of echocardiographic findings in African-American, Hispanic, and white men and women aged >60 years. Am J Cardiol 87:1131–1133, 2001.
34. Aronow WS, Ahn C, Kronzon I, et al: Prognosis of congestive heart failure in patients aged > or = 62 years with unoperated severe valvular aortic stenosis. Am J Cardiol 72:846–848, 1993.
37. Aronow WS, Ahn C, Shirani J, et al: Comparison of frequency of new coronary events in older adults with mild, moderate, and severe valvular aortic stenosis with those without aortic stenosis. Am J Cardiol 81:647–649, 1998.
40. Braunwald E: On the natural history of severe aortic stenosis. J Am Coll Cardiol 15:1018–1020, 1990.
42. Aronow WS, Kronzon I: Prevalence and severity of valvular aortic stenosis determined by Doppler echocardiography and its association with echocardiographic and electrocardiographic left ventricular hypertrophy and physical signs of aortic stenosis in elderly patients. Am J Cardiol 67:776–777, 1991.
55. Livanainen AM, Lindroos M, Tilvis R, et al: Natural history of aortic valve stenosis of varying severity in the elderly. Am J Cardiol 78:97–101, 1996.
64. Brown ML, Pellikka PA, Schaff HV, et al: The benefits of early valve replacement in asymptomatic patients with severe aortic stenosis. J Thorac Cardiovasc Surg 135:308–331, 2008.
67. Bonow RO, Carabello BA, Chatterjee K, et al: ACC/AHA 2006 practice guidelines for the management of patients with valvular heart disease: executive summary. A report of the American College of Cardiology/American Heart Association task force on practice guidelines (writing committee to revise the 1998 guidelines for the management of patients with valvular heart disease). Developed in collaboration with the Society of Cardiovascular Anesthesiologists. Endorsed by the Society for Cardiovascular Angiography and Interventions and the Society of Thoracic Surgeons. J Am Coll Cardiol 48:598–675, 2006.
72. Belkin RN, Khalique O, Aronow WS, et al: Outcomes and survival with aortic valve replacement compared with medical therapy in patients with low-, moderate-, and severe-gradient aortic stenosis and normal left ventricular ejection fraction. Echocardiography 28:378–387, 2011.
79. Asimakopoulos G, Edwards MB, Taylor KM: Aortic valve replacement in patients 80 years of age and older. Survival and cause of death based on 1100 cases: collective results from the UK heart valve registry. Circulation 96:3403–3408, 1997.
95. Valhanian A, Alfieri O, Andreotti F, et al: Guidelines on the management of valvular heart disease (version 2012). Eur Heart J 33:2451–2496, 2012.
101. Smith CR, Leon MB, Mack MJ, et al: Transcatheter versus surgical aortic -valve replacement in high-risk patients. N Engl J Med 364:2187–2198, 2011.
103. Kodali SK, Williams MR, Smith CR, et al: Two-year outcomes after transcatheter or surgical aortic-valve replacement. N Engl J Med 366:1686–1695, 2012.
114. Aronow WS, Kronzon I: Correlation of prevalence and severity of aortic regurgitation detected by pulsed Doppler echocardiography with the murmur of aortic regurgitation in elderly patients in a long-term health care facility. Am J Cardiol 63:128–129, 1989.
118. Aronow WS, Ahn C, Kronzon I, et al: Prognosis of patients with heart failure and unoperated severe aortic valvular regurgitation and relation to ejection fraction. Am J Cardiol 74:286–288, 1994.
127. Aronow WS, Ahn C, Kronzon I, et al: Congestive heart failure, coronary events, and atherothrombotic brain infarction in elderly blacks and whites with systemic hypertension and with and without echocardiographic and electrocardiographic evidence of left ventricular hypertrophy. Am J Cardiol 67:295–299, 1991.
129. Henry WL, Bonow RO, Borer JS, et al: Observations on the optimum time for operative intervention for aortic regurgitation. I. Evaluation of the results of aortic valve replacement in symptomatic patients. Circulation 61:471–483, 1980.
168. Aronow WS, Schwartz KS, Koenigsberg M: Correlation of murmurs of mitral stenosis and mitral regurgitation with presence or absence of mitral annular calcium in persons older than 62 years in a long-term health care facility. Am J Cardiol 59:181–182, 1987.
169. Aronow WS, Koenigsberg M, Kronzon I, et al: Association of mitral annular calcium with new thromboembolic stroke and cardiac events at 39-month follow-up in elderly patients. Am J Cardiol 65:1511–1512, 1990.
174. Kaplan S, Aronow WS, Lai HM, et al: Patients with echocardiographic aortic valve calcium or mitral annular calcium have an increased prevalence of moderate or severe coronary artery calcium diagnosed by cardiac computed tomography. Int J Angiol 16:45–46, 2007.
180. Varma R, Aronow WS, McClung JA, et al: Prevalence of valve calcium and association of valve calcium with coronary artery disease, atherosclerotic vascular disease, and all-cause mortality in 137 patients undergoing hemodialysis for chronic renal failure. Am J Cardiol 95:742–743, 2005.
202. Aronow WS, Ahn C, Kronzon I: Echocardiographic findings associated with atrial fibrillation in 1,699 patients aged >60 years. Am J Cardiol 76:1191–1192, 1995.
204. Aronow WS, Kronzon I: Correlation of prevalence and severity of mitral regurgitation and mitral stenosis determined by Doppler echocardiography with physical signs of mitral regurgitation and mitral stenosis in 100 patients aged 62 to 100 years with mitral annular calcium. Am J Cardiol 60:1189–1190, 1987.
208. Aronow WS, Ahn C, Kronzon I, et al: Association of mitral annular calcium with prior thromboembolic stroke in older white, African-American, and Hispanic men and women. Am J Cardiol 85:672–673, 2000.
211. Aronow WS, Schoenfeld MR, Gutstein H: Frequency of thromboembolic stroke in persons greater than or equal to 60 years of age with extracranial carotid arterial disease and/or mitral annular calcium. Am J Cardiol 70:123–124, 1992.

44 Cardiac Arrhythmias

Wilbert S. Aronow

VENTRICULAR ARRHYTHMIAS

The prevalence of complex ventricular arrhythmia (VA) in older adult patients without cardiovascular disease detected by 24-hour ambulatory electrocardiogram (ECG) was 50% in men and women,[1] 31% in men and women,[2] 30% in men and women,[3] 20% in men and women,[4] 16% in women and 28% in men,[5] and 33% in men and women.[6] The prevalence of complex VA detected by 24-hour ambulatory ECG was 55% in older adults with hypertension, valvular heart disease, or cardiomyopathies,[5] 68% in older adults with coronary artery disease (CAD),[5] and 55% in 843 older adults with heart disease.[6,7] Complex VA was present on a 1-minute strip of an ECG in 2% of 104 older adults without cardiovascular disease and 4% of 843 older adults with cardiovascular disease.[6] In older adults with cardiovascular disease, there is a higher prevalence of ventricular tachycardia (VT) and of complex VA in those who have an abnormal left ventricular (LV) ejection fraction,[8] echocardiographic LV hypertrophy,[9] or silent myocardial ischemia.[10]

Prognosis of Ventricular Arrhythmias

No Heart Disease

Nonsustained VT or complex VA diagnosed by 24-hour ambulatory ECG[3,11,12] or by 12-lead ECG with 1-minute rhythm strips[6] in older adults with no clinical evidence of heart disease were not associated with an increased incidence of new coronary events. Exercise-induced nonsustained VT[13] or complex VA[14] in older adults with no clinical evidence of heart disease also was not associated with an increased incidence of new coronary events. Therefore, asymptomatic nonsustained VA and complex VA in older adults without heart disease should not be treated with antiarrhythmic drugs.

Heart Disease

In older adults with heart disease, nonsustained VT[3,10,12] or complex VA[3,6,10,12] increased the incidence of new coronary events. At 2-year follow-up of 391 older adults with heart disease, the incidence of new coronary events was increased 6.8 times in older adults with VT and an abnormal LV ejection fraction and 7.6 times in older adults with complex VA and an abnormal LV ejection fraction.[3] At 27-month follow-up of 468 older adults with heart disease, the incidence of primary ventricular fibrillation (VF) or sudden cardiac death was increased 7.1 times in older adults with VT and echocardiographic LV hypertrophy and 7.3 times in patients with complex VA and echocardiographic LV hypertrophy.[12] At 37-month follow-up of 404 older adults with heart disease, the incidence of new coronary events was increased 2.5 times in older adults with VT and silent ischemia and 4.0 times in older adults with complex VA and silent ischemia.[10]

General Therapy

Underlying causes of complex VA should be treated when possible. Treatment of congestive heart failure (CHF), LV dysfunction, digitalis toxicity, hypokalemia, hypomagnesemia, myocardial ischemia (by antiischemic drugs such as β-blockers or by coronary revascularization), hypertension, LV hypertrophy, hypoxia, and other conditions may eliminate or reduce the severity of complex VA. Such patients should not smoke or drink alcohol and should avoid drugs that may cause or increase complex VA.

All older adults with CAD should be treated with aspirin,[15-17] β-blockers,[16-22] angiotensin-converting enzyme (ACE) inhibitors,[16,17,23-28] and statins[16,17,29-35] unless there are contraindications to these drugs.

Age-related physiologic changes may affect absorption, distribution, metabolism, and excretion of cardiovascular drugs.[36] Numerous physiologic changes that occur with aging affect pharmacodynamics, resulting in changes in end-organ responsiveness to cardiovascular drugs.[36] Drug interactions between antiarrhythmic drugs and other cardiovascular drugs are common, especially in older adults.[36] Important drug-disease interactions also occur in older adults.[36] Class I antiarrhythmic drugs are more proarrhythmic than class III antiarrhythmic drugs. Except for β-blockers, all antiarrhythmic drugs can cause torsade de pointes VT (polymorphous appearance associated with a prolonged QT interval).

Class I Antiarrhythmic Drugs

Class I antiarrhythmic drugs are sodium channel blockers. Class Ia antiarrhythmic drugs have intermediate channel kinetics and prolong repolarization; these drugs include disopyramide, procainamide, and quinidine. Class Ib antiarrhythmic drugs have rapid channel kinetics and shorten repolarization slightly; these drugs include lidocaine, mexiletine, phenytoin, and tocainide. Class Ic antiarrhythmic drugs have slow channel kinetics and have little effect on repolarization; these drugs include encainide, flecainide, lorcainide, moricizine, and propafenone. None of the class I antiarrhythmic drugs have been demonstrated in controlled, clinical trials to decrease sudden cardiac death, total cardiac death, or total mortality.

Table 44-1 shows the effect of class I antiarrhythmic drugs on mortality in patients with heart disease and complex VA.[37-43] A meta-analysis of six double-blind studies of patients with chronic atrial fibrillation who underwent direct-current cardioversion to sinus rhythm showed that the mortality rate at 1 year was higher in patients treated with quinidine (2.9%) than in patients treated with a placebo (0.8%).[44]

Of 1330 patients in the Stroke Prevention in Atrial Fibrillation (SPAF) study, 127 were treated with quinidine, 57 with procainamide, 34 with flecainide, 20 with encainide, and 7 with amiodarone.[45] The adjusted relative risk of cardiac mortality was increased 1.8 times and the adjusted relative risk of arrhythmic death was increased 2.1 times in patients receiving antiarrhythmic drugs versus no antiarrhythmic drugs.[45] In patients with a history of CHF, the adjusted relative risk of cardiac death was increased 3.3 times and the adjusted relative risk of arrhythmic death was increased 5.8 times in patients taking antiarrhythmic drugs versus no antiarrhythmic drugs.[45]

An analysis was made of 59 randomized, controlled clinical trials including 23,229 patients that investigated the use of class I antiarrhythmic drugs after myocardial infarction (MI).[46] The class I antiarrhythmic drugs investigated included aprindine, disopyramide, encainide, flecainide, imipramine, lidocaine, mexiletine, moricizine, phenytoin, procainamide, quinidine, and tocainide.

TABLE 44-1 Effect of Class I Antiarrhythmic Drugs on Mortality in Patients With Heart Disease and Complex Ventricular Arrhythmias

Study	Results
International Mexiletine and Placebo Antiarrhythmic Coronary Trial[37]	At 1-year follow-up, mortality was 7.6% for mexiletine and 4.8% for the placebo.
Cardiac Arrhythmia Suppression Trial I[38,39]	At 10-month follow-up, mortality for arrhythmia or cardiac arrest was 4.5% for encainide or flecainide versus 1.2% for the placebo; mortality was 7.7% for encainide or flecainide versus 3.0% for the placebo; adverse events, including death, were more frequent in older adults taking encainide or flecainide.
Cardiac Arrhythmia Suppression Trial II[39,40]	At 18-month follow-up, mortality for arrhythmia or cardiac arrest was 8.4% for moricizine versus 7.3% for the placebo; 2-year survival rate was 81.7% for moricizine versus 85.6% for the placebo; adverse events, including death, were more frequent in older adults taking moricizine.
Aronow et al[41]	At 2-year follow-up, mortality was 65% for quinidine or procainamide versus 63% for no antiarrhythmic drug; quinidine or procainamide did not reduce sudden death, total cardiac death, or total mortality in older adults with ischemic or nonischemic heart disease, abnormal or normal LV ejection fraction, and presence or absence of VT.
Moosvi et al[42]	Two-year sudden death survival was 69% for quinidine, 69% for procainamide, and 89% for no antiarrhythmic drug; 2-year total survival was 61% for quinidine, 57% for procainamide, and 71% for no antiarrhythmic drug.
Hallstrom et al[43]	At 108-month follow-up, the adjusted relative risk of death or recurrent cardiac arrest on quinidine or procainamide versus no antiarrhythmic drug was 1.17.

LV, Left ventricular; *VT*, ventricular tachycardia.

TABLE 44-2 Effect of β-Blockers on Mortality in Patients With Heart Disease and Complex Ventricular Arrhythmias

Study	Results
Hallstrom et al[43]	At 108-month follow-up, the adjusted relative risk of death or recurrent cardiac arrest for β-blockers versus no antiarrhythmic drug was 0.62.
Beta Blocker Heart Attack Trial[47-49]	At 25-month follow-up, propranolol reduced sudden cardiac death by 28% in patients with complex VA and by 16% in patients without VA; propranolol decreased total mortality by 34% in patients aged 60–69 years.
Norwegian Propranolol Study[50]	High-risk survivors of acute MI treated with propranolol for 1 year had a 52% decrease in sudden cardiac death.
Aronow et al[51]	At 29-month follow-up, compared with no antiarrhythmic drug, propranolol caused a 47% reduction in sudden cardiac death, a 37% decrease in total cardiac death, and a 20% borderline significant decrease in total death.
Cardiac Arrhythmia Suppression Trial[52]	Patients on β-blockers had a reduction in all-cause mortality of 43% at 30 days, of 46% at 1 year, and of 33% at 2 years and a decrease in arrhythmic death or cardiac arrest of 66% at 30 days, of 53% at 1 year, and of 36% at 2 years; β-blockers were an independent factor for reduced arrhythmic death or cardiac arrest by 40% and for decreased all-cause mortality by 33%.

LV, Left ventricular; *MI*, myocardial infarction; *VA*, ventricular arrhythmia; *VT*, ventricular tachycardia.

Mortality was increased in patients receiving class I antiarrhythmic drugs versus patients receiving no antiarrhythmic drugs (OR = 1.14).[46] None of the 59 studies showed that the use of a class I antiarrhythmic drug decreased mortality in patients after MI.[46]

On the basis of the available data, none of the class I antiarrhythmic drugs should be used to treat VT or complex VA in older adult or younger patients with heart disease.

Calcium Channel Blockers

Calcium channel blockers are not useful in the therapy of complex VA. Although verapamil can terminate a left septal VT, hemodynamic collapse can occur if intravenous verapamil is given to patients with the more common forms of VT. An analysis was made of randomized, controlled clinical trials (N = 20,342) that investigated the use of calcium channel blockers after MI.[46] Mortality was insignificantly increased in patients receiving calcium channel blockers than in patients receiving no antiarrhythmic drugs (odds ratio [OR] = 1.04).[46]

On the basis of the available data, none of the calcium channel blockers should be used to treat VT or complex VA in older adult or younger patients with heart disease.

β-Blockers

An analysis of 55 randomized, controlled clinical trials including 53,268 patients that investigated the use of β-blockers after MI showed that mortality was decreased in patients who received β-blockers versus a placebo (OR = 0.81).[46] β-Blockers caused a greater decrease in mortality in older patients than in younger patients.[18-21,47] Table 44-2 indicates the effect of β-blockers on mortality in patients with heart disease and complex VA.[43,47-52]

The decrease in mortality as a result of the use of β-blockers in older adults with heart disease and complex VA is due more to an antiischemic effect than to an antiarrhythmic effect.[53] β-Blockers also abolish the circadian distribution of sudden cardiac death or fatal MI,[54] markedly decrease the circadian variation of complex VA,[55] and abolish the circadian variation of myocardial ischemia.[56] Based on the available data, β-blockers should be used to treat older and younger patients with heart disease and complex VA if there are no contraindications to the use of β-blockers.

Angiotensin-Converting Enzyme Inhibitors

ACE inhibitors have been demonstrated to reduce sudden cardiac death in some studies of patients with CHF.[24,57] ACE inhibitors should be used to reduce total mortality in older and younger patients with CHF,[24,26,57,58] an anterior MI,[25] and an LV ejection fraction of 40% after MI.[23,26,59] ACE inhibitors should be administered to treat older adult and younger patients with CHF with abnormal LV ejection fraction[24,26,57,58] or with normal LV ejection fraction.[60,61]

On the basis of the available data, ACE inhibitors should be used to treat older and younger patients with VT or complex VA associated with CHF, an anterior MI, or an LV ejection fraction of 40% after MI if there are no contraindications to the use of

ACE inhibitors. β-Blockers should be administered in addition to ACE inhibitors in treating these patients.[59]

Class III Antiarrhythmic Drugs

Class III antiarrhythmic drugs are potassium channel blockers, which prolong repolarization manifested by an increase in QT interval on the ECG. These drugs are effective in suppressing complex VA, including nonsustained VT, by increasing the refractory period. However, antiarrhythmic aggravation can occur, especially torsade de pointes.

Table 44-3 shows the effect of class III antiarrhythmic drugs on mortality in patients with heart disease.[62-67] None of the class III antiarrhythmic drugs have been found in a double-blind, randomized, placebo-controlled clinical trial to decrease mortality in patients with heart disease and complex VA.

In 481 patients with VT, D,L-sotalol caused torsade de pointes (12 patients) or an increase in VT episodes (11 patients) in 23 patients (5%).[68] On the basis of the available data, β-blockers are preferred to the use of D,L-sotalol in treating older adult and younger patients with heart disease and VT or complex VA.

Amiodarone is very effective in suppressing VT and complex VA associated with heart disease.[64,65,67,69] However, the incidence of adverse effects from amiodarone approaches 90% after 5 years of therapy.[70] In the Cardiac Arrest in Seattle: Conventional Versus Amiodarone Drug Evaluation study, the incidence of pulmonary toxicity was 10% at 2 years in patients receiving 158 mg of amiodarone daily.[69] Amiodarone can also cause hyperthyroidism, hypothyroidism, and cardiac, dermatologic, gastrointestinal, hepatic, neurologic, and ophthalmologic adverse effects.

Because amiodarone has not been demonstrated to reduce mortality in older adult or younger patients with VT or complex VA associated with prior MI or CHF and has a very high incidence of toxicity, β-blockers are preferred to the use of amiodarone in treating these patients. Some data suggest that patients receiving amiodarone plus β-blockers have a better survival time than patients receiving amiodarone.[71]

Invasive Intervention

If patients have life-threatening VT or VF resistant to antiarrhythmic drugs, invasive intervention should be conducted. Patients with critical CAD and severe myocardial ischemia should undergo coronary artery bypass graft surgery to reduce mortality.[72]

Surgical ablation of the arrhythmogenic focus in patients with life-threatening VT can be curative. This treatment includes aneurysmectomy or infarctectomy and endocardial resection with or without adjunctive cryoablation based on activation mapping in the operating room.[73-75] However, the perioperative mortality rate is high. Endoaneurysmorrhaphy with a pericardial patch combined with mapping-guided subendocardial resection frequently cures recurrent VT with a low operative mortality and improvement of LV systolic function.[76] Radiofrequency catheter ablation of VT has also been beneficial in the management of selected patients with arrhythmogenic foci of monomorphic VT.[77-79]

Automatic Implantable Cardioverter-Defibrillator

The automatic implantable cardioverter-defibrillator (AICD) is the most effective treatment for patients with life-threatening VT or VF. Table 44-4 indicates the effect of the AICD on mortality in patients with ventricular tachyarrhythmias.[80-86] Tresch and colleagues[74,75] showed in retrospective studies that the AICD was very effective in treating life-threatening VT in older adult and younger patients. The Canadian Implantable Defibrillator study found that patients most likely to benefit from an AICD were those with two of the following factors: age (70 years), LV ejection fraction (35%), and New York Heart Association (NYHA) function class III or IV.[87]

TABLE 44-3 Effect of Class III Antiarrhythmic Drugs on Mortality in Patients With Heart Disease

Study	Results
Julien et al[62]	At 1-year follow-up, mortality was not different in patients after MI on D,L-sotalol versus a placebo.
Waldo et al[63]	At 148-day follow-up, mortality in patients after MI was increased by D-sotalol (5.0%) versus a placebo (3.1%).
Singh et al[64]	At 2-year follow-up of patients with CHF and complex VA, survival was not different for amiodarone versus a placebo.
Canadian Amiodarone MI Arrhythmia Trial[65]	At 1.8-year follow-up of patients after MI with complex VA, mortality was not different for amiodarone versus a placebo.
European MI Amiodarone Trial[66]	At 21-month follow-up of patients after MI, mortality was not different for amiodarone (13.9%) versus a placebo (13.7%).
Sudden Cardiac Death in Heart Failure Trial[67]	At 45.5-month follow-up, compared with a placebo, amiodarone caused an insignificant (6%) increase in mortality, and implantable cardioverter-defibrillator therapy significantly reduced mortality by 23%.

CHF, Congestive heart failure; *MI,* myocardial infarction; *VA,* ventricular arrhythmia.

TABLE 44-4 Effect of the Automatic Implantable Cardioverter-Defibrillator on Mortality in Patients With Ventricular Tachyarrhythmias

Study	Results
Multicenter Automatic Defibrillator Implantation Trial[80]	At 27-month follow-up, the AICD caused a 54% reduction in mortality.
Antiarrhythmics versus Implantable Defibrillators Trial[81]	Compared with drug therapy, the AICD caused a 39% decrease in mortality at 1 year, a 27% reduction in mortality at 2 years, and a 31% decrease in mortality at 3 years.
Canadian Implantable Defibrillator Study[82]	Compared with amiodarone, at 3 years, total mortality rate was insignificantly decreased by 20% and the arrhythmic mortality was insignificantly reduced by 33%.
Cardiac Arrest Study Hamburg[83]	Propafenone was stopped at 11 months because mortality from sudden death and cardiac arrest recurrence was 23% for propafenone versus 0% for an AICD.
Cardiac Arrest Study Hamburg[84]	Compared with amiodarone or metoprolol, the 2-year mortality was decreased 37% by an AICD.
Multicenter Unsustained Tachycardia Trial[85]	Compared with electrophysiologic guided antiarrhythmic drug therapy, the 5-year total mortality was borderline significantly decreased 20% by an AICD and the 5-year risk of cardiac arrest or death from arrhythmia was decreased 76% by an AICD.
Multicenter Automatic Defibrillator Implantation Trial II[86]	At 20-month follow-up, compared with medical therapy, the AICD caused a 31% significant reduction in mortality.

AICD, Automatic implantable cardioverter-defibrillator.

In MADIT-II, the reduction in sudden cardiac death in patients treated with an AICD was significantly reduced: by 68% in 574 patients younger than 65 years, by 65% in 455 patients aged 65 to 74 years, and by 68% in 204 patients aged 75 years.[88] The median survival in 348 octogenarians treated with AICD therapy was greater than 4 years.[89]

At 26-month follow-up, survival was 91% for patients treated with metoprolol plus an AICD versus 83% for patients treated with D,L-sotalol plus an AICD.[90] An observational study in 78 patients with CAD and life-threatening VA treated with an AICD showed at the 490-day follow-up that the use of lipid-lowering drugs reduced recurrences of life-threatening VA.[91] At the 33-month follow-up of 1038 patients (mean age, 70 years) who had AICDs, use of β-blockers significantly reduced the frequency of appropriate AICD shocks.[92] At the 32-month follow-up of 965 of these patients, all-cause mortality was significantly reduced: 46% by use of β-blockers, 42% by use of statins, and 29% by use of ACE inhibitors or angiotensin receptor blockers.[93] These data support the use of β-blockers, statins, and ACE inhibitors or angiotensin receptor blockers in the treatment of patients with AICDs.

The American College of Cardiology/American Heart Association (ACC/AHA) guidelines recommend that class I indications for treatment with an AICD are (1) cardiac arrest due to VT or VF not caused by a transient or reversible cause; (2) spontaneous sustained VT; (3) syncope of undetermined origin with clinically relevant, hemodynamically significant sustained VT or VF induced at electrophysiologic study when drug therapy is ineffective, not tolerated, or not preferred; (4) nonsustained VT with CAD, prior MI, LV systolic dysfunction, and inducible VF or sustained VT at electrophysiologic study that is not suppressed by a class I antiarrhythmic drug; (5) patients with prior MI (at least 40 days previously) with an LV ejection fraction less than or equal to 35% who are in NYHA class II or III; (6) patients with prior MI (at least 40 days previously) with an LV ejection fraction less than 30% who are in NYHA class I; and (7) patients with nonischemic dilated cardiomyopathy with an LV ejection fraction less than or equal to 35% who are in NYHA class II or III.[94]

The 2009 updated ACC/AHA guidelines for treatment of CHF with class I indications recommend use of an AICD in (1) patients with current or prior symptoms of CHF and reduced LV ejection fraction with a history of cardiac arrest, VF, or hemodynamically destabilizing VT; (2) patients with CAD at least 40 days after MI, an LV ejection fraction equal to or less than 35%, NYHA class II or III symptoms on optimal medical therapy, and an expected survival greater than 1 year; and (3) patients with nonischemic cardiomyopathy, an LV ejection fraction equal to or less than 35%, NYHA class II or III symptoms on optimal medical therapy, and an expected survival greater than 1 year; and (4) may be used in patients receiving cardiac resynchronization therapy for NYHA class II or ambulatory class IV symptoms despite recommended optimal medical therapy.[95,96]

ACC/AHA class IIa indications for treatment with an AICD are (1) unexplained syncope, significant LV dysfunction, and nonischemic cardiomyopathy; (2) sustained VT and normal or near normal LV function; (3) hypertrophic cardiomyopathy with one or more major risk factors for sudden cardiac death; (4) prevention of sudden cardiac death in patients with arrhythmogenic right ventricular dysplasia/cardiomyopathy who have one or more risk factors for sudden cardiac death; (5) reduction of sudden cardiac death in patients with long-QT syndrome who have syncope and/or VT while using β-blockers; (6) nonhospitalized patients awaiting cardiac transplantation; (7) Brugada syndrome with syncope; (8) Brugada syndrome with documented VT that has not resulted in cardiac arrest; (9) patients with catecholaminergic polymorphic VT with syncope and/or documented sustained VT on β-blockers; and (10) cardiac sarcoidosis, giant cell myocarditis, or Chagas disease.[94]

During 1243 days mean follow-up of 549 patients, mean age 74 years, who had an AICD for CHF, 163 (30%) had appropriate AICD shocks, 71 (13%) had inappropriate AICD shocks, and 63 (12%) died. [97] Stepwise logistic regression analysis showed that significant independent prognostic factors for appropriate AICD shocks were smoking (OR = 3.7) and statins (OR = 0.54) , for inappropriate AICD shocks were atrial fibrillation (OR = 6.2) and statins (OR = 0.52), and for time to mortality were age (hazard ratio [HR] = 1.08 per 1-year increase), ACE inhibitors or angiotensin receptor blockers (HR = 0.25), AF (HR = 4.1), right ventricular pacing (HR = 3.6), digoxin (HR = 2.9), hypertension (HR = 5.3), and statins (HR = 0.32).[97]

During implantation and during the 38-month follow-up observation of 1,060 patients (mean age, 70 years) who had AICDs, complications occurred in 60 patients (5.7%).[98] In a registry of 5,399 AICD recipients for primary or secondary prevention, rates of appropriate AICD shocks were similar among patients aged 18 to 49, 50 to 59, 60 to 69, 70 to 79, and 80 years and older.[99]

ATRIAL FIBRILLATION

Atrial fibrillation (AF) is the most common sustained cardiac arrhythmia. The prevalence of AF increases with age.[100-103] The prevalence of AF in 2101 patients (mean age, 81 years) was 5% in patients aged 60 to 70 years, 13% in patients aged 71 to 90 years, and 22% in patients aged 91 to 103 years.[101] Chronic AF was present in 16% of older adult men and in 13% of older adult women.[101] The prevalence of chronic AF in a study of 1563 patients (mean age, 80 years) living in the community and seen in an academic geriatrics practice was 9%.[103]

AF may be paroxysmal or chronic. Episodes of paroxysmal AF may last from a few seconds to several weeks. Spontaneous conversion of paroxysmal AF to sinus rhythm occurs in 68% of patients having AF of less than 72 hours' duration.[104]

Predisposing Factors

Factors predisposing to AF include alcohol, atrial myxoma, atrial septal defect, cardiomyopathies, chronic lung disease, conduction system disease, CHF, CAD, diabetes mellitus, drugs, emotional stress, excessive coffee, hypertension, hyperthyroidism, hypoglycemia, hypokalemia, hypovolemia, hypoxia, myocarditis, neoplastic disease, pericarditis, pneumonia, postoperative state, pulmonary embolism, systemic infection, and valvular heart disease. Table 44-5 lists the increased prevalence of echocardiographic findings

TABLE 44-5 Echocardiographic Findings in 254 Patients With Chronic Atrial Fibrillation and 1445 Patients With Sinus Rhythm, Mean Age 81 Years

Variable	Higher Prevalence in Atrial Fibrillation
Rheumatic mitral stenosis	17.1 times
Left atrial enlargement	2.9 times
Abnormal LV ejection fraction	2.5 times
Aortic stenosis	2.3 times
≥ 1+ mitral regurgitation	2.2 times
≥ 1+ aortic regurgitation	2.1 times
LV hypertrophy	2.9 times
Mitral annular calcium	1.7 times

Adapted from Aronow WS, Ahn C, Kronzon I.[105]
LV, Left ventricular.

in 254 older adult patients with chronic AF compared with 1445 older adult patients with sinus rhythm (mean age, 81 years).[105] In the Framingham Heart Study, low serum thyrotropin levels were independently associated with a 3.1 times increase in the development of new AF in older adults.[106]

Associated Risks

The Framingham study showed that the incidence of death from cardiovascular causes was 2.0 times higher in men and 2.7 times higher in women with chronic AF than in men and women with sinus rhythm.[107] The Framingham study also demonstrated that after adjustment for preexisting cardiovascular conditions, the odds ratio for mortality in patients with AF was 1.5 in men and 1.9 in women.[108] At the 42-month follow-up of 1359 patients (mean age, 81 years) with heart disease, patients with AF had a 2.2 times higher probability of developing new coronary events than those with sinus rhythm after controlling for other prognostic variables.[109] In 106,780 Medicare beneficiaries (65 years of age) from the Cooperative Cardiovascular Project treated for acute MI, AF was present in 22%.[110] Compared with sinus rhythm, older adults with AF had a higher in-hospital mortality (25% vs. 16%), 30-day mortality (29% vs. 19%), and 1-year mortality (48% vs. 33%).[110] AF was an independent predictor of in-hospital mortality (OR = 1.2), 30-day mortality (OR = 1.2), and 1-year mortality (OR = 1.3).[110] Older adults who developed AF while they were hospitalized had a worse prognosis than older adults who already had AF.[110]

AF is an independent risk factor for thromboembolic (TE) stroke, especially in older patients.[100,101] In the Framingham study, the relative risk of stroke in patients with nonrheumatic AF compared with patients in sinus rhythm was 2.6 times higher in patients aged 60 to 69 years, 3.3 times higher in patients aged 70 to 79 years, and 4.5 times higher in patients aged 80 to 89 years.[100] AF was an independent risk factor for TE stroke in 2101 patients, mean age 81 years, with a relative risk of 3.3.[101] The 3-year incidence of TE stroke was 38% in patients with AF and 11% in patients with sinus rhythm.[101] The 5-year incidence of TE stroke was 72% in patients with AF and 24% in patients with sinus rhythm.[101]

AF was present in 313 of 2384 patients (13%), mean age 81 years.[111] AF was present in 201 of 1024 patients (17%) with LV hypertrophy and in 112 of 1360 patients (8%) without LV hypertrophy.[111] At the 44-month follow-up, both AF (risk ratio [RR] = 3.2) and LV hypertrophy (RR = 2.8) were independent risk factors for new TE stroke. The higher prevalence of LV hypertrophy in older adults with chronic AF contributes to the higher incidence of TE stroke in older adults with AF.

At the 45-month follow-up of 1846 patients, mean age 81 years, both AF (RR = 3.3) and 40% to 100% extracranial carotid arterial disease (ECAD) (RR = 2.5) were independent risk factors for new TE stroke.[112] Older adults with both chronic AF and 40% to 100% ECAD had a 6.9 times higher probability of developing new TE stroke than those with sinus rhythm and no significant ECAD.[112]

Symptomatic cerebral infarctions were present in 22% of 54 autopsied patients aged 70 years or older with paroxysmal AF.[113] Symptomatic cerebral infarction was 2.4 times more common in older patients with paroxysmal AF than in older patients with sinus rhythm.[113] AF also causes silent cerebral infarction.[114]

AF is a predisposing factor for CHF in older patients. As much as 30% to 40% of LV end-diastolic volume may be attributable to left atrial contraction in older patients. Absence of a coordinated left atrial contraction decreases late diastolic filling of the left ventricle because of loss of the atrial kick. A rapid ventricular rate associated with AF also shortens the diastolic filling period, which further decreases LV filling.

A retrospective analysis of the Studies of Left Ventricular Dysfunction Prevention and Treatment Trials found that AF was an independent risk factor for all-cause mortality (RR = 1.3), progressive pump failure death (RR = 1.4), and death or hospitalization for CHF (RR = 1.3).[115]

AF was present in 132 of 355 patients (37%), mean age 80 years, with prior MI, CHF, and an abnormal LV ejection fraction.[116] AF was present in 98 of 296 patients (33%), mean age 82 years, with prior MI, CHF, and a normal LV ejection fraction.[116] In this study, AF was an independent risk factor for mortality with a risk ratio of 1.5.[116]

A rapid ventricular rate associated with chronic or paroxysmal AF may cause a tachycardia-related cardiomyopathy, which may be an unrecognized curable cause of CHF.[117,118] Control of a rapid ventricular rate by radiofrequency ablation of the atrioventricular (AV) node with permanent pacing caused an improvement in LV ejection fraction in patients with medically refractory AF.[119]

Clinical Symptoms

Older adults with AF may be symptomatic or asymptomatic with their arrhythmia detected by physical examination or by an ECG. Examination of a person after a stroke may lead to the diagnosis of AF. Symptoms may include palpitations, skips in heartbeat, fatigue on exertion, exercise intolerance, cough, dizziness, chest pain, and syncope. A rapid ventricular rate associated with loss of atrial contraction reduces cardiac output and may cause hypotension, angina pectoris, CHF, acute pulmonary edema, and syncope, especially in older adults with mitral stenosis, aortic stenosis, or hypertrophic cardiomyopathy.

Diagnostic Tests

When AF is suspected, a 12-lead ECG with a 1-minute rhythm strip should be obtained to confirm the diagnosis. If paroxysmal AF is suspected, a 24-hour ambulatory ECG should be obtained. All patients with AF should have an M-mode, two-dimensional, and Doppler echocardiogram to determine the presence and severity of cardiac abnormalities causing AF and to identify risk factors for stroke. Appropriate tests for noncardiac causes of AF should be performed when clinically indicated. Thyroid function tests should be performed because AF or CHF may be the only clinical manifestations of apathetic hyperthyroidism in older adults.

General Treatment Measures

Along with drug therapy, treatment of AF should include therapy of the underlying disorder (such as hyperthyroidism, pneumonia, or pulmonary embolism) when possible. Surgical candidates for mitral valve replacement should undergo surgery if it is clinically indicated. If mitral valve replacement is not performed in patients with significant mitral valve disease, elective cardioversion should not be performed in patients with AF. Precipitating factors such as CHF, hypoxia, hypokalemia, hypoglycemia, hypovolemia, and infection should be treated immediately. Alcohol, coffee, and drugs (especially sympathomimetics) that precipitate AF should be avoided. Paroxysmal AF associated with the tachycardia-bradycardia (sick sinus) syndrome should be treated with permanent pacing in combination with the use of drugs to slow a rapid ventricular rate associated with AF.[120]

Control of Very Rapid Ventricular Rate

Immediate direct-current cardioversion should be performed in patients who have paroxysmal AF with a very rapid ventricular rate associated with an acute MI, chest pain caused by myocardial ischemia, hypotension, severe CHF, or syncope. Intravenous verapamil,[121] diltiazem,[122] or β-blockers[123-126] may be used to immediately slow a very rapid ventricular rate associated with AF.

Control of Rapid Ventricular Rate

Digitalis glycosides are ineffective in converting AF to sinus rhythm.[127] Digoxin is also ineffective in slowing a rapid ventricular rate associated with AF if there is associated hyperthyroidism, fever, hypoxia, acute blood loss, or any condition involving increased sympathetic tone.[128] However, digoxin should be used for slowing a rapid ventricular rate in AF unassociated with increased sympathetic tone, the Wolff-Parkinson-White syndrome, or hypertrophic obstructive cardiomyopathy, especially if there is LV systolic dysfunction. The usual maintenance oral dose of digoxin administered to patients with AF is 0.25 to 0.5 mg daily, with the dose decreased to 0.125 to 0.25 mg daily for older adults who are more susceptible to digitalis toxicity.[129]

Oral verapamil,[130] diltiazem,[131] or a β-blocker[132] should be added to the therapeutic regimen if a rapid ventricular rate associated with AF occurs at rest or during exercise despite digoxin. These drugs act synergistically with digoxin to depress conduction through the AV junction. In a study of digoxin 0.25 mg daily, diltiazem-CD 240 mg daily, atenolol 50 mg daily, digoxin 0.25 mg plus diltiazem-CD 240 mg daily, and digoxin 0.25 mg plus atenolol 50 mg daily, digoxin and diltiazem as single drugs were least effective and digoxin plus atenolol was most effective in controlling ventricular rate in AF during daily activity.[133]

Amiodarone is the most effective drug for slowing a rapid ventricular rate associated with AF.[134,135] However, its adverse effect profile limits its use in the treatment of AF. Oral doses of 200 to 400 mg of amiodarone daily may be administered to selected patients with symptomatic life-threatening AF refractory to other drug therapy.

Therapeutic concentrations of digoxin do not decrease the frequency of episodes of paroxysmal AF or the duration of episodes of paroxysmal AF detected by 24-hour ambulatory ECG.[136,137] In fact, digoxin has been demonstrated to increase the duration of episodes of paroxysmal AF, a result consistent with its action in reducing the atrial refractory period.[136] Therapeutic concentrations of digoxin also do not prevent a rapid ventricular rate from developing in patients with paroxysmal AF.[136-138] Therefore, digoxin should be avoided in patients with sinus rhythm with a history of paroxysmal AF.

Nondrug Therapies

Radiofrequency catheter modification of AV conduction should be performed in patients with symptomatic AF in whom a rapid ventricular rate cannot be slowed by drug therapy.[139,140] If this procedure does not control the rapid ventricular rate associated with AF, complete AV block produced by radiofrequency catheter ablation followed by permanent pacemaker implantation should be performed.[141,142] In 44 patients, mean age 78 years, radiofrequency catheter ablation followed by pacemaker implantation was successful in ablating the AV junction in 43 of 44 patients (98%) with AF and a rapid ventricular rate not controlled by drug therapy.[142]

In patients with CHF and chronic AF, AV junction ablation with implantation of a VVIR pacemaker was superior to drug therapy in controlling symptoms in a randomized, controlled study of 66 patients.[143] Surgical techniques have also been developed for use in patients with AF in whom a rapid ventricular rate cannot be slowed by drug treatment.[144-146] Appropriate indications for using an implantable Atrioverter in the treatment of AF need further investigation.[147]

Randomized studies have demonstrated that circumferential pulmonary vein radiofrequency ablation was more effective than antiarrhythmic drug therapy in preventing recurrence of AF (93% vs. 35%) in 198 patients at 1 year[148] and (87% vs. 37%) in 67 patients at 1 year.[149] There are no long-term follow-up data showing a reduction in stroke risk in patients apparently cured of AF with radiofrequency catheter ablation. Anticoagulation therapy still needs to be administered to these patients who are at increased risk of developing TE stroke. Left atrial appendage closure with the Watchman device is a reasonable alternative to consider for patients at high risk for TE stroke but with contraindications to oral anticoagulant therapy.[150]

Tachycardia-Bradycardia Syndrome

Paroxysmal AF associated with the tachycardia-bradycardia (sick sinus) syndrome should be treated with a permanent pacemaker in combination with drugs to decrease a rapid ventricular rate associated with AF.[120] Ventricular pacing is an independent risk factor for the development of chronic AF in patients with paroxysmal AF associated with the tachycardia-bradycardia syndrome.[151] Patients with paroxysmal AF associated with the tachycardia-bradycardia syndrome and no signs of AV conduction abnormalities should be treated with atrial pacing or dual-chamber pacing rather than with ventricular pacing because atrial pacing is associated with less AF, fewer TE complications, and a lower risk of AV block than is ventricular pacing.[152]

Wolff-Parkinson-White Syndrome

Direct-current cardioversion should be performed if a rapid ventricular rate in paroxysmal AF associated with the Wolff-Parkinson-White syndrome is life-threatening or fails to respond to drug treatment. Drug treatment for paroxysmal AF associated with the Wolff-Parkinson-White syndrome includes propranolol plus procainamide, disopyramide, or quinidine.[153] Digoxin, verapamil, and diltiazem are contraindicated in patients with AF associated with the Wolff-Parkinson-White syndrome because these drugs shorten the refractory period of the accessory AV pathway, causing faster conduction down the accessory pathway. This results in a marked increase in ventricular rate. Radiofrequency catheter ablation or surgical ablation of the accessory conduction pathway should be considered in patients with AF and fast AV conduction over the accessory pathway.[154]

Slow Ventricular Rate

Many older adults are able to tolerate AF without the need for treatment because the ventricular rate is slow as a result of concomitant AV nodal disease. These patients should not be treated with a drug that depresses AV conduction. A permanent pacemaker should be implanted in patients with AF who develop cerebral symptoms such as dizziness or syncope associated with ventricular pauses greater than 3 seconds that are not drug-induced, as documented by a 24-hour ambulatory ECG. If patients with AF have drug-induced symptomatic bradycardia and the causative drug cannot be discontinued, a permanent pacemaker must be implanted.

Elective Cardioversion

Elective direct-current cardioversion has a higher success rate of converting AF to sinus rhythm than does medical cardioversion.[155] Unfavorable conditions for elective cardioversion of chronic AF to sinus rhythm include duration of AF greater than 1 year, moderate to severe cardiomegaly, echocardiographic left atrial dimension greater than 45 mm, digitalis toxicity (contraindication), slow ventricular rate (contraindication), sick sinus syndrome (contraindication), mitral valve disease, CHF, chronic obstructive lung disease, recurrent AF despite antiarrhythmic drugs, and inability to tolerate antiarrhythmic drugs. Elective cardioversion of AF either by direct current or by antiarrhythmic drugs should not be performed in asymptomatic older adults with chronic AF.

Antiarrhythmic drugs that have been used to convert AF to sinus rhythm include amiodarone, disopyramide, dofetilide, encainide, flecainide, ibutilide, procainamide, propafenone, quinidine, and sotalol. None of these drugs are as successful as direct-current cardioversion (which is 80% to 90% successful) in converting AF to sinus rhythm. All of these drugs are proarrhythmic and may aggravate or cause cardiac arrhythmias.

Encainide and flecainide caused atrial proarrhythmic effects in 6 of 60 patients (10%).[156] The proarrhythmic effects included conversion of AF to atrial flutter with a 1-to-1 AV conduction response and a very rapid ventricular rate.[156] Flecainide has induced VT and VF in patients with chronic AF.[157] Antiarrhythmic drugs, including amiodarone, disopyramide, flecainide, procainamide, propafenone, quinidine, and sotalol, caused cardiac adverse effects in 73 of 417 patients (18%) hospitalized for AF.[158] Class Ic drugs such as encainide, flecainide, and propafenone should be avoided in patients with prior MI or LV systolic dysfunction because these drugs may cause life-threatening ventricular tachyarrhythmias in these patients.[39]

Ibutilide and dofetilide are class III antiarrhythmic drugs that have recently been used to try to convert AF to sinus rhythm. Twenty-three of 79 patients (29%) with AF treated with intravenous ibutilide converted to sinus rhythm.[159] Polymorphic VT developed in 4% of patients taking ibutilide in this study.[159] All of these patients had abnormal LV systolic function. Eleven of 75 patients (15%) with AF treated with intravenous dofetilide converted to sinus rhythm.[160] Torsade de pointes occurred in 3% of patients treated with intravenous dofetilide.[161] After 1 month, 22 of 190 patients (12%) with CHF and AF had sinus rhythm restored with dofetilide compared with 3 of 201 patients (1%) treated with a placebo.[161] Torsade de pointes developed in 25 patients (3%) treated with dofetilide and in none of the patients (0%) treated with a placebo.[161] Direct-current cardioversion of AF has a higher success rate in converting AF to sinus rhythm and a lower incidence of cardiac adverse effects than any antiarrhythmic drug. However, pretreatment with ibutilide has been shown to facilitate transthoracic cardioversion of AF.[162]

Unless transesophageal echocardiography has shown no thrombus in the left atrial appendage before cardioversion,[163] oral warfarin therapy should be administered for 3 weeks before elective direct-current cardioversion or drug cardioversion of patients with AF to sinus rhythm.[164] Anticoagulant therapy should be administered at the time of cardioversion and continued until sinus rhythm has been maintained for 4 weeks.[164] After direct-current or drug cardioversion of AF to sinus rhythm, the left atrium becomes stunned and contracts poorly for 3 to 4 weeks, predisposing to TE stroke unless the patient is receiving oral warfarin.[165,166] The maintenance dose of oral warfarin should be titrated by serial prothrombin times so that the INR is 2.0 to 3.0.[164] A controlled, randomized, prospective clinical trial is needed to compare conventional anticoagulant treatment before cardioversion of AF with a transesophageal echocardiography–guided strategy.[167]

Use of Antiarrhythmic Drugs to Maintain Sinus Rhythm

The efficacy and safety of antiarrhythmic drugs after cardioversion of AF to maintain sinus rhythm have been questioned. It has not been demonstrated that patients cardioverted from AF to sinus rhythm have a decreased incidence of subsequent TE stroke. A meta-analysis of six double-blind, placebo-controlled studies of quinidine involving 808 patients who had direct-current cardioversion of chronic AF to sinus rhythm found that 50% of patients receiving quinidine and 25% of patients receiving a placebo were in sinus rhythm at 1 year.[44] However, the mortality was higher in patients treated with quinidine (2.9%) than in patients treated with a placebo (0.8%).[44] In a study of 406 patients, mean age 82 years, with heart disease and complex VA, the incidence of adverse effects causing drug cessation was 48% for quinidine and 55% for procainamide.[41] The incidence of total mortality at 2-year follow-up was insignificantly higher in patients receiving quinidine or procainamide than in patients not receiving an antiarrhythmic drug.[41]

In another study, 98 patients were randomized to sotalol and 85 patients to quinidine after direct-current cardioversion of AF to sinus rhythm.[168] At 6-month follow-up, 52% of sotalol-treated patients and 48% of quinidine-treated patients were in sinus rhythm.[168] At 1-year follow-up of 100 patients with AF cardioverted to sinus rhythm, 30% of 50 patients randomized to propafenone and 37% of 50 patients randomized to sotalol remained in sinus rhythm.[169]

Of 1330 patients in the SPAF study, 127 patients were receiving quinidine, 57 procainamide, 34 flecainide, 20 encainide, 15 disopyramide, and 7 amiodarone.[45] Patients taking an antiarrhythmic drug had a 2.7 times increased adjusted relative risk of cardiac mortality and a 2.3 times increased adjusted relative risk of arrhythmic death compared with patients not taking an antiarrhythmic drug.[45] Patients with a history of CHF taking an antiarrhythmic drug had a 4.7 times increased relative risk of cardiac death and a 3.7 times higher relative risk of arrhythmic death than patients with a history of CHF not taking an antiarrhythmic drug.[45]

A meta-analysis of 59 randomized, controlled studies comprising 23,229 patients, including older adults, that investigated the use of aprindine, disopyramide, encainide, flecainide, imipramine, lidocaine, mexiletine, moricizine, phenytoin, procainamide, quinidine, and tocainide after MI showed that the mortality was higher in patients receiving class I antiarrhythmic drugs (OR = 1.14) than in patients not receiving an antiarrhythmic drug.[45] None of the 59 studies demonstrated a decrease in mortality among patients receiving class I antiarrhythmic drugs.[45]

Ventricular Rate Control

Because maintenance of sinus rhythm with antiarrhythmic drugs may need serial cardioversions; exposes patients to the risks of proarrhythmia, sudden cardiac death, and other adverse effects; and needs the use of anticoagulant treatment in patients in sinus rhythm who have a high risk of recurrence of AF, many cardiologists, including myself, prefer the treatment strategy, especially in older adults, of ventricular rate control plus anticoagulant treatment in patients with AF. β-Blockers such as propranolol (10 to 30 mg tid or qid) can be administered to control VA[50] and following conversion of AF to sinus rhythm. If AF recurs, β-blockers have the additional advantage of slowing the ventricular rate. β-Blockers are also the most effective drugs in preventing and treating AF after coronary artery bypass graft surgery.[170] In a double-blind, randomized placebo-controlled study of 394 patients receiving metoprolol CR/XL or a placebo after cardioversion of persistent AF, metoprolol was more effective than a placebo in preventing recurrence of AF and in decreasing the ventricular heart rate when AF recurred.[171]

The Atrial Fibrillation Follow-Up Investigation of Rhythm Management (AFFIRM) study randomized 4060 patients, mean age 70 years (39% women), with paroxysmal or chronic AF of less than 6 months duration and with high risk for stroke to either maintenance of AF with ventricular rate control or to an attempt to maintain sinus rhythm with antiarrhythmic drugs after cardioversion.[172] Patients in both arms of this study were treated with warfarin. All-cause mortality at 5 years was insignificantly increased (15%) in the maintenance of sinus rhythm group compared with the ventricular rate control group (24% vs. 21%).[172] TE stroke was insignificantly reduced in the ventricular rate control group (5.5% vs. 7.1%), and all-cause hospitalization was significantly reduced in the ventricular rate control group (73% vs. 80%).[172] In both groups, the majority of strokes occurred after warfarin was stopped or when the international normalized ratio (INR) was subtherapeutic. There was no significant difference in quality of life or functional status between the two treatment groups.[172] In septuagenarian patients in the AFFIRM study, a rate-control strategy was associated with significantly lower mortality and hospitalization compared with a rhythm control strategy.[173] Data from the AFFIRM study showed increased mortality among patients taking digoxin according to one analysis[174] but not in a propensity-matched analysis in which this author was a coinvestigator.[175]

The Rate Control Versus Electrical Cardioversion for Persistent Atrial Fibrillation study Group randomized 522 patients with persistent AF after a previous electrical cardioversion to receive treatment aimed at ventricular rate control or rhythm control.[176] Both groups were treated with oral anticoagulants. At 2.3-year follow-up, the composite end point of death from cardiovascular causes, heart failure, TE complications, bleeding, implantation of a pacemaker, and severe adverse effects of drugs was 17.2% in the ventricular rate control group versus 22.6% in the rhythm control group.[176] In this study, women randomized to rhythm control had a 3.1 times significant increase in cardiovascular morbidity or mortality versus women randomized to ventricular rate control.[177]

The 2-year mortality was similar in 1009 patients with AF and CHF treated with rate control or rhythm control.[178] During 19-month follow-up of 110 patients with a history of AF treated with antiarrhythmic drug therapy, recurrent AF was diagnosed by ECG recordings in 46% of the patients and by an implantable monitoring device in 88% of the patients.[179] AF lasting longer than 48 hours was detected by the monitoring device in 50 of the 110 patients (46%). Nineteen of these 50 patients (38%) were completely asymptomatic.[179]

RISK FACTORS FOR THROMBOEMBOLIC STROKE

Risk factors for TE stroke in patients with AF include age,[100,180-183] diabetes mellitus,[181] echocardiographic left atrial enlargement,[184,185] echocardiographic LV systolic dysfunction,[183,185,186] echocardiographic LV hypertrophy,[183,184] ECAD,[112] history of CHF,[181,186,187] prior MI,[180,181,184,188] hypertension,[181,184,186,187] mitral annular calcium,[180,189] prior arterial thromboembolism,* rheumatic mitral stenosis,[183,184] and women older than 75 years.[186] Table 44-6 lists independent risk factors for new TE stroke in 312 patients with chronic AF, mean age 84 years.

TABLE 44-6 Risk Factors for New Thromboembolic Stroke in 312 Older Adults With Chronic Atrial Fibrillation

Variable	Risk Ratio
Age	1.03/yr increase
Prior stroke	1.6
Abnormal LV ejection fraction	1.8
Mitral stenosis	2.0
LV hypertrophy	2.8
Abnormal LV ejection fraction	1.8
Serum total cholesterol	1.01 per 1 mg/dL increase
Serum high-density lipoprotein cholesterol	1.04 per 1 mg/dL decrease

Adapted from Aronow WS, Ahn C, Kronzon I, et al.[183]
LV, Left ventricular.

*References 101, 107, 181-183, 186, 187, and 190.

In the SPAF study involving patients (mean age, 67 years) with nonrheumatic AF, recent CHF (within 3 months), a history of hypertension, prior arterial thromboembolism, echocardiographic LV systolic dysfunction, and echocardiographic left atrial enlargement were independently associated with new TE events.[185,187] The incidence of new TE events was 18.6% per year if three or more risk factors were present, 6.0% per year if one or two risk factors were present, and 1.0% per year if none of these risk factors were present.[185] In the SPAF III study, patients (mean age, 72 years) were considered to be at high risk for developing TE stroke if they had a previous thromboembolism, CHF, or abnormal LV systolic function; if they had a systolic blood pressure higher than 160 mm Hg; or if they were women older than 75 years of age.[186]

Antithrombotic Therapy

Prospective, randomized studies have shown that warfarin was effective in reducing the incidence of TE stroke in patients with nonvalvular AF.[181,186,190-196] Analysis of pooled data from five randomized controlled trials demonstrated that warfarin decreased the incidence of new TE stroke by 68% and was more effective than aspirin in decreasing TE stroke.[181] Nonrandomized observational data from an older adult population, mean age 83 years, found that 141 patients with chronic AF treated with oral warfarin to achieve an INR between 2.0 and 3.0 (mean INR was 2.4) had a 67% decrease in new TE stroke compared with 209 patients with chronic AF treated with oral aspirin.[197] Compared with aspirin, warfarin caused a 40% decrease in new TE stroke in patients with prior stroke, a 31% reduction in new TE stroke in patients with no prior stroke, a 45% decrease in new TE stroke in patients with an abnormal LV ejection fraction, and a 36% reduction in new TE stroke in patients with a normal LV ejection fraction.[197]

At 1.1-year follow-up in the SPAF III study, patients with nonvalvular AF considered to be at high risk for developing TE stroke randomized to therapy with oral warfarin to achieve an INR between 2.0 and 3.0 had a 72% decrease in ischemic stroke or systemic embolism compared with patients randomized to therapy with oral aspirin 325 mg daily plus oral warfarin to achieve an INR between 1.2 and 1.5.[186] Adjusted-dose warfarin caused an absolute decrease in ischemic stroke or systemic embolism of 6.0% per year.[186] In the Second Copenhagen Atrial Fibrillation, Aspirin, Anticoagulation (AFASK) study, low-dose warfarin plus aspirin was also less effective in decreasing stroke or a systemic TE event in patients with AF (7.2% after 1 year) than was adjusted-dose warfarin to achieve an INR between 2.0 and 3.0 (2.8% after 1 year).[198]

Analysis of pooled data from five randomized controlled trials showed that the annual rate of major hemorrhage was 1.0% for the control group, 1.0% for the aspirin group, and 1.3% for the warfarin group.[181] The incidence of major hemorrhage in patients taking adjusted-dose warfarin to achieve an INR of 2.0 to 3.0 in the SPAF III study (mean age 72 years) was 2.1%.[186] In the Second Copenhagen AFASK study, the incidence of major hemorrhage in patients, mean age 73 years, was 0.8% per year for patients taking adjusted-dose warfarin to achieve an INR between 2.0 and 3.0 and 1.0% per year for patients treated with aspirin, 300 mg daily.[198] The incidence of major hemorrhage in older adults, mean age 83 years, was 4.3% (1.4% per year) for patients with chronic AF taking warfarin to maintain an INR between 2.0 and 3.0 and 2.9% (1.0% per year) for patients with chronic AF treated with aspirin, 325 mg daily.[197]

In the SPAF III study, 892 patients, mean age 67 years, at low risk for developing new TE stroke were treated with oral aspirin, 325 mg daily.[199] Mean follow-up was 2 years. The incidence of new ischemic stroke or systemic embolism (primary events) was 2.2% per year.[199] The incidence of new ischemic stroke or systemic embolism was 3.6% in patients with a history of hypertension and 1.1% in patients without a history of hypertension.[199]

In the Anticoagulation and Risk Factor in Atrial Fibrillation study, women off warfarin had significantly higher annual rates of thromboembolism (3.5%) than men (1.8%).[200] Warfarin was associated with significantly lower adjusted TE rates for both women (60% reduction) and men (40% reduction) with similar annual rates of major bleeding (1.0% and 1.1%, respectively).[200]

The Atrial Fibrillation Clopidogrel Trial with Irbesartan for the Prevention of Vascular Events (ACTIVE W trial) demonstrated in patients with AF that the annual risk of first occurrence of stroke, noncentral nervous system systemic embolus, MI, or vascular death was 3.93% in 3371 patients randomized to warfarin to maintain an INR between 2.0 and 3.0, and 5.60% in 3335 patients randomized to clopidogrel 75 mg daily plus aspirin 75 to 100 mg daily, with a 44% significant decrease in the primary outcome attributed to warfarin.[201] The incidence of major bleeding was insignificantly (10%) higher in patients treated with clopidogrel plus aspirin than in patients treated with warfarin.[201]

On the basis of the available data, older adults with chronic or paroxysmal AF who are at high risk for developing TE stroke or who have a history of hypertension and who have no contraindications to anticoagulation therapy should receive long-term oral warfarin to achieve an INR of 2.0 to 3.0.[164,202] Hypertension must be controlled. Whenever the person has a prothrombin time taken, the blood pressure should also be checked. The physician prescribing the dose of oral warfarin should be aware of the numerous drugs that potentiate the effect of warfarin causing an increased prothrombin time and risk of bleeding.[36] Older adults with AF who are at low risk for developing TE stroke or who have contraindications to therapy with long-term oral warfarin should be treated with aspirin 325 mg orally daily.

New Antithrombotic Drugs

In the Randomized Evaluation of Long-Term Anticoagulation Therapy (RE-LY) study, 18,113 patients, mean age 72 years, with nonvalvular AF and a risk of stroke were randomized to the direct thrombin inhibitor dabigatran 150 mg bid or 110 mg bid or to warfarin to maintain an INR between 2.0 and 3.0.[203] Median follow-up was 2.0 years. The primary outcome was stroke or systemic embolism. Compared with warfarin, dabigatran 150 mg bid reduced the primary outcome 34%, reduced all-cause mortality from 4.13% per year to 3.64% per year, and had a similar incidence of major bleeding.[203] Compared with warfarin, dabigatran 110 mg bid had a similar incidence of the primary outcome and of all-cause mortality but reduced major bleeding per year from 3.36% to 2.71%.[203] The U.S. Food and Drug Administration (FDA) approved the 150-mg dose of dabigatran but not the 110-mg dose of dabigatran for treating AF because the 150-mg dose reduced TE events better than warfarin.[204] The FDA approved a 75-mg dose bid of dabigatran in patients with an estimated glomerular filtration rate between 15 and 29 mg/mL/1.73 m^2 although patients with an estimated glomerular filtration rate less than 30 mg/mL/1.73 m^2 were excluded in the RE-LY trial.[204] Dabigatran does not have an antidote.

In the Rivaroxaban Once Daily Oral Direct Factor Xa Inhibition Compared With Vitamin K Antagonism for Prevention of Stroke and Embolism Trial in Atrial Fibrillation (ROCKET AF), 14,264 patients, mean age 73 years, with nonvalvular AF at increased risk for stroke were randomized to the direct factor Xa inhibitor rivaroxaban 20 mg daily or to warfarin to maintain an INR between 2.0 and 3.0.[205] Median follow-up was 707 days. The primary outcome was stroke or systemic embolism. The primary end point and major bleeding were similar in both treatment groups. Significant reductions in intracranial hemorrhage (0.5% vs. 0.7% per year) and in fatal bleeding (0.2% vs. 0.5%) occurred in the rivaroxaban group.[205] Rivaroxaban does not have an antidote.

In the Apixaban versus Acetylsalicylic Acid [ASA] to Prevent Stroke in Atrial Fibrillation Patients Who Have Failed or Are Unsuitable for Vitamin K Antagonist Treatment (AVERROES) study, 5,599 patients, mean age 70 years, with nonvalvular AF at increased risk for stroke for whom vitamin K antagonist therapy was unsuitable were randomized to the direct factor Xa inhibitor apixaban 5 mg bid or to aspirin 81 to 324 mg daily.[206] Mean follow-up was 1.1 years. The primary outcome was stroke or systemic embolism. Compared with aspirin, apixaban reduced the primary outcome 55% from 3.7% per year to 1.6% per year, reduced mortality 22% from 4.4% per year to 3.5% per year, reduced first hospitalization for cardiovascular causes from 15.9% per year to 12.6% per year, and did not increase major bleeding or intracranial hemorrhage.[206]Apixaban has no antidote.

In the Apixaban for Reduction in Stroke and Other Thromboembolic Events in Atrial Fibrillation (ARISTOTLE) trial, 18,201 patients, mean age 70 years, with nonvalvular AF and at least one additional risk factor for stroke were randomized to apixaban 5 mg bid or to warfarin to maintain an INR between 2.0 and 3.0.[207] Median follow-up was 1.8 years. The primary outcome was ischemic or hemorrhagic stroke or systemic embolism. Compared to warfarin, apixaban reduced ischemic or hemorrhagic stroke by 21% from 1.60% per year to 1.27% per year, all-cause mortality 11% from 3.94% per year to 3.52% per year, major bleeding 31% from 3.09% per year to 2.13% per year, and hemorrhagic stroke 49% from 0.47% per year to 0.24% per year.[207] Edoxaban is another effective direct factor Xa inhibitor that works as well as warfarin to prevent stroke or systemic embolism in patients with nonvalvular AF. Compared to warfarin, edoxaban resulted in significantly lower rates of bleeding and death from cardiovascular causes. Edoxaban has not yet been approved by the FDA.[208]

ATRIAL FLUTTER

Atrial flutter is usually paroxysmal and only rarely chronic. Untreated patients with atrial flutter and no disease of the AV junction usually have a 2 : 1 AV conduction response with an atrial rate of approximately 300 beats per minute and a ventricular rate of 150 beats per minute. Over time, atrial flutter usually degenerates into AF.

Management of atrial flutter is similar to management of AF. Direct-current cardioversion is the treatment of choice for converting atrial flutter to sinus rhythm.[209] Atrial flutter treated with intravenous ibutilide in 38% of 78 patients converted to sinus rhythm.[160] Atrial flutter treated with intravenous dofetilide in 54% of 16 patients converted to sinus rhythm.[151] Atrial pacing may also be used to try to convert atrial flutter to sinus rhythm.[210]

Intravenous verapamil,[121] diltiazem,[122] or β-blockers[123-126] may be used to immediately slow a very rapid ventricular rate associated with atrial flutter. Oral verapamil,[130] diltiazem,[131] or a β-blocker[132] should be added to the therapeutic regimen if a rapid ventricular rate associated with atrial flutter occurs at rest or during exercise despite digoxin. Amiodarone is the most effective drug for slowing a rapid ventricular rate associated with atrial flutter.[135] Digoxin, verapamil, and diltiazem are contraindicated in patients with atrial flutter associated with the Wolff-Parkinson-White syndrome because these drugs shorten the refractory period of the accessory AV pathway, causing more rapid conduction down the accessory pathway. Drugs such as quinidine should never be used to treat patients with atrial flutter who are not being treated with digoxin, a β-blocker, verapamil, or diltiazem because a 1 : 1 AV conduction response may develop.

Patients with atrial flutter are at increased risk for developing new TE stroke.[211,212] Anticoagulant therapy should be administered before direct-current cardioversion or drug cardioversion of patients with atrial flutter to sinus rhythm using the same guidelines as for converting AF.[164-167,202] Patients with chronic atrial flutter should be treated with oral warfarin with the INR maintained between 2.0 and 3.0[164,202] or with dabigatran,[203] rivaroxaban,[205] or apixaban.[207]

Radiofrequency catheter ablation of atrial flutter is a highly successful procedure, especially when the right atrial isthmus is incorporated in the atrial flutter circuit.[213,214] Demonstration of bidirectional isthmus block after catheter ablation predicts a high long-term success rate.[214] A second radiofrequency catheter ablation may be needed in up to one third of patients, especially in those with right atrial enlargement.[213] Radiofrequency catheter ablation was successful in converting 63 of 70 patients (90%), mean age 78 years, with atrial flutter to sinus rhythm.[142]

ATRIAL PREMATURE COMPLEXES

The prevalence of frequent atrial premature complexes (APCs) diagnosed by 24-hour ambulatory ECG in older patients was 18% in 729 older women and 28% in 643 older men in the Cardiovascular Health study[7] and 28% in 407 patients, mean age 82 years.[8] Although frequent APCs may trigger a paroxysm of AF, atrial flutter, or supraventricular tachycardia (SVT), they are of no clinical significance when found incidentally and should not be treated. If a supraventricular tachyarrhythmia is triggered by frequent APCs, a β-blocker should be administered.

SUPRAVENTRICULAR TACHYCARDIA

The ventricular rate in paroxysmal SVT usually ranges between 140 and 220 beats per minute and is extremely regular. The prevalence of short bursts of paroxysmal SVT diagnosed by 24-hour ambulatory ECG in 1476 patients, mean age 81 years, with heart disease was 33%.[182] At 42-month follow-up of 1359 patients, mean age 81 years, with heart disease, paroxysmal SVT was not associated with an increased incidence of new coronary events.[109] At 43-month follow-up of 1476 patients, mean age 81 years, paroxysmal SVT was not associated with an increased incidence of new TE stroke.[182]

Sustained episodes of SVT should first be treated by increasing vagal tone by carotid sinus massage or the Valsalva maneuver or by facial immersion in cold water. If vagal maneuvers are unsuccessful, intravenous adenosine is the drug of choice.[215] Intravenous verapamil, diltiazem, or β-blockers may also be used. If these measures do not convert SVT to sinus rhythm, direct-current cardioversion should be used.

Most patients with paroxysmal SVT do not require long-term therapy. If long-term therapy is required because of symptoms due to frequent episodes of SVT, digoxin, propranolol, or verapamil may be administered.[216] These drugs are the initial drug of choice for AV nodal reentrant and AV reentrant SVT, the most common forms of SVT. For SVT associated with the Wolff-Parkinson-White syndrome, flecainide or propafenone may be used if there is no associated heart disease.[217] If heart disease is present, quinidine, procainamide, or disopyramide plus a β-blocker or verapamil should be used.[217] Radiofrequency catheter ablation should be used to treat older patients with symptomatic, drug-resistant SVT and should be considered an early treatment option.[142,218] Radiofrequency catheter ablation was successful in converting 60 of 66 patients, mean age 78 years, with SVT to sinus rhythm.[142]

ACCELERATED ATRIOVENTRICULAR RHYTHM

Accelerated AV junctional rhythm, also called nonparoxysmal AV junctional tachycardia (NPJT), is a form of SVT and is caused by enhanced impulse formation within the AV junction rather than by reentry.[219] This arrhythmia is usually due to recent aortic or mitral valve surgery, acute MI, or digitalis toxicity. The ventricular rate usually ranges between 70 and 130 beats per minute. Treatment of NPJT is directed toward correction of the underlying disorder. Hypokalemia, if present, should be treated with potassium. Digitalis should be stopped if digitalis toxicity is present. β-Blockers may be given cautiously if this is warranted by clinical circumstances.

PAROXYSMAL ATRIAL TACHYCARDIA WITH ATRIOVENTRICULAR BLOCK

Digitalis toxicity causes 70% of cases of paroxysmal atrial tachycardia (PAT) with AV block. Digoxin and diuretics causing hypokalemia should be stopped in these patients. Potassium chloride is the treatment of choice when the serum potassium is low or low-normal. Intravenous propranolol will cause conversion to sinus rhythm in approximately 85% of patients with digitalis-induced PAT with AV block and in approximately 35% of patients with PAT with AV block not induced by digitalis.[220] By increasing AV block, propranolol may also be beneficial in slowing a rapid ventricular rate in PAT with AV block.

MULTIFOCAL ATRIAL TACHYCARDIA

Multifocal atrial tachycardia (MAT) is usually associated with acute illness, especially in older patients with pulmonary disease. MAT is best managed by treatment of the underlying disorder. Intravenous verapamil has been reported to be effective in controlling the ventricular rate in MAT, with occasional conversion to sinus rhythm.[221] However, the author found intravenous verapamil not very effective in treating MAT.[222] The tendency of intravenous verapamil to aggravate preexisting arterial hypoxemia also limits its use in the group of patients most likely to develop MAT.[221]

BRADYARRHYTHMIAS

With aging, there is a loss of specialized muscle cells (called P cells) within the sinus node, which are responsible for initiating impulse formation. By age 75 years, the sinus node may consist of less than 10% P cells.[223] A progressive increase in the amount of collagen within the sinus node also occurs with aging.[224] There is an age-related reduction in conducting cells in the His bundle and both bundle branches, which are the distal parts of the cardiac conduction system. Diseases associated with aging, such as CAD, hypertension, and valvular heart disease, also adversely affect the cardiac conduction system.

Numerous drugs can cause bradyarrhythmias and conduction disturbances. Hypothyroidism, hyperkalemia, hypokalemia, and hypoxia can also depress cardiac impulse formation and conduction. Drugs and endocrine and metabolic disorders causing reversible cardiac impulse formation and conduction abnormalities must be considered before deciding to implant a permanent pacemaker.

A 12-lead ECG with a 1-minute strip may detect bradyarrhythmias caused by sick sinus syndrome, AV block, right and left bundle branch block, bifascicular block, and trifascicular block. ECG manifestations of sick sinus syndrome include severe sinus bradycardia, sinus pause or arrest, sinus exit block, sinus node reentrant rhythm, AF or atrial flutter with a slow ventricular rate not drug-induced, failure of restoration of sinus rhythm after cardioversion for tachyarrhythmias, a longer than 3-second pause after carotid sinus massage, and a tachycardia-bradycardia syndrome. The tachycardia-bradycardia syndrome is characterized by paroxysmal AF, atrial flutter, or SVT followed by periods of sinus bradycardia, sinus arrest, or sinoatrial block.

Dyspnea, weakness, fatigue, falls, angina pectoris, CHF, episodic pulmonary edema, dizziness, faintness, slurred speech, personality changes, paresis, and convulsions in older patients may be caused by bradyarrhythmias. Death may result from prolonged ventricular asystole. Older patients with symptoms that may be due to bradyarrhythmias should have a 12-lead ECG with a 1-minute rhythm strip. Since ECG abnormalities may be intermittent, a 24-hour ambulatory ECG may need to be performed.

In a prospective study of 148 patients, mean age 82 years, with unexplained syncope, 24-hour ambulatory ECG diagnosed bradyarrhythmias with pauses greater than 3 seconds requiring permanent pacemaker implantation in 21 patients (14%).[2] Of these 21 patients, 8 had sinus arrest, 7 had advanced second-degree AV block, and 6 had AF with a slow ventricular rate not drug-induced. At 38-month follow-up after pacemaker implantation, recurrent syncope developed in only 3 of the 21 older patients (14%).[2]

In some older patients without clinical evidence of heart disease and recurrent episodes of unexplained syncope, a patient-activated memory loop event recorder may be used to capture the ECG tracings preceding and during syncope.[225] Older patients with unexplained syncope and heart disease should undergo an electrophysiologic study.[225] Box 44-1 shows class I indications for permanent pacemaker implantation.[94] Modes of pacing, pacemaker codes, and pacemaker follow-up are discussed in detail elsewhere.[226]

BOX 44-1 Class I Indications for Permanent Pacing

A. Third-degree atrioventricular (AV) block with:
   1. Symptomatic bradycardia
   2. Arrhythmias and other medical conditions that require drugs that cause symptomatic bradycardia
   3. Pauses = 3.0 seconds or any escape ventricular rate <40 beats per minute in awake, symptom-free patients
   4. After catheter ablation of AV junction
   5. Postoperative AV block not expected to resolve after surgery
   6. Neuromuscular diseases with AV block
B. Second-degree AV block with symptomatic bradycardia
C. Chronic bifascicular and trifascicular block with:
   1. Intermittent third-degree AV block
   2. Type II second-degree AV block
   3. Alternating bundle branch block
D. After acute myocardial infarction with:
   1. Persistent second-degree AV block in His-Purkinje system with bilateral bundle branch block or third-degree AV block within or below His-Purkinje system
   2. Transient second- or third-degree infranodal AV block and associated bundle branch block
   3. Persistent and symptomatic second- or third-degree AV block
E. Sinus node dysfunction
   1. Sinus node dysfunction with symptomatic bradycardia
   2. Symptomatic chronotropic incompetence
F. Prevention and termination of tachyarrhythmias
   1. Symptomatic recurrent supraventricular tachycardia terminated by pacing after drugs and catheter ablation fail to control arrhythmia or cause intolerable side effects (downgraded to class IIa indication)
   2. Symptomatic recurrent sustained ventricular tachycardia as part of an automatic defibrillator system
G. Prevention of tachycardia
   1. Sustained pause-dependent ventricular tachycardia, with or without prolonged QT, in which efficacy of pacing is documented
H. Hypersensitive carotid sinus and neurally mediated syncope
   1. Recurrent syncope caused by carotid sinus stimulation; minimal carotid sinus pressure induces asystole >3 seconds in absence of any drug that depresses sinus node or AV conduction

Adapted from Epstein AE, DiMarco JP, Ellenbogen KA, et al.[94]

KEY POINTS: VENTRICULAR ARRHYTHMIAS

- β-Blockers are the only antiarrhythmic drugs that reduce mortality in patients with heart disease and complex ventricular arrhythmias
- Class I indications for an implantable cardioverter-defibrillator
- Cardiac arrest due to ventricular tachycardia (VT) or ventricular fibrillation (VF) not caused by a transient or reversible cause
- Spontaneous sustained VT
- Syncope of undetermined origin with clinically relevant, hemodynamically significant sustained VT or VF induced at electrophysiologic study when drug therapy is ineffective, not tolerated, or not preferred
- Nonsustained VT with coronary artery disease, prior myocardial infarction (MI), left ventricular (LV) systolic dysfunction, and inducible VF or sustained VT at electrophysiologic study that is not suppressed by a class I antiarrhythmic drug
- Patients with prior MI at least 40 days previously with an LV ejection fraction less than or equal to 35% who are in New York Heart Association (NYHA) class II or III
- Patients with prior MI at least 40 days previously with an LV ejection fraction less than 30% who are in NYHA class I
- Patients with nonischemic dilated cardiomyopathy with an LV ejection fraction less than or equal to 35% who are in NYHA class II or III

For a complete list of references, please visit www.expertconsult.com.

KEY REFERENCES

3. Aronow WS, Epstein S, Koenigsberg M, et al: Usefulness of echocardiographic abnormal left ventricular ejection fraction, paroxysmal ventricular tachycardia, and complex ventricular arrhythmias in predicting new coronary events in patients over 62 years of age. Am J Cardiol 61:1349–1351, 1988.
10. Aronow WS, Epstein S: Usefulness of silent ischemia, ventricular tachycardia, and complex ventricular arrhythmias in predicting new coronary events in elderly patients with coronary artery disease or systemic hypertension. Am J Cardiol 65:511–522, 1990.
12. Aronow WS, Epstein S, Koenigsberg M, et al: Usefulness of echocardiographic left ventricular hypertrophy, ventricular tachycardia and complex ventricular arrhythmias in predicting ventricular fibrillation or sudden cardiac death in elderly patients. Am J Cardiol 62:1124–1125, 1988.
17. Smith SC, Jr, Benjamin EJ, Bonow RO, et al: AHA/ACCF secondary prevention and risk reduction therapy for patients with coronary and other atherosclerotic vascular disease: 2011 update. A guideline from the American Heart Association and American College of Cardiology Foundation. J Am Coll Cardiol 58:2432–2446, 2011.
32. Heart Protection Study Collaborative Group: MRC/BHF heart protection study of cholesterol lowering with simvastatin in 20,536 high-risk individuals: a randomised placebo-controlled trial. Lancet 360:7–22, 2002.
33. Aronow WS, Ahn C: Incidence of new coronary events in older persons with prior myocardial infarction and serum low-density lipoprotein cholesterol > or = 125 mg/dl treated with statins versus no lipid-lowering drug. Am J Cardiol 89:67–69, 2002.
35. Stone NJ, Robinson J, Lichtenstein AH, et al: ACC/AHA guideline on the treatment of blood cholesterol to reduce atherosclerotic cardiovascular risk in adults. A report of the American College of Cardiology/American Heart Association Task Force on Practice Guidelines. J Am Coll Cardiol 2013. published online November 12, 2013.
41. Aronow WS, Mercando AD, Epstein S, et al: Effect of quinidine or procainamide versus no antiarrhythmic drug on sudden cardiac death, total cardiac death, and total death in elderly patients with

heart disease and complex ventricular arrhythmias. Am J Cardiol 66:423–428, 1990.
51. Aronow WS, Ahn C, Mercando AD, et al: Effect of propranolol versus no antiarrhythmic drug on sudden cardiac death, total cardiac death, and total death in patients greater than or equal to 62 years of age with heart disease, complex ventricular arrhythmias, and left ventricular ejection fraction (40%). Am J Cardiol 74:267–270, 1994.
59. Aronow WS, Ahn C, Kronzon I: Effect of beta blockers alone, of angiotensin-converting enzyme inhibitors alone, and of beta blockers plus angiotensin-converting enzyme inhibitors on new coronary events and on congestive heart failure in older persons with healed myocardial infarcts and asymptomatic left ventricular systolic dysfunction. Am J Cardiol 88:1298–1300, 2001.
67. Bardy GH, Lee KL, Mark DB, et al: Amiodarone or an implantable cardioverter-defibrillator for congestive heart failure. N Engl J Med 352:225–237, 2005.
79. Channamsetty V, Aronow WS, Sorbera C, et al: Efficacy of radiofrequency catheter ablation in treatment of elderly patients with supraventricular tachyarrhythmias and ventricular tachycardia. Am J Ther 13:513–515, 2006.
88. Goldenberg I, Moss AJ: Treatment of arrhythmias and use of implantable cardioverter-defibrillators to improve survival in elderly patients with cardiac disease. Clin Geriatr Med Heart Fail 23:205–219, 2007.
92. Kruger A, Aronow WS, Lai HM, et al: Prevalence of appropriate cardioverter-defibrillator shocks in 1,038 consecutive patients with implantable cardioverter-defibrillators. Am J Ther 16:323–325, 2009.
93. Lai HM, Aronow WS, Kruger A, et al: Effect of beta blockers, angiotensin-converting enzyme inhibitors or angiotensin receptor blockers, and statins on mortality in patients with implantable cardioverter-defibrillators. Am J Cardiol 102:77–78, 2008.
94. Epstein AE, DiMarco JP, Ellenbogen KA, et al: ACC/AHA/HRS guidelines for device-based therapy of cardiac rhythm abnormalities: executive summary. A report of the American College of Cardiology/American Heart Association Task Force on Practice Guidelines (Writing Committee to Revise the ACC/AHA/NASPE 2002 Guideline Update for Implantation of Cardiac Pacemakers and Antiarrhythmia Devices). J Am Coll Cardiol 51:2085–2105, 2008.
95. Yancy CW, Jessup M, Bozkurt B, et al: 2013 ACCF/AHA guidelines for the management of heart failure: executive summary. A report of the American College of Cardiology Foundation /American Heart Association Task Force on Practice Guidelines. Developed in collaboration with the American College of Chest Physicians, Heart Rhythm Society, and International Society for Heart and Lung Transplantation. Endorsed by the American Association of Crdiovascular and Pulmonary Rehabilitation. J Am Coll Cardiol 62:1495–1539, 2013.
97. Desai H, Aronow WS, Ahn C, et al: Risk factors for appropriate cardioverter-defibrillator shocks, inappropriate cardioverter-defibrillator shocks, and time to mortality in 549 patients with heart failure. Am J Cardiol 105:1336–1338, 2010.
105. Aronow WS, Ahn C, Kronzon I: Echocardiographic findings associated with atrial fibrillation in 1,699 patients aged >60 years. Am J Cardiol 76:1191–1192, 1995.
172. The Atrial Fibrillation Follow-Up Investigation of Rhythm Management (AFFIRM) Investigators: A comparison of rate control and rhythm control in patients with atrial fibrillation. N Engl J Med 347:1825–1833, 2002.
173. Shariff N, Desai RV, Patel K, et al: Rate-control versus rhythm-control strategies and outcomes in septuagenarians with atrial fibrillation. Am J Med 126:887–893, 2013.
182. Aronow WS, Ahn C, Mercando AD, et al: Correlation of paroxysmal supraventricular tachycardia, atrial fibrillation, and sinus rhythm with incidences of new thromboembolic stroke in 1476 old-old patients. Aging (Milano) 8:32–34, 1996.
184. Aronow WS, Gutstein H, Hsieh FY: Risk factors for thromboembolic stroke in elderly patients with chronic atrial fibrillation. Am J Cardiol 63:366–367, 1989.
197. Aronow WS, Ahn C, Kronzon I, et al: Effect of warfarin versus aspirin on the incidence of new thromboembolic stroke in older persons with chronic atrial fibrillation and abnormal and normal left ventricular ejection fraction. Am J Cardiol 85:1033–1035, 2000.
200. Fang MC, Singer DE, Chang Y, et al: Gender differences in the risk of ischemic stroke and peripheral embolism in atrial fibrillation. The Anticoagulation and Risk Factors in Atrial Fibrillation (ATRIA) study. Circulation 112:1687–1691, 2005.
202. Fuster V, Ryden LE, Cannom DS, et al: ACC/AHA/HRS focused updates incorporated into the ACC/AHA/ESC 2006 guidelines for the management of patients with atrial fibrillation. A report of the American College of Cardiology Foundation/American Heart Association Task Force on Practice Guidelines and the European Society of Cardiology Committee for Practice Guidelines. J Am Coll Cardiol 57:e101–e198, 2011.

45 Syncope

Rose Anne Kenny, Jaspreet Bhangu

INTRODUCTION

Definition

Syncope is a transient loss of consciousness (TLOC) due to transient global cerebral hypoperfusion and is characterized by rapid onset, short duration, and spontaneous complete recovery. TLOC is a term that encompasses all disorders characterized by self-limited loss of consciousness, irrespective of mechanism. By including the mechanism of unconsciousness—transient global cerebral hypoperfusion—the current syncope definition excludes other causes of TLOC such as epileptic seizures and concussion, as well as certain common syncope mimics such as psychogenic pseudosyncope.[1]

Epidemiology

Syncope is a common symptom, experienced by up to 30% of healthy adults at least once in their lifetime.[2] Syncope accounts for 3% of emergency department visits and 1% of medical admissions to a general hospital.[3,4] Syncope is the seventh most common reason for emergency admission of patients older than 65 years.[5] The cumulative incidence of syncope in a chronic care facility is close to 23% over a 10-year period, with an annual incidence of 6% and recurrence rate of 30% over 2 years. The age of first faint, a commonly used term for syncope, is younger than 25 years in 60% of persons, but 10% to 15% of individuals have their first faint after the age of 65 years.[6-8]

Syncope due to a cardiac cause is associated with higher mortality rates, irrespective of age.[9] In patients with a noncardiac or unknown cause of syncope, older age, a history of congestive cardiac failure, and male gender are important prognostic factors of mortality.[10] It remains undetermined whether syncope is directly associated with mortality or is merely a marker of more severe underlying disease.[2] Figure 45-1 details the age-related difference in prevalence of benign vasovagal syncope compared to other causes of syncope

The Irish Longitudinal Study on Ageing (TILDA; www.tilda.ie) is a population-based study of people aged 50 years and over that has incorporated questions on syncope and falls in addition to a broad spectrum of health, social, and economic questions. A number of community-dwelling adults ($N = 8163$), mean age 62 years (range, 50 to 106 years), were asked whether they experienced fainting in their youth, throughout their life, or over the past 12 months. A total of 23.6% had one or more episodes in the previous 12 months, of which 4.4% were syncope and 19.2% were falls (Table 45-1). Although the prevalence of syncope rose with age, the increase in falls was much more remarkable; in particular, the increase in nonaccidental or unexplained falls was most striking. Unwitnessed syncope most commonly presents as an nonaccidental or unexplained fall, supporting the rising prevalence of atypical syncope with advancing years.

The General Practitioners' Transition Project in the Netherlands has demonstrated that the age distribution of patients presenting to their physician with syncope shows a peak in females at 15 years of age and a second peak in older patients (see Figure 45-1).[11] The Framingham Offspring study has similarly demonstrated a bimodal peak of first syncope in those in their the mid-teens and the second in those older than 70 years.[9]

The true prevalence of syncope is underestimated due to the phenomenon of amnesia for TLOC. Amnesia has been reported in patients with vasovagal syncope (VVS) and carotid sinus syndrome (CSS)[12-14] but is likely to be present in all causes of syncope. The overlap between syncope and falls also leads to underreporting (see Table 45-1 and Figure 45-1).

Pathophysiology

The temporary cessation of cerebral function that causes syncope results from transient and sudden reduction of blood flow to parts of the brain responsible for consciousness (brain stem reticular activating system). The predisposition to VVS starts early and lasts for decades. Other causes of syncope are uncommon in young adults, but are much more common as persons age.[15,16]

Regardless of the cause, the underlying mechanism responsible for syncope is a drop in cerebral oxygen delivery below the threshold for consciousness. Cerebral oxygen delivery, in turn, depends on cerebral blood flow and oxygen content. Any combination of chronic or acute processes that lowers cerebral oxygen delivery below the consciousness threshold may cause syncope. Age-related physiologic impairments in heart rate, blood pressure, cerebral blood flow, and blood volume control, in combination with comorbid conditions and concurrent medications, account for the increased incidence of syncope in older adults. Blunted baroreflex sensitivity manifests as a reduction in the heart rate response to hypotensive stimuli. Older adults are prone to reduced blood volume due to excessive salt wasting by the kidneys as a result of a decline in plasma renin and aldosterone levels, a rise in atrial natriuretic peptide level, and concurrent diuretic therapy.[15] Low blood volume, together with age-related diastolic dysfunction leading to low cardiac output, coupled with inadequate heart rate responses to stress, increases susceptibility to orthostatic hypotension and VVS.[17] Cerebral autoregulation, which maintains a constant cerebral circulation over a wide range of blood pressure changes, is altered in the presence of hypertension and possibly by aging; the latter factor is still controversial.[18] In general, it is agreed that sudden mild to moderate declines in blood pressure can affect cerebral blood flow markedly and render an older person particularly vulnerable to presyncope and syncope. Syncope may thus result from a single process that markedly and abruptly decreases cerebral oxygen delivery or from the accumulated effect of multiple processes, each of which contributes to reduced oxygen delivery.

Causes of Syncope in Older Adults

Reflex syncope and orthostatic hypotension (OH) are the most frequent causes of syncope in all age groups and clinical settings and responsible for most episodes in younger patients. However, cardiac causes of syncope, structural and arrhythmic, become more common in older patients and are responsible for one third of syncope in patients seen in the emergency room and chest pain unit.[1,19-21] The prevalence of unexplained syncope varies according to diagnostic facilities and age from 9% to 41% (see Table 45-1). In the older patient, history may be less reliable, and multiple causes of syncope may also be present (Box 45-1).[5,20,22-24] Multimorbidity and polypharmacy are more common in older patients with syncope and can add to the

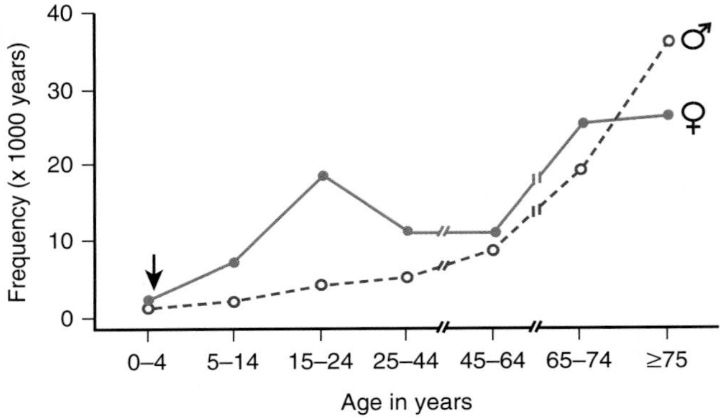

Figure 45-1. Frequency of the complaint of fainting as reason for encounter in general practice in the Netherlands. Data were obtained from the general practitioners' transition project. *(From Wieling W, Ganzeboom KS, Krediet CT, et al: [Initial diagnostic strategy in the case of transient losses of consciousness: the importance of the medical history]. Ned Tijdschr Geneeskd 147:84–854, 2003.).*

TABLE 45-1 Prevalence of Syncope and Falls in a Population Study

	Age (yr)			
Previous Year %	**50-64**	**65-74**	**75+**	**Total**
Syncope	4.17	4.74	4.84	4.42
Falls	17.46	19.46	24.43	19.19
Non-accidental/unexplained falls	7.61	9.41	11.58	8.87

Adapted from Finucane C, O'Connell MDL, Fan CW, et al: Age-related normative changes in phasic orthostatic blood pressure in a large population study: findings from the Irish Longitudinal Study on Ageing (TILDA). Circulation 130:1780–1789, 2014.

complexity of identifying an attributable cause of events (Figures 45-2 and 45-3).[25-27]

Multifactorial Causes. Previously, up to 40% of patients with recurrent syncope remained undiagnosed, despite extensive investigation, particularly older patients, who have marginal cognitive impairment and for whom a witnessed account of events is often unavailable. More recently, diagnostic yield for all ages has improved with the application of guidelines.[28] Although diagnostic investigations are available, the high frequency of unidentified causes in clinical studies may occur because patients failed to recall important diagnostic details,[14,29] because of the stringent diagnostic criteria used in clinical studies or, probably most often, because the syncopal episode resulted from a combination of chronic and acute factors rather than from a single obvious disease process.[22] A multifactorial cause likely explains most cases of syncope in older adults who are predisposed because of multiple chronic diseases and medication effects superimposed on the age-related physiologic changes described earlier.[30] Common factors that in combination may predispose to or precipitate syncope include anemia, chronic lung disease, chronic heart failure, and dehydration. Medications that may contribute to or cause syncope are listed in Table 45-2.

Individual Causes. Common causes of syncope are listed in Box 45-1. The most frequent individual causes of syncope in older patients are neurally mediated syndromes, including CSS, orthostatic hypotension, and postprandial hypotension, as well as arrhythmias, including tachyarrhythmias and bradyarrhythmias.

BOX 45-1 Causes of Syncope

REFLEX SYNCOPAL SYNDROMES

Vasovagal faint (common faint)
Carotid sinus syncope
Situational faint

- Acute hemorrhage
- Cough, sneeze
- Gastrointestinal stimulation (swallow, defecation, visceral pain)
- Micturition (postmicturition)
- Postexercise
- Pain, anxiety

Glossopharyngeal and trigeminal neuralgia

ORTHOSTATIC

Aging
Antihypertensives
Autonomic failure

- Primary autonomic failure syndromes (e.g., pure autonomic failure, multiple system atrophy, Parkinson disease with autonomic failure)
- Secondary autonomic failure syndromes (e.g., diabetic neuropathy, amyloid neuropathy)

Medications (see Table 45-1)
Volume depletion

- Hemorrhage, diarrhea, Addison disease, diuretics, febrile illness, hot weather

CARDIAC ARRHYTHMIAS

Sinus node dysfunction (including bradycardia-tachycardia syndrome)
Atrioventricular conduction system disease
Paroxysmal supraventricular and ventricular tachycardias
Implanted device (pacemaker, implantable cardioverter defibrillator) malfunction
Drug-induced proarrhythmias

STRUCTURAL CARDIAC OR CARDIOPULMONARY DISEASE

Cardiac valvular disease

- Acute myocardial infarction, ischemia
- Obstructive cardiomyopathy
- Atrial myxoma
- Acute aortic dissection
- Pericardial disease, tamponade
- Pulmonary embolus, pulmonary hypertension

CEREBROVASCULAR

- Vascular steal syndromes

MULTIFACTORIAL

These disease processes are described in the next section. Disorders that may be confused with syncope and that may or may not be associated with loss of consciousness are listed in Table 45-3.

Presentation

Manifestations in this age group are challenging, and often recognition is the first step to optimizing management and care of these patients. To start with, syncope in the older patient is underrecognized, particularly in acute-care settings, because the presentation is frequently atypical. The older patient is less likely to have a warning or prodrome prior to syncope, commonly has amnesia for loss of consciousness, and frequently experiences an unwitnessed event,[12] thus presenting with a fall rather than

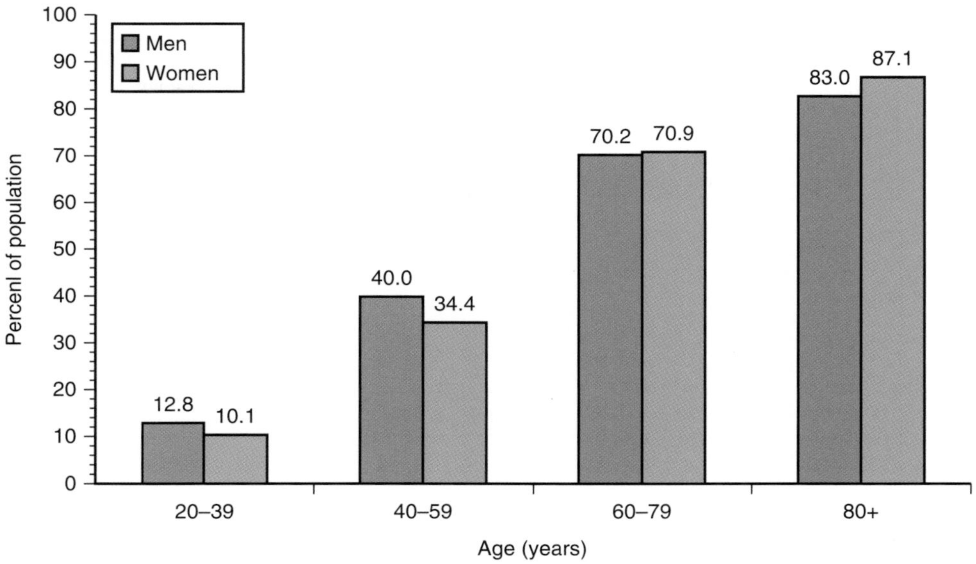

Figure 45-2. Prevalence of cardiovascular disease in adults. *(Adapted from Go AS, Mozaffarian D, Roger VL, et al; American Heart Association Statistics Committee and Stroke Statistics Subcommittee: Heart disease and stroke statistics—2013 update: a report from the American Heart Association. Circulation 127:e6–e45, 2013.)*

TABLE 45-2 Drugs That Can Cause or Contribute to Syncope

Drug	Mechanism
Diuretics	Volume depletion
Vasodilators • Angiotensin-converting enzyme inhibitors • Calcium channel blockers • Hydralazine • Nitrates • α-Adrenergic blockers • Prazosin	Reduction in systemic vascular resistance and venodilation
Other antihypertensive drugs • α-Methyldopa • Clonidine • Guanethidine • Hexamethonium • Labetalol • Mecamylamine • Phenoxybenzamine	Centrally acting antihypertensives
Drugs associated with torsades de pointes • Amiodarone • Disopyramide • Encainide • Flecainide • Quinidine • Procainamide • Solatol	Ventricular tachycardia associated with a prolonged QT interval
Digoxin	Cardiac arrhythmias
Psychoactive drugs • Tricyclic antidepressants • Phenothiazines • Monamine oxidase inhibitors • Barbiturates	Central nervous system effects causing hypotension; cardiac arrhythmias
Alcohol	Central nervous system effects causing hypotension; cardiac arrhythmias

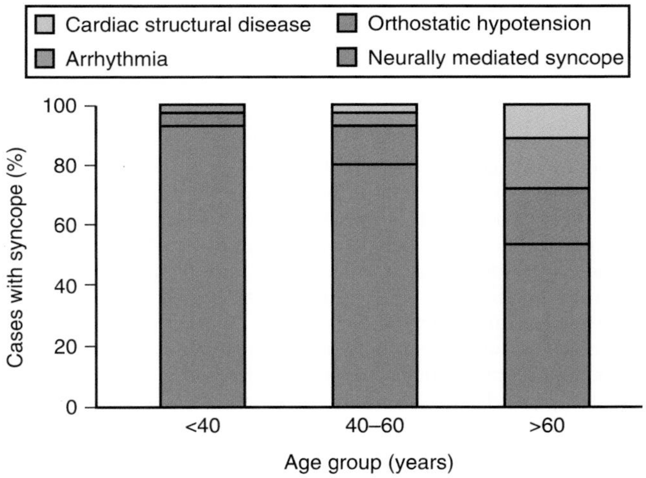

Figure 45-3. Causes of syncope by age. *(From Parry SW, Tan MP: An approach to the evaluation and management of syncope in adults. BMJ 340:c880, 2010.)*

TABLE 45-3 Differential Diagnosis of Syncope in the Older Adults

Conditions With LOC or Partial LOC	Conditions Without LOC
Epilepsy	Cataplexy
Metabolic disorders, including hypoglycemia, hypoxia, hyperventilation with hypocapnia	Drop attacks
Vertebrobasilar TIA	Falls
Intoxication (e.g., alcohol, medication overdose [sedatives, analgesics])	TIA (anterior circulation)

LOC, Loss of consciousness; *TIA*, transient ischemic attack.

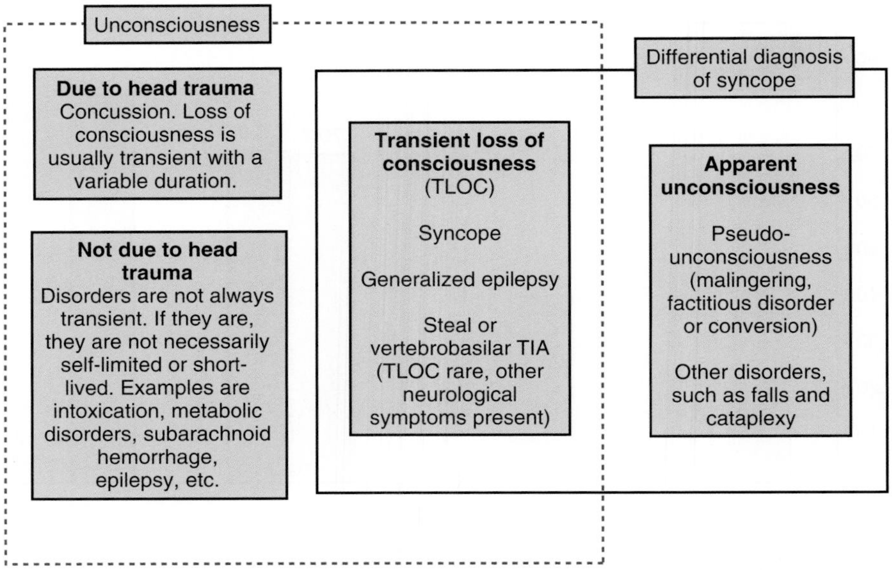

Figure 45-4. Syncope in relation to real and apparent loss of consciousness.

TLOC.[14,22,31] These events are typically described as nonaccidental (not a trip or slip) or unexplained falls. Therefore, history alone cannot be relied on when assessing the older patient. Injurious events such as fractures and head injuries are also more common, further emphasizing the importance of thorough early investigation and diagnosis.[32]

The underlying mechanism of syncope is transient cerebral hypoperfusion. In some forms of syncope, there may be a premonitory period in which various symptoms (e.g., lightheadedness, nausea, sweating, weakness, visual disturbances) warn of an impending syncopal event.[33] Often, however, loss of consciousness occurs without warning or recall of warning.[14,29] Recovery from syncope is usually accompanied by almost immediate restoration of appropriate behavior and orientation. Amnesia for loss of consciousness occurs in many older adults and in those with cognitive impairment. The postrecovery period may be associated with fatigue of varying duration. In younger patients, nausea, blurred vision, and sweating predict noncardiac syncope, but only dyspnea predicts cardiac syncope in older patients.[33]

Syncope and falls are often considered two separate entities with different causes. Recent evidence suggests, however, that these conditions may not always be distinctly separate.[34] In older adults, determining whether patients who have fallen have had a syncopal event can be difficult. At least half of syncopal episodes are unwitnessed, and older patients may have amnesia for loss of consciousness.[14] Amnesia for loss of consciousness has been observed in 30% of patients with CSS who present with falls and 25% of all patients with CSS, irrespective of presentation.[35] Emerging evidence has suggests a high incidence of falls in addition to traditional syncopal symptoms in older patients with sick sinus syndrome and atrioventricular conduction disorders. Thus, syncope and falls may be indistinguishable and may, in some cases, be manifestations of similar pathophysiologic processes. Specific causes of syncope are presented in the following sections.[36]

Evaluation

The initial step in the evaluation of syncope is to consider whether there is a specific cardiac or neurologic cause or whether the cause is likely multifactorial.[1,37,38] The starting point for the evaluation of syncope is a careful history and physical examination. A witness account of events is important to ascertain, when possible.[39,40] Three key questions should be addressed during the initial evaluation:

- Is loss of consciousness attributable to syncope?
- Is heart disease present or absent?
- Are there important clinical features in the history and physical examination which suggest the cause?

Differentiating true syncope from other nonsyncopal conditions associated with real or apparent loss of consciousness is generally the first diagnostic challenge and influences the subsequent diagnostic strategy. A strategy for differentiating true syncope and nonsyncope is outlined in Figures 45-4 and 45-5. The presence of heart disease is an independent predictor of a cardiac cause of syncope, with a high sensitivity of 95% but a low specificity of 45%.[41]

Patients frequently complain of dizziness alone or as a prodrome to syncope and unexplained falls. Four categories of dizzy symptoms—vertigo, dysequilibrium, lightheadedness, and others—have been recognized. The categories have neither sensitivity nor specificity in older, as in younger, patients. Dizziness, however, may more likely be attributable to a cardiovascular diagnosis if associated with pallor, syncope, prolonged standing, palpitations, or the need to lie down or sit down when symptoms occur.

Initial evaluation may lead to a diagnosis based on symptoms, signs, or electrocardiographic findings. Under such circumstances, no further evaluation is needed and treatment, if any, can be planned. More commonly, the initial evaluation leads to a suspected diagnosis (see Figure 45-3), which needs to be confirmed by directed testing.[3,42] If a diagnosis is confirmed by specific testing, treatment may be initiated. On the other hand, if the diagnosis is not confirmed, patients are considered to have unexplained syncope and should be evaluated following a strategy such as that outlined in Figure 45-5. It is important to attribute a diagnosis, if possible, rather than assume that an abnormality known to produce syncope or hypotensive symptoms is the cause. To reach a diagnosis, patients should have symptom reproduction during investigation and preferably alleviation of symptoms with specific intervention. It is not uncommon for more than one

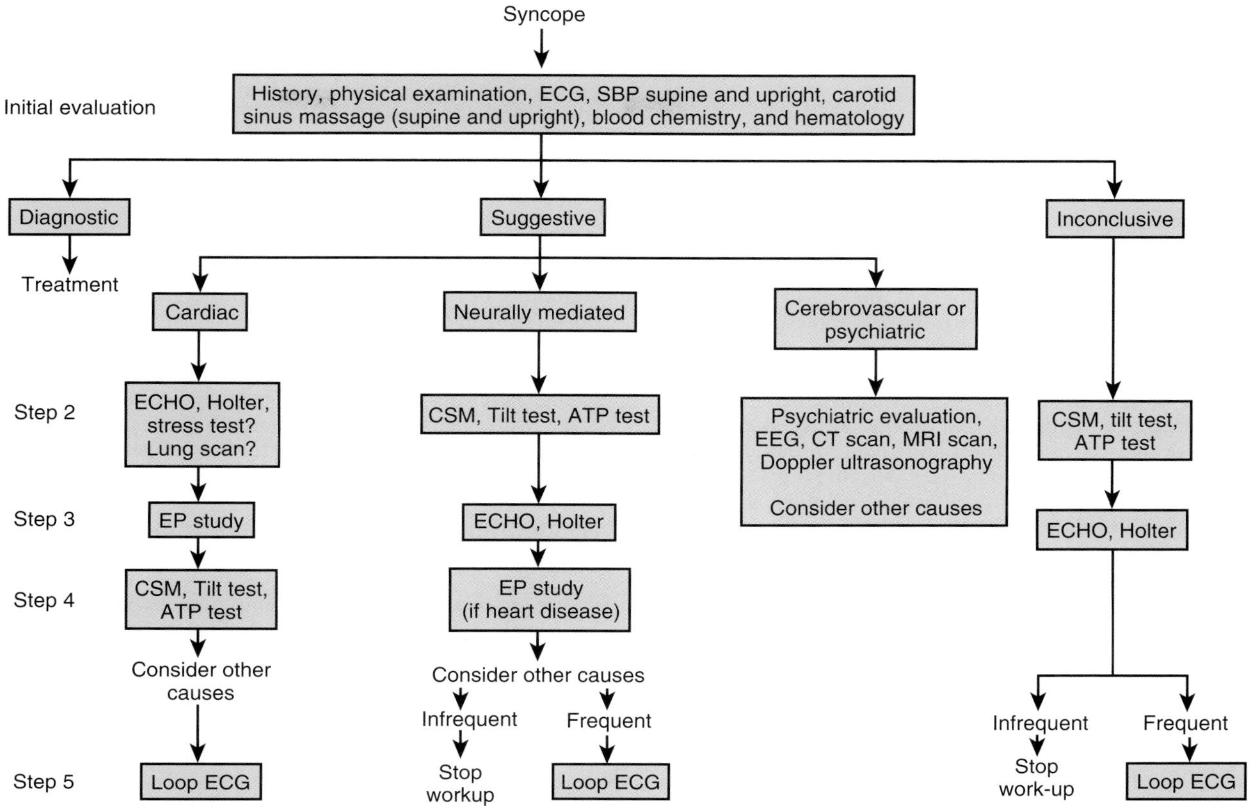

Figure 45-5. An approach to the evaluation of syncope for all age groups. *ATP test,* Adenosine provocation test; *CSM,* carotid sinus massage; *ECG,* electrocardiogram; *ECHO,* echocardiogram; *EEG,* electroencephalography; *EP study,* electrophysiologic study; *SBP,* systolic blood pressure.

predisposing disorder to coexist in older patients, rendering a precise diagnosis difficult. In older adults, treatment of possible causes without clear verification of an attributable diagnosis may often be the only option.

An important issue in patients with unexplained syncope is the presence of structural heart disease or an abnormal electrocardiogram (ECG). These findings are associated with a higher risk of arrhythmias and a higher mortality at 1 year.[43] In these patients, cardiac evaluation, consisting of echocardiography, stress testing, and tests for arrhythmia detection (e.g., prolonged electrocardiographic and loop monitoring, electrophysiologic study) are recommended. The most alarming electrocardiographic sign in a patient with syncope is probably alternating complete left and right bundle branch block or alternating right bundle branch block with left anterior or posterior fascicular block, suggesting trifascicular conduction system disease and intermittent or impending high-degree atrioventricular (AV) block. Patients with bifascicular block (right bundle branch block plus left anterior or left posterior fascicular block, or left bundle branch block) are also at high risk of developing high degree AV block. A significant problem in the evaluation of syncope and bifascicular block is the transient nature of high-degree AV block and, therefore, the long periods required to document it by electrocardiography.

In patients without structural heart disease and a normal ECG, evaluation for neurally mediated syncope should be considered. The tests for neurally mediated syncope consist of tilt testing and carotid sinus massage.

The presentation, evaluation, and management of other common causes of syncope are presented in the following sections. These may occur as the sole cause of a syncopal episode or as one of multiple contributing causes.

ORTHOSTATIC HYPOTENSION

Pathophysiology

Orthostatic or postural hypotension is arbitrarily defined as a 20-mm Hg fall in systolic blood pressure or a 10-mm Hg fall in diastolic blood pressure on assuming an upright posture from a supine position. Orthostatic hypotension implies abnormal blood pressure homeostasis and is a frequent observation in older adults. Prevalence of orthostatic hypotension varies between 4% and 33% among community-living older persons depending on the method used. Higher prevalence and larger falls in systolic blood pressure have been reported with increasing age and often signify general physical frailty. Prevalence of OH in older community-dwelling adults is 30%[44] and increases to more than 50% in geriatric ward patients,[45] making its diagnosis highly relevant. Orthostatic hypotension is an important cause of syncope, accounting for 14% of all diagnosed cases in a large series. In a tertiary referral clinic dealing with unexplained syncope, dizziness, and falls, 32% of patients older than 65 years had orthostatic hypotension as a possible attributable cause of symptoms.

A recent population-based study that used beat-to-beat measurement of orthostatic blood pressure has demonstrated a significant age gradient for orthostatic blood pressure; in 7% of 50- to 55-year-olds systolic and diastolic blood pressures failed to stabilize by 2 minutes after standing compared with 41% of those

80 year of age and older.[46] Failure of stabilization was associated with falls, depression, and global cognitive impairment.[46-49]

Causative Factors

Aging

The heart rate and blood pressure responses to orthostasis occur in three phases: (1) an initial heart rate rise and blood pressure drop; (2) an early phase of stabilization; and (3) a phase of prolonged standing. All three phases are influenced by aging. The maximum rise in heart rate and the ratio between the maximum and minimum heart rates in the initial phase decline with age, implying a relatively fixed heart rate, irrespective of posture. Despite a blunted heart rate response, blood pressure and cardiac output are adequately maintained on standing in active, healthy, well-hydrated and normotensive older adults because of decreased vasodilation and reduced venous pooling during the initial phases and increased peripheral vascular resistance after prolonged standing. However, in older adults with hypertension and cardiovascular disease who are receiving vasoactive drugs, these circulatory adjustments to orthostatic stress are disturbed, rendering them vulnerable to postural hypotension.[50] More recent research has suggested that the velocity of the initial orthostatic heart rate response at 10 and 20 seconds predicts mortality and morbidity.[51]

This age-related gradient may reflect autonomic dysfunction, increased arterial stiffness, and muscle pump defects.[52] Traditionally, orthostatic hypotension is defined as a reduction in systolic blood pressure (BP) of at least 20 mm Hg or in diastolic BP of at least 10 mm Hg within 3 minutes of standing [53] Orthostatic intolerance refers to symptoms and signs with an upright posture due to circulatory abnormality.[1] Syndromes of orthostatic intolerance that may cause syncope include the following: initial orthostatic hypotension, during which symptoms of lightheadedness and dizziness or visual disturbance are experienced seconds after standing; classic orthostatic hypotension, during which dizziness, presyncope, fatigue, weakness, palpitations, and visual and hearing disturbances are experienced; delayed orthostatic hypotension, during which there is a prolonged prodrome, frequently followed by rapid syncope; delayed orthostatic hypotension and reflex syncope, during which a prolonged prodrome is always followed by syncope; reflex syncope triggered by standing, during which there is a classic prodrome and triggers, always followed by syncope; and postural orthostatic tachycardia syndrome, during which there is symptomatic heart rate (HR) increases and instability of BP without syncope.[1] Many older patients with orthostatic hypotension also have postprandial hypotension. Causes of orthostatic hypotension include volume depletion or disturbance of the autonomic nervous system, resulting in failure in the vasoconstrictor compensatory mechanisms induced by an upright posture.[54]

Hypertension further increases the risk of hypotension by impairing baroreflex sensitivity and reducing ventricular compliance. Hypertension increases the risk of cerebral ischemia from sudden declines in blood pressure. Older adults with hypertension are more vulnerable to cerebral ischemic symptoms, even with modest and short-term postural hypotension, because the threshold for cerebral autoregulation is altered by prolonged BP elevation. In addition, antihypertensive agents impair cardiovascular reflexes and further increase the risk of orthostatic hypotension.[55,56]

Medications

Drugs are important causes of orthostatic hypotension (see Table 45-2). Ideally, establishing a causal relationship between a drug and orthostatic hypotension requires identification of the culprit medicine, abolition of symptoms by withdrawal of the drug, and rechallenge with the drug to reproduce symptoms and signs. Rechallenge is often omitted in clinical practice in view of the potential serious consequences. In the presence of polypharmacy, which is common in older adults, it becomes difficult to identify a single culprit drug because of the synergistic effect of different drugs and drug interactions. Thus, all drugs should be considered as possible contributors to orthostasis.[57,58]

Other Conditions

A number of non-neurogenic conditions are also associated with postural hypotension. These conditions include myocarditis, atrial myxoma, aortic stenosis,[59] constrictive pericarditis, hemorrhage, diarrhea, vomiting, ileostomy, burns, hemodialysis, salt-losing nephropathy, diabetes insipidus, adrenal insufficiency, fever, and extensive varicose veins. Volume depletion for any reason is a common sole or contributing cause of postural hypotension and, in turn, syncope.

Association With Primary Autonomic Failure Syndromes

There are three distinct clinical autonomic syndromes associated with orthostatic hypotension—pure autonomic failure (PAF), multiple system atrophy (MSA), or Shy-Drager syndrome (SDS)—and autonomic failure associated with idiopathic Parkinson disease (IPD). PAF, the least common condition and a relatively benign entity, was previously known as idiopathic orthostatic hypotension. This condition presents with orthostatic hypotension, defective sweating, impotence, and bowel disturbances. No other neurologic deficits are evident, and resting plasma epinephrine levels are low. MSA is the most common of these and has the poorest prognosis. Clinical manifestations include features of dysautonomia and motor disturbances due to striatonigral degeneration, cerebellar atrophy, or pyramidal lesions. Additional neurologic deficits include muscle atrophy, distal sensorimotor neuropathy, pupillary abnormalities, restriction of ocular movements, disturbances in rhythm and control of breathing, life-threatening laryngeal stridor, and bladder disturbances. Psychiatric manifestations and cognitive defects are usually absent. Resting plasma epinephrine levels are usually within the normal range but fail to rise on standing or tilting.

The prevalence of orthostatic hypotension in Parkinson disease (PD) rises with advancing years and with the number of medications prescribed. Cognitive impairment, in particular abnormal attention and executive function, is more common in PD with orthostatic hypotension, suggesting a possible causal association with hypotension, including watershed hypoperfusion and infarction. Orthostatic hypotension in PD can also be due to autonomic failure and/or to side effects of antiparkinson medications.

Secondary Autonomic Dysfunction

Autonomic nervous system involvement is seen in several systemic diseases. A large number of neurologic disorders are also complicated by autonomic dysfunction, which may involve several organs and lead to a variety of symptoms in addition to orthostatic hypotension. These include anhidrosis, constipation, diarrhea, impotence, retention of urine, urinary incontinence, stridor, apneic episodes, and Horner syndrome. Among the most serious and prevalent conditions associated with orthostasis due to autonomic dysfunction are diabetes, multiple sclerosis, brain stem lesions, compressive and noncompressive spinal cord lesions, demyelinating polyneuropathies (e.g., Guillain-Barré syndrome), chronic renal failure, chronic liver disease, and connective tissue disorders.

Presentation

The clinical manifestations of orthostatic hypotension are due to hypoperfusion of the brain and other organs. Depending on the degree of fall in BP and cerebral hypoperfusion, symptoms can vary from dizziness to syncope associated with a variety of visual defects, from blurred to complete loss of vision. Other reported ischemic symptoms of orthostatic hypotension are nonspecific lethargy and weakness, suboccipital and paravertebral muscle pain, low backache, calf claudication, and angina. Several precipitating factors for orthostatic hypotension have been identified, including speed of positional change, prolonged recumbency, warm environment, raised intrathoracic pressure (e.g., from coughing, defecation, micturition), physical exertion, and vasoactive drugs.[60]

Evaluation

The diagnosis of orthostatic hypotension involves a demonstration of a postural fall BP after active standing. Reproducibility of orthostatic hypotension depends on the time of measurement and on autonomic function. The diagnosis may be missed on casual measurement during the afternoon.[61] The procedure should be repeated during the morning after the older adult maintains a supine posture for at least 10 minutes. Sphygmomanometer measurement will detect hypotension, which is sustained. Phasic BP measurements are more sensitive for detection of transient falls in BP. Where possible, these methods should be used. Active standing is more appropriate than head-up tilt because the former more readily represents the physiologic α-adrenergic vasodilation due to calf muscle activation.[62] Once a diagnosis of postural hypotension has been made, evaluation involves identifying the cause(s) of orthostasis mentioned earlier.

Management

The goal of therapy for symptomatic orthostatic hypotension (Table 45-4) is to improve cerebral perfusion. There are several nonpharmacologic interventions that should be tried initially. These include avoidance of precipitating factors for low BP, elevation of the head of the bed at night by at least 20 degrees, and application of graduated pressure from an abdominal support garment or compression stockings. Medications known to contribute to postural hypotension should be eliminated or reduced. Studies in a small number of patients have suggested benefit from implantation of cardiac pacemakers by increasing HR during postural change. However, the benefits of tachypacing on cardiac output in patients with maximal vasodilation are short-lived, probably because venous pooling and vasodilation dominate. A large number of drugs have been used to raise BP in orthostatic hypotension, including fludrocortisone, midodrine, ephedrine, desmopressin (DDAVP), octeotride, erythropoietin, and nonsteroidal antiinflammatory drugs. Fludrocortisone (9-alpha-fluhydrocortisone), 0.1 to 0.2 mg, causes volume expansion, reduces natriuresis, and sensitizes α-adrenoceptors to noradrenaline. In older adults, the drug can be poorly tolerated in high doses and for long periods. Adverse effects include hypertension, cardiac failure, depression, edema, and hypokalemia. Midodrine is a direct-acting sympathomimetic vasoconstrictor of resistance vessels. Treatment is started at a dose of 2.5 mg three times daily and requires gradual titration to a maximum dose of 45 mg/day. Adverse effects include hypertension, pilomotor erection, gastrointestinal symptoms, and central nervous system toxicity. Side effects are usually controlled by dose reduction. Midodrine can be used in combination with low-dose fludrocortisone, with good effect. DDAVP has potent antidiuretic and mild pressor effects; intranasal doses of 5 to 40 μg at bedtime are useful. The main side effect is water retention. This agent can also be combined with fludrocortisone, with a synergistic effect.

Drug treatment for orthostatic hypotension in older adults requires frequent monitoring for supine hypertension, electrolyte imbalance, and congestive heart failure. One option for treating supine hypertension, which is most prominent at night, is to apply a glyceryl trinitrate (GTN) patch after going to bed, remove it in the morning, and take midodrine with or without fludrocortisone 20 minutes before rising. This is effective, provided that the older person remains in bed throughout the night. Nocturia is therefore an important consideration. To capture these coexistent diurnal BP variations of supine hypertension and morning orthostasis, 24-hour ambulatory BP monitoring is preferred for the management of postural hypotension. Postprandial hypotension due to splanchnic vascular pooling often coexists with orthostatic hypotension in older patients.

TABLE 45-4 Management of Orthostatic Hypotension in Older Adults

Identify and treat correctable causes.
Reduce or eliminate drugs causing orthostatic hypotension (see Table 45-2).
Avoid situations that may exacerbate orthostatic hypotension.
• Standing motionless
• Prolonged recumbency
• Large meals
• Hot weather
• Hot showers
• Straining at stool or with voiding
• Isometric exercise
• Ingesting alcohol
• Hyperventilation
• Dehydration
Raise the head of the bed to a 5- to 20-degree angle.
Wear waist-high, custom-fitted, elastic stockings and an abdominal binder.
Participate in physical conditioning exercises.
Participate in controlled postural exercises using the tilt table.
Avoid diuretics and eat salt-containing fluids (unless congestive heart failure is present).
Drug therapy
• Caffeine
• Fludrocortisone
• Midodrine
• Desmopressin
• Erythropoietin

VASOVAGAL SYNCOPE

Pathophysiology

The normal physiologic responses to orthostasis, as described earlier, are an increase in HR, rise in peripheral vascular resistance (increase in diastolic blood pressure), and minimal decline in systolic BP to maintain an adequate cardiac output. In patients with VVS, these responses to prolonged orthostasis are paradoxical. The precise sequence of events leading to VVS is not fully understood. The possible mechanism involves a sudden fall in venous return to the heart, rapid fall in ventricular volume, and virtual collapse of the ventricle due to vigorous ventricular contraction. The net result of these events is stimulation of ventricular mechanoreceptors and activation of the Bezold-Jarisch reflex, leading to peripheral vasodilation (hypotension) and bradycardia. Several neurotransmitters, including serotonin, endorphins, and arginine vasopressin, play an important role in the pathogenesis of VVS, possibly by central sympathetic inhibition, although their exact role is not yet well understood.[63]

Healthy older adults are not as prone to VVS as younger adults. Due to an age-related decline in baroreceptor sensitivity, the paradoxic responses to orthostasis (as in VVS) are possibly less marked in older adults. However, hypertension, atherosclerotic cerebrovascular disease, cardiovascular medications, and impaired baroreflex sensitivity can cause dysautonomic responses during prolonged orthostasis, in which BP and HR decline steadily over time, and render older adults susceptible to VVS. Diuretic- or age-related contraction of blood volume further increases the risk of VVS.[64]

Presentation

The hallmark of VVS is hypotension and/or bradycardia sufficiently profound to produce cerebral ischemia and loss of neural function. VVS has been classified into cardioinhibitory (bradycardia), vasodepressor (hypotension), and mixed (both) subtypes, depending on the BP and HR response. In most patients, the manifestations occur in three distinct phases—a prodrome or aura, loss of consciousness, and postsyncopal phase. A precipitating factor or situation is identifiable in most patients. Common precipitating factors include extreme emotional stress, anxiety, mental anguish, trauma, physical pain or anticipation of physical pain (e.g. anticipation of venesection), warm environment, air travel, and prolonged standing. The most common triggers in older adults are prolonged standing and vasodilator medication. Some patients experience symptoms in specific situations such as micturition, defecation, and coughing. Prodromal symptoms include extreme fatigue, weakness, diaphoresis, nausea, visual defects, visual and auditory hallucinations, dizziness, vertigo, headache, abdominal discomfort, dysarthria, and paresthesias. The duration of prodrome varies greatly, from seconds to several minutes, during which some patients take actions such as lying down to avoid an episode. Older patients may have poor recall for prodromal symptoms. The syncopal period is usually brief, during which some patients develop involuntary movements, usually myoclonic jerks, but tonic clonic movements also occur. Thus, VVS may masquerade as a seizure. Recovery is usually rapid, but older patients can experience protracted symptoms such as confusion, disorientation, nausea, headache, dizziness, and a general sense of ill health.

Evaluation

Several methods have evolved to determine an individual's susceptibility to VVS such as the Valsalva maneuver, hyperventilation, ocular compression, and immersion of the face in cold water. However, these methods are poorly reproducible and lack correlation with clinical events. Using the strong orthostatic stimulus of head-up tilting and maximal venous pooling, VVS can be reproduced in a susceptible individual.[65] Head-up tilting as a diagnostic tool was first reported in 1986[66] and, since then, validity of this technique in identifying susceptibility to neurocardiogenic syncope has been established. Subjects are tilted head up for 40 minutes at 70 degrees. HR and BP are measured continuously throughout the test. A test is diagnostic or positive if symptoms are reproduced, with a decline in BP of greater than 50 mm Hg or less than 90 mm Hg. This may be in addition to significant HR slowing. As with CSS, the hemodynamic responses are classified as vasodepressor, cardioinhibitory, or mixed. The cardioinhibitory response is defined as asystole in excess of 3 seconds or HR slowing to less than 40 beats/min for a minimum of 10 seconds. Orthostatic hypotension, VVS, and carotid sinus hypersensitivity may overlap, particularly in older patients.[67]

The sensitivity of head-up tilting can be further improved by provocative agents that accentuate the physiologic events leading to VVS. One agent is intravenous isoproterenol, which enhances myocardial contractility by stimulating β-adrenoreceptors. Isoproterenol is infused prior to head-up tilting at a dose of 1 μg/min and gradually increased to a maximum dose of 3 μg/min to achieve a HR increase of 25%. Although the sensitivity of head-up tilt testing improves by about 15%, the specificity is reduced. In addition, as a result of the decline in β-receptor sensitivity with age, isoproterenol is less well tolerated and less diagnostic and has a much higher incidence of side effects. The other agent that can be used as a provocative agent and is better tolerated in older adults is sublingual nitroglycerin, which, by reducing venous return due to vasodilation, can enhance the vasovagal reaction in susceptible individuals. Nitroglycerin provocation during head-up tilt testing is thus preferable to other provocative tests in older patients.[65,68] The duration of testing is shorter, cannulation is not required, and sensitivity and specificity are better than for isoproterenol.

Because syncopal episodes are intermittent, external loop recording will not capture events unless they occur approximately every 2 to 3 weeks. Implantable loop recorders (Reveal; Medtronic) can aid diagnosis by tracking bradyarrhythmias or tachyarrhythmias, causing less frequent syncope. To date, no implantable BP monitors are available, with the exception of intracardiac monitors, which are not recommended for the diagnosis of a benign condition such as VVS.[69,70]

Management

Avoidance of precipitating factors and evasive actions such as lying down during prodromal symptoms have great value in preventing episodes of VVS. Withdrawal or modification of culprit medications is often the only necessary intervention in older adults. Doses and frequency of antihypertensive medications can be tailored by information from 24-hour ambulatory monitoring. Older patients with hypertension who develop orthostatic or vasovagal syncope while taking antihypertensive drugs present a difficult therapeutic dilemma and should be treated on an individual basis.

Many patients experience symptoms without warning, necessitating drug therapy. A number of drugs are reported to be useful in alleviating symptoms. Fludrocortisone (100 to 200 μg/day) works by its volume expanding effect. Studies have suggested that serotonin antagonists such as fluoxetine (20 mg/day) and sertraline hydrochloride (25 mg/day) are also effective, although further trials are necessary to validate this finding. Midodrine acts by reducing peripheral venous pooling and thereby improving cardiac output and can be used alone or in combination with fludrocortisone, but with caution. Elastic support hose, relaxation techniques (e.g., biofeedback), and conditioning using repeated head-up tilt as therapy have been used as adjuvant therapies. Permanent cardiac pacing is beneficial in some patients who have recurrent syncope due to cardioinhibitory responses.[71]

POSTPRANDIAL HYPOTENSION

The effect of meals on the cardiovascular system was determined from postprandial exaggeration of angina, which was demonstrated objectively by deterioration of exercise tolerance following food. Postprandial reductions in BP manifesting as syncope and dizziness were subsequently reported, leading to extensive investigation of this phenomenon. In healthy older adults, 60 minutes after a meal of varying compositions and energy content, systolic BP falls by 11 to 16 mm Hg and HR rises by 5 to 7 beats/min. However, the change in diastolic BP is not as consistent. In older adults with hypertension, orthostatic hypotension, and autonomic failure, the postprandial BP fall is much greater and without the corresponding rise in HR.[72] These responses are marked if the energy and simple carbohydrate content of the meal is high. In most fit and frail older adults, most postprandial hypotensive episodes go unnoticed.[73] When systematically evaluated, postprandial hypotension was found in over one third of nursing home residents.

Postprandial physiologic changes include increased splanchnic and superior mesenteric artery blood flow at the expense of peripheral circulation and a rise in plasma insulin levels without corresponding rises in sympathetic nervous system activity. Vasodilator effects of insulin and other gut peptides, including neurotensin and vasoactive intestinal peptide (VIP), contribute to hypotension. The clinical significance of a fall in BP after meals is difficult to quantify. However, postprandial hypotension is causally related to recurrent syncope and falls in older adults. A reduction in the simple carbohydrate content of food and/or replacement with complex carbohydrates or high-protein, high-fat, and frequent small meals, are effective interventions for postprandial hypotension. Drugs useful in the treatment of postprandial hypotension include fludrocortisone, indomethacin, octreotide, and caffeine. Given orally along with food, caffeine prevents hypotensive symptoms in fit and frail older adults but should preferably be given in the mornings because tolerance develops if it is taken throughout the day.[74]

CAROTID SINUS SYNDROME AND CAROTID SINUS HYPERSENSITIVITY

Pathophysiology

CSS is an important but frequently overlooked cause of syncope and presyncope in older adults.[16] Episodic bradycardia and/or hypotension resulting from exaggerated baroreceptor mediated reflexes or carotid sinus hypersensitivity characterize the syndrome. It is diagnosed in persons with otherwise unexplained recurrent syncope who have carotid sinus hypersensitivity. The latter is considered to be present if carotid sinus massage produces asystole exceeding 3 seconds (cardioinhibitory), fall in systolic BP exceeding 50 mm Hg in the absence of cardioinhibition (vasodepressor), or a combination of the two (mixed).[75,76]

Epidemiology

Up to 30% of healthy older adults have carotid sinus hypersensitivity. The prevalence is higher in the presence of coronary artery disease or hypertension. Abnormal responses to carotid sinus massage are more likely to be observed in individuals with coronary artery disease and in those on vasoactive drugs known to influence carotid sinus reflex sensitivity, such as digoxin, β-blockers, and α-methyldopa. Other hypotensive disorders such as VVS and orthostatic hypotension coexist in one third of patients with carotid sinus hypersensitivity. In centers that routinely perform carotid sinus massage in all older patients with syncope, CSS is the attributable cause of syncope in 30%.[77] This figure needs to be interpreted within the context of these centers evaluating a preselected group of patients who have a higher likelihood of CSS than the general population of older adults with syncope. The prevalence in older adults presenting with syncope is unknown.

CSS is virtually unknown before the age of 50 years; its incidence increases with age thereafter. Men are more commonly affected than women, and most have coronary artery disease or hypertension. CSS is associated with appreciable morbidity. Approximately 50% of patients sustain an injury during symptomatic episodes, including a fracture. In a prospective study of falls in nursing home residents, a threefold increase in the fracture rate in those with carotid sinus hypersensitivity was observed. Carotid sinus hypersensitivity can be considered as a modifiable risk factor for fractures of the femoral neck. CSS is not associated with an increased risk of death. The mortality rate in patients with the syndrome is similar to that of patients with unexplained syncope and the general population matched for age and gender. Mortality rates are similar for the three subtypes of the syndrome.[78]

The natural history of carotid sinus hypersensitivity has not been well investigated. In one study, most of those with abnormal hemodynamic responses but without syncopal symptoms (90%) remained symptom-free during a follow-up period of over 1 year, whereas half of those who presented with syncope had symptom recurrence. More recent neuropathologic research has suggested that carotid sinus hypersensitivity is associated with neurodegenerative pathology at the cardiovascular center in the brain stem.[79,80]

Presentation

The syncopal symptoms are usually precipitated by mechanical stimulation of the carotid sinus, such as head turning, tight neckwear, neck pathology, and vagal stimuli, such as prolonged standing. Other recognized triggers for symptoms are the postprandial state, straining, looking or stretching upward, exertion, defecation, and micturition. In a significant number of patients, no triggering event can be identified. Abnormal response to carotid sinus massage (see later) may not always be reproducible, necessitating repetition of the procedure if the diagnosis is strongly suspected.

Evaluation

Carotid Sinus Massage

Carotid sinus reflex sensitivity is assessed by measuring HR and BP responses to carotid sinus massage. Cardioinhibition and vasodepression are more common on the right side. In patients with cardioinhibitory CSS, over 70% have a positive response to right-sided carotid sinus massage, alone or in combination with left-sided carotid sinus massage. There is no fixed relationship between the degree of HR slowing and the degree of fall in BP.

Carotid sinus massage is a crude and unquantifiable technique and is prone to intraobserver and as interobserver variation. More scientific diagnostic methods using neck chamber suction or drug-induced changes in BP can be used for carotid baroreceptor activation but have not been validated for routine clinical use. The recommended duration of carotid sinus massage is from 5 to 10 seconds. The maximum fall in HR usually occurs within 5 seconds of the onset of massage (see Figure 45-2).

Complications resulting from carotid sinus massage include cardiac arrhythmias and neurologic sequelae. Fatal arrhythmias are extremely uncommon and have generally only occurred in patients with underlying heart disease who have been undergoing therapeutic rather than diagnostic massage. Digoxin toxicity has been implicated in most cases of ventricular fibrillation. Neurologic complications result from occlusion of or embolization from the carotid artery. Several authors have reported cases of hemiplegia following carotid sinus stimulation, often in the absence of hemodynamic changes. Complications from carotid sinus massage however, are uncommon. In a prospective series of 1000 consecutive cases, no patient had cardiac complications and 1% had transient neurological symptoms which resolved. Persistent neurologic complications were uncommon, occurring in 0.04%.[81] Carotid sinus massage should not be performed in patients who have had a recent cerebrovascular event or myocardial infarction.

Symptom reproduction during carotid sinus massage is preferable for a diagnosis of CSS. Symptom reproduction may not be possible for older patients with amnesia because of loss of consciousness. Spontaneous symptoms usually occur in the upright position. It may be worthwhile to repeat the procedure with the patient upright on a tilt table, even after demonstrating a positive response when the patient is supine. This reproduction of symptoms aids in attributing the episodes to carotid sinus hypersensitivity, especially in patients with unexplained falls who deny loss of consciousness. In one third of patients, a diagnostic response is only achieved during upright carotid sinus massage.

Management

No treatment is necessary in persons with asymptomatic carotid sinus hypersensitivity.[82] There is no consensus, however, on the timing of therapeutic intervention in the presence of symptoms. Considering the high rate of injury in symptomatic episodes in older adults, as well as the low recurrence rate of symptoms, it is prudent to treat all patients with a history of two or more symptomatic episodes. The need for intervention in those with a solitary event should be assessed on an individual basis, taking into consideration the severity of the event and patient's comorbidity.

Treatment strategies in the past included carotid sinus denervation achieved surgically or by radioablation. Both procedures have largely been abandoned. Dual-chamber cardiac pacing is the treatment of choice in patients with symptomatic cardioinhibitory CSS. Atrial pacing is contraindicated in view of the high prevalence of sinoatrial and atrioventricular block in patients with carotid sinus hypersensitivity. Ventricular pacing abolishes cardioinhibition but fails to alleviate symptoms in a significant number of patients because of aggravation of a coexisting vasodepressor response or development of pacemaker-induced hypotension, referred to as pacemaker syndrome. The latter occurs when ventriculoatrial conduction is intact, as is the case for up to 80% of patients with the syndrome. Atrioventricular sequential pacing (dual chamber) is thus the treatment of choice and, because this maintains atrioventricular synchrony, there is no risk of pacemaker syndrome. With appropriate pacing, syncope is abolished in 85% to 90% of patients with cardioinhibition.

In a study of cardiac pacing in older adults who fall (mean age, 74 years) who had cardioinhibitory carotid sinus hypersensitivity, falls during 1 year of follow-up were reduced by two thirds in patients who received a dual-chamber system.[77] Syncopal episodes were reduced by half. Over 50% of patients in the aforementioned series had gait abnormalities, and 75% had balance abnormalities that would render them more susceptible to falls under hemodynamic circumstances, thus further suggesting the multifactorial nature of many falls and syncopal episodes.[83]

Treatment of vasodepressor CSS is less successful due to poor understanding of its pathophysiology. Ephedrine has been reported to be useful, but long-term use is limited by side effects. Dihydroergotamine is effective but poorly tolerated. Fludrocortisone, a mineralocorticoid widely used in the treatment of orthostatic hypotension, is used in the treatment of vasodepressor CSS with good results, but its use is limited in the longer term by adverse effects. A small randomized controlled trial has suggested good benefit with midodrine (an α-agonist). Surgical denervation of the carotid artery may be a valid treatment option.[84,85]

Cardiac Syncope

One third of cases of syncope in older patients are caused by cardiac disorders[20] (see Figure 45-3). There is a higher morbidity and mortality associated with cardiac syncope.[9,86] Cardiac syncope is characterized by little or no prodrome, occurrence when supine or during exercise, and association with palpitations or chest pain.[87] However, the older patient may not recall these symptoms. Heart disease is an independent predictor of cardiac syncope, with a sensitivity of 95% and specificity of 45% [37] The prevalence of cardiac disease, including structural heart disease and arrhythmias, rises dramatically with age (see Figures 45-2 and 45-3),[26,27,88] and cardiac syncope should be considered when the surface ECG is abnormal or left ventricular systolic dysfunction is present.[87]

Diagnosis

The gold standard for the diagnosis of cardiac syncope is symptom rhythm correlation— contemporaneous HR and rhythm recording during syncope. Cardiac monitoring may also identify diagnostic abnormalities, such as asystole in excess of 3 seconds and rapid supraventricular tachycardia (SVT) or ventricular tachycardia (VT).[89-91] The absence of an arrhythmia during a recorded syncopal event excludes arrhythmia as a cause unless the patient has a dual diagnosis. In patients older than 40 years with recurrent unexplained syncope who do not have structural heart disease or an abnormal ECG, the attributable cause of syncope is bradycardia in over 50% of them.[40,92-94]

Cardiac Monitoring

Prompt hospital admission or intensive monitoring is recommended when cardiac disease is present in the setting of syncope (Table 45-5). Although telemetry or inpatient monitoring is indicated if the patient is at high risk of a life-threatening arrhythmia, as per the electrocardiographic abnormalities detailed in Table 45-4, the diagnostic yield from telemetry is low, 16% in one series.[95]

Diagnostic yield from Holter monitoring is only 1% to 2% in unselected populations.[1] Incidental arrhythmias are much more common in older adults; for example, atrial fibrillation occurs in one in five men older than 80 years.[96] External loop recorders have a higher diagnostic yield in older patients but some of them may have difficulty operating the devices,[97,98] and automated arrhythmia detection is therefore preferred.[99] Normal ambulatory electrocardiography (e.g., Holter, external loop) in the absence of symptoms does not exclude a causal arrhythmia,[87] and monitoring for longer intervals is imperative to capture rhythm during symptoms. Diagnostic rates are much higher in older patients using an implantable loop recorder (ILR)[100,101] and are helpful in up to 50% of patients with syncope and unexplained falls.[102-104] Early insertion of ILRs in older adults is important to consider in view of the disproportionately high number of cardiac causes of syncope in this group.[102] This approach is also more cost-effective.[105,106] Difficulties with ILRs include the inability to activate the device, particularly if patients have cognitive impairment. However, automated recordings and remote monitoring have a much improved diagnostic yield.[107] Magnetic resonance imaging (MRI) brain scans have been increasingly used for investigation of other symptoms in older adults; therefore, MRI-compatible devices should always be used.

Echocardiography. Echocardiography (ECHO) should be performed in syncope patients in whom a structural abnormality is suspected. The prevalence of structural cardiac abnormalities increases with age.[88] The test is of most benefit in older patients with aortic stenosis[108] and to evaluate the ejection fraction. Cardiac arrhythmias are evident in up to 50% of patients with an ejection fraction of less than 40%.[109]

Ambulatory Blood Pressure Monitoring. Patterns of BP behavior, including postprandial hypotension, hypotension after medication ingestion, orthostatic- and exercise-induced hypotension, and supine systolic hypertension, can be readily identified by this investigation. Modification of timing of meals and medications is guided by BP patterns.[24]

Exercise Stress Testing. Exercise stress testing is indicated to investigate cardiac disease and is useful for patients who present with exercise-induced syncope.[1] However, it is not always possible in older patients, who may alternatively require angiography to investigate their cardiac status.

Electrophysiologic Study. Electrophysiologic study is indicated in the older nonfrail patient with syncope when a cardiac arrhythmia is suspected.[24] Diagnosis is based on confirmation of an inducible arrhythmia or conduction disturbance.[110] The benefit

TABLE 45-5 Management of Cardiac Syncope

Recommendations	Class*	Level*
Syncope due to cardiac arrhythmias must receive treatment appropriate to the cause	I	B
Cardiac Pacing		
Pacing is indicated in patients with sinus node disease in whom syncope is demonstrated to be due to sinus arrest (symptom—ECG correlation) without a correctable cause	I	C
Pacing is indicated in sinus node disease patients with syncope and abnormal CSNRT	I	C
Pacing is indicated in sinus node disease patients with syncope and asymptomatic pauses ≥ 3 s (with the possible exceptions of young trained persons, during sleep and in medicated patients)	I	C
Pacing is indicated in patients with syncope and second degree Mobitz II advance or complete AV block	I	B
Pacing is indicated in patients with syncope, BGBB, and positive EPS	I	B
Pacing should be considered in patients with unexplained syncope and BBB	IIa	C
Pacing many be indicated in patients with unexplained syncope and sinus node disease with persistent sinus bradycardia itself asymptomatic	IIb	C
Pacing ins not indicated in patients with unexplained syncope without evidence of any conduction disturbance	III	C
Catheter Ablation		
Catheter ablation is indicated in patients with symptom—arrhythmia ECG correlation in both SVT and VT in the absence of structural heart disease (with exception of atrial fibrillation)	I	C
Catheter ablation may be indicated in patients with syncope due to the onset of rapid atrial fibrillation	IIb	C
Antiarrhythmic Drug Therapy		
Antiarrhythmic drug therapy, including rate control drugs, is indicated in patients with syncope due to onset of rapid atrial fibrillation	I	C
Drug therapy should be considered in patients with symptom—arrhythmia ECG correlation in both SVT and VT with catheter ablation cannot be undertaken or had failed	IIa	C
Implantable Cardioverter Defibrillator		
ICD in indicated in patients with documented VT and structural heart disease		
ICD in indicated when sustained monomorphic VT is induced at EPS in patients with previous myocardial infarction		
ICD should be considered in patients with documented VT and inherited cardiomyopathies or channelopathies		

Recommendations from the European Cardiac Society Taskforce on Syncope Cardiac Syncope; adapted from Moya A, Sutton R, Ammirati F, et al: Guidelines for the diagnosis and management of syncope (version 2009): the Task Force for the Diagnosis and Management of Syncope of the European Society of Cardiology (ESC). Eur Heart J 30:2631–2671, 2009.

AV, Atrioventricular; *BBB,* bundle branch block, *CSNRT,* corrected sinus node recovery time; *ECG,* electrocardiogram; *EPS,* electrophysiologic study; *ICD,* implantable cardioverter defibrillator; *SVT,* supraventricular tachycardia; *VT,* ventricular tachycardia.

*Class of recommendation.

is dependent on pretest probability based on the presence of organic heart disease or an abnormal ECG.[111]

An electrophysiologic study has the advantage of providing diagnosis and treatment in the same session (transcatheter ablation).[24] It is most effective for the following: identification of sinus node dysfunction in the presence of significant sinus bradycardia of 50 beats/min or less; prediction of impending high-degree AV block in patients with bifascicular block; and for the determination of inducible monomorphic VT (in patients with a previous myocardial infarction) and inducible SVT with hypotension in patients with palpitations.[24]

Management

The management of cardiac syncope is dependent on the specific cardiac diagnosis, as outlined in Table 45-5.[1]

Challenges in the Older Patient

Frailty. For older adults who have frailty, carefully considered and individualized decisions need to be made that incorporate the trade-offs of potential benefits against the increased risk of harm, particularly the possible burdens of intensive investigations and realistic opportunities to improve quality of life.[112]

Unwitnessed Events in the Older Adult. In the older adult, a witness account may not be available for falls or syncopal events in up to 40% of patients.[13]

Medications, Polypharmacy, and Syncope. Polypharmacy is more common in older adults. Some of the most frequently prescribed syncope-related medications used in combination are are antihypertensives, antianginals, antihistamines, antipsychotics, tricyclic antidepressants, and diuretics. These cause bradycardia, QT interval prolongation, orthostatic hypotension, and VVS. Drug interactions can also cause syncope, particularly in the older patient with multiple comorbidity and polypharmacy.[113] A temporal association between onset or change of medication and symptoms may be evident, although progression of age-related physiologic changes may cause syncope, even with long-standing established medications.[24]

The TILDA study has reported an increased risk and frequency of syncope with the use of tricyclic antidepressants.[57] The side effect most frequently reported is hypotension, but bradycardia and tachycardia have also been reported.[114,115]

Cognition. Cognitive impairment rises with age; 20% of people older than 80 years have established dementia,[115] rising to 40% in those older than 90 years.[116] Cognitive impairment is characterized by memory problems, attention difficulties, and executive dysfunction; hence, compliance with cardiac monitoring systems may be compromised.

Cognitive impairment is particularly high in older patients with carotid sinus hypersensitivity.[117] Likewise, patients with some subtypes of dementia, such as Lewy body or Alzheimer dementia, have a higher prevalence of syncope, orthostatic hypotension, and carotid sinus hypersensitivity. Establishing a causal relationship between symptoms and arrhythmia or hypotension is particularly difficult in these patients, given that the history is not reliable and events are often unwitnessed.[12,31,118]

There is emerging evidence that low BP may cause or exaggerate cognitive dysfunction,[119] possibly because cerebral hypoperfusion is associated with cerebral damage via small vessel arteriosclerosis and cerebral amyloid angiopathy, as well as exaggerated white matter disease.[120]

Dual Diagnosis. In the older patient, multiple causes of syncope may be present, including cardiac factors (e.g., bradyarrhythmias, SVT tachyarrythmias, ventricular tachyarrhythmias, long QT) and reflex syncope or autonomic impairment (see Box 45-1).[23] Attributing a cause in the context of multiple abnormalities is not always possible, and treatment of all possible causes is recommended. In one series of patients with syncope, mean age 66.5 ± 18 years, 23% had a dual diagnosis. The principal predictors of dual diagnosis were advanced age and treatment with α-receptor blockers and benzodiazepines. The most frequent dual diagnoses were orthostatic hypotension and vasovagal syndrome; 2.8% of these patients had a triple diagnosis, and these were the oldest old.[121]

Focal Neurology With Syncope. Transient ischemic attacks or stroke and syncope are considered mutually exclusive presentations. However, one recent series has reported that 5.7% of syncope patients experience focal neurologic events at the time of syncope or presyncope.[122,123] Awareness of this phenomenon is important to prevent misdiagnosis of stroke and an inappropriate increase of antihypertensive medications, which would further exacerbate hypotensive symptoms.

SUMMARY

The prevalence of syncope rises with age and is challenging because of atypical presentation, overlap with falls, and poor recall of events. Oder adults are less likely to have a prodrome and may have amnesia for loss of consciousness and unwitnessed events. Cardiac causes and dual pathology are more common, and compliance with newer monitoring technologies is inadequate. Consequent morbidity and mortality are higher than in younger patients. A high index of suspicion for cardiovascular causes of falls and dual pathology will help determine the diagnosis and early target intervention.

Syncope is a common symptom in older adults due to age-related neurohumoral and physiologic changes plus chronic diseases and medications that reduce cerebral oxygen delivery through a number of mechanisms. Common individual causes of syncope encountered by the geriatrician are orthostatic hypotension, CSS, VVS, postprandial syncope, sinus node disease, AV block, and ventricular tachycardia. Algorithms for the assessment of syncope are similar to those for young adults, but the prevalence of ischemic and hypertensive disorders and cardiac conduction disease is higher in older adults, and the cause is more often multifactorial. A systematic approach to syncope is needed, with the goal being to identify a single likely cause or multiple treatable contributing factors. Management is then based on removing or reducing the predisposing or precipitating factors through various combinations of medication adjustments, behavioral strategies, and more invasive interventions in select cases, such as cardiac pacing, cardiac stenting, and intracardiac defibrillators. It is often not possible to attribute a definitive cause of syncope in older adults, who frequently have more than one possible cause, and pragmatic management of each diagnosis is recommended.

KEY POINTS

- Syncope is experienced by up to 30% of adults in their lifetime with a rising incidence in those older than 70 years.
- Vasovagal syncope, orthostatic hypotension, and carotid sinus syndrome are the most common cause of syncope in older adults.
- Cardiac causes of syncope, including structural heart disease and arrhythmia, occur with higher frequency in older patients.
- Up to 40% of older patients have more than one cause for syncope, and multimorbidity plays a large role in the underlying cause of syncope in older adults.
- Syncope is a common cause of falls in older adults, and up to 60% of patients have amnesia for of consciousness, making the diagnosis of syncope challenging
- Standardized, guideline-based evaluation of patients who experience syncope provides the highest diagnostic yield for determining the underlying cause.

For a complete list of references, please visit www.expertconsult.com.

KEY REFERENCES

1. Moya A, Sutton R, Ammirati F, et al: Guidelines for the diagnosis and management of syncope (version 2009): the Task Force for the Diagnosis and Management of Syncope of the European Society of Cardiology (ESC). Eur Heart J 30:2631–2671, 2009.
2. Ganzeboom KS, Mairuhu G, Reitsma JB, et al: Lifetime cumulative incidence of syncope in the general population: a study of 549 Dutch subjects aged 35-60 years. J Cardiovasc Electrophysiol 17:1172–1176, 2006.
9. Soteriades ES, Evans JC, Larson MG, et al: Incidence and prognosis of syncope. N Engl J Med 347:878–885, 2002.
14. Parry SW, Steen IN, Baptist M, et al: Amnesia for loss of consciousness in carotid sinus syndrome: implications for presentation with falls. J Am Coll Cardiol 45:1840–1843, 2005.
16. Brignole M: Distinguishing syncopal from non-syncopal causes of fall in older people. Age Ageing 35(Suppl 2):ii46–ii50, 2006.
19. Olde Nordkamp LR, van Dijk N, Ganzeboom KS, et al: Syncope prevalence in the ED compared to general practice and population: a strong selection process. Am J Emerg Med 27:271–279, 2009.
21. Ungar A, Mussi C, Del Rosso A, et al: Diagnosis and characteristics of syncope in older patients referred to geriatric departments. J Am Geriatr Soc 54:1531–1536, 2006.
34. Parry SW, Steen N, Bexton RS, et al: Pacing in elderly recurrent fallers with carotid sinus hypersensitivity: a randomised, double-blind, placebo controlled crossover trial. Heart 95:405–409, 2009.
35. McIntosh SJ, Lawson J, Kenny RA: Clinical characteristics of vasodepressor, cardioinhibitory, and mixed carotid sinus syndrome in the elderly. Am J Med 95:203–208, 1993.
38. Panel on Prevention of Falls in Older Persons, American Geriatrics Society and British Geriatrics Society: Summary of the Updated American Geriatrics Society/British Geriatrics Society clinical practice guideline for prevention of falls in older persons. J Am Geriatr Soc 59:148–157, 2011.
46. Finucane C, O'Connell MDL, Fan CW, et al: Age-related normative changes in phasic orthostatic blood pressure in a large population study: findings from the Irish Longitudinal Study on Ageing (TILDA). Circulation 130:1780–1789, 2014.
53. Consensus Committee of the American Autonomic Society, American Academy of Neurology: Consensus statement on the definition of orthostatic hypotension, pure autonomic failure, and multiple system atrophy. Neurology 46:1470, 1996.
65. Bartoletti A, Alboni P, Ammirati F, et al: 'The Italian Protocol': a simplified head-up tilt testing potentiated with oral nitroglycerin to assess patients with unexplained syncope. Europace 2:339–342, 2000.
66. Kenny RA, Ingram A, Bayliss J, et al: Head-up tilt: a useful test for investigating unexplained syncope. Lancet 1:1352–1355, 1986.
69. Brignole M, Sutton R, Menozzi C, et al: Early application of an implantable loop recorder allows effective specific therapy in patients with recurrent suspected neurally mediated syncope. Eur Heart J 27:1085–1092, 2006.
77. Kenny RAM, Richardson DA, Steen N, et al: Carotid sinus syndrome: a modifiable risk factor for nonaccidental falls in older adults (SAFE PACE). J Am Coll Cardiol 38:1491–1496, 2001.
102. Brignole M, Menozzi C, Maggi R, et al: The usage and diagnostic yield of the implantable loop-recorder in detection of the mechanism of syncope and in guiding effective antiarrhythmic therapy in older people. Europace 7:273–279, 2005.
115. Ballard C, Shaw F, McKeith I, et al: High prevalence of neurovascular instability in neurodegenerative dementias. Neurology 51:1760–1762, 1998.
118. Cummings SR, Nevitt MC, Kidd S: Forgetting falls. The limited accuracy of recall of falls in the elderly. J Am Geriatr Soc 36:613–616, 1988.

46 Vascular Surgery

Charles McCollum, Christopher Lowe, Vivak Hansrani, Stephen Ball

INTRODUCTION

As the prevalence of atherosclerosis increases with advancing age, it is hardly surprising that specialists in geriatric medicine frequently find vascular disease in their patients. For many, their overall degree of frailty is such that neither detailed investigation nor vascular surgery will be indicated. However, vascular surgeons now routinely perform procedures in octogenarians and will increasingly do so as the population ages.

Older adults suffer a range of vascular conditions. This chapter focuses on the four vascular problems of greatest concern to geriatricians: (1) limb ischemia; (2) abdominal aortic aneurysm; (3) carotid disease; and (4) chronic venous insufficiency, venous ulcers, and the swollen leg.

ARTERIAL DISEASE OF THE LIMB

Background

Most older adult patients with peripheral artery disease (PAD) have chronic symptoms rather than acute leg symptoms. The spectrum ranges from intermittent claudication to critical limb ischemia (CLI) with rest pain, ulceration, gangrene, and the threat of limb loss (Figure 46-1). Vascular intervention is rarely indicated for intermittent claudication in older adults unless it significantly impairs quality of life. CLI is the tipping point in arterial insufficiency where stenosis and/or occlusion of the limb arteries, often at multiple levels, lowers the downstream perfusion pressure to the extent that nutritional flow to tissues is severely compromised, impairing wound healing or threatening tissue viability.[1] Without urgent revascularization, tissue necrosis may occur within days or weeks and lead to major limb amputation. In contrast to intermittent claudication, where intervention is never urgent or even essential, CLI is an absolute indication for investigation with a view to angioplasty or surgery to restore adequate perfusion to the tissues of the foot.

Acute limb ischemia is also common in older adults and can involve the upper or lower limb. There may be little or no significant arterial disease previously with embolization due to atrial fibrillation. Acute ischemia is often secondary to acute thrombosis in patients with PAD. Acute ischemia usually requires immediate (within 2 to 3 hours) investigation and treatment.

Peripheral Artery Disease

Epidemiology

As chronic PAD is often missed in older adults, its prevalence cannot be estimated reliably; however, the prevalence of intermittent claudication is approximately 7% in patients aged 70 years or older.[2] The incidence of CLI is thought to be in the range of 500 to 1000 per million in Europe and the United States with prevalence of approximately 1% in patients aged 60 to 90 years.[1]

Intermittent Claudication

Intermittent claudication has a benign prognosis as perfusion of the tissues at rest is normal, but the peripheral arteries cannot deliver the 10-fold increase in blood flow required by exercising skeletal muscle. Only 10% of patients with claudication require vascular reconstruction, and with conservative care, most improve or remain stable.

However, the risk of myocardial infarction and stroke in this group is similar to that of individuals with established coronary artery disease. A reduced ankle-brachial (pressure) index (ABI) as a result of PAD is associated with a three- to six-fold increase in cardiovascular mortality and all-cause mortality independent of the Framingham Risk Score.[2] Managing cardiovascular risk is more important for most patients with claudication than investigation with a view to a vascular procedure. Management includes smoking cessation, optimization of blood pressure and diabetic control, and statin and platelet inhibitory therapy.

Critical Limb Ischemia

Rest pain, ulceration, and gangrene indicate that tissue perfusion has begun to decompensate. Without prompt diagnosis and treatment, the outlook for patients with CLI is poor. Untreated CLI is associated with major amputation, disability, and death. Even following arterial reconstruction, 20% to 25% of patients will have died within a year and 25% to 30% will have suffered major amputation. Only 25% will be alive and free from signs and symptoms of CLI.[2,3]

Evaluation and Diagnosis The clinical history is critical; the pain of intermittent claudication is felt in the muscle, reproducibly develops with similar levels of exercise, and recovers within minutes of resting (without needing to sit down). CLI is associated with tissue loss and ischemic rest pain. Rest pain invariably occurs in the toes or forefoot unless there is acute limb ischemia involving the calf or even the whole leg. In individuals with CLI, elevation of the limb usually aggravates symptoms while dependency usually brings some degree of relief.[4]

Insonating blood flow in the ankle arteries using a handheld Doppler instrument and measuring the ABI is a simple bedside test that should replace the palpation of pulses, which is subjective and unreliable.[1] In patients with leg pain, an ABI of 0.8 is more than 95% sensitive to PAD, but an exercise test is needed to exclude PAD; an ABI of greater than 0.9 after exercise effectively excludes PAD as a cause of symptoms or a threat to wound healing.[5] It can be used as a first-line test in geriatric clinics or on the wards. Symptoms of CLI rarely develop in patients with an ABI greater than 0.5, but falsely high ABI may be measured in patients with calcified calf arteries. Any elevated ABI greater than 1.2 with a monophasic Doppler signal is almost certainly false because of calf artery calcification; symptomatic patients should be referred for a vascular opinion. If there is discrepancy between clinical signs and ABIs, particularly in patients with diabetes or chronic renal failure, further investigation should be dictated by clinical symptoms and signs. The inability to detect flow in the ankle arteries by Doppler, or measure an ankle arterial pressure, suggests very severe ischemia that needs emergent treatment.

Noninvasive imaging by the vascular laboratory through the use of duplex Doppler ultrasound, computed tomographic angiography (CTA), or magnetic resonance angiography (MRA) has replaced invasive catheter digital subtraction angiography for most diagnostic purposes and for the planning of some interventions.

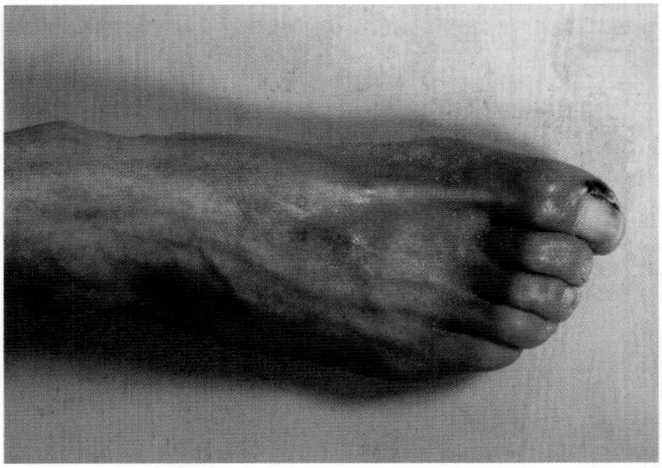

Figure 46-1. Critically ischemic foot with characteristic hyperemia ("sunset foot") and tissue loss.

Duplex Doppler Ultrasound

Duplex ultrasound is now the first line of investigation for PAD and in general should be undertaken in all patients with symptoms sufficient to justify possible intervention. High-definition ultrasound is used to image the anatomy of the artery and any arterial disease and is combined with color Doppler to detect blood flow and quantify the severity of any stenosis.[6-8] Duplex is operator dependent and is best undertaken by experienced clinical vascular scientists. Images can be limited by vessel calcification, and visualization of the iliac arteries is often unsatisfactory because of overlying bowel gas. Duplex ultrasound is ideal for imaging the carotids, abdominal aorta, and all the arteries in the limbs. Results can be used for planning procedures such as angioplasty and stenting.[9,10]

Magnetic Resonance Angiography

MRA is now widely available, avoids radiation, and allows detailed three-dimensional reconstruction of the entire arterial tree. The gadolinium contrast used carries little risk of contrast-induced nephropathy when used in recommended doses,[11] although caution is still advised in patients with severe acute or chronic renal insufficiency (estimated glomerular filtration rate [eGFR] < 30).[12] MRA is the imaging modality of choice for planning of endovascular and surgical procedures when duplex imaging is insufficient, and it is particularly useful in assessing iliac disease (Figure 46-2). The sensitivity of MRA for segmental stenosis greater than 50% is 95% with a specificity of 96%, but the severity of stenoses are frequently overestimated.[13] It is contraindicated in patients with pacemakers and other metallic implants, may not be tolerated by patients with claustrophobia, and is inaccessible for some very obese patients. When MRA is not possible, CTA is the alternative.

Computed Tomographic Angiography

Modern multidetector computed tomography scanners deliver high-quality arterial imaging with lower doses of radiation. The advantages of CTA over MRA include image acquisition with no signal "dropout" in previously stented vessels, patients' preference for CTA, and less risk of overestimating the severity of stenosis. One disadvantage of CTA is that interference due to arterial calcification can obscure luminal narrowing or occlusion. The risk of contrast-induced nephropathy is an issue in older adult patients with chronic kidney disease, although this can be mitigated by prehydration.[11] MRA is far easier to interpret, which is why it is more widely used than CTA to take images of PAD.

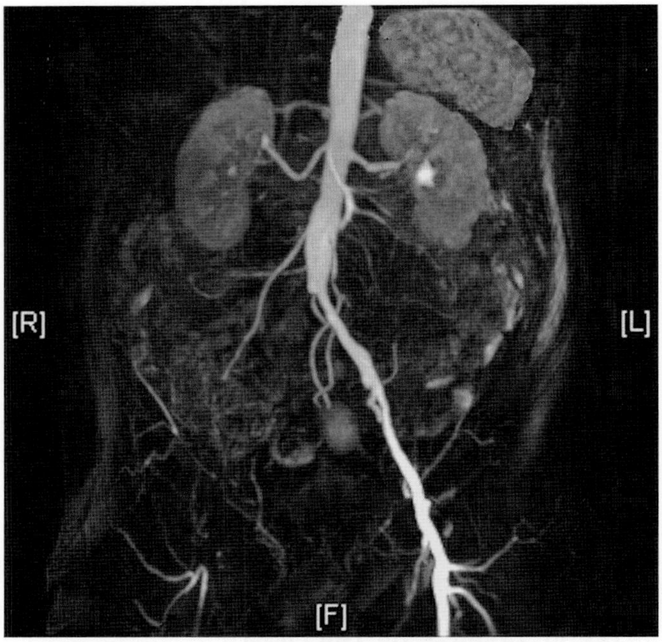

Figure 46-2. Magnetic resonance angiogram demonstrating occlusion of the right iliac system with the common femoral artery bifurcation filled via collateral circulation.

Treatment

All patients should be advised on managing cardiovascular risk. Statins reduce cardiovascular events in patients with PVD[14] and can also prevent plaque instability and thrombosis by moderating endothelial function and inflammatory changes in the arterial wall.[15] Platelet-inhibitory therapy is mandatory unless contraindicated, with clopidogrel being the initial drug of choice. Patients with claudication should be advised to stop smoking, lose weight if appropriate, and exercise with a view to improving their general fitness. Surgery or angioplasty for intermittent claudication should almost never be offered before a period of optimized medical care of at least 3 to 4 months. Vasodilator drugs such as naftidrofuryl are of minimal value and should probably be avoided.[2,16]

It is vital to recognize the onset of CLI, which requires urgent evaluation and treatment. Recent developments in endovascular therapy, such as drug-eluting balloons and stents, allow treatment of more complex lesions and also treatment of patients previously unfit for bypass surgery. However, because multilevel disease is usual in CLI, combined open surgery and endovascular procedures have become commonplace; for a patient with both iliac and femoral artery disease, the "inflow" can be treated by iliac angioplasty (with a stent if necessary) while the disease in the common or superficial femoral artery is treated surgically during the same procedure. For patients with superficial femoral artery disease and a life expectancy of greater than 2 years, the evidence is that a surgical "bypass first" approach achieves better long-term survival and limb salvage that an "angioplasty first" approach.[17]

Acute Limb Ischemia

The classic symptoms of sudden onset pain, pallor, pulselessness, loss of sensation, and loss of function indicate a surgical emergency. Sensory loss and loss of muscle function are the only signs

47 Venous Thromboembolism in Older Adults

Hamsaraj G.M. Shetty, Philip A. Routledge

INTRODUCTION

Venous thromboembolism (VTE) is the third most common cardiovascular disease and an important cause of morbidity and mortality. Older people account for nearly two thirds of episodes.[1] Between 65 and 69 years of age, annual incidence rates per 1000 for deep vein thrombosis (DVT) and pulmonary embolism (PE) are 1.3 and 1.8, respectively, and rise to 2.8 and 3.1 in individuals aged between 85 and 89 years. Older men are more likely than women of similar age to develop PE. About 2% develop PE and 8% develop recurrent PE within 1 year of treatment for DVT.[2]

VTE causes 25,000 to 32,000 deaths in hospitalized patients in the United Kingdom. It accounts for 10% of all hospital deaths. This, however, is likely to be an underestimate because many hospital deaths are not followed by a postmortem examination. The cost of managing VTE in the United Kingdom is estimated to be approximately 640 million pounds.[3] About 25% of patients treated for a DVT subsequently develop debilitating venous leg ulceration, the treatment of which is estimated to cost 400 million pounds in the United Kingdom.[3] The most serious complication of VTE is PE, which untreated has a mortality of 30%. With appropriate treatment, mortality is reduced to 2%.[3] The diagnosis of VTE is often delayed until the occurrence of a clinically obvious (and occasionally fatal) PE. The diagnosis of PE is more often missed in older people and is sometimes made only at postmortem.

The Virchow triad (named after Rudolf Virchow, 1821–1902) describes the three main predisposing factors for development of thrombosis. The first is alteration in blood flow, which may be reduced in people with heart failure (a common problem in older people) and in less mobile individuals. The second factor, injury to the vascular endothelium, is more relevant to arterial thromboembolism than to VTE. The third factor, hypercoagulability, is important because increases in clotting factor concentration, platelet and clotting factor activation, and a decline in fibrinolytic activity have all been reported in older people.[4]

Risk Factors

The risk factors for VTE are well recognized (Box 47-1). Many of these (e.g., poor mobility, hip fractures, stroke, and cancer) are more frequently present in older people, who are also more likely to be hospitalized. Hospitalization is associated with an increased risk of VTE: the incidence is 135 times greater in hospitalized patients than in the community. The risk of VTE is greatest in medical inpatients, and it is estimated that 70% to 80% of hospital-acquired VTEs occur in this group. About a third of all surgical patients develop VTE before prophylactic treatments are used. A particular high-risk group is orthopedic patients. Without prophylaxis, 45% to 51% of orthopedic patients develop DVT. It is estimated that in Europe approximately 5000 patients per year are likely to die of VTE following hip or knee replacement, when prophylactic treatments are not given. Atypical antipsychotic agents are commonly prescribed in older people. The rate of hospitalization for VTE has been reported to be increased in association with risperidone (adjusted hazard ratio [AHR], 1.98; 95% confidence interval [CI], 1.40-2.78), olanzapine (AHR, 1.87; CI, 1.06-3.27), clozapine and quetiapine fumarate (AHR, 2.68; CI, 1.15-6.28).[5]

Clinical Presentation and Diagnosis

Deep Vein Thrombosis

Unilateral swelling of a leg is the most common feature in older patients with DVT.[6] Calf pain may sometimes be present. A history of recent hospitalization for orthopedic surgery, stroke, or for some other illness is common. There may occasionally be a history of anorexia, weight loss, or other symptoms suggestive of an underlying neoplasm.

It is well recognized that the clinical diagnosis of DVT can be difficult because the physical signs may often be absent or subtle, and the diagnosis may be more difficult in older people. Some individuals may be unable to complain about a swollen leg because of dementia, delirium, or dysphasia. In addition, other conditions mimicking DVT, such as a ruptured Baker cyst, are also more likely to occur in this age group. The clinical diagnosis of DVT relies on observing a swollen, warm, lower limb, which may sometimes be associated with engorged superficial veins. The Wells score attempts to take all relevant circumstances, symptoms, and signs into account and has been recommended as a useful initial screening test to ascertain whether DVT is likely or unlikely.[7] Calf tenderness may also be present. If there is a difference of more than 2 cm in circumference between the two lower limbs, DVT must be excluded by appropriate investigations, unless there is another obvious explanation.

Doppler ultrasonography has a sensitivity of 96% and specificity of 98% for a proximal DVT and so it is the investigation of first choice to diagnose a DVT. Contrast venography may be necessary in selected patients, especially if clinical suspicion is high and the Doppler scan is negative. Estimation of the concentration of D-dimer (a fibrin degradation product of thrombolysis), especially when combined with a clinical probability score such as the two-level DVT Wells score[8] (Table 47-1), can be clinically useful. Wells and coworkers have shown that DVT can be ruled out in a patient who is judged clinically unlikely to have DVT and who has a negative D-dimer test. They suggest that that ultrasound testing can be safely omitted in such patients.

In patients with suspected DVT and a "likely" two-level DVT Wells score, the National Institute of Health and Care Excellence (NICE) guidelines recommend proximal leg vein ultrasound scanning within 4 hours and, if the result is negative, a D-dimer test should be performed. If the proximal leg vein ultrasound scan cannot be done within 4 hours, a D-dimer test should be performed. If the test results are positive, an interim 24-hour dose of a parenteral anticoagulant should be administered and, thereafter, a proximal leg vein ultrasound scan carried out within 24 hours.[8] The guidelines further recommend that the proximal leg vein ultrasound scan should be repeated 6 to 8 days later for all patients with positive D-dimer test results and a negative proximal leg vein ultrasound scan. In those patients in whom DVT is suspected and with an "unlikely" two-level DVT Wells score, a D-dimer test should be carried out, and if the result is positive,

BOX 47-1 Risk Factors for Venous Thromboembolism

LOW RISK

- Minor surgery (<30 min) + no risk factors other than age
- Minor trauma or medical illness

MODERATE RISK

- Major general, urologic, gynecologic, cardiothoracic, vascular, or neurologic surgery + age > 40 yr or other risk factor
- Major medical illness or malignancy
- Major trauma or burn
- Minor surgery, trauma, or illness in patients with previous deep vein thrombosis (DVT) or pulmonary embolism (PE) or thrombophilia

HIGH RISK

- Prolonged immobilization
- Aged older than 60 years
- Previous DVT or PE
- Active cancer
- Chronic cardiac failure
- Acute infections (e.g., pneumonia)
- Chronic lung disease
- Lower limb paralysis (excluding stroke)
- Body mass index > 30 kg/m^2
- Fracture or major orthopedic surgery of pelvis, hip, or lower limb
- Major pelvic or abdominal surgery for cancer
- Major surgery, trauma, or illness in patients with previous DVT, PE, or thrombophilia
- Major lower limb amputation

TABLE 47-1 Two-Level Deep Vein Thrombosis Wells Score

Clinical Feature	Points	Patient Score
Active cancer (treatment ongoing, within 6 months, or palliative)	1	
Paralysis, paresis, or recent plaster immobilization of the lower extremities	1	
Recently bedridden for 3 days or more or major surgery within 12 weeks requiring general or regional anesthesia	1	
Localized tenderness along the distribution of the deep venous system	1	
Entire leg swollen	1	
Calf swelling at least 3 cm larger than asymptomatic side	1	
Pitting edema confined to the symptomatic leg	1	
Collateral superficial veins (non-varicose)	1	
Previously documented deep vein thrombosis (DVT)	1	
An alternative diagnosis is at least as likely as DVT	−2	
CLINICAL PROBABILITY SIMPLIFIED SCORE		
DVT *likely*	2 points or more	
DVT *unlikely*	1 point or less	

Reproduced with permission from National Institute for Health and Care Excellence: Venous thromboembolic diseases: the management of venous thromboembolic diseases and the role of thrombophilia testing (NICE guidelines [CG144]), June 2012. http://www.nice.org.uk/guidance/cg144. Accessed September 26, 2015.

either a proximal leg vein ultrasound scan should be conducted within 4 hours of being requested or an interim 24-hour dose of a parenteral anticoagulant (if a proximal leg vein ultrasound scan cannot be carried out within 4 hours) should be administered and a proximal leg vein ultrasound scan (carried out within 24 hours of being requested) should be offered.[8]

Pulmonary Embolism

Sudden onset of dyspnea is the most common presenting feature of PE in older people. Sudden onset of a pleuritic chest pain, cough, syncope, and hemoptysis are other common presenting symptoms. In an older patient with stroke or recent orthopedic surgery, onset of any of these symptoms should greatly increase the suspicion of underlying PE. Because of high incidence of cardiovascular disease and age-related decline in cardiovascular function in general, older people are less likely to tolerate cardiovascular decompensation because of moderate or severe PE. They are, therefore, more likely to have syncope after a PE.[9] Patients with smaller PEs can have very nonspecific symptoms and thus the diagnosis is often missed in this group.

Clinical features will depend on the severity of the PE. In patients with a moderate to severe PE, tachycardia, hypotension, cyanosis, elevated jugular venous pressure, right parasternal heave, loud delayed pulmonary component of the second heart sound, tricuspid regurgitation murmur, and pleural rub may be present. However, in patients with smaller PEs, clinical examination may be normal, except possibly for a sinus tachycardia. Unexplained tachycardia in a patient who is potentially at risk for VTE should alert the clinician to the possibility of PE.

Arterial blood gas analysis is a useful initial test in patients with suspected PE. Presence of hypoxia, or worsening of preexisting hypoxia, makes the diagnosis more likely, unless there are other comorbid conditions to account for it.

An electrocardiogram (ECG) may show sinus tachycardia, S wave in lead I, Q wave and T inversion in lead III, right bundle branch block or a right ventricular strain pattern. In patients with severe PE, a P "pulmonale" may be seen. New onset of atrial fibrillation also can be a feature of PE.

A chest radiograph may show elevated hemidiaphragm, atelectasis, focal oligemia, an enlarged right descending pulmonary artery, or a pleural effusion. Many older patients have coexistent cardiac failure or chronic pulmonary diseases, which can also cause some of the radiographic abnormalities associated with PE.

Computed tomography pulmonary angiography (CTPA) is increasingly being used as the diagnostic test for detecting a PE. A meta-analysis has indicated that the rate of subsequent VTE detection after negative CTPA results is similar to that following conventional pulmonary angiography.[10] One randomized, single-blind, noninferiority trial demonstrated that CTPA is equivalent to a ventilation/perfusion (V/Q) scan in ruling out PE. In the study, CTPA also diagnosed PE in significantly more patients.[11] The British Thoracic Society has recommended CTPA as the initial lung imaging modality of choice for nonmassive PE.[12] It has largely replaced the V/Q scan as the investigation of first choice in older patients because of its greater ability to detect PE even in patients with coexistent cardiac and respiratory disease.

The NICE guideline recommends that in patients in whom a PE is suspected and with a "likely" two-level PE Wells score[8,13] (Table 47-2), an immediate CPTA or, if not available, immediate interim parenteral anticoagulant therapy followed by an urgent CTPA should be offered. A proximal leg vein ultrasound scan should be considered if the CTPA is negative and a DVT is suspected. In patients in whom a PE is suspected and with an "unlikely" two-level PE Wells score, a D-dimer test should be offered and, if the result is positive, an immediate CTPA or immediate interim parenteral anticoagulant therapy followed by a CTPA if a CTPA cannot be carried out immediately.

TABLE 47-2 Two-Level Pulmonary Embolism Wells Score

Clinical Feature	Points	Patient Score
Clinical signs and symptoms of deep vein thrombosis (DVT) (minimum of leg swelling and pain with palpation of the deep veins)	3	
An alternative diagnosis is less likely than PE	3	
Heart rate > 100 beats/min	1.5	
Immobilization for more than 3 days or surgery in the previous 4 weeks	1.5	
Previous DVT/pulmonary embolism (PE)	1.5	
Hemoptysis	1	
Malignancy (on treatment, treated in the last 6 months, or palliative)	1	
Clinical Probability Simplified Scores		
PE *likely*	More than 4 points	
PE *unlikely*	4 points or less	

Reproduced with permission from National Institute for Health and Care Excellence: Venous thromboembolic diseases: the management of venous thromboembolic diseases and the role of thrombophilia testing (NICE guidelines [CG144]), June 2012. http://www.nice.org.uk/guidance/cg144. Accessed September 26, 2015.

Treatment

Proximal (sometimes called "above-knee") DVTs are associated with very high risk of a PE and can cause progressive, painful swelling of the affected leg and even venous gangrene, if untreated. The immediate priority is to prevent a PE, which potentially can be fatal. Low-molecular-weight heparins (LMWHs) should be given subcutaneously for 5 days or until the international normalized ratio (INR) is in the therapeutic range (INR 2 to 3) as a result of concurrent oral vitamin K antagonist (VKA) therapy. Warfarin is the most widely used VKA internationally. It is continued for at least 3 months after the first episode. Fondaparinux is an alternative to LMWHs. Unfractionated heparin (with dose adjustments based on the activated partial thromboplastin time [APTT]) is advocated for initial treatment in people with severe renal impairment, since LMWHs and fondaparinux are predominantly excreted by the kidneys.[14] The NICE guideline also recommends consideration of unfractionated heparin in patients with an increased risk of bleeding.[8]

Because older patients are more sensitive to the effects of VKAs such as warfarin, they are more likely to be over-anticoagulated during initiation of the treatment using non-tailored induction doses. Use of a tailored induction dosing regime is likely to reduce this possibility. One such regimen[15] uses a first dose of 10 mg and subsequent doses are adjusted daily thereafter, depending on the INR. Another induction regimen that has been shown to be safe and accurate in hospitalized patients older than 70 years involves giving 4 mg of warfarin daily for 3 successive days.[16] The recommended target INR for treatment of VTE is 2.5 (range, 2 to 3).[14]

The orally administered direct thrombin inhibitor (dabigatran) and anti-Xa antagonists (apixaban and rivaroxaban) are also licensed for use in VTE. Dabigatran[17] and rivaroxaban[18] are recommended by NICE as an option for treating PE and preventing recurrent DVT and PE in adults. (Apixaban has not yet been appraised by NICE for the treatment and secondary prevention of DVT or PE.) They are administered in fixed doses and produce anticoagulant effect within 2 to 3 hours of intake. Routine monitoring of their anticoagulant effect is not necessary. At present they do not have any specific antidotes and are more expensive than warfarin. Unlike warfarin, all non-warfarin oral anticoagulants are in part excreted by the kidney and require dose reductions depending on renal function.[19] Dabigatran should be avoided if the estimated glomerular fraction rate (eGFR) is less than 30 mL/min/1.73 m^2 or, in the case of rivaroxaban and apixaban, less than 15 mL/min/1.73 m^2.[19]

In patients with active cancer and a confirmed proximal DVT or PE, LWMH should be offered. This therapy should be continued for 6 months and then the risks and benefits of continuing anticoagulation reassessed.[8] In patients with active malignancy and VTE who are not treated with an LMWH, VKAs such as warfarin have been recommended, by the American College of Chest Physicians, over dabigatran or rivaroxaban for long-term therapy.[14]

Guidelines from NICE distinguish between a "provoked" DVT or PE and an "unprovoked" episode.[8] A provoked DVT/PE occurs in individuals who, within the previous 3 months, have had a transient but major clinical risk factor for DVT or PE. Such risks include surgery, trauma, and significant immobility. NICE defines significant immobility as being bedbound, unable to walk unaided, or being likely to spend a substantial proportion of the day in bed or in a chair, situations that are more likely to exist for older individuals.

The NICE guideline recommends that clinicians consider prescribing a VKA such as warfarin beyond 3 months to patients with an unprovoked PE, taking into account the patients' risk of VTE recurrence and whether they are at increased risk of bleeding. For patients with unprovoked proximal DVT, NICE recommends that clinicians consider extending the VKA beyond 3 months if their risk of VTE recurrence is high and there is no additional risk of major bleeding. In both cases the guideline recommends that the clinician discuss with the patient the benefits and risks of extending their oral anticoagulant treatment.[8] Patients who have a major, nonreversible risk factor such as cancer are at high risk of recurrence and therefore should be considered for long-term anticoagulant therapy.[20]

Anticoagulation is not normally recommended for patients with below-knee DVT who are considered to be at low risk for proximal extension. They can be monitored by serial imaging of the deep veins for 2 weeks.[14]

Practical Aspects of Oral Anticoagulant Therapy in Older Adults

Older people are more sensitive to the anticoagulant effect of warfarin. This is probably due to a combination of pharmacodynamic and pharmacokinetic factors.[21,22] Warfarin dose requirement declines with age. In one study, patients aged younger than 35 years required a mean of 8.1 mg/day, more than twice as much to maintain the same INR as in patients older than 75 years.[22] The relationship between age and warfarin requirements is, however, rather weak.[22] In one study, warfarin clearance (wholly by metabolism since no warfarin is excreted unchanged in the urine) was shown to decline with age.[23]

Chronologic age, especially over the age of 80 years, appears to be a risk factor for bleeding in patients receiving anticoagulants.[24,25] Hemorrhagic complications due to warfarin are more likely to occur in the first 90 days of anticoagulant therapy (especially in the first month), either because of poor control of anticoagulation or the unmasking of an underlying lesion, such as a peptic ulcer or malignancy. High INRs (>4.5), poor control of anticoagulation, and inadequate patient education regarding anticoagulant therapy are also likely to increase the risk of bleeding.

Studies have reported a log-linear relationship between the intensity of anticoagulation and the risk of bleeding.[26] Risk of

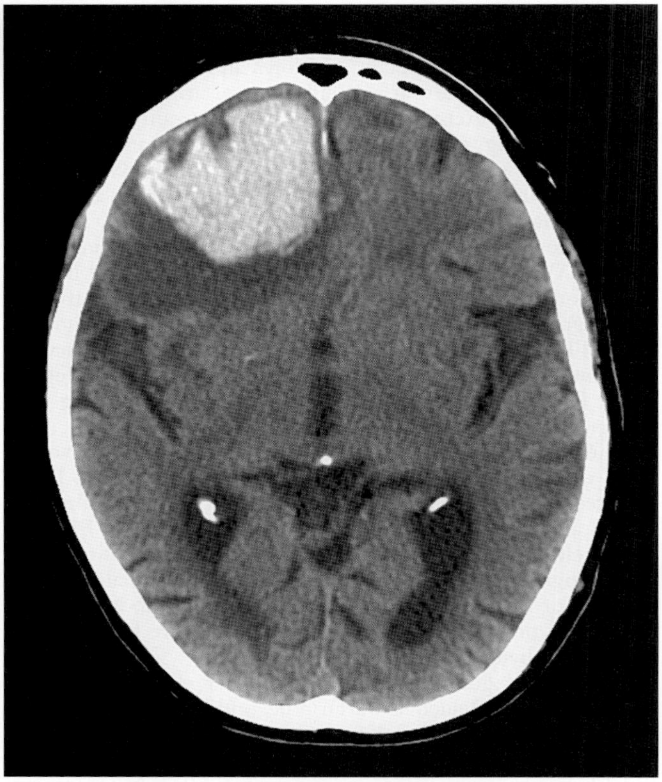

Figure 47-1. Computed tomography scan of head showing intracerebral hemorrhage.

bleeding rises threefold between INRs of between 2 and 3, and further threefold between 3 and 4.[27] Because a high INR is one of the most important risk factors for bleeding in older people, the aim of treatment should be to maintain the lowest intensity of anticoagulation consistent with effective treatment or prophylaxis.

Polypharmacy is common in older people and increases the chances of drug interactions that can result in over-anticoagulation. Using caution with medications that are well known to enhance anticoagulant effect (e.g., antibiotics [particularly macrolides], amiodarone, etc.) and adjusting the dose of warfarin appropriately will reduce the likelihood of over-anticoagulation and consequent bleeding.

Fatal hemorrhages tend to be intracranial and are more likely to occur in older people[27] (Figure 47-1). Older adults are more predisposed to intracranial bleeding because of the increased prevalence of leukoaraiosis and other cerebrovascular diseases. Older people are also more likely to have falls and so are at a greater risk of developing subdural hematomas.

Hemorrhage associated with anticoagulant therapy should always be investigated to exclude an underlying pathologic condition, even if the bleeding occurred when the INR was high. Unexplained anemia in an anticoagulated patient may well be due to occult bleeding (e.g., retroperitoneal hemorrhage). Sometimes atypical bleeding sites and presenting symptoms may pose diagnostic difficulties (e.g., alveolar hemorrhage [suggested by unexplained anemia or dyspnea]).

Management of Over-Anticoagulation and Bleeding

Because of the high risk of bleeding associated with excessive anticoagulation, measures to bring the INR down to the therapeutic range should be instituted as soon as possible. If the INR is less than 8 (and depending on the indication for anticoagulation), warfarin is temporarily discontinued and reinstituted once the INR has fallen to less than 5, providing there is no bleeding or only minor bleeding. If the INR is over 8 and there is no bleeding or minor bleeding, temporary discontinuation of warfarin is also recommended, but if the patient has other risk factors for bleeding, low-dose vitamin K either orally (0.5 to 2.5 mg) or intravenously (0.5 mg) will help to bring it within the therapeutic range in most patients.[28] Anaphylactoid reactions with intravenous vitamin K have rarely been reported, but their incidence seems to be lower with newer preparations and when the dose is administered very slowly. In patients with major bleeding, warfarin should be discontinued and anticoagulation reversed urgently with prothrombin complex concentrate (factors II, VII, IX, and X), or fresh frozen plasma if the concentrate is not available. In addition, vitamin K_1 (5 to 10 mg) by slow intravenous injection is recommended to sustain the reversal. Urgent reversal of anticoagulation is particularly important in patients with intracerebral bleeding as it will prevent the continued expansion of the hematoma (the latter is associated with an even poorer outcome).

Monitoring Vitamin K Antagonist Therapy

Close monitoring of VKA therapy will reduce the likelihood of over- or under-anticoagulation. Computer dosing software systems can help to maintain optimal control and thus significantly reduce the risk of bleeding and thromboembolic events, as well as highlighting non-attendance, triggering recall and review, and facilitating audit. Prescribers should also discuss with the patient the risks, benefits, and implications of long-term warfarin treatment.[29]

Inferior Vena Cava Filters

In patients who have contraindications for anticoagulation, and those who bleed or continue to have thromboembolism during anticoagulant therapy, placement of an inferior vena cava (IVC) filter has been undertaken. The PREPIC study, which included 400 patients with proximal DVT, with or without PE, followed up for 8 years, reported a significant reduction in the incidence of symptomatic PE but an increase in the incidence of DVT in patients treated with an IVC filter compared with those who received standard anticoagulant therapy. There was no significant difference in the development of postphlebitic syndrome or mortality between the two groups.[30] Complications of IVC filters include misplacement or embolization of the filter, vascular injury or thrombosis, pneumothorax, and air embolus. In view of the risk of IVC filter blockage as a result of thrombosis, it is recommended that a course of anticoagulant therapy should be commenced once the risk of bleeding has resolved. A limited number of small studies have reported no IVC thrombosis with the use of retrievable IVC filters.[31] NICE recommends that a temporary IVC filter should be offered to patients with proximal DVT or PE who cannot have anticoagulation treatment. The filter should be removed when the patient becomes eligible for anticoagulation treatment.[8]

Treatment of Pulmonary Embolism With Hemodynamic Instability

Massive PE may result in acute cor pulmonale or cardiogenic shock. This is more common in older patients. Such patients should be managed in an intensive therapy unit unless they have a terminal illness or a poor quality of life. In addition to cardiovascular and respiratory resuscitation, treatment options for patients with hemodynamic instability include thrombolysis. The most commonly used thrombolytic agent is recombinant tissue plasminogen activator. Intracranial hemorrhage occurs in about

3% of patients treated with thrombolytic agents. In patients with massive PE who have contraindications for thrombolysis, or when it has failed, catheter-assisted thrombus removal or surgical pulmonary embolectomy can be attempted. Despite these measures, mortality is very high in patients with PE complicated by cardiogenic shock.

Prevention

As noted previously, the risk of developing VTE increases in hospitalized older patients. Patients with stroke, patients with hip fractures, and patients who have had orthopedic surgery are at particularly high risk. In such patients, prophylaxis implementation rates have been reported to range between 13% and 64%. Prophylactic treatments are particularly underused in medical patients. A very large multinational cross-sectional survey designed to assess the VTE risk in an acute hospital setting reported 51.8% of patients to be at risk (64.4% surgical, mean age 60 years, and 41.5% medical patients, mean age 70 years). Of these, 58.5% of surgical and only 39.5% of medical patients were receiving appropriate thromboprophylaxis.[32]

In hospitalized acutely ill medical patients, unfractionated heparin (UFH), LMWH, and fondaparinux have all been shown to be effective in preventing VTE. LMWH is more effective than UFH.[33]

In patients undergoing total hip and knee replacements, LMWH, fondaparinux, apixaban, dabigatran, and rivaroxaban are all effective in preventing VTE.

Graduated Compression Stockings and Intermittent Pneumatic Compression

Graduated compression stockings (GCS) reduce the risk of VTE in surgical patients, but they are not superior to LMWHs. Ideally, they should be used in contribution with LMWHs, but in patients who are at high risk of bleeding, they can be used on their own. Because most older patients have peripheral vascular disease, the GCS should be used with extreme caution: inappropriate use has been known to cause ischemic complications. Use of thigh-length GCS in patients admitted to hospital with acute stroke is ineffective in preventing the occurrence of symptomatic or asymptomatic proximal DVT.[34]

Intermittent pneumatic compression reduces the risk of DVT (absolute risk reduction, 3.6%; 95% CI, 1.4-5.8) and mortality in immobile, hospitalized, older stroke patients.[35] After proximal DVT, approximately 60% of patients develop postthrombotic syndrome (PTS). A randomized, double-blind, placebo controlled trial with compression stockings did not show a reduction in the incidence of PTS.[36] Continued treatment with LMWH for 6 months after the diagnosis of DVT may reduce the risk of PTS.[37]

Prognosis

A population-based cohort study of patients with VTE found that the overall probable and definite (in parentheses) cumulative percentage of VTE recurrence at 7, 30, and 180 days and 1 and 10 years was 1.6% (0.2%), 5.2% (1.4%), 10.1% (4.1%), 12.9% (5.6%), and 30.4% (17.6%), respectively. The risk of recurrence was greatest in the first 6 to 12 months after the initial VTE. Independent predictors of first overall VTE recurrence included increasing age and body mass index, neurologic disease with paresis, malignant neoplasm, and neurosurgery.[38]

A prospective international registry, which studied clinical predictors for fatal PE in patients with VTE, has reported 3-month mortality and fatal PE rates of 8.65% and 1.68%, respectively. Patients with symptomatic nonmassive PE at presentation were found to have a 5.42-fold higher risk of fatal PE compared with patients with DVT without symptomatic PE ($P < .001$). The risk of fatal PE was 17.5 times higher in patients having a symptomatic massive PE. Other independent risk factors for fatal PE were immobilization for neurologic disease, age greater than 75 years, and cancer.[39]

Long-term complications of VTE include postthrombotic syndrome and chronic thromboembolic pulmonary hypertension.

CONCLUSION

VTE continues to be an important cause of morbidity and mortality in older people. There have been major advances in its diagnosis and treatment over the past 15 to 20 years. LMWHs and VKAs such as warfarin are effective in treatment and prevention. Orally administered factor Xa inhibitors and direct thrombin inhibitors are also therapeutic options. Whatever treatment is advocated in the future, prompt clinical diagnosis and carefully monitored institution of therapy (taking into account what is known about the pharmacology of these therapeutic agents in older people) will optimize efficacy and reduce morbidity and mortality from VTE.

KEY POINTS

- Venous thromboembolism (VTE) is an important cause of mortality in hospitalized patients and is more common in older adults.
- Risk factors for VTE, such as immobility, hip fracture, and stroke are more common in older people.
- In an older patient with stroke or recent orthopedic surgery, sudden onset of dyspnea, chest pain, or syncope should markedly increase the suspicion of underlying pulmonary embolism (PE).
- Computed tomography pulmonary angiography (CTPA) is the initial lung imaging modality of choice for nonmassive PE.
- For prevention and initial treatment of both deep vein thrombosis (DVT) and PE, low-molecular-weight heparins are the drugs of first choice.
- Older people are more sensitive to the anticoagulant effect of warfarin.
- Studies have reported a log-linear relationship between the intensity of anticoagulation and the risk of bleeding.
- In patients with massive PE, treatment options include thrombolysis or thromboembolectomy.
- Orally administered factor Xa inhibitors and direct thrombin inhibitors are available for prevention and treatment of VTE.
- Prompt clinical diagnosis and carefully monitored institution of therapy will reduce morbidity and mortality from VTE in the aging population.

For a complete list of references, please visit www.expertconsult.com.

KEY REFERENCES

8. National Institute for Health and Care Excellence: Venous thromboembolic diseases: the management of venous thromboembolic diseases and the role of thrombophilia testing (NICE guidelines [CG144]), 2012. http://www.nice.org.uk/guidance/cg144. Accessed September 26, 2015. Detailed clinical guidelines with key references.
13. Wells PS, Anderson DR, Rodger M, et al: Derivation of a simple clinical model to categorize patients' probability of pulmonary embolism: increasing the models utility with the SimpliRED D-dimer. Thromb Haemost 83:416–420, 2000.
14. Kearon C, Akl EA, Comerota AJ: Antithrombotic therapy for VTE disease: antithrombotic therapy and prevention of thrombosis, 9th ed: American College of Chest Physicians evidence-based clinical practice guidelines. Chest 141(Suppl):e419S–e494S, 2012.

15. Fennerty A, Dolben J, Thomas P, et al: Flexible induction dose regimen for warfarin and prediction of maintenance dose. BMJ 288:1268–1270, 1984.
16. Siguret V, Gouin I, Debray M, et al: Initiation of warfarin therapy in elderly medical inpatients: a safe and accurate regimen. Am J Med 118:137–142, 2005.
19. Heidbuchel H, Verhamme P, Alings M, et al: European Heart Rhythm Association practical guide on the use of new oral anticoagulants in patients with non-valvular atrial fibrillation. Europace 15:625–651, 2013. Valuable paper with very useful practical information about using new oral anticoagulants.

48 Asthma and Chronic Obstructive Pulmonary Disease

Paul Hernandez

DISEASES OF AIRFLOW OBSTRUCTION

Two common chronic lung diseases found in older adults are characterized by expiratory airflow obstruction on lung function testing: asthma and chronic obstructive pulmonary disease (COPD). In most cases, it is possible to distinguish asthma from COPD on the basis of a thorough clinical assessment (Table 48-1).[1,2] This discrimination is important, as certain aspects of management of the two conditions differ. A significant proportion of older individuals share features of both conditions to such an extent that they may be diagnosed with a relatively newly defined entity by the Global Initiative for Asthma (GINA) and Global Obstructive Lung Disease (GOLD) committees: asthma-COPD overlap syndrome (ACOS).[1,2] Individuals with ACOS tend to have greater symptom burden, more frequent exacerbations, and greater health care resource consumption.[1,2]

ASTHMA IN OLDER ADULTS

Introduction

Asthma is a common chronic lung disease that affects individuals of all ages. Previously, asthma was considered a disease primarily of children and young adults. Recent epidemiologic studies have dispelled this notion. The increased prevalence of asthma in older adults is the result of increased survival of children and young adults with asthma, a higher number of people with adult-onset asthma, and increased awareness among clinicians.[3] Despite the recent attention placed on asthma as a lung disease that can affects older adults, underdiagnosis and misdiagnosis are still common.[4] Clinically, asthma at older ages is associated with greater morbidity, greater mortality, and higher health care costs than in younger individuals. The presence of multiple morbidities and frailty contribute to diagnostic confusion and complicates management. More research is needed to help clinicians confront this growing challenge.

Asthma was defined by consensus in the 2014 GINA report as "a heterogeneous disease, usually characterized by chronic airway inflammation. It is defined by the history of respiratory symptoms such as wheeze, chest tightness, shortness of breath, and cough that vary of time and intensity, together with variable expiratory airflow limitation."[1] Many different asthma phenotypes exist, including allergic asthma, non-allergic asthma, late or adult-onset asthma, occupational asthma, and asthma with fixed airway obstruction (often misdiagnosed as COPD). Although allergic asthma, in particular, more commonly has its onset in childhood, any of the asthma phenotypes can be seen in older people.

Epidemiology

Globally, asthma is conservatively estimated to affect 300 million people of all ages and ethnicities with wide variability in prevalence from country to country, ranging from 1% to 18% of the population.[1,3,5-7] The prevalence of asthma has been rising for several decades, in parallel with increases in rates of allergy and changes (modernization and urbanization) in living conditions of the world's population. In the United States, population survey estimates of the prevalence of physician-diagnosed asthma in older adults have ranged from 4% to 11%, disproportionally affecting women.[8] Most surveys have relied on subjects reporting a physician diagnosis of asthma, which has its limitations, particularly in older adults. Asthma may be underdiagnosed because of misclassification as other conditions (e.g., COPD, heart disease), underreporting of symptoms by older individuals, and underuse of objective tests (e.g., spirometry) to confirm a clinical diagnosis. Asthma can also be overdiagnosed; a randomly sampled population study of physician-diagnosed asthma in Canada found no objective evidence of current asthma in one third of subjects studied.[9] Older age at time of asthma diagnosis was associated with an overdiagnosis of asthma. Despite these limitations of epidemiologic studies, it is apparent that asthma affects a significant percentage of older individuals and that the numbers are expected to continue to rise over the coming years.

Asthma in older people places a high burden on both patients and society. Older adults with asthma have higher rates of hospitalization and proportionally increased health care costs compared to younger adults and children with asthma.[10] In part, this relates to the complexity of management of asthma in the setting of multiple comorbidities. According to the U.S. Centers for Disease Control and Prevention, asthma deaths in older adults account for more than 50% of asthma fatalities annually, with an approximately 5.8 asthma deaths per 100,000 reported in the years 2001 through 2003.[4,5] Mortality rates have been estimated to be fourfold higher in individuals older than 65 years compared to adults with asthma who are younger than 65 years, with a tendency for higher mortality rates in women.[10]

Pathophysiology

Asthma is a heterogeneous condition that develops from complex interactions among genotypic and environmental factors. A number of candidate genes have been identified that predispose to asthma. Environmental risk factors that play a role in asthma pathogenesis include the amount and timing of exposure to indoor and outdoor allergens, tobacco smoke, respiratory tract infections, air pollution, occupational sensitizers and irritants, and diet.[1]

Asthma is a chronic inflammatory airway disease involving many inflammatory cells and mediators. Although the clinical expression of asthma can be variable and episodic, airway inflammation is typically a constant feature of the disease. The key inflammatory cells in asthma include mast cells, eosinophils, T lymphocytes, and macrophages. Neutrophils play a role in certain asthma phenotypes (e.g., smokers, severe and late-onset asthma). Numerous cellular mediators are released by inflammatory and structural cells in asthma, including cytokines (e.g., interleukin [IL]-4, IL-5, IL-13), cysteinyl leukotrienes, chemokines, histamine, and nitric oxide, which amplifies the inflammatory response through recruitment and activation of additional inflammatory cells. Structural airway changes are characteristic of asthma. Airway narrowing results from increased airway smooth muscle contraction, thickening of airway wall (e.g., smooth muscle

TABLE 48-1 Differentiating Asthma and Chronic Obstructive Pulmonary Disease (COPD)

Feature	Asthma	COPD
Age of onset	Usually < 40 years	Usually > 40 years
Exposure history	Unrelated	Smoking > 10 pack-years, or other inhaled noxious substances
Atopy, allergies	Frequent in patient or family members	Unrelated
		Unrelated
Symptoms	Intermittent, variable	Persistent
Sputum production	Infrequent	Common
Clinical course	Stable, with exacerbations	Progressive, with exacerbations
Lung function	May be normal, ± reversibility and bronchial hyperresponsiveness	Persistent airflow obstruction, incompletely reversible
Chest radiography	Normal	Hyperinflation
Sputum inflammation	Usually eosinophilic	Usually neutrophilic

Data from Global Initiative for Asthma: Global strategy for asthma management and prevention 2014, http://www.ginasthma.org/; Global Initiative for Chronic Obstructive Lung Disease: Global strategy for the diagnosis, management and prevention of COPD 2015, http://www.goldcopd.org.

hypertrophy, basement membrane thickening, edema, and inflammatory cell infiltration), and mucus hypersecretion. Another important feature of asthma is airway hyperresponsiveness, an exaggerated bronchoconstriction response to various stimuli.[11]

The adaptive changes of the immune system with aging have implications for the pathophysiology of asthma. Traditionally, atopy (immunoglobulin E [IgE] sensitization to at least one antigen) or allergy was thought to be associated more strongly with asthma in childhood than with late-onset asthma.[12] Total IgE levels and antigen-specific sensitization fall with normal aging.[8,13] The Epidemiology and Natural History of Asthma[14] study examined asthma in older (>65 years old) compared to younger individuals; older individuals with asthma had lower total IgE levels, fewer positive skin prick tests, and less atopic clinical conditions (e.g., allergic rhinosinusitis or atopic dermatitis).[14] However, some recent studies have shown that older individuals with asthma are more likely to demonstrate allergen sensitization than older individuals without asthma, albeit to a lesser extent than younger individuals with asthma.[15] The most common aeroallergens (e.g., cat, dust mite, cockroach) to which older individuals with asthma are sensitized, not surprisingly, varies based on characteristics (e.g., urban vs. rural) of the population studied. The role and importance of atopy in asthma pathogenesis in older adults clearly needs further investigation. There is also a reduction in T lymphocyte number and activity with aging; the resultant immunosenescence diminishes the effectiveness of vaccinations and increases susceptibility to viral and bacterial infection.[8] Respiratory tract infection is an important cause of poor asthma control and exacerbations in older adults. Whether respiratory tract infections, particularly viral, are important in asthma pathogenesis in older adults, as has been proposed in children, needs further study.

Diagnosis

The diagnosis of asthma is based on clinical assessment (i.e., history and physical examination) and objective testing. Asthma symptoms tend to vary over time (often worse at night or early morning) and in intensity. Typical symptoms include wheeze, dyspnea, chest tightness, cough, and, to a lesser extent, sputum production that occur spontaneously or may be triggered by various stimuli (e.g., air quality, aeroallergens, respiratory tract infections, exercise, scents).[1] During physical examination of people with asthma, they may exhibit normal breathing or they may show signs of airflow obstruction (e.g., wheeze, prolonged expiratory phase), hyperinflation (e.g., shortened tracheal length, barrel chest, diminished breath sound intensity), or, during severe exacerbations, increased respiratory difficulty (e.g., tachypnea, tachycardia, pulsus paradoxus, cyanosis, diaphoresis, accessory muscle use, changes in mental status). The physical examination is often more relevant to assess for conditions that may mimic asthma symptoms.

BOX 48-1 Differential Diagnosis of Asthma in Older Adults

- Lung diseases
  - Chronic obstructive pulmonary disease (COPD)
  - Asthma-COPD overlap syndrome (ACOS)
  - Bronchiectasis
  - Interstitial lung disease
- Heart disease
  - Congestive heart failure
- Upper airway diseases
  - Chronic rhinosinusitis
  - Vocal cord dysfunction
- Hyperventilation
- Deconditioning

Asthma symptoms may be poorly perceived, underreported, or misinterpreted to relate to other causes in older adults. History should include assessment of risk factors for asthma, such as presence of personal or family history of atopy and occupational history. The differential diagnosis for asthma in older people is broad, as many other conditions manifest with typical symptoms of asthma (Box 48-1). Differentiating asthma from COPD can be difficult at times (see Table 48-1). Overcoming the diagnostic challenge of asthma in older adults requires careful clinical assessment and additional objective tests beyond pulmonary function tests (PFTs) not typically required in children or young adults.

Objective testing is required to confirm a clinical suspicion of asthma. PFTs are used to demonstrate variable airflow obstruction and/or bronchial hyperresponsiveness, hallmark features of asthma. Unfortunately, PFTs may be difficult to perform in some older individuals because of physical or cognitive impairments or they may be difficult to interpret because of poor reliability of predicted normal values in this age group. Newer techniques to reliably measure pulmonary function (e.g., forced oscillometry) are being developed and validated that require less cooperation and effort on the part of the patient.[16]

Pulmonary Function Tests

PFTs are essential to confirm a clinical suspicion of asthma in all ages, especially in older adults. Reversible airflow obstruction is a cardinal feature of asthma; however, it may be absent in individuals with mild disease or who are well controlled on treatment. Spirometry, a simple and widely available yet underutilized PFT is used to evaluate for the presence of reversible airflow obstruction. Spirometry assesses the volume of air forcibly inhaled and exhaled as a function of time. Spirometry reports provide tabular numerical values and graphical representations of volume versus time and flow versus volume. International standards for spirometry equipment, technical personnel performing the test, test procedure, quality measures, reference values, test interpretation, and reporting have been well described.[17,18] It is important that PFT laboratories choose reference values that are derived from the age range of their patient population.

Airflow obstruction can be confirmed on spirometry by demonstrating a reduction in the ratio of the forced expiratory volume at 1 second (FEV_1) to forced vital capacity (FVC). It is important to use the lower limit of normal (below the fifth percentile of the predicted value) rather than a fixed ratio (i.e., 0.70) to determine abnormality. This is especially true in older adults, as the FEV_1/FVC ratio decreases with normal aging. Data from the Third National Health and Nutrition Examination Survey (NHANES-III) in the United States showed that among healthy older adults who had never smoked, one fifth of those with observed FEV_1/FVC% above the NHANES-III fifth percentile had FEV_1/FVC% ratios less than 70%.[19] Patients with mild airflow obstruction involving predominantly peripheral, small airways may have a preserved FEV_1 and FEV_1/FVC but reduced mid and terminal forced expiratory flows (FEF25%-75%, FEF75%) resulting in a concave shape to the expiratory limb, compared to normal shape, of the flow-volume spirogram (Figure 48-1).

Testing for reversibility of expiratory airflow obstruction or excessive variability in lung function can be achieved in a number of ways.[1] Spirometry can be done before and shortly after (10 to 15 minutes) the administration of a short-acting bronchodilator (e.g., 200 to 400 µg inhaled salbutamol). An increase in FEV_1 of at least 12% *and* 200 mL from baseline confirms reversibility. Alternatively, patients can be taught to use a simple handheld device to measure and record peak expiratory flow (PEF) twice daily over a period of weeks. Average daily diurnal variability in PEF more than 10% over a 2-week period or an increase in PEF more than 20% after 4 weeks of treatment for asthma confirms excessive variability in lung function.

Some individuals with asthma do not have evidence of variable or reversible airflow obstruction; in these individuals, it may be necessary to test for bronchial hyperresponsiveness (BHR) to confirm a diagnosis of asthma.[1] Bronchial challenge testing can be safely achieved in older adults by a number of means, including the inhalation of methacholine, histamine, mannitol, and hypertonic saline, or by eucapnic hyperventilation. Methacholine bronchoprovocation, the most commonly used clinical test, involves inhalation of progressively greater concentrations of methacholine with regular measurement of spirometry. A positive test is a greater than 20% fall in FEV_1 compared to baseline at a set concentration of methacholine (e.g., < 8 mg/mL). BHR is more prevalent in older adults, independent of other associated factors, including prechallenge lung function, smoking exposure, and atopy.[20] BHR is associated with an increase in respiratory symptoms, rate of lung function decline, and mortality. Although BHR is not specific for asthma, in the absence of treatment with antiinflammatory medications, a negative test is useful to rule out asthma as a cause of current respiratory symptoms.

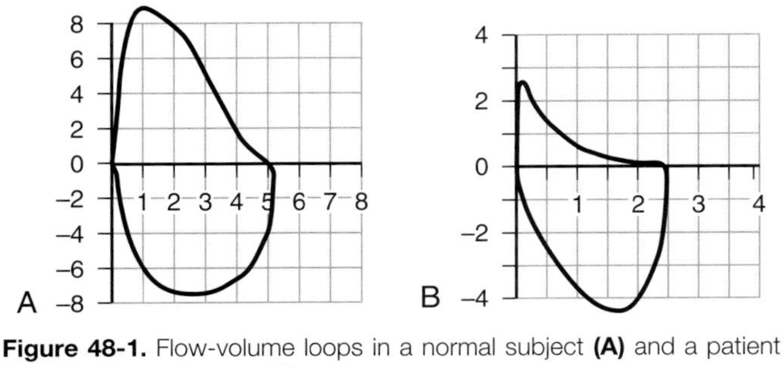

Figure 48-1. Flow-volume loops in a normal subject **(A)** and a patient with airflow obstruction **(B).**

Other PFTs are rarely indicated to assess for asthma or obstructive lung disease.[18] Lung volumes may reveal a pattern of hyperinflation (increased functional residual capacity) and gas trapping (increased residual volume [RV]; increased ratio of RV to total lung capacity [TLC]). Diffusing capacity and respiratory muscle strength are not usually affected by asthma. Measurements of lung volume, gas exchange, and respiratory muscle strength are of greater utility to assess for other respiratory conditions in the differential, for example, to assess for restrictive pattern with impaired gas exchange in patients with interstitial lung disease.

Other Laboratory Tests

Atopy can be assessed with allergy skin tests or a blood test for specific IgE. Atopic individuals may have an increase in eosinophils on differential complete blood count. Although the presence of atopy increases the likelihood of asthma as the cause of respiratory symptoms, it is not sensitive or specific for asthma. Awareness of atopy can be helpful when counseling patients regarding allergen avoidance. Other investigations are primarily used in suspected asthma to assess for conditions in the differential (see Box 48-1). These tests include chest imaging (chest radiograph, chest computed tomography scan) to assess for parenchymal lung disease, and electrocardiogram and echocardiogram to assess for heart disease (e.g., congestive heart failure). Additional investigations may be required based on the presenting symptoms and signs.

Management

Long-term goals of asthma care have been described by GINA (Box 48-2).[1] Management of asthma in older adult patients does not differ from the approach taken with younger adults. A management approach that aims to achieve control of asthma symptoms will also help to prevent asthma exacerbations. An alternative approach to asthma management, less applicable in primary care because of the lack of access to the testing required, involves the adjustment of treatment based on noninvasive measurements of airway inflammation.[1,21,22] A number of international and national asthma guidelines recommend that in management of moderate to severe asthma in specialized asthma care centers, induced sputum cell counts, specifically eosinophils, can be used to titrate antiinflammatory medication.[1,21,22] Despite the greater ease of measurement, some guidelines caution against the use of fractional concentration of exhaled nitric oxide as a noninvasive marker of airway inflammation because of its poor specificity in the monitoring of asthma management.[1,21]

Regular assessment of asthma control and future risk for exacerbations and lung function loss is essential in the management of asthma. Asthma control can be assessed clinically by enquiring about asthma symptoms and the need for rescue medication.[1,21] GINA has recommended four simple questions to determine the level of asthma symptom control over the preceding 4 weeks

BOX 48-2 Global Initiative for Asthma Goals of Asthma Care

Achieve control of asthma symptoms.
Maintain normal activity levels.
Minimize the risk of exacerbations.
Minimize lung function loss.
Minimize risk of treatment side effects.

TABLE 48-2 Global Initiative for Asthma Assessment of Asthma Symptom Control

In the Past 4 Weeks, Has the Patient Had ...	Response
Daytime asthma symptoms more than twice a week?	Yes__ No __
Nighttime awakening because of asthma?	Yes__ No __
Reliever medication needed more than twice a week?	Yes__ No __
Activity limitation due to asthma?	Yes__ No __
Level of Asthma Symptom Control	**Number of Yes Responses**
Well controlled	None
Partially controlled	1-2
Poorly controlled	3-4

(Table 48-2). Other national asthma guidelines include questions about time missed from work (or school in children), frequency of exacerbations, and monitoring of lung function using PEF meter or spirometry relative to the individual's usual best values to assess asthma control.[21] Risk factors for asthma exacerbations beyond poor asthma control include past history of recent or severe (e.g., requiring intensive care unit admission or intubation) exacerbations, poor baseline lung function, inadequate treatment with inhaled corticosteroids (ICSs), comorbidities (including obesity, smoking, allergen sensitization), and poor psychosocial situation.[1]

A bigger challenge clinically than assessing asthma control is assessing asthma severity. This cannot be done at the time of initial assessment. Instead, assessment of asthma severity is done retrospectively over months and is based on the medication burden required to achieve symptom control once other barriers have been managed (e.g., comorbidities, adherence, and inhaler technique). As for the level of symptom control, asthma severity may fluctuate over time. However, management decisions are not based on severity of disease but rather on the goals of asthma care (see Box 48-2).

GINA recommends a stepwise approach to asthma management that combines nonpharmacologic and pharmacologic treatments with adjustments based on clinical assessment and response to therapy.[1] Individuals with asthma should become partners in their own care, necessitating an understanding of their disease and its treatments and an awareness of patient preferences by the health care providers. Good communication and collaboration between individual with asthma and health care providers are essential. Collaborative self-management education, ideally delivered by a trained respiratory educator, will provide patients with knowledge, skills, and self-efficacy to achieve the best clinical outcomes. Essential components of such a program include a written action plan to recognize and self-manage asthma worsening or exacerbation, environmental control, identification and avoidance of triggers, proper inhaler technique, monitoring of control (symptoms ± PEF), and better understanding of the disease and medications used to treat asthma.[1,21,22] Compared to usual care, self-management education has been shown to reduce hospitalizations (relative risk [RR], 0.64; 95% confidence interval [CI], 0.50-0.82); emergency department visits (RR, 0.82; 95% CI, 0.73-0.94); unscheduled doctor visits (RR, 0.68; 95% CI, 0.56-0.81); days off work or school (RR, 0.79; 95% CI, 0.67-0.93); and nocturnal asthma (RR, 0.67; 95% CI, 0.0.56-0.79).[23]

Asthma medications are categorized as relievers, controllers, or add-ons. All patients should have access to a *reliever* medication, a fast-onset bronchodilator for rapid relief of asthma symptoms. Individuals who require only a low-dose ICS (a controller medication) to maintain asthma control should have a short-acting β_2-agonist (SABA) inhaler as a reliever (Figure 48-2, steps 1 and 2). Individuals with more severe asthma who require an ICS plus an add-on controller (e.g., long-acting β-agonist [LABA] inhaler) to maintain asthma control (see Figure 48-2, steps 3, 4, and 5) have the option of choosing a LABA that is also fast-acting (e.g., formoterol). In this instance, there is the option to use a *s*ingle ICS/LABA inhaler as both *m*aintenance *a*nd *r*eliever *t*herapy (SMART) without the need for a separate SABA inhaler as a reliever.[1,21]

The primary *controller* medication in asthma is ICS, essential to treat airway inflammation characteristic of this condition. Regular ICS use results in better asthma control, improved lung function, and improved health-related quality of life and reduces the likelihood of exacerbation and asthma-related death. Numerous ICSs are available; GINA and other guidelines provide guidance by categorizing the dose range for each ICS as low, medium, and high.[1,21,22] After achieving initial asthma control for 3 months, the lowest dose of ICS necessary to maintain control should be sought. This minimizes the risks of long-term ICS use, which includes local (e.g., oropharyngeal candidiasis, dysphonia) and systemic (e.g., ecchymosis, osteoporosis, cataracts, suppression of hypothalamic-pituitary axis) adverse effects. To further reduce the potential for adverse effects from ICSs, patients should be taught proper inhaler technique; for example, a pressurized metered-dose inhaler should be used with a spacer or valved-holding chamber, and the mouth should be rinsed after drug inhalation.

Leukotriene receptor antagonists (LTRAs) are oral antiinflammatory controller medications. LTRAs are less effective than ICSs for controlling asthma but are an alternative in patients who cannot tolerate or refuse to take ICSs. LTRAs are also used as *add-on* medications when asthma control cannot be achieved with a low-dose ICS (see Figure 48-2, steps 3, 4, and 5), particularly in individuals with concomitant allergic rhinosinusitis.

The preferred *add-on* medication for older patients with asthma is LABA, usually given in combination with an ICS in the same inhaler. The ICS/LABA combination inhaler increases adherence and reduces the risk of treating asthma with LABA monotherapy for maintenance, a strategy associated with increased asthma mortality,[24] overusing ICS and LABA in separate inhalers. Theophylline is another class of oral add-on bronchodilator medication. The usefulness of theophylline in older adults is limited because of the need to monitor serum drug levels, potential for drug-drug interactions, and serious adverse effects, including gastrointestinal intolerance, cardiac arrhythmias, and seizures. Omalizumab is a monoclonal anti-IgE antibody indicated in the treatment of moderate to severe allergic asthma. It is administered by subcutaneous injection every 2 to 4 weeks in a dosing regimen based on total IgE level and body weight. In a very small minority of individuals with severe, poorly controlled asthma, oral corticosteroids (e.g., prednisone) are required as chronic add-on maintenance therapy. With chronic use of systemic corticosteroids, there is risk for many side effects, including osteoporosis, diabetes mellitus, cataracts, myopathy, and increased susceptibility to infections. Systemic corticosteroids are most useful in the treatment of moderate to severe acute exacerbations of asthma. Individuals with moderate to severe, poorly controlled asthma who require add-on therapy beyond ICS/LABA and LTRA should be referred to an asthma specialist.

In individuals with severe asthma that remains poorly controlled despite addressing nonpharmacologic issues and maximizing pharmacotherapy, bronchial thermoplasty may be a treatment option. Bronchial thermoplasty, an intervention delivered via the fiber optic bronchoscope, has been shown to reduce the frequency of severe asthma attacks and emergency department visits.[25] There is uncertainty regarding the long-term benefits of bronchial thermoplasty, as it is a treatment that is not widely available and has not been studied in older adults.

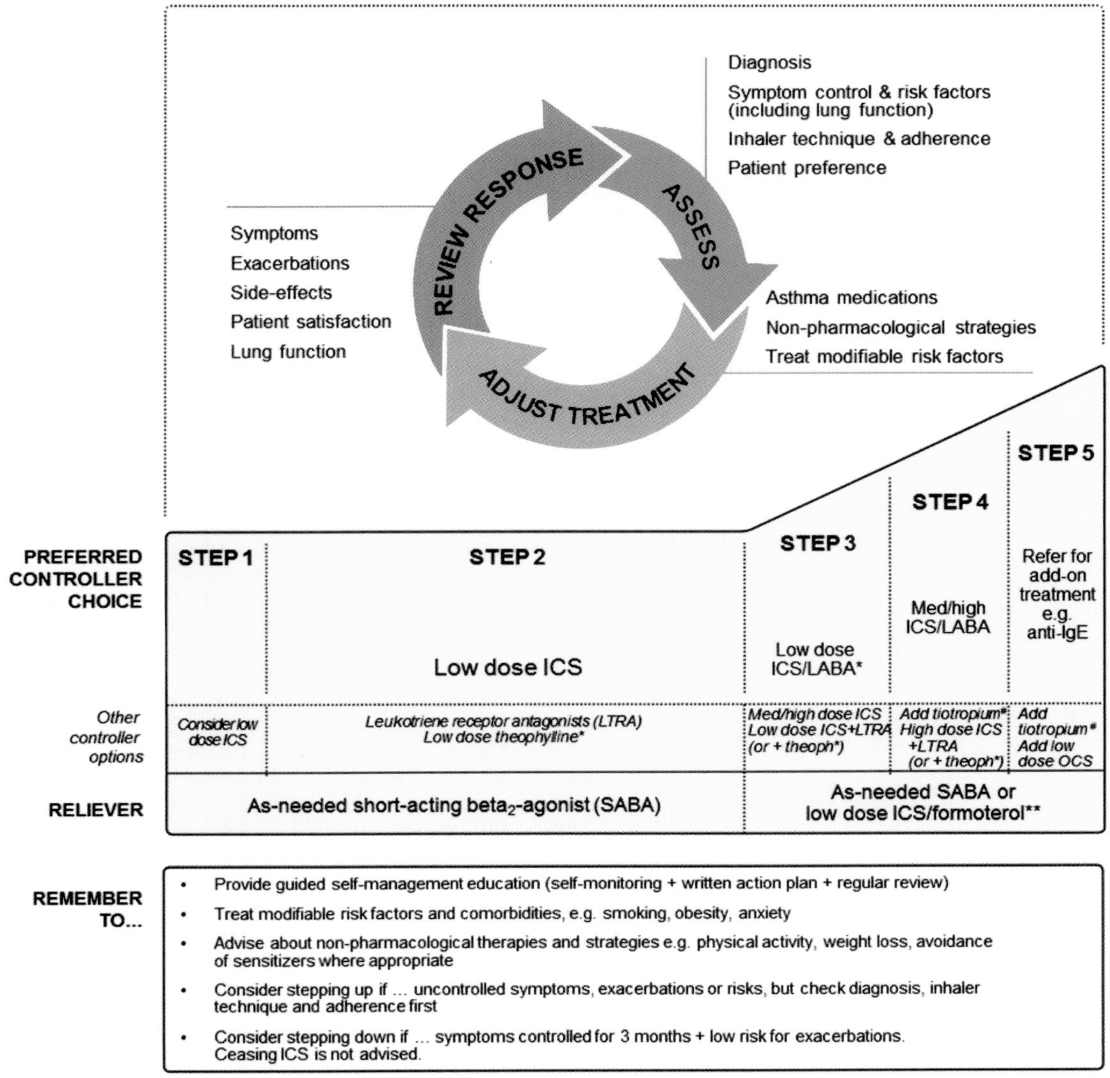

ICS: inhaled corticosteroids; LABA: long-acting beta$_2$-agonist; med: medium dose; OCS: oral corticosteroids; anti-IgE: anti-immunoglobulin E therapy. See Box 3-6 for low, medium and high doses of ICS for adults, adolescents and children 6–11 years.

* For children 6–11 years, theophylline is not recommended, and the preferred Step 3 treatment is medium dose ICS.

** Low dose ICS/formoterol is the reliever medication for patients prescribed low dose budesonide/formoterol or low dose beclometasone/formoterol maintenance and reliever therapy.

Tiotropium by soft-mist inhaler is an add-on treatment for patients with a history of exacerbations; it is not indicated in children <18 years.

See Chapter 3 Part D (p.50) for management of exercise-induced bronchoconstriction.

Figure 48-2. Global Initiative for Asthma guidelines step-wise treatment algorithm. *Anti-IgE,* Anti-immunoglobulin E; *ICS,* inhaled corticosteroid; *LABA,* long-acting β_2-agonist; *LTRA,* leukotriene receptor antagonist; *OCS,* oral corticosteroid; *SABA,* short-acting β_2-agonist. *(Global Strategy for Asthma Management and Prevention 2015, © Global Initiative for Asthma [GINA] all rights reserved. Available from* http://www.ginasthma.org.*)*

There are a few special considerations when treating asthma in older adults. The presence of multiple comorbid illnesses may pose diagnostic challenges and affect treatment choices. Treatment of comorbid illnesses may require medications that are contraindicated or that complicate asthma, for example, β-blockers required for ischemic heart disease. Frailty and cognitive impairment may result in improper inhaler technique and poor drug delivery. Complex treatment regimens and polypharmacy can contribute to poor adherence. Cognitive impairment may also result in poor perception of asthma symptoms and limit the value of self-management education management strategies. Despite these challenges, the TENOR study demonstrated that older patients with asthma had lower health resource use and better health-related quality of life than younger adults with asthma, despite having worse lung function.[14] With good management, older adults with asthma can achieve good outcomes.

CHRONIC OBSTRUCTIVE PULMONARY DISEASE IN OLDER ADULTS

Introduction

COPD is a major cause of morbidity and the fourth leading cause of death among adults worldwide.[3] The predominant risk factor for development of COPD is cigarette smoking. The 2015 GOLD report defined this chronic lung disease as "a common preventable and treatable disease, characterized by persistent airflow limitation that is usually progressive and associated with an enhanced chronic inflammatory response in the airways and the lung to noxious particles and gases. Exacerbations and comorbidities contribute to the overall severity in individual patients."[2] The definition emphasizes a few characteristic features of COPD that deserve mention:

- "Treatable and preventable" despite the progressive, irreversible nature of this condition, there is hope for individuals with COPD. Treatment can improve the burden of this illness at all disease stages, and through primary and secondary prevention (e.g., smoking cessation), there is the chance to alter the natural history of COPD.
- "Chronic inflammatory response … to noxious particles" highlights the importance of cigarette smoking in the pathogenesis. Although the type of inflammation in COPD differs from that of asthma, this is an inflammatory disease affecting airways and lung parenchyma.
- "Comorbidities contribute to the overall severity" underlines the growing awareness that COPD is not just a lung disease, and therefore successful management requires identification and treatment of multiple morbidities that often coexist in the individual with COPD.

The removal of any mention of diagnostic terms associated with past COPD definitions that were based on either the symptom of chronic, productive cough (i.e., chronic bronchitis) or anatomic changes (i.e., emphysema) reflects the shift to a more functional definition that is easier to operationalize in clinical practice and research.

Epidemiology

Studies have revealed wide variability in COPD prevalence by country, with estimates ranging from 4% to 20% of adults older than 40 years.[3] This variability may reflect differing study methodologies and definitions of COPD, age of population, and exposure to risk factors in the population studied. Burden of Obstructive Lung Disease (BOLD) is a population-based study in which participants from many countries (38 completed or in progress in 2015) complete standardized questionnaires and high-quality postbronchodilator spirometry so that the researchers can assess the prevalence, risk factors, social and economic burden of COPD.[26] The application of rigorous sampling and assessment methods has revealed the discord between prevalence statistics generated from administrative databases or population surveys and the reality. For example, in Canada, based on the methodology from BOLD, the overall prevalence of COPD in the Canadian Obstructive Lung Disease (COLD) study was 11.6% (95% CI, 9.9-13.3), two to three times greater than the prevalence reported by Statistics Canada from previous community health surveys.[27] COPD often goes underdiagnosed until advanced stages of the disease; as a result, prevalence is generally underestimated in surveys that rely on self-reported doctor diagnosis without objective measurement of lung function.

As with many other chronic diseases, age is a major risk factor for COPD. The Latin American Project for the Investigation of Obstructive lung Disease (PLATINO) study reported that the prevalence of COPD in five major Latin American cities increased with age; in adults aged 40 to 49 years, prevalence ranged from 2.2% to 8.4%; in adults aged 50 to 59 years, prevalence was 4.5% to 16.2%; and in adults 60 years and older, prevalence was 18.4% to 30.3%.[28] Similarly, in Australia, the BOLD study reported that the diagnosis of non–fully reversible airflow obstruction (e.g., COPD) increased with age: 40 to 54 years, 6.0%; 55 to 74 years, 16.6%; 75 years and older, 40.0%.[29] In the Australian study, prevalence of COPD was similar between men and women in the younger adult age group but much greater in men than in women in older adults; in contrast, in the PLATINO study, men outnumbered women in all age groups.

Cigarette smoking is the major risk factor for COPD. The global tobacco epidemic is alarming; death from COPD related to smoking is estimated at 1 million persons annually and is expected to continue to rise.[30] There is a lag of many years, often decades, before the inflammatory response and lung injury caused by smoking manifests clinically as COPD. This contributes to the underdiagnosis and delayed diagnosis of COPD. Prevalence of COPD globally reflects smoking rates from decades past, particularly in developed countries where inhalation of other noxious substances (e.g., smoke from indoor solid fuels used for heating and cooking) is a less common cause of COPD. COPD prevalence is expected to continue to increase worldwide for many decades, particularly in Asia and Africa, as a result of increased smoking rates and population aging.

Morbidity and health care costs related to COPD increase with age and presence of comorbidities. The Global Burden of Disease Study reported the burden of chronic conditions, including COPD, based on sum of life years lost due to premature mortality and years lived with disability (i.e., the disability adjusted life years).[31] In 1990, COPD was the twelfth leading cause of disability adjusted life years lost worldwide and is projected to be seventh in 2030.[31,32] In terms of mortality, COPD was the sixth leading cause of death worldwide in 1990 and projected to be fourth in 2030.[31,32] The projected increased mortality globally is largely accounted for by increasing prevalence of COPD among woman and in underdeveloped countries.

The economic burden of COPD is enormous and growing. In United States, in 2008 the annual direct costs related to COPD were $29.5 billion and indirect costs were $20.4 billion.[2] Care of patients hospitalized for acute exacerbation of COPD (AECOPD) accounts for the greatest proportion of total direct health care costs and increases with increasing disease severity.[33] In Canada, AECOPD is the number one cause for hospitalization among ambulatory-care sensitive chronic conditions in adults.[34] Individuals with COPD hospitalized for another reason have higher age-adjusted mortality and length of stay compared to individuals without COPD.

Pathophysiology

COPD is a chronic lung disease resulting from inflammation, fibrosis, and destruction of small and large airways, lung parenchyma, and lung vasculature. Inflammation results from chronic exposure to inhaled noxious substances and can continue long after the exposure stops (e.g., after smoking cessation). The type of inflammatory response in COPD differs from that in asthma; the predominant inflammatory cells are $CD8^+$ T lymphocytes, neutrophils, and macrophages.[35] These inflammatory cells release various mediators that amplify the inflammatory response through chemotaxis of other inflammatory cells and release of proinflammatory cytokines and growth factors. Individuals who develop COPD are prone to an imbalance in proteases (e.g., elastase) and antiprotease (e.g., α_1-antitrypsin) and between oxidants and antioxidants that can contribute to inflammation, fibrosis, and tissue destruction.[35]

The earliest pathologic change in COPD is thought to be inflammation of the small airways less than 2 mm in diameter (e.g., bronchiolitis).[36,37] Because small airways make only a minor contribution to the overall resistance to expiratory airflow as assessed on standard PFTs (e.g., spirometry), these changes are often "silent" and undetected clinically.[38] In larger airways, mucous gland hypertrophy, mucus hypersecretion, epithelial changes, and mucociliary dysfunction result in poor mucus clearance, increased frequency of productive cough (e.g., chronic bronchitis), and increased risk for bronchial infection. Alveolar wall destruction results in enlarged airspaces distal to terminal bronchioles (e.g., emphysema). Reduced elastic recoil from loss of lung parenchymal attachments to airways (from emphysema) results in further small airway narrowing and collapse. With progressive expiratory airflow limitation, air is trapped distal to small airways, resulting in lung hyperinflation and gas trapping.

Vascular injury, particularly of small muscular pulmonary arteries, is common in COPD. The combination of vascular changes, expiratory airflow limitation, and emphysema can result in significant ventilation perfusion (V/Q) abnormalities.[39] As COPD progresses, these V/Q abnormalities manifest clinically as a reduction in diffusing capacity on PFTs and abnormalities on arterial blood gases (e.g., hypoxemia and/or hypercapnia). In advanced stages of disease, cor pulmonale and pulmonary hypertension may develop.[35]

Lung function loss occurs in the normally aging lung and is similar to that observed in COPD as a consequence of alveolar enlargement without wall destruction, so-called senile emphysema.[40] Aging hallmarks that contribute to age-related COPD pathogenesis and progression include epigenetic alterations, loss of proteostasis, mitochondrial dysfunction, senescence, and altered adaptive immune responses.[40]

As indicated, COPD is also characterized by extrapulmonary, systemic manifestations (Box 48-3). Systemic inflammation, chronic hypoxemia, malnutrition, adverse effects of medications, physical inactivity, social isolation, and shared common risk factors (e.g., cigarette smoking) all play a role. Even in clinically stable patients, blood levels of markers of systemic inflammation are elevated, including C-reactive protein, fibrinogen, tumor necrosis factor-α (TNF-α), and IL-6.[35] Malnutrition is a common finding in patients with moderate to severe COPD and is an independent risk factor for mortality.[41] Fat mass and fat-free mass are depleted; it is believed that weight loss, in particular, skeletal muscle mass loss, is associated with elevated proinflammatory cytokines (IL-6 and TNF-α).[42] Resting energy expenditure is also elevated in patients with COPD and contributes to the negative energy balance, which may be reversed by nutritional supplements when coupled with an exercise training program.[42]

Acute Exacerbation of Chronic Obstructive Pulmonary Disease

The slow, progressive course of COPD can be punctuated by acute events associated with worsening of symptoms beyond the usual day-to-day variability for that individual, referred to as AECOPD. Typical symptoms of AECOPD last for at least 2 days and include increased dyspnea and change in sputum (i.e., volume, purulence, and/or viscosity).[43] Other possible manifestations include increased wheeze and cough, symptoms of an upper respiratory tract infection, fever, tachypnea, tachycardia, worsening lung function, and increase in systemic markers of inflammation. Operational definitions of AECOPD for clinical trials and epidemiologic studies often require individuals to recognize the event and change their usual COPD management, either on their own or on the advice of a health care professional. However, based on cohort studies in which subjects record daily symptom diaries and lung function at home, it is apparent that as many as 50% of AECOPD events go unreported and untreated but still have a negative impact on outcomes.[44] Severity of AECOPD events are categorized as mild (unreported or not requiring new medications), moderate (managed on outpatient basis with addition of antibiotics and/or systemic corticosteroids), or severe (leading to hospitalization).[2] These events are usually precipitated by a viral or bacterial respiratory tract infection or exposure to air pollutants. AECOPD events are associated with more rapid decline in lung function and health-related quality of life, increased mortality, and increased consumption of health care resources.[45] Up to 50% of the total cost of care of COPD results from treatment of AECOPD requiring hospitalization.[33] Evidence-based recommendations for prevention and management of AECOPD have been published.[2,45]

BOX 48-3 Common Systemic Manifestations and Comorbidities of Chronic Obstructive Pulmonary Disease

Cachexia
Skeletal muscle wasting and dysfunction
Osteopenia and osteoporosis
Cardiovascular disease
Lung cancer
Glaucoma and cataracts
Metabolic syndrome
Depression and anxiety

Diagnosis

The clinical diagnosis of COPD relies on the presence of risk factors, elucidation of typical symptoms and signs, and confirmation of non–fully reversible expiratory airflow obstruction (i.e., reduced postbronchodilator FEV_1/FVC) on spirometry. Risk factors for COPD should be sought on history, including age, exposure to noxious inhaled substances (e.g., cigarette smoke, occupational dusts), and family history of COPD. Typical symptoms of COPD include dyspnea, exercise intolerance, cough, sputum production, wheeze, and frequent or severe respiratory tract infections. These historical factors have been combined in targeted case-finding tools for diagnosing COPD, such as the Canadian Lung Health Test (Box 48-4).[46]

Physical examination to detect signs of airflow obstruction and hyperinflation has low sensitivity, particularly in mild disease.[47] Airflow obstruction can result in prolonged forced expiratory time, prolongation of the expiratory phase of breath sounds, and wheeze on chest auscultation. Signs of hyperinflation include shortened cricothyroid-sternal notch length, increased anteroposterior diameter of the chest (e.g., barrel chest), hyperresonance to percussion, and diminished breath sound intensity on auscultation. The absence of signs of COPD in an individual

BOX 48-4 Canadian Lung Health Test

Are you a smoker or ex-smoker? Are you older than 40 years of age?

1. Do you cough regularly?
2. Do you cough up phlegm regularly?
3. Do even simple chores make you short of breath?
4. Do you wheeze when you exert yourself (exercise, go up stairs)?
5. Do you get many colds, and do your colds usually last longer than your friends' colds?

If you answered yes to one or more of these five questions, you should undergo spirometry.

with risk factors and typical symptoms of COPD should not deter the clinician from arranging for spirometry to confirm the diagnosis. In advanced disease, signs of systemic manifestations and complications of COPD, such as peripheral muscle wasting and signs of right-sided heart failure, may be evident.

Pulmonary Function Tests and Other Laboratory Investigations

As in asthma, spirometry is an essential test in making the diagnosis of COPD. Spirometry should be performed before and after administration of a short-acting bronchodilator. Reduced post-bronchodilator FEV_1/FVC confirms the presence of non–fully reversible airflow obstruction. It is important to use the 95% confidence interval for this ratio rather than a fixed ratio (e.g., <0.70) to define the lower limit of normal; otherwise, airflow obstruction will be overdiagnosed, especially in older adults. As demonstrated in the first Lung Health Study, the presence of reversibility on spirometry is a common finding in COPD and alone does not imply a diagnosis of asthma or predict the rate of future loss of lung function.[48]

Other PFTs may be used to fully characterize the individual patient with COPD. Lung volumes may demonstrate evidence of hyperinflation (i.e., increased functional residual capacity) and gas trapping (i.e., increased RV and RV/TLC). Diffusing capacity is often reduced, particularly in the emphysematous COPD phenotype. Abnormalities on arterial blood gases may be evident in advanced disease; in the absence of comorbidities, severe hypoxemia and hypercapnia occur in COPD only at the stage of severe airflow obstruction (e.g., FEV_1 < 50% predicted).

Field and laboratory tests of exercise capacity can be used to quantify the severity of exercise intolerance and response to therapy in COPD. A 6-minute walk test is an easy field test to perform without the requirement of expensive laboratory equipment and provides additional clinical information (e.g., oxygen desaturation with exertion, locus of symptom limitation during exercise) and prognostic information.[49] A laboratory-based, cardiopulmonary exercise test also provides an objective assessment of maximum oxygen uptake and can detect presence of dynamic hyperinflation.[49]

Chest roentgenogram may reveal evidence of hyperinflation, including low, flat diaphragms, increased retrosternal airspace, and hyperlucency of the lungs.[50] A computed tomography scan is rarely indicated in patients with COPD but has greater sensitivity than plain radiographs for detection of emphysema and, to a lesser extent, chronic bronchitis.[50] Chest imaging has its greatest value in working up the differential diagnosis of COPD (e.g., congestive heart failure) or to assess for comorbid conditions (e.g., lung cancer, bronchiectasis).

Management

Once the diagnosis is established, the goals of COPD management include slowing disease progression, alleviating symptoms, improving exercise tolerance, and preventing and treating exacerbations to improve patient health status and reduce mortality.[46] Good communication among the individual with COPD, informal caregivers, and health care professionals is essential to establish individual patient goals of care. Comprehensive non-pharmacologic and pharmacologic treatments are provided in a step-wise fashion to achieve those goals, based on disease severity.

Disease severity in COPD is determined by an assessment of level of disability, burden of COPD-related symptoms, degree of airflow obstruction, and frequency and severity of acute exacerbations.[2,46] Dyspnea and exercise intolerance can be simply assessed using the Medical Research Council scale for breathlessness, ranging from 1 (no limitation) to 5 (breathlessness while dressing/undressing or resulting in patient being unable to leave the house).[51] Overall symptom burden can be assessed using a validated tool such as the 8-item, COPD Assessment Test score.[52] FEV1% predicted measured during spirometry is used to categorize severity of airflow obstruction as mild (≥80% predicted), moderate (≥50% to <80% predicted), severe (≥30% to <50% predicted), or very severe (<30% predicted).[2] COPD prognosis relates to a number of factors that have been combined in composite scores, the best known being the BODE index: *b*ody mass index as an assessment of nutritional status; *o*bstruction assessed by FEV_1% predicted; *d*yspnea assessed by the modified Medical Research Council dyspnea scale; and *e*xercise capacity assessed by distance walked on a 6-minute walk test.[41]

Ideally, all individuals with COPD should become collaborative partners in their own care. COPD self-management education, delivered by a trained respiratory educator, provides patients with knowledge, skills, and self-efficacy to achieve the best clinical outcomes. Components of a self-management program for COPD, such as Living Well With COPD (http://www.livingwellwithcopd.com/), include a written action plan to recognize and self-manage acute exacerbations, learn proper inhaler technique, adopt a healthy lifestyle, and gain a better understanding of the disease and medications used to treat COPD. Compared to usual care, self-management education in adults with COPD has been shown to significantly reduce hospital admissions due to COPD (by 39.8%), emergency department visits (by 41.0%), and unscheduled physician visits (by 58.9%), while improving health-related quality of life.[53,54] However, on a cautionary note, there have been inconsistent results from other studies. A study of a comprehensive care management program designed to reduce the risk for COPD hospitalization conducted in 20 Veterans Affairs hospital-based outpatient clinics in the United States was stopped prematurely by the safety monitoring board because of unanticipated excess mortality with no reduction in hospitalization.[55]

Smoking cessation is an essential secondary prevention to slow progression in established COPD. The Lung Health Study demonstrated that complete smoking cessation is necessary to maximally slow the accelerated loss of lung function associated with cigarette smoking that is characteristic of COPD.[56] A U.S. Public Health Service–sponsored clinical practice guideline on treating tobacco use and dependence recommended that even brief individual, group, and telephone smoking cessation counseling sessions are effective.[57] There is no evidence, however, of benefit from hypnosis or acupuncture as smoking cessation interventions. In contrast, a number of pharmacologic treatments have been shown in clinical trials to increase quit rates when used in conjunction with smoking cessation counseling. Currently available treatment options include nicotine replacement therapy delivered by various routes (i.e., transdermal patch, gum, and inhaler), the antidepressant bupropion, and varenicline, a partial agonist of nicotinic acetylcholine receptors.[57]

Optimal integrated care of a chronic condition like COPD, which can be associated with systemic manifestations and multiple comorbidities, often requires a complex intervention such as pulmonary rehabilitation. Pulmonary rehabilitation has been jointly defined by the American Thoracic Society and European Thoracic Society as "a comprehensive intervention based on a thorough patient assessment followed by patient tailored therapies that include, but are not limited to, exercise training, education, and behavior change, designed to improve the physical and psychological condition of people with chronic respiratory disease and to promote the long-term adherence to health-enhancing behaviors."[58] Components of pulmonary rehabilitation include aerobic and strength exercise training, behavioral change and collaborative self-management education, and nutritional and psychosocial support delivered by a multidisciplinary health care team. Pulmonary rehabilitation can be effectively delivered in a hospital, community, or home setting. Typically, participants attend exercise and education sessions as a small group two to five times per week for 6 to 12 weeks. Some programs also provide ongoing maintenance sessions for pulmonary rehabilitation graduates. When added to usual care of COPD, pulmonary rehabilitation has been clearly shown in multiple randomized clinical trials to improve dyspnea, exercise tolerance, and health-related quality of life, while reducing anxiety and depression.[58,59] Pulmonary rehabilitation has also been shown to reduce number of hospital days and mortality in individuals who have recently (<4 weeks) suffered an AECOPD.[60]

Pharmacotherapy

Bronchodilators are the main pharmacotherapy used for symptom relief in older adults with COPD. Bronchodilators decrease airflow obstruction, hyperinflation, and gas trapping. The resultant reduction in dyspnea and improved exercise tolerance translate into improved health-related quality of life. Inhaled long-acting bronchodilators have also been shown to reduce frequency of AECOPD. There is no evidence, however, that bronchodilators slow the rate of lung function loss in older adults with COPD.[2] Three classes of bronchodilators are available: inhaled β_2-agonists, inhaled anticholinergics (or antimuscarinics), and theophyllines. As with asthma, theophyllines, which are weak bronchodilators, are of limited value in older adults because of problems with frequent and serious side effects, drug-drug interactions, and the need to monitor blood levels.

The inhaled route is preferred for bronchodilators, although attention to choice of delivery device and proper inhaler technique is essential to ensure optimal medication delivery, especially in older adults. Inhalation of drug can be achieved through various devices, including pressurized metered-dose inhalers, preferably used with a spacer or valve-holding chamber; breath-actuated dry powder inhalers; or nebulizers. Short-acting (i.e., 4- to 6-hr) and long-acting (i.e., 12- to 24-hr) medications are available for both classes of inhaled bronchodilators, β_2-agonists and anticholinergics. Additive effects on lung function improvement are seen when the two classes of inhaled bronchodilators are combined.

Inhaled bronchodilators are generally very well tolerated. Adverse effects of inhaled β_2-agonists can include tremor (particularly in older adults), sinus tachycardia and other cardiac rhythm disturbances, restlessness, hypokalemia, and mild hypoxemia. Typical adverse effects of inhaled anticholinergics include dry mouth, metallic taste, glaucoma (if medication directed into the eyes), tachyarrhythmia, and, in rare cases, prostatic symptoms.

Unlike in asthma, ICSs are not used alone in the treatment of COPD. ICSs have no effect on rate of lung function decline in COPD.[2] When used to treat COPD, an ICS is given in combination with a LABA; the combination of an ICS with a LABA has been shown to improve lung function, symptoms, exercise tolerance, and health-related quality of life, while reducing frequency of AECOPD.[2] The risks of long-term ICS use include local (e.g., oropharyngeal candidiasis, dysphonia) and systemic (e.g., ecchymosis, osteoporosis, cataracts, suppression of hypothalamic-pituitary axis, pneumonia) adverse effects.

A number of noninhaled pharmacologic treatments may be prescribed with the goal to reduce the future risk of AECOPD rather than to provide symptom relief. All individuals with COPD without contraindication should receive an annual influenza vaccination.[45] Pneumococcal vaccine should also be administered, although the evidence that this will result in reduction in number of AECOPD events is lacking compared to influenza vaccination.[45] Individuals with COPD who continue to suffer frequent AECOPD events despite optimal inhaled maintenance medication may benefit from the addition of an oral medication. Selective phosphodiesterase-4 inhibition with an oral once-daily medication (e.g., roflumilast) has also been shown to reduce the number of AECOPD events in individuals with moderate to severe COPD. Unlike nonselective phosphodiesterase inhibitors (i.e., theophyllines), adverse effects are less problematic but include gastrointestinal intolerance and weight loss.[45] Macrolide antibiotics have been investigated as chronic immune-modulator medications in COPD and have been demonstrated to reduce the number of AECOPD events. However, patient selection criteria and long-term safety and efficacy are uncertain with this class of oral medications for treating COPD. Concerns exist related to possible emergence of antibiotic-resistant organisms and adverse effects, including QT prolongation and hearing loss.[45] Oral mucolytic agents (e.g., *N*-acetylcysteine, carbocysteine) have also been shown to reduce risk of AECOPD with relatively few adverse effects.[45] Of note, statins are not effective in reducing the risk of AECOPD; however, because of the presence of cardiovascular risk factors, many individuals with COPD will meet established criteria for treatment with this class of medication.[45] Although indicated in the acute management of moderate to severe AECOPD, there is no role for chronic use of oral corticosteroids in the treatment of COPD.[2,45]

Severe α_1-antitrypsin deficiency is a rare, heritable cause of emphysema and COPD resulting from an imbalance between proteases (e.g., lung neutrophil elastase) and antiproteases (e.g., α_1-antitrypsin). There is low-grade evidence that weekly intravenous augmentation therapy will reduce mortality, preserve lung density on computed tomography scan, and reduce the rate of lung function decline.[61] However, this therapy is expensive and not widely available.

Long-term oxygen therapy is indicated in the treatment of chronic hypoxemia in COPD. The benefit of long-term oxygen therapy has been established based on two randomized clinical trials showing a reduction in mortality when used for at least 15 hours per day.[62,63] Criteria for long-term oxygen therapy is based on results of room air arterial blood gases done when the individual is clinically stable showing an arterial oxygen pressure (PaO_2) of less than 55 mm Hg and oxygen saturation less than 88% or a PaO_2 between 55 and 59 mm Hg with evidence of cor pulmonale or polycythemia.[2]

Dyspnea is a cardinal symptom of COPD. Despite optimal nonpharmacologic and pharmacologic management, some individuals with COPD will have persistent, severe dyspnea that negatively affects their quality of life. The Canadian Thoracic Society published a clinical practice guideline recommending a "dyspnea ladder," a comprehensive step-wise approach to dyspnea management in COPD.[64] At the top of the ladder, long- and short-acting opioid medications are indicated in the treatment of severe dyspnea refractory to other nonpharmacologic and pharmacologic treatments in COPD. Protocols have been suggested by the Canadian Thoracic Society for dosing of opioids and management of potential adverse effects.[64]

Surgery for Chronic Obstructive Pulmonary Disease

Various surgical interventions have been explored in the palliative management of severe COPD. Lung volume reduction surgery (LVRS) involves the resection of areas of emphysematous lung to improve mechanics and function of the remaining, more normal lung. Following pulmonary rehabilitation, when compared to usual care, LVRS was shown in the National Emphysema Treatment Trial to improve mortality in the subgroup of subjects with heterogeneous emphysema predominantly affecting upper lobes and low baseline exercise capacity.[65] Bronchoscopic lung volume reduction (BLVR) achieved through the placement of endobronchial valves has been proposed as an alternative to LVRS. BLVR has been shown to induce small changes in lung function, functional exercise capacity, and health-related quality of life.[66]

BOX 48-5 Poor Prognostic Factors in Chronic Obstructive Pulmonary Disease

Severe airflow obstruction
Poor exercise tolerance
Severe dyspnea
Poor nutritional status
Requiring long-term oxygen therapy
Pulmonary hypertension
Frequent or severe acute exacerbations

Bullectomy, the resection of giant bullae, may be considered when bullae occupy at least half a hemithorax and are compressing relatively normal adjacent lung.[67] COPD is currently the most common indication for lung transplantation. Individuals with COPD and very poor prognosis (i.e., assessed by the BODE score) associated with very severe airflow obstruction or gas exchange, acute hypercapnia during AECOPD, or pulmonary hypertension are potential candidates for lung transplantation.[68] Older age is no longer an absolute contraindication to lung transplantation; however, survival is lower in recipients older than 65 years, likely because of the presence of comorbidities.[68]

Advanced Care Planning

Individuals with advanced COPD report lower health-related quality of life than individuals with lung cancer and receive less support from the health care system.[69] At all grades of frailty, COPD worsens prognosis.[70] High symptom burden, social isolation, fear of abandonment, emotional and financial strain, and uncertainty about events at the end of life place a heavy burden on individuals with advanced COPD and their informal caregivers. Compared to people with lung cancer, the illness narratives of frail older adults with COPD tend to focus more on fear of dependence than on fear of dying.[71] Innovative models of integrated care have been investigated to address this unmet need for individuals living and dying with advanced COPD.[72] An essential component of these integrated care models is timely and ongoing communication to identify patient values and treatment preferences and to choose informed substitute decision makers to improve care throughout their illness, including at the end of life. All individuals with COPD particularly those with advanced disease and features suggesting a poor prognosis (Box 48-5),[46] should be offered the opportunity to discuss and develop an advanced care plan.

KEY POINTS

- Asthma and chronic obstructive pulmonary disease (COPD) are common disorders associated with significant morbidity and mortality in older adults.
- Recognizing the role of inflammation in the pathogenesis of asthma and COPD is important in the management of both disorders.
- COPD is a systemic disease associated with extrapulmonary manifestations and systemic inflammatory response.
- The symptoms and signs of airway disease in older adults can be nonspecific and overlap considerably with other common disorders in this age group.
- The Global Initiative for Asthma (GINA) and Global Obstructive Lung Disease (GOLD) guidelines are valuable resources in the management of asthma and COPD in older adults.

For a complete list of references, please visit www.expertconsult.com.

KEY REFERENCES

1. Global Initiative for Asthma: Global strategy for asthma management and prevention 2014. http://www.ginasthma.org. Accessed March 16, 2015.
2. Global Initiative for Chronic Obstructive Lung Disease (GOLD): Global strategy for the diagnosis, management and prevention of COPD, 2015. http://www.goldcopd.org. Accessed March 24, 2015.
8. Yáñez A, Cho S-H, Soriano JB, et al: Asthma in the elderly: what we know and what we have yet to know. World Allergy Organ J 7:8, 2014.
10. Tsai CL, Lee WY, Hanania NA, et al: Age-related differences in clinical outcomes for acute asthma in the United States, 2006-2008. J Allergy Clin Immunol 129:1252–1258, 2012.
14. Slavin RG, Haselkorn T, Lee JH, et al: Asthma in older adults: observations from the epidemiology and natural history of asthma: outcomes and treatment regimens (TENOR) study. Ann Allergy Asthma Immunol 96:406–414, 2006.
15. Hanania NA, King MJ, Braman SS, et al: Asthma in the elderly: current understanding and future research needs—a report of a National Institute on Aging (NIA) workshop. J Allergy Clin Immunol 128(Suppl):S4–S24, 2011.
26. Buist AS, McBurnie MA, Vollmer WM, et al: International variation in the prevalence of COPD (the BOLD study): a population-based prevalence study. Lancet 370:741–750, 2007.
32. Mathers CD, Loncar D: Projections of global mortality and burden of disease from 2002 to 2030. PLoS Med 3:e442, 2006.
37. Hogg JC, Chu F, Utokaparch S, et al: The nature of small-airway obstruction in chronic obstructive pulmonary disease. N Engl J Med 350:2645–2653, 2004.
40. Meiners S, Eickelberg O, Königshoff M: Hallmarks of the ageing lung. Eur Respir J 45:807–827, 2015.
53. Bourbeau J, Julien M, Maltais F, et al: Reduction of hospital utilization in patients with chronic obstructive pulmonary disease: a disease-specific self-management intervention. Arch Int Med 163:585–591, 2003.
56. Anthonisen NR, Connett JE, Murray RP: Smoking and lung function of Lung Health Study participants after 11 years. Am J Respir Crit Care Med 166:675–679, 2002.
58. Spruit MA, Singh SJ, Garvey C, et al: An official American Thoracic Society/European Respiratory Society statement: key concepts and advances in pulmonary rehabilitation. Am J Respir Crit Care Med 188:e13–e64, 2013.
70. Galizia G, Cacciatore F, Testa G, et al: Role of clinical frailty on long-term mortality of elderly subjects with and without chronic obstructive pulmonary disease. Aging Clin Exp Res 23:118–125, 2011.

49 Nonobstructive Lung Disease and Thoracic Tumors

Ben Hope-Gill, Katie Pink

Respiratory disease is a major cause of morbidity and mortality, affecting 1 in 10 of the population older than 65 years.[1] The presentation and management of respiratory disease often differs in older adults. This chapter provides some insight into these differences while reviewing current evidence.

RESPIRATORY INFECTIONS

Respiratory infection is common in older adults. Age-related factors include declining lung function and structural changes to the chest wall and muscles that result in reduced chest wall compliance.[2] In addition, mucociliary function declines with age and the immune system can be depressed. With increasing age there is an increase in oropharyngeal colonization with potential respiratory pathogens and also an increased incidence of microaspiration.[3] Malnutrition, in particular hypoalbuminemia, has also been associated with increased risk of infection in older adults.[4] Finally, institutionalization leads to greater exposure to respiratory pathogens.

INFLUENZA

Influenza tends to occur in seasonal epidemics each winter. In the United States, influenza causes 20,000 to 40,000 deaths per year. Although 60% of cases of influenza occur in adults younger than 65 years, more than 80% of deaths due to seasonal influenza occur in adults aged 65 years and older.[5-7] Older people are more likely to be hospitalized[8] and to experience significant functional decline.[9] In addition, complications such as infective bronchitis and secondary bacterial pneumonia occur more frequently in older adults, most commonly due to *Staphylococcus aureus* and *Streptococcus pneumoniae* infection.[10] In addition, cerebrovascular and cardiovascular deaths can be precipitated by influenza infection.[11] The 2009 influenza A pandemic (H1N1) caused higher rates of illness in children and young adults and lower rates of illness in adults aged 60 and older when compared to traditional seasonal influenza.[12] This was felt to be related to exposure of this age group to antigenically similar influenza viruses earlier in life.

Vaccination

National guidelines in the United Kingdom recommend influenza vaccination for all adults aged older than 65 years and those in long-term care.[13] The aim is to reduce complications from influenza. In the United States, vaccination is recommended for everyone over the age of 6 months.[14] A Cochrane review, however, has highlighted the paucity of good evidence supporting this approach.[15] Only one randomized control trial was identified that adequately assessed efficacy and effectiveness of vaccination in adults older than 65 years, and this was not adequately powered to detect any effect on complications. It did show an effect against influenza symptoms. That result was obtained even though some evidence suggests that the antibody response to vaccination is attenuated in frail older adults.[16] A further Cochrane review could not find evidence to support the vaccination of health care workers in preventing influenza in adults older than 60 years living in long-term care facilities.[17]

In the United States national vaccination uptake is less than 50%,[18] and in the United Kingdom and Europe only a minority of those eligible for vaccination receive it.[19,20] Possible explanations include patient concerns regarding side effects, frustration that previous vaccination has not prevented influenza-like illness, and the deferment of vaccination by doctors when patients have a mild upper respiratory tract infection.[21]

Treatment

Neuraminidase inhibitors (zanamivir, oseltamivir) have been the subject of debate with regard to their effectiveness at preventing and treating influenza.[22] Oseltamivir was widely prescribed during the 2009 H1N1 pandemic. These agents must be taken within 48 hours of the onset of symptoms. Current U.K. guidelines recommend their use for at-risk groups, including adults aged older than 65 years when national surveillance schemes indicate influenza is circulating or in localized outbreaks within institutions.[23] Clinical trials have suggested that these agents may reduce symptom duration by 1 or 2 days and decrease hospitalization and death rates in older adults.[24,25] Further studies are required. The neuraminidase inhibitors are well tolerated and the safety profile among older adults is similar to that in younger adults. The most common adverse effects are nausea, vomiting, and abdominal pain. Zanamivir may cause bronchospasm.[26] Amantadine and rimantadine are only effective against influenza A and are associated with toxic side effects and with rapid emergence of drug-resistant variants.[26,27] Specific studies in the older adult population are lacking.[28] Routine use of these agents is not recommended.[23]

In the United Kingdom, the National Institute for Health and Care Excellence (NICE) guidance recommends that postexposure prophylaxis with oseltamivir or zanamivir be given to all adults living in residential care facilities, regardless of vaccination status, during localized outbreaks.[29] A recent systematic review found that individuals in care homes that received chemoprophylaxis were significantly less likely to develop influenza than those in homes with no intervention.[30] In the community setting, postexposure prophylaxis is only recommended for high-risk adults (including those older than 65 years) if they have not been vaccinated or if the circulating strain of influenza is known to be different from the vaccination strain.[29] Amantadine is not recommended for use as a postexposure prophylaxis.

PNEUMONIA

Community-acquired pneumonia has an incidence of 5 to 11 in 1000 in the adult population.[3,31-33] People older than 75 years have a six times greater risk compared with those younger than 60 years.[33-36] Older adults in residential care are particularly vulnerable.[3,31,37] This is largely explained by the greater prevalence of frailty in this population. Chronic obstructive pulmonary disease (COPD), diabetes, heart failure, malnutrition, malignancy, and dysphagia are all risk factors for pneumonia in late life.[3,31,38] Mortality is 5.7% to 14% and increases with age. In the United States, pneumonia is the ninth leading cause of death.[39-42]

The most common causative organism is *Streptococcus pneumoniae*. Other pathogens include *Haemophilus influenzae*, viruses (commonly influenza, parainfluenza, respiratory syncytial virus), gram-negative bacilli, and *Staphylococcus aureus*. In older adults, infections with "atypical" organisms such as *Mycoplasma* and

BOX 49-1 Pneumonia Severity Prediction; CURB-65 Score

- **C**onfusion of new onset (or worsening of existing state for those with background cognitive impairment)
- Serum **U**rea > 7 mmol/L
- **R**espiratory rate ≥ 30/min
- **B**lood pressure (systolic BP < 90 mm Hg or diastolic BP ≤ 60 mm Hg)
- Age ≥ **65** years

A score is awarded for each variable present. A score of 3 or higher represents severe pneumonia.

Legionella are less common.[39,40] Infection with gram-negative bacilli and anaerobic organisms may occur after aspiration.[3,31,43] There is no conclusive evidence that the pathogens associated with nursing home–acquired pneumonia are different from those associated with other older adults in the United Kingdom, although studies in North America have reported an increased incidence of gram-negative bacilli and *S. aureus*.[44-46]

Many older persons often show frailty syndromes when they become ill, such as functional decline, delirium, and falls. Lethargy and anorexia are other common presenting symptoms.[3,31] For example, a chest x-ray will demonstrate pneumonia in nearly a quarter of older adult patients with acute confusion and no clinical signs.[47] Fever is less likely to be present in older patients.[3,31,48,49] The presence of tachypnea is an important clinical sign in this population.[49]

A number of scoring systems can be used to assess severity in community-acquired pneumonia, including the Pneumonia Severity Index and the CURB-65 score.[50,51] Current British Thoracic Society (BTS)[32] and American Thoracic Society (ATS)[52] guidelines recommend the use of the CURB-65 score (Box 49-1) because of its simplicity and strong predictive power for severe pneumonia. Those patients with a low score (0-2) have a low mortality risk and may be suitable for community-based treatment with oral antibiotics.[51] However, this may not be appropriate for some very frail older adults or for those with psychosocial concerns. As Isaacs insisted, the degree of monitoring that an older person requires is a good guide to who requires admission.[53]

Management

The investigation and management of community-acquired pneumonia are discussed in guidelines published by both the BTS and the ATS.[52] Initial empirical treatment is with broad-spectrum antibiotic therapy against *Pneumococcus* and "atypical" organisms. Current recommendations suggest the combination of amoxicillin plus a macrolide antibiotic for patients with moderately severe pneumonia. An alternative for penicillin-allergic patients is a fluoroquinolone with enhanced pneumococcal activity, such as levofloxacin.[32] Local antibiotic resistance patterns need to be taken into account. Intravenous antibiotic therapy is only required in patients with severe pneumonia or in patients who are unable to take oral preparations. Antibiotic-associated colitis and *Clostridium difficile* infection are particular concerns with intravenous antibiotics.[54-56] There is evidence that in patients with severe pneumonia, delay in the administration of the first antibiotic is associated with increased mortality.[57-59]

Following an episode of pneumonia, it is important to ensure that radiologic changes resolve, particularly in older adults and smokers who are at increased risk of an underlying malignancy. Radiologic clearance is slower in older people.[32,40] As always, the principle of only ordering tests for which a positive result will be acted on holds.

Nosocomial Pneumonia

The incidence of hospital-acquired pneumonia increases significantly with age[60] and the mortality rate can be as high as 50%.[3,31] Treatment regimes should cover gram-negative anaerobic bacteria. *Pseudomonas* species and methicillin-resistant *Staphylococcus aureus* (MRSA) should also be considered.

Vaccination

Polysaccharide pneumococcal vaccination is recommended for all adults older than 65 years.[32,52] Reimmunization is unnecessary. Despite strong evidence of pneumococcal vaccination efficacy in preventing invasive pneumococcal disease, there is no evidence that routine vaccination prevents all-cause pneumonia or mortality.[61]

TUBERCULOSIS

The incidence of tuberculosis (TB) is now declining in the Western world, although it continues to rise in Africa because of the HIV pandemic. World Health Organization (WHO) surveillance data from 2012 showed an incidence of 3.6 cases per 100,000 population in the United States and 15 cases per 100,000 population in the United Kingdom.[62] In those born in either the United Kingdom or the United States, the incidence of active TB increases with age, with a doubling of the incidence in adults older than 80 years.[63] Most cases in older adults represent reactivation of previous disease.[63] This may be precipitated by an age-related reduction in cell-mediated immunity or secondary to other factors such as malnutrition, alcoholism, cancer, diabetes mellitus, HIV infection, or treatment with corticosteroids.[2] A significant proportion (up to one fifth) of cases are related to new transmission of TB.[64]

TB is particularly common among care home residents in the United States[65] with the incidence of active TB being two to three times higher than in those living in the community[66,67] because of reactivation of disease and institutional outbreaks.[68]

Presentation

The presentation of TB in older adults can be insidious and nonspecific; weight loss, weakness, or a change in cognitive function is sometimes the only manifestation.[2,69] Dyspnea is often present, whereas hemoptysis and fever are observed less frequently.[64,65] It is important to consider TB if a patient has a cough or pneumonia that incompletely responds to conventional treatment.

The chest radiographic changes of TB are similar in all age groups, although in older people cavitary disease is less common.[65] Miliary TB is likely in older adults, although the diagnosis is frequently missed.[2] The presence of radiographic manifestations of previous TB infection in an older patient with nonspecific infective symptoms should alert physicians to exclude reactivation. Extrapulmonary TB is uncommon and is often difficult to diagnose. Sites involved include the genitourinary tract, the central nervous system, the lymphatics, and bone. Extrapulmonary TB is more common in children and older people.[70]

Investigation

Pulmonary TB is usually diagnosed by culturing *Mycobacterium tuberculosis* from sputum. Guidelines suggest that three sputum samples should be sent for culture.[71] In older patients it may be difficult to obtain spontaneous sputum samples, and sputum induction or bronchoscopy with bronchial washings may be required. The presence of acid-fast bacilli (AFB) on Ziehl-Neelsen staining (smear positive) suggests the diagnosis of pulmonary TB; however, *M. tuberculosis* can take up to 6 weeks to be cultured using conventional techniques. It is important to remember that AFB smear positivity alone does not distinguish *M. tuberculosis* from nontuberculous mycobacterial infection (NTM). Rapid culture techniques, including polymerase chain reaction (PCR) or gene probe analyses, allow earlier diagnosis. Once a patient has been diagnosed with TB, HIV testing should be performed.[72]

Patients with suspected TB are usually investigated as outpatients; however, smear-positive older adult care home residents should be isolated to prevent transmission.[67] If admitted to the hospital, patients should be isolated until their sputum status is known. If multidrug-resistant tuberculosis (MDR-TB) is suspected, patients should be managed in a negative air pressure room. Patients who are smear positive need to remain isolated until they have completed 2 weeks of antituberculous treatment.[67,71]

Tuberculin Skin Test

The tuberculin skin test measures cell-mediated immunity against TB. It is positive in both active and latent disease and also in people who have received bacillus Calmette-Guérin (BCG) immunization. False negatives can occur in immunocompromised patients because of anergy. Anergy prevalence increases with age because of a decline in cellular immunity, and the value of the tuberculin skin test is therefore reduced.[63] It is mainly used in the diagnosis of latent TB.

Interferon-γ Tests

Interferon-γ blood tests detect tuberculosis infection by measuring interferon-γ release from T cells in response to antigens that are highly specific to *Mycobacterium tuberculosis* but are absent from the BCG vaccine. In the United Kingdom they are primarily used to confirm the diagnosis of latent TB in the presence of a positive tuberculin skin test, or in those people for whom a skin test is less reliable (e.g., previous BCG vaccination).[71]

Management

Recommendations for antituberculous therapy do not differ in older people. Initial empirical therapy should consist of a four-drug regime for 2 months (rifampicin, isoniazid, pyrazinamide, ethambutol), followed by a two-drug regime for 4 months (rifampicin and isoniazid). Extrapulmonary TB is treated in the same way, with the exception of TB meningitis, which requires 12 months of treatment.[71] Directly observed therapy may be useful in selected individuals who are at risk of poor compliance. Contact tracing is an important aspect of management, and current recommendations are available in national and international guidelines.[71]

MDR-TB (resistance to rifampicin and isoniazid) is uncommon in the older adult population in the United Kingdom and United States. This is probably because active TB in older adults usually results from reactivation of latent infection that was acquired when there was no effective antituberculous chemotherapy.[63]

Older patients often show a greater incidence of drug toxicity and intolerance. They are more likely to be coprescribed other medication, and this increases the likelihood of drug interactions. Rifampicin, in particular, can reduce the levels of many medications through induction of the cytochrome P450 system. The use of isoniazid has been associated with increased levels of some anticonvulsants and benzodiazepines.[68]

Rifampicin, isoniazid, and pyrazinamide are all associated with gastrointestinal side effects and hepatotoxicity. Hepatic toxicity is increased in older patients.[73] Ethambutol can cause a loss of visual acuity and color discrimination and close monitoring is required in elderly patients whose visual acuity may already be impaired. Isoniazid can cause peripheral neuropathy, particularly in patients with coexisting renal failure. This can be prevented by pyridoxine. Finally, rifampicin may cause bodily fluids to become discolored orange.

Latent TB

Latent TB is defined as a positive tuberculin skin or interferon-γ test, with a normal chest x-ray and no symptoms of TB. Individuals who are identified as having latent TB through contact screening should be offered chemoprophylaxis. In the United States all residents of care homes are screened for latent TB on admission.[74] Those with latent TB are treated with chemoprophylaxis. Treatment regimes comprise either isoniazid alone for 6 months or isoniazid and rifampicin combined for 3 months.[67] It is important to identify and treat latent TB prior to immunosuppressant treatment, particularly anti–tumor necrosis factor-α (anti-TNFα) therapy.[75]

Prognosis

In 2012 in the United Kingdom there were 261 deaths from active TB, 72% of which occurred in adults older than 65 years of age.[76] Many older patients will have long-term sequelae from tuberculous infection. Pulmonary fibrosis is a recognized complication, as is pleural thickening and restrictive lung disease from pleural infection. Historical surgical techniques have also led to chest wall deformities. These patients with restrictive lung disease are at risk of hypercapnic respiratory failure and may require home noninvasive ventilation.[77]

NONTUBERCULOUS MYCOBACTERIAL INFECTION

Pulmonary infection with nontuberculous mycobacteria has become increasingly recognized, including in older adults.[78] Predisposing factors include chronic lung diseases, such as COPD and bronchiectasis, as well as immunosuppression, particularly HIV infection. Clinical and radiologic features are similar to those of pulmonary TB. Treatment can be difficult because of drug intolerance. Guidelines on the diagnosis and treatment of nontuberculous mycobacteria have been published by both the BTS and the ATS.[79,80]

BRONCHIECTASIS

Bronchiectasis is characterized by the permanent dilation of bronchi, with chronic airway inflammation and excess sputum production. The prevalence of non–cystic fibrosis bronchiectasis in the United States is estimated to be 51 per 100,000 population. The prevalence increases markedly with age (4/100,000 aged 18 to 34 vs. 272/100,000 aged 75 years and older).[81] The advent of high-resolution computed tomography (HRCT) scanning means milder forms of bronchiectasis are now being identified.

Bronchiectasis is often a sequela of childhood infections such as pertussis, measles, TB, and severe pneumonia.[82] Bronchiectasis is increasingly being recognized as a complication of COPD. A causative factor cannot be identified in many cases; these are termed *idiopathic bronchiectasis*. Causes and investigation of bronchiectasis are outlined in Table 49-1.

Management

The aims of treatment are to reduce symptoms, promptly treat exacerbations, and prevent disease progression. A multidisciplinary approach with input from physiotherapists, respiratory nurses, and dieticians is particularly important for older patients. Bronchodilators are effective in treating associated airflow

TABLE 49-1 Causes and Investigation of Bronchiectasis

All-Age Causes of Bronchiectasis	(% Prevalence)
Idiopathic	(53%)
Postinfectious	(29%)
Allergic bronchopulmonary aspergillosis	(11%)
Immune deficiency	
- Total humoral	(11%)
- Total neutrophil function	(1%)
Rheumatoid arthritis	(4%)
Ulcerative colitis	(2%)
Ciliary dysfunction	(3%)
Young syndrome	(5%)
Cystic fibrosis	(3%)
Aspiration/gastroesophageal reflux	(4%)
Panbronchiolitis	(<1%)
Congenital	(<1%)
Investigation of Bronchiectasis	
HRCT	
Spirometry with bronchodilator reversibility	
Sputum culture and AFB culture	
Total IgE, *Aspergillus*-specific IgE and IgG	
Serum Igs	
Antipneumococcal antibody titers	
Rheumatoid factor	
CF genotype, sweat test	
Serum α_1-antitrypsin levels	

AFB, Acid-fast bacilli; *CF,* cystic fibrosis; *HRCT,* high-resolution computed tomography; *Ig,* immunoglobulin.

Adapted from Pasteur MC, Helliwell SM, Houghton SJ, et al: An investigation into causative factors in patients with bronchiectasis. Am J Respir Crit Care Med 162(4 Pt 1):1277–1284, 2000.

TABLE 49-2 Causes of Unilateral Effusion

Transudative Effusions	Exudative Effusions
Very Common	Common
- Left ventricular failure	- Malignancy
- Liver cirrhosis	- Parapneumonic effusion
- Hypoalbuminemia	
- Peritoneal dialysis	Less common
- Pulmonary infarction	- Rheumatoid arthritis
Less common	- Autoimmune disease
- Hypothyroidism	- Benign asbestos effusion
- Nephrotic syndrome	- Pancreatitis
- Mitral stenosis	- Post-MI syndrome
- Pulmonary embolus	
Rare	Rare
- Constrictive pericarditis	- Yellow nail syndrome
- Urinothorax	- Drugs
- Superior vena cava obstruction	- Fungal infections

MI, Myocardial infarction.

BOX 49-2 Light's Criteria for Classification of Unilateral Pleural Effusion

The pleural fluid is an exudate if one or more of the following criteria are met:

- Pleural fluid protein divided by serum protein > 0.5
- Pleural fluid lactate dehydrogenase (LDH) divided by serum LDH > 0.6

obstruction, and mucolytics are useful to aid sputum clearance.[83] Many people advocate daily physiotherapy with postural drainage or cough augmentation, particularly during exacerbations. Inhaled corticosteroids may be useful in improving lung function and reducing exacerbation frequency.[84,85] Surgery remains an option for selected patients with localized disease or those with troublesome hemoptysis. Bronchial artery embolization is an alternative treatment strategy for patients with hemoptysis.[86]

Acute exacerbations should be treated promptly with antibiotics. Regular oral or nebulized antibiotics may be necessary for those individuals who have frequent exacerbations. Prophylactic azithromycin has antiinflammatory and antimicrobial properties and has shown promise in reducing exacerbation frequency in bronchiectasis.[87] Caution is required when initiating this drug because of the small risk of prolongation of the QT interval, which can be linked to sudden cardiac death, particularly in older adults with heart disease.[88] Microbiologic investigations are commonly challenging to interpret, due to chronic airway colonization by a variety of organisms, most often *Haemophilus influenzae*. *Pseudomonas aeruginosa* infection is often difficult to treat and may require more prolonged courses of combination intravenous antibiotics.[85]

PLEURAL EFFUSION

The investigation and management of pleural effusions are summarized in guidelines from the BTS and are beyond the scope of this chapter.[89] Investigation in older adults does not differ from investigation in younger individuals. Practice has changed so that all pleural taps are performed under ultrasound guidance by a practitioner qualified in pleural ultrasound.[90] A diagnostic pleural tap will differentiate exudative from transudative effusions and will often ascertain the cause (Table 49-2). Lights criteria should be used to classify effusions with pleural fluid total protein content between 25 and 35 g/dL, particularly in older adults in whom a single pleural fluid protein value is less reliable (Box 49-2). Other parameters that may be diagnostically useful include pleural fluid cytology, culture and sensitivity, pleural fluid glucose, pH and cell profile, depending on the clinical scenario. If the cause of an exudative effusion remains unclear after pleural fluid analysis, a computed tomography (CT) scan of the thorax, abdomen, and pelvis is advised. This is most useful if performed before full drainage of the effusion. If diagnostic uncertainty still remains after a CT scan, then medical thoracoscopy should be considered. Thoracoscopy is more sensitive than blind Abrams pleural biopsy and is well tolerated in patients of all ages. It is a useful diagnostic technique, allowing direct visualization of the pleura, and has the added advantage of offering fluid drainage and pleurodesis in a single procedure.[89]

PNEUMOTHORAX

The incidence of pneumothorax in the United Kingdom is 24 in 100,000 men per year and 9.8 in 100,000 women per year. The age distribution is biphasic, with peaks seen in the 20- to 24-year and 80- to 84-year age groups,[91] which is attributed to primary and secondary spontaneous pneumothorax, respectively. Older patients tend to have secondary pneumothorax related to underlying chronic lung disease, most commonly COPD.

Individuals with pneumothorax usually have acute dyspnea that is often out of proportion to the size of the pneumothorax. Pleuritic chest pain occurs less frequently than in younger patients.[92] The diagnosis is usually confirmed on a chest x-ray; however, in rare cases a CT scan of the thorax may be necessary to differentiate a pneumothorax from complex bullous lung disease.[93]

The treatment of pneumothorax in older adults is as per the BTS guidelines.[90] Adults with symptomatic secondary pneumothoraces need hospital admission and intercostal drain insertion. Small (<1 cm) or asymptomatic pneumothoraces may be managed with aspiration or even close observation.[93]

Indications for surgical intervention include persistent air leak, second ipsilateral pneumothorax, and first contralateral pneumothorax. The aims of surgery are to resect or suture the bleb that caused the pneumothorax and to perform pleurodesis to prevent recurrence. Thoracoscopy and video-assisted thoracic surgery (VATS) can be performed safely in the older adult population with a low morbidity and mortality.[94,95] In those patients who are either unable or unwilling to undergo surgery, chemical pleurodesis can be attempted; however, recurrence rates are high with this approach.[93]

INTERSTITIAL LUNG DISEASE

Interstitial lung disease (ILD), or idiopathic interstitial pneumonia, is a term used to describe a heterogeneous group of disorders of the lung parenchyma characterized by varying patterns of inflammation and fibrosis.[96] One of the most important distinctions among the idiopathic interstitial pneumonias is between idiopathic pulmonary fibrosis (IPF) and the other interstitial pneumonias.[96] Figure 49-1 outlines the current classification system.

The diagnosis of ILD is complex and older adult patients with suspicious features should be referred for a specialist respiratory opinion. Clinical, radiologic, and pathologic features frequently overlap, which makes accurate diagnosis difficult. Therefore, diagnosis should be undertaken in the context of a multidisciplinary team meeting comprising respiratory clinicians, thoracic radiologists, and pathologists with expertise in the evaluation of ILD. The diagnostic process requires a comprehensive clinical and physiologic evaluation followed by HRCT scanning in most cases. Surgical biopsy is recommended if clinical or radiologic features are not typical and preclude accurate diagnosis and if the patient is fit enough for a surgical procedure.[97] Although surgical lung biopsy is generally well tolerated, specific studies in older adults are lacking.[98] Video-assisted thoracoscopic biopsy is increasingly being performed in place of open lung biopsy. Transbronchial biopsy is less invasive, but, with the exception of sarcoidosis, samples are usually nondiagnostic. A history of systemic involvement (eye, joint, skin) or the presence of serum autoantibodies may suggest an underlying connective tissue disorder. It is particularly important to distinguish IPF from other ILDs as prognosis is poorer and the approach to treatment is different in this condition.[99]

IDIOPATHIC PULMONARY FIBROSIS

Idiopathic pulmonary fibrosis (previously termed *cryptogenic fibrosing alveolitis*) is the most common form of interstitial pneumonia. The diagnosis requires either a radiologic or pathologic diagnosis of usual interstitial pneumonia (UIP). Estimates on the prevalence of IPF range from between 1.25 and 23.4 cases per 100,000 population in Europe to as high as 63 per 100,000 population in the United States using wide case definitions.[100] It is a disease of older adults with increasing prevalence with age (especially older than 75 years). Indeed, symptom onset is uncommon before age 50.

Patients typically have progressive breathlessness and an irritating dry cough. Clinical examination will reveal digital clubbing in 25% to 50% of patients and fine end-inspiratory crackles, usually in a posterobasal distribution, on auscultation of the chest.[96,101,102] Lung function tests typically show a restrictive deficit with a reduction in vital capacity, total lung capacity, and transfer factor. Chest x-ray changes include reticulonodular shadowing with reduced lung volumes. HRCT appearance is pivotal to establishing the diagnosis. Typical HRCT features of UIP include subpleural reticulation with honeycombing and traction bronchiectasis with basal predominance and minimal ground glass change or nodularity. Surgical lung biopsy is not required in patients with characteristic clinical and radiologic features of UIP but should be considered in the presence of atypical features.[96,97,102]

The prognosis of IPF is poor. Median survival from diagnosis is less than 3 years.[96,102] However, the course of the disease can be highly variable in individual patients with some declining rapidly and others remaining more stable.

Management

The increase in clinical trial data regarding drug treatment of IPF has increased the treatment options available for patients with this devastating condition. Prior to the PANTHER study,

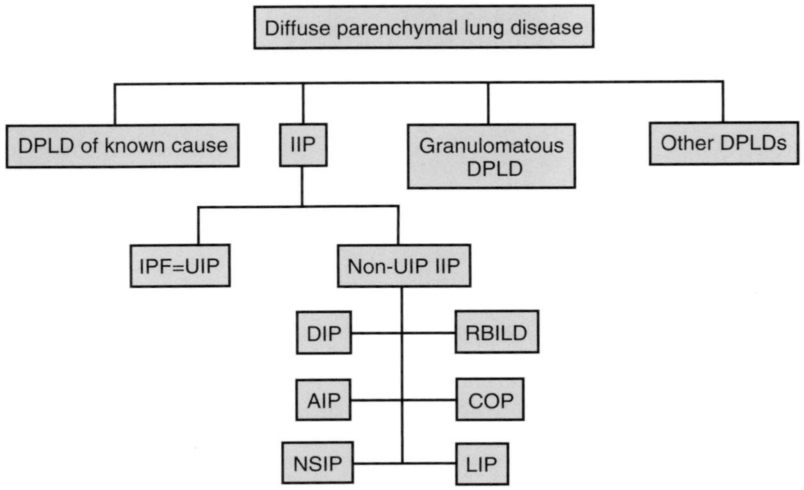

Figure 49-1. Classification of diffuse parenchymal lung disease. *AIP,* Acute interstitial pneumonia; *COP,* cryptogenic organizing pneumonia; *DIP,* desquamative interstitial pneumonia; *DPLD,* diffuse parenchymal lung disease; *IIP,* idiopathic interstitial pneumonia; *IPF,* idiopathic pulmonary fibrosis; *LIP,* lymphocytic interstitial pneumonia; *NSIP,* nonspecific interstitial pneumonia; *RBILD,* respiratory bronchiolitis–associated ILD; *UIP,* usual interstitial pneumonia.

many clinicians used a combination of azathioprine, corticosteroids, and *N*-acetylcysteine in an attempt to slow disease progression. The triple therapy arm (azathioprine plus prednisolone plus *N*-acetylcysteine) of this large randomized study was stopped prematurely in 2011 when it was established that patients receiving triple therapy were more likely to die or experience serious adverse events compared to those receiving a placebo.[103] The trial continued to investigate single-agent *N*-acetylcysteine versus a placebo. However, results have subsequently shown no benefit from lone treatment with *N*-acetylcysteine compared with a placebo at slowing disease progression.[101]

Pirfenidone is a costly drug that has antiinflammatory and antifibrotic effects. Several randomized placebo controlled trials have shown a reduction in the rate of decline in lung function (forced vital capacity), and pooled data have demonstrated an improvement in survival.[104-106] In the United Kingdom, NICE guidelines recommend it as an option in patients with a forced vital capacity between 50% and 80% predicted; however, NICE stipulates that for patients treated by the National Health Service, pirfenidone should be discontinued if there is physiologic evidence of significant disease progression.[107]

Two phase III clinical trials of the tyrosine kinase inhibitor nintedanib showed evidence of significant slowing of disease progression in patients with IPF. The role of nintedanib in relation to pirfenidone therapy for treating IPF has not yet been established; however, it is likely that within the next few years there will be a range of treatment options and the possibility of combination therapy for patients with this condition.[107]

Patients younger than 65 years should be considered for referral for lung transplantation.[108] Best supportive care includes oxygen therapy, pulmonary rehabilitation, and palliative care, and patients should be actively managed. Treatment of coexisting gastroesophageal reflux should be considered as there is some evidence that microaspiration may be associated with IPF; the precise role of antireflux therapy, however, has not been established.[109] Given the increasing complexity of the assessment and management of IPF, patients should be cared for by clinical teams with expertise in the diagnosis and management of ILD.

DRUG-INDUCED INTERSTITIAL LUNG DISEASE

Drug-induced ILD is most prevalent in older people by virtue of their greater lifetime drug exposure. The most commonly prescribed causative agents are amiodarone, methotrexate, angiotensin-converting enzyme (ACE) inhibitors, and nitrofurantoin. Treatment involves withdrawal of the causative agent and immunosuppressive therapy in some cases.

CONNECTIVE TISSUE DISEASE

Autoimmune disorders, including rheumatoid arthritis, Sjögren syndrome, systemic lupus erythematosus (SLE), systemic sclerosis, and polymyositis, are all associated with lung fibrosis. Respiratory symptoms may precede other manifestations of the disease. The association between rheumatoid arthritis and interstitial fibrosis is strongest in older people. The mean age of onset is in the fifth or sixth decade. The incidence, clinical presentation, prognosis, and response to therapy vary depending on the underlying disorder and the histologic pattern of disease. In general, ILD associated with the collagen vascular disorders has a better prognosis and response to treatment than IPF.[110] Corticosteroids and other immunosuppressive agents are used, but care must be taken with older patients, in whom significant adverse effects are more common.[111] Immunosuppressant therapy is associated with significant toxicity, including myelosuppression and hepatic toxicity. Drug interactions are also a particular problem because of frequent comorbidities and polypharmacy. For example, the concomitant use of allopurinol with azathioprine leads to increased azathioprine levels.[112]

SARCOIDOSIS

Sarcoidosis is a multisystem disorder that most frequently affects the lungs. Case series suggest that it is less common in older adults, who represent between 7.8% (adults older than 65 years) and 17% (adults older than 50 years) of patients.[113,114] The presenting symptoms usually include breathlessness and cough although symptoms may be nonspecific, with a decline in general health.[115] Löfgren syndrome is rarely seen in adults aged over 50 years.[114] A study of late-onset sarcoidosis suggested a higher incidence of asthenia, uveitis, and skin lesions than in younger patients.[116] In contrast, erythema nodosum and chest x-ray abnormalities occurred less frequently. Serum ACE levels are of limited value diagnostically, particularly in older adults who have an increased incidence of renal failure and diabetes (which are associated with raised serum ACE levels).[115,117] Diagnosis should be confirmed histologically whenever possible.[118] The course of the disease seems to be similar in younger and older patients.[115,116] Corticosteroids are used to treat selected patients with pulmonary involvement and should be supervised by clinicians with expertise in the management of sarcoidosis. Other indications for systemic corticosteroid use in sarcoidosis include hypercalcemia, ocular disease, and cardiac, neurologic, or renal involvement.

PULMONARY VASCULITIS

The vasculitides are broadly subclassified according to size of vessel involvement, clinical features, and associated conditions. Small vessel vasculitis is further subdivided according to the presence or absence of antineutrophil cytoplasmic antibodies (ANCAs). The incidence of ANCA-associated vasculitis is increasing. Wegener granulomatosis is a small vessel, systemic necrotizing vasculitis with a peak age of onset at 55 years. Clinical presentation in older adults is similar to that seen in younger adults, although ear, nose, and throat involvement is observed less frequently.[119-121] Some studies suggest older adult patients have an increased incidence of renal and neurologic involvement at diagnosis,[121] but this is not a consistent finding.[119,120] Diagnosis may be difficult because of the presence of coexistent disease such as COPD that influences clinical and radiologic features.[112] Circulating ANCA levels are positive in the majority of patients with renal involvement but are frequently negative in more limited disease. Biopsy of affected organs is recommended to confirm the diagnosis.

Therapy is subdivided into phases with different treatment regimes for remission induction and maintenance therapy. Several large-scale multicenter trials have provided clarification regarding the most appropriate treatment regimes. The combination of oral corticosteroids and cyclophosphamide will induce remission in 90% of patients. Even so, relapse rates are high and survival is worse after age 60.[119-121] Renal involvement is also associated with a poorer prognosis. A reduction in immunosuppressant dose in older adults has been shown to be effective and to reduce the risk of leucopenia.[122,123] Death usually results from uncontrolled vasculitis or systemic infection.

HYPERSENSITIVITY PNEUMONITIS

Hypersensitivity pneumonitis is caused by an immunologic reaction to the inhalation of organic antigens. It is often associated with the formation of systemic precipitating antibodies. Common precipitating antigens include bird proteins (bird fancier's lung) and thermophilic actinomycetes (farmer's lung). Most commonly it presents as a chronic illness related to repeated exposure, but an acute form is also recognized. In approximately half of patients, a causative antigen cannot be identified. Management centers on antigen avoidance although in some patients, disease progression occurs despite this management strategy. Corticosteroids can be used to improve lung function, although their effect on long-term outcome is unclear. Other immunosuppressants, such as azathioprine, are used for their steroid-sparing effect in chronic cases.

OCCUPATIONAL LUNG DISEASE

Pneumoconiosis

Pneumoconioses are pulmonary diseases caused by the inhalation of mineral dusts. Common causative mineral dusts include coal dust, silica, beryllium, and asbestos.

Coal Workers Pneumoconiosis

Because of a steady reduction in the numbers of underground coal miners in Western Europe and the United States, the incidence of coal workers pneumoconiosis has fallen in those geographic areas. Other countries still employ large numbers of miners. In the United States there were 8111 deaths from coal workers pneumoconiosis between 1998 and 2007 of which 90% occurred in adults older than 65 years.[124] Dust exposure results in inflammation and fibrosis of the lung parenchyma. Coexistent COPD is common. Simple pneumoconiosis is usually asymptomatic and is identified as nodular shadowing on a chest x-ray. Progressive massive fibrosis is associated with exertional breathlessness and a cough (often productive of black sputum) and may lead to cor pulmonale and respiratory failure. Chest x-ray features include fibrotic masses, usually in the upper zones, on a background of simple coal workers pneumoconiosis.

Asbestosis

Asbestosis is a fibrotic lung disease caused by exposure to asbestos dust. Diagnosis depends on a reliable history of significant asbestos exposure (usually a 10- to 20-year exposure period in an environment with more than 25 fibers/mL of asbestos in the atmosphere). Markers of exposure, such as pleural plaques or pleural thickening, are almost always present. Occupations at greatest risk include shipyard workers, asbestos factory workers, plumbers, insulation workers, and industrial electricians. There is a latency period of 15 to 20 years between exposure and the development of asbestosis; hence it is predominantly a disease of middle to old age. The incidence of asbestosis increased during the first decade of the twenty-first century in both the United Kingdom and the United States.[125,126] Treatment is supportive and patients should be informed of their eligibility for compensation.

LUNG CANCER

Lung cancer is the most common malignancy worldwide and is the leading cause of cancer deaths. It is predominantly a disease of older people with more than 90% of cases being diagnosed in patients older than 60 years and about 40% of cases being diagnosed in patients older than 75 years.[127] Most patients have advanced disease at presentation and, as a result, the survival rate is poor. In the United Kingdom, the 1-year survival rate is approximately 30%, with a 5-year survival rate of only 9%.[128] In the United States, the 5-year survival rate is higher (16.8%).[129] Guidelines on the diagnosis and management of lung cancer have been published by the American College of Chest Physicians[130] and the National Institute for Care Excellence in the United Kingdom.[131] Tobacco smoking has been firmly established as the most important risk factor for developing lung cancer. Other occupational and environmental carcinogens also increase the risk. Radon exposure (arising from radioactive decay of uranium 238 in the Earth's crust) is a recognized risk factor in miners,[132] and there is also evidence that residential radon exposure increases the risk of developing lung cancer.[133,134]

Presentation and Investigation

Most cases of lung cancer have presenting symptoms of breathlessness, recurrent chest infections, chest pain, hemoptysis, or weight loss. Other cases may be diagnosed as an incidental finding on routine chest x-ray. The aims of investigation are to make a definitive diagnosis and to stage the cancer appropriately so that treatment decisions can be made. A staging CT scan of the thorax, followed by bronchoscopy or endobronchial ultrasound, is the usual approach. In patients with peripheral tumors, percutaneous CT-guided biopsy is more likely to obtain a histologic diagnosis. Bronchoscopy is well tolerated in all age groups, with a low risk of significant complications.[118] Endobronchial ultrasound-guided transbronchial needle aspiration (EBUS-TBNA) has the advantage of being able to accurately stage the mediastinal lymph nodes in addition to obtaining histologic diagnosis. A recent study has confirmed its safety and tolerability in an older adult population.[135] In very frail patients, invasive investigation may not be appropriate and a clinical diagnosis of lung cancer may suffice. Positive emission tomography (PET) scanning is indicated for any patients who are being considered for potentially curative treatment. It also has a role in the investigation of the solitary pulmonary nodule. The specificity of PET is not high, and many benign inflammatory lesions produce false-positive results.[131]

Non–small cell lung carcinoma (NSCLC) (including adenocarcinoma, squamous cell carcinoma, and large cell carcinoma) accounts for 85% of all new diagnoses. Small cell lung carcinoma accounts for the remaining 15%.[131,136] The TNM system is now used to stage all lung cancers.[137] This has replaced the old classification of small cell lung carcinoma whereby disease was classified into limited (confined to one hemithorax, including ipsilateral mediastinal and supraclavicular nodes) or extensive disease (spread beyond the hemithorax).[131]

Management

Treatment decisions in lung cancer cases are based on the stage of disease, histology, the presence of comorbid diseases, and performance status (Table 49-3); they should not be based on chronologic age. Despite this, there is evidence that older patients are undertreated and are underrepresented in clinical trials, making evidence-based decision difficult.[138-140] When assessing patients, it is useful to perform a comprehensive geriatric assessment, including measures of functional status, comorbidity, cognitive state, and nutritional status.[141] Aging is associated with a physiologic decline in organ function and a number of changes in drug pharmokinetics and pharmodynamics. These changes result in differences in treatment tolerance between older and younger patients.[136] Clinical trials specifically designed for the older adult population are needed, although over the past 10 years some progress has been made.[141]

TABLE 49-3 WHO Performance Status Score

Grade	Explanation of Activity
0	Asymptomatic
1	Symptomatic but ambulatory (able to perform light work)
2	In bed less than 50% of day (unable to work but able to live at home with some assistance)
3	In bed more than 50% of day (unable to care for self)
4	Bedridden

NON–SMALL CELL LUNG CARCINOMA

Surgery

Surgery is the treatment of choice for all patients with resectable (stage I/II) NSCLC who are fit enough for the procedure. A number of studies have confirmed the feasibility of surgical treatment in older adults, including octogenarians. However, evidence suggests that fit older adult patients are less likely to be offered surgery than are younger patients with more comorbidities. VATS techniques are increasingly used.[94]

Adjuvant Chemotherapy

Postoperative chemotherapy should be offered to patients with a good performance status and histologic evidence of locally advanced disease (T1-3, N1-2).[131] A trial of patients older than 70 years has shown a significant survival benefit with adjuvant chemotherapy (although not for patients older than 80 years) with similar tolerability compared with younger patients.[142] The risk/benefit ratio in patients older than 80 years has not been adequately studied, and the use of adjuvant chemotherapy remains controversial.[141]

Radical Radiotherapy

Radical radiotherapy is indicated in early stage disease if all of the disease can be encompassed in a radiotherapy field.[131] Older patients are frequently unable to undergo surgery because of comorbidities or reluctance to proceed. In these cases radical radiotherapy is effective, with reported mean survival times of 20 to 27 months and 5-year survival rates of 15% to 34% in patients older than 70 years. Treatment outcomes and toxicity rates do not differ with age.[143] Continuous hyperfractionated accelerated radiotherapy (CHART) is high-dose radiotherapy given three times a day for 12 days. A large randomized trial has shown an improvement in 2-year survival from 20% with conventional radiotherapy to 29% with CHART.[144]

Stereotactic Ablative Radiotherapy

Stereotactic ablative radiotherapy (SABR) is a form of high-precision radiotherapy that can be used to treat very early (stage I) lung cancer. It is given over a short period of time and is associated with minimal damage to surrounding structures. It is therefore an attractive option in older adults and those with poor baseline lung function.[141]

Radiofrequency Ablation

Radiofrequency ablation is a new radiologic technique for treating selected early lung cancers in patients unsuitable for surgical resection. An electrode is inserted into the mass through which electric current is passed to ablate the tumor cells. Pneumothorax is the main complication.[145]

Locally Advanced Disease

Patients with locally advanced NSCLC (stage II-III) should be considered for combined chemo/radiotherapy.[131] Combined treatment may offer a survival benefit but needs to be balanced against the increased risk of toxicity. Conflicting evidence exists regarding this approach in older patients. Treatment outcomes are comparable to those of younger patients; however, there is a higher risk of toxicity in older patients.[146] For patients with an impaired performance status or severe comorbidity, radiotherapy alone is an alternative.[147,148]

Palliative Chemotherapy

Chemotherapy is the mainstay of treatment for patients with advanced disease (stage III-IV).[131] A standard regimen would include a platinum-based chemotherapy agent with a single third generation agent (e.g., carboplatin/cisplatin plus vinorelbine/gemcitabine/paclitaxel/docetaxel). This has a modest survival benefit (increase in median survival by 1.5 months, 10% improvement in 1-year survival) compared with supportive care alone.[131,149] Platinum-based chemotherapy is efficacious in older individuals; however, it is associated with significant toxicity (nephrotoxicity, ototoxicity, neurotoxicity).[150] Furthermore, the survival benefit of chemotherapy is limited to patients with a good performance status (WHO 0-1).[148] It is therefore only an option in fit older patients.[141]

Epidermal Growth Factor Receptor Tyrosine Kinase Inhibitors

Knowledge of cancer biology has enabled the development of new agents that specifically block pathways involved in oncogenesis. Gefitanib and erlotinib are selective inhibitors of epidermal growth factor receptors (EGFRs) that have demonstrated activity in patients with NSCLC.[151] These agents are well tolerated and are first-line treatments for those patients with an EGFR mutation.[141] A recent trial enrolled very old patients (older than 80 years) or patients with poor performance status[3-4] and demonstrated significant benefit even in these patients.[152]

Palliative Radiotherapy

Radiotherapy can be used to improve symptoms, particularly hemoptysis, chest pain, dyspnea, and cough. Older patients tolerate radiotherapy well and gain equivalent palliation compared with their younger counterparts.[153] Performance status does not influence benefit from radiotherapy.

SMALL CELL LUNG CARCINOMA

Small cell lung carcinoma is an aggressive form of cancer and tends to metastasize early. As a result, chemotherapy is the mainstay of treatment. Two thirds of patients have widespread disease at presentation. The median survival is only 2 to 4 months without treatment.[154] Surgery can be considered in early stage disease (T1-2a).[131]

Limited Stage Disease

In limited stage disease (T1-4, N0-3, M0), response rates to chemotherapy are between 70% and 80%, with a median survival of 12 to 16 months. Only 4% to 5% of patients can be considered cured.[155] The standard treatment for limited disease small cell lung cancer is four to six cycles of a platinum-based chemotherapy regimen (commonly etoposide plus carboplatin) combined with thoracic radiotherapy. In patients who achieve complete remission, prophylactic cranial irradiation is offered. Prophylactic cranial radiotherapy has been shown to reduce the incidence of brain metastases and is associated with a slight survival benefit (5.4% at 3 years).[156]

Many trials have looked at chemotherapy regimens for older patients with small cell lung carcinoma. Standard regimens remain the most effective and are therefore the treatment of choice despite their significant toxicity.[157] Comprehensive geriatric assessment is essential for appropriate patient selection.[158] For frailer patients, less aggressive regimens can be used. Such regimens include dose reduction, shortened treatment duration, and single-agent chemotherapy.[131,155]

Thoracic radiotherapy is associated with considerable toxicity (bone marrow and esophageal), particularly in older patients. Sequential chemoradiotherapy is less toxic than a standard concurrent approach. A meta-analysis of thoracic radiotherapy trials showed a small but significant survival benefit (5.4% ± 1.4% at 3 years) from treatment. However, this effect was lost in patients older than 70 years.[159] Recent guidelines support the use of thoracic radiotherapy in fit older adults (WHO performance status, 0-2) with close attention paid to treatment-related toxicity.[157]

Extensive Disease

Response rates to chemotherapy are between 60% and 70%, with a median survival of 7 to 11 months. Virtually no patients survive to 5 years.[155] Chemotherapy alone is the standard treatment of extensive disease; radiotherapy has only a palliative role. Dual-agent platinum-based regimens are the most effective, and usually six cycles are given. Quality of life should be the goal. There is evidence that prophylactic cranial radiotherapy in extensive small cell lung carcinoma reduces the incidence of symptomatic brain metastasis and improves overall survival (1-year survival rate 27.1% vs. 13.3%).[160]

Palliative Care

Supportive care is particularly important in the treatment of lung cancer as most patients have incurable disease. Symptom control, psychological support, and social requirements should all be addressed. A multidisciplinary approach is recommended, involving respiratory physicians, palliative care teams, oncologists, physiotherapists, occupational therapists, and dietitians.[131]

MALIGNANT MESOTHELIOMA

Pleural mesothelioma has been increasing in incidence in the United Kingdom since the 1960s. The annual number of deaths from mesothelioma is predicted to rise until the 2020s.[161] In 2011 there were 2570 new diagnoses of mesothelioma in the United Kingdom.[162] Asbestos exposure is the cause of 85% of cases.[163,164] The latency period is typically long, with a mean of 41 years (range, 15 to 67 years).[164] As a result, mesothelioma is typically a disease of older men; 46% of new diagnoses in 2011 were in individuals aged 75 years or older.[162] The prognosis is poor, with a median survival of 14 months from symptom onset.[164] Patients with mesothelioma may be eligible for compensation if they are able to verify occupational exposure to asbestos.

Presenting symptoms are classically chest pain and dyspnea, which is related to pleural fluid or thickening. Mesothelioma of the peritoneal cavity can also occur. A CT scan of the thorax may identify pleural nodules or diffuse thickening. Pathologic diagnosis can be made by examination of pleural fluid cytology (sensitivity of 60% to 76%[163,165]); however, a pleural biopsy is usually required. Medical thoracoscopy (or VATS procedure) is the procedure of choice to diagnose mesothelioma because of its superior sensitivity compared with blind Abrams needle biopsy (90% vs. 43%).[166,167]

Management

The management of mesothelioma is largely palliative. Dyspnea is relieved by drainage of pleural fluid and pleurodesis. Palliative chemotherapy can be given to patients who have a good performance status although there is no randomized control trial evidence to show that chemotherapy confers better quality of life and survival than active supportive care alone.[163] Pemetrexed in combination with cisplatin was licensed for treatment of malignant mesothelioma after a randomized control trial showed a survival benefit compared with cisplatin alone (median survival time 13.2% vs. 9.3 months).[168] Combination treatment was associated with a higher incidence of significant toxicity. Pemetrexed can be efficacious and well tolerated in older adult patients,[169] although trials have not specifically addressed its use in older adults with mesothelioma.

The role of surgery in mesothelioma remains controversial, especially in frail older adults. In any case, radical surgical resection (extrapleural pneumonectomy) is associated with a relatively high risk of morbidity and mortality and does not have a significant beneficial impact on survival.[167,170] Debulking surgery is effective in preventing fluid recurrence and may be associated with increased survival although this has not been established in a randomized control trial.

Radiotherapy can be used as a palliative treatment to provide pain relief. It also can be used as part of the management strategy when extrapleural pneumonectomy is performed. Prophylactic radiotherapy is administered to scars produced by biopsy, pleural drainage, or both. A randomized trial has shown that this prevents the risk of seeding of malignant cells,[171] although more recent trials have questioned this.[172,173]

KEY POINTS

- Age-related changes to the lungs predispose older adults to higher rates of respiratory disease.
- Respiratory infections, diffuse parenchymal lung disease, and thoracic tumors are common in older adults.
- Most respiratory illness in older adults requires a multidisciplinary team approach to care, including geriatric physicians and respiratory physicians.
- Management strategies require a careful evaluation of performance status, comorbidity, and concurrent medication.
- Respiratory disease is diverse and frequently presents nonspecifically in older adults. Accurate diagnosis usually requires careful systematic evaluation.

For a complete list of references, please visit www.expertconsult.com.

KEY REFERENCES

3. Simonetti AF, Viasus D, Garcia-Vidal C, et al: Management of community-acquired pneumonia in older adults. Ther Adv Infect Dis 2(1):3–16, 2014.
32. Lim WS, Baudouin SV, George RC, et al: BTS guidelines for the management of community acquired pneumonia in adults: update. Thorax 64(Suppl 3):iii1–iii55, 2009.
34. Kaplan V, Angus D, Griffin M, et al: Hospitalized community-acquired pneumonia in the elderly: age- and sex-related patterns of care and outcome in the United States. Am J Respir Crit Care Med 165(6):766–772, 2002.
64. Cruz-Hervert LP, García-García L, Ferreyra-Reyes L, et al: Tuberculosis in ageing: high rates, complex diagnosis and poor clinical outcomes. Age Ageing 41(4):488–495, 2012.
67. American Thoracic Society/Centers for Disease Control and Prevention/Infectious Diseases Society of America: Controlling tuberculosis in the United States. Am J Respir Crit Care Med 172(9):1169–1227, 2005.
68. Thrupp L, Bradley S, Smith P, et al: Tuberculosis prevention and control in long-term-care facilities for older adults. Infect Control Hosp Epidemiol 25(12):1097–1108, 2004.
79. Griffith D, Aksamit T, Brown-Elliott B, et al: An official ATS/IDSA statement: diagnosis, treatment, and prevention of nontuberculous mycobacterial diseases. Am J Respir Crit Care Med 175(4):367–416, 2007.
82. Nicotra M, Rivera M, Dale A, et al: Clinical, pathophysiologic, and microbiologic characterization of bronchiectasis in an aging cohort. Chest 108(4):955–961, 1995.

90. Havelock T, Teoh R, Laws D, et al: Pleural procedures and thoracic ultrasound: British Thoracic Society pleural disease guideline 2010. Thorax 65(Suppl 2):ii61–ii76, 2010.
93. MacDuff A, Arnold A, Harvey J, et al: Management of spontaneous pneumothorax: British Thoracic Society pleural disease guideline 2010. Thorax 65(Suppl 2):ii18–ii31, 2010.
96. American Thoracic Society, European Respiratory Society: American Thoracic Society/European Respiratory Society International Multidisciplinary Consensus Classification of the Idiopathic Interstitial Pneumonias. Am J Respir Crit Care Med 165(2):277–304, 2002.
97. Bradley B, Branley HM, Egan JJ, et al: Interstitial lung disease guideline: the British Thoracic Society in collaboration with the Thoracic Society of Australia and New Zealand and the Irish Thoracic Society. Thorax 63(Suppl 5):v1–v58, 2008.
102. National Institute for Health and Care Excellence: Idiopathic pulmonary fibrosis (NICE guidelines [CG163]). https://www.nice.org.uk/guidance/cg163, 2013. Accessed September 25, 2015.
103. The Idiopathic Pulmonary Fibrosis Clinical Research Network: Prednisolone, azathioprine and N-acetylcysteine for pulmonary fibrosis. New Engl J Med 366:1968–1977, 2012.
107. National Institute for Health and Care Excellence: Pirfenidone for treating idiopathic pulmonary fibrosis (NICE technology appraisal guidance [TA282]). https://www.nice.org.uk/guidance/ta282, 2013. Accessed September 25, 2015.
108. Orens J, Estenne M, Arcasoy S, et al: International guidelines for the selection of lung transplant candidates: 2006 update—a consensus report from the Pulmonary Scientific Council of the International Society for Heart and Lung Transplantation. J Heart Lung Transplant 25(7):745–755, 2006.
112. Langford C: Vasculitis in the geriatric population. Rheum Dis Clin North Am 33(1):177–195, 2007.
113. Stadnyk A, Rubinstein I, Grossman R, et al: Clinical features of sarcoidosis in elderly patients. Sarcoidosis 5(2):121–123, 1988.
120. Hoganson D, From A, Michet C: ANCA vasculitis in the elderly. J Clin Rheumatol 14(2):78–81, 2008.
122. Haris Á, Polner K, Arányi J, et al: Clinical outcomes of ANCA-associated vasculitis in elderly patients. Int Urol Nephrol 46(8):1595–1600, 2014.
130. Alberts WM: Introduction to the third edition: Diagnosis and management of lung cancer, 3rd ed: American College of Chest Physicians evidence-based clinical practice guidelines. Chest 143(5 Suppl):38S–40S, 2013.
131. National Institute for Health and Care Excellence: Lung cancer: the diagnosis and treatment of lung cancer (NICE guidelines [CG21]). https://www.nice.org.uk/guidance/cg121, 2011 Accessed September 25, 2015.
135. Evison M, Crosbie PA, Martin J, et al: EBUS-TBNA in elderly patients with lung cancer: safety and performance outcomes. J Thorac Oncol 9(3):370–376, 2014.
141. Pallis AG, Gridelli C, Wedding U, et al: Management of elderly patients with NSCLC; updated expert's opinion paper: EORTC Elderly Task Force, Lung Cancer Group and International Society for Geriatric Oncology. Ann Oncol 2014.
163. British Thoracic Society Standards of Care Committee: BTS statement on malignant mesothelioma in the UK, 2007. Thorax 62(Suppl 2):ii1–ii19, 2007.

50 Classification of the Dementias

Richard Camicioli, Kenneth Rockwood

OVERVIEW

Dementia is a critical public health problem worldwide, especially as populations age. As a consequence, physicians dealing with a range of other age-associated problems can expect to see such problems in patients with dementia. Dementia diagnosis is evolving. Here, we review recent developments in the syndromic approach to dementia, and then highlight aspects of its differential diagnosis.[1] Dementia generally has been defined in terms of multifocal cognitive impairment sufficient to impair function and typically is distinguished from cognitive decline of lesser severity and impact. Since the seventh edition of this book was published in 2010, several changes in dementia conceptualization have been proposed. These include a new lexicon and several new sets of diagnostic criteria,[2-6] as well as growing support for the claim that "subjective cognitive impairment," even "subjective memory complaints," are important risks for developing dementia.[7] Especially important have been the proposals to diagnose what previously were understood as dementing illnesses, notably Alzheimer disease, without dementia being present. Even so, the new criteria must be considered in light of potential challenges raised by prospective, community-based autopsy studies. As detailed next, pathologic changes consistent with pathologically defined entities, including Alzheimer disease (plaques and tangles), Parkinson disease (α-synuclein/Lewy bodies), and cerebrovascular disease (large and small vessel strokes, white matter changes), can be seen in patients with cognitive decline short of dementia. Moreover, such pathologic changes often overlap in individuals. Furthermore, these studies show that some individuals can have clinical dementia without clear pathologic markers.

LIMITATIONS OF CURRENT CLASSIFICATION

The syndrome of dementia remains largely as it always has been. The fifth edition of the American Psychiatric Association's *Diagnostic and Statistical Manual of Mental Disorders* has renamed dementia as a "Major Neurocognitive Disorder."[8] Although there are many important details for research,[9] including an attempt to provide a common language for the description of overlapping aspects of dementia, delirium, and depression, the new criteria require validation and appear to have little practical impact on how to proceed. Awaiting more widespread adoption of this inclusive term, we will stick with *dementia* in this chapter. It remains the case that, as they age, most people find that their memory is not as good as it used to be. Many fewer actually have dementia.[10] Where to draw the line between memory complaints and dementia—and how many lines to draw—is controversial, highlighting the artificiality of the definition as a purely discrete entity.[11] In addition, other aspects of behavior, such as neuropsychiatric problems (including depression) and mobility difficulties, precede dementia and are associated with cognitive decline, highlighting the restrictive nature of current classifications based mainly on cognitive criteria.[12] Nevertheless, making a diagnosis of the dementia syndrome in relation to the severity of cognitive impairment and a clinically important impact on activities of daily living remains practical. It recognizes that care needs are present or anticipated, and it assists in linking cognitive and behavioral syndromes to pathology.

Against this traditional approach is the view that waiting until the disease is clinically evident is to wait too long. This desire to get at the dementing illnesses before their clinical onset motivates the new criteria (especially the proposal for preclinical diagnosis), which hold that to do so is to wait past a time when intervention might alter the clinical course of dementia, perhaps even preventing it entirely. We will consider this, and the prospect of disease-modifying drugs, later.

Turning to other limitations of the how dementia is approached as a syndrome, the issue of the onset of clinically important change is another area of potential controversy. Delirium is considered a syndrome of acute onset with fluctuating attention and an identifiable cause. Delirium does not always reverse.[13] Indeed, persisting delirium is now recognized as a state that not uncommonly merges with dementia, likely reflecting shared elements of pathophysiology in relation to neurodegenerative and inflammatory processes.[14] Whether this is because the delirium causes the chronic, persistent, cognitive impairment or simply because the delirium occurred in the setting of dementia (or predementia), or whether many delirium symptoms that fall short of meeting delirium criteria are signaling an at-risk state for which our current descriptions are inadequate, is not clear.[15] Acute onset of dementia can occur and does not always indicate delirium.

Especially in the emerging era of presymptomatic diagnosis of dementing illnesses, the issue of how best to consider multiple causes requires consideration anew. An important challenge is the realization that the specificity of cause, symptoms, and neuropathology is much fuzzier than had been appreciated, especially in very old people.[16] Dementia chiefly happens not just in older adults but, as is becoming clear from an emerging body of evidence, it arises largely in people who have many health deficits.[17-20] Despite many patients having distinct symptomatic profiles in relation to the type of dementia that they have, as age increases, overlap of symptoms is common.[21] This overlap also extends to the underlying neuropathology, something that especially has been revealed by prospective, community-based studies. The fact that autopsy series in community-dwelling older adults show that many have mixed pathologies[22] (up to three quarters in some series) has implications, especially for our understanding of mechanisms.[23] Interpretations vary as to how often dementia arises as a result of complex constellations of underlying neuropathology versus the simple fact of cumulative damage.[24] Whether neuropathology under these circumstances will retain its iconic "gold standard" status or whether it will be viewed best as an aspect of construct validation (another factor to be considered) is debatable.[25] Other consequences arise. From a clinical standpoint, DSM-V modifications have been argued to be most in line with this new reality and are held to provide clinicians with a common language that can thereby be used to describe overlapping symptoms and set these in the context of distinct profiles.[26] Against this background, it remains to be seen how much sense it makes to view patients with single-gene mutations in early-onset dementia as offering "proof of concept" for disease-modifying therapy that might avoid late life dementia in people with a panoply of causes. Very early attempts at combining biomarkers (e.g., within cerebrospinal fluid [CSF] or across modalities) showed that dementia tests are not exempt from trade-offs in sensitivity and specificity.[27]

An additional challenge to the interpretation of the many causes that give rise to dementia in older people is overlapping pathology, which may be more the rule in older adults where Alzheimer pathology can overlap with vascular or Lewy bodies and other age-related changes. Furthermore, each of these pathologic markers can be present in patients who are apparently cognitively intact. Further challenging the present understanding is that older people can decline cognitively without obvious brain changes other than atrophy, at least as detectable by current techniques.

DEMENTIA DEFINITIONS

General criteria for dementia (and its congeners) include the DSM-V criteria and International Classification of Diseases, 10th revision (ICD-10) criteria; each features the requirements of both cognitive impairment (in more than one domain of cognition) and functional impairment. Memory impairment is specified as a domain for ICD-10. Competing sets of criteria for vascular dementia have been supplanted by a proposal from the Society for Vascular Cognitive Impairment (VASCOG).[28] Current dementia with Lewy bodies criteria include the presence of distinctive clinical features, such as REM sleep behavior disorder, and laboratory findings such as decreased dopamine transporter binding.[29,30] Even so, although the criteria have increased in specificity, this has come at a cost of less sensitivity; interestingly, one proposed remedy has been the use of composite scores, reflecting a general theme of paying attention to both quantitative and qualitative aspects of dementia diagnosis, especially in late life. The definition of Parkinson dementia has been addressed,[31] although its main distinction in relation to Lewy body dementia (how long motor symptoms preceded cognitive ones) is artificial. Criteria for frontotemporal lobar degeneration that predict pathologic findings have also been put forward.[32] Recent criteria for the behavioral variant of frontotemporal dementia have been validated in autopsy series, with individual items showing moderate-substantial interrater reliability.[33] Similarly, subtypes of primary progressive aphasias, which have varied pathologies, have been related to autopsy findings, albeit with imperfect clinical-pathologic correlation.[34]

RISK FACTORS

Age

Age is the most potent risk factor for most dementias,[35] including Alzheimer disease, dementia with Lewy bodies, and Parkinson disease with dementia and vascular cognitive impairment/dementia. Since age is associated with each of these, overlapping pathology is common.[22,23,36] Despite the obvious relationship with age, the now obsolete NINCDS-ADRD criteria placed age limits, with a lower limit of 40 years of age and upper limit of 90 years of age, for a diagnosis of Alzheimer disease.[37] This highlights why those criteria needed updating: dementia appears to affect most people aged 90 years and older and to arise from multiple causes.[16] In familial Alzheimer disease, onset in the 30s is not unheard of and even though more unusual disorders such as childhood metabolic disorders become more common, Alzheimer remains an important consideration in younger cases. Although a number of genetic and metabolic conditions cause dementia in younger people, these will not be covered.[38]

Frontotemporal dementias (FTDs) are a group of clinically defined syndromes associated with dementia, typically with onset younger than age 65 and with recognized variants.[32,33,34,39] However, many patients with FTD syndromes, including frontotemporal lobar degeneration, progressive nonfluent aphasia, semantic dementia, corticobasal ganglionic degeneration, and frontotemporal dementia with motor neuron disease, have onset in old age, where clinical features such as memory problems may be confused with Alzheimer disease, which itself can have focal presentations, with prominent executive dysfunction, apraxia, or visuospatial deficits.[40,41] Additional distinct pathologic entities, including argyrophilic grain disease[42] and hippocampal sclerosis,[43] have been recognized as entities that overlap phenotypically with more common dementias. Given their predilection for medial temporal lobe involvement, not surprisingly, memory impairment is evident, which leads to confusion with Alzheimer disease.[44] Their distinction from other pathologic disorders such as the FTD syndromes is not clear.

Family History and Genetics

Young-onset dementia is more often associated with a strong family history consistent with autosomal dominance. For example, familial Alzheimer disease and FTD typically occur in the younger age range, but late-onset individuals are not that unusual in practice. Patients with frontotemporal dementias are more likely to have a family history.[45] Gene carriers with common mutations associated with frontotemporal dementia, including progranulin, *MAPT*, and *C9orf72*, can have a long prodromal phase, leading to confusion with psychiatric disorders or mild cognitive impairment states.[46] The range in age of onset can vary within a family with a genetic family history, and sometimes family history is not known. In Alzheimer disease, mutations in the *presenilin 1* (*PSEN1*) gene predominate among patients who are younger than 60 years of age but can have a range in age of onset.[47] A family history, with dementia occurring in more than one first-degree relative, is not uncommon, even in old age. A history of more than one first-degree relative is more common in young-onset dementia than in those with onset in the oldest old age range (>80 years). Although the apolipoprotein E4 (*ApoE4*) allele is a risk factor for Alzheimer dementia, it does not account for all of the increased risk associated with family history. It now has been established that several genes are implicated in late-onset Alzheimer disease, where their roles typically are small but act in combination, including with APOE loci variants.[48,49]

Gender is a factor that affects the differential diagnosis on an epidemiologic basis, with men more likely to have vascular dementia and Lewy body dementia and women more likely to have Alzheimer disease.[50] More than a genetic factor, gender influences behavior (i.e., exposure to environmental risk factors) and hormonal levels, which could influence dementia risk. Moreover, women may be at greater risk for autoimmune disorders.

Psychiatric Disorders

Neuropsychiatric symptoms may precede a dementia diagnosis and are more common in people with mild cognitive impairment than in cognitively intact older people.[51] Neuropsychiatric symptoms can increase the risk of progression from a mild cognitive impairment state to dementia.[52] Depression has been identified as a risk factor for dementia, and a depression syndrome of dementia has been identified.[53] Even so, disentangling the two can be complicated. Reactive depression can occur as a consequence of a dementia diagnosis. Given that depression is common in older adults, occurrence of dementia with depression might occur by chance. However, common causes (i.e., cerebrovascular disease, dementia with Lewy bodies, and Alzheimer disease) can lead to both depression and dementia, and several studies have shown that depression precedes dementia.[54]

Neuropsychiatric symptoms are common in all of the dementias. Psychosis, specifically visual hallucinations, is a core criterion for dementia with Lewy bodies and commonly occurs in Parkinson disease, where symptoms of psychosis can precede dementia or occur in the setting of dementia.[55,56] Delusions, notably paranoia, are commonly seen in adults who have Alzheimer disease, and impaired insight and judgment, as well as other behavioral problems, are central symptoms of frontotemporal dementia and are commonly seen in adults who have vascular dementia.[57]

Other Risk Factors

As noted, the overall level of health is an important risk for dementia: in older adults, dementia is strongly associated with more health deficits and with frailty (defined either as a syndrome or as a state).[17-20] Note also that, especially considering frailty as a syndrome, some of the neuropathologic markers of dementia are also associated with phenotypic features of frailty.[58] Cardiovascular disease–related risk factors (i.e., hypertension, diabetes, smoking, hypercholesterolemia) increase the risk of late life dementia.[59] It is not clear if vascular risk factors cause damage via stroke or ischemia that lowers cognitive reserve or if they incite a pathologic cascade that leads to accelerated cognitive decline. Related risk factors are educational attainment and physical activity level, which have been associated with dementia risk but are confounded by socioeconomic status, which in turn affects general health, especially cardiovascular health.[60]

Head trauma is another fairly consistently identified risk factor for late life dementia, which may similarly affect brain function.[61] Chronic traumatic encephalopathy is receiving increased attention as a potentially preventable cause of dementia.[62] Both acute cerebrovascular events and head injury in older people can be associated with global cognitive decline and can accelerate the course of an established dementia. Data regarding mild cognitive impairment are less clear.

DEMENTIA ASSOCIATED WITH OTHER DISORDERS

Numerous disorders can cause dementia because of effects on brain function. Approximately 7% to 10% of dementias can come on suddenly, often indicating a cerebrovascular event or other medical problem.[63] When onset is abrupt, it is possible that the onset marks a delirium, and investigations and interventions should proceed accordingly. Although the differential diagnosis of delirium can overlap with that of dementia, and people with dementia are at risk for delirium, the two should be considered distinct. The disorders discussed in this section can give rise to prolonged illness that can lead to confusion with degenerative disorders. In some cases they are treatable and can potentially be cured, although this is unusual.[64,65] Strictly speaking, such disorders are among issues that should be excluded for a patient to meet criteria for a degenerative dementia; however, sometimes they can cause irreversible change in the absence of a neurodegenerative disorder.

Alcohol/Drugs/Toxins

Alcohol is an important covert cause of dementia worldwide. Abuse of alcohol is underrecognized in general, and it should be screened for.[66] Direct effects of alcohol on central nervous system function can produce syndromes such as Wernicke encephalopathy (nystagmus, restricted extraocular movements, ataxia) and Korsakoff syndrome (with persistent executive and memory dysfunction), which are recognizable causes of cognitive impairment since they often present in association with other examination features in the setting of alcohol abuse. This clinical picture can also occur in the absence of alcohol exposure with severe malnutrition where similar imaging and clinical changes are present,[67] with involvement of the medial thalami and the periventricular region of the third ventricle, the periaqueductal area, the mammillary bodies, the tectal plate, and, in rare cases, the dorsal medulla.[68] It can be difficult to separate effects of chronic exposure of alcohol from other effects, such as effects on vascular risk and brain injuries, for which people with alcohol abuse are at increased risk. Associated lifestyle habits (e.g., smoking) and socioeconomic status can also compound risk for dementia in a population prone to alcohol abuse. Lower levels of intake of alcohol are reported to be protective, but it is difficult to separate this from other factors.[69]

Although alcohol is a common cause of hepatic disease, including cirrhosis, hepatic dysfunction from any cause can lead to an encephalopathy and cognitive impairment. Although in principle reversal of liver damage will lead to normalization of cognitive function, this may not always be the case. Direct effects of toxins such as manganese accumulation and unmeasured substances may be responsible for neurologic dysfunction in the setting of hepatic dysfunction.[70]

Medications for various conditions have been associated with chronic cognitive impairment. Particular drugs include corticosteroids, anticholinergic medications, benzodiazepines, psychiatric medications, and antiepileptic medications, among others. Drugs should be discontinued if they might be temporally associated with cognitive decline. Aging is associated with pharmacokinetic and pharmacodynamic changes that might lead to a chronic medication becoming toxic without clearly being temporally associated with cognitive decline. Accidental overdosing due to forgetfulness can also contribute to amplified effects of medications.[71]

Other toxins, especially metals such as aluminum, mercury, bismuth, and lead, have been associated with cognitive dysfunction. Toxins affecting cholinergic or mitochondrial function (e.g., pesticides) or those causing white matter damage (e.g., solvents) can be related to chronic cognitive impairment. Metals such as copper, zinc, and iron are involved in normal cellular processing and have been examined in relation to dementia.

Autoimmune and Inflammatory Disorders

Autoimmune and inflammatory causes are rare but treatable causes of dementia in older adults.[72] Vasculitis can cause dementia through ischemic damage. All forms of vasculitis (e.g., small vessel or large vessel) can lead to progressive neurologic dysfunction. There are often clues to the diagnosis, such as systemic complaints, headache, and sometimes evidence for an associated autoimmune disease. Large vessel vasculitides such as giant cell (temporal) arteritis, Churg-Strauss syndrome, polyarteritis nodosa, Wegener granulomatosis, Behçet syndrome, and Sjögren syndrome often show evidence for systemic disease and inflammatory markers (increased C-reactive protein and sedimentation rate). Serologic investigations can identify vasculitis associated with other autoimmune disorders; however, primary central nervous system vasculitis can cause progressive cognitive decline unassociated with other markers.[73] Angiography and brain biopsy may be necessary to diagnose inflammatory disorders causing dementia, although evidence for an inflammatory process can often be identified by examining spinal fluid (elevated cell count, increased immunoglobulin synthesis, elevated protein level). A sedimentation rate or C-reactive protein can be associated with a chronic inflammatory process of any cause, but also specifically with giant cell arteritis. Immunoglobulins are elevated in inflammatory disorders, but monoclonal elevation can be associated with multiple myeloma.

Limbic encephalitis on an autoimmune basis can present as an acute or a subacute dementia. It can be paraneoplastic or nonparaneoplastic. Imaging findings can mimic prion disease, but distinct changes, including high signal change on magnetic resonance imaging (MRI), are important to recognize. As with other autoimmune dementias, nonspecific CSF changes can be evident.

Specific serum or CSF abnormalities can confirm the diagnosis. Practically, such patients should be examined and investigated for the presence of a neoplasm, recognizing that a purely autoimmune process may cause a clinically indistinguishable syndrome and that these disorders are treatable. Thus care must be taken to not simply rely on the presence of antibodies but to consider the level of the antibody titers and the possibility of false positive results.[74] Inflammatory disorders can also lead to a hypercoagulable state, which can be seen in association with anticardiolipin or antiphospholipid antibodies, sometimes with evidence for a lupus anticoagulant. Sneddon syndrome is characterized by livedo reticularis associated with hypercoagulability, which typically occurs in younger people but can also occur in older people.[75] Antinuclear antibodies, extractable nuclear antibodies, antiphospholipid or anticardiolipin antibodies or a lupus anticoagulant, as well as physical examination findings, may point to an autoimmune or collagen vascular disorder. Nonvasculitic autoimmune meningoencephalitis is a relatively recently recognized cause of dementia, sometimes, but not necessarily, associated with collagen vascular disorders such as Sjögren syndrome, antiphospholipid antibody syndrome, systemic lupus erythematosus, mixed connective tissue disease, or Hashimoto encephalitis.[76,77] In some patients brain biopsy may be warranted, which may be justifiable given that it is treatable. Drugs, notably nonsteroidal antiinflammatory medications, can be associated with a meningoencephalitis, which can mimic a subacutely progressive dementia.[78] Sarcoidosis is a great mimicker among inflammatory disorders. It can have ocular, central, and peripheral nervous system involvement. Since it can present at any age, it should be considered in the differential diagnosis of dementia in older people.[79]

Endocrine Disorders

Metabolic and endocrine dysfunctions are common, but occasionally they are associated with potentially treatable causes of dementia.[80] Thyroid disorders, including hyperthyroidism and hypothyroidism, are associated with chronic cognitive impairment, and hence screening for thyroid dysfunction is recommended by most consensus guidelines. Autoimmune thyroid disease is associated with Hashimoto encephalitis, which is a treatable cause of dementia, with an abrupt or insidious onset, elevated antithyroid antibodies, and response to steroids.[81] Thyroid disease has also been identified as a risk factor for dementia.

Hyper- and hypoparathyroidism have been associated with cognitive impairment. Hyperparathyroidism is associated with hypercalcemia, which itself can lead to cognitive dysfunction. Hypoparathyroidism is commonly caused by surgical removal of the parathyroid glands, and treatment with calcium replacement and vitamin D are necessary. Parathyroid dysfunction is common in patients with renal failure. Parathyroid disorders can be associated with brain calcification. Recent studies have implicated vitamin D deficiency in cognitive decline and dementia; whether this reflects lack of outdoor activity, leading to lower levels of sun exposures; dietary factors; or an independent risk factor is not clear.[82]

Secondary or primary adrenal dysfunction can lead to cognitive dysfunction. Clues such as a history of steroid treatment or electrolyte abnormalities are often present. Assessment of adrenal function and possibly empirical therapy should be considered.

Diabetes is diagnosed by the presence of sustained hyperglycemia, which increases risk for cerebrovascular disease, but it can also lead to cognitive dysfunction without intervening cerebrovascular events.[83] Other secondary consequences include hyperlipidemia. Moreover, treatment of diabetes can lead to hypoglycemic episodes. Whether recurrent mild hypoglycemia causes direct nervous system damage is not clear, but severe and prolonged episodes clearly can cause permanent brain dysfunction. The metabolic syndrome defined by the presence of truncal obesity, hyperglycemia, high triglycerides, low HDL, and hypertension may increase the risk of cognitive impairment, but separating the effects of each component and elucidating direct from indirect (e.g., via strokes or accelerating progression of Alzheimer pathology) may be challenging.[84] Moreover, recent work suggests that the impact of the metabolic syndrome is strongest in people younger than 70 years of age, suggesting a loss of specificity in the setting of accumulating age-related deficits.[17]

Head Trauma and Dementia in Older Adults

Head injury is a risk factor for dementia. Although profound head trauma can clearly cause cognitive impairment, and repeated severe injury can lead to a dementia (e.g., dementia pugilistica), the mechanisms by which (and if) less severe head injury leads to cognitive impairment is not as clear.[85] Whether minor head injuries can trigger dementia also is not clear.[62]

In older people, subdural hematoma is a consequence of head injury but can occur spontaneously.[86] Anticoagulant use is a risk factor for hemorrhage and is a clear indication for brain imaging in patients with cognitive decline. Other states, such as renal failure, should be kept in mind. Relatively rapid progression, focal signs, and gait impairment are indicators that should prompt imaging. The decision to image can be challenging in patients with an existing dementia, but intervention can lead to improvement in function and should be considered in the case of superimposed subdural hematoma.

Infectious Disorders

Acute infections of any kind can lead to delirium, for which dementia is an important risk factor and which, in turn, is a risk for dementia.[87] Chronic infection of the nervous system can be associated with progressive cognitive decline without obvious systemic manifestations. Among these, HIV and syphilis are diseases for which serologic testing is diagnostic, although CSF examination is needed to confirm central nervous system involvement.[88] Although these disorders are more likely considerations in younger patients, it is important to realize that they can occur at any age. Given successful chronic treatment for HIV infection, more people will be living into old age and hence at risk for dementia.[89] Testing for syphilis was recommended routinely in the past and should be considered when appropriate. A search for chronic systemic infections by chest x-ray, urinalysis, and spinal fluid examination should be done if there are clinical clues or rapid onset. In addition, HIV has a worldwide reach and is an important contributor to cognitive dysfunction on a global scale.

Other chronic central nervous system infections such as cryptococcosis and tuberculosis should be considered in atypical patients with dementia, especially with rapid progression. Although these often occur in the setting of immunosuppression, where other opportunistic infections occur (e.g., toxoplasmosis, *Nocardia*, aspergillosis), they can occur without obvious predisposing factors. Another progressive infection that can cause insidious cognitive decline in a setting of immune incompetence is primary multifocal leukoencephalopathy. This generally presents as a patchy white matter disease.

Whipple disease, Lyme disease, West Nile virus, and listeriosis are unusual infectious disorders with central nervous system predilection. Both Whipple disease and Lyme disease can be associated with a chronic course. West Nile and other viral encephalopathies generally occur as acute illnesses. Viral encephalitis can have insidious presenting symptoms and can cause sufficient brain damage that leads to dementia. These often have additional clinical features and risk factors (including exposures), which raises the index of suspicion. A more rapid course suggests an acute infection such as herpes simplex, whose suspicion should prompt treatment with acyclovir. Whipple disease is associated with other neurologic findings (see later discussion) on examination, such as vertical gaze palsy and parkinsonism, and is important to consider in unusual subacute central nervous system disorders since it is treatable.[90]

Prion disease can occur at any age. It can occur in sporadic, genetic, and iatrogenic or infectious forms. Although sporadic Creutzfeldt-Jakob disease (CJD) is common in older adults, some genetic mutations associated with CJD can have late life onset and specific polymorphisms can affect the clinical presentation. CJD leads to a rapidly progressive dementia, usually with other clinical findings, including myoclonus, visuospatial impairment, and cerebellar ataxia, parkinsonism/pyramidal signs, and akinetic mutism being features of the diagnosis.[91] Laboratory evidence for CJD includes electroencephalogram (EEG) findings of periodic sharp waves, MRI changes on T2, FLAIR or diffusion weighted scans, and CSF evidence for elevation of the 14-3-3 protein. MRI changes are both sensitive and specific and complement CSF examination,[92] whereas EEG changes are not sensitive but, in the appropriate clinical setting, are highly suggestive. CSF proteins including14-3-3 and others (such as tau) may be helpful in differential diagnosis but need to be interpreted in clinical context.[93,94] MRI, EEG, and CSF examinations remain useful in ruling out other clinical mimics such as nonconvulsive seizures or chronic infections. Additional mimics include lithium or other drug toxicity, dementia with Lewy bodies, vasculitis of the central nervous system, autoimmune limbic encephalitis, and nonvasculitic autoimmune encephalopathy.

Metabolic Disorders and Nutritional Deficiencies

Most guidelines recommend assessment of metabolic conditions in the setting of dementia. Although criteria for degenerative conditions require exclusion of a potentially contributory condition, a common scenario is the co-occurrence of metabolic and degenerative conditions. With this in mind, assessment of complete blood count, glucose, electrolytes, renal function, liver function, vitamin B_{12}, and thyroid-stimulating hormone (TSH) is commonly recommended. Including calcium, magnesium, and phosphates in the electrolyte assessment can uncover abnormalities contributing to cognitive impairment. Similarly, folate (B_9) levels and those of other B vitamins, such as thiamine (B_1), riboflavin (B_2), niacin (B_3), and pyridoxine (B_6), have sometimes been associated with cognitive impairment but are usually normal and are not tested for routinely.[95]

Hepatic and renal dysfunction can be associated not only with delirium but also with a chronic picture of cognitive impairment. Although conditions leading to dysfunction in these organs, such as alcohol in the case of hepatic dysfunction or diabetes in the case of renal dysfunction, can also lead to cognitive impairment, toxin accumulation as a consequence of hepatic or renal dysfunction can directly affect cognition. Hepatic dysfunction can lead to manganese accumulation, which is associated with parkinsonism and cognitive impairment. Hyperammonemia on the basis of hepatic dysfunction can be associated with a chronic encephalopathy, even in the absence of elevated transaminases or bilirubin. It is increasingly recognized that patients with renal failure on dialysis can have dementia, which has important implications for decision making.[96] In dialysis patients, cognitive impairment can be a consequence of secondary hyperparathyroidism, which can also occur from other causes, such as surgical removal of the parathyroid glands.[97]

Neoplastic and Paraneoplastic Disorders

Direct effects of central nervous system neoplasms are usually self-evident and can be sought out using imaging if there are systemic clues or a history of a malignancy. Physical examination signs generally progress along with cognitive dysfunction. Occasionally patients do not have a prior history, making this possibility one of the important reasons for brain imaging. Some primary central nervous system neoplasms, such as lymphomas or gliomas, can present relatively insidiously, though they often present acutely (seizure or stroke mimic) or subacutely and imaging might not declare their presence or they can be nonspecific. Angiocentric lymphomatosis is an example in which proliferating cells are perivascular and imaging may be normal.[98] Although central nervous system lymphomas are often seen in the setting of immunosuppression on the basis of medications or HIV, they can occur independent of these risk factors.

Indirect effects of malignancy can be associated with paraneoplastic syndromes that include dementia-like presenting symptoms. As noted, limbic encephalitis is associated with central nervous system–directed antibodies, which can occur in the absence of a neoplasm.[99]

Chemotherapy and central nervous system radiation therapy for malignancy can complicate the picture by causing central nervous system effects that can be immediate and direct, or delayed. Radiation-induced leukoencephalopathy can sometimes be confused with recurrence or emergence of central nervous system malignancy.

Respiratory and Sleep Disorders

Hypoxemia and hypercarbia have direct effects on cognitive function; hence, pulmonary problems such as chronic obstructive pulmonary disease should be considered in the assessment of both acute and chronic cognitive decline. Acute anoxic injury is a well-recognized form of brain damage, and selective vulnerability of specific cell groups such as hippocampal neurons is recognized. Sleep apnea is another sleep problem that should be considered in the differential diagnosis of patients with day-to-day fluctuations in cognitive complaints. Sleep apnea alone is associated with problems on cognitive test performance.[100] Recent studies have shown sleep apnea to be a risk factor for cerebrovascular disease, which provides another mechanism for causing cognitive impairment.

Altered sleep patterns may be a risk factor for dementia; moreover, disruption of sleep is common in dementia.[101] Increased sleep fragmentation is common in aging and exaggerated in Alzheimer disease. Insomnia and hypersomnolence can occur in the course of a number of dementias and can be challenges to family members. Familial fatal insomnia is a prion disease associated with dementia that can also occur sporadically. REM sleep behavior disorder is a common symptom in synucleinopathies such as dementia with Lewy bodies, and these are included as supportive criteria for diagnosis.

Structural Lesions and Normal Pressure Hydrocephalus

Structural lesions of all types provide deficits that are localization related. The presence of rapid progression, focal features (including gait impairment and incontinence, which suggest frontostriatal damage), and risk factors for structural lesions (e.g., evidence of systemic malignancy, anticoagulation, or renal disease) merits cerebral imaging. In patients with existing cognitive impairment, the search for an additional structural cause may be necessary in cases of rapid decline. One consequence of structural problems near sites of ventricular drainage is hydrocephalus, which should be differentiated from normal pressure hydrocephalus (NPH).[102]

NPH is a specific entity in which hydrocephalus is present in the setting of the clinical triad of progressive dementia, gait difficulty, and urinary urgency and incontinence. Since each of these clinical symptoms/signs is common in older people for various reasons, it is plausible to have all three occur by chance. Moreover, cerebrovascular disease can affect the same frontostriatal circuits affected in NPH. The presence of comorbid central nervous system disease does not preclude improvement from shunting in individual patients; however, coexistent Alzheimer pathology may be associated with lack of improvement after shunting.[103] Currently the presence of the clinical triad with imaging evidence for hydrocephalus is necessary for the diagnosis. Improvement with lumbar puncture removal of a large volume of CSF, continuous external lumbar drain, or increased compliance on infusion into the lumbar space may be helpful in predicting patients who will improve from shunting. Clinical features such as long-standing clinical features, especially dementia, and the presence of verbal memory impairment make improvement less likely.

CLINICAL EXAMINATION FEATURES IN DIFFERENTIAL DIAGNOSIS

Aging is associated with physical changes that need to be differentiated from those of age-related disease. Features on the neurologic examination can assist in the differential diagnosis of degenerative dementias, as well.[104] Although patients with Alzheimer disease and frontotemporal dementia often have normal basic neurologic examinations, subtle findings such as slowing are often present early on. Over time and in subsets of patients, features such as extrapyramidal signs (bradykinesia and rigidity, often without resting tremor) can develop. Cerebrovascular disease commonly coexists with Alzheimer disease; hence, focal pyramidal findings (including the Babinski sign) and gait impairment can confound the diagnosis.

Autonomic Dysfunction

Older people can have autonomic problems such as postprandial hypotension, which can be exaggerated in the setting of systemic disorders such as diabetes or antihypertensive medication. Autonomic dysfunction is more commonly seen in dementia with Lewy bodies and in Parkinson disease with or without dementia.[105] This can be identified by history and confirmed by autonomic testing. Cardiac metaiodobenzylguanidine (MIBG) nuclear medicine scan abnormalities consistent with denervation can be seen in dementia with Lewy bodies and Parkinson disease and can add support to the diagnosis. Autonomic dysfunction can be seen in people with vascular disease in relation to risk factors such as diabetes. Multiple system atrophy, which is characterized by autonomic dysfunction, parkinsonism, and cerebellar dysfunction, is associated with executive dysfunction, which, if severe enough, can lead to dementia. Prion disease has also been associated with autonomic dysfunction.

Ocular and Visual Findings

Pupillary irregularities and abnormalities in accommodation, impaired pursuit movements, and diminished upgaze are seen in aging. Dementing disorders associated with eye movement abnormalities include Huntington disease, which is associated with an inability to perform saccades. Patients need to move their head (head thrusts) during saccades. Impaired downgaze, which can be overcome with oculocephalic head maneuvers, is characteristic of progressive supranuclear palsy. Dementias affecting the frontal lobes, including progressive supranuclear palsy, can affect initiation of saccades.[106] Opsoclonus (rapid nonstereotyped irregular involuntary eye movements) is seen in postviral encephalitis and as a paraneoplastic syndrome. Rhythmic eye movements associated with jaw and palate movements (oculomasticatory myorhythmia) is characteristic of Whipple disease. Nystagmus is characteristic of multiple system atrophy and other disorders affecting the brainstem and cerebellum.

Visuospatial impairment on a cortical basis is common in Alzheimer disease, dementia with Lewy bodies, and CJD, particularly the Heidenhain variant, which has predominant visuospatial impairment. This can occur early in the course of Alzheimer disease and indicates a phenotypic variant with some (but not absolute) diagnostic confidence.[41]

Pyramidal Disorders

Pyramidal (upper motor neuron) signs (decreased fine motor function, spastic increase tone, brisk reflexes, upgoing plantar responses) are common in people with cerebrovascular disease affecting the gray or white matter as well as in amyotrophic lateral sclerosis (motor neuron disease), which is also associated with lower motor neuron signs (weakness, wasting, fasciculations), which can be associated with progressive cognitive decline. Motor neuron disease can also be seen in frontotemporal dementia. Upper motor neuron signs are also seen in multiple system atrophy. Structural lesions of the nervous system often cause upper motor neuron signs.

Parkinsonian Disorders

Parkinsonism is defined by two signs among rest tremor, rigidity, and bradykinesia. These signs are nonspecific but are seen in Parkinson disease, dementia with Lewy bodies, progressive supranuclear palsy, multiple system atrophy, vascular parkinsonism, and NPH and occur in late Alzheimer disease and frontotemporal dementias. Thus parkinsonian features are very helpful in the differential diagnosis of dementia. Although gait impairment can occur early in Parkinson disease, it is more common in the other parkinsonian disorders noted and, if present at the time of diagnosis, provides a diagnostic trigger that the diagnosis is not Parkinson disease.

Cerebellar Signs

Cerebellar dysfunction can also lead to gait ataxia. It is prominent in alcohol-related dementia and, along with parkinsonism, can be seen in CJD. The cerebellar variant of multiple system atrophy, which can be associated with executive dysfunction, is also characterized by nystagmus on extraocular motility testing, appendicular dysmetria, and gait ataxia along with autonomic features.

Neuropathy and Other Lower Motor Neuron Findings

Evidence of neuropathy can be seen in a number of systemic problems associated with dementia, such as alcoholism, diabetes, renal dysfunction, and vitamin B_{12} deficiency. More ominously, rapidly progressive lower motor neuron problems can indicate a process involving the subarachnoid space (e.g., infection, carcinomatous meningitis). Neuropathy can be seen in paraneoplastic syndromes.

Gait Impairment

Balance and gait are integrated functions that involve all levels of the nervous system and require intact musculoskeletal and cardiorespiratory function; therefore, impaired balance or gait in the setting of dementia provides important clues to the differential diagnosis and raises concern for systemic disorders that might be contributing to cognitive dysfunction. Gait and balance impairment impact mobility and safety and need to be addressed if they are causing functional impairment. Dementias associated with gait impairment include Parkinson disease with dementia, vascular dementia, dementia with Lewy bodies, and NPH.[107]

Seizures and Myoclonus

Seizures increase in frequency with aging, often in association with central nervous system disease and metabolic insults. It is always important to consider reversible causes of seizures. Intermittent nonconvulsive seizures can mimic dementia by affecting cognitive function. Conversely, drugs used to treat seizures can affect cognitive function. It is important to also recognize that people with dementia can have coexistent seizures and to treat them appropriately.

Myoclonus is defined as rapid jerking movements associated with motor activation (positive myoclonus) or loss of activation (negative myoclonus). Myoclonus is common in CJD but can also be seen in other disorders associated with cognitive dysfunction, such as Alzheimer disease and corticobasal ganglionic degeneration. Apraxia refers to deficits in performing complex motor tests in the setting of intact comprehension and basic sensory and motor function. Apraxia and overlapping features with primary progressive aphasia and frontotemporal dementia are characteristic of the corticobasal syndrome, which can be caused by corticobasal ganglionic degeneration, where it is typically asymmetric, or even Alzheimer disease, where it typically occurs late in the course of disease. Jerking movement might be a clue to the presence of seizures as well and thus must be interpreted in clinical context.

Other Hyperkinetic Movements

Chorea is evident in the setting of some dementias. Huntington disease and its phenocopies exhibit chorea.[108] Patients with acquired disorders such as thyroid disease or antiphospholipid antibody syndrome or patients with strokes can also exhibit chorea. Postural tremor is common in dementia with Lewy bodies, and recent studies have suggested that it can be associated with an increased risk of cognitive decline.[109]

LABORATORY INVESTIGATIONS IN DEMENTIA

Laboratory investigations in dementia can be looked at from two perspectives; one is to obtain positive evidence for a diagnosis. A brain biopsy can provide proof of the presence of an entity associated with dementia.[110] This must be kept in clinical context since the diagnosis is based on the presence of a clinical picture accompanied by pathologic evidence. In living patients, other laboratory tests can provide strong evidence for the cause of dementia in an individual.

The second reason for laboratory investigation is to identify conditions that can contribute to cognitive dysfunction in older adults. To do this, clinicians must understand not only the natural history of degenerative dementias, including atypical presentations, but also the ways in which systemic problems interact with older people with and without dementia. An example is vascular dementia caused by an acute stroke in a location that makes sense with the clinical picture. Another example is identification of a potentially reversible metabolic or infectious problem, which, when reversed, leads to reversal of dementia. Although reversible dementia was emphasized until the 1990s, since the publication of reviews drawing attention to the relative rarity of reversible dementia, enthusiasm for reversible dementia has been tempered.[64,65] This too came about with the move from the long tradition of seeing Alzheimer disease as a "diagnosis of exclusion" in which a long list of competing diagnoses must be "ruled out" to the recognition of more characteristic staging. Covert causes of cognitive impairment form the basis for recommendation of laboratory testing formed by consensus groups.[2-6,111-113] In many cases, disorders so identified do not account for the full clinical picture in a patient with dementia, yet it still can help with improving a patient's function and, hence, quality of life. This highlights the importance of identifying and considering treatment of "treatable" conditions even in a patient in whom a degenerative dementia might be considered. Treatments need to be addressed in the context of a patient's overall prognosis.

SUMMARY

In summary, dementia is a syndrome with a range of causes and contributing conditions. A framework for diagnosing degenerative dementias must take into consideration the possibility of other coexisting conditions that can contribute to cognitive dysfunction in older adults. To do this, clinicians must understand not only the natural history of degenerative dementias, including atypical presentations, but also the ways in which systemic problems interact with older people with and without dementia.

KEY POINTS

- Dementia is generally defined as multifocal cognitive impairment that is sufficient to impair function. It is distinguished, although not always without arbitrariness, from cognitive decline of lesser severity and impact.
- The differential diagnosis of dementia is a long process, but as people age, a diagnosis of Alzheimer disease, commonly in the presence of cerebrovascular disease, becomes more likely.
- This approach of starting with what is common and looking for features that make this diagnosis less likely is distinct from the long tradition of seeing Alzheimer disease as a "diagnosis of exclusion" in which a long list of competing diagnoses must be "ruled out."

For a complete list of references, please visit online only at www.expertconsult.com.

KEY REFERENCES

3. McKhann GM, Knopman DS, Chertkow H, et al: The diagnosis of dementia due to Alzheimer's disease: recommendations from the National Institute on Aging-Alzheimer's Association workgroups on diagnostic guidelines for Alzheimer's disease. Alzheimers Dement 7(3):263–269, 2011.
4. Albert MS, DeKosky ST, Dickson D, et al: The diagnosis of mild cognitive impairment due to Alzheimer's disease: recommendations from the National Institute on Aging-Alzheimer's Association workgroups on diagnostic guidelines for Alzheimer's disease. Alzheimers Dement 7(3):270–279, 2011.
5. Sperling RA, Aisen PS, Beckett LA, et al: Toward defining the preclinical stages of Alzheimer's disease: recommendations from the National Institute on Aging-Alzheimer's Association workgroups on diagnostic guidelines for Alzheimer's disease. Alzheimers Dement 7(3):280–292, 2011.
6. Dubois B, Feldman HH, Jacova C, et al: Advancing research diagnostic criteria for Alzheimer's disease: the IWG-2 criteria. Lancet Neurol 13(6):614–629, 2014. Erratum in: Lancet Neurol 13(8):757, 2014.
8. American Psychiatric Association: Diagnostic and statistical manual of mental disorders, fifth edition (DSM-5), Washington, DC, 2013, American Psychiatric Association.
28. Sachdev P, Kalaria R, O'Brien J, et al: Diagnostic criteria for vascular cognitive disorders: a VASCOG statement. Alzheimer Dis Assoc Disord 28(3):206–218, 2014.
29. McKeith IG, Dickson DW, Lowe J, et al: Diagnosis and management of dementia with Lewy bodies: third report of the DLB Consortium. Neurology 65:1863–1872, 2005.
31. Emre M, Aarsland D, Brown R, et al: Clinical diagnostic criteria for dementia associated with Parkinson's disease. Mov Disord 22(12): 1689–1707, 2007.
32. Rascovsky K, Hodges JR, Knopman D, et al: Sensitivity of revised diagnostic criteria for the behavioural variant of frontotemporal dementia. Brain 134:2456–2477, 2011.

39. Chare L, Hodges JR, Leyton CE, et al: New criteria for frontotemporal dementia syndromes: clinical and pathological diagnostic implications. J Neurol Neurosurg Psychiatry 85(8):865–870, 2014.
111. Knopman DS, DeKosky ST, Cummings JL, et al: Practice parameter: diagnosis of dementia (an evidence-based review). Report of the Quality Standards Subcommittee of the American Academy of Neurology. Neurology 56(9):1143–1153, 2001.
112. Hort J, O'Brien JT, Gainotti G, et al: EFNS guidelines for the diagnosis and management of Alzheimer's disease. Eur J Neurol 17(10):1236–1248, 2010.
113. Filippi M, Agosta F, Barkhof F, et al: EFNS task force: the use of neuroimaging in the diagnosis of dementia. Eur J Neurol 19(12): e131–e140, 1487–1501, 2012.

51 Neuropsychology in the Diagnosis and Treatment of Dementia

Margaret Sewell, Clara Li, Mary Sano

INTRODUCTION

The aging of the U.S. baby boomer population has given rise to a significant increase in the prevalence of Alzheimer disease, the most common form of dementia in adults older than 65 years. One in three Americans aged 85 and older has Alzheimer disease, and by 2050, up to 16 million are predicted to have Alzheimer disease.[1] Dementia is defined as significant impairment in cognitive functioning (serious enough to interfere with daily life) that is not accounted for by other medical conditions. Mild cognitive impairment (MCI) is a condition of significant cognitive deterioration from a presumed higher level without functional impairment, which may be a prodromal stage of dementia. Neuropsychologists can assist in characterizing cognitive loss and providing diagnostic differentiation, thereby supporting early detection of cognitive change in individuals with dementia. Despite the fact that detection is possible even at early stages, nearly half of older primary care patients remain undiagnosed and untreated, partly because health care providers do not have time or access to assessment and may lack places to refer patients for needed support services.[2] This chapter reviews indications for neuropsychological evaluation, discusses new diagnostic criteria and methods of assessment, and describes how test results can direct treatment planning.

INDICATIONS FOR NEUROPSYCHOLOGICAL ASSESSMENT

A neuropsychological evaluation can be helpful in distinguishing pathologic cognitive performance from normal aging by examining patterns of performance across cognitive domains. Signature patterns of cognitive strengths and weaknesses, including assessed activities of daily living (ADLs), may support the diagnosis of specific types of dementia or MCI and may be useful in predicting the course or progression of cognitive disease to help determine whether a patient is safe to live alone or manage his or her finances. This is important because compared with normal controls, those with MCI and dementia have elevated mortality rates.[3]

CHANGES IN DIAGNOSTIC CRITERIA TO DETECT MILDER IMPAIRMENT

New diagnostic criteria for Alzheimer disease have been proposed,[4-6] each specifying a slightly different role for neuropsychological testing (Table 51-1). The revised diagnostic criteria reflect significant scientific advances in genetics and biomarkers for Alzheimer disease pathology. Evidence that neuropathology may precede symptoms, has led to criteria for presymptomatic stages.[5,7] The National Institute of Neurological and Communicative Disorders and Stroke–Alzheimer's Disease and Related Disorders Association (NINCDS-ADRDA) criteria, used primarily to guide research, require the presence of gradual episodic memory impairment confirmed with neuropsychological testing, with supportive features, including the presence of at least one Alzheimer disease biomarker.[5]

The National Institute on Aging–Alzheimer's Association (NIA-AA) provides criteria for Alzheimer disease, MCI, a clinical diagnosis for and a categorization of MCI due to Alzheimer disease used for research,[8] and research guidelines for an asymptomatic, preclinical phase.[9] The criteria for probable Alzheimer disease first require meeting criteria for a general dementia. These criteria require cognitive and behavioral symptoms that (1) interfere with functional abilities or usual activities, (2) represent a decline from previous function, and (3) are not explained by delirium or other psychiatric disorder. Evidence of cognitive impairment can be assessed through clinical examination or by neuropsychological testing and must include impairment in two or more cognitive domains. In the current criteria, attention is brought to a wide range of impairments, including language, visuospatial, and executive deficits, along with mood-related or behavioral symptoms. Special mention is given to language, because expressive aphasias often thought to be focal in nature can progress to be part of a general dementia syndrome. In addition, changes in behavior, personality, and comportment are now considered a "cognitive domain" and can include agitation, apathy, and social withdrawal. Although memory impairment may be the most common deficit, it is not required for the dementia diagnosis. The diagnosis of Alzheimer disease continues to use the distinction of probable and possible Alzheimer disease to rate the level of confidence based on clinical presentation. Probable Alzheimer disease has four criteria: three of inclusion (slow, insidious onset; evidence of worsening of cognition; and at least one amnestic or nonamnestic cognitive deficit) and one of exclusion (the presence of vascular disease or other dementia). NIA-AA recommends that comprehensive neuropsychological testing be used in complicated cases when a standard office exam and cognitive screen such as the Mini Mental State Examination (MMSE) are not sufficient to provide a clear diagnosis.

The NIA-AA defined core clinical criteria for a diagnosis of MCI described by Albert et al.[8] These criteria include (1) cognitive complaint or cognitive problems suspected by family, friend, or care provider; (2) impairment in one or more cognitive domains; (3) relative independence in functional abilities; and (4) not demented. The diagnosis of MCI due to Alzheimer disease, often used in research, requires biomarker evidence of neurodegeneration, or amyloid or tau accumulation.

The *Diagnostic and Statistical Manual of Mental Disorders*, fifth edition (DSM-5), provides definitions for major and mild neurocognitive disorders (NCDs). Diagnostic criteria require evidence of a cognitive decline ("significant" for major and "modest" for mild) from a previous level of functioning in one or more cognitive areas (e.g., memory, executive functioning) based on report by the patient or family and "preferably" documented by neuropsychological test performance.[6] Functional decline is required for major NCD, defined as needing help with everyday activities such as bill paying or shopping. Functional decline is not required for minor NCD, although extra effort or time may be needed to complete daily activities. Mild NCD captures the diagnosis of MCI (which was previously coded as cognitive disorder not otherwise specified), and the criteria overlap with those for MCI due to Alzheimer disease as outlined in the NIA-AA diagnostic guidelines.[8]

Once criteria for major or mild NCD are met, additional diagnostic criteria are provided to identify specific subtypes classified according to cause (e.g., Alzheimer disease, substance use, human immunodeficiency virus [HIV] infection).

TABLE 51-1 New Diagnostic Criteria

Criteria for Probable Alzheimer Disease	DSM-5 2013	Research Criteria: *NINCDS–ADRDA 2007*	Research Criteria: NIA-AA 2011
Insidious onset	X	X	X
Onset over months to years		X	X
Progressive decline	X	X	X
Deficits are not explained by delirium or other medical or psychiatric conditions	X	X	X
Social/occupational impairment	X		X
Presence of episodic memory deficit	X	X	
Cognitive deficits in at least two domains	X		X
Neuropsychological testing required for diagnosis?	Preferably	X	Only if routine history and mental status testing are inconclusive
Abnormal PET or MRI scan		Supportive feature*	For research purposes
Genetic markers?	X Required only if there is evidence of multiple causes and no clear evidence of progression and decline in memory and another cognitive domain	Supportive feature*	For research purposes
Abnormal cerebrospinal fluid marker required?		Supportive feature*	For research purposes

DSM-5, Diagnostic and Statistical Manual of Mental Disorders, fifth edition; *MRI,* magnetic resonance imaging; *NIA-AA,* National Institute on Aging–Alzheimer's Association; *NINCDS-ADRDA,* National Institute of Neurological and Communicative Disorders and Stroke–Alzheimer's Disease and Related Disorders Association; *PET,* positron emission tomography.

*At least one supportive feature is required for diagnosis of probable AD.

CLINICAL INTERVIEWING

A clinical interview lays the groundwork for both test selection and interpretation of the neuropsychological results. Informants, often caregivers or family members, are helpful as they can often provide critical information regarding the onset and course of symptoms. Reporting by a person with memory problems may not be accurate,[10] and informant reports have been shown to relate to objective test deficits.[11] Careful questioning can help diagnosticians identify features of specific types of dementia (insidious or precipitous course, falls, significant apathy, profound language decline, sudden behavioral changes) and other medical conditions that cause cognitive impairment (e.g., sleep apnea, drug and alcohol abuse, depression, misuse of prescription medications).

SCREENING AND BRIEF COGNITIVE ASSESSMENTS IN THE DIAGNOSIS OF DEMENTIA

In the primary care setting, brief screens can help physicians identify those at greatest risk for cognitive impairment (e.g., indicators include age, education, history of stroke, presence of diabetes, depression, and a need for help with finances).[12] In their comprehensive review of brief screening instruments to identify cognitive impairment in older adults, Lin and colleagues[13] identified the following instruments as reliable in the detection of dementia: the MMSE, Clock Drawing Test, Memory Impairment Screen, Abbreviated Mental Test, Short Portable Mental Status Questionnaire, Free and Cued Selective Reminding Test, 7-Minute Screen, Telephone Interview for Cognitive Status, and the Informant Questionnaire on Cognitive Decline in the Elderly.

As a group, these instruments have demonstrated reasonable ability to distinguish normal cognition from dementia, although their ability to distinguish milder states such as MCI from normal aging is inconsistent.[13] However, one recent study found that the Montreal Cognitive Assessment was better at distinguishing normal cognition from MCI than the MMSE.[14]

Patients with suspected dementia or MCI who pass the screen can be referred for full neuropsychological testing that can better capture the subtle effects of MCI.[15]

The challenge is in persuading physicians in primary care, in the context of time constraints and reimbursement issues, of the value of using any of these instruments and of the value of early diagnosis, as it may be difficult to identify the care services of those with positive screens.[16]

In summary, cognitive screening and brief cognitive assessments in the primary care setting can be useful for detecting frank dementia and may be administered by those with a minimal amount of training to identify those in need of further evaluation. In clinical practice, neuropsychological testing remains the most accurate method to identify and characterize very early symptoms and distinguish them from other types of cognitive impairment.

Assessment of Cognitive Impairment and Dementia

A comprehensive neuropsychological battery to determine the presence and nature of a dementia includes tests of memory, language, attention, visuospatial function, motor function, executive function, and depression. Tests are most often administered with paper and pencil, although computerized versions (e.g., NeuroTrax MindStreams,[17] Cogstate, MicroCog, and Cambridge Neuropsychological Test Automated Battery[18]) are becoming increasingly available. The decision to rely on computerized testing when diagnosing older adult patients needs to be determined on a case-by-case basis because the technology may be unfamiliar or frustrating to seniors.[19]

In the context of the clinical history, results are then examined for typical patterns that may suggest different types of cognitive impairments. Additionally, the presence of neuropsychiatric symptoms and level of independence with ADLs and instrumental ADLs (IADLs) are often assessed. ADLs include highly overlearned tasks such as dressing, toileting, and grooming, whereas IADLs refer to more complex tasks with greater cognitive demand, such as managing money, cooking, and shopping. Additional structured questionnaires may be used with either patients or informants to assess specific subsets of symptoms, such as fluctuating cognition, behavioral changes, or anxiety.

Despite the perception that psychological testing is lengthy and expensive, testing is tailored to the ability of the patient and the cost is covered by Medicare. Tests can be selected to assess the major domains of cognition affected in dementia and that address specific concerns raised in the clinical interview. Because reaching a diagnosis of dementia includes documenting a decline from a previous level of functioning, it is necessary to estimate premorbid

TABLE 51-2 Commonly Used Neuropsychological Tests

Domains to Be Assessed	Tests Used With Age-Corrected and/or Education Norms for Adults Older Than 65 Years
Premorbid ability	North American Reading Test (NART)
	Vocabulary (WAIS-IV)
Verbal memory	Rey Auditory Verbal Learning Test (RAVLT)
	California Verbal Learning Test (CVLT)
	Logical Memory Test (from WMS-IV)
	CERAD Word List Test
Visual memory	Visual Reproduction (from WMS-IV)
	Rey Complex Figure Drawing Test (RCFT)
Simple attention	Digit Span (from WAIS-IV)
	Trail-Making Part A
Language	Animal Naming Test (ANT)
	Controlled Oral Word Association Test (COWAT)
	Boston Naming Test (BNT)
Executive function	Trail-Making Part B
	Wisconsin Card Sort Test (WCST)
	Stroop
	Similarities (from WAIS-IV)
Visuospatial	Coding (from WAIS-IV)
	Rey Complex Figure Test (RCFT)
	Clock Drawing Test
Motor	Grooved Pegboard Test
	Finger Tapping Test
Mood	Geriatric Depression Scale (GDS)
	Hamilton Depression Rating Scale (HDRS)
	Beck Anxiety Inventory (BAI)

WAIS-IV, Wechsler Adult Intelligence Scale, fourth edition; *WMS-IV,* Wechsler Memory Scale, fourth edition.

level of functioning. This can be accomplished through a careful review of educational and occupational history, tests of vocabulary that tend not to decline even in the presence of dementia, or, for those with at least 8 years of formal education, word reading tests that use a formula that takes into account education and number of reading errors to provide a crude estimate of premorbid verbal IQ.[20] However, individuals with particularly high or low levels of formal education may leave doubt about how to interpret cognitive complaints. Well-established normative data on cognitive tests can provide a method for evaluating cognitive performance and detecting a change when baseline data or assessment of premorbid functioning is not available.

A summary of commonly used tests may be found in Table 51-2.

Major and Minor Neurocognitive Disorders due to Alzheimer Disease

A substantial amount of research has indicated that Alzheimer disease is associated with a particular pattern of cognitive deficits that distinguish it from normal aging[21] and, in some cases, from other forms of dementia. Specifically, the ability to learn and retain verbal information distinguishes those with mild Alzheimer disease from healthy older adults.[22-27] Verbal memory is most commonly assessed with either word lists (e.g., California Verbal Learning Test [CVLT], Rey Auditory Verbal Learning Test [RAVLT]) or stories (e.g., Logical Memory). Normative data for initial and delayed recall as well as cued recognition are available. Performance on verbal memory tests is marked by difficulty in both the free and cued recall of recently learned information.[28] However, in patients with early-onset Alzheimer disease, initial learning may be preserved, although, compared with normal controls, deficits in both acquisition and consolidation of information may still be present, as well as evidence of a shallower learning curve.[29,30] Deficits in both encoding and delayed recall become more severe as the disease progresses.[31] Examination of specific patterns of responses on delayed recall suggests that normal controls tend to recall words equally from the beginning and end of a list whereas individuals with Alzheimer disease rely heavily on words only from the end of the list (recency effect); this suggests that individuals with Alzheimer disease, not having transferred the information from primary to secondary memory, have not really "learned" the words at all.[32,33] The sensitivity of Alzheimer disease patients to interference[34] is evidenced by a high number (relative to normal controls) of intrusions (e.g., when words from a second list appears while patient is attempting to recall words from a previously learned list) and repetitions.[35] This finding is observed on tests of both word lists and stories.[36] The very earliest cognitive impairments associated with Alzheimer disease are usually to episodic memory, complex attention, and organizational skills.[37] Visual memory may also be assessed, although there is some evidence that visuospatial skills naturally deteriorate with age, making these tasks less discriminatory. However, some studies have identified nonverbal memory impairments in very mildly impaired Alzheimer disease patients compared with normal controls on the delayed recall portion of the Rey Complex Figure Test (RCFT).[38]

Dysexecutive functioning is often an early symptom to appear, although usually after episodic memory impairments.[39] Those with Alzheimer disease exhibit poorer cognitive flexibility, problem solving, parallel processing, planning, set shifting, and abstract thinking compared with normal older adults. These deficits, which worsen as the disease progresses, are captured in tests such as phonemic fluency, similarities, go/no-go type tests, card sorting, and trail-making. Deficits in this area have been consistently related to poor functional ability,[40] trouble with managing finances,[41] and higher need for care.[42]

Certain language abilities are also impaired in adults with early Alzheimer disease. Impaired language domains include naming, assessed with a picture naming task such as the Boston Naming Test ([BNT], a test of 60 pictures encompassing high- and low-frequency words), and fluency, measured by assessing the rate of word production for a given letter (phonemic fluency) or within a given category, such as naming animals or vegetables (semantic fluency). Naming is impaired early,[43] and, unlike healthy older adults who also have benign "senior moments," those with Alzheimer disease often do not benefit from prompting, either semantic (giving hints about what the object is) or phonemic (saying the beginning of the sound of the word). Performance on the BNT can discriminate among normal controls, patients with MCI, and patients with Alzheimer disease.[44,45] However, the BNT may be less discriminatory among those with low education or from diverse cultural backgrounds. Naming and fluency deficits worsen as Alzheimer disease progresses.[46] Semantic fluency test performance (e.g., naming as many animals as possible in 60 seconds) is impaired very early in Alzheimer disease, relative to phonemic fluency.[47,48] Some suggest[49] that animal naming is more difficult because of impairment of semantic knowledge required for any category test. However, in patients with early Alzheimer disease, basic comprehension and verbal expression are intact.

Simple attention (measured, e.g., by Digit Span) is usually preserved in early Alzheimer disease. However, tasks that require divided attention (Trails B) or selective attention (the Stroop test) are often impaired in the Alzheimer disease patient[50] and may reflect working memory deficits and difficulties processing and responding to several pieces of information simultaneously. Divided attention may be intact in patients who have very mild Alzheimer disease,[51,52] although problems are worsened at the moderate stages of the illness.[53]

For those with early Alzheimer disease, visuospatial functioning is often well preserved, relative to memory, language, and executive function. However, deficits may be seen on visuoconstructional tests such as clock drawing and complex geometric figure drawing.[54] Deficits in visuospatial abilities have been associated with wandering and driving difficulties.[55] Performance on tests of visuospatial functioning (e.g., the copy portion of RCFT) may be lowered by executive deficits such as planning and organization, rather than by visual spatial impairment. Other tests of visuospatial function that do not have a high executive demand, such as the Judgment of Line Orientation Test, may be a more accurate measure of pure visuospatial ability.

In summary, a typical early-onset Alzheimer disease profile, in the absence of significant depression, might reveal (1) moderately impaired initial learning with significantly impaired delayed recall on tests of verbal memory, (2) relatively well-preserved performance on phonemic fluency in the context of impaired semantic fluency and naming, (3) intact simple attention, (4) impaired performance on executive functioning tests measuring cognitive flexibility and planning, and (5) very mildly impaired performance on tests of visuospatial and visuoconstructional ability.

Mild Cognitive Impairment

MCI (with amnestic and nonamnestic subtypes) has been characterized as a transitional phase between the cognitive changes associated with normal aging and dementia.[56] Criteria include a cognitive complaint by the patient (or observation of one by a family member or care provider), and objective decline on neuropsychological testing in the context of intact ability to manage daily affairs, if less efficiently.[8] Conversion rates for this group of MCI patients to Alzheimer disease may range from 12% to 15% a year to 80% at 6 years,[57] although there is not a consensus about prevalence rates (with ranges from 10% to 20% in those older than age 65) because of differences in samples and diagnostic criteria employed[13] and the tests used to detect impairment.[58,59] Early detection of a specific dementia such as Alzheimer disease is desirable because this can allow for earlier intervention.[60] Poor performance (usually defined as >1.5 standard deviations below age-adjusted norms) on standardized tests of verbal memory (e.g., delayed recall of word lists) or executive ability (e.g., Trails B, Stroop Interference Test) has been shown in numerous studies to be a sensitive predictor of progression to Alzheimer disease in those with amnestic MCI[50,51,61-63] and in discriminating amnestic MCI from Alzheimer disease.[64] In some studies[65] but not all,[61] naming and semantic fluency tests have also distinguished between amnestic MCI patients who convert to Alzheimer disease and those who do not. Other studies[66] have observed that when memory scores were used in isolation to predict conversion from MCI to Alzheimer disease, sensitivity and specificity were low, but the addition of tests from other domains, particularly executive function, produced higher predictive accuracy.

In summary, patients with MCI present with subjective cognitive complaints but with minimal functional decline; neuropsychological testing can identify cognitive impairment relative to normal controls, and these cases are at heightened risk for converting to Alzheimer disease.

Vascular Neurocognitive Disorders

Vascular disease is the second most common cause of cognitive loss and dementia (Alzheimer disease is the first), and it is estimated to account for approximately a third of all dementia cases. As is the case with Alzheimer disease, the DSM-5 criteria for vascular neurocognitive disorders include both a major cognitive disorder and a mild classification. The major classification includes deficits in one or more domains, including complex attention, executive function, learning and memory, language, perceptual-motor, and social cognition, based on concerns of the patient or informant or on testing. These must be accompanied by interference with independent function and must not occur solely in a state of delirium or be attributable to another condition. Probable major vascular neurocognitive disorder is comparable to what has been described as vascular dementia.[67] The mild classification stipulates mild deficit with no loss of independence. This condition, previously described as vascular cognitive impairment (VCI), was characterized by cognitive complaints observed by the patient or others, and was associated with impairment in a wide range of neuropsychological functions.[68,69] Reports of longitudinal follow-up of such cases yields relatively high rates of dementia with many ultimately diagnosed as Alzheimer disease (35%) or mixed Alzheimer disease and vascular dementia (15%).[70] The evidence for vascular causation includes the presence of cerebrovascular disease, identified from history, physical examination, and/or neuroimaging, of sufficient severity to account for the neurocognitive deficit. Accurately identifying VCI or dementia requires careful attention to historical information. The onset may be both rapid and temporally related to a stroke-like event, or it may be gradual with a progression that is described as stepwise. The classification of "probable" is used when cognitive impairment occurs in temporal proximity to a focal event such as a stroke or transient ischemic attack and when there is imaging evidence of cerebrovascular involvement. The "possible" designation is used when only one criterion (imaging or temporal proximity) is met or when vascular risk factors are invoked.

Several studies of group comparisons with Alzheimer disease subjects suggest that when individuals with vascular dementia are clinically diagnosed, the vascular dementia group often has less severe memory impairment. The pattern that is often reported within vascular dementia is one in which working memory is more likely to be impaired than delayed recall, a pattern that is the opposite of that of Alzheimer disease.[71] Cued recall and recognition of previously learned material is generally intact, unlike in Alzheimer disease. A recent study suggests that subclinical vascular disease characterized by small vessel disease and white matter hyperintensities has a specific effect on the learning curve but not necessarily on retention.[72] Executive function is commonly impaired in patients with vascular dementia, and the deficit may be disproportional to other cognitive deficits such as memory.[73] Language deficits such as naming and verbal fluency impairments are common, particularly with subcortical and thalamic infarcts. Although verbal fluency may be impaired, the distinctive pattern of preserved phonemic fluency and impaired semantic fluency seen in Alzheimer disease is uncommon.[74] In fact, some studies suggest that in contrast to patients with Alzheimer disease, patients with vascular dementia have worse phonemic fluency scores relative to semantic fluency,[75,76] a finding that may be reflective of executive function impairment. Another area reported to be impaired in vascular dementia is psychomotor speed and measures of attention. Although focal deficits can be responsible for some such impairment, they may be exacerbated by depression, which is a common concomitant of vascular dementia.[77]

In summary, vascular dementia and VCI may have a less robust episodic memory deficit with the possibility of a range of impairments. The likelihood of executive function deficit and depression are higher than in patients with Alzheimer disease. Although the precision of diagnosing vascular dementia and other cognitive syndromes is hampered by the breadth of the possible deficits, it is important to consider vascular condition and risks because many are remediable and may improve cognition through general health benefits without curing the underlying dementia.

Major Neurocognitive Disorder due to Frontotemporal Lobar Degeneration

Frontotemporal lobar degeneration (FTLD) represents approximately 10% of all dementia cases, but it disproportionately affects younger people as reflected by the fact that more than half of

FTLD cases are 45 to 64 years old.[78] Numerous terms have been proposed to describe this complex group of conditions associated with pathology in the frontal and anterior temporal areas, including *frontotemporal dementia* and *Pick disease*,[79] among others. FTLD represents a spectrum of interrelated but distinct disorders that includes two clinical variations: behavioral variant and primary progressive aphasia (the latter with three subtypes: nonfluent, semantic, and logopenic).

Behavioral Variant Frontotemporal Degeneration. Behavioral variant frontotemporal degeneration (FTD) is the most common variant of FTLD and is characterized by early personality and behavioral changes, including apathy, impulsivity, hyperorality, and inappropriate social interaction.[80] The striking early behavioral symptoms necessitate a differential diagnosis not just among dementias but between dementia and psychiatric illness.[81] It is important to distinguish Alzheimer disease from behavioral variant FTD because course, treatment, and prognosis may differ. Specifically, the efficacy of cholinesterase inhibitors is perceived to be highest in Alzheimer disease and poorest in FTLD. Perceived efficacy is affected more by who is treated than by what is used.[82]

Efforts to distinguish behavioral variant FTD from Alzheimer disease patients using neuropsychological tests have been inconsistent, in part because of small sample sizes, different stages of illness, and varying diagnostic criteria. Neuropsychological profiles in behavioral variant FTD patients are overall, compared with Alzheimer disease patients, characterized by poor executive and language function. Regarding memory function, performance on the delayed recall of word list tests is better preserved in behavioral variant FTD patients relative to those with Alzheimer disease.[83] Studies have suggested that, on language tests, those with behavioral variant FTD are more impaired than those with Alzheimer disease on tests of verbal fluency. Specifically, Rascovsky and colleagues[84] found that compared with Alzheimer disease patients, those with autopsy-confirmed FTD exhibited more impairment on verbal fluency tests (both semantic and phonemic) perhaps because of the significant executive demand of search strategies. Some have observed more impaired phonemic fluency compared with semantic fluency in those with behavioral variant FTD,[85] the converse of the pattern typically observed in Alzheimer disease. On tests of executive function, behavioral variant FTD patients may be proportionately worse than those with Alzheimer disease on tests of cognitive set switching and cognitive flexibility than memory tests.[86] Visuospatial skills are relatively intact in comparison to other cognitive deficits,[87] although visuospatial tasks that include significant executive ability such as organization and planning (e.g., the RCFT) may prove difficult. Clock drawing and block design may be better measures of visuospatial ability in individuals with behavioral variant FTD.

Primary Progressive Aphasia. Primary progressive aphasia (PPA) is a variant of FTLD that describes isolated and severe progressive language impairments (fluency or comprehension) not caused by stroke. Although the nomenclature is inconsistent and researchers do not always agree on the clinical presentations, three subtypes of PPA have been described, namely, semantic, nonfluent, and, more recently, logopenic. Expanded classification and research criteria have been proposed[88] to update Mesulam's original classification and diagnostic criteria for PPA.[89]

The core features of *semantic variant PPA*, characterized by atrophy in the left anterior temporal lobe, are progressive and severe problems with confrontation naming and single-word comprehension[90] in the relative absence of other cognitive difficulties early in the disease. Among individuals with semantic variant PPA, scores on category fluency may be worse than those on letter fluency, and scores on naming may be worse than those on comprehension.[91] Later in the illness, despite profound deficits in semantic memory and meaning, expressive language may retain its fluency (e.g., normal prosody and volume) but often grows increasingly empty.[92] Early in the illness, visuospatial, attentional, and executive abilities generally remain intact. Regarding memory function, one study observed poor delayed recall but normal new learning in those with semantic variant PPA.[93]

Nonfluent variant PPA is associated with damage in the left perisylvian language areas and is characterized by effortful, halting speech accompanied by significant word retrieval difficulty in the context of preserved single-word comprehension. Among individuals with nonfluent PPA, performance is profoundly impaired on tests of verbal fluency. Some researchers[94] argue that category and letter fluency tests can help distinguish among semantic PPA, nonfluent PPA, and Alzheimer disease, with Alzheimer disease patients least impaired and nonfluent PPA patients most impaired on letter fluency. Hodges and colleagues[93] observed that a simple "repeat and point" test was effective in distinguishing semantic PPA from nonfluent PPA, with poor performance by semantic PPA patients on pointing (comprehension) and poor performance by nonfluent PPA patients on repeating. There is evidence of slower executive functioning performance in those with nonfluent PPA compared to patients with either semantic variant PPA or Alzheimer disease.[85] However, compared with patients with behavioral variant FTD, those with nonfluent PPA do better on tests of executive function and attention.[95] Episodic memory scores are generally intact early in the illness,[94] although because of the nature of the illness (poor expressive language), nonverbal tests of memory may be more useful.

Core features of *logopenic variant PPA* include word retrieval difficulties and impaired repetition of sentences. Testing in patients with suspected logopenic variant PPA is characterized by severe impairment on digit and letter span tests, in the context of slow speech and intact grammar and articulation.[96] Although this subgroup is still not fully understood, some studies[97] have observed that certain neuropsychological tests (e.g., Peabody Picture Vocabulary Test and Northwest Anagram Test) can distinguish those with the logopenic variant from both semantic and nonfluent variants, with the logopenic group performing better than either of the other groups on these tests.

In summary, FTLD is a group of related disorders that is associated with an early age of onset and a precipitous course. The behavioral variant is associated with marked behavioral changes and poor executive functioning in the context of relatively spared memory and visuospatial skills. The language variants of PPA include semantic, nonfluent, and logopenic subgroups; some initial research in this area suggests the possibility of distinct patterns of deficits on tests of verbal fluency, naming, and executive functioning.

Major and Minor Neurocognitive Disorder due to Parkinson Disease

Parkinson disease dementia (PDD) develops in 20% to 40% of Parkinson patients.[98] The onset is typically insidious, with variable rates of progression, and the dementia must follow the onset of motor symptoms by at least 1 year.[99] Furthermore, neuropsychiatric symptoms, including hallucinations and depression, are frequent.[100] MCI-associated Parkinson disease (PD-MCI), like Alzheimer disease, frequently progresses to dementia.[101,102] One meta-analysis of more than 1000 PD patients[103] observed that nearly 26% had PD-MCI.

PDD is consistent with a typical subcortical pattern, namely, impairments in attention (including working memory and divided attention), executive function (particularly planning and set shifting), and visuospatial function. Compared with other impairments, language function is relatively well preserved.[104] Most research concurs that episodic memory deficits are milder in

PDD than Alzheimer disease and that the problems are caused by deficits in retrieval more than encoding and storage.[105-107] This is illustrated by evidence of poor free and delayed recall but retained ability to recall previously learned information when prompted. Compared to patients with Alzheimer disease, patients with PDD exhibit poor executive functioning, which is evidenced by poor performance on tests of initiation/perseveration and card sorting.[108] Deficits on attention tests distinguish PDD from Alzheimer disease,[109] particularly on tasks that require divided attention.[110] Visuospatial task performance may be more impaired in PDD than Alzheimer disease, including pentagon copy.[111] Patients with PDD exhibit cognitive slowing, but measuring this is often complicated by the fact that most tests have some motor component,[112] making it difficult to distinguish the physical from the cognitive. It is also important to measure depression because it occurs in up to 50% of Parkinson patients and its presence may exacerbate poor neuropsychological test performance.[113] The presence of depression is associated with more significant cognitive impairment even in those Parkinson patients without dementia.[114]

In summary, the dementia associated with Parkinson disease is characterized by high rates of depression and by a subcortical pattern of poor attention, poor visuospatial and executive functioning, slowed processing speed, and relatively spared memory and language abilities.

Major and Minor Neurocognitive Disorder due to Lewy Body Disease

The complex relationship between the role of Lewy body pathology in Lewy body disease (LBD) and its relationship to PDD is not fully understood.[111] The primary triad of symptoms associated with LBD includes fluctuating cognition (e.g., attention and alertness that vary noticeably day to day), gait disturbance or Parkinson-like symptoms of bradykinesia and rigidity, and visual hallucinations. Other symptoms may include rapid eye movement sleep behavior disorders and frequent falls. Accurate diagnosis is critical because LBD is associated with a dangerous sensitivity to neuroleptic medications.[115] The cognitive changes observed in PDD and LBD are so similar that the two disorders are only clinically distinguished by the timing of the onset of symptoms: the motor symptoms in LBD patients occur no more than 1 year prior to the onset of dementia and frequently after the onset of dementia, whereas motor symptoms in PDD patients must precede dementia by at least 1 year.[98]

Characterizing LBD with neuropsychological testing can be difficult because the cognitive deficits so closely resemble those of PDD.[105] Memory is impaired, although not as severely as in Alzheimer disease, and, as in PDD, the problem is more one of retrieval than encoding.[116] Taken together, studies suggest that LBD patients, compared with Alzheimer disease patients, exhibit more severe deficits in executive functioning, visuospatial functioning, and attentional abilities.[117-119] Poor visuospatial function appears to be a significant predictor of cognitive decline in those with LBD but not Alzheimer disease.[120] In LBD, poor performance on tests of visuoperceptual and spatial functions may be related to the fact that these individuals are vulnerable to visual hallucinations.[101] Although it is difficult to distinguish LBD from PDD with neuropsychological testing, a handful of studies have observed poorer performance by LBD patients on tests of attention, visuoperceptual skills, and executive function, controlling for illness severity.[121] Recent research[122] suggests that even at the MCI level, those with LBD-MCI perform worse on tests of memory, executive functioning, and visuospatial function than do those with PD-MCI.

In summary, LBD is difficult to distinguish from PDD and Alzheimer disease through use of neuropsychological testing, although the cognitive impairments, which usually precede any Parkinsonian symptoms, are more likely to resemble PDD and be accompanied by fluctuating attention and visual hallucinations.

Depression and Dementia

Older adults may present symptoms of forgetfulness and apathy that relate to depression, dementia, or both. In the past, the term *pseudodementia*[123] was used to describe depression in older adults because the symptoms of forgetfulness and confusion mimicked dementia. Distinguishing dementia from depression is critical because of the comparative success with which depression can be treated. Although, for many patients, the cognitive deficits remain after depressive symptoms are successfully treated,[124] the pattern of cognitive performance associated with neurodegenerative disease is distinct and detectable. Patterns from test performance results have emerged that may distinguish depression from early dementia and, in conjunction with clinical history, may help predict which nondemented depressed patients are at high risk for developing dementia.

In patients with depression, significant cognitive impairment is more common in older adults than in younger adults,[125,126] and the severity of cognitive impairment on neuropsychological tests falls somewhere between normal controls and those with early Alzheimer disease. Older adult patients experiencing a first-time depression exhibit problems with executive function and attention, with less relative memory impairment, compared to either those with recurrent depression or normal controls.[127] Older depressed adults without dementia perform poorly on tests of psychomotor speed and various aspects of executive function compared to those without depression.[125,128] Some have observed that the cognitive deficits associated with depression fit a more subcortical than cortical pattern,[129] with the preservation of language, memory, and praxis relative to Alzheimer disease patients. On tests of verbal memory, depressed patients perform better than Alzheimer disease patients, with less impairment in retention and recognition of previously learned material.[130] Regarding language, a meta-analysis of fluency in depressed older adult patients observed that Alzheimer disease patients were more impaired on both phonemic and semantic fluency than depressed patients, although the relative severity of semantic fluency impairment in Alzheimer disease patients remained.[131]

The relationship between depression and Alzheimer disease is complex.[132] The issue centers on whether depression in late life (whether recurrent or initial onset) may herald incipient dementia[133,134] or whether the presence of depression is a risk factor for the later development of dementia.[135,136] Many studies have examined factors that may clarify this distinction, including the proximity of depression and dementia,[137] whether the depression onset is early or late,[125] the presence of vascular illness,[138] whether psychotropic treatment is effective,[139,140] the effect of chronic life-long depression,[141] and gender.[142] Some research suggests that specific neuropsychological profiles may predict which depressed patients are at high risk for developing dementia. In a small retrospective study, Jean and colleagues[143] observed in a group of older depressed patients that baseline performance on tests of attention and memory were more impaired in those with subsequent dementia, with additional deficits in orientation in those who went on to develop Alzheimer disease and in executive and visuospatial function in those who developed LBD or vascular dementia. Repeated neuropsychological evaluations may be useful in those with depression with cognitive complaints; results from one large prospective study[144] suggest that cognitive functioning will continue to decline in depressed patients who eventually develop dementia and showed that baseline neuropsychological test performance was lower in those depressed patients who went on to develop dementia.

In summary, although the relationship between depression and Alzheimer disease is complex and not fully understood, a

TABLE 51-3 Patterns of Cognitive Impairment by Domain and Dementia

	Episodic Memory	Attention	Language	Executive	Visuospatial	Behavioral Symptoms
Alzheimer disease	(I)	Simple (P) Divided (I)	Phonemic (P) Semantic (I) Naming (I)	(I)	Simple (P) Complex (I)	Early apathy, late psychotic symptoms
Mild cognitive impairment—amnestic	Immediate and Delayed recall (I); Recognition (I)	Simple (P) Divided (P)	(P)	(P)	(P)	(P)
Vascular dementia	Immediate and Delayed recall (V) Recognition (P)	Simple (P) Divided (I)	(I)	(I)	(P)	Depression
Behavioral variant FTLD	(V)	Simple (P) Divided (I)	(I)	(I)	(P)	Disinhibition, apathy, hyperorality, inappropriate social interaction
Semantic variant PPA	(P)	(P)	(I) Comprehension (I) Fluency	(P)	(P) (I) Visual agnosia	(P)
Nonfluent variant PPA	(P)	(P)	(I) Fluency (P) Comprehension, (I) Expressive speech	(P)	(P)	(P)
Parkinson disease dementia	(V) Immediate and Delayed recall (P) recognition	(I)	(P)	(I)	(I)	Depression, possible hallucinations, psychomotor slowing
Dementia with Lewy bodies	(V) Immediate and Delayed recall (P) Recognition	(V)	(V)	(I)	(I)	Hallucinations, delusions
Depression	(V) Immediate and Delayed recall (P) Recognition +	(V)	(V) Fluency (P) Naming	I/V	(P)	Psychomotor slowing, apathy

FTLD, Frontotemporal lobar degeneration; *I,* impaired; *P,* preserved; *PPA,* primary progressive aphasia; *V,* variable.

clinical presentation of depression, particularly with symptoms of apathy and cognitive complaints, warrants neuropsychological evaluation. The results, particularly if measured on more than one occasion, may help in determining whether the patient has depression, dementia, or both.

A summary of the pattern of cognitive deficits associated with different dementias and depression may be found in Table 51-3.

TEST RESULTS USED TO GUIDE TREATMENT PLANNING AND AS OUTCOME MEASURES IN RESEARCH

Neuropsychologists are also called on to determine functional abilities, including task-specific decisional capacity. Neuropsychological evaluations of memory and executive functions (e.g., planning and reasoning) are important in this area as they document the cognitive strengths and weaknesses that help determine a patient's current ability to drive, make medical decisions, manage medication, live alone, and handle financial responsibilities.

Level of independence with ADLs and IADLs should always be evaluated, either informally or with standard measures. Impairment in these areas has a dramatic impact on both the patient and caregiver, affecting quality of life, caregiver burden, and decisions regarding nursing home placement. Decline in ability to manage IADLs may happen relatively early in most forms of dementia and is related to deficits in memory, sustained attention, and problem solving. Most patients in the mild to moderate stages of Alzheimer disease experience some difficulty with medication management, cooking, and shopping.[145]

In the dementia research setting, cognitive testing is used as an outcome measure to assess the effectiveness of new pharmacologic and nonpharmacologic treatments and interventions. Performance differences between active and placebo conditions are used to gauge the efficacy of agents in combination with other global and functional measures (e.g., ADLs, behavioral symptoms). Repeated neuropsychological testing may also be used to assess an intervention in longitudinal studies or the cognitive impact of a medical procedure or treatment.

CHALLENGES TO NEUROPSYCHOLOGICAL ASSESSMENT IN OLDER ADULTS

There are several challenges to neuropsychological assessment in older adults. First, sensory impairment, common in older adults, may interfere with testing. Because many tests present stimuli visually or orally, serious hearing and visual loss can make test administration and performance interpretation difficult. Direct assessment and sample items are often used to ensure sensory capacity is adequate for the test. Another challenge is mobility limitations, as arthritis in hand joints or tremor can slow performance on timed tests and thus limit the validity of such procedures. This can be overcome, in some cases, by measuring differences in time for low and high cognitive demand tests rather than depending on the absolute time of a single test.

Low literacy (defined as not reading in any language) as a result of low levels of formal education or life-long disability can also impede testing but can be addressed by selecting assessment tools that use oral presentation, pictures, or other stimuli that do not require reading or knowledge of an alphabet. In this situation, it is important to rely on normative data of comparable individuals in order to have confidence about deficits. When this is not available, physicians must depend on clinical experience.

Language and culture can also challenge selection and interpretation of testing. Ideally patients should be assessed in the language in which they are most competent by an evaluator who is equally competent in the language. Translation can be used, but adequate normative samples against which to compare performance are sparse. Cultural specificity in test items can compromise scoring. For example, literal translations may not provide the same complex meaning as demonstrated in the original version, but experienced translators can help overcome these pitfalls.

SUMMARY

Neuropsychological testing is a valuable tool in the identification and description of many cognitive disorders and can aid in the differential diagnosis of normal aging, MCI, Alzheimer disease and other dementias, and depression. Furthermore, test results may help answer critical clinical questions regarding the safety of a patient who continues to drive, live alone, or manage finances.

The variability among neuropsychological profiles is most apparent in the first several years of the illness, underscoring the importance of early evaluation and diagnosis. Knowledge of a dementia diagnosis early on can improve health outcomes in several ways: by initiating pharmacologic treatment during the time of illness in which it works best, by providing clinical research opportunities to families that could lead to better treatment, and by giving patients the opportunity, while they still retain decisional capacity, to prepare for the future by creating advance directives and making decisions about finances and other family matters.

A frank and empathic discussion may also help alleviate the guilt and blame that occurs when the patient or caregiver has been under the erroneous impression that the cognitive deficits would disappear if only one "tried harder." The role of the informal caregiver cannot be underestimated, and given that psychosocial interventions for caregivers are effective[146] and may delay institutionalization,[147] an early and accurate diagnosis of a loved one may open the door for the caregiver to adjust to the role of caregiving[148] and seek both support and education.

KEY POINTS

- Diagnostic criteria for dementia have been revised to reflect a shifting focus to the minimally symptomatic stages of illness.
- Neuropsychological testing is an effective way of identifying very early cognitive impairments and distinguishing them from normal aging, mild cognitive impairment, and various types of dementia using relatively brief batteries of tests.
- Neuropsychologists can assist in characterizing the causes and consequences of cognitive loss, determine decisional capacity, and distinguish between dementia and comorbidities such as depression.
- Patients who present with cognitive impairments in the context of either motor symptoms (e.g., gait changes) or behavioral symptoms (disinhibition) should be referred for a neuropsychiatric evaluation.
- Early diagnosis of a dementia may improve treatment effectiveness, future planning, and quality of life for both patient and caregiver.
- Poor performance on verbal memory tests (both encoding and retrieval) is common in Alzheimer disease, but nonamnestic deficits may also be early signs. Non-Alzheimer dementias may be characterized by other cognitive or behavioral impairments such as language (semantic, nonfluent, or logopenic variant primary progressive aphasia), executive function (Parkinson disease dementia, vascular dementia), personality changes (behavioral variant frontotemporal degeneration), and psychotic symptoms (Lewy body disease).
- Performance on neuropsychological tests and measures of activities of daily living and instrumental activities of daily living are used as outcome variables in the development of pharmacologic and nonpharmacologic treatments for dementia.

For a complete list of references, please visit www.expertconsult.com.

KEY REFERENCES

4. Jack CR Jr, Albert MS, Knopman DS, et al: Introduction to the recommendations from the National Institute on Aging-Alzheimer's Association workgroups on diagnostic guidelines for Alzheimer's disease. Alzheimers Dement 7:257–262, 2011.
5. Dubois B, Feldman HH, Jacova C, et al: Research criteria for the diagnosis of Alzheimer's disease: revising the NINCDS-ADRDA criteria. Lancet Neurol 6:734–746, 2007.
8. Albert MS, DeKosky ST, Dickson D, et al: The diagnosis of mild cognitive impairment due to Alzheimer's disease: recommendations from the National Institute on Aging-Alzheimer's Association workgroups on diagnostic guidelines for Alzheimer's disease. Alzheimers Dement 7:270–279, 2011.
15. Langa KM, Levine DA: The diagnosis and management of mild cognitive impairment: a clinical review. JAMA 312:2551–2561, 2014.
19. Sano M, Egelko S, Ferris S, et al: Pilot study to show the feasibility of a multicenter trial of home-based assessment of people over 75 years old. Alzheimer Dis Assoc Disord 24:256–263, 2010.
22. Salmon DP, Bondi MW: Neuropsychological assessment of dementia. Annu Rev Psychol 60:257–282, 2009.
50. Blacker D, Lee H, Muzikansky A, et al: Neuropsychological measures in normal individuals that predict subsequent cognitive decline. Arch Neurol 64:862–871, 2007.
60. Sano M: Neuropsychological testing in the diagnosis of dementia. J Geriatr Psychiatry Neurol 19:155–159, 2006.
68. Hachinski V, Iadecola C, Petersen RC, et al: National Institute of Neurological Disorders and Stroke-Canadian Stroke Network vascular cognitive impairment harmonization standards. Stroke 37:2220–2241, 2006.
71. Misciagna S, Masullo C, Giordano A, et al: Vascular dementia and Alzheimer's disease: the unsolved problem of clinical and neuropsychological differential diagnosis. Int J Neurosci 115:1657–1667, 2005.
73. Graham NL, Emery T, Hodges JR: Distinctive cognitive profiles in Alzheimer's disease and subcortical vascular dementia. J Neurol Neurosurg Psychiatry 75:61–71, 2004.
77. Park JH, Lee SB, Lee TJ, et al: Depression in vascular dementia is quantitatively and qualitatively different from depression in Alzheimer's disease. Dement Geriatr Cogn Disord 23:67–73, 2007.
84. Rascovsky K, Salmon DP, Ho GJ, et al: Cognitive profiles differ in autopsy-confirmed frontotemporal dementia and AD. Neurology 58:1801–1808, 2002.
85. Gregory CA, Hodges JR: Clinical features of frontal lobe dementia in comparison to Alzheimer's disease. J Neural Transm Suppl 47: 103–123, 1996.
89. Mesulam MM: Primary progressive aphasia—a language-based dementia. N Engl J Med 349:1535–1542, 2003.
95. Perry RJ, Hodges JR: Differentiating frontal and temporal variant frontotemporal dementia from Alzheimer's disease. Neurology 54: 2277–2284, 2000.
97. Mesulam M, Wieneke C, Rogalski E, et al: Quantitative template for subtyping primary progressive aphasia. Arch Neurol 66:1545–1551, 2009.
104. Mayeux R, Chen J, Mirabello E, et al: An estimate of the incidence of dementia in idiopathic Parkinson's disease. Neurology 40:1513–1517, 1990.
105. Emre M: Dementia associated with Parkinson's disease. Lancet Neurol 2:229–237, 2003.
110. Salmon DP, Galasko D, Hansen LA, et al: Neuropsychological deficits associated with diffuse Lewy body disease. Brain Cogn 31:148–165, 1996.
124. Bhalla RK, Butters MA, Mulsant BH, et al: Persistence of neuropsychologic deficits in the remitted state of late-life depression. Am J Geriatr Psychiatry 14:419–427, 2006.
125. Butters MA, Whyte EM, Nebes RD, et al: The nature and determinants of neuropsychological functioning in late-life depression. Arch Gen Psychiatry 61:587–595, 2004.

127. Rapp MA, Dahlman K, Sano M, et al: Neuropsychological differences between late-onset and recurrent geriatric major depression. Am J Psychiatry 162:691–698, 2005.
133. Devanand DP, Sano M, Tang MX, et al: Depressed mood and the incidence of Alzheimer's disease in the elderly living in the community. Arch Gen Psychiatry 53:175–182, 1996.
144. Ganguli M, Du Y, Dodge HH, et al: Depressive symptoms and cognitive decline in late life: a prospective epidemiological study. Arch Gen Psychiatry 63:153–160, 2006.
146. Mittelman MS, Haley WE, Clay OJ, et al: Improving caregiver well-being delays nursing home placement of patients with Alzheimer disease. Neurology 67:1592–1599, 2006.

52 Alzheimer Disease

Jared R. Brosch, Martin R. Farlow

Alzheimer disease (AD) is the most common cause for dementia affecting older adults. The illness was first described by Alois Alzheimer in 1906 in a 51-year-old woman with well-described features of dementia. After death, her brain was examined and found to have numerous cortical plaques and tangles, characteristic of the illness.[1] The disease was thought to be rare for 6 decades until its clinical and neuropathologic features were recognized to be largely identical to those occurring in older dementia patients.[2]

The illness is the most frequent cause of dementia in the United States, currently afflicting as many as 5.2 million mostly older adults.[3] The incidence doubles every 6 years after the age of 50 years. As the over-80 population has rapidly grown, with improved health care leading to longer survival, it is estimated that the prevalence of AD in the United States by 2050 will increase to 13.8 million Americans, with 7.0 million older than 85 years.[4] This disabling disease is the most common cause of neurodegeneration and is the major condition leading to nursing home placement. The economic costs are huge, with direct health care, nursing home costs, and caregiving costs at home globally totaling greater than $315 billion.[5] Only symptomatic therapies are currently available, but no known therapy delays or halts disease progression. If a drug or lifestyle alteration (e.g., diet, exercise) could be found that delayed functional deterioration by as little as 1 to 2 years, it would substantially reduce the costs to families and society.[6]

PATHOLOGY AND MECHANISMS OF DISEASE

In AD, the illness begins with atrophy in the entorhinal cortex and hippocampus and, as clinical symptoms worsen, there is spread to most areas of the cortex, except for the occipital lobes.[7]

Microscopic examination of cortical sections from the brain of a patient with AD reveals global loss of neurons and increased numbers of extracellular amyloid plaques.[8] The amyloid plaques are diffuse and possibly benign, because similar deposits may be found in normal older adults, and compact, often associated with neuritic changes, possibly caused by effects of the deposited amyloid or by smaller oligomers of the β-amyloid protein on surrounding dendrites and axons (Figure 52-1). β-Amyloid proteins are also frequently found deposited diffusely in cerebral blood vessel walls. In addition to β-amyloid plaques, intracellular lacy fibrillar accumulations of material are present in neurons, called neurofibrillary tangles (NFTs; Figure 52-2).[9] NFTs are composed of paired helical filaments largely consisting of abnormally hyperphosphorylated tau. These are the defining features originally described by Alzheimer 102 years ago.

The amyloid plaques are made of β-amyloid proteins of various lengths, from 39 to 42 amino acids long.[10] The β-amyloid 1-40 amino acid type is in plasma and cerebrospinal fluid (CSF), but the 1-42 form comprises the major component of the cores of these amyloid plaques. The β-amyloid proteins are derived from a larger transmembrane protein that is widely present in the brain, the amyloid precursor protein (APP). They are cleaved from APP by the β-secretase and γ-secretase enzymes, which have been characterized and are active targets for drug therapy.[11]

Mutations have been found to be associated with familial AD, as will be described later in this chapter, in the genes coding for the β-amyloid proteins and for the presenilins, which likely are a component of γ-secretase.[12] Studies of the effects of these mutations in cell lines and transgenic animals that develop amyloid deposits and plaques in their brains, similar to patients with AD, have provided insights into how these proteins normally function and how, when disturbed by mutation, their functions are altered, leading to dementia. Those findings should provide insights into sporadic AD and, using these models, several drugs have been developed to reduce production of the β-amyloid proteins or speed their metabolism and clearance. It is hoped that these drugs will also be effective for sporadic AD.

Interestingly, although considerable evidence has suggested that β-amyloid and its toxic effects on the brain may initiate the cascade of pathophysiologic processes that leads to AD, the progression of dementia correlates more closely to numbers of NFTs or number of synapses lost.

Clearly, a cascade of processes involving different mechanisms, including inflammation and disturbed calcium homeostasis, occurs as AD progresses (Figure 52-3). Neurotransmitter systems are differentially affected. The cholinergic system is susceptible to early dysfunction, and increasing cholinergic deficiency has been correlated with clinical progression. As AD progresses, the glutaminergic, noradrenergic, and serotonergic systems deteriorate, causing further cognitive losses and often behavioral abnormalities. Therapeutic research since the late 1980s has focused on correcting these neurotransmitter deficits, with some modest success and resulting clinical benefits.

Extracellular amyloid plaques and intraneuronal NFTs in the cortex are the cardinal features of AD. Stereotypic spread of the NFTs, as originally described by Braak and Braak (1991),[7] defined a basis for neuropathologic criteria for AD staging that is still useful today. NFTs are found in the entorhinal cortex and adjacent areas of the hippocampus. Braak stages I and II typically are not associated with clinical symptoms. In stages III and IV, NFTs have spread to the limbic regions, and cognitive deficits are present. By stages V and VI, NFTs have spread to other regions of the cortex except the occipital cortices, and the severity of the dementia is worse.

Newer criteria assessing plaque and tangle densities have been developed. Khachaturian criteria count numbers of amyloid plaques in a 1-mm^2 field of the neocortex, with numbers adjusted for age.[13] The Consortium to Establish a Registry for Alzheimer's Disease criteria count plaques in three designated brain regions using defined stains.[14] The Reagan criteria assess plaques and tangle numbers in a highly specified way and appear to have generally high correlation in confirming the diagnosis of AD and assessing disease stage.[15]

Substantial evidence has suggested that plaques and tangles can be found in great numbers in many older adults with normal cognitive functioning, and that considerable overlap exists in plaque and tangle pathology between very old normals (>90 years) and those in this age range with dementia, reemphasizing the necessity for clinicopathologic correlation in diagnosis.[16] Although these pathologic features correlate less well in the oldest old, the presence of neocortical atrophy remains a strong associated factor for Alzheimer dementia at any older age.[17]

EPIDEMIOLOGY AND GENETICS

Aging is the biggest risk factor for AD. Rarely, patients in their 20s and 30s have been reported to have AD, but the onset of

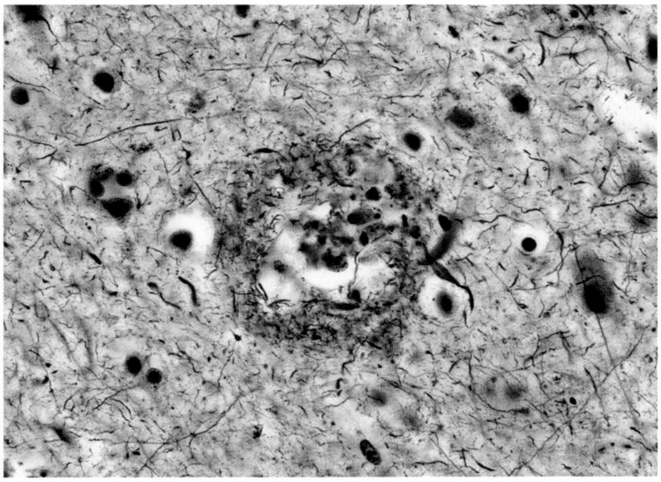

Figure 52-1. Neuritic plaques revealed by silver stain from cortex of patient with Alzheimer disease (×400).

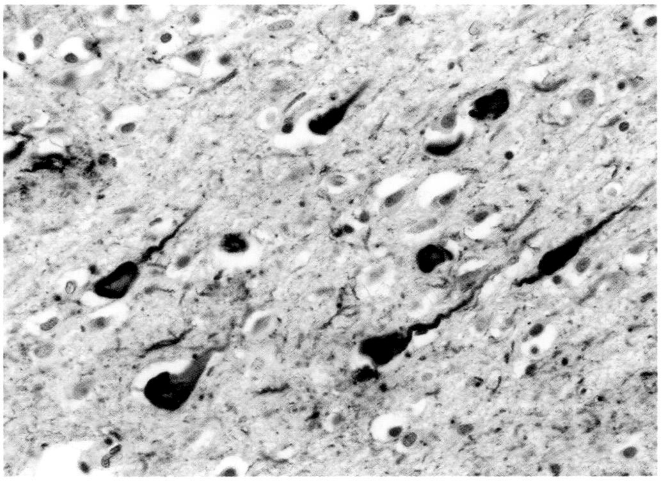

Figure 52-2. Neurofibrillary tangles in cortical section of brain from patient with Alzheimer disease.

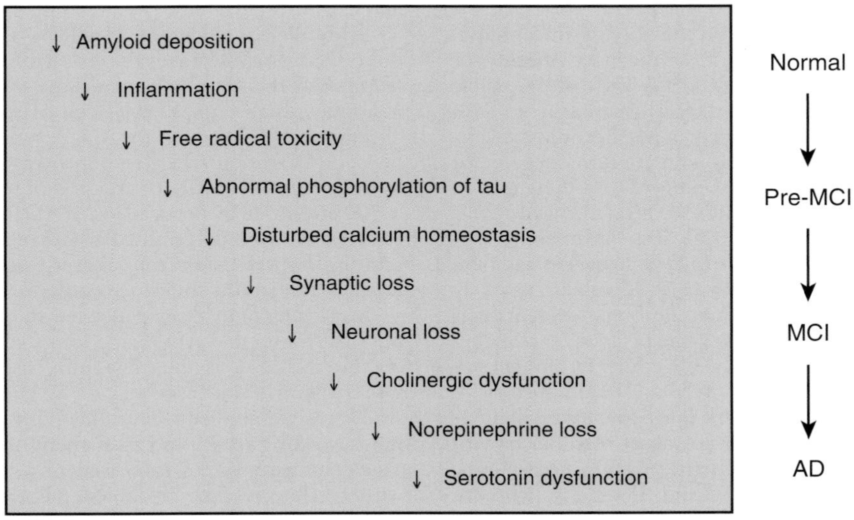

Figure 52-3. The cascade of mechanisms in Alzheimer disease (AD). Shown is the hypothetical cascade of processes occurring as Alzheimer disease progresses. The specific abnormalities are well established, but their order with regard to causality remains controversial. *MCI,* Mild cognitive impairment.

clinical symptoms is uncommon until the 50s, with yearly probability of incidence rapidly increasing to age 65 to 75 years, when 1% to 5% of the general population is affected. By age 75, the prevalence is as high as 15% in the United States, and by age 85, it has been estimated to afflict 35% to 50% in the oldest old.[18] Studies have suggested that the prevalence continues to climb, with most older adults by their 90s showing clinical signs of at least early dementia. However, in these oldest old with dementia, underlying brain pathology may differ little from age-matched normal subjects other than that demented patients have greater neuronal losses, and their rate of disease progression may be relatively slow. Therefore, even though these patients meet current clinical criteria for AD, it is unclear that they really have the same illness and may have a larger contribution from underlying vascular disease.[19]

The second most common risk factor for AD is family history, with approximately 20% of patients with AD having two or more first-degree relatives affected. The pattern of inheritance is typically autosomal dominant. In families with AD, several genetic mutations have been identified that are causative for the disease. Almost all the known mutations cause presenile forms of the disease. A few dozen families with onset of AD predominantly in their 40s and 50s have mutations in the APP gene, usually in the region of the gene that codes for the β-amyloid proteins. It is thought that these mutations result in abnormal β-amyloid metabolism, with resultant chronically higher levels of the protein leading to AD.[20]

The other mutations causing early-onset familial disease have been localized to the presenilin-1 (PS-1) gene on chromosome 14 and the presenilin-2 (PS-2) gene on chromosome 1. Again, only a few dozen families have been found in which PS-2 gene mutations are associated with AD, whereas more than 160 different mutations in the PS-1 have been found in several hundred families to cause AD and occasionally other symptoms, such as spasticity, seizures, or ataxia.[21,22] The presenilins are part of a complex that acts functionally as γ-secretase.[12] As noted, γ-secretase slices APP to produce β-amyloid.

Increased levels of β-amyloid are also found in AD patients with PS-1 or PS-2 mutations.[20] These mutations are the most commonly known cause of autosomal dominant familial AD, but they still cause less than 1% of all cases of AD. Even in patients with a family history of onset of dementia in those younger than 65 years, these mutations are causative in less than 10%. An early-onset patient with AD is more likely to have one of these mutations if there is a family history of other affected family members having a similar early age of onset. Other than aid in confirming the diagnosis or risk for AD in a limited number of these relatively rare families, the major importance of these mutations has been to create transgenic animals that have been useful in the following: unraveling disease mechanisms; hastening the development of new drugs and testing procedures; and finding other novel therapeutic approaches, such as targeted immunologic stimulation by β-amyloid vaccination or administering monoclonal antibodies targeted to the β-amyloid proteins to accelerate their degradation.

The major genetic risk factor identified for AD in late-onset, sporadic, and familial patients is the ε4 polymorphism of the apolipoprotein E (ApoE) gene.[23] ApoE is one of the major cholesterol- and lipid-carrying proteins in peripheral blood. In the brain and spinal fluid compartments, it is the only significant lipid transport protein and also functions as a transport protein for β-amyloid. It comes as types ε2, ε3, and ε4, with the ε2 allele being relatively uncommon. The ε4 allele is carried by 15% to 20% of the general population and the ε3 allele by almost everyone else. The 1% to 2% of individuals who are homozygous for the ε4 allele have a 50% risk of developing AD by their mid to late 60s. Those who are heterozygous for the ε4 allele have a 50% risk of developing AD by their mid to late 70s.[23] Women heterozygous for ε4 are more likely to develop AD at an earlier age than men.[24] Individuals who carry only the ε2 or ε3 allele are likely not to develop AD in their 80s or not at all. Some evidence has suggested that inheriting the ε2 allele may be protective, reducing the risk for AD. Inheritance of the ε4 allele confers a similar risk for AD, regardless of whether or not there is a family history.

Determination of the ApoE genotype in a patient with dementia improves diagnostic specificity in the subset of subjects with the ε4 genotype, but it is arguable whether diagnostic accuracy is improved enough to be clinically helpful. If subjects who are homozygous or heterozygous for ε4 and do not develop dementia in their at-risk age range, current evidence suggests that their future risk of dementia is no greater than that of an age-matched, non-ε4 carrier in the general population for developing AD. Therefore, presymptomatic ApoE ε4 genotyping for future risk for AD is currently not recommended. Interestingly, ApoE ε4 patients have been found to recover less completely from head trauma, so a more prominent history of head trauma may be a pseudomarker for carrying the ApoE ε4 polymorphism.[25] It has been found that in individuals with mild cognitive impairment (MCI), the ApoE ε4 genotype is associated with a significantly greater risk for conversion to AD,[26] and ε4-carrying patients with MCI were more responsive to donepezil therapy.[27] Clinical disease progression after conversion to AD is not influenced by the ApoE genotype, so the ApoE ε4 protein may be more influential in the earlier biologic stages of the illness. However, once disease spreads and the cascade of destructive pathophysiologic processes begins, the ApoE genotype no longer influences the rate of progression. Considerable evidence in late-onset AD has suggested that there are multiple genetic polymorphisms that may play a role in increasing the risk for some patients to develop the illness.[28,29]

Other factors that influence risk for AD are gender and education. Women are at greater risk for AD, even with adjustment for their longer survival to an older age. In the past, this greater risk for AD has been suggested by several epidemiologic studies to be due to postmenopausal estrogen deficiency, and estrogen replacement was believed to be primary prevention for AD. However, the Women's Health Initiative Memory Study of estrogen in older women has shown that estrogen replacement may increase, rather than decrease, the risk for dementia.[30,31]

In several studies, increased education has been associated with reduced overall risk for AD and/or later onset of the illness. It has been hypothesized that better educated individuals have a greater cognitive reserve, so the underlying biologic process of disease must progress further for clinical symptoms to develop.[32,33] However, the protective effects of cognitive training and mental exercises have not demonstrated convincing benefits in delaying disease onset. Interestingly, several studies have suggested that physical exercise may be protective and decrease brain atrophy and/or delay disease progression.[34] A large, multicenter, randomized controlled trial investigating exercise in AD is currently underway, and results will be available after 2018.[35]

Epidemiologic studies and small pilot trials have suggested that nonsteroidal antiinflammatory drugs (NSAIDs) prevent or delay progression in AD.[36] However, several large double-blind, placebo-controlled trials have indicated no significant reduction in risk for AD with NSAIDs but have shown a significantly increased risk for gastrointestinal symptoms, such as hemorrhage, and cardiovascular disease, including stroke.[37,38]

A number of studies and trials have suggested that the metabolic syndrome increases the risk for AD.[39] Specifically the main features of the metabolic syndrome-diabetes mellitus or insulin resistance, high cholesterol level, hypertension, and obesity-are all suggested risk factors for AD. Several prospective studies have been investigating whether improving or treating these factors individually will reduce conversion of normal or MCI individuals to AD and/or delay progression of AD in subjects already affected. It remains to be determined whether these approaches, such as treating hypertension and treating insulin resistance with glitazones and statins to reduce cholesterol, are effective.

A growing body of evidence has found an association between physical frailty and AD incidence. A study of 823 patients demonstrated that each unit change in baseline frailty score led to a more than 9% increased risk of developing AD.[40] Frailty in this study was a composite score involving grip strength, body mass index, walking speed, and assessment of fatigue. An autopsy study also demonstrated an increased risk of AD pathology, with or without the presence of clinical dementia, in those with higher frailty scores.[41] Frailty is also associated with mild cognitive impairment and has an impact on quality-of-life scores in those with AD.[42,43]

EPIDEMIOLOGY AND GENETICS

Aging is the biggest risk factor for AD. Rarely, patients in their 20s and 30s have been reported to have AD, but the onset of clinical symptoms is uncommon until the 50s, with yearly probability of incidence rapidly increasing to age 65 to 75 years, when 1% to 5% of the general population is affected. By age 75-85 the prevalence is otherwise as high as 18% in the United States, and over age 85, it has been estimated to afflict 33% to 42%.[4] Studies have suggested that the prevalence continues to climb, with most older adults by their 90s showing clinical signs of at least early dementia. However, in these oldest old with dementia, underlying brain pathology may differ little from age-matched normal subjects other than that demented patients have greater neuronal losses, and their rate of disease progression may be relatively slow. Therefore, even though these patients meet current clinical criteria for AD, it is unclear that they really have the same illness and may have a larger contribution from underlying vascular disease.[19]

The second most common risk factor for AD is family history, with approximately 20% of patients with AD having two or more

TABLE 52-4 Laboratory Evaluation of Patients With Dementia

Type of Study	Examples
Basic studies, excluding reversible with specific indication from history for causes of dementia or examination	Complete blood count (CBC)
	Chemistry or metabolic panel (SM-17)
	Thyroid function tests (thyroid-stimulating hormone [TSH])
	Vitamin B_{12}, folate levels
	Computed tomography (CT) or magnetic resonance imaging (MRI)
	HIV testing
	Sedimentation rate
	Hemoglobin A1C (Hb A1C)
	Urinalysis
	Chest X-ray
	Urine or plasma for drugs or heavy metals
Adjuvant studies to aid diagnosis	
Other tests as indicated by history or physical or neurologic examination	Single-photon emission computed tomography (SPECT)
	Positron emission tomography (PET)
	Lumbar puncture with cerebrospinal fluid for β-amyloid

transient, is greatly appreciated by patients and their caregivers, and the benefits fully justify performing an evaluation for reversible conditions.

A second purpose of the laboratory evaluation is to aid differential diagnosis of the neurodegenerative and vascular dementias (e.g., AD, dementia with Lewy bodies or Parkinson dementia, vascular dementia, frontotemporal dementia [FTD]). Accurate diagnosis of the cause of the dementia can guide counseling patients, families, and caregivers regarding the course and prognosis. Accurate diagnosis of dementia is also important in guiding therapeutic choices. There is evidence from double-blind, placebo-controlled trials suggesting some efficacy for available drugs in all the irreversible dementias mentioned, except FTD.

Metabolic abnormalities can worsen cognitive deficits. Relatively minor deviations out of the normal range can exacerbate mental impairment in older adults, particularly those with some other preexisting cause for the cognitive impairments or dementia. Metabolic and endocrine causes are all potentially reversible.

Hyperkalemia may occur in many patients taking diuretics for the treatment of hypertension or with congestive heart failure, as well as in those taking steroids. Hypernatremia may be found in patients with dehydration, which can occur in impaired older patients who are dependent on others for fluid intake; hyponatremia may occur in association with a variety of chronic illnesses or medications; and hypocalcemia and hypercalcemia are found more rarely but also can affect cognitive functioning and should be screened for.

The most common reversible endocrine cause for dementia in older adults is hypothyroidism. Diabetes mellitus, which is increasing rapidly in the United States, is another cause that has reversible and irreversible aspects. Unrecognized intermittent hyperglycemia or hypoglycemia may cause cognitive impairment, which is reversible. The longer term effects of diabetes mellitus on vessel walls may result in subcortical ischemic vascular disease, directly causing vascular dementia and also being a risk factor for AD.

Chronic diseases of the major organ systems may all secondarily cause cognitive impairment. These chronic illnesses include acute and chronic pulmonary disease, such as asthma, chronic obstructive pulmonary disease, and pulmonary fibrosis; liver disease, such as hepatitis and cirrhosis; cardiac disease, such as congestive heart failure and arrhythmias; chronic central nervous system (CNS) infections, such as tuberculosis, *Cryptococcus*, and other fungal infections; HIV; CJD; Whipple disease; and syphilis. Most patients will have other symptoms or signs, and lumbar puncture to obtain CSF for testing is usually required for diagnosis. Older patients with urinary tract infections and upper respiratory infections may also have reversible cognitive impairments. Subclinical or partial seizures may mimic dementia, with intermittent worsening confusion or automatisms such as lip smacking suggesting the diagnosis.

Polypharmacy in older adults is arguably the most common reversible cause of cognitive impairment. A partial list of the drug categories that are the biggest offenders includes anticholinergics, antihypertensives, antidepressants, antianxiety drugs, antipsychotics, analgesics, and hypnotics. If suspected, their use may be eliminated or the lowest dosage necessary to control symptoms should be used.

In evaluating for potentially reversible causes of dementia, space-occupying masses or other structural abnormalities in the brain may be identified by brain imaging with techniques such as computed tomography (CT) or magnetic resonance imaging (MRI). Most frequent abnormalities identified might include ischemic changes, including strokes, normal pressure hydrocephalus, subdural hematomas and hygromas, tumors such as large meningiomas, and gliomas or brain metastases from unidentified primary tumors.

Selective frontal or temporal atrophy on an MRI or CT scan may suggest FTD, and multiple large vessel strokes or smaller subcortical strokes may suggest vascular dementia. Discrimination of FTD from AD in individual patients may be difficult using clinical examination and CT or MRI. Functional imaging measuring blood flow or metabolism by single-photon emission computed tomography (SPECT) or positron emission tomography (PET) may be better able to discriminate FTD from AD and other forms of dementia.

Behavioral Symptoms

Behavioral disturbances are common in AD and increase as the illness declines to the more severe stages. Dysfunctions in the cholinergic and glutaminergic systems are associated with cognitive impairment in AD but, with disease progression, abnormalities in other neurotransmitter systems can be demonstrated that likely underlie the onset of behavioral or psychiatric symptoms.[56] For example, aggressiveness has been associated with dysregulation in the γ-aminobutyric acid–ergic, serotonergic, and noradrenergic systems. Similarly, depressive symptoms have been associated with loss of neurons in the medial raphe nuclei and locus ceruleus, with consequent depletion of serotonin and noradrenalin. Treatment approaches have been guided by these observations. Major therapeutic targets in patients with AD include agitation, depression, anxiety, and insomnia or disturbances in day-night sleep cycles. Treatment of these symptoms may be difficult, and none of the drugs currently used to treat these symptoms has been approved by the U.S. Food and Drug Administration (FDA) for treating behavioral symptoms in AD.

Double-blind, placebo-controlled trials are limited, but available data have suggested that substantial placebo effects occur with treatment of most of these symptoms, and that many commonly used drugs have modest effects. Treatment of behavioral symptoms is of great importance to family members and caregivers because they are difficult to manage and are one of the principal factors for nursing home placement.

Aggressive or assaultive behaviors are relatively common in AD, with roughly 20% of patients in the community and up to 50% of nursing home patients committing physical assaults. Verbal attacks are reported to occur in 50% of patients with AD. Hallucinations occur in as many as 30% of patients at home and in 50% of nursing home patients. Changes in the environment, such as being moved to a new locale, having a new caregiver, or simply as the result of disease progression, may precipitate all the previously listed symptoms. A comparative study has suggested limited efficacy for the most commonly used drugs for agitation.[57]

The atypical neuroleptics, despite evidence suggesting some increased risk for stroke with chronic use, are still most useful in patients with AD for treating agitation.[58,59]

In the absence of approved drugs or a convincing clinical trial evidence base for treating patients with behavioral symptoms, the following general therapeutic approach should be followed. Target symptoms for treatment should be identified before therapy begins. Typical symptoms include wandering, physical aggression, restlessness, agitation, pacing, screaming, disinhibition, delusions, hallucinations, misidentification, sleep disturbances and, often, depression. Iatrogenic causes such as anticholinergic and pain medications should be excluded, infections and other new illnesses, as well as potential sources of pain should be eliminated and possible changes in the environment should be investigated. For the identified target symptoms, drug treatment should be started and advanced slowly. When symptoms are controlled, periodic attempts should be made to wean the medications.

Biologic Markers of Diagnosis of Disease Progression

No biomarkers are currently sensitive and specific enough to establish the diagnosis of AD reliably, but some have potential utility as adjuncts to the clinical evaluation. The NIA-AA criteria have incorporated several biomarkers in establishing a diagnosis of probable AD with evidence of AD pathophysiologic process (see Figure 52-2). A high probability of AD pathology is demonstrated if abnormalities in β-amyloid deposition and neuronal injury are shown in biomarker data. β-Amyloid deposition is established if the β-amyloid level is low in the CSF or if there is a positive amyloid PET scan. Neuronal injury is proven with high CSF tau levels, decreased fluorodeoxyglucose-PET (FDG-PET) uptake in the temporoparietal cortex, or disproportionate atrophy in the mediobasolateral temporal lobe and medial parietal cortex on a structural MRI scan. These biomarkers are widely used as a secondary assessment to support efficacy claims for antidementia drugs in clinical trials (Figure 52-4). Serial MRI scans may be more widely used clinically to assess disease progression if one of the investigational drugs currently under study delays disease progression. Both MRI spectroscopy and ^{18}FDG-PET detect metabolism changes associated with AD (Figure 52-5), but lack of longitudinal data and high cost have limited their broad adoption.

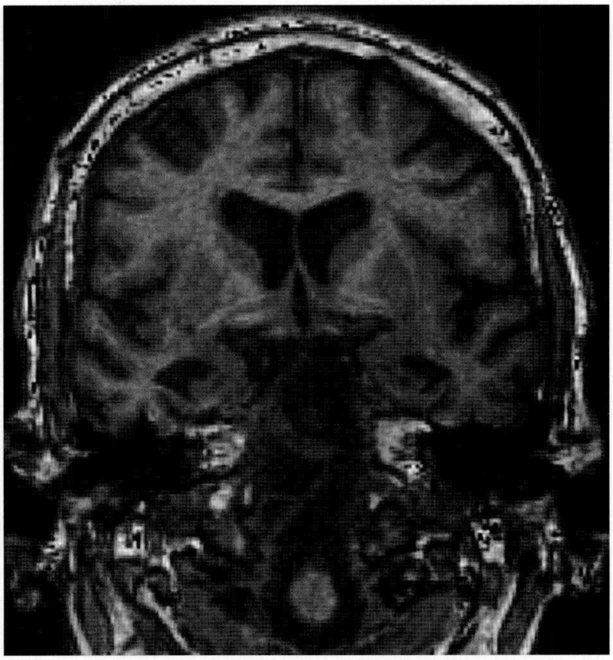

Figure 52-4. MRI study with coronal view through the hippocampal region illustrating moderately severe mediotemporal atrophy and milder global atrophy typical for Alzheimer disease.

An agent-labeling amyloid, Pittsburgh compound B (PIB), has been demonstrated to label amyloid deposits reliably in the brains of patients with AD (Figure 52-6). Unfortunately, 10% to 20% of normal older adults by the age of 65 years show PIB positivity, and the percentage of normal adults with significant PIB positivity progressively increases to 50% for normal patients in their mid-80s.[60] However, in those with amnestic MCI, PIB positivity appears to predict earlier conversion to dementia, and the absence of PIB positivity appears to be strong evidence against progression to AD.[61] In 2012, the FDA approved a compound, florbetapir, that uses radioactive fluorine, which has a longer half-life than PIB. The drug and imaging scan have become available in large centers, but have similar clinical limitations as PIB imaging.[62] Currently, the scan is not currently approved for reimbursement by most insurance companies, including Medicare. It is now being used in many clinical trials as a marker of abnormal amyloid metabolism, as per the NIA-AA criteria noted earlier.

Beyond structural MRI and PET (FDG and amyloid PET), several other imaging modalities to aid in the diagnosis of AD are under investigation. In an abnormal resting state, functional MRI demonstrates mesial temporal lobe cerebral blood flow (CBF) and a greater change in CBF in patients at risk for developing AD.[63] Diffusion tensor imaging (DTI) is a technique that has been used to study AD changes in subcortical white matter tracts. Changes in white matter tracts in the parahippocampal region, lateral temporal lobe, fornix, prefrontal white matter, and corpus callosum have been shown to be characteristic in 335 scans carried out in Europe.[64] SPECT scans are similar to PET scans in that they measure gamma ray emission. SPECT imaging is less expensive than PET scans because the equipment and radioisotopes are less expensive and more widely available. SPECT imaging has been shown to have high specificity in detecting abnormal hippocampal radiotracer uptake in MCI patients who go on to develop AD compared to those who do not.[65] In vivo imaging of tau deposition is an important new modality that is likely to become an important adjunct to available procedures. Tau deposition is strongly associated with cognitive decline. Amyloid PET gives only a partial picture of the in vivo pathophysiologic process in AD. PET tracers that bind tau will not only aid in the diagnosis of AD but will also help guide tau-based therapeutics.[66]

β-Amyloid 1-42 protein levels in CSF from patients with AD are lower than those in age-matched controls.[67] Similarly, tau protein levels and phospho tau levels are significantly higher in AD than in normal older patients.[68] Unfortunately, abnormal β-amyloid and tau levels occur in other neurodegenerative diseases such as CJD and DLBD, and some overlap occurs with normal aging. Combining these two measures improves the accuracy of diagnosis, but it is unclear that CSF β-amyloid and tau measurements improve the specificity of clinical diagnosis enough to justify lumbar puncture in most patients.

In general, biologic markers for AD and disease progression have become more widely available in clinical practice but cost limitations and lack of disease-modifying therapies continue to hinder their usefulness. Ultimately, the investigation of a number of markers in plasma and CSF in large prospective longitudinal studies, such as the Alzheimer's Disease Neuroimaging Initiative, may yield more sensitive and specific biologic markers for AD.

TREATMENT

Current therapies for AD treat cognitive or behavioral symptoms but have not been shown to delay the biologic progression of disease. The development of a therapy to delay or prevent the onset of dementia and delay disease progression remains an actively pursued but so far elusive goal.

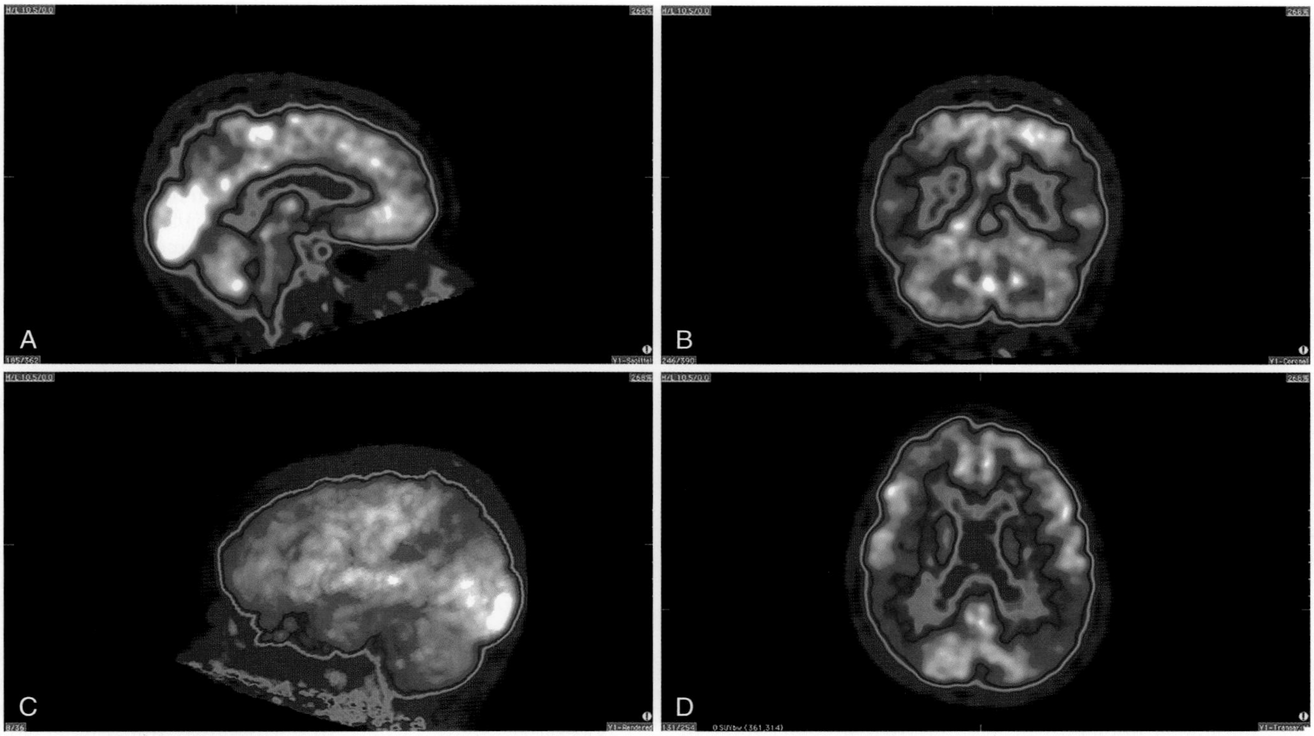

Figure 52-5. Views from a PET 18-fluorodeoxyglucose study in a patient with Alzheimer disease. The images demonstrate decreased signal or metabolism in the posterior parietal regions, as may characteristically be seen with this illness. **A,** Mid sagital view demonstrating decreased posterior cingualte/parietal hypometabolism. **B,** Coronal view demonstrating decreased metabolism in parietal lobe. **C,** Sagital view through temporal and parietal lobes. **D,** Axial view illustrating hypometabolism in post parietal lobe.

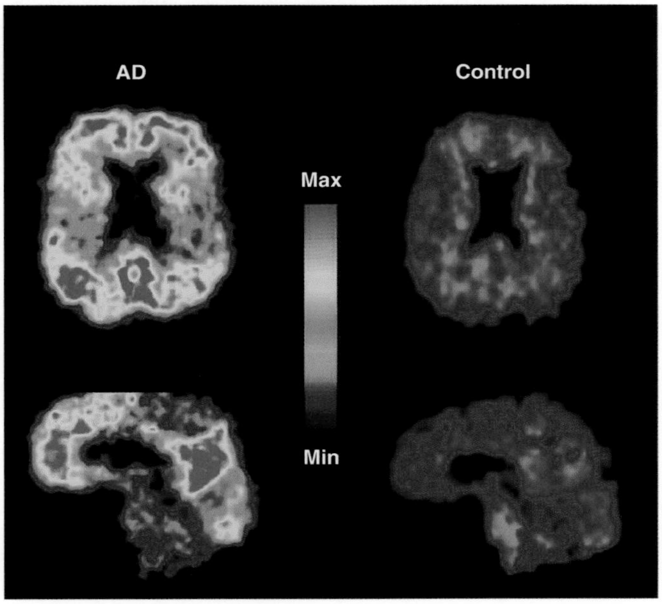

Figure 52-6. Agent-labeling amyloid, Pittsburgh compound B, illustrating significant uptake in the frontal and parietal regions in a patient with Alzheimer disease.

Pharmaceutical Agents

Currently available drugs for AD modestly improve some aspects of cognition and function in ADLs, and have some less well-established beneficial effects on behavioral disturbances (Table 52-5).[69-73] Significant benefits are seen only in a minority of patients, and stabilization and temporary reduction of symptomatic decline are the best results achieved in most other patients. Families and caregivers need to be cautioned against unrealistic expectations. Benefits always need to be weighed against adverse effects when deciding whether a drug dose should be increased or whether the antidementia medication should be continued at all.

TABLE 52-5 Clinical Trial Evidence for Drugs Approved for Treatment of Alzheimer Disease

Study	Treatment or Placebo: Dose (mg)	No. of Subjects	Treatment, Effect
Donepezil	Placebo	153	
Rogers et al,	5 mg	152	2.5
1998[69]	10 mg	150	2.9
Rivastigmine	Placebo	235	
Corey-Bloom	1-4 mg	233	21
et al, 1998[70]	6-12 mg	231	3.8
Galantamine	Placebo	213	
Raskind et al,	24 mg	212	1.6
2000[71]	32 mg	211	3.4
			SIB
Memantine	Placebo	126	
Reisberg et al, 2003[72]	20 mg	126	5.7
Memantine + donepezil	Placebo	201	
Tariot et al, 2004[73]	10 mg D + 20 mg M	203	3.3

SIB, Severe impairment battery (1-100); Alzheimer disease assessment scale cognitive component (1-70).

Cholinesterase Inhibitors

Recognition that cholinergic deficiency, including progressive loss of cholinergic neurons in a brain region known to be involved in learning and memory, has led to the development of the cholinesterase inhibitors. Tacrine, the first cholinesterase inhibitor successfully developed to treat AD, caused liver toxicity and thus required frequent blood testing to monitor liver function. It had a very short half-life, which made four times daily dosing necessary; this was very difficult for AD patients and their caregivers to comply with. It never was used widely in clinical practice. Donepezil is a cholinesterase inhibitor that more selective for acetylcholinesterase, rivastigmine inhibits acetylcholinesterase and butyrylcholinesterase, and galantamine inhibits cholinesterase but also modulates acetylcholine effects on nicotinic receptors. The clinical significance of these differences in the cholinesterase inhibitor is unknown. Double-blind, placebo-controlled trials have demonstrated that donepezil, rivastigmine, and galantamine mildly improve cognition, function in ADLs, and behavior in some patients with mild to moderate-stage AD for periods of between 6 and 18 months (see Table 52-5).[74] Donepezil and rivastigmine have also proven effective for treating patients with moderate- to severe-stage dementia. Donepezil was approved for severe-stage AD in 2006[75] and rivastigmine in 2013.[76]

When therapy is initiated, all cholinesterase inhibitors need to be titrated to decrease adverse effects and achieve the maximum tolerated dose to optimize benefits. If adverse effects occur, doses may be skipped or the dosage reduced until they abate or lessen, and higher dosages may again be tried at a later time. In general, the effects on cognition, function in ADLs, and behavior potentially may be accompanied by and weighed against adverse effects such as nausea, vomiting, and diarrhea, which also increase with dose.

Finding the optimal balance between adverse and beneficial drug effects in the individual patient is the goal. If patients are intolerant of one cholinesterase inhibitor, they may tolerate another, so a trial of switching to an alternative medication sometimes is appropriate. Both the AD 2000 Collaborative Group Study and Alzheimer's Disease Cooperative Studies–Mild Cognitive Impairment Trial have suggested that donepezil, and by implication the other cholinesterase inhibitors, may be less effective after 18 to 24 months.[27,77] Neuropathologic studies, however, have suggested that central cholinergic deficits in MCI may be less than in AD.[78] The AD 2000 study design included periodic withdrawal, suggesting that the conclusion reached in each of these studies—that the efficacy of cholinesterase inhibitor therapy wanes after 18 to 24 months—may not be generalizable. Substantial open-label follow-up data are available for all the cholinesterase inhibitors suggesting, but not proving, continued beneficial effects for 5 years or longer. However, these data are uncontrolled and have been biased by selective dropouts.

The schedule for withdrawing these drugs is a major concern. As a general principle, they should be stopped when the patient is no longer benefiting from their use, but this may be difficult to assess those with late-stage disease. In severely affected patients, the drugs should be withdrawn when patients are no longer able to interact meaningfully with family or caregivers.

Medications Acting on the Glutamatergic System

Memantine belongs to a second class of drugs that works by partially antagonizing glutamate at the *N*-methyl-D-aspartate (NMDA) receptor, which may improve symptoms in AD by two different mechanisms of action. First, the regulation of glutamate effects improves signal transmission, improving the efficiency of neurotransmission and, presumably, at a clinical level relieves cognitive symptoms. Second, memantine may prevents excess calcium entrance into the neurons following glutamate stimulation, thus potentially having neuroprotective effects. In patients with moderate- to severe-stage disease, as demonstrated in previous clinical trials, memantine mildly improves cognitive deficits, function in ADLs, and behavior. Adverse clinical effects with memantine are fewer than with the cholinesterase inhibitors, and one large double-blind, placebo-controlled trial in AD patients on established donepezil has suggested that there may be fewer rather than more side effects when memantine is added, as well as an additive symptomatic benefit. Trials in patients with milder stage AD have demonstrated less consistent benefits. Memantine is currently not recommended for use in this population. With memantine, as with the cholinesterase inhibitors, symptomatic benefits may be difficult for caregivers to judge in some patients, so they should be counseled about realistic expectations regarding the potential magnitude of benefits with this therapy. As with the cholinesterase inhibitors, memantine should be continued until the patient is judged to be no longer benefiting or has no meaningful personal interactions.

Previously Accepted Therapies: Ineffective?

Vitamin E was reported to delay functional deterioration, nursing home placement, and death by approximately 25% in those with moderate- to severe-stage AD in a large double-blind, placebo-controlled trial.[79] However, these results were obtained only after adjusting for group differences in cognitive functioning at baseline, and no cognitive benefits were seen in the group taking vitamin E. The vitamin E group in the Alzheimer's Disease Cooperative Study Group–Mild Cognitive Impairment study showed no benefit versus placebo,[27] and other studies have also suggested risks concerning thrombosis with the vitamin E dose of 2000 U used in these studies. Vitamin E is no longer broadly recommended as a therapy for AD.

Similarly, several epidemiologic studies have suggested that estrogens and NSAIDs may delay the onset of AD.[36] However, several large double-blind, placebo-controlled studies have suggested that estrogens and NSAIDs used as prophylactically in normal older adults and in patients with AD may have greater risks than benefit.[80-82]

More Targeted Therapeutic Approaches

Broad acceptance of the β-amyloid hypothesis as a target for therapy and the availability of transgenic animal models known to develop amyloid plaques has made reducing β-amyloid the major focus in developing drugs to delay disease progression. More detailed understanding of AD metabolism has led to the development of β- and γ-secretase inhibitors that block the formation of β-amyloid from the APP by interfering with the enzymes that slice it from the larger APP. Studies of γ-secretase inhibitors have not been promising, but β-secretase studies are underway that are targeting β-amyloid products in mild AD and in patients with MCI. To date, there have been several drugs used to test the β-amyloid hypothesis (passive vaccination and infusion of active antibodies against amyloid) that have not proven to be effective in clinical trials.[83,84]

Despite early failures of the β-amyloid hypothesis, several ongoing clinical trials using antibodies against various regions of the β-amyloid peptide continue to be pursued by various pharmaceutical companies. Many of the early trials have shown excellent tolerance for the medications and some evidence hinting at stabilization of cognitive function. Current hypotheses revolve around earlier treatment with these medications, and research studies include these three well-funded trials targeting asymptomatic individuals[85]:

- The Dominantly Inherited Alzheimer Network (DIAN) trials involve patients with identified genetic mutations that will be treated with one of two antiamyloid monoclonal antibody infusions.

- The Alzheimer's Prevention Initiative Autosomal Dominant AD trial also targets patients with a specific *PSEN1* mutation and treatment with the antiamyloid drug crenezumab.
- The Anti-Amyloid treatment in Asymptomatic AD (A4 trial) targets presymptomatic older patients who have biomarkers suggesting underlying pathophysiologic changes of AD.

Clinically, few drugs are being tested on tau protein–based targets, but this is an active area of interest. It is possible that a combination of drugs targeting several targets may be the ultimate solution to halting and/or reversing AD. Only time will tell.

Acknowledgment

This work was supported in part by grant PHS P30 AG10133 from the National Institutes of Health and the National Institute of Aging.

KEY POINTS

- The diagnosis of probable Alzheimer disease is determined by a clinical process rather than a laboratory test.
- The major risk factors for Alzheimer disease are older age, ApoE ε4 genotype, and lifestyle (metabolic syndrome).
- It is unclear whether determination of the ApoE ε4 genotype in a patient with dementia improves diagnostic specificity enough to be clinically useful.
- Several different disease mechanisms associated with Alzheimer disease have been identified that are targets for drug therapy.
- Symptomatic treatment with cholinesterase inhibitors is effective for patients with mild-, moderate-, and severe-stage Alzheimer disease.
- Symptomatic treatment with memantine is effective in moderate-to-severe stage Alzheimer disease, and benefits are seen with memantine added to cholinesterase inhibitors.
- Mutations associated with familial Alzheimer disease have led to the creation of transgenic animals that have greatly facilitated therapeutic research.
- Amyloid-labeling agents using PET imaging are being evaluated for their predictive, diagnostic, and risk factor utility regarding Alzheimer disease.
- Behavioral symptoms in Alzheimer disease are common, and most therapies are unapproved and at best marginally effective.
- Several promising treatments for Alzheimer disease identified in epidemiology studies have failed in clinical trials.

For a complete list of references, please visit www.expertconsult.com.

KEY REFERENCES

8. Braak H, Braak E, Bohl J: Staging of Alzheimer-related cortical destruction. Eur Neurol 33:403–408, 1993.
14. Mirra SS, Heyman A, McKee D, et al: The consortium to establish a registry for Alzheimer's disease (CERAD). Part II: Standardization of the neuropathological assessment of Alzheimer's disease. Neurology 41:479–486, 1991.
23. Saunders AM, Strittmatter WJ, Schmechel D, et al: Association of apolipoprotein E allele epsilon 4 with late-onset familial and sporadic Alzheimer's disease. Neurology 43:1467–1472, 1993.
44. American Psychiatric Association: Diagnostic and statistical manual of mental disorders (DSM-V), ed 5, Washington DC, 2013, American Psychiatric Association.
46. McKhann GM, Knopman DS, Chertkow H: The diagnosis of dementia due to Alzheimer's disease: recommendations from the National Institute on Aging-Alzheimer's Association workgroups on diagnostic guidelines for Alzheimer's disease. Alzheimers Dement 7:263–269, 2011.
48. Sperling RA, Aisen PS, Beckett LA: Toward defining the preclinical stages of Alzheimer's disease: recommendations from the National Institute on Aging-Alzheimer's Association workgroups on diagnostic guidelines for Alzheimer's disease. Alzheimers Dement 7:280–292, 2011.
57. Schneider LS, Tariot PN, Dagerman KS, et al: Effectiveness of atypical antipsychotic drugs in patients with Alzheimer's disease. N Engl J Med 355:1525–1538, 2006.
62. Yang L, Rieves D, Ganley C: Brain amyloid imaging-FDA approval of florbetapir F18 injection. N Engl J Med 367:10, B85–B87, 2012.
66. Villemagne VL, Fodero-Tavoletti MT, Masters CL, et al: Tau imaging: early progress and future directions. Lancet Neurol 14:114–124, 2015.
69. Rogers SL, Farlow MR, Doody RS, et al: A 24-week, double-blind, placebo-controlled trial of donepezil in patients with Alzheimer's disease. Neurology 50:136–145, 1998.
77. Courtney C, Farrell D, Gray R, et al: Long-term donepezil treatment in 565 patients with Alzheimer's disease (AD2000): randomised double-blind trial. Lancet 363:2105–2115, 2004.

53 Vascular Cognitive Disorders

Perminder S. Sachdev

The term *vascular cognitive disorder* (VCD) refers to a heterogeneous group of disorders in which the salient feature is the presence of cognitive impairment primarily attributable to cerebrovascular disease (CVD). The conceptualization of this disorder has had a checkered history, with a variety of terms used to describe overlapping conditions. VCD is used not only for vascular dementia, including poststroke and multi-infarct dementia, but also for cognitive impairment of vascular origin that does not meet dementia criteria. VCD is recognized as the second most common cause of dementia after Alzheimer disease (AD), with varied clinical, neuropathologic, and neuroimaging manifestations. There is also considerable interest in the role of vascular injury in the pathogenesis and clinical manifestations of AD. Experimental work has shown a functional and pathogenetic synergy between the vascular endothelium and neural cells, and the dysfunction of the neurovascular unit has been a focus to understand the pathomechanisms of cognitive impairment. The fact that vascular risk factors are modifiable has led to the claim that VCD may be a preventable form of dementia.

HISTORICAL OVERVIEW AND TERMINOLOGY

The long-standing concept of hardening of the arteries or cerebral atherosclerosis as a cause of senility[1] was challenged in the 1960s by the neuropathologic studies from Newcastle-Upon-Tyne, England, which suggested that vascular dementia (VaD) was related to multiple brain infarctions exceeding a certain threshold and was distinct from AD as a cause of dementia.[2] The concept was further elaborated in a 1974 paper, which stated that "...when vascular disease is responsible for dementia it is through the occurrence of multiple small or large cerebral infarcts."[3] This led to the widespread use of the term *multi-infarct dementia* (MID) as being synonymous with VaD.[3] The last 2 decades have witnessed a major challenge to this narrow conceptualization of VaD, with an expanded concept that includes not only multiple cortical and/or subcortical infarcts, but also strategic single infarcts, noninfarction white matter lesions, hemorrhages, and hypoperfusion as possible causes of VaD.[4]

The broader VaD construct was, however, also considered to be inadequate to represent the full spectrum of cognitive dysfunction of vascular origin for a number of reasons. First, the focus on dementia precluded the inclusion of milder forms of cognitive impairment that failed to reach the threshold of dementia but were nevertheless important, especially for prevention. Second, growing neuropathologic evidence has indicated that most dementias have a neurodegenerative, usually due to AD pathology, and vascular basis,[5] and that these pathologies appear to act synergistically.[6] Third, most diagnostic criteria for dementia required the presence of memory impairment[7,8]; this was at odds with the clinical experience of the varied cognitive profile of VaD, with memory being relatively spared, especially in the early stages of the disease.[9] This led to the introduction of the construct vascular cognitive impairment (VCI),[10] which includes a broad spectrum of clinical profiles, from mild cognitive impairment to dementia, as well as individuals in whom cognitive impairment showed mixed primary neurodegenerative and vascular features or mixed features.[11] The VCI construct provides a dimensional approach to cognitive impairment of vascular origin, recognizing that the impairment can range from mild to very severe. The underlying pathology is varied, including single strategic infarcts, multiple infarcts, and noninfarct white matter lesions or leukoaraiosis, hypoperfusion, or hemorrhage; the vascular lesions can coexist with other brain pathologies.[11] It also affords greater attention to opportunities for primary and secondary prevention.[4,10,11]

The VCI construct is not without its limitations. The term *impairment* is used in medicine to indicate a reduction or loss of function in any domain of functioning and is applied as a statistical construct based on normative data or demonstration of disability, but is not used to denote a disorder. Moreover, VCI has sometimes also been used in the literature to denote mild cognitive impairment (MCI) due to vascular factors, equating VCI with vascular MCI. Hence, the use of VCD recognizes that there is often a need for a categoric diagnosis, which encompasses mild impairment, predementia, and dementia syndromes at the same time.[12,13] It can embrace many syndromes and diseases and also acknowledges the fact that patients with CVD also have noncognitive syndromes, such as depression, anxiety, and psychosis, which need to be distinguished from cognitive disorder. So-called functional impairment is seen as a consequence of the disorder. The use of the plural form, disorders, acknowledges that VCD comprises many diseases, each with varying severity and patterns of dysfunction.[13]

EPIDEMIOLOGY

The prevalence and incidence of VCD vary, depending on the diagnostic criteria applied and the population studied. In 11 population-based European studies conducted in the 1990s, the age-standardized prevalence of VaD was estimated to be 1.6% compared to 4.4% for AD.[14] The prevalence of VaD increased from 0.3% in those aged 65 to 69 years to 5.2% in those aged 90 years and older. VaD accounted for 15.8% of all cases of dementia in these studies.[14] The Canadian Study of Health and Aging used a broader concept of VCI and estimated that approximately 5% of people older than 65 years had VCI, with 2.4% having VCI (not dementia), 0.9% having mixed dementia (vascular and neurodegenerative), and 1.5% having VaD.[15] The incidence of VaD reportedly ranges from 6 to 12 cases/1000/year in those older than 70 years.[16] The prevalence of VaD is much higher in poststroke patients, with 6% to 32% being reported in various clinical samples 3 months after a stroke.[17-19] Dementia is 3.5- to 5.6-fold more frequent in stroke patients than in stroke-free controls. Poststroke dementia (PSD) has a complex cause, with a varying combination of large and small vessel disease, as well as nonvascular pathology such as AD contributing to the picture. Many stroke patients, up to 10% in some studies,[17,18] have cognitive impairment sufficient to diagnose dementia prior to the stroke. In a longitudinal study, the 10-year risk of dementia after stroke was estimated at 19.3%, compared to 11.0% in nonstroke controls,[20] suggesting that a stroke doubles the risk of incident dementia, although this excess risk diminishes with time and does not apply to those older than 85 years.[21]

Vascular lesions are common in autopsy studies of dementia cases, with approximately one third showing significant vascular pathology,[22,23] although this does not indicate the clinical relevance of such pathology. A review of pathologic studies, however, has shown a wide range in prevalence of VaD, from 0.03% to

85.2%, with a median figure of about 11%.[23] Vascular brain lesions are also common in population-based autopsy series. In the U.S. Adult Change in Thought study,[24] microinfarcts were common in nondemented (29%) and demented (63%) individuals, as were cystic infarcts (23% and 36% respectively), and the presence of two or more microinfarcts increased the risk of dementia 4.8 times (95% confidence interval [CI], 1.91 to 10.26). Other population-based neuropathologic studies[5,25,26] have also highlighted the importance of vascular lesions, in particular microinfarcts, in the development of dementia. Consequently, VCD is generally referred to as the second most common form of cognitive impairment after AD.

Geographic variations in the prevalence of VCD have been noted, but the data are inconclusive. VaD was previously reported to be more common than AD in some Eastern Asian countries,[27] but more recent data have shown a reversal. In the Hisayama Study from Japan,[28] the incidence of vascular dementia was 12.2/1000 person-years for men and 9.0/1000 person-years for women, whereas for AD it was 5.1 and 10.9/1000 person-years, respectively. In the last 3 decades, the ratio of VaD to AD in Japan has shifted from 2 : 1 to 1 : 1, probably due to better control of vascular risk factors and stroke prevention.[29] Reports from China have suggested a similar trend, with more recent studies reporting a higher prevalence of AD than VaD.[30] Data from other developing countries are limited, but it has been suggested is that although AD is the most common cause of dementia, VaD is relatively more common than in industrialized countries.[27]

CAUSES AND PATHOPHYSIOLOGY

Because the essential feature of VCD is that cognitive deficits are attributable to CVD, and the latter is extremely varied, the clinical manifestations and causes of VCD are very heterogeneous. One approach to the pathophysiology of VCD has been to examine the contributions made by large vessel disease, small vessel disease, noninfarct ischemic changes, and small and large hemorrhages. The parenchymal lesions associated with these factors are summarized in Table 53-1.

Large Vessel Disease

VCD has traditionally been associated with large vessel disease leading to one or more strokes, generally referred to as MID or PSD, although the cognitive impairment is not always above the threshold for dementia (see later). The pathologic lesion is atherosclerosis of large extracranial or intracranial vessels, which causes ischemia through a reduction of blood flow (hemodynamic cause) or artery to artery embolism. The most commonly affected extracranial site is the bifurcation of the common carotid artery, with the aortic arch and proximal subclavian and vertebral arteries also being commonly affected.[31] Severe carotid stenosis is common; intracranial atherosclerosis as a cause of stroke is less common in whites but more common in Asian and African American populations.[32] Large artery atherosclerosis, however, accounts for only 30% of strokes; cardioembolic events (25% to 30% of strokes) and small vessel disease (25%) are also commonly responsible.

PSD is defined as cognitive impairment from any cause following stroke that is significant enough to affect daily function; it may be vascular, neurodegenerative, or mixed. The prevalence of PSD varies, depending on diagnostic criteria used, age of the study population, and delay between stroke and cognitive evaluation.[33] In the Framingham Study, the rate of dementia in people with a history of stroke was approximately double that of the nonstroke population but, if cognitive impairment without dementia is included, the rates are much higher.[18,20,34]

Risk factors for MID and PSD may be patient-related or stroke-related. Vascular risk factors such as hypertension, diabetes, hyperlipidemia, and smoking have shown an inconsistent association,[18,34] whereas age, low education, and preexisting cognitive impairment or dependency have shown a more consistent association.[18,33,34] The relationship between preexisting cognitive impairment and risk of PSD has been seen as robust, likely reflecting some combination of the effects of stroke, effects of chronic ischemia, and presence of preexisting neurodegenerative impairment. A report from the Rotterdam Study has brought this into question, however.[35] It may be that the number of vascular risk factors is more important than any one individual factor in predicting PSD.[18] Neuroimaging features such as global cerebral atrophy and mediotemporal lobe atrophy are associated with a higher risk of PSD.[36] Although mediotemporal atrophy has been proposed as a marker of preexisting neurodegenerative disease in these cases, it is also present in VaD and in patients without preexisting clinical evidence of dementia.[37]

It was previously believed that a certain threshold of tissue loss, put at 50 mL of cerebral tissue by the Newcastle group,[2] was necessary for dementia to manifest. This is no longer considered to be the case, and much smaller lesions can produce cognitive disorders, including dementia.[18] Stroke characteristics are nevertheless important. Dementia is usually associated with supratentorial lesions, left hemispheric lesions, or anterior and posterior cerebral artery lesions, and multiple infarcts are commonly implicated, although these may not always be large artery infarcts.[33] Most often, cognitive impairment in association with vascular disease results from the cumulative effects of several cortical infarcts of varying size and number—the basis of cortical MID as described by Hachinski and colleagues in 1974.[3] The infarcts of MID occur predominantly in the cortical and subcortical arterial territories and distal fields. Single strategic infarcts in the cortex (hippocampus, angular gyrus) or subcortex (thalamus, caudate, globus pallidus, basal forebrain, fornix, genu of the internal capsule) can result in characteristic PSD cognitive syndromes. For example, angular gyrus infarction is associated with an acute onset of fluent dysphasia, visuospatial disorientation, agraphia, and memory loss that can be mistaken for AD.[38] However, many reports of dementia following single strategic infarcts do not necessarily exclude small vessel disease or associated AD pathology.

Large vessel disease seldom occurs in isolation because neuroimaging evidence of small vessel disease is ubiquitous in older adults with varying degrees of clinical significance, and some degree of Alzheimer-type, Lewy body disease, and other neurodegenerative pathology may be coexisting. The presence of white matter lesions (leukoaraiosis), lacunes, microbleeds, hippocampal sclerosis, and cerebral atrophy should all be taken into consideration.

TABLE 53-1 Parenchymal Lesions of Vascular Cause Associated With Vascular Cognitive Disorders

Disease	
Large vessel disease	Multiple infarcts
	Single strategically placed infarct
Small vessel disease	Multiple lacunar infarcts in white matter and deep gray matter nuclei
	Ischemic white matter change
	Dilation of perivascular spaces
	Cortical microinfarcts
	Cortical and subcortical microbleeds
Hemorrhage	Intracerebral hemorrhage
	Multiple cortical and subcortical microbleeds
	Subarachnoid hemorrhage
Hypoperfusion	Hippocampal sclerosis
	Laminar cortical sclerosis

Small Vessel Disease

Small vessel disease (SVD) includes leukoaraiosis, subcortical infarcts, incomplete infarction and microbleeds. It is much more common than large vessel disease and may be the most common cause of VCD.[39,40]

White Matter Lesions

Leukoaraiosis (literally, thinning of the white matter)—white matter lesions (WMLs)—describes diffuse, confluent, white matter abnormalities, which are low density on computed tomography (CT) and hyperintense on T2-weighted magnetic resonance imaging (MRI) and fluid-attenuated inversion recovery (FLAIR). The latter are usually referred to as white matter hyperintensities (WMHs). Increasing sensitivity of MRI has resulted in less specificity and predictive validity of leukoaraiosis, which can now be detected in more than 90% of older adults[41,42] and nearly 50% of individuals in their late 40s.[43] Just as the term *leukoaraiosis* does not presuppose pathology, white matter changes are not specific to infarcts but may also occur with leukodystrophies, metastases, and other inflammatory conditions.[44] Leukoaraiosis may be present at varying degrees, from small punctate hyperintensities to large confluent lesions. The major neuropathologic features found in leukoaraiosis in association with VCI include axonal loss, enlargement of perivascular spaces, gliosis, and myelin pallor.[44] They are caused by arteriosclerosis, lipohyalinosis, and fibrinoid necrosis of small vessels, in particular the long perforating arteries, with or without occlusion.[23] Importantly, WMLs are more extensive in the periventricular regions and extend to the deep white matter but spare areas protected from hypoperfusion, such as the subcortical U-fibers and external capsule, claustrum, and extreme capsule.[45] Whether periventricular and deep white matter lesions are distinct in their cause, presentation, or rate of progression is not well understood.[46]

The association between leukoaraiosis and cognitive and functional decline appears robust,[47,48] but the cognitive domains affected have not been clearly established. The Sydney Stroke Study showed a particular association with information processing speed and frontal executive functioning.[48,49] The Framingham Study showed an association between the presence of leukoaraiosis and executive function, new learning, and visual organization.[50] In general, confluent lesions appear to have a more reliable relationship with cognitive impairment.[18] WMLs progress over time, with the Sydney Stroke Study showing a rate of progression of 13%/year in nonstroke older adults. The baseline WML load was the best predictor of the rate of progression.[51] Decline in cognition is, however, not consistently related to this increase, and appears to be better explained by measures of atrophy.[18] Visual and volumetric quantitative measurement scales for leukoaraiosis have been developed but are limited in their utility as outcome measures by ceiling effects.[52]

With the development of newer MRI techniques, such as diffusion tensor imaging (DTI), it has been demonstrated that white matter that appears normal on T2-weighted images may also have abnormal anisotropy or diffusivity, which relates to neuropathology,[53] and may have relevance for cognitive function.[54] Abnormalities on DTI are, however, not delineated well enough at present to be incorporated into diagnostic criteria or be used clinically.

Lacunes

VCD may also be associated with lacunar infarction, although there is a lack of consensus on the specific number and location of the lacunes required for a VCD diagnosis. It is well recognized that one or two lacunes are not uncommon in older adults with no cognitive impairment and may be incidental findings.[55] More than two lacunes outside the brain stem would generally be regarded as necessary to support a diagnosis of VCD.[56] Single lacunes placed strategically in the striatum or the thalamus, usually above a certain size of threshold,[57] may produce a VCD, but a temporal relationship between lacunar infarction and the cognitive syndrome must be present to be able to attribute VCD to a single lacune. Single lacunes may also be sufficient when associated with extensive periventricular and deep white matter lesions.[58] The Newcastle neuropathologic criteria for VaD [59] have suggested more than three lacunar infarcts as being sufficient evidence, but this must be considered along with other vascular pathologies, in particular WMLs that are generally present concurrently. Lacunes are best detected on T1- or T2-weighted MRI scans using a FLAIR sequence on a 1.0-T scanner or greater. A lacune has usually been regarded as a lesion between 3 and 15 mm in size, a definition favored by the STRIVE criteria,[60] but definitions vary, with a maximum diameter from 1 to 2 cm.[61,62]

Microinfarcts

Microscopic infarcts, less than 1 mm in size, are common in the brains of older adults, but are not visible on gross neuropathologic examination or MRI on a 3-T scanner. There is good evidence for their pathophysiologic importance in autopsy studies.[59] With new developments in high-field MRI, it may be possible to image microinfarcts in patients in the future.[63]

Dilated Perivascular Spaces

Infarctions should be distinguished from dilated perivascular spaces (PVSs); the neuroimaging characteristics are described in the STRIVE criteria.[60] Although dilated perivascular or Virchow-Robin spaces may represent an early stage of CVD with underlying microvascular degeneration,[59] they have not commonly been considered a feature supporting VCD,[64] thereby needing further study.

Microbleeds

Cerebral microbleeds (CMBs) may be a manifestation of SVD and are seen as susceptibility artifacts on certain MRI sequences, such as T2* gradient-recalled echo and susceptibility weighted imaging. They are common in community-dwelling older adults, from 7% in younger adults (45 to 55 years) to 36% in those older than 80 years.[65] Their prevalence is elevated in AD, in which they have been associated with cerebral amyloid angiopathy, and is markedly increased in individuals with multiple lacunar strokes or vascular dementia, in which they are associated with hypertensive arteriopathy.[66] Microbleeds associated with hypertension are seen in the deep nuclei and brain stem, and those with AD are generally lobar in location. CMBs have been associated with cognitive dysfunction in a number of domains, although the relationship between location and the type of cognitive deficits is inconsistent.[66-68] Because microbleeds are not uncommon in cognitively normal older adults, attribution of the VCD to these, especially VaD, should follow a careful exclusion of other causes of cognitive impairment and only if many of these lesions are present. More data are needed in relation to the standard measurement of CMBs, and their diagnostic and prognostic significance before CMBs are routinely applied in clinical assessments.[67]

Hemorrhages

Cognitive disorders have been associated with subdural hemorrhage (SH) and subarachnoid hemorrhage (SAH), the presence of which on an MRI scan should alert the diagnostician to their possible significance. Cognitive deficits have been reported in 19% to 62% of patients following SAH,[69] and their severity is related to the severity of SAH,[70] although other factors such as older age, the presence of arterial vasospasm and delayed cerebral infarction, increased intracranial pressure, intraparenchymal and intraventricular hemorrhages, hydrocephalus, and location of the aneurysm are all important.[69] Subdural hemorrhage is an uncommon cause of cognitive disorder, with reports that about 50% of older adults with chronic SH have cognitive deficits,[69] which may be progressive and not always reversible with surgical drainage.[71] Because SH is usually a result of trauma and not vascular pathology, it should be not be regarded as a VCD. SAH is due to vascular pathology, and its associated cognitive deficits are appropriately regarded as VCD. Multiple hemorrhages or hemorrhagic infarcts are often associated with VCD, with common causes being sporadic or hereditary conditions associated with cerebral amyloid angiopathy (CAA)[72] and other genetic disorders,[73] although hypertension may have a role. VCD has also been associated with cortical and subcortical microbleeds, which may be related to hypertension or CAA, as described earlier.[67]

Brain Atrophy

Gray matter atrophy may show a stronger association with cognitive impairment than strategic infarcts and subcortical vascular disease.[74] Cortical atrophy predicts cognitive decline independently of vascular burden on neuroimaging.[75] In particular, mediotemporal atrophy (MTA) shows an association with cognitive dysfunction, especially memory.[76] MTA was initially thought to indicate underlying neurodegenerative pathology because of the predilection of pathology in the mediotemporal lobes of those with AD. However, MTA may also result from vascular pathology,[77] and reduced hippocampal volumes have been reported in VaD in the absence of AD pathology at autopsy.[78] Thalamic volume has also shown an association with the degree of cognitive impairment.[76]

Hippocampal Sclerosis

Cognitive impairment and dementia are sometimes associated with hippocampal sclerosis (HS) in older adults. This usually presents as slowly progressive memory impairment, resembling AD, and the diagnosis is confirmed on pathology. HS is characterized by severe neuronal loss with reactive gliosis in the CA1 sector of the hippocampus. With MRI, the findings are of hippocampal atrophy, often asymmetric, without necessarily the hyperintense signal on T2-weighted imaging seen in younger people with HS. The pathogenesis is multifactorial, with ischemic injury often playing a major role.[79]

Cerebral Amyloid Angiopathy

Cerebral amyloid angiopathy is a heterogeneous group of sporadic and, more rarely, hereditary diseases in which amyloid proteins aggregate in the vessel walls of leptomeningeal and cortical arteries, arterioles, capillaries and, less commonly, veins.[80] CAA is associated with a spectrum of clinical presentations, including transient ischemic attacks (TIAs), stroke, seizures, migraine, and cognitive impairment and behavioral symptoms. Clinical presentations include lobar hemorrhage, subarachnoid hemorrhage, cortical infarction, and cognitive profiles similar to those of subcortical ischemic vascular disease. CAA is a prevalent finding in dementia with vascular and neurodegenerative pathology, but has also been found in clinically asymptomatic patients in autopsy studies.[5,23] T2-weighted MRI often reveals evidence of prior cerebral microhemorrhage, but its significance in a given patient with cognitive impairment is unclear and needs to be correlated with other clinical and imaging characteristics.[80] Positron emission tomography (PET) scans using Pittsburgh compound B or other tracers allows labeling of vascular and parenchymal amyloid.

Genetic Causes

VCDs have been associated with a number of mendelian disorders. Cerebral autosomal dominant arteriopathy with subcortical infarcts and leukoencephalopathy (CADASIL) is a hereditary microangiopathy associated with mutation in the Notch3 gene on chromosome 19.[81] The clinical presentation consists of migraine with aura, mood disturbance, recurrent subcortical strokes, and progressive cognitive decline.[82] Although a comparatively rare cause of VCD, it deserves special mention for two reasons. First, it is generally considered to be a model of pure VCD because generally the onset occurs between the ages of 40 and 50 years, when comorbid AD pathology is rare. Second, the use of cholinesterase inhibitors in those with CADASIL has shown statistically significant improvement in some measures of executive function. This provides a basis for cholinergic therapy for VCD. Cholinergic mechanisms appear to play a critical role in cerebral perfusion.[83] The best diagnostic criteria for CADASIL are the modified NINDS-AIREN (National Institute of Neurological Disorders and Stroke Association Internationale Pour la Recherche et l'Enseignement en Neurosciences) criteria for subcortical ischemic VaD.[84]

Other genetic cerebrovascular disorders include cerebral autosomal recessive arteriopathy with subcortical autosomal recessive leukoencephalopathy (CARASIL), hereditary endotheliopathy with retinopathy, nephropathy, and stroke (HERNS), pontine autosomal dominant microangiopathy and leukoencephalopathy (PADMAL), retinal vasculopathy with cerebral leukodystrophy (RVCL), and collagen type IV, alpha1 (COL4A1)–related disorders.[81]

Although harboring the ε4 genotype of the apolipoprotein E (Apo E) gene increases the risk of AD, its role in VCD is less clear, although data have been presented for its association with WMLs and VCD.[85] Because WMLs show moderate to high heritability, the search for other genes is currently being undertaken.[85]

Other Factors

The occurrence of dementia in an individual with CVD is also influenced by other factors. Age and education have consistently emerged as two such factors.[40] The effect of age, however, may be seen as representing an accumulation of deficits over time and the body's response in terms of reparative processes. In this context, the cumulative deficit model of frailty has been applied to dementia,[86] with vascular disease being one such deficit as part of a larger whole, albeit a very important one in the case of VCD. This research[87] has suggested that multiple deficits involving diverse organs and functions such as vision, hearing, arthritis, bowel and bladder function, dentition, and skin, which add up to a frailty index, predict dementia, just as they predict mortality, delirium, and disability.[88] This suggests that the presence of dementia, whether it is related to vascular or other diseases, is attributable to cumulative deficits, greater biologic age of the organism, and possibly aberrant repair processes.[86]

SUBTYPES OF VASCULAR COGNITIVE DISORDERS

Subcategories of VCD have been described, but they have been used inconsistently because overlap between the subcategories is common. Most patients with VCD have a combination of cortical and subcortical lesions, referred to as corticosubcortical VCD. This term subsumes cortical VCD, because it is rare for vascular lesions to be exclusively cortical. It also partially subsumes the older term *multi-infarct dementia*, which is characterized by multiple cortical and subcortical infarcts, although multiple infarcts can also be exclusively subcortical and lead to VCD. VCD may also be subcategorized according to cause as being largely ischemic or hemorrhagic. Another subcategory is poststroke VCD, although this has a complex cause with a varying combination of large and small vessel disease, as well as nonvascular pathology such as AD contributing to the picture.

It is now well recognized that VCD may be exclusively due to subcortical vascular lesions, and various attempts have been made to characterize subcortical VCD.[40,58,59] The pathologic basis of this is SVD leading to multiple lacunes, WMLs, and noninfarct white matter changes. VCD may therefore be related predominantly to WMLs of vascular origin, which has sometimes been referred to as Binswanger disease. However, the historical usage of this term has made it controversial.[40] Pure subcortical VCD with a slowly progressive course that simulates AD but does not have the characteristic brain amyloid burden of AD has recently been documented.[89] A special case of subcortical VCD is thalamic dementia due to infarctions located in the thalamus, with relatively little involvement of other brain structures.[90]

The clinical hallmark of subcortical VD or subcortical ischemic vascular disease (SIVD) is a profile of a dysexecutive syndrome, with no (or minimal) memory impairment, commonly accompanied by psychomotor slowing and seen in the presence of subcortical, including white matter, injury. It is clear that lesions in the prefrontal subcortical circuit (including the prefrontal cortex, caudate, pallidum, and thalamus) or thalamocortical circuit may manifest as the subcortical syndrome. More commonly, however, the profile is accompanied by memory impairment that is more than minimal.[91] In any case, these lesions are also associated with increased risk of stroke and dementia. Although it has been proposed that this profile is associated with more rapid cognitive decline, even when controlling for other vascular risk factors, this view has been disputed.[92]

OVERLAPPING AND INTERACTIVE EFFECTS OF VASCULAR AND NEURODEGENERATIVE DISEASES

Both CVD and AD pathologies are common in the brains of older adults, and mixed pathologies account for most dementia cases in community-dwelling older people,[5] exceeding pure AD and pure VCD. This could simply be the concurrence of two common pathologies, with an additive effect on cognitive function, as was shown in the Nun Study, where the clinical expression of AD pathology was greatly enhanced by the presence of infarcts.[6] However, there has been increasing evidence that vascular disease promotes AD and vice versa, suggesting interactive and reciprocal amplifying effects of the two pathologies.[93]

Vascular factors have been implicated in the pathogenesis of AD based on evidence from many sources. Risk factors for CVD, such as hypertension, diabetes, insulin resistance, obesity, hyperlipidemia, hypercholesterolemia, and smoking, have been reported to increase the risk of AD independently of stroke,[94,95] even though the correlation of these factors is greater with VCD and less so with AD.[96] Cerebrovascular function is reduced in the early stages of AD and in those with mild cognitive impairment at risk of developing dementia due to AD.[93] There has been accumulating evidence that hypoperfusion and hypoxia promote β-amyloid (Aβ) production and thereby amyloid plaque formation.[97] The vascular pathway is also important for the clearance of Aβ from the brain, because it is transported along the perivascular pathway through a transvascular transport system.[98] Recent evidence has also shown the acceleration of tau pathology in transgenic Alzheimer mice with vascular lesions.[99]

All these findings suggest that vascular factors have an important role in the pathogenesis of AD. On the other hand, AD pathology is known to lead to cerebrovascular lesions. CAA is present in 82% to 98% of AD patients.[80] Apo E 4, a major genetic risk factor for AD, is known to disrupt the blood-brain barrier (BBB) through its proinflammatory activation.[93] According to the amyloid hypothesis of AD, Aβ oligomers are toxic to brain cells. It is possible that these oligomers are independently toxic to the pericytes and/or endothelial cells, thereby compromising the neurovascular unit and the BBB.

In understanding the effect of vascular pathology on neuronal dysfunction, it is important to place an emphasis on the neurovascular unit, which is comprised of vascular cells, including endothelium and mural cells (e.g., brain capillary pericytes, arterial and/or venous vascular smooth muscle cells), glial cells (e.g., astrocytes, microglia, oligodendroglia), and neurons.[93] Recent studies have shown that pericytes regulate BBB permeability and play a major role in maintaining the cerebrovascular integrity at the level of brain capillaries, which in turn prevents various potentially neurotoxic and vasculotoxic macromolecules in the blood, such as Aβ, from entering the central nervous system (CNS). The BBB is compromised in hypoxic injury as well as in AD. The neurovascular unit also regulates the afferent and efferent arms of the immune system in the brain, with immune cells being involved in vascular homeostasis.

A number of factors therefore come into play in linking cerebral blood vessels with grey and white matter damage in an interactive process. Risk factors predispose the brain to oxidative stress, leading to endothelial dysfunction, which reduces resting blood flow in marginally perfused cerebral regions, disrupts the BBB, and causes myelin damage. Tissue edema due to BBB dysfunction exacerbates the tissue hypoxia and activates inflammation, leading to the production of cytokines and adhesion molecules in vascular cells, reactive astrocytosis, and activated microglia.[93] Hypoxia, inflammation, and oxidative stress combine to damage the oligodendroglia, which starts a vicious cycle of tissue damage. Apo E and Aβ interact in this process, thereby completing the link between AD and CVD pathologies. The joint role of the two pathologies in producing cognitive dysfunction is summarized in Figure 53-1.

CLINICAL FEATURES

VCD is a clinical diagnosis. A detailed account is sought from the patient and family or caregiver about the onset and progression of cognitive domains affected (e.g., memory, speed of thinking or acting, mood, function), vascular risk factors (e.g., hypertension, hyperlipidemia, diabetes mellitus, alcohol or tobacco use, physical activity), and evidence of CVD in the form of gait disturbance, urinary incontinence,[11,13,61] a history of atrial fibrillation, coronary artery bypass surgery or angioplasty stenting, angina, congestive heart failure, peripheral vascular disease, TIAs or strokes, and endarterectomy. Other elements of the medical history, such as hypercoagulable states, migraine, and depression, may also be helpful.[61] The physical examination should include blood pressure, pulse, body mass index (BMI), waist circumference, and examination of the cardiovascular system for evidence of arrhythmias or peripheral vascular disease, neurologic examination for focal neurologic signs, and assessment of gait initiation and speed.[11]

Subjective Report

A clinical concern for a cognitive disorder may stem from the patient or knowledgeable other person (informant; e.g., family, caregiver), physician, or other professional that there has been a decline in cognitive functioning. The individual has to rely on others to plan or make decisions, has had to abandon complex projects, repeats self in conversation, needs frequent reminders to orient to the task at hand, has significant difficulties with expressive or receptive language, has difficulty in navigating in familiar environments, or has a clear disturbance in body schema, calculation ability, reading or writing. In mild cases, the disturbance is more subtle, and the individual, although still independent, may perform tasks with greater effort than before and resort to compensatory strategies.

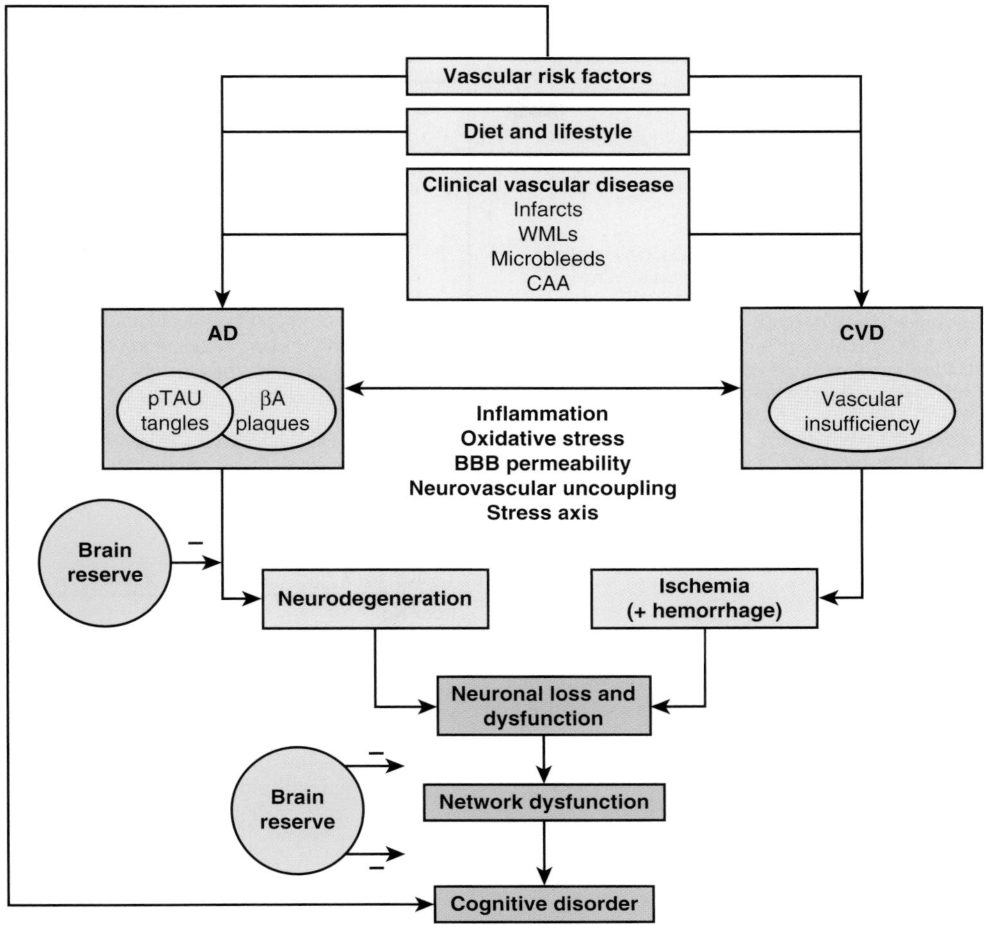

Figure 53-1. Proposed model for the vascular origins of dementia and interaction with Alzheimer pathology. AD, Alzheimer disease; βA, β-amyloid protein; BBB, blood-brain barrier; CAA, cerebral amyloid angiopathy; CVD, cerebrovascular disease; pTau, phosphorylated tau protein; WMLs, white matter lesions.

The classic description of MID was that of an acute stepwise or fluctuating decline in cognition, with intervening periods of stability and even some improvement.[3,10] This pattern is temporally related to cerebrovascular events of infarction, hemorrhage, or vasculitis, and the temporal relationship is not difficult to establish clinically. The cognitive impairment is at its peak soon after a stroke and may show significant improvement over the next 3 months; persistence beyond this period is generally considered necessary for the cognitive disorder to be diagnosed.[100] Further improvement may occur beyond the 3 months, but its rate is much slower.[101] Many individuals with VCD do not, however, present with this picture and show a gradual onset with slow progress, rapid development of deficits followed by relative stability, or some other complex presentation.[11] VCD with a gradual onset and slow progression is generally due to small vessel disease leading to lesions in the white matter, basal ganglia, and/or thalamus. The gradual progression in these cases is often punctuated by acute events, which leave subtle neurologic deficits such as focal weakness, unilateral incoordination, asymmetric reflexes, unsteadiness, small step gait, or parkinsonian signs.[40]

Cognitive Assessment

The pattern of cognitive deficits in VCI is as broad as the construct itself.[9] Single strategic infarcts can have characteristic cognitive profiles, whereas subcortical lesions (and, less commonly, cortical lesions) are often associated with a cluster of features termed the *subcortical syndrome*, which includes abnormalities of information-processing speed, executive function, and emotional lability that are not recognized by standard cognitive assessments, such as the Mini-Mental State Examination (MMSE).[102] Screening with subsets of tests such as the five-word immediate and delayed recall, six-item orientation task, and phonemic fluency tests from the Montreal Cognitive Assessment (MoCA)[102] is currently recommended,[61] with administration of the entire MoCA, Trail Making Test, or semantic fluency test if time allows. Cognitive test batteries recommended for 5- and 30-minute assessments, according to the harmonization criteria,[61] are listed in Table 53-2.

Subcortical lesions are often associated with impairments of executive function, which is broadly defined as the ability to sequence, plan, organize, initiate, and shift between tasks. Although executive dysfunction has proven useful and sensitive for the evaluation and even prediction of disease progression, this is not specific to VCI. Even though clinicians who evaluate patients for VCD and executive dysfunction more generally are justly skeptical about relying on the MMSE as a global screening measure of cognition, tests of executive function are not adequate, in isolation, for assessing VCD.

Memory impairment, especially the ability to learn new information and retain it over time, is an early disturbance in AD, but is relatively spared in VCD, especially in the early stages.[9,18,91]

TABLE 53-2 Neuropsychological Protocols for Assessment of Vascular Cognitive Disorders*

Protocol	Tests
30-Min test protocol	Semantic fluency (animal naming) Phonemic fluency (controlled oral word association test) Digit symbol coding from the Wechsler Adult Intelligence Scale, third edition Hopkins verbal learning test Center for Epidemiologic Studies—Depression Scale Neuropsychiatric Inventory, Questionnaire Version (NPI-Q) Supplemental—Mini-Mental State Examination (MMSE), Trail Making Test†
5-Min protocol	Montreal Cognitive Assessment (MoCA) subtests • Five-word memory task (registration, recall, recognition) • Six-item orientation • One-letter phonemic fluency

*Recommended for harmonization of the assessment.[61]
†Supplemental—the rest of the MoCA, semantic fluency (animal naming) test, Trail Making Test, and MMSE to be administered at least 1 hour before or after the above tests.

This is inconsistent with many criteria sets for the diagnosis of VaD, which require memory impairment as a necessary feature, something that has been remedied in the recent *Diagnostic and Statistical Manual of Mental Disorders*, fifth edition (DSM-V),[103] criteria and the newly proposed VASCOG (International Society of Vascular Behavioral and Cognitive Disorders) criteria.[13]

Establishing a Predominantly Vascular Cause for the Cognitive Disorder

Because some degree of vascular pathology is very common in the brains of older adults, how much pathology, as observed on neuroimaging or neuropathology, is sufficient to account for the observed cognitive deficits? There is no simple answer to this vexing question. Expert clinical judgment is frequently necessary for such a determination and, when vascular and Alzheimer pathologies are combined, this may become a moot point. The determination relies on the history, physical examination, and neuroimaging. Neuroimaging is critical for increased certainty in the diagnosis, and its lack can result in significant diagnostic inaccuracy by overlooking silent brain infarction and WMLs. Neuroimaging is also important to rule out some less common causes, such as brain tumor or normal pressure hydrocephalus (NPH), and it may be important to distinguish vascular dementia from AD or frontotemporal degeneration as the cause of the cognitive impairment.

CT or MRI may be used, with the latter being more sensitive. Attempts have been made to define the minimal radiologic evidence necessary. The California criteria[100] require two or more ischemic strokes, with at least one infarct outside the cerebellum for a diagnosis of VaD. The NINDS-AIREN criteria[104] require multiple large vessel strokes or a single strategically placed infarct (angular gyrus, thalamus, basal forebrain or posterior carotid artery, or anterior carotid artery territories), multiple basal ganglia and white matter lacunes, or extensive periventricular WMLs. The SIVD criteria[58] require extensive confluent WMLs, along with lacunar infarcts. It must also be pointed out that the terminology used to describe neuroimaging abnormalities also varies, and there was a recent attempt to standardize the reporting of neuroimaging abnormalities in relation to small vessel disease.[60] The neuroimaging criteria proposed in the VASCOG criteria for VCD[13] are listed in Box 53-1.

BOX 53-1 Presence of Significant Neuroimaging (MRI or CT) Evidence of Cerebrovascular Disease

One of the following VASCOG criteria[13]:

1. One large vessel infarct sufficient for mild VCD; two or more large vessel infarcts generally necessary for VaD
2. An extensive or strategically placed single infarct, typically in the thalamus or basal ganglia, may be sufficient for VaD
3. Multiple lacunar infarcts, more than two, outside the brain stem; one or two lacunes may be sufficient if strategically placed or in combination with extensive white matter lesions
4. Extensive and confluent white matter lesions
5. Strategically placed intracerebral hemorrhage, or two or more intracerebral hemorrhages
6. Combination of the above

CT, Computed tomography; *MRI,* magnetic resonance imaging; *VaD,* vascular dementia; *VCD,* vascular cognitive disorder.

TABLE 53-3 Hachinski Ischemic Score

Item No.	Description	Value
1*	Abrupt onset	2
2*	Stepwise deterioration	1
3*	Fluctuating course	2
4	Nocturnal confusion	1
5	Preservation of personality	1
6	Depression	1
7	Somatic complaints	1
8*	Emotional incontinence	1
9	History of hypertension	1
10*	History of stroke	2
11	Associated atherosclerosis	1
12*	Focal neurologic symptoms	2
13*	Focal neurologic signs	2

The entries with an asterisk (*) are included in the modified score. The recommended cut-off scores in dementia patients are 4 for Alzheimer disease and 7 for multi-infarct dementia.
Adapted from Hachinski VC, Iliff LD, Zilhka E, et al: Cerebral blood flow in dementia. Arch Neurol 32:632–637, 1975; and Hachinski V, Oveisgharan S, Romney AK, Shankle WR: Optimizing the Hachinski Ischemic Scale. Arch Neurol 69:169–175, 2012.

DIAGNOSTIC CRITERIA

An earlier approach to the diagnosis of VaD, in particular its differentiation from Alzheimer dementia, was the use of the Hachinski Ischemic Score (HIS),[105] designed primarily for MID, with 13 items and a recommended cut-off score of 4 for AD and 7 for VaD and a sensitivity of 89% and specificity of 89%[106] (Table 53-3). Recently, a shortened version of the HIS was published, with five composite question items or seven single-question items, which performed as well or better than the original HIS instrument.[107]

Diagnostic criteria have been published for VaD, and it is only recently that the term *vascular neurocognitive disorder* was adopted by DSM-V[103] and *vascular cognitive disorder* by the VASCOG group.[13] Commonly used diagnostic criteria for VaD in the past included the NINDS-AIREN criteria,[104] Alzheimer's Disease Diagnostic and Treatment Centers (ADDTC) criteria,[100] DSM-IV criteria,[7] and International Classification of Diseases tenth edition (ICD-10) criteria[8] (Table 53-4). These diagnostic criteria show little association with each other, making comparisons difficult,[36,108] and do not include mild VCD, which may account for up to half of those with VCD.[109] Furthermore, the

TABLE 53-4 Comparison of Diagnostic Criteria for Vascular Cognitive Disorders

Diagnostic Criteria	Requirements for Diagnosis	Comments
DSM-IV—vascular dementia[7]	Course characterized by stepwise decline in cognition and function Focal neurologic signs and symptoms or laboratory evidence of focal neurologic damage are judged to be related to the clinical presentation	Requires memory impairment as one of the cognitive domains affected Definitions lack detail; influenced by concept of multi-infarct dementia No neuroimaging features Does not include mild disorder
ADDTC criteria for ischemic vascular dementia[100]	At least one infarct outside the cerebellum Evidence of two or more strokes by history, neurologic signs, or neuroimaging Or, in the case of a single stroke, a clear demonstration of a temporal relationship between the stroke and cognitive presentation	Temporal relationship not defined Requirement for neuroimaging evidence of stroke is too confined—small vessel disease, including leukoaraiosis, not included
ICD-10[8]	Patchy distribution of cognitive deficits and focal neurologic signs Cerebrovascular disease must be judged to be causally related to the dementia	Definitions lack detail Does not include mild disorder
NINDS-AIREN[104]	Cognitive decline in memory *and* two other cognitive domains severe enough to interfere with activities of daily living *and* clinical and radiographic evidence of cerebrovascular disease *and* a relationship between neuroimaging and clinical presentation (onset of dementia within 3 months following stroke or abrupt onset of cognitive impairment or fluctuating stepwise progression of cognitive decline)	Requirement for cognitive domains affected less permissive compared with ADDTC criteria Requirement for neuroimaging evidence of CVD—more strict Does not include mild disorder Temporal relationship with cerebrovascular event—strict
DSM-5 criteria[103]	Mild and major neurocognitive disorders based on subjective report, objective testing, and level of interference with independent functioning Criteria for vascular cause, including exclusion criteria Memory impairment not obligatory for diagnosis	New terminology, yet to be fully accepted
VASCOG criteria[13]	Vascular mild cognitive disorder and vascular dementia based on subjective report, objective testing, and level of interference with independent functioning. Criteria for vascular cause, including exclusion criteria Memory impairment not obligatory for diagnosis	Introduced the concept of vascular mild cognitive disorders Reliability and validity of the criteria yet to be fully examined

ADDTC, Alzheimer's Disease Diagnostic and Treatment Centers; DSM-V, *Diagnostic and statistical manual of mental disorders*, ed 5; ICD-10, International Classification of Diseases, 10th version; NINDS-AIREN, National Institute of Neurological Disorders and Stroke Association Internationale Pour la Recherche et l'Enseignement en Neurosciences.

time lines for temporal association have not been reflected by empirical data. In a Mayo Clinic population-based neuropathologic study, in which 13% of those studied had pure VaD without major evidence of AD, it was required that dementia following a known stroke resulted in high specificity but low sensitivity of autopsy-verified cases.[110]

More recently, a number of efforts have been made to present a new set of criteria that take recent developments in the field into consideration. The process started with the development of harmonization standards as consensus recommendations from the NINDS and Canadian Stroke Network (CSN) that aimed to establish screening protocols and data sets for clinical practice and research,[61] followed by the publication of DSM-IV criteria[103] and, more recently, the VASCOG criteria.[13] The last two recognize that VCD is multifactorial, its presentation is different from that of AD, cognitive and functional impairment lie on a continuum from normal to mild disorder to a dementia (or major neurocognitive disorder in DSM-V), and neuroimaging increases the certainty of diagnosis. The VASCOG criteria are summarized in Box 53-2.

BOX 53-2 Types of Vascular Lesions Associated With Vascular Cognitive Disorders

1. Atherosclerosis
2. Cardiac, atherosclerotic and systemic emboli
3. Arteriolosclerosis
4. Lipohyalinosis
5. Amyloid angiopathy
6. Vasculitis—infectious and noninfectious
7. Venous collagenosis
8. Arteriovenous fistulae—dural or parenchymal
9. Hereditary angiopathies—cerebral autosomal dominant arteriopathy with subcortical infarcts and leukoencephalopathy, CADASIL[81]; cerebral autosomal recessive arteriopathy with, for example, subcortical autosomal recessive leukoencephalopathy, CARASIL
10. Giant cell arteritis
11. Berry aneurysms
12. Miscellaneous vasculopathies—fibromuscular dysplasia, moya-moya
13. Systemic microangiopathies without vascular inflammatory cell infiltrates
14. Cerebral venous thrombosis

CARASIL, Cerebral autosomal recessive arteriopathy with subcortical autosomal recessive leukoencephalopathy.

NEUROPSYCHIATRIC SYMPTOMS

Given the injury to prefrontal brain regions, neuropsychiatric symptoms are common in those with VCD.[111] Depression, psychosis, agitation, and apathy are of particular interest. Depression is the most extensively studied affective syndrome in VCD. Poststroke depression is common and, in clinical settings, figures of 21.6% for major and 21% for minor depression have been cited.[112] In addition, criteria for a so-called vascular depression have been proposed, but have yet to be fully accepted.[113] The relationship of bipolar disorder with SVD remains uncertain. Psychotic symptoms are common in VaD, with one review[114] reporting that 37% of patients experienced psychotic symptoms, of which 19% to 50% experienced delusions, 14% to 60% visual hallucinations, and 19% to 30% delusional misidentification. Apathy is common in VCD, with the point prevalence in VaD calculated to be 33.8% and the prevalence in stroke patients ranging from 22.5% to 56.7%.[115] Apathy is common in CADASIL, with one study reporting a prevalence of 41%.[116]

NEUROPATHOLOGY

A definitive diagnosis of VCD warrants neuropathologic verification.[23] This will confirm the clinical or radiologic evidence of vascular brain injury or detect such an injury not detected by brain imaging (e.g. small lacunes, microinfarcts, selective neuronal loss). It identifies the type of underlying cerebrovascular lesions, such as arteriolosclerosis or cerebral amyloid angiopathy. Box 53-3 lists the vascular lesions associated with VCD. Neuropathologic examination also ascertains the presence of other brain pathology relevant to cognitive dysfunction. For example, if the pathologic examination reveals plaques and neurofibrillary tangles of sufficient severity to suggest AD as the major cause of cognitive impairment, a diagnosis of VCD cannot be sustained, although a dual cause can still be determined. The same is true for other pathologic findings. The heterogeneity of vascular pathology has made it difficult to establish validated criteria for VCD. Some attempts have been made to characterize and quantify vascular brain pathology[23,59,117] and harmonize criteria,[61] but have thus far not achieved general consensus. Neuropathology on autopsy does not elucidate the relationship between vascular lesions and clinical presentation and cannot therefore be used as a test of 100% sensitivity and specificity.[118]

Biomarkers

The heterogeneity of VCD has made the development of reliable nonimaging biomarkers extremely challenging. Some suggested cerebrospinal fluid (CSF) biomarkers of CVD are the albumin index as a marker of damage to the BBB, sulfatide for demyelination, neurofilament for axonal degeneration, and matrix metalloproteinases for vascular disease.[61] Because none of these is specific to VCD, they are not currently recommended for use for this diagnostic purpose. CSF markers for AD are, however, better developed, with lower levels of Aβ42 and elevated levels of tau or phosphorylated tau being indicative of AD pathology.[119,120] These, along with amyloid imaging using PET, may help determine AD as the main or contributory cause of the cognitive disorder. Their use is encouraged in clinical trials and research studies of VCD to rule out AD. Other neuroimaging procedures to determine the rate of brain atrophy, hippocampal or mesial temporal atrophy, cerebral blood flow, and cerebral metabolic rate may be useful in the differential diagnosis in some cases, but their status as

BOX 53-3 Proposed VASCOG Criteria for Vascular Mild Cognitive Disorder and Vascular Dementia (or Major Cognitive Disorder)

PRESENCE OF A COGNITIVE DISORDER

Mild Cognitive Disorder

A. Acquired decline in one or more cognitive domains, as evidenced by the following:
   1. Concerns of a patient, knowledgeable informant, or clinician of mild levels of decline from a previous level of cognitive functioning; *and*
   2. Evidence of modest deficits on objective cognitive assessment based on a validated measure of neurocognitive function
B. The cognitive deficits are not sufficient to interfere with independence (i.e., instrumental activities of daily living are preserved), but greater effort, compensatory strategies, or accommodation may be required to maintain independence

Dementia (or Major Cognitive Disorder)

A. Evidence of substantial cognitive decline from a documented or inferred previous level of performance in one or more of the domains outlined above. Evidence for decline is based on the following:
   1. Concerns of the patient, knowledgeable informant, or clinician of significant decline in specific abilities *and*
   2. Clear and significant deficits in objective assessment based on a validated objective measure of neurocognitive function
B. The cognitive deficits are sufficient to interfere with independence

EVIDENCE FOR PREDOMINANTLY VASCULAR CAUSE OF COGNITIVE IMPAIRMENT

A. One of the following clinical features:
   1. The onset of the cognitive deficits is temporally related to one or more cerebrovascular events (CVEs). The evidence of CVEs is one of the following:
      a. Documented history of a stroke, with cognitive decline temporally associated with the event
      b. Physical signs consistent with stroke
   2. Evidence for decline is prominent in speed of information processing, complex attention and/or frontal executive functioning in the absence of history of a stroke or transient ischemic attack. One of the following features is also present:
      a. Early presence of a gait disturbance (small step gait [*marche petits pas*] or magnetic, apraxic-ataxic, or parkinsonian gait); this may also manifest as unsteadiness and frequent, unprovoked falls
      b. Early urinary frequency, urgency, and other urinary symptoms not explained by urologic disease
      c. Personality and mood changes—abulia, depression, or emotional incontinence
B. Presence of significant neuroimaging (MRI or CT) evidence of cerebrovascular disease (CVD)

EXCLUSION CRITERIA

A. History
   1. Early onset of memory deficit and progressive worsening of memory and other cognitive functions such as language (transcortical sensory aphasia), motor skills (apraxia), and perception (agnosia) in the absence of corresponding focal lesions on brain imaging or history of vascular events
   2. Early and prominent parkinsonian features suggestive of Lewy body disease
   3. History strongly suggestive of another primary neurologic disorder
B. Neuroimaging: absent or minimal cerebrovascular lesions on CT or MRI
C. Other medical disorders severe enough to account for memory and related symptoms
   a. Other disease of sufficient severity to cause cognitive impairment, eg, brain tumor, multiple sclerosis, encephalitis
   b. Major depression, with a temporal association between cognitive impairment and the likely onset of depression
   c. Toxic and metabolic abnormalities sufficient to account for cognitive abnormalitiies
D. For research: the presence of biomarkers for Alzheimer disease (cerebrospinal Aβ and pTau levels or amyloid imaging at accepted thresholds) excludes diagnosis of probable VCD, and indicates AD with CVD

Adapted from Sachdev P, Kalaria R, O'Brien J, et al: Diagnostic criteria for vascular cognitive disorders. Alzheimer Dis Assoc Disord 28:206–218, 2014.
CT, Computed tomography; *MRI,* magnetic resonance imaging; *VCD,* vascular cognitive disorder.

biomarkers of AD is uncertain.[59] Emerging markers include carotid intimal-medial thickness and arterial stiffness, which are associated with arterial aging and may serve as risk markers of VCD.[121]

DISEASE PROGRESSION

Because of its heterogeneity, the progression of VCD shows considerable variability. PSD generally carries a poor prognosis.[33] Risk factors for progression and functional decline include age, previous cognitive impairment, polypharmacy, hypotension during acute stroke, depression, and medial temporal atrophy. If dementia is not present immediately after stroke, up to one third of patients have a change in their diagnostic category (NCI [no cognitive impairment], CIND [cognitive impairment, no dementia], dementia) within 1 year.[122]

Patients with mild VCD show less rapid progression than those with dementia, but the presence of certain baseline features such as prior history of stroke and memory impairment coupled with functional impairment may indicate an increased risk of progression to incident dementia.[122] Medial temporal atrophy and thalamic atrophy appear to be more important than white matter hyperintensities in predicting cognitive impairment and dementia after stroke.[123] Most people with VCD show clinical progression that is readily detectable. Current cognitive and functional assessments such as the MMSE, Disability Assessment for Dementia (DAD), and Functional Rating Scale (FRS) may be less responsive to deterioration in the severe stages of VCI.[124] Compared with AD, those with VCI may show more prominent progression of affective symptoms such as depression.[124]

Longitudinal studies of WMLs have shown substantial progression. In normal aging populations with early confluent to confluent lesions, the rate of progression ranges from 0.23 to 1.33 cm^3/year.[125] In hypertensive individuals, the rate is higher, and it is much higher in CADASIL.[126] The frequency of new lacunes ranges from 1.6% to 19.0% over 3 to 5 years in different studies,[127] with the Dijon Stroke Registry showing an incidence of lacunes of 16.7% over 5 years.[127] The incidence of microbleeds varies strongly with age. The progression of SVD on neuroimaging markers has not been clearly correlated with the progression of cognitive deficits.

PREVENTION

Primary Prevention

Because many risk factors for VCD have been identified, it is arguable that VCDs are at least partially preventable. Data for this have gradually accumulated over the last 2 decades and were summarized recently.[121] In relation to lifestyle risk factors (e.g., diet, physical activity, alcohol intake, obesity, smoking), there is reasonable evidence that adequate physical activity, weight control, smoking cessation, and moderation of alcohol intake are advisable.[121] Higher education has been found to be a protective factor in VCD, as for dementia in general. Complex cognitive activity has been examined as a protective factor against cognitive decline, and it may again be nonspecific and unrelated to the cause of the cognitive decline.[128] Treatment of depression is recommended, although the evidence that it predisposes to cognitive decline is still equivocal.[121]

Of the physiologic risk factors, hypertension has received the greatest attention. Hypertension increases the risk of stroke and thereby of VCD.[129] There is evidence from observational and intervention studies that treatment of midlife hypertension reduces the risk of dementia, including VCD, and the longer the duration of treatment, the stronger the protective effect.[121] The evidence for the benefit of treating hypertension in the very old is, however, uncertain. The evidence that any particular class of antihypertensive drugs is more protective than others is inconclusive. It is reasonable to treat hyperglycemia and hypercholesterolemia to reduce the risk of VCD, but the benefits of treating inflammation are uncertain.[121] It is also important to attend to concomitant vascular disease. Because stroke poses a major risk for VCD, stroke prevention and its prompt treatment, followed by rehabilitation, including cognitive training, should be emphasized in any measures used to prevent VCD. Treatment of atrial fibrillation with an anticoagulant is also important, and diseases of the coronary or peripheral arterial circulation and clinically detectable renal and cardiac failure have all been associated with cognitive impairment and should be addressed, although the link with cognitive decline is less well established.

Secondary Prevention

There have been major advances in the treatment of acute stroke[130] and the prevention of recurrent stroke, including treatment of risk factors, use of antiplatelet agents and anticoagulants, and surgical intervention,[131] and these should be implemented. The use of neuroprotective agents in stroke patients have, however, been disappointing.[132] Even after the development of a VCD, attention to risk factors discussed for primary prevention is relevant for the potential slowing of future decline.

There have been a few studies that examined interventions to slow the progression of SVD. In the Perindropril Progression Against Recurrent Stroke Study (PROGRESS), the MRI substudy showed that a more intensive blood pressure–lowering regimen might reduce the rate of progression of WMLs.[133] In a secondary analysis of the Study on Cognition and Prognosis in the Elderly trial, patients treated with the angiotensin receptor blocker candesartan showed a reduced risk of white matter hyperintensities, possibly related to blockage of AT1 and activation of AT2 receptors.[134] The benefit of statins on WMLs is equivocal. In regard to lowering of homocysteine levels, the VITATOPS MRI substudy showed that the use of B vitamins was associated with reduced progression of WMLs in those with severe SVD.[135]

TREATMENT

Symptomatic Treatment

The effects of treatment in VaD are modest. Cholinesterase inhibitors have been examined. Galantamine was studied in VaD, AD, and a mixed group, and there was less decline in cognition, function, and behavior in the drug group, driven by the mixed subgroup.[136] A subsequent study showed a global benefit with galantamine in pure VaD, but not for daily functions.[137] With donepezil, some cognitive benefit was found, but global and functional efficacy were not consistent in the two studies.[138,139] Rivastigmine has been less well studied, with a suggestion of beneficial effects on executive function.[140] In a study of donepezil in CADASIL patients, there was no beneficial effect, although secondary analysis showed a benefit in executive function.[141] Two studies with memantine, an *N*-methyl-D-aspartate antagonist, showed some improvement in cognition but without global or functional benefit.[142,143] A meta-analysis has concluded that only small benefits of uncertain clinical meaningfulness were available using cholinesterase inhibitors or memantine.[144] Although some patients experience clinical benefit, no clinical features predicting treatment response have been found. The case for cholinergic inhibition is mixed, even though cholinergic mechanisms appear to play a critical role in cerebral perfusion.[83] A Cochrane review of VaD trials has concluded that donepezil studies provide the best benefit for cognitive improvement in pure VaD and galantamine in mixed dementia, but the benefits of rivastigmine and memantine were not proven.[123,145] However, the studies that most persuasively assembled groups of pure VaD patients[145] had small effect sizes, no dose response, limited evidence for convergence of treatment effects within and across trials, and no clear translation into what physicians might look for in usual care.[145]

Other drugs that have been tried in VaD include nimodipine, piracetam, huperzine A, cytidine diphosphocholine, and vinpocetine, but with no beneficial effects.[121] Nimodipine and huperzine A may, however, have a role in SVD and deserve further study.[121] Sertraline has been shown to have a beneficial effect on executive function in VCD in a small study.[146]

KEY POINTS

- Vascular cognitive disorder (VCD) is an umbrella term that includes vascular dementia (including poststroke, multi-infarct dementia, and subcortical ischemic dementia), and mild cognitive disorder of vascular origin that does not meet the criteria for dementia. The plural term *vascular cognitive disorders* is often used.
- The clinical diagnostic criteria for VCD are evolving. The VASCOG criteria were recently proposed to encompass the spectrum of vascular cognitive disorders.
- VCD is a clinical diagnosis, with neuroimaging necessary to increase the certainty of the diagnosis. Neuropathology plays a supportive role.
- The cause is varied, with large vessel disease, small vessel disease, intracranial hemorrhage, brain atrophy, and venous disease all contributing. The clinical presentation and longitudinal course are therefore very variable.
- Treatment of VCD is symptomatic and often unsatisfactory. Cholinesterase inhibitors and *N*-methyl-D-aspartate (NMDA) antagonists have only limited evidence for use, although some of this may represent underrecognition of mixed dementia in Alzheimer disease trials.
- VCD is potentially preventable through management of risk factors, although empirical evidence for prevention is somewhat limited.

For a complete list of references, please visit www.expertconsult.com.

KEY REFERENCES

3. Hachinski VC, Lassen NA, Marshall J: Multi-infarct dementia: a cause of mental deterioration in the elderly. Lancet 304:207–209, 1974.
5. Neuropathology Group, Medical Research Council Cognitive Function and Aging Study: Pathological correlates of late-onset dementia in a multicentre, community-based population in England and Wales. Neuropathology Group of the Medical Research Council Cognitive Function and Ageing Study (MRC CFAS). Lancet 357:169–175, 2001.
6. Snowdon DA: Brain infarction and the clinical expression of Alzheimer disease. The Nun Study. JAMA 277:813–817, 1997.
9. Looi JCL, Sachdev PS: Differentiation of vascular dementia from AD on neuropsychological tests. Neurology 53:670–678, 1999.
11. O'Brien JT, Erkinjuntti T, Reisberg B, et al: Vascular cognitive impairment. Lancet Neurol 2:89–98, 2003.
13. Sachdev P, Kalaria R, O'Brien J, et al: Diagnostic criteria for vascular cognitive disorders. Alzheimer Dis Assoc Disord 28:206–218, 2014.
21. Savva GM, Stephan BCM: Epidemiological studies of the effect of stroke on incident dementia: a systematic review. Stroke 41:e41–e46, 2009.
23. Jellinger KA: Morphologic diagnosis of "vascular dementia"—a critical update. J Neurol Sci 270:1–12, 2008.
40. Román GC, Erkinjuntti T, Wallin A, et al: Subcortical ischaemic vascular dementia. Lancet Neurol 1:426–436, 2002.
45. Pantoni L, Garcia JH: Pathogenesis of leukoaraiosis: a review. Stroke 28:652–659, 1997.
49. Sachdev PS, Brodaty H, Valenzuela MJ, et al: Progression of cognitive impairment in stroke patients. Neurology 63:1618–1623, 2004.
60. Wardlaw JM, Smith EE, Biessels GJ, et al: Neuroimaging standards for research into small vessel disease and its contribution to ageing and neurodegeneration. Lancet Neurol 12:822–838, 2013.
61. Hachinski V, Iadecola C, Petersen RC, et al: National Institute of Neurological Disorders and Stroke-Canadian Stroke Network vascular cognitive impairment harmonization standards. Stroke 37:2220–2241, 2006.
67. Cordonnier C, Al-Shahi Salman R, Wardlaw J: Spontaneous brain microbleeds: systematic review, subgroup analyses and standards for study design and reporting. Brain 130:1988–2003, 2007.
72. Attems J, Jellinger K, Thal DR, et al: Sporadic cerebral amyloid angiopathy. Neuropathol Appl Neurobiol 37:75–93, 2011.
84. Benisty S, Hernandez K, Viswanathan A, et al: Diagnostic criteria of vascular dementia in CADASIL. Stroke 39:838–844, 2008.
89. Lee JH, Kim SH, Kim GH, et al: Identification of pure subcortical vascular dementia using ^{11}C-Pittsburgh compound B. Neurology 77:18–25, 2011.
93. Iadecola C: The pathobiology of vascular dementia. Neuron 80: 844–866, 2013.
100. Chui HC, Victoroff JI, Margolin D, et al: Criteria for the diagnosis of ischemic vascular dementia proposed by the state of California Alzheimer's Disease Diagnostic and Treatment Centers. Neurology 42:473–480, 1992.
104. Roman GC, Tatemichi TK, Erkinjuntti T, et al: Vascular dementia: diagnostic criteria for research studies. Report of the NINDS-AIREN International Workshop. Neurology 43:250–260, 1993.
107. Hachinski V, Oveisgharan S, Romney AK, et al: Optimizing the Hachinski Ischemic Scale. Arch Neurol 69:169–175, 2012.
121. Gorelick PB, Scuteri A, Black SE, et al: Vascular contributions to cognitive impairment and dementia: a statement for healthcare professionals from the American Heart Association/American Stroke Association. Stroke 42:2672–2713, 2011.
145. Malouf R, Birks J: Donepezil for vascular cognitive impairment. Cochrane Database Syst Rev (1):CD004395, 2004.

54 Frontotemporal Lobar Degeneration

Kristel Sleegers, Christine Van Broeckhoven

INTRODUCTION

Frontotemporal lobar degeneration (FTLD) is a neurodegenerative condition that selectively affects the frontal and anterior temporal lobes of the brain, resulting in progressive shortfalls in behavior and language. More than a century ago Arnold Pick, a Czechoslovakian neurologist and psychiatrist, first published a report on FTLD. He described a 71-year-old man who developed dementia with sensory aphasia and behavioral symptoms.[1] Autopsy demonstrated severe atrophy of the frontotemporal lobes, swollen ("ballooned") achromatic neurons, and argyrophilic inclusions within frontal neurons consisting of insoluble filaments of the microtubule associated protein tau, a protein crucial for intraneuronal transport and structural integrity of the cell. These tau-positive inclusions were later referred to as Pick bodies, and their presence was necessary for pathologists to come to a diagnosis of Pick disease. Gradually, the eponym was taken over by clinicians to diagnose patients with a dementia syndrome with disinhibited behavior. Today, after two decades of progress in clinical, pathologic, genetic, and cell biologic research, we recognize that FTLD is highly heterogeneous in its clinical presentation, pathologic substrate, and cause.[2]

The increasing understanding of this causal heterogeneity is causing a shift in perspective from one that focuses on differences in clinical manifestation to one that is based on distinct proteinopathies. This distinction will be crucial in the diagnosis and management of these diseases, as well as for development of biomarkers and a curative treatment where none currently exists.

EPIDEMIOLOGY

FTLD is the third most common cause of neurodegenerative dementia, after Alzheimer disease (AD) and dementia with Lewy bodies.[3] FTLD is mostly considered an early onset dementia, but reported onset ages vary from 21 to 89 years. Epidemiologic data are sparse, particularly on the older adult population, and estimates of prevalence and incidence vary widely. This can be explained, in part, by the heterogeneity of FTLD, regional differences in the contribution of genetic causes of FTLD, and evolving diagnostic criteria. Estimates of the proportion of patients with an onset after 65 years range from 25% to 70%.[4,5] The incidence of FTLD in people aged 65 years or older ranges from 3.44 to 16.7 patients per 100,000 patient-years, compared to 0.64 to 4.1 per 100,000 patient-years in the group aged 64 or younger.[5-7] FTLD does not appear to affect males and females differently.[8] Disease duration is generally shorter than for other neurodegenerative diseases such as AD[5,9] and is estimated to be, on average, 6 to 7 years but may be as long as 35 years.[10] Although data on risk factors for FTLD are sparse, positive family history has long been recognized as a major risk factor for FTLD (see section Genetics).

CLINICAL PRESENTATION

The most frequent and best recognized clinical presentation of FTLD is frontotemporal dementia, also called behavioral variant FTLD (bvFTD), which typically presents with changes in personality, behavior, and social comportment[11] and is associated with atrophy of the prefrontal and anterotemporal cortex. Less frequently, FTLD presents with language dysfunction in the context of a primary progressive aphasia (PPA), which can further be subdivided into a semantic variant (svPPA) and an agrammatic or nonfluent aphasia (nfvPPA).[12] The nonfluent variant is characterized by dysfunction of expressive language and is associated with asymmetric atrophy of the left frontal and temporal cortices. On the other hand, the pattern of atrophy in svPPA is bilateral, although often asymmetric, affecting the middle and inferotemporal cortex, and language dysfunction mainly consists of impaired word comprehension. Of the clinical variants of FTLD, bvFTD is the most common, with an estimated frequency of 57% among FTLD patients. nfvPPA is estimated to occur in 24% and svPPA in 19% of all FTLD patients.[13] Notwithstanding clear distinctions, considerable clinical overlap exists between these disorders, likely reflecting the expanding distribution of pathologic changes in different brain regions.

Individuals with bvFTD typically exhibit an insidious change of personality and behavioral abnormalities, such as loss of social awareness, poor insight, and blunting of affect. Other prominent symptoms include disinhibition, antisocial behavior, poor impulse control, and stereotypical or ritualized behavior, such as foot tapping or more complex behavioral routines, or repetitive use of a phrase,[14,15] reflecting the topography of neurodegeneration. Behavioral symptoms seem to be most severe in patients with right hemisphere involvement.[16] Cognitive impairment may be less prominent initially and mainly involves working memory and executive function. Cognitive changes include impaired attention, abstraction, problem solving, planning and organization and perseveration. Visuospatial skills are remarkably spared until late stages of the disease. Frequently, dietary changes are reported, such as cravings for sweets and gluttony, leading to weight gain in many patients. Apathy can be another prominent feature, often reflecting involvement of the medial frontal and anterior cingulate regions. Language changes may include echolalia, perseveration, and eventually mutism.[15] During the course of the disease motor symptoms may develop, such as parkinsonian signs (akinesia and rigidity in ≈14%) or symptoms of motor neuron disease (MND) (4%-17%).[4]

In patients with svPPA, communication is mainly impaired by difficulties in recognizing and understanding the meaning of words. Use of substitute words and semantic paraphasias is frequent in otherwise grammatically flawless speech.[17] Loss of word comprehension is part of a more widespread loss of semantic knowledge of faces and emotions, facts, and objects. This puts additional strain on daily activities, for example, by inability to recognize ordinary household objects.[14] svPPA patients often display disinhibited or compulsive behavior, which may be more prominent than in bvFTD.[14] Episodic memory is relatively spared, but memory for autobiographic events is often affected.

In contrast to svPPA, patients with nfvPPA display decreased fluency of speech, while comprehension of single words is usually intact. Symptoms include word-finding difficulties, changes in pronunciation, grammatical errors, anomia, phonemic paraphasias, stuttering, and apraxia of speech.[14] Semantic and episodic memories are preserved. Awareness of language deficits may

TABLE 54-1 Clinical, Genetic, and Pathologic Correlations in Frontotemporal Lobar Degeneration

Clinical Presentation	% of FTLD	Associated Genes		Comorbidities			Neuropathologic Subtypes				
				Parkinsonism	MND	IBM PDB	FTLD-tau	FTLD-TDP	FTLD-FUS	FTLD-UPS	FTLD-ni
bvFTD	57%			+	+	+/–	++	++	+	+/–	+/–
		C9orf72	++	+	++			type B > A		+/–	
		GRN	+	+				type A			
		MAPT	+	+			+				
		VCP	+/–		+/–	+		type D			
		CHMP2B	+/–	+/–	+/–					+	
nfvPPA	24%			+	+/–		++	+			
		C9orf72	+								
		GRN	++	+				type A			
		MAPT	+	+			+				
svPPA	19%			+/–	+/–		+/–	++ (type C)			
		Rarely genetic									

bv, Behavioral variant; *FTLD,* frontotemporal lobar degeneration; *FUS,* fused in sarcoma; *IBM,* inclusion body myopathy; *MND,* motor neuron disease; *nfv,* agrammatic or nonfluent variant; *ni,* no inclusions; *PDB,* Paget disease of the bone; *PPA,* primary progressive aphasia; *sv,* semantic variant; *TDP,* TAR DNA-binding protein; *UPS,* ubiquitin proteasome system.
Number of + signifies relative frequency of the observation; +/– indicates rare observation.

explain socially withdrawn behavior and depression. Changes in behavior tend to occur later in the disease, and numerous patients eventually develop corticobasal syndrome (CBS) or progressive supranuclear palsy (PSP).

Although FTLD may clearly present with one of the three disorders, in the natural course of the disease patients will invariably develop symptoms of the other FTLD syndromes. Moreover, overlap with symptoms of Parkinson disease (PD), CBS, PSP, amyotrophic lateral sclerosis (ALS), or AD is not exceptional (Table 54-1).[18] This may be due to progressive involvement of other brain regions in the disease process, but also to comorbidity, especially in older adult patients.

NEUROPATHOLOGY

FTLD derives its name from the characteristic atrophy of frontal and temporal cortices. Patterns of atrophy differ between FTLD patients, however, strongly correlating with the different clinical phenotypes. Five distinct neuropathologic phenotypes are currently distinguished to underlie neurodegeneration in FTLD, based on the presence or absence of characteristic intracellular protein inclusions and their major constituents, which can be detected upon microscopic examination and immunohistochemistry (see Table 54-1).[19]

The first neuropathologic phenotype to be described is characterized by abnormal accumulations of hyperphosphorylated microtubule associated protein tau in neuronal and glial cells. This subtype, currently referred to as FTLD-tau, is found in less than 50% of FTLD autopsies.[20] The three most common pathologies in this category are Pick disease, corticobasal degeneration (CBD) and PSP.[21] Hallmarks of Pick disease are the neuronal cytoplasmic inclusions of hyperphosphorylated tau called Pick bodies. In the adult brain, six isoforms of tau exist, three of which contain three microtubule-binding domains (3R) and three of which contain four binding domains (4R), at a 1:1 ratio.[22] The tau protein aggregates in Pick bodies predominantly consist of 3R tau. CBD and PSP are characterized by protein inclusions consisting primarily of 4R tau. CBD is morphologically further characterized by neuritic thread pathology and astrocytic plaques, with a predominance of forebrain pathology. PSP can be recognized by severe atrophy of subcortical nuclei and hallmark tufted astrocytes.[21]

More than 50% of autopsies show ubiquitin immunoreactive neuronal inclusions that are tau negative.[3] In most patients these inclusions consist of ubiquitinated, hyperphosphorylated TAR DNA-binding protein with molecular weight 43kDa (TDP-43).[23] This phenotype, called FTLD-TDP, is further categorized in four subtypes (type A, B, C and D), based on the pattern and preponderance of neuronal cytoplasmic and intranuclear inclusions.[24] FTLD-TDP can be found in bvFTD, nfvPPA, svPPA, and FTLD with motor neuron disease, with an imperfect correlation between pathologic subtype and clinical presentation,[21] although FTLD-TDP type C seems to present predominantly with svPPA, and type D is typical for a clinical syndrome involving inclusion body myopathy, Paget disease of the bone, and frontotemporal dementia (IBMPFD).[24] Correlations between various genetic causes of FTLD and the FTLD-TDP subtypes have been reported (see Genetics).

A third neuropathologic phenotype, observed in 5% to 10% of FTLD cases, demonstrates ubiquitin immunoreactive neuronal inclusions that consist of fused in sarcoma (FUS) protein, therefore called FTLD-FUS.[25] Three subtypes of FTLD-FUS are recognized, atypical FTLD-U (aFTLD-U), basophilic inclusion body disease (BIBD), and neuronal intermediate filament inclusion disease (NIFID). aFTLD-U gives rise to a well-defined clinical presentation with early onset and severe psychobehavioral deficits. BIBD is characterized by basophilic neuronal inclusions but is clinically heterogeneous, including ALS. Neuronal inclusions observed in NIFID are immunoreactive for neuronal intermediate filaments. The associated clinical phenotype is FTLD with pyramidal or extrapyramidal symptoms.[26]

In a minority of FTLD patients, neuronal or glial protein deposits are observed that have not been characterized to date, delineating a subtype referred to as FTLD–ubiquitin proteasome system (FTLD-UPS). Infrequently, neuropathologic examination does not reveal protein deposits, therefore defined as FTLD with no inclusions (FTLD-ni).

GENETICS

About 40% of FTLD patients have a positive family history, and in 20% to 30% the mode of inheritance is autosomal dominant.[10] First-degree relatives of patients with FTLD have a 3.5 times increased risk of developing FTLD.[27] Mutations in three genes—progranulin (*GRN*),[28,29] chromosome 9 open reading frame 72 (*C9orf72*),[30-32] and microtubule associated protein tau (*MAPT*)[33]—account for the majority of autosomal dominantly inherited FTLD (see Table 54-1).

The most common genetic cause of FTLD is a pathogenic expansion of a non-coding repeat of six nucleotides (G_4C_2) in *C9orf72*. Identified in 2011, after 5 years of molecular genetic research on families with a mixed phenotype of FTLD and ALS, the discovery of this pathogenic hexanucleotide repeat expansion rapidly explained almost 30% of FTLD, 50% of ALS, and nearly 90% of FTLD-ALS cases.[34,35] In FTLD patients with a *C9orf72* repeat expansion, the most frequent clinical subtype is bvFTD. In addition to an increased frequency of symptoms of ALS, parkinsonism is observed in up to 25% of expansion carriers.[36,37] In unaffected individuals the hexanucleotide repeat ranges from 2 to 24 repeat units, whereas in affected patients the expanded repeat sequence can consist of thousands of repeat units.[34] Although the normal function of *C9orf72* remains elusive, three mechanisms have been postulated to bring about neurodegeneration in *C9orf72* repeat expansion carriers. These include reduced transcription of *C9orf72* due to location of the repeat expansion in a genomic region important for regulation of *C9orf72* expression,[30,35] RNA toxicity due to sequestration of RNA-binding proteins and repeat-containing RNA molecules,[30] and abnormal translation of the expanded repeat, resulting in the formation of aggregation-prone dipeptide repeat proteins.[38] Evidence exists to support all three mechanisms, suggesting they all contribute to neuronal death. Neuropathologically, *C9orf72* repeat expansions are mainly associated with FTLD-TDP type B pathology although other pathologic subtypes have been reported.[39] The characteristic dipeptide repeat aggregates are invariably present, suggesting this precedes TDP pathology in *C9orf72*-mediated FTLD.

The prevalence of *MAPT* mutations in FTLD ranges from 5% to 20%, the wide range reflecting geographic differences due to local founder effects. The most frequent clinical presentation is bvFTD, but *MAPT* mutation carriers may also present with parkinsonism or symptoms consistent with PSP or CBS.[40] The mutation spectrum is wide, including missense and silent mutations, small deletions, splice site mutations, and possibly copy number variations (Alzheimer Disease and Frontotemporal Dementia Mutation Database [http://www.molgen.vib-ua.be/FTDMutations]).[41] Pathogenic *MAPT* mutations bring about neuronal loss through altered interaction between tau protein and the microtubule network, tau filament formation, and/or changes in ratio of 3R and 4R tau isoforms.[42] *MAPT* mutations are typically associated with FTLD-tau, although not all FTLD-tau can be explained by currently known *MAPT* mutations. It should be noted that most molecular genetic screenings to date have focused on only those parts of the gene known to be involved in microtubule binding or splicing.

GRN mutations occur at a similar frequency as *MAPT* mutations, although relative frequencies can differ between populations as a result of founder effects.[10] *GRN* mutations show a considerable clinical heterogeneity, even within families. The clinical spectrum includes bvFTD and nfvPPA, but also AD, PD, and CBS.[10] Symptoms of MND are less likely. Pathogenic *GRN* mutations lead to a loss of function through a reduction in functional progranulin.[2] Progranulin is a widely expressed secreted precursor protein with functions ranging from cell growth to inflammatory response. Given the reduction in functional progranulin protein in mutation carriers, progranulin is postulated to have a role in neuronal survival or neuroinflammation.[2] The neuropathologic phenotype of *GRN*-mediated FTLD is FTLD-TDP type A.[24] The pattern of atrophy is often asymmetric, correlating with differences in clinical presentation. Predominant left-sided atrophy is typically found in patients with a clinical presentation of PPA, whereas right-sided atrophy correlates with bvFTD.

In addition, several infrequent (<1%) causes of FTLD have been reported. Mutations in valosin-containing protein (*VCP*) cause FTLD as part of the autosomal dominant syndrome IBMPFD,[43] with the neuropathologic substrate FTLD-TDP type D.[24] Mutations in chromatin-modifying protein 2B (*CHMP2B*)[44] disrupt the endosomal secretory complex, because of accumulation of mutant protein on the surface of enlarged vesicular structures. Intraneuronal inclusions observed in brains of *CHMP2B* carriers are tau, TDP-43, and FUS negative, and account for part of the neuropathologic subtype FTLD-UPS.[45] Homozygous mutations in the gene encoding triggering receptor expressed on myeloid cells 2 (*TREM2*; 6p21.1) have been correlated with frontotemporal dementia in consanguineous families,[46-48] possibly in the context of Nasu-Hakola disease. In rare instances, mutations are identified in genes predominantly involved in other neurodegenerative diseases such as AD.[41]

Of note, not all patients with a positive family history carry a mutation in one of these genes, indicating that additional genetic causes or risk factors remain to be identified. One putative risk gene, *TMEM106B*, has been reported in a genome-wide association, but its role in disease is still unclear.[49] On the other hand, causal mutations in *GRN* and *C9orf72* are also quite frequently found in patients without evidence of an autosomal dominant pattern of inheritance, reflecting age-related penetrance or presence of modifying factors. On average, *MAPT* and *VCP* mutation carriers have the youngest age at onset (<50 years), followed by *C9orf72* repeat expansion carriers (mean onset age 55 years), *GRN* mutation carriers (mean onset age 59 years) and *CHMP2B* (mean onset age 65 years),[41] but onset age can be highly variable, even within one family, and may range from the second to the eighth decade.

DIAGNOSTIC WORKUP

It can be difficult to reach a clinical diagnosis of FTLD; diagnostic delay is estimated between 3 and 4 years.[50] Because of insidious changes in behavior and personality, patients are often initially referred to a psychiatrist. A neurologic examination, with emphasis on detailed cognitive and behavioral assessment, combined with neuropsychologic testing and neuroimaging, provide the foundations for a clinical diagnosis of FTLD. It is important to exclude other (potentially reversible) causes of cognitive and behavioral deficits, such as normal pressure hydrocephalus, tumors, hypothyroidism, alcohol abuse, and large or small vessel disease.

The most recent (2011) diagnostic criteria for bvFTD[11] require the presence of a slow progressive deterioration of behavior and/or cognition, affecting at least three of the following six symptoms: early disinhibition; apathy or inertia; loss of empathy or sympathy; perseverative, stereotyped, or compulsive behavior; hyperorality and dietary changes; and a neuropsychologic profile demonstrating deficits in executive function with relative sparing of memory and visuospatial skills. A distinction is made between possible bvFTD (when the previously mentioned criteria are met), probable bvFTD when supported by neuroimaging, and definite bvFTD when supported by histopathologic evidence or presence of a known pathogenic mutation.

Likewise, the most recent (2011) diagnostic criteria for PPA[12] recognize three levels of diagnostic certainty: clinical PPA, imaging-supported PPA, or PPA with definite pathology in case of histopathologic or genetic evidence. A clinical diagnosis of nfvPPA requires at least one of the two core symptoms, agrammatism or apraxia of speech, and at least two additional features that can include impaired comprehension of syntactically complex sentences, spared single-word comprehension, and/or spared object knowledge. A clinical diagnosis of svPPA requires the presence of two core features, that is, impaired confrontation naming and impaired single-word comprehension. Three additional features should be present, such as impaired object knowledge, surface dyslexia/dysgraphia, spared repetition, and/or spared speech production.

Neuropsychologic Testing

The Mini-Mental State Examination (MMSE)[51] has limited use in diagnosing FTLD. In patients with bvFTD, MMSE scores may be normal even when the patient already requires nursing home care.[52] On the other hand, language may be impaired, hindering a proper MMSE test of patients with svPPA or nfvPPA.[14] Other neuropsychologic test results should be interpreted with caution, especially when only the (quantitative) test scores are considered. Failure to perform on a neuropsychologic test may be due to various reasons, which are not reflected in the overall score. Especially in bvFTD, behavioral abnormalities such as impulsive behavior and perseveration can affect test performance [15] such that the neuropsychologic test scores would not differentiate from other neurodegenerative disorders such as AD. However, when taking into account the qualitative errors during testing, diagnostic accuracy for bvFTD may increase from 71 to 96%.[53] A large meta-analysis of cognitive tests discriminating between AD and bvFTD showed that measures of orientation, memory, language, visuomotor function, and general cognitive ability discriminated best but that overlap in test performance was still considerable, indicating that a differential diagnosis should not be based on neuropsychologic tests alone.[54]

Several, more easily applicable clinical and behavioral assessment scales exist that are not (or are less) burdensome to the patient and that perform relatively well in distinguishing patients with FTLD from patients with other neurodegenerative diseases; these instruments include the Middelheim Frontality Score,[55] the Philadelphia Brief Assessment of Cognition,[56] and the Frontal Behavioral Inventory (for caregivers).[57]

Neuroimaging

The three clinical FTLD syndromes show different patterns of gray matter atrophy on volumetric structural MRI, which can also be distinguished from AD and other related disorders, such as PSP and CBS.[18] Furthermore, other structural causes of behavioral abnormalities, such as tumors or small or large vessel disease, can be excluded. In the early stages of disease, structural MRI may show cortical volume within normal limits. Functional neuroimaging with positron emission tomography or single photon emission computed tomography might already reveal a pattern of hypoperfusion in frontal and/or temporal lobes.[58] Other neuroimaging modalities such as diffusion tensor imaging have been suggested to improve diagnostic discrimination.[59] Molecular imaging with an amyloid β ligand can support discriminating FTLD from AD.[60] Development of tau imaging tracers for in vivo diagnosis of FTLD-tau is in progress.[61,62]

Genetic Testing

The only way to obtain certainty regarding the underlying disease entity during life is when a mutation screening of the genes implicated in FTLD reveals a pathogenic mutation. Because of the genetic heterogeneity of FTLD, algorithms for diagnostic genetic testing have been developed,[63,64] guided by local mutation frequencies, correlations between genes and clinical presentations, and presence of comorbid features like ALS or parkinsonism. For example, based on mutation frequency, *C9orf72* screening should be performed first, unless there is concomitant CBS or PSP (suggestive of *GRN* or *MAPT*), or Paget disease of bone or inclusion body myopathy, which are predictive of a *VCP* mutation. Concomitant symptoms of ALS argue against a *GRN* mutation, whereas a clinical presentation of nfvPPA is suggestive of *GRN*.[10,40] *MAPT* mutations are highly penetrant so arguably need not be screened for in sporadic patients.[65] A caveat here is that the presence of ALS or PD may be misinterpreted because of clinical heterogeneity when examining family history. Furthermore, high variability in onset age may obscure an autosomal dominant pattern of inheritance. Technologic progress has made it feasible to perform genetic screenings for these genes simultaneously, which will greatly facilitate genetic diagnostic testing for FTLD.

Genetic testing should always be paired with counseling because in addition to producing diagnostic certainty, the results of genetic testing also have a profound impact on family members, especially in the current absence of a targeted cure for FTLD. It is important to remember that mutation carriers can be asymptomatic until late in life.[10] This complicates the interpretation of a positive test in the context of presymptomatic screening. Moreover, incomplete knowledge of the causes of FTLD complicates the interpretation of a negative test, and conversely it is possible that mutations of unclear pathogenic significance are found. Therefore, presymptomatic screening is not straightforward in absence of a known genetic cause in an affected relative.

Biochemical Markers

The role of cerebrospinal (CSF) fluid or blood-based biomarkers in positive diagnosis of FTLD is still limited, but genetic and neuropathologic breakthroughs are expected to change this in the near future. Commercially available assays that measure levels of total tau, hyperphosphorylated tau, and amyloid beta simultaneously in CSF add to the differential diagnosis between AD, LBD, and FTLD, but CSF tau levels may be normal in FTLD patients.[66] Normal CSF tau levels have even been reported in *MAPT* mutation carriers.[67] In contrast, *GRN*-mediated FTLD can be reliably detected in serum and plasma because of the characteristic reduction of circulating progranulin protein resulting from loss of function mutations.[68] This can already be detected in a presymptomatic stage, extending the future utility of this test once a treatment for *GRN*-mediated FTLD is available. In addition, if future treatment is aimed at remediating loss of progranulin, treatment efficacy and safety can be monitored with the same assay. Assays for TDP-43 are under development, but their clinical usefulness needs to be investigated further.[69]

TREATMENT AND STRATEGIES

Although currently no curative treatment exists for FTD, treatment options exist to diminish the burdensome (behavioral) symptoms associated with the disease, to significantly improve patient care and quality of life. Both pharmacologic and nonpharmacologic symptomatic approaches exist. Strategies for symptomatic treatment of FTLD are derived from other disorders with behavioral disturbances, such as AD. Studies addressing the efficacy and safety of these symptomatic medications in FTLD are limited. Most evidence comes from case reports and open-label studies of very small patient groups. The decision to prescribe any of these medications should be carefully considered for each patient, but especially in older adults, in light of interaction with other medication and comorbidity.

Selective serotonin reuptake inhibitors (SSRIs; fluoxetine, fluvoxamine, sertraline, and paroxetine) may counteract social abnormalities (such as depression, anxiety, disinhibition, impulsivity, and sexually inappropriate and stereotyped behavior), but they are also reported to suppress eating abnormalities (such as decreased satiety and food cravings).[14,70] Although the use of SSRIs in FTLD is plausible given the association of these behavioral abnormalities and changes in cortical serotonin levels,[70] the results of the few existing trials have been inconsistent.[71,72]

Other behavioral features such as agitation and psychosis are often treated with neuroleptic medication, but the traditional neuroleptic agents have undesirable side effects, such as parkinsonism or somnolence, particularly in older patients. Extrapyramidal side effects may be less pronounced when patients take atypical antipsychotic drugs, but increased mortality during use of atypical antipsychotics has been reported in older adults.[70] On the other hand, a study specifically addressing this issue suggested these drugs are well tolerated by older adults.[73] Anticonvulsant drugs are sometimes given to treat aggression, but side effects (including confusion) limit their use in older adults.[74] No placebo-controlled trials exist.[70]

Acetylcholinesterase inhibitors (rivastigmine, donepezil, galantamine) used to treat symptoms of AD are being examined for use in FTLD patients, even though the cholinergic system seems to be relatively unaffected in FTLD compared with AD.[70] Studies on the efficacy of cholinesterase inhibitors give inconsistent results.[14,70] Overall, cholinesterase inhibitors appear not to have an effect on cognition. Memantine, a drug that targets the glutamatergic system in AD, has been tested in a trial; results showed no changes in behavior and worsening of cognitive performance.[75]

Behavioral symptoms tend to be more distressful early in the disease, both for the patient and for those surrounding the patient. But as the pathologic process progresses, patients gradually display more apathy and less behavioral disturbance, allowing withdrawal of symptomatic treatment in advanced stages.[14]

Similar to pharmacologic treatments, the nonpharmacologic management of a patient should be tailored to his or her specific symptoms and should be adapted, when needed, during the course of the disease. Interventions include structuring of the environment and the establishment of daily schedules to reduce the chance of agitation, controlled access to food for patients with food cravings, and help in planning and avoiding of complex multistep activities for patients with executive dysfunction.[74]

When language dysfunction is prominent, focus should be on optimizing communication, for example, by speaking slowly in short sentences in cases of impaired comprehension and by employing picture cards or computer-assisted devices in cases of reduced fluency.[74] Other nonpharmacologic approaches should be targeted to reduce physical discomfort, such as reducing the risk of falls, physical therapy, prevention of decubitus ulcers in bedridden patients, and prevention of aspiration pneumonia, especially in patients with gorging behavior.[74] Special attention should also be given to caregivers of FTLD patients. The symptoms of FTLD (inappropriate behavior, agitation, and psychosis) can cause considerable distress for caregivers and are unknown to many people so community support for caregivers may fall short.[76]

The discovery of FTLD genes has been instrumental in identifying novel molecular targets for drug development. Several drugs aiming at modifying tau pathology are in the phase of clinical trial, and preclinical studies targeting *C9orf72* and *GRN* mediated FTLD show promising results.[77-79] Ultimately, management should be fitted to the underlying disease entity, because this will be the only possibility to cure the disease.

KEY POINTS

- The main presenting symptoms of FTLD are changes in personality, changes in behavior, or language dysfunction.
- FTLD is a clinically, genetically, and pathologically heterogeneous disorder.
- FTLD has a strong genetic component, with three major genetic causes (*C9orf72, MAPT,* and *GRN*) and two rare genetic causes (*CHMP2B* and *VCP*) currently known.
- Distinction of the different molecular entities (FTLD-tau, FTLD-TDP, FTLD-FUS, or other) will increasingly be important when medicine aimed at treating the cause of the disease becomes available.
- Currently only symptomatic treatment strategies exist; these treatments can improve quality of life but can have adverse side effects, so their use in older adult patients should be carefully considered.
- Biomarkers and drugs specific for the different molecular entities are in early stages of development.

For a complete list of references, please visit www.expertconsult.com.

KEY REFERENCES

2. Sleegers K, Cruts M, Van Broeckhoven C: Molecular pathways of frontotemporal lobar degeneration. Annu Rev Neurosci 33:71–88, 2010.
11. Rascovsky K, Hodges JR, Knopman D, et al: Sensitivity of revised diagnostic criteria for the behavioural variant of frontotemporal dementia. Brain 134:2456–2477, 2011.
12. Gorno-Tempini ML, Hillis AE, Weintraub S, et al: Classification of primary progressive aphasia and its variants. Neurology 76:1006–1014, 2011.
19. Mackenzie IR, Neumann M, Bigio EH, et al: Nomenclature and nosology for neuropathologic subtypes of frontotemporal lobar degeneration: an update. Acta Neuropathol 119:1–4, 2010.
20. Sieben A, Van Langenhove T, Engelborghs S, et al: The genetics and neuropathology of frontotemporal lobar degeneration. Acta Neuropathol 124:353–372, 2012.
28. Baker M, Mackenzie IR, Pickering-Brown SM, et al: Mutations in progranulin cause tau-negative frontotemporal dementia linked to chromosome 17. Nature 442:916–919, 2006.
29. Cruts M, Gijselinck I, van der Zee J, et al: Null mutations in progranulin cause ubiquitin-positive frontotemporal dementia linked to chromosome 17q21. Nature 442:920–924, 2006.
30. DeJesus-Hernandez M, Mackenzie IR, Boeve BF, et al: Expanded GGGGCC hexanucleotide repeat in noncoding region of C9ORF72 causes chromosome 9p-linked FTD and ALS. Neuron 72:245–256, 2011.
31. Gijselinck I, Van Langenhove T, van der Zee J, et al: A C9orf72 promoter repeat expansion in a Flanders-Belgian cohort with disorders of the frontotemporal lobar degeneration-amyotrophic lateral sclerosis spectrum: a gene identification study. Lancet Neurol 11:54–65, 2012.
32. Renton AE, Majounie E, Waite A, et al: A hexanucleotide repeat expansion in C9ORF72 is the cause of chromosome 9p21-linked ALS-FTD. Neuron 72:257–268, 2011.
33. Hutton M, Lendon CL, Rizzu P, et al: Association of missense and 5'-splice-site mutations in tau with the inherited dementia FTDP-17. Nature 393:702–705, 1998.
34. Cruts M, Gijselinck I, Van Langenhove T, et al: Current insights into the C9orf72 repeat expansion diseases of the FTLD/ALS spectrum. Trends Neurosci 36:450–459, 2013.
62. Villemagne VL, Okamura N: In vivo tau imaging: obstacles and progress. Alzheimers Dement 10:S254–S264, 2014.
63. Goldman JS, Rademakers R, Huey ED, et al: An algorithm for genetic testing of frontotemporal lobar degeneration. Neurology 76:475–483, 2011.
64. Van Langenhove T, van der Zee J, Gijselinck I, et al: Distinct clinical characteristics of C9orf72 expansion carriers compared with GRN, MAPT, and nonmutation carriers in a Flanders-Belgian FTLD cohort. JAMA Neurol 70:365–373, 2013.
77. Tsai RM, Boxer AL: Treatment of frontotemporal dementia. Curr Treat Options Neurol 16:319, 2014.

55 Delirium

Eamonn Eeles, Daniel Davis, Ravi Bhat

INTRODUCTION

Delirium represents an acute disorder of consciousness. Serially time-ordered, organized, and with reflective awareness of self and the environment, consciousness also represents an experience of graded complexity and quality. It follows that disturbance of consciousness as part of delirium is accompanied by impairments in arousal, attention, thinking, perception, and memory.[1] A temporary dissolution of the mind poses grave vulnerability through impaired communication of personal needs and flawed execution of function amid a cocktail of aberrant behavior. Frailty and illness collide, and so disturbance in mobility, falls and fractures, and pressure ulceration add to the burden of illness. Although delirium can persist, usually it resolves in the setting of good premorbid cognition in community-dwelling older adults. Even so, its legacy can be far reaching and often negatively impacts all measured clinical outcomes (risk of dementia, functional decline, institutionalization, and mortality) and is most capricious in cases of persistent delirium.[2,3]

Delirium is derived from the Latin *dēlīrāre*, meaning "out of the furrow," and has long been recognized as a disturbance in the train of thinking.[4] Indeed, the meaning of delirium has undergone much iteration over the past 200 years, but descriptions of delirium from medical text,[5] philosophical verse,[6] and even fables[7] have maintained considerable stability over time and space.

As delirium most commonly develops in frail older adults, it most frequently arises in hospitals and long-term care facilities. It should be widely accepted that delirium sufferers are among the sickest and most vulnerable patients in hospitals and management is often poor.[8] Patients with delirium are also the first to suffer when care standards fall. Delirium remains fervently and stubbornly underrecognized. This undoubtedly contributes further to the burden of morbidity.

Evolution of the Delirium Concept and Diagnostic Criteria

Disturbance of consciousness is a characteristic feature of delirium that distinguishes it from the classical form of Alzheimer disease. It has been the hardest feature to operationalize.[4] Greiner's development of the concept "clouding of consciousness" in delirium[9] can be understood in the context of the nineteenth-century view of impairments in consciousness represented as "organic" brain disease.[10] "Clouding" has come to refer to both a state of lowered arousal between alertness and coma[11] and a denseness of the medium in which psychic events occur.[12] Geschwind's influential views,[13] based mainly on studies of delirium in younger adults,[14] paved the way for operationalization of delirium as an attentional disorder in modern classificatory systems.[15] However, disturbance of attention is not the only cognitive disorder seen in, neither is it the sole preserve of, delirium.[16] So how does the role of consciousness relate to delirium, and how may this assist physicians with diagnosis?

One way of describing consciousness is the state in which all waking thoughts are marshaled and temporally organized and expressed. There is no thought content that, in the study of delirium symptoms, has not in some way been disrupted. Unless there is a recess of consciousness beyond sentinel thought, then it follows that disturbance of consciousness must be axiomatic to a diagnosis of delirium.[17] Consciousness embodies a duality of reflection, subserved through a parallel but binary functional network. Experientially, conscious thought is divided into reflection (default mode) and goal-related (task positive) states, respectively. Functional magnetic resonance imaging (MRI) data would suggest a reversible reduction in resting state connectivity in relation to delirium status to support this premise and reduced task induced deactivation of DMN regions.[18] These perspectives on the relationship between consciousness and delirium provide a conceptual model for research in delirium. Temporally ordered awareness, and consciousness, is a macrostate property whose construct belies definition and prediction according to the component parts.[19] In other words, the condition of consciousness is imbued by central nervous system (CNS) complexity but cannot easily be explained by it. At the event horizon, where consciousness breaks down and the status of delirium is conferred, all such higher function is perturbed with loss of temporal ordering of information being key.[20] Reduced intercortical connectivity is attributed to loss of CNS hierarchy. Lower order, reflexive structures within the primitive brain and limbic system are then left to drive behavior.[21]

Conventionally, attention was related also with consciousness level (arousal) in the International Classification of Diseases (ICD) and earlier iterations of the *Diagnostic and Statistical Manual of Mental Disorders* (DSM). Both attention and arousal are hierarchically related: it is possible to have full arousal but profound inattention (in hypervigilance), but the converse is not true.[22] It is interesting that the fifth edition of the DSM (DSM-5) has abrogated consciousness in favor of its handmaiden, awareness.[23] There are implicit threats that inclusion of awareness, displacement of low arousal states and consciousness from a diagnosis of delirium may bring.[22] To redress this diagnostic schism, it is important to consider alternative ways in which consciousness, as it relates to delirium, can be operationalized. Arousal still remains an important construct in explaining the spectrum of behavior in delirium.

Clinical Features

Abnormal arousal ranges from the hyperalert-hyperactive state often accompanied by hallucinations, illusions, and delusions (so-called hyperactive delirium) to a state of somnolence and hypoalertness (so-called hypoactive delirium).[24] Whereas the archetypal image of delirium is the hyperactive state with psychosis, older patients are more likely to experience mixed states (lying in bed or fluctuating between states of hyperalertness and somnolence).[25] "Activated" features are overrepresented on screening and diagnostic criteria, leaving hypoactive delirium most vulnerable to underrecognition[26,27] if placid behavior had not already succeeded in this. The subtype of delirium that is most easily missed may also be associated with the worst outcome.[28] An approach to recognition is to systematizing psychomotor behavior or, more inclusively, arousal. Concentrating on the core features common to all subtypes is a practical solution not without merit. We can posit that inability to engage represents severe inattention and acute low-arousal states equate with inattention and cognitive disruption. These phenomena are as much a delirium that is indistinguishable from delirium diagnosed on the basis of cognitive testing and interview. Not only is this approach conceptually grounded, but it also offers a means of unifying the spectrum of divergent behavior as part of the syndrome.

Cases in which attention is testable offer a portal to consciousness and shine a light on the presence or absence of delirium.[29] Staff involved in daily care of older people often have difficulty in formally assessing inattention and thus may not recognize delirium.[30] Interviewing a patient over a 2-minute period can be a simple way to assess attention, and the Edinburgh Delirium Test Box (and smartphone app) has been developed for this purpose.[31]

Altered arousal detected through use of tools such as the modified Richmond Agitation Sedation Scale (m-RASS) may be fairly specific to delirium,[32] particularly when attention is difficult to quantify.

Time disorientation is commonly measured best by nursing staff in hospitals[33]; is a useful guide to the presence and severity of dementia or delirium in older hospital patients[34]; and, when present at admission, is a risk factor for delirium at follow-up.[35]

What is the impact of these disruptions in conscious flow on an individual level? Many patients experience temporal dislocation (i.e., simultaneously encountered past and present) entwined with the misperception of imagination as reality.[36] Commonly, patients recount visions of a frightening, morbid, or sinister nature. Within psychosis, hallucinations (visual or auditory) and delusions may be elicited and can be disturbing to patients and those around them. Delusions and hallucinations may evoke recall distress in those who remember their delirium, even after recovery.[36]

Acuity of onset, usually over hours to days, in conjunction with fluctuation, is a core feature of, but not peculiar to, delirium.[37] Triangulation of history (from patients, relatives, clinical staff)—to characterize the presentation, recognize the duration of onset, and probe for possible triggers—is mandatory.

Differential Diagnoses

Most patients who arrive at the hospital with acute dementia have, or will develop, delirium (32% to 89%).[38] Because the clinical features may be similar, behavioral changes in an individual with dementia can mistakenly be normalized by the contribution of environmental change or perceived as a natural sequela of dementia (or indeed aging itself). Greater than expected (although what constitutes an "expected" amount is difficult to standardize) deterioration in cognition, along with new onset of hallucinations and delusions, is suggestive of a delirium superimposed on dementia (DSD) that has not been captured by rating scales.[39] The core problem with DSD is that the reference standards for delirium and dementia[23,40] propose the syndromes as being mutually exclusive. It is clear this is far from common experience. Few of the assessment tools for delirium even included dementia patients,[39] although validation studies for more recently developed scales report the diagnostic accuracy in participants with and without dementia.[41,42]

Variability in symptoms is also a characteristic of dementia with Lewy bodies (DLB), and the psychopathologic similarities of visual hallucinations and disrupted sleep cycle add another masquerade.[43] Avoidance of typical psychotropic agents, in any patient with Parkinsonian features, helps prevent characteristic neuroleptic sensitivity associated with the disorder. Depression and delirium may share negative symptoms and even a broad range of cognitive deficits. The mood and behavioral changes observed as part of the delirium syndrome, particularly hypoactive delirium, may account for the tendency to misdiagnose the two conditions. Rapidity of onset, relative inattention, and impaired arousal in the acute hospital setting usually reliably guides clinicians to a diagnosis of delirium. Also not to be ignored are the less frequent but potent causes of delirium that arise from primary CNS disorder that can be classified broadly into lesions or infection, particularly when the clinical picture is associated with focal neurologic signs, fever, or both. Acute cognitive decline may be observed also in patients with strategic infarct dementia.[44]

It is worth noting specialized investigation for those disorders where overlap or cause by a CNS disorder is suspected. The electroencephalogram (EEG) offers an adjunct to clinical assessment. Well described and replicated, the pattern of "diffuse slowing"[45] on EEG can help to distinguish a delirium from the following conditions: DSD,[46] temporal lobe epilepsy, depression, and nonconvulsive status epilepticus.[47] The EEG is useful in defining more peculiar CNS causes of delirium, such as limbic encephalitis and Creutzfeldt-Jacob disease.[48] Although the EEG is still valid for use in an older population,[49] a level of patient compliance is required that is not reliably achievable in patients in a delirious state. It therefore remains a diagnostic adjunct to the more challenging differential diagnoses outlined but does not replace the less invasive and more responsive focus of robust, bedside clinical and cognitive assessment.

Behavioral and psychological symptoms of dementia are also difficult to distinguish from DSD, compounded by the fact that neither has a reference-standard definition in the DSM or ICD.[23,40] A pragmatic approach would maintain that acute change in cognitive, arousal, or perceptual symptoms in existing dementia should prompt the search for a general medical precipitant.[50]

Prevalence

Delirium afflicts most acutely hospitalized, frail, older patients. In-hospital reported rates of delirium vary widely, typically 20% to 30%,[51] and are a propensity of the magnitude of the frailty and illness severity burden. The emergency department mixes increasing presentations of older patients with acute illness[52] and extrapolates to a prevalence of delirium of between 7% and 20%.[53] Clinicians who are more removed from the distal consequences of delirium in the emergency department setting often fail to undertake cognitive assessment.[54] Even when cognitive assessment is performed, it does not always register with a diagnosis of delirium or affect management. System pressures within an emergency department, through the prism of patient flow, do not readily enhance the landscape of care for patients with delirium. Overbearing management as a substitute for deft clinical problem solving does little to aid those "butterflies at the wheel" at risk of delirium.[55] Optimization of care aligned to the needs of the older patient in the emergency department is not insurmountable; an education program with geriatrician support has been advocated as a simple way of improving care delivery,[56] and recent work suggests delirium is finally emerging as a priority in the emergency department.[22,57]

The orthogeriatric population is host to a 4% to 53% postoperative incidence of delirium following hip fracture.[58] Similarly, the intensive care unit is a potent conflagration of illness severity as to be inevitably bound with delirium and a prevalence of 80% in older patients.[59]

Delirium also transgresses beyond the acute sector, most commonly as a continuous episode through discharge from hospital.[60] Even at conservative estimates, delirium and subsyndromal delirium still represent a significant and largely unexplored health burden in postacute facilities.[61]

Many, if not most, individuals dying from chronic illness, regardless of location, experience confusion.[62] An inability to separate those who die with delirium, as opposed to those who die from delirium, possibly conflates the bleak survival figures.[63] As yet, nothing within the delirium syndrome offers the ability to distinguish a temporarily recoverable process from a "terminal drop." However, in late stages of dementia, a phase of chronic delirium often may not resolve even after due diligence to cause, earning the epithet "delentia."[2]

Multicomponent intervention strategies have had little impact on outcomes in the palliative care setting,[64] and contemporary studies are needed. An interdisciplinary and consensus-driven focus is advised with goals of treatment not adding to the burden of the dying process.

DELIRIUM AND DEMENTIA: PATHOPHYSIOLOGY

An emerging literature indicates that delirium is a strong predictor of new-onset dementia as well as acceleration of existing cognitive decline.[65] This is consistent across different settings: after hospitalization[66]; in those with dementia[67,68]; in postoperative patients[69]; after critical care[70]; and in community populations.[61,65] Prospectively linking delirium with permanent decrements in cognitive function challenges the construct of dementia because it suggests that dementia pathophysiology may be affected by processes outside the brain.

Experimental Models

It is convenient to consider two mechanisms for brain injury in the context of acute illness: direct and indirect.[71] Direct brain insults include hypoxemia, stroke, trauma, or medications. In such conditions, brain dysfunction evidently arises as a direct consequence of the pathologic process.

Usually, acute pathology arises in the periphery (e.g., infection/inflammation, pain). A unifying idea is that aberrant stress responses have an impact on brain and brain function.[71,72] There are a number of routes through which systemic processes in the periphery can have an effect on the brain. Inflammatory mediators can interact directly with neurons in areas where the blood-brain barrier is deficient, neurohumoral connections communicate directly through the vagus nerve, and endothelial glial cells can transmit cytokine signals into the brain parenchyma.

Neuroendocrine axes responsible for managing the normal stress response can become pathologically disrupted such that delirium is precipitated, sustained, or both. For example, glucocorticoid regulation through the hypothalamic-pituitary-adrenal (HPA) axis is vital, because sustained high levels may lead to chronic activation of low-affinity receptors, and this, in itself, is cytotoxic (e.g., Cushing disease). Reciprocally, it is known that chronic neurodegeneration in the limbic system leads to dysregulation of the HPA axis so the higher order control of the cortisol response can become exaggerated. Together, these situate neuroinflammatory and neuroendocrine mechanisms as "aberrant stress mediators."

At a cellular level, it is understood that neurodegenerative conditions such as Alzheimer disease can initiate responses from microglia, the resident monocyte/macrophage system in CNS.[73] Morphologically activated microglia can adopt a wide number of functional phenotypes, determined by a range of conditions. Crucially, microglial responses to neurodegeneration are on a spectrum from M1 (classical macrophage activity) to M2 (growth-repair functions). Thus, these immunologic phenotypes may be deleterious (enhancing neurodegeneration) or beneficial (clearing amyloid deposits). In animal models, microglia have been shown to migrate to new amyloid plaques.[74] In vitro, microglial receptors (e.g., Toll-like receptor 4) can contribute to innate immunity through clearing amyloid plaques.[75] Although the regulatory mechanisms are not completely understood, it appears that the predominant response to amyloid is not overly aggressive and, indeed, may be antiinflammatory in part; taken together, these result in microglial priming. Microglial priming is a key concept and represents a state whereby glia are morphologically activated but not proinflammatory. However, this primed state can result in phenotypic switching in response to an inflammatory challenge. One such murine model of delirium based upon a primed neurodegenerative state exhibits a delirium-like syndrome only in conjunction with an exaggerated proinflammatory cytokine response to peripheral inflammatory challenge. Furthermore, microglia express cyclooxygenase-1, and prostaglandin-mediated cognitive dysfunction can be blocked by nonsteroidal antiinflammatory drugs, suggesting therapeutic opportunities.[76]

Cerebrospinal Fluid Biomarkers

A range of biomarkers have been considered in cerebrospinal fluid (CSF) studies of delirium, although generally, studies have been small and with little overlap.[77] Age and concomitant dementia are always likely to be major confounders, and this is not always adequately addressed. Nonetheless, at least in perioperative hip fracture, there is some preliminary evidence that stress (cortisol), inflammation (interleukins [IL-1β, IL-6, IL-8]), and direct astrocyte injury (calcium-binding protein B [S100B]) are involved.[78] Interestingly, in the major study to examine CSF β-amyloid 1-42, tau, and phosphorylated-tau, levels were not associated with delirium status, perhaps suggesting that postoperative delirium arises through pathophysiologic pathways distinct from Alzheimer disease altogether.[79]

Neuroimaging

Many attempts to image people with concurrent delirium are unsuccessful. In addition, there is a more general bias selecting younger and fitter participants amenable to scanning, especially if using intensive protocols such as MRI.

Studies to date have been small, with significant heterogeneity in populations.[80] The largest prospective cohort examined neuroimaging correlates of delirium after critical illness.[81] Longer duration of delirium was associated with smaller brain volume and more white matter disruption, and both of these correlated with worse cognitive scores 1 year later. Further, white-matter hyperintensities have been shown to be associated with delirium after elective cardiac surgery.[82]

Clinical Models

Delirium arises from the synchronized assault of multiple interacting factors. Causation in medicine is often associated with the idea of a single cause that arose from the success of the germ theory in the nineteenth century.[83]

Given the conceptual limitations, development of a model of delirium has been refined to incorporate predisposing and precipitating factors.[84] Consistently identified, independently associated predisposing factors include older age, male gender, visual impairment, dementia and cognitive impairment, depression, functional dependence, immobility, alcoholism, increased comorbid conditions, previous stroke, and azotemia and share frailty as an underlying theme. Similarly, independently associated precipitating factors include medications, such as sedative hypnotics and narcotics in toxicity or withdrawal, similarly for delirium tremens; severe acute illness; infections, especially urinary tract infections; metabolic abnormalities, especially hyponatremia; hypoxemia; shock; anemia; pain; physical restraint use; bladder catheter use; any iatrogenic event; intensive care unit treatment; surgeries; and high number of procedures in hospital.[85] From this list it is then possible to identify individuals who are predisposed to delirium upon whom preventative interventions have been successfully implemented.[86] However, this model, although superficially similar to the vulnerability-stress models used in psychiatry,[87] has implicit assumptions that may not hold true in the context of delirium. Risk factors such as male gender are useful in predicting delirium but, unlike vulnerabilities, do not provide a template for causal mechanism. Moreover, the temporal separation between predisposing and precipitating factors may be relatively short, making isolation of vulnerability and stress an arbitrary distinction. Finally, the model fails to account for the many dynamic interactions between illnesses, physiologic states, and interventions that typically occur in the setting of delirium.

So how may we speculate on cause in delirium and under what conceptual framework? Illness can be considered as the somatic anomaly and its current or potential manifestations.[88] In older patients, each somatic anomaly individually is not sufficiently provocative enough to generate a delirium. Therefore, global health measures pertinent to an older population, such as frailty, may provide a summative insight to risk that is perhaps easier to conceptualize with regard to the entity of delirium. Frailty appears to be associated with elevated rates of delirium,[89] but this is debatable according to the phenotypic model of frailty.[90] Thus, geriatric syndromes, such as delirium, arise when frail individuals with multiple deficits are on the brink of failure. When complex systems fail, it is their highest order functions that manifest disturbance. Consciousness is one such high-order function within a complex system yielding to failure in the context of frailty. Cognitive chaos is observed where functional integration of the CNS unravels and reflexive but poorly formed urges take to the streets.[19] This accounts for why delirium symptoms are so broad and why tracking other higher state variables, such as mobility and balance, as markers of delirium progress makes sense. If the classical (as in systemic level) conceptual framework for delirium relates to complex system dynamics, then what is observed at a quantum and cellular level?

Investigations into biomarkers for delirium are still in their infancy, although some have focused on putative pathophysiologic links between delirium and dementia in clinical populations.[72,73,74,76,91] Insofar as the biologic mediators of delirium may result in permanent neuronal damage, four systems have come to attention: specific Alzheimer pathology, S100B, cortisol, and inflammatory cytokines.

In a cohort of individuals with hip fracture, postoperative delirium was strongly associated with premorbid cognitive decline, although this was not associated with CSF β-amyloid 1-42, tau, and phosphorylated-tau levels.[92] This study was underpowered to detect mediating pathways between premorbid cognitive impairment, biomarkers of Alzheimer pathology, and subsequent delirium. Nonetheless, consistent with the Vantaa study of epidemiologic pathology, postoperative delirium might be understood as arising through pathophysiologic pathways distinct from Alzheimer disease.

S100B, a marker of astrocyte damage, has been shown to be elevated in delirium, both in plasma and in CSF.[93,94]

The HPA axis may be dysregulated in delirium and dementia. Chronic hypercortisolemia is directly cytotoxic (e.g., cognitive impairment in Cushing disease), and aberrant stress responses may be a core feature of delirium.[95] Moreover, neurodegeneration in the limbic system may lead to inappropriately sustained cortisol after a stress response, and delirium itself is associated with elevated CSF cortisol levels.[96]

Although these studies are small and require cautious interpretation, this accumulating evidence lends support for the impact of delirium itself contributing to, and/or being a mediator of, permanent cognitive impairment.

Prevention of Delirium

Landmark multicomponent intervention studies by Inouye and coworkers[97] built on their predictive model to address risk factors for delirium in medical patients. The Yale Delirium Prevention Trial comprised optimizing multiple states including orientation, promoting early mobilization, preventing sleep deprivation, prescribing minimal psychotropic drugs, addressing vision and hearing, and correcting hydration. Improvement in rates of delirium, by approximately one third, followed. These earlier multicomponent prevention studies have been replicated in numerous other cohorts of medical patients with broadly generalizable results[98] and are at least cost-neutral to implement.

The evidence for prevention of delirium is compelling where the patient population is less heterogeneous, such as a surgical setting. A large study of proactive geriatric consultation versus usual care was undertaken in the setting of hip fracture.[99] The recommendations made—essentially basic aspects of good care—achieved a reduction of 33% in cases of delirium compared with usual care. Multicomponent intervention strategies have been integrated into what is expected as a standard of care.[100]

Reorientation strategies may be a potent intervention.[101] It appears that the closer the reorientation is embedded within the medium of familiarity, as family-provided reorientation strategies have shown, the greater the therapeutic margin will be.[102] By extension, the most potent reorientation strategy would be management of a patient in his or her own home and may represent a light on the hill for future delirium management.

The role of drugs in prevention is debatable, with some support for haloperidol and second-generation antipsychotics. Melatonin has recently been shown to not reduce delirium among patients in intensive care.[103] The major trial for cholinesterase inhibitors resulted in early termination because of increased mortality in the intervention arm,[104] although convincing trials outside the critically ill population have yet to be conducted.

The role of life course approaches to risk of delirium has received scant attention. Pluripotent strategies, such as exercise and nutrition, reduce the incidence of both dementia and burden of frailty with primary prevention of delirium a sound clinical, research, and epidemiologic focus.

Delirium Evaluation

Untreated delirium represents an excess risk of adverse event through pressure ulcers, falls, and fractures. In delirium, as with other geriatric syndromes, multiple common pathologies associated with aging, and their treatments, are most often responsible and can be evaluated in the main without redress to invasive procedures. First, recognizing that delirium is a sensitive marker of illness should trigger a sensible and proportionate screen for underlying causes, namely, medications (toxicity), medications (withdrawal), medications (recreational), infections, cardiac or organ failure, metabolic issues, endocrine factors, or some combination of these.[105] The presence of multiple comorbidity and polypharmacy challenges standardized treatment regimens. An individualized approach to management of the cause in a frail, older patient should be considered.

The role of ergonomic screening tools in the detection of delirium is elevated given that underrecognition remains, and the many tools, including the most commonly cited instrument, the Confusion Assessment Method,[106] require formal training and a degree of experience to actualize the published psychomotor performance.[107] An abundance of screening tools abound but simple, easy-to-administer and still valid instruments are relatively sparse. The 4AT[42] is one such new tool that has encouraging psychometric properties, can be used without prior training, and can be interpreted even when patients are unable to participate (i.e., at low arousal states). Other tools such as the SQiD[108] and SQeeC[109] are novel, brief, and promising for their respective ease of use, and further research is awaited.

Drug Treatment

The role of cholinesterase inhibitors in delirium has been studied with the intent of correcting the central cholinergic deficit described as part of the syndrome. Donepezil has failed to demonstrate a benefit in terms of reduction in the incidence of delirium although larger studies are called for.[104] Most recently, haloperidol was found to reduce the incidence of delirium in a surgical population.[110] However, inconsistent findings in the literature with respect to haloperidol, both in terms of prevention and management, twinned with potential side effects, thwart its recommendation for use in standard practice.[111] Atypical antipsychotics such as quetiapine, by contrast, offer less in the way of extrapyramidal side effects and are associated with a reduction in duration of delirium symptoms.[112] Metabolic complications and association with increased risk of stroke remain important considerations with some of the atypical drugs. Impairment in enzymes of drug metabolism in delirious individuals should also temper dosaging strategies.[113] Other agents, such as dexmedetomidine, ketamine, and clonidine, are candidate therapies in the critically ill cohort.[114] It remains that drugs are not an alternative for best care and should be deliberated over only when adequate nonpharmacologic management strategies have been implemented or when a crisis forces the hand of pharmacotherapy.

Management of Delirium

Multicomponent intervention strategies have been developed to correct the multifactorial cause of delirium (Table 55-1). Approach to management, in patients with delirium who may not be able to express their requirements, is best summarized as an adaptation, intuition, and redressing of Maslow hierarchy of (unmet) needs. A moment of reflection to consider why such a perspective is warranted is worthwhile. Sensory impairment is an example of a defined risk factor targeted in management strategies (and prevention).[97,98] To fulfill place orientation, one needs to assimilate sensory information to construct a geographic reference. Sensory deficits, such as visual impairment, are accrued with advancing age, so as to be almost saturated in a population of octogenarians. Visual loss may be compensated for in a person's familiar environment, with reinforced cues to maintain orientation. However, the hospital presents myriad novel sensory stimuli that adversely interact with protagonist deficiencies. Inability to selectively process this overstimulating external information as part of attention deficit within delirium can lead to misperception of sensory signals and resultant hallucinations or illusions to compound a fragmented internal map. The individual, by way of disorganized thinking, may also be rendered unable to express his or her level of spatial orientation or be oblivious to its relevance. It then becomes clear how optimization of sensory function (e.g., by making sure the patient has a clean pair of glasses) is an important standard of care in older hospitalized patients.

However, most management studies exploring multicomponent intervention principles, à la prevention studies, have been equivocal in terms of outcome.[115,116] Delirium, in a surgical setting

TABLE 55-1 Priorities (Consensus, Evidence-Based, and Speculative) for the Prevention, Management, and Advancement of the Treatment of Delirium

Community-Based Prevention	Hospital-Based Prevention	Hospital-Based Management	Postdischarge Management	Clinical Research Opportunities
Hospital avoidance strategies	Implementation of basic standards (e.g., screening for delirium) Minimization of iatrogenesis†	Implementation of basic standards (e.g., review of medications)†	Responsive, proportionate, and holistic follow-up†	Pragmatic research into optimizing care delivery
Identification and management of frailty	Multicomponent interventions to address frailty‡ Reorientation‡ Nutrition‡ Multidisciplinary care† Physiologic correction‡ Sensory optimization‡ Minimization of ward transfers† Avoidance of polypharmacy‡	Multicomponent interventions to address frailty† Reorientation† Nutrition† Multidisciplinary care† Physiologic correction† Sensory optimization† Minimization of ward transfers† Reduction of drug burden†	Identification and management of frailty Reduction and cessation of antipsychotics	The interaction between frailty, interventions to ameliorate frailty, and delirium Transference from basic science models to trials of newer therapies Validation of delirium models using advanced imaging
Pleiotropic interventions (e.g., exercise/ nutrition)	Monitor and promote early mobilization‡	Monitor and promote early mobilization†	Review of the primary triggers for delirium and other state variables (e.g., mobility)	Delirium, mobility, and response to physical therapy
Early diagnosis and management of dementia	Screening for dementia†	Screening for delirium resolution and residual cognitive impairment	Screening for subsyndromal delirium or dementia†	The interaction between dementia, including non-Alzheimer dementia, and delirium
Education of nursing home facilities and staff	Education of nursing and medical staff†	Education of medical and nursing staff†	Caregiver support and education	The role of education of nonmedical staff, families,* and general public using multimedia solutions
Integrated geriatric care for planned major surgery	Targeted drug treatments (e.g., melatonin for sleep disturbance)‡ Family-based screening/ reorientation‡	Delirium units Supported early discharge Family-based screening/ reorientation† Management in the nursing home with CGA capability	Adaptive and versatile methods of follow-up such as telemedicine	The role of novel and targeted interventions and models of care supported by assistive technologies
Public health awareness	Audit of care and cycle of care improvement†	Audit of care and cycle of care improvement†	Public health awareness/ NGO engagement	Development of key indicators in the management of delirium

*Speculative role.
†Consensus role.
‡Evidence-based role.

at least, is amenable to reduction in duration and severity, but these benefits do not extend to the medical population. Good geriatric care may hasten recovery from delirium with sustained cognitive outcomes at 1 year[116] but with debatable longer term and cost-effectiveness value. Delirium units have been shown to reduce mortality, but further studies are needed.[117]

Consensus-based guidelines in the management of delirium have occupied this deficiency.[118] Experts have a high level of agreement over recommendations even if their application is often weak. DSD, or the elephant superimposed on the room, remains insufficiently considered.

Why Delirium Is So Poorly Managed and Future Directions

Delirium is poorly recognized. The failure to identify delirium as a clinical diagnosis may be a function of its mercurial and protean presentation but is rarely due to a surfeit of understanding of delirium.[105] Recognition, particularly early detection, remains pivotal and can improve outcomes. Interventions for other disorders that visibly affect patient outcome have revolutionized how such conditions are perceived, such as thrombolysis in stroke. Delirium may lack such a single dramatic intervention. Reinforcement, or even justification of, therapeutic nihilism occupies the void and gives rise to the purity of impotence.

Understanding the needs of the known delirious patient may be a further challenge. Aberrant attribution of behavior to aging; lack of awareness of screening tools, with frequent reliance on levels of orientation only; insufficient knowledge of cognitive disorders; poor use of collateral nursing history; and the caregiver toll have an impact on recognition of delirium.[119] Philosophical orientation of nurses to health and aging may influence recognition. In one study, nurses using a healthful perspective (i.e., regarding "good health" in aging as normal) were most likely to differentiate between acute confusion and chronic confusion.[120] Among doctors, trainee physicians recognize that delirium is common, serious, distressing, and treatable.[121] However, they lacked confidence in their diagnostic and management skills. Delirium education may thus have to address both teaching of clinical skills and enhancing the ability to question stereotypes. Educational strategies provide an improved knowledge base for clinicians and translate to better detection rates for delirium.

The Problem Is Not With Our Stars

In delirium, we are less like ourselves and occupy a self that is abroad in the world. If what makes us notionally self and a fellowship with humanity—in other words, consciousness—has been lost, albeit transiently, then what are the implications? If, in the moment of illness, an individual "deviates from the furrow" from what is recognizably and acceptably human, does this offer a reason why care is different or even an excuse for it? If the traits that make us identify with humanity (i.e., communication, empathy, and autonomy) are lost in the individual with delirium, this opens the possibility of mechanistic dehumanization. The target may be viewed, counter to Immanuel Kant's theory of morality, as a means to an end.[122] In this sense, the scenario described by the Francis report wherein patients with delirium were given antipsychotics to quell their behavior (rather than an approach to understand and manage the causes) can be viewed as a failure facilitated by dehumanization.[8] The categorical imperative was breached; patient-drug interaction was the means by which the end, improved behavior, was sought rather than an understanding and treatment of the causes of behavioral change. At an institutional level, such practices may be considered as a window to the soul of the cultural attitudes of individual hospitals.[123] Only by recognizing that despite the loss, usually transient, of sentience, patients retain inviolable human characteristics, encapsulated by the trait of dignity. Their human needs are often accentuated by their lack of agency and sickness combined, while external signals to their deficiency may be less apparent. A systematic approach to considering and addressing unmet needs may help the unwary practitioner to practically deal with what can be a challenging management situation.

FUTURE DIRECTIONS

Delirium as a Disorder of Arousal

DSM-5 affords an opportunity to examine the fundamental construct of delirium. The specific mention of arousal is important. While coma should not be regarded as delirium, all other states of abnormal arousal are described as indicating de facto inattention. Acute illness, underlying dementia, and superimposed delirium all interact to affect level of arousal. The extent to which each has an impact on cognitive and functional outcomes urgently warrants research.

Clinical Assessment

The plurality of available assessment scales probably suggests that no one tool is suitable for all purposes. Understanding how the diagnostic accuracy of any tool varies with setting and degree of training is crucial. An attempt to test clinical models of delirium at a functional level and with novel techniques is important. Also key is the proportion of comorbid dementia in the assessment population, and there is increasing tendency to report this in validation studies. Formal cognitive testing is often not possible because of low arousal, but few tools operationalize this. Head-to-head comparisons in the context of randomized controlled trials will help determine which scales work best in practice. For the whole field, greater detail in each publication on the operational approach for any reference standard is strongly desirable.[124]

Pathophysiology

There is no doubt that more experimental work is required, but the development of meaningful cognitive and behavioral animal models to explore possible hypotheses has not been straightforward. There is likely to be a range of existing animal research in fields relevant to delirium but not engaged with clinical investigations. Examples might include neuroinflammation in sepsis, vasculopathy in the blood-brain barrier, and microbiome impact on encephalopathy. Experimental researchers in these areas may not even be aware of the clinical construct of delirium; this unawareness can lead to missed opportunities for translational collaboration. Ultimately, there is a need for an infrastructure to engage and cross-fertilize with experimental researchers in a wide range of fields.

Public Health Directions

The public health impact of dementia is widely acknowledged and the relevance of delirium's role in highlighting cognitive impairment will become more prominent. Dementia care within acute hospitals needs to be closely aligned with delirium care. Delirium/dementia-friendly hospitals will be the norm. Crucially, studies demonstrating that delirium care is cost-effective will be a potent driver to change. Innovative practices in delirium education will also help, as will a more conscious approach to knowledge translation.[125,126]

Public Engagement

Thankfully, awareness of delirium is increasing among health professionals. However, there have not been any large-scale attempts to engage the public on delirium. The term is hardly used among patients and reasons for this are not clear. Greater efforts from the scientific and clinical research communities, perhaps in conjunction with aging-related third sector organizations, to increase public understanding are necessary. Such efforts will be rewarded by highlighting need for research funding and also improving standards of care.

KEY POINTS

- Delirium is a common and underrecognized disorder among institutionalized and frail older patients.
- Understanding delirium as a disorder of consciousness content assists with appreciating clinical disturbance in arousal, time perception, and attention.
- Standardized screening tools that are valid and easy to administer are essential.
- Delirium prevention and management are achieved through multifactorial interventions that reflect addressing the common problems encountered in older individuals.
- Education strategies improve knowledge and recognition of delirium and should be tailored to the health professional.
- A growing understanding of the science of delirium is emerging, and targeted candidate therapeutic agents are a focus of future research.

For a complete list of references, please visit www.expertconsult.com.

KEY REFERENCES

4. Lipowski LZ: Delirium: Acute confusional states, New York, 1990, Oxford University Press.
11. Plum F, Posner JB: The diagnosis of stupor and coma, ed 3, Philadelphia, 1982, FA Davis.
18. Choi SH, Lee H, Chung TS, et al: Neural network functional connectivity during and after an episode of delirium. Am J Psychiatry 169:498–507, 2012.
20. Bhat R, Rockwood K: Delirium as a disorder of consciousness. J Neurol Neurosurg Psychiatry 78:1167–1170, 2007.
22. European Delirium Association, American Delirium Society: The DSM 5 criteria, level of arousal and delirium diagnosis: inclusiveness is safer. BMC Med 12:141, 2014.
36. Bhat R: Psychotic symptoms in delirium. In Hassett A, Ames D, Chiu E, editors: Psychosis in the elderly, London, 2005, Taylor & Francis, pp 135–148.
42. Bellelli G, Morandi A, Davis DH, et al: Validation of the 4AT, a new instrument for rapid delirium screening: a study in 234 hospitalised older people. Age Ageing 43:496–502, 2014.
45. Romano J, Engel GL: Delirium I. Electroencephalographic data. Arch Neurol Psychiatry 51:356–377, 1944.
61. Davis DH, Barnes LE, Stephan BC, et al: The descriptive epidemiology of delirium symptoms in a large population-based cohort study: results from the Medical Research Council Cognitive Function and Ageing Study (MRC CFAS). BMC Geriatr 14:87, 2014.
63. Eeles EM, Hubbard RE, White SV, et al: Hospital use, institutionalisation and mortality associated with delirium. Age Ageing 39:470–475, 2010.
65. Davis DH, Muniz Terrera G, et al: Delirium is a strong risk factor for dementia in the oldest-old: a population-based cohort study. Brain 135(Pt 9):2809–2816, 2012.
66. Witlox J, Eurelings LSM, De Jonghe JFM, et al: Delirium in elderly patients and the risk of postdischarge mortality, institutionalization, and dementia: a meta-analysis. JAMA 304:443–451, 2010.
72. Cunningham C, Wilcockson DC, Campion S, et al: Central and systemic endotoxin challenges exacerbate the local inflammatory response and increase neuronal death during chronic neurodegeneration. J Neurosci 25:9275–9284, 2005.
76. Hshieh TT, Fong TG, Marcantonio ER, et al: Cholinergic deficiency hypothesis in delirium: a synthesis of current evidence. J Gerontol A Biol Sci Med Sci 63:764–772, 2008.
77. Hall RJ, Shenkin SD, Maclullich AM: A systematic literature review of cerebrospinal fluid biomarkers in delirium. Dement Geriatr Cogn Disord 32:79–93, 2011.
84. Inouye SK, Charpentier PA: Precipitating factors for delirium in hospitalized elderly persons. Predictive model and interrelationship with baseline vulnerability. JAMA 275:852–857, 1996.
90. Joosten E, Demuynck M, Detroyer E, et al: Prevalence of frailty and its ability to predict in hospital delirium, falls, and 6-month mortality in hospitalised older patients. BMC Geriatr 14:1, 2014.
94. Van Munster BC, Korevaar JC, Korse CM, et al: Serum S100B in elderly patients with and without delirium. Int J Geriatr Psychiatry 25:234–239, 2010.
100. O'Mahony R, Murthy L, Akunne A, et al: Guideline Development Group: Synopsis of the National Institute for Health and Clinical Excellence guideline for prevention of delirium. Ann Intern Med 154:746–751, 2011.
106. Inouye SK, van Dyck CH, Alessi CA, et al: Clarifying confusion: the confusion assessment method. A new method for detection of delirium. Ann Intern Med 113:941–948, 1990.
109. Lin S, Eeles E, Pandy S, et al: Screening in delirium: a pilot study of two screening tools, the Simple Query for Easy Evaluation of Consciousness (SQeeC) and Simple Question in Delirium (SQiD). Australas J Ageing 2015. [Epub ahead of print].
112. Tahir TA, Eeles E, Karapareddy V, et al: A randomized controlled trial of quetiapine versus placebo in the treatment of delirium. J Psychosom Res 69:485–490, 2010.
116. Pitkälä KH, Laurila JV, Strandberg TE, et al: Multicomponent geriatric intervention for elderly inpatients with delirium: a randomized, controlled trial. J Gerontol A Biol Sci Med Sci 61:176–181, 2006.

56 Mental Illness in Older Adults

Chris Fox, Yasir Hameed, Ian Maidment, Ken Laidlaw, Andrea Hilton, Naoko Kishita

INTRODUCTION

Mental illness is common in older adults, and those who have a concurrent physical illness are particularly vulnerable. Although these conditions tend to be underdetected and undertreated, their outcome with appropriate management is often excellent. This chapter reviews the main mental health disorders aside from dementia.

DEPRESSION AND ANXIETY IN OLDER ADULTS

Despite the commonly held negative stereotypes of aging as mainly loss and decrepitude, and despite depression and anxiety being major causes of mental health problems in later life, rates of late-life depression and anxiety are paradoxically lower than rates reported for younger or middle-aged adults.[1-3] Rickards[4] and Leiberman[5] estimate depression prevalence of between 20% and 45% and 25% and 40%, respectively, in community-dwelling populations of older people. Depression prevalence rates are elevated when taking account of medical conditions.[2,6] Nevertheless, even in these cases, depression is not an inevitable outcome. For example, the prevalence of depression after stroke is 33%.[7] Depending on methods of sampling and measurement, prevalence of depression in Parkinson disease is reported as high as 75%.[8] However, this high prevalence estimate should be tempered by the clinical challenge of an accurate diagnosis of depression in Parkinson disease because of symptom overlap.

In a systematic review of community-based studies assessing prevalence of late-life depression, Beekman and colleagues[9] calculated an average prevalence rate of 13.5% for clinically relevant depression symptoms. More recently, McDougall and coworkers[10] reported an estimated prevalence of depression among people aged 65 years and older of 8.7% from a large epidemiologic study conducted across England and Wales, with a prevalence rate for severe depression of 2.7%. There does not appear to be a relationship between age and prevalence of depression, whereas factors associated with increased rates of depression were being female, experiencing medical comorbidity and disability, and levels of social deprivation. Wilson and associates[11] reported elevated prevalence (21%) rates of depression in very old people (80 to 90 years) living alone.

The Centers for Disease Control and Prevention note that, contrary to popular belief, older people experience less frequent occurrence of mental distress, with lifetime histories of depression at 10.5% and anxiety at 7.6% that are lower than those reported for depression and anxiety (19.3% and 12.7%, respectively) in adults in midlife (50 to 64 years).[12]

Depression rates may also be elevated in those populations who reside in institutional settings.[3] Thakar and Blazer[13] reported rates of depression as high as 35% in residents in long-term care (LTC) facilities in the United States and note that depression is very often underrecognized. Seitz and colleagues[14] carried out a literature review of the prevalence of psychiatric disorder in LTC and identified 26 studies of depression prevalence and reported rates of 5% to 25%, with a median prevalence rate of 10%. Depressive *symptoms* were more prevalent, ranging from 14% to 82%, with a median prevalence rate of 29%. This suggests that depression may be elevated in residents in LTC, but perhaps arriving at a formal diagnosis of depression is more difficult in the context of an LTC facility. Likewise, providing treatment for depression in an LTC facility can be challenging.[15] As yet, there is no robust evidence base for the application of structured psychological therapies for depression in LTC,[13] although the evidence, such as it is, suggests that older people may benefit from a psychosocial approach to emotional distress.[15]

In effect, rates of depression in community-dwelling older adults are surprisingly uncommon when considering the challenges that can be posed by age. Moreover, the prevalence of depression is lower in older adults compared to adults of working age.[16]

Blazer[1] suggests three protective factors associated with aging explain the low rate of depression in later life. These factors are better emotional regulation skills through selectively optimizing positives, increased wisdom through learning to deal with adversity and uncertainty, and resilience as a result of coping better with stressful events. Jorm[3] suggests that depression and anxiety rates reduce with age because of a multitude of factors, such as decreased emotional responsiveness (evidence suggests that levels of neuroticism decrease with age); increased emotional control (older people have developed skills in coping strategies that result in better emotional stability); and psychological immunization (people develop a resilience and resistance to depression through exposure to adverse life events).

The relationship between depression and dementia is a complex one. Depression can contribute to development of dementia or worsening of cognitive problems in dementia. In a large retrospective cohort study involving more than 35,000 participants, researchers found that depression in midlife was associated with increased risk of later dementia by 20% and later life depression by 70%. Having midlife and later life depression increased the risk of dementia by 80%.[17] Dementia, especially at an early stage, can lead to depression. This is especially true when the patient has good insight and realizes the impact of this degenerative and terminal illness on quality of life and stress on caregivers. Vascular dementia and Alzheimer dementia are more associated with depression than are other types of dementia.

Anxiety may be more common in later life than depression, but anxiety disorders are much less common than anxiety symptoms.[18,19] Furthermore, it may be less common for older people to receive a diagnosis of an anxiety disorder on its own,[18] but it may be more likely as a comorbid diagnosis with depression. Until relatively recently, there were no specific psychometrically robust measures of anxiety in older people.

Generalized anxiety disorder (GAD) and specific phobias are the most common anxiety disorders.[19] Wolitzky-Taylor and coworkers[19] in a comprehensive review, reported the prevalence for all anxiety disorders in later life from 4.5 to 14.2%, and cite the Epidemiological Catchment Area study prevalence as being 5.5% and thus lower than in adults of working age. Wolitzky-Taylor and associates[19] report prevalence of GAD between 1.2% and 7.3% in the studies in their sample, and lifetime prevalence for GAD is estimated at 3.6%. However, a full understanding of late-life anxiety prevalence is challenging because of variable methodologic quality, sampling issues, operational definitions, and the entry age for which anxiety in later life is identified (in some studies this is defined as 55 years). Some anxiety disorders in later life appear uncommon; for example, the prevalence of obsessive compulsive disorder (OCD) is reported as only 0.8% to 1.0%. Of note for understanding anxiety disorders in later life is that conditions such as GAD appear to be of long duration and, unlike depressive disorders, are less likely to spontaneously remit.[20]

Bryant and colleagues[18] examined the prevalence for late-life anxiety disorders and symptoms in community-dwelling and clinical samples. The most common anxiety disorders are specific phobias (1.4% to 25.6%) and GAD (1.3% to 7.1%), with a low prevalence for panic disorder. However, Bryant and coworkers[18] comment that data on panic disorder are sparse, but when symptoms are measured, rates can be as high as 26.2%. As with previous reviews, reported prevalence rates vary considerably, with prevalence for anxiety disorders in community-dwelling older people of between 1.2% and 14% and prevalence for anxiety symptoms in community samples between 15% and 52.3%. Because symptom reporting is variable, it is not possible to be sure that samples are comparable. It is not surprising that prevalence rates are higher in clinical samples, reported as between 15% and 56%. Clinical samples also vary because of the overlap between anxiety symptoms and physical symptoms, as well as lack of valid psychometric tools for assessing anxiety disorders, which makes accurate diagnosis challenging. Nonetheless, it should be evident that there is a higher prevalence of anxiety symptoms in physically ill hospitalized older people and that the presence of anxiety (disorders and symptoms) is associated with an increased risk of poorer outcome.[18]

Posttraumatic stress disorder (PTSD) in later life is an interesting condition with a different course linked to the life history of individuals and, in some cases, cohorts. In a contemporary review, Bottche and associates[21] divide PTSD into late or early life acquired symptoms. PTSD in older people acquired earlier in life may be more common in veterans or in holocaust survivors, whereas PTSD symptoms acquired later in life are more likely to occur after accidents or natural disasters. Overall lifetime prevalence rates of PTSD are lower in older (3.9%) than in younger (6.1%) or middle-aged adults (6.2%), but when considering higher risk populations such as those with war trauma experience, prevalence rates are much higher (3% to 56%). High rates of PTSD are reported in holocaust survivors (24.2%). Data about the lifetime course and outcome of PTSD following early traumatization remain inconclusive.[21]

Management of Mood Disorders in Older Adults

The management of depression in physically ill older adult patients is essentially the same as for depression in general. Antidepressant and psychological therapy are equally effective in older and younger adults, although in pharmacotherapy, medical comorbidities and the possibility of adverse consequences or interactions between antidepressants and other drug treatments must be considered carefully. Antidepressant prescribing for depressed older people appears to have increased in recent years, perhaps because of the perceivably superior safety profile of selective serotonin reuptake inhibitors (SSRIs).

Drugs associated with depression include propranolol, β-blockers, antiparkinson drugs, cimetidine, clonidine, estrogens and progesterone, tamoxifen, and dextropropoxyphene. Depression is also associated with malignant and cerebrovascular disease; myocardial infarction; and thyroid, parathyroid, and adrenal endocrine disturbance.

Removal of depression-causing medication and treatment of illnesses associated with depression may improve mood. Antidepressants should be given at adequate doses for a minimum of 4 weeks before concluding they are ineffective and changing to a different class. If response is poor, consider whether the patient is adhering to the treatment and increase to a higher dose.

Coupland and colleagues[22] reported a cohort study investigating classes of antidepressant drugs. All classes were associated with increased risks of adverse events, but there were differences in the type and frequency of serious effects across medication classes. The SSRIs were associated with an increased risk of falls (hazard ratio [HR], 1.66; 95% confidence interval [CI], 1.58 to 1.73), and citalopram, escitalopram, and fluoxetine were also associated with hyponatremia (HR, 1.52; 95% CI, 1.33 to 1.75). Trazodone, mirtazapine, and venlafaxine were associated with higher risks of all-cause mortality and several potentially life-threatening events, including attempted suicide or self-harm and stroke or transient ischemic attack. The study showed that low-dose tricyclic antidepressants remain popular—at least in the United Kingdom (31.6% of all antidepressant prescriptions)—and did not have the highest hazard ratio for any of the adverse outcomes reported. Important interactions between unknown patient factors and drug choice could still have occurred. For example, medication such as venlafaxine is typically used in more severe or treatment-resistant depression (which may be indicative of severe medical comorbidity). Trazodone and mirtazapine are more likely to be prescribed to patients with serious sleep disturbance or agitation, factors that again are often linked with more serious physical ill health. As the dose of tricyclic antidepressants increased, the risks of all-cause mortality, falls, seizures, and fractures increased. For most adverse outcomes, the high-risk periods were during the month after starting or stopping antidepressants.

Depression in older adults frequently fails to respond to initial treatment. Pharmacologic strategies for treatment-resistant depression may be useful despite the toxicity risk. Nortriptyline, lithium, and bupropion were found to be useful additive treatments in cases where an SSRI is the initial treatment. Older people require careful monitoring for effectiveness and adverse effects, with provision of information (to the patient and caregiver) about the risks of falls, confusion, agitation, and increased suicidal ideation. Although people with dementia are at an increased risk of developing depression, the evidence for efficacy of antidepressants in these patients is poor.[23]

Pathologic crying, or more rarely pathologic laughing, can be a distressing feature of depression, and there is evidence that SSRIs can be efficacious in reducing symptoms within days of commencing therapy.

The safety profile of electroconvulsive therapy (ECT) in older patients with depression is very good. A wide spectrum of clinical responses has been demonstrated, including reduction of anxiety symptoms. ECT is at least as effective in adults aged 60 and older as those aged 18-60 years and may positively influence outcome. Unilateral electrode placement appears as effective as bilateral in older patients, but there is evidence that unilateral electrode placement is associated with fewer memory-related side effects in this age group.

Psychological treatments are underused in older age. This is partly because their availability is often limited. There is also a misconception that older people lack the psychological flexibility to benefit from psychotherapeutic interventions.[24] Older adults appear to respond particularly well to cognitive therapy for depression; this is effective both in an individual setting and (more economically) in groups.[24] The focus is often on real or threatened losses (bereavement, physical health, financial security) and on fears of impending death.[24] Brief, highly focused cognitive behavioral therapies such as problem-solving therapy are being advocated increasingly for older people, including those with some degree of cognitive dysfunction. These approaches may be effective when used in people at high risk to prevent, as well as treat, depression in older age.[24]

Another brief talking therapy, interpersonal psychotherapy, has also been shown to be effective in older people. Collaborative care has emerged as a helpful approach toward integrating primary and secondary care teams and combining the use of a range of treatment modalities. Tailored collaborative care is associated with substantial benefits (compared with treatment as usual) in terms of improvement in depressive symptoms, better physical functioning, and enhanced quality of life.

Suicide in Older Adults

The highest suicide rates are found in males aged 75 years and older. Suicide among older adults in North America is almost twice as common as in the rest of the population, and this finding is replicated in most other countries. About 90% of those who commit suicide have at least one diagnosable mental illness. The most common psychiatric disorder associated with completed suicide is depression.[25]

Men who commit suicide more commonly use violent methods (e.g., hanging or guns), whereas women more commonly use overdoses or self-poisoning methods.[26] Older people are more successful when it comes to completed suicide compared to younger people. Factors that may explain this include more physical fragility and illness in older people and higher chance of social isolation (therefore, they are unlikely to be interrupted or stopped). In addition, research has shown that older people are more determined to die when they attempt suicide and are less impulsive than younger people. Any suicidal attempt or gesture by an older person should be taken very seriously. Multiple physical and mental illnesses increase the risk of suicide. Physical illnesses such as epilepsy, chronic obstructive pulmonary disease, congestive heart failure, and mental health disorders (e.g., anxiety, depression, and bipolar disorders) are specifically associated with higher rates of suicide.[27] Other factors associated with suicide in older adults include bereavement, substance misuse, increasing social isolation, deteriorating physical health, and pain.

Attempted suicide closely resembles completed suicide in older adults. Psychiatric illness, particularly depression, is prominent in most cases. Minor depression and personality dysfunction are associated with suicide attempts of relatively low intent and higher levels of psychosocial stresses. Hopelessness persisting after remission of other depressive symptoms is associated with suicide attempts and completed suicide. On the other hand, personality disorders and substance misuse disorders may have a lower prevalence in older populations and are therefore less associated with completed suicide compared to younger populations. Suicide is much more closely associated with depression in older than in younger subjects, and the best predictor of suicidality is the current severity of depression. The increased rate of suicide in those experiencing physical ill health is mediated by depression.

Somatoform Disorders

Somatoform disorders are those in which physical symptoms occur in the absence of any or sufficient organic pathology to account for them and include conversion disorder, somatization disorder, pain disorder, and hypochondriasis. They are not due to malingering or fabricated symptoms, and the patient experiences the symptoms presented. Psychological contributory factors can usually be identified. They are considered as anxiety disorders and can present outside psychiatry in medical settings.

The two main classification systems in psychiatry—the International Classification of Diseases, tenth edition (ICD-10) and the *Diagnostic and Statistical Manual of Mental Disorders*, fifth edition (DSM-5)—differ slightly in their definitions and subcategorizations of somatoform disorders. The ICD-10 diagnosis of somatoform disorders (F45) defines the main feature of these disorders as "repeated presentation of physical symptoms together with persistent requests for medical investigations."[28] Additional features are that patients with somatoform disorders will not be reassured by normal test results and, even if physical cause is found, it does not explain the severity of the emotional distress or the preoccupation. The ICD-10 includes the following subcategories for somatoform disorders: somatization disorder; undifferentiated somatoform disorder; hypochondriacal disorder; somatoform autonomic dysfunction; persistent somatoform pain disorder; other somatoform disorders; and somatoform disorder, unspecified. The DSM-5 groups somatoform disorders under one heading called "somatic symptom and related disorders" and defines these disorders as presenting with "excessive thoughts, feelings, or behaviors related to the somatic symptoms or associated health concerns."

The symptoms are not required to be "medically unexplained," and the main factor is the complaints of distressing and chronic somatic symptoms that are associated with significant emotional response.[29]

Prevalence

The estimated prevalence of somatoform disorders in the general population is approximately 6%.[30] Prevalence figures in the older adult population are variable depending on clinical settings. (Hospital-based studies show higher prevalence compared to community-based samples.) Older people often develop exaggerated bodily complaints in the context of physical illness. Physically ill patients may also have generalized anxiety or panic symptoms. The common medical disorders producing anxiety symptoms are endocrine, cardiovascular, pulmonary, and neurologic conditions. A thorough history should help to establish the temporal relationship of psychiatric symptomatology and the onset of medical illness. Although the onset of somatoform disorder is usually in early life and runs a chronic course, somatizing patients avoid psychiatrists in youth and adulthood and so it is not uncommon for them to arrive at a clinic for the first time in older adulthood.[31] There is evidence that somatizing presentations are common among older primary care attendees.[32]

Studies provide various estimates for the prevalence of somatoform disorders in the older adult population depending on their methodologies and clinical settings. The prevalence varies from 1.5% to 13%.[33] The Epidemiological Catchment Area study from the United States suggests the prevalence is the same and rare (0.1%) throughout adult life when the disorder is defined as having 12 or more unexplained medical symptoms. Rates of persistent fatigue are also similar across age groups and occur in more than a quarter of adults of all ages.[34]

These patients usually have clear symptoms of depression or anxiety. Their bodily complaints tend to be restricted to one or two body organs or systems, and they are preoccupied with the possibility of serious physical illness. They demand investigation rather than treatment. In contrast, hypochondriacal preoccupation presenting for the first time in older adults is unlikely to be secondary to anxiety and depression. Hypochondriasis is a persistent, unrealistic preoccupation with the possibility of having at least one serious disease in which normal sensations and appearances are often misinterpreted as abnormal and as signs of disease and the patient cannot accept reassurances from doctors. Older adult patients only rarely present with conversion reactions (e.g., paralysis) or dissociative amnesia in response to stressful experience. Treatment of associated psychiatric conditions may lead to improvement in somatic attributions.[32]

Some studies suggested an association between early traumatic experiences and higher prevalence of somatization in older adults. These somatic symptoms were thought to be manifestations of complex PTSD.[35] Somatoform disorder is associated with higher use of health services. Women have double the risk of somatoform disorders compared to men.[36]

Management

Treatment of somatic disorders should not only focus on medication but also incorporate psychosocial support and psychotherapy.[37] There is good evidence to suggest that psychotherapy is effective in patients with severe somatoform disorder (compared to treatment as usual).[38,39] Somatoform disorders are associated with high occurrence of other psychiatric comorbidity (anxiety and affective disorders), and these should be treated accordingly. St. John's wort was also found to be helpful in reducing the severity of somatoform disorders, but cautious use is recommended because of its potential to interact with other drugs. It may be a useful option in patients who prefer to avoid psychotropic medication or when those medications are contraindicated.[40]

KEY POINTS

- Somatoform disorders describe multiple physical symptoms without an identifiable organic cause. The symptoms are real and experienced by the patient (which is a key difference from malingering or fabricated symptoms).
- Somatoform disorders are usually associated with mental health problems (especially depression, anxiety, or panic symptoms). Establishing the temporal relationship between the somatic and psychiatric symptoms can be difficult.
- Management involves addressing the comorbid psychiatric symptoms and incorporating psychological, social, and spiritual (if applicable) interventions as part of multidisciplinary and holistic care.

PSYCHOTIC DISORDERS

Late-Life Psychosis

Schizophrenia-like psychotic illness later in life, not caused by or resulting from an organic or affective disorder, has been variously termed *paraphrenia*, *late paraphrenia*, and *late-onset schizophrenia*. In 2000, the International Late-Onset Schizophrenia Group defined the terms *late-onset schizophrenia* and *very late-onset schizophrenia* for schizophrenia-like illnesses with onsets between age 40 and 60 and after age 60 years, respectively. The term *late-onset schizophrenia* is used to describe these conditions within this chapter. More circumscribed delusional disorders also occur in late life; these are referred to as *late-life delusional disorders*. In addition, the challenges posed by patients with long-standing psychotic illness (usually schizophrenia) who "graduate" to old age are also considered.

Late-Onset Schizophrenia

The original concept of late-onset schizophrenia referred to the first onset of persecutory delusions and associated hallucinations after the age of 60 years in the absence of an affective or organic psychosis.[41] It may thus be viewed as schizophrenia or a schizophrenia-like illness in older adults. Table 56-1 provides a summary of the phenotypic differences according to age.

Epidemiology

Although the incidence of schizophrenia is highest in people aged 16 to 25 years, there is a second peak in incidence in those aged older than 65.[42] Almost a quarter of the affected patients develop schizophrenia at the age of 40 years or older.

The prevalence of nonaffective psychosis in people aged older than 65 years has been reported as 2.3% in women and 1.7% in men.[43] Data from general medical practices regarding patients with treated schizophrenia (1997-1998) indicate that prevalence peaks in women in the 65- to 74-year age group compared with the 45- to 54-year age group in men, reflecting the higher prevalence of late-onset schizophrenia in women. The incidence of late-onset schizophrenia has been reported at 12.6/100,000/year.[44] Incidence is positively correlated with age, with first admission data suggesting an increase of 11% for every 5-year increase in age.[45] In the United Kingdom, African-Caribbean older people are more likely than white British older people to be in contact with services for a new diagnosis of psychosis.[46] Prevalence of late-onset schizophrenia is likely to be underestimated by community surveys and treatment data, as those affected are far less likely than the rest of the population to cooperate with survey investigators and often refuse treatment. They may only be treated compulsorily and in the context of particularly severe behavioral disturbance or when the illness affects their physical health.

TABLE 56-1 Schizophrenia-Like Psychosis at Different Ages of Onset

Onset ->	Typical (15-40)	Middle Age (41-65)	Very Late (>65)
F:M ratio	0.6:1	2:1	Up to 8:1
Poor premorbid function	++	+	–
Family history of schizophrenia	++	++	–
Sensory deficits	–	–	+
Negative symptoms	+++	++	–
Thought disorder	+++	+++	–
Brain structural (strokes/tumors)	–	–	+
Dose antipsychotic	+++	++	+
Tardive dyskinesia risk	+	+	++

Causation

About 10% of the relatives of patients developing schizophrenia in middle age also have the disease; this is similar to the proportion for patients with early-onset schizophrenia.[47] In family studies of late-onset schizophrenia, however, the rate of schizophrenia in first-degree relatives is much lower.[48] Standardized instruments were not used in the late-onset schizophrenia studies, however, so the data are not directly comparable to those from fully operationalized family studies of younger subjects.

The influence of personality, social, and environmental factors in association with genetic predisposition is clearly complex.[49] Patients with late-onset schizophrenia are often socially isolated and live alone.[50] They are more likely to have paranoid or schizoid premorbid personalities that are characterized by suspicion, sensitivity to setback and disappointment, and preoccupation with what others think about them.[51] Their isolation is often long-standing and may well be secondary to personality traits. They are predominantly unmarried women without close family or personal attachments. Those who do marry often end up divorced or separated. However, premorbid educational, occupational, and psychosocial functioning is less impaired in patients with late-onset compared to early-onset schizophrenia.[51] Fertility is reduced. The consequent social isolation, which is often increased by sensory isolation and retirement, can result in increasing preoccupation with their internal world.

Recent evidence from cohort studies suggests that a history of psychotic symptoms, cognitive problems, poor physical health, visual impairment, and negative life events are risk factors for late-onset psychosis.[52]

In terms of sensory impairment, there is a confirmed association between deafness and very late-onset schizophrenia in particular.[51] These patients frequently have a conductive hearing loss acquired in early life to such a degree as to impair social interaction, resulting in "social deafness."[53] Visual impairment may be present but is probably no more common than in normal older adults.[41] Patients with late-onset schizophrenia have been found to come from the lower social classes or socioeconomic groups[50]; this may result from social deterioration secondary to the disease, as also occurs in younger people with schizophrenia.

Presentation and Clinical Features

Patients often arrive for medical services because they complain to the police and neighbors with bizarre accusations over a period of time or because of concern triggered by extreme self-neglect or odd behavior. There are no qualitative differences between the positive symptoms of early-onset schizophrenia and those of late-onset schizophrenia. The clinical presentation of late-onset schizophrenia is quite varied. Patients are in clear consciousness. Usually their mood is normal, although occasionally a secondary depressive mood is found. The history may be difficult to elicit from patients with late-onset schizophrenia because they tend to be suspicious and hostile.

Delusions are a central feature. Persecutory delusions are particularly common. Sexual themes are common in women. The patient may accuse a man or men of entering her bed at night and molesting her sexually. Delusions of influence and passivity phenomena are frequently reported.[54] Patients may describe their bodies as being controlled, or they may complain that some power affects them and they are made to do things against their will. Thought insertion, withdrawal, and broadcasting, however, are fairly rare, and formal thought disorder is almost nonexistent.

Hallucinations are frequently experienced.[50] Those with late-onset schizophrenia experience a great number of different types of hallucinations. Auditory hallucinations are the most common and usually have an accusatory and/or insulting content. The voices speak in the second or the third person with "running commentary" occasionally encountered. Hallucinations of bodily sensation are also found. Patients complain of being vibrated, raped, or forced to have sexual intercourse. Olfactory hallucinations often relating to poisonous gas are encountered. Visual hallucinations are rare in late-onset schizophrenia and, if present, should raise the strong suspicion of an underlying organic state. Comorbid depression and suicidal ideation are common.

It is not only social and sensory isolation that can make people vulnerable to psychosis but also a more vulnerable brain. Older adults' cognitive function is often mildly impaired at initial presentation, to a much lesser degree than found in dementia but significantly more than in psychiatrically healthy age-matched controls.[53] Decline is usually slowly progressive, with only a small group of patients entering the dementia range at 3-year follow-up.

Studies of older adults with psychosis have found lower quality of life to be associated with depression, positive and negative symptoms, cognitive deficits, physical disorders, and poorer perceived health, as well as social factors including loneliness and financial strain.[55]

Brain Imaging Studies

Structural neuroimaging findings in late-onset illness are similar to those found in patients with early-onset schizophrenia. A representative computed tomography (CT) study has reported increased mean ventricle-to-brain ratio with cortical sulci appearances remaining within normal limits.[53] Single-photon emission computed tomography (SPECT) studies have found reduced regional cerebral blood flow (rCBF) in late-onset psychotic patients compared to controls, appearances that are similar to those found in early-onset schizophrenia.[56] Magnetic resonance imaging (MRI) has demonstrated increased periventricular hyperintensities and thalamic signal hyperintensities in late-onset schizophrenia, which have led to the suggestion that cerebrovascular disease may be significant in the pathogenesis of the condition,[57,58] although these findings have not been consistently replicated[59] and may reflect the overrepresentation of individuals with cerebrovascular disease risk factors.

A number of studies using positron emission tomography (PET) scanning have shown increased basal ganglia dopamine D2 receptors in late-onset schizophrenia.[60] However, these findings have not been consistently replicated, particularly in drug-naive subjects, suggesting that some of the differences initially reported may reflect treatment rather than disease-induced receptor alteration.

Neuropsychologic Testing

Patients with late-onset schizophrenia have been shown to perform less well on the Mental Test Score and Digit Copying Test than age-matched controls. Deficiencies have also been shown on full-scale IQ tests, tests of frontal lobe function, and verbal memory tasks.[53] The presence of brain abnormalities was not associated with particularly low neuropsychologic test scores. When patients with late-life schizophrenia are compared to those with young-onset disease, they have less neuropsychologic deficit in abstraction and cognitive flexibility but more global impairment.

Assessment, Treatment, and Course

The initial management of late late-onset schizophrenia involves assessment and engagement.[50] Patients should be assessed at home because they are unlikely to comply with outpatient appointments and because their psychotic symptoms may be strongly triggered by cues within their normal environment and less obvious away from it. If hospital admission is needed, it commonly results in an apparent complete remission followed by relapse on return home. Access to the home of a patient with late-onset schizophrenia can be difficult. This can lead to assessment under the Mental Care Act (in the United Kingdom) or involvement of the courts and police according to local country legislation.

Late-onset schizophrenia may run a chronic course,[61] but recent studies have shown remission rates of 48% to 60% after treatment. Attempts at treatment should begin in the community wherever possible, with hospital admission reserved for patients with particularly severe or dangerous behavioral disturbance or poor self-care. Medication, psychosocial intervention, and ECT have all been reported to produce temporary remission. Adequate antipsychotic treatment produces improvement in psychotic symptoms but not much improvement to the patient's pretreatment level of social functioning. Dosages are much lower than those used in younger patients with schizophrenia because people with late-onset schizophrenia are often very sensitive to extrapyramidal side effects.[62] Patients do better (in terms of side effects, efficacy, and negative symptoms) with atypical antipsychotics, but risperidone and olanzapine are relatively contraindicated in those with cardiovascular morbidity or diabetes. A good response to antipsychotics has been found in patients with very late-onset schizophrenia-like psychosis,[63-66] even better than in late-onset schizophrenia[63] and older adult early-onset schizophrenia patients.[63,64] Patients are often not adherent to medication, particularly if they live alone. Even when compliance is assured, many patients with late-onset schizophrenia remain psychotic, although they may be less distressed by their symptoms and less disturbed in their behavior.[60,67] Community psychiatric nursing involvement has been shown effective. There is conflicting evidence regarding whether depot medication improves adherence.[46]

An attempt should be made to correct remediable physical or environmental contributory factors, particularly through alleviating sensory or social isolation. A flexible approach is required, and patients' characteristic insistence on remaining isolated (as they have often been for much of their lives) must be respected. Patients' requests for rehousing should be resisted if they are secondary to delusional beliefs; if symptoms improve or even abate in a new home setting, this is usually only a temporary respite. Consideration of capacity is important to prevent self-neglect or financial abuse. Old "tormentors" reemerge, and new ones may be acquired. Antipsychotic medication is a vital component of the total therapeutic package but is far from the whole answer; improvisation and ingenuity in engaging these patients and then retaining them in long-term follow-up is crucial to maintain both compliance and an optimal level of social functioning and to reduce risk of symptomatic relapse.

Late-Life Delusional (Paranoid) Disorder

It has been estimated that 4% of the community-living older adult population experience some persecutory delusions.[68] Such beliefs are commonly associated with a neuropsychiatric disorder. A primary delusional disorder is present when there is evidence of persistent, nonbizarre delusions that are not attributable to another psychiatric disorder or any organic cause.[69] Delusional disorder refers to persistent delusions without evidence of schizophrenia, schizophreniform, or mood disorders. Hallucinations are not prominent. There is no evidence of organic dysfunction. The distinction between such disorders and late-onset schizophrenia reflects the relative absence of schizophrenia-like features other than delusions in the late-life delusional group. Delusional disorder occurs in middle as well as late life. Men tend to be affected earlier than women (40 to 49 years vs. 60 to 69 years).

Pathogenesis and Causation

An increased prevalence of schizophrenia has been observed in families of patients with late-life delusional disorder.[70] Individuals with avoidant, paranoid, or schizoid personality disorders may be more susceptible to developing a delusional disorder. There is an association between hearing loss and delusional disorder in older adults.[71] Immigration or low socioeconomic status may also predispose individuals to delusional disorder.[72] There is an increased frequency of women, immigrants, and children of immigrants with somatic delusions diagnosed as part of a delusional disorder. There may be an association of early life trauma and the failure to reproduce progeny with the development of delusions in later life.[73]

Management and Outcome

The optimal approach to treating older adults with delusional disorder encompasses drug treatment, psychotherapy, and environmental change.[74] Antipsychotics may be effective in decreasing the intensity of the delusions, but (as in late-onset schizophrenia) nonadherence is a common problem and allocation of a community mental health worker may be important if the person is willing to engage with services. Intramuscular depot neuroleptics may be preferable. Antidepressant drugs and ECT have been used with variable success in delusional patients, particularly those with coexistent depressive symptoms. The provision of alternative explanations for patients' delusional beliefs may be a useful psychotherapeutic approach. There are few outcome data available, but the overall outcome is often poor.[69]

Graduates

The term *graduates* is used to refer to patients with long-standing mental illness who have "graduated" to elderly status.[75] Many graduates entered a mental hospital when relatively young and remained in institutional care for much of their lives, only returning to the community to live independently or in group homes when the large psychiatric hospitals closed in the 1990s.

The largest subgroup is composed of graduates who have schizophrenia. Most of the remainder have primary diagnoses of affective psychoses, learning disability, or personality disorder. Disability in the graduate population is varied. Some patients may require total nursing care, whereas others remain physically fit and relatively competent in daily living skills. Many have some degree of cognitive impairment. There are associations between negative symptoms (social withdrawal, slowness, underactivity, poverty of speech, lack of interest, and poor self-care), cognitive deficit, and structural brain abnormality. This highlights the issue of the long-term cognitive effects of schizophrenic illness. Some of the deficits of chronic schizophrenia are probably integral to the illness process and may manifest at a relatively early stage in the evolution of the illness over time. In addition, increasing social disability may be secondary to the deleterious effects of institutional care on the capacity to return to independent living. It has been suggested that in some patients a phenomenon of "burnout" in schizophrenia (an amelioration of positive symptoms after the age of 55) may occur, but this is still disputed.[76] The lowered prevalence of positive symptoms in this group may be a result of reduced exposure to the stresses and strains of everyday life rather than either the effects of medication or the natural history of schizophrenia.

Patients with schizophrenia have high rates of obesity, hypertension, diabetes, and cigarette smoking (and, therefore, cardiovascular and respiratory disease) compared to the non-schizophrenic population. Consequent to this, and to higher rates of suicide, their life expectancy is reduced by 20%.[77] Among those living in institutional settings, there is a high prevalence of physical disability and handicap. This increases with age but is not confined to older adult patients or those with the longest duration of stay. The presence of neurologic abnormalities referred to as "soft" neurologic signs—including disorders of posture and tone, disturbances in motor performance, inappropriate activity, abnormal movements, automatic movements, and difficulties in speech production—seem to be intrinsic to the schizophrenic process and cannot be attributed to hospitalization, physical treatment, or undiagnosed neurologic illness.[78]

The care of graduate patients encompasses elements of good practice within older adult psychiatry, psychiatric rehabilitation, and medicine of older adults.[75] The needs of graduates are very different from those of patients with severe dementia, and they should not be cared for in the same settings. Patients' skills should be identified and cultivated as part of a rehabilitative process, in the context of working toward an improved quality of life by improving the physical and social environment. Residential options in the community are varied and should be determined by the individual's present and likely future physical and mental health needs. Medication regimens often need review, and many patients benefit from cautious reduction or withdrawal of antipsychotic drugs that have often been prescribed in substantial amounts over the years.

Depressive Psychosis

Epidemiology

Depressive psychosis is common in inpatient settings and causes great suffering and disability. Kivela and Pahkala[79] reported a 1% point prevalence of psychotic depression in older people of both sexes in a Finnish community study and a 2.7% prevalence of nonpsychotic depression.[80] Ohayon and Schatzberg[81] found a 0.3% point prevalence of psychotic depression versus 1.3% of nonpsychotic depression in the older population in five European countries. Kessing,[82] in a large epidemiologic study in Denmark incorporating both outpatient and inpatient settings, found that patients with a late-onset (>65 years) first depressive episode had a higher prevalence of psychosis than their early-onset counterparts (28.2 vs. 20% in outpatient settings and 52.6 vs. 38.6% in inpatient settings).

Clinical Features

Psychotic depression and nonpsychotic depression differ in significant ways.[83-86] Parker and coworkers[86] found significantly higher levels of psychomotor disturbance (agitation or retardation) in patients with psychotic depression.[84] Others, including Baldwin[83] and Lee and associates,[86] did not find such differences in psychomotor disturbance. The severity of depression is worse in psychosis. Patients with psychotic depression have higher rates of feelings of guilt or deserved punishment. Delusions of paranoid and somatic types are the most prevalent, followed by those of guilt.[83,84] About one third of deluded patients experience hallucinations, mainly auditory.[84] Suicidal behavior appears to be higher,[85] and suicidal ideation is more severe.[87]

Flint and colleagues[88] found that patients older than 60 years exhibited significantly lower comorbidity with current or past panic disorder, social anxiety, or PTSD. Gournellis and coworkers[89] compared younger (younger than 60 years) with older (older than 60 years) patients and both early-onset and late-onset psychotic major depression patients. Both groups of older patients exhibited higher severity levels of hypochondriasis and physical impairment compared with the younger group. Moreover, late-onset patients, compared with younger patients had more gastrointestinal symptoms, physical impairment, and delusions of somatic and impending disaster content but less frequent delusions of guilt and paranoid content. The older early-onset depressive psychosis patients have an intermediate position between the young and older late-onset patients with regard to hypochondriacal ideation; gastrointestinal symptoms; and delusions of somatic, guilt, and paranoid content.

Neuropsychological Features

Studies suggest a specific disturbance in executive functioning with impairment of psychomotor speed, which is indicative of a more global neuropsychological impairment, associated with cortical atrophy in frontal and temporal regions.[90] Other studies have found a more global cognitive impairment in the domains of general intelligence, attention, memory, visuospatial abilities, language function, psychomotor speed, and executive function.[91,92]

Risk Factors and Neurobiologic Correlates

Family studies: there is disagreement if family history of depression is increased[87] or remains the same.[84,85,93]

Genetic studies: Zubenko and associates[94] reported that the apolipoprotein E4 allele frequency was nearly four times higher in psychotic depression compared to nonpsychotic depression.

Enzyme studies: serum dopamine-β-hydroxylase activity has been found to be significantly lower in depressive psychotic patients than in nonpsychotic patients.[95] This might be a risk factor for psychosis through increased central dopaminergic activity.

Neuroimaging studies: two MRI studies[87,96] have reported that older people with depressive psychosis have smaller frontal lobe volumes, smaller temporal lobe volumes,[87] more brainstem atrophy, and a more enlarged third ventricle,[87] along with more hyperintensities in the pontine reticular formation.[87] These differences were associated with more impaired frontal lobe function and mental processing speed, poorer physical health,[87] and more vascular risk factors.[93]

Treatment

Treatment of the Acute Phase: Antidepressant Monotherapy. Treatment response rates to antidepressant monotherapy are poor, with inconsistent estimates of 18%,[7] 23%,[87] and 44%.[98]

Treatment of the Acute Phase: Combination Therapy. Meyers and colleagues[99] found olanzapine-sertraline was well tolerated and equally effective in both younger and older adults. Moreover, it was more effective than the combination olanzapine-placebo. However, both age groups experienced important metabolic side effects (increases in weight and triglyceride and cholesterol levels), especially the younger group. Older patients were more likely to fall.[100]

Combination Therapy Versus Monotherapy. Kok and colleagues[101] found no differences between psychotic and nonpsychotic depression with regard to efficacy or tolerability of an antidepressant-antipsychotic combination. Mulsant and coworkers[98] reported a higher, although nonsignificant, efficacy of a nortriptyline-perphenazine combination compared with a nortriptyline-placebo combination (50% vs. 44%). Meyers and associates,[99] in a 12-week study, found that an olanzapine-sertraline combination was superior to an olanzapine–placebo combination. Flint and Rifat[102] reported 25% efficacy of a nortriptyline-perphenazine combination, which rose to 50% after lithium coadministration. ECT has been reported up to 88% effective in this group of patients.

Maintenance and Continuation Treatment. In older adult patients with depressive psychosis who had achieved remission with ECT, relapse rates over 6 months did not differ between patients receiving nortriptyline plus perphenazine and those receiving nortriptyline plus placebo.[103] Patients receiving the active combination suffered from more extrapyramidal symptoms, falls, and tardive dyskinesia. Navarro and coworkers[104] found that patients receiving monthly maintenance ECT plus nortriptyline had a lower risk of relapse and recurrence than the nortriptyline subgroup at the end of the first year and a significantly better outcome at the end of a 2-year follow-up.

There is strong evidence that ECT in older patients with depressive psychosis is highly effective. The combination of a first-generation antipsychotic plus a tricyclic antidepressant and a tricyclic antidepressant monotherapy are equally effective, although the latter has fewer adverse effects.

Course and Outcome

Older patients with depressive psychosis experience more relapses and recurrences over a 2-year period.[105-107] Studies vary, with Murphy[108] finding only 10% of older people with PMD achieved full remission and almost a quarter died during a 1-year follow-up. By contrast, Baldwin,[97] in a 42- to 104-month retrospective follow-up study, failed to detect any differences between older-age psychotic depression and nonpsychotic depression patients regarding clinical course, relapse rate, or mortality.

Mania

Mania is characterized by elevation of mood and is associated with activity disturbance. It can be isolated or can be part of a relapsing condition with depressive episodes commonly known as bipolar disorder.

Epidemiology

A community 35-year incidence survey conducted in the United Kingdom found that the incidence of mania peaks in early adult life, with a tenth of new-onset cases of mania occurring after the age of 60 years.[109] This contrasts with studies based on psychiatric admission data, which suggest a stable incidence rate across age groups. Bipolar affective disorder is not uncommon in older adults[110]; prevalence rates range from 0.1% to 0.4%. However, it accounts for only 5% of patients admitted to geropsychiatric inpatient units.[111]

Older patients with mania typically had their first manic episode in their mid to late 50s.[112] People with mania of earlier onset are underrepresented in these hospitalized samples; possible explanations for this include effective treatment with lithium, burnout after many years, and higher mortality rates among younger patients with bipolar disorder. In approximately half of older patients with mania, the first episode of mental illness is depression,[113] with many years of latency before mania becomes manifest.

Clinical Features

Bipolar disorders are characterized by cycles of elevation and lowering of mood that does not fade with age.[114] Many of the clinical features of mania are similar to those found in younger patients, but dramatic physical overactivity, violence, criminal behavior, infectious euphoria, and grandiosity are less common in older patients.[115] Clinical experience suggests that mixed mood states are more commonly found in older subjects, but this has not been substantiated in a controlled study.[116] Adverse life events, particularly episodes of illness, more commonly appear to precipitate mania in older subjects. Subjective confusion or perplexity is relatively prominent in older adults. First-episode mania in very late life with no previous psychiatric history is often associated with comorbid neurologic disorder.

A manic episode has a duration of at least 1 week with elevated, expansive, or irritable mood. The mood disturbance is associated with manic symptoms, which can include inflated self-esteem or grandiosity, decreased need for sleep (e.g., one feels rested after only 3 hours of sleep), more talkative than usual or pressure to keep talking, flight of ideas or subjective experience that thoughts are racing, attention easily drawn to unimportant or irrelevant items, increase in goal-directed activity (either socially or sexually), psychomotor agitation, and excessive involvement in pleasurable activities that can cause harm (e.g., engaging in unrestrained spending, sexual indiscretions, or unwise business investments).

Secondary Mania

This concept refers to an episode of mania causally associated with medical illness, exogenous substances, and organic cerebral dysfunction.[115] First-onset mania in older adults should be considered to have an underlying organic cause until proven otherwise. The frequent presence of some degree of nonprogressive cognitive impairment in secondary mania reflects its heterogeneous origin. Even if no acute cause is discovered, there is still a greater prevalence of coexisting neurologic illness. Stroke is the most characteristic precipitant of secondary mania, and long-standing cerebrovascular disease is also overrepresented, with white matter hyperintensities often found on MRI scans. Family history and prior psychiatric disturbance are uncommon in secondary mania.

Treatment of Mania in Older Adults

The drug treatment of older adult patients with mania is similar to that of younger patients, but drug doses will generally be smaller. Neuroleptics are the mainstay of acute treatment. In secondary mania, treatment is also directed at the underlying medical cause. First-line prophylactic treatment is with lithium, although the risks of neurotoxicity are higher, even at relatively low serum lithium levels. The acute antimanic effect may also be useful in older adults. The anticonvulsants carbamazepine and sodium divalproate and atypical antipsychotics are increasingly widely used for their mood-stabilizing effects, but few data about their use in older people with mania have been reported. Olanzapine and risperidone are contraindicated in people with dementia because of increased risk of stroke. Family involvement is important in ongoing management. The risk of marital and family breakup is high. The range of skills available within a multidisciplinary team is often needed to deal with the complexities of managing bipolar disorder in older adults.

Comorbidities are common, with an average of two comorbid medical conditions and relatively high medication use. Comorbid conditions in older adults with bipolar disorder should be assessed to enable tailored treatment to optimize the general condition of these patients.[117]

Outcome

The acute and long-term outcome is similar to that in younger patients. Mania with first onset in old age may, however, have a poorer prognosis than mania recurring in old age, perhaps because of the greater likelihood of comorbid physical disease or cognitive impairment.[116]

PERSONALITY DISORDERS IN OLDER ADULTS

Personality disorders are generally recognizable by adolescence or earlier and continue throughout most of adult life. They become less obvious in middle life or old age, but, as in younger people, the diagnosis is only applicable where there has been long-standing dysfunction from the beginning of adult life.[118] Some lifelong obsessive or schizoid personality traits may worsen in old age, possibly as a result of experiencing increasing stress and adversity or as a way of adapting to losses in old age[119] and may present for the first time as a person who has interpersonal difficulties becomes dependent on others. Borderline personality disorder (BPD) has a low prevalence in older adults.

Despite some studies concluding that personality disorder symptoms “burn out,” “fade,” or “disappear” as patients age,[120] some report that functional impairment persists even when full criteria for a personality disorder are no longer met.[121] Drake and Valliant[122] reported that interpersonal impairment continues throughout the lifespan. Thus, it is possible that personality disorder presentation changes over time but continues to have a negative impact on psychosocial functioning; however, it is currently unclear how far this applies.[123,124]

Trappler and Backfield[124] reported on three patients (older than 50 years) with BPD and noted a broad range of borderline traits. Rosowsky and Gurian[125] compared eight older adult patients (aged 64 years) with BPD to controls and found less identity disturbance and impulsivity (including self-harm, risk taking, and substance use) in the older adults.

Shea and associates[126] divided patients into three age groups based on age at study entry: 18 to 24, 25 to 34, and 35 to 45 years. The patients were followed for 6 years for improvement in both psychosocial functioning and BPD symptoms. Here, younger and older subjects showed roughly equal improvement, although the oldest age group showed a change in direction from improvement to worsening functioning midway through the 6-year follow-up. In this case, the authors suggested the change constituted a reappearance of difficulties with advancing age generally, rather than only in a subgroup as originally suggested by Stone.[127] However, analyses emphasized differences in course rather than fundamental differences at baseline, such as specific criteria met; results also did not assess differences in specific aspects of functional impairment. A second study[128] evaluated group differences between patients with BPD, patients with other personality disorders, and subjects with no personality disorders in three age groups: 20 to

30, 31 to 40, and 41 to 50 years. Results showed less suicidality and impulsivity in older groups but comparable levels of distress and anxiety for BPD at all ages. However, patients older than 50 were not included in these analyses. Demographic differences, axis I comorbidity, or differences in functional impairment also were not assessed. Thus, it remains unclear what clinical qualities might uniquely characterize older BPD patients at intake.

Older adults were more likely to endorse chronic emptiness and less likely to endorse impulsivity, self-harm, and affective instability. Older adults also reported fewer substance use disorders, more lifetime hospitalizations, and higher social impairment.[129]

Global well-being, life satisfaction, and capacity to cope with illness and loss in old age are also critically influenced by personality and its adaption to old age.[130] Personality traits may be critical in adapting to the adverse life events all too often encountered by older people.

Epidemiology

An individual's personality is essentially stable over time.[130] Introversion has, however, been shown to increase with age,[131] whereas extraversion, neuroticism, and openness to experience decrease.[132] Older people tend to have higher scores on scales for orderliness, social conformity, and emotional stability and lower scores for activity and energy.[133] A decline in sociopathy and criminality has been documented.[134] Few large-scale studies of personality disorder in older adults have been performed. An early epidemiologic survey[135] reported a prevalence of 3.6% to 10.6% for personality disorder in people aged 65 years and older. More recent surveys of older community-living individuals using standardized diagnostic schedules have found lifetime prevalence rates for personality disorders ranging between 2.1% and 18%; a more recent meta-analysis reported an overall prevalence of 10% of those older than 50 years.[136,137] The mental health of older male prisoners is reported to be worse than that of younger prisoners, with 45% having a psychiatric illness with a prevalence of personality disorders of 30%.[138] Older adults who experienced childhood adversity were found to have a greater risk of personality disorder (odds ratio, 2.11; 95% CI, 1.75 to 2.54), which was not moderated by age.[139]

Comorbidity

People with personality disorders are vulnerable to other psychiatric illnesses. In particular, there is an association between personality disorder and affective illness, although the first episodes of depression or anxiety disorders usually occur before old age. People with late-onset schizophrenia often have premorbid schizoid or paranoid traits.

Senile Self-Neglect (Diogenes Syndrome)

Patients with this syndrome (also known as senile self-neglect or senile squalor syndrome) often come initially to departments of geriatric medicine. They usually exhibit gross self-neglect and domestic neglect, often accompanied by hoarding and social withdrawal. Although the most common diagnosis is dementia, others are depressed, have a paranoid psychosis, or abuse alcohol. Rarely patients have an obsessional disorder. Several studies have reported that approximately one third to one half have no psychiatric illness and tend to have higher than average intelligence.[140] For others, the syndrome can be understood as an expression of abnormal personality traits, in reaction to stress and loneliness or as the end stage of long-standing reclusiveness. Some authors have suggested that frontal lobe degeneration or obsessive compulsive disorder tends to be present if those patients are investigated thoroughly, although this is usually difficult to diagnose as patients are uncooperative.[141] Most people with Diogenes syndrome live alone, but a number of cases of folie à deux have been reported. The prognosis of such cases is not good. Compulsory hospitalization is difficult to accomplish, and mortality is high; apparently successful rehabilitation is usually followed by relapse.[142] Daycare might maintain an individual, but some form of institutional care usually becomes necessary. The Mental Capacity Act may prove helpful to manage patients if they lack capacity and their neglect is significantly impairing their health.

Outcome of Personality Disorder in Older Adults

Clinical experience suggests that personality disorder symptoms become less intrusive and cause less impact on patients, their families, and health care professionals by the time the person reaches old age.[118] Formal long-term follow-up studies, however, are sparse. Immature personality disorders, including antisocial, impulsive, histrionic, dependent, and narcissistic disorders, usually improve with time. Mature personality disorders, including anancastic, paranoid, schizoid, and schizotypal types, tend to persist into later life. Deterioration may become evident in the obsessive-compulsive patient as increased rigidity, in the paranoid patient as more suspiciousness and isolation, and in the schizotypal/schizoid patient as more social withdrawal and anxiety.

Patients with BPD tend to improve (or not survive) as they age, and thus rarely is BPD found in older adults. Good global outcome in such patients is associated with high intelligence, attractiveness, artistic talent, and coexisting obsessive-compulsive traits.[143] The highly subjective "likeability" seems also to confer good prognosis. Poor outcome is associated with a history of parental brutality, impulsivity, poor premorbid functioning, and coexistent schizotypal/antisocial personality disorder.[144]

In patients with antisocial personality disorder, there is a tendency toward spontaneous remission so that these individuals are rarely encountered after the age of 60.[118] Patients with schizotypal and schizoid personality disorder rarely seek treatment, so little is reported on their long-term outcome, but the outlook is probably poor.[145] There is also little information on the outcome of histrionic, narcissistic, obsessive-compulsive, and depressive personality disorders.[118]

Management of Personality Disorder in Older Adults

There has been little formal study of treatment approaches to personality disorder in older adults.[118] The management of coexisting psychiatric illness is as discussed previously, and many of the traits are less expressed in behavior when these are treated. The psychotherapeutic treatment of older adult patients may be unpromising for individuals with long-standing personality disorders who may have particular difficulty in resolving a lifetime of failed relationships and missed opportunities. Cognitive analytic therapy, which is about interpersonal understanding rather than using an illness model, is a therapeutic approach used to search for the meaning behind symptoms and offers a narrative reconstruction of an individual's life story.[146] It is used to generate a written reformulation and diagrams and has been used to help older people with narcissistic and borderline traits.[146] The use of medication in older adults with personality disorders has not been formally studied.

ALCOHOL DISORDERS

Epidemiology and Causation

Recent evidence suggests that alcohol misuse and dependence in older people is prevalent but is poorly recognized and poorly treated for various reasons. Generally there is lack of awareness about magnitude of this problem in older adults. In addition, there is the barrier of stigma associated with substance misuse, which may prevent the patient and professionals from exploring harmful drinking. Furthermore, there is lack of dedicated and specialist substance misuse services for older patients.[147] Among older adults, sociodemographic factors associated with alcohol use disorders include being male, socially isolated, single, and separated or divorced. Older adults with insomnia or chronic pain, those previously dependent on alcohol, and those with current depression or dementia seem particularly vulnerable to developing alcohol-related problems in old age.[148] Persisting social problems perpetuate the cycle of loneliness and further drinking.[149] Estimated prevalence of alcohol misuse or dependence in older people has varied depending on the setting and methodology of each study.[150] In general, community studies report lower prevalence compared to hospital-based studies.

The surveys, which are cross-sectional, do not take into account that drinking less may be a cohort rather than an age effect, whereby those who are currently older may always have had a relatively low intake. New cohorts of older people may drink more than those who started drinking in the 1920s.[151]

The prevalence of alcohol-use disorders in older people is approximately 1% to 3%.[152] The results from the National Epidemiological Survey of Alcohol and Related Conditions showed that in patients aged 65 years and older, 2.36% of men and 0.38% of women met criteria for alcohol abuse.[153] The National Health Interview Survey showed that in a sample of people aged 60 years and older, 50% of men and 39% of women reported daily drinking for the year before the survey. Binge drinking once a month or more was reported in 5.9% of men and 0.9% of women in that age group.[154] In hospital settings, the prevalence of substance misuse is approximately 10-fold more compared to community studies.[155] These prevalence estimates are mirrored in European countries, with some differences among countries (western European countries had higher prevalence compared to eastern countries). Also, the prevalence is greater in males and in people of higher socioeconomic status.[156] The problem does not seem to be largely confined to developed countries, as studies from developing countries, which were thought to be largely "dry," are now showing higher prevalence.[157] Risk factors for alcoholism are listed in Box 56-1.

BOX 56-1 Risk Factors for Alcoholism

- Family history
- Previous substance misuse
- Personality traits/disorders
- Factors that may increase exposure to/consumption of substances
  - Chronic painful illness
  - Insomnia
  - Long-term prescribing
  - Stress
  - Loneliness
  - Depression
  - Substance availability
- Factors that may increase the effects and misuse potential of substances
  - Pharmacokinetic and pharmacodynamics factors
  - Chronic medical conditions
  - Use of other medications

Modified from Atkinson RM: Substance abuse in the elderly. In Jacoby R, Oppenheimer C, editors: Psychiatry in the elderly, Oxford, England, 2002, Oxford University Press, pp 799–834.

Recommended Alcohol Consumption

Substantial evidence supports lowering the recommendation for alcohol intake for older people to reflect physiologic and pathologic changes associated with aging. The Royal College of Psychiatrists recommended an upper limit of an average of 1.5 units a day (averaged over a week). It also suggested defining binge drinking for older adults as the intake of more than 4.5 units for men and 3 units for women in a single session.[159]

Categories of alcohol misuse:

Hazardous drinking is defined as a level of alcohol intake that increases the risk of harm for the person or others. This is mostly seen as a public health problem rather than posing a risk to the individual.[160]

Harmful use is used to describe alcohol consumption that results in actual harm to the physical and mental health.[161]

Alcohol dependence is a cluster of symptoms characterized by craving for alcohol and the development of tolerance (need to drink higher amount to achieve the same effect). Preoccupation with alcohol and continued use despite harmful effects is also seen.[162]

Early Versus Late Alcohol Misuse Pattern

The pattern of alcohol use disorders in older people is broadly divided into two categories, namely, early and late onset. Early onset is characterized by misuse of alcohol starting at a younger age and continuing to old age. Two thirds of older adults with alcohol misuse fall into this category, and they have higher physical and mental health comorbidities.

Late onset describes alcohol use disorders occurring in late adulthood (fourth and fifth decades). The onset of a drinking problem is frequently related to adverse life events or physical and mental health problems (e.g., depression, loneliness, or loss of employment). People in this category may have fewer physical and mental health problems, and their chance of recovery may be higher.[163]

Clinical Features

The diagnosis of alcohol abuse may be difficult because the presentation may be masked, unsuspected, or atypical.[164] In a general medical setting, the prevalence is higher and the index of suspicion should be raised.[165] In particular, alcohol abuse should be suspected in the assessment of otherwise unexplained falls.

Alcohol abuse may be accompanied by a wide range of neuropsychiatric complications. Patients can have cognitive impairment, problems related to mixed intoxication with drugs, or unrecognized withdrawal states.[166] Alcohol abuse is also associated with functional psychiatric disorder, particularly depression.[167] Up to one third of older adults who break the law either abuse alcohol or are dependent on it, and they are often under the influence of alcohol when the crime is committed.[168] The benign course of "normal" drinking seems very different, however, from that of the problem drinkers in old age who often come for medical help when brain damage or social breakdown supervenes. A past history of alcohol-related problems is associated with both depression and dementia in later life. Depression and anxiety are major comorbid diagnoses. There is a strong association between alcohol misuse and suicidal attempts in both sexes.[169] It is estimated that 25% of patients with dementia also have alcohol misuse disorder and 20% of older adults with depression have comorbid alcohol misuse.[159] Psychiatric comorbidities of substance misuse are common in older people (including intoxication and delirium, withdrawal syndromes, anxiety, depression, and cognitive changes or dementia).

Screening Tools

Alcohol abuse in older people is often undetected,[170] particularly in patients with medical conditions, and screening at-risk groups may help physicians identify individuals at risk of alcohol abuse.[148] Various short questionnaires used to screen for alcohol misuse have been used and validated in older people. These include the CAGE questionnaire,[171] the Michigan Alcohol Screening Test–Geriatric Version (MAST-G),[172] Short Michigan Alcoholism Screening Test–Geriatric Version (SMAST-G),[173] and Alcohol Use Disorders Identification Test (AUDIT).[174] The sensitivities and specificities of these instruments vary. The CAGE has low validity, whereas MAST-G has high specificity and sensitivity for older people in various clinical settings, including outpatient clinics and elderly care homes.[175]

Alcohol and Cognitive Impairment

Alcohol is one of the common causes of cognitive impairment in older people after degenerative neurologic diseases (e.g., dementia), stroke, traumatic brain injury, and medication misuse.

The effect of alcohol on the brain is complex with a dual neurotoxic and neuroprotective effect depending on the amount consumed. Significant evidence exists based on neuroimaging and longitudinal studies showing that excessive alcohol consumption in older people is associated with increased risk of cognitive impairment and dementia. On the other hand, weaker evidence suggests that a low or moderate level of consumption may have a protective effect against cognitive decline and dementia. This has to be interpreted cautiously because of the heterogeneous methodologies and lack of standardization of the studies suggesting this association.[176]

Primary alcoholic dementia occurs when alcohol is the primary causative factor, whereas the term alcohol-related dementia is used when alcohol is contributing to the cognitive impairment and is not an essential factor in the cause.[177] A useful cognitive screening tool that can be used in older people with suspected substance misuse is the Montreal Cognitive Assessment. It is a brief and easy test that does not require specific training to administer.[178]

Management

When an individual is recognized as having an alcohol-related problem, several services may need to be involved. Home visits are often invaluable in the initial assessment.[179] Hospital admission may be needed to break the drinking routine, reduce risks associated with acute alcohol withdrawal,[180] and allow for full physical and psychiatric assessment. Alcohol withdrawal symptoms become more severe with age, and detoxification is more likely to be complicated by intercurrent illness. Withdrawal seizures occur within 24 hours, if at all. Tremor, tachycardia, hypertension, anxiety, nausea, and insomnia are prominent features of the alcohol withdrawal syndrome in older adults.

The patient should be nursed in a calm, well-lit environment. Shorter-acting benzodiazepines are preferred for sedation. The dosage for older patients undergoing detoxification should begin at about one third of that used for a fit younger person and should then be titrated against the clinical response. A long-term management plan needs to be formulated with either abstinence or controlled drinking as a goal. Older people respond better to social intervention than to intensive confrontation. Alcohol is often an occupation, and drinkers' social contact may be entirely with other drinkers.

Thus, part of the plan has to involve consideration of where and how someone who wishes to be an ex-drinker will spend the day. Amelioration of social stresses, group socialization, family work, medical treatment, and management of depression are all part of the approach needed.

Cognitive therapy, sometimes delivered through alcohol services, is often used. Those who wish to continue to drink and are eating little will often take thiamine, which may help protect them from Korsakov syndrome. Disulfiram is not recommended in older people because of increasing medical risks involved with ingesting alcohol while taking the drug.[181]

KEY POINTS

- Alcohol use disorders in older adults are prevalent but poorly recognized and treated.
- There are significant comorbid physical (e.g., chronic pain) and psychiatric disorders (e.g., depression) associated with excessive alcohol use in older people.
- Recommended daily alcohol intake should be lower for older people; the most conservative figure is not more than 1.5 unit of alcohol a day (averaged over a week).
- Excessive alcohol use is associated with variable degrees of cognitive impairment, some of which can be reversible upon reducing alcohol intake to "safe" or recommended level.
- Montreal Cognitive Assessment (MOCA) is a useful cognitive screening tool in older people with suspected coexisting alcohol use disorder.
- Management involves safe reduction and detoxification with close monitoring of physical health. An inpatient detoxification may be preferable due to the high prevalence of physical health problems.
- Holistic care with addressing psychological and social needs

CONCLUSION

This chapter has considered some of the key issues outside dementia in relation to mental health disorders in older people. There remains a dearth of research in these areas, and recommendations from younger patients may not apply. What is clear is that there is link with physical ill health and frailty in these disorders and prompt recognition and management could reduce the development of increasing dependency.

For a complete list of references, please visit www.expertconsult.com.

KEY REFERENCES

14. Seitz D, Purandare N, Conn D: Prevalence of psychiatric disorders among older adults in long term care homes: a systematic review. Int Psychogeriatr 22:1025–1039, 2010.
17. Barnes DE, Yaffe K, Byers AI, et al: Midlife vs late-life depressive symptoms and risk of dementia. Arch Gen Psychiatry 69:493–498, 2012.
19. Wolitzky-Taylor KB, Castriotta N, Lenze EJ, et al: Anxiety disorders in older adults: a comprehensive review. Depress Anxiety 27:190–211, 2010.
22. Coupland C, Dhiman D, Morriss R, et al: Antidepressant use and risk of adverse outcomes in older people: population based cohort study. BMJ 343:d4551, 2011.
29. American Psychiatric Association: Diagnostic and statistical manual of mental disorders, ed 5, Washington, DC, 2013, American Psychiatric Association.
33. Hilderink PH, Collard R, Rosmalen JGM, et al: Prevalence of somatoform disorders and medically unexplained symptoms in old age populations in comparison with younger age groups: a systematic review. Ageing Res Rev 12:151–156, 2013.
52. Brunelle S, Cole MG, Elie M: Risk factors for the late-onset psychoses: a systematic review of cohort studies. Int J Geriatr Psychiatry 27:240–252, 2012.

100. Flint A, Laboni A, Mulsant B, et al: Effect of sertraline on risk of falling in older adults with psychotic depression on olanzapine: results of a randomized placebo-controlled trial. Am J Geriatr Psychiatry 22:332–336, 2014.
111. Aziz R, Lorberg B, Tampi RR, et al: Treatments for late-life bipolar disorder. Am J Geriatr Pharmacother 4:347–364, 2006.
117. Dols A, Rhebergen D, Beekman A, et al: Psychiatric and medical comorbidities: results from a bipolar elderly cohort study. Am J Geriatr Psychiatry 22:1066–1074, 2014.
124. Trappler B, Backfield J: Clinical characteristics of older psychiatric inpatients with borderline personality disorder. Psychiatr Q 72:29–40, 2011.
139. Raposo SM, Mackenzie CS, Henriksen CA, et al: Time does not heal all wounds: older adults who experienced childhood adversities have higher odds of mood, anxiety, and personality disorders. Am J Geriatr Psychiatry 22:1241–1250, 2014.
147. O'Connell H, Chin AV, Cunningham C, et al: Alcohol use disorders in elderly people—redefining an age old problem in old age. BMJ 327:664–667, 2003.
152. Caputoa F, Vignolib T, Leggioc L, et al: Alcohol use disorders in the elderly: a brief overview from epidemiology to treatment options. Exp Gerontol 47:411–416, 2012.
178. Nasreddine ZS, Phillips NA, Bédirian V, et al: The Montreal Cognitive Assessment, MoCA: a brief screening tool for mild cognitive impairment. J Am Geriatr Soc 53:695–699, 2005.

57 Intellectual Disability in Older Adults

John M. Starr

DEFINITION AND CAUSES

Intellectual disability (ID) is the current term used to describe what in the United Kingdom has been known as learning disability and in the United States as mental retardation. The World Health Organization's International Classification of Diseases (ICD-10) still uses the term *mental retardation*, and its report on healthy aging in this population uses the term *intellectual disabilities*. In Australia the 1986 Victorian Act of Parliament defines intellectual disability in the following way:

> *Intellectual disability in relation to a person over the age of five years means a significant sub-average general intellectual functioning existing concurrently with deficits in adaptive behavior and manifested during the developmental period. (Intellectually Disabled Persons Services Act, 1986)*

The threshold at which general intellectual functioning is considered "subaverage" is often fixed at an IQ of 70, two standard deviations below the mean IQ. Controversially in 1992 the American Association on Intellectual and Developmental Disabilities (AAIDD) loosened this threshold to include people with IQs in the range of 70 to 75. The AIDD also required deficits in 2 out of 10 assessed areas of adaptive functioning. This definition was adapted by the American Psychiatric Association's *Diagnostic and Statistical Manual of Mental Disorders*, fourth edition (DSM-IV). In 2002 the AAIDD reinstated the IQ 70 threshold and required deficits in conceptual, social, and practical adaptive skills to be present. Areas covered by these skills include communication, personal care, home life, social skills, community utilization, self-governance, health and safety, functional academic skills, work, and leisure activities. These changes in definition have implications for epidemiologic data collection, but the key concept of ID remains. An IQ less than 70 is necessary but is, in itself, inadequate for the diagnosis to be made. For the diagnosis to be made, there must be evidence of both a developmental disorder (with onset during childhood) and deficits in adaptive behavior.

Further classification of ID can be made within the broad definition. The Diagnostic Criteria for Psychiatric Disorders for Use with Adults with Learning [Intellectual] Disabilities (DC-LD)[1] describes the mental health of a person with ID in terms of ID severity, ID causes, and related mental disorders (developmental disorders, psychiatric illness, personality disorders, problem behaviors, and other disorders). Severity is grouped according to IQ: 50 to 69, mild ID; 35 to 49, moderate; 20 to 34, severe; and less than 20, profound. The Swedish model of ID classification developed by Kylen[2] is often helpful in clinical situations where IQ is not known:

Severe: Communication is based on simple nonverbal signs, no verbal communication, no concept of time or space. Equivalent to IQ less than 10.

Moderate: Limited verbal skills. Limited understanding of local space. Can structure thoughts in relation to individual experiences. Equivalent to IQ 10 to 40.

Mild: Basic literacy and mathematical skills present. Can rearrange, structure, and perform concrete cognitive operations. Equivalent to IQ 41 to 70.

Severity may also be broadly estimated in terms of functional abilities:

Mild: Social and work skills adequate to work at a minimum wage

Moderate: Requires significant support to be able to work in a protected environment

Severe: Can partially contribute to his or her economic support with total supervision

In addition, the DC-LD includes appendices that relate to medical factors influencing health status and contact with health services. The latter are highly relevant because developmental disorders that affect the brain, giving rise to ID, often affect other body systems also.

The cause of ID is frequently unknown in older adults but can be considered along conventional lines of external causes (infection, injury, poisoning), internal disorders (endocrine, metabolic), perinatal insults, and congenital conditions (chromosomal abnormalities, gene mutations). The latter are of particular relevance to the health of older adults with ID as specific syndromes are associated with risk of particular physical disorders and diseases. Common syndromes seen in older adults include Down syndrome (DS), Angelman syndrome, fragile X syndrome, Klinefelter syndrome, Turner syndrome, and Williams syndrome. Table 57-1 provides a brief description of these. It is worth noting that, given the preceding definition of ID, by no means does everyone with one of these syndromes fulfill the diagnostic criteria for ID; this is particular true of women with Turner syndrome, who have a tendency for nonverbal cognitive deficits but are often of average intelligence.

Just as there is a considerable overlap between congenital syndromes, such as DS and ID, there is a similar overlap between ID and autism. The diagnosis of autism depends on (1) abnormal social development, (2) communication deficits, and (3) restricted and repetitive interests and behavior. Approximately three quarters of people with autism have a nonverbal IQ less than 70 and hence also fulfill diagnostic criteria for ID, but in autism social and communication skills are worse than expected for any given nonverbal IQ.

EPIDEMIOLOGY OF INTELLECTUAL DISABILITY AND AGING

Prevalence

In 2001 the World Health Organization reported,

> *The prevalence figures [of ID] vary considerably because of the varying criteria and methods used in the surveys, as well as differences in the age range of the samples. The overall prevalence of mental retardation is believed to be between 1% and 3%, with the rate for moderate, severe and profound retardation being 0.3%.*[3]

Extrapolating these figures to the United Kingdom provides estimates of approximately 175,800 people with moderate-to-profound ID and between 586,000 and 1,465,000 with mild ID.[4] For Finland the equivalent estimates are 15,300 and between 51,000 and 127,500, respectively. Population-based surveys in Finland have estimated moderate-to-profound ID prevalence at

TABLE 57-1 Characteristics of Common Syndromes Associated With Intellectual Disability

Syndrome Name	Chromosomal Abnormality	Phenotypic Appearance*
Angelman syndrome	15q11-q13 in the maternally contributed chromosome (cf. Prader-Willi syndrome has same deletion in paternal chromosome); a few cases due to paternal chromosome 15 disomy and a few due to putative single gene mutation on chromosome 15	Microcephaly, ataxic gait, strabismus, scoliosis
Down syndrome	Vast majority trisomy of chromosome 21; a few have trisomy 21 mosaicism; small proportion translocation of chromosome 21	Flat facial profile, epicanthic fold, relative hyperglossia, single palmar crease
Fragile X syndrome	X-linked, semi-dominant disorder with reduced penetrance Number of fragile sites on X-chromosome identified, two important for intellectual disability around X27.3	Broad forehead with long face, large ears, strabismus, high arched palate, macroorchidism, scoliosis, joint hyperextensibility
Klinefelter syndrome	XXY and XXY mosaicism with variants XXXY or XXYY	Taller than average, microorchidism, youthful appearance, gynecomastia
Turner syndrome	XO, partial deletion of second X chromosome, XO mosaicism	Short stature, premature ovarian failure, high arched palate, low-set ears, webbed neck, strabismus, cubitus valgus, scoliosis, short fourth metacarpals
Williams syndrome	Deletion of *CLIP2, GTF2I, GTF2IRD1, LIMK1,* and other genes from chromosome 7	"Elfin" features of upturned nose, widely spaced eyes, wide mouth with full lips, small chin, high levels of empathy and anxiety

*The phenotypic features are "typical" and may not be evident in all people with the syndrome. Similarly, many phenotypic features are found in unaffected individuals.

TABLE 57-2 Common Adult Medical Problems in Various Intellectual Disability Syndromes

Study	Country	Dates	Incidence Changes (per 10,000 Live Births)
Krivchenia E, et al: Am J Epidemiol 137:815–828, 1993	United States	1970–1989	Increase in all groups except urban white population where incidence decreased due to terminations of pregnancy; 11.7 average over whole period
Carothers AD, et al: J Med Genet 36:386–393, 1999	Scotland	1990–1994	Decrease from 10.8 to 7.7
Merrick J: Down Syndr Res Pract 6:128–130, 2001	Israel	1964–1997	Decrease from 24.3 to 10, but unchanged when terminations of pregnancy included
Verloes A, et al: Eur J Hum Genet 9:1–4, 2001	Belgium	1984–1998	Decrease following, but not fully explained by, prenatal screening from 12.6 to 6.2 live births
Nazar HJ, et al: Rev Med Chile 134:1549–1557, 2006	Chile	1972–2005	Increase, 3.36 average over whole period
Morris JK, Alberman E: Br Med J 339:3794, 2009	United Kingdom	1989–2008	Live births fell by 1% over 19 years; overall prenatal and postnatal diagnoses rose by 71%

no more than 0.2% and overall ID prevalence at just over 1%.[4] The situation is similar for the United Kingdom.[4] Notably, Finnish prevalence rates estimated from national registers is a little lower at 0.7%, perhaps indicating that not all people with ID are known to Finnish health or social services.[5] Within overall prevalence figures there is considerable variation by age. In the Finnish national register survey, the rates were 0.53% for individuals aged 15 years and younger, 0.70% for those aged 16 to 39 years, 0.92% for those 40 to 64 years old, and 0.38% for those 65 years and older.[5] Variation in Finland between age groups was attributed to changes in incidence, mortality, diagnostic practices, and benefit provision. Changes in diagnostic practices have been discussed in the previous section and benefit provision is specific to Finland, but changes in ID incidence and mortality have been tracked across the world. A meta-analysis of 52 population-based studies also estimated prevalence at just over 1%, falling with age.[6]

Incidence

Estimation of ID incidence is problematic given that ID is, by definition, a developmental disorder and thus there is no single point at which it is recognized. In view of this, DS is often used as a proxy because it is the largest single cause of ID. However, its use as a proxy is far from ideal because risk is clearly associated with maternal age and consequent prenatal screening that has been widely introduced. Table 57-2 summarizes secular trends in DS incidence from various countries. Overall DS incidence appears to have been rising prior to the introduction of prenatal screening. This resulted in a decrease that is projected to be offset by increasing mean maternal age. Overall, there seems little to indicate a great change in ID incidence per 1000 live births, and numbers of people with ID may track the overall birth rates in different countries.

Mortality

Mortality has had the greatest impact on ID prevalence, especially in older age groups. In 1900 a child with DS would expect to survive to approximately 9 years of age. In the United States median age at death for children with DS increased from 25 years in 1983 to 49 years in 1997.[7] Mean life expectancy for a child born with DS in the United Kingdom in 2011 was 51 years, with a median life expectancy of 58 years.[8] The improvement likely reflects improved socioeconomic circumstances, improved correction of congenital cardiac abnormalities, and perhaps changing attitudes to treating people with ID. There is only a minor difference in life expectancy for people with DS compared with other causes of ID.[9] Identification of common causes of death in people with ID is made difficult by poor death certificate completion. For example, many people in the United States had either ID or DS listed as a primary cause of death, which is inappropriate.[9] However, as the ID population ages, the causes of death are thought to resemble those in the general population more and more closely. Those with mild ID survive longer, and there is some equivalence to this observation in the general population, where people with low IQs within the normal range suffer premature mortality largely attributable to cardiovascular disease.[10] Current trends suggest that people with ID can expect to live to 60 to 65 years, and an increasing proportion will survive beyond this age.

BIOLOGIC AGING IN INDIVIDUALS WITH INTELLECTUAL DISABILITY: SYNDROMIC AND NONSYNDROMIC

Even with recent improvements, the life expectancy of people with ID is considerably less than that of the non-ID population. This raises the question as to whether ID is associated with accelerated biologic aging. The measurement of biologic age usually depends on identifying suitable biomarkers of aging. Criteria for such biomarkers have been proposed[11]:

1. They must reflect some basic biologic process of aging rather than disease.
2. They must have high cross-species reproducibility.
3. They must change independently of chronologic time.
4. They must be obtainable antemortem.
5. They must be measurable over a short period compared to the life span of the organism.

One such biomarker is telomere length.[12] There is a paucity of data on telomere length in ID in general, but there is evidence for telomere shortening in DS[13] though this appears to be downstream from cellular redox status[14] as is also likely in the general population.[15] In cri-du-chat syndrome there is often a deletion of the short arm of chromosome 5 where the telomerase reverse transcriptase (*hTERT*) gene is localized (5p15.33). Reconstitution of telomerase activity by ectopic expression of *hTERT* extends telomere length, increases population doublings, and prevents the end-to-end fusion of chromosomes.[16] It may thus be one element contributing to the syndrome's phenotypic features. Whether this is the case or not, accelerated telomere shortening occurs with aging in this syndrome.[17] At least a further 5% of ID is attributable to similar subtelomeric deletions or copy number variations[18] and these, too, can influence telomere length. Telomere length is thus a potentially useful index of accelerated biologic aging in ID, but whether it contributes to aging itself or is only a correlate remains unclear. Moreover, telomere shortening is subject to syndrome-specific effects. Beyond the cellular level, various physiologic biomarkers are also affected in ID. Physiologic variables are long recognized as indices of biologic age.[19] The limited data available indicate that people with DS have accelerated biologic aging but that people with nonsyndromic ID do not.[20,21] In summary, the evidence suggests that syndromic biologic aging dominates over any accelerated biologic aging that might be associated with ID in general and that different ID syndromes are likely to have different aging profiles depending on the specific genetic changes underlying them.

AGE-RELATED DISEASE: SYNDROMIC AND NONSYNDROMIC PATTERNS

People with ID exhibit considerable morbidity. A study of 346 people aged 20 to 50 years in North Sydney found they had a mean 2.5 major problems and 2.9 minor problems each with 42% of these undiagnosed prior to the study, and of the 58% already known, only 49% were being managed adequately.[22] A study of 1371 adults aged 40 years and older in New York State found that increased age was associated with higher prevalence of cardiovascular disease, cancer, respiratory disease, musculoskeletal disorders, infections, and visual and hearing impairments; gastrointestinal disease was not associated with age but with being male, more severe ID, cerebral palsy, and obesity.[23] Compared with the non-ID population, there was less cardiovascular disease and musculoskeletal disease, except osteoarthritis, and people with DS did not have solid neoplasias. However, these data may reflect underdiagnosis and lifestyle factors such as the low rate of cigarette smoking among people with ID. A similar age-related pattern of disease was found in southern Holland.[24] The pattern may change as fewer people with ID live in institutions: there is evidence from the United Kingdom that poor diet, reduced physical activity, and obesity risk factors are greater in women with ID who are more able and independent.[25] In addition to the general tendency for high levels of morbidity, which is associated with both age and degree of ID severity, specific syndromes carry their own particular risks (Table 57-3). The most common syndrome in older adults with ID is DS, and discussion of the various problems in people with DS can provide a general approach to such problems in other syndromes.

TABLE 57-3 Secular Trends in Down Syndrome Incidence

Syndrome	Cardiovascular Problems	Neurologic Problems	Sensory Problems	Other Problems
Angelman		Seizures common, ataxia, absence of speech	Otitis media	Respiratory infections, obesity
Down	Septal defects, valvular disease	Seizures in ≈10%, Alzheimer-type dementia	Cataracts, hearing loss	Osteoporosis, hypothyroidism, blood dyscrasias, atlantoaxial instability
Fragile X	Septal defects, valvular disease	Seizures can occur	Cataracts, coloboma	Joint instability, hernias
Myotonic dystrophy		Myotonia with muscle weakness		
Rubinstein-Taybi	Septal defects, valvular disease	Seizures can occur	Cataracts, optic nerve abnormalities, hearing loss	Renal abnormalities (absent/extra kidneys), cryptorchidism
Smith-Lemli-Opitz	Septal defects, valvular disease		Visual and hearing loss	Low cholesterol levels, multiple organ abnormalities
Smith-Magenis	Septal defects, valvular disease	Sleep disturbance, self injury, aggression, peripheral neuropathy	Hyperacusis, wax buildup	Multiple organ abnormalities, hypothyroidism, immunoglobulin deficiency
Williams	Septal defects, valvular disease, hypertension	Cerebrovascular disease		Multiple organ abnormalities, hoarse voice, hypothyroidism, constipation

Down Syndrome: Effects on Systems

Cardiovascular: Late Effects of Congenital Heart Disease, Hyperlipidemia

Congenital heart disease is common in many ID syndromes as multiple genes contribute to its etiology; DS is a common cause of ID-associated congenital heart disease. Nowadays there is no reason why children with DS and congenital heart defects should not have surgical correction.[26] Complications of uncorrected congenital heart disease, such as Eisenmenger syndrome and infective endocarditis, are thus becoming rare. In addition, persistent atrial septal defects are associated with increased risk of cerebral embolic events. However, many people with DS are not under regular follow-up once they become adults and may continue to have problems with arrhythmias. In particular, right bundle branch block is not uncommon after surgery. This is usually of no relevance until some form of left bundle branch block occurs when progression to complete heart block becomes more likely. There may also be residual hypoxemia due to persisting right-to-left shunts. Again, this generally is of no consequence until some extra stress to the system occurs, such as a general anesthetic. Some residual shunts may also be associated with a degree of pulmonary hypertension. Lifestyle factors and associated obesity put adults with DS at increased risk of hyperlipidemia. It is unclear how much impact this has on cardiovascular disease risk in this population, but there is evidence for a deleterious effect on cognition (see the next section).

Neurologic: Dementia, Epilepsy, Vision and Hearing Loss

Dementia is three to four times more prevalent among adults with ID than the similarly aged general population.[27] The prevalence in DS is substantially higher. Forty percent of those older than 50 years acquire an Alzheimer-type dementia with the typical neuropathologic features present in nearly everyone by the age of 40 years.[28] Dementia incidence in those older than 50 is 18%,[29] indicating the very short survival once the condition is diagnosed. Despite similar neuropathologic features, clinical manifestation of dementia often differs in DS with frontal lobe symptoms, such as deficits in executive functioning characterized by planning problems, personality changes, and development of problem behaviors being present at an early stage. It is natural to attribute any such changes to the onset of a dementing illness in DS because dementia is so common, but other conditions, even something as simple as constipation, can also occur with similar atypical symptoms. A full health assessment, with attention to physical factors, is therefore necessary. Epilepsy is common in ID, including DS, and may signal the onset of dementia in older adults; this may be especially the case for late-onset myoclonic epilepsy. People with more severe ID are at increased risk of seizures. Seizures are usually controllable with monotherapy. In other syndromes, seizures can be far more difficult to control.

Visual problems in DS may be associated with development; approximately 60% of children with DS require glasses. People with DS have a flat nasal bridge, which can result in their glasses slipping. Strabismus is also common. In later life, cataracts are highly prevalent, nearly 30% in those aged 65 and older.[30] Hearing impairment is also common and, similar to visual impairment, may date from childhood. Hearing impairment may result from a buildup of ear wax, but hearing aids are often needed for both conductive and sensorineural deficits.

Gastrointestinal: Dentition, Gastroesophageal Reflux, Constipation

Although not associated with either aging or mortality, gastrointestinal complaints are frequent in individuals with DS. In the general population dental status is an index of socioeconomic status and so poor dentition may reflect this in DS where conventional socioeconomic measures are often unhelpful. It may also reflect both severity of ID (affecting oral hygiene) and age. Chronic gingivitis and especially periodontitis is highly prevalent in DS and is associated with cardiovascular disease, respiratory disease, and diabetes. Gingival hyperplasia is sometimes found in people who are taking phenytoin for epilepsy. Obesity is common in DS and is associated with gastroesophageal reflux (GERD) and cholelithiasis. A Dutch study of 77 adults with ID aged 60 years or older found 9% had GERD, 10% symptomatic cholelithiasis, and 57% chronic constipation; the latter was far more common in those with mild ID compared with moderate or severe ID.[31] Only the minority of adults with GERD complained of typical symptoms; most had insomnia or behavioral changes.

Endocrinologic: Hypothyroidism, Testosterone and Estrogen Deficiency

Approximately one quarter of people with DS develop hypothyroidism, many in childhood or early adulthood. Other forms of endocrine failure are also more common. Women with DS are twice as likely to experience early menopause, compared with the general population,[32] with a median age of approximately 46 years. Those women who experience menopause earlier are also at increased risk of developing dementia at a younger age.[33] This may reflect some general biologic aging phenomenon, or it may be associated with a specific lack of estrogen. It is unclear whether age at menopause relates to IQ as is the situation in the general population.[34] Men with DS tend to have elevated follicle-stimulating hormone (FSH) and luteinizing hormone (LH) levels with low testosterone levels. There is a lack of trials of testosterone replacement therapy in men with DS, so it is unclear whether testing gonadal hormone levels is useful.

Musculoskeletal: Arthritis, Metabolic Bone Disease

Osteoarthritis is common in DS and, similar to other conditions, may be associated with obesity. Osteoporosis is also common and may, in part, relate to hypothyroidism and gonadal hormone failure. In one screening of community residents with ID, aged 40 to 60 years, 21% had osteoporosis and 34% osteopenia.[35] People with DS appear to benefit from vitamin D and calcium treatment as much as the general population.[36]

Dermatologic: Eczema, Acne, and Diseases of the Scalp

Eczema, acne, and yeast-associated folliculitis are all common in individuals with DS. The latter may reflect some subtle deficiency of cellular immunity as also reflected by increased prevalence of fungal infections of the nails.[37] There is evidence of altered T-cell function, especially in older men with DS.[38] An immunologic cause may also underpin the increased incidence of alopecia, as suggested by the high prevalence of autoimmune thyroid disease. Adults with DS may have low neutrophil counts with a tendency of lymphocyte counts also to be on the low side.[37]

ASSESSMENT OF THE HEALTH OF OLDER ADULTS WITH INTELLECTUAL DISABILITY

The preceding sections indicate that older people with ID have an increased disease load and usually suffer from multiple pathologic conditions. Disease load increases with ID severity and hence particularly affects those people with more communication problems. Partly for this reason, disease often goes undetected. When assessing the health of someone with ID, it is worth recalling the North Sydney experience in which half of major medical problems were unknown and of the half that were already known about, half were inadequately managed.[22]

The Multidisciplinary Setting of Assessment

People with ID are usually at the center of a complex support system. It is usually worth taking time to elucidate this together with identifying all the health and social care professionals involved, as this often provides useful information. Typical professional contacts might include social workers, clinical psychologists, speech and language therapists, community nurses, psychiatrists with an interest in ID, occupational therapists, audiology services, and community dentists. In some countries people with ID have formal legal representatives; for example, in Scotland a welfare guardian can be appointed under the Adults with Incapacity Act. Although information gathering is very important, such information may not always be reliable. For example, when 589 adults with ID were being discharged from a large Scottish institution, the nurses who had been looking after them thought 49% of the adults had perfect vision, whereas actual ophthalmologic assessment showed that only 0.8% did.[39] Similarly, the nurses thought 74% of the adults had perfect hearing, whereas audiologic assessment found this was the case for only 11%.

Brief Physical Health Screening Tools

Many of the brief physical health screening tools available were designed to be administered by nurses. They are usually based on making medical diagnoses and are not designed to assess atypical presentation of disease. Wilson and Haire provided the prototype for this kind of assessment, largely applying methods of examination used in the non-ID population, which, as in other studies, noted the large number of health problems that had gone undetected prior to screening.[40] These assessments were originally designed to detect threats to health. For example, routine physical examination of the chest is performed because respiratory infection is a major cause of death in people with ID.[41-43] However, even in the general population, chest examination[44] has poor sensitivity and specificity. The same can be said for many aspects of routine physical examination, such as abdominal examination[45] and musculoskeletal examination.[46] In addition, older adults with ID do not always find conventional medical examinations easy to tolerate. Explaining the relevance of various elements, such as chest percussion, can be difficult. In addition, physical examination can trigger recall of experiences of physical or sexual abuse. Screening tools are therefore best used to provide a checklist for information gathering as a background for fuller assessment.

User-Led Physical Health Assessments

One way to find a workable way to assess the health of older people with ID is to find out what they consider to be health and what kinds of assessment they find acceptable. The comprehensive health assessment program (CHAP) is one such example developed in Australia and validated by randomized control trial with its acceptability to participants assessed.[47,48] The CHAP is a development from the Cardiff health check that was also subject to a randomized control trial[49]; its validation is thus reassuring as to the validity of carer-answered items since other assessments have found carer responses to be unreliable, as noted earlier. Although acceptable to people with ID, the CHAP was not designed to align with their particular priorities for health. This alignment is essential because at present people with ID feel that the partnership between them and their physician is far from equal.[50] Moreover, government policies are beginning to require this; for example, NHS Scotland directives recommend attention to these "critical factors":

- Component parts of the health screen which must be relevant to the particular health needs of persons with learning disabilities (rather than the general population)
- The acceptability of the health screen to persons with learning disabilities and their carers[51]

When older adults are asked about their understanding of health, three key themes emerge:

1. Being able to do things and participate in activities
2. Nutrition;
3. Hygiene and self-care[52]

Moreover, their concept of health is much closer to the World Health Organization's definition in that it incorporates aspects of well-being beyond the mere absence of disease.[53] Appropriate health assessments need to capture these positive aspects, therefore, by asking questions related to the key health themes in addition to the standard medical checklists designed to identify disease. Similarly, examination needs to incorporate measures germane to the health themes rather than merely aiming to identify disease. It is not surprising that such aspects of assessment are welcomed by adults with ID,[52] and several have been validated in this population. Figure 57-1 provides a template user-led health assessment that includes independently validated items that are both generally acceptable and feasible.[54] In practice it takes an average of 20 to 30 minutes to complete, and this tends to be a little quicker in those with more severe ID who find some of the items very difficult (e.g., peak flow). Indeed, it is sensible to note the severity of ID in conjunction with the assessment and, where this is unknown, use the Swedish classification developed by Kylen.[2] The assessment provides a good baseline against which changes in health status can be assessed. To work out foot size to which shoe size can be compared, the chart in Table 57-4 can be used by measuring foot length (draw a line on a piece of paper at the heel and toes); allow one half size either way. It is not uncommon for older adults with ID to have shoes larger than their measured size because their feet are often disproportionately wide.

Mental Health Assessment

Assessing mental health may fall to specialists in the psychiatry of ID. However, it is useful for physicians to be able to diagnose delirium and dementia in older adults with ID. The principles of diagnosing delirium in people with ID are no different from those in the general population. The ICD-10 diagnostic criteria comprise (1) impairment of consciousness and attention, (2) global disturbance of cognition, (3) psychomotor disturbance, (4) sleep/wake cycle disturbance, and (5) emotional disturbance. Generally the diagnosis applies to symptom duration of less than 6 months. The challenge is being able to make the diagnosis in people with severe or profound ID in whom there is usually a background disturbance of all five criteria. Here a fluctuating course can be a helpful indicator of the presence of delirium. Similarly, psychomotor disturbance, unexplained hypo- or hyperactivity, is also a useful pointer. Emotional disturbance is likely to be expressed nonverbally by changes in behavior.

Similarly, the diagnosis of dementia in people with ID can also require considerable clinical skill. The key diagnostic criterion is demonstrating cognitive decline from baseline and this usually requires two detailed clinical psychology assessments. Several assessment tools are available; one that spans the general and ID population is the Severe Impairment Battery.[55] Having demonstrated cognitive decline, a hierarchic approach can be adopted to determine the causes: this comprises considering (1) physical illness, (2) effects of medication, (3) sensory loss, (4) environmental change or life events, and (5) mental illness.[27] This is not to say that the diagnosis of dementia cannot be made in the presence

Medical information

Age ______ Sex ______ Cause of LD ___________

Known medical problems

1 ______________ 2 ______________

3 ______________ 4 ______________

5 ______________ 6 ______________

Medication

1 ______________ 2 ______________

3 ______________ 4 ______________

5 ______________ 6 ______________

Allergies ______________

Smoking ______________ **Alcohol** ______________

Residence and support ______________

Hobbies/interests ______________

____

Systems inquiry

Respiratory SOBOE Wheeze Cough ____

GI GERD symptoms Constipation Weight loss ____

Fecal incontinence never / occasional / frequent / always

GU urinary incontinence never / occasional / frequent / always

Menstruation Previous pregnancies ______

Trauma/falls in the last year ______________

Vision

Recognizes parents, staff, etc.	Y/N
Recognizes shapes	Y/N
Names/matches colors	Y/N
Gets lost in house, street, etc.	Y/N
Can climb stairs, see curbstone	Y/N
Can walk in the dusk	Y/N
Recognizes houses, cars, etc. when moving	Y/N
Can find small object on patterned tablecloth	Y/N
Gazes at lights	Y/N
Is visual attention fleeting	Y/N

Sleep

Hours per night Wakes at night During day ____

Physical activity

Hours of moderate/severe per week ______________

Socioeconomic

Number of pairs of outdoor shoes ______________

Townsend disability scale

Are you able to... Score (0, no difficulty; 1 with difficulty; 2 unable)

1 Cut your own toenails? ______________

2 Wash all over or bathe? ______________

3 Get on a bus? ______________

4 Go up and down stairs? ______________

5 Do the heavy housework? ______________

6 Shop and carry heavy bags? ______________

7 Prepare and cook a hot meal? ______________

8 Reach an overhead shelf? ______________

9 Tie a good knot in a piece of string? ______________

TOTAL ______________

Physical assessment

Height cm Pubis-feet cm

Weight kg Waist cm Hip cm

Teeth Missing Decayed Filled

Vision Range of EOMs normal / abnormal

Funduscopy

Hearing (End expiratory whisper out of direct view 1m from ear)

Objects	Left	Right
Key		
Ball		
Pen		
Comb		
Bag		
Tape		

Otoscopy Normal / Abnormal

Cardiovascular

Pulse BP sitting BP standing

Heart sounds pp's edema

Respiratory

Cervical lymphadenopathy Thoracic kyphoscoliosis Yes / No

PEFR L/min

Neurologic

Grip strength Sit / stands 20 secs

Resting tremor Yes / No Foot vibration sense Left Right

Feet Size Size of footwear

Nails in good condition

Figure 57-1. A template user-led health assessment for older adults with ID. *EOMs*, Extraocular movements; *GERD,* gastroesophageal reflux disease; *GI,* gastrointestinal; *GU,* genitourinary; *LD,* learning disability; *PEFR,* peak expiratory flow rate; *SOBOE,* shortness of breath on exertion.

TABLE 57-4 Foot Size Chart*

Inches (US)	cm	Men	Women	UK	Europe	Mondopoint
8	20.3	2	3	1	33.0	21.3
8⅙	20.7	2½	3½	1½	33.6	21.7
8⅓	21.2	3	4	2	34.3	22.2
8½	21.6	3½	4½	2½	34.9	22.6
8⅔	22.0	4	5	3	35.5	23.0
8⅚	22.4	4½	5½	3½	36.2	23.4
9	22.9	5	6	4	36.8	23.9
9⅙	23.3	5½	6½	4½	37.5	24.3
9⅓	23.7	6	7	5	38.1	24.7
9½	24.1	6½	7½	5½	38.7	25.1
9⅔	24.6	7	8	6	39.4	25.6
9⅚	25.0	7½	8½	6½	40.0	26.0
10	25.4	8	9	7	40.6	26.4

*Sizes depend on foot length (biggest foot with sock on).

of any of these five possible contributors to cognitive decline; indeed, not infrequently such potential contributors coexist with dementia. Nevertheless, it is generally worthwhile addressing reversible causes of cognitive decline (e.g., sensory loss) whenever possible. As noted earlier, behavioral changes may predate any clinically evident cognitive decline.

COMMUNICATION

The General Medical Council's *Tomorrow's Doctors*[56] lists 14 basic duties of a doctor, the first 8 of which are especially pertinent when caring for older adults with ID:

- Make the care of your patient your first concern.
- Treat every patient politely and considerately.
- Respect patients' dignity and privacy.
- Listen to patients and respect their views.
- Give patients information in a way they can understand.
- Respect the rights of patients to be fully involved in decisions about their care.
- Keep your professional knowledge and skills up to date.
- Recognize the limits of your professional competence.

Carers and other members of the multidisciplinary team, such as nurses and speech language therapists, can be particularly helpful if you feel you are reaching the limits of your own professional competence in communicating with people with ID. Most older adults with ID will be on the mild end of the spectrum and thus be able to communicate verbally. It is important to take account of any sensory loss, which is common, and to provide an appropriate environment to facilitate communication. Plenty of time should be available. It is good practice to use plain language and keep sentences short, with just one idea per sentence. Conditional sentences are best avoided. It is also helpful to use concrete rather than abstract terms, supporting this with nonverbal aids whenever possible. If you are drawing a body part, remember to put this in context of the external human figure. Pictures of sunrises or beds may help with eliciting duration of symptoms. Just as with other communication, it is sensible to check what has been understood by asking people with ID to explain things in their own words. Various organizations produce easy-to-read information on common health topics, which can be helpful. For example, the Royal College of Psychiatrists have produced a Books Beyond Words series.

HEALTH PROMOTION

Health promotion is predicated on having appropriate health targets. Typically targets are set aiming for equity with the non-ID population based on evidence for effective interventions[57] and cover these areas:

- Dental health
- Hearing and vision
- Nutrition and growth
- Prevention and treatment of chronic constipation
- Epilepsy review
- Thyroid screening
- Identify and treat mental health problems
- GERD and *H. pylori* eradication
- Osteoporosis
- Medication review
- Vaccination
- Provision of exercise opportunities
- Regular physical assessment and review
- Breast and cervical cancer screening

In addition to these general recommendations, there may be syndrome-specific actions to be considered. User-led concepts of health (functional ability and participation, nutrition, self-care and hygiene) are likely to be useful in structuring health promotion for older adults with ID. Communication is key to good health promotion. For example, if a health promotion campaign endorses a negative stereotype of obesity, people with ID may identify with the stereotype and feel "unhealthy" as a consequence. It would be preferable to deliver a clear positive message about healthy eating and exercise instead. Perhaps the most important task of health promotion is to communicate with carers, and any social or health care professionals involved in the care of an older adult with ID, the importance of enhancing functional abilities, participation, and self-care.

INTELLECTUAL DISABILITY AND FRAILTY

People with ID are more likely to be frail, whether frailty is defined by a phenotype or deficit accumulation approach.[58] In both cases, frailty develops at younger ages and is more severe than in the general population. It is also commonly associated with disability[59,60] and with the earlier onset of conditions such as a range of chronic diseases, hearing loss, depression, and falls, leading, in this context, too, to the suggestion that it represents a form of accelerated aging.[61] Among people aged 50 years and older, frailty is also associated with a greater requirement for health care.[62] Physical fitness (measured with items such as manual dexterity, visual reaction time, balance, comfortable and fast walking speed, muscular endurance,[63] cardiorespiratory fitness, grip strength, and muscular endurance) has been found to be associated with decline in daily functioning.[64] This suggests that interventions to improve physical fitness might have a role in mitigating risk in relation to function decline and perhaps also to health care use. It is notable also that, as with frail older adults in the general population, frailty is also associated with a greater risk of prescription errors, suggesting that preventive maneuvers need also to be targeted at mitigating risks related to routine care.

KEY POINTS

- There is a rapid increase in the number of adults with intellectual disability surviving into old age.
- Diagnosis requires an IQ of less than 70 together with evidence of a developmental disorder and deficits in adaptive behavior.
- Severity of intellectual disability can be estimated according to verbal skills.
- Health status is influenced by the degree of intellectual severity and specific syndromic associations.
- Older adults with intellectual disability envisage health in terms of (1) being able to do things and participate in activities, (2) nutrition, and (3) hygiene/self-care.
- User-led health assessments are feasible and relate closely to conventional health outcomes.
- Dementia is common in older adults with intellectual disability. Diagnosis is aided by a hierarchic approach that considers (1) physical illness, (2) effects of medication, (3) sensory loss, (4) environmental change or life events, and (5) mental illness.
- Frailty is also common in people with intellectual disability and occurs at younger ages and with greater severity. Improving physical fitness can reduce later ill-health, disability, and health care use.

For a complete list of references, please visit www.expertconsult.com.

KEY REFERENCES

1. Royal College of Psychiatrists: OP48. DC-LD: Diagnostic criteria for psychiatric disorders for use with adults with learning disabilities/mental retardation, London, 2001, Royal College of Psychiatrists.
2. Kylen G: En begavningsteori, Stockholm, 1985, Stiftelsen ala.
3. World Health Organization: The World Health Organization Report 2001—Mental health: new understanding, new hope, Geneva, 2001, World Health Organization.
6. Maulik PK, Mascarenhas MN, Mathers CD, et al: Prevalence of intellectual disability: a meta-analysis of population-based studies. Res Devel Disabil 32:419–436, 2011.
21. Carmeli E, Kessel S, Bar-Chad S, et al: A comparison between older persons with Down syndrome and a control group: clinical characteristics, functional status and sensorimotor function. Down Syndr Res Pract 9:17–24, 2004.
22. Beange H, McElduff A, Baker W: Medical disorders in adults with mental retardation. Am J Ment Retard 99:595–604, 1995.
23. Janicki MP, Davidson PW, Henderson CM, et al: Health characteristics and health services utilization in older adults with intellectual disability living in community residences. J Intellect Disabil Res 46:287–298, 2002.
24. van Schrojenstein Lantman-de Valk HMJ, van den Akker M, Maaskant MA, et al: Prevalence and incidence of health problems in people with intellectual disability. J Intellect Disabil Res 41:42–51, 1997.
25. Robertson J, Emerson E, Gregory N, et al: Lifestyle risk factors and poor health. Res Dev Disab 21:469–486, 2000.
27. Strydom A, Livingston G, King M, et al: Prevalence of dementia in intellectual disability using different diagnostic criteria. Br J Psychiatr 191:150–157, 2007.
37. Prasher V: Screening of medical problems in adults with Down syndrome. Down Syndr Res Pract 2:59–66, 1994.
39. Kerr AM, McCulloch D, Oliver K, et al: Medical needs of people with intellectual disability require regular reassessment, and the provision of client- and carer-held reports. J Intellect Disabil Res 47:134–145, 2003.
41. Jones RG, Kerr MP: A randomized control trial of an opportunistic health screening tool in primary care for people with intellectual disability. J Intellect Disabil Res 41:409–415, 1997.
47. Lennox N, Rey-Conde T, Bain C, et al: The evidence for better health from health assessments: a large clustered randomised controlled trial. J Intellect Disabil Res 48:343, 2004.
49. Jones RG, Kerr MP: A randomized control trial of an opportunistic health screening tool in primary care for people with intellectual disability. J Intellect Disabil Res 41:409–415, 1997.
52. Fender A, Marsden L, Starr JM: What do older adults with Down's syndrome want from their doctor? A preliminary report. Br J Learning Disabil 35:19–22, 2007.
53. Starr JM, Marsden L: Characterisation of user-defined health status in older adults with intellectual disabilities. J Intellect Disabil Res 52:483–489, 2008.
54. Fender A, Marsden L, Starr JM: Assessing the health of older adults with intellectual disabilities: a user-led approach. J Intellect Disabil 11:223–239, 2007.
59. Evenhuis HM, Hermans H, Hilgenkamp TI, et al: Frailty and disability in older adults with intellectual disabilities: results from the healthy ageing and intellectual disability study. J Am Geriatr Soc 60:934–938, 2012.
60. Schoufour JD, Mitnitski A, Rockwood K, et al: Predicting disabilities in daily functioning in older people with intellectual disabilities using a frailty index. Res Dev Disabil 35:2267–2277, 2014.
61. Lin JD, Lin LP, Hsu SW, et al: Are early onset aging conditions correlated to daily activity functions in youth and adults with Down syndrome? Res Dev Disabil 36C:532–536, 2014.
62. Schoufour JD, Evenhuis HM, Echteld MA: The impact of frailty on care intensity in older people with intellectual disabilities. Res Dev Disabil 35:3455–3461, 2014.
63. Hilgenkamp TI, van Wijck R, Evenhuis HM: Feasibility of eight physical fitness tests in 1,050 older adults with intellectual disability: results of the healthy ageing with intellectual disabilities study. Intellect Dev Disabil 51:33–47, 2013.

58 Epilepsy

Khalid Hamandi

INTRODUCTION

Epileptic seizures are typically short lived and transitory but nonetheless have the potential for considerable disability because of the unpredictable nature of attacks, the risk of injury they bring, and neurologic impairment from repeated seizures and adverse effects of treatment.[1] Driving is restricted, and there is social embarrassment, stigma, and impact on employment.[2-4] Fundamental questions regarding the neurobiology of epilepsy, reasons for its development, factors that make seizures start and stop, and the variable response to treatments remain unanswered.

Epilepsy in older adults needs special consideration.[5] An older adult with presenting symptoms that suggest a diagnosis of epilepsy can be a considerable clinical challenge.[5,6] Diagnosis rests on the history of events obtained from the patient and a reliable witness. There are no clinical signs that can be elicited in a clinic, beyond directly observing a seizure, to support the diagnosis, and tests can have normal results or show nonspecific abnormalities that catch the unwary. The differential diagnosis of collapse or altered consciousness in older adults is wide. A previous diagnosis of epilepsy made earlier in life might not explain new or ongoing attacks and the term *known epileptic* (seen in some medical records) should be avoided.

Older people with a diagnosis of epilepsy can be considered as falling into four groups:

1. Those with new-onset seizures in late life
2. Those with an established diagnosis of epilepsy with seizures persisting or recurring in late life
3. Those with new-onset attacks in late life that have been misdiagnosed as epilepsy
4. Those with an established diagnosis of epilepsy with new or ongoing attacks that are not caused by epilepsy

DEFINITION

An epileptic seizure is the clinical manifestation of an abnormal synchronous neuronal discharge. Epilepsy is defined as a tendency toward recurrent epileptic seizures. A diagnosis of epilepsy is not appropriate after a single event.[7] In older adults the likelihood of further seizures can be more likely when the seizure has occurred as a result of a structural brain lesion.[8-10] Traditionally the ability to predict who will develop epilepsy after a first seizure was deemed insufficient to warrant the label or treatment. In 2014 the International League Against Epilepsy (ILAE) published new proposals for the operational definition of epilepsy, which included "one unprovoked (or reflex) seizure and a probability of further seizures (at least 60%), occurring over the next 10 years." A seizure occurring at least 1 month after a stroke was provided as an example in this new operational definition.[11] The proposals have undergone much discussion and scrutiny within the epilepsy community. For example, what is the evidence base, and how does one calculate recurrence risk after one seizure even in the presence of intracranial pathology? The level of adoption of these new proposals remains to be seen.

EPIDEMIOLOGY

Epilepsy is the third most common neurologic condition in old age after dementia and stroke.[11] The incidence is two to three times higher than that seen in childhood.[6] A community study, the United Kingdom General Practice Survey of Epilepsy and Epileptic Seizures, found that 24% of newly diagnosed cases of definite epilepsy occurred in people aged older than 60 years.[9,12] A significant rise in incidence with increasing age has been confirmed in several studies, from an overall incidence of 50 per 100,000, to 70 to 80 per 100,000 in adults older than 60 years and 160 per 100,000 in adults older than 80 years[13-16] (Figure 58-1). The prevalence of epilepsy is generally taken as between 5 and 10 cases per 1000 persons, with a lifetime prevalence of 2% to 5%.[17] Rates are dependent on case ascertainment and agreement on definitions used, for example, active epilepsy (ongoing seizures) versus controlled epilepsy.[18]

In light of these data, there would appear to be relative underprovision in specialist care for older people with epilepsy. The reasons for this are unclear, but possible explanations include a lesser perceived impact on lifestyle in older people with epilepsy compared to their younger counterparts, or less focus on the condition in older patients in light of more pressing clinical issues such as associated or unrelated comorbidities.[19]

CLASSIFICATION

Epilepsy classification might be considered by generalists as overly complex. This need not be the case if the principles behind the classification schemes are better understood. The current classification of epilepsy was developed by the ILAE Commission on Classification and Terminology.

There are two parallel schemes: one for epileptic seizures[20] and another for epilepsy syndromes.[21] In 2010 the ILAE proposed a further revision, mostly around terminology to reflect new concepts (discussed in detail in the following sections).[22]

Accurate syndromic classification helps direct treatment decisions and provide information on prognosis. Classification is also important for epidemiologic studies and service needs assessments. Furthermore, rigorous attempts at classification benefit the whole diagnostic process and reduce, or identify, previous epilepsy misdiagnoses. A good understanding of epilepsy syndromes that occur in childhood or early adult life remain useful when dealing with older patients because seizure risk can persist throughout life, patients may carry a diagnostic label that may not be correct, and questions regarding the continuation of long-standing medication may be raised. Several areas of confusion seem to arise in epilepsy classification in the nonspecialist setting. Typically confusion arises from the use of outdated terminology or from the failure to distinguish between terms intended to describe seizure types and those intended to designate epilepsy syndromes or some causal substrate.

Epilepsy is not a specific disease but a heterogeneous group of disorders manifesting the neuroanatomic and pathophysiologic substrate causing the seizures. A useful schema from the

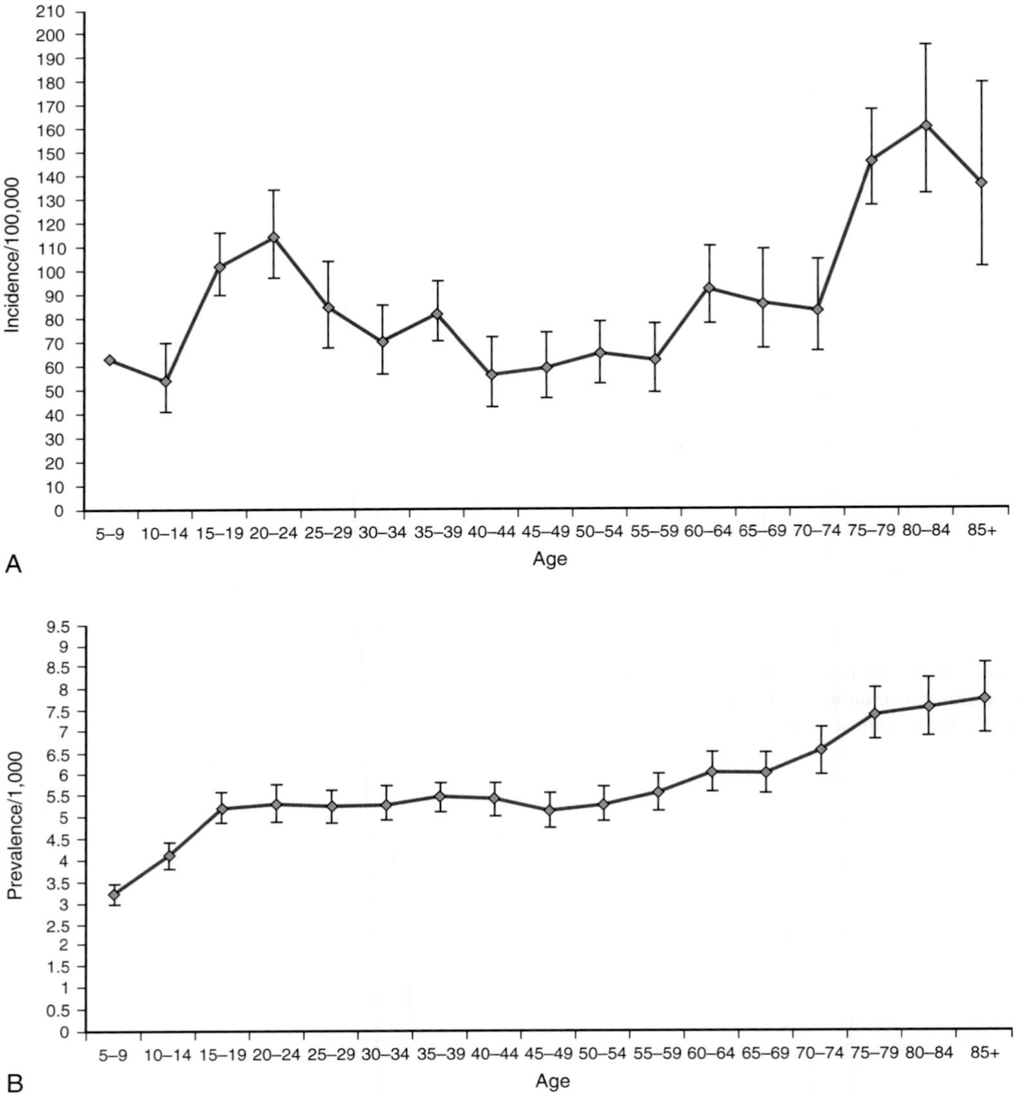

Figure 58-1. A, Age-specific incidence of treated epilepsy per 100,000 persons. **B,** Age-specific prevalence of treated epilepsy per 1000 persons. *(Source: Wallace H, Shorvon S, Tallis R: Age-specific incidence and prevalence rates of treated epilepsy in an unselected population of 2,052,922 and age-specific fertility rates of women with epilepsy.* Lancet *352:19–26, 1998, with permission.)*

ILAE considers five parts, or axes, organized in a hierarchic fashion allowing the integration of available and new information.[23] The five axes are as follows:

Axis 1: Ictal phenomenology—describing in detail the seizure event

Axis 2: Seizure type—localization within the brain and precipitating stimuli for reflex seizures should be specified when appropriate

Axis 3: Syndrome—with the understanding that a syndromic diagnosis may not always be possible

Axis 4: Cause—includes a specific disease, genetic defects or pathologic substrates causing seizures

Axis 5: Impairment—optional but often useful additional diagnostic parameter that can be derived from an impairment classification adapted from the World Health Organization's International Classification of Impairment, Disability and Handicap (ICIDH-2)

This five-axis scheme has not been adopted widely in a formal sense. However, it remains a useful framework for clinicians who have patients with epilepsy, and it is used in some form by most epileptologists and epilepsy clinics. It can be applied in any setting, essentially considering in each case (1) the seizure type, (2) brain area or areas involved, and (3) the cause or syndrome.[24] The precise terminology, and how it is applied, remains under debate and is likely to continue until the precise mechanisms and causes of epileptic seizures are defined to replace what are, in many cases, concepts and descriptions. The long-running debate of how best to classify epilepsy continues.[23]

Shortcomings of Existing Classification Schemes

Changing lists of descriptive entities inevitably cause confusion. A simplified system based on causation rather than descriptive terminology would be preferred, particularly with advances in imaging and genetics.[25] However, knowledge is insufficiently complete for a reliable causative classification to allow this at this stage. Perhaps the main limitation of the ILAE classification scheme is its poor dissemination among nonepilepsy specialist health care professionals. Revisions in the classification scheme and the rationale behind the revisions tend to be published in specialist journals and as such remain relatively inaccessible to nonepilepsy specialists. Given that epilepsy is so commonly encountered, this is one area that should be addressed.

The terms *grand mal* and *petit mal* are still commonly heard from patients and some practitioners; they are, however, outdated terms and should be avoided. Although they may provide a reference to a seizure type, they give little indication of the true seizure semiology, the possible pathophysiology, or even a secure diagnosis. Patients may use the term *grand mal* to refer to any big episode, either a complex partial seizure or a generalized tonic-clonic seizure. Similarly, *petit mal* can be used to refer to any brief alteration of consciousness and needs additional history to define the event further.

Despite any shortcomings in epilepsy classification, those involved in the care of patients with epilepsy, or episodes that might be attributed to epilepsy, should familiarize themselves with the current scheme and in particular the principles behind it.

EPILEPTIC SEIZURES

The International Classification of Epileptic Seizures (ICES) was developed by a panel of international experts examining video recordings of clinical and electroencephalographic seizures[20] and linked to Axis 2 of the ILAE publication described earlier.[23] It is based on a consensus of opinions. Box 58-1 shows the current recommended classification of epileptic seizures. By design the categories are descriptive. The first level of this system distinguishes between *generalized seizures*, a seizure whose initial semiology indicates, or is consistent with, "originating at some point within, and rapidly engaging, bilaterally distributed networks. Such bilateral networks can include cortical and subcortical structures, but do not necessarily include the entire cortex"[22]; and *focal seizures*, a seizure whose initial semiology indicates, or is consistent with, involvement of more localized or lateralized brain area.

BOX 58-1 International League Against Epilepsy (ILAE) Task Force Seizure Classification

- Generalized seizures
  - Tonic-clonic (in any combination)
  - Absence
    - Typical
    - Atypical
    - Absence with special features
    - Myoclonic absence
    - Eyelid myoclonia
  - Myoclonic
    - Myoclonic
    - Myoclonic atonic
    - Myoclonic tonic
  - Clonic
  - Tonic
  - Atonic
- Focal seizures
- Unknown
- Epileptic spasms

Adapted from Berg AT, Berkovic SF, Brodie MJ, et al. Revised terminology and concepts for organization of seizures and epilepsies: report of the ILAE Commission on Classification and Terminology, 2005-2009. Epilepsia 51:676–685, 2010.

Generalized Seizures

These are categorized into absence, myoclonic, tonic, clonic, or tonic-clonic events. Absence seizures can be subcategorized into typical absence and atypical absences. Typical absences are seen in idiopathic generalized epilepsy (see later section). They occur in childhood-onset syndromes but can persist into old age. (Typical absence seizures of childhood were previously referred to as petit mal, but this term is now considered obsolete.) They consist of an alteration of consciousness. Occasionally there is associated eye flickering, but other motor manifestations are rare. Attacks are brief; they last usually less than 30 seconds. Characteristic electroencephalogram (EEG) findings are of generalized spike wave discharges of 3 to 5 Hz. Myoclonic jerks are brief muscular jerks affecting the limbs and, less commonly, the trunk. The term *myoclonic jerk* comes under the heading of generalized seizures. However, myoclonic jerks do occur in focal epilepsy, affecting one limb or side; if strictly following the ILAE scheme, these would be classified as focal motor seizures.

Focal Seizures

These are separated into motor, somatosensory or special sensory, autonomic, and psychic. The term *localization-related*, previously proposed for focal seizures, is cumbersome and not widely adopted. The terms *focal* and *partial* remain in more common use. For the past few decades, focal seizures have been separated into simple partial seizures (consciousness is preserved, awareness is maintained) or complex partial seizures (consciousness is lost). The preservation or loss of consciousness is very relevant in the clinical setting, as it indicates a level of impairment caused by seizures. A seizure aura, often taken to be the warning before a seizure, is a simple partial seizure that may immediately precede a complex partial seizure or secondary generalization. Auras can occur in isolation (i.e., a simple partial seizure). Auras are typically short lived, lasting from seconds to a few minutes but rarely longer.

Temporal Lobe Seizures

These are perhaps the most familiar of all focal seizure types. Seizures either arise from mesial temporal structures, part of the limbic system (e.g., the hippocampus), or from the temporal neocortex. Symptoms at onset include epigastric discomfort, "butterflies" or a rising sensation, abnormal taste, experiential phenomena such as déjà vu, and psychic features, fear, or euphoria. These symptoms are usually short lived, lasting from seconds to a few minutes, and can occur in isolation without progression to the loss of awareness of secondary generalization. Patients will often recall these initial symptoms as seizure auras. A complex partial seizure of temporal origin will typically manifest with orofacial automatism (e.g., lip smacking or repeated swallowing). This is an extremely useful piece of history from a witness, and specific inquiry is helpful. In addition, there may be limb automatisms and typically there is dystonic posturing. Patients typically feel tired with the need to sleep after an attack.

Frontal Lobe Seizures

Frontal lobe seizures vary greatly because of the size of the frontal lobe and the many functions it subserves. The semiology of frontal lobe seizures depend on the origin and spread of the epileptogenic focus.[26] The frontal lobe contains the primary motor cortex, supplementary motor cortex, prefrontal cortex, and the limbic and paralimbic cortices.

In general, frontal lobe seizures manifest with prominent motor features. There may be forced head version or forced eye deviation. Limb involvement can include tonic, clonic, or postural movements or bilateral vigorous motor automatisms, for example, bicycling. Sometimes bizarre motor movements are seen; occasionally patients can retain consciousness even with jerking in all four limbs. These features can lead to an incorrect diagnosis of nonepileptic seizures. A "Jacksonian march" refers to a march or spread of the focal motor seizure in a predictable and sequential manner from a distal limb to proximal areas or from leg to arm. The term *Todd paresis* refers to a transient hemiparesis that can last a day or more occurring after a secondary generalized focal motor seizure.

Occipital Seizures

Occipital onset seizures manifest, as would be expected, with visual phenomena. Typically these are vivid or formed hallucinations. They are distinct from migraine aura in that colors are vivid and evolve over seconds rather than the several minutes of a migraine aura. They may involve flashing balls of light or revolving bright colors. Other manifestations include well-formed hallucinations, which are of a short duration of seconds to minutes and may evolve to secondary generalized seizures.

Parietal Seizures

Parietal lobe seizures are rare.[27] The parietal lobes are involved in the processing and integration of sensory and visual information. Stereotyped episodes that involve pain, numbness and tingling, heat, or pressure sensations suggest parietal lobe seizures.

EPILEPSY SYNDROMES

The International Classification of Epilepsies and Epilepsy Syndromes (ICEES)[21] supplements the ICES. Some epilepsy categories represent pure disease entities, whereas others represent a spectrum of clinical forms (e.g., idiopathic generalized epilepsy).

The concepts of generalized and focal are no longer recommended in the classification of syndromes. Classification is based on causative concepts: idiopathic, epilepsy occurring alone (Greek *idios*) without apparent underlying pathology; symptomatic, with a known underlying cause; and cryptogenic, with an unknown but suspected underlying cause. The most recent ILAE revision proposes the following change in terminology: idiopathic is to be referred to as genetic, symptomatic as structural/metabolic, and cryptogenic as unknown.[22] Again, the extent of adoption of all aspects of this new terminology remains to be seen.

Idiopathic Generalized Epilepsy

Idiopathic (or genetic) generalized epilepsy (IGE) is characterized by one or more of the following seizure types: typical absences, myoclonic jerks, and generalized tonic-clonic seizures; interictal and ictal generalized spike or polyspike and wave on EEG. The term *genetic generalized epilepsy* has been proposed by the ILAE[22] and is now seen in many publications and is used clinically, but wide-scale adoption of the term in favor of IGE is probably best left until the true genetic architecture of the epilepsies is understood.[26] Further syndromic subclassification of IGE is made on the prevalence of the different seizure types and EEG features. The inclusion of age of onset and diurnal seizure patterns are proposed by some. The main subgroups seen in adults with epilepsy are the following:

- Juvenile myoclonic epilepsy
- Juvenile absence epilepsy
- Epilepsy with generalized tonic-clonic seizures on awakening

It still remains debated whether different clinical manifestations represent different ends of a biologic continuum or a group of distinct syndromes.[28] The typical onset age of IGE is childhood or early adult life. However, a later onset form is recognized,[29,30] and there are case reports of classical IGE presenting for the first time in older adults.[31,32]

The term *idiopathic* refers to a disorder unto itself, *sui generis* (i.e., without other neurologic abnormality) and *not* etiology unknown. The risk of seizures in individuals with IGE usually continues into old age. A late presentation of absence status in four patients older than 60 years with a prior diagnosis of IGE and absence seizures that resolved in their second decade has been reported.[33] Response to appropriate antiepileptic drug (AED) treatment is good in most, but not all. One study of epilepsy patients with IGE older than age 60 found a small subgroup who experienced an exacerbation of seizures in old age.[34]

Symptomatic Epilepsy

Symptomatic epilepsy is the predominant cause of new-onset seizures in older adults.[19,35] Symptomatic epilepsy means a cause is known or can be reasonably postulated. In the absence of an imaging abnormality, a history of a prior brain injury (e.g., from intracranial infection [meningitis or encephalitis] or trauma) can be sufficient to attribute a cause to new-onset seizures. The term *remote symptomatic* is used for patients who develop seizures some years after a significant brain injury, in contrast to *acute symptomatic* in which epilepsy is a presentation of new brain dysfunction. In older adults, the likelihood of finding abnormalities, particularly leukoaraiosis, on magnetic resonance imaging (MRI) is high.[36] The relationship of such abnormalities to epilepsy, and why some develop seizures and other not, remains unclear.[37]

MAKING THE DIAGNOSIS

Epilepsy can present with disparate symptoms. Similarly, several other conditions can present with features that may be mistaken for epileptic seizures. The key feature in epilepsy is that episodes are typically stereotyped, unchanged over a long period of time, and usually short lived. The following episodic manifestations occurring in isolation, or in combination, can be caused by epilepsy:

- Loss of awareness or consciousness
- Generalized convulsive movements
- Drop attacks
- Focal movements—jerks, posturing, semipurposeful movements, rarely thrashing, bicycling or motor agitation
- Sensory episodes—tingling, pain, burning
- Vocalization—formed speech, incomprehensible words, screams, or laughter
- Psychic experiences
- Episodic phenomena from sleep
- Prolonged confusion or fugue state

The importance of gathering a careful history before making a diagnosis of epilepsy cannot be overstated. The history should include a description of events from the patient and, crucially, a firsthand description from a witness. Overreliance on a secondhand statement such as "It looked like a fit" is likely to lead to a misdiagnosis. There is no single test to make a diagnosis of epilepsy, and time taken by an experienced clinician in taking a careful history cannot be circumvented. In each case, an account of the circumstances, time of day, situation, prodrome or warning, detailed account of the attack, the semiology and duration of the attack, rate and nature of recovery, and associated symptoms or signs (e.g., headache or confusion) are needed.

Direct questions about the attack itself and other previous attacks are helpful, but care should be taken not to lead the

TABLE 58-1 Features That Help Distinguish Syncope from Epileptic Seizures

Features	Usual Difference: Faints	Usual Difference: Fits	Modification in Older Patients
Posture	Usually occur in the upright position	Not position dependent	Faints in older people are not always position dependent because they are often due to significant, position-independent, pathology.
Onset	Gradual	Sudden	Loss of consciousness may be quite abrupt in syncope in an older person; complex partial seizures may have a gradual onset.
Injury	Rare	More common	A syncopal attack may be associated with significant soft tissue or bony injury in an older person.
Incontinence	Rare	Common	An individual prone to incontinence may be wet during a faint; partial seizures will not usually be associated with incontinence.
Recovery	Rapid	Slow	A fit may take the form of a brief (temporal lobe) absence; a faint associated with a serious arrhythmia may be prolonged.
Postevent confusion	Little	Marked	A prolonged hypoxic episode due to a faint may be associated with prolonged postevent confusion.
Frequency	Usually infrequent with a clear precipitating cause	May be frequent and usually without precipitating cause	Faints associated with cardiac arrhythmias, low cardiac output, postural hypotension, or carotid sinus sensitivity may be very frequent.

history; these questions are best left until the patient and witness have given a free account of the event or events in question. Useful features that are worth inquiring about directly, if not first offered, include head or eye deviation, the nature of limb movements, posturing, jerks or automatisms, and whether movements are rhythmic or synchronous and how they evolved over time. Asking a witness about repeated swallowing or lip smacking can be revealing. Any change of color, breathing pattern, and sweating need to be ascertained along with an account of the recovery period, its duration, and any subsequent symptoms such as headache, confusion, or altered behavior. It is always useful to ask about possible prior attacks that the patient may not associate with their current event; for example, a patient presenting after his or her first generalized tonic-clonic seizure may not make the link between previous experiences of focal seizures, common examples being epigastric sensations, déjà vu, or abnormal tastes or smells. Classically tongue biting and incontinence were thought to strongly indicate an epileptic seizure. This is not always the case. Urinary incontinence can occur during syncope, and injury to the tip of the tongue can occur in syncope although if the sides of the tongue or inner cheek are severely bitten, this usually indicates that a generalized tonic-clonic seizure has taken place.[38]

The past medical history should include inquiries about previous history of head injury, intracranial infection, stroke, dementia, and cardiac history. Family history, medication history, and social history are important as in any other presentation. Specific inquiry should go into living arrangements, driving, occupation, and hobbies or pastimes.

DIFFERENTIAL DIAGNOSIS

The two main differential diagnoses of epileptic seizures to consider are syncope and psychogenic or nonepileptic attacks. Manifestations of both epileptic seizures and syncope may differ in older adults compared to the young, making diagnosis difficult or increasing misdiagnosis. Other rarer conditions leading to blackouts or altered consciousness to consider are hypoglycemia (common in older people with diabetes), other metabolic disorders, structural abnormalities at the skull base affecting the brain stem, and lesions affecting cerebrospinal fluid circulation. Transient cerebral ischemia or transient ischemic attacks (TIAs) are usually easily separated from epileptic events by their frequency and time course. They rarely present with loss of consciousness and TIAs are typically less frequent and do not remain stereotyped over long periods of time. One exception is focal seizures affecting the hand seen in critical cortical ischemia. This is described in more detail later in this chapter.

Syncope

Syncope is the most common cause of episodes of loss of awareness. Syncope is covered in greater detail in Chapter 45. Aspects of an attack should not be taken in isolation and given undue emphasis as elements of epileptic seizures can occur in syncope. Key features of syncopal episodes versus epileptic seizures are the precipitating factors, warning symptoms, a brief loss of consciousness, and rapid recovery, although there can be greater variation in older people (Table 58-1). Features that may mimic seizures include head turning, automatisms, urinary incontinence, and relatively minor tongue biting.[39] Injury can occur from a syncopal fall, although this is less common because people tend to crumple to the floor rather than the fall stiffly as in an epileptic seizure.

In cardiac syncope, attacks occur without warning; there is abrupt unprovoked collapse with brief unconsciousness and rapid recovery. They are not situational and there is less often a prodrome than in vasovagal syncope. Cardiac syncope should be strongly suspected in those with a history of structural heart disease, previous myocardial infarction, rheumatic fever, or heart murmur.

Psychogenic Attacks

Episodes that outwardly appear similar to epileptic seizures but are not caused by ictal electric discharges in the brain are referred to by a number of terms: nonepileptic attacks, nonepileptic seizures, psychogenic nonepileptic attacks (PNEAs) or seizures, or the less favored pseudoseizures.[40] The prevalence of PNEA appears lower in older adults, although no studies have examined ascertainment bias or reporting bias. In a study of video-EEG monitoring in older people (>60 years), PNEA was diagnosed in 10 of 34 patients who had recorded events during the monitoring period[41]; this series came from 71 patients older than 60 years who had undergone video-EEG monitoring out of a total of 440 over a 7-year period. Another study[42] reported a diagnosis of PNEA was made in 7 of 16 patients older than 60 years undergoing video-EEG monitoring; this was from a total of 834 admitted for long-term video-EEG monitoring. Further study of long-term video-EEG monitoring over an 8-year period identified 39 patients admitted for evaluation older than age 60 years, 13 of whom were diagnosed with PNEA on the basis of video-EEG.[43] Nevertheless, PNEA remains an important differential diagnosis in older adults, particularly when apparent medically refractory epilepsy is encountered.[41]

PNEA probably arises as a result of patients responding to psychosocial stress with unexplained somatic symptoms that come to medical attention,[42,44,45] and PNEA is associated with a number of distinct pathologic personality profiles that could be used to tailor therapy.[46] Somatoform disorders, anxiety disorders, mood disorders, and a reinforced behavior pattern are all features associated with PNEA. In one study, a subgroup of older patients with PNEA were more likely to be male and more likely to have a history of traumatic experience related to ill health.[47] Suspicion of PNEA should be raised where there are unusual features to the attacks, associated physical or mental ill health, adverse social circumstances, or bereavement prior to presentation. Confidently securing a diagnosis of PNEA usually requires long-term video-EEG monitoring, an investigation that would appear to be of limited access to the older adult population in most centers.

The Cochrane database review in 2007, and again in 2014, found insufficient evidence to recommend specific treatments for PNEA and stressed the need for new randomized trials to assess treatment interventions.[48] One of the first aims of treatment following a diagnosis of PNEA should be to reduce unnecessary medical interventions or hospital admissions.

Transient Epileptic Amnesia

Transient epileptic amnesia (TEA) has been used to describe recurrent episodes of transient amnesia in the absence of overt seizures.[49] TEA needs to be distinguished from transient global amnesia (see next subsection). In TEA there is evidence for a diagnosis of epilepsy based on one or more EEG abnormalities, co-occurrence of other clinical features of epilepsy (e.g., automatisms or olfactory hallucinations), and clear-cut response to antiepileptic medications.[50] Other features include interictal memory disturbance manifested by accelerated forgetting, remote autobiographic amnesia (i.e., patients demonstrate a patchy but dense loss of memories for important personal events from the remote past), and topographic amnesia (i.e., difficulty navigating their way around new or familiar route).[51,52] It is not clear whether episodes of TEA represent ongoing ictal activity or a postictal phenomenon. Whether TEA is a sufficient diagnostic entity to be regarded as a distinct syndrome[53] or another manifestation of temporal lobe seizures in older adults remains to be clarified.

Transient Global Amnesia

Transient global amnesia (TGA) is a condition of transient loss of memory function that has been described for over 40 years.[54,55] It is more common in middle to late life. Episodes of TGA have a characteristic presentation. There is usually, but not always, a history of provoking factors; these can include one or more of the following: vigorous exercise, acute emotional stress, or change in temperature. During an attack, patients appear mildly agitated and repeatedly question or engage in searching behavior. Attacks typically last several hours but less than 24 hours. During an attack, patients retain self-awareness and long-term memory and can perform familiar tasks or navigate a familiar environment, but they appear unable to lay down any new memories and appear amnesic of all recent events during the attack. Once an attack is over, patients regain some memory about the event but remain amnesic for the central period of the episode. Attacks are usually isolated, but there is a 6% recurrence rate. The clinical presentation is usually so characteristic that, once seen, it is not easily mistaken for epilepsy. There is no evidence to support an epileptic cause or transient arterial ischemic events.[56] A popular hypothesis is that of venous congestion in bilateral temporal lobes as a result of internal jugular vein valve insufficiency and sudden rises in intrathoracic pressure.[57]

If attacks are recurrent, have associated features (e.g., automatisms), and result in symptoms of memory impairment afterward, the diagnosis of TEA should be considered.

Psychogenic Amnesia

Psychogenic amnesia or dissociative fugue is rare and typically triggered by stressful or adverse life events. Careful clinical evaluation may reveal inconsistencies in the presentation that alert the practitioner to a conversion disorder. Features include extensive loss of autobiographic memories (including self-identity) in the context of preserved new learning, absence of repetitive questioning, and the ability to continue normal activities of daily living.

Parasomnias

Parasomnias are disorders that manifest around or during sleep. They are sometimes mistaken for epileptic seizures. The classification of parasomnias is changing as new information emerges.[58] They include REM parasomnias and periodic limb movements. An accurate history is usually sufficient to distinguish these from epilepsy. Occasionally video monitoring can be helpful.

Transient Ischemic Attacks

TIA symptoms tend to be negative (i.e., a loss of function). Epileptic seizures invariably produce positive symptoms. One rare exception is that of apparent focal motor seizures caused by critical cortical ischemia from carotid artery stenosis, or shaking limb TIA (SLTIA) (Figure 58-2). First described in 1962,[59] a handful of cases of SLTIA are reported in the literature.[60-62] Events usually involve shaking of the upper limb that does not spread to the face. Episodes can be short-lived or prolonged. They are typically provoked by maneuvers that appear to decrease cerebral perfusion, such as rising from a bed or a chair, or hyperextending the neck. Shaking does not respond to antiepileptic medication or

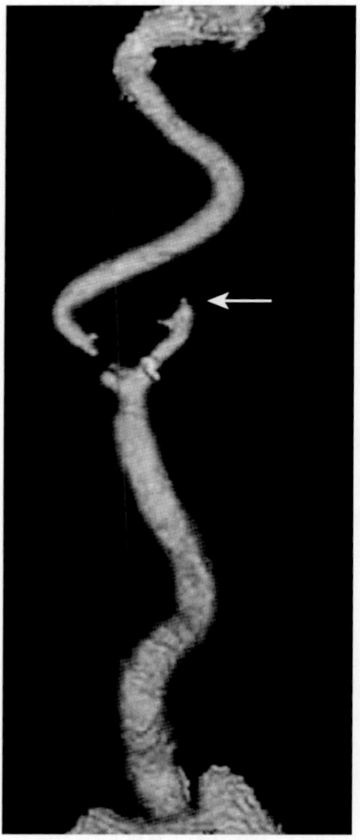

Figure 58-2. Computed tomography angiogram in a 79-year-old patient with recurrent episodes of right arm shaking, worse on standing, shows occlusion of the left internal carotid artery.

benzodiazepines. The EEG during attacks is normal. The abnormal movements respond to measures that restore adequate cerebral perfusion (i.e., carotid endarterectomy or correcting relative hypotension). Single photon emission tomography studies support the hypothesis that SLTIAs are due to hypoperfusion rather than recurrent thromboembolic events.[63]

OTHER CONSIDERATIONS

Convulsive Status Epilepticus

Convulsive status epilepticus (CSE) is defined as 30 minutes or more of either continuous seizure activity or consecutive seizures without regaining consciousness between them. CSE has a bimodal distribution with highest rates in infants and older adults. It is associated with significant morbidity and mortality. Increasing age and underlying causes are predictors of higher mortality.[64-66] Acute or remote symptomatic stroke is a common cause of status epilepticus (SE) in older adults.[67,68]

CSE is a medical emergency. Treatment algorithms for CSE are the same for older adults as for younger adults. There may be local variation in treatment algorithms, but general principles are similar. Practitioners treating medical patients in the acute setting should familiarize themselves with local guidelines. Initially, general resuscitation measures are required; drug treatment with intravenous benzodiazepines should start as soon as the diagnosis is suspected; and care should be taken to avoid respiratory depression, particularly in older adults. If there is no response to intravenous benzodiazepines, the next drug of choice is usually phenytoin, given as an infusion after an initial loading dose. If there is a failure to respond to phenytoin, sedation with an anesthetic agent is necessary. Concurrent EEG monitoring is essential, in conjunction with a search for an underlying cause. Sedation is usually maintained for at least 24 hours while therapeutic levels of an anticonvulsant are instigated.

Nonconvulsive Status Epilepticus

Nonconvulsive status epilepticus (NCSE) is relatively common, making up a third of all cases of SE. NCSE increases in incidence with age.[69] In older adults it also more difficult to diagnose, presenting as an acute or subacute prolonged confusional state. The presentation can be subtle. A high index of suspicion is required, and EEG is essential to make the diagnosis.[70] In the absence of coma, aggressive treatment should be avoided. A prospective study of 25 older patients with NCSE found that treatment with intravenous benzodiazepines was associated with an increased risk of death, and admission to the intensive care unit prolonged hospital stays without improving the outcome.[71] NCSE should be considered in those who suffer neurologic deterioration after stroke or subarachnoid hemorrhage.[72,73] NCSE is an EEG diagnosis, and EEG criteria for the diagnosis of NCSE continue to be developed.[74]

Sudden Unexplained Death in Epilepsy

Sudden unexplained death in epilepsy (SUDEP) is a term used when sudden death occurs in someone with epilepsy with no obvious cause of death found at postmortem.[75] SUDEP accounts for 7% to 17% of epilepsy deaths.[76] It seems likely that either cardiac or respiratory arrest in the context of a generalized tonic-clonic seizure causes SUDEP and that the causation is patient and seizure dependent.[76]

Risk factors for SUDEP include the presence of generalized tonic-clonic seizures, being alone in bed during a seizure, severe epilepsy, structural brain lesion, and younger onset of epilepsy and young age[77]; reporting bias might explain the last two factors. Sudden death in older adults is not necessarily an unusual occurrence. By definition, SUDEP requires that no other cause of death is found at postmortem. Attributing sudden death in older adults to SUDEP is unlikely in the presence of other comorbidities, whereas sudden death in otherwise healthy young persons with epilepsy should be fully investigated. It is not known whether the same mechanisms for SUDEP operate across all age groups, with older adults equally susceptible, or whether older adults are somehow immune from this condition. How to measure the occurrence of SUDEP in older adults may prove difficult.

Immune-Mediated Limbic Encephalitis

New-onset seizures in older adults associated with mood change, personality change, and/or cognitive impairment should prompt consideration of immune-mediated limbic encephalitis. Mention is made of this condition here, as it is an important differential diagnosis to consider, is easily tested for, and responds well to immune therapy. The limbic encephalitides can be separated into paraneoplastic[78] and autoimmune,[79] the latter being a diagnosis after a thorough search for occult malignancy but also based on emerging knowledge of the different antibody subtypes. The two commonly encountered antibodies are to *N*-methyl-D-aspartate (NMDA) receptors, and to the voltage-gated potassium channel complex (VGKC-complex). The latter are associated with a very characteristic seizure type—brachiofacial seizures in which there is tonic contraction of one arm and hemiface over seconds, sometimes repeated several hundred times in a day.[80] These seizures are poorly responsive to AEDs, but complete remission is seen following early treatment with immune therapy with high-dose steroids, intravenous immunoglobulins, or both. Brain MRI shows characteristic high signal change on FLAIR imaging in medial temporal lobe structures, sometimes misdiagnosed as low-grade tumors.[81] Further work continues in identifying other likely pathognomonic antibodies and raises the issue of immune-mediated mechanisms in other epilepsies.[82]

CAUSES

Cerebrovascular Disease

Cerebrovascular disease is the most common cause for epilepsy in older adults[83]; it accounts for 30% to 50% of epilepsy cases in older adults[35] and 75% of symptomatic epilepsies. Poststroke seizures and epilepsy are considered as early (occurring within 2 weeks of stroke) or late (occurring after 2 weeks). A study of 6044 hospital admissions with acute stroke reported 3.1% had epileptic seizures within 24 hours of the stroke, and 8.4% had seizures within the first 24 hours after a subarachnoid hemorrhage or intracerebral hemorrhage.[84] In the United Kingdom, the standard mortality ratio was highest for people with epilepsy and cerebrovascular disease.[85]

Cortical involvement of infarct is a risk factor predilection for developing seizures, and there may be an association with the site of infarction and development of epilepsy.[86] In a large multicenter study, a worse outcome and increased in-hospital complication rate were associated with prophylactic AED use after subarachnoid hemorrhage.[87] Patients who suffer SE of cerebrovascular origin were found to have twice the risk of death at 6 months than patients with stroke and not SE,[88] although the independent effect of SE on mortality after stroke is controversial.[89]

Cerebral Tumors

Older patients with new-onset seizures should have cerebral imaging to exclude a structural cause (Figure 58-3). Benign tumors (e.g., meningiomas) can also present with epilepsy. Surgery for these tumors depends on their location and the fitness of the patient. Typically meningiomas are indolent.

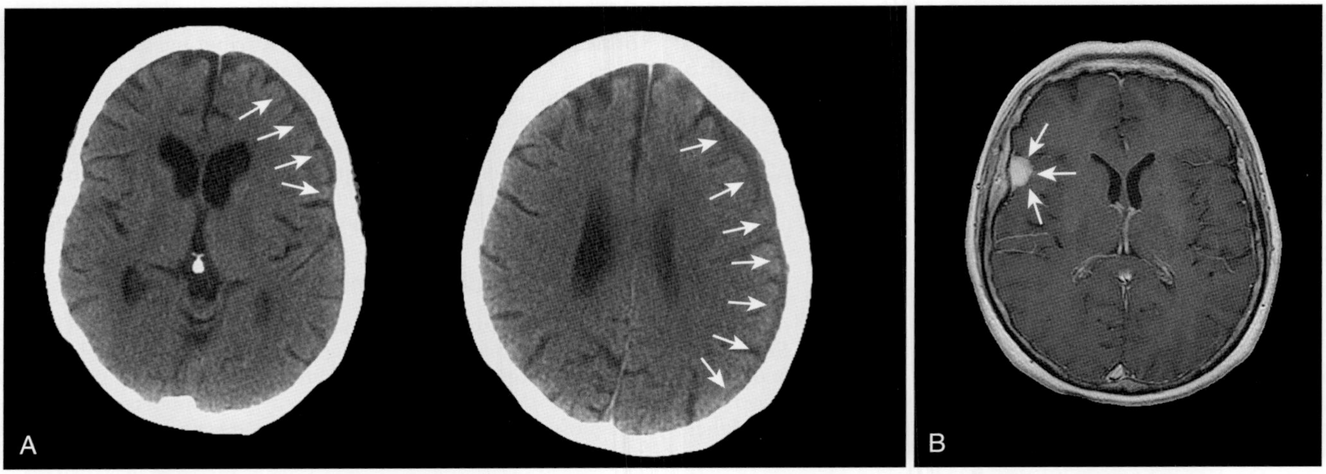

Figure 58-3. Causes of epilepsy. A, Computed tomographic scan of head showing a subdural hematoma in a 68-year-old woman with focal motor seizures affecting the left hand. **B,** Gadolinium enhanced T1-weighted axial magnetic resonance imaging showing right temporal meningioma presenting with simple partial seizures in a 60-year-old woman.

However, they can be slow growing, and the small risk of malignant transformation supports the option of surgery in younger patients with peripheral lesions.

Neurodegenerative Disease

Alzheimer disease is associated with a sixfold increase in unprovoked seizures.[90] The history of seizures in these situations invariably needs to be from the caregiver. A further study found that 21% of patients developed seizures after a diagnosis of dementia of Alzheimer type.[91]

Other Causes

Any structural, inflammatory, immune, or vascular intracerebral process can lead to epileptic seizures. Other causes include trauma; intracranial infection, in particular herpes simplex encephalitis and pneumococcal meningitis; subdural hematoma; paraneoplastic syndromes; limbic encephalitis; and malformations of cortical development (see Figure 58-3).

Provoked Seizures

One or more provoked seizures do not require a diagnosis of epilepsy. Provoked seizures can be caused by metabolic or toxic disturbance. It is important to recognize provoked seizures, as these typically do not warrant treatment with AEDs and driving eligibility may vary.

INVESTIGATION

In older people, routine hematology, biochemistry, plasma glucose, calcium, and liver function should be checked. The mainstay of investigation includes the ECG, EEG, and neuroimaging. Particular attention should be paid to the effect of "normal" aging on brain imaging and neurophysiology. This includes atrophy on computed tomography (CT), atrophy and nonspecific white matter change on MRI, and EEG slowing.

Electrocardiography

The electrocardiogram (ECG) is a simple, quick, inexpensive, and noninvasive test. It should be performed in all patients after a first episode of loss of consciousness, even if the history is strongly suggestive of an epileptic seizure. The ECG should be examined in detail for evidence of conduction abnormalities.[92] More advanced investigation for cardiac or vasovagal syncope should also be considered depending on the history (see Chapter 45).

Electroencephalography

The EEG should be used judiciously. The EEG is a primary investigation in epilepsy. Nevertheless the diagnosis of epilepsy remains a clinical one with EEG providing a supporting role. It is not appropriate as a screening tool or means of excluding epilepsy in those with suspected syncope.[93] Indiscriminate use of the EEG and its reporting can lead to the overdiagnosis of epilepsy.[94] Interpretation of the EEG requires a skilled neurophysiologist. Nonspecific findings can catch the unwary (Figure 58-4). The gold standard for classifying the seizure is simultaneous video-EEG monitoring, but access to such facilities may be restricted.

Long-term video-EEG is useful tool in the investigation of epilepsy in patients of all ages.[95-98] It is primarily used for the following indications:

- Diagnostic clarification of epilepsy versus nonepileptic attacks
- Localization of seizure onset (of practical use only in younger patients being considered for epilepsy surgery)
- Determining seizure frequency in suspected partial or nocturnal seizures

It is notable that published series on the use of video-EEG in older people in large epilepsy centers have reported that patients older than 60 years comprise only 2% to 17% of adult admissions to the monitoring units.[93,96,98]

Neuroimaging

The two standard neuroimaging modalities used in epilepsy are CT and MRI. All cases of new-onset seizures in adults should have brain imaging to exclude a structural lesion. The choice between CT and MRI rests on the cost and practicalities of each technique versus the expected yield leading to a change in management.

CT involves the reconstruction of x-rays taken in multiple planes to produce an image and, as such, involves a radiation dose.

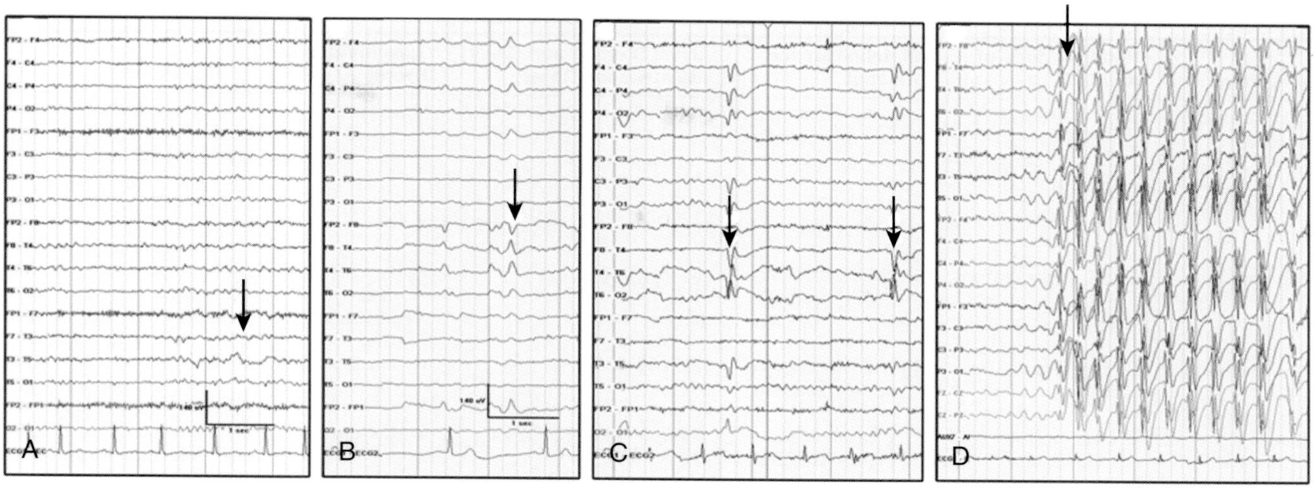

Figure 58-4. Electroencephalogram features. A, Left temporal slow activity, a nonspecific feature. **B,** Right temporal sharp waves in 78-year-old man supporting diagnosis of complex partial seizures. **C,** Focal spikes in teenager with benign epilepsy with centrotemporal spikes. **D,** Generalized spike wave activity in young adult with idiopathic generalized epilepsy, an unequivocal "epileptiform" discharge.

Modern CT scanners are quick, and brain images are acquired within a matter of minutes. The CT bore is relatively open and only the head needs enter. CT is therefore most appropriate in the acute or emergency setting, particularly if the patient is unwell and needs close monitoring, and for patients with claustrophobia or who have difficulty lying flat. CT is superior to MRI for identifying intracranial hemorrhage and for identifying areas of calcification. MRI involves the subject lying in a strong magnetic field with superimposed time-varying magnetic field gradients. MRI takes longer than CT, typically 10 to 20 minutes for a full series of brain images. The subject needs to lie still for the duration of the scan because images are degraded by even a small amount of motion. The scanner bore is relatively narrow and long; patients enter the bore head first, covering most of their body. Patients with claustrophobia and patients unable to lie flat will not tolerate MRI. The advantage of MRI over CT is its much higher image resolution and tissue contrast, hence the ability to detect subtle abnormalities that might cause epilepsy. This is perhaps of greater relevance in young adults with medically refractory seizures being considered for epilepsy surgery. Surgical resection of a benign lesion to treat epilepsy is rarely advantageous in older adults, and the pursuit of subtle benign lesions causing epilepsy is unlikely to alter their management.

ANTIEPILEPTIC DRUG THERAPY

To the nonspecialist there can be a bewildering array of new drugs to treat epilepsy. Twelve AEDs have been developed and licensed worldwide since 1989. By convention, drugs that were available before this time are known as standard AEDs, and those available after 1990 are referred to as newer AEDs. Studies of AEDs in older adults are scant and tend to concentrate on the those aged 65 to 74 years.[99] Benefits and side effects tend to be extrapolated from studies in younger patients. Key points to consider when prescribing AEDs in older adults are the increased risk of side effects; drug-drug interactions; altered protein binding, hepatic metabolism, and renal clearance; and the need for a careful review of already prescribed drugs. When commencing a new AED, a low starting dose and slow titration are recommended.

Standard AEDs are acetazolamide, carbamazepine, clobazam, clonazepam, ethosuximide, valproic acid, phenobarbital, phenytoin, and primidone. The new AEDs include eslicarbazepine, gabapentin, felbamate, lamotrigine, levetiracetam, oxcarbazepine, perampanel, pregabalin, rufinamide, tiagabine, topiramate, vigabatrin, and zonisamide. Of these, felbamate and vigabatrin should not be used because of the risk of severe adverse effects, namely, potentially fatal liver failure or aplastic anemia with felbamate, and retinal damage with irreversible visual field constriction with vigabatrin. These adverse effects were not recognized until a few years following widespread use of the drugs. This highlights the need for postmarketing surveillance of, and adverse reaction reporting on, all new drugs. Standard and newer AEDs commonly used in adults are summarized in Table 58-2.

The currently recommended first-line AEDs are valproic acid for generalized epilepsy and carbamazepine or lamotrigine for focal epilepsy. In many older patients, phenytoin still forms the mainstay of treatment.[100,101] Some older adults with lifelong epilepsy may still be taking phenobarbital or primidone; it is not appropriate to replace these with newer AEDs in patients who are stable.

The newer AEDs are first licensed as add-on therapy (based on results of randomized trials of "add-on" treatment of new drug versus placebo), added to the patient's existing AED regimen. Direct head-to-head comparisons of standard and newer AEDs are lacking. Recent efforts to address this imbalance include the U.K. study of the Standard and New Antiepileptic Drugs (SANAD) study, comparing sodium valproate against new AEDs in generalized seizures and carbamazepine against new AEDs in focal epilepsies. Valproic acid was found to be most effective in IGE,[102] while lamotrigine was favored over carbamazepine for focal epilepsies.[103] The trial did not include a number of later but now important AEDs (e.g., levetiracetam, zonisamide, and pregabalin), and further studies are needed.

A large multicenter study comparing lamotrigine, gabapentin, and carbamazepine in 593 older patients with newly diagnosed epilepsy found lower adverse events in those randomized to lamotrigine or gabapentin compared to carbamazepine, without significant difference in seizure-free rates at 12 months.[102] A subsequent study comparing lamotrigine and sustained release carbamazepine in 185 patients aged older than 65 years did not find a significant difference between lamotrigine and carbamazepine, but there was a trend toward greater efficacy with carbamazepine and lower adverse effects with lamotrigine.[104] A smaller study found similar efficacy but better tolerability of lamotrigine over

TABLE 58-2 Main Antiepileptic Drugs Indicated for Epilepsy in Older Patients and Their Key Features

Drug Name	Putative Mode of Action	Metabolism and Kinetics	Usual Starting and (Daily Maintenance Dose)	Typical Adverse Events	Key Points
Carbamazepine* (1963)	Sodium channel inhibition	Hepatic metabolism; active metabolite	100-200 mg (400-1800 mg)	Hyponatremia rash	First line for focal seizures Can worsen MJ and absences in IGE Wide drug interaction, including warfarin and other AEDs Hyponatremia
Clobazam	GABA augmentation	Hepatic metabolism; active metabolite	10 mg (10-30 mg)	Idiosyncratic rash (rare)	More commonly used as short-term adjunct
Clonazepam	GABA augmentation	Hepatic metabolism	0.5 mg (1-6 mg)	Idiosyncratic rash (rare)	More commonly used as short-term adjunct
Eslicarbazepine* (2012)	Sodium channel inhibition	Hepatic metabolism; active metabolite	400 mg (400-1200 mg)	Hyponatremia rash	Chemical structure similar to carbamazepine Once a day dosing
Gabapentin (1993)	Calcium channel modulation	Not metabolized, urinary excretion unchanged	300 mg (1800-3600 mg)	Weight gain	More commonly used for neuropathic pain
Lamotrigine (1991)	Sodium channel inhibition	50% protein bound, hepatic metabolism	25 mg (100-400 mg)	Idiosyncratic rash Stevens-Johnson syndrome (rare)	First line for focal seizures Rapidly withdraw if rash occurs
Levetiracetam (1999)	Synaptic vesicle protein modulation	Urinary excretion	250 mg (750-3000 mg)	Tiredness Mood disturbance	Mood disturbance, including irritability, short temper
Phenobarbital* (1912)	GABA augmentation	Hepatic metabolism; 25% excreted unchanged	30 mg (30-180 mg)	Drowsiness Mood change Osteomalacia	Rarely initiated today If withdrawal considered, needs to be slow
Perampanel	Glutamate AMPA antagonist	Hepatic (CYP3A4 not CYP450)	2 mg (6-12 mg)	Dizziness Somnolence Irritability	Once-a-day dosing Long half life Take just before bed to avoid impact of peak dose side effects of unsteadiness
Pregabalin (2004)	Calcium channel modulation	Hepatic metabolism (saturation kinetics) 90% protein bound	50 mg (100-600 mg)	Drowsiness Weight gain	Can worsen MJ and absences in IGE Dose-dependent side effects
Primidone* (1952)	GABA augmentation	Hepatic metabolism	125 mg (500-1500 mg)	Idiosyncratic rash	Rarely initiated If withdrawal considered, needs to be very slow
Oxcarbazepine* (1990)	Sodium channel inhibition	Hepatic metabolism	150-300 mg (900-2400 mg)	Idiosyncratic rash Hyponatremia	Similar structure to carbamazepine
Tiagabine (1996)	GABA augmentation	Hepatic metabolism	5 mg (30-45 mg)	Increased seizures; nonconvulsive status	
Topiramate* (1995)	Glutamate reduction; sodium-channel modulation; calcium-channel modification	Mostly hepatic metabolism, with renal excretion	25 mg (75-200 mg)	Weight loss Kidney stones Impaired cognition Word finding difficulty	Dose-dependent side effects
Valproic acid (1968)	GABA augmentation	Hepatic metabolism; active metabolites	200 mg (400-2000 mg)	Hepatotoxicity (rare) Encephalopathy (rare)	First line for generalized seizures
Zonisamide (1990)	Calcium channel inhibition	Urinary excretion	50-100 mg (200-600 mg)	Idiosyncratic rash	Similar chemical structure to topiramate

AED, Antiepileptic drug; *GABA,* γ-aminobutyric acid; *IGE,* idiopathic generalized epilepsy; *MJ,* myoclonic jerk.
*Induces hepatic enzymes and therefore affects plasma levels of other drugs undergoing hepatic metabolism (e.g., warfarin).

carbamazepine in poststroke epilepsy,[105] and another study found switching to lamotrigine was associated with an improvement on side effect profile.[106]

Adverse Effects

All AEDs have side effects. These can be dose dependent or idiosyncratic. Dose-dependent side effects can be minimized by using a low starting dose with slow titration. Idiosyncratic side effects cannot be predicted and usually necessitate rapid drug withdrawal. Idiosyncratic side effects include rash, blood dyscrasias, bone marrow impairment, liver failure, and Stevens-Johnson syndrome.

Dose-dependent side effects most commonly affect the central nervous system. They typically include dizziness; drowsiness; lack of energy or weakness; unsteadiness or incoordination; mood disturbance that includes depression, hostility, anger, irritability, and nervousness; cognitive effects that include confusion, difficulty concentrating or paying attention, and abnormal thinking; speech or language problems; and difficulty falling asleep or staying asleep. Gastrointestinal side effects include nausea, abdominal pain, and diarrhea. Side effects can include frequency or urgency of micturition and effects on sexual function. Dose-dependent side effects are typically worsened by polytherapy,[107] and the lowest dose of AED that controls seizures should be the aim. Taking more than three AEDs in combination is rarely helpful, and those on several AEDs should have medication rationalized as best as possible.

Patients should be cautioned specifically regarding common or potentially serious side effects (see Table 58-2). It is helpful if patients have a rapid access point or contact number for advice in case side effects develop so that drugs are neither stopped suddenly nor continued with potentially harmful consequences. Some side effects occur when starting or raising the dose of an AED and wear off after a few days. Recurrent or unpleasant side effects need to be identified and addressed early.

Long-term adverse effects include osteoporosis. Osteoporosis is more common in women taking AEDs. Calcium and vitamin D levels should be measured in women taking enzyme-inducing AEDs every 2 to 5 years, and bone densitometry can be used to assess the risk of osteoporosis. Vitamin D and calcium supplementation can be taken in an attempt to correct any deficiencies. Bone fracture rates in epilepsy are two to three times that of the general population,[108] and screening for bone health in epilepsy is recommended.[109]

Drug-Drug Interactions

Drugs that undergo hepatic metabolism are altered by hepatic enzyme-inducing AEDs (see Table 58-2). Those with the least risk for interactions are levetiracetam, gabapentin, and pregabalin,[110] although it remains to be seen how this translates in clinical practice. Enzyme-inducing AEDs should be considered carefully in patients already on medication, all prescribed drugs should be reviewed, and warfarin can be a particular concern.

Although there is a long-held belief that antidepressants lower the seizure threshold and are proconvulsant, there is little evidence to support this view.[111] Depression is common in patients with epilepsy and, where present, should be treated appropriately. The risk of seizures is dose dependent, and new antidepressants, particularly at low doses, are considered safe in most cases. Antidepressants least likely to affect AED levels are citalopram, escitalopram, venlafaxine, duloxetine, and mirtazapine.[110]

Therapeutic Plasma Monitoring

With the exception of phenytoin, monitoring plasma drug levels is generally not helpful in managing AED therapy. Laboratory reference ranges are of little value in dose adjustments, which should be done according to clinical response and dose-related side effects. A cross-sectional study of 92 nursing home residents in the United States found lower carbamazepine doses and serum concentrations than in younger adults. The daily dose was significantly lower for the oldest age group (>85).[112]

Withdrawing Antiepileptic Drugs

Should AEDs be withdrawn in older patients with late-onset seizures who have been seizure free for a period of time? What about people entering older age who have taken AEDs most of their lives with seizure freedom? Studies that address drug withdrawal have been done in younger populations.[113,114] Conditions that lead to increased risk of relapse after drug withdrawal include focal epilepsy, generalized tonic-clonic seizures, the presence of cerebral pathology, and an abnormal EEG. Many of these conditions apply to older adults with new-onset seizures. The severity and frequency of seizures and the patient's view on taking medication can influence decisions to withdraw AEDs. It is difficult to extrapolate recurrence risk from population studies to individual patients.

Worthy of special note is the older person who has been on lifelong treatment with phenobarbital or primidone. Both are barbiturates and very difficult to withdraw without potential for recurrence of seizures. If withdrawal of one of these agents is being considered, then it should be with specialist advice and the drug slowly titrated down over many months, for example, 10% of the initial daily dose every 6 weeks.

THE IMPACT OF EPILEPSY

Epilepsy is a chronic disease. It is associated with stigma and public misconceptions. A questionnaire-based survey of a small number of older patients with epilepsy found their main concerns to be the impact on driving and transportation and medication side effects.[115] Other concerns included personal safety, social embarrassment, employment, and memory loss (Box 58-2).

In a study of more than 1000 adults with epilepsy in the United States, using U.S. Census Bureau data for comparison, respondents received less education, were less likely to be employed or married, and came from lower income households.[116] Uncertainty and fear of having a seizure were listed as the worst things about having epilepsy. Lifestyle, school, driving, and employment limits were also listed as major problems, and, when asked to rank a list of problems, cognitive impairment was ranked highest. A study using a health-related quality-of-life questionnaire in older adults found lower scores in those with epilepsy compared to those without the condition. AED side effects and depression were thought to be the main reasons.[117] Another study concluded that fear of even infrequent seizures could affect quality of life in older adults.[4] Cognitive impairment is a major concern and is higher in those on more than one AED.[118,119]

For patients with epilepsy, motor vehicle licensing is usually restricted until a defined seizure-free interval has passed.[120] This varies from country to country. Medical practitioners need to be familiar with their own licensing authority regulations.[121]

Beyond driving restrictions, a commonsense approach should be taken to further restrictions on activity. Day-to-day activities should otherwise not be limited. Patients with severe or frequent seizures may develop a fear of public places or of being left alone; physicians should be mindful of this.

BOX 58-2 The Impact of Epilepsy

- Seizures
  - Time lost
  - Injury
  - Social disruption/embarrassment
  - Hospital admission
  - Cognitive decline
  - Driving
  - Hobbies
  - Social interactions
  - Grandparenting
- Diagnosis
  - Stigma
  - Misconceptions
  - Fear
- Medication
  - Acute adverse events
  - Long-term side effects
  - Drug-drug interactions
- Underlying disorder
  - Neurologic decline

SERVICES FOR PATIENTS WITH EPILEPSY

Older patients with epilepsy or with blackouts should be seen by a specialist with an interest in the condition. Not all older patients will have access to specialist services. Syncope is the main differential diagnosis, and not only epilepsy specialists and geriatricians but all physicians who treat patients with blackout should be aware of different presentations. An epilepsy service should work closely with cardiologists, neuroradiologists, and neurophysiologists. One area that appears lacking is access to video-EEG. Epilepsy nurse specialists have important roles in long-term follow-up and information provision and can provide rapid access to specialist advice.[122-125] The role of a wider multidisciplinary team dedicated to epilepsy, which includes input on all aspects of social care (e.g., social and occupational services), has not been well characterized.

AREAS FOR RESEARCH

"The observation made in previous editions of this textbook that geriatric epileptology is a relatively underdeveloped and under-researched field remains true. The outstanding research agenda is substantially the same" (Raymond Tallis, *Brocklehurst's Textbook of Geriatric Medicine and Gerontology*, ed 7).

There remains much to be learned about how and why seizures start and stop. Research in this area is predominantly in younger people and in animal experimentation. Are there differences in seizure mechanisms in older adults? Why is there such a disparity between IGE and symptomatic epilepsy across the extremes of age? How common is misdiagnosis? How common is PNEA? It is easily missed without an index of suspicion and access to appropriate investigation.

Do seizures have more adverse physical effects in old people, or is the converse true? Is there such a thing as SUDEP in older people? How frequent are fractures and other significant injuries? What are the cognitive impairments associated with repeated seizures? Is this cause or effect? The main themes of many social epilepsy review articles are women with epilepsy, pregnancy, driving, and lifestyle issues. What are the information needs of the older person with epilepsy?

When to Use Antiepileptic Drugs

Should a physician treat a single, unprovoked tonic-clonic seizure in an older patient or wait for two or more seizures? The ongoing Multicenter Epilepsy and Single Seizure (MESS) study should help to answer this question. What are the chances of recurrence where there is no overt cause? How easy are seizures to control in old age? More prospective studies are needed to answer these questions.

The Role of the Newer Generation of Antiepileptic Drugs

What is the place of the new-generation anticonvulsants in the de novo treatment of onset seizures in older adults? Studies addressing this question should focus not simply on the traditional endpoints such as seizure control. The newer AEDs may offer additional advantages in reducing subtle adverse effects on gait and mobility, especially because "minor" effects of this sort, in frail older people, may translate into significant disability.

The Organization of Epilepsy Services

How best should we provide a service for older adults who have seizures? What are the elements of an optimal overall comprehensive service? Who should provide it? How should we evaluate it? If we had answers to these questions, our management of seizures in old age would be considerably better than it is now.

KEY POINTS

- The most important step in the management of a person with suspected seizures is to determine whether or not the events are indeed epileptic fits.
- All adult patients with new-onset or suspected seizures should have brain imaging.
- About 80% of people with onset of seizures late in life will be controlled with the first choice drug. Drug-drug interactions are an important consideration in older people.
- The management of established epilepsy goes far beyond drug treatment. Key elements are reassurance, education, information, and support.
- Aside from phenytoin treatment, anticonvulsant blood level monitoring is not routinely indicated for most antiepileptic drugs.
- Older patients with seizures require initial specialist assessment and should have access to continuing specialist services, in line with recommendations for younger people.

For a complete list of references, please visit www.expertconsult.com.

KEY REFERENCES

2. Baxendale S, O'Toole A: Epilepsy myths: alive and foaming in the 21st century. Epilepsy Behav 11:192–196, 2007.
11. Fisher RS, Acevedo C, Arzimanoglou A, et al: ILAE official report: a practical clinical definition of epilepsy. Epilepsia 55:475–482, 2014.
22. Berg AT, Berkovic SF, Brodie MJ, et al: Revised terminology and concepts for organization of seizures and epilepsies: report of the ILAE Commission on Classification and Terminology, 2005-2009. Epilepsia 51:676–685, 2010.
42. Reuber M, Elger CE: Psychogenic nonepileptic seizures: review and update. Epilepsy Behav 4:205–216, 2003.
43. Kellinghaus C, Loddenkemper T, Dinner DS, et al: Non-epileptic seizures of the elderly. J Neurol 251:704–709, 2004.
53. Butler CR, Graham KS, Hodges JR, et al: The syndrome of transient epileptic amnesia. Ann Neurol 61:587–598, 2007.
54. Hodges JR, Warlow CP: Syndromes of transient amnesia: towards a classification. A study of 153 cases. J Neurol Neurosurg Psychiatry 53:834–843, 1990.
60. Baquis GD, Pessin MS, Scott RM: Limb shaking—a carotid TIA. Stroke 16:444–448, 1985.
69. Walker MC: Treatment of nonconvulsive status epilepticus. Int Rev Neurobiol 81:287–297, 2007.
71. Litt B, Wityk R, Hertz SH, et al: Nonconvulsive status epilepticus in the critically ill elderly. Epilepsia 39:1194–1202, 1998.
79. Irani SR, Vincent A, Schott JM: Autoimmune encephalitis. BMJ 342:d1918, 2011.
80. Irani SR, Michell AW, Lang B, et al: Faciobrachial dystonic seizures precede Lgi1 antibody limbic encephalitis. Ann Neurol 69:892–900, 2011.
81. Willis MD, Jones L, Vincent A, et al: VGKC-complex antibody encephalitis. QJM 107:657–659, 2014.
92. Marsh E, O'Callaghan P, Smith P: The humble electrocardiogram. Pract Neurol 8:46–59, 2008.
94. Benbadis SR, Tatum WO: Overinterpretation of EEGs and misdiagnosis of epilepsy. J Clin Neurophysiol 20:42–44, 2003.
100. Leppik IE: Choosing an antiepileptic. Selecting drugs for older patients with epilepsy. Geriatrics 60:42–47, 2005.
109. Sheth RD, Harden CL: Screening for bone health in epilepsy. Epilepsia 48(Suppl 9):39–41, 2007.
115. Martin R, Vogtle L, Gilliam F, et al: What are the concerns of older adults living with epilepsy? Epilepsy Behav 7:297–300, 2005.
119. Hermann B, Seidenberg M, Sager M, et al: Growing old with epilepsy: the neglected issue of cognitive and brain health in aging and elder persons with chronic epilepsy. Epilepsia 49:731–740, 2008.

59 Headache and Facial Pain

Gerry Saldanha

INTRODUCTION

Worldwide, headache disorders are one of the most prevalent medical complaints. This will continue because of the changing demographic of aging populations and because people experience headaches more commonly in their later years. Headaches are often more severe in older people, and secondary causes occur with increased incidence. Primary headache disorders (migraine, tension-type headache, and cluster headache) may persist into old age, although incidence and prevalence are reduced. The management of older patients is often complicated by comorbidities and the medications that may be prescribed for those conditions.

Headache is frequently underdiagnosed and undertreated, and many do not seek medical advice.[1] *The International Classification of Headache Disorders*, now in it third edition,[2] has further refined the diagnostic criteria for headaches and facial pains, thus improving the quality of clinical trials and diagnostic rigor in the clinic. Although this has obviously benefited the sufferers of headache, most published data are from younger cohorts, and few clinical trials recruit older people.

Few epidemiologic studies have been carried out to estimate the size of the headache problem. In one year in the United States, 70% of the general population had a headache, 5% of whom sought medical attention.[3] Less is known about the frequency of headache in the older adult population, although in a large population-based study carried out in East Boston,[4] some 17% of patients older than 65 years reported frequent headache, with 53% of women and 36% of men reporting headache in the previous year. Headache prevalence in the older adult age group ranges from 5% to 50%.[5,6] Overall, headache appears to be less frequently reported in the older adult population[5] and shows a decline with age.[4,8] Most studies show that the prevalence of primary headache syndromes declines with increasing age.[8-11] One obvious limitation of these studies is that none is longitudinal and so may not differentiate an effect of aging from cohort or period effects. In addition, older adult patients may be less complaining, or the emergence of other, more serious problems may have suppressed reporting of a benign symptom such as headache.

In older adults headache is more likely to represent organic pathology.[12] A clinic-based retrospective case record study[13] concluded that, although it was less likely that older people would attend a hospital outpatient clinic for diagnosis of headache, there was a 10-fold increase in the likelihood of finding organic pathology. Recruitment bias is a problem in these studies. Nevertheless, it is likely that headache is a more serious complaint from the older adult patient.

A large lifetime prevalence study[14] that used a population-based questionnaire found that although migraine and tension-type headache appeared to decrease with increasing age, chronic tension headache has significantly higher prevalence rates in the older adult population. Medication overuse remains an important factor in the cause of chronic daily headache in older adults, especially in patients who have been subject to frequent migraine headache.[15]

Headache remains an extremely common condition of older people; much of it has benign origin, but more care needs to be taken with older patients to rule out underlying pathology, especially when they present for the first time.

PRIMARY HEADACHE DISORDERS

Migraine

Migraine is an episodic disorder that is diagnosed from the history; it commonly starts around puberty but can start at *any* age.[16] Epidemiologic studies are difficult to carry out and are dogged by numerous problems.[17] Only 5% of migraineurs consult specialists,[18] so clinic-based studies will suffer from referral bias. It is clear that a significant proportion of the burden of migraine headache is undiagnosed and untreated, more so in older adults. A number of population-based studies have been carried out.[10,18-29]

Rasmussen and colleagues[27] did not find a decrease in migraine prevalence with increasing age, in contrast to the findings of Stewart and coworkers,[25] who also showed that it is uncommon for migraine to start in a person's later years.[10] The female preponderance of migraineurs persists in this age group.[16] Migraine headaches tend to improve with increasing age.[30]

Symptoms and Diagnosis of Migraine

Migraine is classified into two main forms: migraine with aura (formerly referred to as "classic migraine") and migraine without aura (formerly referred to as "common migraine"), based on criteria of the International Headache Society (IHS).[31] Other varieties of migraine include ophthalmoplegic, retinal, basilar, and familial hemiplegic. Complications of migraine include migrainous infarction (a neurologic deficit not reversible by 7 days) and status migrainosus (an attack of headache or aura lasting more than 72 hours). Migraine aura can exist without headache, and the same patient may, at different times, experience headache with aura, headache without aura, or aura without headache.[32,33]

To diagnose migraine without aura, five attacks are needed, each lasting 4 to 72 hours and having two of the following four characteristics: unilateral location, pulsating quality, moderate or severe intensity, and aggravation by routine physical activity. In addition, the attacks must have at least one of the following: nausea or vomiting or photophobia and phonophobia. Migraine without aura is more common than migraine with aura and is usually more disabling.

Migraine with aura is diagnosed when there have been at least two attacks with any three of the following features:

- One or more fully reversible aura symptoms
- Aura developing over more than 4 minutes
- Aura lasting less than 60 minutes
- Headache following aura with a free interval of less than 60 minutes

A simpler working definition for the clinical diagnosis of migraine was proposed by Solomon and Lipton.[34] A positive diagnosis could be made on any two of the following four symptoms:

- Unilateral headache
- Pulsating quality

- Nausea
- Photophobia and phonophobia

A similar headache must have occurred in the past, and structural disease must have been excluded. Migraine attacks generally are divided into five phases: the prodrome (hours or days before the headache), the aura (migraine with aura), the headache, the headache termination, and the postdrome phase.[32] Symptoms of the prodrome may include mental, neurologic, or general (constitutional, autonomic) symptoms. Individuals may experience depression, euphoria, irritability, restlessness, mental slowness, hyperactivity, and drowsiness. General symptoms may include a feeling of coldness, sluggishness, thirst, anorexia, diarrhea, constipation, fluid retention, and food cravings. Photophobia and phonophobia may also occur.

The aura is a group of neurologic symptoms that precede or accompany the attack. They may be visual, sensory, or motor and may also cause language or brainstem disturbance. Headache usually occurs within 60 minutes of the end of the aura,[31] but it may begin with the aura. Most patients have more than one type of aura and progress from one type to another in subsequent attacks. Common visual symptoms are the positive phenomena, such as hemianopic photopsia (flashes of light) and teichopsia or fortification spectra. Scotomata may follow. Complex visual distortions and hallucinations are reported but are more common in younger people.[35] Somatosensory phenomena, typically paresthesias with anatomic march of symptoms, may occur, and motor disturbance may result in hemiparesis. Aphasia has also been reported.[8,36] Migraine aura symptoms may therefore be characterized by both positive and negative symptoms. Acephalgic migraine is an entity characterized by the neurologic dysfunction of the aura but without headache. This is strictly a diagnosis of exclusion, especially in older people. These so-called migraine accompaniments may occur for the first time in the older age group[37,38] and can be easily confused with transient ischemic attacks (TIAs) except in the most classic of cases. Migraine with aura and acephalgic migraine can be confused with TIAs, and vice versa. Headache occurred with 36% of TIAs in one series[39] and is more common in vertebrobasilar ischemia.[40,41] Migrainous aura in older adults presents a particularly difficult diagnostic dilemma. Transient hemiparetic or hemisensory symptoms occurring in older people for the first time should be assumed to be vascular (i.e., TIA) in cause until proven otherwise. Alternating hemisensory/paretic symptoms are more likely to be migrainous but still could have an embolic cause. Investigation including carotid Doppler studies and echocardiography will be necessary to manage potentially treatable embolic sources. Visual disturbance is more likely to be helpful as fortification spectra and colored zigzag lines are unlikely to occur in straightforward TIAs and are almost always migrainous in origin. Migraine with aura may occur for the first time in older adults, although, in general, new-onset migraine in the older age group is unusual[13,42] and may reflect the development of vascular change. It is often helpful in these cases to elicit a previous history of common migraine earlier in life.

The headache of migraine is typically throbbing in nature and exacerbated by exercise.[43] The pain may be unilateral in 60% of cases but bilateral at the outset in up to 40%.[8] Unilateral headache may later become bilateral during the attack. The intensity is moderate to severe, and pain may radiate down the neck to the shoulder. Some 40% of migraineurs report short-lived jabs of pain lasting seconds and having a needle-like quality, the so-called ice pick pains.[44]

The common accompanying symptoms of nausea and vomiting may make it difficult for the patient to take oral medication. Photophobia and phonophobia are common; many patients retire to a dark and quiet room for rest. Constitutional, mood, and mental changes are universal,[8] and patients are usually left feeling lethargic for a period after the attack.

Basilar migraine is a variant characterized by brainstem dysfunction such as ataxia, dysarthria, diplopia, vertigo, nausea and vomiting, and alteration in cognition and consciousness. Headache is invariable. In older adults these symptoms should be assumed to be of vascular origin until proven otherwise.

Ophthalmoplegic migraine is rare and can be confused with the presentation of berry aneurysm. Attacks of migraine-like pain occur around the eye with oculomotor nerve dysfunction and dilation of the pupil. The ophthalmoplegia may last from hours to months. The differential diagnosis includes orbital inflammatory disease and diabetic mononeuropathy.

Migraine attacks may vary in frequency from a few each year to several each week. Trigger factors include certain foods, red wine,[45] hormone replacement treatment in postmenopausal women,[46] irregular meals, and a change in sleep habit.[47] Environmental triggers include flickering lights, noise, rapidly altering visual stimuli, and even certain types of weather. Head injury and stress may lead to migraine attacks.

Treatment of Migraine

Once the diagnosis has been established, reassuring the patient may suffice. Any obvious precipitating cause such as diet, lack of sleep, or environmental factors should be discussed. Relaxation therapy may be helpful, but special diets have little place in management.

Pharmacotherapy includes treatment of the acute attack and consideration of prophylactic therapy. It should be remembered that changing biology in older adults will influence response to medication.[48] Gastric emptying slows, delaying absorption of medication; hepatic blood flow is reduced and so is glomerular filtration rate, affecting drug metabolism, usually leading to increased half-life. In general, therefore, pharmacotherapy should be started with caution in older adults, who are often taking medications for other comorbidities. Acute treatment should be started by the patient at the outset of an attack and is best limited to simple soluble analgesics such as paracetamol or aspirin (Table 59-1). Combination analgesics such as co-proxamol should be avoided, if possible, because of side effects and risk of medication overuse leading to so-called transformed migraine. For a more severe headache, nonsteroidal antiinflammatory drugs (NSAIDs) are used.[49] Ibuprofen (200 mg tid) may be obtained in the United Kingdom without prescription, or naproxen (250 mg tid) by prescription, or diclofenac (75 mg bid). This group of drugs should be administered with caution in the older adult population because of the increased risk of gastrointestinal hemorrhage, especially when there is a past history of peptic ulceration[50,51] or renal insufficiency.

TABLE 59-1 Drugs for Use in the Treatment of Migraine*

Migraine Attack Treatments	Migraine Prophylaxis
Soluble aspirin	Propranolol and other β-blockers
Soluble paracetamol	Tricyclic antidepressants
Antiemetics such as domperidone	Pizotifen
Suppositories	Topiramate
Nonsteroidal antiinflammatory drugs	Calcium channel antagonists
Sumatriptan (subcutaneous or oral)	Methysergide
Other triptans	Sodium valproate
Medihaler ergotamine and other ergotamine preparations	
Combination analgesia	

*Care must be taken with possible interactions with preexistent treatments and conditions such as asthma (if β-blockers are to be prescribed). Medications are listed in order of preference.

For moderate to severe migraine not responding to simple analgesia, sumatriptan can be tried. The initial dose is 50 mg orally and can be increased to 100 mg if there is no response. Subcutaneous self-administration is the preferred route when there is significant nausea or vomiting. Sumatriptan is a $5HT_1$ agonist and is thought to act as a selective cerebral vasoconstrictor. Up to 80% of patients obtain relief from headache within 2 hours after an injection[52] and up to 65% after a tablet dose.[53] The advantage is that the drug may be administered at any point during an attack and repeated if necessary. Flushing, tingling in the neck and head, and chest tightness can occur in up to 5% of patients.[54] Because sumatriptan may cause coronary vasoconstriction, it is contraindicated in patients with ischemic heart disease or uncontrolled hypertension. Special care in some older people is required because the loss of subcutaneous fat may lead to intramuscular injection and more rapid absorption. A recent study failed to demonstrate increased risk of stroke, myocardial infarction, cardiovascular death, ischemic heart disease, or overall mortality in older adults.[55] Pharmacotherapy should be combined with rest and sleep. A number of newer triptans have been licensed for use in migraine treatment and may be selected depending on the individual patient.[56]

Ergotamine preparations are best reserved for occasional (>1 month interval) severe headaches. They are potent vasoconstrictors and are best avoided in patients with a history of vasoocclusive disease, peripheral vascular disease, or hypertension, and those receiving β-blockers or with a history of Raynaud phenomenon. Patients should be strongly encouraged to avoid overuse of these drugs, because this can lead to resistant medication-misuse headache. Admission for drug withdrawal may be required when this occurs.

The accompanying symptoms of nausea and vomiting are often as disabling as the headache and require treatment in their own right. Metoclopramide is the most commonly used antiemetic, and by promoting gastric emptying, it aids absorption of coadministered medication. However, it can cause extrapyramidal side effects, especially in older people. Domperidone is less likely to cause this problem, as it does not cross the blood-brain barrier, but it does not aid gastric emptying.

Prophylactic therapy is indicated when there is severe recurrent headache causing disruption to daily life—as a guide, more than two severe headaches per month. Various drugs are used, including β-blockers, antidepressants, serotonin antagonists, calcium channel blockers, and, on occasion, anticonvulsants. Treatment is started at a low dose and built to maintenance. Possible side effects should be discussed and the regimen kept as simple as possible because many patients in this age group are likely to have coexistent medication. Patients should be weaned from therapy every 4 to 6 months.

Of the β-blockers, propranolol, metoprolol, and atenolol have all been shown to be effective in up to 60% to 80% of patients, producing a greater than 50% reduction in attack frequency.[57,58] Atenolol (50 to 100 mg daily) has a better side effect profile than propranolol (20 to 160 mg daily). Patients may complain of fatigue, dizziness, nightmares, and cold extremities. Care should be taken when there is peripheral vascular disease and in combination with ergotamine.

The tricyclic antidepressants have been used in migraine prophylaxis, although the evidence for their efficacy is largely based on anecdotal reports or uncontrolled trials. Their effect in headache may be independent of their antidepressant effect.[57,59] Amitriptyline is most commonly used, although fluoxetine has fewer anticholinergic side effects and causes less weight gain.[60] Paroxetine may be a suitable alternative when anxiety is a factor.[61] Because of their common side effect of drowsiness, the tricyclics are administered at the lowest effective dose at bedtime and slowly increased as necessary. Older people are more vulnerable to the muscarinic side effects. The typical starting dose for amitriptyline should be 10 mg, increasing to 150 mg if needed.[62]

Sodium valproate (0.6 to 2.5 g daily) is well tolerated, and there is clinical trial evidence of efficacy.[63] Side effects of valproate include tremor, ataxia, and, less commonly, an extrapyramidal syndrome. Topiramate now has a license for use in migraine prophylaxis; the use of anticonvulsants for migraine prophylaxis has been reviewed.[64]

Calcium channel antagonists are not licensed for migraine prophylaxis in the United Kingdom but have been shown to be of benefit.[57] The mechanism of action of these compounds in migraine is uncertain and side effects are common, including edema, flushing, dizziness, and, not infrequently, an initial increase in headache frequency. Improvement of headache may require several weeks of treatment.[65]

Of the serotonin antagonists, the two most commonly prescribed are pizotifen and methysergide. Pizotifen is a $5HT_2$ antagonist that is usually commenced in a dose of 0.5 mg at night and increased in stepwise manner to a dose of 4.5 mg. It has mild antidepressant activity but unfortunately stimulates appetite and leads to weight gain if diet is not controlled. It can produce beneficial effects in 40% to 79% of patients.[66] Methysergide is also a $5HT_2$ antagonist with some affinity for the $5HT_1$ receptor. It is effective prophylaxis in up to 60% of migraineurs, possibly with better results in those with migraine with aura.[67] Side effects are common and include myalgia, weight gain, nausea, and hallucinations (especially after the first dose). The complication of retroperitoneal, endocardial, and pulmonary fibrosis is rare and prevented by stopping treatment for 3 to 4 weeks every 4 to 6 months. The starting dose is 1 mg at night but may be increased to 6 mg daily in divided dosage.

Feverfew (*Tanacetum parthenium*) is an herbal remedy long used for headache treatment. It has limited effect, and the side effects include mouth ulceration and loss of taste.[68,69]

Newer treatments for migraine include the approval of onabotulinumtoxin type A for the prophylaxis of chronic migraine. This drug was approved after the PREEMPT clinical trials[70] and, to date, the safety data are encouraging.[71] Patients should be selected carefully and published injection protocols adhered to.

Tension Headache

Tension-type headache may be broadly classified into infrequent episodic tension-type headache, frequent episodic tension-type headache (at least 10 episodes occurring over 1 to 15 days a month), and chronic tension-type headache (headache occurring on more than 15 days per month).[31] The clinical features include the following:

- Pressing/tightening (nonpulsating) quality
- Mild or moderate intensity
- Bilateral location
- No aggravation when walking up or down stairs or doing similar routine physical activity

There should *not* be photophobia and phonophobia, although either alone is permitted within the definition. Patients should *not* experience nausea or vomiting (although the IHS criteria allow for nausea but not vomiting in the diagnosis of chronic tension-type headache).

In both types of headache, there may be pericranial muscle tenderness with or without increased electromyographic activity, although this does not assume that muscle tension is the cause of the headache.[72] In all age groups, tension-type headache is the most common form of headache, peaking in the 30s and 40s.[73] Chronic tension-type headache is more common in the older age groups than is episodic tension-type headache, and only 5% of patients with chronic tension-type headache report onset after the age of 60 years.[74] Within all age groups, tension headache remains most common in females with a 1-year period prevalence of 27.1% in females and 25.6% in males in one large telephone-based study.[27,73]

The pain of tension-type headache is usually described as a constant ache, which is infrequently pulsatile. Patients may describe a tight band about the head or a sensation of wearing a tight cap. There may be associated stiffness of the neck and upper back; in contrast to migraine, the pain is usually of lesser intensity. Scalp tenderness may lead to avoidance of hair brushing. This symptom is also recorded in migraineurs, and it may persist for some days after the headache has subsided.[75]

The headache may be unilateral or bilateral, commonly occipital or frontal but may involve any site. It can be relieved by changing position.

Patients with episodic tension headache may experience pericranial muscle tenderness with palpable nodules.[76] Depression, anxiety, and other psychological factors are important in the pathogenesis of tension headache, although, not infrequently, patients may initially deny any role.

Depression is common in the community at large, and in an average family practice in the United Kingdom it is the fourth most commonly diagnosed disorder.[77] The headache associated with depression can have features described for tension-type headache, and the headaches are often present for years or even throughout the patient's life. The headache is typically diurnal, usually worse in the morning and in the evening. There may be identifiable emotional, physical, and psychic complaints. These problems merit attention in their own right, especially in older adults when organic pathology is more likely anyway. The presence of severe depression in older people can be easily overlooked. Other headaches associated with depression can be described more bizarrely, with almost a delusional tone. Such headaches may indicate a serious psychiatric disorder and should lead to urgent psychiatric referral.

Treatment includes reassurance, simple analgesia as abortive treatment for the acute attack, and treatment of any psychopathology that may be present. Simple analgesia such as paracetamol should be used for acute attacks of pain. NSAIDs are more likely to be associated with side effects in older adults, such as gastric erosions and renal and hepatic complications.[78] Frequent episodic tension-type headache and chronic tension-type headache may require the use of prophylaxis—tricyclics such as amitriptyline remain the most useful drugs, especially when there is sleep disorder. The latter is especially useful when sleep disturbance is a prominent symptom.[79] Fluoxetine (20 mg daily) is less sedating. Paroxetine (10 mg daily) may be helpful when there are additional anxiety symptoms. Monoamine oxidase inhibitors should be avoided if possible. Psychiatric help may be appropriate, although patients often initially reject this suggestion. Relaxation therapy and biofeedback may also have a role.

The mixed headache syndrome—migraine and tension-type headache in the same patient—usually responds to treatment with tricyclic antidepressants with the addition of analgesia for acute episodes. There are no specific data on the prognosis of tension-type headache in older people, although there is a tendency for improvement with increasing age.[80] It is important to continually bear in mind that secondary headache is more common in older patients and that careful evaluation of the history and examination and a lower threshold for investigation should be applied in older adults with apparent nonspecific headache.

Chronic Daily Headache

The syndrome of chronic daily headache (CDH) accounts for 40% of patients seen in headache clinics[81] and worldwide is estimated to affect 3% to 5% of the population.[82] Only 5% reported their chronic headache as starting after 60 years of age.[74] CDH is defined as 15 or more headache days a month for 3 months or more.

BOX 59-1 Chronic Daily Headache Subtypes

Chronic tension-type headache
Transformed migraine
Drug-induced headache
Nondrug-related headache
Medication overuse headache
New daily persistent headache
Posttraumatic headache

There are several subtypes of CDH (Box 59-1), with chronic migraine presenting five times more commonly than chronic tension-type headache to the specialist headache clinic.[83] The features of tension-type headache are discussed elsewhere in this section. Medication overuse is probably the third most common form of chronic headache after chronic tension-type headache and chronic migraine and is thought to affect up to 1% of the world population.[84,85] The free availability of analgesics containing caffeine, codeine, barbiturates, and tranquilizers over the counter has been implicated as one cause of this syndrome.[86,87] The management of this syndrome can be particularly challenging and hinges on the discontinuation of analgesic overuse, the possibility of going "cold turkey," and the use of suitable alternatives for weaning and prophylaxis.[88] In a proportion of patients the headache may revert to its original episodic form, but in the remainder the avoidance of analgesic overuse will require the initiation of prophylaxis.[89] Suitable prophylactic treatment such as amitriptyline in an initial dose of 10 mg at night increased to 75 mg as tolerated is effective, with improvement seen at 2 to 14 days. The drug should be continued at an effective dose for 6 months and then withdrawn slowly over 3 months. Caution should be exercised in those with glaucoma and prostatism. Anticonvulsant drugs used in migraine prophylaxis may be effective, and sodium valproate, gabapentin, and, more recently, topiramate have been used with favorable results.[90,91] Patient and physician education is especially important in prevention and management of this difficult headache syndrome.

Episodic migraine may evolve into CDH. In one study, 489 of 630 patients (78%) with CDH had a clear preceding history of episodic migraine.[92] This so-called transformed migraine may be caused by excessive use of opioid and simple analgesics, barbiturates, ergot compounds, caffeine, and frequent use of triptans. Headaches are often more severe on waking owing to a drug-free withdrawal period overnight effectively causing rebound. Hemicrania continua is side-locked headache that often has autonomic symptoms and shows an exquisite response to indomethacin.[93,94]

The differential diagnosis includes headaches arising from the neck, temporal arteritis, mass lesions, and visual acuity problems. Because tension-type headache is often associated with depression, sleep disorder, and situational life events, especially in the older adult population, the treatment of CDH must include behavioral, psychological, and social aspects.

Cluster Headache

This condition, although most common in young adults, may have its onset in the seventh decade when the clinical features are the same.[95,96] The IHS classification divides the condition into episodic and chronic cluster headache, the latter being more common in the older adult population.[97] A review of the literature suggests a lifetime prevalence of 124/100,000,[98] with a higher male preponderance in the young but more females older than 60 years affected than males.[99]

Cluster headache is characterized by bouts of severe pain and autonomic activation. The pain is constant, often described as "boring" in nature, and patients are restless in contrast to those with migraine who lie quietly. The pain is often centered around one eye, and there may be ipsilateral lacrimation, nasal congestion, and rhinorrhea. There is usually conjunctival injection, and there may be associated ptosis, meiosis, and eyelid edema. The pain may spread to the whole side of the face. Bouts of pain occur one to three times per day with alarm-clock regularity, commonly an hour or so after going to sleep, and last from 15 minutes to a few hours (with a usual duration of 45 to 90 minutes). The headache may start and end abruptly, and in some patients there may be interictal discomfort.[100] The cluster period typically lasts for 1 to 2 months and then subsides. During the cluster attacks, alcohol is a potent precipitant, usually setting off an attack within an hour of ingestion, as are vasodilator drugs such as nitrates. One study examined the association of alcohol dehydrogenase genotypes and cluster headache but with only preliminary findings.[101] The chronic form continues without remission often for many years.

Treatment is symptomatic. Oxygen at 100% is useful in the emergency department and can be given at home. It is important that a high flow valve is used with a nonrebreather mask capable of delivering 7 to 10 L/min. More practically, sumatriptan by subcutaneous injection is the drug of choice for acute attacks.[102] However, it should be remembered that many patients may have cardiovascular disease, which limits the use of this drug. Nasal sumatriptan may be used but appears to be less effective.[103] Preventive treatments may be considered in terms of short-term measures and longer duration treatment for those with a more chronic course to their clusters. Steroids (e.g., prednisolone 1 mg/kg daily for a week and reducing by 10 mg a week) may shorten a cluster period, but relapse often occurs and so they may be used with other forms of prophylaxis.[104] Verapamil is the drug of choice for all forms of cluster headache prophylaxis[105] and compares favorably with lithium,[106] particularly in view of the plethora of potential neuropsychiatric side effects of the latter. Doses of verapamil range from 240 mg to 960 mg bid in divided dose. Because this drug can cause heart block, a baseline electrocardiogram (ECG) should be taken, an initial dose of 80 mg tid commenced, and then every 10 days or so the dose should be increased in 80-mg increments until attacks are suppressed or side effects prevent further titration. An ECG should be done after each increment. Sodium valproate may be tried in resistant cases.[107] Lithium carbonate given in standard psychiatric doses (600 to 1200 mg) and monitored accordingly is useful in chronic cluster headache but less so in episodic cluster headache. One small trial demonstrated benefit of melatonin 10 mg for prophylaxis.[108] In rare cases, surgical intervention is attempted. Percutaneous radiofrequency trigeminal gangliorhizolysis and posterior fossa trigeminal sensory rhizolysis have been performed but are of unproven benefit. Surgery can cause a reduction in facial sensation and corneal hypoesthesia with increased risk of corneal ulceration.[109]

Cluster headache is an underdiagnosed cause of recurrent paroxysmal cranial pain in the older adult population. It may not have the usual classic features in this age group. Treatment may need to be given empirically when there is doubt. Furthermore, symptomatic cluster-like headache may accompany other conditions such as glaucoma and sinusitis.

Chronic paroxysmal hemicrania (Sjaastad headache), a rare variant of cluster headache, differs in the brevity (3 to 45 minutes) and frequency (up to 40 times a day) of the attacks. The invariable response to indomethacin forms part of the diagnostic criteria.[2]

FACIAL NEURALGIAS

Trigeminal Neuralgia

Diagnosis

Trigeminal neuralgia is diagnosed clinically. It rarely begins before the age of 30 years,[110,111] has a prevalence of 0.1 to 0.2/1000 and an incidence of up to 20/100,000/year after the age of 60 years, and the female-to-male ratio is 3 : 2.[112] Higher incidences are reported[113] up to 28.9/100,000/year in the Netherlands.[114] The symptoms are pathognomonic. The pain is periodic, of high intensity, and lancinating, lasting from 20 to 30 seconds and followed by a period of relief lasting a few seconds to a minute, which may be followed by further paroxysms of pain. The pain usually commences in the maxillary and mandibular divisions of the trigeminal nerve, and in fewer than 5% of cases it begins in the ophthalmic division. In some 10% to 15% of cases, all the divisions are involved and the symptoms may be bilateral in 3% to 5%.[100] Apart from the quality and characteristic site of pain, the patient can usually identify trigger factors such as brushing the teeth, washing the face, shaving, biting, chewing, or even a gust of cold wind on the face. Avoidance behavior is common. The most recent Classification of Headache Disorders[2] includes the diagnostic category of classical trigeminal neuralgia with concomitant persistent facial pain, previously known as atypical trigeminal neuralgia or trigeminal neuralgia type II. The prognosis for remission in this form is less good, and in fewer cases is it possible to demonstrate neurovascular compression (see later). Central sensitization has been proposed as a factor.[115,116]

The pain of trigeminal neuralgia may occur daily for weeks or months followed by remission of varying periods. Unfortunately there is a tendency for the disorder to deteriorate, with increased frequency of attacks increasingly resistant to treatment. Clinical examination should be normal, and any loss of facial sensation should be promptly investigated, preferably with gadolinium-enhanced magnetic resonance imaging (MRI) of the brain and trigeminal system, to rule out a compressive lesion of the nerve. Autonomic symptoms are not present in this condition. The presence of autonomic activation and pain primarily in the first division of the nerve is more likely to represent one of the trigeminal autonomic cephalalgias than trigeminal neuralgia.

Cause

Proximal nerve root demyelination due to mechanical irritation of proximal trigeminal nerve root is believed to be the pathophysiology of this condition. The proximal nerve roots lie within central nervous system (CNS) nerve tissue, which extends several millimeters from the surface of the pons. Animal laboratory data, however, are more consistent with a central mechanism mediated by the loss of segmental inhibition within the spinal trigeminal sensory nucleus. To reconcile these observations, Fromm and associates[117] proposed that spontaneous peripheral activity from the irritated nerve, in the presence of the failure of the normal central inhibitory mechanisms, may cause paroxysmal bursts of neuronal activity within the trigeminal nucleus and its thalamic relays, perceived as neuralgia by the patient. This has been likened to a form of "sensory reflex epilepsy."[118] Some evidence for the peripheral component of this hypothesis comes from the common finding of vascular loops (arterial or venous) in association with the nerve root in a majority of symptomatic patients.[119,120] Other compressive pathology should be considered, including schwannoma, lymphoma, meningioma, and a variety of other tumors and infiltrative lesions. Pathologic specimens reveal focal demyelination within the proximal (CNS) part of the root. It is proposed that ephaptic transmission of spontaneously generated ectopic impulses results in symptoms.[121] Because vessels tend to become more ectatic with age, this may explain why the condition is more common in older people.

Treatment

The treatment of this condition is initially medical.[122-124] Occasionally the symptoms are so severe that hospital admission is required to control symptoms and prevent a downward spiral of increasing pain, dehydration, and depression. This is particularly the case for older and infirm individuals.

Of the few high-quality randomized controlled trials, most have enrolled small numbers in single centers. A 2007 review confirmed that carbamazepine remains the first-choice drug, and pain relief is usually obtained within 4 to 24 hours.[125] The initial dose of 100 mg tid is increased every 48 hours in a stepwise manner until symptom relief or side effects occur. Patients should be warned of the potential for drowsiness, rash, and unsteadiness. A baseline full blood count is recommended because leukopenia occurs commonly and agranulocytosis rarely; treatment should be stopped immediately if the latter occurs. Although carbamazepine is usually effective at blood levels of 25 to 50 mg/L, the dose can be titrated to the maximum tolerated in resistant cases. Therapy should be maintained until the patient has been free of pain for at least 4 weeks, after which slow reduction of dose by decrements of 100 mg of carbamazepine each week may allow for complete withdrawal of the drug. For patients who experience limited efficacy or side effects, oxcarbazepine should be tried. This is a prodrug of arbamazepine and does not utilize the hepatic cytochrome system, thereby resulting in fewer drug interactions. Recent guidelines have suggested that lamotrigine and baclofen may be effective if carbamazepine and oxcarbazepine fail.[126,127] A small open label trial of pregabalin demonstrated positive results.[128] Combination therapy may be necessary but may aggravate drowsiness. Alternatively, phenytoin, clonazepam, or sodium valproate can be added. Polypharmacy should be avoided if possible because of additional side effects and problems with compliance.

Surgical intervention should be considered if medical treatment fails. Up to 50% of patients may eventually require some form of surgical treatment. Early referral should be considered when symptomatic control with pharmacotherapy proves difficult. There are two main options, rhizotomy or microvascular decompression.

Percutaneous treatments, including balloon compression, radiofrequency rhizotomy, and glycerol rhizolysis, are relatively safe and simple. Patients require only light anesthesia, and the procedure is carried out under radiographic screening control. Selective root lesioning is achieved if a stimulating electrode is employed, and this reduces the side effects (discussed later). Acute pain relief can be accomplished in more than 90% of patients, and this can be maintained in the long term with repeated treatments if necessary.[129] Glycerol, injected into the Meckel cave, acts as a neurotoxin. Atypical trigeminal neuralgia responds less well to treatments in general.

The main side effect is sensory loss (usually less with glycerol injection). Corneal hypoesthesia is a problem and may result in ulceration. Rarely there may be masseter weakness. Both forms of treatment have about 90% success, and the patient can be discharged home within 24 hours. Unfortunately, the reported recurrence rates are about 25%. In a study comparing glycerol rhizolysis and posterior fossa exploration, freedom from pain at 5 years was 59% and 68%, respectively.[130] Cheng and coworkers have recently reviewed the literature on these treatments.[131]

Gamma knife radiosurgery is the least invasive treatment but with unknown long-term outcomes as few data are available beyond 5 years of treatment. Rates of pain relief of 70% have been reported at 6 months after treatment; the effects are often delayed and facial numbness may occur.[132]

Microvascular decompression involves major neurosurgery with a posterior fossa approach. This procedure was pioneered by Jannetta.[133] If a blood vessel is found in close association with the trigeminal root or deforming it, it is mobilized and a small sponge of polyvinyl chloride is interposed between the nerve and the vessel. This procedure is generally well tolerated by older patients who are otherwise medically fit for surgery.[134] Recurrence rates of up to 24% at 30 months after the procedure were reported in one study.[135] Overall, the recurrence of pain after any surgical procedure was 19% with a minimum 5-year follow-up, with microvascular decompression providing the greatest relief and patient satisfaction.[136]

Glossopharyngeal Neuralgia

This syndrome has the same symptom characteristics as trigeminal neuralgia, but the pain is felt in the region of the tonsil and ear. Trigger factors include swallowing, coughing, and talking, and the distribution of the pain is in the sensory territory of the glossopharyngeal nerve and the auricular and pharyngeal branches of the vagus nerve. Rarely the patient may become unconscious during an attack because of asystole.[35] Neurologic examination is normal unless the syndrome is secondary to pathology such as neoplasm, infection, or inflammatory disease.

Treatment is the same as for trigeminal neuralgia with carbamazepine as first-choice pharmacotherapy. The medical treatment of this condition is less successful than in the case of trigeminal neuralgia, and surgery is more often undertaken.[137] If there is no improvement, microvascular dissection of the intracranial section of the glossopharyngeal nerve and upper two rootlets of the vagus can be undertaken.[138,139]

Postherpetic Neuralgia

Postherpetic neuralgia occurs following 10% of attacks of shingles, but this figure rises to 50% in adults older than 60 years.[140] The most common site is the ophthalmic division of the trigeminal nerve. The virus has a predilection for the trigeminal (23% of cases[141]) and upper cervical ganglia, and in the acute stages the herpetic eruption is seen in the appropriate distribution. The Ramsay Hunt syndrome is caused by herpetic infection of the facial nerve. Excruciating pain may precede the eruption of vesicles by 1 to 3 days. The latter are seen over the external auditory meatus and mastoid process and may occur with edema and redness of the ear, making examination difficult. Occasionally, other cranial nerves may be affected with involvement of the trigeminal nerve, leading to loss of sensation on the face and numbness of the palate occurring when the ninth nerve is affected. A careful search for vesicles around the ear and in the mouth will make the diagnosis clear. There may also be involvement of the fourth, sixth, and oculomotor nerves,[142] with the possibility of long-term paralysis.

The syndrome of postherpetic neuralgia is characterized by a constant burning or aching pain with occasional stabbing components and occurs following healing of the rash. It may take several weeks or months to emerge. There is sensory loss over the affected area, and invariably allodynia develops.

Treatment is symptomatic.[143] Antiviral therapy such as acyclovir was shown to provide marginal evidence for reduction of pain incidence at 1 to 3months following zoster onset. Famciclovir reduced the duration of the neuralgia but not its incidence, as did valacyclovir. Steroids had no effect on postherpetic neuralgia.[144,145] Amitriptyline taken at the onset may reduce the incidence of postherpetic neuralgia, but more trials need to be undertaken.[144] Acyclovir (800 mg five times daily) may be prescribed if the rash is extensive or if there is a threat to eyesight. Opiate analgesia may be required. Once neuralgia is established, amitriptyline is of proven benefit,[146,147] and carbamazepine may help to control the stabbing component of the pain. Relief of pain may be gained in up to 80% of cases. Nortriptyline and desipramine may be better tolerated, causing less sedation; the former has been shown to be as effective as amitriptyline.[148] Transcutaneous electrical nerve stimulation (TENS) may sometimes be useful. Topical capsaicin cream has had variable success.[149,150] Topical lidocaine patch 5% has been shown to be efficacious in patients with evidence of allodynia. The patch can be cut to any shape and placed over active lesions; the main side effect seems to be mild local skin irritation. Both gabapentin and pregabalin are licensed for the treatment of this condition,[151,152] which is notoriously difficult to treat and may require multidisciplinary input.[153]

PERSISTENT IDIOPATHIC FACIAL PAIN

Previously described as atypical facial pain, this syndrome occurs rarely in older people. It is defined as cranial pain that that does not follow dermatomal boundaries or conform to any of the known patterns of headache or cranial neuralgia. It is defined as pain that is present daily for more than 2 hours for more than 3 months.[2] The diagnosis can be made only after the exclusion of organic pathology, including dental and sinus disease.[154] Many patients are believed to be depressed[39] and receive tricyclic antidepressants, generally with a good result.[155] Lance and Goadsby[100] have proposed an organic basis to this syndrome. However, tricyclics remain the treatment of choice, together with the judicious use of baclofen. Occasionally the pain may have a throbbing vascular nature, and, when intermittent, it is worth considering a diagnosis of facial or "lower half" migraine.[156] In one study from Germany of 517 migraine sufferers, pain involved the head and lower half of the face in 8.9% of patients.[157] In this case, a trial of a β-blocker or sumatriptan may be useful.

HEADACHE ARISING FROM THE NECK

Cervical spondylosis, affecting the neck vertebrae, has a strong association with aging.[158] Disc degenerative disease leads to a loss of intervertebral height with narrowing of the central canal exacerbated by facet joint arthrosis and posterior ligamentous fibrosis. Intervertebral foramina may become narrowed, leading to radiculopathy. Thus, spondylotic changes may compress cervical nerves or the spinal cord to produce a syndrome of cervical spondyloradiculopathy with or without myelopathy. Symptomatic cervical spondylosis is more common in men than in women and produces symptoms typically in the fifth and sixth decades. Neck pain and headache may result, and although most of the population older than 40 years has radiologic changes consistent with cervical spondylosis without symptoms, in those with symptomatic disease (brachialgia or myelopathy), 40% reported headache as a chief symptom and 25% reported it as a major symptom.[159] The mechanism of cervicogenic headache remains uncertain and is hotly debated.[160] It may be defined as headache arising from the structures of the neck, unilateral, and possibly exacerbated by neck movement. It is proposed that the convergence of sensory afferents from cervical structures with descending trigeminal pathways in the upper cervical segments of the spinal cord allows for bidirectional referral of pain between the neck and trigeminal receptive fields of the face and head.[161] However, overall cervical spondylosis is an uncommon cause of headache.

The head pain resulting from cervical degenerative disease is frequently occipital in distribution but may radiate to the vertex or even the frontal area. The greater occipital nerve (C2) provides much of the sensory input from the back of the head, and irritation of this nerve typically causes occipital headache. The pain is usually described as constant, not throbbing, and of moderate intensity. Associated muscle tenderness, perhaps secondary to spasm, may be present, and this may make differentiation from tension headache difficult. It is disputed whether the cervical spine itself gives rise to headache per se, but headache may arise as a secondary phenomenon because of muscle spasm in the neck.[158] Movements of the cervical spine may aggravate the headache, and examination will reveal reduced range of movement and suboccipital tenderness with muscle spasm. Headache arising from the cervical spine is often unilateral and may be exacerbated by digital pressure on neck muscles and on head movement. There may be posterior to anterior ipsilateral radiation of the pain. It is interesting that mild migrainous features such as photophobia, nausea, and vomiting may be present.[2]

Treatment is usually conservative with NSAIDs or simple analgesics. Cervical collars are of uncertain worth and, if used, should be combined with referral to a physiotherapist for neck exercises. Surgery is considered when there is myelopathy or radiculopathy, especially when it is progressive.

Lesions of the bones of the upper cervical spine and base of skull can give rise to occipital ache by pressure on the cervical nerves. Myeloma, osteomyelitis, metastatic tumor, and erosive inflammatory disease such as rheumatoid arthritis can all cause headache and neurologic deficit. Paget disease can cause basilar invagination with traction on the upper cervical nerves and/or hydrocephalus, both of which may result in headache.[159] A plain skull x-ray will usually rule out these possibilities if suspected.

SINUS DISEASE AND DENTAL DISEASE

Head and facial pain may be referred from the cranial sinuses. Experiments have shown that inflammation of the sinus lining is rarely painful[162] but that pain arises from inflammation of the ducts and ostia of the sinuses or inflammation of the nasal turbinates.[35] Disease of the frontal sinuses causes ache localized over these sinuses; that of the antrum is usually referred to the maxillary region and into the zygomatic or temporal areas. Headache associated with sphenoidal and ethmoidal disease is felt mainly behind the eyes and over the vertex of the skull. Sinus headache is frequently overdiagnosed in the primary care setting, and many patients satisfy criteria for tension-type headache and migraine.[163] A sensible approach is to carefully elicit a history of symptoms compatible with nasal acute sinus inflammation (purulent nasal discharge, local pain over the relevant sinus) in addition to headache. Chronic sinusitis rarely causes headache. Migraine is more likely to be the cause of recurrent headache than sinusitis, even in the presence of rhinitic symptoms.[164,165]

The pain of sinus disease is usually deep-seated and dull, aching, and nonpulsatile. Adopting a recumbent position may relieve the headache of sinus disease, so these headaches are less prominent at night than during the day. Pain may be exacerbated by shaking the head or adopting a head-down position. Coughing or straining also exacerbates the pain by raising intracranial venous pressure.

The treatment of sinusitis is symptomatic with decongestants and analgesia, but unremitting pain may indicate a more sinister cause and merits further investigation.

Dental disease is referred to the distribution of the trigeminal nerve. In general, upper jaw disease is referred to the maxillary division and lower jaw disease to the mandibular division. The cause of such pain is usually obvious, but continued facial pain may merit referral to a maxillofacial surgeon. Examination of the patient with facial pain includes assessment of the teeth and a search for tooth sensitivity with percussion.

VASCULAR DISORDERS AND HEADACHE

Giant Cell Arteritis

(See also Chapter 72.)

This condition is rare in people younger than 50 years, with incidence rising 10-fold between the sixth and ninth decades. Population-based studies suggest that up to 40% to 60% of patients develop polymyalgia rheumatica in addition to giant cell arteritis.[166] The female-to-male ratio is approximately 4:1, and the prevalence varies from 7/100,000 in 50-year-olds to 70/100,000 in octogenarians.[167] The reported rates are highest in Scandinavian countries and lower in Mediterranean and Asian countries, and there is an association of HLA-DRB1*04.[168] Headache is the most common symptom (85% at some point in the disease),[169] but is only reported as the initial symptom in a third of patients.[170] It is usually severe (but may be mild), is persistent, may throb, and disturbs sleep. The headache may have phenotypic features of primary headache disorders such as migraine or cluster headache.[171,172] The pain is usually bitemporal but may be unilateral, frontal, or generalized. Scalp tenderness is common, and patients may avoid grooming the hair. Jaw claudication (facial pain when chewing), first described by Horton,[173] is virtually pathognomonic of this condition and may affect up to half of patients,[174] and infarction of the tongue can follow. Vascular claudication may affect the arms and even the muscles of deglutition. Constitutional symptoms such as fatigue and malaise, lethargy, anorexia, and a low-grade fever are reported in up to 63% of patients.[175]

Sudden visual loss may affect up to 20% of cases and is an early manifestation.[176,177] This is a result of ischemia of the posterior ciliary arteries (and, less commonly, ischemia of the retinal artery) and secondary ischemic optic neuropathy, or infarction of the choroid. Patients may complain of nonpainful amaurosis fugax, a shade covering the eye, sudden total visual loss, or transient diplopia (involvement of extraocular muscles). Left untreated, the second eye usually becomes affected within 1 to 2 weeks. It is interesting that patients with optic complications had lower clinical and laboratory markers of inflammation, were less likely to be anemic, and were more likely to be HLA-DRB1*04 positive.[178] Patients who have other ischemic complications were more likely to experience retinal ischemia.

Giant cell arteritis affects the proximal aorta and its extracranial arteries, that is, large and medium-sized muscular arteries with a prominent internal elastic membrane and vasa vasorum. The inflammation is most severe at the junction of the intima and media of vessels, disrupting the elastic lamina. Intradural vessels do not have a lamina, so intracranial inflammation is rarely seen.[179] The affected vessels become nodular, tortuous, and swollen. The superficial temporal artery may become palpable, tender, and pulseless. There is medial necrosis with formation of granulomatous tissue and invasion of lymphocytes and giant cells. Often there is thrombosis of the lumen. Extracranial vascular complications may occur, including mononeuropathies and peripheral neuropathy. (Complications of treatment, such as steroid-induced myopathy, should not be forgotten.) Cerebrovascular disease is rare because of the predilection for extradural vessels; if present, it tends to affect the vertebral circulation preferentially and carries a higher mortality risk.[180,181]

Although temporal artery biopsy remains the gold standard, unfortunately the pathology is not continuous, and "skip lesions" mean that there is a good chance that a temporal artery biopsy will be negative. A minimum biopsy length of 1 cm can help to minimize the risk of false negatives.[182] There is no consensus on the role of bilateral biopsies, either simultaneous or sequential. Although a biopsy is desirable, treatment should not be delayed in clinically suspicious cases; biopsy specimens may show changes even 2 weeks after initiation of steroid treatment.[183] Color Doppler ultrasonography of the temporal arteries has been demonstrated to show good specificity but variable sensitivity.[184,185]

The erythrocyte sedimentation rate (ESR) is a vital diagnostic test but can be normal in up to 10% of cases.[186-188] The mean value in one study was 89 mm/hr with a value of less than 40 mm/hr seen in less than 5% of cases.[189] C-reactive protein is believed to be a more sensitive indicator of disease activity in giant cell arteritis, although ESR remains the time-honored marker.[190] The combination of elevated ESR and C-reactive protein improves the diagnostic yield.[191] A study carried out at the Mayo Medical Center of 525 consecutive patients undergoing temporal artery biopsy demonstrated that the absence of jaw claudication, elevated ESR, and temporal artery tenderness with the presence of synovitis had a 95% predictive rate of negative temporal artery biopsy.[192] Nonspecific abnormalities include a mild normochromic normocytic anemia and leukocytosis. Plasma fibrinogen levels are elevated, as are other acute-phase proteins. Liver function tests are often abnormal, with an elevated alkaline phosphatase and elevated transaminases. An elevated creatine phosphokinase does not occur and should lead to a search for an alternative diagnosis.

If clinical suspicion is high, the patient should be commenced on high-dose corticosteroids immediately because failure to act may cost the patient loss of vision. Prednisolone (60 to 80 mg) is given usually with rapid clinical effect. In the presence of visual or focal neurologic symptoms, high-dose intravenous methylprednisolone should be prescribed. Guidelines have been proposed as recently as 2010.[193] Failure of the symptoms to respond within 24 to 48 hours should lead to review of the diagnosis. High-dose steroids are maintained for 2 to 4 weeks and then tapered gradually (by a maximum of 10% of the total daily dose every 2 weeks) depending on the ESR and the patient's symptoms. Alternate day steroid regimens are associated with a higher treatment failure rate and should be avoided.[194] Hasty dose reduction should be avoided, and most patients will take up to 6 months to reduce to a level of less than 10 mg/day. A typical tapering regimen would involve reduction by 10 mg every 2 weeks to 20 mg, then by 2.5 mg every 2 weeks to 10 mg/day, and then by 1 mg per month assuming that no relapse occurs.[193] The addition of NSAIDs can reduce minor recurrent symptoms.[195] Patients will need treatment for many months and most for several years; relapse is most common in the first year after stopping steroids, especially when the dose is reduced to 5 to 10 mg daily.[196,197] After stopping treatment, the patient's ESR and symptoms should be monitored for at least 6 months to a year in case of relapse. Visual loss because of a relapse is unusual after a lengthy course of steroids. Osteoporosis prophylaxis may be necessary. There is some evidence from retrospective studies that combining low-dose aspirin with steroid therapy (where there is no contraindication, and with a proton-pump inhibitor) may lower the risk of ischemic complications, even though thromboembolic occlusion is not thought to be the cause.[198,199]

Any older person with malaise, arthralgia, depression, and vague headache should be considered a possible case until proven otherwise.

Cerebrovascular Disease and Hypertension

Headache is a common accompaniment to cerebrovascular disease[200,201] and may occur before, during, or after TIA or stroke. The pain is often throbbing in nature and exacerbated with effort. Usually it is lateralized to the side of ischemia. It occurs most frequently when there is parenchymal hemorrhage (57%) but also with TIAs (36%), thromboembolic infarct (29%), and lacunar infarction (17%). It appeared that posterior circulation events (44%) were more frequently associated with headache than anterior circulation events (31%).[202] This study was before the computed tomography (CT) era, so it may be that hemorrhagic strokes were included in the data. A more recent study, however, reached similar conclusions.[203]

Headache does not occur more frequently in the hypertensive than in the normotensive general population unless it is of extreme degree or associated with rapid rises of blood pressure, as in pheochromocytoma.[204] Occasionally, however, migraine has undoubtedly been aggravated by the occurrence of hypertension.

Carotid and Vertebral Artery Dissection

Extracranial arterial dissection is a more common cause of stroke and headache in younger persons, but it also is a cause of headache and cerebrovascular ischemia in older people. The anterior circulation is more commonly affected.[205] Carotid artery dissection and occlusion give rise to ipsilateral pain involving the face and forehead and occasionally the neck. The pain is described as burning or throbbing but can be sudden and stabbing and may be mistaken for subarachnoid hemorrhage (discussed later). Horner syndrome may be present ipsilateral to the involved

60 Stroke: Epidemiology and Pathology

Christopher Moran, Velandai K. Srikanth, Amanda G. Thrift

STROKE EPIDEMIOLOGY

This chapter is concerned with the study of patterns and risk factors associated with stroke and the pathologic changes observed in stroke. The major types of stroke are ischemic stroke (due to cerebral vessel occlusion) and hemorrhagic stroke (due to bleeding from cerebral vessel). In epidemiologic tradition, stroke has been defined as "rapidly developing clinical signs of focal disturbance of cerebral function lasting more than 24 hours (unless interrupted by surgery or death) with no apparent cause other than of vascular origin."[1] However, this definition has since evolved with the use of modern radiologic techniques (e.g., diffusion-weighted magnetic resonance imaging [DW-MRI]) that are more sensitive to early infarction in patients suffering transient symptoms lasting less than 24 hours. The American Heart Association has recently adopted a position defining ischemic stroke—or central nervous system (CNS) infarction—as "brain, spinal cord, or retinal cell death attributable to ischemia, based on either pathological, imaging, or other objective evidence of focal ischemic injury in a defined vascular distribution, or clinical evidence of focal ischemic injury based on symptoms persisting ≥24 hours or until death, and other etiologies [are] excluded."[2] Those who suffer transient sudden focal neurologic symptoms less than 24 hours of presumed vascular origin, but without demonstrable infarction on sensitive brain imaging, are considered as having a transient ischemic attack (TIA). The impact of the these revisions to stroke and TIA definitions on prior and future estimates of prevalence, incidence, mortality, and risk factors have yet to be fully understood.

In the following sections, we summarize the current knowledge about the epidemiology and pathology of stroke, with implications particularly for older adults with frailty.

Burden of Stroke

From a population level, the burden of stroke can be measured in three different ways—by measuring mortality, prevalence, or incidence. Each method has its advantages and limitations.

Stroke mortality figures usually include all individuals with stroke recorded as the primary cause of death on their death certificates. Systematic and long-term collection of these data allows assessment of trends over time and comparisons among countries. Mortality figures are subject to limitations, including imprecision in death certification and incomplete assessment of the overall burden of stroke; between 45% and 60% of people with stroke survive beyond 5 years.[3-5]

Stroke prevalence studies can be used to assess health in survivors and assist with the planning of community health care resources, but may not provide an accurate reflection of the population burden of stroke because of issues such as selection and survival bias. Carefully conducted stroke incidence studies provide the best source of information on the burden of stroke, allowing a better understanding of the empirical relation among incidence, mortality, and survival. For example, changes in stroke mortality may attributable to changes in stroke incidence, case fatality (reflecting changes to stroke severity or poststroke management), or a combination of both.

Comparison between identically conducted stroke incidence studies in the same population will help determine where the changes have occurred. Such repeat incidence studies are expensive and labor-intensive because of the strict ideal criteria required for their conduct.[6-9] Because of this, most stroke incidence studies in the past decade were undertaken in high-income countries, but there are several now being carried out in low and middle-income countries. Recent comprehensive reviews of the global burden of stroke summarizes many of these studies and shows some marked differences in stroke burden between high-income and low- and middle-income countries.[10-12]

Stroke Mortality

According to the Global Burden of Diseases Study, stroke and ischemic heart disease collectively contributed to 1279 million deaths in 2010, or one in four deaths worldwide, compared with one in five in 1990.[13] According to the World Health Organization (WHO), stroke is the second most common single cause of death in the world after ischemic heart disease.[14] In 2012, an estimated 6.7 million deaths from stroke occurred worldwide; these deaths comprised approximately 11.9% of all deaths.[14] The contribution of stroke to mortality varies by income level of countries. In 2012, approximately 43% of these deaths occurred in low- to middle-income countries, 55% in upper middle-income countries, and only 22% in high-income countries.[14] The greater number of strokes deaths occurring in low- and middle-income countries than in high-income countries is attributable to their larger population (≈fourfold that of the population in high-income countries).[15]

There are now substantial data on time trends in stroke mortality rates from low-, middle-, and high-income countries. In a comprehensive systematic review, Krishnamurthi and Feigin and colleagues have summarized trends in annual mortality rates by age and country income status from 1990 to 2010.[10,11] They showed that overall, stroke mortality rates declined over this period, irrespective of a country's income status. The age-adjusted annual mortality rate/100,000 population for ischemic stroke fell significantly from 63.8 (95% confidence interval [CI], 56.5 to 66.0) to 40.3 (95% CI, 38.2 to 43.1) in high-income countries and from 50.1 (95% CI, 42.0 to 64.1) to 43.1 (95% CI, 38.3 to 51.9) in low-income countries. Mortality rates for hemorrhagic stroke also fell from 32.7 (95% CI, 29.9 to 35.7) to 20.3 (95% CI, 18.6 to 22.9) in high-income countries and from 80.4 (95% CI, 63.7 to 96.9) to 61.9 (95% CI, 52.5 to 72.3) in low-income countries.

These declines were observed for all age categories, but were more pronounced in those aged 75 years and older, with up to a 40% reduction in rates in these older age groups (Table 60-1). However, mortality overall from stroke was much greater in those 75 years and older than in those younger than 75 years. In the WHO Monitoring Trends and Determinants in Cardiovascular Disease (WHO MONICA) project, Sarti and associates have provided evidence to suggest that declining case fatality rates may underlie the observed changes in mortality.[16] These observations have been supported by reductions in the mortality incidence rates observed by Krishnamurthi and coworkers from 1990 to 2010 in most countries.[10] The reasons underlying reduced case fatality rates are most likely to be improvements in stroke care, with earlier and more appropriate diagnoses, rapid acute treatments, and increasing presence of organized stroke units.

TABLE 60-1 Global Trends in Age-Adjusted Annual Stroke Incidence and Mortality*

Age Group, Stroke Type, and Effect Measure	High-Income Countries		Low- and Middle-Income Countries	
	1990	*2010*	*1990*	*2010*
AGE < 75 YR				
Ischemic Stroke				
Incidence	110.8 (95% CI, 103.1-118.5)	100.5 (95% CI, 94.0-107.2)	101.88 (95% CI, 89.20-116.42)	106.90 (95% CI, 93.62-121.41)
Mortality	18.57 (95% CI, 16.07-19.49)	11.86 (95% CI, 10.47-12.69)	18.08 (95% CI, 14.57-24.39)	14.71 (95% CI, 12.90-18.75)
Hemorrhagic Stroke				
Incidence	41.9 (95% CI, 38.9-45.2)	38.5 (95% CI, 35.6-41.2)	61.64 (95% CI, 52.84-71.54)	75.68 (95% CI, 64.93-88.74)
Mortality	20.95 (95% CI, 18.82-22.83)	12.29 (95% CI, 11.12-13.74)	49.36 (95% CI, 39.54-59.56)	36.53 (95% CI, 31.01-42.71)
Total Stroke				
Incidence	152.7 (95% CI, 142.3-163.2)	138.9 (95% CI, 130.6-148.2)	163.5 (95% CI, 142.4-187.2)	182.5 (95% CI, 158.9-209.6)
Mortality	39.5 (95% CI, 35.8-42.4)	24.2 (95% CI, 22,3-26.3)	67.4 (95% CI, 63.5-77.0)	51.2 (95% CI, 44.4-55.0)
AGE ≥ 75 YR				
Ischemic Stroke				
Incidence	2824.4 (95% CI, 2627.6-3018.4)	2344.0 (95% CI, 2197.0-2503.8)	2367.5 (95% CI, 2026.7-2735.5)	2575.4 (95% CI, 2240.7-2850.2)
Mortality	1511.4 (95% CI, 1353.6-1565.1)	950.1 (95% CI, 905.5-1030.6)	1075.7 (95% CI, 915.7-1336.5)	949.9 (95% CI, 838.6-1128.4)
Hemorrhagic Stroke				
Incidence	417.5 (95% CI, 385.9-450.8)	380.1 (95% CI, 351.4-409.6)	713.8 (95% CI, 603.3-847.4)	859.4 (95% CI, 729.2-1012.6)
Mortality	407.1 (95% CI, 380.5-462.1)	275.1 (95% CI, 253.8-320.3)	1072.9 (95% CI, 819.3-1329.5)	874.8 (95% CI, 736.8-1026.6)
Total Stroke				
Incidence	3241.9 (95% CI, 3020.9-3458.8)	2724.1 (95% CI, 2553.9-2899.8)	3081.4 (95% CI, 2631.0-3562.0)	3434.8 (95% CI, 2979.2-3952.1)
Mortality	1918.5 (95% CI, 1746.9-2031.9)	1225.1 (95% CI, 1155.4-1393.9)	2148.6 (95% CI, 2009.7-2459.4)	1824.7 (95% CI, 1590.7-1947.8)

Estimates were obtained from data provided by the authors of the Global Burden of Disease Study 2010.[10,11] *Figures in parentheses are the 95% confidence interval (CI) of the point estimates.*
*Per 100,000 person-years between 1990 and 2010.

However, it is not yet clear if case fatality rates are higher among those with prestroke frailty, which is common in older adults. In preliminary analyses, a frailty index derived from a combination of prestroke health conditions, function, walking ability, and blood test results was associated with a 16% increased risk of dying in hospital after an acute stroke.[17] These results, although intuitive, need to be supported by more substantive evidence.

Prevalence and Incidence of Stroke and Subtypes

A number of stroke prevalence studies have been conducted around the world. Stroke prevalence (per 100,000 population, standardized to the world population older than 65 years) appears least in rural South Africa (1,539/100,000), United States (4,536/100,000) and New Zealand (4,872/100,000), whereas a greater prevalence was evident in L'Aquila, Italy (6,812/100,000), Newcastle, England (>7,000/100,000), and Singapore (7,337/100,000).[18-21] Interestingly in Singapore, prevalence rates among Malays (5,396/100,000) appeared less than those of Chinese (7,829/100,000) or Indian (6,871/100,000) descent, although this difference was not statistically different.[21] Differences in environmental or genetic risk factor profiles, poststroke care, or both may influence these geographic variations in prevalence.

Stroke is a heterogeneous condition with two main subtypes, ischemic and hemorrhagic stroke. Depending on the study region, the more common ischemic stroke (IS) accounts for 63% to 84% of all strokes, whereas intracerebral hemorrhage (ICH) accounts for 7% and 20% of all strokes.[18] The proportion of hemorrhagic strokes appears to be greater in nonwhite populations and among those living in low- and middle-income countries compared with white populations in high-income countries.[22-25] Within the category of ischemic stroke, there are further subtypes that are classified based on clinical signs alone or on actual stroke mechanisms (e.g., large vessel disease, cardioembolism, small vessel disease).[26,27] The most frequently used classification system in large-scale, population-based epidemiologic studies is based on clinical features alone, as devised by the investigators of the Oxfordshire Community Stroke Project, which differentiates stroke into total or partial anterior infarction, posterior infarction, and lacunar infarction.[27] The advantage of this classification system is that it does not require expensive investigations ,which may be unavailable in low-income countries or less freely available in middle-income countries. The disadvantage of such a system is that the actual subtype of ischemic stroke may be erroneous because at least 10% of those classified as "lacunar" infarctions (implying small vessel disease) will have a proximal source of embolus from large vessels or the heart.[28]

Prevalence studies also provide a measure of the impact of stroke on survivors and the consequent health burden on patients, caregivers, and society at large. Declining stroke case fatality and mortality rates translate into an increased prevalence, resulting in an increased burden of stroke to those communities affected. Importantly, about 50% of stroke survivors are likely to require assistance in everyday activities. Frail older adults who suffer strokes are most at risk of poststroke functional decline, with one preliminary report suggesting an 8% increased risk of major physical disability in those with a higher prestroke score on a frailty index.[17] Stroke[29] and frailty[30] are each also associated with a greater prevalence of cognitive impairment, and hence it is likely that the burden of cognitive impairment will be greater among frail older adults suffering strokes than among others. Thus, frailty may be an important marker of particularly vulnerable stroke patients who are likely to require enhanced health care, rehabilitation, and support systems to maintain their functional status.

Incidence of Stroke and Transient Ischemic Attack

Until a few years ago, most incidence studies of stroke conducted according to so-called ideal criteria had been undertaken in high-income regions, such as Europe, Australia, and the Americas,[18,24,31-39] with Barbados being an exception.[40] More recently, stroke incidence estimates have been generated for low-, middle-, and high-income countries (see Table 60-1).[10,11] It must be noted, however, that there are a large number of regions in the world where there is a lack of high-quality data from which to infer accurate estimates of incidence or mortality.[12] Bearing this in mind, data from the Global Burden of Disease Study have shown that the age-standardized incidence/100,000 person-years for ischemic stroke is estimated to range from as low as 51.9 (Qatar) to as high as 433.9 (Lithuania; estimates for hemorrhagic stroke ranged from as low as 14.6 (Qatar) to as high as 159.8 (China).[10] There also appears to be substantial regional variation by stroke type, with ischemic stroke incidence highest among Eastern Europe and hemorrhagic stroke incidence highest among Central and East Asia.[10]

Examination of trends over time has shown that overall stroke incidence declined significantly, particularly in the 1970s and 1980s, in high-income countries.[35,41-46] This decline in high-income countries appears to have continued over the last decade (1990-2010), with a 13% and 19% overall reduction in ischemic and hemorrhagic stroke incidence, respectively[10] However, in low- and middle-income countries during the same period, there was a nonsignificant increase (6%) in the incidence of ischemic stroke, but a significant increase (19%) in the incidence of hemorrhagic stroke. These upward trends in stroke incidence in low- and middle-income countries were observed among those younger than 75 years and those 75 years of age and older (see Table 60-1). The most likely explanation for the differences in trends in stroke incidence between high- and low-income countries is the epidemiologic transition occurring in the latter. Increasing life expectancy, industrialization, and urbanization have led to a shift in risk factor profiles (e.g., increasing rates of hypertension, diabetes, smoking) in low- and middle-income countries to resemble those historically observed in high-income countries. Such factors, in addition to genetic differences, may largely explain the rising incidence of hemorrhagic stroke in these regions.

The actual incidence of TIA is harder to determine accurately in a population because of the transient nature of symptoms and the presence of other conditions that may mimic a TIA, such as migraine and seizures. However, in parallel to stroke, the annual rates for TIA have also declined among those 65 years of age and older in high-income regions such as Rochester, Minnesota,[47] France,[48] Belgium,[49] and Australia.[50] In France and Australia, an increase was observed in TIA incidence among those younger than 65 years, possibly reflecting increased awareness of the risk of stroke in this age group over time or diagnostic misclassification of TIA mimics.[48,50] There are presently no published systematic estimates of TIA incidence in low- and middle-income populations.

Costs of Stroke

Globally, on a societal level, stroke is responsible for approximately 2% to 4% of total health care costs. The costs of stroke have been estimated by using a variety of bottom-up and top-down approaches in a number of Western countries. Using a bottom-up approach, the estimated 12-month cost of stroke in Australia in 1997 was $420 million.[51] Acute hospitalization (28%) and inpatient rehabilitation (27%) comprised most of these costs. The average cost per case was $14,361during the first 12 months and $33,658 over a lifetime, with overall lifetime costs being greater for ischemic stroke than for intracerebral hemorrhage (ICH).[51,52] There are also significant economic costs attributable to informal caregiving. Dewey and colleagues[53] carried out an economic analysis to determine the total 12-month costs associated with informal care for first-ever strokes. They estimated that the total costs of informal care for first-ever strokes comprised between 4% and 7% of total stroke-related costs during the first year and between 14% and 23% of costs over a lifetime. This demonstrates the considerable burden placed on the families of people with stroke. Long-term costs associated with stroke have been recently estimated by Gloede and associates.[54] In this analysis, compared with cost estimates at 3 or 5 years after stroke, the costs for hemorrhagic stroke were substantially greater at 10 years (by 24%), whereas those for ischemic stroke remained relatively constant. The exact reasons for the increase in long-term direct costs for hemorrhagic stroke remain as yet unexplained, but may involve increasing costs of hospital care, medication use, and residential care, among others.

Risk Factors for Stroke

During the last half of the twentieth century, a large number of major nonmodifiable and modifiable stroke risk factors were identified from studies conducted in high-income countries. In addition to these data, there have recently been substantial risk factor data emerging from low- and middle-income countries.[55]

Nonmodifiable Risk Factors

Nonmodifiable risk factors are those that cannot be altered by intervention. These include factors such as advancing age, male gender, ethnicity, socioeconomic status, family history, and genetic conditions. Age is strongly associated with stroke incidence, with incidence rising from 10 to 30/100,000 person-years in those younger than 45 years of age to 1,200 to 2,000/100,000 person-years in those aged 75 to 84 years.[18] Within each age group, stroke incidence is greater among men than women.[31,56] In the older age groups, however, the overall number of strokes is often greater in women than men simply because of the larger number of women surviving to these ages. Even in high-income countries, people living in greater socioeconomic disadvantage have a greater incidence of stroke. Those living in the most disadvantaged areas of Melbourne, Australia, had incidence rates of stroke that were almost double (366/100,000/year) that of those living in the least disadvantaged areas (200/100,000/year).[57] Similar differences have been seen in other parts of the world, including Sweden[58] and the United Kingdom,[59,60] although in some studies it is unclear whether differences are attributable to ethnicity rather than socioeconomic status.

Modifiable Risk Factors

Modifiable risk factors are those that can be altered through treatment or by changes in behavior. By reducing the prevalence of these risk factors, it is therefore possible to reduce the incidence or recurrence of the disease. Such established and modifiable risk factors in high-income countries include hypertension, smoking, diabetes, and atrial fibrillation. There are also other less well-established risk factors and protective factors, including alcohol consumption, regular exercise, obesity, oral contraception, hormone replacement, and illicit drug use. In a major multinational study (INTERSTROKE) performed in urban areas in low- and middle-income countries, a cluster of risk factors, including hypertension, smoking, diabetes, central adiposity, excessive alcohol intake, low physical activity, poor diet, psychosocial stress, and depression, accounted for up to 90% of the population-attributable risk for stroke.[55] It is possible that such risk factors interact with each other in many different ways in contributing to the risk of stroke rather than being independent of each other, and such interactions may be different between different age groups. It is also possible that risk factors may be different in those living in rural populations below the poverty line. Because the INTERSTROKE study excluded those who did not undergo imaging studies, possibly because they could not afford it, the study did not include this population group.[61]

Hypertension, a condition that is highly prevalent with increasing age, is one of the most clearly recognized and probably the most important risk factor for stroke at a population level. In a meta-analysis of about 13,000 strokes in 450,000 individuals, in which prospective cohorts were studied to assess the influence of diastolic blood pressure (BP) on the risk of stroke, the authors showed that for each 10-mm Hg increase in diastolic BP, the risk of stroke increased by 1.84 (95% CI 1.80 to 1.90).[62] In the same collaborative study, the strength of the association between usual BP and risk of death from stroke was shown to decline to some extent with increasing age. However, stroke is so much more common in older adults than in middle-aged adults that the absolute annual difference in stroke death associated with a given difference in BP increases with increasing age.

Atrial fibrillation is associated with a high stroke risk and accounts for a major part of the population-attributable risk of stroke, particularly in older adults. The incidence and prevalence of atrial fibrillation has increased markedly over the past 2 decades.[63] Importantly, the risk of stroke in people with atrial fibrillation is greater in older adults than in younger adults.[59] In the Framingham Study, the risk attributable to atrial fibrillation increased significantly from 1.5% for those aged 50 to 59 years to 23.5% for those aged 80 to 89 years.[64]

Diabetes mellitus may be responsible for up to 20% of the population-attributable risk fraction in the developed world.[64] However, it is uncertain whether the risk attributable to diabetes mellitus or other factors such as dyslipidemia change significantly with increasing age.

Numerous studies have been undertaken to assess the association between smoking and stroke.[65] Evidence for an association between smoking and the risk of stroke is strengthened by the demonstration of a positive dose-response relationship. In addition, smoking cessation is associated with a reduced risk of stroke when compared with current smoking. In the Honolulu Heart Program, smokers who continued to smoke at the year 6 of follow-up were at an increased risk of stroke, whereas those who had ceased smoking at the year 6 of follow-up showed a reduced risk of stroke.[66] This provides some further support that smokers can reduce their risk of ischemic stroke after smoking cessation.

TABLE 60-2 Relative Population Impact of Treating Selected Risk Factors for Ischemic Stroke

Risk Factor	Prevalence	Relative Risk (Range)	Relative Impact
Hypertension	~20% men ~15% women	2.5-8.0	High
Atrial fibrillation (age, yr)		2.0-6.0	High in older age groups with additional risk factors
≥40	~2.0%		
≥65	~5.0%		
Men ≥ 75	~10%		
Women ≥ 75	~6.0%		
Smoking	~25% men ~20% women	1.5-6.0	High
Hypercholesterolemia*	~15% men ~15% women	1.5	Low
Diabetes	~5%	1.5-4.0	Low
Heavy alcohol consumption†	~2.5%	2.0-2.5	Low

*Hypercholesterolemia is defined as a plasma cholesterol level ≥6.5 mmol/L.

†Heavy alcohol consumption is defined as drinking on average ≥five standard drinks/day.

PREVENTION OF STROKE

If the impending increase in burden of stroke is to be minimized or even reduced, prevention strategies must be improved considerably. The main aim of primary and secondary prevention strategies for stroke is to reduce stroke incidence and recurrence. The effectiveness of prevention strategies is influenced by three important characteristics of each risk factor for stroke—whether the risk factor is modifiable, strength of the association, and prevalence of the risk factor in the population. The strength of the association is indicated by the relative risk or odds ratio of the exposure variable. Higher relative risks indicate stronger associations. The prevalence of a risk factor is the proportion of people in the population in whom the factor is present. The more common the risk factor in the population, the greater is its prevalence. Together, the relative risk and prevalence give an indication of how useful these factors are as targets for prevention strategies (Table 60-2).

Declines in stroke incidence in high-income countries have largely been attributed to improvements in the primary prevention of stroke. The introduction of BP-lowering agents with increasing efficacy and improvement in living standards provide plausible explanations for these declines. Significant decreases in systolic and diastolic BP, cholesterol levels, and prevalence of smoking were reported by the Oxford Vascular Study investigators during the 20-year interval in which incidence rates of stroke were seen to decline by 29%.[35] More modest declines in incidence among other studies may reflect the fact that other risk factors, such as an aging population, obesity, and diabetes mellitus, may be increasing, despite aggressive approaches to reducing hypertension, hypercholesterolemia, and smoking.[46] Primary prevention efforts should be now be particularly focused on reducing stroke incidence in low- and middle-income countries, given the rising incidence in these regions and their large populations. Primary prevention may involve a mass approach or high-risk approach.

Mass Approach

The mass or population approach to prevention involves changing risk factors at a population level. This may involve media and education campaigns to alter risky behaviors on a population basis or may involve government legislation. This approach may result in an overall small reduction in the risk factor on an individual basis, but may have a significant impact on the whole population.

Reducing BP levels within the population is an important strategy for reducing stroke risk. This could be achieved by various means, including reducing salt intake and promotion of exercise. It is estimated that people consume, on average, approximately two to three times more salt than is recommended.[67] Reducing salt intake by 50% would reduce BP in hypertensive and normotensive individuals[68] and also has been estimated to reduce stroke incidence by 22%[69] and stroke mortality by up to 25%.[70] Of the salt we consume, 80% is hidden in processed foods; thus, reducing the amount of salt added to food during its production would have an enormous public health impact.[71] A reduction in only 20% of the salt content of processed foods could lead to a significant drop in BP levels in the population. Encouraging governments to legislate such changes in the food industry remains a major barrier. Other cost-effective, population-wide prevention strategies may be tobacco and alcohol control via increased taxation and the regulation of accessibility and the promotion of healthy diets and exercise.

High-Risk Approach

The high-risk individual approach involves identifying people at high risk of stroke and introducing treatment strategies or minimizing risky behaviors. They may be identified through mass screening campaigns or opportunistic screening during other health consultations and could be encouraged to cease smoking, introduce exercise, or reduce alcohol or fat intake. Risk factors could also be modified in high-risk individuals by treatment with medications, such as antihypertensive agents to reduce BP levels or use of lipid-lowering drugs to reduce cholesterol levels.

In a meta-analysis conducted by the Blood Pressure Lowering Treatment Trialists' Collaboration, those treated with antihypertensive medication had a 28% to 38% lower incidence of stroke, depending on the agent used.[72] Although improvements have been made in the identification and treatment of hypertension, significant improvements in both these areas still need to be made, particularly in developing regions of the world.[73]

Another high risk approach is to target people who have already had a stroke because they are at increased risk of stroke recurrence. Among those who survive an initial stroke, up to 20% suffer another event within 5 years.[74] Controlling hypertension can reduce the incidence of recurrent stroke by up to 28%.[75] Furthermore, this reduction in risk has been observed in normotensive and hypertensive individuals with stroke.[76] Other prevention strategies that have demonstrated effectiveness in those with a previous stroke include the use of antiplatelet agents such as aspirin, dipyridamole, ticlopidine, or clopidogrel and the use of anticoagulants in those with atrial fibrillation.

Combined Approach to Prevention

To maximize the prevention of stroke, a combined approach to prevention should be used. This includes population and high-risk primary prevention approaches, as well as targeting those who have already had a stroke (secondary stroke prevention). The high-risk approach may involve screening patients for particular risk factors opportunistically and then providing treatment for those at high risk. To complement this strategy, the population approach should also be used. This might be achieved by educating people via mass media campaigns or government legislation.

PATHOLOGIC MECHANISMS UNDERLYING STROKE

Ischemic Stroke

Atherosclerosis is the most common cause of cerebral infarction caused by large and medium vessel disease and is mediated by thrombotic and embolic complications. Atherosclerosis is an almost universal feature of large and medium-sized arteries in older adults and is most severe in the aortic arch and at points of bifurcation (e.g., carotid bifurcation) and confluence (e.g., basilar artery). In large extracranial vessels, thrombus tends to complicate the ruptured or eroded unstable atherosclerotic plaque.[77] Such plaques are characterized by a large necrotic core covered by a thin, inflamed, fibrous cap similar to coronary arterial plaque.[78] Exposure of the thrombogenic plaque core causes activation of platelets and triggering of the coagulation cascade. The resulting thrombus occludes the vessel in situ or, more commonly, probably dislodges as an embolus and occludes a distal smaller vessel. Rupture of unstable plaques appears to be less common in intracranial vessels, in which atherosclerosis may more commonly mediate stroke by low-flow effects or by acting as luminal narrowings at which the emboli impact. On occasion, intracranial or extracranial vessel occlusion may occur as a result of dissection of the lumen; the most commonly seen sites are the vertebral and carotid arteries.

Small, deep (lacunar) infarcts are likely to be due to two important causes.[79] The first is small vessel atherosclerosis and the second is a complex destructive lesion of small arteries (so-called lipohyalinosis) characterized in the acute phase by fibrinoid necrosis and in the healed phase by the loss of wall architecture, collagenous sclerosis, and mural foam cells.[79] The etiopathogenesis of lipohyalinosis is uncertain but may be linked to inherited and acquired disorders of small vessel tone or it may be a postocclusive phenomenon.[80]

Ischemic strokes crossing arterial boundaries may occur due to cerebral venous sinus thromboses. Cerebral veins and venous sinuses may become thrombosed when a variety of constitutive and acquired factors, local and systemic, promote hypercoagulability and/or venous stasis.[81] However, in many cases, the pathogenesis is uncertain.

The size, shape, and location of occlusive arterial infarcts conform more or less to individual arterial supply zones, with variations dependent on interindividual differences in vascular anatomy, adequacy of collaterals, preexisting vascular disease, and other factors. Hemorrhagic transformation of initially pale ischemic infarcts is relatively common following spontaneous or therapeutic lysis of thromboemboli.[82] Bleeding may be severe enough to mimic a primary intracerebral hemorrhage.[83] The distribution of infarction in global cerebral circulatory insufficiency is diverse, but commonly involves spinal as well as cerebral arterial border zones and selectively vulnerable brain regions, such as the CA1 zone of the hippocampus; neocortical layers 3, 5, and 6; cerebellar Purkinje cells; and basal ganglia.[83,84] Venous infarcts characteristically do not conform to arterial supply zones and are often accompanied by subarachnoid and intracerebral hemorrhage and massive brain swelling.

Irrespective of size or location, brain infarcts are areas of ischemic coagulative necrosis of all cellular elements, ultimately becoming fluid-filled cavities.[85] Temporary or less severe ischemia may produce areas of so-called incomplete infarction,[86] characterized by death of only the most vulnerable cells, in particular neurons, representing perhaps a neuropathologic substrate of TIAs.[87] The ultimate fate of affected brain depends not only on the severity and duration of ischemia, but also on how selectively vulnerable is the region and its component neurons and on the degree and duration of reperfusion (delayed neuronal death).[88] The marginal zone of brain around the doomed ischemic core has cerebral blood flow levels between these thresholds of synaptic transmission and membrane failure. This penumbra, nonfunctional yet viable, is the focus of potential therapeutic salvage.[89] A better understanding of the cascade of ischemic neuronal damage[90] may yet provide effective stroke therapy targets, and it has been increasingly speculated that the future of stroke treatment lies in rapidly instituted combination therapy with thrombolytic, neuroprotective and, ultimately, perhaps regenerative or trophic agents such as the use of stem cells.

Hemorrhagic Stroke

The most common type of hemorrhagic stroke remains the classic, spontaneous, hypertensive hemorrhage, characteristically in the basal ganglia, thalamus, lobar white matter, cerebellum, and pons, in approximate descending order of frequency.[91] The pathogenesis has been difficult to study, but circumstantial evidence has indicated the same, or closely related, lesion to that causing lacunar infarction,[92] with which it colocalizes and shares a common risk factor profile. Thus, a destructive lesion characterized by fibrinoid necrosis and associated with hypertension is considered by many to be the underlying vascular lesion in most cases.[93] In older adults, an increasingly recognized form of spontaneous brain hemorrhage is due to cerebral amyloid angiopathy, in which bleeds are typically lobar, superficial, and multiple.[94] The mechanism of amyloid-related bleeds, their relation to classic hypertensive bleeds, and the contribution of amyloid angiopathy to cognitive decline in Alzheimer disease are not definitively understood.

Intracerebral hemorrhage is more often acutely fatal than ischemic stroke due largely to its mass effect and the consequent potential for raised intracranial pressure and reduced cerebral perfusion. Hematomas, however, tend to dissect and separate brain tissue, with relatively less direct parenchymal damage. Therefore, should the patient survive and the hematoma be cleared by phagocytic cells to leave a blood-stained, slitlike cavity, the prognosis for recovery may be better than that for cerebral infarcts of similar size and location.

KEY POINTS

- There are two main subtypes of stroke, ischemic and hemorrhagic stroke.
- According to the World Health Organization (WHO), stroke is the second most common single cause of death in the world after ischemic heart disease.
- Frail older adults who suffer a stroke are most at risk of poststroke functional decline.
- Established and modifiable risk factors in high-income countries include hypertension, atrial fibrillation, smoking, and diabetes. Less well-established risk factors include alcohol consumption, physical inactivity, obesity, oral contraception, hormone replacement, and illicit drug use.
- A combined approach of population and high-risk primary prevention approaches, as well as targeting those who have already had a stroke (secondary stroke prevention), is most likely to deliver maximal benefit in reducing global stroke burden.

For a complete list of references, please visit www.expertconsult.com.

KEY REFERENCES

10. Krishnamurthi RV, Feigin VL, Forouzanfar MH, et al: Global and regional burden of first-ever ischaemic and haemorrhagic stroke during 1990-2010: findings from the Global Burden of Disease Study 2010. Lancet Glob Health 1:5e259–e281, 2013.
11. Feigin VL, Forouzanfar MH, Krishnamurthi R, et al; Global Burden of Diseases, Injuries, Risk Factors Study 2010 (GBD 2010); GBD Stroke Experts Group: Global and regional burden of stroke during 1990-2010: findings from the Global Burden of Disease Study 2010. Lancet 383:245–254, 2014.
18. Feigin VL, Lawes CM, Bennett DA, et al: Stroke epidemiology: a review of population-based studies of incidence, prevalence, and case-fatality in the late 20th century. Lancet Neurol 2:143–153, 2003.
26. Adams HP Jr, Bendixen BH, Kappelle LJ, et al: Classification of subtype of acute ischemic stroke. Definitions for use in a multicenter clinical trial. TOAST. Trial of Org 10172 in Acute Stroke Treatment. Stroke 24:135–141, 1993.
27. Bamford J, Sandercock P, Dennis M, et al: Classification and natural history of clinically identifiable subtypes of cerebral infarction. Lancet 337:1521–1526, 1991.
35. Rothwell PM, Coull AJ, Giles MF, et al: Change in stroke incidence, mortality, case-fatality, severity, and risk factors in Oxfordshire, UK from 1981 to 2004 (Oxford Vascular Study). Lancet 363:1925–1933, 2004.
62. Prospective Studies Collaboration: Cholesterol, diastolic blood pressure, and stroke: 13,000 strokes in 450,000 people in 45 prospective cohorts. Lancet 346:1647–1653, 1995.
73. Feigin VL, Krishnamurthi R: Stroke prevention in the developing world. Stroke 42:3655–3658, 2011.
79. Donnan G, Norrving B, Bamford J, et al, editors: Subcortical stroke, ed 2, Oxford, England, 2002, Oxford University Press.
83. Caplan L: Intracerebral hemorrhage revisited. Neurology 38:624–627, 1988.

61 Stroke: Clinical Presentation, Management, and Organization of Services

Christopher Moran, Thanh G. Phan, Velandai K. Srikanth

INTRODUCTION

Stroke and transient ischemic attacks (TIAs) are the most common clinical manifestations of disease of cerebral blood vessels. Other manifestations of cerebrovascular disease are subclinical and include cerebral white matter lesions, "silent" brain infarcts, and cerebral microbleeds. This chapter focuses mainly on stroke and TIA, with less emphasis on subclinical cerebrovascular disease. In terms of therapy, the chapter does not deal with primary prevention but, rather, with acute treatment, recovery, and secondary prevention.

Stroke and TIAs are the leading causes of acute neurologic admissions to hospitals throughout the world and tend to predominantly affect older people. Stroke is the second leading single cause of death worldwide.[1] Approximately one third of stroke patients die within the first 6 months, and approximately 60% die within 5 years after stroke.[2] Stroke ranks as the sixth most important cause of disability among survivors.[3] Increasingly, in the developed world, patients admitted with stroke tend to be frail and have multiple comorbidities. The impact of a stroke on frail older people can be particularly devastating, often leading to a move from their home environment to residential care facilities. It is important to adopt a cohesive and multidisciplinary approach to minimize long-term stroke-related disability and enhance quality of life for the affected person. In the past decade significant improvements in stroke care, based on clinical trial evidence, have been made, and these improvements have resulted in measurable reductions in mortality and disability.

DEFINITIONS

Stroke and Transient Ischemic Attack

The American Heart Association recently defined ischemic stroke (or central nervous system infarction) as "brain, spinal cord, or retinal cell death attributable to ischemia, based on *either* pathologic, imaging, or other objective evidence of focal ischemic injury in a defined vascular distribution, *or* clinical evidence of focal ischemic injury based on symptoms persisting ≥24 hours or until death, and other etiologies excluded."[4] Intracerebral hemorrhage is the term applied to sudden focal neurologic symptoms and brain imaging evidence of brain parenchymal hemorrhage. TIAs refer to transient sudden focal neurologic symptoms lasting less than 24 hours and being of presumed vascular origin but without demonstrable infarction or hemorrhage on brain imaging. The type of brain imaging used can make a major difference as to whether a person is diagnosed as having a TIA or stroke. Computed tomography (CT) scans, although sensitive to intracerebral hemorrhage, are relatively insensitive to the presence of early or small infarctions. The use of acute diffusion-weighted magnetic resonance imaging (DWI-MRI) allows the detection of small infarcts in patients who may otherwise be labeled as having a TIA. Nonspecific symptoms such as faintness, loss of consciousness, dizziness, confusion, or falls are highly unlikely to be due to a TIA or stroke, unless they are accompanied by focal neurologic symptoms.[5] Acute delirium, a common syndrome affecting older people, is unlikely to last only a few hours and is almost always not secondary to a TIA, although it can be an uncommon presentation of acute stroke.[6]

Subclinical Cerebrovascular Lesions

Subclinical cerebrovascular lesions are abnormalities detected on MRI brain scans of older people in the absence of a history of acute stroke. They include silent brain infarcts, cerebral white matter lesions, and cerebral microbleeds.[7] Silent brain infarcts are usually small subcortical infarcts seen in approximately 10% of the general population older than 65 years, which occur more frequently with increasing age and in the presence of traditional vascular risk factors such as hypertension, smoking, hypercholesterolemia, and diabetes mellitus.[7] White matter lesions are visible as hyperintense (bright) signals seen on fluid-attenuated inversion recovery (FLAIR) sequences of MRI scans almost ubiquitously in people aged older than 65 years (their severity increasing with age) and in those with a history of hypertension.[7] Cerebral microbleeds are small hypointense (dark) lesions seen on susceptibility weighted imaging MRI sequences and represent hemosiderin deposits adjacent to small vessels. Hypertension, low cholesterol, and the apolipoprotein epsilon 4 (ApoE4) allele are associated with the presence of cerebral microbleeds.[8] All three manifestations of subclinical cerebrovascular disease commonly coexist in severe forms in frail older people, can lead to insidious cognitive and motor decline, and increase the risk of both ischemic and hemorrhagic stroke.[7]

STROKE TYPES

Strokes are either ischemic (80%) or hemorrhagic, each having different pathophysiologic mechanisms and treatments. The mechanisms of arterial occlusion are predominantly those of artery-to-artery embolism and cardioembolism rather than in situ vessel thrombosis. In the absence of arterial venous malformation, aneurysm and cavernous angioma, intracerebral hemorrhage occur in approximately 15% of all cases of stroke, and are either due to hypertensive small vessel disease or amyloid angiopathy.[9] Distinguishing ischemic and hemorrhagic stroke is important as their treatments are quite different (thrombolysis and antiplatelet/anticoagulant treatments are used for the former). Some infarcts have hemorrhagic components and may be mistaken for primary intracerebral hemorrhage (Figure 61-1). Separation of these two types of stroke requires careful consideration of the clinical features and their imaging findings.[10]

Ischemic Stroke Subtypes

The most commonly used classification for ischemic stroke in observational epidemiology is the Oxfordshire Community Stroke Project (OCSP). This classification is based on clinical features and not advanced imaging findings, and hence it is not particularly useful in correctly identifying stroke mechanisms. In clinical trials, the most commonly used criteria for classification are the Trial of Org 10172 in Acute Stroke Treatment (TOAST) criteria.[11] This is a classification of subtypes using a combination of clinical features and results of ancillary diagnostic studies.

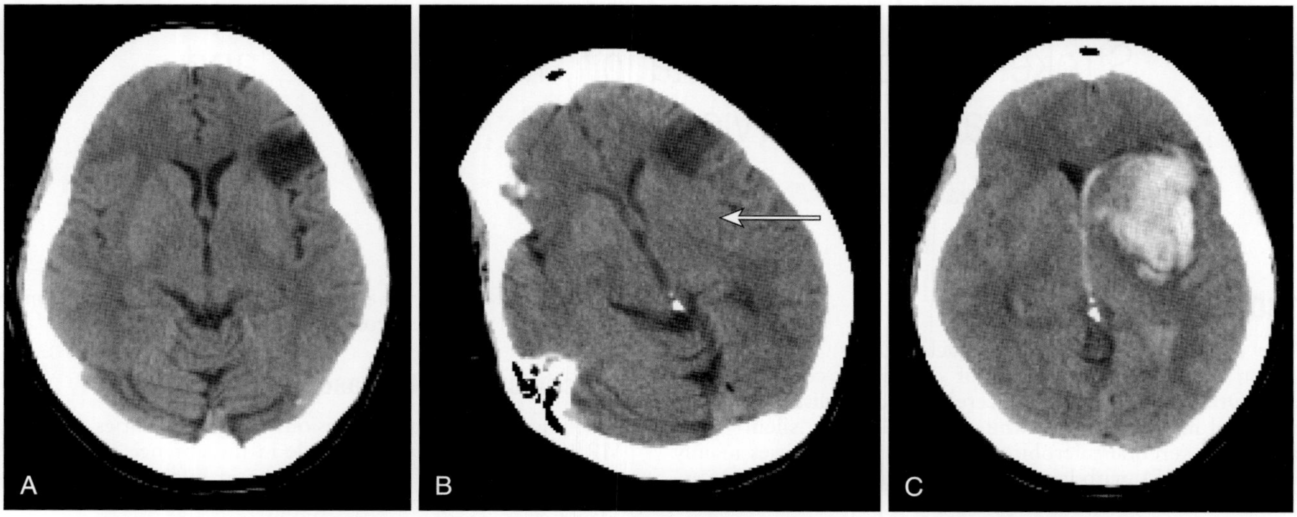

Figure 61-1. Hemorrhagic infarct and not primary intracerebral hemorrhage. An 83-year-old female had resolving right hemiparesis but residual right hemianesthesia **(A).** Twelve hours later she redeveloped right hemiparesis with obscuration of the left lentiform nucleus (*solid arrow* in **B**). Her blood pressure was elevated at 230/120 mm Hg. She deteriorated overnight with the final CT scan, performed 24 hours **(C)** after admission, looking indistinguishable from a primary intracerebral hemorrhage.

"Possible" and "probable" diagnoses can be made based on the physician's certainty of diagnosis based on all available clinical information. The TOAST classification denotes five categories of ischemic stroke: (1) large-artery atherosclerosis, (2) cardioembolism, (3) small vessel occlusion, (4) stroke of other determined cause, and (5) stroke of undetermined cause.[11] A feature of this classification is that stroke is attributed to the offending carotid artery if the level of stenosis of that artery is greater than 50%. However, patients can have thromboembolic disease from carotid artery even when the level of stenosis is less than 50%. The degree of stenosis is important when deciding on whether carotid endarterectomy is required, rather than excluding large artery atherosclerosis as a mechanism.

CLINICAL PRESENTATION OF STROKE AND TRANSIENT ISCHEMIC ATTACK

The clinical features of TIA and stroke are the results of ischemia affecting eloquent brain areas. The classical patterns of stroke presentations are dealt with later in this chapter but cannot be exhaustively covered in this chapter alone. (For a detailed examination of this topic, see *Stroke Syndromes*, edited by Bogousslavsky and Caplan.[12]) However, it must be borne in mind that very old patients (>80 years of age) can have atypical presenting symptoms[13] (e.g., falls or reduced mobility) and often have prestroke frailty, and a reasonable index of suspicion for stroke must be maintained for such people.

Clinical Features of Stroke

Motor weakness is the most common presenting feature in stroke, affecting about 80% of patients. The pattern of weakness is a clue to the location of the stroke lesion. Unilateral face, arm, and leg weakness often indicates involvement of the middle cerebral artery (MCA) territory, whereas bilateral weakness may indicate posterior circulation involvement. Pure unilateral motor weakness without cortical signs suggests involvement of the subcortical motor tracts (a "lacunar" syndrome). The presence of ideomotor dyspraxia (a disorder of higher cortical disorder of motor initiation) can sometimes mimic motor weakness. Weakness of the articulatory and swallowing muscles can lead to symptoms of dysarthria and dysphagia, respectively, and can occur from strokes affecting both anterior and posterior circulations.

Over 60% of stroke patients admitted to the hospital suffer some form of tactile sensory impairment, and smaller proportions either suffer loss of proprioception or have cortical sensory impairment.[14] Sensory abnormalities may be associated with delayed but debilitating poststroke pain syndromes.[15]

Higher cortical deficits that have the most important adverse impact on patients are dysphasia (usually dominant hemisphere stroke) and hemineglect. Broca aphasia (also termed expressive aphasia or motor aphasia) is most commonly caused by strokes involving the left frontal opercular and central cortex, with or without involvement of the subcortical striatocapsular region. It is characterized by effortful speech, word-finding difficulty, phonemic errors, and agrammatism, but comprehension is relatively preserved. Sensory aphasia with relatively fluent speech but poor language comprehension is usually associated with strokes involving the superior temporal lobe and includes Wernicke aphasia and conduction aphasia, among others. Global aphasia refers to severe impairment of motor speech, and comprehension and is usually a consequence of a major left MCA stroke.

Hemineglect is characterized by a reduction in attention to stimuli and events on one side of the body and can occur with either right or left hemisphere stroke.[16] Hemineglect may affect visual, auditory, and somatosensory perceptual systems and is associated with poor outcome.[17] Visual symptoms may arise from lesions affecting the visual pathway anywhere from the retinal to the occipital cortex. Retinal or ophthalmic artery occlusion occurs as a result of embolism from the carotid system and can lead to monocular blindness. Visual field defects are common, leading to either hemianopia or quadrantanopia, depending on the site of the lesion and the extent of damage to the optic radiation. Ocular movement abnormalities are commonly seen in stroke affecting the brainstem, but also less commonly seen with cerebellar and cerebral lesions. Diplopia is usually associated with eye movement abnormality and can be quite disabling. Detection and characterization of visual deficits in stroke patients are of extreme importance, given their potential impact on daily life and complex activities such as driving.

Vertigo or a disordered perception of motion of either the patient or the environment can be caused by strokes involving the vertebrobasilar circulation and is often accompanied by nystagmus. Ataxia of the trunk or limbs may be caused by strokes affecting the cerebellum and adjacent brainstem. Several auditory symptoms may also be associated with brainstem strokes including sudden hearing loss, hyperacusis, tinnitus, and auditory hallucinations.

Stroke is very commonly associated with neurocognitive syndromes at acute presentation as well as in the medium to long term.[18] Close to 50% of survivors have some form of cognitive impairment at 3 months after stroke[19]; this can occur as a result of the effects of the stroke itself, or it may be a sign of worsening or unmasking of preexisting cognitive decline. Stroke is strongly associated with a twofold increase in the risk of dementia after stroke with the presence of prestroke cognitive decline explaining a large proportion of these cases.[20] Up to 30% of patients may also suffer from depressed mood in the medium to long term after stroke.[21] Urinary and fecal incontinence are common and disabling effects of stroke. The prevalence of urinary incontinence among survivors of stroke ranges from 36% to 83% within the first year.[22] Incontinence may be a direct consequence of loss of neurogenic control or due to functional incapacitation secondary to immobility or cognitive loss, and is a marker for increased mortality after stroke and overall poor outcome among survivors.

Clinical Features of Transient Ischemic Attack

Features compatible with anterior circulation TIA commonly include unilateral motor, sensory or sensorimotor impairment, dysphasia, and amaurosis fugax. The diagnosis of amaurosis fugax is based on the patient's report of a transient unilateral visual loss, described on closer questioning as "a curtain coming down" over the affected eye with inability to see through this curtain. Features of posterior circulation TIA include vertigo and/or diplopia, or loss of balance, or unilateral weakness.

INVESTIGATIONS FOR STROKE

Brain Imaging

Diagnosis of Hemorrhage

Computed tomography (CT) should be performed to exclude intracranial hemorrhage. Hemorrhage in the basal ganglia and pons suggests that hypertension may be the likely cause, whereas hemorrhage in cortical (lobar) locations suggests the possibility of amyloid angiopathy as the primary causal mechanism.

Recognition of Ischemic Changes on Computed Tomography Scans

Early ischemic changes such as parenchymal hypoattenuation and diffuse swelling of the hemisphere[23] are present in the first 6 hours in approximately one half to three quarters of patients with MCA territory infarction.[24]

MRI Findings in Stroke

Signal change on DWI-MRI reflecting altered water diffusion can reveal bright signal abnormalities within minutes of ischemia in the majority of patients with ischemic stroke.[25] The signal change on DWI becomes less bright after 10 days.[26] Hemorrhage, on the other hand, contains paramagnetic material and has a dark signal on T2-weighted images. The evolution of magnetic resonance (MR) signal changes in intracerebral hemorrhage is complex and the reader is referred to the description by Atlas and Thulborn.[27]

Evaluating Tissue at Risk

Stroke pathophysiology can now be inferred from dynamic scanning by tracking a bolus of intravenous contrast with sequential acquisition of CT or MR images. These CT or MR perfusion images enable analysis of cerebral perfusion deficit. For MR images, the salvageable tissue is represented by the difference between the poorly perfused region and the region of restricted diffusion (infarct core).[28] For CT perfusion images (Figure 61-2), the infarct core is represented by the most poorly perfused region on CT perfusion images (either cerebral blood volume or relative cerebral blood flow images). The abnormally perfused region is defined by the mean transit time or cerebral blood flow maps. These dynamic scanning methods are used to guide thrombolysis therapy.

Diagnosis of Stroke Mechanism

Vascular Imaging

Extracranial ultrasound can provide evidence of carotid artery and vertebral artery disease, but it has certain limitations. Ultrasound is operator dependent, and assignment of degree of carotid artery stenosis is also dependent on blood flow velocity in that artery. Consequently, a critically narrow artery on one side can lead to compensatory elevation of velocity in the contralateral artery leading to erroneous misclassification of the contralateral artery as critically stenosed. Ultrasound assignment of carotid artery stenosis as moderate (50% to 70% stenosis) can either mean that the artery is between 50% and 70% or greater than 70% stenosed, and a near occlusion can mean near occlusion, complete occlusion, or critical stenosis. A rule of thumb is that when the ultrasound suggests more than 50% stenosis and the patient is fit for carotid endarterectomy, a second test such as CT angiography (CTA) or contrast-enhanced MR angiography (MRA) may be necessary to clarify the exact degree and nature of the stenosis. CTA is performed by rapid injection of contrast bolus and acquiring the images during the arterial phase of contrast arrival in the brain and thus provides coverage from the aortic arch to the circle of Willis. MRA techniques are either "bright blood" or "black blood" techniques depending on the signal intensity of blood. Contrast-enhanced MRA is performed by fast injection of an intravascular contrast agent (gadolinium) and acquiring images during the arterial phase of contrast arrival. CTA and MRA have largely replaced digital subtraction angiography for investigation of carotid artery disease.[29,30]

Cardiac Investigations

An electrocardiogram (ECG) can facilitate identification of atrial fibrillation (AF), which requires anticoagulation for stroke prevention. Ambulatory cardiac monitoring is a useful tool that can assist in detecting paroxysmal AF, which may not show up on an ECG. However, a single episode of monitoring may be insufficient to detect AF, and recent studies indicate a need for longer and more frequent monitoring, which may become feasible with evolving technology.[31,32] Echocardiography can assist in relatively uncommon situations where valvular heart disease or endocarditis is clinically suspected as mechanisms underlying ischemic stroke. However, its routine use is controversial. It is rare to find an abnormality on an ECG that would lead to anticoagulation in patients with normal ECG results and cardiovascular examination. Routine echocardiography may lead to the chance finding of patent foramen ovale, which may further confuse clinical decisions, as the evidence is lacking for endovascular therapy in such situations.[33-35] Complex aortic arch atheroma confers a fourfold increased risk of stroke.[36] While transesophageal echocardiography is superior to transthoracic echocardiography for the

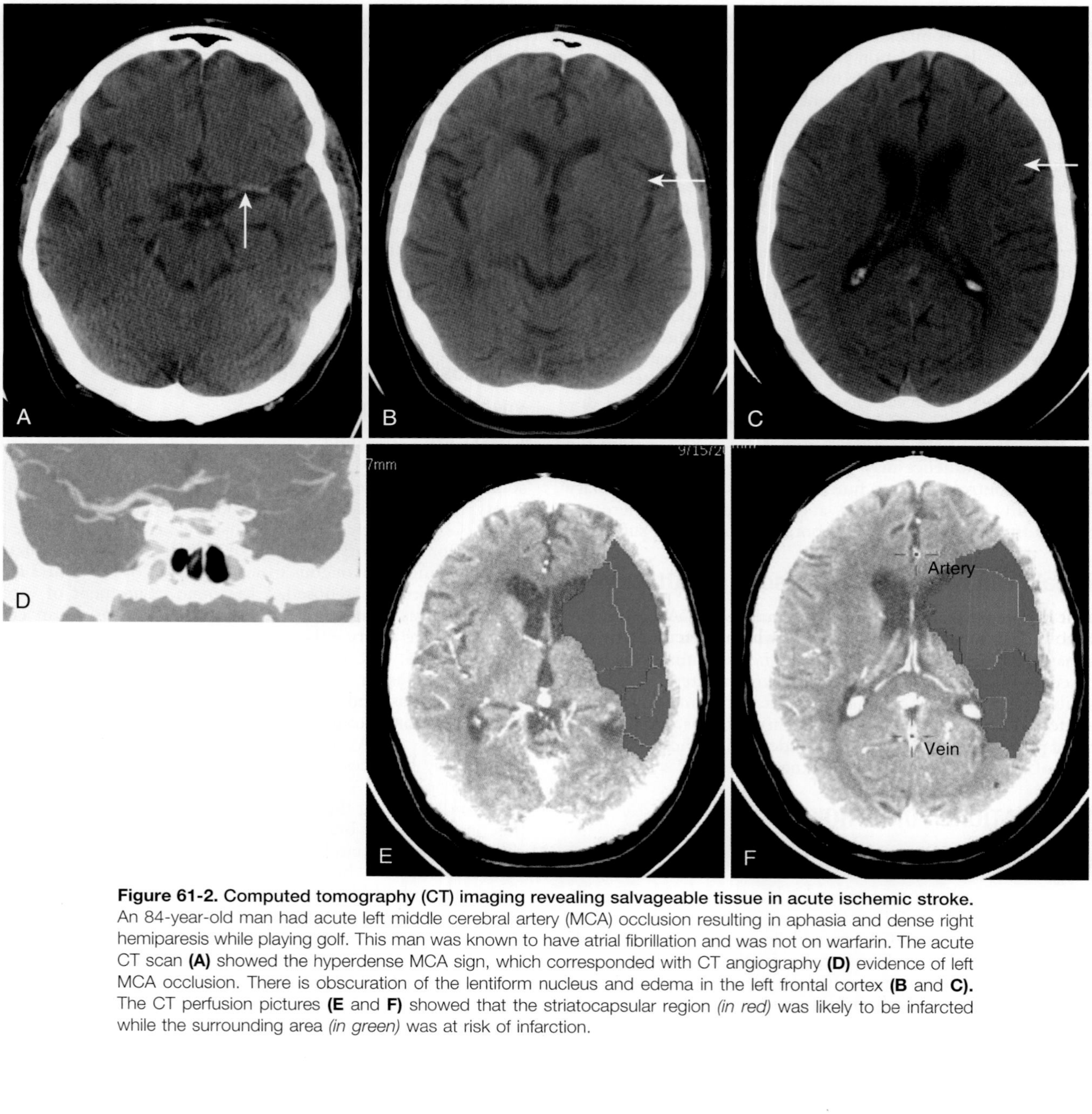

Figure 61-2. Computed tomography (CT) imaging revealing salvageable tissue in acute ischemic stroke. An 84-year-old man had acute left middle cerebral artery (MCA) occlusion resulting in aphasia and dense right hemiparesis while playing golf. This man was known to have atrial fibrillation and was not on warfarin. The acute CT scan **(A)** showed the hyperdense MCA sign, which corresponded with CT angiography **(D)** evidence of left MCA occlusion. There is obscuration of the lentiform nucleus and edema in the left frontal cortex **(B** and **C).** The CT perfusion pictures **(E** and **F)** showed that the striatocapsular region *(in red)* was likely to be infarcted while the surrounding area *(in green)* was at risk of infarction.

detection of aortic arch atheroma,[37] there is no evidence at this time whether warfarin may be more useful than routine antiplatelet therapy in patients with arch atheroma.[36]

Blood Tests for the Diagnosis of Stroke Risk Factors

Blood tests may be of some use in assessing stroke risk in the acute setting, but their actual use is relatively limited for this purpose. Serum cholesterol levels dip acutely after stroke and return to "true" values approximately 12 weeks after stroke onset.[38] Similarly, acute phase hyperglycemia may occur in stroke patients irrespective of diabetes mellitus, and hence it is advisable to conduct definitive testing for this a few weeks after stroke. Inflammatory markers such as erythrocyte sedimentation rate and high-sensitivity C-reactive protein can be performed to examine the possibility of temporal arteritis or subacute bacterial endocarditis, but more often these markers are useful in determining the course of poststroke infections. Routine testing for antiphospholipid antibody levels is unhelpful because of its high prevalence in people older than 40 years,[39] poor specificity for stroke risk,[39,40] and lack of utility in determining therapy.[41] In older patients, a full blood count can be helpful to exclude uncommon thrombotic disorders such as thrombocythemia or polycythemia rubra vera, but it is unlikely that a routine search for other rare thrombophilic causes of stroke will be useful.

Management of Stroke Patients

Organized Stroke Unit Care

The implementation of organized stroke units has been the most important advance in acute stroke management. A collaboration of stroke unit trialists demonstrated that organized stroke units need to treat approximately 25 patients to prevent one from dying or being dependent.[42] Outcomes were also better in patients admitted to a discrete ward under the care of a dedicated multidisciplinary team, compared with a roving stroke service visiting patients on general medical wards.[43] The consistent characteristics of effective stroke units appear to be (1) a comprehensive approach to medical problems, impairments, and disabilities; (2) active and careful management of physiologic abnormalities; (3) early mobilization; (4) skilled nursing care; (5) early setting of rehabilitation plans; and (6) early assessment and planning of discharge needs with involvement of caregivers.[44] Appropriate fluid and nutritional support in the acute phase with either intravenous fluids or nasogastric feeding are also important in those who have significant dysphagia and risk of aspiration. Early nasogastric feeding, within the first week after stroke, has been associated with reduced mortality but with an increase in dependency on others for activities of daily living.[45] Therefore, percutaneous endoscopic gastrostomy should be reserved for only those who require long-term care and need assisted feeding because of severely impaired swallowing. The early detection and treatment of pyrexia and infectious complications is a major contributor to the effectiveness of stroke unit care.[46] A protocol-driven approach in stroke units can also facilitate the standard use of intermittent pneumatic compression devices to prevent venous thromboembolism, with recent evidence supporting their superiority in ischemic stroke compared with low-molecular-weight heparin or graduated compression stockings.[47] There is no evidence of benefit of the use of heparin or its derivatives in the prevention of venous thromboembolism in patients who have acute ischemic stroke.[48] Nursing care should incorporate avoidance of pressure areas, urinary catheters, and bed rest because these contribute significantly to the development of complications such as sepsis and deep venous thrombosis. Blood pressure reduction should be generally avoided in the acute phase (except in selected situations such as before thrombolysis or in people with hemorrhagic strokes and mass effect) because of concerns about interfering with cerebral autoregulation; if performed, it should be done cautiously and in well-monitored situations. A very important component of stroke unit care is the conduct of regular (weekly) formal multidisciplinary meetings, which serve as forums for the entire team to discuss various aspects of individual patient care and set early plans for rehabilitation and discharge.[44] There is emerging evidence that prestroke frailty is an important determinant of poststroke complications and outcome.[49,50] Stroke unit care provides the ideal setting for careful multidisciplinary decision making regarding the use of acute thrombolysis, blood pressure control, medication management, treatment of infection, and early mobilization while taking into account degree of frailty.

Treatment of Acute Ischemic Stroke

Three specific interventions have been shown to be effective in randomized trials for the acute treatment of ischemic stroke; these are antiplatelet agents,[51] tissue plasminogen activator (tPA), and endovascular therapy.[52-54] Neuroprotective agents have largely failed to show benefits in acute stroke therapy.

The International Stroke Trial (IST) and Chinese Aspirin Stroke trial (CAST) clearly demonstrated the efficacy of aspirin (160 to 300 mg) as an acute stroke therapy for ischemic stroke.[51,55] Of several trials that studied the efficacy of low-molecular-weight heparin in acute ischemic stroke, none showed superiority over aspirin but with increased risk of intracranial hemorrhage.[56] The introduction of recombinant tPA has led a paradigm shift in reversing the neurologic deficit caused by acute ischemic stroke.[52,53] It is postulated that the mechanism of action of tPA is lysis of the thrombus/embolus leading to recanalization of the arterial lumen and salvage of the ischemic brain tissue. The beneficial effect of tPA was greatest in those treated within 3 hours of stroke onset, may be beneficial up to 6 hours,[57] and is now recommended for use within 4.5 hours after onset. The most important adverse effect of tPA is symptomatic intracerebral hemorrhage in about 6% of cases. Symptomatic intracerebral hemorrhage accounts for most of the early excess deaths among those treated with tPA (odds ratio, 3.72; $P < .0001$), and its risk rises with age, high blood pressure, and very severe neurologic deficits.[1] Despite concerns regarding an increased risk of bleeding in older people, those older than 80 years appear to receive similar benefits from tPA as those younger than 80 years.[57-59] Research is also under way to identify thrombolytic agents with lower risk of hemorrhage which may be safer to use in older age groups.[60] However, there are some important caveats to using thrombolysis in older patients. The presence of a significant preexisting dementia or extreme frailty (particularly in those already living in high-level residential care) may be cause for concern and be relative contraindications to thrombolysis. Older patients with extensive cerebral white matter lesions or microbleeds visualized on brain imaging may be more likely to develop thrombolysis-related intracranial hemorrhage.[61] Treatment decisions in such frail older patients must be based on individually estimated risks and benefits.

In addition to intravenous thrombolysis, there has been a significant advance with respect to the introduction of endovascular therapy for acute ischemic stroke. In 2015, there were five published randomized controlled trials in people aged 18 to 80 years, showing a large benefit for clot extraction with a stent retriever device in addition to intravenous therapy for proximal arterial occlusion in the anterior circulation compared with intravenous therapy alone.[54] Benefits included a greater number of patients discharged with no disability, reduction in disability, and reduced length of stay. The 2015 American Heart Association/American Stroke Association (AHA/ASA) guidelines recommends this therapy as having class 1, level A evidence for the treatment of acute ischemic stroke resulting from occlusion of the MCA.[54]

Acute Treatment of Intracerebral Hemorrhage

At present, there are no specific treatment options with proven efficacy for intracerebral hemorrhage. Surgical intervention for decompression may also be considered in patients with cerebellar hematoma. Recently, results from a large clinical trial in acute hemorrhagic stroke showed that rapid intensive reduction of blood pressure was safe, without benefit for the primary outcome of death or disability, and a possible benefit for reducing dependence.[62] Further evidence from other trials of acute blood pressure reduction[63] and antifibrinolytic agents in acute hemorrhagic stroke are awaited.[64,65]

Stroke Recovery

Most patients who survive a stroke make some functional recovery. Recovery may be intrinsic, which involves a degree of return of neural control (early recovery), or adaptive, in which alternative strategies are used to overcome disability (delayed recovery). Although the exact neural mechanisms underlying stroke recovery are still poorly understood, emerging evidence suggests that the plasticity of the adult brain may play a role. It is postulated that recovery from brain injury occurs because of restoration of function in damaged neural structures (restitution) and by the development of new pathways in the unaffected areas of brain, which take over the lost function (substitution).[66] The highest rate of recovery usually occurs in the first few weeks after stroke, with lesser amounts occurring over the next 12 months.[67] Measurable recovery seldom occurs after 12 months, although there are the occasional exceptions to this rule. The degree of recovery depends largely on the severity of the initial deficit, with the likelihood of complete recovery lower in those with severe initial deficit. It is often difficult to make predictions of recovery in individual patients except those with very mild stroke. Multidisciplinary rehabilitation is a critical component of stroke care and is aimed at restoring functional independence and reducing impairment. A wide range of rehabilitation interventions are available for stroke patients and in different settings (hospital, home, community), and a detailed discussion is outside the scope of this chapter. The reader is referred to a recent excellent review by Langhorne, Bernhardt, and Kwakkel.[68] Recovery may be affected adversely by the development of stroke-related complications and importantly by the presence of comorbidity and frailty.[69] The impact of physical therapy (such as muscle strengthening) intuitively may appear beneficial for frail stroke patients, general muscle weakness being a common feature of frailty, but there is a paucity of evidence to support this contention at the present time. Results of a small clinical trial show that the presence of frailty dampened the effect of a psychosocial intervention in older stroke patients, and in some, was even harmful.[70] The specific rehabilitation approaches that may be suitable for frail older stroke patients with multiple comorbidities are yet to be clearly defined.

Secondary Stroke Prevention

Secondary prevention refers to the treatments that may be used to prevent a recurrent stroke or a first stroke after a TIA. There have been significant advances in secondary prevention in the past decade based on results from several large-scale randomized controlled trials.

Antiplatelet Therapy

Antiplatelet therapy forms the cornerstone for secondary stroke prevention. Aspirin appears to be the drug of choice for arterial noncardioembolic ischemic stroke and is as effective as warfarin in this setting.[71,72] The addition of dipyridamole (200 mg bid) to aspirin provides an additional stroke reduction of 1% per year over aspirin alone.[73,74] The drawback to the aspirin-dipyridamole combination is many patients drop out of therapy because of vasodilatory headache caused by dipyridamole.[73,74] The combination of aspirin and dipyridamole appears to have equivalent efficacy to clopidogrel alone, and AHA/ASA guidelines recommend aspirin, aspirin-dipyridamole, or clopidogrel in the secondary prevention of stroke.[75] While the combination of aspirin and clopidogrel provides additive benefit in acute coronary syndrome, there is uncertainty whether this combination offers better stroke protection than clopidogrel alone.[76] In Chinese patients with TIA and minor stroke, early combination therapy with clopidogrel and aspirin for the first 21 days, followed by aspirin alone, appeared superior in reducing risk of stroke within 90 days,[77] but these results are yet to be reproduced in non-Asian populations. In addition, several trials are currently under way to test the efficacy of newer antiplatelet agents such as ticagrelor and prasugrel.

Anticoagulation

Warfarin has clearly been shown to be effective for secondary prevention in patients with AF[78] but not in cases of intracranial artery stenosis.[79] The annual risk of intracranial hemorrhage associated with warfarin is relatively low, approximately 2%.[80] The risk of falling is often cited as the reason for not starting warfarin in the very old although the benefits of stroke prevention in this high-risk group may still outweigh the risk of bleeding in older patients.

Newer oral anticoagulants are now available that do not require monitoring. The caveat is that they are licensed for use in patients with nonvalvular AF and thus patients need to have an ECG before these medications are prescribed. One study showed that dabigatran (a direct thrombin inhibitor) at a dosage of 110 mg bid was noninferior to warfarin in the prevention of stroke in those with AF, whereas at the dosage of 150 mg bid, dabigatran was superior to warfarin for stroke prevention.[81] Rivaroxaban, a factor Xa inhibitor, was shown to be noninferior to warfarin in preventing stroke in those with AF,[82] whereas another factor Xa inhibitor, apixaban, was shown to be superior to warfarin.[83] Both of these factor Xa inhibitors had a lower risk of intracranial hemorrhage than did warfarin. In a recent meta-analysis of trials of these new anticoagulants, their use in people older than 75 years was not associated with excess bleeding, and they were either noninferior or more efficacious than warfarin.[84] The principal issue that remains to be solved with the new anticoagulants is the development of reliable assays of anticoagulant activity, which are critical to prevent or treat bleeding complications.

Blood Pressure Reduction

Blood pressure reduction has assumed great importance in secondary stroke prevention. A systematic review of various classes of antihypertensives found that the magnitude of the reduction of stroke risk in those with hypertension was directly related to the degree of systolic blood pressure lowering.[85] The angiotensin-converting enzyme inhibitor perindopril and the diuretic indapamide showed a significant reduction in the risk of stroke among both hypertensive and nonhypertensive individuals with a history of stroke or TIA.[86] In this study, the combination therapy arm produced larger blood pressure reductions and larger risk reductions than did single drug therapy with perindopril alone. This finding regarding the benefit of perindopril with or without indapamide has been confirmed in patients older than 80 years[87] with the caveat that it was performed in the setting of primary prevention and patients had systolic blood pressure higher than 160 mm Hg. There is no evidence that the effect is limited to angiotensin-converting enzyme inhibitor; trial results published in 2008 showed that angiotensin receptor blocker (telmisartan) is as effective.[88] Commencing antihypertensive agents in the acute stroke setting must also be done cautiously given recent evidence suggesting that lowering of blood pressure acutely post-stroke may be harmful.[89] Overall, successful secondary prevention hinges heavily on blood pressure control, whether it is achieved with lifestyle modifications or medication, with the latter often being required. Although antihypertensive therapy is a key strategy in the secondary prevention of stroke, the optimal magnitude of blood pressure reduction required to prevent recurrent stroke in older people is not clear. Systolic hypertension is a management dilemma in frail older stroke patients who may appear to warrant treatment, but treatment is often complicated by the side effects, such as increased risk of falls. Some such patients may have substantial carotid artery stenosis and may require slightly higher blood pressure to ensure adequate cerebral perfusion. Given such concerns, the AHA/ASA recently recommended a systolic brachial blood pressure target of 150 mm Hg for stroke prevention in people older than 60 years.[90]

Lipid-Lowering Agents

3-Hydroxy-3-methylglutaryl–coenzyme A (HMG-CoA) reductase inhibitors (statins) provide an absolute risk reduction in stroke of approximately 2% over 5 years.[91] In addition to the results from this trial, which focused on patients up to 75 years old, data from secondary prevention trials involving statins in heart disease suggests a benefit in patients older than 80 years.[92] There is a small increase in the risk of hemorrhagic stroke with statins that is outweighed by the overall benefit, and this increased risk is associated with having an initial hemorrhagic stroke, being older, and having poorly controlled blood pressure but not with having low cholesterol levels.[93] Statins for stroke prevention in the very old must be used cautiously and preferably at lower doses.

Carotid Endarterectomy and Endovascular Therapy

Carotid endarterectomy is one of the most effective secondary prevention measures for the prevention of recurrent ischemic stroke in patients with 70% to 99% symptomatic internal carotid artery stenosis.[94,95] In a pooled analysis of large trials, the benefit of carotid endarterectomy appeared to be magnified in older patients given their greater overall risk of stroke.[96] There is no justification for withholding carotid endarterectomy for patients older than 75 years who are deemed medically fit to undergo surgery. Surgical intervention within 2 weeks of stroke is recommended because the risk benefit from surgery declines with time.[96]

Endovascular therapy (angioplasty and stenting) of the carotid artery appears less suitable. Two European trials in patients with symptomatic carotid stenosis suggested that angioplasty and stenting were less effective than endarterectomy and had higher perioperative risks.[97,98] By contrast, a U.S. trial in which symptomatic and asymptomatic patients participated has shown equivalence between the two modes of therapy.[99] For patients older than 70 years of age, endovascular stenting was associated with higher perioperative complications than was carotid endarterectomy,[100] which is the recommended intervention for older people.[101]

Recent studies have also found no benefit from endovascular closure of a patent foramen of ovale[35,102] compared with usual medical therapy with antiplatelet medications.

ORGANIZATION OF STROKE SERVICES

Given the rapid advances in stroke care in the past decade, it is now recognized that there needs to be a well-organized network of stroke services in order to deliver such care effectively to stroke patients, and this often requires integration of hospital and community services. Most evidence for benefit from organized stroke units in hospitals is seen for comprehensive stroke units, which are those combining acute care and rehabilitation.[103] The core requirements of a comprehensive stroke unit are a well-staffed multidisciplinary team of physicians, nurses, and therapists, whose work is coordinated through regular meetings, and the presence of protocol guided care pathways.[103] Nursing, in particular, is an integral part of any stroke service, particularly given the constancy of nursing provision in any phase of stroke care. A key person within a stroke service is the "stroke nurse manager," whose role involves acute triaging and delivery of acute treatment; coordination of care on the ward; liaison between stroke team, patients, and their caregivers; and external organizations involved in stroke care. Development of community-based support networks and rehabilitation services (home-based or outpatient) is important to develop in the context of an integrated stroke care service. Such community services will enable early-supported discharge from hospitals and ongoing support for patients after leaving the hospital.

Outpatient service models for stroke and TIA have flourished in the past 5 years. These are clinics that aim to attend quickly to patients presenting with a TIA with the knowledge that the risk of stroke is highest in the first few days after a TIA.[104] Studies have shown that such urgent evaluation of patients with TIA or minor stroke leads to a dramatic reduction in the risk of recurrent ischemic event at 90 days by up to 80%.[104-106] The principal focus of the clinic would be to assess and institute appropriate secondary prevention strategies such as antiplatelet therapy, blood pressure control, and lipid lowering, keeping in mind that patients with AF and carotid stenosis may need special and rapid attention. Such clinics, if well organized, have the potential to prevent unnecessary hospital admission of TIA patients and can provide substantial cost savings to the health care system.[106]

KEY POINTS

- Stroke is the second leading single cause of death worldwide and the sixth most important cause of disability among survivors.
- Organized stroke units are essential for acute stroke management.
- Three specific interventions have been shown to be effective in randomized trials for the acute treatment of ischemic stroke: tissue plasminogen activator, endovascular therapy, and antiplatelet agents.
- Multidisciplinary rehabilitation is a critical component of stroke care and is aimed at restoring functional independence and reducing impairment.
- A greater body of evidence is required to refine stroke prevention therapies (blood pressure reduction, anticoagulation) in frail older people.

For a complete list of references, please visit www.expertconsult.com.

KEY REFERENCES

11. Adams HP, Jr, Bendixen BH, Kappelle LJ, et al: Classification of subtype of acute ischemic stroke. Definitions for use in a multicenter clinical trial. TOAST. Trial of Org 10172 in Acute Stroke Treatment. Stroke 24:35–41, 1993.
12. Bogousslavsky J, Caplan LR, editors: Stroke syndromes, ed 2, Cambridge, MA, 2001, Cambridge University Press.
13. Muangpaisan W, Hinkle JL, Westwood M, et al: Stroke in the very old: clinical presentations and outcomes. Age Ageing 37:473–475, 2008.
18. Moorhouse P, Rockwood K: Vascular cognitive impairment: current concepts and clinical developments. Lancet Neurol 7:246–255, 2008.
19. Srikanth VK, Thrift AG, Saling MM, et al: Increased risk of cognitive impairment 3 months after mild to moderate first-ever stroke: a community-based prospective study of nonaphasic English-speaking survivors. Stroke 34:1136–1143, 2003.
21. Hackett ML, Yapa C, Parag V, et al: Frequency of depression after stroke: a systematic review of observational studies. Stroke 36:1330–1340, 2005.
22. Williams MP, Srikanth V, Bird M, et al: Urinary symptoms and natural history of urinary continence after first-ever stroke—a longitudinal population-based study. Age Ageing 41:371–376, 2012.
42. Govan L, Weir CJ, Langhorne P: Organized inpatient (stroke unit) care for stroke. Stroke 39:2402–2403, 2008.
43. Langhorne P, Dey P, Woodman M, et al: Is stroke unit care portable? A systematic review of the clinical trials. Age Ageing 34:324–330, 2005.
44. Langhorne P, Pollock A: What are the components of effective stroke unit care? Age Ageing 31:365–371, 2002.
47. Dennis M, Sandercock P, Reid J, et al: Effectiveness of intermittent pneumatic compression in reduction of risk of deep vein thrombosis in patients who have had a stroke (CLOTS 3): a multicentre randomised controlled trial. Lancet 382:516–524, 2013.
51. CAST: randomised placebo-controlled trial of early aspirin use in 20,000 patients with acute ischaemic stroke. CAST (Chinese Acute Stroke Trial) Collaborative Group. Lancet 349:1641–1649, 1997.
52. Tissue plasminogen activator for acute ischemic stroke. The National Institute of Neurological Disorders and Stroke rt-PA Stroke Study Group. N Engl J Med 333(24):1581–1587, 1995.
54. Powers WJ, Derdeyn CP, Biller J, et al: 2015 AHA/ASA focused update of the 2013 guidelines for the early management of patients with acute ischemic stroke regarding endovascular treatment: a guideline for healthcare professionals from the American Heart Association/American Stroke Association. Stroke 2015.

55. The International Stroke Trial (IST): a randomised trial of aspirin, subcutaneous heparin, both, or neither among 19435 patients with acute ischaemic stroke. International Stroke Trial Collaborative Group. Lancet 349:1569–1581, 1997.
59. Mishra NK, Ahmed N, Andersen G, et al: Thrombolysis in very elderly people: controlled comparison of SITS International Stroke Thrombolysis Registry and Virtual International Stroke Trials Archive. BMJ 341:c6046, 2010.
68. Langhorne P, Bernhardt J, Kwakkel G: Stroke rehabilitation. Lancet 377:1693–1702, 2011.
84. Sardar P, Chatterjee S, Chaudhari S, et al: New oral anticoagulants in elderly adults: evidence from a meta-analysis of randomized trials. J Am Geriatr Soc 62:857–864, 2014.
87. Beckett NS, Peters R, Fletcher AE, et al: Treatment of hypertension in patients 80 years of age or older. N Engl J Med 358:1887–1898, 2008.
90. Kernan WN, Ovbiagele B, Black HR, et al: Guidelines for the prevention of stroke in patients with stroke and transient ischemic attack: a guideline for healthcare professionals from the American Heart Association/American Stroke Association. Stroke 45:2160–2236, 2014.
94. Clinical alert: benefit of carotid endarterectomy for patients with high-grade stenosis of the internal carotid artery. National Institute of Neurological Disorders and Stroke Stroke and Trauma Division. North American Symptomatic Carotid Endarterectomy Trial (NASCET) investigators. Stroke 22:816–817, 1991.
104. Rothwell PM, Giles MF, Chandratheva A, et al: Effect of urgent treatment of transient ischaemic attack and minor stroke on early recurrent stroke (EXPRESS study): a prospective population-based sequential comparison. Lancet 370:1432–1442, 2007.

62 Long-Term Stroke Care

Anne Forster

Stroke is an ancient disease, recognized since the time of Hippocrates, when the term *apoplexy* was used to describe someone being suddenly struck down. The lay term *stroke* emerged in the seventeenth century, and this term has only more recently replaced apoplexy in the medical literature.[1]

Despite centuries of reports of this condition and early understanding of its cause, rigorous scientific exploration was slow to gain momentum. However, in the past 50 years, an acceleration in stroke research has had an impact on the care of people with this common condition worldwide. The journal *Stroke* was first published in the 1970s. The first addition of the UK Clinical Guidelines for Stroke (1997) was the forerunner for other national guidelines. These in turn led to the development of audit tools to support a continued cycle of service improvements. Other developments have been more recent: stroke research only began to flourish in China in the early twenty-first century,[2] the World Stroke Organization was established in 2006, and the European Stroke Organisation came into existence in 2007.

Methodologic and technologic advances have underpinned this more dynamic approach to stroke care. The methods of trial evaluation, including health economic analysis, have been massively refined and enhanced and a supportive infrastructure has been developed. The Cochrane Library, founded in 1993, created a platform for worldwide dissemination of research.[3] The Stroke Review Group was among the first to be registered in the library, which, as of 2015, contained 176 active reviews.

Despite advances in identification and reduction of risk, stroke remains a major illness. Annually, 15 million people worldwide suffer a stroke. Of these, 5 million die and another 5 million are left permanently disabled, placing a burden on family and community.[4] At least 900,000 people living in England have had a stroke, of whom 300,000 live with moderate to severe disability.[5] Stroke is the leading cause of serious, long-term disability in the United States.[6] Stroke is an age-related condition, although people of any age can be affected; approximately 25% of strokes occur in people younger than age 65,[7] and 5 in 100,000 children suffer a stroke.[8]

The burden of stroke is considerable at a population, societal, and individual level. Costs are estimated at £7 billion a year in the United Kingdom, with £2.8 billion direct costs to the National Health Service (NHS) in the United Kingdom, £2.4 billion in informal care costs, and £1.8 billion in income lost to productivity and disability.[5] Unplanned visits from the doctor and hospital readmissions contribute to the economic burden and cause stress and discomfort to the patient. Poststroke hospitalization rates are significantly higher than for a matched nonstroke cohort.[9] One study reported that less than 15% of surviving stroke patients had not been readmitted to hospital in 5 years.[10] Cumulative risk of recurrent stroke at 10 years is 39%.[11]

STROKE CARE PATHWAY

The achievements in stroke research have clarified the stroke care pathway. Stroke must be treated as a medical emergency and requires rapid screening and assessment in order to instigate appropriate treatment strategies within the hyperacute stage of onset. This should be followed by assessment by the multidisciplinary team (occupational therapists, physiotherapists, speech therapists, and nurses) and transfer, if required, to a stroke rehabilitation unit.[12] For patients with mild to moderate disability, discharge home with the support of an early supported discharge team is recommended.[13] The robust evidence that rehabilitation in a stroke rehabilitation unit saved lives and reduced disability was a game-changer in terms of the care provided to stroke patients and their caregivers.[14] With the recent advent of perhaps more glamorous treatment options in the acute stage of stroke, the crucial importance of appropriate rehabilitation must not be overlooked. The benefits of treatment in a stroke rehabilitation unit are retained for up to 10 years after the stroke incident.[15] This treatment option should be provided to all people, as benefits are reported regardless of age, sex, and disability levels.

LONG-TERM RECOVERY

Despite these advances, long-term recovery can be poor. Many stroke survivors and their caregivers feel abandoned as service support (if provided) is gradually withdrawn in the weeks following the event.[16] Although some information is available from long-term cohort studies, this lack of routine follow-up for all stroke survivors also limits the generalizable data available to inform our understanding of the long-term consequences of stroke.

The South London Stroke Register, established in 1995, is the largest stroke register in the United Kingdom. Although their data should be considered in the context of the services available and the demographic profile of participants included, useful insights into the scale of the challenges following stroke is provided. From a cohort of 3373 stroke survivors, 20% to 30% had poor outcomes over a range of physical, social, and psychological domains.[17] Rates of inactivity remained stable until year 8, when they increased. Rates of cognitive impairment fluctuated until year 8, when they also increased. Similar levels of anxiety and depression were reported in a smaller, 10-year cohort of 416 patients in Sweden, but their levels of physical activity were more positive, with over 50% reporting the same level of physical activity as prestroke.[18]

It is reported that up to 40% of stroke survivors have loss of function of the upper limb at 1 year post stroke, 80% have reduced mobility, 40% have problems with swallowing, and 33% have aphasia.[12] Deficits in memory, attention and concentration, perception, spatial awareness (neglect), apraxia, and executive functioning are also consequences of stroke. Prevalence is difficult to estimate as their presentations may overlap; studies have used a range of outcome measures, which makes summarization difficult; and subtle cognitive problems (e.g., difficulty in scanning a page) may be missed by commonly used screening tools. Each impairment may have a considerable effect on a stroke survivor's recovery, adversely influencing their ability to engage in physical and social activities. It is important to consider such impairments and appropriately assess, even if reviewed some months or even years after stroke, as they may have been overshadowed by more obvious physical disabilities in the acute stages. Visual field defects should also be considered.[19] There are consistent reports that approximately one third of stroke survivors experienced some anxiety and depression at any one time.[20]

PREDICTIVE MODELS

The domains of The World Health Organization's International Classification of Functioning, Disability and Health (ICF) can provide a meaningful way of understanding these poststroke needs and inform development of service models.[21] Numerous published studies have highlighted the relationships between these domains on the poststroke outcomes of mood disability and quality of life,[22-25] but no definitive predictive models have been created to inform service delivery. Reduction in walking ability may lead to loss of independence in personal activities of daily living, as well as causing social isolation, and is strongly associated with psychological and cognitive factors.[24] Resumption of valued activities (as identified by the person who has experienced the stroke) positively influences health-related quality of life, which may not necessarily relate to level of functional recovery.[26] The caregivers of patients with poor physical and emotional states are likely to have poorer emotional outcomes themselves.[27]

Unmet Needs

The range of problems experienced by stroke survivors and their caregivers often translates into unmet needs defined as "expressed needs that are not satisfied by current service provision."[28] The needs are multifaceted and influenced by a range of social and environmental factors. A survey of more than 1250 participants investigated the prevalence of unmet needs in community-dwelling stroke survivors 1 to 5 years after stroke in the United Kingdom. Nearly half of respondents had one or more unmet long-term need. These needs related to information provision (54%), mobility problems (25%), falls (21%), incontinence (21%), and pain (15%).[29] Over half reported a reduction in leisure activities. Similar patterns of need have been reported in younger and older stroke survivors, more and less disabled, and different geographic settings.[30] Level of need may not necessarily be related to level of functional recovery.[31] Although the level of need is generally high, it is important to recognize that some stroke survivors report no needs. Whether this is because they genuinely have no needs, or because they have accepted their current situation, or because they have no realistic expectation that any identified needs will be successfully met has not been fully explored.

Information Needs

The most commonly reported unmet need is for information, even months or years after the event.[32] A Cochrane review indicates that active involvement of participants, for example, through opportunity to ask questions in a more educational format, is beneficial.[33] The needs of stroke survivors and their caregivers may differ. For the latter, a trajectory of information needs has been proposed with information on stroke and practical training skills provided in the early stages, to a focus on their own needs to participate in social activities, followed by support for planning for the future in the later adaption phases.[34] It is important to consider a strategy for information and educational provision for survivors of stroke and their families across the stroke care pathway and ensure that this is clearly documented and delivered rather than rely on opportunistic delivery.

Views of Patients and Their Caregivers

Many qualitative reports have highlighted the daily struggle for stroke patients and their caregivers. A systematic review and synthesis of 40 qualitative studies on adjusting after stroke from stroke survivors' and caregivers' perspectives presents a detailed and complex picture of fluctuating adjustment and acceptance, influenced by personal, interpersonal, and structural issues (e.g., interaction with health professionals, public awareness of the consequences of stroke).[35] Trajectories of recovery have been identified, indicating some survivors progress though disruption to adjustment and acceptance, whereas others experience cycles of disruption, adjustment, and acceptance, and others continue to experience disruption and decline. This can be exacerbated by a mismatch of the expectations and understandings between the health and social care professionals involved in the delivery of care and the stroke survivors and their caregivers. Realignment of a sense of self and undertaking and contributing to meaningful activity are of importance in the adjustment process, which may continue for years.[36]

Evidence Base

There is a relatively small evidence base for interventions delivered to stroke survivors and their caregivers in the long term, with most evidence focused on the early stages of poststroke recovery. To identify components of an intervention that could be feasibly delivered in the community, an overview of stroke reviews in the Cochrane library was undertaken.[37] The focus was on participants who were at least 6 months post stroke at the start of intervention delivery. Outcomes of interest were those of importance to stroke survivors and their caregivers: perceived health status, participation, quality of life, and mood. Interventions were noninvasive and feasible for delivery in the community without medication or highly specialized equipment. Where there were statistically significant effects across the measures used in a domain, and these were derived from many trials with many participants with no serious risk of bias, the intervention was considered effective on this outcome. Where there was a statistically significant effect but with limitations due to number of participants, differences between measures of the same domain, or serious risk of bias, this was qualified as limited evidence of an effect.

Twenty-eight reviews were identified (which included 352 studies). Ten reviews reported a perceived health status outcome with information provision, inspiratory muscle training, fitness training, and tele-rehabilitation and qualified as limited evidence of an effect. Nine reviews reported mood, with limited evidence of improvements found for information provision and fitness training. Only one of the included reviews (information provision) recorded participation as an outcome with no evidence of effect. The same review reported a small effect on quality of life. Limited evidence from one study reported in two reviews suggested teaching procedural knowledge could reduce caregivers' depressive symptoms and improve perceived health status. However, this intervention, which was tested in single-center study, has recently been evaluated in a large, multicenter trial in which the positive results were not replicated.[38]

A comprehensive review of community-based interventions aiming to reduce depression and/or improve participation and health-related quality of life was undertaken by Graven and colleagues. Of 54 studies identified, less than half were aimed at participants over a year after stroke.[39] These reported evidence for the effectiveness of exercise and physical training[40-44] and some short-term benefits of physiotherapy.[45-46] Analysis of nine randomized controlled trials produced insufficient evidence of benefits of gait training for chronic stroke patients.[45-47] It seems more appropriate to use scarce therapy resources for targeted interventions (e.g., for fall prevention) rather than create a therapy-dependent service.

The importance of maintaining fitness is increasingly emphasized. A Cochrane review based on 45 randomized controlled trials showed that physical fitness (cardiorespiratory) training after stroke has beneficial effects on disability, walking endurance and speed, with minimal adverse events.[48] Another systematic review summarized 28 studies, which included 920 participants who were predominantly mild to moderately disabled, able to walk, and at least 1 year after their stroke. This review concluded that interventions that are aerobic, or have an aerobic component, can improve fitness even though the interventions provided did not meet the guidance of 30 minutes of moderate intensity physical activity most days of the week.[49] Increased physical activity is also beneficial.[50-51]

There are purposely developed courses available (e.g., www.exerciseafterstroke.org.uk and www.laterlifetraining.co.uk), but rollout is limited. This may be due to apprehension of patients because of fear of risks, or lack of knowledge of benefits, or limited awareness of health professionals.[52] Similarly, weekly exercise classes and circuit classes report some benefits in enhancing walking capacity (distance walked in 6 minutes).[53]

Psychological and Emotional Support

The psychosocial consequences of stroke have been highlighted, yet successful models for the provision of psychological support remain elusive. Provision of psychological support involving routine assessment of patients and then input gradated according to need is recommended, but evidence for effectiveness is limited.[12] Such a model does, however, provide the flexibility to assess and address specific problems (e.g., cognitive disorders) within an overarching framework. For some cognitive disorders (e.g., memory problems), compensatory strategies such as pager systems, diaries, and electronic organizers may be helpful.[12] A recent synthesis of six Cochrane reviews (1550 patients) relating to rehabilitation for poststroke cognitive impairment (attention deficits, memory deficits, spatial neglect, perceptual disorders, executive dysfunction, and motor apraxia) concluded insufficient research evidence, or evidence of insufficient quality, to support clear recommendations for clinical practice.[54]

Self-Management

Programs of self-management are promoted in other long-term conditions,[55] and an extensive review[56] concluded that supporting self-management can have benefits for attitudes and behaviors, quality of life, clinical symptoms, and use of health care resources. At present, the optimal timing and format of such programs for stroke survivors are unknown.[57] Few studies have been undertaken after the early phase of stroke care. A systematic review of self-management programs designed for people who have had strokes identified 15 studies (9 of which were randomized controlled trials) in which significant treatment effects in favor of the self-management program were reported in 6. However, all of these studies had been undertaken within the first three months after stroke.[58]

The heterogeneity of stroke survivors suggests that a more supported model of self-management might be appropriate for this client group. The mode of delivery is uncertain. A study by Harrington and colleagues,[59,60] with patients a median of 10 months post stroke, combined a self-management/education program with an exercise intervention and reported a significant improvement in social and physical integration in the community.[60] There is also benefit from the peer support available in such settings.[61] However, compliance can be problematic and strategies need to be developed to promote adherence.[62,63]

POSTSTROKE COMPLICATIONS

The heterogeneity of the stroke population is reflected in the variety of poststroke complications. These complications include urinary incontinence, deep vein thrombosis, seizures, osteoporosis, central poststroke pain, and fatigue.[64]

Incontinence

It is suggested that 15% of stroke survivors remain incontinent at the 1-year follow-up.[65] A Cochrane review[66] identified 12 trials of interventions to promote continence in people after a stroke. Sample size was generally small and a variety of professional-led, behavioral, pharmaceutical, and complementary therapy (acupuncture) interventions were reported. Evidence was insufficient to make definitive recommendations, although professional input through structured assessment and management of care and specialist continence nursing may reduce symptoms. Research evaluating a systematic voiding program is ongoing.[67]

Fatigue

The prevalence of fatigue after stroke is difficult to ascertain because of the variability of outcomes used in reported studies but may be as high as 77%.[68] The cause of fatigue after stroke is uncertain but is likely to be multidimensional. Pharmacologic and nonpharmacologic treatment options have been evaluated with limited success. Some benefits were reported in a small trial (83 participants more than 4 months post stroke) that combined cognitive therapy and graded exercises.[69]

Falls

Falls are common after stroke.[70] Although there is a large generic literature relating to falls, effective interventions specifically for stroke patients in the chronic stage have not yet been identified.[71] Pragmatically, it would seem reasonable to ensure that fall prevention measures (e.g., environmental reviews) are taken to protect stroke patients from injury.

Driving

Many of the impairments persisting after a stroke impinge on a stroke survivor's ability to drive. This is an activity of central importance to many stroke survivors, positively influencing mood and reducing social isolation.[72] Approximately one third may return to driving after 6 months,[73] increasing to 50% at 5 years.[74] Many stroke survivors will require driving specific rehabilitation (and possibly adaptations to their car) to regain the appropriate skills.[73] Approaches to retraining have been well described in a Cochrane review.[74] The review of four studies (245 participants total) concluded that there was no evidence that a driving intervention was more effective than no intervention.

Oral Health

Recently attention has been drawn to the importance of oral health after stroke, as stroke-related motor and cognitive impairments may cause stroke survivors to lose the ability to undertake and/or maintain oral hygiene. This has consequence for oral health but may also link to aspirant pneumonia. Detailed review and meta-analysis have indicated a poorer oral health status among patients with stroke compared to healthy controls, including greater tooth loss, higher dental caries, and poorer periodontal status. If poor poststroke oral hygiene becomes established, the longer it continues the poorer the outcomes will be.[75]

RESIDENTS OF CARE HOMES

Approximately one fifth[76] to one quarter[5] of all care home residents have a history of a stroke. It has been reported that care home residents spend the majority of their time inactive,[77] with low levels of interaction with staff. The risks of sedentary behavior are increasingly emphasized.[78] Encouraging residents to be more active could deliver benefits in terms of physical and psychological health and quality of life.[78] Yet it is reported that only 10% of care home residents receive physiotherapy, and just 3% receive occupational therapy.[79] While this research is now rather old, these services are unlikely to have increased markedly. A large Cochrane review of physical rehabilitation for residents of care homes (67 trials with a total of 6300 residents) concluded that it is feasible to reduce disability, but the effects were small and little information was available on whether benefits were sustained.[80] However, provision of a 3-month program of physiotherapy and occupational therapy for care home residents with stroke did not produce benefits.[81] Supporting a whole-home cultural approach to decreasing sedentary behavior may be more beneficial then time-limited professional-led interventions.

CAREGIVERS OF STROKE SURVIVORS

More than half of stroke survivors are dependent on others for some assistance with activities of daily living. This assistance is commonly provided by family members, who may consequently become stressed and anxious. The health-related quality of life of caregivers fluctuates over time as they adjust to their new role and identity.[82,83] Their psychological well-being may become less linked to the patient's physical ability and more influenced by the patient's cognitive, behavioral, and emotional changes over time.[84]

This burden of care has an important effect on the physical and psychosocial well-being of caregivers, with up to 48% of caregivers reporting health problems, two thirds a decline in social life,[85] and many reporting high levels of strain. Caregivers and family support have a large part to play in poststroke recovery, not only in supporting the stroke survivors (without being overprotective) but also in ensuring that their own health and well-being are maintained. Effective training of caregivers, therefore, should not only improve their own health but also the recovery and adjustment of the stroke patient.[86]

A number of interventions have been evaluated, which have been grouped around three main themes: support and information; interventions that reinforce personal strengths, resources, and coping skills of caregivers; and teaching procedural knowledge and practical skills.[87] A single-center study of the latter reported positive benefits, but these were not replicated in a larger, multicenter trial.[38] This intervention was delivered while the patient was in hospital. It may be that skill training and support are more applicable after discharge, with access to additional help and ongoing support.

VOCATIONAL REHABILITATION

In a comprehensive review of the social consequence of stroke for working-age adults (70 studies with a total of 8810 participants), the proportions of stroke survivors returning to work varied from 0% to 100%, with a mean of 44%.[88] Studies used different methods and time points after stroke, which affects the generalizability of these results. Work is an important component of people's lives, and stroke survivors should be appropriately supported to return to work whenever possible. Effective interventions are likely to be tailored to the individual and therefore are difficult to evaluate in randomized trials.

Whereas returning to work may not be a goal for all, poststroke survivors identify the importance of intellectual stimulation and participating in meaningful activities. But these abilities are reduced for many survivors. Six months after a stroke, approximately 50% of stroke patients consider that they have no meaningful daytime activity[89]; this is reported after an apparently mild stroke,[90] and more than 25% of survivors younger than 45 years report being intellectually unfulfilled.[30]

POSSIBLE SERVICE MODELS

Although stroke survivors, their caregivers, health professionals, and policy makers recognize a need to improve the long-term stroke outcomes and, in particular, to avoid the common experience of abandonment and isolation, service models to address these issues successfully have not yet been identified. The role of a liaison support worker to provide advice and guidance is attractive, but only small benefits that are restricted to mild to moderately disabled stroke survivors have been reported.[91]

The importance of regular professionally led reviews has been recommended,[92] and more recently tools to assess the needs of stroke survivors and their caregivers have emerged.[93,94] But assessment alone will not redress the reported poor long-term outcomes. Linking needs and resources is key. It is likely that some stroke survivors will have a range of complex needs that require individualized case management.[95] Others may have specific clinical problems (e.g., incontinence, painful shoulders) that require appropriate evidenced-based treatment. Given pressures on resource use, programs of supported self-management that include access to relevant information and mechanisms to enhance social networks may be successful in improving long-term outcomes, but these programs will require rigorous evaluation.

KEY POINTS

- Among the 15 million people worldwide each year who have a stroke, 5 million are left permanently disabled, placing a requirement on family and community.
- Despite advances in acute stroke care, long-term recovery can be poor, and stroke survivors and their caregivers can feel abandoned.
- Problems experienced by stroke survivors commonly relate to mobility impairment, falls, incontinence, fatigue, and pain and often translate into unmet needs that include psychosocial aspects.
- Long-term stroke needs do not necessarily relate to the degree of functional recovery.
- More than half of stroke survivors are dependent on others for assistance with activities of daily living. This assistance is commonly provided by family members, who may become stressed and anxious.
- Individualized care based on problem-based approaches, and which embeds maintenance of fitness, psychosocial well-being, and caregiver support, is consistent with the limited evidence base available.

For a complete list of references, please visit www.expertconsult.com.

KEY REFERENCES

12. Intercollegiate Stroke Working Party: National clinical guideline for stroke, ed 4, London, 2012, Royal College of Physicians.
13. Langhorne P, Taylor G, Murray G, et al: Early supported discharge services for stroke patients: a meta-analysis of individual patients' data. Lancet 365:501–506, 2005.
17. Wolfe C, Crichton S, Heuschmann P, et al: Estimates of outcomes up to ten years after stroke: analysis from the prospective South London Stroke Register. PLoS Med 8:e1001033, 2011.
18. Jönsson A, Delavaran H, Iwarsson S, et al: Functional status and patient-reported outcome 10 years after stroke: the Lund Stroke Register. Stroke 45:1784–1790, 2014.
20. Hackett M, Yapa C, Parag V, et al: Frequency of depression after stroke: a systematic review of observational studies. Stroke 36:1330–1340, 2005.
23. Patel M, Tilling K, Lawrence E, et al: Relationships between long-term stroke disability, handicap and health-related quality of life. Age Ageing 35:273–279, 2006.
26. Sturm J, Donnan G, Dewey H, et al: Determinants of handicap after stroke: the North East Melbourne Stroke Incidence Study (NEMESIS). Stroke 35:715–720, 2004.
29. McKevitt C, Fudge N, Redfern J, et al: Self-reported long-term needs after stroke. Stroke 42:1398–1403, 2011.
33. Forster A, Brown L, Smith J, et al: Information provision for stroke patients and their caregivers. Cochrane Database Syst Rev (16): CD001919, 2008.
38. Forster A, Dickerson J, Young J, et al: A structured training programme for caregivers of inpatients after stroke (TRACS): a cluster

randomised controlled trial and cost-effectiveness analysis. Lancet 382:2069–2076, 2013.

39. Graven C, Brock K, Hill K, et al: Are rehabilitation and/or care co-ordination interventions delivered in the community effective in reducing depression, facilitating participation and improving quality of life after stroke? Disabil Rehabil 33:1501–1520, 2011.
45. Green J, Forster A, Bogle S, et al: Physiotherapy for patients with mobility problems more than 1 year after stroke: a randomised controlled trial. Lancet 359:199–203, 2002.
48. Saunders D, Sanderson M, Brazzelli M, et al: Physical fitness training for stroke patients. Cochrane Database Syst Rev (9):CD003316, 2013.
54. Gillespie D, Bowen A, Chung C, et al: Rehabilitation for post-stroke cognitive impairment: an overview of recommendations arising from systematic reviews of current evidence. Clin Rehabil 29:120–128, 2015.
58. Lennon S, McKenna S, Jones F: Self-management programmes for people post stroke: a systematic review. Clin Rehabil 27:867–878, 2013.
66. Thomas LH, Cross S, Barrett J, et al: Treatment of urinary incontinence after stroke in adults. Cochrane Database Syst Rev (1): CD004462, 2008.
67. Thomas LH, Watkins CL, French B, et al: Study protocol: ICONS: identifying continence options after stroke: a randomised trial. Trials 12:131, 2011.
71. Verheyden GS, Weerdesteyn V, Pickering RM, et al: Interventions for preventing falls in people after stroke. Cochrane Database Syst Rev (5):CD008728, 2013.
91. Ellis G, Mant J, Langhorne P, et al: Stroke liaison workers for stroke patients and carers: an individual patient data meta-analysis. Cochrane Database Syst Rev (5):CD005066, 2010.
93. Forster A, Murray J, Young J, et al: Validation of the longer-term unmet needs after stroke (LUNS) monitoring tool: a multicentre study. Clin Rehabil 27:1020–1028, 2013.
94. World Stroke Organization: Post stroke checklist (PSC): improving life after stroke. http://www.worldstrokecampaign.org/learn/the-post-stroke-checklist-psc-improving-life-after-stroke.html. Accessed November 23, 2014.

63 Disorders of the Autonomic Nervous System

Roman Romero-Ortuno, K. Jane Wilson, Joanna L. Hampton

This chapter focuses on the consequences of aging on autonomic cardiovascular control. The neurobiology of aging and the effects of aging on gastrointestinal and urinary tract function are detailed in other sections in this book.

The chapter first provides a brief summary of autonomic pathways involved in cardiovascular control, and the methods used to assess their function. The chapter then reviews the effect of aging on the different components involved in autonomic cardiovascular control, including alterations in afferent and efferent function and in end-organ responsiveness. The integrated effect of these changes on the response of older people to daily stresses of life (i.e., response to upright posture and to food ingestion) is discussed. The final part of the chapter outlines primary and secondary disorders of the autonomic nervous system that are clinically relevant in older people and reviews the clinical management of orthostatic hypotension.

BASIC CONCEPTS OF AUTONOMIC PHYSIOLOGY

Autonomic Pathways

Autonomic regulation depends on three main components. Afferent fibers continuously sense changes in blood pressure (baroreceptors), blood oxygenation, and other chemical signals (chemoreceptors), pain (sensory afferents), and cortical stimulation. These signals are integrated in brainstem centers that ultimately modulate sympathetic and parasympathetic outflows, which are transmitted to target organs via efferent fibers. The baroreflex provides an example of these pathways (Figure 63-1). This is a redundant system, with input from multiple independent afferent pathways that ensure maintenance of cardiovascular regulation even after partial damage.[1,2] The afferent limb of this reflex includes pressure-sensitive receptors located in the walls of cardiopulmonary veins, the right atrium, and within almost every large artery of the neck and thorax, but particularly within the carotid sinus and aortic arch. Stimulated by stretch, these low- and high-pressure baroreceptors monitor venous and arterial pressures, respectively, and relay that information to brainstem centers. Information from the venous and aortic arch baroreceptors is carried centrally via fibers that course within the vagus nerve (X cranial nerve). Carotid sinus baroreceptor nerve activity is relayed centrally first via the carotid sinus (Hering) nerve, then through the glossopharyngeal nerve (IX cranial nerve) before arriving at the same brainstem centers.

Afferent fibers from these multiple baroreceptors have their first synapse in the nucleus tractus solitarius of the medulla oblongata.[3] This nucleus inhibits sympathetic tone and is crucial to baroreflex function. Destroying it (e.g., by experimental lesion[4] or neurologic damage)[5] leads to loss of baroreflex function, resulting in episodes of hypertension and tachycardia.[6] In addition to the afferent input arising from the baroreceptors, the nucleus tractus solitarius also receives modulating input from many other cardiovascular brain centers, such as the area postrema.[7] The nucleus provides excitatory inputs to the caudal ventrolateral medulla, which in turn inhibits the rostral ventrolateral medulla,[8,9] where the pacemaker neurons that produce sympathetic tone are believed to be located.[10] Rostral ventrolateral medulla neurons project to the preganglionic sympathetic neurons in the intermediolateral column of the spinal cord that send fibers outside the central nervous system. Parasympathetic activity is also modulated by the nucleus tractus solitarius, through projections to preganglionic parasympathetic neurons in the nucleus ambiguus and the motor nucleus of the vagus (see Figure 63-1).

The importance of autonomic mechanisms in the regulation of blood pressure is most evident when they fail. Damage of baroreflex afferents (e.g., as a consequence of radiation or surgery), leads to labile blood pressure that is very difficult to control.[6] At the other extreme, degeneration of central or efferent structures, as seen in patients with primary autonomic failure, leads to disabling orthostatic hypotension.[11,12] In the most severe cases, patients are only able to stand for a few seconds before profound orthostatic hypotension causes loss of consciousness (i.e., orthostatic syncope). These disorders are described later in this chapter.

METHODS USED TO TEST AUTONOMIC FUNCTION

Posture (Orthostatic) Test

Perhaps the most informative and simplest autonomic evaluation is the posture test. The patient's blood pressure and heart rate are measured after 5 to 10 minutes in the supine position and repeated after the subject stands motionless for 3 to 5 minutes. There is value in repeating measurements at each of these time points, as one single measurement may or may not be informative. Ideally, beat-to-beat plethysmography is the most informative, but if this is not available, then repetitive manual measurements of both heart rate and blood pressure will enable a clearer assessment and lead to a more accurate diagnosis, especially in cases where the autonomic failure is mild to moderate rather than severe.[13]

Virtually all patients with severe autonomic failure will have an immediate fall in blood pressure on standing. Other autonomic conditions associated with delayed orthostatic hypotension may require a 30-minute stand test to make the diagnosis,[14] but they are usually not associated with widespread autonomic neuropathy. Older patients may find it extremely tiring to stand for 30 minutes unassisted and a passive tilt test, during which data is recorded continuously and the patient is supported physically, will increase the tolerance of completing the test.

Heart rate is crucial in interpreting blood pressure changes. Patients with severe autonomic failure characteristically have no or little (about 10 to 15 beats/min) increase in heart rate despite profound orthostatic hypotension. A greater increase in heart rate usually indicates that other conditions (e.g., volume depletion or medications) are contributing to orthostatic hypotension.

Orthostatic Hemodynamic Assessment With Sphygmomanometer

Routinely, clinicians use the auscultatory or oscillometric method with a sphygmomanometer. In 1996, a consensus committee of the American Autonomic Society and the American Academy of Neurology defined orthostatic hypotension as a drop of at least 20 mm Hg in systolic blood pressure and/or 10 mm Hg in diastolic blood pressure within the first 3 minutes of orthostasis.[15] This definition was intended primarily for clinical situations where orthostatic blood pressure changes are measured with a

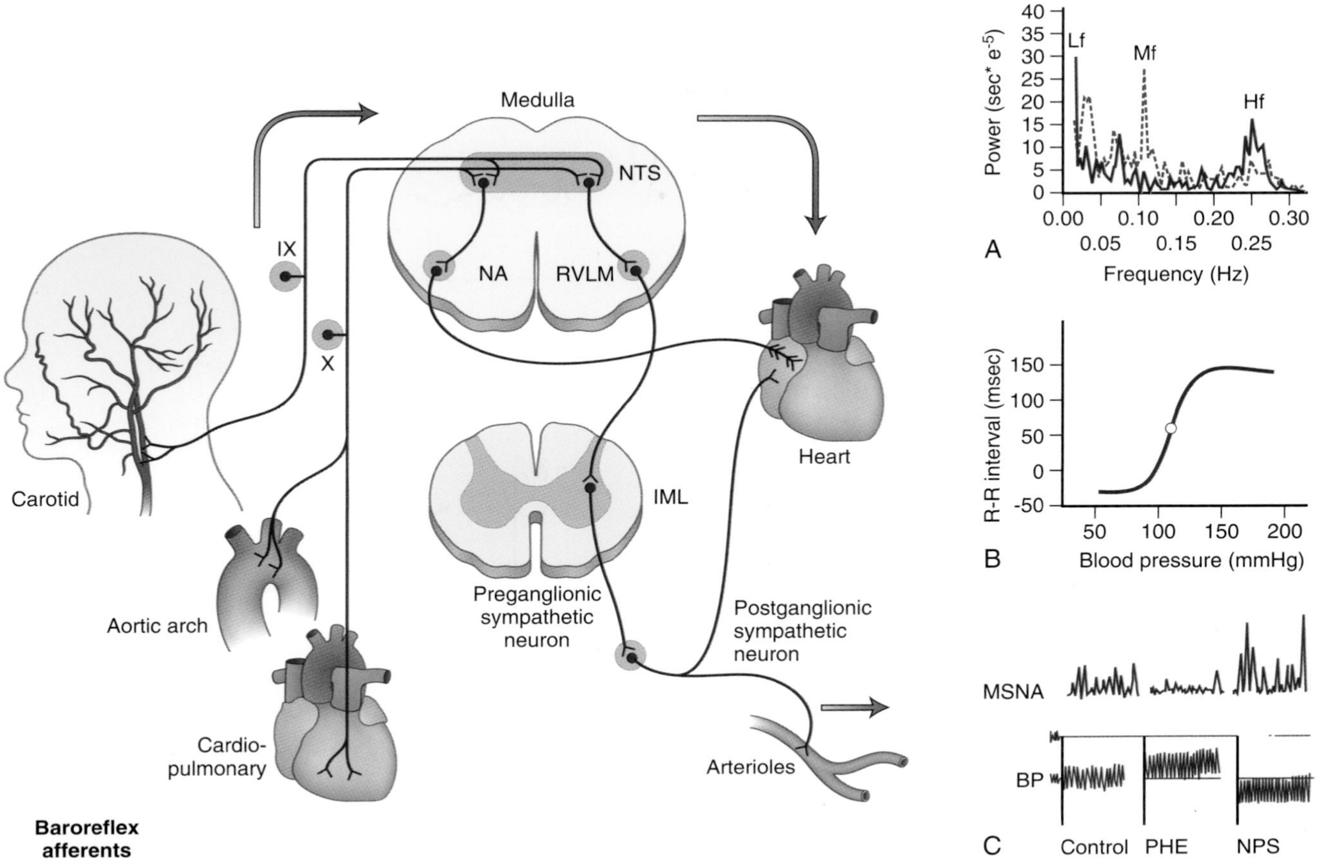

Figure 63-1. Simplified anatomic/functional scheme of baroreflex function. Afferent fibers located in the right atrium and in the cardiopulmonary veins (low-pressure baroreceptors) and in the aortic arch and carotid sinus (high-pressure baroreceptors) are activated by stretch and relay this information through the vagus (X) or glossopharyngeal (IX) nerves to the nucleus tractus solitarii (NTS) of the brainstem. The NTS provides excitatory inputs to the caudal ventrolateral medulla, which in turn inhibits the rostral ventrolateral medulla (RVLM)[8,9] (for simplicity the NTS is shown as projecting direct inhibitory pathways to the RVLM), where pacemaker neurons that originate sympathetic tone are believed to be located. These cell bodies send their efferent projections through the intermediolateral column of the spinal cord (IML). Baroreflex function can be simplified as follows: an increase in blood pressure is detected by arterial baroreceptors, which increase their firing into the NTS; activation of the NTS leads to a greater inhibitory output to the RVLM; inhibition of pacemaker cells in the RVLM results in a compensatory reduction in sympathetic tone. Conversely, a decrease in blood pressure results in decreased firing in the NTS, withdrawal of the inhibitory influence of this nucleus on the RVLM, and a compensatory increase in sympathetic tone. Parasympathetic activity is also modulated by the NTS, through projections to the nucleus ambiguus (NA). An increase in blood pressure will lead to activation of the NTS and of the NA, with increased parasympathetic activity. Methods to assess baroreflex function include **(A)** spectral analysis, by correlating spontaneous changes in blood pressure and heart rate and **(B)** by the neck barocuff method. Results obtained by these methods are influenced by afferent baroreceptor input, brainstem pathways, and end-organ responsiveness. Baroreflex modulation of sympathetic activity can be assessed with **(C)** microelectrode recording of postganglionic efferent sympathetic nerve activity (MSNA). In this example, blood pressure increment with phenylephrine (PHE) produced a baroreflex-mediated decrease in MSNA, and blood pressure reduction with nitroprusside (NPS) produces a baroreflex-mediated increase in MSNA.

sphygmomanometer or automatic oscillometric blood pressure monitors.[16,17]

Orthostatic Hemodynamic Assessment With Beat-to-Beat Monitoring

The introduction of new noninvasive beat-to-beat finger arterial blood pressure monitors led to concerns that the consensus definition of orthostatic hypotension, originally intended for the sphygmomanometer,[15] may lack clinical relevance when applied to beat-to-beat data.[18,19] Some orthostatic hypotension definitions based on continuous hemodynamic assessment include *initial* orthostatic hypotension and can only be measured with continuous noninvasive monitoring.[20] Initial orthostatic hypotension is defined as a transient blood pressure decrease, within 15 seconds after standing, of more than 40 mm Hg in systolic blood pressure and/or more than 20 mm Hg in diastolic blood pressure, with symptoms of cerebral hypoperfusion.[21]

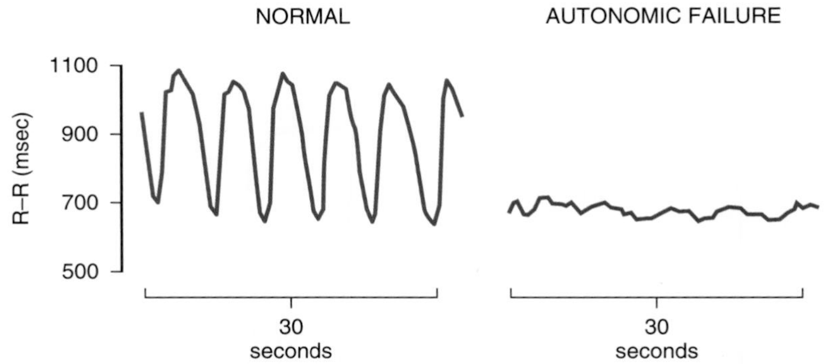

Figure 63-2. Successive electrocardiographic R-R intervals during paced breathing in a normal subject (*left*) and in a patient with autonomic failure (*right*).

The advantage of using continuous noninvasive measurement of finger arterial blood pressure over the conventional sphygmomanometer or the oscillometric measurement method is that the former provides continuous patterns of response that can be visualized and analyzed, not only for blood pressure but also for derived hemodynamic parameters. As a result, three different orthostatic response patterns have been recognized and studied in adults and older people, based on the morphology of the blood pressure recovery after standing[20,22,23]; these three patterns are the quick recovery pattern, which is the normal physiologic response; the slow recovery pattern, which is known to occur in pathologic conditions such as carotid sinus denervation[24] or carotid sinus hypersensitivity[25-27]; and the failure to recover pattern, which is classically observed in patients with autonomic failure.[28] These three "morphologic" patterns of orthostatic blood pressure response have been characterized in research studies using a cluster analysis technique.[29-31]

Noninvasive Autonomic Tests

Heart rate responses to deep breathing (i.e., respiratory sinus arrhythmia) and to the Valsalva maneuver are simple yet informative autonomic tests. They require real-time monitoring of the heart rate. Respiratory sinus arrhythmia is assessed during controlled breathing at a rate of six deep breaths per minute (Figure 63-2). The expiratory/inspiratory (E/I) ratio is calculated by dividing the longest R-R interval by the shorted R-R in inspiration. This E/I ratio decreases progressively with age. Subjects younger than 40 years usually have a ratio less than 1.2 (Figure 63-3). Having the subject blow against a 40 mm Hg pressure for 12 seconds induces a Valsalva maneuver. A 5- to 10-mL syringe can be used as a mouthpiece, which is connected to a sphygmomanometer to monitor pressure. A small leak should be introduced into the system to ensure the subject uses thoracic effort. The increase in intrathoracic pressure produces a transient fall in blood pressure with narrowing of the pulse pressure during phase II (strain), whereas the blood pressure overshoots above baseline values during phase IV (after release) (Figure 63-4). In autonomic failure, the blood pressure continues to fall during phase II and the normal overshoot is absent during phase IV. Thus, appropriate evaluation of the Valsalva response requires continuous recording of blood pressure, which can be accomplished noninvasively with finger plethysmography (Finapres, Portapres, or Task Force Monitor) or tonometry of the radial artery (Colin). Even if the blood pressure cannot be monitored, heart rate responses are useful. The blood pressure changes described previously produce reciprocal baroreflex-mediated changes in the heart rate. The heart rate increases during the hypotensive phase II of the Valsalva maneuver and decreases during the blood pressure overshoot of phase IV. Valsalva ratio is defined as the maximum heart rate during the maneuver divided by the lowest heart rate obtained within 30 seconds of the peak heart rate.[32] As with the E/I ratio, the Valsalva ratio decreases with age and results should be interpreted accordingly (see Figure 63-3). Normal reference ranges have been suggested.[33]

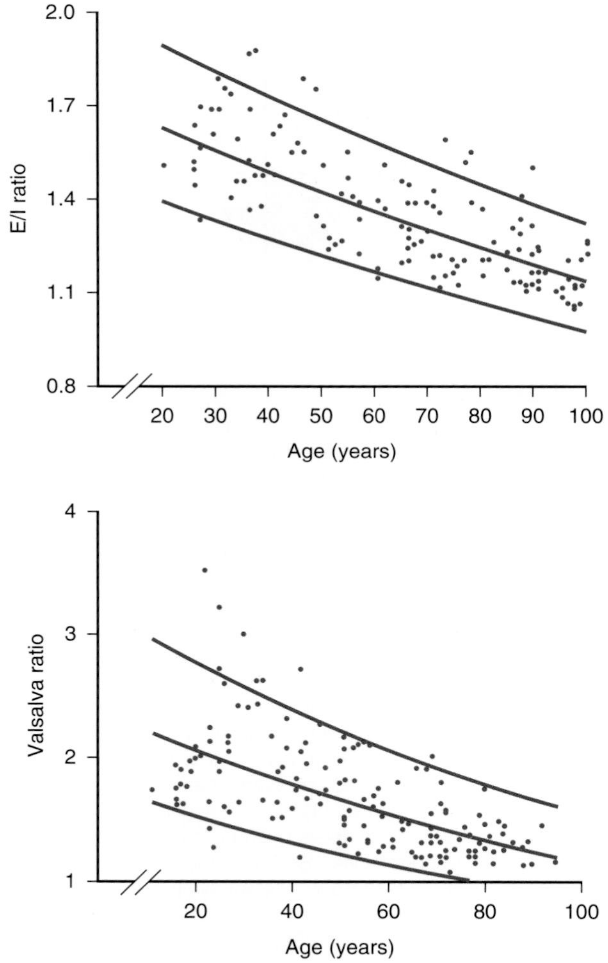

Figure 63-3. Top, Expiratory/inspiratory (E/I) ratio during paced breathing in normal subjects according to age. Linear regression and confidence limits are shown. **Bottom,** Valsalva ratio in normal subjects according to age. Linear regression and confidence limits are shown.

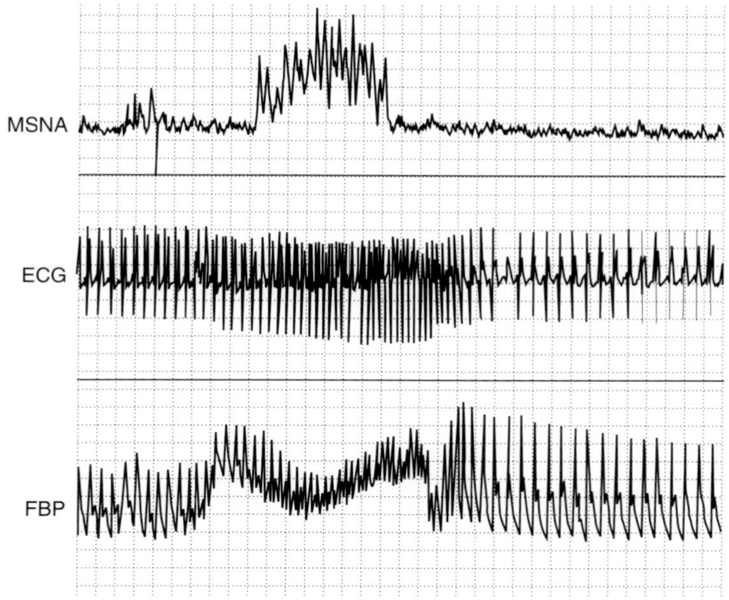

Figure 63-4. Muscle sympathetic nerve activity (MSNA), electrocardiogram (ECG), and finger blood pressure (FBP) during Valsalva maneuver in a normal subject.

Spectral Analysis of Heart Rate and Blood Pressure

Blood pressure and heart rate are kept within a relatively narrow range because of autonomic baroreflex mechanisms. Within this narrow range, however, blood pressure shows substantial variability. Most of this variability is not random but, rather, follows natural rhythmic patterns, which can be studied using spectral analysis techniques. Importantly, these patterns are modulated by the respiratory frequency. In particular, respiration frequency influences heart rate variability, and this interaction is under baroreflex control via the vagus nerves. The "respiratory peak" of heart rate variability, evident in the high-frequency spectrum, can be used to assess cardiac parasympathetic function.

Respiration also modulates blood pressure, but this is mediated through mechanical events and does not reflect autonomic mechanisms and is not affected by autonomic blockade.[34] In contrast, blood pressure exhibits a lower frequency rhythm (Mayer waves). This is mediated in part by sympathetic modulation of vascular tone. There is substantial interindividual variability in the spectral analysis of heart rate and blood pressure, making these methods less suitable for the diagnosis of individual patients with less than severe autonomic impairment. Nonetheless, population studies have shown that impaired heart rate variability as shown by spectral analysis of heart rate is an independent predictor of mortality in patients after myocardial infarction[35] and in patients with diabetes mellitus. Independent of disease status, heart rate variability has been found to be impaired in people with physical frailty.[36]

Assessment of Baroreflex Function

Several methods can be used to quantify the changes in heart rate (or R-R interval) produced by unit change of blood pressure. These methods require the simultaneous monitoring of blood pressure and heart rate. Baroreflex function can be assessed by measuring the reciprocal changes in blood pressure and heart rate that occur spontaneously, or during the phase IV of the Valsalva maneuver. Blood pressure can be increased with phenylephrine or decreased with nitroprusside and the gain of the baroreflex expressed as the change in R-R interval per unit of blood pressure (expressed in msec/mm Hg) during the linear portion of this relationship. Each of these methods provides slightly different normative values of baroreflex gain. It is important to note that changes in blood pressure affect all baroreflex afferents, including carotid sinus and aortic high-pressure receptors and low-pressure receptors located in the venous circulation. The carotid sinus reflex can be selectively investigated by producing positive and negative pressure to the neck, to simulate decreases and increases in intracarotid pressure, respectively. All of these methods rely on instantaneous changes in heart rate, which depend exclusively on the parasympathetic limb of the baroreflex. The sympathetic limb of the baroreflex can be assessed by relating changes in blood pressure to reciprocal changes in muscle sympathetic nerve activity (MSNA).

Biochemical Assessment of Sympathetic Function

Plasma norepinephrine levels provide a useful measure of sympathetic activity. It is particularly useful when measuring acute changes to standard stimuli. For example, upright posture doubles the plasma level in norepinephrine. Patients with autonomic impairment have a blunted response. Basal norepinephrine, however, varies depending on the underlying pathology. It is low in patients with primary autonomic failure and normal or slightly decreased in patients with multiple system atrophy (MSA) (see later discussion). In contrast, patients with volume depletion have an enhanced norepinephrine response to upright posture.

Estimation of Norepinephrine Spillover

Despite the usefulness of plasma norepinephrine measurements, it is noteworthy that only a small percentage of the norepinephrine released by noradrenergic nerves actually reaches the circulation. Most of it is taken back into nerve terminals by the norepinephrine transporter (i.e., reuptake) or is metabolized. Norepinephrine clearance can be measured by infusing a known amount of titrated norepinephrine. During steady-state infusion, it is assumed that clearance of titrated norepinephrine reflects clearance of endogenous norepinephrine. Once clearance is calculated, the norepinephrine appearance rate into the circulation (spillover) can be estimated. A comprehensive review of the advantages and limitations of this technique is beyond the scope of this chapter and can be found elsewhere.[37]

Muscle Sympathetic Nerve Activity

Nerve activity can be recorded directly by introducing a recording electrode into an accessible peripheral nerve. Afferent and efferent fibers can be recorded using this technique. Sympathetic efferent activity can be selectively recorded by careful placement of the electrode. The peroneal nerve at the level of the knee is commonly used to measure postganglionic sympathetic nerve activity. Although there is considerable interindividual variability in MSNA, baseline recordings expressed as sympathetic bursts per minute are highly reproducible in a single individual between different recording sites and when measured on different occasions. MSNA effectively monitors central sympathetic outflow and is tightly modulated by the baroreflex. Stimuli that increase blood pressure by activating central sympathetic outflow produce an increase in MSNA. Conversely, stimuli that increase blood pressure directly, such as an injection of phenylephrine, will produce baroreflex-modulated suppression of MSNA. This recording is also exquisitely sensitive to sympathetic withdrawal. For example, sympathetic activity disappears during neurogenic syncope.[38]

EFFECTS OF AGING ON COMPONENTS OF AUTONOMIC CARDIOVASCULAR CONTROL

Baroreflex Function

There is a progressive decline in baroreflex sensitivity with aging[39] as a result of both vascular and neural deficits. Cardiovagal baroreflex gain (i.e., the reciprocal heart rate changes produced by changes in arterial pressure) declines with age, but the ability of the cardiopulmonary baroreflex to inhibit sympathetic nerve traffic has been reported to be well preserved with age in healthy adults. Hence vagal, but not sympathetic, baroreflex gains vary inversely with individuals' age and their baseline arterial pressures.[33] There is no correlation between sympathetic and vagal baroreflex gains.[40]

Cardiac Parasympathetic Function

Cardiac vagal innervation decreases with age, as clearly shown by a progressive reduction in respiratory sinus arrhythmia (see Figure 63-3). Experimental evidence suggests that long-term physical activity attenuates the decline in cardiovagal baroreflex gain by maintaining neural vagal control,[41] but among older adults, the level of fitness does not prevent the decrease in cardiac vagal function, suggesting that age-related decline in cardiac vagal function cannot be completely prevented by physical activity.[42]

Systemic Sympathetic Function

MSNA increases progressively with age, likely because of increased central nervous system drive (Figure 63-5). Sympathetic nerve traffic increases in a region-specific manner; outflow to skeletal muscle and the gut increases but decreases to the kidney.[43] The increase in central sympathetic outflow results in higher levels of plasma norepinephrine with age, but reduced norepinephrine clearance appears to play a role as well.[44,45] It is suggested that age-related elevations in whole-body and abdominal adiposity can explain why basal MSNA increases with age in healthy humans.[46] The relation between body fat and MSNA is observed in both young and older populations.[47] Tanaka, Davy, and Seals[46] showed that although body mass index (BMI) was similar in groups of younger and older subjects, both total body fatness and abdominal adiposity were greater in the older subjects and were directly related to baseline levels of MSNA. Data indicate that circulating concentrations of leptin are related to both adiposity and MSNA.[48] Thus, age-associated elevations in total and abdominal adiposity may be linked to increases in MSNA, at least in part, via elevations in leptin levels. In contrast to sympathetic neuronal activity, adrenaline secretion from the adrenal medulla is greatly reduced with age, and adrenaline release in response to acute stress is attenuated in older men. Plasma adrenaline concentration remains normal, however, because of reduced plasma clearance.

End-Organ Responsiveness

The number of β-adrenergic receptors in lymphocytes remains steady in older age,[49] and there are higher neurotransmitter levels. However, β-adrenergic responses to norepinephrine are blunted with progressive aging, probably because of β-adrenergic receptor downregulation in response to higher circulating levels of norepinephrine, a defect in G protein receptor complexes and reduced adenyl cyclase activity.[50,51] Depressed β_1 responses lead to impaired cardioacceleration and reduced cardiac contractility. Reduced β_2 responses produce increased vascular tone because α_1 vasoconstriction ability remains unchanged. The combination of age-related vascular stiffening and depressed β-adrenergic function results in reduced arterial baroreflex sensitivity[52] in older subjects.[53,54] Blood pressure in older subjects is sustained by increased peripheral vascular tone, despite depressed cardioacceleration. Because of a higher reliance on vascular resistance, dehydration and vasodilator medications pose a high risk for hypotension and syncope in older subjects. Vasovagal syncope is commonly seen in older adults whose symptoms include presyncope, falls, or syncope.[55] Postjunctional α-mediated vasoconstriction is also impaired in older adults.[56]

Vascular Changes

Aging stiffens blood vessels[57] and alters vasomotor function. In older patients, coronary vasodilation capacity is reduced because of reduced nitric oxide release by the senescent endothelium. Conversely, endothelin release by the endothelium is increased in older people, promoting vasoconstriction.[58] These alterations increase susceptibility to myocardial ischemia, particularly during increased demand stresses such as tachyarrhythmias,[59] and can also impair cerebral autoregulation, increasing susceptibility to syncope. Other age-dependent cardiovascular alterations that can increase predisposition to syncope are increased left ventricular afterload and myocyte hypertrophy. These alterations lead to impaired diastolic filling and chronic ischemia that may predispose patients to cardiac arrhythmias and decrease ventricular volume that may manifest as syncope. Decreased preload volume, precipitated by vasodilators, dehydration, or blood pooling can dramatically reduce cardiac output and precipitate syncope. Susceptibility to atrial fibrillation increases with age because of reductions in pacemaker cells, progressive fibrosis of the cardiac conduction system, and concomitant cardiovascular diseases that alter atrial morphology. In older patients, impaired diastolic filling and a reduction of up to 50% in cardiac output can develop during atrial fibrillation and lead to syncope and unexplained falls.[60]

Neuroendocrine Changes

Plasma renin and aldosterone levels fall with age,[61,62] and atrial natriuretic peptide increases fivefold to ninefold.[63] The vasopressin response to hypotension may also be reduced.[64] These changes

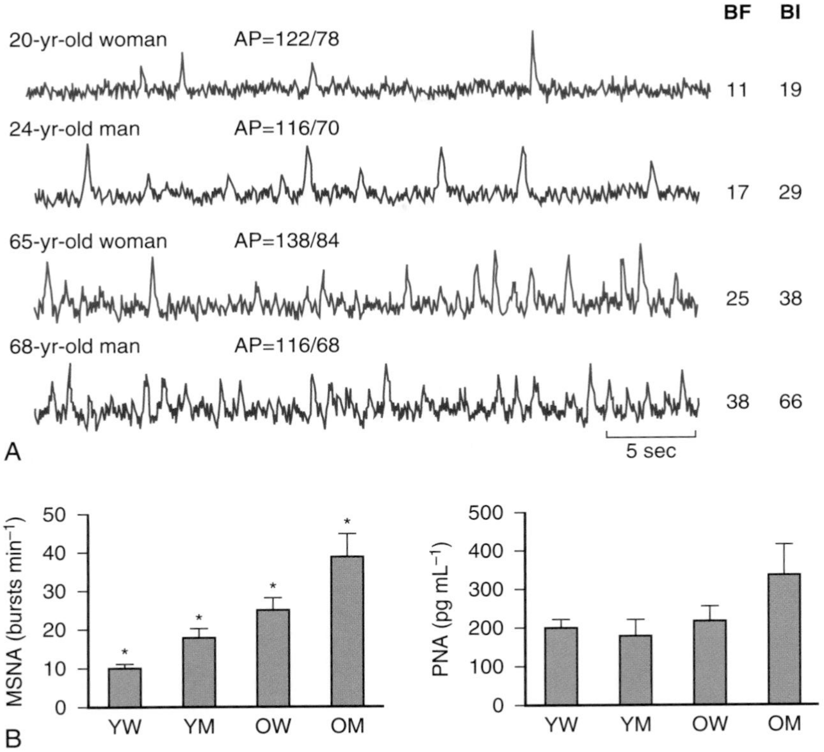

Figure 63-5. Age-associated increases in muscle sympathetic nerve activity (MSNA). A, MSNA from four healthy adult humans under supine resting conditions *(top to bottom):* young woman, young man, older woman, older man. MSNA burst frequency (BF; bursts min^{-1}) and burst incidence (BI; bursts [100 heart beats]$^{-1}$) are higher in the neurograms of the older adults in both sexes. However, the female subjects demonstrate lower MSNA than the males at each age. **B,** Mean ± SEM; values for MSNA in four groups of subjects: young women (YW), young men (YM), older women (OW), and older men (OM). MSNA was at least twice as great in the older compared with the younger subjects of the same sex. At each age, however, MSNA was significantly lower in the women. These age and sex differences in MSNA were not reflected in the corresponding antecubital venous plasma noradrenaline concentrations. *$P < .05$ versus all other groups. *AP,* Arterial blood pressure; *PNA,* plasma noradrenaline concentration. *(From Seals DR, Esler MD: Human ageing and the sympathoadrenal system. J Physiol 528:407–417, 2000).*

make sodium and water conservation less effective and intravascular volume depletion more frequent, thus increasing the tendency for syncope. In addition, many older people have an impaired thirst response to increases in osmolality and do not consume sufficient fluids to prevent hypovolemia.

EFFECTS OF AGING ON AUTONOMIC RESPONSE TO STRESS

The most frequent autonomic stress is the cardiovascular adaptation to upright posture and other physiologically induced changes in intravascular volume. Vascular and neurogenic dysfunction and a host of medications can cause orthostatic hypotension in older patients. In the Cardiovascular Health study,[65] the prevalence of orthostatic hypotension was 18% in subjects aged 65 years or older, although only 2% reported dizziness on standing. There was a modest association with systolic hypertension when supine, with carotid stenosis greater than 50%, and with the use of oral hypoglycemic agents; a weak association with the use of β-blockers; and no association with other antihypertensive drugs. In other reports, however, as expected, the use of antihypertensive medications was significantly related to postural hypotension in older people,[66] and discontinuing antihypertensive medications led to an improvement of orthostatic hypotension.[67]

Orthostatic Hypotension

Older people have impaired defenses against the fluid shifts that normally accompany upright posture; therefore, they have a lower threshold for developing symptomatic orthostatic hypotension compared with younger people. A variety of symptoms develop with a reduction in blood flow to the brain. Typically, patients complain of visual disturbances (e.g., blurring, tunneling, or darkening of vision), dizziness, light-headedness, giddiness, feeling faint, and a dull neck and shoulder ache (coat hanger pain). When orthostatic hypotension is pronounced and cerebral blood flow decreases below a critical level (approximately 25 mL/min per 100 g), syncope (i.e., loss of consciousness) may occur.

A decrease in baroreceptor sensitivity is probably involved in the mild, frequent postural hypotension seen in older people. One study, for example, showed a diminished response to tilt (a baroreceptor-mediated response) but not to non–baroreceptor-mediated stimuli, such as the cold pressor test or isometric exercise.[68] The reduced baroreceptor response in older people (when compared with younger controls) was seen in both hypertensive and normotensive subjects. Insults that would be compensated for in the young may induce symptomatic hypotension in older people. For example, drug-induced orthostatic hypotension is the cause of recurrent dizzy spells or syncope in 12% to 15% of older patients and should always be suspected.[69] Diuretics, calcium antagonists, angiotensin-converting enzyme (ACE) inhibitors, and nitrates are frequently prescribed for older patients for the management of hypertension, congestive heart failure, or ischemic heart disease. Other pharmacologic agents frequently associated with orthostatic hypotension include phenothiazines, antidepressants (including selective serotonin reuptake inhibitors), treatments for Parkinson disease (PD), antipsychotic agents, sedatives, and narcotics. It is also important to note that the more types of these drugs an older person is taking, the greater is the risk of orthostatic hypotension.[67]

Similarly, prolonged bed rest is a common complication of ill health in older people and an important cause of cardiovascular deconditioning. Several mechanisms contribute to decreased orthostatic tolerance and syncope after prolonged bed rest.[70] Bed rest reduces extracellular fluid volume, and the skeletal muscle wasting impairs the lower limb muscle pump that usually facilitates venous return in the upright posture. Under normal conditions, important mechanical adjustments to counteract orthostatic pooling of the blood are the muscle and respiratory pumps. Skeletal muscle tone has critical bearing on the volume of blood displaced into the legs when standing. Because intramuscular pressure is decreased after prolonged bed rest, venous pooling occurs and venous return to the heart is easily compromised in the standing posture. Thus, skeletal muscle atrophy caused by prolonged bed rest should be considered as a primary or aggravating factor in any patient with symptoms of light-headedness on standing or documented orthostatic hypotension. If the problem persists after adequate measures are taken, a pathologic impairment of autonomic function should be considered. The occurrence of orthostatic hypotension in older people is predictive of mortality.[71] A study of 3522 Japanese-American men, aged 71 to 93 years, found that orthostatic hypotension, defined as a decrease in systolic blood pressure by 20 mm Hg or a decrease in diastolic blood pressure by 10 mm Hg, was present in 7%, increased with age, and was an independent risk factor for all cause mortality.[71]

Frailty in older adults is characterized by cumulative decline in many physiologic systems leading to decreased physiologic reserve and vulnerability to stressors.[72] As such, studies have suggested that orthostatic hypotension could be a marker of frailty. A study showed that the physical frailty phenotype was associated with impaired orthostatic heart rate response and a tendency toward lower systolic blood pressure recoverability during the 30-second period after standing.[73] Using a frailty index approach, Rockwood, Howlett, and Rockwood suggested that orthostatic hypotension might be a marker of the system dysregulation seen in frailty.[74]

Postprandial and Heat-Induced Hypotension

Postprandial hypotension and heat-induced hypotension are common causes of falls and syncope in older people.[75,76] In normal subjects, eating, especially carbohydrates, leads to splanchnic vasodilation and hot weather produces cutaneous vasodilation, but there is little change in arterial pressure because of a compensatory increase in sympathetic vasoconstrictor outflow. In older people, as in patients with autonomic failure, both eating and hot weather significantly lower blood pressure (even in the supine position) because these patients cannot compensate for the vasodilation with an appropriate increase in sympathetic outflow.[77,78] Among older residents of nursing homes, 24% to 36% have a 20 mm Hg or greater fall in systolic blood pressure within 75 minutes after eating a meal.[79] In patients with autonomic failure, postprandial hypotension occurs within 30 minutes of meal ingestion, lasts about 1.5 to 2 hours, and can be profound; blood pressure can fall 50 to 70 mm Hg. Thus, it is important to consider the timing of meals when measuring blood pressure in these patients. The initial syncopal episode in patients with chronic autonomic failure is frequently triggered by postprandial hypotension.

DISORDERS OF THE AUTONOMIC NERVOUS SYSTEM IN OLDER PEOPLE

Neurally Mediated Syncopal Syndromes

The most frequent cause of hypotension and syncope in otherwise normal subjects is neurally mediated syncope, also known as reflex syncope. This umbrella term encompasses carotid sinus hypersensitivity, vasovagal syncope, and a number of benign syncopal syndromes, which are triggered by specific actions such as swallowing, voiding, defecating, laughing, weightlifting, and brass instrument playing.[13] Syncope triggered by anxiety or emotion (e.g., fainting at the sight of blood) also fits into this category, as does syncope after vigorous exercise. It is very important, however, to distinguish between syncope during exercise and syncope after exercise, as the former should not be considered a reflex syncope (and needs full cardiac workup). Neurocardiogenic syncope is generally, although not exclusively, observed in patients with no evidence of structural heart disease. Prodromal symptoms include dizziness, blurred vision, nausea, an increasingly hot feeling, and diaphoresis. This syncope results from acute vasodilation and bradycardia.

Neurally mediated syncope is an acute hemodynamic reaction produced by a sudden change in autonomic nervous system activity.[80] The normal pattern of autonomic outflow that maintains blood pressure in the standing position (increased sympathetic and decreased parasympathetic activity) is acutely reversed. Parasympathetic outflow to the sinus node of the heart increases, producing bradycardia, while sympathetic outflow to blood vessels is reduced, resulting in profound vasodilation.

Classic neurally mediated syncopal syndromes are triggered after compression of carotid baroreceptors in the neck (carotid sinus syncope),[38] following rapid emptying of a distended bladder (micturition syncope)[81] or distention of the gastrointestinal tract.[82] Glossopharyngeal or trigeminal neuralgia can induce syncope by a similar mechanism,[83,84] but both are rare. In several clinical types of neurally mediated syncope, the trigger locus is easily identified, but frequently neurally mediated syncope occurs with no obvious trigger. Although in these cases the source of abnormal afferent signals was believed to be sensory receptors in the heart (i.e., neurocardiogenic or "ventricular" syncope),[85,86] neurally mediated syncope has recently been induced in patients with heart transplants in whom the ventricle is likely to be denervated.[87] Perhaps sensory receptors in heart transplant patients are in the arterial tree rather than the ventricle. Similarly, the threshold to trigger neurally mediated syncope can be lowered by a reduction in cardiac preload caused by reduced intravascular volume or excessive venous pooling. Intravascular volume depletion is common in older people because conservation of sodium and water is less effective, renin and aldosterone levels fall, atrial natriuretic peptide increases, and the vasopressin response to hypotension may be reduced. Moreover, many older adults have an impaired thirst response to increases in osmolality and are prone to hypovolemia, particularly during febrile illnesses. Excessive venous pooling occurs postprandially in the splanchnic circulation, in the skin during exposure to heat, and in the lower limbs because of muscle atrophy when standing after prolonged periods of bed rest, significantly increasing susceptibility to syncope.

Despite the diverse trigger mechanisms of these different types of neurally mediated syncope, the efferent reflex response is remarkably similar. There is an increase in parasympathetic efferent activity to the sinus node, producing bradycardia or even a few seconds of sinus arrest, and a decrease in sympathetic activity responsible, at least in part, for the fall in blood pressure.

Bradycardia is not the only or even the main cause of hypotension because neither atropine nor a ventricular pacemaker (both of which prevent bradycardia) is able to prevent hypotension and syncope. Blood pressure falls mainly because of vasodilation. The mechanisms responsible for vasodilation are not completely understood. Studies using microneurography and measurements of circulating norepinephrine have shown that sympathetic efferent activity decreases.[88-90] Sympathetic "withdrawal," however, seems an incomplete explanation for profound vasodilation. Norepinephrine fails to increase, but vasopressin, endothelin-1, and angiotensin II vasoconstrictor peptides, important to maintain blood pressure (which should partially compensate for the fall in sympathetic activity), increase normally during neurally mediated syncope.[89] To explain the profound fall in blood pressure, β-mediated vasodilation induced by a rise in adrenaline has been postulated.[91] Nitric oxide–mediated vasodilation due to a rise in cholinergic activity may be involved.[80] In summary, current understanding of neurally mediated syncope shows inappropriate reduction in sympathetic nerve activity and norepinephrine release. There is an appropriate increase in epinephrine, angiotensin II, vasopressin, and endothelin release, and preliminary evidence suggests that nitric oxide synthesis is activated.

Baroreflex Failure

The most common cause of baroreflex failure is iatrogenic damage during neck surgery or radiation therapy of neural structures that carry afferent input from the baroreceptors. Atheroma can also cause baroreceptor failure.[92] Neurologic disorders involving the nucleus tractus solitarius, where these afferents have their first synapse, can also produce baroreflex failure. In a few cases, the underlying cause is not found. Baroreflex function is impaired in essential hypertension and can be transmitted as a genetic trait.[93] It is not clear if these cases of baroreflex failure of unknown cause represent the extreme of the spectrum of baroreflex impairment in essential hypertension. Ketch and coworkers describe "four faces of baroreflex failure": hypertensive crisis, volatile hypertension, orthostatic tachycardia, and malignant vagotonia,[94] the most common of which is volatile hypertension or severe labile hypertension. Wide fluctuations of blood pressure are observed, with systolic blood pressure ranging from 50 to 280 mm Hg. Other symptoms that may be observed include hypotension, headache, diaphoresis, and emotional instability. The hypertensive crises are accompanied by tachycardia and are to the result of sympathetic surges, as documented by notable increases in plasma norepinephrine. Treatment with sympatholytics may provide some benefit, attenuating these surges of hypertension and tachycardia, but adequate blood pressure regulation is seldom achieved in the absence of functional baroreflexes. Of interest is that virtually all reported cases are due to bilateral lesions, whereas unilateral lesions are usually clinically silent. This clinical observation underscores the redundancy of the baroreflex system and its importance in cardiovascular regulation.

Chronic Autonomic Failure

Autonomic failure is divided into primary and secondary forms. Primary autonomic failure is caused by a degenerative process affecting central autonomic pathways (MSA) or peripheral autonomic neurons (pure autonomic failure). Secondary autonomic failure results from destruction of peripheral autonomic neurons in disorders, such as diabetes, amyloidosis, and other neuropathies, and very rarely by an enzymatic defect in catecholamine synthesis (dopamine β-hydroxylase deficiency). In chronic autonomic failure (either primary or secondary), orthostatic hypotension and syncope are caused by impaired vasoconstriction and reduced intravascular volume. Vasoconstriction is deficient because of reduced baroreflex-mediated norepinephrine release from postganglionic sympathetic nerve terminals and low circulating levels of angiotensin II caused by impaired secretion of renin. In patients with autonomic failure and central nervous system dysfunction (i.e., MSA), impaired endothelin and vasopressin release also contribute to deficient vasoconstriction in the standing position.

Primary Autonomic Failure

Primary autonomic failure includes several neurodegenerative diseases of unknown cause: pure autonomic failure (PAF), in which autonomic impairment (i.e., orthostatic hypotension, bladder, and sexual dysfunction) occurs alone; MSA (previously designated Shy-Drager syndrome), in which autonomic failure is combined with an extrapyramidal and/or cerebellar movement disorder; PD, in which autonomic failure is combined with an extrapyramidal movement disorder; and diffuse Lewy body disease (DLBD), in which autonomic failure is combined with an extrapyramidal movement disorder and severe cognitive impairment.

Recent findings suggest that the same neurodegenerative process underlies MSA, PD, DLBD, and PAF, as accumulation of α-synuclein in neuronal cytoplasmic inclusions occurs in all of these disorders.[95] A gene encoding for α-synuclein, a neuronal protein of unknown function, is mutated in autosomal dominant PD.[96] Nonfamilial PD does not have the mutation, but α-synuclein accumulates in Lewy bodies in these patients, suggesting a toxic role for aggregates of this protein.[97] It is interesting that cytoplasmic inclusions in MSA also stain positive for α-synuclein,[98] and Lewy bodies in PAF are strongly α-synuclein positive.[99] Thus, abnormalities in the expression or structure of α-synuclein or associated proteins may cause degeneration of catecholamine-containing neurons. α-Synuclein, therefore, is an important component of intraneuronal inclusions in PAF, PD, DLBD, and MSA neurodegenerative disorders, all of which affect the autonomic nervous system to a variable degree.[95] Thus, these disorders are best classified as α-synucleinopathies. It is not surprising, therefore, that there is overlap in the clinical presentation of these disorders, and the clinical differences may reflect the type of deposits (forming Lewy bodies or not) and the localization of these deposits within the nervous system. These similarities and differences are discussed later.

Pure Autonomic Failure

PAF is a sporadic, adult-onset, slowly progressive degeneration of the autonomic nervous system characterized by orthostatic hypotension, bladder and sexual dysfunction, and no other neurologic deficits. Neuropathologic reports of patients with pure autonomic failure showed α-synuclein–positive intraneuronal cytoplasmic inclusions (Lewy bodies) in brainstem nuclei and peripheral autonomic ganglia.[99,100] These patients are otherwise normal, and their prognosis is relatively good. Complications are usually those related to falls.

Multiple System Atrophy

Multiple system atrophy is a term introduced by Graham and Oppenheimer in 1969 to describe a group of patients with a disorder of unknown cause affecting extrapyramidal, pyramidal, cerebellar, and autonomic pathways. MSA includes the disorders previously designated striatonigral degeneration (SND), sporadic olivopontocerebellar atrophy (OPCA), and Shy-Drager syndrome (SDS). The discovery in 1989 of glial cytoplasmic inclusions in the brain of patients with MSA provided a pathologic marker for the disorder (akin to Lewy bodies in PD) and confirmed that SND, OPCA, and SDS are the same disease with different clinical expression.[101] MSA is a progressive neurodegenerative disease of undetermined cause that occurs sporadically and causes parkinsonism, cerebellar, pyramidal autonomic, and urologic dysfunction in any combination.[102,103] Given the ages of onset, many people with MSA also have cognitive impairment, which can make them an awkward fit in clinics geared more toward diagnosing and treating motoric and autonomic dysfunction. The extent to which co-occurrence might represent a causal relationship remains unclear.

Because parkinsonism is the most frequent motor deficit in MSA, these patients are regularly misdiagnosed as suffering from PD. Data from PD brain banks showed how frequently the diagnosis of PD was incorrect; up to 10% of these brains turn out to have MSA.[104] Indeed, even case 1 of James Parkinson's original description (1817), upon which much of his description of *paralysis agitans* was based, was probably suffering from MSA.

Life expectancy among people who have MSA is shorter compared with life expectancy of people with PD. Ben-Shlomo and colleagues[105] analyzed 433 published cases of pathologically proven MSA over a 100-year period. Mean age of onset was 54 years (range, 31 to 78) and survival 6 years (range, 0.5 to 24). Survival was unaffected by gender, parkinsonian, or pyramidal features, or whether the patient was classified as having SND or OPCA. Survival analysis showed a secular trend from a median duration of 5 years for publications between 1887 and 1970 to 7 years between 1991 and 1994. These figures may be biased toward the worst cases, however.

Parkinson Disease

Autonomic dysfunction in PD is rarely as severe as in patients with MSA. A subgroup of patients with PD, however, have severe autonomic failure even early in the course of the disease. In most cases, autonomic failure occurs late in the course of the illness and is associated with levodopa and dopamine agonist therapy. In patients with PD, Lewy bodies are found in central and in peripheral autonomic neurons, and autonomic dysfunction in this disorder may be caused by both preganglionic and postganglionic neuronal dysfunction.

Diffuse Lewy Body Disease

The clinical presentation of patients with DLBD is that of PD, but dementia often dominates the clinical picture. Autonomic dysfunction is frequent in dementia with Lewy bodies, and the severity is intermediate between that of MSA and PD.[106]

Differential Diagnosis Among the α-Synucleinopathies

During the early stages of MSA, autonomic deficits may be the sole clinical manifestation, thus resembling PAF, but after a variable period of time, sometimes several years, extrapyramidal or cerebellar deficits or both invariably develop. In PD, extrapyramidal motor problems are the presenting feature, but later in the disease process, patients may suffer severe autonomic failure, making the clinical distinction with MSA difficult. Complicating the distinction further, some MSA cases display motor deficits before autonomic failure is apparent. In clinical practice, all of these possibilities lead to two main diagnostic problems. First, it cannot be determined whether a patient who has autonomic failure as the only clinical finding and is believed to have PAF will develop more widespread nonautonomic neuronal damage and turn out to have MSA. Second, it may be difficult to establish if a patient with autonomic failure and a parkinsonian movement disorder has PD or MSA. Clinically, the classic parkinsonian resting tremor of unilateral predominance is rarely seen in patients with MSA, in whom bradykinesia and rigidity predominate. Also, with rare exceptions, patients with MSA do not respond as well to antiparkinsonian medications, and the progression of disease is faster.

In addition to clinical criteria, several tests have been used to distinguish between PD, PAF, and MSA. For example, vasopressin release in response to hypotension and growth hormone secretion in response to clonidine are blunted in MSA but preserved in PAF and PD, because brainstem-hypothalamic-pituitary pathways are only affected in MSA.[107-109]

Plasma norepinephrine concentration while supine is frequently normal in MSA but low in PAF because postganglionic neurons are normal in MSA.[110] A sphincter electromyogram shows denervation in MSA because the Onuf nucleus in segments S2-S4 of the spinal cord is affected in MSA but is normal in PD.[111]

There are also important differences in cardiovascular control between MSA, PAF, and PD with autonomic failure. Although patients with MSA have substantial central nervous system degeneration, the brainstem centers where sympathetic tone originates (most likely the rostroventrolateral medulla) and distal pathways are intact. In support of this postulate, supine plasma norepinephrine is normal or slightly decreased in MSA, but this residual sympathetic activity is not baroreflex-responsive, hence their inability to maintain upright blood pressure. Furthermore, interruption of this residual sympathetic activity with the ganglion blocker trimethaphan leads to a profound decrease in supine blood pressure in MSA. In contrast, supine plasma norepinephrine is very low in PAF, and treatment with trimethaphan produces small or no changes in blood pressure, indicating that the lesion is distal to brainstem centers.[112]

Similarly, sympathetic cardiac innervation is selectively affected in PD and PAF but is intact in MSA. Several studies using single photon emission computed tomography (SPECT) imaging with ^{123}I metaiodobenzylguanidine (MIBG)[113-115] and positron emission tomography (PET) with 6-[^{18}F] fluorodopamine[116] have shown abnormal cardiac sympathetic innervation in patients with PD, while it was normal in patients with MSA.[117] In PD, reduced myocardial sympathetic innervation as revealed by MIBG scintigraphy is associated with clinical symptoms of autonomic impairment and this association is more pronounced in men than in women.[118] More recent evidence suggests that the autonomic dysfunction is generalized and predominantly preganglionic in MSA and postganglionic in PD.[119]

Brain Imaging

In patients with MSA, magnetic resonance imaging (MRI) of the brain can frequently detect abnormalities of striatum, cerebellum, and brainstem.[120-124] Striatal abnormalities in MSA include putaminal atrophy and putaminal hypointensity (relative to pallidum) on T2-weighted images and slit-like signal change at the posterolateral putaminal margin. The striking slit-like signal change in the lateral putamen corresponds to the area showing the most pronounced microgliosis and astrogliosis, and the highest amount of ferric iron, at necropsy. This abnormal intensity is frequently asymmetric (Figure 63-6).

Infratentorial abnormalities in patients with MSA seen on MRI include atrophy and signal change in the pons and middle cerebellar peduncle. The pontine base and the middle cerebellar peduncle may appear as high signal intensity on T2-weighted images and as low intensity on T1, suggesting degeneration and demyelination.

Most if not all of these tests produce results that are frequently ambiguous, and accurate methods to distinguish PD from other diseases with extrapyramidal involvement, particularly MSA, are needed. It is argued that because the diagnosis of

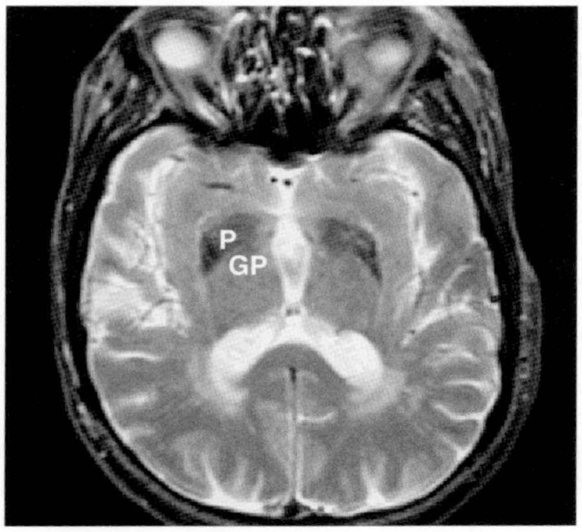

Figure 63-6. Moderate putaminal (P) hypointensity relative to the globus pallidus (GP) in a patient with parkinsonian multiple system atrophy (MSA-P), axial T2 weighting, 1.5 tesla MRI.

MSA during life is based on clinical features, it can only be made with possible or probable certainty and that definite diagnosis requires pathologic confirmation. Routine brain MRI has some diagnostic value when the clinical diagnosis of parkinsonism is uncertain.[125]

Treatment

There are no known treatments targeted at the underlying degenerative disorder or therapies that will modify the course of any of these disorders. Treatment outcomes of the motor abnormalities in MSA patients remain dismal. As mentioned earlier, these patients often do not respond to antiparkinsonian medications. Of the autonomic abnormalities, orthostatic hypotension is often treated successfully. An outline of treatment strategies is included later in this chapter.

Secondary Autonomic Failure

Cholinergic Failure

Botulism and the Lambert-Eaton myasthenic syndrome impair the release of acetylcholine in both somatic and autonomic nerves, producing muscle weakness and cholinergic dysautonomia. Botulism is an ascending, predominantly motor polyneuropathy with cranial nerve involvement, beginning 12 to 36 hours after ingesting food contaminated with the neurotoxins of the anaerobic bacteria *Clostridium botulinum*. The toxin impairs the presynaptic calcium-associated release of acetylcholine, leading to symptoms of cholinergic failure: dry eyes, dry mouth, blurred vision, dizziness, paralytic ileus, urinary retention, and anhidrosis. Treatment is supportive; respiratory failure and cardiac arrhythmia can occur. Recovery is often protracted, with autonomic dysfunction lasting as long as 6 months after onset.

The Lambert-Eaton myasthenic syndrome is an autoimmune disorder, most commonly paraneoplastic, associated with small cell lung carcinoma. Autoantibodies to voltage-gated calcium channels, most commonly the P/Q type, have been found in these patients. Electrophysiologic and pharmacologic studies have reproduced the functional effects of the Lambert-Eaton myasthenic syndrome in passively immunized mice and confirmed that anti-P/Q-type calcium channel antibodies inhibit transmitter release from autonomic neurons and are likely to be responsible for the autonomic dysfunction in this syndrome. Dry mouth, erectile dysfunction, proximal muscle weakness, and depressed tendon reflexes are characteristic. The risk of developing cancer is estimated to be 62% over the 2 years following diagnosis; this risk decreases over time.[126,127] Autonomic dysfunction is worse in older patients with a carcinoma[128] but improves with treatment of the underlying carcinoma.[129]

Pandysautonomias

Pandysautonomias involve both sympathetic and parasympathetic neurons. Pandysautonomic neuropathies can be divided into preganglionic (most frequently demyelinating) and postganglionic (most frequently axonopathic). These neuropathies are acute or subacute with gradual but often incomplete recovery of autonomic function.[130,131] Patients have blurred vision, dry eyes and mouth, nausea, vomiting, abdominal pain, diarrhea, constipation, and loss of sweating.

The acute pandysautonomias are uncommon in older people and affect almost exclusively healthy young individuals. Those with a protracted course and incomplete recovery are, more frequently, postganglionic axonal.[130,132] The preganglionic demyelinating pandysautonomia with variable involvement of the somatic nervous system is part of a spectrum ranging from pure pandysautonomia—with minimal somatic deficits—to classic Guillain-Barré syndrome[133] and profound muscle weakness and may have a better outcome than the postganglionic axonopathic pandysautonomia. The cause of these pandysautonomias is unknown but a postinfectious or other immune-mediated process is postulated. In some cases they are paraneoplastic,[134,135] and many patients have autoantibodies to ganglionic acetylcholine receptors. Patients with anti-Hu antibody-related paraneoplastic syndrome having progressive dysautonomia have also been described, both with acute onset and a subacute course of neurologic symptoms. Autonomic symptoms may improve with treatment of the underlying cancer.

Signs of autonomic hyperactivity or hypoactivity are present in one third to two thirds of patients with the acute inflammatory demyelinating polyradiculoneuropathy or Guillain-Barré syndrome.[136,137] Most cases have mild autonomic hypoactivity with resting tachycardia because of decreased parasympathetic activity and ileus. Urinary retention is less common. With autonomic hyperactivity, sweating is excessive and there can be alternating hypertension or hypotension and alternating bradycardia or tachycardia. Mortality is increased with significant dysautonomia.[138]

Chronic small fiber (postganglionic) neuropathies can be metabolic (e.g., diabetes or amyloidosis), inherited (e.g., Fabry disease), or infectious (e.g., HIV). Autonomic dysfunction in both amyloid and diabetes tends to involve all organs. Autonomic failure (orthostatic hypotension and a fixed heart rate) may be the presenting feature. More frequently, patients show a mixed pattern of distal small fiber autonomic and sensory neuropathy or predominantly small fiber sensory neuropathy with only mild autonomic involvement.[134,139] The autonomic symptoms may accompany, precede, or follow the somatic neuropathy.[140,141] Alternating diarrhea and constipation, explosive diarrhea, urinary retention, anhidrosis, or gustatory hyperhidrosis may be present. Erectile dysfunction is the most common autonomic symptom in diabetes,[142,143] and sudomotor changes may be the earliest sign in diabetic neuropathy.[144-147]

Pandysautonomias are commonly associated with the acquired immunodeficiency syndrome (AIDS),[148-150] often combined with a distal sensory polyneuropathy.[151,152] Autonomic symptoms such as bladder and sexual dysfunction are present in up to 60% of patients.

Mild, chronic (or subacute) autonomic neuropathies or ganglionopathies, affecting both sympathetic and parasympathetic fibers, are sometimes associated with Sjögren syndrome.[134] Tonic pupils, sudomotor dysfunction, and cases of severe pandysautonomia have been reported.[153]

Autoimmune Autonomic Ganglionopathy

Acetylcholine is the neurotransmitter in sympathetic and parasympathetic autonomic ganglia, activating nicotinic receptors. Antibodies against the alpha-3 subunit of the ganglionic acetylcholine receptor (α3-AChR Ab) have been identified and proposed to play a causal role in cases of dysautonomia.[154,155] Clinical presentation may be typical of classic acute pandysautonomia following a viral type of illness or can be indistinguishable from pure autonomic failure. Reports show complete (but in some cases transient) recovery in a few patients with acute pandysautonomia that were treated early with intravenous immunoglobulin therapy[156,157] or plasma exchange.[158,159] Although encouraging, it is difficult to establish a definitive treatment of this condition based on case reports, and it is likely that some form of immunosuppression will be needed to manage these patients. Nonetheless, the reports do provide preliminary evidence of the causal role of these antibodies in causing autonomic impairment.

MANAGEMENT OF ORTHOSTATIC HYPOTENSION

Pathophysiology-Guided Therapy

Maintenance of blood pressure in the standing position requires a sustained increase in peripheral vascular resistance (i.e., vasoconstriction) and adequate intravascular volume. In patients with chronic autonomic failure, orthostatic hypotension is due to deficient baroreflex-mediated vasoconstriction and also because of reduced intravascular volume and consequently reduced venous return.

Deficient Vasoconstriction

In autonomic failure, vasoconstriction is mainly deficient because of reduced baroreflex-mediated norepinephrine release from postganglionic sympathetic nerve terminals and lack of activation of postsynaptic α-adrenergic receptors in the vascular wall. Also contributing to blunted orthostatic vasoconstriction in these patients are low circulating levels of angiotensin II resulting from deficient renal sympathetic innervation and reduced secretion of renin. In patients with autonomic failure and central nervous system dysfunction (e.g., MSA), impaired endothelin and vasopressin release are also likely to contribute to the deficient vasoconstriction.

Reduced Intravascular Volume

There are several reasons for reduced extracellular fluid volume in patients with autonomic failure. Impaired sympathetic activation directly decreases sodium reabsorption in the kidney.[160] It also inhibits renin secretion so that aldosterone is low, which again contributes to a decrease in renal sodium reabsorption. Other hormones involved in fluid homeostasis are also impaired in autonomic failure. For example, hypophyseal vasopressin release in response to hypotension is markedly reduced in patients with autonomic failure caused by central nervous system lesions (e.g., MSA). Low vasopressin levels prevent water conservation, contributing to intravascular volume depletion.

Anemia is a common complication of autonomic failure, likely the result of inadequate erythropoietin levels.[161-163] Although basal erythropoietin synthesis is not reduced in autonomic failure, the increase in erythropoietin synthesis in response to anemic hypoxia appears to be blunted in these patients. The modest decrease in red blood cell mass is another factor contributing to reduced intravascular volume.

Initial Clinical Management of Orthostatic Hypotension

A complete medication history should be obtained to identify and possibly eliminate agents that can cause orthostatic hypotension. Polypharmacy is a common occurrence in older patients, and many classes of medications can contribute to hypotension, including antihypertensives, diuretics, antimuscarinics, and treatments for PD. Levodopa and dopamine agonists exacerbate orthostatic hypotension, especially during the first weeks of treatment. Gradual dosage increases when initiating therapy or dose reductions in established patients can minimize this adverse effect. Dietary sodium and water intake should be maximally increased in these patients. Patients also should be instructed not to lie prone. Lying flat when sleeping results in accelerated sodium loss from pressure natriuresis and reduced renin release, leading to loss of intravascular volume. This leads to overnight volume depletion and worsening of orthostatic hypotension in the morning. Elevating the head of the bed by 6 to 9 inches may be helpful although the evidence for this in patients with autonomic failure is poor. In healthy volunteers, there is some evidence that sleeping with the bed tilted by 18 inches reduces the drop in blood pressure on standing.[164] The beneficial effect of nocturnal head and torso elevation results from lessening supine hypertension, thus reducing "pressure natriuresis" by the kidney and, in some patients, by increasing renin secretion.

Patients should be educated about the hypotensive effects of alcohol, large meals, hot weather, and after physical exertion. Isotonic exercise produces less hypotension than isometric exercise, and exercise in a swimming pool prevents blood pressure reductions. In patients with autonomic failure, eating can significantly lower blood pressure because the splanchnic vasodilation induced by food is not appropriately compensated by vasoconstriction in other vascular beds. In some patients, hypotension only occurs postprandially. Thus, patients should be advised to eat frequent, small meals with low carbohydrate content and to minimize their alcohol intake. Caffeine taken with breakfast may be helpful as it has some vasoconstrictor actions, but it is also a diuretic and these opposing effects may negate its usefulness. Hot baths should be avoided, and patients should be especially careful during warm weather because heat-induced vasodilation still occurs, but sympathetic vasoconstriction is impaired. Straining at stool with a closed glottis (i.e., producing a Valsalva maneuver), playing wind instruments, and singing can be particularly dangerous for patients with hypotension. A high-fiber diet is encouraged to prevent constipation. The use of knee-high compressive stockings is not effective, but waist-high stockings with grade 2 compression (grade 2 is equivalent to 30 to 40 mm Hg pressure) and/or abdominal binders may be an effective, albeit sometimes poorly tolerated, countermeasure for orthostatic hypotension. This is because the greatest proportion of blood pooling occurs within the splanchnic circulation.[165]

Pharmacologic Treatment of Orthostatic Hypotension

Only patients with symptomatic orthostatic hypotension should be treated pharmacologically. Perhaps because of adaptive cerebral autoregulatory changes, some patients with autonomic failure tolerate very low arterial pressures when standing without experiencing symptoms of cerebral hypoperfusion. Blood pressure levels change throughout the day and from one day to another. Thus, the patient's normal cycle of blood pressure and orthostatic symptoms should be identified by means of a 24-hour ambulatory blood pressure monitor before treatment is initiated. The treatment strategy is based on counteracting the underlying pathophysiology, by increasing intravascular volume (e.g., fludrocortisone, desmopressin, erythropoietin), potentiating the pressor effects of endogenous norepinephrine and angiotensin (fludrocortisone), or using short-acting pressor agents (e.g., midodrine) to improve upright blood pressure.

Fludrocortisone

Fludrocortisone is a synthetic mineralocorticoid that is practically devoid of glucocorticoid effect.[166] Its action leads to sodium and water retention, but this effect is not targeted to the intravascular space and is only transient. It is postulated that its effectiveness in improving orthostatic hypotension is due to potentiation of the pressor effects of endogenous vasoconstrictors such as norepinephrine and angiotensin II. Therapy with fludrocortisone (Florinef) is typically initiated with a dose of 0.1 mg per day. At least 4 to 5 days of treatment are necessary for a therapeutic effect to be evident. The most clinically relevant side effect to watch for is the development of hypokalemia. Fludrocortisone increases extracellular and intravascular volume by increasing sodium reabsorption by the kidney, thus increasing cardiac output and standing blood pressure. The dose of fludrocortisone should be increased slowly and doses greater than 0.3 mg are not effective. Body weight, blood pressure, and the possible development of heart failure because of volume overload should be monitored. Weight gain of 2 to 5 pounds is expected. A certain degree of pedal edema should not be of concern. Indeed, it may be necessary to support the venous capacitance bed. A small study demonstrated that up to one third of older patients stopped taking fludrocortisone because of side effects.[167]

Desmopressin

Desmopressin (DDAVP) is a synthetic vasopressin analogue, which acts specifically on the V2 receptor (renal tubular cell) responsible for the antidiuretic effect of the hormone. At the dose given, DDAVP has no vasoconstrictor effect because it does not activate the V1 receptor, which is in vascular smooth muscle. Nocturnal intranasal administration of DDAVP reduces nocturnal polyuria and raises standing blood pressure in the morning without worsening supine hypertension.[168] The problems with the use of DDAVP are the risk of hyponatremia and fluid retention. Treatment with this drug, therefore, should always be started with caution, and serum sodium should be monitored.

Recombinant Erythropoietin

Anemia is a common complication of autonomic failure.[161] Because blood pressure in autonomic failure is extremely sensitive to even small changes in intravascular volume, modest decreases in red blood cell mass and blood viscosity can exacerbate orthostatic hypotension. Studies in patients with autonomic failure have shown that reversing the anemia using recombinant erythropoietin increases upright blood pressure and ameliorates symptoms of orthostatic hypotension.[161,162,169] Erythropoietin, a polypeptide hormone produced mostly by the kidney, plays a central role in the regulation of red blood cell production. The synthesis of erythropoietin is controlled by a feedback mechanism based on an oxygen sensor. When oxygen delivery to the kidney decreases, as with blood loss or chronic anemia, the synthesis of erythropoietin by renal interstitial cells increases.[170] The hormone is released into the bloodstream and stimulates red cell progenitors in the bone marrow, thereby increasing red cell production. In some patients with autonomic failure, chronic anemia does not produce an adequate increase in serum erythropoietin levels[162]; this is seen in renal disease, malignancy, and other chronic disorders.

A likely mechanism for the increase in blood pressure following erythropoietin treatment is an increase in intravascular volume and blood viscosity because of increased red blood cell mass. In patients with renal failure receiving erythropoietin treatment, however, no correlation was found between increased blood pressure and increased hematocrit[171]; this suggests additional mechanisms for the hypertensive effect of the hormone.

Midodrine

When volume expansion is not sufficient to control symptoms, a pressor agent may be added. The pressor agent of choice is now midodrine, a selective α_1-adrenergic agonist, which is well absorbed after oral administration and does not cross the blood-brain barrier.[172] Midodrine is effective in increasing orthostatic blood pressure and ameliorating symptoms in patients with orthostatic hypotension.[173] Because a single dose of midodrine increases pressure for only 4 hours, it can be prescribed two or three times daily, depending upon the physical activity of the patient and can be avoided later in the day because it increases supine blood pressure. An advantage of a pressor agent over fludrocortisone is that its blood pressure raising effect lasts only a few hours. Thus, it can be administered specifically when the patient needs it, typically before breakfast and before lunch and preceding physical activity.[173] Recumbent hypertension is a common side effect, but standing up readily lowers blood pressure. The dose of midodrine should be titrated slowly starting with 2.5 mg bid or tid. The dose can be quickly increased to 10 mg bid or tid based on the blood pressure response. Most patients with orthostatic hypotension require chronic treatment with fludrocortisone, and adding midodrine allows a lower dose of fludrocortisone to be used. This combination treatment may reduce the long-term complications associated with chronic mineralocorticoid administration. Piloerection and scalp itching are frequent side effects of midodrine.

Pyridostigmine

By inhibiting cholinesterase enzymes that degrade acetylcholine, pyridostigmine facilitates neurotransmission at the level of the autonomic ganglia. This results in an increase in blood pressure that is proportional to residual sympathetic tone. Thus, pyridostigmine has the advantage of preferentially increasing blood pressure on standing, without worsening supine hypertension.[174] On average, it is not as potent as other short-acting pressor agents, but it can be effective in a given patient. The most common side effects of pyridostigmine are nausea, vomiting, and diarrhea, which can limit its effectiveness in patients with orthostatic symptoms.

Atomoxetine

Residual sympathetic tone can also be harnessed in these patients by prolonging the actions of synaptic norepinephrine by inhibiting its reuptake with atomoxetine.[175] In patients with MSA and residual sympathetic tone, atomoxetine can be a potent pressor agent even at very low doses. In contrast, it has little if any effect in patients with pure autonomic failure.

Droxidopa

Droxidopa is a precursor of norepinephrine that has been available for some time but was only approved by the U.S. Food and Drug Administration in February 2014.[176] There is some trial evidence to show that it is effective in reducing symptoms and increasing postural blood pressures in patients with neurogenic orthostatic hypotension (e.g., PD, MSA, and PAF).[177]

Other Agents

Several other agents have been used in the treatment of orthostatic hypotension in autonomic failure. The somatostatin

BOX 63-1 Stepwise Approach to the Management of Orthostatic Hypotension in Older People

- Remove aggravating factors:
  - Replace volume depletion
  - Review drugs (e.g., diuretics, tricyclic antidepressants, vasodilators, antihypertensives, antimuscarinics, insulin in diabetics with autonomic impairment)
- Patient education:
  - Avoid inactivity/prolonged bed rest/deconditioning
  - Avoid large meals
  - Reduce alcohol
  - Maneuvers such as leg crossing to increase cardiac output on standing
- Nonpharmacologic treatment:
  - Liberalized salt intake (but beware of concurrent supine hypertension)
  - Head tilted up during the night
  - Waist-high grade 2 compression stockings
  - Exercise/physical activity as tolerated
- Pharmacologic treatment:
  - Sodium chloride 1 g with meals
  - Fludrocortisone 0.1-0.3 mg/day
  - Midodrine 2.5-10 mg tid PRN
- Pragmatic use of "sick day rules":
  - Advise patients to omit diuretics and antihypertensive drugs if they develop problems likely to cause volume depletion (e.g., diarrhea and vomiting)

analogue octreotide[178,179] is sometimes effective in improving orthostatic hypotension. Clonidine, an α_2-adrenergic agonist, has been used with occasional success in patients with severe pure autonomic failure by inducing peripheral vasoconstriction.[180] Conversely, the α_2-adrenergic antagonist yohimbine is often useful in less severe patients by increasing residual sympathetic tone.[181]

Treatment of Supine Hypertension

Some centers advocate the use of intermediate acting β-blockers such as atenolol or centrally active agents such as clonidine at bedtime in addition to raising the head of the bed to prevent supine hypertension. However, none of these regimens has been rigorously tested.[182]

Treatment of Related Conditions

Supine Hypertension and Diurnal Blood Pressure Variation

In addition to orthostatic hypotension, two distinct features of autonomic failure are hypertension when the patient is supine and notable diurnal variation in blood pressure. The mechanism responsible for supine hypertension is unclear. It is surprising that despite low norepinephrine and low angiotensin levels, systemic vascular resistance is increased in patients with autonomic failure when they are supine. The nocturnal supine hypertension causes pressure natriuresis. The subsequent reduction in extracellular fluid volume aggravates orthostatic hypotension in the morning. Patients with chronic autonomic failure frequently have elevated supine blood pressure and may be incorrectly diagnosed with arterial hypertension. This group of patients can be very difficult to treat, and a pragmatic approach is recommended. First, the diagnosis should be confirmed with a 24-hour ambulatory blood pressure monitor. Second, patients should be treated according to the severity of symptoms from their orthostatic hypotension. A balance must be struck between overly aggressive management of the supine hypertension to avoid the risk of orthostatic hypotension resulting in falls and subsequent significant morbidity.[30]

Postprandial Hypotension

Although the precise mediators of postprandial hypotension have not been fully characterized, adenosine and insulin are prime suspects. It is not surprising that treatment of postprandial hypotension is targeted at these mediators. Caffeine, an adenosine receptor antagonist, and octreotide, which blocks the release of insulin, are effective in preventing postprandial hypotension.[183,184] Some patients with diabetic autonomic neuropathy may not tolerate octreotide because of gastrointestinal side effects. Acarbose, an α-glucosidase inhibitor, also prevents postprandial hypotension, likely through its ability to prevent the quick rise in insulin levels that occurs after meals.[185]

Summary

Evaluations of antihypertensive therapy and nonpharmacologic interventions are the first steps in treating orthostatic hypotension. Hypotensive therapy should be discontinued if possible. Salt and fluid intake should be increased, and patients should be instructed to elevate the head of the bed and never to lie flat. Education about the effects of eating, hot weather, bathing, exercise, and rising quickly from a prone position will assist in effective behavior modification. If pharmacotherapy is needed, fludrocortisone, midodrine, and erythropoietin (for anemia) may be helpful in normalizing blood pressure regulation.

KEY POINTS

- Dysautonomia is common with age and with a variety of illnesses, which can be grouped as instances of primary autonomic failure (chiefly neurodegenerative) and secondary autonomic failure.
- Age-related changes in the autonomic nervous system are not uniform.
- Routine clinical tests of the integrity of the autonomic nervous system rely on orthostatic changes in blood pressure, heart rate responses to deep breathing, and assessment of baroreflex function in response to a Valsalva maneuver.
- Orthostatic hypotension and neutrally mediated syncope are the most common manifestations of autonomic impairment in older adults.
- A heart rate response to standing less than 10-15 beats/min despite profound orthostatic hypotension is a sign of autonomic failure; greater than this suggests volume depletion and/or medication side effects.
- The successful treatment of orthostatic hypotension in older adults requires a multifaceted approach.

For a complete list of references, please visit www.expertconsult.com.

KEY REFERENCES

6. Robertson D, Hollister AS, Biaggioni I, et al: The diagnosis and treatment of baroreflex failure. N Engl J Med 329:1449–1455, 1993.
13. The European Society of Cardiology Guidelines for the diagnosis and management of syncope reviewed by Angel Moya, MD, FESC, Chair of the Guideline Taskforce with J. Taylor, MPhil. Eur Heart J 30:2539–2540, 2009.
15. Consensus statement on the definition of orthostatic hypotension, pure autonomic failure, and multiple system atrophy. The Consensus Committee of the American Autonomic Society and the American Academy of Neurology. Neurology 46:1470, 1996.

18. Wieling W, Schatz IJ: The consensus statement on the definition of orthostatic hypotension: a revisit after 13 years. J Hypertens 27:935–938, 2009.
23. Wieling W: Laboratory assessment of disturbances in cardiovascular control. In Kenny RA, editor: Syncope in the older patient: causes, investigations and consequences of syncope and falls, London, 1996, Chapman & Hall Medical, pp 47–71.
26. Kerr SR, Pearce MS, Brayne C, et al: Carotid sinus hypersensitivity in asymptomatic older persons: implications for diagnosis of syncope and falls. Arch Intern Med 166:515–520, 2006.
27. Mulcahy R, Jackson SH, Richardson DA, et al: Circadian and orthostatic blood pressure is abnormal in the carotid sinus syndrome. Am J Geriatr Cardiol 12:288–292, 301, 2003.
29. Romero-Ortuno R, Cogan L, Foran T, et al: Continuous noninvasive orthostatic blood pressure measurements and their relationship with orthostatic intolerance, falls, and frailty in older people. J Am Geriatr Soc 59:655–665, 2011.
30. Romero-Ortuno R, O'Connell MD, Finucane C, et al: Insights into the clinical management of the syndrome of supine hypertension–orthostatic hypotension (SH-OH): the Irish Longitudinal Study on Ageing (TILDA). BMC Geriatr 13:73, 2013.
31. Cooke J, Carew S, Quinn C, et al: The prevalence and pathological correlates of orthostatic hypotension and its subtypes when measured using beat-to-beat technology in a sample of older adults living in the community. Age Ageing 42:709–714, 2013.
65. Rutan GH, Hermanson B, Bild DE, et al: Orthostatic hypotension in older adults. The Cardiovascular Health Study. CHS Collaborative Research Group. Hypertension 19:508–519, 1992.
72. Clegg A, Young J, Iliffe S, et al: Frailty in elderly people. Lancet 381:752–762, 2013.
73. Romero-Ortuno R, Cogan L, O'Shea D, et al: Orthostatic haemodynamics may be impaired in frailty. Age Ageing 40:576–583, 2011.
74. Rockwood MR, Howlett SE, Rockwood K: Orthostatic hypotension (OH) and mortality in relation to age, blood pressure and frailty. Arch Gerontol Geriatr 54:e255–e260, 2012.
92. Hayat A, Whittam D: Baroreceptor failure related to bilateral carotid artery disease: an uncommon cause of labile hypertension. Intern Med J 44:105–106, 2014.
95. Fanciulli A, Strano S, Colosimo C, et al: The potential prognostic role of cardiovascular autonomic failure in alpha-synucleinopathies. Eur J Neurol 20:231–235, 2013.
103. Gilman S, Wenning GK, Low PA, et al: Second consensus statement on the diagnosis of multiple system atrophy. Neurology 71:670–676, 2008.
118. Guidez D, Behnke S, Halmer R, et al: Is reduced myocardial sympathetic innervation associated with clinical symptoms of autonomic impairment in idiopathic Parkinson's disease? J Neurol 261:45–51, 2014.
125. Meijer FJ, Aerts MB, Abdo WF, et al: Contribution of routine brain MRI to the differential diagnosis of parkinsonism: a 3-year prospective follow-up study. J Neurol 259:929–935, 2012.
164. Fan CW, O'Sullivan E, Healy M, et al: Physiological effects of sleeping with the head of the bed elevated 18 in. in young healthy volunteers. Ir J Med Sci 177:371–377, 2008.
167. Hussain RM, McIntosh SJ, Lawson J, et al: Fludrocortisone in the treatment of hypotensive disorders in the elderly. Heart 76:507–509, 1996.
182. Logan IC, Witham MD: Efficacy of treatments for orthostatic hypotension: a systematic review. Age Ageing 41:587–594, 2012.

64 Parkinsonism and Other Movement Disorders

Jolyon Meara

Movement disorders in older adults can be broadly classified into the akinetic-rigid hypokinetic conditions, in which voluntary movement is reduced, and hyperkinetic conditions, in which excess involuntary movements called dyskinesias are present (Box 64-1). Dyskinesias can be further classified into tremor, dystonia, tics, myoclonus, and chorea. This distinction is as not absolute as, for example, in Parkinson disease (PD), the most common akinetic-rigid syndrome, involuntary movements are often present. Akinetic-rigid syndromes are usually associated with poor mobility and difficulty with walking because of the presence of a gait apraxia.

Movement disorders are common in older age and are a significant cause of impairment, disability, and handicap.[1] Once diagnosed, these disorders can often be effectively treated. These conditions often present in older people at an advanced stage, and it is not uncommon in older patients acutely admitted into the hospital for other conditions to make the diagnoses of hitherto unrecognized essential tremor, parkinsonism, orofacial dyskinesia, or drug-induced movement disorder.

AKINETIC-RIGID SYNDROMES

The akinetic-rigid syndromes are a group of disorders characterized by parkinsonism, which results from the combination of akinesia, rigidity, and, often but not always, tremor (Box 64-2). Parkinsonism is often associated with impaired balance and a gait apraxia leading to falls and impaired mobility. Levodopa-responsive parkinsonism of unknown cause that has particular clinical features, a characteristic clinical progression, and Lewy body neuropathology in the substantia nigra is called *idiopathic parkinsonism* or *PD* and accounts for approximately 70% of cases of parkinsonism.[2,3] Other causes of parkinsonism include drugs, vascular disease, and, much less frequently, multisystem degenerative conditions, which include progressive supranuclear palsy, multiple system atrophy, and corticobasal degeneration. With increasing age, not only does the risk of parkinsonism increase but also the likelihood of parkinsonism having a cause other than PD.

PARKINSON DISEASE

Although PD can present at any age, it rarely occurs outside of old age.[4] Cross-sectional prevalence studies of PD and parkinsonism show at least two thirds of subjects to be older than 70 years. PD is usually insidious in onset and may have a long symptomatic phase before eventual diagnosis, with symptoms being mistakenly attributed by patients and their physicians to the inevitability of "old age." The rate of progression in PD is strongly related to age at onset rather than to disease duration, which explains the often rapidly disabling motor deterioration associated with dementia seen in subjects with onset beginning after 70 years of age (late-onset disease). Minimal signs of parkinsonism may result from normal aging changes in the basal ganglia or incidental Lewy body changes, making the diagnosis of PD in older people even more difficult.[5]

Clinical Features

Classically PD has been considered a disorder of voluntary motor control, which in young subjects is a reasonable assumption. However, the increasing realization of the widespread nature of neuropathology in PD, coupled with our increasing recognition of nonmotor symptoms, has now led to the concept of PD being a multisystem multiorgan disorder.[6] Nonmotor symptoms are increasingly common with disease progression and older age at disease onset and therefore are a major feature of PD in older subjects.[7,8,9] Cognitive impairment, often progressing to dementia, is the most powerful factor that determines quality of life in older people with PD. Late-onset PD is probably best thought of as being primarily a dementia associated with poor mobility and a high risk of falls.[10,11]

Neuropathology

PD is characterized by cell loss and gliosis in the substantia nigra and other pigmented brainstem nuclei that are often visible to the naked eye on sectioning the midbrain.[12,13] Aging also results in cell loss in the substantia nigra, although the distribution of cell loss is very different from that seen as a result of PD.[14] Surviving cells in the substantia nigra contain typical inclusions in the cytoplasm called Lewy bodies, which are now known to be largely an aggregation of a protein called α-synuclein.[15] Most cases of PD diagnosed in life are found to have Lewy bodies in the substantia nigra.[16] However, Lewy body pathology in the substantia nigra does not necessarily lead to the clinical picture of PD, and conversely, largely from the studies of familial parkinsonism, other pathologies not involving Lewy bodies can give rise to a clinical picture typical of PD.[17,18] Lewy bodies are also found in other specific brain sites outside the brainstem, including the cerebral cortex, olfactory bulb, and enteric plexi.[19,20] Lewy bodies can be found in up to 10% of postmortem examinations in older subjects with no apparent history of parkinsonism in life (incidental Lewy body disease). It is unclear whether such individuals, if they had survived, would have developed PD or, because of protective mechanisms, were able to contain the disease process in a subclinical state.[21] The role of the Lewy body in the pathology of PD is still unknown, and it is unclear whether the Lewy body represents a defense mechanism or the result of the primary disease process.

PD also involves the ascending serotonergic, noradrenergic, and cholinergic projections to the cortex and basal ganglia.[22] Clinicopathologic studies have demonstrated that coexisting neuropathology within the striatum and in other areas of the brain is extremely common in older subjects with histologically confirmed PD.[23] Braak and colleagues have proposed that the primary degenerative process in PD, based on the assumption that the presence of Lewy bodies indicates neuronal loss, begins not in the substantia nigra but in the olfactory tracts, lower brainstem, and enteric nervous tissue.[24] This model fits well with the increasing recognition that rapid eye movement (REM) sleep disorders, hyposmia, and constipation may precede the motor symptoms of PD by several years. The proposed pattern of disease progression also indicates the potential for interaction with environmental agents via the olfactory system and gut.

Motor Features

Akinesia is the central motor abnormality in PD that refers to a lack of spontaneous voluntary movement, slowness of movement

BOX 64-1 Classification of Movement Disorders

AKINETIC-RIGID STATES

Parkinsonism

HYPERKINETIC STATES

Tremor
Chorea
Dystonia
Myoclonus
Complex movement disorders
Drug-induced movement disorders (tardive dyskinesia)

BOX 64-2 Causes of Parkinsonism

PRIMARY PARKINSONISM

Parkinson disease (idiopathic/sporadic parkinsonism)

SECONDARY PARKINSONISM

Drug-induced parkinsonism
- Neuroleptic drugs
- Calcium blocker cinnarizine

Vascular parkinsonism (pseudoparkinsonism)
- Multi-infarct states
- Single basal ganglia/thalamic infarct
- Binswanger disease

Multisystem degenerative diseases
- Progressive supranuclear palsy
- Multiple system atrophy (striatonigral type)
- Corticobasal degeneration
- Alzheimer disease
- Wilson disease (young-onset parkinsonism)
- Dementia with Lewy bodies
- Neurofibrillary tangle parkinsonism

Toxins
- MPTP
- Manganese

Familial parkinsonism

Postinfectious parkinsonism
- Creutzfeldt-Jakob disease
- AIDS
- Postencephalitis (encephalitis lethargica)

Miscellaneous causes
- Hydrocephalus
- Posttraumatic
- Tumors

Metabolic causes (postanoxic)

AIDS, Acquired immunodeficiency syndrome; *MPTP,* 1-methyl-4-phenyl-1,2,2,6-tetrahydropyridine.

(bradykinesia), and faulty execution of movement.[25] Marsden brilliantly described akinesia as the "failure to execute automatic learned motor plans."[26] Voluntary movements tend to be of low amplitude and to show increased fatigability. There is a particular difficulty with sequential and concurrent self-paced movements. When asked to oppose the index finger to the thumb in a tapping motion, patients often start with reasonably fast, large-amplitude movements, but the speed and amplitude then rapidly decrease and the movement fades away. Akinesia in the lower limb is best tested by asking the patient to tap the heel of the foot on the floor as rapidly as possible; in this situation, akinesia can be heard as well as seen. Older patients often find bedside tests for akinesia difficult to execute and may perform poorly because of cognitive impairment, painful arthritis, restricted joint range, and muscle weakness. Action tremor from any cause can interfere with the quality of normal hand and finger movements, and this can make the assessment of akinesia difficult in the presence of essential or dystonic tremor.

Rigidity is an increased resistance of muscle to passive stretch felt by the examiner. Clinically, rigidity is best detected at the wrist joint. The patient is asked to relax as fully as possible while the examiner makes flexion and extension movements of the wrist joint with the patient's forearm supported. Passive movements of the head can be used to detect axial rigidity. Parkinsonian rigidity is not velocity-dependent and is present to the same degree at all joint positions in flexion and extension ("lead-pipe" rigidity). Activation procedures, akin to the Jendrassik maneuver to enhance tendon jerks, can bring out "activated rigidity" that was not previously present. Transient activated rigidity may be a normal finding in anxious individuals. Activated rigidity in the neck muscles may be the first sign of rigidity in PD. Tremor in the upper limb due to any cause will result in a ratchet-like quality of intermittent resistance at the wrist joint called cogwheel rigidity that is not specific to PD.

Tremor, usually of the hand, is the presenting feature of PD in approximately 70% of cases. Hand tremor characteristically occurs at rest when the postural muscles are relaxed and has a frequency of approximately 4 to 6 Hz. In an anxious patient, postural tremor can easily be misidentified as a resting tremor. Most patients with PD manifest a range of resting, postural, and action tremors. A resting tremor of the hand involving the thumb and index finger described as "pill-rolling" and often brought out when the patient is observed walking is very suggestive of PD or drug-induced parkinsonism. Tremor usually begins insidiously in one hand before spreading to the leg on the same side. After a further delay of sometimes a year or more, the opposite hand and leg become affected. In rare cases, PD can present with tremor alone (tremor-dominant PD) with variable degrees of mild rigidity and akinesia found on examination. Tremor-dominant PD is a slowly progressive disorder and can be very difficult to distinguish from essential and dystonic tremors. Individuals with a diagnosis of PD recruited into trials of neuroprotection in PD, who are subsequently found to have no evidence of nigrostriatal dysfunction on positron emission tomography (PET) and single-photon emission computed tomography (SPECT) scans, may well have dystonic tremor.

Postural balance can be assessed clinically by asking the patient to stand and then gently pushing the patient forward from behind, with the other hand in front to prevent a fall. Falls or feelings of imbalance strongly suggest the presence of impaired righting reflexes, even if this is not evident at the time of examination. Axial motor disturbances leading to gait disturbance, dysphagia, and dysarthria are a feature of late-onset PD and often respond poorly to drug treatment.

In older people with PD, the severity of clinically elicited motor signs, the benchmark of disease severity in clinical research trials, is often poorly correlated with functional impairment and handicap in daily living. For example, despite the bedside demonstration of severe akinesia in the clinic, one patient still managed to make breakfast that day, albeit slowly, and was able to make the arduous journey to the hospital.

Nonmotor Features

Nonmotor symptoms, particularly hyposmia, sleep disorder, and constipation, may predate the onset of motor symptoms by many years. Nonmotor features of PD are varied and, with disease progression, dominate the clinical picture.[9,27] In late-onset PD, nonmotor features are usually advanced by the time of diagnosis and progress more rapidly than in earlier-onset disease. Autonomic system involvement leads to postural hypotension, urinary incontinence, sexual dysfunction, constipation, and abnormalities of sweating.[28] The progression of PD pathology in the cerebral cortex leads to a range of neuropsychiatric and cognitive problems, including dementia, psychosis, hallucinations, apathy, and depression.[29,30] Sensory symptoms, usually painful in nature and involving the lower limbs, also occur and are difficult to treat successfully. A rating scale for nonmotor symptoms has been developed, but, like so many assessment scales, it is more useful in research settings than in clinical practice.[31]

Dementia and cognitive impairment are common problems in the management of PD in older adults.[32] The cause most frequently appears to be Lewy body pathology in the cerebral cortex.[29] Dementia that develops a year or more after parkinsonism is described as PD dementia (PDD), whereas dementia present at the start of the illness is called *dementia with Lewy bodies* (DLB). These two conditions are generally thought to represent two ends of a spectrum of Lewy body disease.[33,34] The situation is more complicated than this with the expansion in the United Kingdom of organized memory clinic care for people with dementia. This has resulted in the identification of individuals with established dementia, who never fulfilled DLB diagnostic criteria, who subsequently develop typical features of PD, and who appear to benefit from cautious levodopa treatment. The risk of dementia in older adults with PD is five times that of age-matched subjects without PD,[11] and after 8 years of follow-up the prevalence of dementia may reach nearly 80%.[10]

Dysthymia, or mild depression, is fairly common in PD,[7,35-37] but major depression is unusual in the absence of previous significant depressive illness. The natural history of depression or depressive symptoms in PD and the response to antidepressant drug treatment has been poorly studied.[38] Apathy is also frequently described in individuals with PD and may be mistaken for depression.[39] A range of nocturnal and daytime sleep disorders is now well described in PD and include REM sleep behavior disorder and excessive daytime sleepiness.[40]

Visual hallucinations are common in PD and occur early in late-onset disease.[41] Rather than simply being side effects of antiparkinsonian medication, visual hallucinations are now thought to be the direct result of Lewy body pathology in the ventral-temporal brain areas, indicating that the second half of the course of the disease has been reached.[42,43] Visual hallucinations have been suggested as a useful marker to distinguish PD from non–Lewy body parkinsonism.[43]

Psychosis in PD usually occurs in older patients with established cognitive impairment or dementia and again indicates the presence of significant cortical disease.[44]

Delirium in PD is also common in older patients with cognitive impairment and is precipitated by the usual suspects commonly invoked in geriatric practice. All antiparkinsonian medications increase the risk of delirium; this risk is greatest with anticholinergics, dopamine agonists, selegiline, and amantadine. Visual hallucinations commonly occur in conjunction with psychosis or delirium. Delirium has a remarkable but unexplained and little researched effect on motor symptoms in PD. Patients with acute delirium are often hyperactive and wander around the ward despite refusing all antiparkinsonian medication for days at a time. As the delirium lifts and medication is reintroduced, motor function again deteriorates to the previous parkinsonian state of frozen immobility.

Clinical Diagnosis

The diagnosis of PD is a two-stage process that remains heavily dependent on clinical skills.[45] First, the symptoms of parkinsonism need to be sought in the history and the signs of parkinsonism established by clinical examination. Progressively small handwriting (micrographia) with the written word disappearing into a shaky line is strongly suggestive of parkinsonism. Difficulty turning over in bed is also a good clue to the early development of axial akinesia. A good witness account, usually from a spouse, is very useful in confirming the often rather general and nonspecific slowing down seen in older patients with PD. The gradual inability to keep up with a spouse on daily routine walks is again a useful early indication of gait disturbance and akinesia. Loss of saliva from the mouth at night (sialorrhea) is also helpful, indicating the presence of akinetic bulbar function. Second, if parkinsonism is detected, consideration has to be given to what type of parkinsonism is present by applying validated clinical diagnostic criteria[23,46] (Box 64-3).

BOX 64-3 Guideline Diagnostic Criteria for Parkinson Disease

A progressive usually nonfamilial disorder with bradykinesia (slowness of initiation of voluntary movement, progressive reduction in speed and amplitude of repetitive movement, and difficulty switching smoothly from one motor program to the next) and at least one of the following:

- Muscular rigidity
- Coarse 4 to 6 Hz resting tremor
- Impaired righting reflexes (not caused by primary visual, vestibular, cerebellar, or proprioceptive dysfunction)

Absolute exclusion criteria are the following:

- Exposure to neuroleptic drugs within the year before the onset of symptoms or exposure to MPTP
- Presence of cerebellar or corticospinal tract signs
- Past history of encephalitis lethargica or viral encephalitis with oculogyric crises
- Stepwise progression or a history of multiple strokes
- Presence of communicating hydrocephalus or a supratentorial tumor
- Presence of severe early autonomic failure
- Supranuclear gaze palsy

Modified from Gibb WRG, Lees AJ: A comparison of clinical and pathological features of young and old-onset Parkinson's disease. Neurology 38:1402–1406, 1988.
MPTP, 1-Methyl-4-phenyl-1,2,2,6-tetrahydropyridine.

In older patients, the diagnosis of parkinsonism can be extremely difficult, even in expert hands, particularly when the clinical picture is complicated by other diseases, cognitive impairment, depression, and atypical features.[47] The diagnosis of parkinsonism in acutely ill frail patients in the hospital should be approached with particular caution because, once the patient has recovered from the acute illness, the apparent signs of parkinsonism may not be present. A confident diagnosis of parkinsonism cannot always be made in older people, and sometimes a trial of levodopa at an adequate dosage (at least 600 mg daily) may be required. The use of DaTSCAN-SPECT imaging of the nigrostriatal tract using a radiolabeled tracer for the dopamine transporter may help distinguish atypical postural and action tremors in older patients and lead to the correct diagnosis of PD, essential tremor, and dystonic tremor.[48,49]

How good are experts at distinguishing PD from other types of parkinsonism? Two important clinicopathologic brain bank studies addressed this problem and demonstrated that diagnostic accuracy for PD at death, when diagnostic accuracy is going to be highest, was only approximately 76%.[23,50] Diagnostic accuracy in later cases referred to a brain bank was shown to have improved to approximately 84%.[51] The use of stringent clinical diagnostic criteria can improve the specificity for correct diagnosis to over 90% but at the expense of a reduced sensitivity of approximately 70% since true but clinically atypical cases are excluded.

BOX 64-4 Subtypes of Parkinson Disease

Early onset (<50 years old) versus late onset (>70 years old)
Tremor dominant versus postural imbalance and gait disorder
Benign slow progression versus malignant rapid progression
Unilateral with or versus bilateral disease with or without axial disease and without impaired balance
Lewy bodies mainly in brainstem (PD) versus Lewy bodies mainly in cortex (DLB)

Modified from Meara J, Bhowmick BK: Parkinson's disease and parkinsonism in the elderly. In Meara J, Koller WC, editors: Parkinson's disease and parkinsonism in the elderly, Cambridge, England, 2000, Cambridge University Press, pp 22–63.
DLB, Dementia with Lewy bodies; *PD,* Parkinson disease.

Clinical Subtypes

Clinical observation suggests that subtypes of PD exist, and yet surprisingly little scientific study of this phenomenon has been undertaken (Box 64-4).[46,52,53] Late-onset disease tends to progress more quickly than early-onset disease (symptoms before the age of 40 years) and is more often associated with cognitive impairment.[54] Patients in the longitudinal DATATOP study who were classified as having rapidly progressive disease were older, had more severe postural imbalance and gait disorder (PIGD group), and exhibited less tremor at study entry than the group with slowly progressive disease. Tremor-dominant disease was associated with less disability, less cognitive impairment, and less depression compared to a group with akinetic rigidity and postural imbalance. The DATATOP analysis suggested that cognitive function and motor deterioration were relatively independent once adjustment for age had taken place.[54] However, patients with late-onset disease appear to become demented sooner than patients with early-onset disease of similar duration.[55] The risk of disabling levodopa-induced dyskinesias appears to be much lower in patients with late-onset compared with early-onset disease. Motor fluctuations are also less evident in late-onset disease with the possible exception of the end-of-dose "wearing off" of drug benefit.

The clinical expression and progression of PD with age is likely to reflect the impact of additional neuropathology from vascular or Alzheimer type pathology as well as effects of cell loss because of aging.[56] Indeed, vascular and Alzheimer type changes in the striatum and cortex may protect older patients from levodopa dyskinesia and motor fluctuations but reduce the therapeutic response to levodopa and increase the risk of cognitive impairment or dementia.

Epidemiology

PD has a strong age-associated risk, and both prevalence and incidence increase exponentially with age.[57,58] Whether the incidence of PD truly falls in extreme old age is still unclear. The apparent drop in incidence in extreme old age may reflect diagnostic difficulties or limitations of case ascertainment in small populations. PD affects all racial groups and, after adjusting crude rates to a standard population and allowing for differences in study methodologies, has a fairly uniform worldwide distribution of approximately 110 per 100,000.[57] Differences in adjusted prevalence rates may still be explained by differential survival, diagnostic bias, and variable mortality rates. Population-adjusted prevalence rates for PD in European subjects older than age 65 years have been reported as 2.3% for parkinsonism and 1.6% for PD.[59] Studies in which all eligible subjects are examined using the total census approach have shown that up to a third or more of subjects ascertained as having PD were medically undiagnosed before the study.[60,61] A longitudinal study of 4341 older subjects initially free of parkinsonism reported an average annual incidence rate of 530 per 100,000 for parkinsonism and 326 per 100,000 for PD.[62]

The strong age-associated risk of PD means that over the next few decades the burden of PD worldwide will increase, particularly in the most populous regions of the Far East and China, where the greatest increase in older people and incident cases of PD will occur.[63] The number of people older than 50 years who have PD is likely to double in the 10 countries with the biggest populations over the next quarter of a century.[63]

Parkinsonism in institutional care has received little research attention despite the fact that 15 years from diagnosis approximately 40% of survivors will need long-term care.[9] The prevalence of parkinsonism appears to be high in hospitals, nursing homes, and residential/retirement homes.[64] A survey in the United States of 5000 nursing home residents older than 55 years reported a prevalence for medically diagnosed PD of nearly 7%.[65] A European study found that 42% of cases of PD in older subjects living in institutions were medically undiagnosed.[66] Nursing home residents with PD tended to be more disorientated, depressed, and functionally disabled than residents without PD.[67,68] Psychosis and dementia are the two main factors increasing the risk of admission to nursing homes of older people with PD.[67,68]

Cause

The cause of sporadic PD is unknown but is likely to represent interaction between environmental agents and genetic susceptibility. Potential mechanisms to explain this interaction are suggested by the Braak hypothesis of disease progression,[24] the existence of environmental neurotoxins such as 1-methyl-4-phenyl-1,2,2,6-tetrahydropyridine (MPTP),[69] and the occurrence of incidental Lewy body disease.

Twin studies suggested that, apart from early-onset disease, genetic mechanisms were relatively unimportant in the causation of PD.[70] However, since then, rare monogenic forms of familial parkinsonism have been described, the most common relating to mutations in the *LRRK2*, *Parkin*, and *PINK1* genes.[71] A total of at least 13 genetic loci have been reported that result in dominantly and recessively inherited parkinsonism, usually of early onset and often with clinical features atypical of PD. These genes are most likely to be involved in protein degradation, oxidative stress responses, and mitochondrial function. Neuropathologic findings resulting from these gene mutations are variable but consistently reveal nigral degeneration with or without Lewy bodies. Even when the clinical picture is indistinguishable from PD, as occurs in *LLRK2* mutations, the pathologic findings can be remarkably varied. Mutations at the *LLRK2* locus result in dominantly inherited PD with reduced penetrance causing an age of onset typical of PD that may account for 1% of "sporadic" cases of PD.[72] Overall, approximately 5% of sporadic incident PD may have a clearly defined genetic basis. The relationship between clinical features and progression in early PD and genetic markers for PD is currently under investigation in the large PROBAND study, which is scheduled to close to recruitment in 2016.

Several environmental agents, such as MPTP and manganese, can cause parkinsonism, but no environmental exposure that is widespread enough and persistent enough over thousands of years to cause sporadic PD has yet been found.

Treatment of Parkinson Disease

In the United Kingdom, despite the fact that a wide range of drugs are available to treat the motor symptoms of PD, in practice dopamine replacement in the form of levodopa is the mainstay of treatment, particularly in older patients. Detailed discussion of their use can be found in reviews of drug therapy.[72-74] Clinical guidance from the National Institute for Health and Care Excellence (NICE) in the United Kingdom (set to be updated in 2016) has also been issued.[75] Worldwide in emerging economies, many drugs for PD are either unavailable or unaffordable. Despite great research efforts, no drug treatment appears to delay disease progression. Drug treatment improves, although rarely abolishes, motor impairment.

Naturally, especially in older patients, drug treatment should be combined with rehabilitative approaches involving physical therapists, occupational therapists, speech and language therapists, and a range of other allied health and welfare professionals.[76-79]

The model of holistic care in PD has been supported by the development of the PD nurse specialist role.[80] Although this development has led to significant improvements in the care of older patients with PD, the findings of a randomized trial of this service were disappointing, probably as a result of the study design and methodology that were used.[81]

Drug Treatment of Motor Features

Levodopa

The most effective and widely available drug treatment for the motor symptoms of PD in older adults remains levodopa combined with dopa decarboxylase inhibitors (co-careldopa/co-beneldopa), and virtually all people are prescribed these drugs at some stage in their disease. As levodopa-induced disabling dyskinesias and motor fluctuations are rare in older people, levodopa treatment should not be delayed, particularly since many such patients will already be significantly disabled by their PD. Side effects of levodopa commonly include nausea and vomiting, dizziness on standing, and daytime drowsiness. Nausea is usually a short-term problem but in older patients can persist and result in a subtherapeutic levodopa dose. Domperidone given half an hour before each levodopa dose is useful in reducing levodopa-induced nausea but should be prescribed carefully given concerns over its long-term cardiac risk profile.[82] Long-term use of domperidone, particularly at a high dose, is best avoided whenever possible, although a small number of patients will require long-term domperidone to control levodopa-induced nausea. Confusion and hallucinations are usually only seen in older patients who already have evidence of cognitive impairment or dementia. Postural hypotension should be assessed before starting levodopa. To avoid falls and injury, patients need to be careful getting out of bed and rising from the table after meals. Many older people will still be driving, so advice should be given about the risk of daytime drowsiness and the need to inform the driving authorities and motor insurers.

To minimize side effects, a "low slow" introduction of levodopa should be adopted. A suggested regime for initiating levodopa treatment in older people is shown in Box 64-5. Although there is no convincing evidence that levodopa accelerates disease progression, it seems sensible to use the minimum dose of levodopa that leads to an acceptable health-related quality of life for the patient. Unfortunately, many older patients are unable to tolerate a maximally therapeutic dose of levodopa. Conversely, occasionally older people are undertreated with levodopa, and the first stage in management is often to gently increase levodopa dosage and closely monitor the response. In drug-naïve patients, it is important to clearly document the response to a 6-week period of adequate levodopa treatment (ideally at least 600 mg daily) as this can help to clarify the clinical diagnosis and can also give some indication of the likely degree of the future control of motor symptoms.

Delayed controlled-release forms of levodopa (Sinemet-CR, Madopar-CR) are available and may have a limited role in selected individuals. Controlled-release preparations may help early sleep disturbance resulting from PD symptoms in the first few hours of the night.[83] Unpredictable absorption may account for the failure of these drugs to reduce levodopa-induced dyskinesias and fluctuations.[84] Dispersible levodopa formulations (Madopar dispersible tablets 62.5/125 containing 50 mg and 100 mg levodopa, respectively) are very useful and have a rapid onset of action due to the ease of absorption but reduced duration of response compared to conventional levodopa. Dispersible formulations can rescue patients from sudden "off" periods and provide a "kick start" before getting up in the morning. Wider use of Madopar dispersible tablets may reduce the need for apomorphine treatment. Patients with dysphagia may also benefit from dispersible formulations. Co-careldopa tablets can be crushed and dissolved effectively in fizzy drinks and will readily pass down a fine bore nasogastric tube. In advanced PD complicated by poor control related to variable drug absorption, levodopa can be administered by duodenal infusion (Duodopa) in highly selected patients. Older patients with advanced disease are unlikely to derive much benefit from this invasive and expensive treatment.

BOX 64-5 Starting Levodopa in Older People

- Take baseline measures of disease state and lying/standing blood pressure.
- Start levodopa as co-careldopa 12.5 mg/50 mg or co-beneldopa 62.5 mg once daily with breakfast for 1 week.
- Increase to one tablet at breakfast and lunch for 1 week and then to one tablet at breakfast, lunch, and tea for a week.
- Continue to slowly build up the levodopa by one tablet each week until reaching two tablets three times daily with food (a total of 600 mg levodopa daily).
- Use domperidone 10 mg half an hour before each levodopa dose if nausea develops (rarely necessary with slow upward titration of levodopa).
- Review to assess motor response and side effects after 4 weeks of 600 mg of levodopa daily.
- Adjust levodopa dose to obtain optimal benefit with the smallest dose possible or minimize side effects by slowly increasing or decreasing dose.
- In nonresponders, slowly increase levodopa as before until limited by side effects.
- Failure to respond to a dose of greater than 1.2 mg levodopa daily in the absence of malabsorption makes a diagnosis of Parkinson disease very unlikely.

Inhibition of Levodopa Metabolism

The effects of levodopa can be boosted by treatment with drugs that inhibit the breakdown of levodopa by the enzymes MAO-B and COMT. Entacapone given at a dose of 200 mg with each daily dose of levodopa prevents the peripheral metabolism of levodopa by COMT and increases the uptake of levodopa in the brain. Entacapone has been shown to increase the duration of the clinical response to levodopa in patients with and without motor fluctuations.[85-87] Entacapone can cause nausea and vomiting, dyskinesias, discoloration of the urine, and diarrhea. Tolcapone, previously withdrawn because of liver toxicity, is now available again in the United Kingdom for specialist-restricted use under close supervision with careful monitoring of liver function. Studies investigating the early use of levodopa and entacapone combined in a single formulation (Stalevo) compared to levodopa alone suggest that entacapone is best prescribed only when needed for specific indications.[88]

Endogenous and exogenous levodopa can also be enhanced by central MAO-B inhibition using selegiline or the newer rasagiline, which, unlike selegiline, is not metabolized to troublesome amphetamine-like metabolites.[89] Both drugs have modest antiparkinsonian effects. The issue of potential neuroprotective effects of both of these drugs is unresolved and on balance appears unlikely, at least by the time of clinical presentation.[90,91] However, rasagiline is a reasonable option in early-stage PD in older adults who are not frail and when neuroprotection may still be relevant. The combination of selegiline and levodopa in older frail subjects appeared to be associated in one study with increased mortality and falls.[92] Whether this also applies to rasagiline is unknown, but this class of drug may be best avoided in more advanced disease and in older patients with cognitive impairment or a history of falls and syncope.

Levodopa-Induced Fluctuations and Dyskinesias

Clinical impressions suggest that motor fluctuations and dyskinesia are common after 5 years or so of levodopa exposure. The DATATOP study in 352 de novo patients reported a prevalence of 50% for motor fluctuations and 33% for dyskinesia after only a mean of 20 months levodopa exposure.[93] However, a study in 618 patients on levodopa treatment reported motor complications in only 22% of the study group after nearly 5 years of follow-up.[84] This difference may reflect methodologic differences between the two studies in the definitions of motor complications. Factors governing the risk of levodopa-induced complications appear to be the age of the patient at presentation, disease severity, and the dose and duration of levodopa treatment. Younger patients presenting before 60 years old appear to be at particular risk of these problems. The risk of these problems, and much more relevantly the risk of *disabling* dyskinesias and motor fluctuations, seems to fall rapidly with increasing age of disease onset.[94] Among adults who are older than 60 years at disease onset, disabling dyskinesias as a result of levodopa are rare. Several strategies can be used to treat these problems when they do arise in older patients.[95] Amantadine has antidyskinetic effects, and more effective drugs to combat this problem are in development.

Dopamine Agonists

Dopamine agonist drugs have a limited role in older adults in whom the risk of disabling levodopa-induced dyskinesias is very low and the risk of disabling side effects is high.[96,97] Dopamine agonists, with the exception of apomorphine, are less effective than levodopa, and side effects in older adults are common, especially postural hypotension, confusion, and psychosis. Impulse control disorder, which is now well described in younger patients given dopamine agonist treatment, is rarely seen in older patients.[98] Monotherapy with dopamine agonist drugs in order to delay the use of levodopa is rarely justified in older patients, although agonists may be useful as adjunctive therapy to levodopa in carefully selected older people. Pergolide and cabergoline are linked with an increased risk of regurgitant heart valves.[99] Dopamine agonist treatment is now effectively restricted to non-ergot agonists such as pramipexole, ropinirole, or rotigotine administered in the form of a transdermal patch. Long-acting forms of pramipexole (prolonged-release pramipexole) and ropinirole (modified-release ropinirole) can be particularly useful in improving motor control over the entire 24-hour period. The rotigotine patch can help in patients undergoing planned or emergency surgery to maintain treatment throughout the operation and in patients unable to absorb drugs orally after bowel surgery.[100]

Apomorphine

Apomorphine is a particularly valuable but underused dopamine agonist that is administered subcutaneously by intermittent injection or continuous infusion.[101,102] Apomorphine has a rapid onset of action and has a magnitude of effect similar to that of levodopa but of much shorter duration. Apomorphine by intermittent injection can be used to rescue patients from distressing motor (immobility, rigidity, tremor) and nonmotor (including sleep disturbance, pain, dyspnea, anxiety, depression, panic, dystonia) symptoms refractory to oral medication. Severe nausea and vomiting are commonly induced by apomorphine and can be controlled by pretreatment for a few days with oral or rectal domperidone. Rotation of injection sites, massage of the skin before and after injection, reduction of apomorphine dose, and good injection technique can reduce the incidence of painful nodules at injection sites. Continuous administration by pump over the waking hours can decrease "off" time by around 50% to 70% and can also reduce levodopa-induced dyskinesias[103] and improve neuropsychiatric symptoms. An effective program of apomorphine treatment requires the expertise and commitment of a PD nurse specialist who can work across the hospital and community interface. Unfortunately, since many older patients are unable to administer apomorphine by injection when they develop an "off" state or manage the pump on their own, the usefulness of apomorphine is limited by the availability of a partner or caregiver to help administer the drug.

Older frail patients with advanced disease who still appear to get reasonable benefit from their oral drugs for at least some period of the day and are adequately supported should be considered for a trial of apomorphine therapy.[103] Apomorphine can lead to hypotension and drowsiness, which can limit its use, and nonresponsive features such as dysarthria, freezing, and postural imbalance will continue to progress. After a time, the benefits of apomorphine will become outweighed by side effects, disease progression, and difficulties of administration and will lead to drug withdrawal. In our practice we have successfully managed selected older patients for up to 5 years on apomorphine therapy with good results over this time.

Drug Treatment of Nonmotor Features

The treatment of nonmotor features remains a major challenge, particularly since dopaminergic drugs often make these worse, and lags far behind our ability to identify them. The research-based evidence supporting most of our attempts at treating nonmotor symptoms is poorly developed. Cognitive impairment, depression, anxiety, autonomic failure, and sleep disturbance can be improved in some patients by using a wide range of drug and nondrug interventions. Depression can respond to selective serotonin reuptake inhibitors such as sertraline[104] and citalopram,[38] and low-dose buspirone can help anxiety. Excessive sweating may be controlled by β-blockers in some patients.[105] Postural hypotension that does not improve after simple measures can sometimes be managed by the careful use of fludrocortisone.[106] Domperidone can also be useful in this situation. Troublesome sialorrhea in some older adults may respond well to intermittent injection of the salivary glands with botulinum toxin.[107] Levodopa-induced neuropsychiatric complications, including hallucinations, delusions, and delirium, may respond to atypical neuroleptic drugs such as clozapine and quetiapine started at a very low dose and slowly increased.[108-110] Further research evidence is needed to determine how useful acetylcholinesterase inhibitors such as rivastigmine and donepezil are in treating cognitive impairment and behavioral disturbances in PD. Daytime drowsiness may respond to modafinil[111,112] and REM sleep behavior disorder to low-dose clonazepam.[113]

Drug Strategies in Advanced Disease and Palliative Care

With time, disabling features of PD dominate the clinical picture and do not respond to dopaminergic drug treatment. These features include dementia, postural imbalance, dysarthria, and dysphagia. Falls become increasingly common, drooling is often a major source of embarrassment, and social isolation and difficulties in communication are common. At this stage in the disease, weight loss can be quite marked, appears out of proportion to the difficulties in nutrition caused by dysphagia, and occurs despite apparent adequate nutritional intake. Patients at this stage are less tolerant of dopaminergic drugs, and the insidious onset and development of cognitive impairment results in hallucinations, confusion, and psychosis. A common early sign of intolerance of levodopa is marked drug-induced drowsiness. Drug treatment at this stage is largely limited by the presence and extent of cognitive impairment. All medication needs to be reviewed, and any drugs with anticholinergic activity or known to cause confusion should be slowly withdrawn. Amantadine, selegiline, and dopamine agonist drugs tend to be poorly tolerated at this stage. If problems persist, the dose of levodopa may also have to be reduced and a balance found between mental clarity and mobility. At some stage, concerns regarding fitness to drive will inevitably emerge in people with PD who drive and cannot be ignored by the patient, family, or doctor. In cases where fitness is uncertain, sometimes the only fair way forward is to embark on a practical assessment of driving skills; this usually helps resolve the situation while maintaining the trust between doctor and patient.

In advanced stages of the disease, drug regimes often need to be simplified using low doses of standard formulation levodopa to try to maintain mobility as far as possible. Severe rigidity may on occasion respond to intermittent apomorphine used at critical times of the day. Patients approaching the stage of palliative care are often residents in nursing homes, particularly if cognitive impairment is advanced. The primary care team supported by the PD nurse specialist needs to work closely together to optimize treatment at this time. Pain can be a significant problem in some patients and may respond to apomorphine. A clear management plan needs to be developed to deal with issues such as the use of antibiotics to treat chest infections, the provision of artificial hydration and feeding, cardiopulmonary resuscitation, and the appropriateness of transfer to acute medical facilities.[114]

Surgical Treatment

Neurosurgery, particularly deep brain stimulation of the subthalamic nucleus, is becoming increasingly used as a treatment option in PD but has little relevance since cognitive impairment, which is the major contraindication to neurosurgery, is frequently already present in older patients.[115,116] Furthermore, neurosurgery is largely directed at improving drug-induced dyskinesia or increasing "off" time in patients with motor fluctuations, neither of which is common in older patients. Furthermore, even in older patients with a good initial response to surgery, rapid disease progression may result in any benefit from neurosurgery being short-lived.

Prognosis of Parkinson Disease in Older Patients

Patients and their families faced with the diagnosis of PD are understandably concerned about what the future holds for them in terms of keeping independent and minimizing disability. As with every chronic progressive disease, it is difficult to predict accurately an individual's prognosis. In older people the prognosis may also be determined by concurrent morbidity. Prognosis needs to be based on a detailed clinical assessment, the physician's clinical experience and judgment, and the application of research-based evidence. One large prospective clinical study of drug treatment in PD indicated that disability scores based on clinical assessment scales tended to return to pretreatment levels by 4 years of follow-up.[117] This study recruited 782 patients who mostly had mild disease, although it is unclear how long symptoms had been present before study entry. The mean age of patients in this study was approximately 62 years old. The Unified Parkinson's Disease Rating Scale (UPDRS) score of subjects requiring the addition of levodopa in the DATATOP study increased by around 7 points per year over the 3-year follow-up, most of the increase being due to deterioration in the motor subscale.[93] A total of 273 (34%) out of the original 800 patients recruited in this study needed to start levodopa treatment after 1-year follow-up. Clinical features associated with more rapid disease progression and a poor prognosis include older age at onset, impaired cognitive function, dominant akinesia-rigidity, and postural imbalance.[54,55] In the absence of poor prognostic features, most older patients at diagnosis could reasonably be told to expect a period of 5 to 6 years of good disease control. Deteriorating cognitive function is likely to determine health-related quality of life more than advancing motor impairment.

Mortality is significantly increased in older patients with PD despite optimum drug treatment, and age-specific mortality rates appear to be increasing as frailer subjects reach older age. Cognitive impairment or dementia has a powerful influence on the survival of older people with PD.[118]

Other Causes of Parkinsonism

Parkinsonism can arise from several causes (see Box 64-2), although these, with the exception of drug-induced parkinsonism, are much rarer than PD. Even though PD is the most common cause of parkinsonism, accounting overall for approximately 70% of cases, this proportion falls with increasing age.

Drug-Induced Parkinsonism

The most common form of secondary parkinsonism, largely the result of the use of neuroleptic (dopamine-blocking) drugs in the treatment of serious mental illness, is drug-induced parkinsonism (DIP), which may still be frequently overlooked in older patients.[119-121] A total of 32% of a series of patients with parkinsonism referred to a neurology clinic were found to have DIP. Older patients, especially women, have increased risk of DIP and may inadvertently be prescribed neuroleptic drugs to treat dizziness (prochlorperazine) and gastric upset (metoclopramide). Other nonneuroleptic drugs such as the calcium channel blocker cinnarizine, tetrabenazine, and very rarely lithium, fluoxetine, paroxetine, and amiodarone can cause DIP. Clinically, DIP is indistinguishable from PD. Over 90% of cases tend to develop within 3 months of starting the offending drug. After withdrawal of the drug, signs of parkinsonism may take several months to resolve. In most older patients with DIP, the signs never resolve, and careful monitoring reveals the subsequent development of PD. Presumably, subclinical PD was "brought out" by the neuroleptic drug. The treatment of DIP involves, whenever possible, stopping the causative drug. When this is not possible, anticholinergic medication can help control symptoms, as can amantadine. The value of levodopa is uncertain, as it can worsen the mental condition for which the neuroleptic drug may have been originally prescribed and may be ineffective because of the dopamine receptor blockade.

Parkinsonism-Plus

Several rare multisystem degenerative conditions, such as progressive supranuclear palsy,[122,123] multiple system atrophy,[124,125] and corticobasal degeneration,[126,127] can present with parkinsonism. Of these, multiple system atrophy can, on occasion, be impossible to distinguish clinically from sporadic PD for the whole length of the natural history of the disease. The response to treatment can also be misleading as multiple system atrophy can respond well to levodopa. Warning signs suggesting the possibility of parkinsonian-*plus* disease are a poor response to levodopa, poor tolerance of levodopa, striking asymmetry of motor signs, early onset of dementia, the presence of pyramidal or cerebellar signs, early onset of falls, rapidly deteriorating mobility, severe autonomic disturbance, and evidence of progressive supranuclear gaze abnormalities.

Vascular Parkinsonism

Parkinsonism can result from vascular disease of the brain presenting with gait apraxia, truncal ataxia, relative sparing of the upper limb, and absence of tremor.[128,129] A history of hypertension and of other vascular risk factors is often present, and brain imaging usually shows widespread deep white matter ischemic changes. In rare cases, strategic infarcts within the basal ganglia can give rise to a condition clinically indistinguishable from PD. The use of DaTSCAN-SPECT may be useful in this situation. Older adults with vascular parkinsonism can benefit from levodopa, so a trial of treatment should be started to assess their response.

HYPERKINETIC MOVEMENT DISORDERS

Essential Tremor

Essential tremor (ET) is the most common involuntary movement disorder and usually presents as a long-standing bilateral persistent postural tremor involving the hands and forearms.[1,130] An action tremor is often also present. The head, voice, and legs may also be involved with decreasing frequency. In approximately 50% of cases, a family history of similar tremor also exists, as does a temporary improvement of tremor after alcohol. Although usually annoying and embarrassing, ET can also result in severe disability and handicap. The prevalence of ET increases with age, reaching a crude figure of 39.2 per 1000 individuals older than 65 years.[130]

ET is commonly misdiagnosed as PD and is also sometimes confused with dystonic and drug-induced tremor. A key factor in helping to distinguish ET from PD is the length of the tremor history, which usually goes back many years but may be difficult to establish. ET worsens with age, so patients with ET can present in old age without an apparent history of preexisting tremor. The distinction between ET and PD in older adults is made more difficult, as a resting tremor can occur in ET and tremor-dominant PD can be associated with a postural rather than resting tremor. Head tremor is rare in PD, although jaw tremor is not infrequently found. A trial of drug therapy may again be needed. In this situation, diagnostic difficulty may be resolved by the use of DaTSCAN-SPECT.[48] The prevalence of PD in patients with ET appears to be slightly higher than that expected by chance alone, although this could reflect the diagnostic difficulties in relation to postural tremors.

Dystonic tremor can be easily confused with ET and tremor-dominant PD, although it tends to be more jerky in nature and is often associated with subtle dystonic posturing of the head.[131] Sometimes a trial of treatment is needed to help distinguish between these two conditions. The treatment of ET is disappointing, although some patients obtain benefit from β-adrenergic drugs such as propranolol or the anticonvulsant primidone. Side effects, especially in older patients, limit the usefulness of these drugs. Severe cases of ET may respond to repeated botulinum toxin injections or bilateral thalamic stimulation. Primary orthostatic tremor, a fast palpable but not visible tremor of the thigh and calf, should also be recognized as a rare cause of unsteadiness on standing.[132]

Dystonia

In older patients, dystonia most commonly presents as task-specific dystonia such as writer's cramp, blepharospasm, torticollis, dystonic head tremor, laryngeal dystonia, or cranial dystonia. Blepharospasm commonly presents in later life and, when severe, may respond to botulinum toxin injections. Blepharospasm can also complicate progressive supranuclear palsy and PD. Dystonia can respond to high-dose anticholinergic medication, although older patients tolerate this poorly.

Chorea

The rapid, often jerky, nonrepetitive and dancelike movements that typify chorea are not uncommonly seen in older patients and require a diagnosis rather than the label of "senile chorea." Drugs are a common cause of this condition, particularly neuroleptics giving rise to tardive chorea. Levodopa also commonly causes choreiform dyskinesias. In older people, chorea can also result from subcortical vascular lesions. Hemiballismus, a high-amplitude form of usually unilateral chorea involving the arm and leg and occasionally the trunk, is seen in older patients as a result of infarction or hemorrhage in the region of the subthalamic nucleus. This movement disorder, when severe, can be life-threatening but is usually self-limiting and responds to neuroleptic drugs and tetrabenazine. Late-onset Huntington disease must always be excluded.[133] In this situation, chorea is usually associated with cognitive impairment. The diagnosis can be confirmed by genetic testing for evidence of an expanded cytosine–adenosine–guanine (CAG) repeat sequence on the short arm of chromosome 4.[133,134] Other rare causes of chorea include systemic lupus erythematosus, neuroacanthocytosis, polycythemia rubra vera, hyperthyroidism, and electrolyte disturbances. Oro-buccal-lingual choreiform dyskinesia is not uncommon in studies of nursing home residents who have never been exposed to neuroleptic drugs and appears to be related to loss of teeth and failure to wear dentures.[135]

Restless Legs Syndrome

The condition of unpleasant deep sensory disturbances in the legs associated with irresistible leg movements on trying to get to sleep increases in prevalence with age.[136,137] Individuals with these symptoms usually also have abnormal leg movements in the early stages of pre-REM sleep. Restless legs syndrome occurs in many other neurologic diseases as well as in medical conditions such as anemia and renal failure and in response to certain drugs such as lithium and tricyclic antidepressants. This condition can respond to levodopa, dopamine agonist drugs, clonazepam, and codeine.

Drug-Induced Movement Disorders

Drugs commonly cause involuntary movements, usually as a result of the indiscriminate and inappropriate use of neuroleptic drugs in older people.[138] A wide range of other drugs have been linked (usually by isolated case reports in the literature) to involuntary movements, although it is often difficult to evaluate the clinical significance of such reports. In addition to parkinsonism and acute dystonic reactions, neuroleptics can also cause a wide range of tardive movement disorders, including an intense and distressing motor restlessness called akathisia.[139] Neuroleptic malignant syndrome can result from the introduction or increase in dose of a neuroleptic drug or from sudden reduction in dopaminergic drug treatment for PD.[140] This syndrome consists of fever, intense rigidity, confusion, autonomic disturbance, and involuntary movements. Rigidity elevates the muscle enzyme creatinine phosphokinase, and rhabdomyolysis can develop with associated renal failure. Mortality from this condition can be high. A similar condition, the toxic serotonin syndrome, can result from the combination of a selective serotonin reuptake inhibitor with a monoamine oxidase inhibitor. Many drugs, including lithium, sodium valproate, amiodarone, tetrabenazine, amphetamine, tricyclic antidepressants, and β-agonists, can cause tremor. Chorea can result from the use of estrogens, lithium, and amphetamines, and myoclonus can result from the use of tricyclic antidepressants and chlorambucil.

KEY POINTS: PARKINSONISM AND OTHER MOVEMENT DISORDERS

- The prevalence of essential tremor, parkinsonism, and drug-induced movement disorders increases significantly with age.
- Movement disorders in older people often remain undetected and are difficult to diagnose, and individuals in whom such a diagnosis is considered should be referred for specialist assessment.
- Accurate diagnosis, comprehensive assessment, and careful documentation of the response to drug therapy and rehabilitation are key factors in the successful long-term management of these disorders.
- Delaying levodopa treatment in older patients with Parkinson disease (PD) is rarely justified given the disabling nature of the condition and the low incidence of disabling levodopa-induced dyskinesias and motor fluctuations in this age group.
- PD is a multisystem multiorgan degenerative disease and nonmotor features, particularly dementia and cognitive impairment, dominate the clinical picture in older subjects and largely determine quality of life.

For a complete list of references, please visit www.expertconsult.com.

KEY REFERENCES

1. Khatter AS, Kurth MC, Brewer MA, et al: Prevalence of tremor and Parkinson's disease. Parkinsonism Relat Disord 2(4):205–208, 1996.
6. Marras C, Lang A: Changing concepts in Parkinson disease. Neurology 70:1996–2003, 2008.
9. Hely MA, Morris JG, Reid WG, et al: Sydney Multicenter Study of Parkinson's disease: non-L-dopa-responsive problems dominate at 15 years. Mov Disord 20:190–199, 2005.
10. Aarsland D, Andersen K, Larsen JP, et al: Prevalence and characteristics of dementia in Parkinson disease: an 8-year prospective study. Arch Neurol 60:387–392, 2003.
11. Hobson JP, Meara RJ: The risk and incidence of dementia in a cohort of elderly subjects with Parkinson's disease. Mov Disord 19:1043–1049, 2004.
16. Hughes AJ, Daniel SE, Ben-Shlomo Y, et al: The accuracy of diagnosis of parkinsonian syndromes in a specialist movement disorder service. Brain 125:861–870, 2002.
31. Martinez-Martin P, Schapira AH, Stocchi F, et al: Prevalence of nonmotor symptoms in Parkinson's disease in an international setting: study using nonmotor symptoms questionnaire in 545 patients. Mov Disord 22:1623–1629, 2007.
63. Dorsey ER, Constantinescu R, Thompson JP, et al: Projected number of people with Parkinson disease in the most populous nations, 2005 through 2030. Neurology 68:384–386, 2007.
71. Gasser T: Update on genetics of Parkinson's disease. Mov Disord 22(Suppl 17):S343–S350, 2007.
73. Goetz CG, Poewe W, Rascol O, et al: Evidence-based medicine review update: pharmacological and surgical treatment of Parkinson's disease: 2001 to 2004. Mov Disord 20:523–529, 2005.
74. Horstink M, Tolosa E, Bonuccelli U, et al: Review of the therapeutic management of Parkinson's disease. Report of the EFNS and MDS-ES. Part II: late (complicated) Parkinson's disease. Eur J Neurol 13:1186–1202, 2006.
75. National Institute for Health and Care Excellence: Parkinson's disease: diagnosis and management in primary and secondary care (NICE guidelines [CG35]), June 2006. www.nice.org.uk/CG035. Accessed October 11, 2015.
78. Keus SHJ, Bloem BR, Hendriks EJM, et al: Evidence-based analysis of physical therapy in Parkinson's disease with recommendations for practice and research. Mov Disord 22:451–460, 2007.

65 Neuromuscular Disorders*

Timothy J. Doherty, Michael W. Nicolle

Aging is associated with substantial decline in neuromuscular performance.[1] This is perhaps best exemplified by age-associated loss of muscle mass and strength, a phenomenon often referred to as sarcopenia (see Chapter 72 for full review of sarcopenia). Neuromuscular disorders are an important cause of disability at all ages but often result in greater impairment and disability in older adults as they are superimposed on age-related impairment of both motor and sensory function of the peripheral nervous system. For example, it is well established from both anatomic and in vivo electrophysiologic studies that aging alone is associated with significant reductions in the numbers of functioning motor neurons and motor axons.[1-4] This appears true for both distal and proximal muscles in the upper and lower limbs, but it may be more severe in distal lower limb muscles. Moreover, these losses of motor neurons (motor units) approach 70% in distal lower limb muscles by 80 years of age and are a major contributing factor to age-related loss of muscle mass, strength, and power (i.e., assessment of dynamic strength or force at a given velocity).[5,6] In healthy older adults, lower limb strength and power are strongly related to functional indices such as gait speed and balance; these factors become of even greater importance in frail older adults.[7-9] What is less well appreciated is the substantial impact on function that occurs when a disorder affecting the motor or sensory system is superimposed on the normal aging process. Often this combination results in significant disability and contributes substantially to the frailty syndrome.[10] For example, an 80-year-old woman with preexisting lower limb weakness following a fall and hip fracture who develops a peroneal nerve palsy superimposed on a diabetic neuropathy will experience much greater disability as a result of these combined problems than a younger counterpart with a simple foot drop from peroneal nerve injury. In cases such as this, in addition to reduced ability to perform activities such as heavier housework or gardening, she would also walk more slowly, may have lost weight, and is likely to have reduced grip strength; muscular weakness might also contribute to a sense of excessive fatigue and increased fall risk. This is one example where a single new problem (foot drop), combined with normal age-related changes, could account for manifestation of the frailty phenotype.

The impact of aging on the sensory system is less well established. Postmortem and biopsy studies show that aging results in losses of dorsal root ganglion cells and a decline in the numbers of sensory axons.[11,12] This is apparent in reduced sensory nerve action potential amplitudes from standard nerve conduction studies in older men and women.[13] This likely translates to impaired sensory function that can impact balance and motor control. As with the motor system, any superimposed disorder will have a greater functional impact.[10]

In addition, given these observations, in some cases, slowly progressive disorders (e.g., inclusion body myositis [IBM], polyneuropathy, or polyradiculopathy) are mistaken for the expected or typical losses of muscle mass, strength, and power associated with aging. Therefore, it is imperative that clinicians appreciate common presenting features of neuromuscular disorders and recognize how they differ from so-called normal or typical aging.

*Material in this chapter contains contributions from the previous edition, and we are grateful to the previous author for the work done.

To this end, this chapter focuses on disorders that are commonly found in older adults, including polyneuropathies, spinal stenosis and neurogenic claudication, myopathies, motor neuron disease (MND), and neuromuscular junction disorders. The general clinical approach is outlined, followed by a discussion of individual disorders and their treatment management.

APPROACH TO THE PATIENT WITH NEUROMUSCULAR DISEASE

History

Weakness, fatigue, atrophy, and altered sensation are the most common presenting symptoms of neuromuscular disease (Table 65-1). An accurate history documenting the onset, pattern, and progression of weakness and sensory loss is crucial in differentiating diagnostic possibilities and may require several meetings with the patient and, in some cases, additional information from a spouse or relatives. In general, most myopathies and disorders of neuromuscular transmission present with proximal weakness and no sensory symptoms. Notable exceptions are myotonic dystrophy type 1 (DM1; also called Steinert disease) and IBM, which may present with predominantly distal weakness. Muscle wasting and loss of reflexes are late manifestations of most myopathies. Alternatively, most neuropathies present primarily with sensory symptoms, earlier loss of reflexes, and distal weakness. Early in the course of polyneuropathies, distal muscle wasting of intrinsic hand and foot muscles is often more impressive than strength loss. Notable exceptions are acute or chronic inflammatory demyelinating polyradiculopathy and diabetic amyotrophy, which may present with mainly proximal weakness (the latter usually accompanied by severe pain at the onset).

Inquiries into the impact of symptoms on sporting abilities, hobbies, occupational history, and military service often help establish the onset and pace of symptoms. Many patients initially ascribe their neuromuscular symptoms to normal aging or painful conditions such as arthritis, and directed questioning is often required. Questions include "How far could you walk 5 years ago?" or "When did you first use a cane or walker?" or "When could you last climb stairs?" More active patients are asked, "When could you last run?" This question is useful because increasing weakness may be present for months, and only the loss or impairment of some well-established task brings it to the patient's attention.

The distribution of weakness is often suggested by the history: difficulties reaching up to a shelf or combing hair suggest upper limb proximal weakness. Proximal lower limb weakness is suggested by difficulty in rising from a low chair or toilet, climbing stairs, and getting in or out of the bathtub. Primary neuromuscular disease rarely presents with falls early in the course, with the exception of IBM, an inflammatory myopathy often associated with asymmetric quadriceps wasting and weakness that may include "buckling" around the knees and falls. Catching the foot on stairs or difficulty in depressing car pedals, turning a key, or opening a jar suggest distal weakness. In myasthenia gravis (MG), power may be reported as normal at rest, with fatigable weakness developing after exercise or later in the day. Fluctuation over

TABLE 65-1 Typical Features of Neuromuscular Disorders Based on Their Localization

Motor neuron	Progressive weakness and atrophy in segmental distribution Bulbar/respiratory involvement Fasciculations Upper motor neuron signs in ALS No sensory involvement
Nerve root	Pain and altered sensation in nerve root distribution Reduced or absent reflexes in same distribution Weakness and atrophy in myotomal distribution
Polyneuropathy	Sensory symptoms with distal to proximal progression Depressed or absent reflexes Distally predominant atrophy and weakness Distal sensory deficits
Neuromuscular junction	Proximal fatigue and weakness No atrophy Absence of sensory symptoms Diplopia, ptosis, bulbar involvement Fatigable weakness of proximal muscles
Muscle	Proximal weakness Weakness > atrophy No sensory involvement Retained reflexes

weeks to months is also suggestive of MG and differentiates it from progressive disorders that may mimic MG, such as MND or mitochondrial myopathies. Speech and swallowing problems (including coughing and choking after ingestion of solids or liquids) and unexplained recurrent pneumonia may suggest bulbar weakness. Weakness of the cervical muscles may lead to head drop, and some patients report the need to use their hand to support the head. Some patients with cervical muscle weakness have neck pain, reflecting prolonged and ineffectual voluntary attempts to keep the head up. The causes of dyspnea are numerous and most often in older adults not primarily related to neuromuscular disorders. However, many neuromuscular disorders involve respiratory musculature. This may manifest as shortness of breath on exertion and especially on lying flat, because of diaphragmatic involvement. Inflammatory myopathies, MND, and neuromuscular transmission disorders should be considered in this setting. Other symptoms suggestive of neuromuscular hypoventilation include disrupted nocturnal sleep, daytime hypersomnolence, early morning mental clouding, and headache as a result of CO_2 retention with associated cerebral vasodilation.

Myalgia is a relatively nonspecific feature seen in some patients with progressive muscular disease. Patients often find myalgia hard to describe and differentiate from joint pain. Prominent myalgia is a feature of many inflammatory myopathies, polymyalgia rheumatica, and the metabolic myopathies. However, pain at rest and lack of pain or cramp with exertion is less suggestive of an underlying defect in muscle metabolism and more suggestive of inflammatory muscle disease, referred pain from joint disease, or a myofascial pain syndrome (fibromyalgia). Uncommonly, myalgia is a presenting feature of the muscular dystrophies, such as fascioscapulohumeral dystrophy. Myotonic dystrophy type 2 (DM2; also known as proximal myotonic myopathy [PROMM]) shares some similarities with DM1 and often presents with muscle pain, stiffness, and proximal weakness. Painful nocturnal muscle cramps can reflect neurogenic diseases, including motor neuron disease/amyotrophic lateral sclerosis (MND/ALS), polyneuropathies, or chronic lumbosacral nerve root injury. Alcohol and drugs, especially those that induce hypokalemia (e.g., diuretics) and those with a structural effect on muscle (e.g., the statins), can induce myalgia. Finally, myalgia may be a prominent symptom in patients with endocrine dysfunction (especially hypothyroidism and hypocalcemia) and those with connective tissue disorders such as systemic sclerosis.

A wide-ranging systemic inquiry is essential in patients with suspected myopathies, as myositis may be a component of many collagen vascular diseases. Both DM1 and DM2 are multisystem disorders whose manifestations are varied and include diabetes, cataracts, cardiac conduction defects, and muscular weakness and wasting. Cardiac involvement is common in many neuromuscular diseases manifesting with cardiac conduction defects or cardiomyopathy or both. Prominent weight loss is a common feature in MND/ALS, reflecting both poor nutritional state and loss of muscle mass.

Many neuromuscular diseases are inherited, and therefore it is important to inquire specifically about family members and, where appropriate, about consanguinity. Premature cardiac and respiratory deaths in family members may reflect complications of an inherited neuromuscular disease or possible associated malignant hyperthermia, if associated with anesthetic exposure. It is often useful to examine first-degree relatives in a family suspected of having an inherited neuromuscular disorder even when the history does not suggest that the older relative is affected, as this can be confirmed by direct examination and has clear genetic implications for the wider family. Myotonic dystrophy, because of its marked variability in expression and the presence of anticipation, may have only minor manifestations (e.g., cataracts and mild weakness) in older adults, compared with major symptoms in siblings. The genetic defect, a trinucleotide repeat expansion, is unstable and can worsen in successive generations, particularly via the female line, leading to a phenomenon known as "anticipation," meaning earlier onset and more severe disease in successive generations.

Sensory symptoms suggest involvement of the dorsal root ganglion, dorsal nerve roots, or sensory fibers (including the central projections such as the dorsal columns). Numbness and paresthesias distally in the toes and feet are the most common presenting symptoms of symmetric polyneuropathies. Symptoms of burning pain, coldness, tightness, and prickling may suggest predominantly small fiber involvement, whereas numbness and loss of balance may indicate predominantly large fiber involvement. The presence of orthostatic hypotension, gastrointestinal disturbance, urinary dysfunction, dryness of the eyes and mouth, and erectile dysfunction in men indicate autonomic involvement. Patchy or asymmetric sensory loss may indicate an underlying vasculitic process or sensory neuronitis. Loss of balance, particularly when in the dark (reducing visual input), may indicate large fiber sensory loss and poor proprioception. Other early clues are difficulty with balance when showering or when walking on uneven surfaces. Again, as with some early motor symptoms, these complaints are often attributed to normal aging and it is not until they are particularly disabling that medical attention is sought or investigation pursued.

Examination

The aim of the examination of the neuromuscular system is to determine the distribution of muscle weakness, sensory loss, and reflex abnormality in order to localize the lesion within the peripheral nervous system (see Table 65-1). Furthermore, it is important to assess the respiratory, cardiovascular, and dermatologic systems for associated abnormalities. The examination may provide clues to the cause and allows for grading of severity. Most acquired and inherited myopathic disorders present symptoms of proximal weakness and wasting (a limb girdle distribution). Selective patterns of muscle involvement may suggest facioscapulohumeral dystrophy (FSHD) or one of the many subtypes of limb girdle muscular dystrophy, but confirmation often relies on DNA analysis or muscle biopsy. A scapuloperoneal distribution of weakness may reflect a myopathic disorder, such as FSHD, or a neurogenic problem, such as spinal muscular atrophy. MG presents with fatigable proximal weakness but without wasting. Lambert-Eaton myasthenic syndrome (LEMS) presents with fatigable proximal weakness and wasting that can be hard to distinguish clinically from a myopathy, although the reduction in deep tendon reflexes and frequent presence of autonomic manifestations in LEMS provides a valuable diagnostic clue. Distal weakness, with involvement of the forearm and hand muscles in the upper limb and the anterior and posterior tibial compartment and intrinsic foot muscles in the lower limb, is commonly due to a peripheral neuropathy or MND/ALS but can also be seen in myotonic dystrophy, IBM, very rare distal forms of spinal muscular atrophy, and in distal myopathies. Weakness of neck flexion and extension (head drop) occurs in myopathic (e.g., DM1, inflammatory myopathy, FSHD), neuromuscular junction (MG), and neurogenic (e.g., MND/ALS) disorders. Paradoxical abdominal movements and indrawing of intercostal muscles on inspiration may indicate respiratory muscle and diaphragm weakness. Identification of isolated mild (grade 4/5 on MRC testing) weakness of the hip flexors is a common observation in older adults and often does not indicate a specific neuromuscular disorder. Therefore, when this is present, before embarking on further investigation, it is important to carefully examine other proximal muscle groups (e.g., hip extensors, shoulder girdle, neck flexors and extensors) looking for patterns of weakness that may indicate a more generalized process. It is also useful to then assess gait and ability to climb stairs or rise from a chair to determine if there are functional consequences.

Having established the pattern of weakness, the symmetry of involvement is often a guide to the underlying cause. Most myopathic diseases result in symmetric weakness. In addition, around a joint, all of the muscles will be involved to about the same degree. IBM is a noteworthy exception to this, as asymmetric forearm flexor or quadriceps involvement is common. In some neurogenic diseases, such as MND/ALS, asymmetry and unequal involvement around a joint are seen, as the weakness tends to follow a segmental pattern of spinal cord involvement, often starting locally and then progressing segmentally.

In primary muscle disorders, tone and reflexes are either normal or mildly reduced. Increased tone and reflexes suggest an upper motor neuron disorder, ALS (which ultimately has combined upper and lower motor neuron involvement), or cervical spondylitic myelopathy, the latter of which is very common in older adults and often goes unrecognized early in its course. Fasciculations are spontaneous, involuntary, visible discrete muscle twitches and reflect motor neuron or motor axon hyperexcitability. Fasciculations are not seen in muscle disease; rather, they reflect neurogenic disorders such as MND/ALS but can be seen in a wide variety of neuropathies, including focal peripheral neuropathies and chronic nerve root disease, in which denervation is a feature. As it is sometimes difficult to differentiate myopathic and neurogenic weakness on symptoms alone, a careful search should be made for fasciculations in all patients who have neuromuscular weakness. Fasciculations may be missed if patients are not undressed fully. The back, abdomen, and tongue should be inspected as well as the limbs. Difficulty is often encountered in observing fasciculations in the tongue; these are best seen with the tongue lying at rest in the floor of the mouth. Pseudofasciculations as a result of anxiety or tremor may be seen in the normal individual when the tongue is protruded.

Myotonia (delayed relaxation) is an uncommon presenting complaint in the older patient and usually signifies myotonic dystrophy, which usually presents in the second or third decade. Joint contractures are occasionally due to inherited muscle disease, whereas foot deformities such as pes cavus reflect longstanding, often genetic, peripheral neuropathies or a slowly progressive upper motor neuron disorder such as hereditary spastic paraparesis.

Depressed or absent reflexes generally indicate a neuropathic disorder, with reflex loss a late sign in muscle diseases. An exception is LEMS, in which the weakness is usually more proximal, especially involving the legs, and reflexes are reduced or absent. The combination of muscle wasting, weakness, and hyperreflexia is typical of ALS but can also be seen with cervical polyradiculopathy and concomitant cervical myelopathy. In these cases, the presence of upper motor neuron signs (e.g., jaw jerk) rostral to the most caudal lower motor neuron signs is a useful observation suggestive of ALS.

Distal, symmetric loss of sensation to pain (pinprick) and temperature are common features of typical, length-dependent neuropathies with small fiber involvement. In older adults, mild loss of vibration sense in the toes is nonspecific, but loss at the ankle or more proximally indicates large fiber involvement, as a result of either peripheral neuropathy or myelopathy with involvement of the dorsal columns. Ankle reflexes that are present or increased in the setting of significant loss of vibration in the legs are a clue to the presence of a myelopathy. Loss of proprioception is often a late finding of large fiber sensory loss, as is a positive result from a Romberg test. Obviously it is important to recognize sensory deficits that follow the distribution of individual peripheral nerves (e.g., median, ulnar, or peroneal nerve) or dermatomes because they indicate a focal mononeuropathy or radiculopathy. The combination of intermittent sensory symptoms in the hands and distal sensory loss in the feet may indicate polyneuropathy, but in older adults carpal tunnel syndrome in combination with multilevel lumbosacral nerve root compression and spinal stenosis should also be considered. As outlined later, electrophysiologic testing is invaluable in sorting these cases out.

Investigations

It is sometimes impossible on the basis of history and examination alone to make an accurate diagnosis in many cases of neuromuscular disease, not least because of the overlap in clinical signs between some neurogenic and myopathic disorders. Confirmation of a neuromuscular diagnosis requires the application of electrophysiologic, pathologic, biochemical, and, increasingly, genetic testing.

With several caveats, measurement of "muscle enzymes" is useful in patients with neuromuscular disease. Serum creatine kinase (CK) appears to be the most sensitive index of muscle necrosis from primary muscle disease and from secondary muscle fiber necrosis because of chronic denervation from neuropathic conditions. The magnitude of CK rise gives some indication of the nature of the pathology: in denervating conditions such as MND/ALS, CK levels are commonly mildly elevated in the 200 to 500 IU/L range and rarely above 1000 IU/L, whereas a more significant increase of 10- to 1000-fold suggests a primary muscle (especially inflammatory myopathy). However, CK levels must be interpreted with caution, as "muscle enzymes" are also found in other tissues. CK consists of three separate isoenzymes: MM, derived from skeletal muscle; MB, derived largely from cardiac muscle; and BB, derived mainly from brain. High CK levels may therefore be seen in patients with acute myocardial injury, large strokes, and, occasionally, hepatic disease, as well as in patients with muscle disease. Even so, given that the major isoenzyme of CK is MM, a high CK level is most likely to reflect neuromuscular disease. Finally, it is also important to appreciate that mild increases in what are typically thought to be liver enzymes, such as aspartate transaminase (AST) and alanine transaminase (ALT), can occur in primary muscle disease (ALT proportionally higher is more indicative of hepatic disease).

Electrophysiology

Electrophysiologic studies are invaluable in the diagnosis of neuromuscular disorders. A detailed discussion of electrophysiologic (electromyographic) techniques in the diagnosis of neuromuscular disease is outside the scope of this chapter but can be found in appropriate textbooks.[14] Nerve conduction studies, in which the conduction velocities and amplitudes of motor and sensory (compound) action potentials in response to electric stimulation of nerves are measured, are used to detect primary pathology of peripheral nerves. Nerve conduction studies are extremely useful in detecting focal nerve injuries such as median neuropathy at the wrist in carpal tunnel syndrome, ulnar neuropathy at the elbow, or common peroneal nerve injury around the fibular head. Reduced amplitudes of motor and sensory studies with normal or mild conduction velocity slowing in the legs are typical of many of the common axonal, length-dependent polyneuropathies (e.g., drug-related, diabetes, idiopathic). Severe conduction slowing and conduction block in multiple nerve segments are important observations as they indicate an acquired demyelinating, often treatable chronic inflammatory demyelinating polyneuropathy.

The most common method for the electrophysiologic assessment of muscle is with concentric or monopolar needle electromyography (NEMG), which detects characteristic patterns that can be used to distinguish neurogenic and myopathic disorders. Normal muscle is electrically silent at rest. In neurogenic disorders resulting in denervation (e.g., ALS), spontaneous activity manifested as positive sharp waves or fibrillation potentials are seen in NEMG studies, and on voluntary activation a reduced interference pattern of the motor unit potentials is seen, reflecting the loss of motor units. By contrast, in many myopathies NEMG reveals small, short-duration motor unit potentials. Electromyography (EMG) studies may also reveal complex repetitive and myotonic (audible as a "dive bomber" or "revving motorcycle" sound) discharges, useful in confirming myotonic disorders, and may suggest a previously unsuspected diagnosis such as DM2 in which weakness predominates and myotonia is often subclinical. Spontaneous activity in the distribution of a nerve root is indicative of a radiculopathy, whereas widespread denervation in multiple regions (e.g. bulbar, cervical, thoracic, and lumbosacral) may indicate MND.

Repetitive nerve stimulation studies are useful in neuromuscular transmission disorders. In both MG and LEMS, a decrement in the compound muscle action potential response occurs with low frequency (2- to 3-Hz) stimulation, which mirrors the clinical phenomenon of fatigable weakness. In LEMS, a characteristic incremental response occurs with high-frequency (20- to 40-Hz) stimulation or after brief maximal voluntary contraction, which mirrors the clinical phenomenon of posttetanic or postcontraction facilitation. Single-fiber EMG (SFEMG) is useful in confirming a neuromuscular junction disorder, particularly in regional forms of MG. It is important to note that whereas SFEMG is highly sensitive for neuromuscular junction disorders (>95%), it is, in turn, very nonspecific with abnormal results possible in any chronic neurogenic condition or myopathy.

Muscle Biopsy

Despite advances in biochemistry, neurophysiology, and genetics, the final diagnosis in patients with muscle disease often requires a muscle biopsy. The development of the technique of needle muscle biopsy, which can be undertaken as a simple outpatient procedure, has made possible one-stop diagnostic neuromuscular clinics with combined clinical, neurophysiologic, and muscle sampling.

The vastus lateralis and deltoid are most commonly biopsied, ideally sampling a muscle that is weak but only moderately affected clinically but not too atrophied, for fear of sampling muscle with only end-stage pathology. Routine histologic stains can be employed on both paraffin-embedded and fresh frozen material and permit assessment of muscle fiber size and morphology and the presence or absence of inflammation. Other stains allow differentiation of muscle fiber types and can be used to study the distribution of cellular enzymes and metabolic reserves.[15] Immunohistochemistry on frozen muscle using antibodies directed against sarcolemmal muscle proteins, such as dystrophin and the sarcoglycans, is crucial in the diagnostic workup of suspected dystrophinopathies and limb girdle muscular dystrophies and permits a more focused search for genetic abnormalities. Western blotting techniques on muscle are often essential in confirming the suspicion of muscular dystrophies. Direct measurement of enzyme activity in fresh muscle is sometimes useful in diagnosing rare metabolic disease such as acid maltase disease and in mitochondrial myopathies where respiratory chain enzymes can be assayed. Electron microscopy of muscle is useful to confirm suspected mitochondrial abnormalities seen on light microscopy and especially to look for intracellular inclusions, which occur in some inherited and acquired muscle disease.

Muscle samples are hard to process, hard to orient, and fast to degrade; for these reasons, the technique of muscle biopsy is unsuitable for routine laboratories. Furthermore, interpretation of muscle biopsies and exclusion of artifactual change is difficult. Therefore, it is important to send muscle samples to special neuromuscular laboratories or to an experienced pathology center. As percutaneous needle and punch biopsies are far less invasive than open procedures, it is possible to use sequential biopsies to follow patients with a muscle disease and monitor response to treatment in individual patients. The smaller sample sizes inherent with these techniques mean that patchy inflammation may be missed.

PERIPHERAL NEUROPATHIES

Peripheral neuropathies are overall the most common neuromuscular disorders found in older adults. It is beyond the scope of this text to provide an in-depth review of all peripheral neuropathies, and the reader is directed to a number of excellent texts.[14,16] This section provides an overview of peripheral neuropathies and specifically addresses diabetic neuropathy because of its high prevalence in older adults.

Typical symptoms of peripheral neuropathy include distally predominant weakness, sensory loss, poor balance, pain, and autonomic dysfunction. Weakness in the majority of polyneuropathies follows a length-dependent pattern and is therefore often more severe in the lower than upper limbs. Weakness tends to become symptomatic in the extensors of the toes and ankles and evertors of the ankle earlier than in the plantar flexors. In the upper limb, difficulties with fine motor tasks such as fastening buttons or picking up coins can be early indications of weakness.

Sensory symptoms of polyneuropathies can be divided into those that indicate involvement of small, thinly myelinated fibers that subserve pain and temperature and those that suggest involvement of large myelinated fibers that are involved in position sense. Common symptoms of small fiber neuropathies include hypersensitivity to footwear or bedclothes, shooting or stabbing pain, difficulty detecting temperature of bath water, and burning sensation. These symptoms usually predominate in the feet, as most neuropathies are length-dependent. Thus, when sensory symptoms reach the level of the knees, they often begin in the hands. Small fiber sensory symptoms of burning, prickling, and allodynia are a common cause of sleep disturbance in older adults. These symptoms should prompt a careful assessment for decreased sensation to pinprick and temperature for consideration of a small fiber–predominant neuropathy.

Large fiber involvement, particularly if it is severe, will typically present with loss of balance and gait difficulty because of the loss of proprioception or position sense. These symptoms often result in mobility limitations[10] in older adults and fear of falling. In particular, patients with balance impairment secondary to peripheral neuropathy tend to avoid crowded areas, such as

BOX 65-1 Peripheral Neuropathies Based on Predominant Symptoms

MOTOR PREDOMINANT

Guillain-Barré syndrome, chronic immune demyelinating polyneuropathy, Charcot-Marie-Tooth disease, multifocal motor neuropathy, motor neuron disease

SENSORY PREDOMINANT

Idiopathic, diabetic symmetric polyneuropathy, paraneoplastic (often ganglionopathy), Sjögren syndrome, paraprotein-associated, connective tissue disease, vitamin E deficiency (very rare)

SMALL FIBER SENSORY ONLY

Diabetic neuropathy, idiopathic (acute or chronic), hereditary sensory and autonomic neuropathy (very rare)

BOX 65-2 Clinical Classification of Diabetic Neuropathies

SYMMETRIC

- Diabetic polyneuropathy
- Diabetic autonomic neuropathy
- Painful diabetic neuropathy

ASYMMETRIC

- Diabetic radiculoplexopathy
- Diabetic thoracic radiculoneuropathy
- Mononeuropathies
- Carpal tunnel syndrome
- Ulnar neuropathy at the elbow
- Peroneal neuropathy at fibular head
- Cranial neuropathies

grocery stores and shopping malls. These symptoms should prompt an examination for decreased sensation to light touch, vibration, and position sense as well as reduction or loss of deep tendon reflexes.

Autonomic symptoms include urinary retention or incontinence, abnormal sweating, constipation and diarrhea, and symptoms of orthostatic hypotension.[17] These symptoms are often initially overlooked as indicative of a neuropathic disorder and prompt assessment for a primary cardiac or central neurologic disorder cause.

Most neuropathies affect both motor and sensory fibers; however, pure or predominantly sensory involvement can be seen in concert with diabetes, malignancies (paraneoplastic neuropathies), and idiopathic sensory neuropathy in older adults. Pure motor involvement may indicate multifocal motor neuropathy (MMN),[18] a rare demyelinating disorder that typically presents initially with focal weakness of upper limb muscles, or may suggest MND. Along the same lines, most neuropathies have symmetric, distally predominant features. Asymmetry may indicate mononeuritis multiplex associated with vasculitis, hereditary neuropathy with liability to pressure palsies, or common focal or entrapment neuropathies. Box 65-1 outlines some common presentations based on the predominant fiber population involved.

Once a pattern of small or large sensory fiber predominance has been established, the absence or presence of motor involvement has been defined, and the symptoms and signs have been determined as symmetric or asymmetric based on the clinical assessment, it is often of considerable value to obtain electrophysiologic studies before other investigations to confirm or extend the clinical characterization. Most expert clinicians agree that is also useful to obtain a fasting blood sugar level, serum creatinine level, electrolyte panel, complete blood count, vitamin B_{12} level, and serum protein electrophoresis (and immunofixation if indicated) as part of the initial workup.[19] Often expensive testing for specific antibodies or genetic testing should await the results of electrophysiologic testing and is often best directed by clinicians and centers with specialized expertise.

Electrophysiologic testing is extremely helpful in tailoring future investigation because it can determine whether the process is predominantly axonal (most common) or demyelinating as well as reveal subclinical motor or sensory involvement. The presence of a demyelinating process is extremely important to establish, as this often indicates a treatable acquired neuropathy (e.g., chronic inflammatory demyelinating polyneuropathy or MMN) or a hereditary neuropathy if there is uniform slowing of conduction velocities. If an axonal neuropathy is present, it is important to determine if it is symmetric (most common) or asymmetric and multifocal, which may indicate an underlying vasculitic process requiring further investigation and treatment.[20]

It is important to note that standard nerve conduction studies examine only large, myelinated fibers. Therefore, the results of the studies may be normal or only mildly affected in small fiber neuropathies (e.g., diabetes).

Diabetic Neuropathy

Diabetic neuropathy is the most common form of peripheral neuropathy in the Western Hemisphere, with increasing prevalence resulting from the growing prevalence of obesity and type 2 diabetes.[21] A number of different classification schemes exist for diabetic neuropathy; a common one is outlined in Box 65-2. The most common form is a mixed but predominantly sensory, motor, and autonomic symmetric diabetic peripheral neuropathy (DPN), which may comprise up to 70% of cases.[15]

A predominantly sensory, often painful, neuropathy comprises the other largest group. Diabetic neuropathy is common and may be present in up to 50% of individuals with type 1 diabetes and 45% of those with type 2 diabetes if comprehensive batteries of testing are used.[21,22] A general rule is that the prevalence of a neuropathy in diabetes increases 1% to 2% for each year a patient has diabetes. In patients with only impaired glucose tolerance, the prevalence figures remain controversial.[23] Risk factors for DPN include the duration and severity of hyperglycemia, smoking, other complications such as retinopathy or nephropathy, and cardiovascular disease. The pathophysiology of DPN remains somewhat controversial but includes axonal injury from hyperglycemia and associated polyol flux, particularly sorbitol through the aldose reductase pathway; microangiopathy and hypoxia; oxidative and nitrative stress from free radicals; and deficiency of growth factors.[15] Indeed, the metabolic syndrome itself may be directly linked to diabetic neuropathy through the combined effects of dyslipidemia, insulin resistance, systemic inflammation, and the activation of the renin-angiotensin-aldosterone system leading to oxidative stress and cellular damage.[21]

Symptomatically, patients with DPN typically have positive neuropathic features such as prickling, tingling, and pins and needles; burning; or, occasionally, shooting sensations. Negative symptoms such as numbness of the toes or feet can paradoxically occur along with the positive features. Many patients experience symptoms mainly at night and experience painful allodynia (pain in response to nonpainful stimuli) from bed sheets; others experience symptoms throughout the day that are related to walking or footwear. True sensory ataxia is less common but can occur with severe involvement. Symptoms may stay confined to the lower extremity but may advance to the hands as they progress to the level of the knees in the lower limb. Early sensory symptoms in the hands should raise the question of a superimposed carpal tunnel syndrome, which has a very high prevalence in those with DPN.[24]

Clinical examination in patients with DPN reveals distal, sensory greater than motor deficits to all sensory modalities and often loss of ankle deep tendon reflexes. Motor deficits are less common, but patients may have weakness of toe extensors and flexors and, in more severe cases, weakness of ankle dorsiflexors.

The most effective intervention to prevent the incidence or limit the progression of DPN is enhanced glucose control. The Diabetes Control and Complications Trial followed more than 1400 individuals with type 1 diabetes for 5 years and reported a 60% reduction in the incidence of DPN in those receiving more frequent insulin dosing.[25] Similarly, Linn and colleagues reported a 70% reduction in DPN in 49 patients treated with enhanced glucose control for 5 years.[26] In contrast, the benefits of enhanced glucose control have been less definitive in those with type 2 diabetes.[21]

Diabetic foot ulcers are of considerable importance when assessing older adult patients with DPN. Diabetic ulcers occur because of a combination of sensory loss and repetitive pressure on bony prominences such as the metatarsal heads or heel. This, in combination with trophic changes caused by the neuropathy, leading to drying and cracking of the skin, leads to chronic tissue injury. Further progression may occur as a result of loss of proprioception leading to abnormal foot position and biomechanics. Careful inspection of the feet on a daily basis, screening for early evidence of sensory deficits, proper footwear with adequate height of the toe box or forefoot, and foot orthoses are all useful in terms of preventing the occurrence of ulceration and reducing the risk of amputation.[27]

Treatment of neuropathic pain associated with DPN has been the topic of numerous well-controlled clinical trials. Well-established guidelines support the use of a number of pharmacologic approaches with the strongest evidence in favor of tricyclic antidepressants, serotonin-norepinephrine reuptake inhibitors, pregabalin, and gabapentin.[28]

Diabetic lumbosacral radiculoplexopathy neuropathy (DLRPN), often referred to as diabetic amyotrophy or proximal diabetic neuropathy, requires special mention because of its higher prevalence in older adults and the severe disability often associated with it. DLRPN is a devastating condition that affects only about 1% of individuals with diabetes, more commonly type 2.[29] It typically presents with severe, asymmetric, acute onset of proximal leg pain and weakness. Frequently it occurs in concert with a large concomitant weight loss. In many cases, affected patients have not been diabetic for a long period of time and have no other end organ complications from DM, including frequent absence of a length-dependent diabetic neuropathy. The symptoms are usually unilateral or asymmetric and involve proximal lower limb segments such as the hip flexors and knee extensors. The condition may spread more distally and to the contralateral side over a few days. Although pain is the most severe initial manifestation, often requiring narcotic analgesia, severe weakness typically develops in the first few days, often severely affecting the hip flexors and knee extensors and also the more distal muscles, including the ankle plantar and dorsiflexors. Gait aids or wheelchairs are often required for mobility.

The cerebrospinal fluid may reveal elevated protein, providing evidence that the disease process is proximal at the level of the spinal roots. Electrophysiologic (EMG) testing reveals axonal injury or denervation in affected muscles, often including the paraspinal muscles, often with severe loss of recruitment implying substantive loss of axons. Given that axonal loss is the mechanism, the time course of recovery is typically many months. In our experience, most of these patients do well and improve gradually, if provided supportive therapy and then treated later with appropriate physical therapy in the form of resistance exercise and gait retraining.

The purported pathophysiologic basis of DLRPN is ischemic injury, possibly secondary to microvasculitis. Given this, immunomodulation may be useful if started early in the course of disease, as has been demonstrated in nondiabetics with idiopathic lumbosacral plexopathy. To date, however, clinical trials in people with diabetes have not supported this theory.[29]

NEUROGENIC CLAUDICATION AND SPINAL STENOSIS

Lumbosacral radiculopathy, specifically multilevel root disease often associated with lumbosacral spondylosis, and associated spinal stenosis is a common, often debilitating problem that typically affects older adults.[30] Symptoms of neurogenic claudication are often sometimes mistaken for polyneuropathy; however, specific features revealed from history, physical examination, and electrodiagnostic testing help distinguish these conditions. The most common symptom of neurogenic claudication secondary to lumbosacral spinal stenosis is back pain and aching pain that refers into the buttocks, hamstrings, thighs, and lower legs that is worsened with walking. Often there is associated numbness and weakness that occurs in association with the pain and discomfort. Typically, contrary to most peripheral neuropathies, the symptoms of pain, numbness, and weakness improve with rest or when seated. Lumbar extension tends to worsen symptoms, and most patients improve with flexion of the spine (e.g., walking while pushing a shopping cart or riding a bicycle, which may be much easier than walking similar durations). This is in contrast to vascular claudication, which tends to produce more localized pain in the calves, no sensory symptoms, and tends to be unaffected by spinal position.[31,32] The physical examination is often uninformative in patients with features of neurogenic claudication. It may reveal reduced or absent ankle jerks if the S1 roots are affected and distal sensory loss in the L5 and S1 distribution. Fixed weakness is uncommon and usually mild.

Imaging with computed tomography (CT) scanning or magnetic resonance imaging (MRI), which shows ligamentous thickening better, typically reveals multilevel degenerative spondylitic disease, foraminal narrowing and encroachment, and central canal narrowing. The latter two are secondary to disc protrusion, thickening of the ligamentum flavum, and facet hypertrophy secondary to degenerative disease. Spondylolisthesis, usually degenerative, also may lead to significant canal narrowing.

Electrodiagnostic testing in patients with neurogenic claudication may reveal reduced distal compound muscle action potentials in the intrinsic foot muscles secondary to chronic axonal injury in the L5 and S1 roots. The sural and superficial peroneal sensory nerve action potentials may be mildly reduced but are typically well preserved because the injury is proximal to the dorsal root ganglion. This pattern of severe motor involvement and mild sensory involvement is sometimes erroneously interpreted as indicative of a polyneuropathy. However, this is the opposite pattern of that seen in the vast majority of polyneuropathies that present with earlier and more severe sensory involvement on nerve conduction studies with less severe motor involvement. Needle EMG of lower limb muscles (tibialis anterior, gastrocnemius, quadriceps) often reveals mild, chronic denervation, reinnervation changes in the form of large-amplitude, long-duration motor unit potentials, and little or no evidence of active denervation, owing to the slowly progressive nature of the root disease.

Conservative treatment is often undertaken initially and includes physiotherapy focusing on spinal flexion and aerobic exercise such as cycling, which tends to be better tolerated than walking. Pain usually responds to nonsteroidal antiinflammatory drugs (NSAIDs) or mild narcotic analgesics (e.g., codeine, tramadol). Patients with severe back and radicular pain may benefit symptomatically from epidural corticosteroid injections.

Surgical intervention should be considered for those who do not respond adequately to nonoperative treatment or if their disability is severe (principally mobility limitations). The typical approach involves laminectomy and partial facetectomy. The role of fusion is less clear but is often recommended when there is stenosis accompanied by spondylolisthesis. Some evidence from randomized controlled trials supports surgery over conservative management, at least in the 2 years following surgery,[32] and the surgical outcomes tend to favor those with greater canal narrowing.[33]

INFLAMMATORY MYOPATHY (MYOSITIS)

Inflammatory myopathy, or myositis, is among the most common muscle disorders presenting acutely or subacutely in older adult patients and can be subdivided into infectious and idiopathic categories. Infectious causes, including viral and bacterial pathogens, are the most common causes of myositis worldwide but tend to be transient monophasic disorders. Idiopathic inflammatory myopathies are a significant cause of chronic neuromuscular disease and constitute a spectrum that includes polymyositis, dermatomyositis, and IBM. Polymyositis and dermatomyositis are related but distinct conditions and are discussed together first.

Causes of Polymyositis and Dermatomyositis

Both polymyositis and dermatomyositis are autoimmune disorders, although the antigenic targets are ill defined. There is strong circumstantial evidence that polymyositis is an autoimmune disorder: like most autoimmune disorders, polymyositis is more common in women; polymyositis may arise or fluctuate in pregnancy; polymyositis is often associated with other organ- and nonorgan-specific autoimmune disorders; a polymyositis phenotype can be triggered by viral illnesses (HIV and HTLV-1) or by certain drugs, especially D-penicillamine; polymyositis responds to immunosuppression and modulation; finally, as further discussed later, muscle biopsies provide evidence of T cell–mediated cytotoxic process directed against unknown muscle antigens. Similarly, dermatomyositis is more common in women, may arise or fluctuate in pregnancy, is often associated with other autoimmune disorders, can be triggered by D-penicillamine, responds to immune therapies, and on muscle biopsy shows damage reflecting a humoral-mediated capillary angiopathy. Dermatomyositis is also more likely to be associated with an underlying cancer.

Clinical Features of Polymyositis and Dermatomyositis

Dermatomyositis presents in childhood or in older adults with a female predominance, as with many other autoimmune disorders. Polymyositis is rare in children; most patients develop the condition in their third to fifth decade.[34] Polymyositis and dermatomyositis present with symptomatic proximal weakness causing functional impairment (neck extensors and flexors, shoulder girdle, trunk and abdominal muscles, and hip and knee extensors and flexors), diffuse myalgias (in up to a third of patients, especially in dermatomyositis), or a rash. Examination reveals symmetric proximal weakness and wasting with preserved deep tendon reflexes, and neck and bulbar weakness are common. The pathognomonic rash of dermatomyositis is a purplish-red butterfly discoloration over the face, often associated with periorbital edema and a heliotrope rash over the eyelids. An additional V-shaped rash may be seen in the sun-exposed areas of the chest as well as a rash over the extensor aspects of elbows and knees. Patients may have a typical rash of dermatomyositis without clinically apparent weakness (amyopathic dermatomyositis), although it is interesting that these same patients have subclinical changes evident on muscle biopsy.[35] Polymyalgia rheumatica, sometimes confused for an inflammatory myopathy, causes myalgia that is often worse in the shoulder girdle but without significant weakness.

Symptomatic myoglobinuria may occur in rare, acute cases of both polymyositis and dermatomyositis and can precipitate acute renal failure.

Polymyositis and dermatomyositis are frequently associated with connective tissue disorders: polymyositis with lupus, Sjögren syndrome, and rheumatoid arthritis; and dermatomyositis with scleroderma and mixed connective tissue disease.[5] Systemic features, including vasculitis of the heart or gut, subcutaneous calcinosis, Gottron nodules around the knuckles, and nail fold capillary changes, are seen in dermatomyositis.[36]

Respiratory muscle weakness occurs rarely in both polymyositis and dermatomyositis, but fibrosing alveolitis is relatively common in dermatomyositis, and it is then often associated with antibodies against Jo-1 (histidyl tRNA transferase synthetase).[37] Aspiration pneumonia can occur in patients with severe bulbar weakness and in patients with dermatomyositis and esophageal involvement.

Dermatomyositis, and perhaps polymyositis, can be associated with an underlying malignancy, although estimates of the frequency of this association vary widely from approximately 5% to 40% in published series.[38] This disparity in part reflects differences in case ascertainment: many case reports are anecdotal and there are few prospective or retrospective studies. Moreover, diagnostic criteria have also differed between reports, and muscle biopsy has not always been employed to confirm the presence of necrosis. Whatever the true incidence of this association, simple investigations, along with a systemic examination (including mammography, a chest radiograph, and an abdominal ultrasound), are appropriate. The underlying malignancies mirror those found in the population of similar age and gender.

Differential Diagnosis of Polymyositis and Dermatomyositis

The clinical diagnosis of dermatomyositis is usually straightforward, although lupus associated with a facial rash and motor neuropathy might cause confusion. Differential diagnosis of polymyositis is wider, as it may be confused with IBM (discussed later), MND, or myasthenia. The weakness in MG often affects deltoids and triceps, whereas the inflammatory myopathies more commonly affect deltoid and biceps. Additionally, in myasthenia, muscle weakness occurs without significant muscle wasting, and in MND both upper and lower motor neuron features are apparent. Finally, as inflammatory myopathies in older adult patients can be confused with muscular dystrophies, it is always prudent to take a family history, particularly in those who have not shown the expected response to immunosuppression.

Investigations of Polymyositis and Dermatomyositis

Serum creatine kinase (CK) is usually, but not always, elevated, often 10 to 50 times the normal value, and this is almost exclusively due to increases in the CK-MM fraction. However, CK values do not correlate well with either myalgia or weakness in patients with polymyositis and dermatomyositis, and in up to 15% of clinically affected individuals CK values are normal. Although the erythrocyte sedimentation rate is also usually elevated, this is nonspecific, and it is not a reliable disease marker. An autoantibody screen is worthwhile given the frequent association with collagen vascular disease. Other appropriate baseline investigations include lung function tests, a chest x-ray, and an electrocardiogram. Particularly in the presence of dermatomyositis, appropriate screening for malignancy is recommended and includes chest x-ray or chest CT, CT or ultrasound of the abdomen and pelvis, mammogram in women, and colonoscopy if indicated.

Neurophysiologic investigations are crucial in the evaluation of patients with suspected myositis. Concentric or monopolar

NEMG studies in polymyositis and dermatomyositis patients usually show myopathic features with small amplitude, short-duration polyphasic "myopathic" discharges but with additional indications of muscle irritability: increased insertional activity and spontaneous activity (including positive sharp waves and fibrillation potentials), reflecting myogenic denervation secondary to muscle fiber necrosis. To increase the sensitivity of EMG, very proximal muscles should be studied, including the hip flexors, thoracic paraspinals, and proximal shoulder girdle muscles. Nerve conduction and repetitive nerve stimulation studies are useful to exclude motor neuropathy and neuromuscular junction disorders, respectively (however, false positive repetitive stimulation can occur, in rare cases, in patients with myositis, with low levels of decrement of less than 20%).

Muscle biopsy is crucial to confirm the diagnosis. As already noted, the biopsy should be performed from a weak but not wasted muscle. Almost invariably the muscle biopsies are abnormal in both polymyositis and dermatomyositis, but if normal and a strong clinical suspicion remains, a second biopsy should be performed as the pathology can be patchy and sampling errors therefore occur. In polymyositis the pathology consists of a T cell–mediated cytotoxic necrosis: initially, $CD8^+$ cells and macrophages surround healthy muscle fibers and subsequently invade them. Muscle fibers show increased HLA class I expression (normally minimal or absent).[39,40] Endomysial fibrosis is common in polymyositis, and massive fibrosis may underlie some apparently treatment-resistant cases.[40] In dermatomyositis, it is thought that circulating antiendothelial antibodies activate complement and C3, triggering further changes in the complement cascade and generating membrane attack complex , which traverses and destroys endomysial capillaries. With destruction and reduced number of muscle capillaries, ischemia or microinfarcts occur in the periphery of the muscle fascicle (watershed area). Finally, as a late event, complement-fixing antibodies, B cells, $CD4^+$ T cells, and macrophages traffic to the muscle.[40] There is often a surprising divergence between clinical and pathologic features in dermatomyositis, and perifascicular atrophy is a useful feature in otherwise bland biopsies.

Treatment of Polymyositis and Dermatomyositis

Treatment of polymyositis and dermatomyositis is largely based on clinical practice and experience. Although there have been many studies of immunotherapy in inflammatory myopathies, they often group together adult and child dermatomyositis, polymyositis, and IBM patients. Most studies are retrospective and uncontrolled, and in several studies subjective measures and reduced CK are defined as a response. To date, there have only been a few small randomized trials of intravenous immunoglobulin in polymyositis and dermatomyositis (see the discussion in Mastalgia[41]).

Oral prednisone remains the drug of first choice for patients with both polymyositis and dermatomyositis. Patients should be started on oral prednisone 1 mg/kg body weight/day.[30] A clinical response should be evident within 3 months in most patients, with a biochemical response (a reduction in the serum CK level) often preceding clinical improvement. Many now advocate the early use of a second-line immunosuppressive agent such as azathioprine or methotrexate, as these have a useful steroid-sparing action in the longer term. Intravenous immunoglobulin is useful as a rescue therapy for patients with acute or severe dermatomyositis, but it has not been proven to work in polymyositis, has been shown to be ineffective in IBM, and is occasionally used at intervals for patients with problems related to steroids. A few patients remain resistant to steroids, and if the diagnosis is secure, cyclophosphamide is a useful alternative agent. It is important to remember that the dose of steroids should be tapered according to the clinical response rather than the CK level. It can be difficult for physician and patient alike to detect subtle improvements, and objective physiotherapy assessments, including myometry, can be useful. Although it is usually possible to taper off the dose of steroids after about 3 months, many patients require a maintenance dose of steroids. In all cases where prednisone is started and is likely to continue beyond 3 months, but especially in older adults, osteoporosis prophylaxis with bisphosphonates, calcium, and vitamin D is essential, as is regular screening for diabetes and hypertension.

The prognosis of both dermatomyositis and polymyositis is generally good, unless associated with an underlying malignancy. Respiratory involvement, especially fibrosing alveolitis, carries a poor prognosis. If patients fail to respond to steroids, IBM may be the diagnosis. Patients should be reevaluated and sometimes rebiopsied.

INCLUSION BODY MYOSITIS

IBM, initially considered to be a rare inflammatory myopathy in older adults, is emerging as the most common cause of new-onset myositis in this age group. The clinical, muscle biopsy, neurophysiologic, and prognostic features of IBM are different from both polymyositis and dermatomyositis.

The pathogenesis of IBM is unclear, but it is most likely a degenerative condition with a secondary immune attack on muscle. IBM may be an immune disorder as there is a modest association with other autoimmune disorders such as diabetes, and muscle pathology shows inflammatory features similar to polymyositis, with $CD8^+$ cells, macrophages, and increased HLA class I expression. However, IBM may be a degenerative condition involving intracellular muscle protein trafficking, as (1) muscle contains increased levels of amyloid, prion protein, and other molecules, as seen in Alzheimer disease, and (2) to date there is no evidence of maintained response to immunotherapy in the vast majority of cases.

IBM usually presents as a painless, profound, insidious, progressive wasting of quadriceps muscles associated with a characteristic genu recurvatum stance and frequent falls. In a minority of patients, weakness and wasting begin in the arms, where wrist and finger flexors are often preferentially affected. It is of note that muscle weakness and wasting is often asymmetric and may develop over many years. Myalgia and myoglobinuria are rare. Between a quarter and a third of patients have profound distal weakness, especially in the forearms, associated with a wasting of the medial flexor compartment, and weakness of finger flexors, particularly the deep ulnar component. This may be mistaken for ulnar neuropathy or MND early in the course of the disease. Deep tendon reflexes are often depressed, out of keeping with the extent of weakness giving rise to confusion with neuropathies. Dysphagia and neck flexion weakness are common in IBM and can affect up to 90% of female patients. IBM is not associated with malignancy, and there is a male preponderance.

The differential diagnosis of IBM is wide: upper limb presentations of IBM may be confused with cervical radiculopathies or MND/ALS.[42] The depressed reflexes seen in most patients with IBM can cause confusion with neuropathies, but the clinical sensory examination is normal. The combination of a weak quadriceps muscle group and a depressed knee reflex may suggest LEMS, but, of course, in IBM no posttetanic potentiation of reflexes is seen. The indolent history in most patients with IBM may suggest an inherited disorder, but the asymmetric weakness and wasting, as well as the pattern of involvement with IBM, reflect its acquired nature.

Several investigations are helpful in patients with suspected IBM. Nerve conduction studies are usually normal but may show features consistent with a mild axonal neuropathy. On EMG studies, myopathic, neurogenic, or, very commonly, a mixed "myogenic-neurogenic" picture is seen, and a high index of clinical suspicion is therefore necessary if the diagnosis is to be considered. CK level may be significantly elevated, but more often it is normal or only mildly elevated reflecting the low turnover of muscle cells in this disorder. Muscle biopsies show inflammatory changes, far more marked than one would expect given the often modest elevation of CK, with an infiltration of $CD8^+$ cells, and macrophages. In addition, muscle fibers may contain eosinophilic inclusions and rimmed vacuoles with basophilic stippling, hinting at a degenerative process. On electron microscopy, characteristic intracellular filamentous inclusions are seen, as in other degenerative conditions. Immunohistochemistry demonstrates an increased expression of "degenerative" proteins, including amyloid precursor protein, prion protein, ubiquitin, and α-synuclein, prompting comparisons between IBM and Alzheimer disease.[43] The lack of response to immunotherapy (discussed later) suggests that the inflammatory changes may be secondary to a degenerative process within the muscle, rather than a primary event.

The outcome of treatment of IBM is disappointing. To date, all attempts at immunosuppression and immunomodulation have failed to induce a consistent and long-lasting benefit. High-dose steroids, methotrexate, azathioprine, cyclophosphamide, and intravenous immunoglobulin have all been tried separately and in various combinations, with inconsistent but largely negative results.[41] Early studies suggested that some patients might benefit from intravenous immunoglobulin, but larger randomized studies failed to substantiate this finding.[44-46] Some evidence shows that exercise is of benefit early in the course of the disease, and many patients benefit from the use of canes and walkers. Patients with severe weakness often require wheelchairs or motorized scooters for mobility. Severe dysphagia may require enteral nutrition in the form of a gastrojejunal feeding tube.

DRUG-INDUCED MYALGIA AND MYOPATHY

A large number of drugs induce muscle symptoms, but a simple classification is not possible,[47] and an overview with important examples of each is given. Clinical and neurophysiologic combinations of a myopathy, a neuropathy, and neuromuscular junction abnormalities often suggest a drug-related toxic or endocrine cause.

Several drugs, including statins, fibrates, and aminocaproic acid, can induce a painful cramping acute or subacute necrotizing myopathy. Most commonly, statins produce myalgia or a mild asymptomatic elevation of the CK level, with no weakness or electrophysiologic abnormalities. However, statins may cause a painful myopathy a few weeks after starting the drug, and this is more common in patients with diabetes, preexistent renal disease, and hepatic disease, especially if on other P450-inhibiting drugs, multiple lipid-lowering agents, or higher than recommended statin doses. Unfortunately, clofibrate and other fibrates can also induce a myopathy; a useful causal clue may be subclinical neurophysiologic evidence of associated neuropathy and myotonia. The underlying mechanisms remain unclear, although secondary mitochondrial dysfunction may be important.[47] Statin- and fibrate-induced myopathies might be confused with inflammatory myopathies; drug-induced myopathies evolve more rapidly and improve, although often slowly, with cessation of the drug. In the presence of a statin-induced myopathy, the CK level is almost always elevated.

Antimalarial agents (including chloroquine), amiodarone, and perhexiline can induce a chronic painless proximal myopathy with vacuolar change and lysosomal inclusions on muscle biopsy. Amiodarone-induced neuropathy is more common than a myopathy, although the two may coexist.

Similarly, vincristine commonly induces a neuropathy, although some patients also have a myopathy. Diuretics and laxatives may induce muscle pains and/or cramps secondary to hypokalemia and occasionally, with very low serum potassium levels, can be associated with a painful or painless vacuolar myopathy.

D-Penicillamine may induce an inflammatory myopathy resembling polymyositis, or a drug-induced MG; both conditions tend to improve on withdrawal of the drug.

Critical-illness neuropathy is well recognized and may be associated with a myopathic counterpart. Its pathogenesis is unclear and is likely to reflect a combination of immobility, high-dose steroid treatment, electrolyte imbalance, sepsis, multiorgan failure, and the toxic effects of antibiotics and paralyzing agents, together with vitamin deficiency.

Excessive alcohol consumption is often associated with neuromuscular disease. Alcohol can induce an acute myopathy, often associated with hypokalemia, and possibly a chronic myopathy, although chronic wasting and weakness is more common because of a toxic neuropathy, as is a small fiber neuropathy with painful burning feet.

ENDOCRINE AND METABOLIC MYOPATHIES

Steroid-Induced Myopathy

Most patients with Cushing disease have clinical and neurophysiologic features of a myopathy.[48] The prolonged use of steroids is also often associated with a chronic, painless myopathy and less commonly an acute painful necrotizing (critical-illness) myopathy. Steroid-induced myopathy is typically associated with obesity, moon facies, and other classic stigmata of glucocorticoid excess. Steroid myopathy can be difficult to recognize in patients receiving steroids for inflammatory muscle disease, although steroids are unlikely to be the culprit unless used for more than 4 weeks, when patients will have other stigmata of glucocorticoid excess. Proximal leg weakness, particularly the hip flexors, is the most common clinical manifestation of a steroid myopathy. NEMG results are usually normal or mildly abnormal, although the presence of fibrillation potentials or positive sharp waves should suggest another cause. As CK levels may be normal in both steroid-induced and inflammatory myopathies, and EMG findings can occasionally be similar, muscle biopsy is sometimes required to distinguish disease activity from iatrogenic myopathy. The pathogenesis of steroid-induced myopathy is complex and involves hypokalemia and alterations in carbohydrate and protein metabolism. Structural changes on muscle biopsy include type 2 fiber atrophy (although this is nonspecific), lipid deposition, and vacuole formation. Using second-line immunosuppressive drugs such as azathioprine to treat the inflammatory disease in question may facilitate treatment, which consists of slowly withdrawing steroids. Unfortunately, patients recover slowly from steroid-induced myopathy. For these patients, an exercise program can be helpful.

Thyroid Dysfunction

Muscle weakness is seen in the vast majority of thyrotoxic patients. Hyperthyroid myopathy may be associated with myalgia and fatigue, and thyrotoxic patients may readily overlook it. Weakness may be proximal or generalized and occasionally involves bulbar and respiratory muscles.[49] Ocular involvement (Graves disease) may occur in patients with hyperthyroidism and reflects both excessive adrenergic activity and inflammatory changes in extraocular muscle and surrounding orbital tissue.[50] Hyperthyroid myopathy is commonly associated with proximal weakness without wasting, resembling that seen in MG. The association of autoimmune disorders means that patients with autoimmune dysthyroid disorders may have myasthenia and vice versa. Dysthyroid ophthalmopathy, where the extraocular muscles are often enlarged, producing restricted extraocular muscle movement, can be confused with ocular myasthenia and can coexist within the same patient. Recognition of such associations is important in targeting treatment. Patients with thyrotoxicosis may also have alterations in deep tendon reflexes and fasciculations, which can mimic MND/ALS and cause diagnostic confusion. Given these potential diagnostic pitfalls, it seems reasonable to recommend initial thyroid function tests and, in some cases, screening for autoantibodies against thyroid tissue, in all patients with neuromuscular disease, although thyroid disease is much less likely to produce a neuropathy.[51] Investigation of serum CK, EMG, and muscle biopsy is usually unhelpful, because there are no specific diagnostic features of the condition, but it may be useful in rare cases where dual pathology is suspected (e.g., polymyositis and thyroid myopathy). Occasionally, thyrotoxicosis is associated with a neuropathy, although mixed neuropathic and myopathic features are seen in EMG. The pathogenesis of thyroid myopathy is complex and likely to involve alterations in both muscle metabolism and electric properties, principally through increased Na^+, K^+-ATPase pump activity. Finally, thyrotoxic periodic paralysis[52] is a rare but well-recognized disorder, more common in individuals of Asian descent. (The periodic paralyses are a group of predominantly inherited neuromuscular disorders in which paralysis is related to electrolyte imbalances.[53])

Hypothyroidism is also frequently associated with neuromuscular manifestations, which may dominate the clinical picture and, in rare cases, may predate the development of overt biochemical abnormalities.[49] A recent prospective study underlies the strength of these associations: in patients with recently diagnosed thyroid dysfunction, 79% of hypothyroid patients had neuromuscular complaints including pain and stiffness and 38% had clinical weakness.[54] Symptoms did not correlate with serum CK levels and improved slowly with L-thyroxine therapy. Muscle biopsy shows glycogen accumulation at the periphery of the muscle fiber. The exact relationship between the muscle biopsy and clinical features remains unexplained. Hypothyroid myopathy may cause diagnostic confusion. First, patients may have delayed relaxation of deep tendon reflexes and occasionally pseudomyotonia (Hoffman syndrome), simulating features of the genetic myotonic disorders. Second, occasionally patients have very high CK levels and marked muscle wasting, simulating an inflammatory or inherited muscle disease.[48]

MOTOR NEURON DISEASE/AMYOTROPHIC LATERAL SCLEROSIS

MND/ALS is a relatively common, progressive, and usually fatal disorder with degeneration of both upper and lower motor neurons of uncertain cause. Death usually occurs as a consequence of respiratory failure. MND/ALS has an incidence of 1 to 3/100,000 and a prevalence of approximately 4 to 6/100,000.

The cause of MND/ALS is unclear, and a number of potential mechanisms have been suggested: excessive glutamate, an influx of calcium, and a subsequent excitotoxic cascade triggering cell damage and apoptosis are likely to be important. Familial syndrome cases may comprise up to 10% of cases. Mutations in the gene for superoxide dismutase (*SOD1*) account for the largest portion of these (20% of familial cases) suggesting that free-radical damage and excessive oxidative stress are potentially important in this subset of patients.[55]

Clinical features of MND/ALS reflect upper and lower motor neuron involvement. Nocturnal cramps are an early feature but rarely prompt patients to consult physicians. MND/ALS often begins in an asymmetric fashion in a single body region (intrinsic hand muscles, arms, legs, trunk, bulbar musculature) but ultimately involves all four regions; bulbar, cervical, thoracic, and lumbosacral. Lower motor neuron features include asymmetric muscle wasting and weakness, fasciculations, and depressed reflexes. Upper motor neuron features include spastic hypertonia, pyramidal weakness, and brisk deep tendon reflexes with extensor plantar responses. A combination of a wasted, weak quadriceps muscle with a pathologically brisk knee jerk is very suggestive of MND/ALS, as is the combination of a wasted and fasciculating tongue with a pathologically brisk jaw jerk. Neck weakness is common in MND and may lead to a head drop. Eye movement disorders, sensory signs (in the absence of entrapment neuropathies), and sphincter involvement are all distinctly rare in MND and should suggest another diagnosis.

Investigations in MND/ALS (1) provide support for the clinical diagnosis and (2) exclude structural or other potentially treatable pathologies. A serum CK level may be modestly increased (<1000 IU/mL) but is nonspecific. Neurophysiologic tests are useful in excluding another neurogenic disorder (e.g., multilevel root disease, multifocal motor neuropathy), myopathic process, or neuromuscular transmission disorder. They are also more sensitive than the clinical exam in demonstrating lower motor neuron involvement, with the neurogenic abnormalities reflecting both denervation and chronic reinnervation. A careful search for nerve conduction block is warranted in patients without upper motor neuron signs, who might have multifocal motor neuropathy, a rare but treatable autoimmune neuropathy frequently associated with antibodies against GM1 ganglioside.[56] Structural imaging, ideally MRI scanning, is sometimes often useful to exclude pathologies such as degenerative disc disease, which may cause both cord and nerve root compression (most commonly secondary to cervical spondyloarthropathy and associated myelopathy) with consequent mixed upper and lower motor neuron signs. Structural imaging is especially important when signs are confined to the limbs and there are no upper or lower motor neuron signs above the cervical involvement.

Unfortunately, no effective therapies are available, and to date, trials with a variety of nerve growth factors have been disappointing. Riluzole, an antiglutamate agent, produces a modest prolongation of life and should be considered at an early stage in all patients with possible MND/ALS.[57] The lack of curative drug therapy should not be taken to imply that nothing can be done to mitigate the impact of the disease. Rehabilitation utilizing the many different skills of the multidisciplinary team should be available at every stage.[57,58] Gastrostomy feeding is useful at an early stage both to maintain the patient's nutritional state and to reduce the chance of aspiration in those with significant bulbar weakness. The role of noninvasive and invasive ventilation in patients with MND remains controversial but overall appears to improve survival and quality of life.[59]

MYASTHENIA GRAVIS

MG is an autoimmune disorder in which neuromuscular transmission is disrupted by antibodies against postsynaptic skeletal muscle proteins, usually the nicotinic acetylcholine receptors (AChRs).[60,61] More recently other targets at the neuromuscular junction, including muscle-specific kinase (MuSK) and low-density agree lipoprotein receptor-related protein 4 (LRP4), have been identified in small numbers of patients.[62-64] The characteristic clinical feature of MG is fatigable weakness, usually involving extraocular, bulbar, axial, and proximal extremity muscles.[60] Therapies for MG are highly effective and include acetylcholinesterase inhibitors, immunosuppression, and temporary immunomodulation. The clinical features and management of MG in the aged person are similar to that in younger individuals. MG may be more common in older adults than was thought, and an increased risk of adverse effects of medications as well as increased likelihood of comorbidities in older adults mandates even more careful monitoring of therapy.[65,66] Thymectomy, although helpful in patients with early-onset MG, may not be beneficial for late-onset MG apart from its role in the removal of a thymoma.[67]

Clinical and Epidemiologic Features of Myasthenia Gravis

The clinical hallmark of MG is fatigable and fluctuating weakness of skeletal muscles.[60] The initial presenting symptoms are often ocular: diplopia and ptosis. Most patients develop generalized weakness subsequently. In 20% to 25% of patients with "ocular MG," the weakness remains restricted to the extraocular muscles.[68,69] In the remainder, generalized weakness can affect bulbar muscles, producing weakness of chewing or facial expression, dysphagia, dysarthria, and neck flexion or extension. Extremity weakness, usually proximal and symmetric, affects arms more than legs. Characteristic in MG is weakness that is worse at day's end and fluctuates in severity over weeks or months.

MG is uncommon, with an estimated prevalence of 80 to 100/1 million and an incidence of about 6/1 million.[70,71] Although myasthenia can present at any age, two peaks of onset define two clinical subgroups.[72-75] In "early-onset" MG, more common in females, onset is between ages 18 and 50 years. "Late-onset" MG, with onset after age 50, is more common in males.[74,76] Epidemiologic evidence suggests that MG is more common in older adults than was thought, and it may be misdiagnosed more commonly.[65,66,72,76-80] In older adults, MG is most often misdiagnosed as a stroke. Although evidence suggests that the incidence of MG is increasing in older adults, whether this is because of an aging population, increased recognition of MG or a true increase in incidence remains to be proven. MG in older adults may be more likely to be pure ocular, AChR antibody positive and not associated with thymic pathology.[72] However, older adult patients appear to respond equally well to treatment, with the prognosis after a myasthenic crisis being similar to that of early-onset patients.[80] "Seronegative" MG, without detectable anti-AChR antibodies, is clinically similar to seropositive MG, responds to the same treatments, and likely has a similar humoral mediation.[81] In a third of seronegative generalized MG patients, antibodies against MuSK are found.[62] Rare nonimmune "congenital myasthenic syndromes" occur when mutations produce a structural abnormality in one of the proteins at the neuromuscular junction.

LEMS is an even rarer disorder, with antibodies against presynaptic nerve terminal voltage-gated calcium channels (VGCCs).[82] It is often paraneoplastic, usually secondary to an underlying small cell lung cancer. The clinical manifestations of LEMS consist of fatigable muscle weakness (mainly affecting the legs and presenting as a gait abnormality), autonomic dysfunction, and depression of the deep tendon reflexes. The diagnosis and treatment of LEMS is similar in many respects to that of MG, with the exception that 3,4-diaminopyridine is a much more effective symptomatic treatment in LEMS than pyridostigmine, which will not be discussed further here.[83,84]

Neuromuscular Transmission and the Pathophysiology of Myasthenia Gravis

Depolarization of the nerve terminal at the neuromuscular junction opens presynaptic VGCCs, allowing calcium influx and the release of acetylcholine from the nerve terminal. Acetylcholine binds reversibly to AChRs on the postsynaptic skeletal muscle surface, resulting in muscle fiber depolarization and eventually muscle contraction. Finally, acetylcholine dissociates and is metabolized by acetylcholinesterase in the synaptic cleft, or it diffuses away from the neuromuscular junction.[85]

In MG, anti-AChR antibodies impair neuromuscular transmission.[86] When action potential generation fails at enough muscle fibers, the clinical result is weakness. Serum anti-AChR antibodies are found in approximately 85% of generalized MG patients, although titers may be lower in older adults.[61,76] The thymus seems to be implicated in the genesis or perpetuation of MG, as most early-onset MG patients have thymic hyperplasia.[87] The other main pathologic alteration, a thymoma, is present in 10% to 20% of all MG patients, in 24% to 38% of late-onset patients, much less commonly in patients with ocular MG, and very rarely in patient with seronegative MG.[88,89] When there is a thymoma, MG tends to be more severe, with a higher mortality.[90] In 10% to 20% of MG patients, especially those older than 50 years, the thymus is atrophic.[91]

Diagnosis

Suspicion for a diagnosis of MG is often delayed as a result of fluctuating weakness.[88] Routine electrophysiologic studies in MG usually produce normal results. Low-frequency (2 to 5 Hz) repetitive nerve stimulation may reveal a "decrement" in the motor amplitude.[85] SFEMG is highly sensitive (>90%) at detecting impaired neuromuscular transmission, but it is less specific.[92,93] Serum anti-AChR antibodies, highly specific for MG, are detected in approximately 85% of patients with generalized MG and in 50% with ocular MG[61] and are almost always present if there is a thymoma. Approximately 5% of seronegative generalized MG patients have antibodies against a different muscle protein, MuSK.[62] MuSK antibodies are found more commonly in female MG patients with prominent bulbar weakness and are not found in patients with purely ocular MG. More recently LRP4 antibodies have been found in smaller numbers of MG patients although it remains to be seen whether there is a specific associated clinical phenotype.[64]

Treatment

Before effective treatment was available, the mortality from MG was high, even worse in late-onset MG or if a thymoma was present. With effective treatment, the mortality from MG has dropped to less than 5%, although bulbar or respiratory muscle weakness continues to be a major source of morbidity.[94,95]

Treatment options include drugs that mask symptoms and more specific therapies to suppress or modulate the aberrant autoimmune response. The choice of specific therapies is dictated by the need for rapid improvement, convenience, expense, and the frequency of adverse effects.

Pyridostigmine (Mestinon) inhibits acetylcholinesterase, increasing acetylcholine at the neuromuscular junction. It does not affect the underlying immune process. Its duration of action is usually 3 to 6 hours but variable, ranging from 2 to 12 hours.[96] A long-acting preparation (Mestinon Supraspan 180 mg) is used at bedtime for patients with significant nocturnal or early morning weakness. Side effects, usually gastrointestinal, are mild. Although usually effective, Mestinon alone is often insufficient, especially in ocular MG. Most patients eventually require treatment with corticosteroids or other immunosuppressives.[97]

The efficacy of immunosuppressive agents is similar, and there may be synergism when used in combination. Prednisone is the most commonly used drug after Mestinon. Although highly effective, it has a significant risk of adverse effects. Low doses have fewer side effects but are less effective and take longer. Immediate high-dose treatment (50 to 100 mg/day) may cause transient worsening in weakness, so a gradual increase in dose is preferable.[98] Maximal benefit can take 4 to 9 months. There are numerous adverse effects, especially with prolonged high-dose corticosteroid therapy and in older adults.[88,99] Osteoporosis, more likely in older adults, especially if on corticosteroids, should be anticipated and prevented with bisphosphonates, calcium, and vitamin D.[100] Once MG is improved, the dose of prednisone is tapered slowly to lessen the chance of relapse, less likely when other immunosuppressives such as azathioprine are also used.[101]

Azathioprine is used as a sole therapy in MG when the situation is less pressing or when there are contraindications to corticosteroids. More commonly, it is added as a steroid-sparing agent. Azathioprine has fewer adverse effects than corticosteroids. However, its use requires monitoring for hepatic and hematologic toxicity, and it has a long delay (12 to 18 months) before optimal benefit. Cyclosporine is one of the few agents shown in a randomized controlled trial to be of benefit in MG.[102] Because it is expensive and has many adverse effects, it is used mainly in patients with severe MG not responding to prednisone and azathioprine. Mycophenolate, in widespread use in MG, seems to be effective, although no more so than other available agents, and has less toxicity. Two trials showed no additional benefit to prednisone, probably because prednisone alone is effective in the short term in mild MG and the trials were too short to demonstrate a steroid-sparing effect.[103,104] Several other immunosuppressive agents, including cyclophosphamide and tacrolimus, have also been used in patients with MG.[105] None has been proven to be superior to the previously mentioned drugs, and they are used mainly when MG is unresponsive to these agents.

Although there is widespread acceptance for thymectomy in MG, the precise indications and surgical approach remain controversial, and a randomized controlled trial is under way to clarify its role in MG.[106] It is generally accepted as effective in early-onset AChR antibody–positive patients with generalized MG. Its role is unproven and even more controversial in seronegative patients and in older adults (in the absence of a thymoma) when the thymus is often atrophic.[67,107] A thymoma is removed to avoid local growth and infiltration of adjacent mediastinal structures, yet it has less effect on the clinical course of MG than removal of a hyperplastic thymus. In MuSK-positive MG patients, the thymus is less pathologically involved, if at all, and the role of thymectomy even more uncertain.[108,109]

Incomplete benefits or delayed benefits from medical treatment are problematic for patients with moderate or severe MG. Plasma exchange and intravenous immunoglobulin are both equally useful when there is significant respiratory and bulbar involvement (a "myasthenic crisis"), as well as before surgery to reduce postoperative complications. Both temporarily improve neuromuscular transmission. Clinical benefit is usually maximal 1 to 2 weeks after treatment begins and lasts for 2 to 8 weeks. Sustained benefit requires immunosuppression. Both are expensive, produce temporary improvement, and are not advisable for the long-term management of most MG patients.[110,111] Numerous reports attest to the efficacy of rituximab, a monoclonal antibody against CD20 expressed on B lymphocytes, in MG. Similar to intravenous immunoglobulin and plasma exchange, benefits are temporary although perhaps longer lasting than these immunomodulatory treatments. It seems to be particularly effective in patients with MuSK antibodies. It is likely to have a place in MG refractory to immunosuppression.[105]

Several other drugs may worsen neuromuscular transmission and are best avoided in a patient with MG.[112] However, many myasthenics can take one or more of these medications without any obvious ill effect. It is important to educate the patient and her or his general physician about this possibility and to consider these medications as a cause of otherwise unexplained worsening.

More is known about the pathogenesis of MG than any other autoimmune disorder. As a result, the treatment of MG is highly successful, although the frequency of adverse effects is often a limiting factor. MG may be more common in older adults, although it is often not diagnosed initially, and older adult patients are more susceptible to the adverse effects of medications. Managing a patient with MG is usually a rewarding experience, with most patients responding to treatment and achieving significant improvement in their symptoms, although the adverse effects of long-term treatment can be significant.

KEY POINTS

- Neuromuscular disorders are common in older adults and may be mistaken for normal biologic aging.
- Most acquired and inherited myopathies present with symmetric proximal weakness.
- Most neuropathies present with distal sensory symptoms and weakness as a late manifestation.
- When weakness and fatigue predominate and sensory symptoms are absent, consider a neuromuscular transmission disorder, motor neuron disease, or a myopathy.
- Consider inclusion body myositis in patients with frequent falls and slowly progressive weakness/wasting of the quadriceps and forearm/finger flexors.

For a complete list of references, please visit www.expertconsult.com.

KEY REFERENCES

1. Doherty TJ: Invited review: aging and sarcopenia. J Appl Physiol 95:1717–1727, 2003.
2. Doherty TJ, Chan KM, Brown WF: Motor neurons, motor units, and motor unit recruitment. In Brown WF, Bolton CF, Aminoff MJ, editors: Neuromuscular function and disease: basic, clinical, and electrodiagnostic aspects, Philadelphia, 2002, WB Saunders, pp 247–273.
7. Bean JF, Kiely DK, Herman S, et al: The relationship between leg power and physical performance in mobility-limited older people. J Am Geriatr Soc 50:461–467, 2003.
9. Rantanen T, Avlund K, Suominen H, et al: Muscle strength as a predictor of onset of ADL dependence in people aged 75 years. Aging Clin Exp Res 14:10–15, 2002.
13. Rivner MH, Swift TR, Malik K: Influence of age and height on nerve conduction. Muscle Nerve 24:1134–1141, 2001.
19. England JD, Gronseth GS, Franklin G, et al: American Academy of Neurology. Practice parameter: evaluation of distal symmetric polyneuropathy: role of laboratory and genetic testing (an evidence-based review). Report of the American Academy of Neurology, American Association of Neuromuscular and Electrodiagnostic Medicine, and American Academy of Physical Medicine and Rehabilitation. Neurology 72:185–192, 2009.
25. The Diabetes Control and Complications Trial Research Group: The effect of intensive treatment of diabetes on the development and progression of long-term complications in insulin-dependent diabetes mellitus. N Engl J Med 329:977–986, 1993.
28. Bril V, England J, Franklin GM, et al: Evidence-based guideline: Treatment of painful diabetic neuropathy: report of the American Academy of Neurology, the American Association of Neuromuscular and Electrodiagnostic Medicine, and the American Academy of Physical Medicine and Rehabilitation. Neurology 76:1758–1765, 2011.
32. Weinstein JN, Tosteson TD, Lurie JD, et al: Surgical versus nonsurgical therapy for lumbar spinal stenosis. N Engl J Med 358:794–810, 2008.
41. Mastaglia FL: Treatment of autoimmune inflammatory myopathies. Curr Opin Neurol 13:507–509, 2000.
58. Miller RG, Jackson CE, Kasarskis EJ, et al: Practice parameter update: the care of the patient with amyotrophic lateral sclerosis: multidisciplinary care, symptom management, and cognitive/behavioral impairment (an evidence-based review): report of the Quality Standards Subcommittee of the American Academy of Neurology. Neurology 73:1227–1233, 2009.
60. Nicolle MW: Myasthenia gravis. Neurologist 8:2–21, 2002.
66. Vincent A, Clover L, Buckley C, et al: Evidence of underdiagnosis of myasthenia gravis in older people. J Neurol Neurosurg Psychiatry 74:1105–1108, 2003.
82. O'Neill JH, Murray NM, Newsom-Davis J: The Lambert-Eaton myasthenic syndrome. A review of 50 cases. Brain 111:577–596, 1988.
92. Oh SJ, Kim DE, Kuruoglu R, et al: Diagnostic sensitivity of the laboratory tests in myasthenia gravis. Muscle Nerve 15:720–724, 1992.

94. Christensen PB, Jensen TS, Tsiropoulos I, et al: Mortality and survival in myasthenia gravis: a Danish population based study. J Neurol Neurosurg Psychiatry 64:78–83, 1998.
103. Sanders DB, Hart IK, Mantegazza R, et al: An international, phase III, randomized trial of mycophenolate mofetil in myasthenia gravis. Neurology 71:400–406, 2008.
104. The Muscle Study Group: A trial of mycophenolate mofetil with prednisone as initial immunotherapy in myasthenia gravis. Neurology 71:394–399, 2008.
105. Silvestri NJ, Wolfe GI: Treatment-refractory myasthenia gravis. J Clin Neuromuscul Dis 15:167–178, 2014.

66 Intracranial Tumors

Caroline Happold, Michael Weller

INTRODUCTION

Intracranial tumors, as most cancers, show an increasing incidence with advancing age, with age-adjusted incidence rates for the most frequent primary brain tumors, glioblastoma and meningioma, peaking in the population aged 65 years and older, according to the most recent data from the Central Brain Tumor Registry of the United States (CBTRUS) statistical report (Table 66-1).[1] In our continuously aging population, brain tumors of older adult patients have therefore become a topic of great relevance over recent decades. Overall, the incidence of specific tumor histologies, the survival prognosis, and mortality differ from those of the younger patient populations. A reduced tolerance to therapy, restricted use of therapies, and diversities in tumor biology have been discussed as possible explanations for the shorter survival of older patients with aggressive brain tumors. However, because most clinical studies in the field of brain cancer excluded older people, few data were relevant to treating these patients and therapeutic recommendations remained controversial. Some relevant information is now available from recent prospective randomized trials that studied older patients with malignant brain tumors.

CLINICAL PRESENTATION

The leading symptom of a progressive intracranial mass is mainly a neurologic deficit in the corresponding localization, irrespective of the histologic subtype of the brain tumor. In general, primary brain tumors occur mainly in the supratentorial region: for gliomas, this comprises the hemispheres, mainly the frontal lobe (≈1/4), the temporal lobe (≈1/5) and the parietal lobe (≈1/10).[1] Therefore, leading symptoms of tumor growth can include personality change and mood disorders (frontal cortex), lateralized sensory or motor symptoms (parietal and motor cortex), epileptic seizures (temporal lobes), and aphasia (mainly left-sided Broca or Wernicke region). Meningiomas, arising from the arachnoid cap cells, usually do not invade the brain but compress the cerebral cortex and can trigger the same symptoms. Neoplasias of the posterior fossa are less frequent; present with gait instability, ataxia, and diplopia; and are most likely to be of metastatic origin in older adults.

More general signs of a space-occupying lesion are headaches, nausea, and morning vomiting and dizziness, all related to an increase in intracranial pressure as a result of the expanding nature of the brain tumor, as well as, especially in cases of malignant tumors and non–central nervous system (CNS) neoplasias such as brain metastases or CNS lymphomas, to the surrounding edema.

Symptoms mostly develop progressively over time, especially in more slowly growing brain tumors, such as meningiomas, where manifestation of a symptom can take months or years. Some benign brain tumors are only discovered incidentally in the context of cerebral imaging for unrelated reasons. On the other hand, aggressively invading brain tumors, as glioblastomas, usually present with subacute neurologic symptoms that develop over days or a few weeks, but they can also manifest with an acute incident, such as a focal or generalized epileptic seizure.

None of the presentations differs significantly in older patients when compared to younger patients, as the local distribution remains stable in all age groups. Yet, especially unspecific symptoms such as apathy or mild cognitive impairment tend to be neglected for longer time periods in older patients, as they are often misjudged as age-related dementing processes or as depression. Moreover, in patients with preexisting brain atrophy, increased intracranial pressure can manifest later than usual in the course of the disease, as the loss of parenchymal volume allows for a larger expansion of the tumor mass without occurrence of early symptoms. Acute manifestations, such as hemiparesis or epileptic seizure, are often misinterpreted as ischemic incidents initially, which strengthens the importance of additional imaging diagnostics beyond clinical assessments.

DIAGNOSTIC

Imaging

The best type of imaging for diagnosing most types of brain tumors is magnetic resonance imaging (MRI), ideally contrast-enhanced MRI, which has proven to be the most sensitive imaging detection technique for brain lesions in general. Although there is no specific diagnostic imaging marker to differentiate tumor entities definitely, there are certain typical features characterizing different tumor types. Meningiomas arise from arachnoid cap cells and therefore grow extraaxially, attached to the dura mater. They are usually highly contrast enhancing and well demarcated. In contrast to these mostly benign tumors, gliomas grow diffusely, infiltrating into the brain parenchyma, usually enhancing more with higher degree of malignancy. Whereas low-grade gliomas usually show no contrast enhancement and manifest as hypointense lesions, the majority of anaplastic gliomas and glioblastomas strongly enhance gadolinium as a correlate of blood-brain barrier disruption. Glioblastomas typically present with additional central necrosis. Yet, these features can be absent in some scans, and the features of CNS lymphomas, brain metastases or even abscesses can resemble those of high grade gliomas. Eventually, no final diagnosis can be made based solely on imaging criteria, and tissue sampling via biopsy or resection is mandatory to evaluate the optimal therapeutic approach.

Computed tomography (CT) scans are often used in urgent situations, when rapid imaging is required. They allow for a good identification of meningiomas attached to the dural base of the skull, where bone infiltration can occur, and can be helpful to assess calcifications in oligodendrogliomas or bleedings in metastases. Still, the poorer imaging quality in comparison to MRI and the irradiation exposure have made the CT scan a second-line choice. However, especially in patients with cardiac pacemakers or metal residua in the body, who cannot undergo magnetic scans, CT scans remain an option.

Lumbar Puncture

The analysis of cerebrospinal fluid (CSF) can be indicated in patients with suspected brain tumors when the detection of floating malignant cells revealed by a cytologic examination might affect the therapeutic approach, for example, in CNS lymphomas or with meningeal spread of metastatic disease (neoplastic meningitis). This examination is not required for the diagnosis of a solid tumor and should not be performed without prior cerebral

TABLE 66-1 Average Annual Age-Adjusted and Age-Specific Incidence Rates per 100,000 for Brain Tumors

Age at Diagnosis	0-19	20-34	35-44	45-54	55-64	65-74	75-84	>84
HISTOLOGY								
Pilocytic astrocytoma	0.84	0.24	0.12	0.09	0.09	0.06	0.06	—
Diffuse astrocytoma	0.27	0.50	0.58	0.61	0.79	1.02	1.14	0.68
Anaplastic astrocytoma	0.09	0.28	0.39	0.46	0.65	0.90	0.92	0.39
Glioblastoma	0.15	0.41	1.23	3.59	8.03	13.09	15.03	8.95
Oligodendroglioma	0.05	0.31	0.47	0.42	0.32	0.22	0.20	0.10
Anaplastic oligodendroglioma	0.01	0.09	0.17	0.18	0.20	0.16	0.10	—
Ependymoma	0.28	0.36	0.48	0.60	0.56	0.56	0.40	0.16
Embryonal tumors (medulloblastoma)	0.65	0.18	0.11	0.09	0.05	0.04	0.04	—
Meningioma	0.14	1.36	4.66	8.79	14.4	25.08	37.49	49.48
Lymphoma	0.01	0.10	0.26	0.44	0.86	1.82	2.27	1.18

Data from www.CBTRUS.org.

imaging because of the rare risk of cerebral herniation and neurologic worsening after acute decompensation resulting from CSF drain.

CLASSIFICATION

Secondary Brain Tumors/Metastases

Cerebral metastases occur in up to 30% of adult patients with systemic tumor diseases, therefore representing an issue seen more commonly in older adults.[2] The most frequent source of brain metastases is the respiratory tract, followed by breast cancer and melanoma.[3-5] Of note, approximately 10% of brain metastases arise from an unknown primary source. Occurrence of brain metastases always indicates a poor prognosis, and median survival from this moment on is significantly reduced to the range of 3 to 6 months,[6] especially when patients have diminished reserve, as is often the case in older adults who have undergone intensive treatment of the primary tumor. In a large database analysis of patients with brain metastases, a new prognostic index, the graded prognostic assessment (GPA), was validated. It includes patient age older than 60 years as one of four prognosis-defining components that limits the median survival time. Whereas the prognostic value of age is often diminished as more factors are taken into account, the GPA was later confirmed for specific subgroups of primary cancers, and patient age was a highly significant factor, especially in the cluster of the most frequent source of brain metastases (the lung cancer patients), for both non–small cell lung cancer and small cell lung cancer.[7,8] Beyond this, therapy of metastases is similar in younger or older patients, depends strongly on the systemic situation control, and can comprise either resection (in cases of a single metastasis) or palliative whole-brain irradiation. In cases of disseminated spread of metastatic tumor cells (neoplastic meningitis), patient age was identified as therapy-independent prognostic factor, with a median overall survival of 3.2 months in patients older than 60 years compared to 6.3 months in patients younger than 60 years.[9]

Primary Brain Tumors

Primary brain tumors are classified according to the World Health Organization (WHO) classification based on their histologic phenotype, including neuroepithelial-derived glial cells, meningeal cells, or even lymphatic cells, as for primary CNS lymphoma, and graded from benign (WHO I) to the more aggressive forms (WHO III, WHO IV) based on their biologic behavior.[5] The two most frequent tumor entities are *meningiomas*, classified as mainly nonmalignant primary brain tumors and accounting for 36.1% of all primary brain tumors, and *gliomas*, accounting for 28% of all and 80% of malignant primary brain tumors, with the WHO grade IV glioblastoma being the most important and lethal subgroup.[1] Both meningioma and glioblastoma, as well as CNS lymphoma, present with a specific peak incidence in older adults, and the age of the patient represents a therapy-independent prognostic factor, depicted for glioblastoma in Table 66-2.

TABLE 66-2 Relative Survival Rates for Glioblastoma by Age Group

Age Group	Patient Number	1-Year Survival (%)	2-Year Survival (%)	5-Year Survival (%)	10-Year Survival (%)
0-19	393	56.0	32.6	18.2	12.6
20-44	2,953	67.2	36.8	17.6	10
45-54	5,448	54.1	22.2	6.5	3.1
55-64	8,004	42.3	15.1	4.1	1.5
65-74	7,495	25.3	8.3	2.0	0.8
>74	6,318	10.6	3.1	0.9	—

Data from www.CBTRUS.org.

Gliomas

Gliomas are the most common malignant primary brain tumors in adults, and higher age represents an independent negative prognostic factor.[1,10] Even less aggressive low-grade gliomas develop a more unfavorable course of disease in older patients, leading to recommendations of an earlier therapeutic approach compared to younger patients, including surgical debulking or radiation therapy, usually up to a total dose of 50.4 Gy. The role of temozolomide (TMZ) chemotherapy for low-grade gliomas in patients of higher age (older than 40 years) versus standard radiation therapy (28 × 1.8 Gy) was investigated in the EORTC 22033-26033 study; data analysis is currently ongoing. Even so, most glial primary brain tumors in older people are the high-grade gliomas, and approximately 50% of glioblastoma patients are older than 60 years.[1] Because of the markedly poor prognosis of this tumor entity, with increasing incidence especially in the geriatric population, glioblastomas are discussed here in more detail.

Glioblastoma remains a fatal disease despite therapeutic advances, and population-based studies have identified age as an important prognostic factor for survival in this tumor entity, with significantly lower median overall survival in the older adult patient population.[11,12] In a landmark clinical study assessing the addition of TMZ, an alkylating chemotherapeutic agent, to the former sole standard of care, irradiation, a beneficial effect on overall survival was demonstrated in a patient cohort of 573 patients between 18 and 70 years of age, with a survival improvement from 12.1 to 14.6 months in the combination arm.[13] Yet, because the subgroup of patients older than 65 years was small and no patients older than 70 years were eligible for inclusion, no recommendations for the older adult patient population could be deduced from this study, making the application of this regimen to this group debatable.[14] Two large Surveillance, Epidemiology, and End Results (SEER) program database analyses from the pre-TMZ era illustrate that older patients tend to be undertreated, being offered fewer treatment options (surgery, radiotherapy, or chemotherapy), reflected in a reduced overall survival of 4 months, and that combination of surgery and radiotherapy was not the standard of care in the patient population older than 70 years.[11,15] In the past decade, the first randomized studies have assessed the role of different therapeutic regimens in the older adult population with glioblastoma. Keime-Guibert and colleagues analyzed the role of an irradiation regimen of 50.4 Gy versus best supportive care alone in a cohort of 85 patients aged older than 70 years and demonstrated an increased median overall survival of 6.7 versus 3.9 months.[16] In the post-TMZ era, the results of two large randomized phase III studies (the NOA-08 trial and the Nordic trial) were reported in 2012,[17,18] both comparing a chemotherapy-based first-line treatment to radiotherapy specifically in the older adult patient population. The NOA-08 trial compared a single-modality dose-dense TMZ regimen (7 days on/7 days off) to the standard radiotherapy with 60 Gy total in patients older than 65 years suffering from high-grade astrocytic glioma (grade III/IV). Results demonstrated the noninferiority of the chemotherapy but at the cost of increased myelotoxicity. The Nordic trial assessed two radiotherapy regimens (standard 60 Gy vs. hypofractionated 34 Gy) and a standard 5 out of 28 days TMZ regimen in patients older than 60 years, with a relevant subgroup of patients older than 70 years. Results were comparable for either TMZ or hypofractionated radiotherapy, with a worse outcome for the standard radiotherapy arm. In summary, both trials confirmed chemotherapy as an option in older patients, and both trials endorsed a higher benefit of the TMZ therapy in patients with tumors with methylguanine DNA methyltransferase (MGMT) promoter methylation. MGMT is a DNA repair protein, and methylation of the MGMT promoter has been proposed as a predictive factor for survival in patients with glioblastomas, as assessed in the patient population from the European Organisation for Research and Treatment of Cancer/National Cancer Institute of Canada (EORTC/NCIC) trial, treated with alkylating chemotherapy.[19] Several later studies confirmed a positive prognostic role for MGMT promoter methylation in older people with glioblastomas,[20,21] and the predictive impact of the promoter methylation was confirmed in these patients.[22] Therefore, the current pattern of care has shifted from radiotherapy as the only option in older glioblastoma patients to a more biomarker-driven therapeutic approach, and MGMT-methylated patients are treated with single-modality TMZ rather than radiotherapy at diagnosis.[14] Other biomarkers that play a more prominent role in the younger patient population are less relevant in the older adult population; for example, *IDH1* mutations, that are prognostic in glioblastoma patients, are virtually absent in older patients.[23] Other age-dependent genetic alterations potentially involved in glioblastoma survival[24] have not been validated as prognostic markers.

Meningiomas

Meningiomas are the most frequent primary brain tumors in adults, accounting for one third of primary intracranial tumors,[25] and incidence rates increase progressively with age.[1] An apparent increase in incidence may result from the wider use of imaging diagnostics, especially in older people, leading to a higher rate of meningioma detection, even in asymptomatic patients. Overall, bioptically benign (WHO I) meningiomas dominate with up to 98.5% of meningiomas reported in some publications[1]; lower percentages have been described in others.[5] Only few meningiomas present with signs of malignancy, being classified as WHO II or WHO III. Of note, age is a relevant factor for survival in those aggressive subtypes: the 10-year survival in the younger patient population was 84.4% (age group 24 to 44 years), whereas it was only 33.5% in the age group older than 75 years.[1] For the WHO I tumor group, therapeutic approaches depend on tumor localization and overall patient condition. Watchful waiting can be an option, especially in asymptomatic patients, as the slow tumor growth might not endanger the patient for decades. Otherwise, surgery is the first therapeutic option, additionally allowing for a histologic confirmation of the benign cause. Once the tumor has been resected, many older patients do not experience a recurrence, given the slow growth of these tumors. Especially in frail geriatric patients with potentially several comorbidities, the risk of anesthesia and perioperative complications must be well balanced against the potential benefits of tumor resection. For patients with unresectable meningiomas (e.g., close to the brainstem or a high-risk functional area) or patients with overall reduced general health status unable to undergo surgery, stereotactic radiotherapy is a valuable and safe option in patients older than 70 years. In a retrospective analysis of 121 patients undergoing stereotactic radiotherapy for meningioma, no treatment-related mortality or toxicity higher than grade II was observed.[26]

Primary Central Nervous System Lymphoma

Primary central nervous system lymphoma (PCNSL), a highly malignant tumor with often unfavorable growth kinetics, occurs at an incidence rate of 0.44/100,000, and approximately half of all patients diagnosed with PCNSL are older than 60 years.[27] Whereas cure can be achieved in younger people, cure is almost never achieved in older adults.[28] The tumor biology seen with PCNSL in older people, as well as their higher susceptibility to the side effects of intense chemotherapeutic regimens, often with whole-brain radiation therapy, has been discussed as the main origin of this difference. Older patients suffering from cancer are, in general, more prone to develop neurocognitive impairment as result of a tumor-specific therapy,[29] and although high-dose chemotherapy including methotrexate is effective for tumor control in older patients, the rate of neurotoxicity, including dementia and ataxia, is unacceptably high. Likewise, whole-brain radiation therapy was shown to promote severe neurotoxicity in a large retrospective review including 174 patients older than 65 years,[30] and the combination of chemo- and radiotherapy enforced short- and long-term toxicity in retrospective analyses.[31,32] This was confirmed more recently in a subgroup analysis of a large prospective clinical PCNSL trial, in which 126 patients older than 70 years (out of 526 patients assessed in total) were reviewed for benefit and toxicity of high-dose methotrexate (HD-MTX)–based chemotherapy and whole-brain radiation therapy with respect to progression-free survival and overall survival.[33] There were lower response rates and higher mortality rates in older people. Shorter duration of response was the major difference between younger and older patients, calling for new concepts of maintenance therapy in the latter. Even so, series of patients treated with HD-MTX monotherapy showed efficient and safe applications in older patients,[34,35] and even a patient cohort older than 80 years tolerated a high-dose chemotherapy regimen.[36] Still, because of the nature of methotrexate (MTX) metabolism, reductions of the total MTX doses might be more often necessary in older patients with reduced glomerular filtration rate.

The role of surgery in the context of PCNSL remains controversial. For decades, a biopsy for histopathologic confirmation of the diagnosis was the only standard operative procedure performed, and the attempt to resection was considered obsolete in this special tumor entity. A recent analysis, however, suggests that a gross total resection may translate into prolonged progression-free and overall survival.[37] This choice should again take all potential surgical risk factors, such as comorbidities, into consideration, but it can be considered as an option for the older adult group as well as younger age groups.

THERAPY

Surgery

Whenever feasible, total tumor resection is the treatment of choice for almost all brain tumors. In some tumors, especially those classified as benign, characterized by a noninfiltrating and slow growth pattern, this approach can be curative. Among those tumors are meningiomas or acoustic neurinomas. For more aggressive tumor entities, the degree of resection is still considered a prognostic factor for progression-free and overall survival.[38] In general, the localization of the space-occupying lesion and aspects of safety with regard to the patient's general health condition are more relevant for the decision making of the extent of surgery than is the patient's age.[38a,38b] No data over the last decades supported higher complication rates for older patients undergoing brain surgery.[39,40] The extent of resection seems to be of importance for geriatric patients as well; several series compared biopsy versus resection and demonstrated a benefit in the patient group with higher extent of resection,[41-43] reflected in a reduced risk of death and prolonged median survival. Yet, no prospective randomized trial has assessed the benefit of surgery on survival of older patients. Moreover, as addressed earlier, the higher rate of coexisting conditions impacting the risk of surgery or anesthesia in older adult patients must be taken into consideration, and recovery can be protracted by complications such as prolonged ventilation requirement or bleeding disorders.

Radiotherapy

Radiotherapy is a central part of brain tumor therapy, and for a long time period, this treatment modality was considered the only first-line therapy in older patients with malignant gliomas. Postoperative radiotherapy was shown early to prolong survival of older patients,[15,44,45] and these observations were confirmed in a randomized clinical trial comparing radiotherapy to best supportive care in glioblastoma patients older than 70 years[16] (Table 66-3). In most cases, the aim of radiotherapy is local tumor control and prolonged survival, especially in patients with malignant tumors, or consolidation in less aggressive tumor entities, such as meningiomas, after incomplete resection. In rare cases, radiotherapy aims at a curative approach, but this generally does not apply to tumor entities of older adult patients. With regard to the best radiation course, a prospective randomized study assessed overall survival in patients older than 60 years with glioblastomas, receiving either the standard 6-week regimen of 60 Gy in 30 fractions, compared to a short-course regimen of hypofractionated radiotherapy with 40 Gy in 15 fractions.[46] No significant difference in median overall survival was seen, establishing hypofractionated radiation schedules as a valid therapeutic alternative in older patients. Especially in patients with aggressive tumors and limited life expectancy, an abbreviated radiation course, allowing for a shorter hospital stay, can translate into improved overall quality of life. Radiation-induced neurotoxicity has to be considered, especially in patients receiving whole-brain radiation, as the risk increases, among other factors, with the age of the patient.[47] In patients with aggressive tumors, the shortened life span reduces the risk for patients to experience significant symptoms of neurotoxicity; yet, in patients with less aggressive tumors, and in patients with PCNSL in particular, leukoencephalopathy and brain atrophy, along with severe cognitive impairment, can occur in the course of the disease and relevantly impact the well-being of the patient.[30,32]

Chemotherapy

Since the publication of the landmark EORTC/NCIC study, which added TMZ to the former standard of care (radiotherapy) and produced results of prolongation of overall survival in all analyzed patient groups, chemotherapy is well established in the treatment of malignant gliomas.[13] Subgroup analysis confirmed this benefit in patients aged 60 to 70 years; despite this, a more detailed analysis indicated that this benefit seems to become less prominent with increasing age,[48] albeit in retrospective, nonprespecified statistical analyses. The optimal regimen of TMZ in the older adult population, which is characterized by age-related comorbidities and most often reduced immunofunction and poor bone marrow reserve, remained unclear, as the data collected in the EORTC/NCIC study was mainly based on younger patients and therefore not directly applicable to the older adult population. In the context of the previously mentioned NOA-08 and Nordic trials, a different TMZ regimen, namely 7/7 (1 week on/1 week off), and the standard 5/28 were used. Although the groups cannot be compared, both showed a survival benefit.[17,18] Because the toxicity of the 7 days on/7 days off regimen was higher than the toxicity in the 5/28 regimen, the use of the latter is recommended.[14] Overall, both studies promoted TMZ chemotherapy in the older adult population with high-grade gliomas. The formerly frequently used nitrosureas, such as lomustine (CCNU), are still considered effective alkylators in brain tumor treatment; yet, as the toxicity profile is higher, their use is mainly restricted to recurrence situations. However, as the dose regimen of lomustine comprises a day 1 of 42 schedule, this option remains of interest if patients with lower mobility, lower cognitive function, or generally reduced health resources may still require treatment; in these cases, medication can be given under surveillance once

TABLE 66-3 Randomized Clinical Trials for Older Patients With Glioblastoma

Study	Patient Number	Patient Age (Yr)	Regimen	Survival	*P* value
Roa et al.[46] (randomized)	100	>60	60 Gy (30 ×2) vs. 40 Gy (15 × 2,6)	5.1 months vs. 5.6 months	.57
Keime-Guibert et al.[16] (randomized)	85	>70	50.4 Gy (28 × 1,8) vs. supportive care	29.1 weeks vs. 16.9 weeks	.002
Wick et al.[17] (phase III)	373	>65	60 Gy (30 × 2) vs. TMZ 7/7	9.6 months vs. 8.6 months	.033
Malmstrom et al.[18] (phase III)	291/123	>60/>70	60 Gy (30 × 2) vs. 34 Gy (10 × 3) vs. TMZ 5/8	6.0/5.2 months vs. 7.5/7 months vs. 8.3/9.0 months	.24/.02 .01/.0001

every 6 weeks. It is tempting to speculate that this approach is more efficient in patients with versus without MGMT promoter methylation. Bevacizumab, a monoclonal antibody to the vascular endothelial growth factor (VEGF), is used frequently in glioblastomas at first progression, since glioblastomas are highly vascularized and express proangiogenic factors to form new blood vessels. In older patients, the use of bevacizumab showed better progression-free survival in two phase II studies assessing the role of bevacizumab in combination with chemotherapy: one in newly diagnosed glioblastomas, one in recurrent glioblastomas. Patients older than 50 years even benefited strikingly better from the addition of bevacizumab to first-line standard radiochemotherapy than the younger group.[49,50] At recurrence, bevacizumab has been shown to be beneficial especially in glioblastoma patients older than 55 years, that were found to express VEGF at higher levels; moreover, these patients required less dexamethasone due to the steroid-sparing effect of bevacizumab, which acts on contrast-enhancing tumor parts as well as on the surrounding tumor edema.[51] Since older patients usually require more medication for several indications, the steroid-sparing effect of bevacizumab may in parallel reduce the side effects of cortisone otherwise required. Caution must be exercised when older patients require anticoagulation or are prone to thromboembolic incidents, as bevacizumab can promote bleeding issues and thrombosis.

Finally, in patients with PCNSL, whereas application of HD-MTX was considered feasible even in older patients in retrospective analyses,[34,35] the only phase III study G-PCNSL-SG-1 found significantly lower response rates and higher myelotoxicity, along with reduced survival rates, in the subgroup of patients older than 70 years (126 patients out of 526). Therefore, application of high-dose chemotherapy has to be performed with caution in the older adult population, weighing the risks individually for each patient, and reductions of the MTX doses should be evaluated when glomerular filtration rates worsen, bone marrow toxicity increases, or other side effects occur.

Supportive Therapy

Besides the primary tumor–specific therapy, patients with brain tumors often require supportive medication to control symptoms related to the invading tumor, the surrounding edema, or even side effects of the therapy itself. Most commonly, steroids are administered to brain tumor patients with large tumor-surrounding edema to reduce mass effects and improve clinical symptoms as headaches or neurologic deficits.[52,53] Usually, dexamethasone is preferred, for its potent glucocorticoid activity and its long half-life. Other indications for steroids include nausea and vomiting caused by chemotherapy,[54] and in the specific case of PCNSL, steroids are considered to be part of the therapeutic concept.[55] With regard to the response to steroids, older patients might respond as well as younger patients.[56] Yet, side effects, such as diabetes, osteoporosis, and psychiatric effects, are common with steroid application, and older patients are usually more prone to experience toxicity, in short-term and long-term steroid regimens because of their higher rate of premorbidity.

As epileptic seizures are a frequent symptom of brain lesions, a significant number of patients require antiepileptic drugs in the course of disease.[57] In this context, it is relevant to choose a compound with low interaction profile (especially in older patients already requiring multiple medications) and without relevant organotoxic side effects and to start at low doses with careful titration. Therefore, most of the older substances are no longer used in the first-line antiepileptic therapy setting. For instance, carbamazepine and phenytoin act as enzyme inducers and valproic acid acts as an enzyme inhibitor, therefore interacting with drugs such as warfarin (Coumadin) and chemotherapeutic agents. Likewise, cardiac and hepatic side effects, as well as induction of osteoporosis, must be considered when prescribing these drug classes; the side effects are therefore endangering older patients more than younger ones. Most importantly, biologic overdosing of these substances can induce severe encephalopathy. Yet, even the newer substances are not free of side effects, and the renal metabolized levetiracetam, which is usually well tolerated in younger patients, can induce severe fatigue and dizziness in older patients, impacting their quality of life. Overall, all patients requiring supportive medication must be monitored for potential harmful side effects, and dose reductions or change of substance might be required.[58-60]

CONCLUSION

Overall, the incidence of primary and secondary brain tumors increases significantly with advancing age. Therefore, a careful assessment of neurologic symptoms and diagnostic completion with an appropriate imaging technique should be performed in any older patient with progressing neurologic deficits, including less typical presentations, like cognitive impairment and confusion. Whenever feasible, histopathologic confirmation of the diagnosis should be sought. In case of symptoms or malignant lesions, treatment should include surgical resection if possible, also in the older adult population. Based on the origin of the tumor, radiotherapy and chemotherapy, alone or in combination, can follow surgery, and adjuvant treatment is no longer restricted to younger patients. When risks of toxicity are well balanced, aggressive treatment in older patients helps improve overall survival.[61] Lately, more clinical randomized trials aim at assessing optimal strategies for the treatment of the continuously increasing population of older patients.

KEY POINTS

- The incidence of brain tumors increases significantly with age.
- Meningioma (benign) and glioblastoma (malignant) are the most common primary brain tumors found in older adult patients.
- The clinical presentation of brain tumors can vary depending on the localization of tumor and can mimic other diseases common in older patients.
- For diagnosis, tumor tissue sampling and histopathologic assessment should always be sought in addition to neurologic examination and imaging studies.
- Benign tumors may be cured by complete surgical resection only. Malignant tumors almost always require a multimodal approach, including surgery, radiotherapy, and chemotherapy.
- Recent studies of malignant gliomas focusing on the older adult population have confirmed a survival benefit with intensive tumor-specific therapy. When risks of toxicity are well balanced, aggressive treatment in older patients might help improve overall survival.
- As older patients often present with comorbidities, side effects of tumor-specific as well as supportive medication must be monitored closely.

For a complete list of references, please visit www.expertconsult.com.

KEY REFERENCES

1. Ostrom QT, Gittleman H, Liao P, et al: CBTRUS statistical report: primary brain and central nervous system tumors diagnosed in the United States in 2007-2011. Neuro Oncol 16(Suppl 4):iv1–iv63, 2014.
3. Barnholtz-Sloan JS, Sloan AE, Davis FG, et al: Incidence proportions of brain metastases in patients diagnosed (1973 to 2001) in the Metropolitan Detroit Cancer Surveillance System. J Clin Oncol 22:2865–2872, 2004.

5. Louis DN, Ohgaki H, Wiestler B, et al: WHO classification of tumours of the central nervous system, Lyon, France, 2007, IARC Press.
13. Stupp R, Mason WP, van den Bent MJ, et al: Radiotherapy plus concomitant and adjuvant temozolomide for glioblastoma. N Engl J Med 352:987–996, 2005.
14. Weller M, van den Bent M, Hopkins K, et al: EANO guideline for the diagnosis and treatment of anaplastic gliomas and glioblastoma. Lancet Oncol 15:e395–e403, 2014.
16. Keime-Guibert F, Chinot O, Taillandier L, et al: Radiotherapy for glioblastoma in the elderly. N Engl J Med 356:1527–1535, 2007.
17. Wick W, Platten M, Meisner C, et al: Temozolomide chemotherapy alone versus radiotherapy alone for malignant astrocytoma in the elderly: the NOA-08 randomised, phase 3 trial. Lancet Oncol 13: 707–715, 2012.
18. Malmstrom A, Gronberg BH, Marosi C, et al: Temozolomide versus standard 6-week radiotherapy versus hypofractionated radiotherapy in patients older than 60 years with glioblastoma: the Nordic randomised, phase 3 trial. Lancet Oncol 13:916–926, 2012.
22. Reifenberger G, Hentschel B, Felsberg J, et al: Predictive impact of MGMT promoter methylation in glioblastoma of the elderly. Int J Cancer 131:1342–1350, 2012.
23. Hartmann C, Hentschel B, Wick W, et al: Patients with IDH1 wild type anaplastic astrocytomas exhibit worse prognosis than IDH1-mutated glioblastomas, and IDH1 mutation status accounts for the unfavorable prognostic effect of higher age: implications for classification of gliomas. Acta Neuropathol 120:707–718, 2010.
24. Batchelor TT, Betensky RA, Esposito JM, et al: Age-dependent prognostic effects of genetic alterations in glioblastoma. Clin Cancer Res 10(Pt 1):228–233, 2004.
30. Ney DE, Reiner AS, Panageas KS, et al: Characteristics and outcomes of elderly patients with primary central nervous system lymphoma: the Memorial Sloan-Kettering Cancer Center experience. Cancer 116:4605–4612, 2010.
33. Roth P, Martus P, Kiewe P, et al: Outcome of elderly patients with primary CNS lymphoma in the G-PCNSL-SG-1 trial. Neurology 79:890–896, 2012.
41. Chaichana KL, Garzon-Muvdi T, Parker S, et al: Supratentorial glioblastoma multiforme: the role of surgical resection versus biopsy among older patients. Ann Surg Oncol 18:239–245, 2011.
46. Roa W, Brasher PM, Bauman G, et al: Abbreviated course of radiation therapy in older patients with glioblastoma multiforme: a prospective randomized clinical trial. J Clin Oncol 22:1583–1588, 2004.
50. Lai A, Tran A, Nghiemphu PL, et al: Phase II study of bevacizumab plus temozolomide during and after radiation therapy for patients with newly diagnosed glioblastoma multiforme. J Clin Oncol 29:142–148, 2011.
60. Saetre E, Perucca E, Isojarvi J, et al: An international multicenter randomized double-blind controlled trial of lamotrigine and sustained-release carbamazepine in the treatment of newly diagnosed epilepsy in the elderly. Epilepsia 48:1292–1302, 2007.
61. Scott JG, Suh JH, Elson P, et al: Aggressive treatment is appropriate for glioblastoma multiforme patients 70 years old or older: a retrospective review of 206 cases. Neuro Oncol 13:428–436, 2011.

67 Disorders of the Spinal Cord and Nerve Roots

Sean D. Christie, Richard Cowie

Most pathologic processes that affect the spinal cord in older adults are related to degenerative diseases of the spinal column or to insufficiency of the cord's blood supply. Even so, old age does not exclude many of the disorders that are more commonly seen in other age groups. In most patients, a definitive diagnosis can be made clinically by taking a directed history and performing a careful examination.

Neurologic assessment of an older adult is sometimes made difficult by failure to obtain a clear history or by the presence of common comorbidities that can challenge interpretation of symptoms and signs. For example, muscle atrophy may mimic neurologic weakness and diminish deep tendon reflexes. Nonetheless, an analysis of how a neurologic disorder has developed and the pattern of neurologic signs should provide a guide to the location of the lesion along the neural axis. A lesion can usually be localized in the cervical, thoracic, lumbar, or sacral segments before specialized neuroradiologic investigation.

CERVICAL RADICULOPATHY AND MYELOPATHY

General Issues

The neuroradiologic sequelae of degenerative disease of the cervical spine were established in the 1950s.[1] The degenerative changes of cervical spondylosis begin with desiccation and fragmentation of the intervertebral discs. As annular elasticity and nuclear hydration become reduced with age, the disc height diminishes. Consequently, extremes of movement are less well tolerated, and the vertebral end plates are subjected to greater stress. Secondary osteophytic spurs then develop circumferentially around the disc, projecting posteriorly into the spinal canal as bony ridges. Parallel degeneration of the hypophyseal (facet) joints combines with spurs from the vertebral bodies to reduce the size of the spinal canal and neural foramina. In most patients, there is progressive loss of movement between vertebrae, although in some cases excessive motion between vertebrae may develop and produce a degree of subluxation. Pathologic changes in the ligamentum flavum cause lack of elasticity and a tendency to buckle, further reducing spinal canal diameter. The compressive effects of the osteophytic spurs and buckled ligamentum flavum on the spinal cord are greatest when the neck is extended.[2] These changes bring about restriction of the natural motion of the spinal cord and nerve roots within the spinal canal.

Repetitive compression and obstruction of the radicular arteries supplying the cord in the neural foramina may further compromise cord function. This effect is aggravated if there is occlusive vascular disease of the proximal arteries in the neck.

Occasionally, acute rupture of a cervical disc can follow sudden twisting or flexion-extension movements of the neck and can produce spinal cord or nerve root compression.[3] The same mechanism can also cause hemorrhage into the spinal cord (hematomyelia). With age, such degenerative changes increase in severity and extent. Epidemiologic studies[4,5] have shown that most degenerative changes are in those who have done heavy labor.

Atomic and radiologic studies show that the neurologic sequelae of cervical spondylosis are more prevalent when the natural size of the spinal canal and neural foramina are restricted.[6] When present, large osteophytic ridges and subluxation of the vertebrae aggravate the situation. The C5-C6 and C6-C7 levels are most commonly affected because these are the points of transition from the more mobile cervical spine to the relatively fixed section in the upper part of the thoracic spine.[5,7]

Clinically, there is generally loss of lordosis, so that the head is held flexed and downward. However, if the natural kyphosis of the thoracic spine is exaggerated, there may be a compensatory extension of the upper cervical spine to maintain forward gaze. Most patients complain of recurrent neck pain and stiffness, together with crepitus on movement. Pain radiates to the occiput, shoulders, and scapula regions.

Radiculopathy

Progressive narrowing of the neural foramina results from osteophytic ridges—the bulging or herniated intervertebral discs and hypertrophy of the facet joints. This produces compression and restriction of movement of the nerve root.

Pain radiates down the arm in the distribution of the nerve root(s) with a deep, boring quality, aggravated by activities such as lifting and reaching. The pain is generally accompanied by paresthesias and some sensory loss in the affected dermatomes. In some patients, sensory symptoms predominate. Muscular weakness is generally mild, but occasionally wasting can occur. The appropriate reflexes are lost.[7]

Cervical Myelopathy

Cervical spondylosis is the most frequent cause of chronic cord compression in older adults. The clinical spectrum is wide, depending on many interrelating factors and the pathogenesis of cord damage. Compression leads to atrophy of the anterior horn cells and lateral and posterior funiculi of the cord.[8] Usually, the onset of symptoms and signs is insidious, and a clinical history can extend for many months or years before help is sought. Most frequently, there is a mixed picture of lower motor neuron features in the arms, together with long tract signs below.[9]

In the upper limbs, complaints of numb clumsy hands with weakness and loss of dexterity are common. Muscle wasting follows segmental anterior horn cell damage, affecting proximal muscles when compression is high in the cervical spine or more distally when compression is lower. The tendon reflexes in the arms are usually lost at the pathologic level of the cord and are exaggerated below. An inverted radial reflex occurs when the site of compression is above the fifth cervical segment, which has been shown to be the most common in older adults.[10] In contrast, there is commonly marked lower limb spasticity where the patient complains of a heavy leaden weakness and a tendency to drag the limb. Some degree of ataxia may be present due to reduction of vibration and joint position sense caused by damage to the posterior columns. Many patients complain of paresthesias and intermittent numbness in the upper and lower limbs.

Occasionally, symptoms may arise abruptly because of severe trauma or sudden extension of the neck in patients with cervical stenosis, such as after a fall. In this situation, a central cord syndrome is common. This scenario produces marked weakness of the upper limbs caused by anterior horn cell damage and a mild spastic weakness of the lower limbs because the peripheral regions of the cord are relatively spared. Frequently, this syndrome is accompanied by allodynia in the upper extremities, particularly the hands, and a suspended sensory loss because the centrally located decussating fibers of the spinothalamic tract are damaged. Very rarely, a hemicord pathology can produce a Brown-Séquard syndrome.

These neurologic disorders can be associated with vertebrobasilar insufficiency, in which symptoms are typically related to rotation and extension of the neck. Because the clinical presentation of spondylotic myelopathy varies, it must be distinguished from other conditions with similar symptoms and signs, including multiple sclerosis, amyotrophic lateral sclerosis (ALS), cerebrovascular disease, cord tumor or syrinx, normal-pressure hydrocephalus, and peripheral neuropathies.

Diagnostic Procedures

Plain radiographs of the cervical spine reveal narrowing of the intervertebral disc space, with sclerosis of adjacent cortical bone, osteophytic spurs, malalignment, and canal diameter. Patients with cervical myelopathy have an average minimal anteroposterior (AP) canal diameter of 11.8 mm,[11] and values less than 10 mm were likely to be associated with myelopathy.[12] An AP canal diameter more than 16 mm rarely produces myelopathic changes.[13] Secondary anterior and posterior osteophytes are demonstrated in Figure 67-1, together with an indication of the size of the spinal canal. Oblique radiographs allow visualization of the neural foramina. However, several authors[14-16] have shown that degenerative changes increase in frequency with age, and that 70% to 90% of those older than 65 years have radiologic abnormalities. In consequence, there is poor correlation between symptomatic and asymptomatic groups and the structural changes revealed on plain radiographs, with problems of sensitivity and especially, of specificity. Rarely, then, do plain radiographs alone dictate therapy.

When the clinical state suggests segmental cord or root compression and surgery is contemplated, specialized neuroradiologic studies are required. Magnetic resonance imaging (MRI), which has largely replaced myelography, reveals degeneration of the intervertebral discs, size of osteophytes, and presence and degree of cord compression (Figure 67-2). MRI also reveals intrinsic cord abnormalities (e.g., syringomyelia, demyelination; see Figure 67-2) and is helpful to exclude other pathologies, including a Chiari malformation and spinal cord tumor. Findings on MRI that correlate with poor functional outcomes include T2 hyperintensities within the spinal cord parenchyma and spinal cord atrophy of a transverse area smaller than 45 mm^2.[17] Unfortunately, MRI scans poorly visualize calcified structures such as osteophytes, and calcified ligaments and discs. Thus, computed tomography (CT) is often performed.

CT[18,19] reveals the size and shape of the vertebral canals and presence of extensive ligamentous calcification, but it cannot give

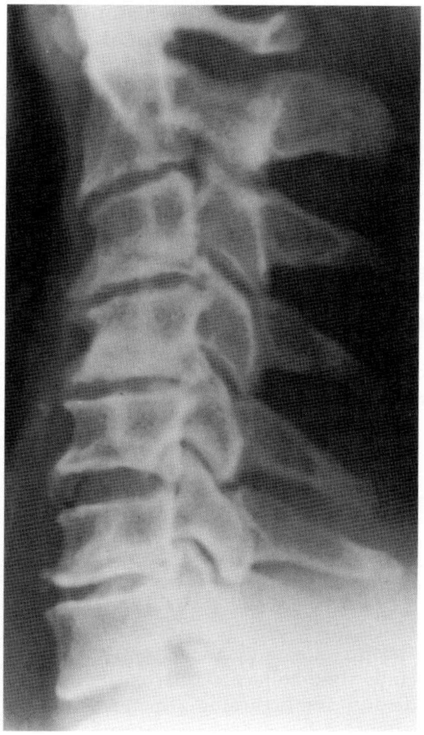

Figure 67-1. Lateral cervical spine radiograph showing widespread spondylosis. Note the loss of disc height and large anterior osteophytes. This patient has a small spinal canal into which project osteophytes at the posterior margin of the C3-C4 of the 4-5 discs.

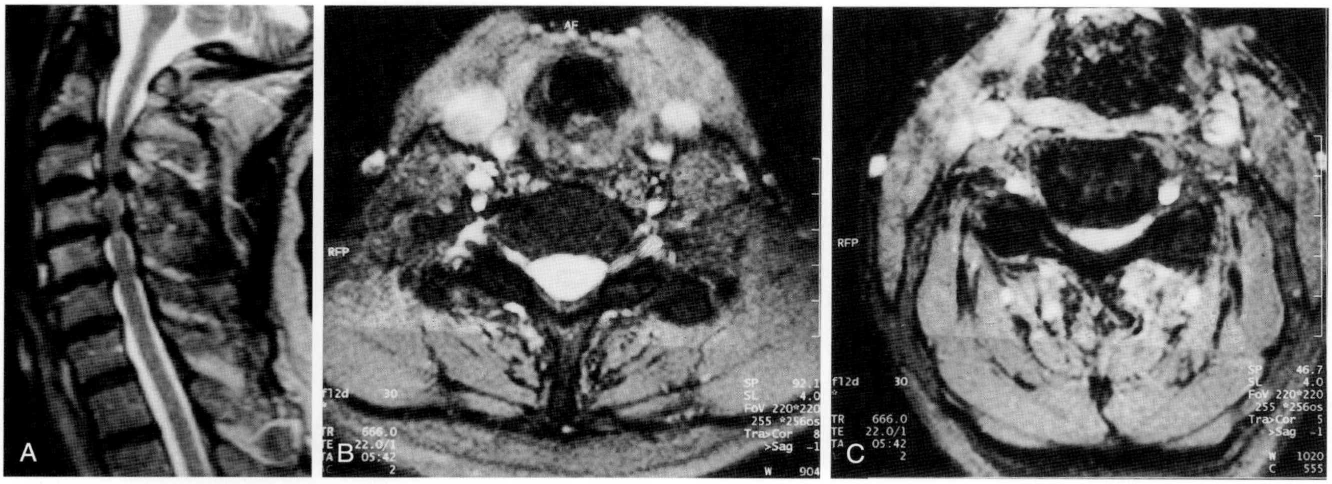

Figure 67-2. A, Lateral MRI scan of the cervical spine showing compression of the spinal cord by posterior osteophytes and buckling of the ligamentum flavum. **B,** Transverse image of normal cervical spine reveals the spinal cord surrounded by cerebrospinal fluid. **C,** Transverse image of the patient seen in **A** showing severe narrowing of the spinal canal and compression of the cord.

details of vertebral displacements, disc protrusions, and corrugation of the bulging longitudinal ligament unless an intrathecal contrast medium has been injected. Myelography is now performed only when MRI is contraindicated, such as in a patient with an implanted pacemaker or neuromodulatory device or in the presence of cerebral aneurysm clips made from materials other than titanium or titanium alloy.[20]

Management

Cervical radiculopathy and associated neck pain improve without surgical intervention in over 90% of cases.[21] Reduction in symptom severity can be achieved through a multimodality approach. This may include analgesia with nonsteroidal antiinflammatory drugs (NSAIDs), opioids, and neuropathic agents such as gabapentin and its derivatives. Physical therapy, including traction, may diminish the severity of symptoms.[22]

Surgical intervention for cervical radiculopathy aims to eliminate the compression on the affected nerve root. The surgical options include anterior and posterior approaches, depending on the location and source of the compression; each carries a good prognosis for neurologic recovery,[23-25] although recovery of muscle wasting is rarely satisfactory. Surgery should be considered when the patient fails to respond to nonsurgical intervention or when neurologic deficits worsen or new deficits arise. Consideration should also be given to patients whose symptoms are so severe they cannot partake in routine daily activities. Finally, the patient must be able to withstand the stress of surgery, including the general anesthetic.

The natural history of myelopathy complicating cervical spondylosis is variable and unpredictable. Many patients run a chronic course characterized by episodes of deterioration separated by periods of stability, whereas others have a more progressive course.[9,26] Most older adults with cervical myelopathy will not need surgical intervention. Often, a nonoperative approach may hasten progression and alleviate symptoms. Noninvasive strategies include rigid collars to restrict small repetitive trauma, NSAIDs, and education regarding avoidance of potential harmful activities.

Surgical treatment is indicated when the myelopathy interferes with daily activities, there is a short progressive history, or there is radiologic evidence of severe cord compression or instability. Anterior decompression of disc and osteophytic spurs is usually carried out when up to three intervertebral levels are affected. Posterior decompression, including laminectomy and laminoplasty, is indicated for more widespread stenosis. In general, the prime objective of surgery has been to halt the decline in neurologic function before further damage to the cord has occurred. However, studies have suggested that there may be a more reliable improvement in neurologic function than previously appreciated.[27]

Prognosis following surgery depends on multiple factors, including duration of symptoms and severity at presentation. A longer duration of symptoms has been shown to diminish functional outcomes following decompression.[28] Likewise, an increasing severity of symptoms at presentation[29] is a poor prognostic factor. Concomitant fusion along with decompression limits motion at the surgical site. This may limit vascular insufficiency associated with movement and prevent further deterioration.[9]

CORD COMPRESSION

Rheumatoid Arthritis

Neck pain and stiffness are common complaints in patients with progressive rheumatoid arthritis (RA). Radiation of pain to the occipital region and cutaneous numbness at the back of the head may occur when the upper cervical nerve roots are compressed. These symptoms may herald the development of atlantoaxial subluxation as a result of destruction of the transverse atlantal ligament by synovitis. There may be rotatory subluxation and vertical migration of the odontoid into the foramen magnum of the skull (cranial settling or basilar impression or invagination). Atlantoaxial subluxation, which occurs in approximately 33% of patients with RA, can be asymptomatic until the slip reaches 8 to 9 mm, at which point spinal cord compression begins. Once myelopathy develops, most patients deteriorate, and 50% die within 6 months. Approximately 20% of patients show subaxial subluxation on cervical radiography, often affecting several segments to produce a so-called staircase deformity of the vertebrae. Compression of the cord and myelopathy are common in this situation.

Most patients present with progressive deterioration of upper limb function, accompanied by tingling, numbness, the Lhermitte phenomenon, gait disturbance, and possibly bladder and bowel dysfunction. It is common for these symptoms to be initially attributed to severe peripheral joint disease and muscle atrophy. Abnormality of spinothalamic function, hyperreflexia and hypertonia, and extensor plantar responses help differentiate the cause from peripheral nerve lesions. Compression of the trigeminal nucleus and tract at the craniocervical junction may produce facial numbness or paresthesias. Lower cranial nerve findings (cranial nerves IX to XII) may be present with cranial settling.

Radiologic assessment requires flexion and extension radiographs of the cervical spine. This is followed by MRI, which will reveal compression or distortion of the spinal cord (Figure 67-3).

Surgical management has to be considered when there is progressive or significant atlantoaxial subluxation or clinical evidence of increasing neurologic morbidity. Because most patients have significant medical problems, such as pulmonary fibrosis, anemia, atrophic skin, and the effects of prolonged steroid or other immunosuppressive therapy, there is significant risk from surgical

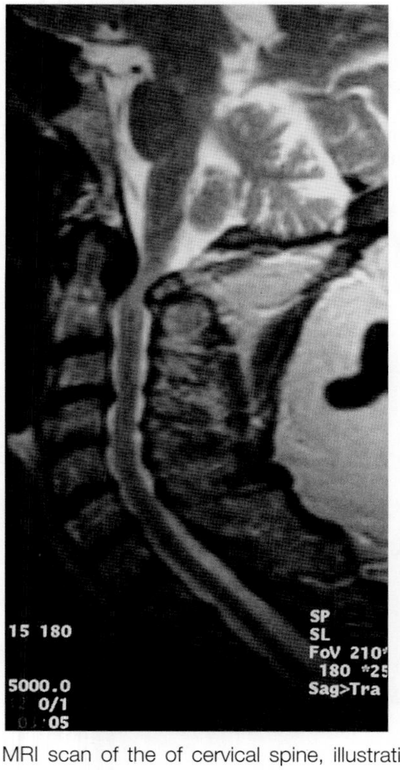

Figure 67-3. MRI scan of the of cervical spine, illustrating pathology attributable to rheumatoid arthritis—cranial settling, cervical stenosis, and subaxial instability.

intervention that needs to be reviewed with the patient and family or caregiver. For some patients, particularly those who are frail, the use of a cervical collar in lieu of surgery may be the best option to manage craniocervical instability, although tolerance of use can be limited.

The surgical approach and procedure may consist of an anterior, transoral, or posterior decompression combined with internal fixation. However, the timing of these interventions remains controversial.[30]

Thoracic Disc Protrusion

The central protrusion of a thoracic intervertebral disc is an unusual cause of cord compression, but one that occurs in older adults because it is associated with degeneration of the disc annulus. Russell[31] has noted that 67% occur between the eighth and eleventh interspaces. Most patients present with a long history of gradually progressive myelopathy, in which sensory and motor symptoms are equally common. However, 49% of patients complain of radicular symptoms of pain and dysesthesiae. Sometimes, the onset is more rapid, leading to a flaccid paraplegia.[32] The presence of a thoracic disc protrusion is generally recognized when MRI is carried out to investigate the progressive neurologic deficit. Cord compression from this source carries a poor prognosis unless surgery is performed. The results of simple decompressive laminectomy are unsatisfactory; a costotransversectomy, transpedicular, or transthoracic approach is recommended.[31,33] Minimal access approaches[34] are better tolerated and may lead to quicker postoperative recovery, particularly in older adults.

Intradural Tumors

Intradural extramedullary tumors cause local compression of the spinal cord and nerve roots. Meningiomas represent approximately 25% of primary spinal cord tumors, and 80% of them occur in women. They are most commonly seen in the sixth decade, and 80% occur in the thoracic spine. Most patients complain of local or radicular pain, the significance of which often goes unrecognized for a long period until progressive spastic paraparesis develops, followed by sensory and bladder dysfunction.[35]

Plain radiographs are rarely helpful. The condition is diagnosed only by myelography or, more commonly, MRI.[36] Results of decompressive surgery are generally good. Levy and colleagues[37] have reported that one third of paraplegic patients are able to walk after tumor excision. Similar successes have been observed in septuagenarians.[38] Neurofibromas are slightly more common than meningiomas, but their peak incidence is in younger age groups, so they are less frequently encountered in older adults.[39] Radicular pain is more common, and enlargement of a neural foramen may be seen on plain radiographs if the tumor extends into the paravertebral tissues. Multiple tumors can be encountered in neurofibromatosis. As with meningiomas, surgical excision should be undertaken and carries a good prognosis for neurologic recovery. However, for older adults or those who are medically unfit, radiosurgery is an option that appears to afford long-term clinical stability.[40]

Metastatic Spinal Tumors

The most common extradural spinal tumors to cause cord compression are those metastasizing from distant carcinomas or primary hematologic tumors. Spread may be arterial, venous via the vertebral venous plexus, or by direct invasion. Although myeloma and carcinomas of the prostate and kidney seem to metastasize preferentially to the spine, in practice the most commonly encountered tumors are those that occur with the greatest frequency. Therefore, primary lung, breast, kidney, and prostate tumors are seen, although in some patients the primary tumor cannot be identified. The thoracic region of the spine is most frequently involved, followed by the lumbosacral and cervical regions.

Most patients present with progressive walking difficulty because of weakness and clumsiness, the significance of which may go unrecognized until the patient is no longer able to bear weight. Many patients have a history of preceding spinal pain, which should always lead to a suspicion of vertebral metastasis in a patient known to have malignant disease. The neurologic deficit may develop very rapidly, with collapse of the vertebra or occlusion of the vascular supply to the cord. An analysis of the level of the sensory deficit helps in assessing the site of the spinal disease and planning the appropriate radiologic investigations. However, plain radiographs of the entire spine and chest should be carried out and may reveal loss of outline of a pedicle, reduction in height of a vertebral body, or soft tissue mass. MRI of the spine is the investigation of choice. However, CT may reveal evidence of bone destruction and allow percutaneous needle biopsy of the lesion.

There has been considerable debate about the value of decompressive surgery because laminectomy alone has produced suboptimal results.[41] As a result, there has been considerable experience with alternate conservative therapies. Commonly, steroids such as dexamethasone are prescribed for their effect on vasogenic edema and to improve tumor-related pain.[42,43] In the 1970s and 1980s, radiotherapy became the mainstay of treatment, and surgical intervention was primarily used as a salvage therapy if patients deteriorated during the procedure. In some centers, radiation remains the initial treatment.[43] However, there has been a resurgence in surgical interest for these patients. This was spearheaded by a randomized-controlled trial by Patchell and associates.[44] This trial compared radiation alone to surgery (circumferential decompression and stabilization) and radiation. The authors showed that the surgical group had improved bladder control and ambulation status compared to the radiation-alone group, and there was no change in survival. Improvements in ambulation and continence are now thought to be appropriate benefits to offset the risks of surgery in patients who are receiving palliative care and have been reported by other groups.[45] However, surgery is not indicated for all patients with metastatic epidural compression. If there is no bony instability and no neurologic compromise, biopsy and radiation treatment are typically offered. Likewise, patients with disseminated disease and an expected survival less than 4 months, those with multiple lesions at multiple levels, very radiosensitive tumors (lymphoma, myeloma), total paralysis longer than 8 hours, or loss of ambulation for 24 hours, or who are medically unfit for surgery may not derive the benefits from surgery.

VASCULAR DISORDERS OF THE SPINAL CORD

The peculiar anatomic arrangement of the arterial blood supply of the spinal cord may protect it from the effects of occlusion of one feeding vessel. The anterior and posterior spinal arteries are fed by radicular arteries, which are branches of vessels arising from the aorta or subclavian arteries. There is generally a large feeding artery in the lower thoracic region, most commonly on the left at T10. A watershed lies at the second thoracic segment of the spinal cord, between areas supplied by thoracic vessels and those from the neck. Interruption of supply can occur in atheroma of the aorta,[46] in a dissecting aneurysm,[47] or as a complication of open and endovascular aortic surgery.[48] The extent and severity of the spinal cord neurologic deficit varies considerably, probably depending on the anatomic variation of the spinal cord vessels in the individual patient.

The syndrome of the anterior spinal artery arises when it is obstructed by thrombus. The onset is sudden, with pain in the back or neck and paresthesias down the arms. The posterior columns receiving a blood supply from the posterior spinal network are preserved so that proprioception and vibration remain intact, whereas thermal and pain appreciation are impaired. In addition, a lower motor paralysis of the arms is associated with spastic paraparesis or paraplegia. In some cases, the presence of cervical spondylosis and an osteophytic ridge has been implicated in local occlusion of the anterior spinal artery.[49] This phenomenon is also recognized in the setting of thrombophlebitis secondary to epidural abscess.[50]

SPINAL CORD INJURY

Acute spinal cord injury (SCI) is a severe and devastating event for the patient, family, and caregiver, regardless of age. However, there has been a perception that older adults fare considerably worse than their younger counterparts. A number of authors have observed an increasing proportion of older patients presenting with acute SCI, with falls (often from standing height) as the leading mechanism of injury in contrast to motor vehicle collisions, which are more common in younger age groups.[51-55] The reasons for these observations are likely multifactorial and include an aging population, alteration in bony structural support secondary to osteopenia or osteoporosis, cervical spondylosis (leading to undiagnosed myelopathic symptoms and predisposing to central cord syndrome), more fragile ambulation status (because of altered sensory mechanisms), osteoarthritis and decreased mobility, neurologic disorders such as Parkinson disease or diabetic peripheral neuropathy, and the effects of polypharmacy.[54]

Several authors have endeavored to reassess the outcomes of SCI in the geriatric setting to evaluate whether current treatment modalities have altered clinical outcomes. In a retrospective review of a prospective cohort, Furlan and coworkers[55] found that patients with SCI 65 years of age and older had a significantly higher mortality rate than younger patients (46.88% vs. 4.86%; $P < .001$). However, they also reported that among survivors, age had no impact on motor or sensory outcomes. This suggests that a significant number of patients (the survivors) could benefit from aggressive treatment and, with a better understanding of predictors of outcome, preferably those that are modifiable, the expected survivors could be identified and treated. Fassett and colleagues[53] conducted a retrospective review of 412 patients older than 70 years treated between 1978 and 2005. They observed an increase in incidence from 4.2% to 15.4%, and the older cohort as a whole tended to have less severe injuries based on the American Spinal Injury Association (ASIA) grading scale. However, the mortality rate in the older patients with severe neurologic impairment was uniformly higher, high enough to yield a statistical difference in mortality between the age groups. Unfortunately, their data did not contain information of preinjury medical conditions. In another study, Krassioukov and associates[51] examined the effect of preexisting conditions on outcomes. In their cohort, the ASIA grade was similar between the younger and older adults; however, the number of preexisting medical conditions was statistically greater in the older group, which correlated to the difference in secondary complications observed between the two groups. When this observation was taken into account, there was no statistical difference in complications or mortality reported to be attributable solely to age. It needs to be borne in mind that this study had relatively small cohorts (28 older adults, 30 younger adults), and the conclusions may differ with more statistical power. Despite this, the authors advocated for an aggressive multidisciplinary approach to SCI in older adults and cautioned against allowing "ageism" to bias treatment.

PAGET DISEASE

Paget disease is a generally progressive disorder of bone that causes neurologic sequelae of the brain, spinal cord, or peripheral nerves, depending on which bones are involved. It is important to recognize these complications, because many respond to treatment of the underlying disorder. In the spine, pagetic changes may affect one or several vertebrae. The disease is characterized by bony destruction followed by repair, which leads to flattening and expansion of the diameter of the vertebral bodies, and thickening of the pedicles and lamina. Bony projections in the vertebral canal cause spinal cord and nerve root compression. Neurologic symptoms may develop suddenly if collapse of a vertebral body occurs.

Spinal cord compression is most common in the thoracic region and generally is slowly progressive, causing a spastic weakness of the lower limbs combined with sensory symptoms and signs. Pain may be due to local bony changes, malignant degeneration, or nerve root compression. In some patients, progressive myelopathy occurs, yet imaging fails to reveal direct compression of the spinal cord. In these patients, progressive ischemia may be the cause of the neurologic deterioration.

When the disease affects the lumbar region, symptoms of single or multiple nerve root compression can develop, producing back pain and sciatica. When the spinal canal is constricted, neurogenic claudication may be the presenting symptom.

Medical treatment of Paget disease aims to reduce osteoclastic activity and thereby diminish the osteoblastic response to increase bone resorption. Typical agents used include calcitonin derivatives and bisphosphonates. Surgical treatment is indicated only when medical treatment fails to control the progression of the neurologic sequelae of the condition. However, control of blood loss from the diseased bone during surgery can be troublesome.[56,57] Decompressive laminectomy was found to improve symptoms in 85% of patients, whereas those who failed to respond usually suffered from malignant degenerative changes. The surgical mortality in this series was 10%.[58]

NEUROLOGIC COMPLICATIONS OF DEGENERATIVE DISEASE OF THE LUMBAR SPINE

Spondylosis of the lumbar spine increases in severity and extent with advancing age, often occurring simultaneously with disease in the cervical region.[4,59] Biochemical and pathologic changes are similar at both sites. Loss of disc height and the development of traction spurs and osteophytes are associated with sclerosis and enlargement of the vertebral bodies. Simultaneous changes in the facet joints occur, with destruction of articular cartilage, laxity of the joint capsule, and osteophytic enlargement of the joint surfaces.[60] This process may be asymmetrical so that rotational subluxation of one vertebra on the other can develop. The lowest intervertebral discs of the lumbar spine are usually affected at the point of transition from the mobile lumbar spine to the fixed sacrum.

A number of discrete neurologic conditions may complicate lumbar spondylosis. These are presented in the following sections.

Acute Nerve Root Entrapment

True herniation of an intervertebral disc can occur in older adults and produce a pattern of symptoms and signs similar to that seen in younger patients.[61] However, compared with the average adult population, older adults have a higher incidence of motor deficits and are more likely to have a sequestrated portion of disc nucleus. Acute root entrapment may also result from compression secondary to rapid expansion of a degenerative spinal synovial cyst.[62]

Chronic Nerve Root Entrapment

Lumbar monoradiculopathy and polyradiculopathy occur in older adults, usually as a result of nerve root compression in the

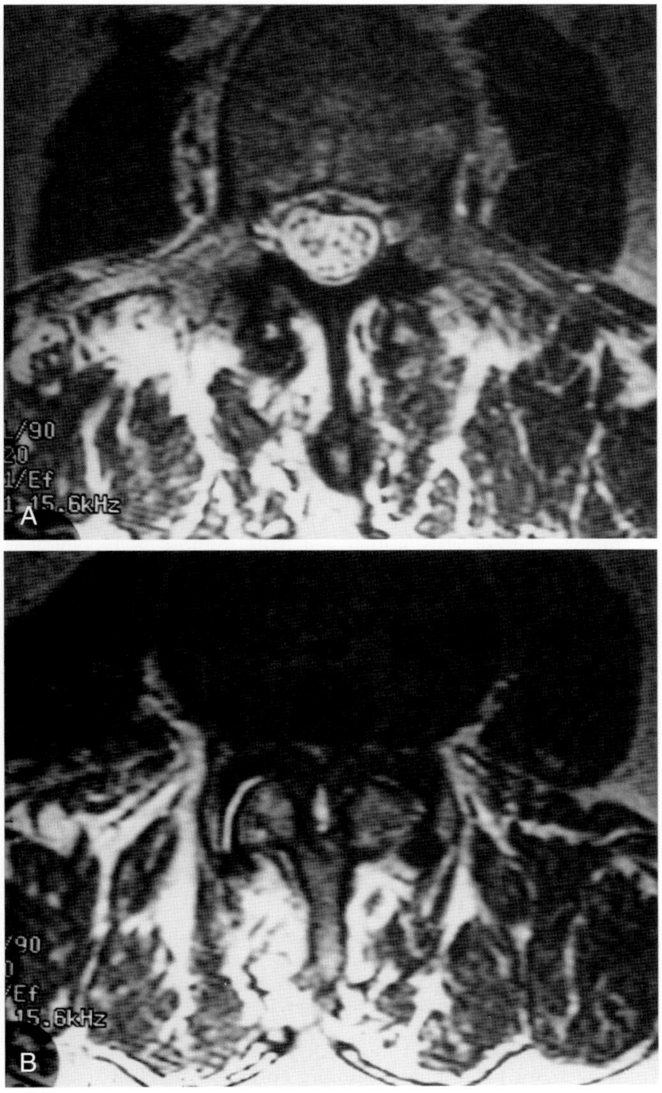

Figure 67-4. MRI scans. **A,** Normal lumbar spine. **B,** Severe spinal canal stenosis.

lateral recess of the spinal canal and in the neural foramen than from disc rupture. As degeneration of the intervertebral disc advances, there is loss of disc height and formation of osteophytes that bulge into the neural foramen; hypertrophy of the facet joint further compromises its capacity. At the same time, partial subluxation of the posterior joint, with upward and forward movement of the superior articular surface, narrows the lateral recess of the spinal canal.[63] At first, extension and rotation of the spine aggravate the process, so that dynamic stenosis (Figure 67-4) may produce intermittent compression and symptoms although, as the condition advances, permanent compression occurs.

Typically, patients complain of pain and stiffness of the back, accompanied by the insidious onset of sciatic pain. These symptoms are generally aggravated by standing or walking and relieved by rest or lying, particularly when the spine is flexed. Patients complain of paresthesias in the legs, which are also precipitated by the same types of activity. In chronic nerve root entrapment caused by stenosis, coughing and straining aggravate the pain, and nerve root stretch tests are generally negative. Some patients show mild weakness of the legs, although objective sensory deficits are rare. The progression of symptoms and signs is generally much slower than for a herniated nucleus pulposis.[64-66]

Nerve root entrapment may complicate degenerative spondylolisthesis. This develops when degeneration of the facet joints and laxity of the disc annulus allow the upper vertebral body to slide forward on the lower. The L4-L5 intervertebral joint is usually affected, but other intervertebral levels can be involved and produce sciatic pain and symptoms of nerve root compression.

Neurogenic Claudication

Narrowing of the central spinal canal can develop as a result of a combination of degenerative hypertrophy of the facet joints, hypertrophy and corrugation of the ligamentum flavum, bulging of the disc and osteophytes, and spondylolisthesis. As the available space in the spinal canal narrows, there is compression of multiple nerve roots of the cauda equina and its circulation. The symptoms of claudication develop. Bilateral leg pain is precipitated by walking or standing and improved with rest, especially when the spine is flexed or when the patient sits or squats.[66]

Patients frequently develop a stooped posture. As the distance walked increases, a heavy leaden weakness builds up in intensity, accompanied by burning paresthesias and fear of the limb giving way.[67] Sometimes neurologic signs are present only after an exercise provocation test on a treadmill. Sharr and coworkers[68] have reported that urinary symptoms due to a neuropathic bladder often complicate central stenosis of the spinal canal.

In older adults, the clinical picture is often confused with the effects of peripheral vascular disease (vascular claudication). In vascular claudication, the pain associated with ambulation is relieved by rest alone and not by flexion of the lumbar spine. Noninvasive vascular studies may help to differentiate the two pathologies.

Investigations

Plain radiographs reveal the extent and severity of degenerative changes of the discs and facet joints. Radiography has been superseded by CT and MRI of the lumbar spine, which reveals the cross-sectional anatomy of the spinal and neural canals and can analyze the degree of degeneration of the disc. However, only MRI can display details of the neural structures adequately.

Radionuclide scanning is generally not helpful because increased uptake is common in areas of osteoarthritis. However, it can exclude spinal infection or neoplasm.

Management

Most older patients do not require surgical decompression, and their symptoms can be controlled by analgesic and antiinflammatory medication and modification of their activities of daily living. Rest and physical treatment, combined with restriction of spinal movement, often produce satisfactory results. However, older adults can withstand surgery well, and age alone is rarely a contraindication to operation.

Surgery is indicated when sciatic pain and other symptoms significantly reduce a patient's physical capability or cannot be controlled by medical treatment. Signs of severe nerve root compression, such as weakness or sensory loss, neurogenic claudication, and cauda equina compression, are firm indications for surgical intervention. The aim of surgery is to decompress the spinal canal and neural foramina, thus freeing the nerve roots. Getty and colleagues[69,70] obtained satisfactory results in 85% of patients after a partial undercutting facetectomy. However, low backache persists after surgery in many patients because of the background degenerative changes, and patients must be advised accordingly.[71,72] However, this effect may be in part related to the surgical approach, because persistent back pain is not reported as commonly following minimal access surgery in older adults.[73]

Approaches to the spine using a minimal access surgical technique (MAST) have become more commonplace and may have a particular role in treatment of the older adult. MAST involves using smaller skin incisions and working through small portals or tubes via a muscle-splitting or muscle-sparing approach, in contrast to the traditional open surgical approaches, which involve stripping the paraspinal muscles off the spine to gain adequate access. These techniques have been shown to minimize surgical trauma and blood loss, reduce postoperative pain, and hasten mobilization and recovery. These advantages may be particularly important when treated a potentially frail population. Rosen and associates[73] have described their experience using a MAST approach for lumbar decompression in a cohort of 50 patients with a mean age of 81 years. They observed no mortality or significant morbidity in their cohort and showed statistical improvement in multiple validated clinical outcome scales, with a mean follow-up of 10 months. In addition to MAST, other approaches, such as dynamic stabilization, have been promising adjuncts to decompressive procedures and are intended to address the issue of concomitant back pain without the need for a surgical arthrodesis.[74,75] However, all these approaches still require the rigors of randomized clinical trials to prove their merits.

KEY POINTS

- Most pathologic processes that affect the spinal cord in older adults are related to degenerative diseases of the spinal column or to insufficiency of the cord's blood supply.
- Surgical treatment is indicated when the myelopathy interferes with daily activities, there is a short progressive history, or there is radiologic evidence of severe cord compression or instability.
- Although myeloma and carcinomas of prostate and kidney seem to metastasize preferentially to the spine, in practice the most commonly encountered tumors are those that occur with the greatest frequency in the community. Therefore, primary lung, breast, kidney, and prostate tumors are seen, although in some patients the primary tumor cannot be identified.
- Typically, patients complain of pain and stiffness of the back, accompanied by the insidious onset of sciatic pain.

For a complete list of references, please visit www.expertconsult.com.

KEY REFERENCES

2. Shedid D, Benzel EC: Cervical spondylosis anatomy: pathophysiology and biomechanics. Neurosurgery 60(Suppl 1):S7–S13, 2007.
7. Abbed KM, Coumans JV: Cervical radiculopathy: pathophysiology, presentation and clinical evaluation. Neurosurgery 60(Suppl 1):28–34, 2007.
17. Mummaneni PV, Kaiser MG, Matz PG, et al: Preoperative patient selection with magnetic resonance imaging, computer tomography and electroencephalography: Does the test predict outcome after cervical surgery? J Neurosurg Spine 11:119–129, 2009.
23. Matz PG, Pritchard PR, Hadley MN: Anterior cervical approach for the treatment of cervical myelopathy. Neurosurgery 60(Suppl 1):S64–S70, 2007.
24. Wiggins GC, Shaffrey CI: Dorsal surgery for myelopathy and myeloradiculopathy. Neurosurgery 60(Suppl 1):S71–S81, 2007.
25. Mummaneni PV, Haid RW, Rodts GE: Combined ventral and dorsal surgery for myelopathy and myeloradiculopathy. Neurosurgery 60(Suppl 1):S82–S89, 2007.
27. Holly LT, Moftakhar P, Khoo LT, et al: Surgical outcomes of elderly patients with cervical spondylotic myelopathy. Surg Neurol 69:233–240, 2008.
32. Sasaki S, Kaji K, Shiba K: Upper thoracic disc herniation followed by acutely progressing paraplegia. Spinal Cord 43:741–745, 2005.
35. Traul DE, Shaffrey ME, Schiff D, et al: spinal-cord neoplasms-intradural neoplasms. Lancet Oncol 8:35–45, 2007.
36. Abul-Kasim K, Thumher MM, McKeever P, et al: Intradural spinal tumors: current classification and MRI features. Neuroradiology 50:301–314, 2008.
40. Dodd RL, Ryu MR, Kammerdsupaphon P, et al: CyberKnife radiosurgery for benign intradural extramedullary spinal tumors. Neurosurgery 58:674–685, 2006.
44. Patchell RA, Tibbs PA, Regine W, et al: Direct decompressive surgical resection in the treatment of spinal cord compression caused by metastatic cancer: a randomised trial. Lancet 366:643–648, 2005.
45. Klimo P Jr, Thompson CJ, Kestle JRW, et al: A meta-analysis of surgery versus conventional radiotherapy for the treatment of metastatic spinal epidural disease. Neuro Oncol 7:64–76, 2005.
47. Trimarchi S, Tsai T, Eagle KA, et al: Acute abdominal aortic dissection: insight from the International Registry of Acute Aortic Dissection (IRAD). J Vasc Surg 46:913–919, 2007.
48. Morales JP, Taylor PR, Bell RE, et al: Neurological complications following endoluminal repair of thoracic aortic disease. Cardiovasc Intervent Radiol 30:833–839, 2007.
52. Pickett GE, Campos-Benitez M, Keller JL, et al: Epidemiology of traumatic spinal cord injury in Canada. Spine 31:799–805, 2006.
53. Fassett DR, Harrop JS, Maltenfort M, et al: Mortality rates in geriatric patients with spinal cord injuries. J Neurosurg Spine 7:277–281, 2007.
54. Jabbour P, Fehlings M, Vaccaro AR, et al: Traumatic spine injuries in the geriatric population. Neurosurg Focus 25:E16, 2008.
55. Furlan JC, Bracken MB, Fehlings MG: Is age a key determinant of mortality and neurological outcome after acute traumatic spinal cord injury? Neurobiol Aging 31:434–446, 2010.
62. Christophis P, Asamoto S, Kuchelmeister K, et al: "Juxtafacet cysts," a misleading name for cystic formations of mobile spine (CYFMOS). Eur Spine J 16:1499–1505, 2007.
73. Rosen DS, O'Toole JE, Eicholz KM, et al: Minimally invasive lumbar spinal decompression in the elderly: outcomes of 50 patients aged 75 years and older. Neurosurgery 60:509–510, 2007.
74. Grob D, Benini A, Junge A, et al: Clinical experience with the Dynesys semirigid fixation system for the lumbar spine: surgical and patient-oriented outcome in 50 cases after an average of 2 years. Spine 30:324–331, 2005.
75. Taylor J, Pupin P, Delajoux S, et al: Device for intervertebral assisted motion: technique and initial results. Neurosurg Focus 22:E7, 2007.

68 Central Nervous System Infections

Lisa Barrett, Kenneth Rockwood

Infections in older adults are associated with significant morbidity and mortality worldwide, pneumonia and influenza ranking 13th in all cause mortality for people aged 65 to 74 years in the United States (http://www.worldlifeexpectancy.com/usa-cause-of-death-by-age-and-gender, accessed November 2014). Despite this fact, few dedicated studies of the distinct clinical presentation and treatment response of infections have been conducted in older individuals. As such, the information in this chapter is almost exclusively based on data from younger populations, together with clinical experience.

BACTERIAL MENINGITIS

Bacterial meningitis is a disease that presents particular challenges in older adults, with higher mortality than in younger adults. In 1973, Fraser, Henke, and Feldman[1] reported that the mean age of death from meningitis increased from 11.5 years in the period 1935 to 1946 to 64 years during the period from 1959 to 1970. In the latter period, more than one half of all deaths from meningitis occurred in those older than 60 years. The incidence of bacterial meningitis rose from 5 cases per 100,000 to 15 cases per 100,000.[1] Surveys from the late 1970s to the 1980s showed an increasing incidence of meningitis in older patients.[2,3] Between 1998 and 2007, although both the incidence and case fatality of bacterial meningitis fell, reflecting further decline from the previous decades, rates were highest in older adults.[4]

Nosocomial meningitis, particularly related to neurosurgical and neurotologic procedures, is also a cause of the increasing meningitis incidence in this older adults.[4,5] Many of these cases occurred in frail older adults.[4]

Bacteria may reach the subarachnoid space by several different mechanisms.[4] Remote focal infections can give rise to bacteremia and seed the meninges. This occurs, for example, in patients who have pneumococcal pneumonia and, less frequently, in patients with pyelonephritis and gram-negative meningitis. Meningitis also develops by way of direct meningeal bacterial inoculation during head trauma or after a neurosurgical procedure. Frail older adult patients are especially prone to falls and head injuries.[6] Meningitis may occur from contiguous spread of infection to the meninges as in patients with otitis media, sinusitis, or mastoiditis. This last mechanism of infection is probably somewhat less common in older adults, compared with younger adults.

Streptococcus pneumoniae remains the most common organism associated with meningitis in older adult patients.[4] Gram-negative bacilli can cause meningitis in older adult patients both by bacteremic spread of infection, such as in urinary tract infection or pneumonia, and as a nosocomial infection after neurosurgery.[7-9] *Escherichia coli* is the most common organism to cause meningitis secondary to bacteremic spread. Gram-negative organisms are responsible for 20% to 25% of cases,[8] implicating infections acquired in health care settings.[10] *E. coli* and *Klebsiella pneumoniae* are the more common gram-negative bacilli to cause meningitis after neurosurgery, but more unusual organisms, particularly *Acinetobacter*, have also been commonly reported.[10,11]

Listeria monocytogenes is also more likely to cause meningitis in older people than in younger adults.[4] Because this infection is T cell mediated, it is possible that known age-associated immune senescence and thymic involution may explain the predisposition of older people to invasive *Listeria* infection. Although *Listeria* accounts for 4% to 8% of all cases of meningitis in older people, it is a much rarer cause of meningitis in young healthy adults.[4] Meningococcal meningitis is the most common cause of meningitis in young adults but a less common cause of meningitis in older people; however, outbreaks have occurred in nursing homes and institutional settings.[12] The incidence of meningococcal meningitis in the older patient population varies from one study to another, mainly reflecting the epidemic nature of the disease. The infection should be considered in older patients who have meningeal signs and have a petechial or macular rash. Often, no focus of infection will be noted.

Skin organisms such as *Staphylococcus aureus* and coagulase-negative staphylococci, as well as gram-negative bacilli, are responsible for most cases of meningitis secondary to head trauma or neurosurgery. *Haemophilus influenzae*, a cause of meningitis in children, is much less common in adults and older people and accounted for approximately 7% of cases between 2003 and 2007. When *H. influenzae* does occur in older patients, it is usually a nonencapsulated variant of the organism.[4] This is in contrast to children, in whom the type B encapsulated organism is most likely to cause infection. Since the introduction of *H. influenzae* type B vaccination, rates of invasive disease have decreased substantially. β-Hemolytic streptococci are a relatively rare cause of meningitis in older people but still cause life-threatening infection and meningitis at the extremes of life.[13]

Diagnosing meningitis in older adults can be challenging. Fever and altered mental status are classic, but appear to lack both sensitivity and specificity, and so other features must be evaluated.[14] As detailed in the chapter on delirium, change in mental status often goes unrecognized, and even when it occurs in older people, can be misattributed to dementia, psychosis, transient ischemia, or stroke. In patients who have undergone neurosurgery, postoperative lethargy may be attributed to an expected postoperative course or postoperative pain medication. Mistaken for a musculoskeletal problem, a stiff neck in an older patient may not arouse the same concern that it would in a young adult.

Patients with contiguous infectious sources may complain of localized findings indicative of the initial site of infection, such as ear or facial pain. Subarachnoid space bacteria will cause an inflammatory reaction in the pia and arachnoid matter manifesting as neck pain and stiffness with protective reflexes that, when present, cause the Kernig and Brudzinski signs. Structures that lie within the subarachnoid space are involved in the inflammatory reaction. Pial arteries and veins may become inflamed and cranial nerve roots damaged.

Delirium may also occur. Confusion, headache, or lethargy is a manifestation of this diffuse, inflammatory process. Papilledema, hydrocephalus, and other focal findings may occur as a result of pus occluding the foramina of Luschka and Magendie, resulting in increased intracranial pressure.

It is common for the clinical features of meningitis in older adults to be subtler than in younger adults. This is a recurring theme in almost all studies that involve older patients with meningitis.[13,15-17] Most studies have found that older adult patients with bacterial meningitis are less likely to have neck stiffness and meningeal signs. Challenges to interpretation of the clinical exam in older patients include the presence of degenerative cervical spine disease and poor neck mobility at baseline. In a classic study, Behrman and colleagues[18] found meningismus present in only 58% of older adult patients with meningitis. Even so, older patients with meningitis typically have more mental status abnormalities and are more likely to have seizures, neurologic deficits, and hydrocephalus. A delay in meningitis diagnosis is frequent, which may explain the high mortality rate in this patient group.[13,19]

Subacute or chronic meningitis, although rare, is more frequently observed in older patients than in other age groups. *Mycobacterium tuberculosis* (discussed later) and *L. monocytogenes* are the most common bacterial causes, and the presentation is most often consistent with basilar meningitis. Individuals may present acutely with decreased level of consciousness, confusion, low-grade temperature, or even seizures, with or without frank meningismus. Often, the patient is not frankly septic but has a moderate inflammatory response that is less fulminant than that observed in other forms of bacterial meningitis. However, a careful history from either the patient or family members will usually provide a subacute picture of chronic headache, decreased appetite, and increased confusion over the course of several weeks. Again, because these symptoms are so nonspecific, it is important to have a high index of suspicion for underlying central nervous system (CNS) infection. New-onset headache in a person without a headache history, especially in the context of constitutional symptoms, should prompt asking about risk factors for tuberculosis (travel, country of origin, personal history of tuberculosis) and listeriosis (undercooked or raw vegetables, outbreak situations, deli meat consumption).

When neck stiffness is the result of meningeal irritation, the neck will resist flexion but can be rotated from side to side. Funduscopic and cranial nerve examination are helpful in identifying associated raised intracranial pressure or brain abscess. Mental status should be carefully described and followed, as increasing lethargy and coma are poor prognostic signs. Examination of the head should include a search for skull fracture, avulsion, or hematoma. Careful otoscopic examination is also a necessity, as otitis media can be missed. Older people can have pneumonia and concomitant meningitis. Indeed, with only mild respiratory symptoms, the physical examination may be the first indication of pneumonia. Cardiovascular examination may detect underlying valvular heart disease predisposing to endocarditis with meningeal seeding. Examination for costovertebral tenderness, decubitus ulcers, and petechial lesions also provide important information about the source and possible causal agent in meningitis.

Timely lumbar puncture is critical to the diagnosis of bacterial meningitis in both young and old individuals. The routine use of neuroimaging (computed tomography [CT]) before lumbar puncture is controversial.[20] A substantial minority of older adult patients with meningitis have focal neurologic findings, and because lumbar puncture is contraindicated in patients with brain abscess, imaging is necessary in these older patients. However, the high mortality rate from meningitis in older adults makes early diagnosis and treatment essential. In consequence, many infectious disease experts now support the strategy of beginning empirical antibiotic therapy pending lumbar puncture, particularly when a delay of hours is anticipated because of imaging delays.[17,21] Some meningitis management guidelines do not always require imaging before lumbar puncture, and this change was associated with a reduction in overall mortality, but follow-up correspondence shows that this is not without controversy.[22-24] In general, if focal neurologic deficits exist or cannot be reasonably assessed, CT before lumbar puncture is reasonable. However, treatment should NOT be delayed pending the diagnostic tests. It is very unlikely that antimicrobial therapy will significantly alter lumbar puncture results within several hours, and enhanced molecular microbiologic techniques can still provide a diagnostic answer if the patient has started antibiotics.

Regarding lumbar puncture, online videos are helpful for novices, even when supervised by experienced operators. Understanding the anatomy is essential, and a series of YouTube videos posted by Raeburn Forbes (www.youtube.com/watch?v=cpl0Zb2p_wA) are a useful resource. A review suggests that small-gauge, atraumatic needles may decrease the risk of headache after diagnostic lumbar puncture, as does reinsertion of the stylet before needle removal.[25]

There is very little literature to suggest that cerebrospinal fluid (CSF) findings differ between older and younger patients with bacterial meningitis. Lumbar puncture will show purulent fluid with white blood cell counts between approximately 500 and 10,000 cells/mm.[3] Polymorphonuclear leukocytes predominate, usually comprising more than 90% of total cell count. Meningitis caused by *L. monocytogenes*, *M. tuberculosis*, or viruses have a mononuclear cell predominance. At least one study has shown that older adult patients with meningitis are more likely to have a diminished CSF cellular response than younger adults,[26] and those with low cell counts but many bacteria on the Gram stain have a poor prognosis. CSF glucose levels are usually low in patients with bacterial meningitis, with CSF to serum glucose ratios less than 50%. Spinal fluid protein is elevated (>50 mg/dL), and very high protein levels are associated with poor prognosis.

CSF Gram stain will be positive for bacteria in 60% to 90% of all patients with meningitis.[14] In a study by Behrman and colleagues,[18] only 50% of older adult patients with meningitis had a positive Gram stain, and the Gram stain is most likely to be negative in patients who have received prior antibiotic therapy. In those patients whose Gram stain is negative, a variety of methods to detect bacterial antigen are now in common use; these include latex fixation, coagglutination, and 16S ribosomal RNA (rRNA) polymerase chain reaction (PCR). Blood cultures are recommended in all patients in whom bacterial meningitis is suspected because almost one half of all older adult patients with meningitis have concomitant bacteremia.[18] In addition, sputum, urine, and wound cultures may be extremely helpful in determining causal agents and source of infection.

The treatment of bacterial meningitis requires prompt initiation of appropriate antibiotic therapy. The antibiotic chosen should be bactericidal for the causal agent and must diffuse across the blood-brain barrier. Table 68-1 lists the causal agent and the antibiotic generally recommended. Information from the history and physical examination, in combination with a careful review of the CSF Gram stain, is the foundation on which the causal agent will be determined and the optimal antibiotic chosen. Although in general a parsimonious approach to consultation serves many frail older adults well, an infectious disease specialist,

TABLE 68-1 Antibiotic of Choice for Bacterial Meningitis

Streptococcus pneumoniae (penicillin MIC < 0.1 μg/mL)	Penicillin
Streptococcus pneumoniae (penicillin resistant; penicillin MIC 0.1-1 μg/mL)	Ceftriaxone
Streptococcus pneumoniae (penicillin resistant; penicillin MIC > 2 μg/mL)	Vancomycin + ceftriaxone
Staphylococcus aureus (methicillin sensitive)	Penicillin
Staphylococcus aureus (methicillin resistant)	Vancomycin
Gram-negative bacilli	Third-generation cephalosporin (see text)
β-Hemolytic streptococci	Penicillin
Listeria monocytogenes	Ampicillin
Neisseria meningitidis	Ceftriaxone
Haemophilus influenzae	Ceftriaxone

MIC, Minimum inhibitory concentration.

when possible, should be involved in the case as the mortality rate from the disease is high and the margin of error is small, and the involvement of an infectious disease specialist appears to be beneficial.[27] The specific epidemiology of the patient's hospital or community will take on increasing importance in determining the antibiotic choice. Given the rising incidence of high-level penicillin-resistant organisms, empirical therapy of pneumococcal and neisserial meningitis should include vancomycin and a third-generation cephalosporin.

In the treatment of gram-negative meningitis, the antibiotic sensitivity pattern of gram-negative bacilli at a particular hospital is also critically important. If the infection has occurred after a neurosurgical procedure, the organisms responsible for previous neurosurgical infections should be noted. If *Pseudomonas aeruginosa* is suspected as the causal agent, ceftazidime is the antibiotic of choice. Cefotaxime or ceftriaxone is generally used for other gram-negative bacilli, including *H. influenzae*. Ampicillin is the drug of choice for *L. monocytogenes*. Once sensitivities are available, penicillin is the drug of choice for methicillin-sensitive staphylococci; vancomycin is the antibiotic of choice for methicillin-resistant staphylococci and most coagulase-negative staphylococci. As noted, ampicillin and vancomycin plus a third-generation cephalosporin is recommended for treatment of meningitis in older people when the causal agent is unknown in order to cover for *Listeria* as well as pneumococci with decreased sensitivity to β-lactam antibiotics.

Staphylococcus aureus can be a particular treatment challenge and is seen in settings both of hematogenous spread[28] and postoperatively, where it can be the most common cause of meningitis after neurosurgery in older adults.[29] Of note is the reported shift from methicillin-sensitive strains to methicillin-resistant *S. aureus* (MRSA) strains[30] in some countries and institutional settings. The latter necessitate use of such medications as linezolid, trimethoprim-sulfamethoxazole, daptomycin, or vancomycin.[31,32]

The role of adjunctive corticosteroid therapy in acute bacterial meningitis in adults with suspected or confirmed pneumococcal meningitis is nuanced. There is discussion that release of bacterial components by the invading pathogen, and the inflammatory reactions that they promote, is the source of secondary systemic and intracranial complications contributing to the high mortality. In consequence, strategies that might inhibit bacterial lysis, or at least not promote it, are being pursued.[33] Included in this is likely to be a reevaluation of the use of corticosteroids as adjuvant treatment and the development of treatment strategies that use antibiotics that are bactericidal but not bacteriolytic.[19] Until further information is available, dexamethasone is associated with decreased sepsis-related mortality in acute *S. pneumoniae* meningitis (de Gans). Therefore, in the empirical setting, dexamethasone 0.15 mg/kg body weight every 6 hours is recommended, with the first dose 15 to 20 minutes prior to the first dose of antibiotics.[34] When cultures are available, if the organism is a bacterium other than *S. pneumoniae* or *M. tuberculosis*, steroids should be discontinued.

Older adult patients with meningitis may be admitted to an intermediate or intensive care unit, where vital signs and neurologic status can be carefully monitored. Some patients are severely dehydrated or volume depleted, and others have septic shock. Colloids or crystalloids may be necessary to improve blood pressure and urine output. In an evolving literature, there is some support for crystalloids, especially with so-called balanced fluids such as Ringer's lactate compared with normal saline, but the generalizability to frail older adults is not known.[35] Inappropriate antidiuretic hormone secretion may accompany CNS infections but should be self-limited if hypotonic solutions are avoided.

The comatose older adult patient requires specialized care in the critical care setting. The patient may need frequent suctioning, particularly if pneumonia is present, secondary to potentially limited pulmonary hygiene in the context of advanced age or underlying structural lung disease such as emphysema. The patient should be turned frequently to prevent decubitus ulcers, and an airbed should be considered in all individuals, particularly those with elevated body mass index, poor preexisting nutritional status, and underlying skin disease. A condom catheter is preferable to a Foley catheter, unless urinary retention develops. In patients who develop relapsing or prolonged fever, a repeat lumbar puncture is necessary. Drug fever, phlebitis, urinary tract infection, intravenous and central lines, and pulmonary emboli are all possible explanations for prolonged fever.

The currently available pneumococcal vaccine is routinely recommended in all patients older than 65 years of age. Although there are no specific data to support the prevention of pneumococcal meningitis in older adults, it is clear that the vaccine decreases the incidence of serious pneumococcal respiratory infection. Because most cases of pneumococcal meningitis in older patients are associated with pneumonia as the initial infection, vaccination in older adult patients would be of benefit in preventing meningitis.

FOCAL LESIONS, CHRONIC MENINGITIS, AND ENCEPHALITIS

Brain Abscess

The classic triad of headache, fever, and focal neurologic symptoms/signs is helpful when present, but it is typically not observed in its entirety very often (e.g., ≈1/5 cases).[36] Although the first symptom in brain abscess is most often a persistent headache, this is very nonspecific and often overlooked, particularly in older adults. Brain abscess more often comes to attention as a mass lesion with focal neurologic deficits.[37] Symptom duration prior to hospitalization can be as long as few weeks, such that insidious onset and progression are quite common. Risk factors for adverse outcomes include a severe change of mental status, neurologic abnormalities on admission, and a short duration between the first symptoms and presentation, suggesting a rapid progression. Common symptoms such as headache, change of mental status, and focal neurologic deficits may be misdiagnosed as cerebral tumors or stroke. It is important to remember that fever is an important positive finding, but normothermia does not rule out infection in older persons. A high index of suspicion for infection should be maintained even without fever.

Generalized seizures prompt hospitalization of many patients with brain abscess, including older adults. Fifty percent of patients with a brain abscess have a focal neurologic sign such as a hemiparesis or focal seizure. Patients may also have diffuse neurologic dysfunction such as a coma, generalized seizure, or neuropsychiatric manifestations. Funduscopic examination may reveal papilledema. Most commonly, but not always, the source of infection in a brain abscess can be discovered.[37] About half the cases arise from contiguous spread (primary infection or as a consequence of surgery, including oral surgery); a further third come about via hematogenous dissemination, notably including infective endocarditis and dental infections.

Streptococcus species (60% to 70%), anaerobic *Bacteroides* species (20% to 40%), Enterobacteriaceae (25% to 30%), and *S. aureus* (15% to 15% posttraumatic or neurosurgery) are the most common causal organisms.[37] The abscessogenic *Streptococcus anginosis* group is also responsible for some proportion of brain abscess, akin to their role in liver and other abscess formation.

As always, the patient's overall state of health can yield a clue, with immunosuppression resulting in an increased likelihood of nonbacterial causes, including *Toxoplasma gondii* and *M. tuberculosis* with human immunodeficiency virus/acquired immunodeficiency syndrome (HIV/AIDS) and fungal abscesses (*Cryptococcus*) in cases of solid organ transplantation.[37] Local epidemiology is always important (e.g., *Histoplasma capsulatum* and *Blastomyces dermatitidis* in an endemic area), as are temporal trends, such as a decline in cases from otitis media and an increase in cases secondary to neurosurgery and trauma.[38]

Unlike the case with bacterial meningitis, where the peripheral white blood cell count is typically markedly elevated, older individuals with brain abscess often have a normal or only slightly elevated white blood cell count. Lumbar puncture reveals the infective organism in only a minority of these cases.[37]

On radiographic imaging, brain abscesses often have a "doughnut" or ring-enhancing appearance. However, this finding is not specific to brain abscesses, and ring-enhancing lesions can also be seen with necrotic tumors and cerebral infarction. Surrounding edema may be seen on CT scan, and symptomatic edema is one indication for corticosteroids.[37] In cases of a single abscess, the most common location is generally that of the frontal lobe or parietal lobe rather than the occipital or temporal lobe. Sites of brain abscesses are often independent from presumed origin of infection, except for the possibility of ear and sinus infections more often leading to abscesses within the frontal brain. Abscess can also be a post-neurosurgical complication following CNS tumor resection, and rarely tumor and infection can present together,[39,40] emphasizing the need for tissue diagnosis.

Surgical aspiration or excision is the only procedure that allows optimal microbiologic documentation, and it should be done without delay.[41] However, some small (<2.5 cm), nonnecrotic lesions or abscesses in vital brain areas[42] may be treated with surgery conserving strategies based on antimicrobials and close follow-up.

Empirical antibiotic therapy should be initiated promptly. Timing in relation to neurosurgery can be controversial, but if the latter cannot proceed within a few hours or if the patient is unstable, immediate antibiotics are proposed.[37] The choice of empirical antimicrobials will depend on the setting and the likely organisms. A third-generation cephalosporin and metronidazole commonly are used where there is no other clearly implicated organism. In the context of postsurgical or traumatic brain abscess, the addition of vancomycin may be considered if MRSA or coagulase-negative staphylococci are possible.

Subdural Empyema

Subdural empyema may arise as a complication of a sinusitis or otitis media, and presenting symptoms often mimic a brain abscess. The presentation may be subtler, and it is necessary to think about the diagnosis in older adult patients with sinusitis and diffuse or nonspecific neurologic symptoms. A contrasted CNS study is indicated, and surgical drainage is mandatory. Antibiotic therapy is targeted at many of the same organisms that cause brain abscess. Length of therapy is generally several weeks with intravenous antibiotics; however, the exact duration of therapy depends on the efficiency of surgical drainage and resolution of the abscess on repeat imaging.

Chronic Meningitis Caused by *Mycobacterium Tuberculosis, Cryptococcus,* and *Coccidioides*

Chronic meningitis is defined as inflammation evolving during weeks to months without resolution of CSF abnormalities.[43] The most common infectious causes of chronic meningitis are *M. tuberculosis* and *Cryptococcus*, although neither is a common problem in North America in general. Tuberculous meningitis (meningitis caused by *M. tuberculosis*) is often an insidious disease and may be especially difficult to diagnose in older people. Nonspecific symptoms of fatigue, anorexia, nausea, and an altered mental status may suggest dementia in older patients, and a miliary picture on chest x-ray may be a useful feature in distinguishing tuberculous meningitis from cryptococcal meningitis. Symptom duration may range from 2 days to 6 months, and hospitalization is often precipitated by change in mental status, headache, or fever. It is worthwhile noting that meningeal signs are present in less than one half of the cases, so it is helpful if meningismus is present but not exclusionary of the diagnosis if it is absent. Ocular palsies, particularly due to involvement of nerve VI, are found in 30% to 70% of cases because of the susceptibility of the lengthy CN VI and the increased intracranial pressure that is almost universally observed in tuberculous meningitis. Magnetic resonance imaging (MRI) with gadolinium enhancement is more useful in diagnosing tuberculous meningitis than is a CT scan, revealing basilar meningeal enhancement, often hydrocephalus and parenchymal hypodensities.[44]

CSF findings often reveal a protein level higher than 50 mg/dL and usually more in the 100 to 500 mg/dL range, as well as a very low glucose level lower than 40 mg/dL. CSF acid-fast positivity varies among studies but can range anywhere from 10% to 80% depending on how many spinal taps were performed and the volume of fluid analyzed. A chest x-ray and purified protein derivative should be routinely obtained. Several attempts have been made to develop a rapid, common, and specific method for diagnosing tuberculous meningitis, and these days, nucleic acid–based tuberculosis detection from large volume (10 to 15 mL) spinal tap is available and has a sensitivity of between 56% to 95%,[45,46] depending on whether the assay was multiplexed or not. It should be noted that these validation studies were not specifically in older adult patients.

Prognosis is influenced by age, duration of symptoms, and neurologic deficits, and mortality is greatest in patients younger than age 5 and older than age 50 (60%). Clinical staging is often based on neurologic status: stage I—rational, no focal neurologic signs or hydrocephalus; stage II—confusion, depression, or focal neurologic deficits; stage III—stuporous or dense paraplegia or hemiplegia. Isoniazid, pyrazinamide, ethambutol, and rifampin penetrate the blood-brain barrier in the context of meningeal irritation to achieve adequate CSF concentrations. However, multidrug-resistant tuberculosis (MDR-TB) may require second-line drugs, and expert consultation with an infectious diseases expert is recommended if the individual has come from a country with high rates of MDR-TB. If MDR-TB is suspected, a molecular test for tuberculosis and rifampin resistance is relatively sensitive and provides quick (<48 hours) results that may help guide second-line therapy.[47]

Adjunctive corticosteroids are recommended for stage II and III disease.[48,49] Prednisone doses begin at 80 mg/day and may be gradually tapered over 4 to 6 weeks as guided by the patient's symptoms. If hydrocephalus is present, ventricular shunting procedures may be necessary.

Cryptococcal Meningitis

Cryptococcal meningitis may present in a manner very similar to tuberculous meningitis. Between 20% and 50% of patients with cryptococcal CNS infection may have no underlying immunodeficiency such as HIV. The meningitis associated with *Cryptococcus* can be persistent, especially in people with HIV/AIDS[50]; however, advanced chronologic age appears not to be a risk factor.[50]

Spinal fluid findings are very similar to those for tuberculosis in that there is a lymphocyte predominance. The India ink test result may be positive in 50% or more of cases. Results of a rapid simple latex fixation test indicate that cryptococcal antigen is often positive in 90% of cases. A CT scan may be helpful to rule out hydrocephalus, which is quite common in cryptococcal meningitis.

Poor prognostic signs for cryptococcal meningitis include a high CSF opening pressure, low CSF glucose level, fewer than

20 white blood cells in the CSF, high titers of cryptococcal antigen in a positive India ink stain, and the presence of HIV disease.

Amphotericin B or the less toxic liposomal formulation is the drug of choice in treating cryptococcal meningitis.[51,52] Flucytosine can serve as a useful adjunct, particularly when trying to lower the dose of amphotericin B to prevent renal insufficiency. However, it has bone marrow suppressive toxicities, and the benefit versus risk should be carefully assessed, particularly in the older adult. There are little data to suggest that flucytosine increases cure and decreases relapse rates outside the context of HIV infection. Fluconazole is particularly useful for maintenance therapy but may also be useful as an acute therapy for patients with cryptococcal meningitis as well, particularly for those patients with less poor prognostic parameters.

Herpes Simplex Encephalitis

Herpes simplex infection is very common and establishes lifelong infection after exposure. Individuals are only intermittently symptomatic, but by the sixth decade, more than 70% of individuals in the United States have evidence of herpes simplex virus type 1 (HSV-1) exposure, and 30% to 70% have serologic evidence of HSV-2 exposure.[53] Not surprisingly, given these high numbers, HSV-associated CNS infections occur in this population. Herpes simplex encephalitis is an uncommon but serious CNS infection, usually caused by reactivation of HSV-1 in older individuals. However, HSV-2 is not unheard of in sexually active individuals older than 60 years.[54] Mortality of untreated biopsy-proven cases is 60% to 80%, with more than 90% of the patients having some form of residual neurologic sequelae, making timely and accurate diagnosis important. This illness occurs in all age groups with an equal number of cases between the sexes. It has no seasonal association, and mortality is higher in patients older than 50 years of age.[55]

The presentation is typically an encephalitis instead of meningitis. Patients may have an abrupt onset of personality change, altered mental status, fever, and headache. Localizing signs such as speech deficits, olfactory hallucinations, temporal lobe seizures, hemiparesis, and visual field defects are common and may suggest the diagnosis, although these tend to be less common in immunocompromised patients.[56] The spinal fluid findings are nonspecific with a prominent lymphocytosis. An elevated number of polymorphonuclear leukocytes may be found early in the disease process but characteristically will later change to a mononuclear site cell predominance as the disease progresses. An elevated red blood cell count can be suggestive of the diagnosis (HSV causes a necrotic process that releases blood into the CSF) but is not required. The electroencephalogram pattern may consist of slow wave complexes at regular 2- to 3-second intervals, usually localized to the temporal lobe. CT scan eventually becomes positive in more than 70% of the patients, but MRI is more sensitive and results are abnormal earlier in the course of the disease.

HSV PCR is helpful in making the diagnosis, although it may be falsely negative at the very beginning of the clinical syndrome. The definitive diagnosis of herpes simplex encephalitis can be made by brain biopsy and appropriate culture and histology, although it is almost never done in the era of molecular testing in resource-rich settings.

Effective therapy usually consists of acyclovir at a dose of 10 mg/kg every 8 hours for 10 days, which must be adjusted for renal function in older adult patients as acyclovir can cause nephrotoxicity, particularly in patients who are dehydrated. In particular, intravenous acyclovir can cause a crystalline nephropathy that may or may not be reversible,[57,58] an effect specific to the intravenous formulation. Valacyclovir offers an oral option that is not as nephrotoxic and, given its high bioavailability, may be very useful in older adult patients with renal compromise. Survival correlates with the patient's level of consciousness at the initiation of treatment; even so, patients treated early can still have devastating consequences.[59] Neurologic sequelae are even higher if treatment is delayed or if the patient is comatose. A high index of suspicion is often required to make the diagnosis and to begin effective therapy for herpes simplex encephalitis.

In rare cases, patients with herpes encephalitis may relapse, and a high index of suspicion should be maintained for distant recurrence in those who have had a previous herpes simplex encephalitis.[52,53] Relapse has occurred up to years later and probably reflects a specific host-virus interaction that is not improved with advancing age.

Other Infectious Encephalitides in Older Persons

West Nile Virus

An important arbovirus in North America since 1999 is West Nile Virus (WNV), which has now been found throughout the United States and Canada, along with Europe, Africa, Russia, Australia, North and South America, and the Middle East. WNV is a mosquito-borne virus that generally causes mild febrile illness but in rare cases (<1%) causes both peripheral and CNS disease and, in some outbreaks, encephalitis.[60-62] It is a summer outbreak–related disease, and often the history of travel or presence in an outbreak area is the only clue to a diagnosis of WNV. Peripheral poliomyelitis-like acute flaccid paralysis is also suggestive of WNV as a cause of encephalitis. Neuroinvasive arboviral infections cause encephalitis 5 to 30 days into the clinical infection, with 5 to 7 days of fever and other nonspecific symptoms of eye pain, facial congestion, and rash before encephalitis develops.[63] A case fatality rate of 4% to 14% was noted and was higher in older adults.[64] Weakness, coma, and coexisting hypertension or diabetes predicted a poor outcome, and more than 50% of individuals had a residual neurologic deficit at 1 year after infection.[65]

CSF findings are nonspecific and typical of other viral encephalitis syndromes, with a lymphocytosis, slightly elevated protein level, and a normal glucose level. MRI findings late in disease may show T2 signals in the thalamus, and an electroencephalogram (EEG) shows the generalized slowing of encephalitis. Serologic blood tests for WNV immunoglobulins G and M (IgG and IgM) antibodies can be ordered and are indicative of the virus, and WNV CSF PCR can be done at referral laboratories.

Care at this point is supportive and aimed at controlling symptoms and seizures. Several trials of immunoglobulin and vaccines are under way, but results are not available at the current time.

Spirochetal Infections

Neurosyphilis

Neurosyphilis is caused by *Treponema pallidum* and can affect the CNS. Although neurosyphilis is often felt to be a late manifestation of syphilis, spirochetes invade the nervous system throughout the entire course of syphilis. In the early stage, it can present with symptoms of meningitis, but syphilitic meningitis may occur at the same time as the rash of the secondary syphilis. Most patients with cerebrovascular involvement have had syphilis for approximately 5 to 10 years. This can manifest as a stroke in a young person. Older adult patients typically have a presentation of paretic neurosyphilis or tabes dorsalis that can present with neuropsychiatric symptoms, including dementia in rare cases.[66]

The interval between infection and manifestation of symptoms often ranges from 20 to 30 years for these syndromes. Men have an increased risk as compared to women. The neurologic examination may be entirely normal with neurosyphilis, and the diagnosis may only be made by a serologic screen testing positive for syphilis and abnormal results on a CSF examination. As the disease progresses, intellectual function can decline and psychotic changes may occur.

Symptoms include irritability, fatigability, personality changes, impaired judgment, depression, confusion, and delusions. Patients may have coarse, movement-induced facial, lingular, and labial tremors. Patients also may have difficulty with distorted handwriting, and abnormal reflexes and focal findings may also occur.[54] Untreated, the disorder is fatal within a few months to 3 or 4 years.

Penicillin treatment can effectively reverse the CSF abnormalities and arrest the disease, but the neurologic outcome depends on the degree of structural CNS damage that had occurred at the time of therapy.[55] CSF findings in general paresis include an opening pressure between 50 mm H_2O and 300 mm H_2O. The cell count is usually less than 100 cells per mm^3 in 90% of cases. The glucose level may be normal or moderately reduced. The protein level is higher than 100 mg/dL in 25% of cases. CSF and blood serologic results are generally positive in more than 95% of cases.[54]

Tabes dorsalis continues to be a common form of CNS syphilis, although the percentage seems to be decreasing. This disease, again, is much more common in men than in women. It has a long incubation period, being as high as 50 years in some patients. The triad of Argyll Robertson pupil, areflexia, and loss of proprioception is characteristic of the disorder. Lightning pains last for a few seconds to minutes at a time and usually occur in the lower extremities. These can be separated by interval-free periods of a few months. Pain sensation is often strikingly impaired compared with that of hot and cold sensation.[55] Reduction or loss of ankle or knee jerks can occur in approximately 80% to 90% of patients. Pupillary abnormalities are noted in 79% of patients and consist of pupils that accommodate but do not react. In older adult patients, diabetes can mimic tabes. Other rare causes mimicking tabes include Wernicke encephalopathy and Charcot-Marie-Tooth disease.

As the disease progresses, sensory ataxia becomes a problem, and many patients have a positive Romberg sign. Less common abnormalities include syphilitic optic atrophy and gastric crises. The majority of patients have abnormal serum and CSF findings. Characteristic CSF findings of tabes usually include a normal opening pressure in 90% of the patients. Only 9% to 10% of patients have a cell count higher than 160. The protein is usually normal to moderately elevated.

The serum rapid plasma reagin (RPR) and *T. pallidum* particle agglutination assay (TPPA) are typically sensitive enough that if both were negative, CSF testing would have low yield. Even so, after decades, and after treatment, diagnosis of late-stage neurosyphilis can be challenging.[67] Patients with only an abnormal protein or cell count might also be strongly considered for penicillin therapy. In patients with signs of neurosyphilis but with an unreactive CSF (normal cells and protein), such as in "burned out" neurosyphilis, the neurologic deficit is probably due to fixed structural damage and will probably not respond. Hypothyroidism, cryptococcal meningitis, and tuberculous meningitis, or other causes of reversible dementia, need to be considered in the differential diagnosis of neurosyphilis.

Despite the uncertainty of diagnosis, if there is reasonable suspicion for neurosyphilis, the treatment is benign enough to warrant therapy in case there is an opportunity to arrest further neurologic deterioration. Individuals should receive penicillin G 24 million units IV daily for 14 days. A fourfold drop in venereal disease research laboratory (VDRL) titer within 1 year is considered sufficient response. Consultation with an infectious disease expert is recommended if an insufficient response is obtained and further therapy is thought to be needed.

KEY POINTS

BACTERIAL MENINGITIS

- Clinical features may be more subtle in older adult patients.
- Cerebrospinal fluid (CSF) findings in older adult patients resemble those of younger adults.
- *Streptococcus pneumoniae* is the most common organism causing meningitis in older adult patients. *Listeria* is more likely to cause meningitis in older adults than in young adults.
- Begin empirical therapy with vancomycin and a third-generation cephalosporin.
- Dexamethasone administration is recommended in adults if pneumococcal meningitis is suspected.
- Modify therapy based on the organism's minimum inhibitory concentration (MIC) to penicillin (rifampin may need to be added if the ceftriaxone MIC > 2 μg/mL).

FOCAL LESIONS

- Brain abscess often presents as a mass lesion.
- Subdural empyema arises as a complication of sinusitis and otitis media.
- CSF findings are nonspecific.
- Ring-enhancing lesions are detected by CT in the majority of patients.
- Often *Viridans streptococcus* and *Streptococcus milleri* are isolated.
- A combination of metronidazole and a third-generation cephalosporin is usually recommended.

TUBERCULOUS MENINGITIS

- Meningeal signs are often absent.
- CSF glucose levels are typically low.
- Ocular palsies (particularly CN VI) are common.
- Acid-fast positivity varies.
- Prognosis is related to clinical stage.
- Steroids and shunts are helpful in managing raised intracranial pressure.

CRYPTOCOCCAL MENINGITIS

- India ink is positive approximately 50% of the time.
- Poor prognostic signs include a high titer of antigen and fewer than 20 white blood cells per high-power field in the CSF.
- ICP may need to be temporarily managed with an external shunt.

HERPES SIMPLEX ENCEPHALITIS

- Begin therapy with high-dose acyclovir pending diagnostic tests.
- An abnormal electroencephalogram can be suggestive of the diagnosis.
- Temporal lobe enhancement on a cranial CT or MRI is highly suggestive of the diagnosis.
- CSF herpes simplex polymerase chain reaction test is very useful in definitively diagnosing the entity.

SPIROCHETAL INFECTIONS

Neurosyphilis

- Often a cause of reversible dementia.
- Older adult patients have tabes dorsalis or paretic syphilis more often than younger patients.
- CSF serologic test result is usually positive.
- Patients who have a positive serum rapid plasma reagin result and an abnormal cell or protein count should be considered for therapy.

LYME DISEASE

- Bell palsy is common.
- Ceftriaxone is the therapy of choice for all forms of central nervous system Lyme disease with the possible exception of facial nerve palsy.

For a complete list of references, please visit www.expertconsult.com.

KEY REFERENCES

4. Thigpen MC, Whitney CG, Messonnier NE, et al: Bacterial meningitis in the United States, 1998-2007. N Engl J Med 364:2016–2025, 2011.
10. Bardak-Ozcem S, Sipahi OR: An updated approach to healthcare-associated meningitis. Expert Rev Anti Infect Ther 12:333–342, 2014.
13. Heckenberg SG, Brouwer MC, van de Beek D: Bacterial meningitis. Handb Clin Neurol 121:1361–1375, 2014.
17. Stockdale AJ, Weekes MP, Aliyu SH: An audit of acute bacterial meningitis in a large teaching hospital 2005-10. QJM 104:1055–1063, 2011.
20. Michael B, Menezes BF, Cunniffe J, et al: Effect of delayed lumbar punctures on the diagnosis of acute bacterial meningitis in adults. Emerg Med J 27:433–438, 2010.
22. Glimåker M, Johansson B, Grindborg Ö, et al: Adult bacterial meningitis: earlier treatment and improved outcome following guideline revision promoting prompt lumbar puncture. Clin Infect Dis 60:1162–1169, 2015.
25. Straus SE, Thorpe KE, Holroyd-Leduc J: How do I perform a lumbar puncture and analyze the results to diagnose bacterial meningitis? JAMA 296:2012–2022, 2006.
34. Van de Beek D, Brouwer MC, Thwaites GE, et al: Advances in treatment of bacterial meningitis. Lancet 380:1693–1702, 2012.
37. Brouwer MC, Tunkel AR, McKhann GM 2nd, et al: Brain abscess. N Engl J Med 371:447–456, 2014.
38. Carpenter J, Stapleton S, Holliman R: Retrospective analysis of 49 cases of brain abscess and review of the literature. Eur J Clin Microbiol Infect Dis 26:1–11, 2007.
56. Tan IL, McArthur JC, Venkatesan A, et al: Atypical manifestations and poor outcome of herpes simplex encephalitis in the immunocompromised. Neurology 79:2125–2132, 2012.
59. Kennedy PG, Steiner I: Recent issues in herpes simplex encephalitis. J Neurovirol 19:346–350, 2013.
66. Zeng YL, Wang WJ, Zhang HL, et al: Neuropsychiatric disorders secondary to neurosyphilis in elderly people: one theme not to be ignored. Int Psychogeriatr 25:1513–1520, 2013.
67. Jantzen SU, Ferrea S, Langebner T, et al: Late-stage neurosyphilis presenting with severe neuropsychiatric deficits: diagnosis, therapy, and course of three patients. J Neurol 259:720–728, 2012.

69 Arthritis in Older Adults

Preeti Nair, Jiuan Ting, Helen I. Keen, Philip G. Conaghan

INTRODUCTION

Rheumatologic diseases are among the most common causes of pain and disability in older people.[1] The prevalence continues to rise with age even in the older adult population, such that by the age of 85 years, the lifetime prevalence of arthritis diagnosed by a general practitioner in the United Kingdom is 65%.[2] Although some conditions are seen in adults of all ages, the clinical presentation and treatment goals will differ in frail older adults with complex comorbidities.[3] It is important to keep in mind the impact of musculoskeletal pain on the individual. Pain is associated with muscle loss, functional limitations, fatigue, sleep disturbance, depressed mood, and poor quality of life, especially in those older than 75.[4]

Although nearly all rheumatic conditions afflict older adults, some are more common in this age group, especially osteoarthritis (OA) and tendon disorders. The most common rheumatic condition in the older adult population are summarized in Table 69-1. However, people commonly present with *more than one* rheumatic condition for example, with combinations of mechanical lower back pain, knee OA, and shoulder tendonitis. A survey of more than 16,000 people older than 55 years reported that the median number of painful joints was four.[5]

Making a Diagnosis of Arthritis

Because there are more than 100 different musculoskeletal conditions, history and examination findings are critical for establishing a "mechanical" or "inflammatory" diagnostic label, thereby guiding the need (or often not) for subsequent investigations. The duration of early morning stiffness is useful: typically, an inflammatory arthritis is associated with more than 60 minutes of morning stiffness, with a clear difference between this morning stiffness and the rest of the day. When people report all-day stiffness, this is unlikely to be true morning stiffness. Typically, an OA joint will produce less than 10 minutes of morning stiffness and is usually associated with disuse stiffness after a period of the mobilization such as sitting. It is not unusual for tendonitis to give 30 minutes of morning stiffness. Mechanical joint pains are usually worse with prolonged usage or weight bearing. The timing of onset of arthritis may be useful in diagnosis: a rapidly painful and swollen joint would raise the question of acute gout, pseudogout, or a septic arthritis. Another important part of history taking is looking for diseases that may be associated with an inflammatory arthritis, such as psoriasis, inflammatory bowel disease, or recent diarrheal infections. There may also be features that suggest that the presenting symptoms are part of a broader connective tissue disease, such as photosensitivity or Raynaud phenomenon. A family history may be useful, although often people don't know what sort of arthritis their family member(s) had. Although uncommon, it is always important to check for "red flag" signs of potential malignancies, especially predominant night pain and associated weight loss or night sweats.

Clinical examination findings are often difficult to interpret, even for experienced clinicians. Modern imaging modalities have highlighted the inaccuracies of clinical examination. The presence of soft-tissue joint swelling or synovitis is not diagnostic in itself of an inflammatory arthritis, as synovitis is common in OA. However, the presence of symmetrical synovitis in multiple small hand joints should raise suspicion of inflammatory arthritis. Bony swelling generally indicates OA.

OSTEOARTHRITIS

Osteoarthritis refers to a clinical syndrome with a variety of causes and outcomes that often differ by joint, but with common pathologic features in the established condition.[6] It is the most common joint problem, with age being the strongest risk factor, and for that reason it is the main focus of this chapter.[7]

The OA process is difficult to define in a succinct phrase because of its complex causes and risk factors and because it impacts patients differently. Definitions traditionally focus on features such as pathology (using radiographic structure), clinical features, or a combination of these. As yet there are no validated diagnostic criteria, although the American College of Rheumatology (ACR) has devised classification criteria that emphasize age, symptoms (including inactivity stiffness), and signs (including crepitus and swelling)[8] (Table 69-2).

Symptomatic OA is more common in women than men, especially in older adults, with a rising prevalence in the Western world. Increases are largely attributable to the aging population[11] and obesity; nearly 1 in 2 people have knee OA by the age of 85 years.[12] Other factors associated with OA initiation include obesity, genes, and epigenetics as well as joint injury or joint overuse (e.g., in certain occupations or elite athletes). The various risk factors, however, may operate differently on individual joints at varying stages of the OA process, depending on personal mechanical factors such as weight and muscle strength and perhaps on the different metabolic and restorative properties of the joint at different ages[13] (Table 69-3).

Pathogenesis and Causes

Despite its varied causal factors, OA is characterized by a remarkably uniform pathologic process of aberrant joint repair ending in joint failure.[7] The process involves decompensation of reparative mechanisms and an imbalance between synthesis and degradation of hyaline cartilage and subchondral bone,[7] resulting in changes affecting the entire joint, including these tissues and the synovium.[14] It is important to note that whereas the historical focus on OA was as a disorder of cartilage, it is now recognized that clinical OA refers to a process involving the whole joint organ, with involvement of all elements of the joint.

Cartilage is a metabolically active tissue, with abundant extracellular matrix (mainly type 2 collagen and proteoglycans) regulated by chondrocytes that, when activated, produce inflammatory cytokines and matrix-degrading enzymes.[15] Chondrocytes also interact with the innate immune system through toll-like receptor expression, activated by molecules that are found in the setting of damage but also by the crystals associated with later-stage OA.[15] It is also hypothesized that a metabolic shift toward catabolism may occur in chondrocytes, as age is associated with increasing levels of advanced glycation end products (which increase oxidative damage) and chondrocytes are known to express receptors for these products.[15]

The importance of the subchondral bone in OA is increasingly being recognized.[16] The active osteocytes in subchondral bone undertake homeostatic remodeling. It has been demonstrated that osteocytes express inflammatory cytokines and proteases in response to mechanical stress.[17] In these areas of stress, where bone is lying under damaged cartilage, the homeostasis may alter such that bone formation predominates, resulting in thickened, stiffened bone. In addition, new blood vessels and nerves infiltrate damaged cartilage, to facilitate new bone formation within the cartilage, and create osteophytes, further contributing to cartilage thinning.[18] This process is considered an aberrant healing process; the extension of articular surfaces may allow redistribution of abnormal joint forces.[19] Magnetic resonance imaging (MRI) has demonstrated the presence of bone marrow lesions, areas of fibrosis, necrosis, and remodeled trabecular bone in about 50% of people with symptomatic OA. These lesions are associated with pain and subsequent compartment-specific cartilage loss.[20]

Synovial inflammation has also been found to be common in imaging studies of OA,[21,22] thought to be reactive to bone and cartilage pathology. Cartilage breakdown products released into the synovial fluid infiltrate the synovium and are irritants[23] resulting in inflammation. This results in the production of inflammatory cytokines and cartilage degradation enzymes, which diffuse

TABLE 69-1 Common Rheumatic Conditions in Older Adults

Category of Condition	Specific Diagnoses
Inflammatory	Gout and other crystal arthritis (i.e., pseudogout), rheumatoid arthritis, septic arthritis
Degenerative	Osteoarthritis, rotator cuff pathology, frozen shoulder, tendonitis
Vasculitis/connective tissue disease	Polymyalgia rheumatica, temporal arteritis
Back pain	Mechanical back pain, degenerative disc disease, osteoporotic vertebral fractures

TABLE 69-2 American College of Rheumatology Classification Criteria for Osteoarthritis

Hip	Knee (Clinical Criteria)	Hand
Pain in the hip and two of the following: ESR < 20 mm/hr Radiographic joint space narrowing Radiographic osteophytes	Pain in the knee and five of the following: Age > 50 <30 min morning stiffness Crepitus Bony enlargement Bony tenderness No synovial warmth	Pain, aching, and stiffness in the hand and three of the following: Fewer than three MCP joints swollen Hard tissue enlargement of two or more DIP joints Hard tissue enlargement of two or more of the following joints: second and third DIP, second and third PIP, both CMC joints Deformity of at least one of the following joints: second and third DIP, second and third PIP, both CMC joints

Modified from references 8, 9, and 10.
CMC, Carpometacarpal; *DIP,* distal interphalangeal; *ESR,* erythrocyte sedimentation rate; *MCP,* metacarpophalangeal joint; *PIP,* proximal interphalangeal.

TABLE 69-3 Risk Factors for Osteoarthritis

Host Factors		Environmental Factors	
Genetic factors	Familial clustering has also been found at the hip and knee[33,34]	Biomechanics	Repetitive ergonomic and biomechanical demands may create joint stresses leading to OA Hemiparesis associated with reduction of expression of OA in the affected limb and overexpression in the remaining functional limb[35] Chopstick use associated with OA of the IP joint of the thumb, second and third MCP, and PIP joints[27]
Age	The strongest identifiable risk factor[36-38]	Trauma	Injuries to the joint, such as dislocations, fractures, ligament ruptures, and meniscal tears[39]
Gender	The age association is strongest in women: possibly a hormonal influence Hand OA has a peak incidence in menopausal women[14]		
Hormones	Controversial Hand OA has a peak in menopausal women; however, the Chingford and Framingham studies suggested estrogen has protective effect[37,40]		
Bone mineral density	Negative relationship between bone mineral density and OA at some sites		
BMI	Obesity is strongly associated with the incidence of knee OA[41] Hand OA[30,42] likely to be related to biomechanical factors		
Joint alignment	Varus deformity of the knee is associated with progressive OA, as is varus/valgus ligamentous instability at the knee joint Developmental problems leading to altered joint biomechanics such as congenital dysplasias		

BMI, Body mass index; *IP,* interphalangeal; *MCP,* metacarpophalangeal joint; *OA,* osteoarthritis; *PIP,* proximal interphalangeal.

into the cartilage stimulating chondrocyte release of proinflammatory cytokines, inhibiting collagen and proteoglycan synthesis,[23] and generally further perpetuating the destructive process.[16] Synovitis is associated with structural progression of the disease[24] and joint replacement.[25]

Risk Factors for Osteoarthritis

OA may be conceptualized as the result of abnormal forces on normal joint tissues, or normal forces on an abnormal joint, or the interplay of both. These interactions are likely to involve host factors (genetics, age, gender) and environmental factors (biomechanics, trauma). It is also possible that some risk factors have not yet been identified. It has been proposed that local biomechanical factors (obesity, joint injury, muscle weakness) initiate damage in OA in joints that are vulnerable because of systemic factors (genetics, age, gender).[7] In OA of the hand, for example, studies have demonstrated handedness and mechanical loading as risk factors, whereas other studies (often focusing on radiographic changes and not symptoms) have found symmetry to be so prevalent that intrinsic factors are likely to be responsible.[26-30] The Hizen-Oshima study[29] found both handedness and symmetry to be associated with OA. Although symmetry was the predominant pattern of involvement in this cohort, the prevalence of index distal interphalangeal joint, thumb interphalangeal joint, and thumb metacarpophalangeal joint involvement was significantly higher in the dominant hand.

Clinical Features

Almost any joint may be affected with OA, but most commonly, OA involves the knees, feet, hands (base of thumb and fingers), and hips. Changes typical of OA are very commonly also seen in the lumbar and cervical spine, but because back pain often involves varying pathologies (including disc degeneration, nerve root compression, and crush fractures, as well as OA changes), the term *peripheral joint OA* is commonly used to separate the OA syndrome in these joints from spinal disease.

There is no widely accepted classification for clinical OA, and it is often described by the distribution of joints involved. For example, disease may be limited to a single joint, such as the knee, or it may be more generalized. Whether subgroups represent specific and pathologically distinct subgroups is uncertain. Currently, generalized OA is considered to be hand OA plus involvement at other sites[31] (generally involvement of three or more joints); however, Kellgren originally coined the term *primary generalized OA* to describe a subset of people with widespread disease (particularly involving the hands and weight-bearing joints such as the knee) on observing a bimodal frequency of joint distribution in his cohort.[28] Dieppe and colleagues have demonstrated a strong positive relationship between age and number of joints affected in individuals with OA. This is likely to be due to a bias of time, meaning that older people recruit new sites with age, and in this study, no distinct subgroups of joint involvement were identified.[32] *Inflammatory OA* is a poorly defined term that refers to a subgroup with a marked inflammatory process affecting hand joints and is sometimes used interchangeably with the term *erosive OA*. Crystal deposition disease is common in advanced OA, often detected clinically as radiographic chondrocalcinosis, and this may cause acute-on-chronic flares of joint pain associated with highly elevated inflammatory markers. A rare subgroup is that characterized by a rapidly destructive process affecting a large joint with radiographic changes that may mimic septic arthritis, sometimes referred to as rapidly progressive OA.[43] Typically, this presents in older women, affects the hip, and may be bilateral.[44] The joint may progress to complete destruction within a year or two. The cause of this rare condition is unknown,[43] but it has recently been associated with the combination of nonsteroidal antiinflammatory drugs (NSAIDs) and anti-nerve growth factor antibodies.[45,46] The hypothesis is that the analgesic effects of NSAID therapy result in increased mechanical loading of the hip, which impairs bone healing.[43] Differential diagnosis requires the exclusion of septic arthritis, crystal disease, and avascular necrosis.

OA usually presents with joint pain made worse with use (considered "mechanical" pain), short-duration stiffness after inactivity (termed *gelling* and commonly confused with the term *locking*), and sometimes audible grating on movement. Examination findings include tenderness on palpation, palpable grating on movement (crepitus), bony enlargement of the joint, effusion, malalignment, and reduction in the range of motion. As OA symptoms progress, muscle loss ensues with associated loss of function and with routine tasks becoming difficult. For example, people with OA of the hand may have trouble writing, turning door knobs, or opening jars. Similarly, older adults with knee or hip OA may have difficulty walking distances, getting out of chairs, or using steps. Additionally OA knee pain can be associated with a sensation of "giving way" (a symptom of muscle weakness), which may result in falls or affect the individual's confidence, which may result in significant physical and mental health risks and contribute to fear and isolation.

PAIN: OA pain is usually related to activity. In early disease, the pain may be episodic, evolving to more continuous pain over years, which may manifest at night, disturbing the person's sleep. The impact of pain and disturbed sleep on psychological health should not be underestimated; depression is common in OA cohorts.[47]

The relationship between pain and imaging-assessed structural abnormalities in OA is complex and not completely understood. Radiographic changes do not correlate well with reported pain. Bone marrow lesions demonstrated on MRI correlate better with pain than radiographic changes.[48] Imaging-detected synovitis has also been associated with OA pain.[49] Such findings are not surprising: both the subchondral bone and synovium are well innervated, unlike the hyaline cartilage, although ingrowth of new nerves and blood vessels has been described in areas of cartilage loss.[50]

STIFFNESS: Stiffness refers to difficulty with, or speed of, joint movement, often after inactivity, such as first thing in the morning or after prolonged sitting. The ACR recognizes morning stiffness of less than 30 minutes duration as part of the diagnostic criteria for OA.[51]

DEFORMITY: The relatively common features of Heberden nodes and Bouchard nodes in OA of the hand is demonstrated in Figure 69-1. Varus, or less commonly valgus deformity, is common with OA structural progression at the knee.

TENDERNESS: Tenderness along the joint line is a common finding in OA. Trochanteric bursitis is common in the presence of quadriceps muscle weakness (and often mistaken for hip OA). Anserine bursitis, medial and distal to the knee, is sometimes seen with OA of the knee.

MUSCLE WASTING AND WEAKNESS: Quadriceps strength, knee pain, and age are more important determinants of functional impairment in older adult patients than the severity of knee OA as assessed radiographically.[52] Difficulty getting out of chairs or cars is a common association with hip and knee OA. Asking the patient to squeeze your hand provides an assessment of grip strength, and assessing their ability to perform a slow straight leg raise (one leg at a time) on a flat couch gives a good indication of quadriceps strength.

SWELLING: There may be palpable bony swelling of osteophytes. Effusions (related to synovial hypertrophy and increased volume of synovial fluid) are not uncommon.

CREPITUS: This is a coarse grating sensation or sound that results from friction between two articular surfaces. It is best appreciated through the range of movement. Although a key feature in criteria, crepitus is a nonspecific sign of joint damage.

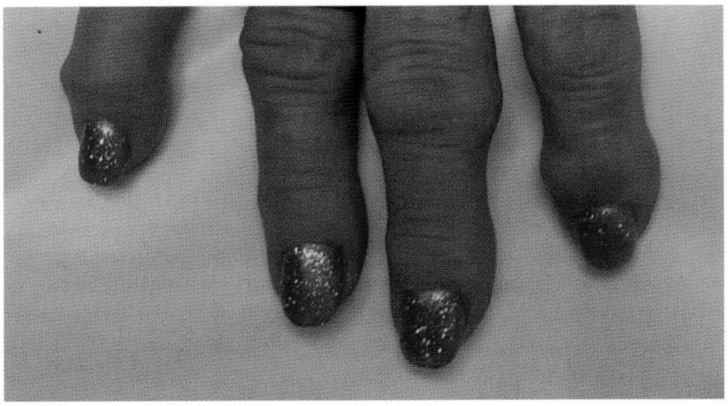

Figure 69-1. The fingers of a patient with primary nodal osteoarthritis of the hands demonstrating Heberden and Bouchard nodes. (Heberden nodes: posterior lateral swelling of the distal interphalangeal joints. Bouchard nodes: posterior lateral swelling of the proximal interphalangeal joints)

Investigations and Diagnosis

A full history and examination is often all that is required to determine the diagnosis and extent and impact of OA on an individual. Investigations are uncommonly required except for differential diagnosis.

IMAGING: The plain x-ray may be useful in differential diagnosis of a painful joint if history and examination are unhelpful. The main radiographic features of OA are loss of joint space, subchondral sclerosis, subchondral cysts, and osteophytosis. Weight-bearing views allow a better assessment of the extent of cartilage loss. It is important to remember that radiographic OA is common in the older adult population and may sometimes be an incidental finding. Overreliance on the radiograph for clinical decision making should be avoided; for example, radiographic OA would not exclude the presence of gout. Clinical judgment should be used to guide the uncommon requirement for other imaging modalities, such as MRI or ultrasound.

LABORATORY FINDINGS: In clinical practice there is no specific laboratory test that can be used to confirm a diagnosis of OA. Unlike in cases of inflammatory arthritis, the acute-phase reactants in patients with OA are expected to be normal.

SYNOVIAL FLUID ANALYSIS: In the presence of an effusion, an arthrocentesis can be a valuable test if inflammatory arthritis is suspected. In OA, the synovial fluid exhibits a low white blood cell count (<1000 cells/mm^3). More importantly, synovial fluid analysis helps to confirm or exclude the presence of monosodium urate or calcium pyrophosphate crystals and also rule out sepsis, bearing in mind that a septic joint may present differently in an older patient as a result of the phenomenon of immunosenescence. Acquiring expertise in joint aspiration is of clinical value.

Management

Several international consensus guidelines for the management of OA are available.[53-58] Therapeutic goals generally involve minimizing pain and disability while maximizing function and quality of life. Common to all guidelines is a holistic approach assessing the impact of OA on the individual. Treatment then incorporates a combination of pharmacologic and nonpharmacologic treatment options, including patient education, exercise programs, self-management, and weight loss strategies if overweight. Management plans should be individualized and consider the patient's perceptions in order to maximize adherence; they must also be devised with consideration given to the potential toxicity of drugs such as NSAIDs and opioids.[55] Key issues in the management of OA are presented in Table 69-4.

Patient Education

Patients should be provided with key information about their prognosis, and misconceptions should be corrected: few people with OA will end up in a wheelchair, and the course of OA is not inevitably progressive. Patients should be encouraged to participate in self-management programs that help increase their understanding of the disease and educate them on treatment options available. Self-management programs may reduce health care utilization,[59] and although they may not have a direct impact on pain or disability, these programs may help improve quality of life; in particular, they may help reduce anxiety and improve self-efficacy.

Exercise

There is a commonly held misconception that exercise may further damage the joints. Although avoidance of high-impact activity is advised, there is good evidence to show that tailored exercise programs can help significantly to reduce pain and disability.[60] There are few contraindications, even in older people, to a "prescription of exercise" that combines stretching, strengthening, and aerobic routines.[61] Exercise not only has a beneficial effect on pain and disability from OA but encourages restorative sleep, improves psychological health, promotes functional independence, and benefits comorbidities such as obesity, diabetes, chronic heart failure, and hypertension.

Optimizing Mechanical Factors

Correcting biomechanical factors is an important management strategy that can be of particular benefit in older adults. The use of a walking stick can help reduce the symptoms of hip or knee OA when held in the contralateral hand.[55] Another example is the use of a hand splint in the setting of base of thumb OA. There are also recommendations on the use of suitable footwear providing shock absorption and adequate arch support. The use of a knee brace in OA of the knee with varus or valgus deformity and instability can not only reduce pain but also reduce the risk of falling.[62] Using a multidisciplinary team approach and referring, when required, to the appropriate discipline, including physiotherapy, occupational therapy, or podiatry, is of great value.

Nonpharmacologic Treatment

Nondrug treatment options should be a consideration in all patients with OA. The simple strategy of thermotherapy with the application of hot or cold packs to the affected joint is safe and low cost, even though evidence regarding effectiveness is limited. A systematic review and meta-analysis published in 2010 showed a short-term benefit of acupuncture in people with OA[63] although a subsequent large trial showed no benefit of acupuncture over sham acupuncture.[64]

Pharmacologic Management

Drug treatment for OA needs individualized consideration as complications related to polypharmacy, drug toxicity, drug interactions, and comorbidities can occur. Generally, the analgesic effect of pharmacotherapy is small, and the evidence suggests that poorly designed trials overestimate the effectiveness of these therapies.[62]

TOPICAL THERAPIES: Topical NSAIDs such as diclofenac and ibuprofen were found to be safer than oral NSAIDs and the plasma concentration is substantially less than an equivalent dose

TABLE 69-4 Key Issues in the Management of Arthritis in Older Adults

OA	Gout	PMR	GCA	RA/SpA
Management should initially encompass pharmacologic and nonpharmacologic treatments. Management should be tailored to the needs and characteristics of the individual. Nonpharmacologic therapies, such as exercise, education, weight loss, splints should be considered as well as pharmacologic therapies. Pharmacologic therapies should be used with a focus on safety: Topical therapies are preferred (topical NSAIDs and capsaicin are safe and efficacious). Paracetamol may be first-line oral therapy. Attention should be paid to gastrointestinal, cardiovascular, and renal risks when prescribing NSAIDs and COX-2 inhibitors. Lowest possible dose for shortest time period. Risks of confusion, falls, and constipation considered when prescribing opioids. Intraarticular corticosteroids are effective for flares of OA or as pain circuit breakers to enable exercises. Surgery has a role, usually for severe symptoms interfering with quality of life.	Treatment of asymptomatic hyperuricemia is not indicated. Always search for a past history of gout attacks. Educate regarding the importance of lifestyle changes (e.g., diet, alcohol, weight loss). Pharmacotherapy of acute attacks: NSAIDs often contraindicated in older adults Colchicine: dose reduction in renal or hepatic impairment, or drugs that interact (statins, diuretics, cyclosporine) Wean oral corticosteroids slowly to prevent flare. Consider intraarticular or intramuscular corticosteroids ULT: Allopurinol is first line, start ≤100 mg daily and titrate up against serum urate. Febuxostat is indicated in allopurinol intolerance. Cover ULT institution with antiinflammatory. Do not stop ULT in an acute attack.	Management should involve a rheumatologist. Consider whether GCA coexists. Should respond promptly and well to prednisolone 10-20 mg/day. Consider steroid-sparing agents if dose reduction is difficult (note: absence of evidence). Consider GI protection and bone protection at initiation of therapy.	Management should involve a rheumatologist. Requires high-dose steroids. Consider steroid-sparing agents (note: absence of evidence). Consider aspirin[68] (note: absence of evidence). Consider GI protection and bone protection at initiation of therapy.	Management should involve a rheumatologist. Management should be holistic, involving education, allied health, and self-management. Begin disease-modifying therapy at diagnosis. Use standard outcome measures to monitor response. Escalate therapy to predefined disease activity targets. Regular monitoring of renal function, LFTs, and CBC is required for drug monitoring. Manage comorbidities (osteoporosis, cardiovascular risks, depression). Comorbidities and polypharmacy may affect pharmacotherapy.

CBC, Complete blood count; *COX-2,* cyclooxygenase-2; *GCA,* giant cell arteritis; *GI,* gastrointestinal; *LFT,* liver function test; *NSAIDs*, nonsteroidal antiinflammatory drugs; *OA,* osteoarthritis; *PMR,* polymyalgia rheumatica; *RA/SpA,* rheumatoid arthritis/spondyloarthritis; *ULT,* urate-lowering therapy.

of oral NSAIDs.[65] Multiple daily applications may limit adherence. The U.K. National Institute for Health and Care Excellence (NICE) guidelines recommend that topical capsaicin may be useful in hand or knee OA, although some days of application may be needed before efficacy is evident.[55]

PARACETAMOL: Historically paracetamol has been commonly used for OA. It lacks contraindications or drug interactions and it is inexpensive. However, a recent meta-analysis suggested only a small analgesic benefit for paracetamol in OA, with questionable clinical significance.[66] A meta-analysis of large observational studies reported some signals of toxicity, particularly in those taking high therapeutic doses; it wasn't clear if this reflected paracetamol or whether paracetamol was highlighting a group using nonprescription NSAIDs (data that are difficult to capture in observational studies).[67]

ORAL NSAIDs: These drugs remain among the most commonly used analgesics for arthritis.[68-69] Systematic reviews indicate that NSAIDs[62] and cyclooxygenase-2 (COX-2) selective agents show consistent good benefits across large numbers of studies.[62] NSAIDs differ in their degrees of COX-1 and COX-2 selectivity; however, all classes of NSAIDs have associations with varying degrees of renal, cardiovascular, and gastrointestinal risk, particularly in the older adult population with comorbidities (Table 69-5). Gastrointestinal risks may be compounded when NSAIDs are used in combination with paracetamol.[70]

TABLE 69-5 Adverse Effects of Nonsteroidal Antiinflammatory Drugs

Type of Adverse Reaction	Example
Gastrointestinal	Indigestion Erosions Peptic ulcer Hemorrhage and perforation Small bowel enteropathy
Hepatic	Hepatocellular damage Cholestasis
Renal	Acute renal failure Interstitial nephritis
Hematologic	Thrombocytopenia Neutropenia Hemolytic anemia
Skin	Photosensitivity Urticaria Erythema multiforme
Chest	Bronchospasm Pneumonitis
Central nervous system	Headache Dizziness Confusion
Cardiac	Increased risk of myocardial infarctions Cardiac failure Hypertension

Although COX-2 inhibitors have lower gastrointestinal side effects, similar to other NSAIDs they are associated with a prothrombotic risk. The NICE recommendations advise the concomitant use of proton pump inhibitors with all NSAIDs.[55] In patients at risk of cardiovascular complications, naproxen seems to have a better cardiovascular profile than other NSAIDs.[71] In general, NSAIDs must be used with caution in frail older adults with OA,[72] given that OA and cardiovascular disease often travel together.[72-74] NSAIDs should be prescribed at the lowest possible dose for the shortest time duration. Great care needs to be taken when prescribing NSAIDs to older people and avoided altogether if possible, especially among those who are frail.

OPIOIDS: Low-dose opioids are recommended in all OA guidelines, even though, like NSAIDs, they carry significant toxicity risks, especially in older adults. The evidence implies the analgesic effect size is bigger than that of simple analgesics.[62] Confusion, constipation, and falls are major issues related to opioid use, especially in a frail population. Modified or slow-release preparations may be useful for night pain, and transdermal preparations may help compliance issues.

INTRAARTICULAR CORTICOSTEROID INJECTIONS: The efficacy of intraarticular corticosteroids has been examined in a Cochrane review, confirming a modest and short-term efficacy of intraarticular corticosteroids in knee OA.[75] There is no evidence to suggest superiority of any one kind of steroid preparation.[71] The risk of infection with an intraarticular steroid injection is very small, although aseptic technique should of course be the norm. There have been concerns regarding cartilage toxicity with repeated injections, although this remains unproven.

OTHER THERAPIES: Several nutraceuticals and food supplements are often used to treat older adults with OA. The best known are glucosamine and chondroitin; the evidence surrounding the efficacy of these agents in OA is mixed, and as a result, most contemporary guidelines do not recommend these therapies.[55,76] There is currently an absence of randomized trial evidence to demonstrate analgesic efficacy of platelet-rich plasma or stem cell therapy in patients with OA, although trials are ongoing.

SURGICAL TREATMENT: Total joint replacement remains a hugely successful procedure, although such replacements often last approximately 20 years and revision procedures (especially in the knee) are complex, so often total joint replacements are not offered to younger patients. Arthroscopy has not been demonstrated to be useful for OA knee symptoms. The 2014 NICE guidelines recommend that surgical intervention should not be offered to people suffering from OA until nonsurgical therapies have been adequately trialled.[55] Surgery should be considered for those who continue to have symptoms that significantly impact their quality of life (rather than using a calculated scoring tool)[77] and be offered before there is prolonged functional limitation that may diminish the benefits of surgery. The decision to refer someone with OA for surgery should not be restricted by patient-specific factors, such as age, smoking, obesity, or gender.[55]

NOVEL TREATMENTS: Several randomized controlled clinical trials have studied the effects of targeting subchondral bone pathology in subjects with OA, using bisphosphonates[78-80] and strontium.[81] These studies have shown mixed effects on pain, and these therapies require further investigation; selection of patients for certain subchondral bone pathologies (e.g., MRI-detected bone marrow lesions) may improve their benefits. More recently investigation has shifted to therapies that have anti-synovitis effects, based on the frequency of synovial inflammation in OA.[82] Studies examining the role of tumor necrosis factor (TNF) blockers have been disappointing.[83] Preliminary data examining the role of methotrexate as an anti-synovitis therapy in knee OA has prompted further randomized controlled trials; results are pending.[84] New approaches to understanding the pathology and pain pathways in OA open up more options, including centrally acting drugs such as duloxetine and tapentadol and peripheral agents such as those targeting nerve growth factor (such as tanezumab[45,46]).

GOUT

Gout is the most common inflammatory arthritis and its prevalence (1% to 2%) has been increasing in recent decades, perhaps reflecting rising uric acid levels in communities. The presentation of gout may differ slightly in the older adult population from what is classically seen in younger community samples: it tends to have a more equal gender distribution and more frequently presents with polyarticular involvement.[85] In older adults it is frequently associated with comorbid conditions such as chronic kidney disease, hypertension, diabetes, and dyslipidemia. This adds complexity to the clinical presentation as well as its management.

Pathogenesis

The clinical picture of gout arises from the deposition of monosodium urate (MSU) crystals in joints and soft tissue. Hyperuricemia is the single most important risk factor for the development of gout, and the progression of asymptomatic hyperuricemia to gout is, in part, a function of the duration and severity of the elevation of serum uric acid—in effect, a reflection of the total body burden of urate. It is important to consider the difference between asymptomatic hyperuricemia and gout: 90% of people with asymptomatic hyperuricemia will not progress to gout, and given current evidence, hyperuricemia does not require urate-lowering therapy.[86]

Large longitudinal cohort studies have shown that a number of dietary factors are associated with the development of gout by affecting the urate pool, including beer, spirits, sugar-sweetened soft drinks, fructose, red meat, and seafood.[87]

When urate levels exceed physiologic saturation thresholds, MSU crystals are formed and elicit an intense inflammatory response, including release of interleukin-1β (IL-1β) by monocytes and macrophages, resulting in a severe painful inflammatory arthritis.[88]

Serum uric acid levels are affected by many factors, and rising or falling levels can trigger acute gout. Consequently, both increase in serum MSU (commonly as a result of dehydration or in increased cellular death following chemotherapy) and a fall in serum MSU as a result of urate-lowering therapy can trigger an attack. Common precipitants are presented in Table 69-6.[89]

Clinical Features

Gout in older people represents a special subgroup where the presentation may be atypical. Gout commonly presents with acute podagra with an exquisitely painful red swollen joint; however, in older adults, it may present with a more systemic presentation, including fevers and delirium, multiple joint involvement, or uncommon site involvement (e.g., the shoulder). An acutely inflamed monoarthritis requires septic arthritis to be excluded. Other differentials include a fracture, calcium pyrophosphate deposition disease ("pseudogout," the other common

TABLE 69-6 Precipitants of Acute Gout in Older Adults

- Changes in serum uric acid concentration
- Alcohol intake
- Dehydration (e.g., resulting from hot weather or long journey)
- Surgery
- Medications (e.g., diuretics, aspirin)
- Comorbidities (e.g., renal failure, cardiac disease)

form of crystal-induced arthritis) and the less common hydroxyapatite-associated arthritis. Clinicians should always ask about a previous episode of podagra, which usually indicates a diagnosis of gout.

Clinically it can be difficult to distinguish acute gout in this setting from sepsis. Typically an acute attack will resolve in 7 to 10 days. In those patients with persistent hyperuricemia, untreated, recurrent flares can occur and even chronic synovitis may develop. In the older age group, gouty tophi (local, organized deposits of urate crystals with associated inflammation) may be the initial manifestation of the disease.[90]

Investigation and Diagnosis

The diagnosis of gout should be confirmed by identification of urate crystals in the synovial fluid or a tophus. However, as this is not always possible, the ACR and the European League Against Rheumatism (EULAR)[91,92] recognize certain clinical features that strongly support the diagnosis of gout. These include rapid development of severe pain, swelling and tenderness that reaches maximum intensity in 6 to 12 hours, recurrent podagra with hyperuricemia, and more than one attack of severe arthritis.

In acute gout, analysis of the synovial fluid from the affected joint usually demonstrates a high inflammatory cell count with predominant neutrophilia. The intensity of the inflammatory attack means that the (very elevated) cell count may mimic that found in infection. Blood testing tends to show high acute-phase reactants. Measurement of serum uric acid may be helpful in supporting the diagnosis if elevated, but it may be paradoxically normal in an acute gout flare.[92]

Imaging may help increase diagnostic certainty. In long-standing disease, plain radiographs may show well-demarcated erosions with overhanging edges, although the sensitivity of plain x-ray is low in early disease.[93] MRI is not usually required but may be useful in identifying tophi in unusual locations.[93] Ultrasound, often the most feasible test, can detect erosions, synovitis, and tophi. The "double contour" sign seen on ultrasound is now recognized to be consistent with gout. The sign occurs when uric acid crystals lying on the cartilage surface form a bright echoic contour, and the cortical bone underlying the cartilage forms another (Figure 69-2). A development in computed tomography (CT) imaging of gout is dual-energy CT, which allows for color identification of the MSU crystals with high specificity; however, it may be less sensitive in the setting of early gout or where the MSU crystal deposits are not very dense.[94]

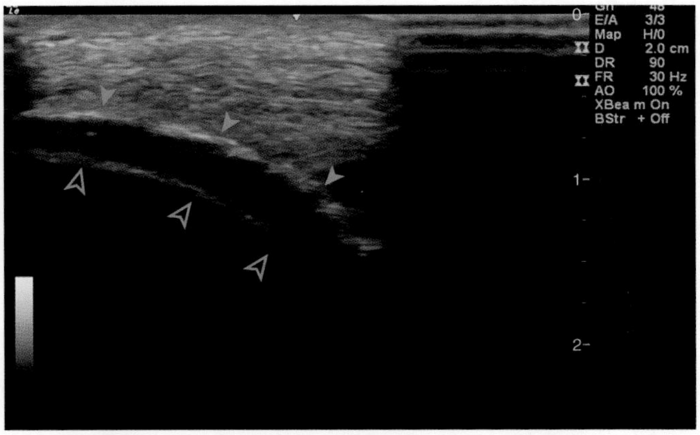

Figure 69-2. A longitudinal ultrasound of the femoral condyle of the knee, showing a "double contour." The bony cortex of the femoral condyle is indicated by the open arrows, and the urate crystals overlying cartilage are indicated by the solid arrows.

Management

Management of gout has three main goals: (1) treatment of an acute flare, (2) ongoing preventive treatment of chronic gout, and (3) prophylaxis against acute flares at the time of initiating urate-lowering therapy. International guidelines have stressed the importance of nonpharmacologic intervention, including education, diet, hydration, exercise, and smoking cessation. Attention to comorbid conditions is essential. Generally, though, in people with recurrent gout, pharmacotherapy is required.

Treatment of an Acute Flare

Treatment should be started as early as possible after the development of symptoms. Both ACR and EULAR guidelines recommend starting antiinflammatory pharmacotherapy within 24 hours of the onset of symptoms.[95] Following treatment with NSAIDs, more than 50% of patients show a major clinical response within 48 hours and 80% after 5 days.[96] There is no evidence to suggest the advantage of any one NSAID over another in terms of safety and efficacy.[97]

Colchicine is commonly the antiinflammatory of choice in gout. Current international guidelines recommend the dosing regimen for colchicine as 1.2 mg stat, followed by 0.6 mg 1 hour later, followed by 0.6 mg once or twice daily as prophylaxis,[98] due to evidence that a low dose is as efficacious and less toxic than previously recommended high doses. Dose adjustments in patients with significant renal or liver disease are required.[98]

Corticosteroids are another effective treatment option for acute gout, especially when NSAIDs and colchicine are contraindicated. International guidelines recommend considering the number and size of joints involved. For involvement of a single large joint, such as the knee, intraarticular injection of corticosteroid (e.g., triamcinolone, 40 mg) is reasonable, whereas if many joints are involved, or injection is contraindicated, oral prednisolone at a dose of 0.5 mg/kg for 5 to 10 days (or for 2 to 5 days with a 7- to 10-day taper) is recommended.[96]

Although NSAIDs, colchicine, and steroids can all be used as first-line treatment of a flare, and indeed may be used in combination, physicians need to be mindful of the challenges of using pharmacotherapy to treat older adults. Although not approved by the U.S. Food and Drug Administration, newer agents, including the IL-1 inhibitors anakinra, canakinumab, and rilonacept, have been shown to be effective therapy for adults with acute gout.[99] The cost-effectiveness of these agents remains unknown.

Ongoing Treatment of Chronic Gout

The key to managing chronic gout and preventing recurrent acute attacks is to lower the serum MSU with urate-lowering drugs.

Allopurinol, a xanthine oxidase inhibitor, is first-line urate-lowering therapy. The EULAR guidelines recommend a treatment target of less than 0.36 mmol/L serum urate concentration for patients with recurrent gout flares,[98] although less than 0.30 mmol/L further reduces risk. Apart from being an effective urate-lowering therapy, allopurinol may also have beneficial effects on renal function, cardiovascular disease, hypertension, and mortality.[100] Although allopurinol is generally well tolerated, it does have a known rare association with the potentially life-threatening allopurinol hypersensitivity syndrome, which is characterized by rash, eosinophilia, leukocytosis, fever, hepatitis, and progressive renal failure. A low starting dose (100 mg/day in any patient and 50 mg/day in those with chronic kidney disease stage 4 or worse) decreases the chance of gout flares and the risk of allopurinol hypersensitivity syndrome.[101]

Febuxostat, also a xanthine oxidase inhibitor, is approved for use as urate-lowering therapy in people with intolerance to allopurinol. Where the previously mentioned agents are ineffective, not tolerated, or contraindicated, the use of uricosuric agents such as probenecid or sulfinpyrazone can be considered; however, these agents have limited efficacy in the setting of moderate to severe renal impairment. Newer agents, including rasburicase and pegloticase (recombinant forms of uricase), have limited use because they are so expensive.

The importance of compliance with ongoing urate-lowering therapy should also be emphasized[98] to achieve best outcomes and prevent a cycle of flare on initiation, followed by cessation. Urate-lowering therapy should NOT be stopped during an acute flare.

Prophylaxis of an Acute Flare during Urate-Lowering Therapy Initiation

It is likely that NSAID therapy while initiating urate-lowering therapy will improve compliance through minimizing the risk of an acute flare. The EULAR guidelines recommend colchicine prophylaxis (0.5 to 1 mg/day) in the initial months of urate-lowering therapy.[98]

CHONDROCALCINOSIS

Chondrocalcinosis refers to the deposition of calcium pyrophosphate crystals in the cartilage, which can lead to arthritis. The term *calcium pyrophosphate deposition* (CPPD) includes several conditions, including an acute inflammatory arthritis, chronic inflammatory arthritis, and OA secondary to CPPD.[102] The condition can present either silently (with chondral calcinosis seen on imaging), as an acute arthritis (historically termed *pseudogout*), a chronic inflammatory process, or as OA. Definitive diagnosis requires the identification of calcium pyrophosphate crystals in synovial fluid, and this process allows exclusion of sepsis in the acutely inflamed joint.[102]

Aging is a key risk factor for the development of CPPD. Other risks include preexisting OA and metabolic conditions such as primary hyperparathyroidism, hemochromatosis, and hypomagnesemia.[102] An older person presenting with CPPD should be screened for these metabolic conditions,[102] but in practice a reversible cause of CPPD is rarely found.

Asymptomatic CPPD requires no intervention. Symptomatic disease management should be holistic, encompassing both nonpharmacologic and pharmacologic therapies.[103] In the setting of an acute inflammatory presentation, cool packs, short-term rest, and intraarticular steroids are recommended.[103] Chronic inflammatory arthritis can be difficult to manage and may require prophylactic NSAIDs; low-dose colchicine; or, in resistant cases, oral steroids or disease-modifying antirheumatic drugs (DMARDs), such as methotrexate or hydroxychloroquine, as anti-synovial therapies.[103]

POLYMYALGIA RHEUMATICA/GIANT CELL ARTERITIS

Polymyalgia rheumatica (PMR) is an inflammatory condition exclusively affecting older adults. It is characterized by symmetrical inflammatory pain of the hip and shoulder girdles, usually associated with high inflammatory markers and an excellent, rapid response to corticosteroids.

Pathogenesis

PMR is associated with giant cell arteritis (also known as temporal arteritis); each is considered an end of a disease spectrum with "pure" PMR having an absence of vascular involvement.[104] Although the pathogenesis is unclear, the concept remains that inflammation is initiated in both conditions following antigen recognition by the dendritic cells or macrophages.[104] The activated dendritic cells or macrophages then secrete inflammatory cytokines, including IL-1, IL-6, and TNF-α, which are responsible for the systemic features of the disease.

Clinical Features

PMR is a clinical syndrome; clinicians tend to consider a response to corticosteroid therapy as a "test of treatment" to establish the diagnosis.[104] Clinically, this can be challenging and presents obvious difficulties in the clinical trial setting. Recently, classification criteria were developed: patients aged 50 years or older presenting with bilateral shoulder pain and elevated C-reactive protein (CRP) and/or elevated erythrocyte sedimentation rate (ESR) can be classified as having PMR in the presence of morning stiffness for more than 45 minutes and new hip pain in the absence of peripheral synovitis or positive RA serology and the absence of a better alternate diagnosis. There may be systemic features, including fever, malaise, and weight loss. Less commonly, patients may also have musculoskeletal problems such as peripheral arthritis, distal hand swelling with pitting edema, and carpal tunnel syndrome,[104] and debate exists as to whether this whether this is PMR or rheumatoid arthritis.

Polymyalgia is associated with giant cell arteritis (GCA) in 10% to 40% of cases. Headache is a prominent symptom in GCA which is usually localized to the temple region and may be associated with scalp tenderness. Visual disturbances and/or jaw claudication are relatively common, and blindness remains a significant risk because of possible involvement of the ophthalmic artery; it is important to take a history for GCA in people presenting with PMR, as GCA management requires more aggressive immunosuppression.[105]

The proximal pain and stiffness syndrome of PMR can occur with many other rheumatologic and inflammatory illnesses, especially in older people. For example, a polymyalgic condition evolving to rheumatoid arthritis is not uncommon in the setting of older adult onset of these diseases.[104] The most common differential diagnosis is that of bilateral rotator cuff disease, which is very common in adults older than 60 years. Some history clues that might help differentiate (nothing is diagnostic) is that patients with tendon disease describe a painful arc and pain when lying on the shoulder in bed. A very uncommon differential diagnosis is polymyositis, which is more likely to present with weakness of the hip and shoulder girdle associated with an elevated creatine kinase, rather than the typical polymyalgic presentation of hip and shoulder girdle morning myalgias in the setting of a normal creatine kinase level.

Investigations

Baseline investigation required to make a diagnosis must include inflammatory markers, chest x-ray, urinalysis, and relevant tests to exclude other causes, including rheumatoid factor and antibodies to cyclic citrullinated peptides (ACPAs).[105] The current EULAR/ACR classification criteria include an algorithm that calls for an ultrasound at first presentation to assess for bursitis, synovitis, and/or tenosynovitis, which are common and often bilateral in patients with PMR.[106]

If GCA is being considered, a temporal artery biopsy is important to assist in the diagnosis but may be negative in a significant number of cases; because of this, the diagnosis is reliant upon the clinician's acumen.[107] Imaging is increasingly being used in GCA to assist in the diagnosis, including ultrasonography and positron emission tomography (PET) scanning. Ultrasonography is likely user dependent, and the sensitivity and specificity values differ among published studies.[108,109]

Management

Despite the lack of high-quality evidence for the management of PMR, EULAR/ACR guidelines based on expert consensus have been published.[110] Recommendations include ensuring relevant mimicking conditions are excluded. Baseline inflammatory marker levels should be measured (to allow objective assessment of response), and assessment should be made at baseline and follow-up of possible steroid-related side effects. The EULAR/ACR guidelines encourage individualized initial steroid regimen, using the lowest possible effective dose, but argue that a lack of evidence precludes identification of a specific dose.[110] British Society for Rheumatology and Australian guidelines recommend the initial use of prednisone, 15 mg and 10 to 20 mg, respectively.[111,112] Generally, it is agreed, the dosage should be gradually tapered once disease control is achieved, with a view to cessation in 1to 2 years. The response is expected to be significant early in the treatment phase, and a lack of significant response should prompt reconsideration of the diagnosis. The EULAR/ACR guidelines recommend a follow-up 2 to 4 weeks after commencing therapy to review response.[110] Many clinicians will use steroid-sparing agents, such as methotrexate or leflunomide, but the evidence to support this practice is somewhat lacking.

For GCA, a higher initial dose of prednisolone at 40 to 60 mg/day is recommended.[65,105] Pulsed glucocorticosteroid therapy is recommended for complicated GCA, including those with visual disturbance.[105,112] Approximately 50% of patients relapse;[113] this may require escalation of steroids, or addition of steroid sparing agents (even though there is no good-quality evidence to support their use). Aspirin is sometimes recommended to reduce the risk of cerebrovascular events in patients with GCA,[105] in the absence of good-quality evidence.

The dose of steroids, duration of therapy, and decision whether to use steroid-sparing agents need to be adjusted according to the individual's presentation. Factors that may influence treatment decisions include disease severity; comorbidities such as diabetes, renal disease, or cardiovascular illness; fracture risk; and adverse events. Bone protection is advised in all patients, and consideration given to gastrointestinal protection.

Key issues in the management of these conditions are presented in Table 69-4.

RHEUMATOID ARTHRITIS

Rheumatoid arthritis (RA) is increasingly becoming a disease of later life. The prevalence varies depending on the demographic studies but is thought to be between 1% and 2%, with increasing prevalence with age.[114-117] Many patients with RA are older than 65 years.

Rheumatoid in older adults may be either "young-onset" RA (in those who have aged) or "elderly-onset" RA. Elderly-onset RA can often be overlooked or ignored by patients and physicians. However, it is important to recognize RA early, as evidence has demonstrated that delays in therapy result in worse outcomes for patients. In older people, it is important to prevent functional deficits, which can be more difficult to manage in patients with existing mobility issues and other comorbidities. The management of RA in older adults is therefore more complex.

Clinical Features

Rheumatoid arthritis usually presents with a symmetrical inflammatory polyarthropathy. It is often insidious in onset and associated with prolonged morning stiffness for more than 60 minutes.[118]

Typically RA involves the small joints of the hands, wrists and metatarsophalangeal joints of feet with sparing of both the distal interphalangeal joints of the hands and feet and the axial joints.[119,120] Less typical presentations include monoarthritis precipitated by joint trauma or PMR-type symptoms[121] preceding development of polyarthritis. Unchecked disease can lead to development of typical deformities such as Z-deformities of the thumb, Boutonniere deformities, swan-necking, ulnar deviation, and joint subluxation.

Systemic symptoms are common and occur in up to one third of patients, with fatigue, mild weight loss, and uncommonly low-grade fevers, which may precede joint involvement by several months.

Extraarticular manifestations can occur at any time in the course of RA and result from the same pathologic process. In previous years, up to 40% of patients developed one or more extraarticular features[122] in the lifetime of disease, the most common of which were rheumatoid nodules, secondary Sjögren's syndrome, and pulmonary fibrosis. With modern management and tight control of inflammation, extraarticular manifestations are now much less common.

Compared with young-onset RA, elderly-onset patients may present atypically. They frequently present with an acute-onset disease, may have less small joint involvement (with the shoulders being commonly involved), a more polymyalgia onset with constitutional features, higher levels of disease activity, a tendency to be seronegative, and they are more often male with a gender ratio approaching 1.[123-126] It has been reported that the outcomes for elderly-onset RA are worse.[127]

Pathophysiology

RA is a heterogeneous condition with several pathways leading to loss of tolerance, autoimmunity, joint inflammation, and subsequent damage. Loss of tolerance leads to formation of inflammatory synovitis that invades and degrades bone and cartilage, leading to bone erosion, tendonitis and tendon rupture, and the traditional deformities once associated with RA.

Understanding is as yet incomplete regarding the cause of loss of tolerance and autoimmunity. It is understood that genetic,[128-130] epigenetic,[131] and environmental factors[132,133] all play some part. In particular, smoking has been linked to loss of tolerance and is a strong risk factor for RA. It is thought that the citrullination of mucosal proteins in the genetically susceptible individual, in the right epigenetic setting, leads to production of antibodies to these modified proteins (ACPAs),[134] which is the first step to loss of tolerance. Gingivitis or chronic lung infections may be the first steps in genetically susceptible people.

Investigation and Diagnosis

RA should be suspected with any inflammatory polyarthritis presentation, particularly with duration of greater than 6 weeks (an acute onset of polyarthritis would suggest an alternative diagnosis and close follow-up is needed). Often clues on history and examination may help to differentiate RA from other inflammatory arthritides. The ACR/EULAR diagnostic criteria for RA may be a useful adjunct for detecting early RA (Table 69-7). Previous 1987 criteria often failed to pick up early RAs, although it was useful for distinguishing between noninflammatory conditions.[135]

The most useful diagnostic tests are the rheumatoid factor and ACPA blood tests. If both are positive, it is more sensitive and specific for RA than either on its own. It is now recognized that ACPAs may be present for many years before onset of clinical RA, and monitoring of these patients over time is important, even when they have nonspecific musculoskeletal symptoms.[136,137]

X-rays of the hands and feet have been the traditional method of imaging in RA and can be used to look for the typical damage associated with RA (erosions and joint space narrowing) to help confirm diagnosis. However, they are often normal at presentation. In cases of diagnostic difficulty, ultrasound or MRI can be helpful to establish presence of synovitis because they are more

TABLE 69-7 Classification Criteria for Rheumatoid Arthritis*

Joint Involvement	Points	Serology†	Points	Acute-Phase Reactants†	Points	Duration of Symptoms	Points
1 Large joint	0	Negative serology	0	Normal CRP and normal ESR	0	<6 weeks	0
2-10 Large joints	1	Low-positive RF or low-positive ACPA	2	Abnormal CRP or abnormal ESR	1	≥6 weeks	1
1-3 Small joints (with or without involvement of large joints)	2	High-positive RF or high-positive ACPA	3				
4-10 Small joints (with or without involvement of large joints)	3						
>10 Joints (at least one small joint)	5						

Modified from Aletaha D, Neogi T, Silman AJ, et al: 2010 rheumatoid arthritis classification criteria: an American College of Rheumatology/European League Against Rheumatism collaborative initiative. Ann Rheum Dis 69(9):1580-1588, 2010.
ACPA, Anti–cyclic citrullinated peptide antibody; *CRP,* C-reactive protein; *ESR,* erythrocyte sedimentation rate; *RF,* rheumatoid factor.
*A score of 6/10 or higher is needed for a diagnosis of rheumatoid arthritis.
†At least one test result is needed for classification.

sensitive than clinical examination in detecting synovitis and more sensitive than x-ray at detecting erosions.[138]

Management

The optimal therapeutic regimen is uncertain, and some available therapies are expensive, meaning that practices may differ between countries and health care systems. The goal of treatment is to minimize synovitis extent and duration, prevent joint damage, and preserve function. Early recognition and diagnosis is absolutely essential, with the immediate initiation of treatment at time of diagnosis, with DMARDs, which have been shown to reduce irreversible injury. The aim is for tight disease control with remission or low disease activity as the accepted target. In older adults, therapies may need to be individualized in the context of comorbidities and polypharmacy. Care should be holistic and involve a multidisciplinary team approach. Involvement of a rheumatologist is essential (see Table 69-4).

Nonpharmacologic Therapies

Nonpharmacologic therapies include patient education, appropriate rest, exercise with involvement of physiotherapist and occupational therapist as needed, and immunizations when appropriate. (Influenza and pneumococcus are recommended, as is hepatitis B for those at high risk; live vaccines are generally not considered safe.) People with RA also get all the other common musculoskeletal problems such as OA and back pain.

Psychosocial interventions are important in the management of RA. Depression is often underrecognized and undertreated in the older adult population and is not an uncommon comorbidity in RA. Cardiovascular disease risk reduction is important as it is an important cause of death in those with RA, particularly in older adults with multiple additional risks.

Osteoporosis is also associated with RA and should be considered and appropriately addressed. Despite this, the risk of major osteoporotic fracture is increased, particularly in older adults.

Appropriate surgical interventions to relieve pain or improve function should be considered in the case of severely deformed joints, although joint surgery to treat RA is performed less often, reflecting modern successful therapeutic approaches.

Pharmacologic Therapies

In parallel with advances in early diagnosis and tight control of inflammation, pharmacologic therapies have improved, especially with the introduction of appropriately dosed methotrexate and biologic DMARDs (bDMARDs).

NSAIDs are still useful in the management of active synovitis, with rapid efficacy, although they carry significant gastrointestinal, cardiovascular, and renal risks in older adults.

Corticosteroids are very useful because of their rapid and powerful antiinflammatory effects. In the short term, while initiating more definitive but slower-acting therapy, corticosteroids can be useful "bridges" to improve symptoms, regain function, and protect structure. They can also be useful in established disease when flares require escalation of therapy but a quick intervention is needed. They also have an important role in preventing structural damage in early disease,[139] particularly until DMARDs take effect. Side effects remain an obstacle limiting long-term use. In older adults with RA, osteoporosis, skin thinning, poor wound healing, myopathy, confusion, and mania can be particularly problematic.[127] However, there has been some evidence to suggest that with doses of less than 10 mg prednisolone daily, the overall benefits of inflammation control may outweigh the detriments of long-term steroid use.[140,141] Using different delivery methods, intramuscular or intraarticular, may allow the clinician more control over the dosage taken and may minimize systemic side effects.

DMARDs. Current management paradigms recommend early initiation at time of diagnosis, with escalation of therapy to achieve the target of clinical remission. DMARDs are long-term therapies; stopping treatment in established RA is associated with a high risk of flares.

Extensive evidence supports the role of DMARD therapies in early RA, but the optimal management regimen is uncertain. Commonly used management paradigms include methotrexate monotherapy[142] (recommended as initial therapy by the ACR), combination DMARD therapy[143](triple therapy with methotrexate, sulfasalazine, and hydroxychloroquine is favored by some),[144] or DMARD in combination with corticosteroids. If remission is not achieved, options include switching DMARDs or adding DMARDs to try and achieve control. The most important message is "treating to target," in which therapy is altered in response to an objective disease activity assessment (such as the Disease Activity Score [DAS]) to try and achieve remission.[145]

Pretreatment evaluation includes a complete blood count; urea, electrolytes, and creatinine; liver function tests; ESR; and CRP. The ACR recommendations for the management of RA indicate that viral hepatitis is a relative contraindication to DMARDs, so consideration should be given to screening prior to DMARD use.[142]

Methotrexate remains the most commonly used DMARD therapy, dosed up to 25 mg once weekly via oral or subcutaneous routes. It has been demonstrated to be effective in older adults,[146]

TABLE 69-8 Current bDMARDs and Small Molecules,* Together with the Inflammatory Arthritides Where They Are Commonly Used

Class	Structure	Agent	RA	AS	PSA
TNF inhibitor	MAB targeting the cytokine	Adalimumab	Y	Y	Y
		Infliximab	Y	Y	Y
		Golimumab	Y	Y	Y
		Certolizumab	Y	Y	Y
	Soluble receptor targeting the cytokine	Etanercept	Y	Y	Y
IL-6 inhibitor	mAb targeting the cytokine	Tocilizumab	Y	N	N
Costimulation blocker	CTLA4-Ig fusion protein targeting CD80 and CD86	Abatacept	Y	N	N
B cell depletion	Chimeric mAb targeting CD20	Rituximab	Y	N	N
T helper cell 17 inhibition	mAb targeting IL-12 and IL-23	Ustekinumab	N	N	Y
Janus kinase inhibition	Janus kinase 1 and 3	Tofacitinib*	Y	N	N
PDE4	Selective inhibitor of the enzyme PDE4	Apremilast*	N	N	Y

AS, Ankylosing spondyloarthritis; *bDMARD,* biologic disease-modifying antirheumatic drug; *CTLA4-Ig,* cytotoxic T lymphocyte antigen-4–immunoglobulin; *IL-6,* interleukin-6; *MAB,* monoclonal antibody; *PDE4,* phosphodiesterase 4; *PSA,* psoriatic arthritis; *RA,* rheumatoid arthritis; *TNF,* tumor necrosis factor.

but it is important to monitor renal function. Because methotrexate is renally excreted, it can accumulate in the setting of progressive renal impairment, leading to myelotoxicity.

Recommendations regarding the monitoring of DMARDs may differ slightly among health systems, countries, and organizations. For example, routine screening for hydroxychloroquine ophthalmologic toxicity is recommended by some organizations but not others. Although the ACR has published guidelines,[142] local practice may differ. There has been little systematic investigation into the safety or efficacy of DMARDs in older adults specifically; however, monitoring more often than is recommended may be required when treating older patients with hepatic or renal impairment or in the context of polypharmacy.[147]

bDMARDs. Biologic DMARDs have revolutionized the treatment of inflammatory arthritis, by targeting very specific aspects of the inflammatory cascade. The commonly used molecules target TNF, IL-6, B cell–specific antigens, and costimulation molecules (Table 69-8). They are rapidly effective and improve both inflammatory signs and symptoms and prevent structural damage.[139,148-153] Whether bDMARDs should be used as first-line therapy in early disease is a matter for debate, but in reality, their widespread use is limited by cost. In practice bDMARDs are often restricted to people who have failed to respond to conventional DMARD therapy. It is important to note that combination therapy, using methotrexate with a bDMARD, often results in superior outcomes and protects against immunogenicity and the development of neutralizing antibodies.[154]

In older people, the main concern about these drugs is the predisposition to infection they bring, particularly herpes zoster, mycobacteria, and other atypical infections, such as encapsulated organisms.[155] Progressive multifocal leukoencephalopathy is an exceedingly rare but devastating infection associated with immunosuppression.[156] Another rare but important side effect to consider is demyelinating disorders, which have been associated with TNF inhibitors.[157] Although the relationship between malignancy and biologics was of great concern, real-life registries have examined the postmarketing use of biologics for many years, and the body of evidence shows no increased incidence of cancer over that associated with having active RA, with the exception of some skin cancers.[155]

There has been little investigation into the specific safety and efficacy of these molecules in older adults; registry data demonstrates that older adults are prescribed bDMARDs less commonly than younger people,[158] and those who are prescribed bDMARDs have more comorbidities than younger controls.[159] However, preliminary evidence regarding the safety of bDMARDs in older adults is reassuring,[160,161] and registry data suggest many clinicians are using bDMARD monotherapy in this age group, allowing disease control without exposure to the toxicities of DMARDs.[159]

These drugs are currently expensive (although less expensive biosimilars are just entering world markets) and associated with significant toxicities. The use of these drugs should be initiated and managed only by a rheumatologist.

Clinical Outcomes

Outcomes for patients with RA have significantly improved over recent decades. In 1987, most people with RA were moderately or severely impaired by 20 years, and the average outpatient had a 30% chance of severe disability.[162] Modern management (including early therapy with DMARDs), the advent of biologics, and utilizing objective outcomes to treat to target have resulted in much better outcomes.[163] More recently, studies have found that 94% of people who have had RA for 10 years or more remain independent in their activities of daily living,[164] and employments rates are becoming similar for people with and without RA.[165,166]

SPONDYLOARTHROPATHY

Spondyloarthritis (SpA), previously known as seronegative spondyloarthropathy, is a label given to a large group of distinct diseases with several overlapping clinical features. The group includes ankylosing spondylitis (AS), non-radiographic axial SpA (similar to AS but not meeting radiographic diagnostic criteria of AS), psoriatic arthritis, reactive arthritis, arthritis associated with ulcerative colitis and Crohn disease, juvenile SpA, and undifferentiated SpA. As a group, these disorders are less common than RA,[167,168] and although older adults may have a form of SpA, they are usually not incident cases.

Pathogenesis

The pathogenesis is incompletely understood. Most of the information that is known relates to AS. Given the commonalities between the different forms of SpA, it is likely that there are related pathogenic mechanisms.[169] SpA tends to differ from RA in that the enthesis is the primary site of pathology, whereas in RA the primary site is the synovium.

Genetics plays a strong role in the pathogenesis of SpA, particularly in AS where it contributes an estimated 90%[170] of heritability, with significant contribution also in other forms of SpA, such as psoriatic arthritis (40%). *HLA-B27* is the major genetic risk factor in SpA, particularly in AS with an estimated 23%[171] contribution; it is present in 90% of people with AS but only 5% of *HLA-B27*–positive people develop AS, suggesting other genetic factors at play. As incident SpA is uncommon in older adults, further discussion of the pathogenesis is beyond the scope of this chapter.

Clinical Features

Common clinical features in SpAs include the following:

1. Inflammatory back pain
   Chronic, lasting more than 3 months
   Insidious onset, improvement with exercise, no improvement with rest, nocturnal pain improving on waking, onset younger than 40 years
   Improves with NSAIDs
   Alternating buttock pain
2. Peripheral arthritis, typically oligoarticular, lower limb and asymmetrical, acute
3. Sacroiliitis
   Characterized by poorly localized, alternating buttock pain
   Typical x-ray changes with joint space narrowing, irregularity, subchondral sclerosis, and ankylosis/fusion
4. Enthesitis (particularly of the Achilles attachment to heel and plantar fasciitis)
5. Dactylitis (inflammation of the tendon sheath leading to typical "sausage digit")
6. Extraarticular features such as uveitis, psoriasis, inflammatory bowel disease
7. *HLA-B27* positivity
8. High CRP, although this does not correlate with disease activity in AS
9. Ankylosis of joints, which may be axial or peripheral

Management

Investigation into management paradigms to achieve optimal outcomes in SpA lags behind RA. AS and psoriatic arthritis are the best studied SpAs. The general aims are similar to those of RA management: (1) to control inflammation in order to improve function and pain, and (2) to prevent subsequent clinical deterioration.[172] Structural changes tend to be irreversible, so prevention is vital.

Once again, regardless of axial or peripheral distribution of disease, education, exercise, physical therapy, rehabilitation, analgesia, and self-management training are helpful for the management of disease. It has been shown that physiotherapy in axial disease in combination with NSAIDs helps to prevent radiographic progression of disease, although the evidence is less clear in other SpAs. Adequate analgesia, which can take the form of oral or intraarticular steroids, for acute flares or even to maintain remission is also important but not ideal because of long-term side effects.

As a general rule, DMARDs are not helpful for the control of axial disease or enthesopathy; NSAIDs are generally first-line pharmacotherapy. Issues regarding NSAID use have been discussed elsewhere in this chapter. In the setting of peripheral arthritis, DMARDs are used; the specific drugs used and the management paradigm are now similar to those applied to RA. Recent evidence supports early DMARD therapy, incorporating a treat-to-target approach to achieve optimal outcomes in patients with psoriatic arthritis.[173]

Should SpA arthritis prove refractory to NSAIDs and exercise (or DMARDs if arthritis is peripheral), then bDMARDs (see Table 69-8) may be instituted. The most effective biologic therapy for patients with SpAs are the TNF inhibitors (see Table 69-8). Issues regarding bDMARD use were discussed earlier in the chapter, but there is little specific evidence relating to the use of these molecules in older adults with SpA.

KEY POINTS

- Management should be tailored to the needs and characteristics of the individual.
- Management should encompass pharmacologic and nonpharmacologic therapies, such as exercise, education, splints.
- Pharmacologic therapies should be used with a focus on safety.
- Attention should be paid to gastrointestinal, cardiovascular, and renal risks when prescribing drugs.
- Management of inflammatory conditions should involve a rheumatologist.
- Consider gastro protection, bone protection, and cardiovascular risk at initiation of therapy in inflammatory diseases.

For a complete list of references, please visit www.expertconsult.com.

KEY REFERENCES

2. Duncan R, Francis RM, Collerton J, et al: Prevalence of arthritis and joint pain in the oldest old: findings from the Newcastle 85+ study. Age Ageing 40:752–755, 2011.
5. Keenan AM, Tennant A, Fear J, et al: Impact of multiple joint problems on daily living tasks in people in the community over age fifty-five. Arthritis Rheum 55:757–764, 2006.
53. Hochberg MC, Altman RD, April KT, et al: American College of Rheumatology 2012 recommendations for the use of nonpharmacologic and pharmacologic therapies in osteoarthritis of the hand, hip, and knee. Arthritis Care Res (Hoboken) 64:465–474, 2012.
55. National Institute for Health and Care Excellence: Osteoarthritis: care and management (NICE guidelines [CG177]), Feb 2014. http://www.nice.org.uk/guidance/cg177. Accessed February 15, 2016.
67. Roberts E, Delgado Nunes V, Buckner S, et al: Paracetamol: not as safe as we thought? A systematic literature review of observational studies. Ann Rheum Dis 75:552–559, 2016.
95. Khanna D, Khanna PP, Fitzgerald JD, et al: 2012 American College of Rheumatology guidelines for management of gout. Part 2: therapy and antiinflammatory prophylaxis of acute gouty arthritis. Arthritis Care Res (Hoboken) 64:1447–1461, 2012.
101. Khanna D, FitzGerald JD, Khanna PP, et al: 2012 American College of Rheumatology guidelines for management of gout. Part 1: systematic non-pharmacologic and pharmacologic therapeutic approaches to hyperuricemia. Arthritis Care Res (Hoboken) 64: 1431–1446, 2012.
103. Zhang W, Doherty M, Pascual E, et al: EULAR recommendations for calcium pyrophosphate deposition. Part II: management. Ann Rheum Dis 70:571–575, 2011.
110. Dejaco C, Singh YP, Perel P, et al: 2015 Recommendations for the management of polymyalgia rheumatica: a European League Against Rheumatism/American College of Rheumatology collaborative initiative. Arthritis Rheumatol 67:2569–2580, 2015.
142. Singh JA, Saag KG, Bridges SL, Jr, et al: 2015 American College of Rheumatology guideline for the treatment of rheumatoid arthritis. Arthritis Care Res (Hoboken) 68:1–25, 2015.
172. Smolen JS, Braun J, Dougados M, et al: Treating spondyloarthritis, including ankylosing spondylitis and psoriatic arthritis, to target: recommendations of an international task force. Ann Rheum Dis 73:6–16, 2014.

70 Metabolic Bone Disease

Roger Michael Francis, Terry Aspray

INTRODUCTION

Bone is a living, dynamic tissue that undergoes constant remodeling throughout life. This is necessary to allow the skeleton to increase in size during growth, respond to the physical stresses placed on it, and repair structural damage caused by structural fatigue or fracture. In addition to its mechanical properties, bone also plays an important role in calcium homeostasis, acting as a mineral reservoir that can be drawn upon to maintain normocalcemia. The skeleton comprises two types of bone: cortical (or compact) and trabecular (or cancellous) bone. Cortical bone is predominantly found in the shafts of the long bones, whereas trabecular bone is mainly located in the vertebrae, pelvis, and the ends of long bones, where it forms a lattice-like structure within an outer shell of cortical bone. Trabecular bone has a larger surface area, undergoes greater remodeling, and is therefore more responsive to changes in calcium homeostasis than is cortical bone. The respective proportion of cortical and trabecular bone varies with the anatomic site, but overall the skeleton is composed of 80% cortical and 20% trabecular bone.

The three major cell types involved in bone remodeling are osteoclasts, osteoblasts, and osteocytes. Osteoclasts are multinucleate cells, derived from macrophage-monocyte precursors, which resorb bone, releasing mineral and removing degraded organic material. Osteoblasts are derived from fibroblast precursors and synthesize bone matrix or osteoid, which is subsequently mineralized around foci of crystal formation known as matrix vesicles. The matrix vesicles are extruded from osteoblasts by exocytosis and contain promoters of crystal formation such as alkaline phosphatase and pyrophosphatase. Osteocytes are mature osteoblasts that become trapped within calcified bone. These are interconnected by long dendritic processes, which may serve as mechanosensory receptors, leading to the production of paracrine factors that regulate bone resorption and formation.

Bone remodeling is initiated by a period of bone resorption lasting about 2 weeks, when osteoclasts erode an area of bone. Osteoblasts are then attracted to the resorption cavity, where, over the subsequent 3 months, new bone matrix is deposited and mineralized. The processes of bone resorption and bone formation are usually closely coupled, but bone formation exceeds resorption during skeletal growth, allowing the skeleton to increase in size and density. Later in life resorption outstrips bone formation, leading to involutional bone loss. Bone remodeling may be influenced by mechanical forces applied to the skeleton, by paracrine factors, and by circulating hormones such as estrogen, testosterone, calcitonin, parathyroid hormone (PTH), and 1,25-dihydroxyvitamin D (1,25[OH]$_2$D).

One of the major regulators of bone remodeling is the receptor activator of nuclear factor kappa B (RANK) and RANK ligand (RANKL) system. RANKL, which is produced by osteoblasts, attaches to RANK on the cell surface of osteoclasts and osteoclast precursors, leading to stimulation of osteoclast differentiation and proliferation. The interaction of RANKL and RANK is blocked by osteoprotegerin (OPG), a soluble decoy receptor produced by osteoblasts and marrow stromal cells. Studies show relationships between circulating concentrations of OPG and bone mineral density (BMD) and it is now apparent that the beneficial effects of osteoporosis treatments may be mediated in part by changes in the RANK, RANKL, and OPG system.[1]

Bone mass changes throughout life in three major phases: growth, consolidation, and involution. Up to 90% of the ultimate bone mass is deposited during skeletal growth, which lasts until the closure of the epiphyses. There is then a phase of skeletal consolidation lasting for up to 15 years, when bone mass increases further until the peak bone mass is achieved in the mid-30s. Involutional bone loss then starts between the ages of 35 and 40 in both sexes, but in women there is an acceleration of bone loss in the decade after the menopause.

OSTEOPOROSIS

Osteoporosis is a skeletal disorder characterized by compromised bone strength, predisposing a person to an increased risk of low trauma or fragility fractures. The three major fragility fractures are those of the forearm, vertebral body, and femoral neck, but fractures of the humerus, tibia, pelvis, and ribs are also common. These fractures are a major cause of mortality, morbidity, and health and social service expenditure in older people, but this is particularly the case with hip fractures. In 2010, 22 million women and 5.5 million men were estimated to have osteoporosis in the European Union alone, with 3.5 million sustaining new fragility fractures of which 620,000 were hip fractures. The associated economic burden of incident and prior fragility fractures was estimated at 37 billion euros, with an expected average increase by 25% over the following 15 years in costs.[2]

There is a strong inverse relationship between bone density and fracture risk, with a two- to three-fold increase in fracture incidence for each standard deviation reduction in BMD. The risk of fracture is also determined by other skeletal risk factors, such as bone turnover, trabecular architecture, skeletal geometry, and previous fragility fracture. However, nonskeletal risk factors for fracture are also important; these include frailty, sarcopenia,[3] postural instability, and conditions associated with falling.[4]

The incidence of fragility fractures increases with advancing age and is higher in women than men, because of their lower peak bone mass, different patterns of cortical and trabecular bone loss, smaller skeletal size, and greater risk of falls. Fractures are also more common in older residents of care homes and nursing homes than in community-dwelling people of the same age, probably because of their higher risk of falls and lower BMD.[5,6]

Prevalence of Osteoporosis

The World Health Organization (WHO) has quantitatively defined osteoporosis as a BMD 2.5 standard deviations or more below the mean value for young adults (T score < −2.5).[7] The prevalence of osteoporosis at the hip in white women in the United States increases from 8% in the seventh decade to 47.5% in the ninth decade.[7] With regard to the probability of fragility fractures, the lifetime risk for a 50-year-old woman in the United Kingdom is 53.2%, compared with 20.7% for a 50-year-old man.[8]

Pathogenesis of Osteoporosis

Bone mass at any age, and therefore the risk of fracture, is determined by the peak bone mass, the age at which bone loss starts, and the rate at which bone loss progresses.

Peak Bone Mass

Osteoporosis and fracture risk are determined in younger life, with the achievement of peak bone mass, which may explain approximately half of subsequent bone mass at the age of 70 years, affected by a number of genetic and epigenetic factors linking maternal health, nutrition, and socioeconomic status with childhood diet, physical activity, diet, and lifestyle.[9] Other potential determinants of peak bone mass include exercise,[10,11] dietary calcium,[12] smoking,[13] and hormonal factors.[14]

Involutional Bone Loss

Bone loss starts between the ages of 35 and 40 in both sexes, possibly related to impaired new bone formation as a result of declining osteoblast function. The onset of bone loss is likely to be genetically determined, and the subsequent rate of bone loss may also be influenced by genetic factors. Recent studies suggest that a number of gene polymorphisms influence BMD and fracture risk. The genes involved include those regulating RANK, Wnt signaling, and other mechanisms involved in bone homeostasis.[15] Although the individual effect of variation in these genes is relatively small, the combined impact of these is similar to other major risk factors for fracture.[15]

Bone loss increases in the decade following menopause in women; this increase occurs as a result of the marked reduction in the circulating estradiol concentrations. Other causes of age-related bone loss include low body weight, smoking, excess alcohol consumption, and physical inactivity. With advancing age, there is a reduction in circulating 25 hydroxyvitamin D (25OHD) and an increase in PTH, which may also contribute to bone loss in older people.

Secondary Osteoporosis

In addition to the factors influencing the attainment of peak bone mass and subsequent involutional bone loss, there are a number of conditions which may accelerate the development of osteoporosis. In older age, the most frequently encountered are oral glucocorticoid therapy, male hypogonadism, hyperthyroidism, myeloma, and the use of antiepileptic drugs.

Clinical Features of Osteoporosis

Osteoporosis is generally considered to be asymptomatic until fractures occur. Fractures of the forearm and hip are usually easy to diagnose, but vertebral fractures may be more difficult to detect clinically. Only 30% of patients come for medical attention after a vertebral fracture, and there are many other causes of acute back pain.[16] Classically, however, a vertebral fracture is associated with an acute episode of back pain lasting for 6 to 8 weeks before settling to a more chronic backache. The pain may radiate anteriorly but rarely radiates to the hips or legs. Individuals with vertebral fractures may also be aware of loss of height of several inches and notice the development of a kyphosis.

Diagnosis of Osteoporosis and Fracture Risk

Before techniques that accurately measure bone density were developed, osteoporosis was usually only diagnosed after a fragility fracture. With the advent of bone densitometry, the term *osteoporosis* is increasingly used to describe reduced BMD. Measurements may be expressed as standard deviation units above or below the mean value for normal young adults or relative to the mean value for control subjects of the same age, to give T and Z scores, respectively. Although accurate measurements of lumbar spine and femoral BMD can be made using dual energy x-ray absorptiometry (DXA), these measurements may be of limited value in some circumstances, such as when degenerative disease in the spine is present. In the investigation of frail older patients with hip and other fragility fractures, many will have osteoporosis and should therefore benefit from treatment, but population-based bone density screening programs cannot be justified, as there is little evidence that such a strategy is effective in the prevention of fragility fractures.[7] The WHO definition of osteoporosis (BMD T score < -2.5) is useful for epidemiologic studies but does not represent a threshold for treatment, which is important, as 70% of women older than 80 years have a T score of less than -2.5, but only a proportion of these will sustain an osteoporotic fracture.[7] Furthermore, although over half of patients with hip fractures have osteoporosis, fewer than 50% of those with other fragility fractures have a T score less than -2.5 on DXA measurement.[17]

As BMD estimation alone is a relatively poor way to predict fracture risk, a range of tools have been developed using clinical risk factors for the assessment risk of both low BMD and high absolute risk of fracture.[18] The most commonly used and validated method is FRAX, which has been developed by WHO and estimates the 10-year risk of major osteoporotic fracture and of hip fracture. Country-specific algorithms use age, gender, and the presence or absence of appropriately weighted risk factors, with or without femoral neck BMD measurements, to estimate fracture risk. The clinical risk factors for fracture used in FRAX, which are partly independent of bone density, comprise low body mass index (BMI), prior fragility fracture, parental hip fracture, current smoking, oral glucocorticoid therapy, alcohol intake, and chronic conditions associated with bone loss, including rheumatoid arthritis. The fracture risk estimate can be made without a BMD measurement and then refined with the results from DXA. In the United Kingdom, QFracture is an alternative algorithm that has been developed using a larger number of clinical risk factors to estimate the same risks of fragility fracture without using BMD,[19] and the National Institute for Health and Care Excellence (NICE) in the United Kingdom recommends that either FRAX or QFracture be used (without BMD) for opportunistic case finding in women older than 65 years and men older than 75 years.[20]

Although case finding might be undertaken using BMD, clinical risk factors, or both, the assessment of fracture risk may be particularly problematic for frail older people, and other tools (including the Garvan fracture risk calculator) may be particularly useful in this situation.[19] Other guidelines have also been developed, which include BMD thresholds for treatment, based on FRAX,[21] but the validity of treatment thresholds based on fracture risk must be evaluated by calibration studies and health economic analysis.[19]

Investigation of Osteoporosis

Because vertebral fractures are not always be easy to diagnose, spine x-rays should be considered in patients with acute back pain, loss of height, or kyphosis, to look for evidence of vertebral deformation, degenerative arthritis, or other pathology. Increasingly, lateral DXA scanning of the spine is entering clinical practice, with vertebral fracture assessment (VFA) as part of routine BMD measurement to identify prevalent vertebral deformity.[22] VFA and spine x-rays are useful in the identification of vertebral deformity and diagnosis of vertebral fracture. However, while spine x-rays are unreliable in the assessment of bone density, they may also show lytic or sclerotic lesions, raising the possibility of

BOX 70-1 Investigations for Secondary Osteoporosis in Older People With Low Trauma Fractures or Low Bone Mineral Density

Full blood count
ESR or CRP
Biochemical profile: including renal function, adjusted serum calcium, and alkaline phosphatase
Thyroid function tests
(Consider) serum testosterone, sex hormone–binding globulin, LH, FSH (men)
Serum and urine electrophoresis (vertebral fractures)
Serum 25OHD and PTH

CRP, C-reactive protein; *ESR,* erythrocyte sedimentation rate; *FSH,* follicle-stimulating hormone; *LH,* luteinizing hormone; *PTH,* parathyroid hormone; *25OHD,* 25 hydroxyvitamin.

TABLE 70-1 Effect of Major Treatment Options on the Risk of Vertebral, Nonvertebral, and Hip Fractures

	Vertebral Fractures	Nonvertebral Fractures	Hip Fractures
Alendronate	A	A	A
Etidronate	A	ND	ND
Risedronate	A	A	A
Raloxifene	A	ND	ND
Strontium ranelate	A	A	(A)
Teriparatide	A	A	ND
Denosumab	A	A	A
Zoledronate*	A	A	A
Ibandronate*	A	(A)	ND
Calcium and vitamin D*	ND	A	A

Modified from references 21 and 24-26.
*Not included in current NICE guidance.
A indicates evidence from randomized controlled trials and/or meta-analysis; (A) reflects that a beneficial effect on fractures risk was found only in post hoc subgroup analysis; ND indicates that fracture reduction has not been demonstrated.

neoplastic disease or degenerative changes, requiring further investigations, which may include isotope bone scan and magnetic resonance imaging (MRI) scan.[16]

In patients with fragility fractures, causes of secondary osteoporosis should be identified by careful history, physical examination, and appropriate investigation (Box 70-1), as specific treatment of underlying conditions such as hyperthyroidism, hypogonadism, and primary hyperparathyroidism increases bone density by up to 15%. Serum 25OHD and PTH measurements may show vitamin D insufficiency and secondary hyperparathyroidism, but these measurements are probably unnecessary if vitamin D, with or without calcium supplementation, is planned.[23] Routine biochemical profile is worthwhile, as hypocalcemia and hypophosphatemia can indicate possible vitamin D deficiency osteomalacia, but these measurements lack diagnostic specificity or sensitivity. Serum 25OHD and PTH measurements are also useful in the further investigation of possible vitamin D deficiency osteomalacia, which is particularly likely in housebound patients or those with previous gastric resection, malabsorption, or the long-term use of antiepileptic drugs. Investigations for secondary osteoporosis should also be performed in patients found to have a BMD below the normal range for their age (Z score < −2.0), to identify modifiable causes of bone loss.

Management of Osteoporosis

All patients with fragility fractures should be given general advice on lifestyle measures to decrease further bone loss, including eating a balanced diet rich in calcium, moderating tobacco and alcohol consumption, and, if possible, maintaining regular physical activity and exposure to sunlight. As bone loss continues into old age in both men and women, the need for specific treatment should be considered in all patients with osteoporosis or fragility fractures. Although most studies of the treatment of osteoporosis have recruited few women older than 80 years, there is no evidence of an attenuated response to treatment with advancing age.

A number of treatments have been shown to increase BMD and decrease the risk of vertebral and hip fractures and the majority of these treatments have been reviewed by both NICE[24-26] and the National Osteoporosis Guideline Group (NOGG).[21] Table 70-1 presents the evidence of clinical effectiveness concluded by the NICE and NOGG working groups, including some agents not reviewed by NICE, specifically calcium and vitamin D supplementation, zoledronate, and ibandronate. More recently, in the absence of "head-to-head" comparison studies, osteoporosis treatments have been evaluated using network meta-analysis, including some of the more recent treatment options. Bisphosphonates, denosumab, and teriparatide were found to be the most effective in reducing the risk of fragility fractures with potentially important differences in fracture risk reduction profiles likely between the agents.[27,28]

Hormone Replacement Therapy

Hormone replacement therapy was previously used in the prevention and treatment of osteoporosis in younger postmenopausal women, but the situation changed with the publication of the results of the Women's Health Initiative Study, which is a study of particular interest for older women, since more than 21% were older than 70 years and were 20 years postmenopause at the time of commencing hormone replacement therapy. Although this study showed a reduction in colon cancer and vertebral, hip, and other fractures, the benefits were outweighed by the increased risk of breast cancer, coronary heart disease, stroke, and thromboembolism.[29]

Raloxifene

Selective estrogen receptor modulators (SERMs), such as raloxifene, have estrogen agonist actions on the skeleton but estrogen antagonist actions on the breast and endometrium. There are a number of SERMs available, including tamoxifen, bazedoxifene, lasofoxifene, toremifene citrate, and raloxifene, which are used as both chemo-preventive agents and treatments for breast cancer and for the prevention and treatment of osteoporosis.[30] In the United Kingdom, raloxifene is licensed for the treatment of osteoporosis. A large study in postmenopausal women with osteoporosis showed that raloxifene increased lumbar spine and femoral neck bone density by 2% to 3% and reduced the risk of vertebral fractures by 30% to 50%, but there is no evidence that it decreases the risk of hip or other nonvertebral fractures. Treatment with SERMs is associated with a decrease in the incidence of breast cancer by 38%; because of this, the U.S. Food and Drug Administration has licensed the drug for breast cancer prevention in women at high risk.[31-33] The main side effect of raloxifene is hot flushes, particularly when used shortly after menopause, but there is also an increased risk of venous thromboembolism. It is generally used in younger postmenopausal women with osteoporosis who are at high risk of vertebral fractures but whose risk of nonvertebral fractures is low.

Bisphosphonates

Bisphosphonates have become the treatment of choice for patients with osteoporosis because of their proven antifracture efficacy and good safety profile. Alendronate and risedronate have been shown in large studies to increase BMD and decrease the incidence of vertebral, hip, and other nonvertebral fractures.[34-36] These oral agents are taken mostly as weekly preparations, which need to be taken on an empty stomach, 30 minutes before food, to ensure that they are absorbed from the bowel. Ibandronate has also been shown to improve BMD and decrease the incidence of vertebral fractures, but, although a post hoc subgroup analysis suggests that it prevents nonvertebral fractures, no reduction in hip fractures has been demonstrated.[37] Ibandronate is available as a monthly oral preparation and a three-monthly intravenous injection. Annual intravenous infusions of zoledronate in women with osteoporosis have been shown to decrease the risk of vertebral fractures by 70% and hip fractures by 41%.[38] A further study in patients with recent hip fracture demonstrated that annual intravenous zoledronate decreases the risk of vertebral and nonvertebral fractures and also reduced mortality by 28%.[39]

Although the antifracture studies with alendronate only recruited patients up to the age of 81 years, there was no evidence of any attenuation of the benefits with advancing age.[40] Risedronate has been shown to decrease fractures in women older than 80 years with treatment resulting in a similar risk to that of untreated patients 10 to 20 years younger.[41] Although there is no definite evidence that risedronate reduces the risk of hip fractures in women in this age group recruited on the basis of clinical risk factors for fracture,[34] there is no reason to suspect it will be ineffective in older women with osteoporosis. Over a third of the patients in the major study of zoledronate in osteoporosis were older than 75 years, suggesting that it is effective even in this older age group.[38]

Oral bisphosphonates are generally well tolerated, but upper gastrointestinal side effects are common. Esophagitis has been reported with oral bisphosphonates, but the risk of this complication may be reduced by following the manufacturers' advice that these agents should be taken with water and recumbency avoided for 30 minutes. Intravenous bisphosphonates may cause an acute phase response, with transient flulike symptoms lasting for a few days. The severity of these symptoms may be reduced by the administration of paracetamol for 3 days starting on the day of bisphosphonate administration. Intravenous zoledronate may also cause symptomatic hypocalcemia, so it is important to ensure that the patient is vitamin D replete before administering this treatment. Increased bone pain has been reported with bisphosphonate treatment but appears to be an uncommon side effect. The major antifracture study of intravenous zoledronate showed an increase in serious atrial fibrillation,[38] but this was unrelated to the timing of infusion. Further meta-analysis of five eligible randomized controlled trials and four observational studies of bisphosphonate therapy has suggested this may be a class effect, with intravenous preparations associated with a greater risk of atrial fibrillation compared with oral preparations.[42] Osteonecrosis of the jaw and delayed dental healing with high-dose intravenous bisphosphonates was first reported in the management of malignancy, but this phenomenon has more recently been seen in patients treated for osteoporosis,[43] and the American Association of Oral and Maxillofacial Surgeons report an incidence of 1.7 to 4 cases per 10,000 patients for oral and parenteral preparations.[44] Atypical femoral fractures have also been reported, in association with bisphosphonates and other antiresorptive medications and an American Society for Bone Mineral Research (ASBMR) task force has highlighted the high relative risk but low absolute risk (3.2 to 50 cases/100,000 person-years) of atypical femoral fractures in patients taking bisphosphonates.[45] This also needs to be seen in context, with a number of other important risk factors, including glucocorticoid therapy, lower limb geometry, and Asian ethnicity. However, duration of therapy also appears to be relevant with an odds ratio per 100 daily doses of 1.3.[46]

Strontium Ranelate

Strontium ranelate is a dual action bone agent that reduces bone resorption and increases bone formation. A large randomized controlled trial of strontium ranelate in postmenopausal women with osteoporosis and at least one vertebral fracture showed increases in BMD of 12.7% in the lumbar spine and 8.6% in the hip after 3 years of treatment.[47] About 50% of this apparent increase is spurious, because of the skeletal incorporation of strontium, which has a higher atomic number than calcium. This study also demonstrated a 41% reduction in the incidence of new vertebral fractures.[47] Another large study of women with osteoporosis showed a 16% reduction in the incidence of nonvertebral fractures with strontium ranelate, but in a post hoc subgroup analysis in women older than 74 years with low BMD (T score < -3.0), there was a 36% reduction in hip fractures.[48] Data from another study suggest that strontium ranelate decreases the incidence of vertebral and nonvertebral fractures in women older than 80 years.[49] Strontium ranelate is available in powder form in sachets, the contents of which are dissolved in water. It should preferably be taken at bedtime, at least 2 hours after eating, to ensure adequate absorption from the bowel. Strontium has been generally well tolerated in clinical trials, but reported side effects include diarrhea and there has been concern over an increased risk of venous thromboembolism and cardiovascular risk, such that withdrawal of its license was threatened. However, it is an attractive treatment option for older patients, with evidence of efficacy in the age group older than 80 and no reported concerns of osteonecrosis of the jaw or atypical femoral fracture which have been reported with antiresorptive medication. Unfortunately, its restriction from use where there are concomitant risks of deep vein thrombosis or prevalent cardiovascular disease limit its widespread utility.[50]

Parathyroid Hormone

The continuously high circulating concentrations of PTH found in primary and secondary hyperparathyroidism is associated with an increase in bone turnover, but bone resorption is stimulated more than bone formation, resulting in loss of bone from the skeleton. In contrast, intermittent administration of PTH stimulates bone formation more than resorption, resulting in an increase in bone mass and density. Recombinant human parathyroid hormone 1-34 (teriparatide) and parathyroid hormone 1-84 have anabolic actions on the skeleton when administered by daily subcutaneous injection. Studies show a larger increase in BMD than that observed with bisphosphonates.[51,52] Teriparatide decreases the incidence of vertebral and nonvertebral fractures, and parathyroid hormone 1-84 reduces the incidence of vertebral fractures, but no reduction in hip fractures has been demonstrated.[52,53] There also appears to be no attenuation of the effects of teriparatide on BMD or fracture reduction with advancing age.[54] These agents are generally well tolerated but may cause transient mild hypercalcemia, nausea, dizziness, and headaches. Because these preparations are much more expensive than bisphosphonates, their use is often restricted to patients with severe osteoporosis or those who fail to respond to bisphosphonates for up to 2 years.

Calcium and Vitamin D

Calcium and vitamin D supplementation has been shown to reduce the incidence of hip and other nonvertebral fractures in older people living in care homes, where vitamin D deficiency and secondary hyperparathyroidism are common.[55] In contrast, recent large studies cast doubt on the role of calcium and vitamin D supplementation in the primary or secondary prevention of low trauma fractures in community-dwelling older people.[56] Nevertheless, meta-analyses show a small reduction in hip fractures with calcium and vitamin D, which is dominated by the effect seen in residents of care homes and with no beneficial effect of vitamin D alone on fracture incidence.[57-59]

Calcium and vitamin D supplementation may cause abdominal bloating, other gastrointestinal symptoms, and change in bowel habit. These may account for the relatively poor compliance and persistence with supplementation. Calcium and vitamin D supplementation is probably most appropriate in older people who are housebound or living in residential or nursing homes, where vitamin D insufficiency and secondary hyperparathyroidism are common and the evidence for benefit is greatest.[57] Many patients receiving treatment for osteoporosis are offered concomitant calcium and vitamin D supplementation. However, it may be better to target nutritional assessment ensuring adequate calcium intake and vitamin D status and offering supplements of vitamin D with or without calcium as required. Most older people are likely to require relatively little added calcium to their diet to achieve the recommended nutritional intake of 700 mg, whereas poor vitamin D status is relatively common[60] and long-term adherence to combined supplementation poor.

Denosumab

Denosumab is a monoclonal antibody directed against RANKL, which it binds with high affinity and specificity. This inhibits the stimulatory action of RANKL on bone resorption. A randomized controlled trial in postmenopausal women with low BMD showed rapid suppression of bone resorption with twice-yearly subcutaneous injections of denosumab, with significant increases in BMD (48) and a reduction in the risk of new radiographic vertebral fracture by 68%, hip fracture by 40%, and nonvertebral fracture by 20%.[61,62] Denosumab has been used in patients with stage 4 and stage 5 chronic kidney disease within clinical trials,[63] and it does not share the side effects associated with the acute phase response seen in potent bisphosphonate therapy. However, there remains a need for caution, particularly with regard to the risk of hypocalcemia associated with all potent antiresorptive agents, and there have been reports of osteonecrosis of the jaw and atypical femoral fractures as seen with bisphosphonates.

Future Treatments

Other novel agents for osteoporosis treatment include antiresorptive cathepsin K inhibitors, which have shown improvements in BMD but fracture reduction and risk data are awaited.[64] Other novel anabolic treatments for osteoporosis include monoclonal antibodies that inhibit the formation or action of sclerostin. Early trials in postmenopausal women with low bone mass have shown an increase in BMD and bone formation with decreased bone resorption.[65] However, the results of larger clinical trials assessing fracture risk are awaited.

Falls Assessment

The risk of fragility fracture is determined by skeletal and nonskeletal factors, including a propensity for falling. Patients who fall and patients who fracture (with or without osteoporosis) share similar risk factors. In a Danish study of a cohort of 1,276,891 men and women older than 65 years followed from 2000 to 2009, an association was found between recognized comorbidities related to falls risk and the incidence of hip and proximal humerus fractures. Although there was a decline in fracture incidence during the study, this was accompanied by a decrease in the incidence of falls risk–related comorbidities, which may explain the overall reduction in fractures.[66] Other data suggest that the use of drugs that increase the risk of falls, such as sedatives and opiates, is associated with an increase in the risk of hip fracture.[67] The epidemiologic evidence is compelling for falls assessment in patients with fragility fractures and for fracture risk assessment in the patients at high risk of falls.[68] Interventions to decrease the risk of falls are likely to be beneficial, and there is some evidence from randomized clinical trials that fractures can be decreased in this population. A recent meta-analysis concluded that exercise interventions significantly reduced the risk of sustaining a fall-related fracture (risk ratio [RR], 0.34; 95% confidence interval [CI], 0.18 to 0.63),[69] and a further meta-analysis found moderate-to-vigorous physical activity to be associated with reduction of hip fracture risk by 45% (95% CI, 31% to 56%) for men and 38% (95% CI, 31% to 44%) for women, hypothesizing that the effect was mediated in part through a decrease in falls risk.[70]

External Hip Protectors

An alternative approach to fracture prevention is to decrease the impact of falls using external hip protectors, which are incorporated into specially designed underwear. A recent meta-analysis, which pooled data from 13 studies (11,573 participants) conducted in nursing or residential care settings, found a reduction in hip fracture risk (RR, 0.81; 95% CI, 0.66 to 0.99). However, some of the studies were assessed to be at high risk of bias. The review concluded that the effectiveness of hip protectors is not clearly established, although they may reduce the rate of hip fractures in frail older people living in nursing care.[71]

Choice of Treatment

All individuals should be given lifestyle advice on diet, exercise, tobacco and alcohol consumption, and exposure to sunlight. In younger postmenopausal women with osteoporosis at high risk of vertebral fractures, raloxifene may be useful, particularly if there is also a significant risk of breast cancer. In older women at high risk of vertebral and nonvertebral fractures, bisphosphonates are currently the treatment of choice. In frail, housebound or institutionalized older people, calcium and vitamin D supplementation should be considered, because of the high prevalence of vitamin D insufficiency and secondary hyperparathyroidism, although many patients may require antiresorptive or anabolic agents, depending on their fracture history and fracture risk. In patients with a past history of recurrent falls, measures should be taken to reduce the incidence of falls. Consideration should also be given to the use of external hip protectors, especially where caregivers are available to encourage compliance with their use.

Frailty

Many older people will be frail and therefore at greater risk of falls and fractures. Physicians are increasingly aware of the interaction between falls risk, osteoporosis, frailty, and sarcopenia. An early observational study linked poorer grip strength (a proxy for sarcopenia) with lower BMD and increased risk of prevalent vertebral fracture in older women, and this observation holds true of middle-aged and older men, using a clinical definition of sarcopenia.[72,73] In another cross-sectional study of 250 women aged 76 to 86 years in the United States, osteopenia/osteoporosis and sarcopenia were more common in frail women than the robust group, and, although the relationship of severe osteopenia/osteoporosis and sarcopenia with frailty was not statistically significant, the likelihood of being frail was much higher in the presence of both of these syndromes (odds ratio [OR], 6.4; 95% CI, 1.1 to 36.8; $P = .037$).[74] In a further prospective study of 152 community-dwelling women, frailty and BMD were assessed at an interval of 12 months. Frailty at baseline predicted a statistically significantly lower hip and spine BMD at follow-up, after controlling for BMI ($P = 0.04$, hip; $P = .007$, spine).[75]

In the Study of Osteoporotic Fracture, a "parsimonious frailty index" was used, based on that of Fried and colleagues, with scores based on weight loss more than 5% in a year, inability to rise from chair, and reduced energy level reported. Using this scoring system, the associated odds ratio for falls and hip fracture for women was 2.4 and 1.8 and for men it was 3.0 and 1.2, respectively.[76,77] There is a clear relationship between these indices of frailty, sarcopenia, and risk of fracture. However, the results of studies of appropriate design and sufficient size are needed to evaluate the effects of interventions, whether physical, nutritional, or pharmacologic, on slowing the rate of progression of frailty and decreasing fracture incidence.

OSTEOMALACIA

Osteomalacia is a generalized bone disorder characterized by an impairment of mineralization leading to accumulation of unmineralized matrix or osteoid in the skeleton. The major cause of osteomalacia in older people is vitamin D deficiency. This is reviewed in some detail in this section, but renal osteodystrophy and hypophosphatemic osteomalacia are beyond the scope of this chapter.

Adequate amounts of calcium and phosphate are essential for mineralization of osteoid to proceed normally, and although vitamin D is important in the homeostasis of calcium and phosphate, the precise role of the vitamin D metabolites in mineralization remains uncertain. The major source of vitamin D is from cutaneous production, following the exposure of the precursor 7-dehydrocholesterol to ultraviolet irradiation. The diet provides much smaller amounts of vitamin D, but this becomes essential when cutaneous production is limited. Vitamin D itself has little biologic activity and is metabolized in the liver to 25OHD, the major circulating form of vitamin D. This undergoes further hydroxylation in the kidneys to form $1{,}25(OH)_2D$, the hormonally active metabolite of vitamin D, which regulates calcium absorption from the bowel, influences bone remodeling, and affects muscle function.

Vitamin D deficiency osteomalacia occurs predominantly because of reduced cutaneous production of vitamin D resulting from lack of exposure to sunlight, increased skin pigmentation, or adherence to cultural or religious dress codes where the skin is covered. It is therefore particularly seen in older people who are housebound and in non-Caucasian immigrants. Vitamin D deficiency osteomalacia is also seen in older people with celiac disease and other causes of malabsorption, as a result of reduced absorption of vitamin D, calcium, and phosphate.

Antiepileptic drugs and severe liver disease are also associated with low serum 25OHD levels and the development of vitamin D deficiency osteomalacia. Antiepileptic drugs induce liver enzymes that metabolize vitamin D to biologically inactive polar metabolites, while liver disease may be associated with impaired 25 hydroxylation of vitamin D. In addition, patients with epilepsy or liver disease may be less exposed to sunlight and thus have reduced cutaneous production of vitamin D.

Osteomalacia in Older People

There is a reduction in serum 25OHD with advancing age, which is mainly due to reduced sunlight exposure, though decreased capacity for cutaneous production, low dietary vitamin D intake, poor absorption, and impaired hepatic hydroxylation of vitamin D may also contribute to this reduction. Serum 25OHD concentrations are lower in individuals living in residential and nursing homes than in people living in the broader community.

Osteomalacia is essentially a histologic diagnosis, so there is little information on the prevalence of vitamin D deficiency in older people. In the United Kingdom, vitamin D deficiency has been defined as a serum 25OHD less than 25 nmol/L,[78] based on the fact that most cases of symptomatic vitamin D deficiency osteomalacia present with a serum 25OHD below this value. Nevertheless, not all individuals with a serum 25OHD of less than 25 nmol/L have histologic evidence of a mineralization defect. The National Diet and Nutrition Survey in the United Kingdom highlights that the prevalence of vitamin D deficiency (serum 25OHD < 25 nmol/L) increases from less than 10% in community-dwelling people aged 65 to 74 years, up to 25% in women older than 85 years and more than 35% in institutionalized older people.[79] This suggests that a significant proportion of older people are at risk of developing vitamin D deficiency osteomalacia, but especially those who are housebound or living in residential or nursing homes.

Clinical Features of Osteomalacia

The presentation of osteomalacia may be variable and the diagnosis may be easily missed in the early stages of the disease because of the vague nature of the symptoms. Patients may complain of aches and pains, aggravated by muscular contraction but tending to persist after rest. Although there is a propensity for fracture in osteomalacia, the soft flexible bone also deforms easily, leading to kyphosis, scoliosis, and deformity of the rib cage, pelvis, and long bones. Patients may also develop a proximal myopathy, causing a waddling gait and difficulties rising from a chair or climbing stairs. Occasionally, the hypocalcemia associated with osteomalacia leads to latent tetany, with paresthesias of the hands and around the mouth, muscle cramps, a *main d'accoucheur* appearance of the hands, and positive Chvostek and Trousseau signs.

Radiology in Osteomalacia

The classic radiologic appearances of osteomalacia are relatively rare and may not be found in the early stages of the disease. Osteomalacic bone is softer than normal and so becomes easily deformed. The intervertebral discs balloon out and deform the adjacent vertebrae to give them a uniformly biconcave codfish appearance. Similar deformity can occur in patients with osteoporosis, but the biconcavity is more regular in osteomalacia than in osteoporosis, where the extent of vertebral deformity is variable. There may be radiologic evidence of deformity of the rib cage, pelvis, and long bones. A characteristic finding in osteomalacia is the Looser zone (also called a pseudofracture), which consists of a large area of osteoid. Looser zones appear as bands of decalcification surrounded by more dense bone, which occur perpendicular to the bone surface, often where nutrient arteries enter bone. Looser zones are seen particularly in the proximal femur, humeral neck, public rami, ribs, metatarsals, and the outer border of the scapula. There may also be radiologic evidence of secondary hyperparathyroidism, with subperiosteal erosions in the metacarpals or phalanges.

Biochemical Findings in Osteomalacia

In vitamin D deficiency osteomalacia, the serum calcium tends to be low because of reduced calcium absorption due to low serum 25OHD and $1{,}25(OH)_2D$ concentrations. The hypocalcemia leads to secondary hyperparathyroidism, which in turn stimulates the renal tubular reabsorption of calcium, leading to a low urine calcium level. The secondary hyperparathyroidism also results in reduced tubular reabsorption of phosphate. Serum phosphate is therefore often low in osteomalacia because of reduced absorption from the bowel and decreased renal tubular reabsorption. The secondary hyperparathyroidism also increases bone remodeling, which is reflected in elevation of the serum alkaline phosphatase level and other biochemical markers of bone turnover. Not all patients with vitamin D deficiency osteomalacia will have hypocalcemia, hypophosphatemia, and raised alkaline phosphatase.[80] Furthermore, these abnormalities may occur individually in the elderly with intercurrent illness, so they lack specificity in the diagnosis of osteomalacia in older people.[81]

Diagnosis of Osteomalacia in Older People

The only definite way of diagnosing osteomalacia is by bone biopsy, but histologic confirmation of the diagnosis is rarely required. A clinical diagnosis can be made in patients with a typical history of bone pain and muscle weakness, particularly if there is radiologic evidence of Looser zones or abnormal biochemical findings such as hypocalcemia, reduced urine calcium level, hypophosphatemia, or a raised alkaline phosphatase level. Measurement of serum 25OHD and PTH is also useful, as the combination of low serum 25OHD and elevated PTH is a strong indicator of the presence of osteomalacia.

Treatment of Osteomalacia

Although vitamin D deficiency osteomalacia can be healed by exposure to ultraviolet light of the appropriate wavelength (290 to 310 nm), vitamin D treatment is more practical. A guideline from the National Osteoporosis Society in the United Kingdom suggests that patients with symptomatic vitamin D deficiency osteomalacia be treated with loading doses of vitamin D, followed by regular maintenance therapy.[23] Loading doses should provide a total of approximately 300,000 IU vitamin D, given either as weekly or daily doses, over a 6- to 10-week period. Vitamin D_3 (cholecalciferol) is preferred over vitamin D_2 (ergocalciferol), as it is cleared less rapidly and is more bioavailable, but the latter may be preferred by vegetarians and patients who wish to avoid vitamin D of animal origin because of religious or cultural beliefs. Oral administration of vitamin D is also recommended, because of unpredictable bioavailability and slower correction of vitamin D deficiency with intramuscular preparations. Maintenance treatment should be instituted 1 month after loading, with doses equivalent to 800 to 2000 IU vitamin D daily. Where correction of vitamin D deficiency is less urgent, maintenance therapy may be started without the use of loading doses. Serum calcium should be checked 1 month after starting vitamin D treatment, in case this has unmasked previously undiagnosed primary hyperparathyroidism.[23]

Treatment of osteomalacia leads to a resolution of the proximal myopathy and any symptoms of hypocalcemia within a few weeks, though the bone pain may take longer to improve. The biochemical abnormalities also persist for up to 6 months after treatment is started, and the bone remains histologically and structurally abnormal during this time. Care should therefore be taken to avoid falls during rehabilitation, as these may easily lead to fractures of the abnormal bone. The serum calcium and phosphate levels return to normal within a few weeks, while the serum alkaline phosphatase level rises further on treatment and may take many months to return to normal. Serum PTH also remains elevated for up to 6 months. Ultimately, radiologic abnormalities such as Looser zones and changes of secondary hyperparathyroidism will resolve on treatment, though deformity will persist despite the remodeling of bone.

PAGET DISEASE

Paget disease of bone is characterized by increased bone turnover, which can involve one or more of the bones in the skeleton. Although the condition may be asymptomatic, it can cause significant morbidity in older people, including bone pain, skeletal deformity, pathologic fractures, deafness, and osteoarthritis.[82]

Prevalence of Paget Disease

The United Kingdom is the country with the highest prevalence of Paget disease in the world, but there is considerable regional variation, with the highest prevalence in North West England.[83] By the eighth decade of life, up to 8% of men and 5% of women in the United Kingdom have evidence of the condition.[84] Studies suggest that Paget disease is also common in most of Europe and in British migrants to Australia, New Zealand, United States, and Canada, but is rare in Scandinavia, Asia, and Africa. There has been a decrease in the prevalence of Paget disease in the United Kingdom and New Zealand over the past three decades, but this trend has not been observed in the United States or Italy.[83] The reason for the decrease in prevalence of Paget disease is unclear, but it may reflect environmental changes or the immigration of people from countries with a low prevalence.

Pathophysiology of Paget Disease

Paget disease is characterized by increased bone resorption mediated by enlarged, hyperactive osteoclasts. These abnormal cells contain characteristic nuclear inclusion bodies, which were previously considered to be of viral origin but may in fact represent protein aggregates due to abnormal autophagy.[83] Osteoclast precursors from patients with Paget disease appear to be particularly sensitive to factors that stimulate bone resorption,[83] including $1,25(OH)_2D$ and RANKL. There is also an increase in osteoblastic activity and new bone formation, which occurs secondary to the elevated bone resorption. The rapid bone turnover leads to the deposition of woven bone, which is more vascular, structurally weak, and prone to deformity and fracture.

The cause of Paget disease remains unclear. There is a significant genetic component to the condition, as about 15% of patients have a family history of the condition. The risk of developing the condition may be sevenfold higher in first-degree relatives of patients with Paget disease.[83] Recent work has identified gene mutations that may contribute to the development of Paget disease and related conditions. The most important of these is in the sequestosome 1 (*SQSTM1*) gene, which encodes for a protein involved in RANK/RANKL signaling. Mutations in the *SQSTM1* gene are found in 20% to 50% of cases of familial disease and 5% to 20% of cases of sporadic disease. A much rarer cause of Paget disease is a mutation in the *VCP* gene, which is associated with hereditary inclusion-body myopathy and frontotemporal dementia.

Although genetic factors may predispose to the development of Paget disease, it is likely that other factors may influence its expression. This is highlighted by the declining incidence of the condition in recent decades, even among those with a genetic predisposition.[83] The clustering of cases of Paget disease within families includes spouses, which suggests not only genetic factors but also a shared environment factor. It has been suggested that Paget disease may result from a slow virus infection, which either causes the disease or triggers it in a susceptible individual. Although paramyxovirus infection has been implicated in the pathogenesis of Paget disease, the results of studies investigating this possibility have been inconclusive.[83] Other factors that have been implicated in the development of Paget disease in susceptible individuals include mechanical forces, low dietary calcium intake or vitamin D deficiency during childhood, and occupational exposure to toxins.

Clinical Features of Paget Disease

The majority of people with radiologic evidence of Paget disease are asymptomatic and do not come to medical attention. In a recent systematic review of 24 studies,[82] bone pain was the most common presenting symptom (52.2%), followed by skeletal deformity (21.5%), deafness (8.9%), and fractures (8.5%). Bone pain in Paget disease may be caused by periosteal stretching, microfractures, or direct nerve stimulation by substances released by osteoclasts during bone resorption. It may also reflect the development of osteoarthritis in adjacent joints, resulting from skeletal deformity and abnormal mechanical loading.

The bones most commonly involved in Paget disease are the pelvis, spine, femur, tibia, and skull,[85] with up to 50% of patients having monostotic disease.[82] Although Paget disease may extend along an individual bone with time, the condition rarely spreads to involve previously unaffected bones.

Paget disease can also cause skeletal deformity, as the abnormal bones thicken, enlarge, and become more flexible. Classically, this causes frontal bossing of the skull, bowing of the long bones, and deformity of the pelvis (protrusio acetabuli). Pagetic bone is more likely to fracture, and fissure fractures can occur on the outer aspect of bowed long bones.

Thickening of the skull may cause compression of the cranial nerves, particularly the auditory nerves, resulting in deafness. Other cranial nerves are only rarely involved in Paget disease. The increased vascularity of Pagetic bone may also result in neurologic deficit because of a "vascular steal" syndrome. Softening of the base of the skull, in rare cases, may lead to basilar invagination, causing brainstem compression. Vertebral involvement can result in crush fractures or, more rarely, spinal cord compression.

A major management problem is the development of secondary osteoarthritis in joints adjacent to involved bone. This may be more disabling than the Paget disease itself and will not respond to treatment of the underlying bone disease. Other complications of Paget disease include high output cardiac failure, as a result of the increased vascularity of the affected bone, which, although often described, is rarely seen. The development of osteosarcoma is also rare, occurring in only 0.25% to 0.30% of cases.[84,85]

Diagnosis and Investigation of Paget Disease

When a diagnosis of Paget disease is suspected, x-rays of the suspicious regions of the skeleton should be performed.[86] These will typically show an increase in size of involved bones and alteration of bone texture, with areas of sclerosis and lucency. There may also be evidence of skeletal deformity, fissure fractures, and osteoarthritis in adjacent joints. Although the radiologic appearances are often said to be pathognomonic, skeletal metastases from occult carcinoma of the prostate or breast should be considered in the differential diagnosis. Computerized tomography, MRI, and bone biopsy may occasionally be required, if the diagnosis remains unknown.[86] The extent of the bone disease should be assessed by isotope bone scan,[86] although x-rays of areas with increased uptake may be advisable, if there is any doubt about the diagnosis. Serum alkaline phosphatase and biochemical markers of bone resorption are often markedly raised in Paget disease, reflecting increased osteoblast and osteoclast activity, respectively, so they may be used to assess the activity of the condition and its response to treatment.

Treatment of Paget Disease

Treatment of Paget disease is directed at suppressing the overactivity of osteoclasts, thereby decreasing bone turnover. Although calcitonin was used for several decades in the management of Paget disease, bisphosphonates have now become the treatment of choice. These agents are generally used in patients with symptomatic Paget disease, but their role in asymptomatic individuals is unclear.[87]

The first bisphosphonate to be used in the management of Paget was oral disodium etidronate, which produced a larger and more prolonged decrease in bone turnover than calcitonin. Unfortunately, the licensed dose of 400 mg etidronate daily for 6 months did not normalize the biochemical markers of bone turnover in the majority of patients. Furthermore, prolonged or higher dose treatment could result in the development of osteomalacia, so the use of etidronate declined when more potent bisphosphonates became available, which did not lead to impaired mineralization.

Oral tiludronate decreased the biochemical markers of bone turnover by at least 50% in 70% of patients but did not normalize it in all cases. The subsequent development of more potent aminobisphosphonates offered the prospect of decreasing bone turnover to normal. Intravenous infusions of pamidronate decrease the biochemical markers of bone turnover by 50% to 80%, resulting in prolonged remission in many patients. Pamidronate may be given by weekly infusion of 30 mg for 6 weeks, or by three fortnightly infusions of 60 mg. The introduction of intravenous pamidronate avoided the potential problems of oral bisphosphonates, such as poor absorption from the bowel, the need to take medication in a fasting condition, and gastrointestinal side effects. These advantages were offset by the need for multiple intravenous infusions and the development of transient flulike symptoms following infusions.

A study compared the effect of a 2-month course of oral risedronate 30 mg daily with etidronate 400 mg daily for 6 months. After 1 year, alkaline phosphatase level was normal in 73% of patients who had taken risedronate, compared with only 18% with etidronate. There was a significant reduction in pain with risedronate, whereas etidronate was associated with nonsignificant improvement. Oral alendronate is licensed for the treatment of Paget disease in the United States but not in the United Kingdom. Alendronate (40 mg daily for 6 months) has also been shown to be superior to etidronate in the management of Paget disease. Nevertheless, the doses of oral bisphosphonates needed to successfully treat Paget disease are associated with significant upper gastrointestinal side effects.

A recent guideline from the Endocrine Society in the United States has recommended intravenous zoledronate as the treatment of choice for Paget disease.[86] Pooled data from two randomized controlled trials with a similar design compared a single intravenous infusion of 5 mg zoledronate with a 2-month course of oral risedronate 30 mg daily.[88] After 6 months, alkaline phosphatase had returned into the normal range in 88.6% of patients receiving zoledronate, compared with 57.9% in the risedronate group. Although pain scores improved in both groups, there appeared to be greater improvement in quality of life with zoledronate than risedronate. A subsequent study followed up 296 patients who had responded to treatment with either zoledronate or risedronate for a further 18 months.[89] In patients treated with zoledronate, the mean alkaline phosphatase remained in the middle of the reference range, whereas it increased in a linear fashion from 6months with risedronate. Intravenous zoledronate causes transient flulike symptoms in 25% of patients, but the severity may be reduced by the use of paracetamol or nonsteroidal antiinflammatory drugs.[86] Zoledronate is potentially nephrotoxic, so it should not be used when the glomerular filtration rate is less than 35 mL/min. It may also cause hypocalcemia in patients with vitamin D deficiency, so the clinician should ensure that the patient is vitamin D replete before administering zoledronate.

Although bisphosphonates decrease bone pain and reduce the activity of Paget disease, there is currently no evidence that any treatment will prevent skeletal deformity, fractures, or other complications of the condition.[87] The choice of bisphosphonate for the management of Paget disease depends on patient preference and tolerability, but the main choice lies between intravenous zoledronate and oral risedronate or alendronate. In patients unable to tolerate bisphosphonates, calcitonin may be beneficial. Although subcutaneous or intranasal calcitonin decreases bone pain and reduces the biochemical markers of bone turnover in Paget disease, the effect on bone turnover is relatively transient, because of the short half-life of calcitonin and the development of neutralizing antibodies in some patients.

KEY POINTS

- The incidence of osteoporosis, osteomalacia, and Paget disease increases with advancing age, contributing to the risk of fracture in older people.
- Fragility fractures are a major cause of excess mortality, morbidity, and health and social service expenditure in older people.
- The risk of fracture is determined by skeletal and nonskeletal risk factors.
- Treatments are available for osteoporosis that improve bone density and reduce the risk of vertebral, hip, and other nonvertebral fractures.
- In addition to the increased risk of fracture, osteomalacia and Paget disease may also cause bone pain and skeletal deformity.
- The most common cause of osteomalacia in older people is vitamin D deficiency, which can be corrected by appropriate supplementation.
- Bisphosphonate treatment in Paget disease reduces bone turnover and decreases bone pain.

For a complete list of references, please visit www.expertconsult.com.

KEY REFERENCES

1. Birch M, Aspray T: The musculoskeletal system: bone. In Abdulla A, Rai GS, editors: The biology of ageing and its clinical implication: a practical handbook, London, 2013, Radcliffe, p xvi.
5. Brennan nee Saunders J, Johansen A, Butler J, et al: Place of residence and risk of fracture in older people: a population-based study of over 65-year-olds in Cardiff. Osteoporos Int 14:515–519, 2003.
7. Assessment of fracture risk and its application to screening for postmenopausal osteoporosis. Report of a WHO study group. World Health Organ Tech Rep Ser 843:1–29, 1994.
8. van Staa TP, Dennison EM, Leufkens HG, et al: Epidemiology of fractures in England and Wales. Bone 29:517–522, 2001.
9. Holroyd C, Harvey N, Dennison E, et al: Epigenetic influences in the developmental origins of osteoporosis. Osteoporos Int 23:401–410, 2012.
17. McLellan AR, Gallacher SJ, Fraser M, et al: The fracture liaison service: success of a program for the evaluation and management of patients with osteoporotic fracture. Osteoporos Int 14:1028–1034, 2003.
21. Compston J, Bowring C, Cooper A, et al: Diagnosis and management of osteoporosis in postmenopausal women and older men in the UK: National Osteoporosis Guideline Group (NOGG) update 2013. Maturitas 75:392–396, 2013.
23. Aspray TJ, Bowring C, Fraser W, et al: National Osteoporosis Society vitamin D guideline summary. Age Ageing 43:592–959, 2014.
28. Murad MH, Drake MT, Mullan RJ, et al: Clinical review. Comparative effectiveness of drug treatments to prevent fragility fractures: a systematic review and network meta-analysis. J Clin Endocrinol Metab 97:1871–1880, 2012.
44. Ruggiero SL, Dodson TB, Fantasia J, et al: American Association of Oral and Maxillofacial Surgeons position paper on medication-related osteonecrosis of the jaw—2014 update. J Oromaxillofac Surg 72:1938–1956, 2014.
45. Shane E, Burr D, Abrahamsen B, et al: Atypical subtrochanteric and diaphyseal femoral fractures: second report of a task force of the American Society for Bone and Mineral Research. J Bone Miner Res 29:1–23, 2014.
57. Ross AC, Taylor CL, Yaktine AL, et al, editors: Dietary reference intakes for calcium and vitamin D, Washington, DC, 2011, National Academies Press.
58. Avenell A, Gillespie WJ, Gillespie LD, et al: Vitamin D and vitamin D analogues for preventing fractures associated with involutional and post-menopausal osteoporosis. Cochrane Database Syst Rev 2:CD000227, 2009.
69. Gillespie LD, Robertson MC, Gillespie WJ, et al: Interventions for preventing falls in older people living in the community. Cochrane Database Syst Rev 9:CD007146, 2012.
76. Ensrud KE, Ewing SK, Cawthon PM, et al: A comparison of frailty indexes for the prediction of falls, disability, fractures, and mortality in older men. J Am Geriatr Soc 57:492–498, 2009.
81. Campbell GA, Hosking DJ, Kemm JR, et al: Timing of screening for osteomalacia in the acutely ill elderly. Age Ageing 15:156–163, 1986.
82. Tan A, Ralston SH: Clinical presentation of Paget's disease: evaluation of a contemporary cohort and systematic review. Calcif Tissue Int 95:385–392, 2014.
84. van Staa TP, Selby P, Leufkens HG, et al: Incidence and natural history of Paget's disease of bone in England and Wales. J Bone Miner Res 17:465–471, 2002.
86. Singer FR, Bone HG, 3rd, Hosking DJ, et al: Paget's disease of bone: an Endocrine Society clinical practice guideline. J Clin Endocrinol Metab 99:4408–4422, 2014.
87. Langston AL, Campbell MK, Fraser WD, et al: Randomized trial of intensive bisphosphonate treatment versus symptomatic management in Paget's disease of bone. J Bone Miner Res 25:20–31, 2010.
88. Reid IR, Miller P, Lyles K, et al: Comparison of a single infusion of zoledronic acid with risedronate for Paget's disease. New Engl J Med 353:898–908, 2005.

71 Orthopedic Geriatrics

Robert V. Cantu

INTRODUCTION

Orthopedic care of older adults, especially those who are frail, presents unique challenges. Frail patients typically have multiple, interacting problems that affect decisions regarding optimal type and timing of treatment. From a strictly orthopedic point of view, inferior bone density and quality compared to younger patients as well as preexisting joint arthropathies can make fixation of fractures challenging and sometimes makes arthroplasty the favored treatment for articular fractures. Increasing evidence suggests coordination of care with an internal medicine or geriatric team provides the best outcomes and minimizes complications.[1] This chapter addresses many of the challenges the orthopedist faces when caring for geriatric patients.

OSTEOPOROSIS

The World Health Organization has defined osteoporosis as a bone mineral density (BMD) value of 2.5 standard deviations or more below the young adult mean.[2] Patients with known osteoporosis are at increased risk for fracture; however, the greatest risk factor for sustaining a fragility fracture is having had a previous one. Most patients with a fragility fracture involving the spine, hip, wrist, or proximal humerus, however, do not meet the BMD definition of osteoporosis.[3] These findings can make it difficult to discern which patients should receive pharmacologic treatment to prevent the risk of fracture. They also suggest patients who have had a previous fragility fracture should receive treatment for osteoporosis, even if their BMD is not 2.5 standard deviations below the mean.

Despite advancements in treatment, osteoporosis afflicts an estimated 323 million people worldwide, and that number is projected to reach 1.55 billion by the year 2050.[4] Fragility fractures result in pain, disability, and medical complications and affect as many as 1 in 3 women and 1 in 12 men during their lifetime. Hip fractures alone are projected to afflict 6.3 million people by the year 2050.[4] The medical expenses following fragility fractures are substantial; for example, the annual cost in Europe has been reported to be an estimated 13 billion euros.[5] The majority of the cost results from hospitalization after the fracture.

The patient who sustains a fragility fracture carries up to a 10-fold increased risk of a second fracture compared to a person who has never had one, with the rate of second fracture within 1 year approaching 20%.[6,7] Despite this risk, many patients who have sustained a fragility fracture are not given any preventive treatment. One study found only 7% of patients admitted with a fragility fracture were receiving osteoporosis treatment, and this number increased only to 13% at the time of discharge.[4] At a minimum, patients who suffer a fragility fracture should be placed on calcium and vitamin D treatment and consideration given to further pharmacologic treatment. An often overlooked part of treatment is a formal gait and balance assessment in physical therapy. Patients who already have difficulty with balance and strength will have even more trouble while recovering from a fracture. Difficulty with gait and balance likely contributes to the high rate of a second fracture within 1 year of the first.

Osteoporosis has a dramatic effect on fracture fixation. Traditional nonlocked plates and screws may not achieve adequate purchase in osteoporotic bone. Locked plates or intramedullary nails should be considered to improve fracture fixation and maintain alignment.[8] Bone cement can be used to augment screw fixation, but care must be exercised to prevent extravasation into soft tissues or into the fracture site. Use of allograft bone struts can help provide increased rigidity to fracture fixation. For some fractures, arthroplasty may provide the best treatment and allow earlier weight bearing and mobilization.

Several authors have looked at whether it is cost-effective to screen for osteoporosis and initiate pharmacologic treatment before the onset of a fragility fracture.[9-12] A study in Australia enrolled 1224 women 50 years and older and categorized them by age group. Dual-energy x-ray absorptiometry scanning was performed on all women and the percentage with osteoporosis was 20% in the 50- through 59-year age group, 46% in the 60- through 69-year age group, 59% in the 70- through 79-year age group, and 69% for those older than 80 years. It was estimated that if all women older than 50 years of age were started on antiresorptive medication, the risk of fracture would decrease by 50% in those with osteoporosis and by 20% in those without osteoporosis. The cost per fracture averted in the 50- through 59-year age group was $156,400, whereas in the older-than-80 age group it was only $28,500. It was concluded that treating all women older than age 50 with antiresorptive medication was not financially feasible. The authors concluded that instituting antiresorptive medication in women older than 60 years with osteoporosis would decrease fractures by 28% and was cost-effective.[13]

GERIATRIC TRAUMA

Although people age 65 and older represent approximately 12% of the population in the United States, they account for 28% of all fatal injuries.[14,15] This segment is also the fastest growing age group. The fact that older trauma patients often are frail can make their treatment more challenging.[16] Cardiopulmonary disease is one of the most common comorbid illnesses and can limit a patient's ability to tolerate surgery and participate in rehabilitation. Neurologic disorders, such as Alzheimer disease and Parkinson disease, are also common and affect mortality rate after injury. Some patients may have residual weakness or contractures from a previous cerebrovascular accident. Any of these disorders can affect gait and balance and limit a patient's ability to comply with weight-bearing restrictions. Endocrine disorders, particularly diabetes, are common in older patients. Diabetic patients often have vascular compromise secondary to small vessel disease and are immunosuppressed. Nonoperative treatment of select fractures may be preferred in these patients, particularly if there is a preexisting diabetic ulcer near the planned operative field.

For multiply injured older adult patients, the injury severity score (ISS) may underestimate the degree of injury and the patient's ability to tolerate it and generally is a poor predictor of mortality.[17] Older adult patients may have a lower ISS than young adults but still be unstable or "in extremis," in the sense that minimal further insult could tip them past the point of recovery. At the same time, failure to stabilize fractures that are causing blood loss and pain may also result in further deterioration. It is this fine line the orthopedic trauma surgeon must walk when treating older patients with multiple fractures. In such cases,

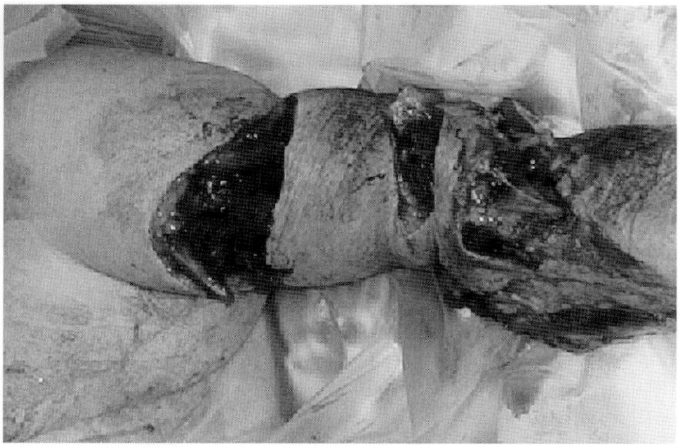

Figure 71-1. Grade IIIC humerus fracture in older trauma patient with multiple injuries. Treatment was immediate amputation.

simple splinting or external fixation of upper extremity fractures and external fixation of lower extremity fractures may represent the best initial treatment.

Few studies have focused specifically on the impact of orthopedic injuries on older trauma patients.[18-22] One retrospective, multicenter study attempted to define factors associated with increased morbidity and mortality rates in older adult patients who had sustained major trauma.[18] Of 326 patients with an average age of 72.2 years, there was an overall mortality rate of 18.1%. Of patients who required fracture stabilization, 77% had this done within 24 hours of admission. The mortality rate for patients who underwent fracture fixation within 24 hours was 11% and for those who had fixation after 24 hours it was 18%, but this difference did not reach statistical significance.[18] The three complications with the highest mortality rates were acute respiratory distress syndrome (81%), myocardial infarction (62%), and sepsis (39%).

For older adult patients with a mangled extremity, early amputation should be considered. Older patients may not be able to withstand the multiple surgeries required to salvage severe open fractures, especially those with vascular insult. If a severely injured limb becomes infected, the cascade of sepsis and multiple system organ failure can proceed quickly. Although it can be a difficult decision, early amputation in an older patient with a mangled extremity can be a life-saving procedure (Figure 71-1).

ANESTHETIC CONSIDERATIONS

Pain management is an important part of orthopedic care in older adults. Early stabilization of fractures is one aspect of pain control that can aid in minimizing narcotic requirements and, in turn, improve respiratory status and mental status. Patients with stabilized fractures can also obtain an upright posture more easily, be weaned from ventilators, and have less delirium; these factors are all critical for survival in older adults. Selective use of nerve blocks or catheters for continuous infusion, such as a femoral nerve block catheter following a femur fracture, can greatly aid in pain relief and minimize narcotic requirements.

Whether spinal or general anesthesia is best for patients with hip fracture remains a matter of debate. A recent retrospective database study of 73,284 patients showed no significant difference in in-hospital mortality, with rates of 2.1% for regional anesthesia and 2.2% for general anesthesia.[23] It is possible that particular patients, such as those with advanced pulmonary disease, may benefit from regional anesthesia. Similarly, for patients with advanced cardiac disease, spinal anesthesia may pose a risk because of the potential for resultant hypotension. When hypotension occurs after spinal anesthesia, it is typically a result of a drop in systemic vascular resistance and not a drop in cardiac output.[24]

An important part of the debate about anesthetic technique, especially for frail older adults who are at increased risk, is the relationship between the type and depth of anesthesia and the occurrence of delirium.[25,26] Although postoperative delirium has long been recognized as a problem, it is commonly not measured as an adverse outcome of surgery, something that is likely to change as the growth in the number of older adults will require that care protocols become better suited to their needs.[27,28]

Part of the preoperative evaluation for many hip fracture patients includes a cardiac risk assessment. For some patients, this results in the acquisition of a transthoracic echocardiogram. In a recent retrospective review of 694 consecutive hip fracture patients, 131 (18.9%) underwent preoperative echocardiogram. It is interesting that no significant difference in mortality was found in-hospital, at 30 days, or at 1 year after surgery between patients who had the echocardiogram and those who did not. None of the patients who had the echocardiogram went on to angioplasty or stent placement. There was a significant difference between the two groups in average time from admission to surgery at 34.8 hours (no echocardiogram) and 66.5 hours (echocardiogram). Length of hospital stay was, on average, 2.24 days longer among the patients undergoing preoperative echocardiogram.[29]

PERIARTICULAR FRACTURES

Treatment of periarticular fractures in older adults often differs from treatment in younger patients. Certain fractures involving the shoulder, elbow, hip, and knee may fare better with arthroplasty rather than open reduction internal fixation (ORIF) in older adults. Several studies have compared ORIF to arthroplasty for displaced femoral neck fractures in older adults.[30-32] The complication rate for those patients undergoing ORIF, including the need for revision surgery, is substantially higher than it is for the arthroplasty group. Controversy exists as to whether hemiarthroplasty or total hip arthroplasty is the best treatment. Some studies seem to favor total joint arthroplasty.[33,34] Dislocation rate is higher, however, with total joint arthroplasty, especially in patients with dementia, with neurologic disorders such as Parkinson disease, or with hemiparesis after a stroke.

Comminuted distal humerus fractures in older adults also may have better outcomes with arthroplasty than with ORIF. Frankle and colleagues reported on 12 patients who underwent ORIF and 12 who underwent total elbow arthroplasty for distal humerus fractures.[35] The total elbow arthroplasty group performed better on the Mayo Elbow Performance Score with 11 excellent and 1 good, compared to 4 excellent, 4 good, 1 fair, and 3 poor in the ORIF group. Müller and coworkers reported on their results with 49 distal humerus fractures in patients older than 65 years treated acutely with total elbow arthroplasty.[36] Inclusion criteria included patients who were "high compliance" and "low demand." Average range of motion at follow-up (average 7 years) was an arc from 24 to 131 degrees. A total of five revision arthroplasties were performed during the follow-up period. The authors concluded that the procedure is recommended when the appropriate inclusion criteria are met.

For periarticular fractures treated with ORIF, the advent of locked plates has allowed for improved fixation, especially in patients with osteoporotic bone. In one retrospective review of 123 distal femur fractures treated with the less invasive surgical stabilization (LISS) system, 93% healed without bone graft, the infection rate was 3%, and there was no loss of distal fixation.[37] In a prospective study of 38 complex proximal tibia fractures treated with the LISS system, 37 of 38 healed with satisfactory alignment, there were no infections, and the average lower extremity measure score was 88.[38] Another review of 77 proximal tibia fractures treated with LISS showed 91% healed without complication.[39] The overall union rate was 97% with an average time to full weight bearing of 12.6 weeks and an infection rate of 4%.

Acetabular fractures are challenging to treat at any age. Helfet and associates were one of the first surgeon groups to report on ORIF of acetabular fractures in older adults.[40] In their review of 18 patients age 60 or older followed for 2 years after surgery, the mean Harris hip score was 90 points. All fractures healed and only one patient had a loss of reduction. Complications included two pulmonary emboli and one missed intraarticular fragment requiring reoperation. The authors concluded that "open reduction and internal fixation of selected displaced acetabular fractures in older adults can yield good results and may obviate the need for early and often difficult total hip arthroplasty."[40]

More recent work has supported primary total hip arthroplasty for select acetabular fractures in older adults[41] (Figure 71-2). To perform arthroplasty in the acute setting may require internal fixation of the fracture to provide enough stability to hold the arthroplasty. Mears and Velyvis have reported their results with this approach in 57 patients with a mean follow-up of 8.1 years and a mean age of 69 years.[41] The mean Harris hip score was 89, and 79% of patients had a good or excellent outcome. The authors concluded that this approach is a viable option for patients with a low likelihood of a favorable outcome with fracture treatment alone.

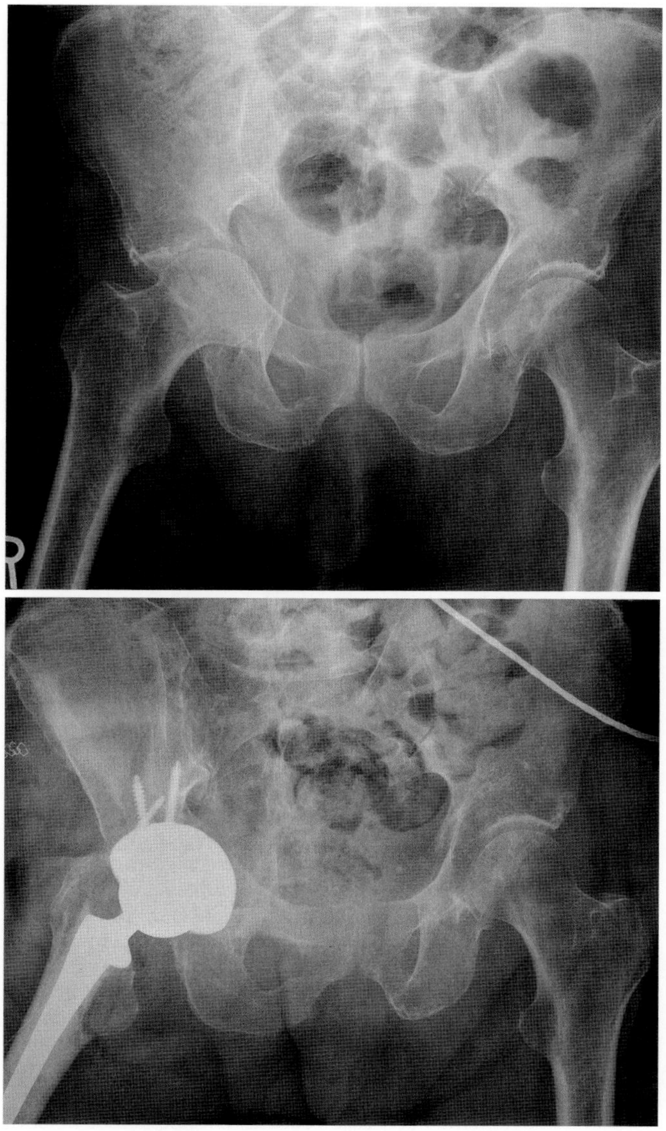

Figure 71-2. Displaced acetabular fracture in older male treated with acute primary total hip arthroplasty.

PERIPROSTHETIC FRACTURES

As the number of patients with total joint replacements continues to rise, so does the number of patients sustaining periprosthetic fractures. These typically occur from low-energy falls, but the bone quality around the prior implant is often of poor quality, making fixation of these fractures challenging. The first step in deciding on the best treatment is to assess the stability of the arthroplasty implants. If the implants are loose, then revision arthroplasty with long stem components is often the best option. The goal is to use stems that extend beyond the fracture by at least two cortical diameters of the bone involved. If the implants are well fixed, then reducing and fixing the fracture is usually the preferred treatment. For certain fractures, such as a supracondylar periprosthetic femur fracture above a total knee replacement, intramedullary nail fixation may be employed, provided the femoral component has an open slot for the nail. Many posterior cruciate ligament–substituting components have a solid metal box and do not allow placement of a nail. In such a scenario, plating may be the best option. The techniques of plating have advanced to the point that most fractures can be treated with indirect reduction to avoid devascularizing the fracture. Plates should overlap the arthroplasty implants to avoid stress risers. Locked plates have provided improved results for many periprosthetic fractures occurring in osteoporotic bone (Figure 71-3).

As increasing numbers of patients have had both total hip and total knee replacements, the rate of interprosthetic fractures is also increasing. The approach to these fractures is similar to that of periprosthetic fractures: first the stability of the implants is

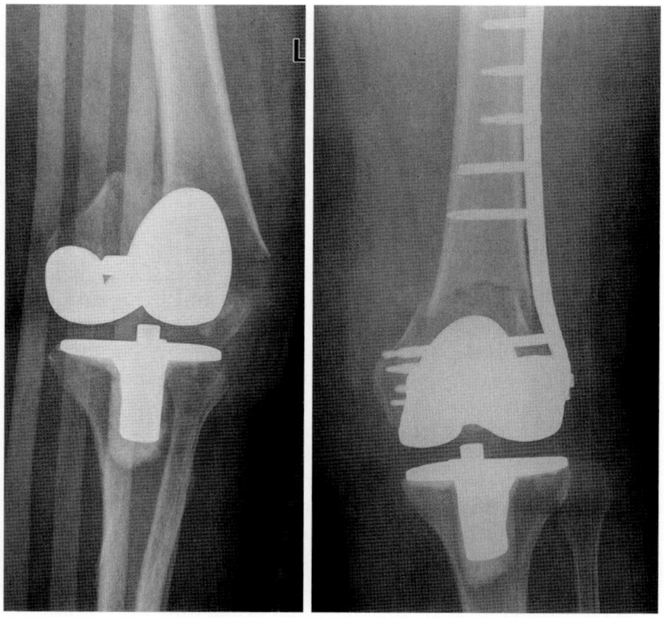

Figure 71-3. Periprosthetic distal femur fracture in osteoporotic bone treated with locking submuscular plate.

determined, and then the best fixation strategy is chosen. Retrograde femoral nails below a total hip implant have been shown to create an increased stress riser in the bone between the nail and the hip implant and should generally be avoided.[42] When possible, plate fixation should overlap the prostheses. It is interesting to note that in biomechanical testing, a well-fixed total knee implant does not increase the risk of interprosthetic fracture.[42]

PREVENTION OF FRACTURES IN OLDER ADULTS

The first step in prevention of fragility fractures is identifying a patient's risk factors. Some risk factors cannot be changed, such as age, family history, or a history of hyperthyroidism, hyperparathyroidism, or rheumatoid arthritis. Many risk factors can be modified, such as avoiding cigarette smoking, sedentary lifestyle, excessive alcohol use, low body mass index, and lack of dietary calcium and vitamin D. Many medications are thought to contribute to osteoporosis; these include glucocorticoids, anticonvulsants, methotrexate, cyclosporin, heparin, and others.

Multiple approaches to preventing osteoporosis and fragility fractures exist. They include nonpharmacologic means, such as a well-balanced diet and exercise, adequate sunlight exposure, not smoking, adequate dietary intake of calcium and vitamin D, and selected use of hip protectors. Exercise seems to be an important modifiable factor in the prevention of fragility fractures. Exercise not only helps prevent osteopenia and osteoporosis but also improves balance and aids in fall prevention in older adults. A multicenter, randomized controlled trial found that group exercise programs were beneficial in preventing falls and improving physical performance in "prefrail" older adult patients.[43] Exercise does not have to be strenuous to achieve results; for example, programs involving the principles of tai chi have been shown to be effective.

Medical treatment of osteoporosis often includes antiresorptive bisphosphonates such as alendronate, risedronate, and ibandronate. Nasal calcitonin and raloxifene have also been used to limit bone resorption. Teriparatide is an anabolic agent that improves bone density by increasing osteoblastic activity as opposed to decreasing osteoclast function like bisphosphonates. The U.S. Food and Drug Administration has withdrawn approval of hormone replacement with estrogen for osteoporosis prevention, except in selected postmenopausal women.[44]

Calcium and vitamin D are relatively inexpensive and have shown benefit in the prevention of osteoporosis. The recommended doses for maximal benefit are 800 IU of vitamin D and 1000 to 1200 mg of elemental calcium. It has been recommended that three types of individuals should take vitamin D and calcium to prevent osteoporosis[1]: patients receiving glucocorticoid treatment,[2] patients with documented osteoporosis,[3] and patients at high risk for calcium or vitamin D deficiency, in particular, older men and women.[45]

Adequate dietary protein seems to be another factor in the prevention of osteoporosis and fragility fractures. Diets deficient in protein can lead to loss of bone mass and decreased bone microarchitecture and strength. Older adult patients who were given a diet with increased protein after a fragility fracture were found to have decreased postfracture bone loss, increased muscle strength, and reduced medical complications during their hospital stay.[46] One author has stated that dietary protein is "as essential" as calcium and vitamin D for bone health and prevention of osteoporosis.[46] Soy protein has been studied prospectively in relation to bone health.[47] Soy protein contains phytoestrogens, which are thought to be beneficial for bone health. In one clinical trial, patients were placed on a diet that included 35 mg of soy protein per day. At the 12-week point, the levels of serum alkaline phosphatase had significantly increased and urinary deoxypyridinoline had decreased. It was concluded that soy protein "can be effective in protecting bone mass."[47]

Hip protectors have been proposed as a relatively inexpensive way to limit hip fractures. A meta-analysis of the Cochrane register of controlled trials concluded that hip protectors are an "ineffective intervention" in the home setting, whereas their utility in nursing or residential care settings is "uncertain."[48] The main reason for their ineffectiveness seems to result from lack of compliance in use.

FRACTURE FOLLOW-UP

The orthopedist may be the only physician a patient sees after a fragility fracture. Close communication between the orthopedist and the patient's internist is needed to implement osteoporosis treatment after a fragility fracture. In a 2006 survey of 140 orthopedists and internists in the United Kingdom, 45% of the internists believed the orthopedist would refer the patient for osteoporosis treatment if it was indicated.[49] When presented with the scenario of a 55-year-old female with a low-energy Colles fracture, 56% of the orthopedists did not request further investigation for osteoporosis. Better awareness of patients at risk for osteoporosis and better communication between the orthopedist and internist as to who will initiate further evaluation and treatment are required to limit the growing burden of fragility fractures.

GERIATRIC-ORTHOPEDIC CO-CARE

Several studies have looked at the effectiveness of co-care between orthopedics and geriatrics regarding inpatient care of older adult patients with orthopedic injuries.[49-51] Most studies have focused on older adult patients with hip fractures. Previous studies have shown mixed results, but many show some advantages. The keys to success seem to be careful targeting of the population, a proactive rather than a reactionary strategy, and attention to improving specific outcomes rather than just a general geriatric assessment. (See also Chapter 37.)

A prospective, randomized trial was carried out on 126 patients 65 years and older admitted to a tertiary academic medical center following a hip fracture.[52] Patients were randomized to either a proactive geriatrics consultation or usual care. The group receiving the geriatrics consultation had a reduction in the incidence of delirium by one third and a reduction in severe delirium by one half.[52] Fisher and colleagues conducted a study of 951 patients, 60 years or older, admitted with a hip fracture over a 7-year period to a single institution. For the first 3 years of the study, patients did not have routine geriatric medicine evaluation, whereas during the final 4 years, there was routine geriatrics consultation. During the second phase, significant reductions in both mortality (4.7% vs. 7.7%; $P < .01$) and rehospitalization rates (7.6% vs. 28%) were seen.[51]

CONCLUSION

Orthopedic care of older adults presents many challenges. Poor bone density can make the goal of stable internal fixation difficult if not impossible in some patients. Comorbid medical conditions can dictate what types of treatment a patient can tolerate. Rehabilitation of injuries may be limited because of the patient's overall physical condition. For some periarticular fractures, performing a joint arthroplasty rather than trying to reconstruct the fracture may result in a more predictable and functional outcome. Shared care between the orthopedist and the internal medicine or geriatric team seems to improve outcomes for many older adult patients. Communication between the orthopedist and the patient's primary care physician is needed to ensure proper osteoporosis management. Each case requires an assessment of both patient and fracture characteristics to determine the most appropriate treatment.

KEY POINTS

- Approximately 1 in 3 women and 1 in 12 men will sustain a fragility fracture.
- Injury severity scores of older patients may underestimate the degree of injury.
- Joint replacement may provide the best treatment for some fractures in older adults.
- Orthopedic and geriatric co-care may improve outcomes for patients with hip fracture.

For a complete list of references, please visit www.expertconsult.com.

KEY REFERENCES

2. Borgstrom E, Johnell O, Kanis JA, et al: At what hip fracture risk is it cost-effective to treat? International intervention thresholds for the treatment of osteoporosis. Osteoporos Int 17:1459–1471, 2006.
6. Astrand J, Karl-Goran T, Tagil M: One fracture is enough! Experience with a prospective and consecutive osteoporosis screening program with 239 fracture patients. Acta Orthop 77:3–8, 2006.
8. Cantu RV, Koval KJ: The use of locking plates in fracture care. J Am Acad Orthop Surg 14:183–190, 2006.
9. Pols HA, Felsenberg D, Hanley DA, et al: Multinational, placebo-controlled, randomized trial of the effects of alendronate on bone density and fracture risk in postmenopausal women with low bone mass: results of the FOSIT study. Fosamax Osteoporosis International Trial Study Group. Osteoporos Int 9:461–468, 1999.
15. DeMaria EJ, Kenney P, Merriam MA, et al: Survival after trauma in geriatric patients. Ann Surg 28:738–743, 1987.
18. Tornetta P, Mostafavi H, Riina J, et al: Morbidity and mortality in elderly trauma patients. J Trauma 46:702–706, 1999.
19. Lonner J, Koval K: Polytrauma in the elderly. Clin Orthop 318:136–143, 1995.
21. Keller JM, Sciadini MF, Sinclair E, et al: Geriatric trauma: demographics, injuries, and mortality. J Orthop Trauma 26:e161–e165, 2012.
30. Tidermark J, Ponzer S, Svensson O, et al: Internal fixation compared with total hip replacement for displaced femoral neck fractures in the elderly. A randomized, controlled study. J Bone Joint Surg Br 85:380–388, 2003.
31. Bhandari M, Devereaux PJ, Swiontkowski MF, et al: Internal fixation compared with arthroplasty for displaced fractures of the femoral neck. A meta-analysis. J Bone Joint Surg Am 85-A:1673–1681, 2003.
33. Rogmark C, Johnell O: Primary arthroplasty is better than internal fixation of displaced femoral neck fractures: a meta-analysis of 14 randomized studies with 2,289 patients. Acta Orthop 77:359–367, 2006.
41. Mears DC, Velyvis JH: Acute total hip arthroplasty for selected displaced acetabular fractures: two to twelve-year results. J Bone Joint Surg Am 84-A:1–9, 2002.
43. Faver MJ, Boscher RJ, Chin A, et al: Effects of exercise programs on falls and mobility in frail and pre-frail older adults: a multicenter randomized controlled trial. Arch Phys Med Rehabil 87:885–896, 2006.

72 Sarcopenia

Yves Rolland, Matteo Cesari, Bruno Vellas

In a paper published in 1997,[1] Irwin Rosenberg described how the term *sarcopenia* (from Greek, *sarx* "flesh" and *penia* "loss") was coined:

> *In 1988, we convened a meeting in Albuquerque, New Mexico to look at various measurements related to the assessment of health and nutrition in elderly populations. … I noted that no decline with age is as dramatic or potentially more significant than the decline in lean body mass. In fact, there may be no single feature of age-related decline more striking than the decline in lean body mass in affecting ambulation, mobility, energy intake, overall nutrient intake and status, independence and breathing. I speculated as to why we had not given this more attention and suggested … we had to give it a name. This would provide recognition by the scientific community and by the National Institutes of Health. … I proposed … sarcomalacia or sarcopenia.*

Since then, the understanding of the aging process has improved, and better and more widely diffused techniques are available for measuring body composition. Nevertheless, the clinical implementation of sarcopenia is still delayed by multiple problems affecting its clear framing and operationalization.[2] To date, sarcopenia is still not recognized as a nosologic entity.

OPERATIONAL DEFINITIONS

Skeletal muscle decline has been operationalized in a number of ways over the years, especially to translate the theoretical concept of the age-related skeletal muscle decline into a clinically meaningful condition of older age. A major challenge has been generating a diagnostic algorithm capable of capturing the two domains of the sarcopenia condition—skeletal muscle mass loss (i.e., a quantitative parameter) and skeletal muscle function loss (i.e., a qualitative parameter). This bidimensional nature of the definition implies the simultaneous assessment as well as the parallel and equivalent consideration of the two factors for the detection of sarcopenia.

The first operational definition of sarcopenia was the one provided by Baumgartner and colleagues[3] in a study of participants recruited in the New Mexico Elder Health Survey and a reference group of young individuals. Sarcopenia was defined as the presence of an appendicular lean mass (weight/height^2) below 7.26 kg/m^2 in men and 5.45 kg/m^2 in women. Subsequently, it was pointed out that the predictive value of the skeletal muscle mass alone for negative outcomes in older adults was not particularly striking.[4,5] At the same time, some studies demonstrated that the best prediction for negative health-related end points was reached when muscle mass was simultaneously considered together with fat mass. For example, Newman and and coworkers,[6] in the Health Aging and Body Composition Study, even proposed a different model of operational definition for sarcopenia based on fat-adjusted appendicular lean mass residuals.

All the early operational definitions available in the sarcopenia literature were particularly focused on quantification of the skeletal muscle mass. Such an approach used the characteristics of a research condition rather than a clinical entity in relation to the condition studied. To more closely approximate the sarcopenia condition to clinical practice, especially for adopting it as a target of interventions against mobility disability), several panels of experts provided operational definitions, including the second (qualitative) domain of the skeletal muscle decline—that is, the muscle dysfunction. Thus, at least four different consensus papers (Table 72-1) were released in a few years proposing to define sarcopenia on the basis of algorithms, simultaneously considering a quantitative estimation of the muscle mass and qualitative estimation of muscle performance.[7-11] Unfortunately, although conceptually similar, the four definitions had key differences. For example, the instrument for quantifying the muscle mass was variable, when specifically indicated. Also, different measures of physical function and muscle strength, with different thresholds of risk, were proposed. Furthermore, the algorithms used to define the sarcopenic individual differently considered the measured components.

Another problem was present from the very beginning. Muscle mass and muscle function have different clinical relevance.[4,5,12] From a geriatric viewpoint, the size of the organ is not particularly relevant, but rather its capacity to sustain the individual at maintaining his or her independent life. Moreover, the age-related declines of muscle mass and muscle function do not follow similar trajectories.[13] The former seems to be relatively more stable over time compared to muscle strength. This might explain why muscle function can discriminate different risk profiles in older adults better. In this context, it is also noteworthy that the combination of quantitative and qualitative parameters in the same algorithm has always been operationalized in an additive way; that is, the two dimensions of sarcopenia are of equal weight in determination of the phenotype and clinical relevance. However, this has been disproved by the growing number of studies demonstrating that the predictive value of sarcopenia definitions for negative health-related events is largely driven by the skeletal muscle quality (physical performance measures) rather than its quantity (skeletal muscle mass).[4,5,12] It is also noteworthy that the clinical relevance of sarcopenia-related parameters is also highly influenced by gender,[12] so that muscle strength parameters seem more predictive of negative outcomes in men, whereas body composition variables, especially those considering adipose tissue, are stronger predictors in women.

With the objective of bypassing all the issues related to the definition of sarcopenia, the Foundation of National Institutes of Health (FNIH) Sarcopenia Project has recently released results from longitudinal observational analyses conducted in a large sample of participants in several cohort studies worldwide.[14] Investigators decided to adopt a different approach compared to what had been proposed in the available consensus definitions. Slow gait speed, which had been previously used as a component of the sarcopenia definitions, became the outcome of models that defined gender-specific optimal cut points for the most predictive parameters of body composition and, separately, muscle strength (Table 72-2).

EPIDEMIOLOGY

After 50 years of age, muscle mass is reported to decline at an annual rate of approximately 1% to 2%, but strength declines at 1.5%/year and accelerates to as much as 3%/year after the age of 60 years.[15] These rates are high in sedentary individuals and twice as high in men as compared to women.[16] However, men, on average, have larger amounts of muscle mass and shorter

TABLE 72-1 Main Operational Definitions of Sarcopenia*

Parameter	International Working Group on Sarcopenia[7]	European Working Group on Sarcopenia in Older People[9]	ESPEN Special Interest Group on Cachexia-Anorexia in Chronic Wasting Diseases[10]	Society of Sarcopenia, Cachexia and Wasting Disorders[8]
Target population	Subjects with clinical declines in physical function, strength, or health status	All persons ≥ 65 yr	Older adults	Persons > 60 yr with clinical declines in physical function, strength, or health status; exclusion of specific muscle diseases, peripheral vascular disease with intermittent claudication, central and peripheral nervous system disorders, and cachexia
Screening	Physical function (4-m usual GS test); if GS < 1.0 m/sec, proceed to BC evaluation	If GS ≤ 0.8 m/sec, proceed to BC evaluation; if GS > 0.8 m/sec, measure hand grip strength; if muscle weakness present, proceed to BC evaluation.		Distance walked during 6-min walk test (cut point, 400 m), or GS < 1.0 m/sec (4- to 6-m track length)
Operative definition	Poor functioning plus poor ALM (assessment by DXA)[3]	Low muscle mass in subjects with GS ≤ 0.8 m/sec or normal GS but low muscle strength	Low muscle mass (≥2 SDs below mean measured in young adults of same gender and ethnic group) plus slow GS (<0.8 m/sec on 4-m track); GS can be replaced by another physical performance measure	Poor functioning plus low ALM (≥2 SDs below mean measured in healthy persons aged 20-30 yr from same ethnic group)

ALM, Appendicular lean mass; *BC,* body composition; *DXA,* dual energy X-ray absorptiometry; *ESPEN,* European Society for Clinical Nutrition and Metabolism; *GS,* gait speed; *SD,* standard deviation.
*Proposed by an international panels of experts; adapted from Cesari M, Fielding RA, Pahor M, et al: Biomarkers of sarcopenia in clinical trials—recommendations from the International Working Group on Sarcopenia. J Frailty Aging 1:102-110, 2012.

TABLE 72-2 Definition of Low Muscle Mass and Poor Muscle Function*

Parameter	Men	Women
Muscle Weakness		
Hand grip strength (recommended)	<26 kg	<16 kg
BMI-adjusted hand grip strength (alternate)	<1.0 kg	<0.56 kg
Low Muscle Mass		
BMI-adjusted ALM (recommended)	<0.789	<0.512
ALM (alternate)	<19.75 kg	<15.02 kg

ALM, Appendicular lean mass; *BMI,* body mass index.
*According to FNIH recommendations—Studenski SA, Peters KW, Alley DE, et al: The FNIH sarcopenia project: rationale, study description, conference recommendations, and final estimates. J Gerontol A Biol Sci Med Sci 69:547-558, 2014.

survival than women, which implies that sarcopenia is potentially a greater health concern in women than in men.

It is difficult to estimate the prevalence of sarcopenia in older adults accurately and definitively due to the multiple ambiguities and controversies existing in its operational definition. Moreover, the need to quantify muscle mass limits the large-scale assessment of the phenomenon. In the New Mexico Elder Health Survey, sarcopenia was found to affect about 20% of men between the ages of 70 and 75 years and about 50% of those older than 80 years; 25% to 40% of women have sarcopenia in the same age ranges.[3] However, Baumgartner later recognized that these estimates, based on a bioelectric impedance equation, might be biased and published revised prevalence estimates based on dual-energy x-ray absorptiometry (DXA) studies; these ranged from 8.8% in women and 13.5% of men aged 60 to 69 years and up to 16% in women and 29% in men older than 80 years.[17] In a healthy, older, community-dwelling population 70 years of age and older in the French Epidemiologie de l'Osteoporose (EPIDOS) study,[18] only 10% of women had sarcopenia based on the Baumgartner's index, but cut-points derived from a different reference group. Using a similar definition, Janssen and coworkers reported retrospectively that 35% of older adults in the population-based National Health and Nutritional Examination Survey III (NHANES III) had a moderate degree of sarcopenia and 10% had a severe degree of sarcopenia.[19] Findings from a separate study by Melton and colleagues using yet another definition has suggested that sarcopenia affects 6% to 15% of persons older than 65 years.[20]

In a recent report,[21] the prevalence of sarcopenia defined according to the European Working Group on Sarcopenia in Older People (EWGSOP) algorithm was found to be influenced by regional and age-related variations. However, the authors estimated its prevalence to be 1% to 29% in community-dwelling populations, 14% to 33% in long-term care populations, and 10% in those in acute hospital care units.

CAUSES

Multiple risk factors and mechanisms contribute to the development of sarcopenia. Lifestyle behaviors such as physical inactivity, poor diet, and age-related changes in hormones and cytokine levels are important risk factors. Postulated mechanisms include alterations in muscle protein turnover, muscle tissue remodeling, loss of alpha motor neurons, and muscle cell recruitment and apoptosis.[22,23] Genetic susceptibility also plays a role and explains individual and group differences in rates of sarcopenia. Each factor in regard to the cause and pathogenesis of sarcopenia potentially contributes differently to the loss of muscle mass, strength, or quality, although the relative influences of each factor on sarcopenia is not yet well understood.

Lack of Physical Activity

Inactivity is an important contributor to the loss of muscle mass and strength at any age.[24-26] Lifelong physical exercise has shown to delay the age-associated skeletal muscle decline.[27] Inactivity results from bed rest studies have indicated that a decrease in muscle strength occurs before a decrease in muscle mass.[28]

Loss of Neuromuscular Function

The neurologic contribution to sarcopenia occurs through a loss of alpha motor neuron axons.[29] Decreased electrophysiologic nerve velocity, related to the dropout of the largest fibers, reduces internodal length, and segmental demyelination occurs with the aging process,[15] but the role of demyelination in sarcopenia seems minor.[30] The central drive that contributes to a decrease in voluntary strength is supposed to be preserved. The progressive denervation and reinnervation process observed during aging that results in fiber type grouping is the potential primary mechanism involved during the development of sarcopenia. From cross-sectional findings, the decline in motor neurons starts after the seventh decade, with a loss of about 50% of alpha motor neurons,[31] and this affects the lower extremities, with their longer axons, more than the upper limbs.[15] The reduction in alpha motor neuron number and in motor unit numbers results in a decline in coordinated muscle action and a reduction in muscle strength. Reinnervation contributes to the final differentiation of nerve fibers and the repartition between the type I fibers (slow oxidative fibers) and type II fibers (fast glycolytic fibers).

During aging, the number of satellite cells and their recruitment ability decrease, with a greater decrease in type II than type I fibers.[32] Satellite cells are myogenic stem cells that can differentiate to new muscle fibers and new satellite cells if activated during the process of regeneration,[33] but this regeneration may lead to imbalance, and the number of type II muscle fibers may decline following damage.

Altered Endocrine Function

There is evidence linking age-related hormonal changes to the loss of muscle mass and muscle strength. However, controversy persists regarding their respective roles and effects on skeletal muscle in adulthood and old age.

Insulin

In young adults, muscle protein synthesis is stimulated by insulin, regardless of glucose tolerance.[34] This anabolic capacity seems to decrease with aging due to insulin resistance (at least partly due to the progressive increase in body and intramyocellular fat mass[20]) and mammalian target of rapamycin complex-1 (mTORC1) signaling.[35,36] The mTORC1 pathway is important to modulate muscle growth by serving as a modulator sensitive to nutritional, hormonal, and exercise stimuli.[37]

Estrogens

There have been conflicting data on the effects of estrogens on sarcopenia. Epidemiologic and interventional studies have suggested that estrogens prevents the loss of muscle mass[38,39] because their decline with age increase the levels of proinflammatory cytokines suspected to be involved in the sarcopenia process, such as tumor necrosis factor-α (TNF-α) and interleukin (IL)-6.[40] Estrogens also increase the level of sex hormone-binding globulin, which reduces the level of serum-free testosterone, so hormone replacement therapy (HRT) should decrease rather than increase muscle mass.[41] Both these mechanisms may play a marginal role involving estrogen during the development of sarcopenia.

Growth Hormone and Insulin-Like Growth Factor 1

Circulating levels and the pulsatile release of growth hormone (GH) are usually decreased in older adults. Therefore, it has been hypothesized that GH might be useful in preventing skeletal muscle decline. Insulin-like growth factor 1 (IGF-1) activates satellite cell proliferation and differentiation and increases protein synthesis in existing fibers.[42] There is also evidence that IGF-1 acts in muscle tissue by interacting with androgens,[43] but there are conflicting results regarding its effect on muscle strength, despite the apparent increase in muscle mass.[44]

Testosterone

Testosterone levels gradually decrease in older men at a rate of 1%/year, and epidemiologic studies have suggested a relationship between low levels of testosterone in older men and loss of muscle mass, strength, and function. The increase in sex hormone–binding globulin levels with age results in lower levels of free or bioavailable testosterone. Clinical and experimental studies have supported the hypothesis that low testosterone levels predict sarcopenia, with low testosterone levels resulting in lower protein synthesis and a loss of muscle mass.[45] Testosterone induces an increase numbers of satellite cells in a dose-dependent manner, which is a major regulating factor of satellite muscle cell function.[43] When administered to hypogonadal subjects or older men with low levels, testosterone[46] increased muscle mass, muscle strength, and protein synthesis. Despite evidence that dehydroepiandrosterone (DHEA) supplementation results in an increase of blood testosterone levels in women and an increase of IGF-1 levels in men, few studies have reported an effect on muscle size, strength, or function.[47]

Vitamin D and Parathyroid Hormone

With aging, 25-OH vitamin D levels decline.[48] Several studies have reported a close relationship between low 1,25-OH vitamin D levels and low muscle mass, low muscle strength, decreased balance, and increased risk of falls.[48] The nuclear 1,25-OH vitamin D receptor has been described in muscle cells,[49] and low levels of vitamin D have been shown to decrease muscle anabolism. Low vitamin D levels may also influence muscle protein turnover through reduced insulin secretion. Low levels of vitamin D are associated with raised parathyroid hormone (PTH) levels, but other studies have suggested that a high PTH level is also independently associated with sarcopenia.[38,50]

Chronic Inflammatory Status

Chronic medical conditions, such as chronic obstructive pulmonary disease (COPD), heart failure, and cancer, are highly prevalent in older adults and are associated with an increased serum level of proinflammatory cytokines and loss of body weight, including lean mass. This condition can occur in younger or older adults is termed *cachexia*.[51] This acute hypercatabolism differs from the long-term, age-related process that leads to sarcopenia. However, aging is also associated with a more gradual, chronic, increased production of proinflammatory cytokines, particularly IL-6 and IL-1, by peripheral blood mononuclear cells. There is some evidence that increased fat mass and reduced circulating levels of sex hormones with aging contribute to this age-related increase in proinflammatory cytokines, which constituted catabolic stimuli.[52-54] Thus, the aging process itself is associated with increased catabolic stimuli, and there is evidence for the hypothesis that cytokines (in particular, TNF-α) predict skeletal muscle decline.[55]

Adipose tissue is an endocrine organ involved in the secretion of proinflammatory cytokines.[56] The close relationship existing between adipose tissue and skeletal muscle justifies the development of the worst case scenario known as sarcopenic obesity, in which the excess of fat mass and reduction of lean mass are present simultaneously.[57-59] Sarcopenic obesity has been reported to predict the onset of disability more than sarcopenia or obesity alone. As for sarcopenia, a unique and clear estimation of the prevalence of the sarcopenic condition is not possible. Several definitions of sarcopenic obesity have been proposed; each is legitimate but differs from the others for the assessment of sarcopenia and obesity. Overall, data have suggested that women tend to have a higher prevalence of sarcopenic obesity compared to men and, even in this case, the condition is strongly associated with age.[60] It has been hypothesized that sarcopenic obesity is associated with increased fatty infiltration of muscle. Fatty infiltration of skeletal muscle is associated with reduced strength and functional status, and it has been hypothesized that infiltration affects muscle function.[61,62] These findings suggest a role of fat mass in the cause of sarcopenia.

Mitochondrial Dysfunction

Mitochondrial function is affected by the cumulative damage to muscle mitochondrial DNA (mtDNA) observed with aging.[63] This results in a reduction of the metabolic rate of muscle cell protein and adenosine triphosphate synthesis and, finally, to the death of the muscle fibers and loss of muscle mass.[64] Probably, low physical activity is an important contributor for mitochondrial dysfunction in older adults. The decline in mitochondrial function with aging might be attenuated by physical activity.[65] some have reported that mitochondrial impairment is only partially reversed after physical training, but does not reach the level of improvement observed in younger adults.[66,67]

Apoptosis

Accumulated mutations in muscle tissue mtDNA are associated with accelerated apoptosis of myocytes, and apoptosis may also be the link between mitochondria dysfunction and loss of muscle mass.[64] Evidence has suggested that myocyte apoptosis is a basic mechanism underlying sarcopenia, and muscle biopsies of older adults show differences associated with apoptosis compared with younger adults.[68] It has also been suggested that type II fibers—those fibers preferentially affected by sarcopenia—may be more susceptible to death via the apoptotic pathway.[69]

Genetic Influences

Genetic factors are major contributors to variability in muscle strength and likely contribute to susceptibility to sarcopenic agents. Genetic epidemiologic studies have suggested that between 36% and 65% of an individual's muscle strength,[70] 57% of lower extremity performance,[71] and 34% of the ability to perform the activities of daily living[72] might be explained by heredity. Sarcopenia and poor physical performance in older adults are also associated with birth weight in men and women, independent of adult weight and height, which suggests that exposure very early in life may also affect risk for sarcopenia in old age in genetically susceptible individuals.[73]

Few studies have explored potential candidate genes that determine muscle strength. In an analysis of the myostatin pathway, a possible muscle mass regulator, linkage was observed to several areas. Several genes were implicated as positional candidate genes for lower extremity muscle strength.[74,75] The actinin–alpha-3 (*ACTN3*) R577X genotype is of interest because it has been shown to influence knee extensor peak power in response to strength training, as has a polymorphism in the angiotensin-converting enzyme (ACE) gene.[76,77] Also, polymorphisms in the vitamin D receptor (VDR) may be associated with muscle strength because of the relationship between vitamin D and its known effect on smooth and striated muscle.[48] Polymorphisms in the VDR have been associated with sarcopenia in older men,[78] muscle strength and body composition in premenopausal women,[79] and muscle strength in older women.[80]

Low Nutritional Intake and Low Protein Intake

Muscle protein synthesis rate is reported to be reduced by 30% in older adults, but there is controversy about how much this reduction is due to nutrition, disease, or physical inactivity, rather than aging.[81,82] It has been recognized by some that protein intake in older adults should exceed the 0.8 g/kg/day recommended intake.[83] Muscle protein synthesis is also decreased in fasting older individuals, especially in specific muscle fractions such as mitochondrial proteins,[84] and thus the anorexia of aging and its underlying mechanisms contribute to sarcopenia by reducing protein intake.

Evidence-based recommendations for optimal protein intake by older adults were recently released by the PROT-AGE Study Group, an international study group endorsed by several scientific organizations and societies.[85] It was noted that to help older adults maintain and regain lean body mass and function, the average daily intake of proteins should be at least in the range of 1.0 to 1.2 g/kg body weight (BW)/day. The group also reinforced the benefits of endurance and resistance-type exercises at individualized levels, suggesting even higher protein intake (≥1.2 g/kg BW/day) for particularly active individuals. The presence of acute or chronic disease, except for severe kidney disease not treated with dialysis, should not prevent the adequate intake of proteins, but should be considered as another reason for increasing the recommended amount of proteins to consume daily.

CONSEQUENCES

Increased clinical and epidemiologic interest in sarcopenia is related to the hypothesis that age-related loss of muscle mass and strength results in decreased functional limitation and mobility disability among older adults. Sarcopenia also plays a predominant role in the cause and pathogenesis of frailty, which is highly predictive of adverse events such as hospitalization, associated morbidity, disability, and death.[86] Sarcopenia has also relevant costs for public health and health care systems.[87] The annual health care cost attributable to sarcopenia has been estimated at $18 billion in the United States alone.[88] Several epidemiologic cross-sectional studies have documented an association between low skeletal muscle mass and physical disability[19] or low physical performance,[62] with the level of disability two to five times higher in the sarcopenic groups. Sarcopenia also results in a decrease in muscular strength and endurance.[1] Sarcopenia, especially the qualitative domain of skeletal muscle decline, is predictive of incident (mobility) disability.[4,12,89]

Part of the theoretical model for sarcopenia involves the positive association between muscle mass and strength and improved functional performance and reduced disability. The relationship between muscle mass and strength is linear,[90] but the relationship between physical performance (e.g., walking speed) and muscle mass is curvilinear.[91] Thus, a threshold defining the amount of muscle mass under which muscle mass predicts poorer physical performance and physical disability should be detectable, but a specific threshold may exist for each physical task. The relationships among strength, muscle mass, and function have important implications regarding the selection of therapeutic approaches. An increase in muscle mass and strength in healthy older adults could have little effect on a specific physical performance, but a small increase in muscle mass among sarcopenic older adults could result in a significant increase in physical performance, despite a relatively small increase in muscle strength. An increase in muscle mass may have no effect on walking speed in healthy older adults but may have a significant impact in very frail older adults. However, differences in functional outcomes and population characteristics are major determinants in the success of interventional studies on sarcopenia, and these differences are attributable, in part, to these methodologic considerations.

TREATMENT AND INTERVENTIONS

Several pharmacologic and nonpharmacologic interventions have been proposed over the years to prevent and/or delay age-related skeletal muscle decline. Considerable evidence has suggested that sarcopenia is a reversible cause of disability and could benefit from intervention.[92-94] However, the effects and ability of these interventions to improve function and prevent disability and reduce age-related skeletal muscle decline in older adults are under debate.

When treating sarcopenia, it could be argued that improving muscle strength or muscle power is more clinically relevant for the outcomes of disability or mobility than increasing muscle mass. However, it is also true that increasing muscle mass is more important for other outcomes, such as protein stores or thermogenesis. The concept that muscle strength and muscle mass are differentially affected by various treatment modalities is supported by experimental and clinical findings. Although behavioral treatment (e.g., physical exercise) increases muscle mass and strength, pharmacologic treatment (e.g., growth hormone) tends to increase muscle mass without significant changes in strength more consistently.

Physical Activity

No pharmacologic or behavioral intervention to reverse sarcopenia has proved to be as efficacious as resistance training. Muscle mass, strength, and muscle quality (strength adjusted for muscle mass) are reported to improve significantly with resistance training in older adults.[95] Robust evidence from several studies has indicated that resistance training such as weight lifting increases myofibrillar muscle protein synthesis,[96,97] muscle mass, and strength, even in frail older adults.[32,98-104] Strength gains result from a combination of improved muscle mass and quality and neuronal adaptation (innervations, activation pattern). However, sarcopenia has been observed in master athletes who maintain resistance training activities throughout their lifetime.[105,106]

The American College of Sport Medicine (ACSM) and American Heart Association (AHA) have suggested that training at 70% to 90% of 1 RM (one repetition maximum) on two or more nonconsecutive days per week is the appropriate training intensity to produce gains in muscle size and strength, even in frail older adults.[106,107] Resistance training in older adults increases strength that is low in absolute terms and similar relative to muscle mass, but the increased muscle size is relatively moderate (between 5% and 10%) compared to the increase in muscle strength. Most of the increase in strength is in neural adaptation of the motor unit pathway,[15] but disuse results in a rapid detraining.[108] Several reports have suggested that maintaining the benefits from resistance training is possible with as little as one exercise program per week.[109]

Whether aerobic training can reduce, prevent, or treat sarcopenia is an important practical question because resistance training is less appealing to many sedentary older adults. Aerobic exercise does not contribute as much to muscle hypertrophy as resistive exercises, but it stimulates muscle protein synthesis,[110] satellite cell activation, and increased muscle fiber area.[111] A possible important aspect of aerobic exercise is that it reduces body fat, including intramuscular fat, which is important for improving the functional role of muscle relative to body weight.

Leisure physical activity is not enough to prevent the decline in muscle mass,[112] but aerobic and resistance activities improve balance, lessen fatigue, increase pain release, reduce cardiovascular risk factors, and improve appetite. Thus, promoting an active lifestyle can prevent the functional effects of sarcopenia, but resistance training is the best approach to prevent and treat sarcopenia, although both training modalities contribute to the maintenance and improvement of muscle mass and strength in older adults.

Interestingly, a recent study by Fragala and associates[113] has shown that hormonal, exercise, and nutritional interventions against muscle weakness and low lean body mass (defined according to the FNIH criteria) can produce meaningful improvements in strength, independently of the quantitative domain of sarcopenia. Moreover, a recent report from the Lifestyle Interventions and Independence for Elders Pilot (LIFE-P) study[114] has shown that a physical activity intervention can improve the physical performance of older adults independently of their baseline status of sarcopenia.

Nutrition

In malnourished older adults, poor protein intake is a barrier to gains in muscle tissue and strength from interventions such as resistance training. Increasing protein intake in older adults, and especially in frail older adults, can minimize the sarcopenic process.[115] However, it is not clear if protein supplementation in the absence of malnutrition enhances muscle mass and muscle strength, because protein supplementation alone or in association with physical training has been unsuccessful.[107] Approaches based on specific nutriments, including essential amino acids (e.g., leucine),[116] have suggested an anabolic effect.[117] It has been reported that essential amino acids stimulate protein anabolism in older adults, whereas nonessential amino acids have no effect in relation to essential amino acids.[118,119] The acute muscle protein synthesis in response to resistance training and essential amino acid ingestion is similar in older and younger adults, but delayed in older adults.[119] In supraphysiologic concentration, leucine stimulates muscle protein synthesis,[116] which may be related to a direct effect of leucine on the initiation of mRNA translation; amino acid supplements are ineffective for muscle protein synthesis if they do not contain sufficient leucine.[120] The quantity and quality of amino acids in the diet are important factors for stimulating protein synthesis, and nutritional supplementation with whey proteins, a rich source of leucine, may be a safe strategy to prevent sarcopenia.[121,122] However, caloric restriction can prevent the loss of muscle mass in animal and perhaps some human studies.[123,124]

The schedule of the protein supplementation is relevant to improving muscle protein synthesis.[85] The feeding pattern is important to optimize muscle protein metabolism. For example, Arnal and coworkers[125] have shown that in older adults, a two-protein pulse feeding pattern is more efficient in improving whole-body protein retention than the same amount of proteins evenly distributed across meals. Nevertheless, the ingestion of large quantities of proteins in a single meal may be difficult to maintain over the long term, especially in older adults. Furthermore, most researchers have agreed that the amount of proteins introduced should be spread equally throughout the day to ensure a greater 24-hour anabolic response.[126]

Prevention of sarcopenia should occur throughout life. The possible influence of specific exposures at critical development periods may have a major impact on the risk of sarcopenia in old age.[73] An adequate diet in childhood and young adulthood affects bone development, and calcium maintenance is required throughout life; this appears to be a reasonable lifestyle and treatment regimen for sarcopenia.

Testosterone

About 20% of men older than 60 years and 50% of men older than 80 years are considered hypogonadic.[127] There are conflicting and inconclusive results of the effectiveness of testosterone therapy on muscle mass and muscle strength in older adults. Testosterone increases muscle mass and strength at supraphysiologic doses in young individuals under resistance training,[128] but such dose levels are not administered to older adults. Some interventional studies have reported a modest increase in lean mass, but most have reported no increase in strength.[107] For the few studies that have reported an increase in strength, the magnitude was lower than through resistance training. Moreover, the anabolic effect of testosterone on lean mass and strength seems weaker in older adults than in younger adults.[107] A meta-analysis[129] has indicated that the benefits of DHEA in older adults are mostly inconclusive to reach a definitive consensus. DHEA does not appear to benefit measures of physical function or performance routinely.

Testosterone is currently not recommended for the treatment of sarcopenia, and side effects associated with other androgens also limit their use. The potential risks associated with testosterone therapy (e.g., increased level of prostate-specific antigen, hematocrit, and cardiovascular risks) compared to the low level of evidence concerning the benefits on physical performances and function explain the recommendations. The administration of high doses of testosterone in randomized controlled trials (RCTs) has been thought to increase the risk of prostate cancer.[130] In 2009, the Testosterone Trial (T-Trial) was funded to examine the efficacy of therapy in 800 older men with low concentrations of testosterone on multiple outcomes, including physical function. The expected results might clarify doubts and improve our knowledge in this field.[131]

Growth Hormone

GH increases muscle strength and mass in younger adults with hypopituitarism but in older adults, who are frequently GH-deficient, most studies have reported that GH supplementation does not increase muscle mass or strength, even in association with resistance training.[107,132] GH increases mortality rate in ill and malnourished persons,[133] and potential serious and frequent side effects, such as arthralgia, edema, cardiovascular problems, and insulin resistance, occur with GH supplementation.[44] To date, there has been little clinical research support for the use of GH supplementation in the treatment of sarcopenia. Previous observations examining the association of IGF-1 with muscle strength and physical performance in older adults have yielded conflicting results.[134] Interestingly, in a study of obese postmenopausal women, the administration of GH alone or in combination with IGF-1 caused a greater increase in fat-free mass and a greater reduction in fat mass than achieved by diet and exercise alone.[135] However, safety issues limit the clinical applications of these findings. Some studies have found that IGF-1 correlates with a risk of prostate cancer in men, premenopausal breast cancer in women, and lung cancer and colorectal cancer in men and women.[136]

Myostatin

Myostatin is a rather recently discovered natural inhibitor of muscle growth,[137] and mutations in the myostatin gene result in muscle hypertrophy in animals and humans.[138,139] Antagonism of myostatin enhanced muscle tissue regeneration in aged mice by increasing satellite cell proliferation.[139] Preliminary results from clinical trials on antagonists of myostatin for the treatment of sarcopenia are expected in the near future.[140]

Estrogens and Tibolone

A review on the effects of estrogen and tibolone on muscle strength and body composition[141] has reported an increase in muscle strength, but only tibolone appears to increase lean body mass and decrease total fat mass. Tibolone is a synthetic steroid with estrogenic, androgenic, and progestogenic activity. HRT and tibolone may both react with the intranuclear receptor in the muscle fibers,[142,143] and tibolone may also act by binding androgen receptors in the muscle fibers and increasing free testosterone and GH levels. However, further research is needed to confirm these findings and the long-term safety of these drugs in older adults. No study has currently confirmed the positive findings in older adults. Moreover, given the well-known side effects associated with the use of these drugs, estrogens or tibolone treatment cannot be recommended as first-choice treatment for sarcopenia.

Vitamin D

Vitamin D supplementation from 700 to 800 IU/day reduces the risk of hip fracture (and any nonvertebral fracture) in community-dwelling and nursing home older adults[144] and the risk of falls.[145] The underlying mechanism may be the increased muscle strength. Janssen and colleagues have reported a histologic muscle atrophy, predominantly of type II fibers, in vitamin D deficiency.[146] The hypothesis that vitamin D may prevent sarcopenia is fascinating, and a growing body of literature has been focused on demonstrating the relationship and mechanisms linking vitamin D to muscle mass and function in older adults.[48]

Angiotensin-Converting Enzyme Inhibitors

Growing evidence has suggested that ACE inhibitors may prevent sarcopenia.[115,147,148] Activation of the renin-angiotensin-aldosterone system may be involved in the progress of sarcopenia. Angiotensin II infused in rats results in muscle atrophy,[149] and several mechanisms such as influences on oxidative stress, metabolic, and inflammation pathways have been suggested through epidemiologic and experimental studies. ACE inhibitors reduce the level of angiotensin II in vascular muscle cell, and angiotensin II may be a risk factor for sarcopenia through the related increase in proinflammatory cytokine production. ACE inhibitors may also improve exercise tolerance via changes in skeletal muscle myosin heavy-chain composition.[150] ACE gene polymorphism also affects the muscle anabolic response and muscular efficiency after physical training.[151] Nevertheless, some reports have provided negative findings about the extracardiovascular actions of ACE inhibitors, in particular concerning their antiinflammatory properties[152] and effects on physical function.[153]

Cytokine Inhibitors

The age-related inflammation process is supposed to be an important factor in the development of sarcopenia, and antiinflammatory drugs may delay its onset and progression. Cytokine inhibitors, such as thalidomide, increase weight and lean tissue anabolism in AIDS patients.[154] TNF-α produces muscle tissue atrophy in vitro. Anti–TNF-α antibodies, given to rheumatoid arthritis patients, may also be an alternative therapeutic opportunity for sarcopenia.[155] However, the benefit-risk balance of these drugs is a major limitation that has not yet been tested in sarcopenic patients. Epidemiologic data have also suggested that consumption of fatty fish rich in the antiinflammatory actions of omega-3 fatty acids may prevent sarcopenia.[156]

Reversal of Apoptosis

Our understanding of the mechanisms of apoptosis suggests that caspase inhibitors may represent a possible future therapy.[63] Apoptosis may be reversible. For example, exercise training reverses the skeletal muscle apoptosis, and caloric restriction reduces apoptosis pathway stimulated by TNF-α.[124,157] Redox modulators such as carotenoids[158] seem to be important factors in influencing loss of muscle strength, functional limitation, and disability. Interest in all these molecules has been suggested by basic research and may be studied in future clinical research projects.

CONCLUSIONS

Improved understanding and treatment of sarcopenia would have a dramatic impact on improving the health and quality of life for older adults, reducing the associated comorbidity and disability and stabilizing rising health care costs. However, continued research is needed to develop a consensus operational clinical definition of sarcopenia applicable in clinical management and clinical and epidemiologic research across populations. Sarcopenia is a complex multifactorial condition; its interrelated underpinnings and onset are difficult to detect and poorly understood. Thus, a comprehensive approach to sarcopenia requires a multimodal approach. Reducing the loss of muscle mass and muscle strength is relevant if physical performance is decreased and disability is increased. Defining targeted older adults for specific treatments in clinical trials is an important issue if the findings and their interpretation are to be inferred to other groups and populations of older adults. An important clinical end point should be the prevention of mobility disability along with reducing, stopping, or reversing the loss of muscle mass, muscle strength, and muscle quality.

Resistance strength training has been the only treatment that affects the muscle aspects of sarcopenia. There are no pharmacologic approaches that provide definitive evidence in the ability to prevent the decline in physical function and sarcopenia. Current and future pharmacologic and clinical trials and epidemiologic studies could radically change our therapeutic approach to understanding and treating mobility and disability in older adults.

KEY POINTS

- Sarcopenia, age-related skeletal muscle decline, is a suitable condition for developing clinical and research studies on aging and the prevention of disability.
- The clinical implementation of sarcopenia is currently limited, also due to a lack of agreement about a unique operational definition.
- Multiple endogenous factors (e.g., loss of neuromuscular function, inflammation, hormonal abnormalities) and exogenous (e.g., sedentary behavior, malnutrition) factors can contribute to the development of the skeletal muscle decline.
- Sarcopenia has been associated with negative health-related outcomes in older adults, in particular disability.
- Interventions against sarcopenia are primarily focused on correcting pathologic abnormalities (e.g., hormonal dysfunction) and promoting healthy lifestyle (e.g., physical activity, appropriate diet).

For a complete list of references, please visit www.expertconsult.com.

KEY REFERENCES

2. Cesari M, Vellas B: Sarcopenia: a novel clinical condition or still a matter for research? J Am Med Dir Assoc 13:766–767, 2012.
7. Fielding RA, Vellas B, Evans WJ, et al: Sarcopenia: an undiagnosed condition in older adults. Current consensus definition: prevalence, etiology, and consequences. International working group on sarcopenia. J Am Med Dir Assoc 12:249–256, 2011.
8. Morley JE, Abbatecola AM, Argiles JM, et al: Sarcopenia with limited mobility: an international consensus. J Am Med Dir Assoc 12:403–409, 2011.
11. Cesari M, Fielding RA, Pahor M, et al: Biomarkers of sarcopenia in clinical trials—recommendations from the International Working Group on Sarcopenia. J Frailty Aging 1:102–110, 2012.
12. Cesari M, Rolland Y, Abellan Van Kan G, et al: Sarcopenia-related parameters and incident disability in older persons: results from the "Invecchiare in Chianti" study. J Gerontol A Biol Sci Med Sci 70:547–558, 2015.
14. Studenski SA, Peters KW, Alley DE, et al: The FNIH sarcopenia project: rationale, study description, conference recommendations, and final estimates. J Gerontol A Biol Sci Med Sci 69:547–558, 2014.
21. Cruz-Jentoft AJ, Landi F, Schneider SM, et al: Prevalence of and interventions for sarcopenia in ageing adults: a systematic review. Report of the International Sarcopenia Initiative (EWGSOP and IWGS). Age Ageing 43:748–759, 2014.
24. Atkins JL, Whincup PH, Morris RW, et al: Low muscle mass in older men: the role of lifestyle, diet and cardiovascular risk factors. J Nutr Health Aging 18:26–33, 2014.
25. Gianoudis J, Bailey CA, Daly RM: Associations between sedentary behaviour and body composition, muscle function and sarcopenia in community-dwelling older adults. Osteoporos Int 26:571–579, 2015.
26. Curtis E, Litwic A, Cooper C, et al: Determinants of muscle and bone aging. J Cell Physiol 230:2618–2625, 2015.
37. Dickinson JM, Fry CS, Drummond MJ, et al: Mammalian target of rapamycin complex 1 activation is required for the stimulation of human skeletal muscle protein synthesis by essential amino acids. J Nutr 141:856–862, 2011.
48. Cesari M, Incalzi RA, Zamboni V, et al: Vitamin D hormone: a multitude of actions potentially influencing the physical function decline in older persons. Geriatr Gerontol Int 11:133–142, 2011.
51. Farkas J, von Haehling S, Kalantar-Zadeh K, et al: Cachexia as a major public health problem: frequent, costly, and deadly. J Cachexia Sarcopenia Muscle 4:173–178, 2013.
60. Zamboni M, Rossi AP, Zoico E: Sarcopenic obesity. In Cruz-Jentoft AJ, Morley JE, editors: Sarcopenia, Chichester, England, 2012, Wiley-Blackwell, pp 181–192.
64. Marzetti E, Calvani R, Bernabei R, et al: Apoptosis in skeletal myocytes: a potential target for interventions against sarcopenia and physical frailty—a mini-review. Gerontology 58:99–106, 2012.
74. Tan LJ, Liu SL, Lei SF, et al: Molecular genetic studies of gene identification for sarcopenia. Hum Genet 131:1–31, 2012.
75. Garatachea N, Lucía A: Genes and the ageing muscle: a review on genetic association studies. Age (Dordr) 35:207–233, 2013.
85. Bauer J, Biolo G, Cederholm T, et al: Evidence-based recommendations for optimal dietary protein intake in older people: a position paper from the PROT-AGE study group. J Am Med Dir Assoc 14:542–559, 2013.
87. Beaudart C, Rizzoli R, Bruyère O, et al: Sarcopenia: burden and challenges for public health. Arch Public Health 72:45, 2014.
113. Fragala MS, Dam TT, Barber V, et al: Strength and function response to clinical interventions of older women categorized by weakness and low lean mass using classifications from the foundation for the national institute of health sarcopenia project. J Gerontol A Biol Sci Med Sci 70:202–209, 2015.
114. Liu CK, Leng X, Hsu FC, et al: The impact of sarcopenia on a physical activity intervention: the Lifestyle Interventions and Independence for Elders Pilot Study (LIFE-P). J Nutr Health Aging 18:59–64, 2014.
126. Calvani R, Miccheli A, Landi F, et al: Current nutritional recommendations and novel dietary strategies to manage sarcopenia. J Frailty Aging 2:38–53, 2013.
129. Baker WL, Karan S, Kenny AM: Effect of dehydroepiandrosterone on muscle strength and physical function in older adults: a systematic review. J Am Geriatr Soc 59:997–1002, 2011.
131. Cook NL, Romashkan S: Why do we need a trial on the effects of testosterone therapy in older men? Clin Pharmacol Ther 89:29–31, 2011.
140. Ebner N, Steinbeck L, Doehner W, et al: Highlights from the 7th Cachexia Conference: muscle wasting pathophysiological detection and novel treatment strategies. J Cachexia Sarcopenia Muscle 5:27–34, 2014.

73 The Pancreas

J.C. Tham, Ceri Beaton, Malcolm C.A. Puntis

BACKGROUND

The pancreas is a retroperitoneal organ located deep to the stomach; it has endocrine and exocrine functions. Some knowledge of its development and structure is necessary as a foundation on which to base an understanding of the diseases that affect it and its changes with age.

Development of the Pancreas

The pancreas begins to develop at day 26 as dorsal and ventral endodermal buds arising from their respective aspects of the primitive tubular foregut. The ventral bud arises together with the embryonic bile duct, and it then migrates posteriorly around the duodenum. Late in the sixth week, the two pancreatic buds fuse to form the definitive pancreas (Figure 73-1).The dorsal pancreatic bud gives rise to part of the head, body, and tail of the pancreas, whereas the ventral pancreatic bud gives rise to the uncinate process and remainder of the head. The two ductal systems fuse, and the proximal end of the dorsal bud duct usually degenerates, leaving the ventral pancreatic duct as the main duct opening at the ampulla. The opening of the dorsal duct, if it persists, forms the accessory duct. The pancreatic endoderm of each bud develops into an epithelial tree that will form the duct system, which drains the exocrine products manufactured in the acini. Endocrine cells arises separately from the ducts and aggregate into the islets.[1]

A failure of migration or fusion of the early pancreatic buds can result in pancreas divisum, which occurs in about 7% of the population. Alternatively, the pancreas can surround the duodenum, resulting in an annular pancreas. Abnormal development of the ventral duct can result in a common channel whereby the junction of the biliary and pancreatic ducts is outside the wall of the duodenum, allowing reflux and mixing of bile and pancreatic juices, which can result in damage to the bile duct in the fetus and a choledochal cyst or damage to the pancreas, causing acute pancreatitis.

Anatomic Relationships

The adult pancreas is a retroperitoneal structure 12 to 15 cm long, extending from the duodenum to the hilum of the spleen. The neck of the pancreas lies anterior to the superior mesenteric vein, and the uncinate process curls around the vein to lie on its right, on the posterior border. Posterior to the head and uncinate process is the inferior vena cava. The splenic artery and vein pass deep to the upper border of the pancreas and provide much of its vascular supply. The right-hand border of the head is closely applied to the concavity of the duodenum, and its superior part is related to the portal vein.

Histology

The pancreas has a lobulated structure, and there are intralobular ducts penetrating the secretory acini, which are flask-shaped structures consisting of typical zymogenic cells. The larger interlobular ducts contain some nonstriated smooth muscle.

The million or so islets of Langerhans are distributed throughout the adult pancreas and consist of endocrine cells. The alpha cells constitute 15% to 20% of the islet cells and produce glucagon. The insulin-secreting beta cells comprise about 65% to 80% of the islet cells, and the delta cells comprise about 3% to 10% of the islet cells and produce somatostatin. The PP (gamma) cells (3% to 5%) produce pancreatic polypeptide, and the epsilon cells (<1%) produce ghrelin.

Exocrine Function

The pancreas secretes 1400 mL/ day of an alkaline, bicarbonate-rich solution containing proenzymes that are converted into active enzymes—proteases, lipases, and glycosidases, such as amylase. In the gut, a proenzyme-like trypsinogen is converted into trypsin by enterokinases; trypsin then in turn releases more trypsin from trypsinogen.

Enzyme secretion is stimulated by cholecystokinin, which is released by the duodenum in response to the presence of food. Secretin, also released from the gut wall, controls the secretion of water and electrolytes, most of which are secreted from the ducts of the pancreas.[2]

Pancreatic exocrine function deteriorates with age; the secretion of bicarbonate and enzymes have been found to be reduced in a group of subjects, average age 72 years, compared with a group whose average age is 36 years.[3] However, 80% to 90% of pancreatic function must be lost before malabsorption becomes apparent; this happens only occasionally in the older patient, in whom other causes of malabsorption are more common.[4]

Endocrine Function

Synthesis and release of insulin from the beta cells of the pancreas is controlled by the level of glucose in the beta cells, which reflects the plasma level. However, overall control of pancreatic function is the result of many complex and interrelated feedback loops. Somatostatin, for example, secreted from the delta cells in response to an increasing blood sugar level, inhibits enzyme release and decreases gut motility. The full complexity of the hormonal control of glucose in the body is as yet not fully elucidated; however, it is clear that there are some functional changes with age.[5]

Age Changes

As well as age-related changes in pancreatic function after the age of 60 years, there are morphologic changes in that the pancreas shrinks and can become more fatty.[6] Patchy fibrosis can also occur in the pancreas from the seventh decade onward, but without the other changes of chronic pancreatitis this age-related focal lobular fibrosis is associated with ductal papillary hyperplasia, which can be premalignant.[7]

TUMORS OF THE PANCREAS

The classification of pancreatic neoplasia can be grouped into two main groups—cystic and solid neoplasia—as shown in the

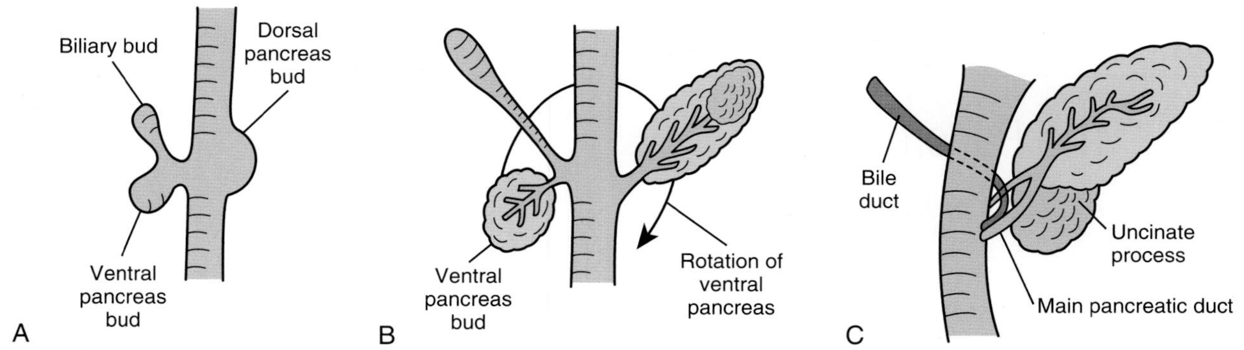

Figure 73-1. Embryology of the pancreas. **A,** The two pancreatic buds form at 26 days development. **B,** Rotation of the ventral pancreas. **C,** At 45 days, the final position is reached, and the ventral and dorsal pancreases have fused.

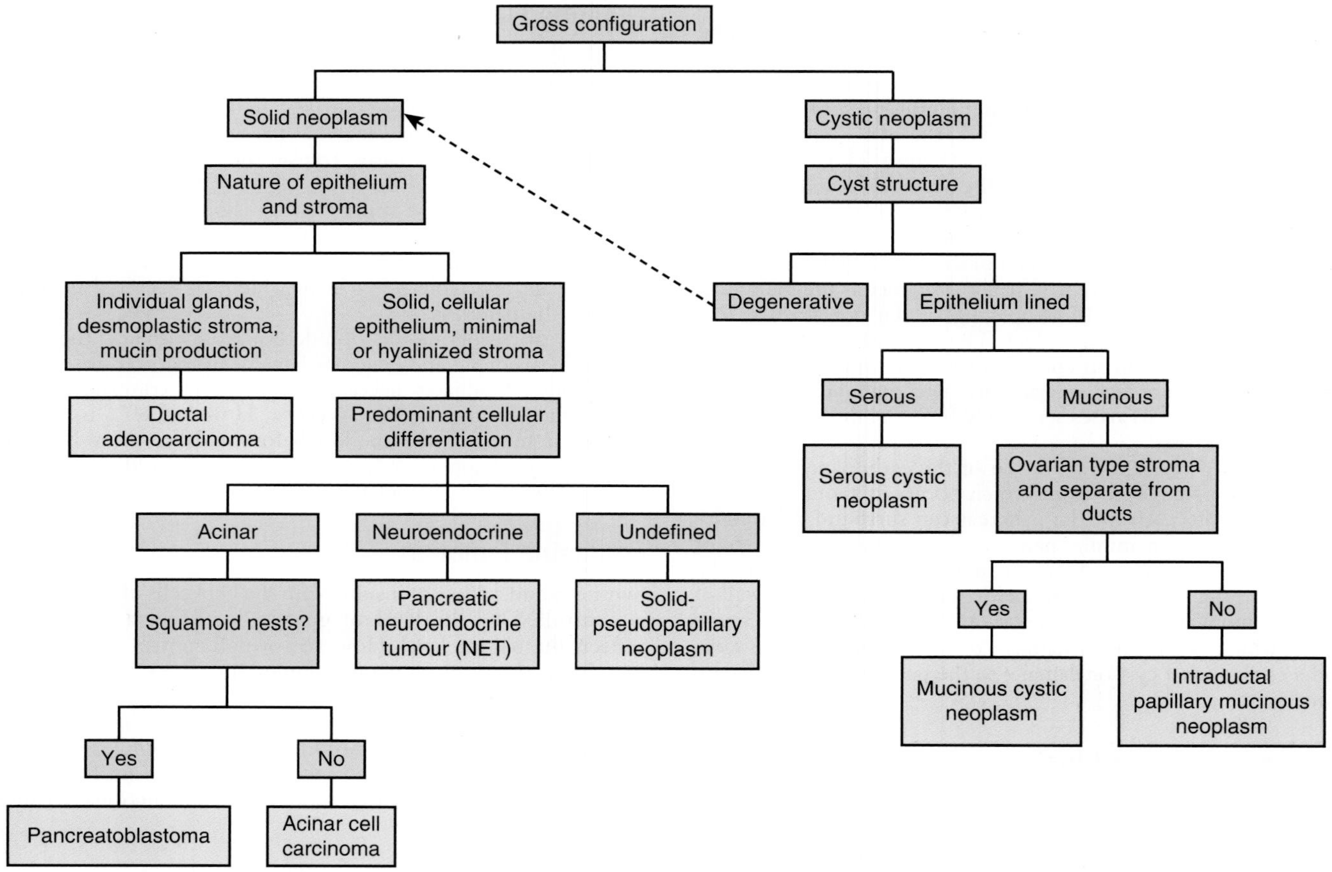

Figure 73-2. Simple algorithm for the diagnostic evaluation of pancreatic neoplasms. *(Adapted from Hruban R, Boffetta P, Hiraoka N, et al: Tumours of the pancreas, In Bosman FT, Carneiro F, Hruban RH, Theise ND, editors: WHO/IRC classification of tumours of the digestive system, ed 4, Geneva, 2010, World Health Organization.)*

algorithm in Figure 73-2. Ductal adenocarcinoma is the most common pancreatic tumor, accounting for 85% of all tumors in the pancreas; it is a malignant tumor with a very poor prognosis.[8] Truly benign tumors such as fibromas, lipomas, and hemangiomas do occur but are exceedingly rare. This chapter will discuss the more common pancreatic neoplasms.

Cystic Tumors

The exact nature of a cystic lesion in the pancreas is still difficult to identify in spite of the use of computed tomography (CT), magnetic resonance imaging (MRI), and ultrasound (US) by transcutaneous and endoscopic techniques. It is often difficult to distinguish an inflammatory lesion from a neoplasm.[9,10] Biopsy is often difficult or inconclusive, and the general advice is to err on the side of resection.[11] During pathologic classification of the tumor, it is important to be sure that the cyst is not a degenerative cyst because this signifies that the underlying tumor is more likely to be a solid tumor, and this will affect management. Immunohistochemistry is useful in differentiating the tumor types. Although these tumors tend to occur more commonly in younger or middle-aged individuals, they also occur up to the seventh and eighth decades and are more likely to be malignant in patients older than 70 years, when resection should be considered.[12]

Serous Cystadenoma

A serous cystadenoma is sometimes known as a serous microcystic tumor. The mean age of presentation is in the sixth decade, and 70% occur in women. The vast majority are benign, and only a handful of cases of malignant serous cystic tumor of the pancreas have been reported.[13]

Mucinous Cystic Neoplasm

This neoplasm accounts for 50% of cystic tumors and is malignant or potentially malignant. It is most common in middle-aged women and should be treated by resection of the affected part of the pancreas.[14]

Intraductal Papillary Mucinous Neoplasm

An intraductal papillary mucinous neoplasm (IPMN) is a tumor that is twice as common in men as in women and has a mean age at presentation in the seventh decade. It is characterized by copious mucous draining at a patulous ampulla from a dilated duct. It has a favorable prognosis following appropriate resection.[15,16]

Lymphoepithelial Cyst

This is a rare epithelium-lined cystic lesion, histologically similar to a branchial cyst.[17]

Cystic Islet Cell Tumors

This tumor results from cystic degeneration of a solid endocrine tumor. Although it is rare, it is important to consider this diagnosis when evaluating a cystic lesion in the pancreas and test for endocrine activity to exclude a functioning tumor, although most of these tumors are nonfunctioning.

Von Hippel–Lindau Syndrome

This is a rare genetic condition with autosomal dominant inheritance. Several types of pancreatic tumors can occur in this condition, including serous cystadenoma, multiple cysts, and endocrine tumors.[18]

Solid Tumors

Ductal Adenocarcinoma

Epidemiology and Age Incidence. Pancreatic cancer is the fifth most common cause of cancer death in the United Kingdom and the seventh most common worldwide.[19] Patients with pancreatic cancer should undergo definitive surgery within days of diagnosis if there is an advanced health care system. However, there is usually a delay of a few weeks prior to surgical treatment. In 2011, the number of deaths from pancreatic cancer in the United Kingdom was 8320, with a rate of 13.2/100,000 population.[19] The incidence of pancreatic cancer in the United Kingdom increases sharply with age, and 96% of patients with pancreatic cancer are 50 years of age or older[20,21] (Figure 73-3).

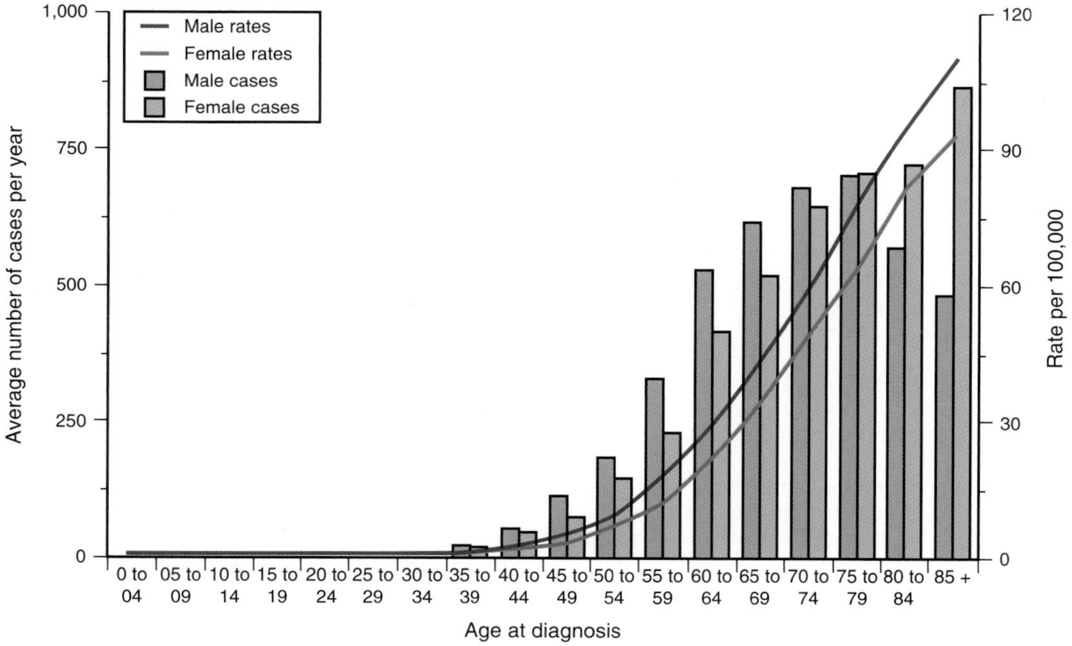

Figure 73-3. Incidence rate of pancreatic cancer in the United Kingdom, 2009-2011. *(From Cancer Research UK: Pancreatic cancer incidence statistics. http://www.cancer researchuk. org/health-professional/cancer-statistics/statistics-by-cancer-type/pancreatic-cancer/incidence. Accessed December 3, 2015.)*

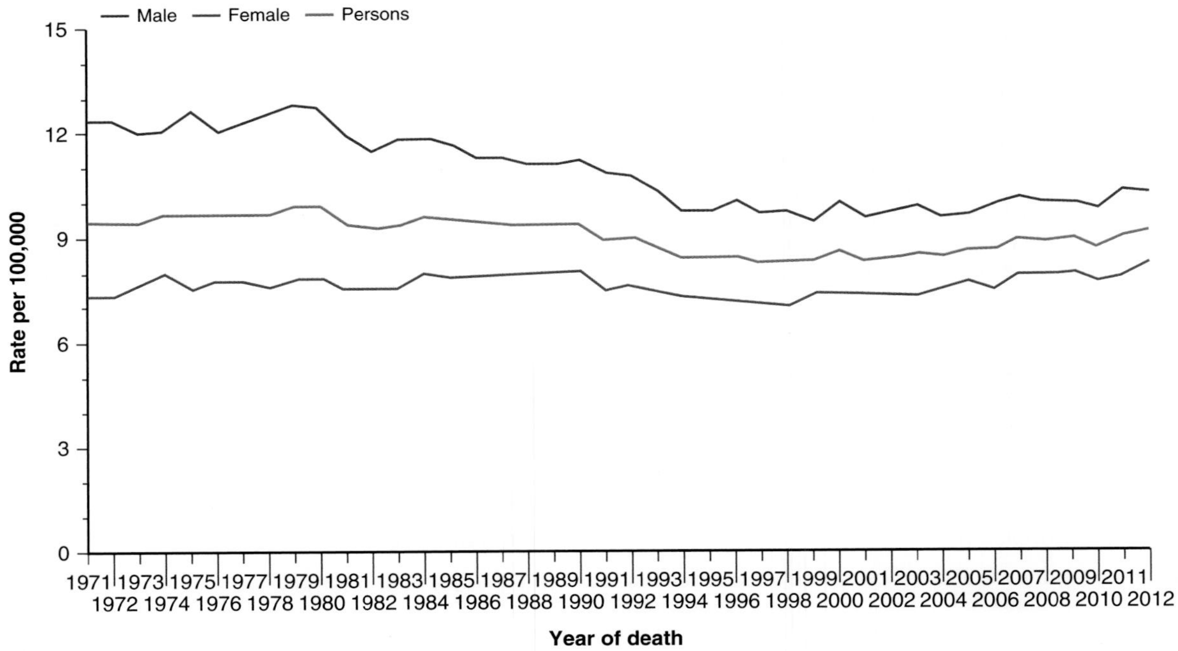

Figure 73-4. European age-standardized mortality rates from pancreatic cancer in the United Kingdom, 1971-2012. *(From Cancer Research UK: Pancreatic cancer mortality statistics.* http://www.cancerresearchuk. *org/cancer-info/cancerstats/types/pancreas/mortality/uk-pancreatic-cancer-mortality-statistics. Accessed December 3, 2015.)*

Pancreatic ductal adenocarcinoma has the lowest 5-year survival rate for all cancers, 3.6% for men and 3.8% for women in the United Kingdom, with a 2% to 9% 5-year survival rate in Europe.[22] The mortality rate is similar to its incidence, reflecting low survival.[19] Fortunately, the mortality rate for pancreatic cancer has decreased in the United Kingdom since the 1970s[19] (Figure 73-4).

Some risk factors that have been reported for pancreatic adenocarcinoma include age, alcohol, blood group A, chronic pancreatitis, diabetes mellitus, exposure to acrylamide, ionizing radiation, obesity, red meat, smoking, possible relationship to increased body mass index (BMI), and genetic factors (e.g., aerodigestive and reproductive cancers, presence of the *BRCA2* gene, familial atypical multiple mole melanoma syndrome, Peutz-Jeghers syndrome, von Hippel–Lindau syndrome, hereditary nonpolyposis colorectal cancer),[23,24] Also, certain infections may result in an increased risk, such as hepatitis, *Helicobacter pylori*, and periodontal disease.[25] However, at present, no definitive causative agents have been discovered as a clear cause of pancreatic cancer.

Presentation. Approximately 85% of patients present with disseminated or locally advanced disease. Symptoms frequently include epigastric or back pain, anorexia, weight loss, and obstructive jaundice.[26]

Pain. Pain can be caused by tumor compression of surrounding structures, tumor size, invasion of pancreatic nerves, and invasion of the anterior pancreatic capsule. Pain intensity at presentation has been found to correlate with survival (29 months for patients without pain, 9 months for those with severe pain).[27] Back pain may predict unresectability and shortened survival after resection.[28]

Weight Loss. Weight loss is a common presenting symptom and can be due to anorexia, catabolic metabolism, or malabsorption; however, weight loss is also a common and nonspecific symptom, especially in older patients.

Jaundice. Sixty percent to 70% of pancreatic adenocarcinomas affect the head of the pancreas. These patients often present with obstructive jaundice due to compression of the biliary tract.[21]

Other. Tumors of the body and tail of the pancreas are frequently associated with late presentation and inoperability. When an older patient presents with a new diagnosis of diabetes mellitus, the presence of an underlying pancreatic cancer should be considered, especially if the patient has other suggestive symptoms. A tumor has been found to be the underlying cause in 1% of patients older than 50 years who have been diagnosed with diabetes.[29] Other presentations may include acute pancreatitis and acute upper gastrointestinal or retroperitoneal hemorrhage.[21]

Diagnosis

The investigations performed in suspected pancreatic cancer are undertaken with the following aims:

- Establishing the diagnosis
- Locating the tumor
- Staging the tumor
- Assessing resectability
- Obtaining a tissue diagnosis

Blood Tests

Serum Antigens. Cancer antigen 19-9 (CA 19-9) is a glycoprotein synthesized by pancreatic cancer cells that is also produced by normal epithelial cells of the pancreas, bile ducts, stomach, and colon.[30] It has been found to have a sensitivity of 70% to 90% and specificity of 75% to 90% for pancreatic cancer, but its level is also elevated in obstructive jaundice, chronic pancreatitis, and biliary and gastrointestinal cancers.[30,31] Although tumor markers cannot actually confirm a diagnosis, they are particularly useful later in the patient's management when a rise in the CA19-9 level, especially if it originally decreased after treatment, may indicate a recurrence. It is not useful as a screening test.[32] Other tumor markers such as carcinoembryonic antigen (CEA) and cancer antigen 125 (CA-125) have limited use due to lower sensitivity and specificity.[31]

However, newer, more sensitive biomarkers are being developed. Serum, bile, salivary, and stool biomarkers based on RNA and new proteins based on proteomic studies, along with those developed as a result of genomic and epigenetic studies, have been shown to be a promising avenue but still require large studies to validate their results.[33]

Imaging

Transabdominal Ultrasound. Transabdominal US is frequently the first-line imaging investigation performed in the older patient presenting with upper abdominal symptoms. The results are variable and are dependent on the operator, patient's body habitus, and presence of overlying gas-filled bowel loops. The sensitivity of diagnosing pancreatic cancer with US ranges from 44% to 95%.[30,34,35] The highest sensitivities have been found in groups in which patients were not scanned on an intention to treat basis, and difficult scans were excluded from the analysis.

Computed Tomography. CT is considered the imaging modality of choice in pancreatic cancer because it can give additional staging information by imaging the chest, abdomen, and pelvis and can provide more detailed information regarding the resectability of pancreatic tumors. Helical CT has been found to be very effective in detecting and staging adenocarcinoma, with a sensitivity of up to 97% for detection and up to 100% accuracy in predicting unresectability, although it is not as good at predicting resectability.[36]

When directly compared with endoscopic ultrasound (EUS) and MRI in a cohort of patients deemed fit for surgery, CT had the highest accuracy in assessing the extent of the primary tumor (73%), locoregional extension (74%), vascular invasion (83%), and tumor resectability (83%).[37] Pancreatic CT should be conducted using a pancreatic protocol modality, which is a multiphase imaging technique that captures images during the noncontrast phase, arterial phase, late arterial phase, and portal venous phase within thin tomograms (3 mm) for precise delineation of any pancreatic lesion and assessment of vascular involvement.[38] The value of CT in predicting resectability, however, can be as low as 38%, with patients predicted to have resectable disease on CT found to be unresectable at laparotomy; the most common causes of unresectability include liver metastases and vascular involvement of the tumor.[36] The contrast medium used for CT is potentially nephrotoxic, patients must be well hydrated, and the serum creatinine level checked because this may be a problem, especially in older patients in whom renal impairment is more common.

Magnetic Resonance Imaging. MRI is comparable to CT in assessing the extent of vascular and lymphatic involvement but may be more sensitive in detecting hepatic and peritoneal disease.[38] Magnetic resonance cholangiopancreatography (MRCP) has been shown to be as diagnostically effective as endoscopic retrograde cholangiopancreatography (ERCP) in patients with symptoms suggestive of pancreatic cancer (84% sensitivity, 97% specificity).[39] MRCP has the added advantage of fewer complications, compared with ERCP, although a number of older patients are unable to tolerate the confined space in an MRI scanner.

Endoscopic Retrograde Cholangiopancreatography. In the diagnosis of cancer of the pancreas, ERCP has a sensitivity and specificity of 70% and 94%[39] and offers the opportunity to obtain a cytologic diagnosis by sampling bile or taking brushings. The value of such sampling can be questionable, however, because a sensitivity of only 60% has been reported, with a specificity of 98%.[40] ERCP can have serious complications, such as pancreatitis, cholangitis, hemorrhage, and death. In addition to being an investigative tool, especially in older patients, ERCP can be used for treatment, such as stent placement, and may be the treatment of choice, rather than resection.

Endoscopic Ultrasound. EUS has been rapidly growing in importance. The high-frequency ultrasound probe positioned in the stomach and duodenum allows high-resolution imaging of the pancreas and surrounding tissue. The accuracy of EUS in evaluating tumor and nodal status has been found to be 69% and 54%, respectively,[41] and EUS has been found to be at least as valuable as CT[42] and equal if not superior to CT for evaluating vascular invasion.[43]

EUS also offers the opportunity of performing fine needle aspiration of the tumor to aid diagnosis. However, in potentially resectable patients, this should generally only be performed via the duodenum rather than the stomach because the duodenum will be removed during resection, and there have been concerns regarding seeding malignant cells in the needle track.

Positron Emission Tomography. Positron emission tomography (PET) exploits the increased glucose metabolism observed in malignant tumors, which has been found by administering a radioactive glucose analogue and then scanning for increased uptake by tumor cells. PET images may be captured concurrently with CT images to aid in localizing any accumulation of tracer. PET is useful in diagnosing small (<2 cm) tumors and has sensitivity and specificity as good as that of EUS, ERCP, and US. It is particularly useful in detecting distant metastasis—for example, cervical nodes.[44] Currently, PET with or without CT is not superior over MRI or CT alone in diagnosing pancreatic cancer but is useful in staging and predicting survival.[45]

Management

Resectable Disease

The only curative treatment for pancreatic cancer is surgical resection, and the proportion of patients considered to be resectable has increased[26] due to the development of new techniques and oncologic management.[46-49] Preoperative imaging is useful for determining clearly inoperable tumors but, at operation, more will be found to be inoperable because of local or distant involvement of other tissue.

For consideration as being resectable on imaging, there should be no involvement of the superior mesenteric artery or celiac axis and no evidence of distant metastasis. Recent consensus has suggested that resection is possible in selected patients with short segment venous occlusion in the superior mesenteric vein or portal venous axis, and possibly even arterial involvement. Such radical surgery does not appear to result in a significant increase in morbidity nor, however, an increase in survival.[49] The absence of improvement in survival rate may be related to undetectable distant metastasis and local spread.[50]

In the jaundiced patient, ERCP for stenting prior to surgery had no benefit on morbidity and mortality compared to the nonintervention group.[51] However, when morbidity is scrutinized, it was noted that in the stent group, the postoperative complications were lower but there was a higher preoperative complication rate; patients had an increased risk of cholangitis.[51]

Surgical options for resecting cancer of the head of the pancreas include distal pancreatectomy, the traditional Whipple pancreaticoduodenectomy, or a pylorus-preserving pancreaticoduodenectomy (PPPD). PPPD involves dividing the bile duct close to the liver hilum, dividing the duodenum 2 cm beyond the pylorus, dissecting the pancreas off the superior mesenteric vein, and dividing the pancreas between the head and neck, with division of the small bowel at the duodenal-jejunal flexure. The reconstruction then involves three anastomoses—restoring gut continuity by a pylorus-jejunal anastomosis, connecting the stump of the bile duct to the jejunum just distal to the pylorus-jejunal anastomosis, and a pancreatic anastomosis. We prefer a pancreaticogastric anastomosis rather than the alternative pancreaticojejunal anastomosis, but the published leakage rate of this technique is up to 10% in some series.[52] Currently, most surgeons use the technique that gives them good results in their hands.

The Whipple procedure differs in that a distal gastrectomy is also performed. It would be expected to cause possible long-term morbidity due to gastric dumping, marginal ulceration, and bile reflux gastritis when compared to the PPPD. There have been questions regarding the adequacy of resection in a PPPD, but a Cochrane review in 2011 demonstrated no significant difference between a Whipple procedure and PPPD in terms of in-hospital mortality, overall survival, and morbidity, apart from shorter operative time in the PPPD.[48]

The overall complication rate for PPPD is around 39%, with mortality ranging from 0% to 7%.[48,53,54] Early complications, including postoperative bleeding and bile leak, have been quoted at rates of 4.8% and 1.2%, respectively, in a meta-analysis.[48]

Other significant early complications of particular importance in older adults due to preexisting comorbidities include cardiac and respiratory complications; older patients have been shown to be treated for significantly more cardiac events following PPPD (13% vs. 0.5%).[55] Late complications related to the nature of the operation include delayed gastric emptying, which occurs in 29% of PPPD patients, and pancreatic fistula in 7.2%.[48] A surrogate marker for significant complications is the necessity for reoperation, which is required in 9.9% of patients.[48] Pancreatic endocrine function is generally maintained,[56] and pancreatic exocrine function should be assessed by measuring fecal elastase levels, because malabsorption will result in malnutrition postoperatively.[57]

Surgery for cancer of the body and tail of the pancreas is less frequently performed because patients usually have only nonspecific symptoms, and a diagnosis is often only made when the tumor is inoperable. When a distal pancreatectomy is possible, it involves dissecting the pancreas off the superior mesenteric vein (SMV), dividing the pancreas, and oversewing the cut end. A splenectomy is also performed in cancer operations to ensure as much oncologic clearance as possible. With the development of more advanced surgical techniques, laparoscopic surgery can now be performed in more complex cases. Compared to open distal pancreatectomy, the laparoscopic procedure is associated with less blood loss and therefore a lower transfusion rate, fewer wound infections, lower morbidity, and shorter hospital length of stay, without any compromise in oncologic outcome.[47]

With advancing technology, robotic surgery has now been tested in pancreatectomy. A recent systematic review on robotic pancreatectomy has suggested that it is comparable to open pancreatectomy and laparoscopic pancreatectomy, with a conversion rate of 14%, mortality rate of 2%, morbidity rate of 58%, and only a 7.3% reoperation rate.[58]

The question of the appropriateness of performing surgery of such magnitude in an older patient is an important one. The patient should be evaluated on an individual basis with regard to comorbidities and fitness for an anesthetic, possibly using assessments such as POSSUM (a multifactorial scoring system)[59] and cardiopulmonary exercise testing (CPEX), which defines the physiologic stress level at which the patient becomes anaerobic.[60] Patients must be made fully aware that their short-term function and nutritional condition may be compromised after a major pancreatic resection.[55]

It has been demonstrated that patients older than 75 years undergoing pancreatic surgery for cancer, when compared with patients younger than 75 years, have an increased mortality rate (10% compared with 7%), are more frequently admitted to the intensive care unit (ICU) unplanned (47% compared with 20%), are treated for more cardiac events (13% vs. 0.5%), are more likely to have a compromised nutritional and feeding status, and are more likely to be transferred for further nursing care prior to discharge home.[55] In older patients, it is particularly important to consider the potential impact of surgery on the quality of life and the need for prolonged rehabilitation. The operative mortality for pancreatic cancer surgery has been shown to increase with advancing age—7% at 65 to 69 years, 9% at 70 to 79 years, and 16% at 80+ years.[61] Some studies, however, when looking at significant predictors of survival, have not found age to be an independent variable.[62,63]

Unresectable Disease

For patients with unresectable disease, the three most important symptoms for palliation are pain, jaundice, and gastric outlet obstruction (GOO). A multidisciplinary team consisting of representatives from surgery, medical oncology, gastroenterology, radiology, and palliative care medicine is essential for the optimal palliation of symptoms.[64]

Pain. The World Health Organization (WHO) approach to pain management in patients with advanced cancer is still recommended,[65] and analgesics should be titrated according to the three-step analgesic ladder: (1) nonopioids, including nonsteroidal antiinflammatory drugs (NSAIDs); (2) weak opioids; and (3) strong opioids. Attention should be paid to the route of administration in pancreatic cancer patients because GOO may be present and the absorption of oral analgesics may be unpredictable.

In patients with severe pain, a celiac plexus block (CPB) with neurolytic solutions may provide analgesia by interrupting visceral afferent pain transmission from the upper abdomen. This can be performed percutaneously, surgically (at the time of laparotomy or bypass), or under EUS guidance. In a prospective, randomized, double-blinded placebo-controlled trial, percutaneous CPB with absolute alcohol has been shown to improve pain relief significantly in patients with unresectable pancreatic cancer compared with opioids, although CPB did not affect quality of life or survival.[66] The major complications from percutaneous CPB include lower extremity weakness, paresthesias, lumbar puncture, and pneumothorax at a rate of 1%. The technique of EUS-guided CPB has become more popular and has been found to be safe and effective in pancreatic cancer.[67,68]

Jaundice. Jaundice can have severe consequences, including intolerable itching, liver dysfunction, and eventually hepatic failure due to bile stasis and cholangitis[69]; relief of the jaundice has been shown to result in a dramatic increase in quality of life.[70] Biliary drainage can be achieved by endoscopic or percutaneous placement of a biliary stent or by a surgical biliary-enteric anastomosis. Biliary stents are plastic (Teflon, polyethylene) or are made of an expandable metal meshwork. Plastic stents are associated with a higher complication rate, including migration, blockage, and infection, although they can be replaced and are less expensive, whereas metal stents have a significantly longer time to first blockage but cannot be removed and are not recommended for patients with a prognosis more than 2 years because of metal fatigue.[69,71] This issue may be more significant in stenting for benign pancreatic disease with jaundice.

Percutaneous stenting is often performed if endoscopic stent placement was difficult or impossible in patients with hilar obstruction, bilateral or multiple strictures, or previous upper gastrointestinal tract surgery. Metal percutaneous stenting provides good palliation, with a procedure-related morbidity of

9%.[72] The choice of an endoscopic or percutaneous approach may depend on local expertise.

A Cochrane review of palliative biliary stents for obstructing pancreatic carcinoma has concluded that based on a meta-analysis, endoscopic stenting with plastic stents appears to be associated with a reduced risk of complications but a higher risk of recurrent biliary obstruction prior to death when compared with surgery.[73] No trials comparing endoscopic metal stents to surgery were identified.

Gastric Outlet Obstruction. A number of patients with unresectable pancreatic cancer will develop functional or mechanical GOO, which can be caused by a dysfunction of gastric or duodenal motility due to celiac nerve plexus infiltration by tumor or duodenal blockage due to tumor infiltration of the wall and lumen. These cases should be fully assessed radiologically with a video contrast meal to assess motility and the existence of tumor blockage prior to planning treatment. For mechanical blockage, surgical gastrojejunostomy can be performed laparoscopically or at open operation. It should, however, be performed at the time of laparotomy or laparoscopy if the intended resection of a pancreatic cancer is not found to be possible, and it may be combined with a biliary bypass. GOO is significantly lower if prophylactic gastrojejunostomy has been performed.[74] Two methods of preempting GOO were studied by comparing two groups that underwent single bypass (hepaticojejunostomy) or double bypass (hepaticojejunostomy and retrocolic gastrojejunostomy). It was found that there was a significantly higher incidence of GOO in the single bypass group (41% vs. 5%), with no significant difference in length of stay, survival, or quality of life.[75]

However, it is pointless trying to drain a stomach that is paralyzed from tumor invasion. Pharmacologic agents such as metoclopramide or erythromycin may occasionally be helpful in this situation.

Endoscopic palliation with a self-expanding metal duodenal stent is an option in GOO. It has been found to be simple and effective, with no complications related to insertion of the stent and a 93% reported improvement in symptoms.[76] Subsequent stent obstruction was observed in 11% of patients.

Chemoradiotherapy

Chemotherapy with or without radiotherapy can be used as an adjuvant treatment in patients following attempted curative resection for pancreatic cancer or as a primary treatment in advanced or metastatic pancreatic cancer. The decision to recommend chemotherapy or chemoradiotherapy for the older patient with pancreatic cancer should be made after careful evaluation of the patient's health status, comorbidities and quality of life, and consideration that physiologic decline and alterations in pharmacodynamics may make the older patient more susceptible to the complications of cytotoxic medication.[77]

The role of adjuvant chemotherapy following curative resection for carcinoma of the pancreas still remains controversial. A meta-analysis of randomized controlled trials has estimated a prolongation of median survival time of 3 months for patients in the chemotherapy group but there was no difference in the 5-year survival.[78] A randomized controlled trial specifically looking at the impact of gemcitabine in patients following gross complete resection of pancreatic cancer demonstrated an improved disease-free survival of 7.5 months, with no difference in overall survival or quality of life.[79]

When comparing chemotherapy alone with combined radiotherapy and chemotherapy, gemcitabine with radiotherapy appears to improve survival compared to gemcitabine alone, but with a higher incidence of significant toxicity.[80] Comparing two different chemoradiotherapy regimens, gemcitabine with radiotherapy patients had longer survival (median, 10.2 to 12.5 months), with no increased complications as compared with 5-fluorouracil (5-FU) with radiotherapy.[81]

The evidence for chemotherapy and chemoradiotherapy specifically in older adults with advanced pancreatic cancer has been limited to retrospective evaluations of patients who had been considered suitable for therapy. Chemotherapy with gemcitabine-based regimens was found to be as acceptable in patients older than 70 as in those younger than 70 years, with no difference in overall survival, but older patients required dose reduction and experienced increased toxicity.[77] Chemoradiotherapy (5-FU and radiotherapy) was also found to be acceptable in those older than 70 years, with no difference in toxicity and an actual increase in median survival for older patients (11.3 vs. 9.5 months).

Other Solid Tumors

Solid Pseudopapillary Neoplasm. These usually occur in young women and are generally benign, but can undergo malignant change. They should be treated by resection, which results in an excellent prognosis.[82]

Acinar Cell Carcinoma. Most of these are malignant and may have pancreatic exocrine enzyme function. This group of carcinomas has a slightly better prognosis compared to ductal adenocarcinoma; the 5-year survival of acinar cell carcinomas ranges from 25% to 50% compared to 3% to 25% for ductal adenocarcinomas.[8]

Neuroendocrine Tumors. Pancreatic neuroendocrine tumors (pNETs) are rare, with an incidence of 1 to 2/1,000,000 population.[83] They have a median age of presentation of 57 years.[84] pNETs are a heterogeneous group of tumors that can be classified according to functionality, tumor localization, rate of proliferation, and metastatic disease.[85] The WHO classification has defined two types of significant pNETs, well-differentiated neuroendocrine tumors (NETs) and well-differentiated neuroendocrine carcinoma (NECs), with NETs comprising 1% to 2% of pancreatic cancers and NECs less than <1%.[8] The 5-year survival rate for NETs is 65%, and the survival rate for NECs ranges from 1 to 12 months.[8]

Management is controversial and includes surgery, chemotherapy, octreotide therapy, interferon-α, and peptide receptor radionuclide therapy. The main goal of surgery is curative resection of tumor, but other indications include relief of symptoms from hormone-secreting tumors or obstruction.[85]

ACUTE PANCREATITIS

Acute pancreatitis is an acute inflammatory process of the pancreas, with variable involvement of the other regional tissues or remote organs.[86] It is a potentially fatal disease, and the incidence in the United Kingdom has been increasing, although the mortality rate has decreased. Incidence and mortality increase with age[87] (Figure 73-5).

Causes

Acute pancreatitis has multiple causes; gallstones (44 to 54%) and alcohol (3 % to 19%) are the predominant causes in the United Kingdom although, in the older population, gallstone disease is the most common cause.[87] Drugs are responsible for a small proportion (≈5%) of cases of acute pancreatitis; because the older patient is more likely to be prescribed medications such as furosemide, NSAIDs, steroids, antibiotics, or cancer drugs, this should be considered as a possible causative factor. Other causes include hypertriglyceridemia, hyperparathyroidism, trauma, and infection. There has been accumulating evidence

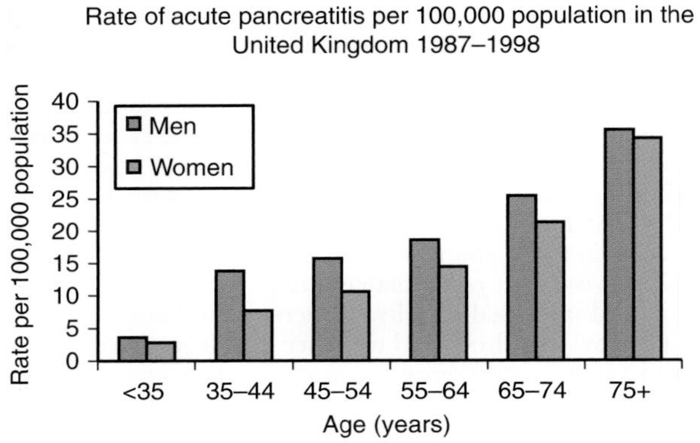

Figure 73-5. Rate of acute pancreatitis by age group. United Kingdom, 1987-1998. *(Data derived from Goldacre MJ, Roberts SE: Hospital admission for acute pancreatitis in an English population, 1963-98: database study of incidence and mortality. BMJ 328(7454):1466-1469, 2004.)*

TABLE 73-1 Glasgow Pancreatitis Scoring System*

Parameter	Value
Albumin	<32 g/L
WCC	>15,000/mm^3
LDH	>600 units/L
AST/ALT	>200 units/L
Glucose	10 mmol/L
Calcium	<2 mmol/L
Urea	>16 mmol/L
pO_2	<8 kPa

ALT, Alanine aminotransferase; *AST,* aspartate aminotransferase; *LDH,* lactate dehydrogenase; pO_2, partial pressure of oxygen; *WCC,* white blood cell count.

*The Glasgow scoring system includes 1 point for each of these parameters.

that the underlying cause of acute pancreatitis is premature intracellular activation of trypsin.[88]

Presentation

Abdominal pain and vomiting are the most common presenting symptoms of acute pancreatitis, and an elevation of the plasma amylase level (to four times normal) will often confirm the diagnosis. The serum amylase level peaks early and then declines over 3 to 4 days, so in a patient presenting late this peak may be missed. A raised serum lipase level is more specific for pancreatitis and persists for slightly longer. The amylase level may be increased for other reasons, such as acute gastrointestinal ischemia, gastrointestinal perforation, or a leaking abdominal aortic aneurysm. It should be noted that these conditions are also more common in the older patient.[89]

Assessment

Immediate assessment should include a clinical evaluation, blood tests (including complete blood count, liver, bone, and renal profiles, blood glucose level), chest x-ray, and any other tests necessary (e.g., echocardiography, spirometry) because of comorbidities present in the older patient. It is important to determine the severity of an attack of acute pancreatitis to help predict outcome and manage the patient in a suitable setting; care in an ICU is recommended for patients with severe acute pancreatitis.[90,91] There are several methods available for assessing severity: the Ranson[92] and Imrie or Glasgow method[93] are specific acute pancreatitis scoring systems based on a range of factors, with a score of 3 or more predicting a severe attack (Table 73-1). APACHE II is based on an assessment of acute physiology and chronic health. It is more complicated to calculate than Imrie or Ranson scores but can give an accurate initial prediction of severity; a score higher than 8 predicts a severe attack.[90] Additionally, it may be used repeatedly to assess the progress of a patient.[94] Trypsinogen activation peptide (TAP)[95] and C-reactive protein (CRP)[96] tests are based on the assay of a single marker and are useful adjuncts to assessing severity. The British Society of Gastroenterology (BSG) guidelines have recommended that APACHE II be performed on admission and the Glasgow score calculated at 48 hours.[90]

Abdominal ultrasound is useful in acute pancreatitis to confirm the presence of gallstones or bile duct dilation. However, gas-filled loops of bowel overlying the pancreas will often diminish the value of these images, so contrast-enhanced US may be more helpful.[97] Early CT is occasionally indicated for diagnosis if clinical or biochemical findings are inconclusive, and an alternative diagnosis needs to be excluded. Abdominal contrast-enhanced CT is most useful in acute pancreatitis 6 to 10 days after admission to look for pancreatic necrosis in patients with persisting organ failure, signs of sepsis or clinical deterioration.[90] A combination of clinical, biochemical, and radiologic evaluation should be used to assess the severity of every pancreatitis case.[98] The Balthazar score is a CT severity index that grades the severity of pancreatitis and extent of necrosis[98]; it differs from the Atlanta classification, which is used to standardize pancreatitis nomenclature in terms of type, severity, and complications.[99]

Management

Approximately 75% of acute pancreatitis is mild and is usually self-limiting, requiring simple supportive management.[100] Severe acute pancreatitis, however, can produce a systemic inflammatory response syndrome (SIRS) and subsequent multiorgan dysfunction syndrome (MODS). The principles of management in severe acute pancreatitis (SAP) are, therefore, to support each organ system and establish appropriate monitoring to detect deterioration or the onset of complications, which may need some form of intervention. Older or obese patients should also be managed in an ICU.[101]

For the management of gallstone pancreatitis, patients with severe pancreatitis and proven choledocholithiasis should undergo ERCP and stone extraction within 72 hours of presentation; those with mild biliary pancreatitis should undergo a cholecystectomy within 2 weeks of initial presentation without prior ERCP.[102] Delays in cholecystectomy should be avoided because there is an increased risk of recurrent pancreatitis.[103] In patients with pancreatitis with concurrent cholangitis, ERCP is recommended, especially when sepsis is not controlled with antibiotics.[102] However, ERCP should only be conducted in carefully selected older patients because the severity of complications is much greater than in younger patients.[104]

Renal System

Adequate and timely intravenous fluid (IV) replacement lowers the risk of developing renal insufficiency and failure. Rapid or aggressive fluid resuscitation can be difficult in the older patient who may have underlying cardiac or respiratory compromise.[105] Hemofiltration or hemodialysis may be necessary if renal failure develops.

Respiratory System

Respiratory failure is the most frequently encountered single-organ malfunction in SAP, and all patients should receive oxygen therapy and monitoring, with oxygen saturation, arterial blood gas sampling, clinical evaluation, and radiologic investigation. Intervention with positive pressure ventilation may be required and, in severe cases, high-frequency ventilation may be indicated.

Cardiac System

Cardiac failure is more commonly seen in those with preexisting cardiac problems, including hypertension, myocardial infarction, and atrial fibrillation, and is therefore more common in older patients. Inotropic support is often needed in these patients.

Gut

Gut anoxia and the inflammatory syndrome can result in intestinal barrier failure and subsequent bacterial translocation, which has been suggested as a factor in the development of infected pancreatic necrosis. Enteral nutrition has been recommended by the BSG guidelines (2005) and the International Association of Pancreatology with the American Pancreatic Association because it may help preserve gut mucosal barrier function[90,91] as compared to parenteral nutrition. Enteral feeding may be nasojejunal or, if the stomach is emptying, nasogastric. If the stomach is not draining, nasogastric aspiration should be used to manage the gastric stasis.[106] A recent meta-analysis has suggested that the enteral route is superior to the parenteral approach in terms of mortality rate, multiorgan failure rate, systemic infection, and necessity of operative intervention for pancreatitis complications.[107] The recommended timing for initiating enteral feed is within 24 hours of hospital admission.[108] In the case of older adults, this aspect bears emphasis, given their greater risk of malnutrition in the hospital.

Other Considerations

The inflammatory response alters capillary permeability and results in edema and hypovolemia.[109] As noted, aggressive IV fluid replacement should be initiated in the patient with SAP,[110] and the cardiovascular response should be monitored with, for example, central venous pressure measurement, Swan-Ganz catheter, pulse contour computer (PiCCO; Philips),[111] and urinary output measurement. Although there is an absence of high-level evidence that the administration of prophylactic antibiotics is beneficial in necrotizing pancreatitis, subgroup analysis in a meta-analysis has stated that imipenem results in a significant reduction in infection rates.[112] However, the use of antibiotics compared to controls showed no significant reduction in mortality.[112]

Older patients can have nonobvious preexisting organ dysfunction, so the risk of complications and mortality may be different in individuals of the same age.[113] Thus, their capacity to tolerate an insult such as SAP is limited, which is reflected by their higher incidence of organ failure (64% vs. 48%).[114]

Management of Pancreatic Necrosis. Nonperfusion of the pancreas on contrast-enhanced CT suggests pancreatic necrosis and, along with the presence of a peripancreatic fluid collection, indicates a poor prognosis.[98] A definition of necrosis was provided in the Atlanta classification, and an attempt to standardize the nomenclature has been published.[99] It is important to determine if the necrosis is infected because sterile necrosis can be left to resolve on its own.[115] Infection may be confirmed by CT- guided needle aspiration. Untreated infected necrosis is almost always fatal, and the necrosis must be débrided and drained at open operation or by a minimally invasive technique.[100,101]

Management of Fluid Collections. Fluid collections, which differ from pseudocysts, can occur within or adjacent to the inflamed pancreas—that is, within the lesser sac or elsewhere in the abdomen, remote from the pancreas. The former is defined as a fluid collection located in or near the pancreas and lacks a defined wall at less than 4 weeks from the episode of pancreatitis, whereas the latter is a collection of fluid following acute pancreatitis, with a defined wall after 4 weeks.[116] There is much controversy in the literature concerning the management of these collections.[86,99] In essence, sterile collections will often resolve, whereas an infected collection (a pancreatic abscess) will need drainage by open operation, endoscopy, or minimally invasive technique; the choice often depends on local expertise and preference.[90,91]

A recent prospective study has suggested that patients with small fluid collections (<4 cm) with mild or no symptoms do not require any intervention other than a follow-up review at 3 months.[116] If the collections have not resolved and the patient becomes symptomatic, percutaneous or surgical intervention can be pursued.

Conclusions

Pancreatitis is more likely to be severe in the older patient, which contributes to the higher mortality rates observed in older patients—2.7 deaths/100 patients in those 45 to 54 years old compared with 18.9% in those 75 years of age or older.[117] Patients with SAP, especially the older patient in whom there may be complicating comorbidities, should be managed in a specialist unit by experienced intensivists and pancreatic surgeons. For patients who survive long term, management of complications such as diabetes and malabsorption caused by destruction of the pancreas will require specialist examination. Attempts must be made to determine the cause of the pancreatitis to try to prevent further attacks. In patients with gallstone pancreatitis, cholecystectomy or ERCP and duct clearance is required.

CHRONIC PANCREATITIS

Chronic pancreatitis is an inflammatory disease resulting in progressive irreversible destruction of the pancreatic parenchyma affecting exocrine and endocrine function. Onset is typically in the fourth decade, with a strong male predominance; presentation in those older than 65 years is rare.[118] Chronic pancreatitis shortens life expectancy by 10 to 20 years and is therefore not typically a disease of the older patient.[118]

Causes and Symptoms

In up to 80% of cases of chronic pancreatitis (CP), the cause is alcohol-related,[119] and long-term alcohol consumption (>35 years) increases the risk of developing CP.[120] The remaining 20% of cases of chronic pancreatitis can be attributed to tropical CP, hereditary CP, pancreatic strictures, pancreas divisum, pancreatic trauma, or idiopathic CP. Idiopathic senile chronic pancreatitis is a subtype of idiopathic CP that presents after the age of 50 years and is more prevalent in older patients.[121] Various theories have been proposed about the mechanisms of cell destruction, inflammation, fibrosis, and atrophy seen in CP, but this is still controversial.

The predominant symptoms of CP include pain, typically remitting and relapsing, exocrine dysfunction characterized by weight loss and malabsorption secondary to steatorrhea, and endocrine dysfunction manifesting as diabetes mellitus. Patients often present with symptoms related to the complications of chronic pancreatitis, which include pseudocysts, ductal calculi, distal bile duct strictures, pancreatic duct strictures, and duodenal stenosis.

Diagnosis

The diagnosis of chronic pancreatitis can be difficult but the clinical history and examination, biochemical tests, and radiologic investigations should be used in combination. Fecal elastase is a useful test to confirm pancreatic exocrine failure and has increasing sensitivity with increasing severity of disease. Other pancreatic exocrine function tests are possible, but are more unreliable and generally are not used.

The role of imaging in CP is diagnostic and therapeutic. US can be used to demonstrate changes in pancreatic tissue and the ductal system; however, CT has greater sensitivity in identifying pancreatic atrophy, pancreatic calcification, dilation of the pancreatic duct, and pseudocysts, which are typically seen in chronic pancreatitis. MRCP is a useful noninvasive method for imaging the biliary and pancreatic ductal system, especially if the pancreatic duct is dilated, and the administration of secretin can improve duct visualization. ERCP can provide similar images and has the advantage of offering therapeutic interventions, including sphincterotomy, dilation of strictures, extraction of calculi, and stenting, although these procedures have a complication rate of 5% to 10%.[122] EUS has become a useful tool for the diagnosis of CP, particularly in the early stages,[123] and is useful therapeutically in celiac plexus blockade, drainage of pseudocysts, and obtaining a tissue diagnosis. The incidence of pancreatic cancer is increased in chronic pancreatitis, and radiologic imaging may be used to distinguish between the two diseases, although this can be difficult. The conclusion is often equivocal,[124] and many patients will be found to be inoperable when they are diagnosed.

Management and Prognosis

The treatment of patients with CP initially involves symptom control, and the goal should be to improve quality of life. Pain should be initially treated with analgesics according to the analgesic ladder but, if this becomes intractable, celiac plexus block can be considered, operatively, percutaneously, or endoscopically.

The main indications for surgery in CP are intractable pain, suspicion of malignancy, and involvement of adjacent organs. It is recommended that surgery should be individualized according to pancreatic anatomy (small or large duct), pain characteristics, exocrine and endocrine function, and medical comorbidities.[125] In the older patient, careful consideration should be given to the risks and benefits of what is potentially major and complicated surgery. Options include gastrojejunostomy, feeding jejunostomy, PPPD, Whipple procedure, total pancreatectomy, lateral pancreaticojejunostomy (Puestow procedure), duodenum-preserving pancreatic head resection (Beger procedure), and local resection of the pancreatic head with longitudinal pancreaticojejunostomy (Frey procedure).

The nutritional status of a patient with CP should be carefully assessed and addressed with appropriate feeding and supplements, and exocrine insufficiency should be managed with enzyme supplements. Endocrine dysfunction may require referral to a diabetologist.

The prognosis for patients with CP is poor, with a 20-year survival of 45% and a significantly worse survival for older patients and those with alcoholic CP.[126]

Pancreatic Ductal Stones as a Consequence of Chronic Pancreatitis

Acute pancreatitis as a result of pancreatic ductal stones is extremely rare. It is usually a result of chronic pancreatitis, and the stone(s) may exacerbate symptoms and complications.[127] Primary pancreatic stones itself is a rare phenomenon, with less than a 1% incidence.[128] The stones usually consist of calcium carbonate crystals that are predisposed to precipitation in chronic pancreatitis. This is a result of an imbalance in buffer chemicals and protein and also obstruction of outflow from the formation of strictures.[129] Resultant complications may include pain and recurrent pancreatitis.

Focus on obtaining proof of calcification is usually aimed at diagnosing chronic pancreatitis and complications as a result of ductal stones, rather than primarily searching for them. Investigations include abdominal x-ray, CT, MRCP, US, and ERCP.[130] Abdominal x-rays are simple and can detect calcification in up to 30% of those with chronic pancreatitis but cannot differentiate between parenchymal calcification and ductal stones.[129] Similarly, CT is a good modality to identify pancreatic calcification, but ERCP or MRCP is better at delineating the pancreatic tree and presence of intraductal stones.[129] Cross-sectional examination of patients with chronic pancreatitis is crucial to exclude concurrent malignancy, as noted previously.[131]

There is no evidence to show that asymptomatic intraductal stones require any treatment. In symptomatic patients, treatment options include symptomatic control with analgesia, endoscopic intervention for stone retrieval, noninvasive stone destruction with lithotripsy, and surgical drainage procedures.[132]

Analgesia that can be used for the control of symptoms ranges from simple analgesia to strong opiates. Adjuvant drugs such as amitriptyline, pregabalin, and gabapentin can be added, along with celiac axis block.[132] This initial management is usually the sole option available to older patients due to their frailty.

ERCP can only be conducted for stone retrieval in patients with three or fewer nonimpacted stones up to 10 mm in diameter and located in the body or head.[130] Stones can be removed by baskets, balloons, or forceps, along with a sphincterotomy.[129] As with any endoscopic procedure, there is the risk of precipitation pancreatitis, cholangitis, hemorrhage, and perforation. ERCP should only be considered in patients if they can tolerate sedation and are lying supine.

Intraductal stones can be pulverized or fragmented using extracorporeal shock wave lithotripsy (ESWL). Because most stones lie close to the ampulla of Vater, ERCP for stone retrieval can be performed but, if it fails, prior fragmentation with ESWL may be useful and sometimes may be the definitive treatment because the stone can be pulverized.[128,133] The success rate is about 58.6% with one or two sessions of ESWL.[133] In 82.8% of patients, a repeat ERCP was found to be necessary to remove the stone(s), and the combination of ESWL with ERCP resulted in 60% to 85% resolution of symptoms.[133,134] One randomized controlled trial has shown that ESWL is the preferred treatment for patients with painful chronic pancreatitis due to intraductal stones. Combining it with ERCP may not be beneficial may add to the cost and increase the risk of complications.[135]

Surgical intervention to treat symptomatic intraductal pancreatic stones are limited and high risk to older patients, especially if they have extensive comorbidities. Careful counseling and strict patient selection are required. The least extensive procedure is the video-assisted thoracoscopic splanchnicectomy.[132,136] The sympathetic nerves from thoracic levels 8 to 12 are identified thoracoscopically and cauterized. The initial success rate is high but declines over time, from 90% relief of symptoms at 6 months to only 49% after 15 months.[136] More invasive procedures, which are probably not appropriate for older adults, include lateral pancreaticojejunostomy (50% recurrence of symptoms, 5% mortality rate) and the various methods of pancreatectomy, as described. However, a randomized controlled trial has shown that the lateral pancreaticojejunostomy is superior to endoscopic intervention in terms of pain relief and requirement for repeated interventions.[137]

KEY POINTS: DUCTAL ADENOCARCINOMA

- Most common malignancy of the pancreas
- Poor survival compared with other cancers
- Patients typically present with epigastric or back pain, anorexia, weight loss, and jaundice
- Diagnosis and staging with CT, MRI, and EUS
- Only surgery curative, but is high risk, particularly in older adults

ACUTE PANCREATITIS

- Increasing incidence and morbidity with age
- Important to assess severity to predict outcome and guide management
- Important to identify cause
- Management is supportive

CHRONIC PANCREATITIS

- Uncommon in older adults
- Typically caused by alcohol
- Imaging with CT, MRCP, and ERCP

For a complete list of references, please visit www.expertconsult.com.

KEY REFERENCES

8. Hruban R, Boffetta P, Hiraoka N, et al: Tumours of the pancreas. In Bosman FT, Carneiro F, Hruban RH, et al, editors: WHO/IRC classification of tumours of the digestive system, ed 4, Geneva, Switzerland, 2010, World Health Organization.
19. Cancer Research UK: Pancreatic cancer mortality statistics. http://www.cancerresearchuk.org/cancer-info/cancerstats/types/pancreas/mortality/uk-pancreatic-cancer-mortality-statistics. Accessed December 3, 2015.
26. Shore S, Vimalachandran D, Raraty MG, et al: Cancer in the elderly: pancreatic cancer. Surg Oncol 13:201–210, 2004.
31. Duraker N, Hot S, Polat Y, et al: CEA, CA 19-9, and CA 125 in the differential diagnosis of benign and malignant pancreatic diseases with or without jaundice. J Surg Oncol 95:142–147, 2007.
37. Soriano A, Castells A, Ayuso C, et al: Preoperative staging and tumor resectability assessment of pancreatic cancer: prospective study comparing endoscopic ultrasonography, helical computed tomography, magnetic resonance imaging, and angiography. Am J Gastroenterol 99:492–501, 2004.
46. Gurusamy KS, Kumar S, Davidson BR, et al: Resection versus other treatments for locally advanced pancreatic cancer. Cochrane Database Syst Rev (2):CD010244, 2014.
50. Gooiker GA, Lemmens VE, Besselink MG, et al: Impact of centralization of pancreatic cancer surgery on resection rates and survival. Br J Surg 101:1000–1005, 2014.
69. Gouma DJ, Busch OR, Van Gulik TM: Pancreatic carcinoma: palliative surgical and endoscopic treatment. HPB (Oxford) 8:369–376, 2006.
77. Maréchal R, Demols A, Gay F, et al: Tolerance and efficacy of gemcitabine and gemcitabine-based regimens in elderly patients with advanced pancreatic cancer. Pancreas 36:e16–e21, 2008.
78. Boeck S, Ankerst DP, Heinemann V: The role of adjuvant chemotherapy for patients with resected pancreatic cancer: systematic review of randomized controlled trials and meta-analysis. Oncology 72:314–321, 2007.
87. Yadav D, Lowenfels AB: Trends in the epidemiology of the first attack of acute pancreatitis: a systematic review. Pancreas 33:323–330, 2006.
90. Working Party of the British Society of Gastroenterology; Association of Surgeons of Great Britain and Ireland; Pancreatic Society of Great Britain and Ireland; Association of Upper GI Surgeons of Great Britain and Ireland: UK guidelines for the management of acute pancreatitis. Gut 54(Suppl 3):iii1–iii9, 2005.
91. Working Group IAP/APA Acute Pancreatitis Guidelines: IAP/APA evidence-based guidelines for the management of acute pancreatitis. Pancreatology 13(Suppl 2):e1–e15, 2013.
98. Balthazar EJ: Acute pancreatitis: assessment of severity with clinical and CT evaluation. Radiology 223:603–613, 2002.
114. Gardner TB, Vege SS, Chari ST, et al: The effect of age on hospital outcomes in severe acute pancreatitis. Pancreatology 8:265–270, 2008.

74 The Liver

Arjun Sugumaran, Joanna Hurley, John Trevor Green

STRUCTURE AND FUNCTION

Many age-related changes in the structure and function of the healthy liver have been shown and may be of importance for clinical practice. Studies have confirmed a decrease in liver size up to 20% to 40% and reduction in hepatic blood flow to 30% to 50%.[1] In addition, a 50% age-related decline in DNA base excision repair in mouse hepatocytes has been reported.[2] Human and animal research has shown that recovery after liver damage is slow in older adult subjects, probably secondary to the previously mentioned factors, but the capacity for regeneration is preserved.[3] Also in the older population, a decrease in mass of functional hepatocytes but increased hepatocyte volume and life span has been observed.[4,5] With regard to hepatocyte structure, there is an increase in the nuclear size and polyploidy; mitochondrial respiratory chain capacity is reduced in humans probably related to accumulation of reactive oxygen species or somatic DNA mutations, but there is also a decreased number of mitochondria seen in the older adult human liver.[6] There are reports of thickening of the endothelial lining by 60% and an 80% decline in the number of endothelial cell fenestrations with increasing age.[7] The resultant implications are impairment of sinusoidal blood flow and hepatic perfusion, as well as reduced uptake of macromolecules such as lipoproteins from the blood,[2] which may contribute to hyperlipidemia and systemic vascular disease.[8] Hepatic secretion of cholesterol has been shown to increase with age, whereas bile flow and bile salt formation are reduced by 50%,[9] which could explain the increased incidence of choledocholithiasis with aging. Kupffer cells (macrophages with a major role in the removal of endotoxins) have impaired phagocytic activity with increasing age and could be the cause for increased susceptibility of older adult patients to sepsis from intraabdominal infection.[10] The term *brown atrophy* is used to describe the macroscopic change seen in the aging liver caused by accumulation of the brown pigment lipofuscin within the lysosomes of hepatocytes; the significance of this in humans is unclear. Studies in rodents suggest that this may contribute to hepatocyte dysfunction by impairing metabolism, secretion, or excretion.[8]

The structural changes with increasing age observed in human and animal studies do not appear to directly reflect any functional degeneration of the older adult liver. Certainly, there are no liver diseases specific to advancing age, unlike diseases of the musculoskeletal and cardiovascular systems.[11] Older adult patients with abnormal liver biochemical tests should be investigated in the same way as younger patients because these changes cannot be attributed to an aging liver. Serum concentrations of most liver enzymes, including serum albumin, remain unaltered,[10] but the effect of malnutrition, infections, or heart failure in older adults should be taken into account. The exception is alkaline phosphatase, which has been reported to increase by approximately 20% between the ages of 20 and 80,[12] probably as a result of leakage from bone into the blood. Values for serum bilirubin in some reports have been shown to be slightly decreased with increasing age, perhaps explained by an effect of reduced cellular muscle mass and decreased hemoglobin concentration.[13]

DRUG AND ALCOHOL METABOLISM

Polypharmacy is common in older adults as a result of multiple comorbidities. The effect of age on hepatic drug metabolism, unlike renal drug excretion, remains controversial, although it is widely perceived that there is a decline in the rate of clearance of drugs undergoing liver metabolism. This is more pronounced among drugs that undergo phase I metabolism. This can result in increased bioavailability of certain drugs that could lead to complications, especially if associated with renal dysfunction. Reductions in liver blood flow and mass with increasing age contribute to a reduced metabolism of rapidly cleared drugs such as propranolol, amitriptyline, verapamil, and morphine,[14] yet metabolism of drugs such as phenytoin and warfarin, cleared in this manner, are unchanged with age.[15] Animal studies have demonstrated impaired enzyme activity with a reduction in microsomal content of cytochrome P450 (CYP) during aging in mice; however, this has not been reproduced in most human studies.[14] Clearance of drugs such as ibuprofen, many benzodiazepines, imipramine, ropinirole, and citalopram have been shown to be reduced by 10% to 50% with increasing age.[15] Several studies of drug metabolism in nonalcoholic fatty liver disease (NAFLD) revealed near uniform downregulation of CYP enzyme 1A2 (CYP1A2), the enzyme that constitutes 13% of the hepatic CYPs and metabolizes 15% of all therapeutic drugs. Some data suggest that drug metabolism can be altered dependent on species, sex, or ethnicity.[16] Differentiation between frail and healthy older adults must be considered when interpreting data of drug metabolism. It has been demonstrated that clearance of paracetamol per unit body weight is significantly reduced in frail older adults when compared with age-matched fit subjects.[17] In addition, a reduction in the clearance of metoclopramide has also been described in frail, but not healthy, subjects older than 65 years.[18] Influence of disease states, environmental factors, and coadministration of other drugs have been postulated as important factors affecting variance of hepatic drug metabolism with aging.[15]

The physiologic effect of alcohol on the aging body differs from that in the young body.[19] Reduced hepatic blood flow, fewer hepatocytes, and reduced body water space result in a prolonged effect of alcohol and comparably higher serum levels in older adults.[20,21] Animal experiments on older rats have revealed decreased alcohol elimination rates, reduced alcohol dehydrogenase activity, and reduced activity of CYP2E1, an important enzyme in the metabolism of alcohol, but to date, this has not been reported in humans.[22]

INVESTIGATIONS

Blood Tests

Liver function tests (LFTs) refer to measurements of serum bilirubin, alkaline phosphatase (ALP), aspartate transaminase (AST), alanine transaminase (ALT), γ-glutamyl transpeptidase (GGT), and albumin, but they should also include the prothrombin time (PT). Mean cell volume (MCV), immunoglobulins, and platelet numbers also provide useful information about liver disease. A

TABLE 74-1 Interpreting Liver Function Tests in Older Adults

Abnormality in Liver Enzymes	Consider
Elevated ALT and AST	Hepatitis A, B, C, and E Alcoholic liver disease Nonalcoholic fatty liver disease Autoimmune hepatitis Hereditary hemochromatosis Medications (e.g., NSAIDs, herbal drugs) Congestive cardiac failure and ischemic hepatitis Celiac disease
Elevated AST only (normal ALT)	Nonhepatic source (Cardiac, skeletal muscle, kidneys, brain, pancreas, lungs, leukocytes, and red blood cells)
Elevated ALP and GGT	Intrahepatic cholestasis (e.g., primary biliary cirrhosis); drugs (e.g., co-amoxiclav, erythromycin); sepsis Extrahepatic cholestasis (e.g., biliary obstruction), stones, strictures, malignancy Hepatic infiltration (e.g., malignancy) IgG4-related cholangiopathy
Elevated GGT only (normal ALP)	Excess alcohol consumption Enzyme-inducing drugs (e.g., barbiturates, phenytoin)[26] Fatty liver, obesity, diabetes mellitus type 2, hypercholesterolemia Renal failure Chronic obstructive pulmonary disease Pancreatic disease Myocardial infarction
Elevated ALP only (normal GGT)	Extrahepatic source—bone Malignancy without liver or bone involvement (e.g., lung) Amyloid, leukemia, granulomas
Isolated raised bilirubin (normal LFTs)	Unconjugated—hemolysis Inherited disorders (e.g., Gilbert syndrome)
Elevated PT only (normal LFTs)	Warfarin Vitamin K deficiency Malabsorption
Low albumin only (normal LFTs)	Malabsorption Malnutrition Urinary and gastrointestinal losses Acute illness

ALP, Alkaline phosphatase; *ALT,* alanine transaminase; *AST,* aspartate transaminase; *GGT,* γ-glutamyl transpeptidase; *IgG4,* immunoglobulin G4; *LFT,* liver function test; *NSAIDs,* nonsteroidal antiinflammatory drugs; *PT,* prothrombin time.

large primary care study found that restricting the LFT panel to ALT and ALP alone would be helpful to diagnose liver disease in the community.[23] In general, conditions affecting the liver cell (hepatocellular disease/hepatitis) cause a rise in AST and ALT, whereas biliary tree disorders (cholestasis) cause raised ALP and GGT. It is important to recognize that these enzymes are also present in other sites of the body, and, when interpreting isolated elevation, extrahepatic sources should always be considered (Table 74-1). Extrahepatic biliary obstruction causing irritation and secondary inflammation of hepatocytes can also result in mildly raised serum transaminase levels,[24] and hepatitis can also lead to a degree of cholestasis with consequent rise in ALP and GGT. In practice, when faced with this situation, it is helpful to recognize the pattern of the so-called dominant distribution of raised enzymes.[25]

If the serum bilirubin level is elevated to greater than twice the upper limit of the normal reference range, then the patient will be clinically jaundiced. Isolated hyperbilirubinemia can be due to hemolysis and Gilbert syndrome where there is absence of enzyme responsible for bilirubin conjugation. It can occur in 5% to 10% of the normal population. Bilirubin can be raised in most types of hepatobiliary pathology,[25] often with an associated rise in liver enzymes. Initial evaluations should determine whether the hyperbilirubinemia is conjugated (direct), as seen in most types of cholestatic liver disease, or unconjugated (indirect), which would indicate hepatocellular damage or other conditions.[26] A low serum albumin level and prolonged PT are sensitive indicators of impaired hepatic synthetic function, seen in both acute and chronic liver disease, and are important prognostic indicators. When interpreting the serum albumin in older adult patients, it must be taken into account that other factors may affect albumin (e.g., malnutrition, renal dysfunction). A prolonged PT may also arise from a deficiency of vitamin K, which is required for synthesis of clotting factors II, VII, IX, and X in the liver. This may be of particular significance in older adults, because dietary insufficiency can exhaust hepatic stores of vitamin K after just 4 weeks. Vitamin K deficiency can be excluded by giving intravenous replacement and then repeating the PT.

Thrombocytopenia is a sign of chronic liver disease caused by portal hypertension that leads to splenomegaly and a resultant increase in sequestration. In cirrhotic patients, gastrointestinal bleeding usually presents with bleeding varices but can lead to iron deficiency anemia. This may be exacerbated by coagulopathy and thrombocytopenia. Hypersplenism can also result in leukopenia and a mild anemia. Serum immunoglobulins help physicians understand liver disease better as a decreased immunoglobulin A (IgA) level can indicate alcohol usage; IgM is raised in patients with primary biliary cirrhosis and IgG is increased in those who have autoimmune hepatitis. A raised MCV usually suggests excessive alcohol, but in older adults, vitamin B_{12} and folic acid deficiency as well as hypothyroidism should be excluded.

The true prevalence of abnormal LFTs in older adults has yet to been clarified. However, research from the early 1980s showed 17% of older adult hospitalized patients had abnormal LFTs, when screened, despite no clinical indication[27]; the most common abnormality was an isolated raised ALP. In the United Kingdom, there is evidence that liver disease may be missed in all age groups as abnormal LFTs are often not investigated.[28] A thorough history is a mandatory part of a "liver screen" and should include the patient's alcohol consumption, current or recent drug use (prescribed or otherwise), risk factors for viral hepatitis, presence of autoimmune diseases, family history of chronic liver disease, and factors such as diabetes, obesity, and hyperlipidemia. Older adult patients with elevated LFT results should be investigated initially with noninvasive serologic tests[29] (Table 74-2). It excludes screen for Wilson disease, which is rarely diagnosed in patients older than 40 years. Liver disease in those with homozygote α_1-antitrypsin deficiency tends to become apparent in the age group of 50 to 60 years but is probably worth including as part of the screen. Serologic screening for celiac disease is also useful as it can cause asymptomatic elevation of transaminase values, which subsequently normalize after the patient is put on a gluten-free diet.[30]

Causes of LFT derangement in patients with a negative liver screen include drugs, sepsis, and other comorbidities. In asymptomatic patients, the most common cause for raised ALT or AST (transaminitis) is steatosis, usually secondary to fatty liver disease in the Western population.[31] Many of the medications taken by older adult patients affect LFTs.[32] This should be borne in mind when reviewing a patient's drug history. In a district general hospital study of hospitalized patients with jaundice, the second most common cause after cancer was found to be sepsis/shock.[33] Other possible causes to consider include alcohol excess, fatty liver, obesity, diabetes, thyroid disease, and Addison disease, which also can cause mild derangement of LFTs. Some expert reviews suggest that, where there is a negative screen, to treat the most likely cause of the abnormal LFTs—that is, alcohol (by abstinence), hepatotoxic drugs (by drug cessation), and NAFLD

TABLE 74-2 Initial Serologic Tests in Older Patients With Abnormal Liver Function Test Results

Screening Test	Disease	Other Clues
Hepatitis A IgM	Hepatitis A	Travel to endemic areas
Hepatitis B surface antigen (HBsAg)	Hepatitis B	Intravenous drug usage Migration status
Hepatitis C virus antibody (HCV antibody)	Hepatitis C	Intravenous drug usage Blood transfusion
Hepatitis E IgM	Hepatitis E	Travel to endemic areas Older adult males, diabetes
Antimitochrondrial antibody (AMA)	Primary biliary cirrhosis	Pruritus, fatigue Female sex Presence of other autoimmune disorders
Smooth muscle antibody (SMA) Liver kidney microsomal antibody (LKM)	Autoimmune hepatitis	Presence of other autoimmune disorders Female sex Raised IgG
Transferrin saturation Ferritin	Hemachromatosis	Diabetes Joint symptoms
Serum α-fetoprotein	Hepatocellular carcinoma	Known chronic liver disease
α_1-Antitrypsin level	α_1-Antitrypsin deficiency	Coexisting lung disease
Anti-tTG antibody	Celiac disease	Malabsorption, anemia
Lipid profile, BMI, BP, Serum glucose, and US	Nonalcoholic fatty liver disease	Comorbidities (e.g., diabetes)

BMI, Body mass index; *BP,* blood pressure; *tTG,* tissue transglutaminase; *US,* ultrasound.

(by weight reduction and diabetes control). After a period of observation, if the LFTs remain abnormal, more detailed investigations should be sought.[26]

Noninvasive means to assess liver fibrosis can be particularly helpful in older adults as it may potentially avoid complications from liver biopsy. Blood test profiles that can predict the stage of liver damage include FibroTest, FibroMeter, Hepascore, FIB-4, and AST-to-platelet ratio index (APRI) panel[34]; the transient elastography (FibroScan) has proven to be superior among these, but combination of tests has been shown to improve accuracy.[35]

Radiology

The role of *abdominal ultrasound* is well established in the evaluation of the liver and biliary tree. It should be the initial imaging for patients with any abnormality of LFTs or where there is a suspicion of liver disease. It is safe and noninvasive and therefore an ideal investigative tool for use in older adult patients. The images require no adaption in interpretation compared to younger patients. Detection of fatty liver is also possible, although ultrasound is unable to accurately quantify the amount of fat present.[24] Ultrasound is also useful in chronic liver disease, particularly to evaluate liver texture and size and for assessing features of portal hypertension such as splenomegaly and abdominal varices. Doppler facilities to detect blood flow provide useful information about portal vein flow, presence of clot, and development of collateral vessels. When performed by an experienced operator, ultrasound is particularly useful in the detection of focal liver lesions.[25] The advent of contrast-enhanced ultrasound has been shown to improve the detection and differentiation of these focal lesions, especially the differentiation of focal nodular hyperplasia from hepatocellular carcinoma.[36] *Spiral computed tomography (CT)* can provide extra detail and is particularly effective in further characterization of focal liver lesions. It can also be used to detect diffuse liver disease because of fat, iron deposition, and cirrhosis as well as to provide further information about other abdominal organs. Caution should be exercised in administering the intravenous contrast agent as it can cause renal failure in patients with underlying reduced creatinine clearance. Even older adult patients with a degree of cognitive impairment may be able to cooperate well with CT scanning, as examinations are now quicker; for example, the entire liver and pancreas can be imaged in one single breath hold.[37] Unenhanced *magnetic resonance imaging (MRI)* of the liver is comparable to enhanced spiral CT in the delineation of focal liver lesions, while avoiding the disadvantage of radiation exposure and the potential nephrotoxic effect of iodinated contrast agent.[38] It has improved the characterization of underlying nodules and fibrotic changes in patients with cirrhosis, particularly when there is sideroblastic nodular regeneration.[39] MRI is also particularly useful in quantifying hepatic iron concentration in patients with hemachromatosis.[38]

Endoscopic retrograde pancreatography (ERCP) used to be a diagnostic procedure to investigate cholestasis but carries the risk of serious complications, including pancreatitis, bleeding, cholangitis, and death. Fortunately, *magnetic resonance cholangiopancreatography (MRCP)* is now widely available in most centers; because it is noninvasive, it remains the investigation of choice for imaging of the pancreatobiliary system. MRCP can pick up cholangiocarcinomas and can demonstrate small common bile duct stones not visualized on ultrasound or CT.[40] After MRCP, physicians can select patients who need intervention with ERCP or simply choose to perform interval scanning, thus avoiding an invasive test. ERCP still has an important role in the management of older adult patients who develop cholangitis secondary to gallstones, as many of these patients will not be candidates for cholecystectomy. *Endoscopic ultrasound* is invaluable for visualization of pancreatic pathologies and delineation of biliary strictures.

One of the most important recent development tools in assessment of liver injury is the invention of FibroScan, or liver ultrasonographic elastography. It can give essential information, such as the presence of advanced fibrosis or cirrhosis, that is equivalent to detail usually obtained from liver biopsy but through noninvasive means.[41] FibroScan is like an ultrasound machine and when the probe is approximated against the liver area, it gives liver stiffness measurement (in kilopascal [kPa]) by using shear wave velocity. The readings are validated to indicate varying degree of liver injury, and research has supplied different ranges of normal and abnormal values dependent on the cause of the liver injury. It is increasingly available in many centers throughout the world and international guidelines recommend treatment decisions for hepatitis B, hepatitis C, and various other liver disorders based on a patient's transient elastography readings. In addition, it can be used as a surveillance tool for patients with NAFLD but with normal LFTs or only transaminitis. Elastography readings of less than 19 kPa have been shown to predict absence of esophageal varices that may help to avoid endoscopies in the older adult population, but this is not yet incorporated into clinical practice.[42] Although the elastography is safe and can possibly help avoid liver biopsy, it is operator dependent and occasionally difficult to interpret results in obese patients. It is also contraindicated in pregnant women or those with pacemakers.

Liver Biopsy

The need for investigation of persistently abnormal LFTs in older adults must depend on clinical context, considering the risks and benefits of liver biopsy and whether the findings will dictate further management. Liver biopsy is not specifically contraindicated in older adult patients, but a 25-year audit from Australia found that increasing age can pose more than 1% risk for major complications following the procedure, particularly in those aged older than 50 years.[43] Most centers perform liver biopsies under ultrasound guidance, so the risk is less compared to blind percutaneous procedures. The patient should be able to understand and cooperate with instructions given by the person performing the liver biopsy and be able to give informed consent.[44] Midazolam can be used as sedation in very anxious patients, but this must be used with caution in older adults. Platelet transfusion and fresh frozen plasma are often administered to correct clotting abnormalities before biopsy to minimize the potential risk of bleeding.[44]

Liver biopsy is indicated to diagnose and assess the severity of either parenchymal disease or focal lesion. In viral liver disease, it stages damage and is useful to plan treatment. In patients with autoimmune hepatitis, among whom 25% are diagnosed after the age of 65,[45] a liver biopsy is indicated for both diagnosis and follow-up.[46] It is not usually indicated for primary biliary cirrhosis or alcoholic liver disease, and its role in NAFLD has not yet been clearly established. Liver biopsy may occasionally be useful in the investigation of liver dysfunction where routine serologic tests are unhelpful or there is an unusual course or severity of illness. If the patient is deeply jaundiced with thrombocytopenia and has other decompensation features, it is better to biopsy via transjugular rather than percutaneous route. It may also be of use in suspected drug reactions, especially herbal medicines. For the assessment of focal liver lesions, the indications for liver biopsy are mainly to exclude hepatocellular carcinoma or cholangiocarcinoma in suspicious nodules that cannot be confidently diagnosed by radiology.[47]

LIVER DISEASES

Liver disease in clinical practice can be classified into acute liver failure (ALF) and chronic liver disease. ALF is a clinical syndrome of acute loss of hepatic function in a patient with no prior history of liver disease.[48] Chronic liver disease is caused by long-standing liver damage and may include complications of cirrhosis, such as ascites and bleeding from varices. Table 74-3 summarizes recognized causes of acute and chronic liver disease. As chronic liver disease is more commonly seen in the older adult population, this will be discussed first.

Liver injury caused by *chronic liver disease* of any origin can result in cirrhosis, defined histologically as a diffuse process with severe fibrosis and nodule formation. As there are no diseases specific to liver aging itself, older patients are affected by the same conditions and have similar clinical manifestations as younger age groups.[49] However, older patients may have more advanced disease when they arrive at the clinic or hospital, and prognosis is poor with increasing age.[50] It is important to recognize that there is a greater mortality rate from other diseases unrelated to the liver, especially pneumonia, in those patients aged 80 years and older who have underlying cirrhosis.[50] In addition, cirrhosis confers a very high risk of operative morbidity and mortality to any patient undergoing abdominal surgery.[51]

TABLE 74-3 Common Causes of Acute and Chronic Liver Disease in Older Adults

Causes of Acute Liver Failure	Causes of Chronic Liver Disease
Acute viral hepatitis A, B, C, and E	Chronic hepatitis B and C
Drug induced	Alcoholic liver disease
Ischemic hepatitis	Nonalcoholic fatty liver disease
Autoimmune hepatitis	Autoimmune liver disease—autoimmune hepatitis, primary biliary cirrhosis, primary sclerosing cholangitis
Portal or hepatic vein thrombosis	Hemochromatosis
	α_1-Antitrypsin deficiency

Cirrhosis has a varied clinical presentation, ranging from asymptomatic individuals with abnormal LFTs to individuals with advanced decompensated liver disease and development of hepatocellular carcinoma (HCC). Recognized stigmata of chronic liver disease include palmar erythema, Dupuytren contracture, clubbing, spider nevi, and gynecomastia.

The prevalence of *chronic hepatitis B virus (HBV)* is declining worldwide, but it is still high in older people of Asian origin. Although acute cases are rare, the natural history of HBV infection appears to be altered in older adults, with a higher risk of progression to chronic infection[52] and a greater likelihood of advanced liver disease than younger patients with the infection.[53] HBV causes liver injury via an immune response against virus-infected hepatocytes. The aim of treatment is to control inflammation and fibrosis by preventing replication of the virus; thus, long-term treatment is required. Drug treatment for HBV (e.g., interferon-α, lamivudine, tenofovir) is available and indicated in patients of all ages with chronic HBV who also have markers of active viral replication (i.e., detectable HBV DNA), elevated transaminase levels, and inflammation/fibrosis on liver biopsy. The decision to treat must consider the presence of other comorbidities and the patient's overall general health. That said, most older adult patients with chronic HBV infection have no evidence of ongoing viral replication, even with advanced liver disease, and therefore are not candidates for antiviral treatment.[53] The increased rate of adverse effects seen with interferon in older patients may render oral antivirals as the agents of choice. The treatment duration can be lifelong, and decisions should be coordinated by experienced specialists. Screening for HCC is of importance where there is a long duration of viral infection, as it develops mainly in patients aged older than 50 with cirrhosis, although it can arise in those with either chronic hepatitis or simple HBsAg carriage.[53] Liver transplantation should be considered for all decompensated hepatitis B patients or in those who have developed HCC.

Chronic hepatitis C virus (HCV) is estimated to affect as many as one in two or three people older than age 80 in some European countries, and it is very common in Asia or Africa.[54] Most older adults with HCV infection acquired it from blood transfusions. The American Association for the Study of Liver Diseases (AASLD) recommends that anyone who received blood transfusion or blood products before 1992 be screened for HCV infection. It is also transmitted by intravenous drug usage, unprotected sex, and tattooing undertaken decades before onset of symptoms. Chronic HCV develops in 55% to 85% of individuals initially infected with HCV,[55] and the progression of fibrosis, clinical presentation of cirrhosis, or development of HCC is more pronounced in those who acquire the infection at an older age.[56-58] The mechanism of this rapid progression in older adults has not been fully established, although factors such as a higher prevalence of the more aggressive genotype 1 among the Western population and impaired immunity have been suggested.[59] Among HCV-infected individuals, cirrhosis becomes more prevalent with age,[59] with studies showing a mean age of 65.4 years for those with cirrhosis.[60] The goals of treatment are to completely eradicate the virus (unlike HBV) and to prevent complications.

The current treatment of choice for active HCV infection is pegylated interferon-α and oral ribavirin. In a recent study, sustained virologic response (meaning the virus is clear for 6 months after stopping treatment) was found to be lower (25%) in patients with genotype 1 hepatitis C infection who were older than 60 years of age, compared to 46% in younger patients.[61] Treatment in older adult patients is controversial because they are more likely to experience adverse effects, including lethargy, confusion, and behavioral change,[62] but guidelines do not stipulate an upper age limit for antiviral therapy. Therapy is contraindicated for patients with reduced life expectancy from severe hypertension, heart failure, coronary artery disease, poorly controlled diabetes, or obstructive lung disease. Adherence to therapy, which is essential to achieving a virologic response, may be suboptimal in older patients.[63] But it is an exciting time for treatment for HCV with the advent of new non–interferon-based daily oral drugs showing a sustained virologic response of up to 85% to 90%. These are direct-acting antivirals that target several sites of nonstructural proteins in the HCV cycle, causing cessation of viral replication.[64] Some of these drugs are approved for treatment in guidelines and should be widely available in the near future. This is a tremendous development as we can safely avoid side effects from interferon and patients can remain virus-free successfully for life. As the drugs are new to market, we do not yet know their long-term effects in older adults, and treatment decisions have to be made on an individual case basis with input from specialist liver centers.

Alcoholic liver disease (ALD) is becoming more common among older individuals. Alcohol is responsible for more than 80% of liver disease in Western countries. The usual maximum recommended level of consumption in most countries is 21 units per week for men and 18 units for women. Alcohol consumption is common in older adults, and the prevalence of alcohol abuse is probably underestimated.[65] Reasons for increased alcohol consumption include associated psychosocial problems, such as loss of spouses, loneliness, and mental health problems that occur with increasing frequency.[19] Although data suggest that most patients with severe ALD present in the fifth or sixth decade of life, a study from the United States reported the peak incidence of alcoholic cirrhosis in the seventh decade among white men.[66] An increased rate of complications and severity of disease at presentation is one important difference in the older adult population, and the presence of other comorbidities may result in the increased capability of alcohol to cause a harmful effect.[67] Those older than 70 years with alcoholic cirrhosis have been shown to have a mortality rate of 75% at 1 year.[68] In older adults, the spectrum of symptoms and signs of ALD do not differ from those seen in younger adults and ranges from asymptomatic elevation in liver enzymes to jaundice and both acute and chronic liver failure. Nonspecific symptoms of ALD, including general malaise and anorexia, are more common with aging.[69] Chronic alcohol ingestion can result in alcoholic fatty liver, which can be reversible even in older adults with abstinence.[19] Patients are living longer because of better therapeutic strategies, and therefore HCC is emerging as a major complication in later life. Alcoholic hepatitis may result from continued or increased alcohol intake, as well as recommencing drinking after a period of abstinence. Severe alcoholic hepatitis results in a potentially life-threatening illness, with deep jaundice, encephalopathy, ascites, and coagulopathy; mortality is up to 30% in 30 days. Underlying cirrhosis may coexist, and signs of decompensated liver disease are common. The prognosis of alcoholic hepatitis is variable; however, ongoing alcohol abuse, the presence of cirrhosis, and severe malnutrition are important prognostic factors and also play a vital role in the allocation of liver transplant.

A raised GGT supports a diagnosis of alcohol-related liver disease when serum AST/ALT levels are elevated at a ratio of 2 : 1, particularly in the presence of a raised MCV. Bilirubin is a useful prognostic indicator and correlates well with the degree of histologic change in alcoholic steatohepatitis.[19] Studies suggest that these brief interventions reduce hazardous alcohol consumption in older adults similar to younger populations.[70] Few clinical studies directly support or refute the hypothesis that withdrawal symptom severity, delirium, and seizures increase with advancing age, but several observational studies suggest that adverse functional and cognitive complications during alcohol withdrawal occur more frequently in older adult patients.[20] Benzodiazepines such as chlordiazepoxide and diazepam are used, based on validated alcohol-withdrawal protocols, with dose and frequency individualized. Older hospital in-patients with concurrent serious illness may have increased sensitivity to adverse effects.[71] β-Blockers, clonidine, carbamazepine, and haloperidol may be used to treat withdrawal symptoms not controlled by benzodiazepines in older adults. Acamprosate has also been used for withdrawal in out-of-hospital settings and shown to reduce craving. Nalmefene is a new opioid system modulator drug approved by various societies for alcohol withdrawal in hospitals. When taken for 6 months, nalmefene has been shown to decrease heavy drinking days by 3.2 days and decrease total alcohol consumption by 14.3 g/day; the effects of nalmefene in older adult patients remain to be seen.[72] Attention to nutrition and replacement of B vitamins via an intravenous route are important in preventing Wernicke and Korsakoff syndromes. For adults with acute alcoholic hepatitis, intensive care management may be indicated. Selected patients may gain benefit from steroid therapy or pentoxifylline, an inhibitor of TNF-α.[73] Management of complications and continued encouragement of abstinence are the mainstay of treatment in patients with alcoholic cirrhosis; liver transplant is the ultimate therapy. Liver transplantation may be the treatment for ALD in selected individuals.[74]

Nonalcoholic fatty liver disease (NAFLD) represents a spectrum of disorders characterized by predominantly macrovesicular hepatic steatosis that occur in individuals in the absence of consumption of alcohol in amounts considered harmful to the liver.[75] This spectrum includes fatty liver and nonalcoholic steatohepatitis (NASH) with inflammation and fibrosis, which can lead to cirrhosis. It is the probable cause of "cryptogenic cirrhosis" in many older adults.[76] Risk factors for underlying NAFLD include obesity (particularly abdominal adiposity), diabetes, hypertension, and raised lipid levels. Older adult patients with NAFLD were found to have more risk factors and more biochemical alterations (higher ALT, low albumin, thrombocytopenia, increased ALT/AST ratio).[77] NAFLD patients older than 65 years of age were found to have a higher percentage of NASH (72% vs. 56%) and advanced fibrosis (44% vs. 25%) compared to younger subjects.[78] For patients with the metabolic syndrome and NASH-associated cirrhosis, liver failure, and not cardiovascular disease, is the main cause of morbidity and mortality.[79] It is estimated that 19% of the U.S. population (28.8 million adults) is affected by NAFLD, and one study from Israel has reported a prevalence of NAFLD, as determined by ultrasound criteria, as high as 46% in a group of patients older than 80 years.[80] Genetic variation in the *PNPLA3* gene has been implicated in increased susceptibility to NAFLD,[81] but environmental influence and increasing incidence of diabetes, ischemic heart disease, hypertension, and obesity pose a high risk for disease progression. Prospective studies are few, but it is thought 10% to 15% of patients will progress to advanced fibrosis and cirrhosis.[82] The overall progression to cirrhosis is slow, but once developed, complications will occur in 45% within 10 years.[83] Older adult patients are therefore likely to constitute a considerable proportion of this cohort. Many patients are asymptomatic; however, initial symptoms can include fatigue, malaise, and right upper quadrant pain. More recently, HCCs were found to develop in noncirrhotic NASH patients and NAFLD is currently the third indication for liver transplant after alcohol and viral hepatitis. The diagnosis can usually be made on the basis of a negative liver screen, mild elevation of transaminases (ALT/AST ratio < 1), evidence of fat on abdominal ultrasound, or features of the metabolic syndrome.[78] Excess alcohol consumption must be excluded. The NAFLD fibrosis score is a validated simple noninvasive tool that can exclude presence of advanced fibrosis with an accuracy of 93%.[84] It is easy to calculate and can prevent the need for a liver biopsy. Slow weight loss by dietary modifications and exercise are recommended to achieve weight loss and improve insulin sensitivity,[75] although this may prove to be challenging in older adults with reduced mobility. Drug treatments for weight loss appear promising, but there may be issues with long-term tolerability relevant to older adult patients; antiobesity surgery is recommended in some centers as a means of controlling weight in NAFLD. Vitamin E and thiazolidinediones are the only group of drugs found to reverse some histologic activity in NAFLD/NASH, and metformin is beneficial in prevention of HCC development. Angiotensin II receptor antagonists should be tried for control of hypertension in this cohort.[75]

Autoimmune hepatitis (AIH) is a chronic necroinflammatory disease of the liver, which can silently progress to cirrhosis.[45] It is characterized by hypergammaglobulinemia (usually IgG) circulating autoantibodies and histologic changes of interface hepatitis. Although it was initially thought to affect predominantly young women, it is now known to have a bimodal distribution with another peak between 50 and 70 years of age.[85] Studies have agreed that approximately 25% of cases of AIH are found in adults older than 65 years.[45] It may present acutely but commonly follows an indolent course in older adults. However, patients older than 60 years have been observed to have a higher rate of cirrhosis at diagnosis. Symptoms can be subtle and may include fatigue, upper abdominal pain, anorexia, and polymyalgia, but a lower rate of arthralgia when compared to younger patients.[45] Autoantibodies such as antinuclear (ANA), anti–smooth muscle (SMA), anti-liver kidney microsomal (LKM), and antisoluble liver/pancreas (SLA/LP) antigens may be positive but are nonspecific. AIH in older adults is almost always characterized by ANA and SMA antibodies, classified as type 1 (classic) disease. The outcomes for older adults with AIH appear to be no worse than they are for younger ones,[52] including those who are untreated.[85] It was traditionally believed that older adult patients had a milder disease course, and controversy existed as to whether treatment was beneficial; however, it is now widely thought that these patients have an excellent prognosis if remission is induced. Treatment failure occurs less commonly in patients older than 60 years compared to younger adults, but it must be recognized by careful monitoring. The preferred initial treatment for severe AIH in older adults is prednisolone in combination with azathioprine.[86] If there is relapse after remission, low-dose prednisolone or azathioprine as maintenance is used although sustained long-term remission free from medication is still possible after relapse and retreatment.[85] However, in older adults, azathioprine is less well tolerated, and use of prednisolone alone in a higher dose is associated with greater frequency of adverse effects. Recently budesonide has been used frequently, as it is well tolerated and does not have all the side effects of prednisolone,[87] but the drawback is that it not licensed to be used in people with cirrhosis. Tacrolimus, mycophenolate mofetil, and rituximab have also been used in difficult-to-treat AIH. Bone protection with bisphosphonates must be instituted early. The incidence of HCC in AIH is low, but caution should be exercised among patients with cirrhosis.

Primary biliary cirrhosis (PBC) is an autoimmune disease that causes destruction of the interlobular and septal bile ducts thereby causing cholestasis, inflammation, fibrosis and cirrhosis.[88] It classically affects middle-aged women, but may manifest in patients older than 65 years in 30% to 40% of cases.[52] Symptom severity at first presentation does not differ in older subjects, although age is known to be an independent adverse prognostic risk factor.[89] Diagnosis can be made by elevated antimitochondrial antibody (AMA) levels in the serum. However, up to 50% have established cirrhosis at diagnosis. When symptoms arise, lethargy and pruritus are characteristic. In late presentation, symptoms and signs of decompensated liver disease can dominate the clinical picture. Jaundice does not become apparent until late in the disease, and serum bilirubin is an important prognostic indicator. Other autoimmune diseases, especially Sjögren syndrome, Raynaud syndrome, or rheumatoid arthritis, may be present. Helpful investigations include raised immunoglobulins, particularly IgM, and raised serum cholesterol. In the presence of symptoms and blood tests highly suggestive of the disease, some hepatologists believe a liver biopsy to be unnecessary, especially in older adult and frail patients, in whom management will not be affected.[47] Liver transplantation is the only effective treatment for patients with end-stage disease, but chance of recurrence is high.[90] Immunosuppressants such as steroids are of no benefit. Ursodeoxycholic acid can improve LFTs and symptoms, but it does not improve overall survival.[91] Obeticholic acid, a bile-acid mimetic that is an agonist for farnesoid X receptor, is currently undergoing human trials for PBC. For pruritus, cholestyramine is the most commonly used agent, but other drugs such as rifampicin, naltrexone, and sertraline can be of benefit. Patients who have marked cholestasis are at risk of malabsorption of fat-soluble vitamins A, D, E, and K and should receive replacement where this occurs. Bone disease such as osteopenia, osteomalacia, and osteoporosis can complicate PBC, so regular dual-energy x-ray absorptiometry (DXA) scans and prophylaxis are indicated.[92]

Hemochromatosis is an inherited autosomal dominant disorder of iron metabolism. Liver damage results from progressive iron deposition, which also affects the pancreas, heart, endocrine organs (pituitary, occasionally thyroid, and adrenals), and joint synovia.[25] It is characteristically diagnosed in men between 40 and 50 years, but in women, because of the protective effect of menstruation, presentation is classically a decade later. Raised serum ferritin and raised transferrin saturation (>60%) are suggestive of the diagnosis. Genetic testing for the *HFE* gene is now widely available, and MRI can be useful in quantification of iron deposits. Liver biopsy is recommended to define or exclude the presence of cirrhosis when biochemical and genetic testing do not give a clear diagnosis and where other causes of liver disease need to be excluded.[44] Presentation can be with symptoms and signs of the complications of chronic liver failure, especially if HCC has developed. The risk of HCC is particularly high in untreated hemochromatosis, estimated at 30%.[24] Venesection should be performed at regular intervals until serum ferritin is less than 50 mg/L. However, older adult patients with underlying heart failure may need smaller volumes of blood removed or less frequent phlebotomy. Iron chelating drugs such as penicillamine, triamterene, and desferrioxamine are occasionally used when phlebotomy alone is not sufficient or cannot be performed very often (e.g., because of concurrent anemia). The aim of treatment is to prevent the onset of cirrhosis and thus HCC. Life expectancy is similar to that of the healthy population if treatment can be achieved before the onset of cirrhosis or diabetes. Transplantation for liver failure remains a viable option, although survival in this group is lower than in those transplanted for other indications.[93] Genetic screening of all first-degree relatives of any age is recommended given the effectiveness of early treatment in preventing complications that significantly reduce life expectancy.

Primary sclerosing cholangitis (PSC) can be diagnosed at any age but is commonly a disease of young males. There is a close association with inflammatory bowel disease, particularly ulcerative colitis. There is also increased risk of developing cholangiocarcinoma. LFTs usually show cholestasis, and AMA is negative. Other autoimmune markers, including antineutrophil cytoplasmic antibody (ANCA), can be positive but are not specific for PSC. MRCP can demonstrate multiple irregular strictures and dilation of the biliary tree showing a beads-on-string appearance. Management involves symptomatic relief of cholestasis, bone disease prophylaxis, and replacement of fat-soluble vitamins. Ursodeoxycholic acid has been tried to modify the course of PSC, but survival benefit was found. Where there are acute episodes of cholangitis, antibiotic treatment is indicated. Balloon dilation or stenting may be undertaken if there is a focal obstructive biliary stricture. Liver transplantation remains the only effective treatment, although there is a high risk of subsequently developing colon cancer in those with ulcerative colitis. Recently, a new entity called IgG4 cholangiopathy has been identified in patients thought to have malignant biliary strictures; it is a benign autoimmune condition diagnosed by raised levels of IgG4 levels, and it responds very well to high-dose steroids.[94] If there are atypical features associated in a patient presumed to have malignant biliary disease, it is worth checking IgG4.

COMPLICATIONS OF CIRRHOSIS

Portal hypertension results from cirrhosis of any cause but can occur acutely following portal vein thrombosis or occlusion of the hepatic vein *(Budd-Chiari syndrome)* that can, in rare cases, present with acute or fulminant liver failure. Although rare in older adults, Budd-Chiari syndrome is a recognized complication of myeloproliferative diseases resulting in a hypercoagulable state. Portal hypertension causes varices, which have important prognostic implications for the patient: 30% will bleed from their varices, irrespective of age, within 2 years of diagnosis. The mortality rate for each bleeding episode is 30% to 50%.[95] Immediate survival after variceal bleeding is similar in older and younger cirrhotic patients, although mid-term and long-term survival rates appear to be worse for the older group.[52] Initial management of a significant bleed requires volume resuscitation of the patient, with care not to precipitate congestive cardiac failure in older individuals. Terlipressin (a vasopressin analogue) to reduce portal blood flow should be used with caution in older adults as it may precipitate an ischemic event, which can be cardiac, mesenteric, or peripheral,[96] and is contraindicated in documented ischemic heart disease. Upper gastrointestinal endoscopy should be arranged urgently; endoscopic treatment using sclerotherapy, or preferably band ligation, has a high success rate of approximately 90% across all age groups.[96] Danis stents (self-expandable removable nitinol stents) and Hemospray (hemostatic agent spray) are additional new endoscopic treatments with proven benefit.[97] If hemostasis cannot be achieved endoscopically, balloon tamponade with either a Sengstaken-Blakemore tube or Minnesota tube can be undertaken to temporarily arrest bleeding. Further management would be to consider transjugular intrahepatic portal systemic shunt (TIPSS) insertion by interventional radiologists. Following TIPSS, there is a greater risk of encephalopathy in older adult patients, and it is recommended that careful assessment be undertaken so the risk of encephalopathy does not outweigh the benefit.[98] It also increases cardiac preload and may precipitate cardiac failure in those with heart disease.[99] Propranolol, a nonselective β-blocker for primary and secondary prevention, has been shown to lessen variceal bleeding and mortality by reducing portal pressure.[96] It should be used with caution in older adults, as they are less tolerant to β-blockers and coexisting heart failure may increase the likelihood of adverse effects. Carvedilol is used in many centers as prophylaxis and has been shown to have a greater impact on portal pressure reduction.

Ascites and peripheral edema are often the first signs of decompensated liver disease,[96] occurring in over half of all patients with cirrhosis over a 10-year period.[100] In a patient with known liver disease, it should not be presumed that the underlying cause of the ascites is cirrhosis. Patients should undergo an ascitic tap, and fluid should be sent for albumin and protein levels, culture and sensitivity, neutrophil count, and, if there is clinical suspicion, amylase and cytology. Patients with cirrhosis generally have low levels of protein or albumin in the ascites. Treatment is aimed at addressing the key underlying factors in the pathogenesis of ascites in cirrhosis formation—portal hypertension and sodium retention. Bed rest is no longer recommended for the treatment of uncomplicated ascites.[100] However, salt restriction is important, and dietary salt should not exceed 90 mmol/day. Food with very low salt content in a hospital setting can be unpalatable,[96] which reduces patient compliance; chili and pepper can be added to food to make up for taste, but recognition and avoidance of malnutrition is important. Vaptans (tolvaptan, satavaptan) have been tried for treatment of ascites and hyponatremia without much benefit and mortality was found to be high, so this cannot be recommended.[101] There is controversy over the role of fluid restriction. Despite sodium retention, some patients have hyponatremia because of impaired free water clearance. Guidelines[100] recommend that water restriction be reserved for those who are clinically euvolemic with severe hyponatremia, who are not taking diuretics and only where there is a normal serum creatinine. In cases where the sodium level is less than 120 mmol/L, diuretics should be stopped. Diuretic therapy remains the mainstay of treatment in patients with ascites. Spironolactone, an aldosterone antagonist, is the first-line drug of choice and can be titrated cautiously to 400 mg once a day with renal monitoring. Amiloride or eplerenone is an alternative. If spironolactone alone does not achieve adequate diuresis, a loop diuretic such as furosemide may be added. Careful monitoring of fluid loss by recording body weight, together with serum urea and electrolytes, should be undertaken, particularly in older adults.[96] Large-volume paracentesis is reserved for patients who initially present with tense ascites. To prevent circulatory dysfunction, volume expansion with intravenous salt-poor human albumin is given concurrently with drainage. Although there are no data on the hemodynamic changes seen during paracentesis specific to older adult patients, it is reasonable to suggest that they should be carefully monitored. TIPSS is a highly effective treatment for refractory ascites; however, it may precipitate encephalopathy, and whether it has a positive impact on overall survival remains to be clarified.

Even with early diagnosis and prompt treatment, *spontaneous bacterial peritonitis (SBP)* carries a mortality rate of 20%.[102] It is diagnosed when the ascitic fluid neutrophil count is higher than 250 cells/mm^3 in the absence of a precipitating cause, such as an intraabdominal or surgically treatable source of sepsis.[100] It is commonly caused by coliforms; however, culture can be negative in many cases. The symptoms are usually nonspecific, especially in older adults where there may be a poor systemic and laboratory response to infection. It should be suspected if there is abdominal pain, fever, or encephalopathy in a patient with ascites or deterioration in blood tests. Third-generation cephalosporins are the antibiotic of choice and will attain high ascitic fluid concentrations.[103] In a third of patients, renal impairment develops, and this is a significant cause of mortality. Treatment with intravenous albumin has been shown to be associated with improvement in circulatory function compared with equivalent doses of fluid as colloid.[104] Continuous prophylactic antibiotics with oral norfloxacin, ciprofloxacin, or Septrin is recommended after an episode of SBP because of the cumulative recurrence rate of 70% at 1 year.[101] SBP is an indicator of poor prognosis and referral for liver transplantation should be considered.

Hepatorenal syndrome (HRS) is a serious complication in patients with advanced cirrhosis and renders a very poor prognosis. Intense vasodilation of the splanchnic circulation causes a relatively low and insufficient cardiac output with effective hypovolemia.[105] Marked vasoconstriction of the renal circulation results in "functional" renal failure with no structural damage to the kidneys.[106] Splanchnic vasoconstrictors such as terlipressin together with albumin infusions are recommended as first-line treatment of HRS. Treatment should continue until there is reversal of HRS, defined as a reduction in serum creatinine below 1.5 mg/dL, commonly seen in week 2,[107] although the optimum duration of treatment is unknown. In most studies of HRS, the incidence of ischemic side effects with terlipressin is approximately 13%,[105] although many studies excluded high-risk patients with ischemic heart disease or arterial disease and also older adults.[108] Alternative therapy with midodrine and norepinephrine have been tried, but results are not as good as with terlipressin. Overall survival of patients with HRS is poor, and liver transplantation again remains the treatment of choice with excellent 3-year survival rates.[109]

The exact underlying pathophysiology of *hepatic encephalopathy (HE)* remains poorly understood, but it is believed that failure to detoxify gut-derived toxins that are normally cleared by the liver is one of the main factors. Elevated circulating levels of ammonia, alteration in neurotransmitter systems, including increased levels of the neuroinhibitor GABA and decreased neuroexcitation, and an altered blood-brain barrier are all thought play an important role.[110] HE is characterized by the development of mental slowing, memory loss, disorientation, worsening somnolence, and occasionally coma in advanced stages.[96] Clinical examination findings include asterixis (liver flap), fetor hepaticus, increased reflexes, or muscular rigidity. Chronic persistent encephalopathy may result in some patients with end-stage liver dysfunction. In its subclinical form, estimated to affect more than 60% of patients with compensated cirrhosis,[96] diagnosis is challenging, in particular in older adult patients where it may be confused with cognitive impairment or early dementia. In addition, older adult patients with subdural hematoma, meningitis, or sepsis from urinary tract infections, cellulitis, or pneumonia may appear to be encephalopathic. One study found a significant proportion of older adult patients with documented liver disease and a presumptive diagnosis of HE had coexisting treatable extrahepatic conditions.[49] When appropriate treatment was administered, including standard therapy for HE, 67% of these patients showed improvement in their encephalopathy. There are also a number of factors that can precipitate HE, and careful identification and treatment of these are important. These factors include gastrointestinal bleeding, electrolyte disturbance, dehydration, drugs (including diuretics), infection, and constipation, especially if older adult patients are noncompliant with laxatives. There is no laboratory test to confirm the diagnosis; ammonia levels may be raised but do not correspond to the severity of symptoms, and electrophysiologic tests are rarely used outside of research. The drawing of a five-pointed star is often useful as constructional apraxia is a common feature of HE and can be assessed at the bedside. Protein restriction used to be recommended, but in view of patient's catabolic state, ascites, and muscle wasting, it is no longer the advice from the major societies. Lactulose is the mainstay of drug therapy. It lowers colonic pH, dissuading replication of ammonia-producing bacteria, reducing absorption of ammonia, and increasing fecal nitrogen elimination by producing osmotic diarrhea.[111] Adverse effects such as diarrhea and abdominal cramps may make it difficult to tolerate in older adults, especially outside the hospital setting. Antibiotics such as neomycin have long-term risks such as ototoxicity and nephrotoxicity. Rifaximin is a new minimally absorbed antibiotic and has been shown to be very effective in preventing exacerbations of encephalopathy and in avoiding hospital admissions. Chronic persistent HE is also an indication for liver transplantation.

Hepatocellular carcinoma (HCC) is a common complication of liver cirrhosis affecting older adults,[112] with median age of diagnosis at 60 years in developed countries. The incidence of HCC among older adults is increasing and mainly contributed by the increase in number of patients with HCV infection and NASH. Five-year survival is poor in all age groups without any treatment. HCC typically presents on a background of known cirrhosis, and it should be suspected in any patient with sudden decompensation. An elevated serum α-fetoprotein (AFP) with characteristic radiologic imaging, especially in the presence of cirrhosis, is widely recognized as diagnostic, although AFP is no longer proposed as a screening marker for HCC. Ultrasound assessment of the liver every 6 months is recommended in all patients with cirrhosis to screen for HCC,[113] as early diagnosis is vital in determining a favorable outcome, especially in older patients. Options in the treatment of HCC in cirrhotic patients include liver transplantation, surgical resection, interventional radiologic techniques, or chemotherapy as assessed by the Barcelona classification of liver cancer (BCLC staging).[114] Data on HCC in patients older than 70 years[115] have shown that it is the advanced stage of HCC and not the patient's age or comorbidities that has the greatest impact on survival rate. Radiofrequency ablation and transarterial chemoembolization are interventional radiologic treatments for HCC used as curative and palliative treatments, respectively, and show good survival rates.[115] They are particularly relevant in older adult patients who are not candidates for liver transplantation but can undergo other effective treatments. These techniques can be applied if patients have early cirrhosis (Child class A or B). Liver transplantation is a viable option if the patients have good performance status and tumor burden within the liver is less.[116]

ACUTE LIVER FAILURE

Because ALF is rare in older adults, little is known specifically about the underlying causes, clinical course, and outcomes in this cohort.[117] It often results in multiorgan failure, with cerebral edema and sepsis being the leading causes of death.[118] ALF commonly occurs initially with malaise or nausea. Jaundice then develops, followed by features of hepatic encephalopathy, and many patients evolve to coma within 1 week or less. Older adult patients with ALF have been described as having a more protracted disease course,[118] and increasing age has been identified as an independent risk factor of mortality from all causes.[119] The presence of other coexisting diseases and smaller functioning liver mass is believed to render them easily susceptible to deteriorating clinically, even to a lesser degree of hepatic necrosis.[116] Impaired regeneration, as described previously, can result in prolonged hepatocyte damage. The spontaneous survival rate for ALF is poor and has been reported as less than 50% for adults of any age.[120] The mortality rate of ALF in the older patients was found to be 85% previously,[116] but recently the survival rate was found to be better in older adults after correction of certain causes.[115] Despite extensive medical investigation, in some cases, the cause remains unknown.

A variety of viral agents can cause acute liver disease. *Acute hepatitis A (HAV)* infection usually begins with a prodromal illness, before the appearance of jaundice. It is typically a self-limiting disease that resolves in the majority of patients within 6 weeks. Although rare in this age group, patients older than 65 years are more susceptible to severe infections and are more likely to have serious complications.[52] In addition, the mortality rate is increased, with the U.K. census data for 1979 to 1985 demonstrating a mortality rate approaching 15% in those older than 75 years.[121] U.S. resident discharge data from the period 2002 to 2011 revealed that more patients admitted with HAV have underlying liver disease and other comorbidities.[122] *Acute HBV and HCV* infections are also rare in adults older than 65 years in the Western world, in part because of the lack of risk factors such as intravenous drug use, high-risk sexual behavior, and the routine screening of donated blood for these viruses. However, sporadic cases and rare outbreaks may still occur.[52] Data from the United States have shown acute HBV still accounts for 3% of all adult ALF cases.[123] Once thought to be a primarily zoonotic disease, *hepatitis E (HEV)* has emerged as an important cause of acute hepatitis in older adults throughout the world. It has an overall mortality rate between 0.5% and 4%. In a U.K. study of sporadic HEV, the majority of cases affected older adult males,[124] and a French study of patients with severe ALF resulting from acute HEV showed a mortality rate for those older than 70 years to be 71%.[125] Many cases of acute HEV present with neurologic (e.g., Guillain-Barré syndrome, neuralgic amyotrophy) and hematologic (e.g., lymphoblastic leukemia) manifestations that may have high morbidity and mortality.[126] Occasionally, HEV can follow a chronic course, especially in immunocompromised patients.[127] Other viruses such as cytomegalovirus, Epstein-Barr virus, and yellow fever are rare but recognized causes of ALF.

Drug-induced ALF occurs with increased frequency in older adults, not only because of increased drug use and polypharmacy but also as a result of accidental or intentional overdose.

Worldwide, the major causative drugs include antituberculous drugs, antibiotics, nonsteroidal medication, and paracetamol (acetaminophen) overdose.[128] Anesthetic drugs of the halothane family cause hepatic failure and death more commonly in older compared to younger patients.[129] Although paracetamol poisoning is predominantly seen in adolescents and young adults, mortality is higher in the older population.[119] In addition, accidental overdose and late presentation are seen more commonly in older adults and are individual risk factors associated with poor prognosis.[119] *N*-acetylcysteine (NAC) is an effective treatment when given within 24 hours of overdose, and it has been shown to decrease the risk of liver injury.[130] It can be used safely in older adult patients. Oral methionine is an alternative drug to be used if patients develop allergic reactions to NAC.

Ischemic hepatitis is thought to more likely occur with older age. One study demonstrated ischemic hepatitis occurring in 1% of older adult patients acutely admitted to the hospital with any complaint.[131] It is often difficult to recognize, as the classical signs of liver failure are not prominent. It is thought to be associated with an episode of hypotensive liver anoxia, which is usually the result of a significant drop in blood pressure.[132] In the absence of any other cause, a striking and reversible rise in serum transaminases (in the order of 10- to 20-fold) is generally accepted as diagnostic in the appropriate clinical setting.[133] A retrospective analysis has indicated that all patients with a clinical diagnosis of ischemic hepatitis had evidence of cardiac disease, usually right sided, suggesting underlying hepatic congestion may be an important part of the pathophysiologic process.[133] Prognosis in ischemic hepatitis is influenced by the underlying condition; in one U.K. study, the mortality rate was found to be one third of older adults.[132]

Autoimmune hepatitis (AIH) can present as an acute severe hepatitis. Belgian data have demonstrated an acute presentation with pronounced jaundice and a biopsy showing severe necrotizing hepatitis present in 19% of the older adult population with ALF (4% of the total study group).[45] AIH should be considered in all older adult patients with ALF and a trial of corticosteroids administered, although some data indicate that it may not affect survival without transplantation.[134]

At present, the mainstay of treatment of older adults with acute liver failure is supportive, to allow time for the liver to recover from the acute insult and eventually regenerate. If the liver has been severely damaged by any of the preceding conditions, emergency transplantation may be indicated. The King's College criteria[135] can be a useful guide for selecting patients for liver transplantation, and urgent discussion with a transplant center should be considered.

FOCAL LIVER LESIONS

Pyogenic liver abscess is common in older adult patients, most often diagnosed after the sixth to seventh decades.[136] Untreated, it is invariably fatal. Biliary tract disorders, such as cholangitis and portal pyemia from intraabdominal sepsis, are common sources of liver abscess; however, few papers have remarked on causes in relation to age. Tuberculosis is not an uncommon cause of pyogenic abscesses, especially in immunocompromised individuals. Data suggest there are no age-related differences with regard to symptoms or laboratory data at presentation.[136] Classical presenting symptoms include abdominal pain, fever, nausea, and vomiting. Examination findings may include a tender liver. Laboratory investigations may reveal an elevated white blood cell count, elevated liver enzymes (especially ALP), raised inflammatory markers, and a low serum albumin. Centrally necrotic liver metastases may sometimes be indistinguishable from abscess on conventional as well as contrast-enhanced ultrasound.[137] Blood cultures can be negative; abscess cultures are often of greater yield, with *Escherichia coli* the most frequently isolated organism across all age groups. The optimal treatment of a pyogenic liver abscess is by complete percutaneous drainage either by needle or indwelling catheter. This is in combination with intravenous antibiotics, which should be continued for 14 days, followed by oral treatment for a minimum of 4 weeks depending on clinical response. A broad-spectrum cephalosporin with metronidazole is usually adequate, but advice from a microbiologist is useful. Surgery is rarely indicated. Progress can be monitored by serial ultrasound, and the search for the underlying cause should be attempted and the cause treated if possible. Active management is well tolerated in older adults, and there appears to be no appreciable difference in mortality rates compared with younger patients except for longer duration of hospitalization.[138] One paper suggested that older patients present with atypical symptoms and have higher recurrence rates.[139]

Liver metastases, particularly of gastrointestinal origin, are common in older adult patients; for example, 35% of those with colorectal carcinoma have liver metastases at presentation.[138] Weight loss, general malaise, and nonspecific abdominal discomfort are common presenting features. However, the finding of metastatic disease can be incidental. Liver biopsy may be indicated where the nature of the primary neoplasm is unknown, and with new immunohistochemistry techniques it may help to indicate the likely primary site and guide further treatment. Lymphoma, for example, resembles hypervascular metastases on ultrasound scanning[36] but has a good prognosis if treated. However, if there is a history of a known primary malignancy, liver biopsy is often not required. Where surgical resection of the metastasis is under consideration, liver biopsy should not be undertaken to minimize risk of seeding. Colorectal metastases have the potential to be cured by liver resection, and increasing numbers of older adult patients are being referred for surgery. A recent meta-analysis comparing laparoscopic versus open hepatectomy with or without synchronous colectomy has shown comparable long-term survival and recurrence of tumor. The hospital stay was much reduced in laparoscopic group as expected, thus leading to improved morbidity.[139] Benign liver lesions include simple cysts, hemangiomas, and focal nodular hyperplasia, which can occur in all age groups. There is no potential for malignant transformation, and patients can be reassured that no treatment is required. The majority of patients are asymptomatic, and these lesions are found incidentally on abdominal imaging but may concern both the patient and the physician. In cysts and hemangiomas, rupture or hemorrhage can occur, causing right upper quadrant discomfort. Mass effect from large lesions can also result in pain, but other causes of pain should be excluded first.[140]

LIVER TRANSPLANTATION

Liver transplantation is the only treatment available for the severe end stage decompensated liver disease and there is growing evidence to suggest that advanced age should not be considered a contraindication. Most centers throughout the world use the Mayo Clinic's model for end-stage liver disease (MELD) score[141] to prioritize patients for transplant in view of the scarcity of donor livers. This is calculated based on the patient's bilirubin, clotting function, and creatinine. More than 10% of patients undergoing liver transplantation in the United States in 2000 were older than 65 years.[142] Data from the United Kingdom[143] and the Mayo Clinic[137] demonstrated no significant difference in survival between age groups within the first 5 years after a transplant. In addition, patients older than 65 years were found to have lower rejection rates, probably because of reduced immune function. After 5 years, survival is significantly worse in older recipients. The mortality in older adult patients after transplant is attributed mainly to development of malignany.[144] In a carefully selected patient, chronologic age alone should not form the basis of refusal for liver transplantation.

KEY POINTS

- There are no liver diseases specific to old age.
- Abnormal liver function tests in older adults should be fully investigated, in the first instance with serologic tests.
- Alcoholic liver disease, nonalcoholic fatty liver disease, and chronic hepatitis C infection are becoming more prevalent in the aging population worldwide.
- No treatment of liver disease is contraindicated by age alone; only by the individual's frailty and comorbidity.
- Liver transplantation for chronic liver disease in selected older adult patients is achieving improved outcomes.

For a complete list of references, please visit www.expertconsult.com.

KEY REFERENCES

3. Schmucker DL, Sanchez H: Liver regeneration and aging: a current perspective. Curr Gerontol Geriatr Res 526379:2011, 2011.
11. Jansen PLM: Liver disease in the elderly. Best Pract Res Clin Gastroenterol 16:149–158, 2002.
14. Woodhouse KW, James OF: Hepatic drug metabolism and aging. Br Med Bull 46:22–35, 1990.
19. Seitz HK, Stickel F: Alcoholic liver disease in the elderly. Clin Geriatr Med 23:905–921, 2007.
20. Meier P, Seitz HK: Age, alcohol metabolism and liver disease. Curr Opin Clin Nutr Metab Care 11:21–26, 2008.
23. Lilford RJ, Bentham LM, Armstrong MJ, et al: What is the best strategy for investigating abnormal liver function tests in primary care? Implications form a prospective study. BMJ Open 3:e003099, 2013.
35. Boursier J, de Ledinghen V, Zarski JP, et al: A new combination of blood test and fibroscan for accurate non-invasive diagnosis of liver fibrosis stages in chronic hepatitis C. Am J Gastroenterol 106:1255–1263, 2011.
45. Verslype C, George C, Buchel E, et al: Diagnosis and treatment of autoimmune hepatitis at age 65 and older. Aliment Pharmacol Ther 21:695–699, 2005.
50. Hoshida Y, Ikeda K, Kobayashi M, et al: Chronic liver disease in the extremely elderly of 80 years or more: clinical characteristics, prognosis and patient survival analysis. J Hepatol 31:860–866, 1999.
61. Silva I, Carvalho Filho R, Feldner AC: Poor response to hepatitis C treatment in elderly patients. Ann Hepatol 12:392–398, 2013.
64. Kim DY, Ahn SH, Han KH: Emerging therapies for hepatitis C. Gut Liver. 8:471–479, 2014.
71. O'Connell H, Chin A, Cunningham C, et al: Alcohol use disorders in elderly people—redefining an age old problem in old age. BMJ 327:664–667, 2003.
78. Noureddin M, Yates KP, Vaughn IA, et al: Clinical and histological determinants of non-alcoholic steatohepatitis and advanced fibrosis in elderly patients. Hepatology 58:1644–1654, 2013.
84. Angulo P, Hui JM, Marchesini G, et al: The NAFLD fibrosis score: a noninvasive system that identifies liver fibrosis in patients with NAFLD. Hepatology 45:846–854, 2007.
89. Newton JL, Jones DE, Metcalf JV, et al: Presentation and mortality of primary biliary cirrhosis in older patients. Age Ageing 29:305–309, 2000.
92. Collier JD, Ninkovic M, Compston JE: Guidelines on the management of osteoporosis associated with chronic liver disease. Gut 50:s1–s9, 2002.
97. Smith LA, Morris AJ, Stanley AJ: The use of hemospray in portal hypertensive bleeding; a case series. J Hepatol 60:457–460, 2014.
101. Dahl E, Gluud LL, Kimer N, et al: Meta-analysis: the safety and efficacy of vaptans (tolvaptan, satavaptan, lixivaptan) in cirrhosis with ascites of hyponatremia. Aliment Pharmacol Ther 36:619–626, 2012.
103. EASL clinical practice guidelines on the management of ascites, Spontaneous bacterial peritonitis and hepatorenal syndrome in cirrhosis. J Hepatol 53:397–417, 2010.
113. Bruix J, Sherman M: Management of hepatocellular carcinoma: an update. AASLD practice guideline. Hepatology 53:1020–1022, 2011.
117. Shiødt FV, Chung RT, Shilsky ML, et al: Outcome of acute liver failure in the elderly. Liver Transpl 15:1481–1487, 2009.
141. Kamath PS, Wiesner RH, Malinchoc M, et al: A model to predict survival in patients with end stage liver disease. Hepatology 33:464–470, 2001.
143. Cross TJS, Antoniades CG, Muieson P, et al: Liver transplantation in patients over 60 and 65 years: an evaluation of long term outcomes and survival. Liver Transpl 13:1382–1388, 2007.

75 Biliary Tract Diseases

Noor Mohammed, Vinod S. Hegade, Sulleman Moreea

GENERAL CONSIDERATIONS

Chapter 74 describes diseases of the liver as they affect older adults. This chapter will examine the related disorders of the biliary tract. Biliary tract disease is suspected when liver function tests (LFTs) are suggestive of cholestasis; the alkaline phosphatase (ALP) level is disproportionately higher than the ratio of the serum transaminase levels of alanine transaminase (ALT) and aspartate transaminase (AST; ALT/AST). A raised ALP level is often associated with a raised bilirubin level, and patients appear clinically jaundiced when the bilirubin concentration in the blood exceeds 51 μmol/L (3 mg/dL). Biliary tract diseases can be divided into intrahepatic and extrahepatic causes (Table 75-1).

Liver Function Tests

Alkaline Phosphatase

ALP is coded by three separate genes and found in many locations in the body—liver, bone, placenta, kidneys, and intestine.[1] Its precise function is unknown. In the liver it appears to downregulate the secretory activities of the intrahepatic biliary epithelium.[2] Its half-life is 7 days, its site of degradation is unknown, and its clearance from serum is independent of the functional capacity of the liver or the patency of the bile ducts.[3] The intestinal contribution (≈10% to 20%) is of limited clinical importance.[4] Subjects older than 60 years have higher ALP values (up to 1.5 times normal) than younger adults, from the liver in older men and from bone in postmenopausal women.[5]

If there is an isolated increase in ALP, it is important to ascertain that this is of liver origin. For practical purposes in older adults, we mainly need to establish whether the raised ALP level is of liver or bone origin. The most practical approach is to measure the γ-glutamyl transpeptidase (GGT) level, whose elevation may also reflect biliary disease. However, GGT is an inducible enzyme that is not completely specific for hepatobiliary disease. It is elevated in people who drink large quantities of alcohol[6] or take medicines such as phenytoin.[7]

ALP isoenzyme levels can be requested with the caveat that the test is heat-labile; bone and liver isoenzymes differ only slightly in electrophoretic mobility, sometimes leading to inconclusive results. 5′-Nucleotidase is a more specific biliary enzyme than GGT but is not measured routinely.[8] Refer to the investigative pathway for raised ALP levels shown in Figure 75-1.

Investigating Cholestatic Jaundice

When a patient is jaundiced with cholestatic LFTs, a thorough history is essential. The key points in the history are duration of jaundice and whether it is associated with abdominal pain, anorexia, weight loss, alcohol intake, and any past medical history of note. The examination is geared to the signs of chronic liver disease, evidence of weight loss, abdominal tenderness, and presence of any mass or organomegaly. Investigations should include a noninvasive liver screen (liver autoantibodies, immunoglobulins, AFP), and an urgent ultrasound (US) examination is requested. If the US scan shows biliary dilation with an obvious cause, further investigation and management will follow accordingly. If there is biliary dilation without any obvious cause, magnetic resonance cholangiopancreatography (MRCP) is requested, proceeding to an endoscopic US scan if necessary. If there is no biliary dilation, intrahepatic causes of cholestasis are the next targets of further investigations; see Table 75-1.

An isolated raised bilirubin level may be seen in older patients and is not an indication of biliary tract disease. It is due to an increase in bilirubin production (e.g., via hemolysis, ineffective erythropoiesis, blood transfusion, resorption of hematomas) or decreased hepatocellular uptake or conjugation (e.g., congenital hyperbilirubinemias). Liver function is otherwise normal, and hyperbilirubinemia is often characterized by a predominant elevation in unconjugated bilirubin levels.

Jaundice resulting from hemolysis is usually mild, with a serum bilirubin level of 68 to 102 μmol/L (4 to 6 mg/dL) because normal liver function can easily handle the increased bilirubin derived from excessive breakdown of red blood cells. Unconjugated bilirubin is not water- soluble and therefore will not pass into the urine—hence, the term *acholuric jaundice*. The urinary urobilinogen level is increased. Causes of hemolytic jaundice are the same as those of hemolytic anemia. Investigations have shown a raised unconjugated bilirubin level but normal serum alkaline phosphatase, transferase, and albumin levels, and serum haptoglobin levels are low.

Most of the congenital and inherited defects are diagnosed in young people; the only condition that could incidentally be found in older patients is Gilbert syndrome, the most common familial hyperbilirubinemia. It is asymptomatic and is usually detected as an incidental finding of a slightly raised bilirubin level, 17 to 102 μmol/L (1 to 6 mg/dL) on a routine check. No signs of liver disease are present. There is a family history of jaundice in 5% to 15% of patients.

Hepatic glucuronidation is approximately 30% of normal, resulting in an increased proportion of bilirubin monoglucuronide in bile. Most patients have reduced levels of uridine 5′-diphosphoglucuronosyltransferase (UDP) glucuronosyl transferase activity, the enzyme that conjugates bilirubin with glucuronic acid.

The major importance of establishing this diagnosis is to inform the patient that it is not a serious disease and prevent unnecessary investigations. Tests show only a raised unconjugated bilirubin level, which is further increased when fasting, during mild illnesses or infections, after surgery, or during consumption of large amounts of alcohol; the reticulocyte count is normal. No treatment is necessary.

Magnetic Resonance Imaging

Magnetic resonance imaging (MRI) is now the investigation of choice for characterization and staging of hepatic, pancreatic and splenic lesions and for imaging the biliary tree using MRCP. It does not involve the use of radiation. MRCP is commonly used for the diagnosis of gallstones, assessment of common bile ducts, intrahepatic ducts, or pancreatic ducts for stenotic lesions or stones, and investigating pancreatitis or abdominal pain of uncertain cause.

A strong magnetic field is used to align rotating hydrogen protons within the tissue being imaged, and T1 and T2 relaxation times are used to create the final image. In T2-weighted images, water appears white and the liver dark, which makes the biliary

TABLE 75-1 Causes of Raised Alkaline Phosphatase Levels*

Intrahepatic Causes	Extrahepatic Causes
Primary biliary cirrhosis (PBC)	Luminal causes—common bile duct stones (choledocholithiasis)
Primary sclerosing cholangitis (PSC)	Mural causes—benign and malignant biliary strictures
IgG4-related sclerosing cholangitis	Extramural causes (e.g., malignant obstruction)
Drug-induced liver injury (DILI) causing cholestasis	
Infiltrative liver diseases (e.g., fatty liver, granulomatous liver diseases, metastatic malignancy, amyloidosis)†	
Viral hepatitis (e.g. hepatitis E)†	
Congestive cardiac failure†	
Infectious hepatobiliary diseases in AIDS (e.g., tuberculosis, cytomegalovirus, microsporidiosis)†	
Biliopathy following liver transplantation†	

*With or without elevated bilirubin levels.
†Not discussed in this chapter.

tree easy to visualize, hence making MRCP the investigation of choice for biliary pathology.

Older patients can find MRI difficult to tolerate because they have to lie supine and still for at least 30 minutes. Noise levels can be high because of vibration of the magnetic coils, and ear plugs or headphones need to be worn. Claustrophobia due to the tight cylindrical scanner can lead to a significant number of patients being unable to complete the test. Sedation can be used to improve compliance. Open coil magnets are increasingly being used for claustrophobic patients and for patients who are too large for the cylindric scanner.

MRI contrast agents (e.g., gadolinium) are safer than the iodinated contrast agents used for CT scanning and rarely cause contrast reactions. However, they can cause contrast nephropathy and, in rare cases, nephrogenic systemic fibrosis in patients with moderate to severe chronic kidney disease.

Contraindications include implanted devices such as cardiac pacemakers, implantable cardioverter-defibrillators (ICDs), nerve stimulators, cochlear implants, and embedded metallic foreign bodies such as intraorbital metallic fragments that may have been present from the working days of the now-retired patients. Transdermal patches need to be removed prior to MRI. There is a risk

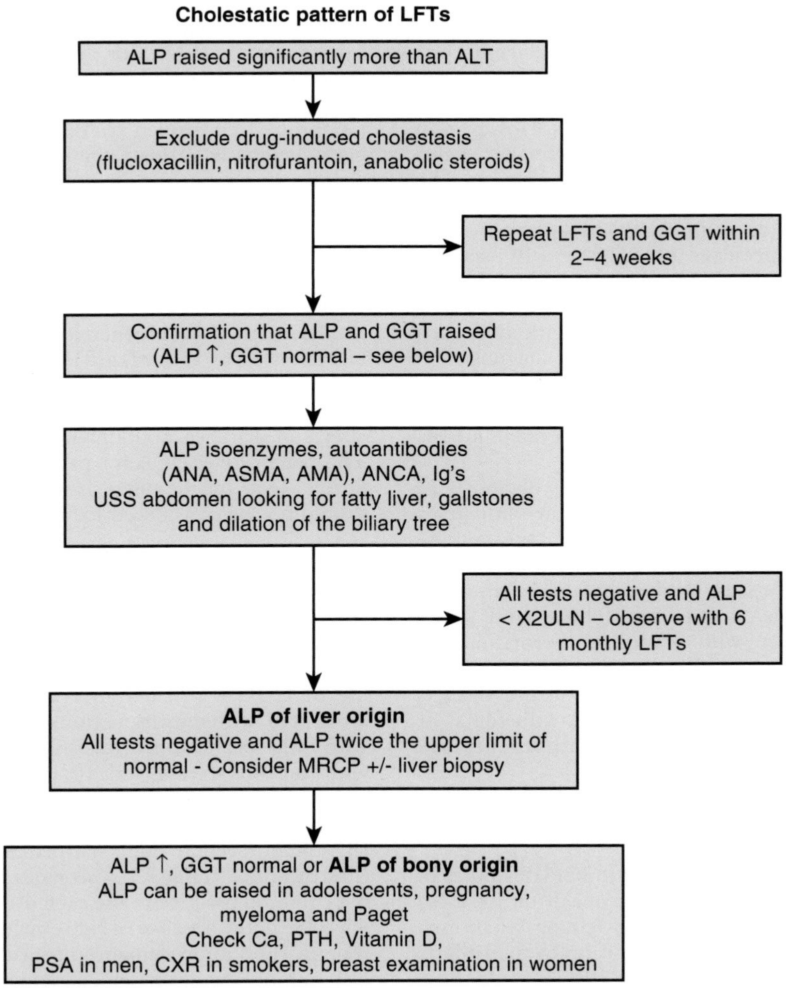
Cholestatic pattern of LFTs
ALP raised significantly more than ALT
Exclude drug-induced cholestasis
(flucloxacillin, nitrofurantoin, anabolic steroids)
Repeat LFTs and GGT within 2–4 weeks
Confirmation that ALP and GGT raised
(ALP ↑, GGT normal – see below)
ALP isoenzymes, autoantibodies
(ANA, ASMA, AMA), ANCA, Ig's
USS abdomen looking for fatty liver, gallstones and dilation of the biliary tree
All tests negative and ALP < X2ULN – observe with 6 monthly LFTs
ALP of liver origin
All tests negative and ALP twice the upper limit of normal - Consider MRCP +/- liver biopsy
ALP ↑, GGT normal or ALP of bony origin
ALP can be raised in adolescents, pregnancy, myeloma and Paget
Check Ca, PTH, Vitamin D,
PSA in men, CXR in smokers, breast examination in women

Figure 75-1. Investigating a raised ALP in general practice. *ALT,* Alanine transaminase; *ALP,* alkaline phosphatase; *AMA,* antimitochondrial antibody; *ANA,* antinuclear antibody; *ANCA,* antineutrophil cytoplasmic antibody; *ASMA,* anti-smooth muscle antibody; *Ca,* calcium; *CXR,* chest x-ray; *GGT,* γ-glutamyl transpeptidase; *LFT,* liver function test; *MRCP,* magnetic resonance cholangiopancreatography; *PSA,* prostate-specific antigen; *PTH,* parathyroid hormone; *ULN,* upper limit of normal.

of contrast nephropathy with gadolinium-based contrast agents in those with advanced chronic kidney disease.

The following are not contraindications and are considered safe for MRI: joint prostheses, coronary or peripheral vascular stents, prosthetic heart valves, sternal wires, inferior vena cava filters, and embolization coils. The composition of intracranial aneurysmal clips needs to be ascertained because most may not be safe during MRI.

PRIMARY BILIARY CIRRHOSIS

Primary biliary cirrhosis (PBC) is an autoimmune cholestatic liver disease of unknown cause, characterized biochemically by a cholestatic pattern of abnormal LFTs, serologically by the presence of antimitochondrial antibody (AMA), and pathologically by apoptotic damage to the biliary epithelial cells lining the small intrahepatic ducts. PBC predominantly affects middle-aged women, with a female-to-male ratio of 10:1 and the median age of disease onset about 50 years.[9] The prevalence of PBC has a considerable geographic and regional variation, ranging from 128 to 180/million in Sweden[10,11] to 150 to 400/million in the United States.[12,13] In the United Kingdom, it ranges from 200 to 250/million, with regional differences.[14,15] The pathogenesis of PBC is characterized by immune cell activation and damage to cholangiocytes, producing intrahepatic bile duct damage. The resulting cholestasis causes direct hepatocyte injury, leading to inflammation, necrosis, and ultimately resulting in liver fibrosis and cirrhosis.

PBC should be suspected in the setting of chronic cholestasis after the exclusion of other causes of liver diseases. However, in older patients, an isolated rise in ALP levels needs further evaluation to rule out other conditions, such as Paget disease. The diagnosis of PBC is conventionally made using the combination of abnormal LFTs (elevation of serum ALP levels of liver origin for at least 6 months), the presence of AMA or PBC-specific serum antinuclear antibodies (ANAs), and/or a liver biopsy. AMAs are the characteristic serologic hallmark of PBC, and a titer of more than 1:40 in the context of cholestatic liver biochemistry is over 95% sensitive and specific for the diagnosis.[16,17] Most patients with PBC have mild elevations of aminotransferase levels (ALT or AST) and increased levels of immunoglobulins (mainly IgM). Serum cholesterol levels are often elevated in PBC patients.

Liver biopsy is not routinely indicated in the diagnosis of PBC nor is it essential before initiating treatment with ursodeoxycholic acid (UDCA). However, it can further substantiate the diagnosis and stage the liver disease. Histologically, PBC is characterized by chronic nonsuppurative cholangitis affecting small intrahepatic bile ducts, mainly interlobular and septal ducts. Focal duct obliteration with granuloma formation has been termed a *florid duct lesion* and, when present, it is considered as pathognomonic of PBC.[18] In later stages of the disease, inflammation is seen in the hepatic parenchyma, with septal or bridging fibrosis eventually leading to cirrhosis, with regenerative nodules.[19]

Genetics of Primary Biliary Cirrhosis

Genome-wide association studies (GWAS) and iCHIP studies of PBC have been undertaken in those of European or Japanese ancestry and have shown that the human leukocyte antigen (HLA) complex makes an important contribution to the genetic basis of PBC. Risk haplotypes associated with PBC include those carrying DRB1*08 and DRB1*04 alleles. Protective haplotypes include those carrying DRB1*11 and DRB1*15 alleles. A total of 27 non-HLA risk loci for PBC have also been identified, harboring highly plausible candidate genes that are mainly involved in innate or acquired immune processes.[20]

Clinical Features

Although most PBC patients are asymptomatic at the time of diagnosis, two characteristic symptoms of the disease, fatigue and pruritus (itch), can occur at any point in the disease course. Although the prevalence of fatigue (up to 78% of patients) and pruritus (20% to 70%) are similar,[21] pruritus is a more specific symptom of PBC than fatigue. Both fatigue and pruritus are complex symptoms, and their cause in PBC remains incompletely understood. Also, for reasons that are currently unknown, neither fatigue nor pruritus correlates with the severity, histologic stage, or duration of PBC. Fatigue is often constant over time but pruritus may diminish in severity, especially during late stages of diseases. A recent study has observed that the intensity of itch depends on the age at disease presentation. In this study, younger patients (<30 years) scored 64% higher in pruritus score than those who presented after 70 years of age.[22] Nocturnal pruritus will affect sleep, worsen fatigue, cause mood changes and cognitive impairment, and impair the overall quality of life. Other features of PBC include dry eyes and/or dry mouth (sicca syndrome), xanthelasma, xanthomata, portal hypertension, osteoporosis, and hyperlipidemia.

Management

UDCA is the only drug licensed by the U.S. Food and Drug Administration (FDA) for the treatment of PBC. UDCA is a bile acid that acts as a choleretic agent, with fewer hepatotoxic properties than endogenous bile acids.[19] In a number of prospective randomized controlled trials, its use at more than 10 mg/kg of body weight (BW)/day has been shown to improve liver biochemistry significantly, slow histologic progression (in those with early stage disease), reduce the risk of developing varices, and improve liver transplant–free survival of patients.[23] However, it has not been shown to be effective in reducing pruritus or improve fatigue. Current guidelines recommend the use of UDCA for patients with PBC who have positive tests for AMAs and elevated liver biochemical markers. The optimal dose of UDCA is 13 to 15 mg/kg BW/day, and it is be used for patients at any stage of PBC, as long as the liver biochemistry is abnormal.[21] UDCA is generally well tolerated, with occasional side effects of diarrhea, abdominal discomfort, nausea, and vomiting. The benefit of UDCA for patients with positive AMA tests and normal liver biochemistry is less clear; therefore, these patients should not be considered for UDCA treatment.

Treatment of Pruritus

It is important to exclude other systemic and dermatologic causes of pruritus, and patients with skin lesions should be referred to a dermatologist. Worsening of pruritus has been reported with the use of UDCA. In such an event, a trial off UDCA should be attempted, with reintroduction of UDCA at a lower dose. Patients with mild localized pruritus should be offered topical treatment with aqueous cream and 1% menthol (emollient and coolant effect). For those with generalized itch, guidelines recommend four specific drugs: cholestyramine (first line) or colesevelam, rifampicin (second line), naltrexone (third line), and sertraline (fourth line).[21] Table 75-2 provides a summary of these drugs. It is a common practice to use each drug as monotherapy for at least 4 weeks (in the absence of side effects) then switching to next-line therapy if no improvement in pruritus occurs. When taking cholestyramine or colesevelam, patients should be advised to separate taking UDCA and any other drugs by at least 3 hours to avoid interference with their absorption. In patients who benefit from cholestyramine but cannot tolerate its side effects, colesevelam should be offered because it has fewer side effects and may have better compliance.

TABLE 75-2 Current Recommendations for Treatment of Pruritus in PBC

Approach	Drug	Mechanism of Action	Dose	Adverse Effects	Comments
First line	Cholestyramine	Bile acid resin	4-16 g/day	Unpleasant taste, bloating, constipation, and diarrhea	Morning dose preferred; separate at least 3 hr from other drugs
	Colesevelam	Bile acid resin	3.75 g/day in two or three divided doses	As above (but less frequent), headache, myalgia	Separate at least 3 hr from other drugs
Second line	Rifampicin (rifampin)	Pregnane X receptor (PXR) agonist and enzyme inducer	150-600 mg/day	Hepatitis, liver failure, hemolysis	150 mg/day when serum bilirubin level < 3 mg/dL; 300 mg/day when serum bilirubin level > 3 mg/dL; regular monitoring of blood count and liver biochemistry
Third line	Naltrexone	Opiate mu receptor antagonist	50 mg/day	Opioid withdrawal–like reaction—abdominal pain, high blood pressure, tachycardia, goose bumps, nightmares	Start at 12.5 mg/day; increase gradually; regular monitoring of liver biochemistry
Fourth line	Sertraline	Serotonin reuptake inhibitor (SSRI)	100 mg/day	Nausea, dizziness, diarrhea, visual hallucinations, increased fatigue	Start at 25 mg/day; increase gradually

In patients with severe, medically refractory pruritus, invasive therapies that have been shown to be effective in case series are narrow-band ultraviolet B (UVB) phototherapy, endoscopic nasobiliary drainage (NBD), plasmapheresis, and molecular adsorbent recirculating system (MARS). Although these interventions are effective, they are not universally available, and the duration of relief from pruritus induced by these invasive therapies is variable, with a need for repeated sessions of treatments to maintain remission of pruritus. Currently, two large multicenter randomized clinical trials have been evaluating the role of ileal bile acid transport (IBAT) inhibitor in treating pruritus in PBC patients (ClinicalTrials.gov identifiers—NCT01899703 and NCT01904058).

Treatment of Fatigue

Fatigue is multifactorial and not a specific symptom of PBC, and other causes of fatigue such as anemia, hypothyroidism, depression, sleep disorder, and vitamin D deficiency should be considered and, when detected, appropriately treated.[21] Currently, there is no effective therapy available for the treatment of fatigue in PBC. Randomized controlled trials have failed to show any benefit with ondansetron (antagonist of serotonin 3 receptor) and fluoxetine (serotonin reuptake inhibitor). An association between fatigue and excessive daytime sleepiness has been shown in patients with PBC.[24] The use of modafinil (a central nervous system stimulant) at doses of 100 to 200 mg/day has been shown to be effective in significantly improving the fatigue in PBC patients with fatigue and daytime somnolence.[25] A staged exercise program and antioxidant vitamins (e.g., ubiquinone, 100 mg/day) have also been suggested to relieve fatigue in PBC.

Liver Transplantation

Liver transplantation is the definitive treatment and has proven survival benefit for PBC patients with advanced-stage disease. Criteria for the recommendation of liver transplantation for a PBC patient are similar to those for other types of end-stage liver diseases. These include decompensated cirrhosis with an unacceptable quality of life or anticipated death within 1 year due to treatment-resistant ascites and spontaneous bacterial peritonitis, recurrent variceal bleeding, encephalopathy, and hepatocellular carcinoma.[18] The post–liver transplantation outcome is favorable, with survival rates above 90% and 80% to 85% at 1 and 5 years, respectively.

PRIMARY SCLEROSING CHOLANGITIS

Primary sclerosing cholangitis (PSC) is a chronic cholestatic disease of unknown cause characterized by inflammation and progressive obliterating fibrosis of the intrahepatic or extrahepatic biliary ducts. It is a slowly progressive disease, eventually leading to biliary cirrhosis and liver failure and complicated by related malignancies, such as cholangiocarcinoma and colorectal cancers. The term *primary* is used to distinguish it from secondary conditions from bile duct strictures causing cholestasis. It is rare (8 to 13 cases/100,000 persons) and affects primarily white men during their fourth or fifth decade of life.[26] However, a Japanese study has suggested a second peak in the seventh decade of life, with a bimodal age distribution.[27] Immune (genetic) and nonimmune (e.g., infections, toxins, ischemic damage, nonsmoking) mechanisms have been postulated as possible causes of PSC. There is a strong association between PSC and inflammatory bowel disease (IBD), which has led to the identification of many shared genetic loci. Coexisting IBD is seen in 75% to 90% of PSC patients, ulcerative colitis (UC) is seen in around 87%, and Crohn disease (CD) in 13%.[28] However, there is no correlation between the severity of PSC and IBD, nor is there a temporal relationship between the onset of the diseases. Furthermore, therapy of IBD has little effect on the course of PSC, and vice versa. Approximately 5% to 30% of patients develop cholangiocarcinoma, with the highest incidence being in the first year of diagnosis; the 5-year survival is only 20% to 40% for resectable disease.[29,30] Individualized treatment for cholangiocarcinoma with liver transplantation and aggressive neoadjuvant chemotherapy has shown promising results. However, the International Liver Cancer Association does not recommend liver transplantation for those with intrahepatic cholangiocarcinoma.[31]

Clinical Features

Patients may be asymptomatic and diagnosed accidentally on routine blood tests. Asymptomatic PSC is found in 20% to 40% of patients investigated for abnormal LFTs. Occasionally, the symptoms have a relapsing and remitting course. Typical symptoms on presentation are jaundice, right upper quadrant pain, pruritus, and fatigue. One third of patients have episodes of acute cholangitis, with recurrent attacks.

Investigations

Liver enzyme levels, and especially ALP levels, are raised in most patients; perinuclear antineutrophil cytoplasmic antibodies (pANCAs) may be detected in 26% to 85% of PSC cases, but they lack specificity for diagnosis. Overlap syndromes with other forms of liver disease have been described. PSC with autoimmune hepatitis-like features has been referred to as autoimmune cholangitis. These patients usually present with high serum ALT levels, modest or no elevations in serum alkaline phosphatase levels, high titers of ANAs and anti–smooth muscle antibodies (SMAs), and histologic liver findings typical of autoimmune hepatitis.

Characteristic stricturing of biliary tracts is seen on MRCP. Dominant strictures develop during the disease course in about 36% to 63% of patients.[32] This leads to further elevation of liver enzyme levels, usually ALP. Dominant strictures develop de novo or are due to diffuse inflammatory periductal fibrosis; more recently, *Candida* has been hypothesized as the causative infective organism.[33,34] These are treated with endoscopic retrograde cholangiopancreatography (ERCP) and biliary stent insertions; however, the development of a dominant stricture is associated with poor outcome.[35] Liver biopsy is rarely required to diagnose PSC. It shows periductal inflammation in the early stages, which then extends to periportal areas, leading to septal fibrosis and necrosis, eventually resulting in frank cirrhosis of the liver.[36]

Treatment

Because there are no targeted treatment options in PSC, medical treatment is aimed at alleviating symptoms and improving the quality of life. Various drugs, including antifibrotic agents such as methotrexate or colchicine, penicillamine, and UDCA, have been used, but none of them have been shown to improve histology. UDCA is the most commonly used drug for the treatment of PSC and has been the only drug shown to improve liver function test results.[37] Studies indicating improvement in liver enzyme levels have shown a possible survival benefit with high doses of UDCA (30 mg/kg BW/day).[38] Systematic reviews assessing the benefits of corticosteroids and penicillamine have not demonstrated an impact on disease progression.[39,40] Bone density and liposoluble vitamin deficiency should be monitored and treated appropriately, particularly in patients with advanced disease. A recent meta-analysis has suggested a possible trend toward lowering the incidence of colorectal cancer in PSC patients treated with low- to medium-dose UDCA.[41]

Pruritus is one of the most common complaints among patients with PSC and can be debilitating. The treatment options are similar to those discussed in the previous section on PBC (see Table 75-2). Currently, liver transplantation is the only life-extending treatment available, with 5-year survival rates of 75% to 85%. However, disease recurrence has been reported in up to 47% of cases, with the presence of IBD being the most important independent predictive factor.[42] The estimated median survival for PSC is about 12 years: for symptomatic patients, there is a reduction in life expectancy, with a mean survival just under 10 years.[43]

AUTOIMMUNE OVERLAP SYNDROMES

Autoimmune hepatitis (AIH) is a chronic hepatitis of unknown cause characterized by hyperglobulinemia, the presence of circulating autoantibodies, and inflammatory changes on liver histology.[44] Up to 18% of patients with AIH may have a variant that overlaps with PBC, PSC, or immunoglobulin G4 (IgG4)-related sclerosing cholangitis (previously termed *autoimmune cholangitis*).[45] Conversely, patients with PBC and PSC may show biochemical or histologic evidence of AIH. The term *autoimmmune overlap syndrome* is used to describe these cases.[46] Detailed descriptions of these syndromes are provided in Chapter 74. Patients with AMA-positive autoimmune PBC overlap respond well to UDCA, 10 to 15 mg/kg BW/day, and glucocorticosteroids, but not those who are AMA-negative.[47] Treatment is started with 20 to 30 mg of prednisolone and calcium and vitamin D for bone protection. Azathioprine (1.5 to 2 mg/kg BW/day) is introduced early as an immunosuppressant and steroid-sparing agent. Prednisolone is tapered off quickly when the ALT level normalizes but is kept at a background level of 5 mg/day for at least 1 year. Bone loss needs to be monitored. There are limited data on the treatment of AIH-PSC overlap syndrome; patients respond less well to corticosteroids alone but may benefit from the addition of azathioprine.[48] There appears to be less of a beneficial long-term outcome with AIH-PSC compared to AIH-PBC in a series from King's College Hospital.[49]

IgG4-RELATED SCLEROSING CHOLANGITIS

IgG4-related sclerosing cholangitis, also termed *autoimmune cholangitis*, is a condition that can present similarly to PSC or even cholangiocarcinoma, but it is important to distinguish between these conditions because the prognoses are completely different. IgG4-related sclerosing cholangitis forms part of the spectrum of the increasingly recognized immune-mediated conditions known as IgG4-related diseases. Other organs that may be affected include the pancreas, salivary glands, lachrymal glands, orbital muscles, and retroperitoneum.[50] The incidence of IgG4-related sclerosing cholangitis is presently unknown but appears to be more common in middle-aged and older men.[51] The pathogenesis is also poorly understood but may involve an autoimmune disorder as well as an allergic component.[52] The diagnosis is made by the measurement of serum IgG4 levels, proceeding to a liver biopsy in the very few cases that do not respond to a trial of steroids. Serum levels of IgG4 are elevated in 60% to 70% patients.[53] Histologically, there is infiltration of the affected organs with IgG4-positive plasma cells and CD4+ T lymphocytes, causing inflammation and fibrosis.[54] Any patient who presents with features of PSC should have serum IgG4 levels measured as part of the workup, which should also include an MRCP. An elevated serum IgG4 level could prompt a trial of steroids because the condition responds well to steroids, and levels of serum IgG4 fall during treatment.[55] The starting dose of prednisolone is not established, but it would be reasonable to use the same drug regimen as for AIH, starting at 40 mg/day and titrating down the dose as the LFT results improve and serum IgG4 levels fall. A response is expected within 2 to 4 weeks of treatment. The use of immunosuppressants as second-line or steroid-sparing agents following normalization of LFTs has not been established but would be similar to the use of azathioprine (1-5-2 mg/kg BW/day) or mycophenolate mofetil (up to 2 g/day), as for AIH. The prognosis of IgG4-related sclerosing cholangitis has not been well defined but, untreated, the disease is likely to progress to cirrhosis and portal hypertension.

DRUG-INDUCED LIVER INJURY CAUSING CHOLESTASIS

Drug-induced liver injury (DILI) can develop following the use of prescription or over the counter drugs as well as with herbal medicines. The annual incidence is estimated to be from 10 to 15/10,000 to 100,000 persons exposed to prescription medications.[56,57] Women may be more susceptible to DILI than men, which may in part be due to their generally smaller size.[59] DILI is characterized by the type of hepatic injury based on the pattern

TABLE 75-3 Classification of Drug-Induced Liver Injury (DILI)

Type	Transaminase	ALT/ALP Ratio (R)
Hepatic (hepatocellular)	ALT ≥ 3 × ULN	R ≥ 5
Cholestatic	ALP ≥ 2 × ULN	R ≤ 2
Mixed	ALT ≥ 3 × ULN ALP ≥ 2 × ULN	R > 2 and R < 5

Adapted from Bjornsson ES, Jonasson JG: Drug-induced cholestasis. Clin Liver Dis 17:191–209, 2013.

ALT, Alanine transaminase; *ALP,* alkaline phosphatase; *R,* ALT/ULN divided by ALP/ULN; *ULN,* upper limit of normal.

BOX 75-1 Common Drugs Causing Liver Injury in Older Adults

- Amitriptyline
- Ampicillin
- Amoxicillin–clavulanic acid
- Anabolic steroids
- Carbamazepine
- Chlorpromazine
- Erythromycin
- Floxacillin
- Haloperidol
- Imipramine

of LFTs—hepatocellular (cytotoxic) injury, cholestatic injury, or a mixed picture. DILI is considered acute if the liver tests have been abnormal for less than 3 months and chronic if they have been abnormal for more than 3months.[58] Hepatocellular injury accounts for most cases of DILI (≈90%).[60] The presence of jaundice (serum bilirubin level > twice the upper limit of normal [ULN]) in association with an ALT level more than three times the ULN is associated with a worse prognosis, known as Hy law, with mortality approaching 14%.[59] In this chapter, we will discuss cholestatic injury, which is defined as an elevated ALP level more than twice the ULN and/or an ALT/ALP ratio less than 2 (Table 75-3)

Histologically, acute cholestatic DILI is called bland or noninflammatory cholestasis when there is evidence of bile plugs in hepatocytes and/or canaliculi, with little inflammation—for example, seen with the use of anabolic steroids.[61] It is called *cholangiolitic inflammatory hepatitis* when there is histologic evidence of prominent cholestasis, portal inflammation, hepatocyte injury, and bile duct proliferation, seen with the use of erythromycin, amoxicillin–clavulanic acid, and angiotensin-converting-enzyme (ACE) inhibitors.[62,63] Chronic cholestatic DILI has features of chronic biliary diseases, such as primary biliary cirrhosis, biliary obstruction, and primary sclerosing cholangitis.[64] Less commonly, prolonged damage can lead to loss of bile ducts and overt ductopenia, which can ultimately lead to cirrhosis and liver failure.[65] Drugs associated with ductopenia include floxacillin, amoxicillin–clavulanic acid, ACE inhibitors, and terbinafine.[66] Common drugs causing cholestatic DILI are shown in Box 75-1.

Treatment

The treatment of cholestatic DILI depends on awareness and recognition of the condition followed by the withdrawal of the suspected offending drug. US is performed to exclude biliary obstruction. There is no specific treatment to reverse cholestasis, and therefore treatment is supportive. Bile acid sequestrants may relieve pruritus. Our practice is to monitor the LFTs every 2 days until they start to improve. The frequency of blood testing can be reduced to twice a week until there is improvement of the cholestasis, and monitoring can then be done weekly until resolution of the episode. In rare cases when the LFTs do not improve or worsen, a liver biopsy may be requested to exclude the complete loss of small bile ducts, histologically *termed ductopenia*. The overall prognosis is good, although complete normalization of the LFTs may take weeks to months.[67] Patients with ductopenia may continue to worsen, and fatalities have been reported. In this case, if the patient is a liver transplantation candidate, referral to a liver transplantation center is recommended.

Patients can be asymptomatic but may have deranged LFTs or present with fever, malaise, anorexia, nausea, and/or jaundice. Patients with cholestasis present with pruritus or excoriations from scratching. The diagnosis is made from the history of exposure to the drug, ruling out other causes of liver disease and the pattern of LFTs. If there is evidence of cholestasis, US is usually requested to exclude biliary obstruction. A liver biopsy is very rarely required but should be considered if diagnostic doubt persists, usually in cases in which the patient fails to improve after withdrawal of the suspected offending drug. Rechallenge is not recommended because it leads to rapid and severe recurrence of the condition. The diagnosis is not always easy to make, because obtaining a reliable drug history can be challenging, and the relationship between exposure to the drug and hepatic toxicity is not always clear. Concomitant liver disease can also confuse the picture. A number of scales (e.g., Council for International Organizations of Medical Sciences [CIOMS] scale, Roussel Uclaf Causality Assessment Method [RUCAM], or U.S. Drug Induced Liver Injury Network [DILIN] scale) have been developed to stratify drug toxicity into objective criteria but none is used routinely in clinical practice.[67,68]

BILIARY CYSTS

Biliary cysts (previously known as choledochal cysts) are cystic dilations of the intrahepatic and extrahepatic biliary tree. They are mainly diagnosed in childhood, presenting with abdominal pain, jaundice, and a palpable mass and confirmed by US or computed tomography (CT).[69] They can be found incidentally in older adults and are asymptomatic. They are more common in women. The incidence varies from 1/50,00 to 100,000.[69] Biliary cysts can lead to ductal strictures, stone formation, cholangitis, secondary biliary cirrhosis, rupture, pancreatitis, and cholangiocarcinoma.

Biliary cysts are classified as types I to V, with type I (involving the common bile duct only) and type IV (involving both the intrahepatic and extrahepatic ducts) accounting for more than 50% and 15% to 35% of cases, respectively.[70] LFTs are within the normal range in asymptomatic cases and show an obstructive picture when complications develop. Biliary cysts are associated with an increased risk of cancer, particularly cholangiocarcinoma, reported to be as high as 30% in types I and IV cysts.[71] Occasionally, they cause occult upper gastrointestinal bleeding (hemobilia), which can be a diagnostic challenge with structurally normal endoscopy, but careful examination of the ampulla may reveal a slow trickle of blood. The diagnosis of a biliary cyst in older adults is usually an incidental finding on US or CT requested for investigation of other abdominal symptoms. If a cyst is suspected based on an US scan, cross-sectional imaging with CT or MRCP is used to delineate the cyst and exclude malignancy. Occasionally, an ERCP or endoscopic ultrasound (EUS) may also be required if there is evidence of biliary obstruction. Cysts with a high malignant potential require surgical management in patients who are fit enough for surgery.[72] If surgery is not an option, cysts can be followed up by annual cross-sectional imaging or re-investigated if symptoms develop or LFTs are deranged.

GALLSTONE DISEASES

Gallbladder stones are found in about 13% to 50% of people aged 70 years, and the percentage increases to 38% to 53% in

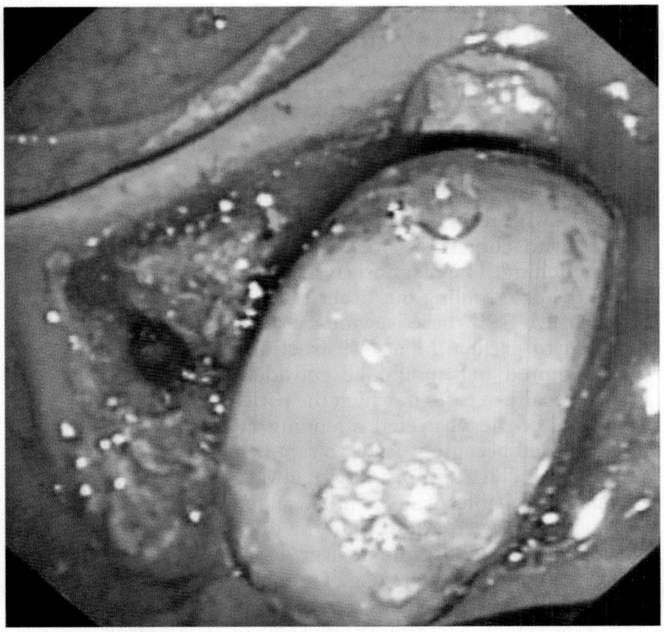

Figure 75-2. Pigmented stone seen with the sludge.

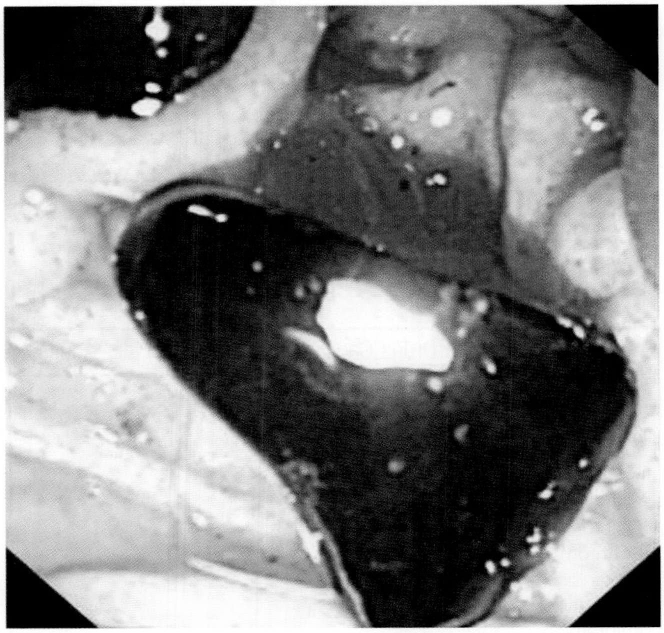

Figure 75-3. Black stone removed en bloc.

those older than 80 years. They occur twice as frequently in women as in men, but this difference decreases with increasing age. Gallstones are of three types, depending on the major constituents—pure cholesterol, pure pigment (which can be black or brown), and mixed. Cholesterol stones are the most frequent, accounting for 80% to 90% of all gallstones in the West. They contain more than 70% cholesterol, often with some bile pigment and calcium.

Impaired gallbladder motility can precede gallstone formation. Intestinal factors, including decreased large bowel transit time, increased colonic gram-positive anaerobic bacteria, increased bile acid–metabolizing enzymes, and higher intracolonic pH values have also been documented.[73]

Black stones are seen in patients with chronic hemolysis (e.g., hereditary spherocytosis, sickle cell disease), when there is an increase in bilirubin levels and also in cirrhosis. Brown pigment stones have layers of cholesterol, calcium salts (mainly palmitate), and calcium bilirubinate. They form in the common bile duct as a result of stasis and infection, usually in the presence of *Escherichia coli* and *Klebsiella*. They are also found with biliary strictures, sclerosing cholangitis, and Caroli syndrome (Figures 75-2 to 75-5).

The most common presentation of gallstone disease is biliary pain. This occurs in the epigastrium and right hypochondrium and does not fluctuate, but persists from 15 minutes up to 24 hours, subsiding spontaneously or with opioid analgesics. It may radiate around to the back in the interscapular region.

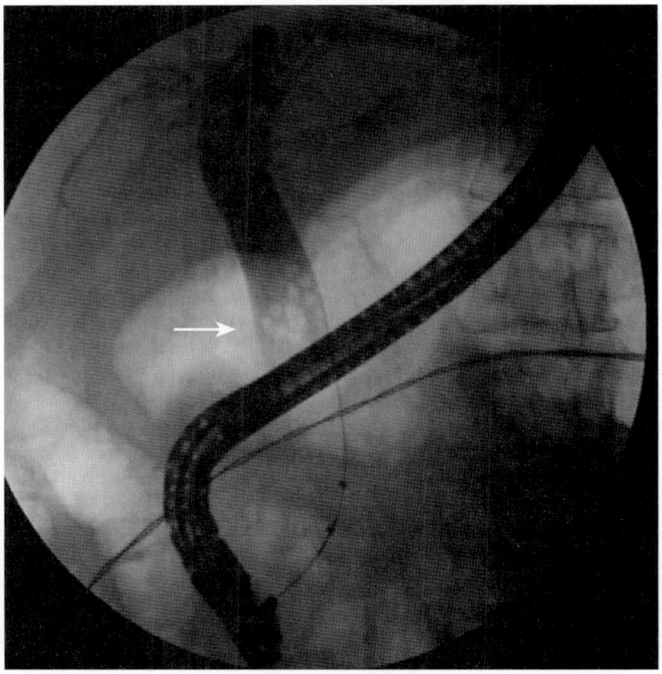

Figure 75-4. Multiple small stones in a distended common bile duct seen as filling defects *(arrow)*.

ACUTE CHOLECYSTITIS

The patient is usually ill with a sudden onset of right upper quadrant pain (which may not radiate to the right shoulder in older patients, as commonly occurs in younger people), high-grade fever, jaundice, nausea, and vomiting. Right hypochondrial tenderness is worse on inspiration (Murphy sign), and thus voluntary guarding, rebound tenderness. and shallow respirations are seen in acute episodes. The presentation of biliary colic in the older patient with diabetes and diabetic neuropathy is usually atypical. In such patients, a condition as serious as gangrenous cholecystitis can present with minimal temperature increases, without significant leukocytosis and few, if any, abdominal complaints. Consequently, clinically significant cholecystitis can be interpreted as an episode of mild biliary colic. A US examination that detects gallstones alone is insufficient for a diagnosis of acute cholecystitis. Additional criteria are as follows:

- Sonographic Murphy sign (focal tenderness directly over the visualized gallbladder)
- Distention of the gallbladder

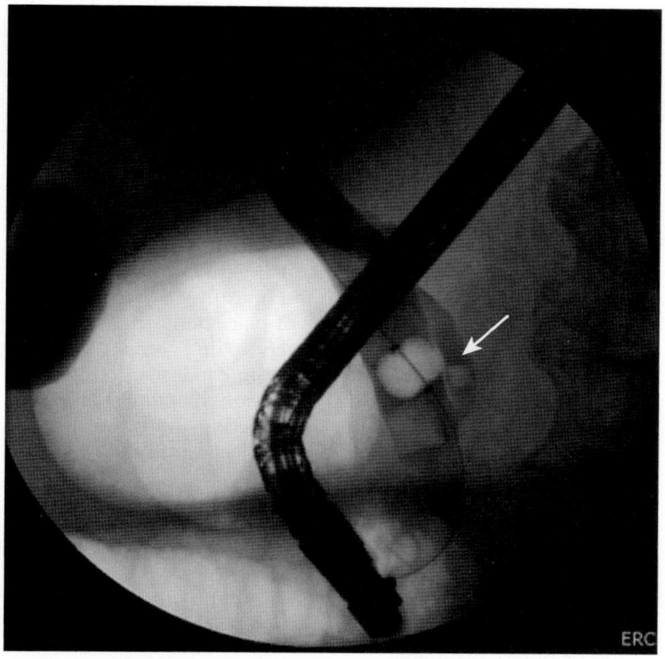

Figure 75-5. Large stones seen in a distended common bile duct *(arrow).*

- Presence of biliary sludge
- Pericholecystic fluid
- Gallbladder wall thickening (but not specific for acute disease)

Common Bile Duct Stones

Common bile duct stones are found in approximately 95% of older patients who present with cholecystitis. Presentation can include one or all of the triad of abdominal pain, jaundice, and fever. The pain is usually severe and is situated in the epigastrium and right hypochondrium; it may be accompanied by vomiting, usually lasts for a few hours, and then clears up, only to return days, weeks, or even months later. The patient is well between attacks. The jaundice is variable in degree, depending on the amount of obstruction. Urine is dark, and the stools are pale. High fever and rigors indicate cholangitis. The liver is enlarged if the obstruction lasts for more than a few hours. Prolonged biliary obstruction or repeated attacks lead to secondary biliary cirrhosis, but this is now rare.

US examination reveals a dilated common bile duct, but stones are detected in only about 75% of cases. MRCP is very useful as an additional diagnostic test, particularly if the bowel hinders good visualization of the common bile duct, and is better than US in detecting stones in the lowest part of the common bile duct. ERCP is usually necessary for duct clearance. If this is not feasible because of large or multiple stones or a technically challenging procedure, plastic stent insertion (single or multiple double-pigtail stents) into the biliary system to gain access and drainage helps settle the sepsis. These stents can then be removed at a later date (usually 3 months), and a further attempt at stone clearance can then be undertaken. In patients with irretrievable common bile duct stones, elective stent exchange every 6 to 12 monthly is a viable treatment option (stent exchange program). If patients are known to have limited life expectancy, in whom the risk of undergoing repeated ERCPs for stent exchanges is deemed higher, stents are placed permanently (expectant management). Unpublished reports comparing the outcomes of these two treatment strategies have suggested that careful selection of subjects is needed for the latter group.[74] Studies on patients managed with indwelling plastic stents have shown that there is reduction of stone size in the follow-up period.[75,76] Rare complications of biliary stones are bilioenteric fistulas (choledochoduodenal and cholecystoduodenal fistulas), generally complicated by recurrent episodes of cholangitis and, rarely, upper gastrointestinal bleeding.[77]

ACUTE CHOLANGITIS

Bacterial infection of the bile ducts is always secondary to bile duct abnormalities. The most frequent causes are common duct stones, biliary strictures, neoplasms, or following ERCP in the presence of large duct obstruction. Symptoms are fever, often with a rigor, upper abdominal pain, and jaundice. Older patients can present with collapse and gram-negative septicemia and renal failure.

Initial therapy of acute cholecystitis and cholangitis is directed toward general support of the patient, including fluid and electrolyte replacement, correction of metabolic imbalances, and antibacterial therapy. In all but mild cases, pain relief with an opiate is required. In the absence of vomiting, the patient can soon tolerate oral fluids, and nasogastric aspiration is not often required.

Antimicrobial therapy is usually empirical. Initial therapy should cover the Enterobacteriaceae, in particular *E. coli*, and anaerobes, especially in older adults and patients with previous bile duct–bowel anastomosis. Antimicrobial therapy includes monotherapy with piperacillin, mezlocillin, third-generation cephalosporins, and ciprofloxacin, depending on the severity of the infection. Caution must be taken when using aminoglycosides for sepsis with renal involvement.

ERCP and sphincterotomy are effective in stone extraction and should be the first therapeutic approach because it is safer than surgery in older adults.[78] Stent insertion may be necessary for a two-stage procedure, as explained earlier.

OTHER DISORDERS

Malignant Obstruction

Malignant obstruction of the biliary tract results from extramural causes, such as carcinoma of the head of the pancreas, or mural causes, such as cholangiocarcinoma, primary carcinoma of the gallbladder, or ampullary tumor. The usual presentation in older adults consists of the insidious painless development of cholestatic jaundice.

Pancreatic Carcinoma

Pancreatic carcinoma is the most common cause of malignant biliary obstruction. Each year, there are approximately 46,000 cases in the United States,[79] 20,000 cases in Japan, and 9,000 in the United Kingdom. Pancreatic cancer affects men and women equally, and 50% of all new cases are diagnosed in those aged 75 years and older. It has the worst survival rate of all cancers, with a 1-year survival of less than 20% and a 5-year survival of only 3%, a figure that has not changed much over the last 40 years. Surgical resection offers the only chance of cure but most patients present with locally advanced or metastatic disease. Pancreatic cancer responds poorly to chemotherapy and a gemcitabine-based regimen only extends survival by a few months.[80]

Cholangiocarcinoma

Cholangiocarcinoma represents less than 3% of gastrointestinal cancers, with an incidence of 1 to 2 cases/100,000 in the United States and an increasing incidence in many developed countries.[81]

There is no association with cirrhosis or viral hepatitis, whereas in the Far East it may be associated with infestation with *Clonorchis sinensis* or *Opisthorchis viverrini*. PSC is a well-recognized risk factor for the development of cholangiocarcinoma. The annual incidence of cholangiocarcinoma in patients with PSC has been estimated to range from 0.6% to 1.5%/year, with a lifetime risk of 5% to 30%. Surveillance is recommended with an annual US or MRCP and the measurement of cancer antigen 19-9 (CA 19-9), but acknowledging that this is not specific for this tumor.[82,83]

Cholangiocarcinomas are classified as intrahepatic, perihilar, or extrahepatic. Intrahepatic tumors are rare (<10%) and seldom present with jaundice. Patients may be asymptomatic, with a raised ALP level, or may present with right upper quadrant pain and weight loss. Perihilar tumors involving the hepatic duct bifurcation are collectively referred to as *calfskin tumors*. Extrahepatic tumors are the most common and tend to present with symptoms and signs typical of obstructive jaundice. The diagnosis is made on CT or MRI but may sometimes require EUS-guided fine-needle aspiration ERCP with brushings for cytology, or CT-guided biopsy. The diagnosis in PSC may be challenging. Local invasion and the proximity of vital structures within the porta hepatis contribute to the difficulty in achieving complete respectability, so that curative surgical resection is rarely possible. Liver transplantation alone is not a current option because of an almost universal likelihood of recurrence.[84] The 5-year survival is poor (20% to 40%), and patients usually die within 6 months.[85-87]

Primary Adenocarcinoma of the Gallbladder

Primary adenocarcinoma of the gallbladder represents less than 1% of all cancers; it occurs chiefly in patients older than 70 years, usually in women, and has striking genetic, racial, ethnic, and geographic characteristics, with an extremely high prevalence in Native Americans and Chileans. Gallstones are usually present, but a definite relationship is uncertain.[88] Polyps larger than 1 cm and that are single, sessile, and echogenic are associated with a higher risk of malignancy. An anomalous junction of pancreaticobiliary ducts, chronic bacterial infections, certain occupational and environmental carcinogens, hormonal changes, and possibly a porcelain gallbladder are additional factors that predispose to cancer. Occasionally, a mass can be palpable in the right hypochondrium. Most cases are discovered during exploration for presumed gallstone disease, and cholecystectomy is performed, if possible. The overall 5-year survival is 5%, and the 1-year mortality is 88%.

Ampullary Tumors

Primary ampullary tumors are rare, with an incidence estimated at 4 to 6 cases/million,[89] and typically present in the seventh decade with cholestatic jaundice. They may ulcerate and produce gastrointestinal hemorrhage or chronic anemia. They develop in adenomas, and there is an increased risk in patients with familial adenomatous polyposis (FAP).[90] The diagnosis is usually made by obtaining tissue via ERCP, and staging is done by CT. Carcinoma of the ampulla can sometimes be resected, with a 5-year survival rate of 40%.

Management of Pancreaticobiliary Malignancy

All but the frailest patients should have their cancer staged to help identify the few who may have a resectable lesion. Staging also helps estimate the prognosis in nonresectable disease, which allows patients and their family and caregivers to deal with the disease. The diagnosis and staging are reached through a combination of CT, MRI, EUS, and ERCP and obtaining tissue for histology. Ideally, all cases should be discussed at a multidisciplinary meeting consisting of physicians, surgeons, radiologists, histopathologists, oncologists, and the palliative care team.

Most of these cancers present late in older adults and tend to be unresectable. The main goal of treatment is to provide palliation of jaundice, avoid early liver failure caused by chronic obstruction, and improve the patient's nutritional and general status.

Jaundice is relieved by the use of plastic or expandable metal biliary stents placed during ERCP or, if ERCP fails, by the percutaneous route. Biliary stenting can be attempted in even the very frail. Plastic stents placed endoscopically have a propensity to clog or occlude within 6 months of placement, thus requiring exchange. Expandable metal stents seem to delay stent occlusion, but they are not removable and are more expensive than plastic stents. However, as a palliative intervention, metallic stents offer a one-step procedure. With tumors affecting the bifurcation of the hepatic ducts, several stents can be placed into the right and left intrahepatic ducts to provide decompression.

Very rarely, palliative surgery can be considered to relieve jaundice by creating a biliary-enteric anastomosis. However, given the morbidity and 30-day mortality (up to 20%) for bypass procedures, nonoperative techniques for palliation are preferred. Duodenal stenoses can be treated with expandable metal stents, which do not preclude further endoscopic management of pancreatic or biliary problems.

KEY POINTS

- Biliary tract disease is suspected when liver function tests suggest cholestasis.
- Biliary tract diseases can be divided into intrahepatic and extrahepatic causes.
- A thorough history, physical examination, obstructive liver enzyme levels, and relevant imaging will lead to diagnosis in most cases; liver biopsy is rarely necessary.
- Biliary malignancies still have a poor prognosis, despite therapeutic advances.
- Liver transplantation is an established treatment of end-stage benign biliary disease.
- Investigation of an isolated ALP can be conducted in general practice (see algorithm).

For a complete list of references, please visit www.expertconsult.com.

KEY REFERENCES

2. Alvaro D, Benedetti A, Marucci L, et al: The function of alkaline phosphatase in the liver: regulation of intrahepatic biliary epithelium secretory activities in the rat. Hepatology 32:174–184, 2000.
9. Griffiths L, Dyson JK, Jones DE: The new epidemiology of primary biliary cirrhosis. Semin Liver Dis 34:318–328, 2014.
13. Lazaridis KN, Talwalkar JA: Clinical epidemiology of primary biliary cirrhosis: incidence, prevalence, and impact of therapy. J Clin Gastroenterol 41:494–500, 2007.
16. Kaplan MM, Gershwin ME: Primary biliary cirrhosis. N Engl J Med 353:1261–1273, 2005.
18. European Association for the Study of the Liver: Clinical practice guidelines: management of cholestatic liver diseases. J Hepatol 51: 237–267, 2009.
19. Lindor K: Ursodeoxycholic acid for the treatment of primary biliary cirrhosis. N Engl J Med 357:1524–1529, 2007.
22. Carbone M, Mells GF, Pells G, et al: Sex and age are determinants of the clinical phenotype of primary biliary cirrhosis and response to ursodeoxycholic acid. Gastroenterology 144:560–569, 2013.
30. Claessen MM, Vleggaar FP, Tytgat KM, et al: High lifetime risk of cancer in primary sclerosing cholangitis. J Hepatol 50:158–164, 2009.
31. Rosen CB, Heimbach JK, Gores GJ, et al: Liver transplantation for cholangiocarcinoma. Transpl Int 23:692–697, 2010.

38. Rupp C, Rossler A, Halibasic E, et al: Reduction in alkaline phosphatase is associated with longer survival in primary sclerosing cholangitis, independent of dominant stenosis.. Aliment Pharmacol Ther 40:1292–1301, 2014.
41. Hansen JD, Kumar S, Lo WK, et al: Ursodiol and colorectal cancer or dysplasia risk in primary sclerosing cholangitis and inflammatory bowel disease: a meta-analysis. Dig Dis Sci 58:3079–3087, 2013.
49. Al-Chalabi T, Portmann BC, Bernal W, et al: Autoimmune hepatitis overlap syndromes: an evaluation of treatment response, long-term outcome and survival. Aliment Pharmacol Ther 28:209–220, 2008.
50. Stone JH, Zen Y, Deshpande V: IgG4-related disease. N Engl J Med 366:539–551, 2012.
57. Chalasani N, Fontana RJ, Bonkovsky HL, et al: Causes, clinical features, and outcomes from a prospective study of drug-induced liver injury in the United States. Gastroenterology 135:1924–1934, 2008.
59. Zhang X, Ouyang J, Thung SN: Histopathologic manifestations of drug-induced hepatotoxicity. Clin Liver Dis 17:547–564, 2013.
65. Lucena MI, Camargo R, Andrade RJ, et al: Comparison of two clinical scales for causality assessment in hepatotoxicity. Hepatology 33:123–130, 2001.
68. Rockey DC, Seeff LB, Rochon J, et al: Causality assessment in drug-induced liver injury using a structured expert opinion process: comparison to the Roussel-Uclaf causality assessment method. Hepatology 51:2117–2126, 2010.
71. Mohammed N, Pinder M, Harris K, Everett S: Endoscopic biliary stenting in irretrievable common bile duct stones: stent exchange or expectant management-tertiary-centre experience and systematic review. Frontline Gastroenterol May 22, 2015, doi:10.1136/flgastro-2015-100566
74. Mohammed N, Godfrey EM, Subramanian V: Cholecysto-duodenal fistula as the source of upper gastrointestinal bleeding. Endoscopy 45(Suppl 2):E250–E251, 2013.
78. Khan SA, Emadossadaty S, Ladep NG, et al: Rising trends in cholangiocarcinoma: is the ICD classification system misleading us? J Hepatol 56:848–854, 2012.
80. Malaguarnera G, Paladina I, Giordano M, et al: Serum markers of intrahepatic cholangiocarcinoma. Dis Markers 34:219–228, 2013.
81. Meyer CG, Penn I, James L: Liver transplantation for cholangiocarcinoma: results in 207 patients. Transplantation 69:1633–1637, 2000.
85. Randi G, Franceschi S, La Vecchia C: Gallbladder cancer worldwide: geographical distribution and risk factors. Int J Cancer 118:1591–1602, 2006.
86. Albores-Saavedra J, Schwartz AM, Batich K, et al: Cancers of the ampulla of Vater: demographics, morphology, and survival based on 5,625 cases from the SEER program. J Surg Oncol 100:598–605, 2009.

75

76 The Upper Gastrointestinal Tract

David A. Greenwald, Lawrence J. Brandt

Symptoms of gastrointestinal disorders are frequently mentioned by older adults during visits to health care providers, and the digestive diseases producing these symptoms are among the most common hospital discharge diagnoses for older patients in the United States.[1,2] As the older adult population expands and their demand for medical care grows, it becomes increasingly important for physicians to be acquainted with the manifestation of diseases of the upper gastrointestinal (UGI) tract in members of this age group.

ORAL CAVITY

The most proximal of the digestive organs has traditionally been considered to be the esophagus; patients with complaints thought to originate within the oral cavity or pharynx were referred to a dentist or specialist in disorders of the ear, nose, and throat. The oral cavity, however, is examined easily by the general practitioner and may reveal the cause of unexplained or apparently unrelated abnormalities; thus, evaluation of the UGI should begin with the mouth.

Mouth and Nutrition

Changes in the oral cavity occasionally limit the ability of older adults to eat and enjoy a normal diet. Problems with eating sometimes are severe enough to cause malnutrition and prompt a search for a wasting illness.[3] The number of general oral health problems has been shown to be a strong predictor of involuntary weight loss in older adults.[4]

A variety of abnormalities of oral structure and function may contribute to malnutrition. The muscles of mastication may become impaired during aging as the result of a decrease in (lean) body mass.[5] Eating occasionally becomes difficult because of tooth loss due to periodontal disease, poor dentition, or loosening of dentures caused by resorption of mandibular bone.[6]

A reduction in food intake by older adults is sometimes related to a change in taste perceptions. The number of taste buds decreases after the age of 45 years, resulting in a decrease in taste sensation, especially the ability to appreciate salty and sweet foods.[7-9] Diminished perception of sour and bitter tastes is associated with palatal defects and typically occurs in patients who wear dentures. Taste sensation may also be altered directly by medications or indirectly affected by a drug's unpleasant flavor. Agents associated with abnormal taste perception, known as dysgeusia, include tricyclic antidepressants, sulfasalazine, clofibrate, L-dopa, gold salts, lithium, and metronidazole. Medications with anticholinergic properties interfere with taste by reducing salivary gland secretions and producing xerostomia. Age alone, however, is not associated with a reduction in stimulated saliva flow in nonmedicated subjects.[10]

Although abnormal perception may lead to deficient nutrition, some primary nutritional disorders may be responsible for dysgeusia and glossitis. For example, vitamin B_{12} and niacin deficiency are associated with a so-called bald or magenta-colored tongue, respectively. Taste sensation and eating habits also are disturbed by processes that interfere with the sense of smell, which typically is diminished substantially by the age of 70 years.[11]

Vascular Lesions

Diminutive vascular lesions of the UGI are poorly understood and rarely reported. The nomenclature for these lesions is confusing; the terms *arteriovenous malformation*, *vascular ectasia*, *angiodysplasia*, and *telangiectasia* are generally used interchangeably, with little regard for their true meaning.

The lips are a frequent site of senescent vascular lesions resembling those of hereditary hemorrhagic telangiectasia (Osler-Weber-Rendu disease [syndrome]), and involvement often includes the UGI. In addition to this form of small vascular abnormality, patients often have sublingual varices, or caviar lesions (Figure 76-1). The walls of these dilated vessels are thick, but the endothelial lining is hypoplastic.[12] In males, sublingual varices may be associated with the occurrence of capillary phlebectasias of the scrotal skin, or Fordyce lesions (Figure 76-2).

Because vascular abnormalities are often responsible for cryptogenic GI bleeding, their presence in the mouth should suggest that similar lesions elsewhere in the GI tract may be responsible for blood loss in such cases.[13] However, not every individual with bleeding vascular lesions of the GI tract has involvement of oral structures, and the presence of oral lesions does not preclude the existence of an unrelated distal bleeding lesion.

Oral Mucosa

A number of abnormalities of the oral mucosa are encountered in older patients. These changes may be the result of medical therapy, signify the presence of a systemic disease, or represent premalignant changes.

Candidiasis

Candidiasis is usually caused by the fungus *Candida albicans*. This organism is part of the normal GI flora, and its presence is not sufficient by itself to produce disease. Mucosal candidiasis occurs only after a change in other constituents of the normal flora or in the presence of an immunologic abnormality. In older patients, the widespread use of antibiotics and immunosuppressive chemotherapy for malignancies is usually responsible for the development of mucosal candidiasis.

The typical oral lesions of candidiasis are soft white plaques that resemble cottage cheese. Characteristically, these plaques can be peeled from the mucosa, leaving the underlying surface raw and bleeding. This observation is important because most other white plaquelike lesions—for example, leukoplakia—cannot be stripped off the mucosa.

A diagnosis of candidiasis is made by smearing scrapings of the lesion on a glass slide, macerating them with 20% potassium hydroxide, and examining this preparation under a microscope for the presence of typical hyphae. A definitive diagnosis can be made by culture on selected media.

Therapy usually consists of reestablishing the normal microbiologic flora by discontinuing antibiotics. In the immunocompromised host and an individual with significant morbidity, topical therapy with nystatin suspensions or troches is usually successful, although treatment with absorbable oral agents such as fluconazole may be required. Antifungal agents may be supplemented

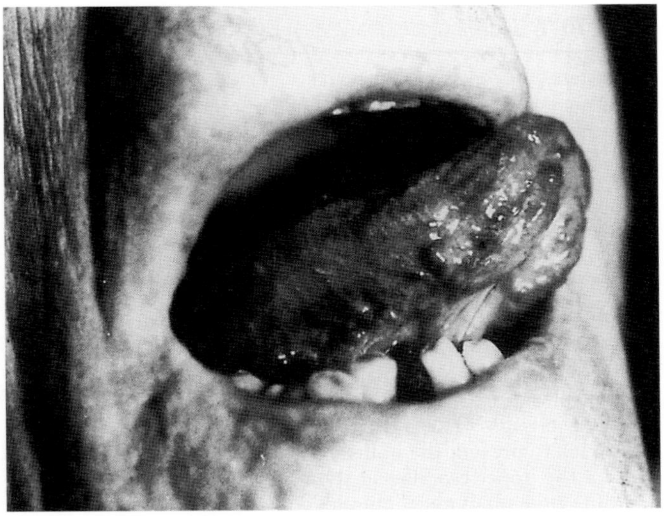

Figure 76-1. Caviar lesion (sublingual varices) in a patient with occult UGI bleeding. *(From Brandt LJ: Gastrointestinal disorders of the elderly, New York, 1986, Lippincott-Raven.)*

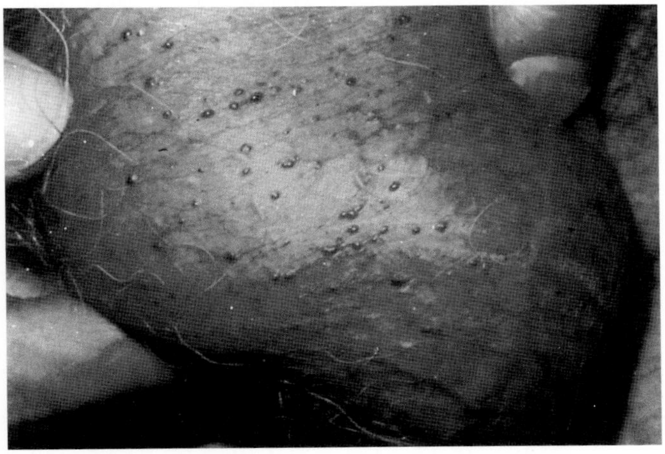

Figure 76-2. Phlebectasias in the scrotum of the same patient as in Figure 76-1. *(From Brandt LJ: Gastrointestinal disorders of the elderly, New York, 1986, Lippincott-Raven.)*

by the use of topical anesthetics to provide symptomatic relief (see later).

Stomatitis

Cancer patients treated with radiation or chemotherapy frequently develop painful inflammation and erosions of the oropharyngeal mucosa. Stomatitis complicating cancer therapy is the direct consequence of drug and radiation toxicity to susceptible, rapidly dividing cell populations of the UGI and an indirect consequence of neutropenia, which impairs regeneration of injured tissues. Radiation to the head and neck also causes xerostomia secondary to fibrosis of the salivary glands. An absence of lubrication by saliva further aggravates mucosal damage, and a lack of salivary immunoglobulin A (IgA) permits the overgrowth of bacteria and fungi. Oral lesions may become infected, contributing to persistent injury, discomfort, and poor nutrition and posing a risk of more widespread infection in immunocompromised individuals.

The initial therapy for stomatitis is promotion of good oral hygiene. Brushing and flossing are contraindicated in neutropenic patients because of the risk of disseminated infection. Instead, mouthwashes containing dilute hydrogen peroxide or a salt and soda solution are used to reduce mucosal bacterial and fungal colonization.

A number of therapeutic mouthwash cocktails have been recommended to relieve symptoms, promote healing, and treat superficial mucosal infection in patients with stomatitis.[14] Some of these cocktails have been tested in controlled trials, but their use is mainly empirical, based on the known analgesic, antibiotic, and protective effects of widely available liquid medicines. Viscous lidocaine (2%) is frequently used as a topical anesthetic, as is diphenhydramine, which is often mixed with oral antacids or kaolin-pectin. Many formulations include sucralfate suspension because it coats damaged epithelium and promotes the production of mucus and protective prostaglandins. Antibiotics used alone or in combination in mouthwash cocktails to treat superficial infection include chlorhexidine gluconate, nystatin, tetracycline, neomycin, vancomycin, and clindamycin. Hydrocortisone and other glucocorticoids have also been added to reduce inflammation, but rapid absorption across the denuded oral mucosa into the systemic circulation may compromise the patient's immune defenses. Artificial saliva replacements (e.g., Salivart, Moi-Stir, Xero-Lube) are also available for patients with xerostomia.

Hairy Tongue

So-called hairy tongue is characterized by hypertrophy of the filiform papillae of the tongue and a lack of normal desquamation. In this condition, the color of the tongue varies from yellow to brown or black, depending on staining by exogenous substances such as tobacco or food and on the presence of various chromogenic microorganisms.[15,16] Hairy tongue is frequently seen in patients who have had extensive radiotherapy to the head and neck. Although these individuals are usually asymptomatic, some complain of nausea, dysgeusia, and halitosis. On occasion, the lingual papillae become so long that they brush against the soft palate, gagging the patient.

Many organisms have been cultured from papillary scrapings from this entity. There is, however, no proof of a cause and effect relationship with any microorganism, and invasion of the lingual epithelium has not been demonstrated. Species of microorganisms that have been isolated are, in all probability, simply colonizing an already abnormal, excessively papillated tongue.

Therapy for this disorder consists of vigorous brushing of the tongue to promote desquamation and remove accumulated debris. In extreme cases, topical treatment with podophyllin, an alcoholic extract of the Mayapple, may result in a dramatic response.

Leukoplakia

The term *leukoplakia* was introduced by Schwimmer in 1877 to describe any white plaque. Today, some authors use this term to refer to histologic zones of hyperkeratosis, acanthosis, and chronic inflammation, whereas others reserve it to describe malignant dyskeratosis and epithelial atypia. Although leukoplakia is considered by many clinicians to be a premalignant condition, its natural history is uncertain because of a lack of uniform definition in case selection. Actually, the term should be abandoned because of its lack of specificity. Any persistent white lesion of the oral mucosa should be biopsied in an attempt to make a specific histologic diagnosis.

Leukoplakia is more common in men than in women and most often occurs during the sixth and seventh decades of life.[17] It can be found anywhere in the oral cavity, although it is most common on the buccal mucosa, tongue, and floor of the mouth. Leukoplakia varies in appearance, partly depending on the age of the lesion. Some investigators consider verrucous patches to be of higher malignant potential than smooth plaques, whereas others believe that granular pinkish-gray to red islands, also called erythroplakia, are most likely to be associated with carcinoma in situ or even invasive malignancy. Such controversy stresses the importance of biopsy in the management of all these lesions. Approximately 10% of patients with leukoplakia have or will develop invasive carcinoma in the lesion.[17-19]

Once the diagnosis of leukoplakia has been substantiated by microscopic examination of a biopsy specimen, therapy is initiated. When dysplasia is present, or when the lesion fails to resolve after a source of physicochemical trauma has been eliminated, treatment consists of ablation.

Epidermoid Carcinoma

Approximately 5% of human cancers arise in the mouth; 95% of oral malignancies are epidermoid carcinomas.[18,19] The lower lip is the most common site of malignancy in the area of the oral cavity. Epidermoid carcinoma of the lip occurs almost exclusively in older men; causative factors include actinic radiation, syphilis, and tobacco use, especially pipe smoking.

Carcinoma of the lip varies in clinical appearance and may be bulky or ulcerated. It metastasizes slowly, usually to the ipsilateral submental or submaxillary lymph nodes. Surgical resection or radiation therapy produces equally good results, with cures in approximately 80% of affected individuals. Successful treatment depends on the duration of symptoms, size of the lesion, and presence of metastases.

Within the oral cavity, half of epidermoid carcinomas originate in the tongue, and the rest arise with equal frequency in the palate, buccal mucosa, floor of the mouth, and gingiva. The disease is seen mainly in older adults and occurs most often in men. Factors suspected to contribute to the development of oral cancer include tobacco, alcohol, nutritional deficiencies, syphilis, and miscellaneous forms of physicochemical trauma, such as irritation from pipe stems and dentures. Almost 90% of patients have a combination of predisposing factors.

Intraoral epidermoid carcinomas display a considerable amount of histologic variation, although lesions tend to be moderately well differentiated. Early carcinomas arising in the tongue typically are painless, even though they may ulcerate. Pain develops later, as the lesions grow, especially if they become secondarily infected. Tumors are usually located on the lateral or ventral surface of the tongue. The site of the primary lesion is of prognostic importance because cancers of the posterior aspect of the tongue tend to be more aggressive. Nodal metastases are located on either or both sides of the neck. Tumors also spread by direct invasion. Early detection is mandatory if patients are to survive for more than 1 year after diagnosis.

Keratoacanthoma is a spontaneously resolving benign lesion that is often mistaken for epidermoid carcinoma.[20] It occurs most frequently in adults 50 to 70 years of age, involves the upper and lower lips equally, and usually presents as a painful umbilicated lesion, seldom more than 15 to 1.5 cm in diameter. It initially appears as a small nodule which reaches full size within 4 to 8 weeks. It persists as a static lesion for another 4 to 8 weeks, after which the keratin core is expelled and the mass resorbed over a period of 6 to 8 weeks. Recurrence is rare.

OROPHARYNX

The oropharyngeal phase of swallowing is exceedingly complex, requiring the participation of multiple distinct structures in the mouth, pharynx, and esophagus, coordinated by six cranial nerves and orchestrated by the swallowing center of the central nervous system. After food has been masticated and moistened with saliva, the tongue initiates swallowing by thrusting the food bolus into the oropharynx. The soft palate prepares for the arrival of the bolus by elevating, so that material from the mouth cannot enter the nasal passages. The glottis also shuts, and the epiglottis tilts downward to prevent the bolus from entering the trachea. Relaxation of the upper esophageal sphincter in association with contraction of the pharyngeal muscles allows propulsion of food into the esophagus (Box 76-1).[21]

BOX 76-1 Causes of Oropharyngeal Dysphagia in Older Adults

Malignancy—pharyngeal carcinoma
Central nervous system disease—tumor, Parkinson disease, stroke
Peripheral nervous system disease—diabetes mellitus
Muscle disease—hypothyroidism
Mechanical—strictures, osteophytes, thyromegaly
Postoperative—laryngectomy
Medications
Motility disorders of the upper esophageal sphincter

Striated muscle involved in the oropharyngeal phase of swallowing, like the muscles of mastication, may be impaired during aging by a decrease in lean body mass. A radiographic study of 100 individuals older than 65 years has suggested that 22 of them had pharyngeal muscle weakness as well as abnormal cricopharyngeal relaxation, with pooling of barium in the valleculae and pyriform sinuses. Several individuals also were noted to have tracheal aspiration of barium. All the subjects, however, were asymptomatic. Thus, although functional changes in the oropharyngeal phase of swallowing may occur with aging, these changes have not been identified as a cause of morbidity in older adults.[22]

Oropharyngeal Dysphagia

Patients with oropharyngeal (cervical or transfer) dysphagia complain of difficulty shifting food from the front of the mouth into the back of the throat or of trouble initiating a swallow once the food bolus has been positioned in the oropharynx. Symptoms may be most severe when the patient attempts to swallow liquids. Signs of transfer dysphagia include nasal regurgitation or the aspiration of oral contents during swallowing as a result of a failure to seal the nasopharynx or trachea by appropriate muscle contraction. Because oropharyngeal dysphagia may be due to a neuromuscular disorder, the patient may display other signs of neuromuscular dysfunction, including dysarthria, nasal speech, cranial nerve dysfunction, weakness, and sensory abnormalities.[23]

A variety of conditions interfere with the transfer of food from the mouth to the esophagus.[24] Mechanical lesions, including tumors, abscesses, and strictures, may block passage of the food bolus or disrupt structures that directly mediate the oropharyngeal phase of swallowing. A neoplasm, infection, or cerebrovascular accident may damage the central nervous system, producing brain stem or pseudobulbar palsy and associated transfer dysphagia. The initiation of swallowing may also be impaired by degenerative diseases of the central or peripheral nervous system, motor end plate, or the muscle itself. Finally, oropharyngeal dysphagia is often caused by a failure of upper esophageal sphincter function. Many of these problems are encountered in older adults.

Cricopharyngeal Achalasia

The term *cricopharyngeal achalasia*, partly derived from the Greek word meaning "absence of slackening," is a misnomer, because the cricopharyngeus muscle of patients with this disorder is capable of relaxing. The problem in cricopharyngeal achalasia is failure of the muscle to function in synchrony with other elements of the swallowing mechanism. As a result, the pharyngeal muscles propel all or part of the food bolus against a closed sphincter, producing symptoms of cervical dysphagia.

When cricopharyngeal achalasia is encountered, it is usually in older adults. Many disorders may cause this problem, but central nervous system diseases predominate. The clinical features are generally those of oropharyngeal dysphagia. Depending on the cause, the onset of symptoms may be sudden, as with a cerebrovascular accident, or intermittent, as with more insidious disorders, such as diabetic neuropathy. The natural history of cricopharyngeal achalasia is also variable, again probably reflecting its many causes—dysphagia may diminish, remain unremitting, or follow a relapsing-remitting course. Most individuals with this disorder have more difficulty swallowing liquids than solids. Many patients have a pulmonary presentation with laryngitis, bronchitis, recurrent pneumonia, bronchiectasis, and pulmonary abscesses as the sequelae of otherwise quiet cricopharyngeal dysfunction.[25] In some patients, symptoms result in such a fear of eating that weight loss, malnutrition, and psychological problems overshadow the motility disorder.

Postintubation Dysphagia

Special mention must be made of cervical dysphagia occurring as a sequela of endotracheal intubation. Unilateral vocal cord weakness is a common complication of endotracheal intubation and, because the vocal cords are important to the formation of a tight laryngeal seal during the oropharyngeal phase of deglutition, patients with vocal cord weakness may experience coughing and aspiration with swallowing. Individuals who have undergone a tracheostomy also may develop symptoms of oropharyngeal dysphagia. Scar formation from a tracheostomy occasionally prevents normal elevation and anterior rotation of the larynx, causing decreased pharyngeal contraction and incomplete upper esophageal sphincter relaxation during swallowing.

Management of Oropharyngeal Dysphagia

Management of oropharyngeal dysphagia depends only in part on its cause. Any underlying disorder, such as parkinsonism, should be treated. If dysphagia persists despite such therapy, or if significant complications result from impairment of the swallowing mechanism, treatment can be directed at the esophagus itself.

Bougienage of the upper esophageal sphincter with mercury-weighted rubber dilators is beneficial to some patients but often gives only temporary relief. This technique is contraindicated by the presence of a pharyngoesophageal diverticulum because of the high risk of perforation (see later).

Many individuals with cricopharyngeal achalasia benefit from surgical interruption of the upper esophageal sphincter.[26] Failure to respond is usually observed in patients with central nervous system disease or peripheral neuropathy, although even they are occasionally relieved of symptoms by this procedure. Serious complications following cervical myotomy are rare. Botulinum toxin injection and balloon dilation also have been used, with limited success. Gastroesophageal reflux or severe distal esophagitis indicating reflux is an absolute contraindication to cricopharyngeal myotomy unless the lower esophageal defect is corrected first.

Pharyngeal Diverticula

Zenker Diverticulum

Zenker diverticulum (Figure 76-3) is a posterior herniation of the hypopharynx through the triangular area just above the upper esophageal sphincter where the oblique and transverse fibers of the cricopharyngeus muscle join. It is seen once in every 1,000 routine upper gastrointestinal series and is more frequent in males. Approximately 85% of cases occur in individuals older than 50 years.[27]

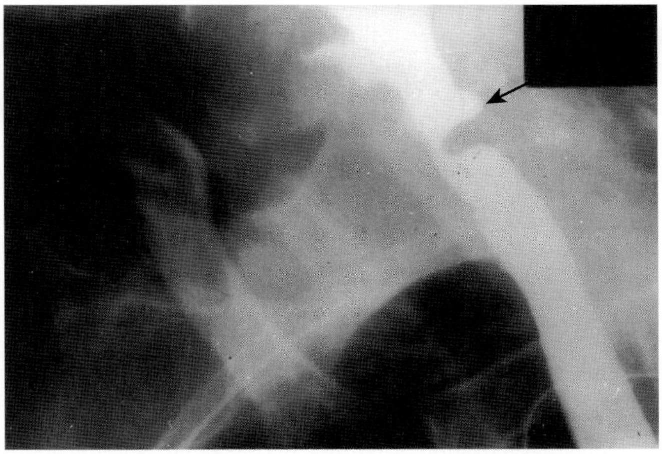

Figure 76-3. Oblique view of a barium-filled esophagus showing a small Zenker diverticulum *(arrow)* proximal to a hypertrophied cricopharyngeus. *(From Brandt LJ: Gastrointestinal disorders of the elderly, New York, 1986, Lippincott-Raven.)*

Symptoms of Zenker diverticulum usually develop insidiously. An annoying irritation in the back of the throat is an early complaint, which may be followed later by the more classic symptoms of oropharyngeal dysphagia. Occasionally, an affected individual complains of a noise like the roar of the ocean or washing machine during swallowing. Postcibal and nocturnal regurgitation of undigested food are common complaints. Obstructive symptoms may be caused by associated cricopharyngeal achalasia or, rarely, by compression of the esophagus by a large diverticulum.

Incoordination and incomplete relaxation of the upper esophageal sphincter during swallowing have been described in association with Zenker diverticulum, lending support to the theory that cricopharyngeal dysfunction leads to high pharyngeal pressures that result in the formation of hypopharyngeal diverticula. Many patients with a Zenker diverticulum, however, have normal function of the upper esophageal sphincter or even reduced upper esophageal sphincter pressure, suggesting that high pharyngeal pressures may be due to stiffening of the pharyngeal muscles with loss of compliance.[28]

Zenker diverticula are usually seen during radiologic examination but, when small, may be missed in the posteroanterior view because of superimposition over the main column of barium in the esophagus. This problem can be avoided by rotating the patient during the study (see Figure 76-3). Endoscopic examination of the UGI in the presence of a hypopharyngeal diverticulum may be associated with an increased risk of perforation; however, this danger is minimized by passage of the instrument under direct vision.

Complications include compression and obstruction of the distal esophagus by a large diverticulum, respiratory difficulties caused by aspiration of diverticular contents, and diverticulitis with perforation. Rarely, carcinoma may develop in a Zenker diverticulum.[29] Worsening of dysphagia, weight loss, and the appearance of blood in regurgitated material suggest the development of a malignant neoplasm.

The therapy for a symptomatic Zenker diverticulum includes surgical excision alone or cricopharyngeal myotomy, with or without removal of the diverticulum.[30] Endoscopic techniques for the treatment of Zencker diverticulum have been well described, with good success rates.[31]

Lateral Pharyngeal Diverticula

Lateral pharyngeal diverticula, or pharyngoceles, occur with increased frequency in older adults and are especially common in men.[32] They develop in the gap between the superior and middle pharyngeal constrictors. Symptoms are the same as those of a Zenker diverticulum. In addition, patients may complain of a neck mass that enlarges with a Valsalva maneuver. Increased intrapharyngeal pressure may be an important causative factor, as exemplified by the frequency of this entity in muezzins and wind instrument players. Surgical repair is safe and effective.

ESOPHAGUS

The muscularis propria of the esophagus is composed of striated muscle fibers proximally and smooth muscle fibers distally. The central nervous system governs the activity of the striated muscle by sequential activation of extrinsic nerves. In humans, the dominant mechanism for control of the smooth muscle of the esophagus is unknown; both central and intramural neural pathways have been demonstrated. Orderly peristaltic contractions of esophageal muscle are necessary for normal esophageal function.

Although no information is available about the effects of aging on the regulation of esophageal muscle activity, alterations in esophageal muscle function have been identified manometrically in older adults. These changes were described first in 1964 by Soergel and colleagues,[33] who referred to motility disturbances in older adults as presbyesophagus. They studied 15 subjects older than 90 years and found a variety of abnormalities; 13 of their patients, however, had diseases known to affect esophageal motility. Subsequent studies have confirmed that in the absence of other disorders, esophageal motility may be abnormal in older adults, but the only manometric change identified in all the published work to date is a reduction in the amplitude of muscle contractions after a swallow.[34-36]

Older adults also may be noted to have disordered motility, or tertiary contractions, on a barium esophagram, but this finding is rarely associated with symptoms.[37] Because motility changes that develop with aging do not appear to have clinical importance, the diagnosis of presbyesophagus should be abandoned. Older patients with dysphagia should be evaluated for the presence of disease processes involving the esophagus, and complaints should not be ascribed to motility changes occurring as a result of advanced age alone.

Dysphagia and Heartburn

Dysphagia and heartburn (pyrosis) are the principal symptoms of esophageal diseases; patients with esophageal disorders, especially older adults, also may complain of respiratory difficulties, painful swallowing (odynophagia), chest pain resembling the pain of myocardial ischemia, regurgitation, and vomiting.[38-40]

Dysphagia is caused by impaired passage of food through the esophagus and is experienced immediately after the act of deglutition. Patients often complain that food "sticks on the way down." Because sensation in the esophagus is referred proximally, lesions at the gastroesophageal junction often appear as symptoms experienced at the level of the sternal notch. When a patient has symptoms that have apparently originated in the area of the proximal esophagus, evaluation of the entire esophagus, often with esophagoscopy and barium radiography, is required.

The pattern of dysphagia frequently suggests the nature of the underlying disease.[41] Schatzki observed that a correct diagnosis can be made after taking a careful history in up to 85% of patients with this complaint.[42] Thus, intermittent dysphagia connotes a motility disorder or a pliant mechanical obstruction, such as an esophageal web. Progressive dysphagia often represents a neoplasm. Individuals who experience difficulty in swallowing liquids and solid foods usually have a primary neuromuscular abnormality and disordered esophageal motility, whereas dysphagia produced only by solid foods is associated with mechanical obstruction of the esophagus.

Heartburn is a manifestation of the reflux of gastric contents into the esophagus and, as its name suggests, is described as being a hot sensation behind the sternum or in the left parasternal area. Pyrosis is relieved by antacids and intensified by bending at the waist or lying supine, especially when the stomach is full. Pyrosis also may be aggravated by some medications, smoking, and ingestion of alcohol, citrus juices, caffeine, chocolate, or peppermint. Discomfort is often accompanied by regurgitation of gastric contents, belching, vomiting, or secretion of saliva (water brash). The nature or extent of esophageal abnormalities associated with gastroesophageal reflux and heartburn cannot be predicted on the basis of the intensity of symptoms, especially in older adults; severe reflux disease, as evidenced by esophageal ulcers, may be present in the absence of substantial symptoms.[43,44]

Motility Disorders

Esophageal Motility Disorders

After individuals with structural lesions have been excluded, over 50% of adults of all ages with a complaint of dysphagia are found to have esophageal motility disorders.[45] These abnormalities may be primary or secondary and are classified according to their manometric signatures. Usually, adults with dysphagia have disordered motility, with nonspecific and inconsistent manometric features.

Nonspecific Secondary Motility Disorders

In older adults, nonspecific disorders of esophageal motility are frequently secondary to a systemic disease. Examples of generalized disorders sometimes responsible for esophageal dysmotility include myxedema, amyloidosis, connective tissue disease, and diabetes mellitus.

Approximately 50% of patients with diabetic neuropathy have abnormal esophageal motility. Findings in these individuals include a decrease in the amplitude of muscle contraction, delayed esophageal emptying, esophageal dilation, and reduced lower esophageal emptying sphincter pressure. In patients with diabetes, the severity of motility changes correlates with the severity of other neuropathic complications; however, affected individuals usually do not have significant dysphagia. Thus, esophageal symptoms in a diabetic must be fully evaluated and not simply attributed to diabetes.

Primary and Secondary Achalasia

Primary achalasia is the second most common motility disorder diagnosed in patients with nonstructural dysphagia, but it is rare in older adults.[46] In those older than 50 years, achalasia is usually secondary to gastric adenocarcinoma (Figure 76-4); pancreatic adenocarcinoma, oat cell carcinoma, reticulum cell sarcoma, and anaplastic lymphoma are responsible for isolated cases.[47,48] Manometric findings in secondary achalasia are identical to those in the primary disorder—absence of esophageal peristalsis, usually in association with an elevation of resting lower esophageal sphincter pressure and failure of the lower esophageal sphincter to relax following an appropriate stimulus. The elevation of resting lower esophageal sphincter pressure typical of achalasia is less pronounced in older adults, who also experience less chest pain in association with this disorder than younger patients.[49]

Patients with both primary and secondary achalasia may experience progressive difficulties in swallowing. Food collects in the esophagus, which may become distended and tortuous, even

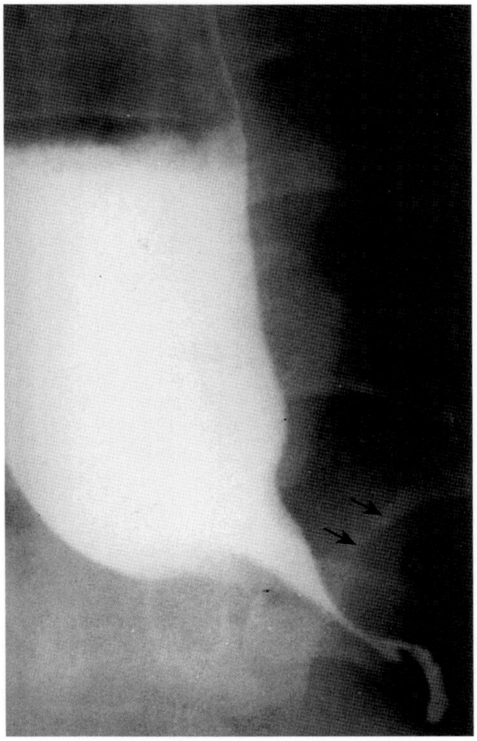

Figure 76-4. Barium esophagram showing tapering of the distal esophagus simulating achalasia. The subtle presence of a mass in the gastric fundus *(arrows)* suggested a diagnosis of carcinoma. *(From Brandt LJ: Gastrointestinal disorders of the elderly, New York, 1986, Lippincott-Raven.)*

when the patient has an underlying carcinoma. In the absence of proximal dilation of the esophagus, a diagnosis of malignancy is favored. When the patient reclines, pooled food flows out of the esophagus back into the pharynx, resulting in coughing and aspiration. Therefore, affected individuals, may present with aspiration pneumonia. In addition to an infiltrate, a chest x-ray may reveal an air-fluid level in the esophagus and absence of the gastric air bubble. Because the presentations of primary and secondary achalasia may be identical, malignancy must be excluded in an older adult with this syndrome. Computed tomography (CT) scans of the chest and upper abdomen, as well as endoscopy with biopsy of the distal esophagus, are recommended.[50] Endoscopic ultrasound may be helpful in differentiating primary from secondary achalasia. Primary achalasia may be treated by pneumatic dilation, surgically, or endoscopically, by peroral endoscopic myotomy (POEM).

The pathogenesis of secondary achalasia is unknown. Submucosal infiltration of the distal esophagus by tumor has been noted in some cases, and normal histology has been found in others.[51] It is possible that in the absence of tumor infiltration, the motility disorder reflects a paraneoplastic neuropathy; manometric and roentgenographic abnormalities may disappear after resection of a gastric carcinoma or therapy for a lymphoma.[52,53]

Diffuse Esophageal Spasm

Although primary esophageal motility disorders usually occur in middle-aged individuals, manometric recordings in older adults with intermittent dysphagia occasionally display the pattern of diffuse esophageal spasm.[38] In this motility disturbance, the patient has simultaneous, repetitive muscle contractions of prolonged duration that occur spontaneously or after a swallow. Normal peristalsis is present most of the time, explaining the intermittent nature of symptoms, which may be triggered by hot or cold foods, pills, or carbonated beverages. The pathogenesis of diffuse esophageal spasm is obscure; on the basis of case reports, some have speculated that in some cases, this disorder represents a stage in the development of achalasia.

Nutcracker Esophagus and Noncardiac Chest Pain

It is usually assumed that in persons free of significant coronary artery disease with chest pain resembling the pain of myocardial ischemia, symptoms are due to an esophageal motility disorder. Such patients, however, rarely have chest pain during esophageal manometry, and provocative testing may be used to precipitate symptoms. Provocative testing with intravenous edrophonium chloride and infusion of acid into the esophagus causes chest pain in about 30% of subjects with a history of noncardiac chest pain.[54] A similar number of patients with noncardiac chest pain have been found to have an esophageal motility disorder, but only 25% of them have symptoms during provocative testing.[44] It is often difficult, therefore, to prove that the esophagus is the source of the patient's complaints.

The most common motility disorder found in patients with noncardiac chest pain is the so-called nutcracker esophagus.[44] This abnormality is characterized by peristaltic muscle contractions of extremely high amplitude and long duration in the distal portion of the esophagus. A defect in esophageal transit can be demonstrated in many affected patients using a radionuclide marker. In one large series of individuals with noncardiac chest pain, 50% of patients with a motility disorder had nutcracker esophagus; other symptomatic individuals were found to have diffuse esophageal spasm.[44] A causal role for these motility defects in the production of chest pain has not been proved. Many patients with noncardiac chest pain have been found to have musculoskeletal disorders.

A number of medications have been used to treat primary esophageal motility disorders, especially diffuse esophageal spasm and nutcracker esophagus. Nitrates, anticholinergics, calcium channel blockers, or sedatives are occasionally effective in relieving symptoms of dysphagia and chest pain; their benefit in this setting, however, has never been evaluated in an appropriately designed trial. Some patients also obtain relief from dysphagia after bougienage. As noted earlier, pneumatic dilation, surgery and endoscopic techniques are the treatment options for primary achalasia.

Hiatus Hernia

The incidence of hiatus hernia (Figure 76-5) increases with each decade of life, from less than 10% of those younger than 40 years to approximately 40% in the sixth and seventh decades and 70% in patients older than 70 years. Symptoms such as pyrosis and regurgitation formerly attributed to the hernia are now known to be due to lower esophageal sphincter dysfunction. Sphincter dysfunction and gastrointestinal reflux are independent of the presence of a hiatus hernia, and the common sliding hiatus hernia is not by itself considered to be pathogenic.

One type of hiatus hernia that deserves special mention is the paraesophageal hernia (Figure 76-6), an uncommon hernia that usually occurs in persons between the ages of 60 and 70 years. Paraesophageal hernias often result in significant complications and therefore are of major importance. These hernias are frequently asymptomatic or cause only nagging discomfort until mechanical entrapment of the herniated stomach occurs. Such a catastrophe is associated with progressive distention of the incarcerated segment, vascular embarrassment, hemorrhage, gangrene, and perforation. In the absence of contraindications, a paraesophageal hernia demands surgical repair.

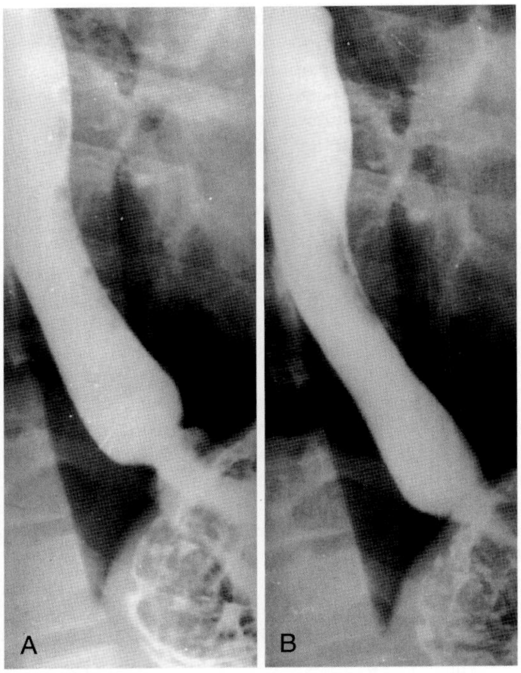

Figure 76-5. Small hiatus hernia **(A)** sliding in and **(B)** out of the thorax. The esophagogastric junction is seen above the diaphragm. *(From Brandt LJ: Gastrointestinal disorders of the elderly, New York, 1984, Lippincott-Raven.)*

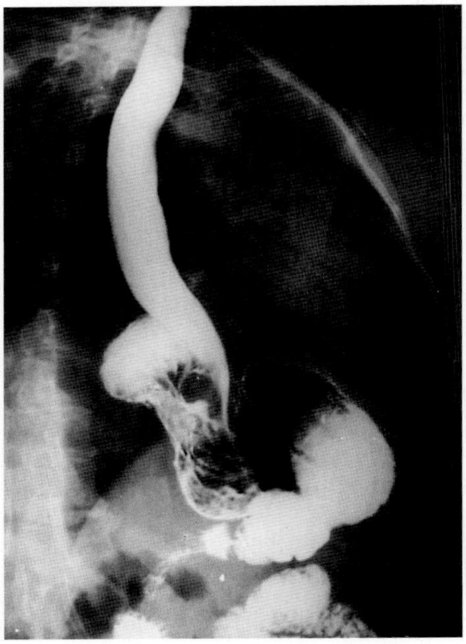

Figure 76-6. Barium esophagram demonstrating a paraesophageal hernia with the gastric fundus above the diaphragm. The esophagogastric junction is at the level of the diaphragm. *(From Brandt LJ: Gastrointestinal disorders of the elderly, New York, 1984, Lippincott-Raven.)*

Reflux Esophagitis

The only notable change in the lower esophageal sphincter seen with aging is a reduction in the amplitude of postdeglutitive contraction or relaxation. Nevertheless, because the secretion of gastrin, which potentiates contraction of the lower esophageal sphincter, increases with age and, because gastric acid secretion declines with age in many individuals, it is unusual for reflux esophagitis to appear for the first time in older adults.[55] The nature or extent of esophageal injury associated with gastroesophageal reflux cannot be predicted on the basis of the intensity of symptoms in older patients.[43] Complications of chronic asymptomatic reflux such as stricture formation may be the initial clinical presentation of esophagitis in about 20% of affected older patients. When an older adult complains of the recent onset of pyrosis, other causes of esophageal symptoms, such as candidiasis, must be considered. The therapy of reflux in older patients is the same as in younger patients; however, attention must be paid to the potential development of adverse effects of medications (see later).[56]

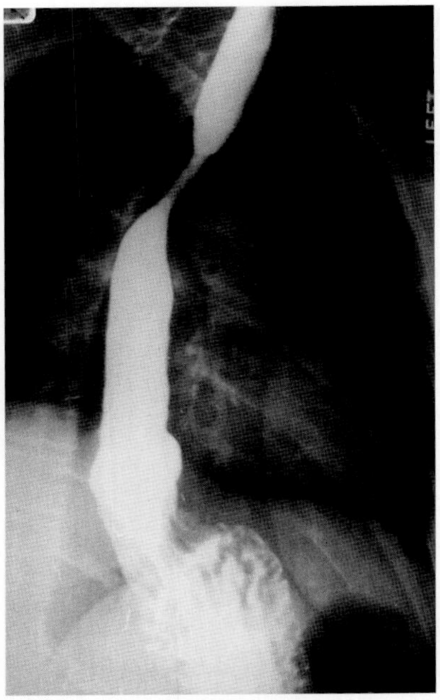

Figure 76-7. Barium esophagram revealing a stricture of the esophagus at the level of the aortic arch in a patient with Barrett's esophagus. A hiatus hernia is also present. *(From Brandt LJ: Gastrointestinal disorders of the elderly, New York, 1984, Lippincott-Raven.)*

Barrett Metaplasia

In patients with Barrett metaplasia, the lower esophagus is lined for a variable distance by columnar epithelium, rather than the usual stratified squamous epithelium.[57] The metaplastic columnar epithelium may be continuous with the columnar epithelium of the stomach and extend in tongues into the distal esophagus, or it may be present in islands surrounded by normal squamous epithelium. The importance of Barrett metaplasia lies in its association with reflux esophagitis, (deep) esophageal ulcers, (high) esophageal strictures (Figure 76-7), and adenocarcinoma. The metaplastic columnar lining is believed to develop as a consequence of gastroesophageal reflux. Esophageal squamous epithelium damaged by exposure to gastric contents is replaced by a specialized columnar epithelium (intestinal metaplasia), a junctional-type epithelium, or a gastric fundic-type epithelium. Each of these three cell types may be seen alone or in combination with the others.

Most cases of Barrett esophagus probably occur in those between the ages of 50 and 70 years; the exact incidence is unknown. The most common symptoms are those related to the reflux of stomach contents, and the entity is diagnosed best by esophagoscopy with multiple biopsies. The presence of specialized columnar epithelium establishes the diagnosis of Barrett esophagus.[57] If the columnar epithelium in the biopsy specimen is one of the other two types, the biopsy must have been made at least 3 cm above the gastroesophageal junction to make the diagnosis. Intestinal metaplasia can be recognized in situ by staining with Alcian blue.

Stricture and neoplasia are long-term complications of Barrett esophagus. There is increasing evidence that cancer arises only in the specialized columnar epithelium. By careful screening using esophagoscopy with directed biopsy every 1 to 2 years, premalignant dysplastic changes can usually be detected.[58,59] The development of severe dysplasia or carcinoma in situ requires treatment, such as ablation (using multipolar electrocoagulation, laser coagulation, or argon plasma coagulation) or resection of the involved esophagus. Destruction of the Barrett epithelium by these techniques is successful initially, but recurrence of the Barrett tissue may occur. Therapy of reflux usually results in symptomatic improvement, but regression of the columnar epithelium does not occur without surgery.

Lower Esophageal Ring

A lower esophageal or Schatzki ring (Figure 76-8) is a thin annular ridge of mucosa projecting perpendicularly into the esophageal lumen at or near the squamocolumnar junction.[60-62] A Schatzki ring may be asymptomatic, found incidentally during evaluation of the UGI for unrelated reasons, or it may cause intermittent episodes of dysphagia and an uncomfortable sticking or pressing sensation due to food lodging above the ring. Episodes commonly occur during hurried meals, meals requiring a great deal of mastication, or meals consumed with alcohol—hence the appellation, steakhouse syndrome. As the lumen of the ring diminishes to less than 12 mm (0.047 inches) in diameter, attacks become more frequent. Attacks usually last several minutes or longer until the patient regurgitates the food bolus or flushes it into the stomach with a beverage.

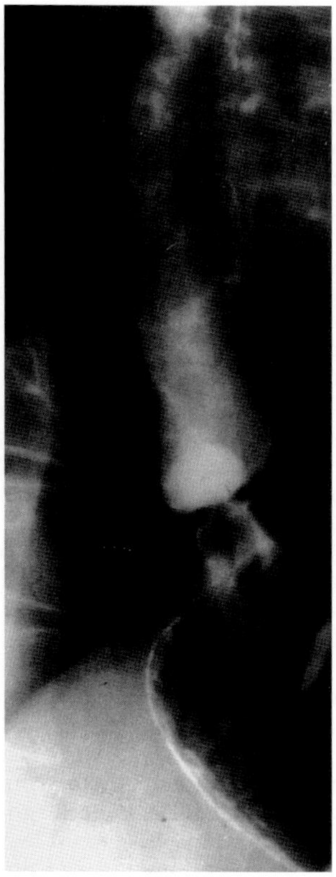

Figure 76-8. A Schatzki ring prevents passage of a barium pill in a patient with intermittent dysphagia. *(From Brandt LJ: Gastrointestinal disorders of the elderly, New York, 1986, Lippincott-Raven.)*

Total obstruction of the esophagus secondary to food impaction frequently brings patients to the emergency department. Relaxation of the esophagus by administration of a small dose of intravenous benzodiazepine or 1 mg of glucagon is occasionally effective in relieving the impaction. Papain solution (meat tenderizer) should not be used to try to digest the meat, because its use has been associated with esophageal perforation. If the impacted bolus does not pass, it must be removed by esophagoscopy. Alternatively, it may be gently nudged into the stomach if a patent lumen can be seen distally, the esophageal mucosa is intact, and there is no bone or other sharp object present. Multiple biopsies to disrupt the ring or dilation with bougies or balloons are techniques used to treat symptomatic rings.

Dysphagia Aortica

Degenerative changes in the aorta may produce compression of the esophagus and dysphagia. Obstruction of the upper esophagus is occasionally caused by a thoracic aneurysm, while the distal esophagus may be squeezed between an atherosclerotic aorta posteriorly and the heart or esophageal hiatus anteriorly. Most patients are women older than 70 years.[63-65] Symptoms are usually prevented by having the patient thoroughly masticate solid foods, but occasionally the obstruction is severe enough to warrant surgical mobilization of the esophagus at the hiatus.[66]

Medication-Induced Esophageal Injury

Esophageal injury can occur as a result of the local caustic effects of medications.[67,68] The most frequent offenders are antibiotics, especially tetracyclines, potassium chloride, ferrous sulfate, nonsteroidal antiinflammatory drugs (NSAIDs), alendronate, and quinidine.

Most patients with medication-induced esophageal injury have no underlying esophageal disorder. Some individuals, however, have nonspecific asymptomatic disorders of esophageal motility, peptic strictures, esophageal compression from left atrial enlargement, a prominent aortic knob, or mediastinal adhesions following thoracic surgery. Pills commonly lodge in the esophagus at the level of the aortic knob or the lower esophageal sphincter without the patient's knowledge. Many cases of pill-induced esophageal injury probably remain unrecognized, with full recovery. The most frequent symptoms of medication-induced esophageal injury are odynophagia and retrosternal pain. Symptoms usually resolve within 6 weeks of stopping the medication or changing to a liquid formulation; however, damage may result in esophageal stricture formation or, occasionally, hemorrhage or perforation. Pills should always be taken with a generous amount of water, and older patients should not take pills immediately before bedtime, because a decrease in salivation and esophageal motor activity accompanies sleeping.[69]

Esophageal Diverticula

Diverticula of the esophagus are much less common than diverticula of other parts of the GI tract. In a review of 20,000 barium studies on the UGI, Wheeler noted only six midesophageal (traction-type) and three epiphrenic (pulsion-type) diverticula, as compared with 1,020 duodenal diverticula.[70] The terms *traction* and *pulsion* refer to commonly accepted theories regarding the pathogenesis of esophageal diverticula. Traction diverticula are thought to be caused by the effects of fibrotic disease in structures contiguous with the esophagus, whereas pulsion diverticula are hypothesized to result from increased intraluminal pressure. Pseudodiverticulosis of the esophagus also has been described.

Midesophageal Diverticula (Traction Diverticula)

Traction diverticula usually occur in the middle third of the esophagus, in which a large group of lymph nodes lies in direct contact with the esophageal wall. Nodal inflammation of this area may lead to periesophagitis, fixation of the esophagus to the lymph nodes, and distortion of the esophageal wall. In the past, tuberculosis was the most common cause of this process; any infection with lymph node involvement, however, may lead to the formation of a traction diverticulum.

Traction diverticula usually occur in patients of middle age or older and are slightly more common in men. They rarely cause symptoms, perhaps because they are small, have a broad neck, and can contract and empty because they contain all the layers of the esophageal wall, including muscle.

Epiphrenic Diverticula (Pulsion Diverticula)

Pulsion diverticula are found in the lower 10 cm of the esophagus, usually on the right wall. Like traction diverticula, they contain all the layers of the esophageal wall; the muscular layer, however, may be quite attenuated.

Epiphrenic diverticula usually develop in men during middle age. Patients may complain of dysphagia or chest pain, but symptoms are probably due to an associated esophageal motor abnormality such as achalasia or diffuse esophageal spasm.[71] The occurrence of an epiphrenic diverticulum without an underlying motility disorder or hiatus hernia appears to be rare.

Many epiphrenic diverticula are asymptomatic and, in these cases no therapy is required.[72] Treatment of esophageal reflux or an underlying motility disorder may afford the patient symptomatic relief.[73,74] In cases of larger diverticula, surgical resection may be necessary.[75]

Intramural Pseudodiverticulosis

In esophageal pseudodiverticulosis, dilation of the excretory ducts of submucosal glands causes multiple small (1- to 3-mm) invaginations of the esophageal wall.[76,77] These defects involve all or segments of the esophagus in a circumferential fashion. Pseudodiverticula are best detected by barium contrast studies; their roentgenographic appearance is characteristic (Figure 76-9). Pseudodiverticulosis is usually diagnosed during the seventh decade of life in patients with dysphagia. In at least 20% of cases, gastroesophageal reflux, motility disorder, or malignancy is found and, in approximately 50% of patients, smears or cultures of the esophageal mucosa reveal *Candida albicans*. Stenoses, or areas of reduced distensibility, are found in up to 90% of cases of pseudodiverticulosis and seem to involve the upper esophagus preferentially. Surprisingly, there is no fixed relationship between the narrowed area and segment involved with pseudodiverticula.

The cause of pseudodiverticulosis is unknown. The term *adenosis* has been used to refer to it because the number of deep esophageal mucous glands is markedly increased. Therapy consists of treatment of associated abnormalities. Coexisting strictures should be evaluated to ensure that they are benign.

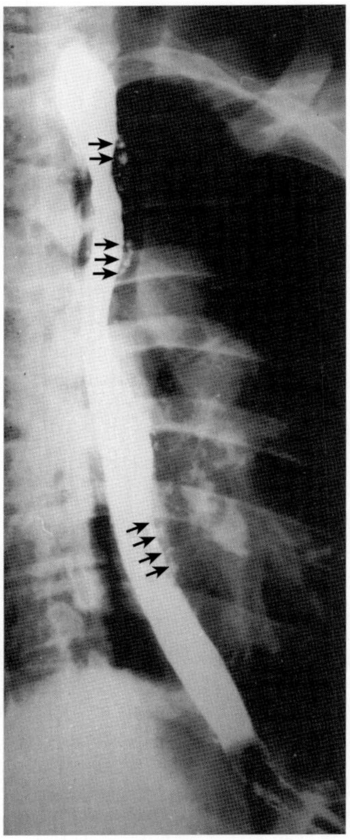

Figure 76-9. Intramural pseudodiverticulosis with multiple outpouchings *(arrows)* on a barium esophagram. *(From Brandt LJ: Gastrointestinal disorders of the elderly, New York, 1986, Lippincott-Raven.)*

Esophageal Candidiasis

Infection of the esophagus is rare in patients without acquired immunodeficiency syndrome, with the exception of infection with *C. albicans*. *C. albicans* is a normal inhabitant of the alimentary tract; the yeast form is found in almost 50% of oral washings and 80% of stool samples.[78] The population of *C. albicans* is suppressed in healthy adults by other intestinal flora. Comparison of fecal specimens from subjects aged 70 to 100 years with those of individuals aged 20 to 69 years have revealed fungi to be more common in the older adults. This finding may be explained by a diminution in esophageal peristalsis, reduction in gastric acid secretion, and age-related alterations in cellular and humoral immunity.

In the absence of antibiotic therapy or an underlying immune disorder, esophageal candidiasis is a disease of older adults. Most cases in this age group, however, occur in association with predisposing conditions, including malignancy, therapy with immunosuppressive or cytotoxic drugs, diabetes mellitus, malnutrition, and treatment with broad-spectrum antibiotics.[79,80]

In the proper clinical setting, dysphagia, odynophagia, substernal burning, or an awareness of food passing down the esophagus should suggest the possibility of candida infection although, even in the presence of infection with *C. albicans*, up to 50% of patients may be asymptomatic. Esophageal candidiasis often results from the extension of oral lesions, and a careful examination of the oral cavity is important for any debilitated patient complaining of esophageal symptoms.

A diagnosis of candida esophagitis may be suggested by an abnormal barium esophagram, although a normal study does not exclude the presence of this organism. Esophagoscopy is the best method for detecting candida infection; raised white plaques, hyperemia, ulceration, and friability are characteristic. The gross appearance of candida esophagitis may be confused with that of exudative esophagitis, and therefore the diagnosis must be confirmed by brushings and biopsies. Typical hyphae are revealed under the microscope in scrapings placed on a glass slide and macerated with 20% potassium hydroxide.

In the appropriate setting, a trial of therapy may be initiated without attempting an invasive diagnosis. As in oral and vaginal candidiasis, therapy usually consists of promoting the reestablishment of normal microbiological flora by discontinuing antibiotics. In an immunocompromised host or an individual with significant morbidity, fluconazole is considered the drug of choice. Odynophagia can be treated with viscous lidocaine or with a swish and swallow preparation of the type used to treat stomatitis (see above). Failure to respond to simple treatment necessitates endoscopic confirmation of the diagnosis and, often, systemic therapy with additional antifungal agents.

Esophageal Neoplasms

Esophageal cancer (Figure 76-10) occurs most frequently after the age of 55 years and is three times more common in men than in women in the United States and two times more common in men than in women in the United Kingdom.[1] In the United States, it accounts for approximately 2% of all reported cancers. Factors associated with the development of esophageal cancer include alcohol and tobacco use, thermal irritation, poor oral hygiene, and esophageal stasis.[1,81,82] Furthermore, an association has been noted with certain esophageal diseases, notably achalasia, Barrett esophagus, lye stricture, and Plummer-Vinson syndrome and with previous gastric surgery.[83-85]

Surveillance, Epidemiology, and End Results (SEER) data have shown an increase in adenocarcinoma by more than 300% from 1975 to 2004; it now represents the most rapidly increasing malignancy in the United States.[86] Esophageal adenocarcinoma is cancer of the gastric fundus or a malignancy that has developed in a segment of Barrett esophagus. Squamous cell carcinoma usually involves the middle third of the esophagus. Local spread occurs early and, because the esophagus dilates so readily, dysphagia, the most common complaint at the time of diagnosis, is a late symptom.

In older adults, an important manifestation of esophageal cancer is an achalasia-like syndrome. Primary achalasia is uncommon in patients older than 50 years. Older adults who present with symptoms of achalasia of less than 1-year duration associated with marked weight loss should be suspected of having a malignancy, usually gastric adenocarcinoma. The pathogenesis of secondary achalasia is unknown; in some cases, the lower esophagus is infiltrated with tumor cells, but in other cases, achalasia may reflect a paraneoplastic process.

The prognosis for esophageal cancer is poor when advanced at diagnosis. Staging is essential, because early-stage lesions can sometimes be successfully treated with electromagnetic radiation (EMR) of a superficial lesion. For advanced lesions, management is directed at relieving progressive obstruction.[87-89] Surgical resection and radiation are the accepted modes of treatment. Surgical resection offers the only chance for long-term survival, but fewer than 50% of all patients presenting with esophageal cancer have a resectable lesion. If there is evidence of nodal or distant metastases, a thoracotomy should be avoided. Thoracic radiation, although useful, may be followed by the development of esophagitis, usually within 3 weeks of initiating therapy and continuing for several weeks after its completion. Chemotherapy may result in symptomatic improvement but does not substantially prolong survival. Combined modality therapy offers advantages over more traditional approaches and may downsize a lesion prior to resection. Palliative therapy with endoscopically placed stents or a thermal ablative technique is often very useful and has improved the quality of life for many patients, albeit without prolonging survival.

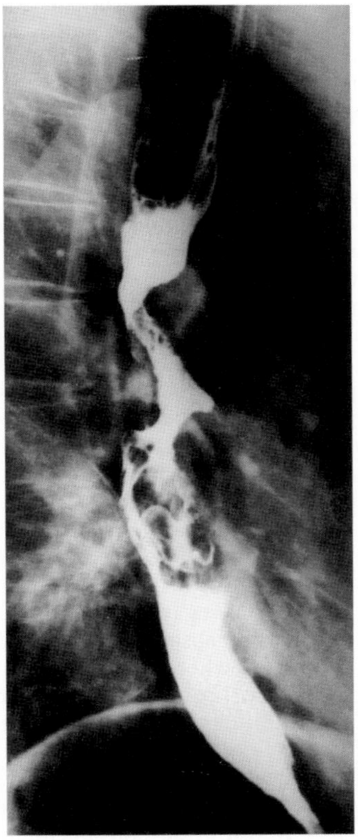

Figure 76-10. Barium esophagram demonstrating an ulcerating esophageal carcinoma. *(From Brandt LJ: Gastrointestinal disorders of the elderly, New York, 1986, Lippincott-Raven.)*

STOMACH

Aging is associated with alterations in the motor and secretory functions of the stomach but, as in other parts of the GI tract, changes in gastric physiology attributable to age alone rarely are responsible for symptoms.

The motor activity of the stomach allows it to behave as two individual, albeit coordinated, organs, one that processes liquids and another that processes solids. The fundus and proximal body of the stomach serve as a reservoir for liquids. In contrast, the distal gastric body and antrum grind solids into small particles and pump them into the duodenum. The actions of both the proximal and distal stomach are controlled by complex neural and hormonal mechanisms. Studies using food labeled with radioactive isotopes have suggested that gastric emptying of liquids is prolonged in older adults, whereas emptying of solids is unaffected by age.[90,91]

Changes in gastric secretion also occur in individuals as they grow older. In the past, almost every study on gastric acid production showed a decline in basal and stimulated acid output with advancing age.[92] Work by Goldschmiedt and associates,[93] however, has suggested that in the absence of *Helicobacter pylori* infection, aging is actually associated with an increase in gastric acid secretion. Previous confusion about the effect of aging on gastric acid secretion was probably related to the high incidence of *H. pylori* infection and chronic atrophic gastritis with secondary achlorhydria in older adults (see later).[94]

Gastric and Duodenal Mucosal Injury

Advances in our understanding of the pathobiology of gastric and duodenal mucosal injury, and improvements in our ability to examine the UGI and detect diseases responsible for mucosal injury, make it important for physicians to use descriptive and diagnostic terminology carefully in clinical practice.[95,96] Unless diagnostic findings are reported with a precision that accurately reflects a current understanding of mucosal injury, the benefits of medical advances made during the past few decades may be lost to patients.

In usual cases of gastric or duodenal mucosal injury, endoscopic inspection often reveals the presence of gross epithelial defects. Small epithelial defects, or erosions, do not penetrate the muscularis mucosae. An ulcer (a discontinuity of or break in the skin) is defined as being larger than 3 mm in diameter and extending a variable distance through the muscularis mucosae, in some cases freely perforating into the peritoneal cavity or penetrating into an adjacent organ. A typical ulcer is composed of four layers or zones—a superficial layer of fibrinopurulent debris overlying a zone of inflammation, a layer of granulation tissue and, at its base, a collagenous scar. Both erosions and ulcers may be sources of bleeding.

Diffuse mucosal erythema, a common finding at endoscopy, in most cases represents microvascular congestion and, although it has been interpreted by many endoscopists as indicating the presence of gastritis, this conclusion is unjustified. Mucosal erythema due to microvascular congestion is caused by a variety of factors and is without any specific causative significance or clinical association.[96] Conversely, patients often have histologic gastritis without the presence of mucosal erythema.

The term *gastritis* implies the presence of inflammation and should not be used unless examination of a biopsy specimen has revealed typical mucosal inflammatory changes, including infiltration of the lamina propria with polymorphonuclear leukocytes and mononuclear cells. Neutrophils are seen early in the course of inflammation (acute gastritis). With the passage of time, mononuclear cells, mainly plasma cells, and eosinophils appear in increasing numbers (chronic gastritis). Most patients with gastritis have a predominance of mononuclear cells in the lamina propria, with a lesser number of neutrophils (chronic active gastritis).[97] The inflammatory changes of gastritis are accompanied by signs of cell injury and regeneration. Cell damage and death cause submucosal hemorrhage and edema and lead to the development of epithelial defects. Hemorrhage and edema may be visible grossly at endoscopy, as well as being evident on microscopic examination of biopsy specimens as erosions and ulcers. In response to injury, the epithelium regenerates by proliferation and differentiation of mucous neck cells, a process that leads to elongation and tortuosity of the gastric pits (foveolar hyperplasia). The vast majority of cases of gastritis are caused by infection with *H. pylori* (type B gastritis). Gastritis also may be due to other less common bacterial infections, granulomatous disease, autoimmune disease (type A gastritis), and hypersensitivity reactions.

Other agents of gastric injury damage the mucosa without exciting an inflammatory response. This gastropathy is sometimes referred to as type C gastritis, an unfortunate misnomer given the noninflammatory nature of the process.[98] Microscopic examination of biopsy specimens from patients with gastropathy typically reveals vascular congestion and edema of the lamina propria, hypertrophy of the muscularis mucosae, and mucosal regenerative changes with foveolar hyperplasia.[99] As in gastritis, cell damage and death are accompanied by submucosal hemorrhage and edema and lead to the development of epithelial defects. The latter changes are all often grossly visible on endoscopy. The most common causes of gastropathy are ingestion of NSAIDs and ethanol.

Helicobacter pylori, Gastritis, and Peptic Ulcer Disease

Infection with *H. pylori*, a spiral gram-negative microaerophilic rod, is the most common chronic bacterial disease in humans. This organism attaches to receptors on the surface of gastric mucous neck cells and is also found on metaplastic gastric epithelium in the duodenum but not on the duodenal mucosa itself or on metaplastic duodenal mucosa in the stomach.[100] *H. pylori* causes alterations in cell structure and function, inflammation, metaplasia, and cell death.[101] A number of virulence factors, including urease, make it possible for the organism to colonize the stomach and produce disease.[102]

H. pylori infection is the most common cause of chronic gastritis (type B antral gastritis) and is one of the two principal causes of peptic ulcer disease, the other being ingestion of NSAIDs. More than 90% of patients with duodenal ulcer and more than 75% of patients with gastric ulcer also have *H. pylori* infection and chronic active gastritis.[1] The relationship between ulcer disease and gastritis was recognized long before the causative role of *H. pylori* in the pathogenesis of peptic ulcer disease was understood. *H. pylori* infection also has been linked to the development of gastric cancer, another gastritis-associated disease.[103]

Infection with *H. pylori* is usually acquired during childhood and usually occurs in persons living under conditions of poverty, crowding, and inadequate sanitation.[104] The prevalence of *H. pylori* infection in the United States and in the nations of western Europe increases with advancing age, a result of the poorer living conditions in these countries during the early years of the twentieth century.[105] Thus, regardless of present socioeconomic status, infection is most prevalent in older individuals. The incidence of peptic ulcer disease also increases progressively with advancing age, reflecting the age-related increase in *H. pylori* infection.

Under experimental conditions, acute infection with *H. pylori* causes transient dyspeptic symptoms accompanied by the development of active antral gastritis.[106] Mucosal inflammation apparently may resolve spontaneously in the minority of patients or become chronic, gradually spreading proximally into the body and fundus of the stomach. As the disease progresses, inflammation extends into the deeper glandular part of the epithelium containing the gastric secretory cells; these include parietal cells, which produce hydrochloric acid and intrinsic factor, chief cells, which produce pepsin, pylorocardiac gland cells, which produce mucus, and endocrine G cells, which produce gastrin. Normal glands are gradually destroyed and replaced by metaplastic glands (intestinal metaplasia) or by atrophic gastric mucosa (atrophic gastritis), a process that takes many years. Atrophic gastritis often is associated with low serum gastrin levels and antibodies to gastrin-secreting cells. Patients with chronic active gastritis frequently also have submucosal hemorrhage, edema, epithelial erosions (erosive gastritis), and peptic ulcers.

Individuals with active gastritis and gastric mucosal atrophy are usually asymptomatic but may complain of intermittent dyspepsia, abdominal pain, distention, nausea and vomiting (nonulcer dyspepsia). The relationship, if any, between symptoms of nonulcer dyspepsia and gastritis is unclear (see later); many persons with dyspepsia do not have gastritis, and many persons with gastritis do not have dyspepsia.[107] Dyspeptic symptoms may be due to the development of a gastric or duodenal ulcer, although at least 50% of patients with acute ulcers are asymptomatic.

H. pylori infection may be diagnosed by a transendoscopic pinch biopsy of the stomach. Microscopic examination of biopsy specimens from infected individuals reveals chronic active gastritis and typical spiral, gram-negative rods in the mucus coating the surface epithelium. The absence of gastritis strongly argues against *H. pylori* infection, whereas its presence suggests that a failure to identify *H. pylori* is due to sampling error. Tissue also may be implanted in commercially available agar plates containing urea and a pH indicator. If *H. pylori* is present in the tissue specimen, bacterial urease will split the urea into bicarbonate and ammonia, raising the pH and producing a color change. Because infection may be patchy, testing several specimens obtained from different parts of the stomach improves the sensitivity of the assay.

Noninvasive diagnosis of *H. pylori* infection can be made by detecting serum antibodies to bacterial antigens. This method of diagnosis is satisfactory—presuming there is no indication for endoscopy—if the patient has not previously been treated with antibiotics to which *H. pylori* is sensitive. Antibody titers decrease gradually after eradication of infection, but qualitative serology remains positive for a number of years, leaving what has been referred to as an immunologic scar. The presence of an immunologic scar makes it impossible to use antibody testing to assess the effectiveness of therapy or occurrence of re-infection. This problem is avoided by using the urea breath test, which is positive only in a setting of active infection. In the urea breath test, the patient is given an oral dose of urea labeled with a stable (^{13}C) or unstable (^{14}C) isotope of carbon. If the patient is infected with *H. pylori*, the urea will be metabolized by bacterial urease to ammonia and bicarbonate, and bicarbonate containing the isotopic tracer will be converted to CO_2 and expired. The presence of labeled CO_2 in samples of expired gas indicates active *H. pylori* infection. A stool assay for detection of *H. pylori* also is available commercially and is widely used.

Simultaneous treatment with a combination of two antibiotics and proton pump inhibitor (PPI) is the most consistently effective means of curing *H. pylori* infection.[108] *H. pylori* is sensitive to a variety of antimicrobial agents, including metronidazole, tetracyclines, macrolides, some quinolones, β-lactams, bismuth preparations, and PPIs. The most commonly used regimen is a combination of amoxicillin, clarithromycin, and PPI. Regimens containing metronidazole are limited by the frequent occurrence of bacterial resistance to this agent. Because of the morbidity caused by *H. pylori* infection, the National Institutes of Health Consensus Development Panel has published guidelines mandating treatment of all *H. pylori*–infected ulcer patients, including those currently without an active ulcer crater or dyspeptic symptoms.[109] The significant treatment failure rate makes it desirable to document cure by conducting a urea breath test or stool assay 4 weeks after completion of therapy. In addition to antibiotic therapy for *H. pylori* infection, patients with acute ulcers should be treated with an antisecretory agent to promote ulcer healing.

Nonsteroidal Antiinflammatory Drugs, Gastropathy, and Peptic Ulcer Disease

NSAIDs are among the most frequently prescribed medicines in the world. Approximately 3 million people in the United States, or 1.2% of the population, take at least one NSAID daily. Uncounted others regularly use over-the-counter NSAID preparations, including aspirin. As a result, NSAID-related morbidity is exceedingly common; each year, 2% to 4% of chronic NSAID users have a serious drug-induced complication involving the GI tract.[110] The use of NSAIDs and complications of NSAID use are most prevalent in older adults.[111-113] In the United Kingdom, NSAID prescription rates for the entire population increased steadily from 1967 to 1985, in direct proportion to the age of the recipient, with progressively more prescriptions being written for progressively older patients.[114] Thus, in 1985, an astonishing 1,400 NSAID prescriptions were written for every 1,000 women in the United Kingdom aged 65 years or older. These chronic NSAID users are estimated to have a two- to threefold greater mortality rate than nonusers because of drug-related GI complications.

Every nonselective NSAID is capable of injuring the GI mucosa and does so in a dose-dependent fashion roughly proportional to its antiinflammatory effects. Virtually 100% of patients who take an NSAID preparation, including aspirin, develop acute gastropathy during the first 1 to 2 weeks of therapy.[115] This gastropathy has the typical histologic features described earlier and characteristically is associated with submucosal hemorrhage and some degree of edema, both of which are often grossly visible at endoscopy. Many NSAIDs, such as aspirin, are weak acids that remain nonionized as the tablets break up and are dispersed in low-pH gastric secretions. Because they are nonionized, NSAIDs easily move across the membranes of epithelial cells and then ionize at the neutral pH of the cytoplasm. In the ionic form, they interact with cell constituents and cause cell damage and death.[116] Dead epithelial cells leave shallow mucosal defects (erosions), which may bleed. Patients often have dyspeptic symptoms during this acute phase of injury.

In a significant minority of chronic NSAID users, mucosal defects enlarge and form true ulcers; approximately 12% to 30% of patients develop a gastric ulcer, and 2% to 19% of patients develop a duodenal ulcer.[117] Older adults seem to be particularly vulnerable to the harmful effects of NSAIDs. In a study of peptic ulcer disease in persons aged 65 years and older, Griffin and coworkers[118] found that almost 30% of ulcers diagnosed in these individuals may have been caused by NSAIDs. The principal mechanism whereby NSAID use leads to the development of peptic ulcers is dose-dependent, systemic inhibition of prostaglandin synthesis. Prostaglandins protect the upper GI mucosa by stimulating the secretion of bicarbonate and mucus, increasing mucosal blood flow and promoting a number of cellular processes crucial to mucosal defense and repair. A decrease in prostaglandin synthesis tips the balance between defensive and aggressive factors in the UGI in favor of those that injure the mucosa, leading to the formation of ulcers and the possible development of complications, including hemorrhage, obstruction, perforation, and penetration into an adjacent organ.

Cyclooxygenase-2 (COX-2)–specific agents have been shown to be equally as efficacious as nonselective NSAIDs in the treatment of osteoarthritis and rheumatoid arthritis, but with significantly fewer GI side effects. These agents have a greater affinity for COX-2 as compared to COX-1; COX-2 is induced in response to inflammation, whereas COX-1 is a constitutive enzyme that functions in a variety of maintenance and housekeeping roles. Many studies have demonstrated a decreased incidence of gastric and duodenal ulcers in patients taking COX-2 selective agents as compared to those using nonselective NSAIDs. The use of COX-2 selective agents is associated with ulceration rates in the GI tract no different than those of placebo.[119]

Various treatment strategies for preventing the development of gastric and duodenal ulcers in patients on chronic NSAID therapy have been tested.[120] Many commonly used medicines are without any demonstrable prophylactic benefit in this setting. Ranitidine and omeprazole have been shown to prevent duodenal but not gastric ulcers in arthritis patients taking NSAIDs.[120-122] Similar results were obtained by Taha and colleagues[123] in arthritis patients treated with prophylactic famotidine; however, in the same study, high-dose famotidine reduced the incidence of duodenal and gastric ulcers.[123] An alternative approach to ulcer prevention in patients who require chronic NSAID therapy is prostaglandin replacement with an oral synthetic prostaglandin E analogue. The prostaglandin E_1 analogue, misoprostol, like famotidine, has been shown to prevent the development of duodenal and gastric ulcers.[124] It also reduces the incidence of bleeding, perforation, and gastric outlet obstruction in patients on chronic NSAID therapy.[112] The use of misoprostol has been limited by its tendency to cause loose stools, abdominal cramps, and flatulence in a significant minority of individuals during initiation of treatment.

The large number of eligible patients makes it impossible to prescribe prophylactic famotidine or misoprostol for every NSAID user or to use COX-2 selective agents in all of them. Instead, an effort should be made to identify and treat those who require chronic NSAID therapy and are at greatest risk for developing a significant NSAID-related complication. Included in this high-risk group are older adults, as well as persons with a history of peptic ulcer disease or previous UGI bleeding, individuals also taking steroids, and patients with cardiovascular disease.[112,113] Once an ulcer develops, a serious complication is often the first sign of its presence in as many as approximately 50% of persons

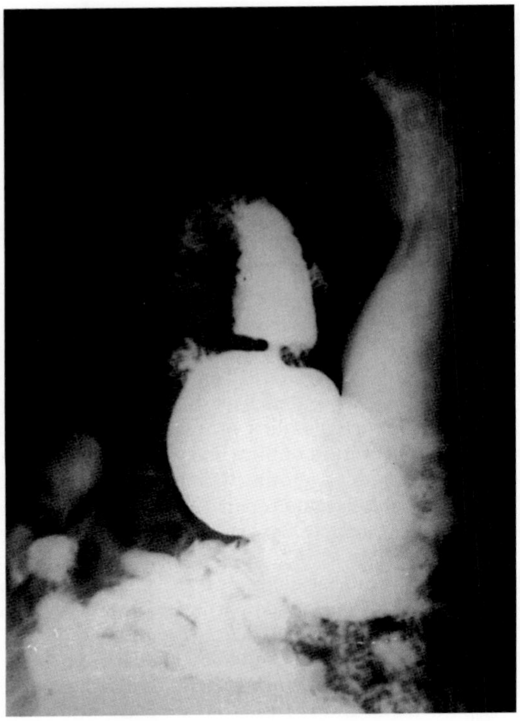

Figure 76-11. UGI revealing a large, benign, geriatric ulcer high on the lesser curvature. *(From Brandt LJ: Gastrointestinal disorders of the elderly, New York, 1986, Lippincott-Raven.)*

with ulcers who have no dyspeptic symptoms. Patients taking NSAIDs who have dyspeptic symptoms require evaluation for ulcer disease as well as possible *H. pylori* infection, and those with ulcers should be treated with an antisecretory agent and antibiotics, if indicated.

Peptic Ulcer Disease in Older Adults

Ulcer disease, whether due to *H. pylori* infection, NSAID use, or some other less common cause, frequently exhibits a virulent course in older adults, with more complications and a higher mortality rate than in younger individuals.[125-127] Duodenal ulcers occur two to three times more frequently than gastric ulcers, but the latter is responsible for two of every three deaths from peptic ulcer disease in older adults, and the death rate increases with advancing age.

The presentation of ulcer disease in older adults tends to be acute, often with bleeding or perforation, but symptoms may be subtle; this is particularly true of gastric ulcers. Gastric ulcers produce chronic blood loss more commonly than duodenal ulcers, and resultant anemia may lead to cardiac or neurologic symptoms. Weight loss and fatigue suggesting malignancy may be the only complaints, a presentation characteristic of giant ulcers. So-called geriatric ulcers (Figure 76-11) high in the cardia may cause misleading symptoms, such as dysphagia mimicking esophageal neoplasm or chest pain suggesting angina. A history of NSAID use is commonly obtained from older patients with peptic ulcer disease.

The complication rate of peptic ulcer disease rises progressively from 31% in patients 60 to 64 years of age to 76% in those 75 to 79 years of age. Surgery should not be withheld or delayed solely because of advanced age because it is often lifesaving in older patients. Bleeding, the most common complication, accounts for half to two-thirds of all fatalities (see later).

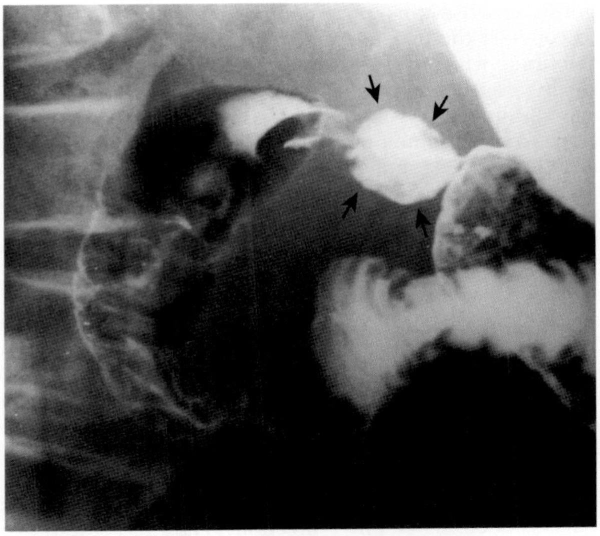

Figure 76-12. UGI series demonstrating a giant duodenal ulcer resembling the duodenal bulb *(arrows). (From Brandt LJ: Gastrointestinal disorders of the elderly, New York, 1986, Lippincott-Raven.)*

Perforation is the second most common complication of peptic ulcers in older adults. The presentation of a perforated ulcer is subtle in this age group, delaying the correct diagnosis and contributing to the high mortality. Gastric outlet obstruction complicates ulcer disease in 10% to 15% of patients older than 60 years, generally occurring in those with a long history of disease; an obstructing malignant lesion must be excluded in such patients.

Duodenal ulcers larger than 2 cm in diameter were once considered a distinct entity because of their poor prognosis, but it is probable that most of these so-called giant duodenal ulcers are caused by *H. pylori* infection or NSAID use, just like smaller lesions. Giant duodenal ulcers usually occur in men older than 70 years who have no prior history of peptic ulcer disease. The most frequent complaint is of abdominal pain radiating to the back or right upper quadrant, suggesting pancreatic or biliary disease. Pain may be relieved by antacids, but aggravated by eating, and is often accompanied by significant weight loss. The ulcer crater is so large that it sometimes is mistaken for the duodenal bulb on a UGI series (Figure 76-12). Although giant duodenal ulcers were often fatal decades ago, today they usually respond to therapy with PPIs and antibiotics when indicated by the presence of *H. pylori* infection.

Giant gastric ulcers have a diameter of over 3 cm.[128,129] They also are most likely caused by *H. pylori* infection or NSAID use. Giant gastric ulcers are slightly more common in males and are usually seen in patients older than 65 years. Pain is not a prominent complaint, but only about 10% of patients are completely free of pain. Pain may radiate to the chest, periumbilical region, or lower abdomen. Morbidity and mortality rates are high, with hemorrhage being the most common complication. These ulcers are usually benign and can be treated with histamine antagonists or PPIs as well as with antibiotics when there is documented *H. pylori* infection. Patients should be followed carefully with endoscopy to demonstrate healing. Candidiasis of the ulcer crater may delay healing and requires adjunctive antifungal therapy.

A number of potential problems must be considered in prescribing acid-suppressive therapy for older patients with peptic ulcer disease. Many antacid preparations contain large amounts of mineral salts, which may produce undesirable effects, such as fluid retention, diarrhea, or constipation. Aluminum hydroxide forms insoluble chelates with a number of drugs, including digoxin, quinidine, and tetracycline, interfering with their absorption. Histamine antagonists variably inhibit the oxidative metabolism of many drugs, prolonging their duration of action. Cimetidine impairs the elimination of, for example, lidocaine, nifedipine, phenytoin, propranolol, quinidine, theophylline, and warfarin. Ranitidine is a less potent inhibitor of mixed-function oxidases than cimetidine, and alterations in drug metabolism caused by ranitidine are usually not associated with pharmacologic effects. Famotidine has no effect on the oxidative metabolism of drugs. Intravenous administration of cimetidine in older patients with impaired renal function may produce mental confusion in a dose-related fashion. Cimetidine may also cause a mild elevation of serum creatinine levels unassociated with impairment of renal function. Ranitidine is a rare cause of hepatitis, and ranitidine and famotidine may cause headache. Sucralfate frequently causes constipation in older adults. The National Institutes of Health Consensus Development Panel has published guidelines mandating antibiotic treatment of all ulcer patients infected with *H. pylori*, including those without an active ulcer crater or dyspeptic symptoms.[109]

Nonulcer Dyspepsia

Patients with nonulcer dyspepsia suffer from chronic, recurrent upper abdominal pain and nausea, which may or may not be related to meals and that occurs in the absence of an ulcer crater.[130] Nonulcer dyspepsia is at least twice as common as true peptic ulcer disease. Most patients with this problem have no recognizable pathologic abnormality, although many have histologic gastritis.[107] Nonulcer dyspepsia is further defined by the absence of reflux esophagitis, disease of the biliary tract or pancreas, or most symptoms of irritable bowel syndrome. The criteria used to select patients for inclusion in clinical studies of nonulcer dyspepsia are very inconsistent, perpetuating confusion about this diagnosis among physicians and patients.[131]

The cause of nonulcer dyspepsia is unknown; numerous explanations have been proposed for this syndrome, including psychosocial factors, altered sensation, abnormal GI motility and compliance, and *H. pylori* infection.[130,131] Gas washout studies have shown that individuals with nonulcer dyspepsia do not have increased gas in their digestive tracts, and therefore complaints of bloating are probably explained by sensitivity to normal volumes of gas; in some individuals, the transit of infused gas is abnormal, suggesting a motility disorder. Gastric antral hypomotility and impaired gastric emptying of solids have been observed in 40% to 50% of patients with nonulcer dyspepsia, and treatment with drugs that affect UGI motility relieves symptoms in many patients.[132-134] Of patients with symptoms of nonulcer dyspepsia, 30% to 50% have chronic active gastritis, even when the gastric mucosa appears grossly normal at endoscopy. It has been suggested that nonulcer dyspepsia is part of the spectrum of disease caused by *H. pylori*, which includes chronic active gastritis, duodenitis, and peptic ulcer disease. The successive development of nonulcer dyspepsia, duodenitis, and duodenal ulcer disease has been termed *Moynihan disease*.[135] *H. pylori* infection, however, has not been shown to be the cause of nonulcer dyspepsia, nor has a definitive relationship between nonulcer dyspepsia and peptic ulcer disease been proven.[136]

In practice, therapy for nonulcer dyspepsia is the same as for peptic ulcer disease, despite the fact that in double-blind, placebo-controlled trials, histamine antagonists and PPIs are only a little better than placebo in treating this disorder, and the role of gastric acid hypersecretion in nonulcer dyspepsia is unproved by formal measurements of basal and peak acid outputs.[137,138] Peptic ulcer disease, NSAID use, *H. pylori* infection, and gastric cancer must be excluded in older patients who present with dyspeptic complaints.

Upper Gastrointestinal Bleeding

Of all cases of acute UGI hemorrhage, 35% to 45% occur in patients older than 60 years and, of these, 50% are caused by peptic ulcer disease.[139-141] Other important causes of gross UGI bleeding in older adults are gastric erosions and esophagitis; these two entities in combination with peptic ulcer disease account for 70% to 80% of hospital admissions for UGI bleeding in older patients.

It is unclear whether older patients with UGI hemorrhage frequently have a long history of underlying acid peptic disease (e.g., chronic peptic ulcer disease) or whether they usually bleed from newly developed lesions. In one series, 36% of older individuals admitted to the hospital with acute UGI bleeding gave no history of preceding symptoms.[139] Alternatively, some patients complain of prior epigastric pain, pain in other parts of the abdomen, anorexia, dyspepsia, pyrosis or, simply, weight loss. Older patients with acute UGI bleeding usually present with hematemesis, although 30% of patients have only melena.[139] Hemorrhage is often seen in persons with chronic medical illnesses, the most common being degenerative joint disease. Therapy with NSAIDs for rheumatologic and other problems has been found to be an important cause of UGI bleeding in older patients.[141,142] Other causes include disease found in younger patients, as well as entities seen almost exclusively in older adults. Geriatric ulcers and giant duodenal ulcers are not associated with an unusually high incidence of hemorrhage, but giant gastric ulcers frequently do bleed.[129]

Aortoenteric fistula is an uncommon cause of GI hemorrhage usually seen in men during the seventh and eighth decades of life. The most common cause is rupture of an arteriosclerotic abdominal aortic aneurysm. Other causes of aortoenteric fistulas include graft-enteric fistula, aortitis, mycotic aneurysm, carcinoma, trauma, foreign body, and peptic ulceration.[143,144] The overwhelming majority of fistulas between the aorta and alimentary tract occur in the duodenum and, as a result, usually produce UGI bleeding. Other reported sites of communication include the esophagus, stomach, distal small bowel, and colon. Most patients experience an initial self-limited or sentinel bleed, followed hours to days later by massive hemorrhage. Mortality is very high but may be reduced by early endoscopic detection of the fistula during investigation of the cause of bleeding. An older patient with an aortic graft who has UGI bleeding, no matter how trivial, must undergo immediate endoscopy because of the possible presence of a graft-enteric fistula.

Another rare cause of massive UGI hemorrhage in older adults is a dilated gastric artery with an overlying mucosal defect, typically located within 2 cm of the cardioesophageal junction. This lesion, called exulceratio simplex, or the ulcer of Dieulafoy, often requires surgical therapy, although it has been treated effectively with thermal therapies, such as electrocautery, laser, and argon plasma coagulation, and mechanical therapies, such as clips and banding.[145,146]

Occasionally, vascular abnormalities of the type found in Osler-Weber-Rendu syndrome (hereditary hemorrhagic telangiectasia) may also be responsible for UGI bleeding in older adults.[147] There may be no history of childhood epistaxis and no family history of similar occurrences, although typical telangiectatic lesions are often found in the oral cavity, lips, nail beds, and skin.

The hospital course of older patients with UGI bleeding is similar to that of younger patients with respect to duration, amount of blood transfused, and frequency of surgery.[148] Older patients, however, suffer significantly more morbidity than younger patients; complications include cardiac, neurologic, and renal disease, sepsis, and reactions to medications and transfusions. Older patients are more likely than younger patients to die during a hospital admission for GI bleeding, especially if peptic ulcer is the cause.

The evaluation and treatment of UGI bleeding in older adults are the same as in younger individuals. Age per se is not a contraindication for surgery; the decision to operate on an individual patient must be made in the context of the clinical setting. Early surgery should be contemplated for older patients who have bled from ulcers, who have signs of major hemorrhage (e.g., hypotension), and when endoscopic findings imply a significant risk of recurrent bleeding.

Volvulus of the Stomach

Volvulus of the stomach is a relatively rare condition usually occurring after the age of 50 years; it requires relaxation of the gastric ligaments for its development.[149,150] Gastric volvulus may be responsible for chronic abdominal symptoms or may be manifested acutely with strangulation and gangrene.

Gastric volvulus is classified according to the axis around which the stomach rotates; torsion about a longitudinal axis formed by a line connecting the cardia and pylorus is known as organoaxial volvulus, and rotation about a vertical axis passing through the middle of the lesser and greater curvatures is referred to as mesenteroaxial volvulus. Approximately 60% of affected patients have the organoaxial type, 30% have the mesenteroaxial type, and 10% have a combination form. Rotation may be partial or complete; complete twists often severely impair gastric blood flow and may cause gangrene, whereas partial twists may be asymptomatic or responsible for chronic symptoms.

Organoaxial volvulus usually has an acute presentation and often is associated with the presence of a large paraesophageal hernia or eventration of the diaphragm. Patients complain of the abrupt onset of upper abdominal or lower thoracic pain. Vomiting gives way to retching, and it is difficult to pass a nasogastric tube beyond the gastroesophageal junction. This group of symptoms and signs has been referred to as the Borchardt triad. Roentgenograms may reveal a gas-filled viscus in the chest or an upside-down stomach in the upper abdomen (Figure 76-13).

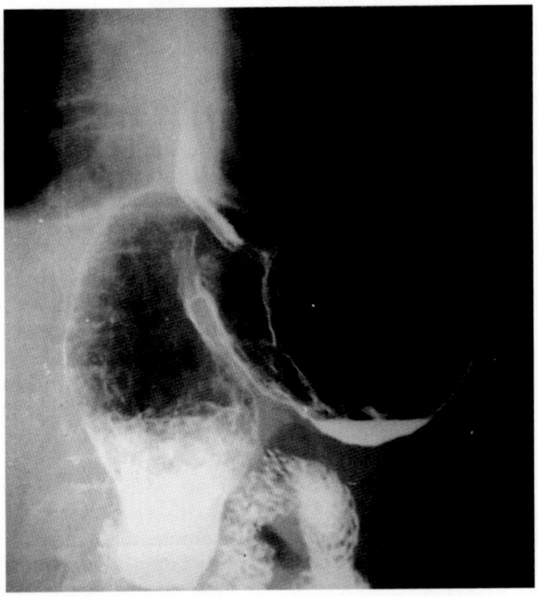

Figure 76-13. An organoaxial volvulus of the stomach identified on a UGI series. *(From Brandt LJ: Gastrointestinal disorders of the elderly, New York, 1986, Lippincott-Raven.)*

Gangrene ensues in approximately 5% of cases, mostly in individuals with a traumatic diaphragmatic hernia. Organoaxial volvulus usually requires surgical correction.

Mesenteroaxial volvulus is often intermittent and incomplete. Affected persons complain of chronic postprandial pain, belching, bloating, vomiting, and early satiety; strangulation is rare. Diagnosis is made by barium roentgenography. Decompression with a nasogastric tube may return the stomach to its normal position. Surgery is indicated for persistent symptoms. Some patients have been successfully treated by fixation of the stomach with two percutaneous endoscopic gastrostomy tubes; these are removed after adhesions fix the stomach to the anterior abdominal wall.

Gastric Tumors

Benign Gastric Tumors

The incidence of benign gastric tumors increases with age. A hyperplastic polyp accounts for 75% to 90% of such growths and typically is a small solitary lesion at the junction of the gastric body and antrum.[151] Hyperplastic polyps are not considered true neoplasms and are not premalignant. They rarely produce symptoms and thus are found incidentally in an evaluation of the UGI tract. In contrast, adenomatous polyps are true neoplasms and account for 10% to 25% of gastric polyps. The mean incidence of malignant change in gastric adenomas has been reported to be from 6% to 75%, probably reflecting their heterogeneity in size, age, and histology (tubular, villous, or mixed).

Gastric polyps may occur in some GI polyposis syndromes, but the only one appearing in older adults is the Cronkhite-Canada syndrome. This disorder is acquired, not inherited, and is characterized by diffuse GI polyposis, protein-losing enteropathy, and ectodermal abnormalities, including hyperpigmentation, alopecia, and dystrophic nail changes. Polyps in this syndrome are hamartomas composed of tubules and mucus-filled cysts.

Mesenchymal tumors, including leiomyomas, fibromas, and tumors of neural origin, account for a significant percentage of benign gastric tumors. Symptoms of these tumors are usually related to their size and not their type. Pain and bleeding are the most common manifestations.

Malignant Gastric Tumors

Gastric Adenocarcinoma. Inexplicably, the incidence of gastric cancer has been decreasing in older adults, whereas relatively more cases are being diagnosed in younger patients.[152] Nevertheless, the vast majority of gastric cancers occur in patients older than 60 years.[1] Carcinoma of the stomach is usually incurable by the time symptoms appear because symptoms often do not develop until the tumor is large. Initial symptoms are often mild and nonspecific. The tendency to treat dyspepsia in older patients without a diagnostic evaluation prompted Sir Heneage Ogilvie to say, in the early 1900s, "in carcinoma of the stomach, alkalis are the undertaker's best friend."

Vague epigastric discomfort, anorexia, early satiety, and weight loss are the most frequent symptoms of gastric cancer. Physical examination may reveal enlarged left axillary and supraclavicular lymph nodes, umbilical nodule, or hard palpable left hepatic lobe. Rarely, the patient develops acanthosis nigricans, dermatomyositis, or an explosive outbreak of skin tags or keratotic lesions (sign of Leser-Trélat), raising the suspicion of a visceral neoplasm. Laboratory abnormalities are nonspecific.

Surgical excision is the only potentially curative treatment for advanced lesions, whereas lesions that are detected early may be suitable for endoscopic resection. Of patients with gastric cancer, 70% to 90% are considered suitable for laparotomy, but only 50% are found to be eligible for potentially curative resections; death occurs in most of these individuals within 1 year. Five-year

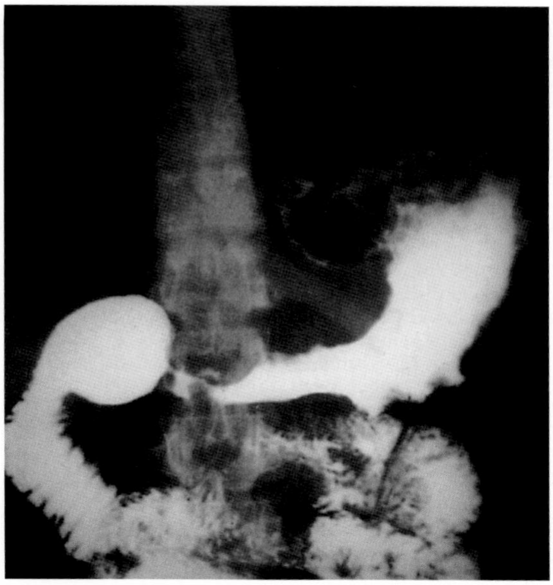

Figure 76-14. UGI series showing a gastric lymphoma with antral narrowing mimicking an adenocarcinoma. *(From Brandt LJ: Gastrointestinal disorders of the elderly, New York, 1986, Lippincott-Raven.)*

survival rates are 5% to 15%. Combined chemotherapy and irradiation may be of some benefit, but irradiation alone is ineffective, except for palliation of bone pain from metastases.

Gastric Lymphoma. The stomach is the most frequent site of primary, extranodal lymphoma and accounts for 50% to 75% of patients with lymphoma of the GI tract. Gastric lymphoma produces nonspecific symptoms, but epigastric pain with weight loss and a palpable mass in a patient who is otherwise well is typical. Radiographically, lymphoma resembles carcinoma in up to two thirds of cases (Figure 76-14). Large ulcerated masses, hyperrugosity, polypoid lesions, or antral narrowing suggests lymphoma. A definitive diagnosis cannot be made from gastroscopic brush cytology and biopsy, and laparotomy may be necessary. Therapy typically is wide excision followed by radiation and leads to a 5-year survival of about 40% to 50%.

SYSTEMIC DISEASES

Diabetes Mellitus

Patients with long-standing diabetes mellitus often have profound abnormalities of GI motility, including delayed gastric emptying of solids.[153] Such abnormalities are frequently without clinical manifestations, although difficulty controlling plasma glucose levels, due to an inconstant and unpredictable rate of gastric emptying, may be a subtle indication of gastroparesis. Gastric atony may be manifested by a gradual onset of upper abdominal fullness, satiety, and vomiting. Gastroparesis and accompanying hypochlorhydria probably underlie the development of gastric bezoars and bacterial and fungal overgrowth in this population.

Diabetic gastroparesis is caused by an abnormality of the autonomic nervous system almost always associated with peripheral or autonomic neuropathy. Metoclopramide has been used to improve gastric motility and relieve symptoms but causes intolerable central nervous system effects, such as tardive dyskinesia, in many patients. Domperidone is effective in many patients, but is not widely available.

Amyloidosis

The GI tract is involved in 50% to 75% of patients with amyloidosis, and in approximately one-50%of these cases the stomach is affected. It is unusual for signs and symptoms of GI involvement to be directly attributable to the amyloidosis per se. Outlet obstruction may be caused by an obstructing mass of amyloid in the distal stomach. Amyloid may also diffusely infiltrate the gastric wall, making surgery difficult, and may be associated with giant gastric ulcers resistant to medical therapy. Prognosis is related to that of the primary disease.

KEY POINTS

- The older adult population has been growing, and their demand for medical care continues to grow, So, it becomes increasingly important for physicians to be acquainted with the manifestation of diseases of the upper gastrointestinal (UGI) tract in members of this age group.
- Abnormalities of the oral mucosa encountered in older patients may be the result of medical therapy, signify the presence of a systemic disease, or represent premalignant changes; these include candidiasis and leukoplakia.
- Oropharyngeal dysphagia, cricopharyngeal achalasia, and postintubation dysphagia are significant clinical issues in older adults, who often have significant swallowing disorders.
- Older patients with dysphagia should be evaluated for the presence of disease processes involving the esophagus, and complaints should not be ascribed to motility changes occurring as a result of age alone.
- Gastroesophageal reflux disease (GERD) and motility disorders of the esophagus are common in older adults; other complaints related to esophageal disease in older adults may mimic symptoms of disease in other systems. Frequent complaints are regurgitation, vomiting, painful swallowing (odynophagia), respiratory difficulties, and chest pain resembling the pain of myocardial ischemia. The differential diagnosis is vast, and the astute clinician needs to consider many possibilities.
- Motor and secretory functions of the stomach are altered with aging but, as in other parts of the GI tract, changes in gastric physiology attributable to age alone rarely are responsible for symptoms. The manifestations of common disorders such as peptic ulcer disease, nonulcer dyspepsia, and upper GI bleeding are often more pronounced in older adults, and these disorders can lead to substantial morbidity in this group.

For a complete list of references, please visit www.expertconsult.com.

KEY REFERENCES

6. Jensen GL, McGee M, Binkley J: Nutrition in the elderly. Gastroenterol Clin North Am 30:313–334, 2001.
22. Plant RL: Anatomy and physiology of swallowing in adults and geriatrics. Otolaryngol Clin North Am 31:477–488, 1998.
25. Achem SR, DeVault KR: Dysphagia in aging. J Clin Gastroenterol 39:357–371, 2005.
30. Law R, Katzka DA, Baron TH: Zenker's diverticulum. Clin Gastroenterol Hepatol 12:1773–1782, 2014.
35. Lee J, Anggiansah A, Anggiansah R, et al: Effects of age on the gastroesophageal junction, esophageal motility, and reflux disease. Clin Gastroenterol Hepatol 5:1392–1398, 2007.
37. Firth M, Prather CM: Gastrointestinal motility problems in the elderly patient. Gastroenterology 122:1688–1700, 2002.
39. Shaker R, Staff D: Esophageal disorders in the elderly. Gastroenterol Clin North Am 30:335–361, 2001.

40. Triadafilopoulos G, Sharma R: Features of symptomatic gastroesophageal reflux disease in elderly patients. Am J Gastroenterol 92:2007–2011, 1997.
43. Richter JE: Gastroesophageal reflux disease in the older patient: presentation, treatment, and complications. Am J Gastroenterol 95:368–373, 2000.
58. Wang KK, Sampliner RE: Diagnosis, surveillance and therapy of Barrett's esophagus. Am J Gastroenterol 103:788–797, 2008.
59. American Gastroenterological Association, Spechler SJ, Sharma P, et al: American Gastroenterological Association medical position statement on the management of Barrett's esophagus. Gastroenterology 140:1084–1091, 2011.
68. Zografos GN, Georgiadou D, Thomas D, et al: Drug-induced esophagitis. Dis Esophagus 22:633–637, 2009.
69. Greenwald DA: Aging, the gastrointestinal tract, and risk of acid-related disease. Am J Med 117(Suppl 5A):8S–13S, 2004.
89. Evans JA, Early DS, Chandraskhara V, et al: The role of endoscopy in the assessment and treatment of esophageal cancer. Gastrointest Endosc 77:328–334, 2013.
90. Soenen S, Rayner CK, Horowitz M, et al: Gastric emptying in the elderly. Clin Geriatr Med 31:339–353, 2015.
113. Laine L: Approaches to nonsteroidal anti-inflammatory drug use in the high-risk patient. Gastroenterology 120:594–606, 2001.
120. Bhatt DL, Scheiman J, Abraham NS, et al: American College of Cardiology Foundation Task Force on Clinical Expert Consensus Documents: ACCF/ACG/AHA 2008 expert consensus document on reducing the gastrointestinal risks of antiplatelet therapy and NSAID use: a report of the American College of Cardiology Foundation Task Force on Clinical Expert Consensus Documents. J Am Coll Cardiol 52:1502–1517, 2008.
121. Scheiman JM: Prevention of NSAID-induced ulcers. Curr Treat Options Gastroenterol 11:125–134, 2008.
125. Linder JD, Wilcox CM: Acid peptic disease in the elderly. Gastroenterol Clin North Am 30:363–376, 2001.
127. Pilotto A, Franceschi M, Maggi S, et al: Optimal management of peptic ulcer disease in the elderly. Drugs Aging 27:545–558, 2010.
129. Zullo A, Hassan C, Campo SM, et al: Bleeding peptic ulcer in the elderly. Drugs Aging 24:815–828, 2007.
130. Tack J, Talley NJ, Camilleri M, et al: Functional gastroduodenal disorders. Gastroenterology 130:1466–1479, 2006.
139. Farrell JJ, Friedman LS: Gastrointestinal bleeding in the elderly. Gastroenterol Clin North Am 30:377–407, 2001.
140. Gostout CJ: Gastrointestinal bleeding in the elderly patient. Am J Gastroenterol 95:590–595, 2000.
152. Sial SH, Catalano MF: Gastrointestinal tract cancer in the elderly. Gastroenterol Clin North Am 30:565–590, 2001.

77 The Small Bowel

Saqib S. Ansari, Sulleman Moreea, Christopher A. Rodrigues

Diseases of the small bowel can be divided into two categories for clinical purposes: (1) diffuse processes, such as celiac disease, that result in the malabsorption syndromes, and (2) discrete diseases, such as small bowel tumors, that produce focal manifestations. Some conditions, such as Crohn disease and radiation enteritis, can cause a combination of malabsorption and focal features. Malabsorption in older adults is not due to aging alone, as the absorption of most nutrients is unaffected with a few exceptions. Lactose malabsorption is common in otherwise healthy older individuals[1,2] and can coexist with other diffuse small bowel diseases. Calcium absorption declines with age because of a higher prevalence of vitamin D deficiency.[3] Lastly, atrophic gastritis is more common in older adults and can adversely affect the absorption of vitamin B_{12} and folic acid. Food-cobalamin malabsorption, the impaired release of the vitamin B_{12} from food, is a result of reduced or absent gastric acid secretion or of the use of acid-suppressing drugs. This is the most common cause of B_{12} deficiency in older people,[4] pernicious anemia and terminal ileal disease/resection being much rarer. Folic acid absorption in the proximal jejunum is also pH dependent and declines with achlorhydria. However, jejunal bacterial overgrowth, another consequence of achlorhydria, can compensate for reduced absorption of the vitamin because of bacterial folate synthesis.[5] Three conditions account for most cases of malabsorption in older individuals: bacterial overgrowth syndrome, celiac disease, and chronic pancreatitis (the latter is actually maldigestion resulting in malabsorption).

Steatorrhea, the typical symptom of fat malabsorption, is much less likely to occur in older adult patients, who may even be constipated despite an increased stool volume. Carbohydrate malabsorption can cause watery diarrhea, abdominal distention, borborygmi, and flatulence. These symptoms are due to the action of bacteria on carbohydrate residues in the colon. The clinical presentation of malabsorption in older adults is nonspecific. It consists of a variable combination of the following: fatigue, poor mobility, anorexia, nausea, diarrhea, anemia, weight loss, depression, and confusion.[6,7] Peripheral edema can result from hypoproteinemia. Vague generalized body ache and muscle weakness can be early clinical indicators of osteomalacia. Vitamin K deficiency may cause bruising, petechiae, and bleeding manifestations. Abdominal discomfort and distention are common, but abdominal pain is relatively rare. Recurrent abdominal pain occurs with chronic pancreatitis, inflammation as in Crohn disease, subacute obstruction as a result of strictures, or chronic mesenteric ischemia.

The diagnosis of malabsorption should therefore be considered in older adult patients with clinical and anthropometric evidence of undernutrition, even in the absence of gastrointestinal (GI) symptoms. A dietary assessment is important in determining whether the malnutrition can reasonably be attributed to inadequate nutrient intake. The details of previous surgical procedures should be ascertained: gastric surgery or intestinal bypass procedures can result in the bacterial overgrowth syndrome, and extensive small bowel resection can cause malabsorption because of a critical reduction in the mucosal absorptive surface area.

INVESTIGATION OF SMALL BOWEL DISORDER

Screening Tests

Routine blood tests are often helpful in the diagnosis of small bowel disease. The full blood count and blood film may show anemia with macrocytosis, an iron-deficient picture, or a dimorphic film. Macrocytosis, leukopenia, and thrombocytopenia suggest megaloblastic anemia. Ferritin, vitamin B_{12}, and red cell folate levels should be measured in patients with suspected malabsorption, even with a normal blood film, as typical changes may not be present in early deficiency. B_{12} deficiency should be further investigated with serologic tests for pernicious anemia (gastric parietal cell and intrinsic factor antibodies), celiac disease (discussed later, a rare cause of isolated B_{12} deficiency), and, if necessary, radiologic or endoscopic evaluation of the terminal ileum. A low B_{12} level with a normal or increased red cell folate level raises the possibility of small bowel bacterial overgrowth. Howell-Jolly bodies in the blood film indicate splenic atrophy, which occurs in association with celiac disease. Osteomalacia results in a raised alkaline phosphatase level with low calcium and phosphate levels and is confirmed by a low serum 25-hydroxycholecaliferol. Vitamin K deficiency prolongs the international normalized ratio (INR). Hypoalbuminemia is a common although nonspecific finding, as it also occurs with poor dietary intake, injury, sepsis, and malignancy. Malabsorption is unlikely if these screening tests are completely normal.

Tests of Absorption

Tests of nutrient absorption such as fecal fat estimation and xylose absorption are no longer used in clinical practice because they are cumbersome to perform, relatively insensitive, and unpopular with patients and professionals. Lactose absorption is the only nutrient absorption test that is widely used.[8] In the standard lactose tolerance test, blood glucose levels are measured before, and 30 and 60 minutes after, the ingestion of 50 g of lactose. A rise of less than 1.1 mmol/L indicates lactose malabsorption, and accompanying (transient) symptoms of abdominal bloating, discomfort, diarrhea, and wind are indicative of intolerance. Alternatively, a lactose hydrogen breath test can be used: after an oral dose of 25 to 50 g lactose, end-expiratory breath samples are collected every 30 minutes for 3 hours. Malabsorption of lactose results in fermentation of the sugar by colonic flora, producing a rise in breath hydrogen. This rise can also occur in patients with small bowel bacterial overgrowth, although usually much earlier than in patients with lactose malabsorption. Approximately 25% of patients will have a false negative test, and hence a trial of a lactose-free diet is reasonable if the diagnosis is suspected clinically.

Radiology and Endoscopy

Double-contrast barium follow-through examination and enteroclysis (small bowel enema) have been used for many years to investigate the small bowel. Enteroclysis is probably more accurate but is more invasive. The role of abdominal ultrasound and computed tomography (CT) scanning is described in the relevant sections.

Advances in magnetic resonance (MR) imaging of the small bowel (MR enterography) now allow excellent visualization of the small bowel noninvasively and without exposure to radiation. MRI is now the investigation of choice for patients with suspected inflammatory bowel disease and small bowel tumors. Older adult patients can find the test difficult to tolerate as they have to lie supine and still for at least 30 minutes. Noise levels can be high because of vibration of the magnetic coils and earplugs or headphones need to be worn. Claustrophobia as a result of the tight cylindrical scanner can lead to a significant number of patients being unable to complete the test. Sedation can be used to improve compliance to the test. Open coil magnets are increasingly being used for claustrophobic patients and for patients who are too large for the cylindrical scanner. MR contrast agents, such as gadolinium, are safer than the iodinated contrast agents used for CT scanning and rarely cause contrast reactions. However, they can cause contrast nephropathy and, in rare cases, nephrogenic systemic fibrosis in patients with moderate to severe chronic kidney disease. Contraindications include implanted devices such as cardiac pacemakers, implantable cardioverter-defibrillators (ICDs), nerve stimulators, cochlear implants, and embedded metallic foreign bodies such as intraorbital metallic fragments that could have been present from the working days of the now retired patients. Transdermal patches need to be removed before MRI is performed. The following are not contraindications and are considered MR safe: joint prostheses, coronary/peripheral vascular stents, prosthetic heart valves, sternal wires, inferior vena caval filters, and embolization coil.[9] The composition of intracranial aneurismal clips needs to be ascertained because most may not be MR safe.

Esophagogastroduodenoscopy (EGD) is the usual method for collecting fluid for culture and for obtaining biopsies from the distal duodenum. The detection of villous atrophy at endoscopy can be improved by viewing the duodenal mucosal surface at high magnification after spraying with indigo carmine.[10]

Wireless capsule endoscopy or video capsule endoscopy is a noninvasive technology that was introduced in 2000.[11] It has made possible the direct visualization of the entire small bowel[12] with a magnification higher than conventional endoscopes, allowing detailed views to the level of individual villi. It consists of a capsule, which is swallowed and propelled by peristalsis, transmitting between two and six images per second via a belt to a data recorder worn by a patient. Approximately 75,000 images are recorded over a 12-hour period, by which time the capsule has usually reached the caecum in most patients. The latest capsule generation has vastly improved image quality and tissue coverage. The data recorder has a built-in real-time viewer that enables live viewing of the capsule progress as it progresses through the small bowel. The images are then downloaded onto a computer workstation and are viewed as a video. The software on which the video is viewed has a built-in Atlas, which has more than 600 small bowel pathology images to aid diagnosis for those who are new to this technology. Capsule endoscopy is currently used for the investigation of obscure GI bleeding (discussed later), of small bowel Crohn disease, in suspected or refractory malabsorption syndromes (e.g., celiac disease), and in suspected small bowel tumors, including screening in familial polyposis syndromes.[13] The major drawbacks of capsule endoscopy are the inability to take biopsies, incomplete visualization of the mucosal surface, and capsule retention requiring surgical or endoscopic removal (1% to 7%). A biodegradable patency capsule without recording facilities is available to ascertain small bowel patency in cases where symptoms suggest possible structuring disease not shown on small bowel barium studies of MR enterography.

Double-balloon enteroscopy (DBE), a technique that can traverse the whole of the small bowel using an enteroscope with an overtube, was first described in 2001. The enteroscope is inserted by either the oral or anal route, so that therapeutic procedures can be carried out.[12,14] General anesthesia is often required for this complex and prolonged technique. The overall diagnostic yield is between 43% and 83%, with a subsequent change in management for 57% to 84% of patients. Complications include postprocedural abdominal pain, pancreatitis, bleeding, and small bowel perforation. Push enteroscopy is currently the most widely available technique for endoscopic examination of the small bowel. The instrument can be inserted 30 to 160 cm beyond the ligament of Treitz and has a channel for biopsies and therapeutic procedures including thermocoagulation of bleeding lesions, polypectomy, and placement of feeding jejunostomy tubes. Lastly, intraoperative enteroscopy, in which the small bowel is "pleated" over an endoscope at laparotomy or laparoscopy, is the most accurate technique but has a significant complication rate.

SMALL BOWEL DISEASES

Celiac Disease

Celiac disease is an immune-mediated small intestinal enteropathy that is triggered by exposure to dietary gluten in genetically predisposed individuals.[15] Dietary gluten in cereals like wheat, barley, and rye leads to characteristic histologic changes, including intraepithelial lymphocytosis, crypt hyperplasia, and, ultimately, villous atrophy. The disease mainly affects the proximal small bowel and decreases in severity distally and may spare the distal jejunum and ileum. A large-scale screening study in subjects from Finland, Italy, the United Kingdom, and Germany found a prevalence of celiac disease of approximately 1%,[16-18] with a recent U.S. study showing a prevalence of 0.71%.[19]

Sixty percent of newly diagnosed patients are adults[20] with a peak incidence in the third decade and a second, smaller peak in the fifth and sixth decades.[21] In a multicenter Italian study, only 60 (4.4%) of 1353 patients with celiac disease were older than 65 years at diagnosis.[22] However, the seroprevalence of celiac disease in an English population of 7257 people aged 45 to 76 years was 1.2% with no significant difference between those younger and older than 65 years of age.[18] In a Finnish population-based study of 2815 individuals, the prevalence of celiac disease in those aged 52 to 74 years was 2.13%, double that in younger adults.[23] The female-to-male ratio in adults is approximately 2 : 1, and this is no different in older adult patients.[18,22] Only 30% to 40% of patients are symptomatic; the rest have clinically silent disease. This variable clinical picture is probably related to the extent of affected bowel. Traditionally patients with celiac disease presented with malabsorption dominated by diarrhea, steatorrhea, weight loss, or failure to thrive,[15] but over time the proportion of newly diagnosed patients with malabsorptive symptoms has decreased.[24] Patients can present with a wide range of symptoms and signs, including anemia, vague abdominal symptoms, neuropathy, ataxia, depression, short stature, osteomalacia, osteoporosis, and lymphoma. Asymptomatic patients are typically diagnosed through screening, which may be initiated because the individual has a related disorder or has symptoms and is a first-degree relative to a patient with celiac disease.

Celiac disease is associated with a number of autoimmune conditions, the most important being insulin-dependent diabetes mellitus, autoimmune thyroid disease, Sjögren syndrome, autoimmune hepatitis, primary biliary cirrhosis, and Addison disease.[21,25-27] Dermatitis herpetiformis can be regarded as an extraintestinal manifestation of celiac disease, as virtually all patients have an enteropathy with characteristic histologic changes. Neurologic disorders such as epilepsy, cerebellar syndrome, dementia, peripheral neuropathy, myopathy, and hyporeflexia have been reported in patients with celiac disease.[28]

Immunoglobulin A (IgA) deficiency affects 2% to 3% of patients with celiac disease and can result in false negative serologic tests. From 90% to 95% of celiac patients have the human leukocyte antigen (HLA) class 2 molecule DQ2, and most of the remainder have DQ8. At least 1 in 10 first-degree relatives are affected.[26]

Diagnosis

Serologic markers are now used routinely for screening patients and high-risk groups with associated disorders or a positive family history. IgA endomysial antibody (EMA) has a specificity of over 98%, but antibody to IgA tissue transglutaminase (tTG) is also very accurate and is a simpler and less expensive test.[25,29]

Patients with an absent tTG or those in whom there is a strong clinical suspicion of celiac disease should have an IgA level test to exclude deficiency—this is routinely carried out by some laboratories. If IgA deficiency is present, tests for IgG tTG or EMA should be carried out. Antibody titers can decrease or disappear with treatment, but this is not a reliable marker of histologic remission.[30,31] Patients with positive serology should have an endoscopy for duodenal biopsies.[32] The diagnosis of celiac disease is readily established in those who, while consuming a gluten-containing diet, have positive serology and a duodenal biopsy with obvious celiac histology (increased intraepithelial lymphocytosis, crypt hyperplasia, and villous atrophy). These changes, accompanied by a clinical response to a gluten-free diet, are adequate to establish the diagnosis.[27,33] Biopsy remains essential for the diagnosis of adult celiac disease and cannot be replaced by serology. To state a definite diagnosis of celiac disease, villous atrophy is required. However, lesser degrees of damage (≥25 intraepithelial lymphocytes but no villous atrophy) combined with positive serology (IgA-EMA or tTG) may also represent celiac disease ("probable celiac disease"), and in these circumstances a trial with a gluten-free diet may be considered to further support the diagnosis of celiac disease.[34]

Follow-up biopsies should be undertaken in patients with celiac disease whose condition does not respond to a gluten-free diet.[34] However, follow-up biopsies are not mandatory in asymptomatic patients on a gluten-free diet with no other worrying features. Rebiopsy after a gluten challenge is rarely carried out now but may be required in cases where there is diagnostic difficulty, such as when the original biopsy was taken while the patient was on a gluten-free diet. The absence of HLA DQ2 and DQ8 virtually excludes the diagnosis and is useful when the patient does not wish to undergo a gluten challenge. Lastly, 5% to 10% of patients have serology-negative disease, and thus histologic confirmation should be undertaken if the likelihood of celiac disease is high (e.g., in symptomatic patients with a positive family history).

Management

The mainstay of management for celiac disease is a lifelong gluten-free diet. Specialist input is central in achieving this, so all patients are referred to a dietitian. It is now generally accepted that patients can take a moderate amount of oats, providing there is no contamination with wheat gluten. Patients are encouraged to join a patient support organization. Patients should have regular clinical follow-up[25,26] for assessment of symptoms and checking for dietary adherence. Annual blood tests should be performed, including full blood count, hematinics, liver function tests, calcium, thyroid function tests, glucose level, and also a vitamin D level at diagnosis.[34] Lactose intolerance can cause apparently resistant disease in some patients. However, milk and milk products are an important source of calcium and should be restricted only if they exacerbate symptoms—ideally after confirming the diagnosis with an objective test. Adult patients with celiac disease should have a calcium intake of at least 1000 mg/day. Patients should receive supplements to correct nutrient deficiencies, as complete recovery of mucosal function can take months. Older adult patients with celiac disease should be given multivitamins and a calcium supplement initially. Bone mineral densitometry should be carried out at diagnosis in all older adult patients with celiac disease. Bone mass improves, but does not normalize, in adult and older adult patients on a gluten-free diet, and other therapeutic measures are often required.[35] Hyposplenism[36] associated with celiac disease may result in impaired immunity to encapsulated bacteria, which increases the risk of infections.[37-39] Vaccination against *Pneumococcus* is therefore recommended.[40] Approximately 5% of patients fail to respond to gluten withdrawal or relapse after an initial remission.[25] Some patients with refractory disease respond to corticosteroids or immunosuppressive agents. Others (a proportion of whom have small intestinal ulcers and strictures [ulcerative enteritis]) have a cryptic T cell lymphoma of the intraepithelial lymphocytes[41] with 5-year survival rates of less than 50%.[25] Patients with ulcerative enteritis often require surgery for complications such as perforation or obstruction.

Neoplasms

The twofold increase in mortality in the first year after diagnosis is largely due to the development of malignant complications.[42] The overall risk of malignancy is less than previously reported[43] and is approximately 30% greater than that of the general population.[42] T cell lymphoma of the small intestine is the most common tumor,[44-46] but there is an increased risk of developing squamous cell carcinomas of the esophagus, mouth, pharynx; adenocarcinoma of the small bowel; and colorectal carcinoma. The incidence of breast[42,45] and lung cancer[42] is decreased. Lymphoma may be the first manifestation of celiac disease, but the diagnosis should also be considered in established patients whose condition is either resistant to, or relapses on, a strict gluten-free diet. Weight loss is the most common symptom, and patients also experience profound lethargy, muscle weakness, abdominal pain, and diarrhea. The prognosis is poor: less than a fifth of patients survive for 30 months.[47] A gluten-free diet has a protective effect against the development of malignancy in celiac disease.[43,45,46]

Bacterial Overgrowth Syndrome

Intestinal bacterial counts normally increase abnormally, and bacterial populations vary in different sections of the GI tract: the jejunum is colonized by gram-positive aerobes and facultative anaerobes, ileal flora contain some strict anaerobes as well, and the colon is heavily populated by predominantly anaerobic bacteria.[48] Malabsorption can occur when the small bowel population increases and becomes more anaerobic. This is partly the result of direct injury to the intestinal mucosa, but uptake or binding of major nutrients and vitamin B_{12} by the proliferating bacteria also play a part.[49] In addition, fat absorption is affected by deconjugation of bile salts by anaerobic bacteria, resulting in impaired micelle formation. Folic acid and vitamin K are synthesized by bacteria, and folate levels are often normal or raised when bacterial overgrowth is present. Two factors are largely responsible for regulating bacterial growth: gastric acid and intestinal motility.[48,49] Gastric acid destroys microorganisms ingested with food and saliva. The interdigestive migrating motor complex, a cyclic fasting motility pattern, regularly propels luminal contents toward the colon, thus preventing stagnation and bacterial overgrowth.[50]

Pathogenesis

The classic disorders associated with bacterial overgrowth are those in which disordered intestinal motility, abnormal reservoirs, or abnormal communications between the proximal and distal intestine result in proliferation of bacteria. Examples of the former are diabetic autonomic neuropathy, late radiation enteropathy, collagen diseases such as scleroderma, and the numerous causes of chronic intestinal pseudo-obstruction. Partial small bowel obstruction due to strictures or adhesions has a similar effect. Abnormal reservoirs that permit stagnation of luminal contents may arise de novo (e.g., small bowel diverticula) or as a result of surgery (e.g., the afferent limb of a Billroth II gastrectomy). Abnormal communications between the proximal and distal intestine result in contamination of the former by denser, more anaerobic bacterial populations. Examples of this group include gastrocolic and jejunocolic fistulas, right hemicolectomy with resection of the ileocecal valve, and surgical bypass of obstructed or diseased intestinal segments. Small bowel bacterial overgrowth in older adults also occurs under conditions that impair gastric acid secretion, such as atrophic gastritis,[49,51] treatment with acid-reducing drugs,[52-54] or after surgery for peptic ulcer disease. Gut immune defenses may be impaired in older adults and thus contribute to their susceptibility to overgrowth.[55]

Clinical Picture

Older adult patients who have bacterial overgrowth with malabsorption typically have presenting symptoms of diarrhea, weight loss, and abdominal bloating associated with hypoalbuminemia and low B_{12} levels. Some anatomic abnormalities associated with bacterial overgrowth (e.g., small bowel diverticula) are more common with increasing age. Most patients who had surgery for peptic ulcer disease before the widespread use of proton pump inhibitors are now elderly. Bacterial overgrowth is thus more common in older adults and is found in 52.5% to 70.8% of patients with symptoms of malabsorption.[6,54,56] It also affects 14.5% to 25.6% of older adults with no GI symptoms.[53,57-59] Some of these individuals are on acid-suppressing medication[53]; others have factors that are associated with slower small bowel transit, such as reduced intake of dietary fiber[53] and physical disability.[59] Subclinical malabsorption is probably present in a proportion who have low albumin and B_{12} levels, and this may also adversely affect bone mineral density.[60]

Diagnosis

The literature on bacterial overgrowth is plagued by the absence of a reliable diagnostic test. Historically, culture of proximal small bowel aspirate (currently usually obtained during EGD) was the gold standard for establishing the diagnosis: proximal jejunal counts greater than 10^5 colony-forming units (CFU)/mL were accepted as abnormal.[48] Although this is probably true for post-surgical patients with blind loops, jejunal bacterial counts in healthy individuals are much lower, in the range of 0 to 10^3 CFU/mL, and a systematic review found no evidence to support culture as a gold standard test.[61] Furthermore, this technique only samples a limited region of the small bowel and may miss overgrowth in the more distal segments. Breath tests were developed as an alternative to the invasive procedure and cumbersome culture techniques were involved.[61,62] However, these tests were largely validated against culture, which raises serious doubts about their reliability.

In the [^{14}C]-glycocholate breath test, 5 to 10 μCi of glycocholic acid, a conjugated bile acid radiolabeled with ^{14}C, is administered with a test meal. Bacterial deconjugation results in separation of [^{14}C]-glycine from cholic acid, and $^{14}CO_2$ produced from the former is measured in breath samples collected over the next 4 to 8 hours. Terminal ileal disease or resection also results in a positive test because the bile acid is not reabsorbed and is then metabolized by colonic flora. The test has largely been abandoned because of its poor sensitivity with a false negative rate of 30% to 40%.

Breath hydrogen measurement after ingestion of 50 to 80 g of glucose or 10 to 12 g of lactulose is an alternative technique that avoids the use of a radioisotope. Metabolism of either carbohydrate by the abnormal bacterial population produces hydrogen, which can be detected by breath testing. The timing of the hydrogen rise is crucial for the lactulose test, as this sugar is not absorbed in the small bowel and produces a second, higher "colonic" hydrogen peak. It is not possible to reliably distinguish the peak produced by small bowel bacterial overgrowth from that due to normal colonic flora without using an oral contrast medium as well. Glucose is thus a better substrate as it is absorbed completely in the proximal small bowel. Furthermore, a small study in healthy volunteers has shown that even a 10-g quantity of lactulose accelerates small bowel transit,[63] and hence the glucose-hydrogen breath test is probably more reliable. Approximately 15% of individuals are colonized by colonic flora, which produce methane, not hydrogen, and false negative tests will occur unless breath methane and hydrogen are both measured.[62] In the [^{14}C]-xylose breath test, elevated $^{14}CO_2$ levels appear in breath samples within 60 minutes of taking 10 μCi of [^{14}C]-xylose with 1 g of unlabeled xylose by mouth. Although the sensitivities and specificities of breath tests are variable, even when compared against culture, they are simple to perform and are probably useful if positive. Until a better test for bacterial overgrowth becomes available, the most practical strategy would be to test, treat, and then retest, in addition to evaluating the clinical response.[61] Patients with confirmed overgrowth should have a small bowel x-ray series to look for abnormal communications or reservoirs.

Management

The conditions underlying bacterial overgrowth (with the exception of strictures and some enteroenteric fistulas) are rarely amenable to surgical correction, and hence antibiotics are the mainstay of treatment.[49] Tetracycline was traditionally used to reduce bacterial flora, but approximately two thirds of patients do not benefit from this drug. Chloromycetin and clindamycin are rarely used now because of their toxicity. Co-amoxiclav and norfloxacin are effective in standard doses given for 7 to 10 days, as is metronidazole in combination with one of the cephalosporins.[64,65] Rifaximin is also effective, and systemic toxicity does not occur because the drug is not absorbed.[66] In some patients, a single antibiotic course produces a satisfactory response lasting for months, but many patients need cyclic courses given at monthly intervals for 4 to 6 months. Octreotide, a long-acting analogue of somatostatin, has been tested in small numbers of patients with connective tissue diseases and chronic intestinal pseudo-obstruction. It improves motility and appears to be highly effective on its own[67] or in combination with erythromycin.[68]

Prokinetic agents (including erythromycin) may play a role in the management of bacterial overgrowth, particularly in older adult patients with prolonged small bowel transit. Probiotics may also be helpful, but further work is required to define their role. Clinicians should avoid using acid-suppressing agents in older adults without a clear indication: apart from their possible role in promoting clinically significant bacterial overgrowth, these drugs can cause food-cobalamin malabsorption and are implicated in an increased susceptibility to *Clostridium difficile* infection.

Crohn Disease

Crohn disease is an idiopathic chronic relapsing disorder, characterized by transmural inflammation and ulceration, occurring in a segmental distribution. Intestinal ulceration ranges from aphthoid erosions to deep fissures, and the course is often complicated by the formation of strictures, abscesses, and fistulas. The disease has a predilection for the terminal ileum, but any region of the GI tract can be affected.

The Montreal classification groups patients according to clinical phenotype, including age at diagnosis, location, and disease behavior.[69] This classification considers three age groups, with those older than 40 years comprising the most advanced group, and the majority of patients have inflammatory disease (70%), followed by stricturing disease (17%) and penetrating disease (13%).[70,71] Penetrating disease includes fistulas, abscesses, or both.

At diagnosis, approximately 28% of patients have terminal ileal involvement only, 50% have ileocolic disease, and 25% colonic disease alone.[72] Small bowel disease is less common in older people.[73] In a study in northern France, 34% of patients older than 60 years had small bowel involvement compared to 64% of younger patients.[70] The prevalence of inflammatory bowel disease is increasing worldwide, and with an aging population, this makes Crohn disease in older adults a growing problem. Although Crohn disease predominantly affects teenagers and young adults, there is also a second smaller peak from the sixth to the eighth decades,[74] although not all studies describe this bimodal pattern consistently.[75,76] Nevertheless, a substantial minority of patients with Crohn disease first develop it in later life. In the French study, 24% of patients were diagnosed with Crohn disease at or above the age of 60 years.[70] In another population-based study from Belgium, 23 of 137 patients (17%) were older than 60 years at diagnosis, with an annual incidence of 3.5 per 100,000 (4.8 per 100,000 in patients younger than 60 years).[77] Smoking, a family history of inflammatory bowel disease, and (in most studies) previous appendicectomy are risk factors for Crohn disease.[76]

Clinical Picture and Investigations

Crohn disease in older adults generally follows clinical pattern similar to that in young people.[78] Main symptoms of Crohn disease include abdominal pain, diarrhea, weight loss, nausea, vomiting, fatigue, fever, abdominal mass, and perianal symptoms. However, it is noted that older adult patients are more likely to have colonic rather than small bowel involvement and thus presenting symptoms of diarrhea and bleeding rather than abdominal pain and vomiting.[79] Diagnostic delay is more common in older than in younger patients with Crohn disease (up to 6 years compared with 2 years).[80-82] This delay may be because of the higher prevalence of conditions that may mimic Crohn disease in older adults, conditions such as diverticulosis, acute ischemic or infectious colitis, or drug-related colitis. Complications of Crohn disease, including stricture formation and penetrating disease, are less common in older adults compared to children.[83]

There is no single definitive test for Crohn disease.[84] The diagnosis is established (and disease activity assessed) by clinical features, inflammatory markers, endoscopic, or radiologic imaging and histology. Standard activity indices incorporating some of these features (Crohn disease activity index [CDAI], Harvey-Bradshaw Index) are used in trials but can also be helpful in clinical practice (e.g., in assessing patients for therapy with anti–tumor necrosis factor [TNF] agents).[85] For example, a CDAI of less than 150 is used to define remission, and severe disease is characterized by a score of higher than 450.[85,86]

A discussion of investigative techniques used in small bowel Crohn disease inevitably overlaps with the investigation of colonic disease. In practice, ileocolonoscopy will probably be the initial investigation of choice. Only a short segment of terminal ileum is examined at colonoscopy, and hence either a double-contrast barium follow-through or enteroclysis is traditionally used to define the extent and severity of small bowel disease. Advances in MRI (including MR enteroclysis) have resulted in improved small bowel visualization,[72,87,88] including the ability to distinguish between inflammatory and fibrotic strictures. MRI has the advantage of not using ionizing radiation and is likely to replace barium studies. CT and ultrasound imaging have been used for many years in patients with Crohn disease to outline phlegmons (inflammatory masses) and abscess cavities and to drain the latter percutaneously. Technical advances have extended the range of both modalities. Ultrasound is now also employed to image the bowel wall and detect strictures. Contrast-enhanced examinations with multislice helical CT scanners have high sensitivity (71% to 83%) and specificity (90% to 98%) in the evaluation of small bowel inflammation.[88] Wireless capsule endoscopy can provide endoscopic images of the entire small bowel.[12,72,88] The diagnostic accuracy of wireless capsule endoscopy is now considered to be superior to that of CT or MR enterography, making it the new gold standard for suspected Crohn disease.[89] As stated previously, wireless capsule endoscopy carries a risk of capsule retention, and a patency capsule may be used to reduce this risk. Push enteroscopy is rarely used in Crohn disease, as the terminal ileum is not visualized with this technique. DBE can be used to take biopsies and do therapeutic procedures such as dilation of strictures.[14,72,88]

Management

Management of late-onset Crohn disease is complex because of problems with misdiagnosis, treatment of comorbid diseases, multiple drug interactions, impaired mobility and cognition, and difficult social and financial issues.[90] Management options for Crohn disease include drug therapy, attention to nutrition, smoking cessation, and, in severe or chronic active disease, surgery.[91] Detailed guidelines (including a series of Cochrane reviews) usually discuss management under two headings: the induction of remission and the maintenance of remission.[92-94]

The medical management of older adult patients with Crohn disease is essentially the same as that in younger patients.[75] However, particular caution is required when using corticosteroids, immunosuppressive agents, and biologic drugs in this age group. One approach to drug therapy is the "start low and go slow" approach, by which patients are regularly reassessed for progression to more aggressive therapy if their response is inadequate.[95]

Sulfasalazine is not effective in small bowel Crohn disease without colonic involvement. Mesalamine preparations coated with a pH-sensitive resin or in ethylcellulose-coated granules start releasing the drug in the small bowel. However, meta-analyses showed that mesalamine was little better than placebo for induction of remission,[96] and the drug was ineffective for maintenance of medically induced remission.[97]

Mesalamine only has a role in reducing the relapse rate after surgical resection.[98]

Budesonide (9 mg daily), a topically active steroid with extensive first-pass metabolism in the liver, is recommended for mild to moderate localized ileocecal disease. Budesonide has a better side effect profile compared to other corticosteroids and does not result in osteoporosis. Prednisolone (40 to 60 mg/day up to 1 mg/kg body weight) is used for severe ileocecal disease and for extensive small bowel disease; more than 80% of patients go into remission or have a partial response by 4 weeks. However, corticosteroids cause many side effects. At 1 year, only 32% of patients will have had a prolonged response, 28% become steroid dependent (i.e., require at least 10 mg/day of prednisolone or budesonide 3 mg/day to prevent recurrence), and 38% require surgery.[99] Steroids have no role in maintaining remission in Crohn disease, although budesonide may delay relapse.

Immunosuppressive agents such as azathioprine (2 to 2.5 mg/kg), 6-mercaptopurine (1 to 1.5 mg/kg), and methotrexate (15 to

25 mg IM/SC weekly with folic acid) are used as steroid-sparing agents. They are effective in maintaining remission and may need to be taken long term. They should be used cautiously in older adult patients given their potential for serious toxicity, although, in clinical trials, 6-mercaptopurine has been tolerated by patients in the seventh decade as well as their younger counterparts.[100] It is important to note that allopurinol can enhance the effects of azathioprine and 6-mercaptopurine and can result in severe bone marrow toxicity.[101]

Antibiotics, including antimycobacterial agents, are not effective as primary therapy for small bowel Crohn disease although the former will be required for septic complications associated with penetrating disease. Monoclonal antibodies against TNF-α (infliximab, adalimumab, certolizumab) are used in refractory disease, in patients who are intolerant to conventional treatment, for maintenance of remission, for fistulating disease, and for some extraintestinal manifestations.[102] These drugs are expensive, and significant adverse effects have been reported, including reactivation of tuberculosis, serious infections, optic neuritis, infusion reactions, and a possible increased risk of developing lymphoma. They increase mortality in patients with class 3 to 4 congestive cardiac failure and are therefore contraindicated in this group.

Malnutrition is common in small bowel Crohn disease and is due to a variable combination of reduced nutrient intake, malabsorption, and increased energy requirements resulting from inflammation, sepsis, or surgery. In most patients, nutrient intake can be increased by using small, frequent, low-fiber meals and supplementary polymeric sip feeds. Some patients benefit from tube feeding, and a few need parenteral nutrition. Enteral nutrition, with either elemental or polymeric diets, can also be used as a primary treatment for Crohn disease but is less effective than corticosteroid treatment[103] and is also less acceptable to patients, despite the absence of side effects.

Patients with Crohn disease are prone to osteopenia and osteoporosis. Bone loss occurs with corticosteroid use, as a direct result of the inflammatory process and also because of malabsorption of calcium and vitamin D in patients with extensive small bowel disease. Reduced bone mineral density is associated with low body mass index, male sex, long-standing disease, ileal resection, and active disease. Comprehensive guidelines for the prevention and management of osteoporosis in inflammatory bowel disease have been published.[35]

Several studies have reported a lower frequency of surgery in older adult patients with Crohn disease compared with younger patients.[104,105] Surgery is required for obstruction as a result of strictures, for suppurative complications, and for disease that is refractory to medical treatment. Older adult patients usually tolerate surgery well. Although postoperative hospital stays are longer because of comorbidity, rates of mortality and of surgical complications are similar to those in younger patients.[106]

Adenocarcinoma of the small bowel can complicate small bowel Crohn disease. Older patients with Crohn disease are at an increased risk of various malignancies, including small bowel, colorectal, stomach, pancreatic, renal cancer, and lung cancers.[107,108] They are also at an increased risk of developing non-Hodgkin lymphoma and skin cancers associated with immunomodulators and anti-TNF therapies.[109]

Small Bowel Ischemia

Small bowel ischemia can be acute or chronic and of arterial or venous origin. Arterial ischemia predominantly affects middle-aged and older people. Mesenteric vein thrombosis accounts for 5% to 10% of patients with acute mesenteric ischemia. It affects a younger cohort of patients (mean age 48 to 60 years) and will therefore not be discussed further.

Acute Arterial Mesenteric Ischemia

Acute arterial mesenteric ischemia[110-112] is caused by embolism, thrombus formation, or nonocclusive ischemia of the superior mesenteric artery (SMA) or its territory. Complete occlusion of the SMA, which supplies the jejunum, the ileum, and the right half of the colon, has catastrophic effects. Patients who survive frequently require long-term nutritional support and may need parenteral nutrition depending on the length of residual jejunum. Embolism accounts for 40% to 50% of cases and usually occurs in older adults with predisposing causes such as atrial fibrillation, left-sided cardiac chamber enlargement, or myocardial infarction. Nonocclusive mesenteric ischemia occurs in 20% to 30% of cases and is due to vasoconstriction of the mesenteric circulation following a low-output state or circulatory collapse, for example, severe congestive cardiac failure, hypotension, cardiac arrhythmias, or following cardiac arrest. Thrombosis (20% to 30%) occurs in the setting of widespread vascular disease, and 20% to 50% of patients have a history of abdominal angina in the preceding weeks to months.

Diagnosis

Patients have severe abdominal pain, but physical examination is initially either normal or reveals only tenderness. This disparity between symptoms and physical signs in an older adult patient with cardiovascular disease or a hypercoagulable state should alert the clinician to the possibility of mesenteric ischemia. Signs of peritonitis, hypotension, vomiting, fever, dark or bright red rectal bleeding, increasing distention, leukocytosis, and metabolic acidosis are features of intestinal infarction. Up to 25% of patients have abdominal distention or GI bleeding without pain, and approximately one third of older adult patients may exhibit an acute confusional state.[113] Leukocytosis and raised serum levels of lactate, amylase, alkaline phosphatase, and phosphate are not reliable markers. Fluid levels, dilated loops of bowel, and "thumbprinting" on plain abdominal films occur in up to one third of patients, but specific radiologic features of infarction, such as gas in the intestinal wall or portal vessels, are rare. CT scanning is more accurate in delineating these changes, can also demonstrate thrombus in the mesenteric vessels, and is useful in excluding other causes of abdominal pain.[114] Duplex ultrasonography has a limited role, but CT and MR angiography are promising approaches that have a high sensitivity and specificity for pathology in the SMA.[115,116] Patients with abnormal films have a poor prognosis as even nonspecific changes usually signify intestinal necrosis. Mesenteric angiography is the gold standard for establishing the diagnosis and should ideally be performed before signs of infarction appear. It can, however, be difficult to differentiate between acute and long-standing vascular changes on an angiogram, particularly in patients with nonocclusive mesenteric ischemia.

Management

Management warrants aggressive measures in the appropriate patients, and initial resuscitation includes monitoring of central pressures, correction of hypovolemia, and inotropic support. Splanchnic vasoconstrictors, mainly norepinephrine (noradrenaline) and digitalis preparations, should be avoided. Broad-spectrum antibiotics are given empirically to treat the septicemia resulting from bacterial translocation across infarcted bowel. Early angiography is the cornerstone of management, even when the decision to operate has been made. The angiographic catheter is left in situ for two reasons: repeat angiography may be required, and the catheter can be used for intraarterial infusion of the vasodilator papaverine. This relieves the associated mesenteric arterial spasm and improves perfusion perioperatively. Patients with established signs of infarction need emergency surgery with resection of infarcted bowel and embolectomy, thrombectomy, or arterial reconstruction. A second-look operation is often indicated 12 to 24 hours later to differentiate between viable and nonviable intestine. Full anticoagulation with heparin is controversial but is generally started 48 hours after embolectomy, thrombectomy, and arterial reconstruction. There are many case reports and small case series of successful thrombolytic[112] and endovascular therapy, including angioplasty, stenting, and mechanical thrombus fragmentation in patients with SMA embolism or thrombosis.[117,118] These forms of therapy are generally only successful if carried out within 12 hours of presentation. The mortality rate of acute arterial mesenteric ischemia is 70% to 90% if the diagnosis is not made before irreversible infarction occurs. The overall mortality has improved since the late 1960s, probably because of earlier diagnosis and aggressive management with intensive care support. In one systematic review, mortality rates for arterial embolism, arterial thrombosis, and nonocclusive ischemia were 54.1%, 77.4%, and 72.7%, respectively.[119] Focal segmental ischemia causes localized infarction, often at multiple sites, and can be due to vasculitis, cholesterol, or atheromatous emboli and various nonvascular diseases. Management consists of surgical resection of the infarcted segment.

Chronic Mesenteric Ischemia

The syndrome of abdominal or intestinal angina is a rare condition that develops as a result of atherosclerosis of the splanchnic circulation.[110-112] Mesenteric blood flow fails to meet the increased metabolic demand that occurs after meals, resulting in pain with or without malabsorption and disordered motility. The pain begins within 30 minutes of a meal and gradually increases to a plateau, which lasts for up to 3 hours. It is located in the upper abdomen, can radiate to the back, and is gnawing or cramping in character. It is sometimes relieved by lying prone or squatting. Constipation, diarrhea, steatorrhea, abdominal bloating, and flatulence may also occur. Patients may miss or restrict meals in order to avoid provoking symptoms (sitophobia), and hence lose weight.

Diagnosis

Clinical assessment often reveals evidence of widespread vascular disease. An abdominal systolic bruit may be present but is a nonspecific finding. Individuals with advanced atherosclerotic disease can have severe stenosis or occlusion of two or even all three main mesenteric arterial trunks and remain asymptomatic. Diagnosis therefore depends on the history as well as on angiographic findings of proximal stenoses in at least two of the main mesenteric trunks, with a collateral circulation indicating chronic ischemia. Occlusion of two vessels is found in over 90%, and three-vessel occlusion in over 50%, of patients with chronic mesenteric ischemia.[112] It is important to exclude atypical angina pectoris and other causes of recurrent abdominal pain, such as biliary pain caused by gallstones and peptic ulcer disease. Duplex ultrasonography, CT, and MR angiography are used to evaluate symptomatic patients before angiography.[120]

Management

Surgical revascularization and percutaneous angioplasty with stenting are the two main therapeutic alternatives, both of which relieve symptoms in most patients. Surgery has higher revascularization rates and lower rates of restenosis or occlusion but also higher perioperative morbidity and mortality associated with longer hospital stays. Endovascular therapy is not feasible in all patients but is particularly suitable for those with short segments of disease. The choice of therapy will therefore be made on an individual basis, as many patients will have widespread vascular disease and other comorbidities.[120-122]

Small Intestinal Neoplasms

Primary small bowel tumors are relatively rare, accounting for only 1% to 2.4% of all GI neoplasms.[123] Approximately two thirds of these tumors are malignant, and the small bowel is frequently involved by metastatic disease, particularly metastatic melanoma.

Benign Tumors

Adenomas, leiomyomas, and lipomas are the most common benign tumors. Adenomas have a slight preponderance for the duodenum and ileum; lipomas are more frequently found in the ileum. Leiomyomas are distributed more evenly in the small bowel but are more commonly found in the jejunum. More than 50% of benign tumors are asymptomatic; the rest manifest with obstruction, intussusception, or occult bleeding. Adenomas and leiomyomas can undergo malignant transformation and should be removed by surgical resection or, in the case of adenomas, by endoscopic resection. Asymptomatic lipomas discovered incidentally can be left in situ, as malignant transformation is unknown.

Malignant Tumors

Data from the Surveillance, Epidemiology, and End Results (SEER) program estimated that 6110 American men and women would be diagnosed with small intestinal cancer in 2008, representing a progressive increase since the 1970s. The age-adjusted incidence for the period 2001 to 2005 was 2.2 per 100,000 for men and 1.6 per 100,000 for women, with a median age at diagnosis of 67 years. The overall 5-year relative survival rate (RSS) for 1996 to 2004 was 57.8%; 31% of patients had localized disease at diagnosis with a 5-year RSS of 77%, 33% had regional spread (5-year RSS, 62.2%), and 29% presented with metastases (5-year RSS, 36%).[124] Adenocarcinomas (35% to 50% of tumors), carcinoid tumors (20% to 40%), lymphomas (14% to 18%), and sarcomas (10% to 13%) are the four major histologic types encountered.[123,125]

Presentation and Diagnosis

Abdominal pain, bleeding, intestinal obstruction, and weight loss are the major manifestations, a palpable abdominal mass being less frequent. Perforation occurs in approximately 10% of cases, periampullary tumors can be accompanied by obstructive jaundice, and diarrhea is more common in patients with lymphoma. With small bowel carcinoids, the carcinoid syndrome, due to the release of serotonin and other vasoactive compounds, causes flushing, telangiectasias, diarrhea, bronchospasm, and, less commonly, right-sided heart failure, but it only occurs when hepatic metastases are present[126,127]; 24-hour urinary 5-hydroxyindoleacetic acid and plasma chromogranin A are appropriate screening tests for carcinoid tumors.

The diagnosis of small bowel malignancy is often delayed because of the nonspecific history and the absence of clinical signs. Enteroclysis is more sensitive than barium follow-through in detecting tumors.[128] Modern multidetector-row CT scanning techniques have significantly improved the detection and staging of these relatively rare tumors.[129] CT scans and barium study results may be normal in patients with small bowel carcinoids, but larger lesions are characterized by fixation, separation, thickening, and angulation with a starburst appearance because of the desmoplastic reaction produced by the tumor. Somatostatin receptor scintigraphy has a sensitivity of up to 90% for detection of the primary tumor and of 61% to 96% for metastases.[126] Wireless capsule endoscopy, push enteroscopy, and DBE have transformed the investigation of small bowel tumors. The proportion of patients in whom the diagnosis is established only at laparotomy has correspondingly decreased.

Adenocarcinoma

The majority (52% to 55%) of adenocarcinomas arise in the duodenum, 18% to 25% in the jejunum, and 13% in the ileum.[104,105] The mean age of presentation is 55 to 65 years. These tumors have a poor prognosis, largely because of late presentation and delayed diagnosis: the overall 5-year survival rate is 26% to 31% with a median survival time of 20 months.[130,131] Surgical resection is curative in the appropriate patients without disseminated disease—usually a Whipple pancreatoduodenectomy for lesions of the first and second parts of the duodenum and segmental resection for tumors at other sites. Chemotherapy and radiotherapy are not effective.

Carcinoid Tumor

The small bowel is the most common site for carcinoid tumors, which are predominantly located in the ileum.[132,133] Duodenal tumors are rare. The mean age of presentation is 64 years, and 40% to 70% of patients have regional or distant (most commonly hepatic) metastases at diagnosis.[126,133] However, carcinoid tumors grow slowly and are compatible with prolonged survival even with incurable disease. The overall 5-year survival rate is 61%, approximately double that of small bowel adenocarcinoma.[133] Surgical resection is the only curative treatment. When liver metastases are confined to one lobe, curative hepatic resection can also be carried out in patients with the appropriate functional reserve. The postoperative mortality of patients who undergo resection of the primary tumor or hepatic metastases is 6% with a 5-year survival of up to 87%.[126] Resection of the primary tumor and regional lymph nodes is even appropriate in some patients with unresectable hepatic secondary tumors, as nodal metastases are associated with intense fibrosis and can compromise the vascular supply of the involved small bowel.[126] The 5-year survival rate of patients with hepatic metastases is 18% to 32%.[127] Treatment options for patients with unresectable disease also include the somatostatin analogues octreotide and lanreotide, interferon, hepatic artery embolization, and chemotherapy. The serotonin receptor antagonists cyproheptadine and ondansetron are used for symptomatic control of the carcinoid syndrome.

Sarcoma

Gastrointestinal stromal tumors (GISTs) are rare soft tissue sarcomas of mesenchymal origin arising from the GI tract.[134,135] These tumors were previously thought to originate from smooth muscle. However, only a minority exhibit the histologic characteristics of true smooth muscle tumors, and most GISTs express the tyrosine kinase growth factor receptor c-KIT, which is detectable by immunostaining for the CD117 cell surface receptor. They are therefore usually clearly distinguishable from leiomyomas and leiomyosarcomas. All GISTs have malignant potential, but tumors smaller than 2 cm in diameter can be regarded as essentially benign. The annual incidence is approximately 10 to 15 per million, and 20% to 30% arise from the small bowel. Most GISTs are diagnosed between the ages of 50 and 70 years. The primary treatment is surgical resection. Conventional chemoradiotherapy is not effective but imatinib, a tyrosine kinase inhibitor, can result in a complete or partial long-term response in up to two thirds of patients with unresectable or metastatic disease.[136,137] Leiomyosarcomas are slightly more common in the jejunum compared to the ileum and less than one fifth involve the duodenum. Surgical resection does not usually entail lymph node resection as these tumors rarely metastasize to the regional lymph nodes.[123]

Lymphoma

Most B cell lymphomas occur in the ileum, whereas the majority of T cell lymphomas are jejunal.[138,139] One quarter of B cell and one half of T cell tumors are multifocal with up to 10 lesions. Two thirds of primary small bowel lymphomas are of the B cell type, the remainder being T cell in origin.[1] Approximately 50% of T cell lymphomas are associated with enteropathy, mainly celiac disease. Twenty percent of B cell lymphomas are low-grade tumors of mucosa-associated lymphoid tissue (MALT lymphomas). Treatment is primarily by surgical resection, but the optimal treatment strategy with adjuvant chemoradiotherapy has not yet been established.[139,140] T cell tumors have a worse prognosis, with 5-year survival rates of 25% compared to 50% for high-grade and 75% for low-grade B cell lymphomas, respectively.[138] The overall 5-year survival in a population-based study of 328 primary small bowel tumors over a 25-year period was 54%.[141]

Obscure Gastrointestinal Bleeding

Obscure GI bleeding is said to occur when bleeding from the GI tract continues despite a normal EGD, colonoscopy, and barium follow-through or enteroclysis.[12,142,143] It accounts for approximately 5% of cases of GI blood loss and can be classified into overt and occult subtypes, depending on whether or not bleeding is clinically evident. Some patients, initially thought to have obscure bleeding, have pathology that is within the reach of conventional endoscopes but has been overlooked.[144] Cameron ulcers (ulcers within a hiatus hernia), Dieulafoy lesions, collapsed esophageal or fundal varices, angioectasias, and gastric antral vascular ectasias can be missed at EGD. Even experienced colonoscopists fail to detect small neoplasms or angioectasias on occasion. Hence, a second-look EGD (and less commonly a colonoscopy) is recommended before assuming that the small bowel is the source of blood loss. Technologic advances that permit endoscopic evaluation of the whole of the small bowel have altered the management of these patients since the early 2000s. The use of radionuclide studies and mesenteric angiography has correspondingly declined. The classification of GI bleeding has also changed, and the conventional terms *upper* and *lower GI bleeding* to denote a source above and below the ligament of Treitz have been replaced. Bleeding above the ampulla of Vater, which is within the reach of an EGD, is termed *upper GI bleeding*. *Mid-GI bleeding* defines a bleeding source in the small bowel from the ampulla of Vater to the terminal ileum and is currently best investigated by wireless capsule endoscopy and enteroscopy. *Lower GI* or *colonic bleeding* is assessed by colonoscopy.

Vascular ectasias are probably the most common reason for mid-GI obscure blood loss in older adults. Nonsteroidal antiinflammatory drug (NSAID)–induced small intestinal ulcers, small bowel tumors, small bowel varices, Crohn disease, and aortoenteric fistulas are the other causes encountered. Radionuclide scans and mesenteric angiography are being replaced by the new modalities. Patients with obscure bleeding should first undergo wireless capsule endoscopy that has a diagnostic yield of 40% to 80%. If negative, a repeat examination should be considered, or, depending on availability, DBE should be carried out (diagnostic yield 75%). Intraoperative enteroscopy, the most accurate (diagnostic yield 70% to 93%) but also the most invasive technique, is usually reserved for critically ill patients with persistent bleeding or when other modalities have failed to reveal the bleeding source. A bleeding vascular lesion in the proximal jejunum may be amenable to therapy via a push enteroscope, but a more distal source (hitherto usually dealt with by surgery) is now accessible via the double-balloon technique.

Nonsteroidal Antiinflammatory Drugs and the Small Bowel

The increasing use of capsule endoscopy has led to the growing recognition of NSAID-induced damage to the distal bowel such as erosions.[145] Most patients with this type of damage are asymptomatic but can show signs of iron deficiency anemia with normal gastroduodenoscopic results or have overt bleeding and even perforation. Less commonly, NDAIDs can cause the formation of diaphragms and strictures that may lead to small bowel obstruction.[146] Cyclooxygenase-2 (COX-2) inhibitors may be more protective than NSAIDs, but mucosal breaks are still seen on capsule endoscopy although their significance is unknown.[147] Colonic erosions and ulceration are also well documented in long-term NSAID users, especially in older adult population.[148] The diagnosis of NSAID-induced small bowel erosions and ulceration is made from the history and by the findings at capsule endoscopy when available. Treatment consists of discontinuation of the offending drug. A full recovery is expected. Strictures may require surgery or endoscopic balloon dilation if located in the terminal ileum.

Bile Acid Diarrhea

Bile acid diarrhea, also known as bile salt malabsorption, is a common cause of diarrhea, but the lack of awareness of this condition results in many undiagnosed cases. Bile acids are required for the absorption of dietary fats. They are produced in the liver, secreted into the biliary system, stored in the gallbladder, and released after meals. More than 90% of bile acids are reabsorbed in the terminal ileum and taken up by the liver, as part of the enterohepatic circulation, and then resecreted. Malabsorption of bile acids results in bile acids reaching the colon, where they stimulate water secretion and intestinal motility, leading to chronic diarrhea. Patients with Crohn disease or other terminal ileal abnormality or resection are particularly at risk of this condition.[149] It is also seen in patients following cholecystectomy,[150] bacterial overgrowth, chronic pancreatitis, and radiation enteropathy. Overproduction of bile acids, rather than malabsorption, can also result in diarrhea, and this is referred to as primary bile acid diarrhea. One study[151] showed that one third of patients with unexplained diarrhea had bile acid diarrhea, and such patients can often be mistaken to have irritable bowel syndrome.[152]

The diagnosis of bile acid diarrhea is easily and reliably made by performing a SeHCAT (selenium homocholic acid taurine) scan. This involves the ingestion of a synthetic analogue of the natural conjugated bile acid taurocholic acid. The retained fraction is assessed by a gamma camera 7 days later, and values less than 15% indicate bile acid diarrhea. Bile acid sequestrants are the main agents used to treat bile acid diarrhea. Cholestyramine and colestipol, which are in powder form, have been used for many years[153] but can be poorly tolerated, causing bloating and flatulence. However, those patients who can tolerate these agents often have immediate results with resolution of symptoms. Colesevelam is a tablet form of bile acid sequestrant that patients seem to tolerate better than the powders.[154] Dietary modifications to a low-fat diet can also be employed to manage symptoms.

KEY POINTS

- Celiac disease, small bowel bacterial overgrowth, and chronic pancreatitis are the main causes of malabsorption in older patients.
- Celiac disease has a prevalence of 1%, and 60% to 70% of patients are asymptomatic.
- Small bowel bacterial overgrowth occurs in 52% to 70% of symptomatic and 14% to 25% of asymptomatic older individuals.
- Crohn disease has a bimodal distribution with a second peak in the older adult population.
- The mortality rate among individuals with acute mesenteric ischemia is very high at 54% to 77%.
- Small bowel tumors are rare and account for only 1% to 2.4% of all gastrointestinal neoplasms.
- Wireless capsule endoscopy and double-balloon enteroscopy have transformed the investigation of small bowel disease.

For a complete list of references, please visit www.expertconsult.com.

KEY REFERENCES

8. Thomas PD, Forbes A, Green J, et al: Guidelines for the investigation of chronic diarrhoea. Gut 52(Suppl 5):v1–v5, 2003.
12. Sidhu R, Sanders DS, Morris AJ, et al: Guidelines on small bowel enteroscopy and capsule endoscopy in adults. Gut 57:125–136, 2008.
15. Ludvigsson JF, Leffler DA, Bai JC, et al: The Oslo definitions for coeliac disease and related terms. Gut 62:43–52, 2013.
27. National Institutes of Health: Consensus Development Conference statement on celiac disease, June 28-30, 2004. Gastroenterology 128(Suppl 1):S1–S9, 2005.
34. Ludvigsson J, Bai J, Biagi F, et al: Diagnosis and management of adult celiac disease: guidelines from the British Society of Gastroenterology. Gut 63:1210–1228, 2014.
35. British Society of Gastroenterology: Guidelines for osteoporosis in inflammatory bowel disease and coeliac disease, 2007. http://www.bsg.org.uk/clinical-guidelines/ibd/guidelines-for-osteoporosis-in-inflammatory-bowel-disease-and-coeliac-disease.html. Accessed November 4, 2015.
54. Elphick DA, Chew TS, Higham SE, et al: Small bowel bacterial overgrowth in symptomatic older people: can it be diagnosed earlier? Gerontology 51:396–401, 2005.
55. Hoffmann JC, Zeitz M: Small bowel disease in the elderly: diarrhoea and malabsorption. Best Pract Res Clin Gastroenterol 16:17–36, 2002.
61. Khoshini R, Dai S, Lezcano S, et al: A systematic review of diagnostic tests for small intestinal bacterial overgrowth. Dig Dis Sci 53:1443–1454, 2008.
69. Satsangi J, Silverberg MS, Vermeire S, et al: The Montreal classification of inflammatory bowel disease: controversies, consensus, and implications. Gut 55:749–753, 2006.
75. Swaroop PP: Inflammatory bowel diseases in the elderly. Clin Geriatr Med 23:809–821, 2007.
79. Hussain SW, Pardi DS: Inflammatory bowel disease in the elderly. Drugs Aging 27:617–624, 2010.
85. National Institute for Health and Clinical Excellence: Guidance on the use of infliximab in Crohn's disease (Technology appraisal guidance [TA40]), 2002. www.nice.org.uk/2009. Accessed October 10, 2009.
86. Strange EF, Travis SPL, Vermeire S, et al: European evidence based consensus on the diagnosis and management of Crohn's disease: definitions and diagnosis. Gut 55(Suppl 1):i1–i5, 2006.
89. Jensen MD, Nathan T, Rafaelsen SR, et al: Diagnostic accuracy of capsule endoscopy for small bowel Crohn's disease is superior to that of MR enterography or CT enterography. Clin Gastroenterol Hepatol 9:124–129, 2011.
90. Katz S, Pardi DS: Inflammatory bowel disease of the elderly: frequently asked questions (FAQs). Am J Gastroenterol 106:1889–1897, 2011.

91. National Institute for Health and Clinical Excellence: Crohn's disease. Management in adults, children and young people (NICE guidelines [CG152]). www.nice.org.uk, 2012.
95. Gisbert JP, Chaparro M: Systematic review with meta-analysis: inflammatory bowel disease in the elderly. Aliment Pharmacol Ther 39:459–477, 2014.
102. Clark M, Colombel J-F, Feagan BC, et al: American Gastroenterological Association (AGA) consensus development conference on the use of biologics in the treatment of inflammatory bowel disease, June 21-23, 2006. Gastroenterology 133:312–339, 2007.
125. Haselkorn T, Whittemore AS, Lilienfeld DE, et al: Incidence of small bowel cancer in the United States and worldwide: geographic, temporal, and racial differences. Cancer Causes Control 16:781–787, 2005.
153. Wilcox C, Turner J, Green J: Systematic review: the management of chronic diarrhoea due to bile acid malabsorption. Aliment Pharmacol Ther 39:923–939, 2014.

78 The Large Bowel

Arnold Wald

ANATOMY

The colon is a large hollow organ derived embryologically from the primitive midgut and hindgut.[1] The appendix and transverse and sigmoid colons have mesenteries, whereas the ascending and descending colons do not. Like the stomach and small intestine, the colon has circular and longitudinal smooth muscle layers but, uniquely, the longitudinal muscle of the colon is separated into three bundles, known as taenia. The configuration of the taenia causes the colon to be divided into haustral folds, which presumably help slow the passage of fecal material and thus facilitate absorption.

The superior mesenteric artery supplies the right colon to the midtransverse colon, whereas the inferior mesenteric artery supplies the left colon.[2] The anorectum derives its blood supply from branches of the internal iliac arteries.[3] In the distal transverse to mid-descending colon, the superior and inferior mesenteric arteries are linked by a series of anastomoses known as the marginal artery of Drummond. This anatomic arrangement increases the vulnerability of this area to ischemic damage.

Innervation of the colon is via the autonomic nervous system and enteric neurons.[4] Parasympathetic innervation is by the vagus nerve in the right colon and by sacral parasympathetics from the second, third, and fourth sacral nerves. Sympathetic innervation is derived from the lowest cervical to the third lumbar nerves via the splanchnic nerves. However, colon function may persist, even after vagal or splanchnic interruption, because of the presence of a well-developed enteric nervous system that can function in the absence of extrinsic innervation.

FUNCTIONS AND SYMPTOMS OF DISORDERS

The principal functions of the colon and rectum are to store fecal wastes for prolonged periods of time and expel them in a socially appropriate manner. Storage is facilitated by adaptive compliance of the bowel and by muscular contractions of colonic smooth muscle, which retard the forward movement of stool, thereby promoting electrolyte and water absorption and reducing stool volume. Forward movement occurs principally by relatively infrequent peristaltic contractions, which move intraluminal contents over long distances. Continence is maintained by the recognition of rectal filling and coordinated function of the anal sphincters and pelvic floor muscles to defer defecation until appropriate. Colonic motility and transit in healthy older adults are similar to those in younger individuals,[5] whereas aging is associated with diminished anal sphincter tone and strength as well as a less compliant rectum.[6] These latter changes may lead to greater susceptibility to fecal incontinence in older adults (see Chapter 105). Fecal incontinence can also be the presentation for other illnesses, in which impaired mobility, dehydration, dyspraxia, or other disorders are the cause. The recognition of this is part of the storied history of geriatric medicine; even so, the diagnosis and management of this socially debilitating problem is often poorest in older adults.[7]

The major symptoms of colonic and rectal disorders are constipation, diarrhea, pain, and rectal bleeding. The conditions that produce these symptoms are not unique to older adults; those occurring with increased frequency in older adults include diverticulosis, neoplasms, ischemic colitis, vascular ectasias, fecal incontinence, constipation, and antibiotic-associated diarrhea and colitis. Inflammatory bowel diseases occur in all age groups, but their onset is less likely in older adults.

DIAGNOSTIC TESTING

Radiologic Contrast Studies

Contrast examination of the large intestine has traditionally been done by using barium sulfate in a single- or a double-contrast technique in which a thickened barium suspension is used to coat the mucosa, followed by insufflation to expand the viscus. Alternatively, water-soluble contrast agents can be used if perforation is suspected.

The single-contrast technique is preferred when studying patients with suspected obstruction, diverticulitis, or fistula, whereas the double-contrast technique is preferred for demonstrating fine mucosal lesions and neoplasms. Although there continues to be some controversy concerning the choice of barium contrast or colonoscopy when investigating colonic diseases, most clinicians favor colonoscopy for its greater sensitivity and opportunity for biopsy and therapy. Contrast studies may be indicated for patients in whom severe stricturing disease or adhesions make colonoscopy hazardous, conditions such as diverticulitis are suspected, if the location and nature of a colonic obstruction require assessment, and if functional and structural information are required. A barium enema should not be attempted when increases in colon pressure may worsen the patient's condition—for example, in patients with suspected toxic megacolon or those with peritoneal signs that suggest ischemic colitis.

When patients complain of constipation or a recent change in bowel habit, barium radiography complements sigmoidoscopy in detecting organic causes, and they are also useful in diagnosing functional megacolon and megarectum. Complete filling of the colon with barium is neither necessary nor desirable in patients with megacolon. However, conventional barium studies provide limited information about colonic motor function in most patients with chronic constipation.[8] Moreover, they are frequently inadequate in frail or hospitalized older patients.[9,10] In general, fluoroscopy of the gastrointestinal (GI) tract has moved from being a first-line study for evaluating GI symptoms to its role as a problem-solving tool.

Imaging Techniques

Abdominal Computed Tomography

This procedure allows visualization of the thickness of the bowel wall, solid viscera within the abdomen, mesenteries, and soft tissues adjacent to the bowel. It offers a modest advance in the diagnosis of diverticulitis by demonstrating inflammation of pericolic fat, abscesses that may contain collections of fluid and gas, and intramural sinus tracts. Fistulas to other organs can be identified when gas is found in the bladder or vagina. It also can identify extension of disease at a distance from the colon, including unsuspected intraabdominal abscesses.

Computed tomography (CT) is also valuable when evaluating and managing complications of Crohn disease, including abscesses, fistulas, involvement of psoas muscles and ureters, and occasionally for percutaneous drainage of collections. Other complications, including sacral osteomyelitis, cholelithiasis, nephrolithiasis, and vascular necrosis of the femoral head associated with corticosteroid therapy, can also be diagnosed.

In appendicitis (and cecal diverticulitis, which is usually misdiagnosed as appendicitis), CT may augment the clinical diagnosis by showing the periappendicular inflammatory process and differentiating phlegmon from abscess.[11] Occasionally, appendicoliths are identified, which are considered pathognomonic of appendicitis when associated with periappendicular inflammatory signs.

CT colonography is a technique devised to detect colon polyps for screening purposes. Detection rates for colonic polyps larger than 6 mm are similar to colonoscopy, but the test has low sensitivity for smaller polyps.[12] The use of three-dimensional evaluation in addition to two-dimensional evaluation may reduce perceptual errors.[13] CT colonography is recommended as an alternative for colon polyp screening in the United States.

Magnetic Resonance Imaging

Although CT remains the most widely used imaging modality for patients with nonbiliary symptoms and nonspecific and acute abdominal pain, magnetic resonance imaging (MRI) has had an increasing role in the evaluation of bowel disease.[14] Its advantages over CT include the absence of ionizing radiation and superior tissue contrast, but it does involve longer acquisition times, increased susceptibility to motion artifact, and higher cost. MR enterography and colonography are the preferred techniques for evaluating small bowel and colonic involvement by inflammatory bowel diseases. MRI may be comparable to endoscopic ultrasound (EUS) in staging rectal cancer but, unlike EUS, it can evaluate stenosing and high rectal tumors while simultaneously imaging the entire pelvis to evaluate for adjacent organ invasion and lymphadenopathy. MRI is also a valuable tool to evaluate anorectal disease, particularly so for perianal fistulas, which may be a complication of Crohn disease, to optimize surgical planning.[15]

Anal and Rectal Endosonography

This procedure accurately delineates the layers of the rectal wall, internal and external anal sphincters, and levator muscles.[16] Endosonography is useful in evaluating pelvic floor structures in many patients with fecal incontinence to detect occult sphincter injuries arising from childbirth or other conditions associated with potential injury to continence mechanisms.[17]

EUS is a rapid, minimally invasive technique used to image rectal polyps and detect focal malignancy within polyps, tumor masses penetrating into the bowel wall, and extramural lesions, such as prostatic tumors and ovarian lesions. Perirectal fistulas and abscesses can also be evaluated, including determination of whether there is destruction of pelvic muscles. It is considered the reference standard for the preoperative staging of rectal and anal cancers, with relatively high accuracy in categorizing tumors and lymph nodes.[18]

Colonoscopy and Flexible Sigmoidoscopy

These procedures are usually performed in the prepared colon, except when evaluating diarrheal illnesses. Colonoscopic examinations provide unparalleled evaluation of the mucosal surfaces and opportunities for biopsy and therapy. These include diagnosis and determining the extent of inflammatory bowel disease, evaluation of patients with overt or occult GI bleeding, evaluation of chronic watery diarrhea, endoscopic sampling and removal of polyps, decompression of sigmoid volvulus or functional megacolon, and ablation of vascular lesions. Colonoscopy is generally done under conscious sedation, whereas flexible sigmoidoscopy often is not. In many older patients, the physician must be aware of their increased sensitivity to sedatives and analgesic medications. Because older adults are susceptible to hypotension and respiratory depression, careful monitoring of the patient during the procedure is especially important. Even in older patients, such procedures are generally safe in experienced hands and when done in units that monitor blood gases and cardiorespiratory functions. Major complications include bleeding and perforation, which should not occur more than once in 1000 routine procedures.

Histopathology

Mucosal biopsies are indicated when evaluating undiagnosed diarrhea, in long-standing ulcerative colitis during surveillance for precancerous dysplasia, when obtaining tissue for viral culture, and in evaluating polypoid or ulcerated lesions. In patients with inflammatory disorders of the colon and rectum, biopsies serve to establish the presence, extent, and distribution of colitis to differentiate ulcerative colitis from Crohn colitis and these disorders from other inflammatory conditions, such as infectious colitis. Biopsies should be obtained from endoscopically normal as well as abnormal areas, because characteristic changes may be patchy and therefore could be missed if too few biopsies are obtained. This is especially true in pseudomembranous, collagenous, and lymphocytic colitides, in which the distal colon may be spared. Because hypertonic phosphate enemas and purgative laxatives may induce mucosal changes that can be mistaken for mild colitis, they should be avoided when evaluating suspected inflammation of the colon.

Fecal Occult Blood Testing

Fecal occult blood tests (FOBTs) identify hemoglobin or altered hemoglobin compounds in the stool. Foods containing peroxidases, such as melon and uncooked broccoli, horseradish, cauliflower, and turnips, may produce false-positive results, whereas reducing agents such as ascorbic acid may decrease sensitivity.[19] Tests that extract the protoporphyrin from hemoglobin, such as HemoQuant, are more specific and quantitative but are also more time-consuming and expensive. Rehydration of Hemoccult slides increases sensitivity but decreases specificity and is not recommended. A weakly positive slide may become negative after 2 to 4 days of storage. Oral iron supplements do not interfere with any of these tests.

The guaiac FOBT is being replaced in many population screening programs for colon cancer and polyps by the fecal immunochemical test (FIT), which detects the intact globin protein portion of human hemoglobin. A labeled antibody attaches to the antigens of any human hemoglobin present in stool, resulting in a positive test. Studies have shown that FIT offers superior sensitivity for advanced colorectal neoplasms (e.g., cancer, advanced adenomas) over that provided by the standard guaiac test.[20] As a result, stool guaiac tests are no longer recommended by any of the U.S. guidelines for colorectal cancer screening.

COLONIC DIVERTICULOSIS

Colonic diverticula are herniations of colonic mucosa through the smooth muscle layers. Diverticula occur in areas of anatomic weakness of the circular smooth muscle created by penetration of blood vessels to the submucosa. They are usually found in the sigmoid and descending colons and rarely, if ever, in the rectum.[21]

This disorder has been recognized with increasing frequency in modern Western countries.[22] Colonic diverticula are present in about one third of persons by the age of 50 years and in about two thirds by the age of 80 years. Dietary fiber insufficiency and the increased longevity of modern Western populations have long been hypothesized to explain the increased prevalence of diverticulosis. Dietary factors may promote increased colonic motor activity and intraluminal pressures, whereas aging may lead to structural weakness of the colonic muscle.[21] However, recent studies have challenged the concept that low-fiber diets and constipation contribute to the development of diverticulosis.[23] Other studies have suggested that genetic factors may play a role.[24] Because diverticula are asymptomatic in most individuals, caution should be taken before attributing nonspecific GI symptoms to them.[25]

Painful Diverticular Disease

Painful diverticular disease is characterized by crampy discomfort in the left lower abdomen. Symptoms are often associated with constipation or diarrhea, as well as with tenderness over the affected areas. These symptoms are similar to those of irritable bowel syndrome and of partial bowel obstruction due to tumors or ischemia. Studies have shown that these patients have altered motor activity in the segments containing diverticula, which are associated with reporting of abdominal pain.[26] In contrast to diverticulitis, there is no fever, leukocytosis, or rebound tenderness.

Diverticulitis

Diverticulitis develops in approximately 10% to 25% of individuals with diverticulosis who are followed for 10 years or more; however, fewer than 20% of these patients require hospitalization. Recent studies have found that among patients with diverticulosis, higher levels of 25-hydroxy vitamin D—25(OH) vitamin D—are associated with a lower risk of diverticulitis.[27] This suggests that screening for (and correcting) low 25(OH) vitamin D levels may reduce the risk for diverticulitis, although this is an unproven hypothesis. Inflammation begins at the apex of the diverticulum when the opening of a diverticulum becomes obstructed (e.g., with stool), leading to micro- or macroperforation of a diverticulum.[28] The presence of a palpable mass, fever, leukocytosis, and/or rebound tenderness indicates an inflammatory process, which often remains localized in the adjacent pericolic tissues but may progress to a peridiverticular abscess.[29] Other complications include fibrosis and bowel obstruction, fistula formation to the bladder, vagina, or adjacent small intestine, and free perforation with peritonitis. The frequency of complications rises significantly with recurrent attacks of diverticulitis.

Making a clinical distinction between painful diverticular disease and diverticulitis carries a sizable rate of error.[28] In an older or debilitated patient, the absence of fever, leukocytosis or rebound tenderness does not exclude diverticulitis.[29]

A disorder characterized by localized inflammation associated with diverticulosis (SCAD [segmental colitis associated with diverticulosis] syndrome) has been described in older symptomatic patients.[30] Symptoms appear after the age of 40 years and are usually characterized by rectal bleeding, diarrhea, and abdominal pain.

Other disorders such as carcinoma, inflammatory bowel disease, and ischemia may mimic symptomatic diverticular disease. Diagnostic studies include barium enema, CT, MRI, ultrasonography, and colonoscopy. In most cases of suspected diverticulitis, barium enema should be delayed for about 1 week to allow some resolution of the inflammatory process. A single-contrast study should be performed cautiously to minimize the risk of perforation. Radiographic findings suggesting diverticulitis include longitudinal fistulas connecting diverticula over segments of colon, fistula into adjacent organs, a fixed eccentric defect in the colon wall, contrast outside the lumen of the colon or diverticulum, and intraluminal defects representing abscesses.[21] CT, MRI, and ultrasonic imaging of the abdomen provide superior definition of colonic wall thickness and extraluminal structures and are the procedures of choice at the time of initial evaluation. Colonoscopy is a less attractive option during an acute episode and is best used to exclude tumors or other conditions if other diagnostic tests are inconclusive.

TABLE 78-1 Medical Treatment of Diverticular Disease

Measure	Painful Diverticulosis	Diverticulitis
Diet	Increased fiber	Reduced fiber (or NPO)
Bulk laxative	Sometimes effective	Not indicated
Analgesic	Avoidance of narcotics	Avoidance of morphine; meperidine best
Antispasmodic	Propantheline bromide (15 mg tid); dicyclomine hydrochloride (20 mg tid); hyoscyamine sulfate (0.125-0.250 mg q4h)	Not indicated
Antibiotic	Not indicated	Oral* Amoxicillin/potassium clavulanate (875/125 mg bid) *or* Ciprofloxacin (500 mg bid) plus metronidazole (500 mg tid) Parenteral Gentamicin or tobramycin (5 mg/kg/day) plus clindamycin (1.2-2.4 g/day) *or* Levofloxacin 500 mg daily plus metronidazole (500 mg q8h) *or* Piperacillin-tazobactam (3.375-4.5 g q6h)

Updated and adapted from Wald A: Colonic diverticulosis. In Winawer SJ, editor: Management of gastrointestinal diseases, Edinburgh, U.K., 1992, Gower Medical, pp 34.1-34.18, with permission.
*Not required in all patients (see text).

The treatment of painful diverticular disease is designed to reduce symptoms based on smooth muscle spasm in contrast to the treatment of diverticulitis, which is designed to treat bacterial infection (Table 78-1). Patients with severe pain, nausea, and vomiting or complications should be hospitalized and given intravenous antibiotics until clinical improvement occurs. The American Society of Colon and Rectal Surgeons has recommended an individualized approach to elective surgery for diverticulitis and laparoscopic management, when possible.[31]

Surgery is recommended for patients with diverticulitis who fail to respond to medical therapy within 72 hours, immunocompromised patients, and those who have fistula to the bladder with pneumaturia and urinary infection or fistula to the vagina with discharge of stool into the vagina. A one-stage operation, in which the diseased segment of bowel is resected and continuity restored by a primary anastomosis, is preferred.[32] In cases of generalized peritonitis or emergent surgery for perforation with abscess or high-grade obstruction, a two-stage procedure requiring a diverting colostomy should be used.[33] Large abscesses can often be drained percutaneously by an interventional radiologist using CT or ultrasonography as a guide.[34] Elective surgery can then be performed after 2 to 3 weeks of antibiotic therapy, often allowing for a single-stage resection.

Emergent surgery is required for generalized peritonitis or persistent high-grade bowel obstruction. Most patients with complicated diverticular disease require surgery, even if clinical recovery occurs, because there is a high risk of recurrent attacks.

In addition to changes in surgical management, recent studies have suggested that a person with uncomplicated acute diverticulitis can be safely managed as an outpatient, and the long-standing recommendation that antibiotics are needed in all patients has been challenged.[24] A survey of Dutch surgeons and gastroenterologists has found that 90% of them manage mild diverticulitis without antibiotics,[35] which is in accordance with recently published Danish national guidelines.[36]

Most patients with SCAD respond to 5-aminosalicylate therapy, with long-term resolution of the disease. On occasion, spontaneous remissions may occur, or persistent, chronically active disease may require resective surgery.[30]

Bleeding

Bleeding associated with diverticula is typically brisk and painless and often arises from the proximal colon. Bleeding is thought to occur when a fecalith erodes into a vessel in the neck of the diverticulum or there is rupture of the penetrating arteriole in its course around the diverticular sac.[21]

An important indication for emergent colonoscopy is to identify the source of bleeding in patients with diverticula, because other lesions not seen by contrast studies may be the actual source. If bleeding is brisk, a bleeding scan or selective mesenteric angiography can locate the site of bleeding; superselective embolization of distal arterial branches has been demonstrated to be highly effective and relatively safe (<25% ischemia rates[37]; see section "Lower Gastrointestinal Bleeding").

APPENDICITIS

Older patients with appendicitis are at increased risk (≈60%) for perforation. They have a higher mortality rate and often do not exhibit a fever or an elevated white blood cell count.[38]

The onset of abdominal pain is abrupt, begins in the midabdomen, relocates to the right lower quadrant, and is often associated with nausea, vomiting, and fever. Physical examination characteristically reveals signs of local peritonitis in the right lower quadrant, and the white blood cell count is frequently elevated. The differential diagnosis includes pyelonephritis, Crohn disease, gastroenteritis, pelvic inflammatory disease, ovarian cyst, and cecal diverticulitis. In older patients, appendicitis may occur in association with colon cancer in which low-grade obstruction results in distention of the appendix and mimics true appendicitis.

If the diagnosis is uncertain, ultrasonography has been shown to have positive and negative predictive values of about 90% for appendicitis and is also useful in identifying another cause of symptoms in patients with right lower quadrant pain.[39] One sonographic criterion for acute appendicitis is visualization of a noncompressible appendix with a diameter more than 6 mm.

INFECTIOUS DISEASES

Clostridium difficile

First described as a cause of diarrhea in 1978, *Clostridium difficile* is responsible for approximately 3 million cases of diarrhea and colitis each year and is the most common cause of hospital-acquired diarrhea in the United States.[40]

The vast majority of cases are associated with two protein exotoxins, A and B, produced by *C. difficile*. Toxin A is an enterotoxin that triggers diarrhea, epithelial necrosis, and a characteristic inflammatory process in animals, whereas toxin B is a cytotoxin in tissue culture but does not by itself cause toxicity in animals.[41] The disease spectrum ranges from mild diarrhea, with little or no inflammation, to severe colitis often associated with pseudomembranes, which are adherent to necrotic colonic epithelium. Acquisition of *C. difficile* occurs most frequently in older adults in hospitals or nursing homes, potentially because of environmental contamination with *C. difficile* and spores carried on the hands of the hospital or institutional staff.[42] Acquisition is often asymptomatic but may have clinical consequences if older patients receive certain antibiotics or chemotherapeutic agents. Other possible risk factors include surgery, intensive care, nasogastric intubation, and length of hospital stay. A smaller number of patients have antibiotic-associated diarrhea but no evidence of *C. difficile* infection.

Although virtually all antibiotics have been implicated, the most common are cephalosporins, ampicillin, amoxicillin, and clindamycin.[43] Less commonly implicated antibiotics are macrolides, sulfonamides, and tetracyclines.[40]

One of the most important developments has been the emergence of a new epidemic strain that is resistant to quinolones such as ciprofloxacin.[44] This strain produces high levels of toxins A and B and also more spores, which can increase risk for contamination; it has spread quickly throughout the United States.[40] Increasingly, quinolones have been commonly associated with *C. difficile* infection (CDI), especially with the epidemic BI strain.

The typical clinical picture of *C. difficile*–associated colitis includes nonbloody diarrhea, lower abdominal cramps, fever, and leukocytosis. Fever is usually low grade although, on occasion, it can be quite high. In severe cases, dehydration, hypotension, hypoproteinemia, toxic megacolon, or even colonic perforation may occur.

In severely ill patients, the diagnostic test of choice is flexible sigmoidoscopy or colonoscopy. Because the distal colon is involved in most cases, flexible sigmoidoscopy is usually satisfactory; however, changes may be confined to the right colon in up to one third of cases, making colonoscopy necessary if less extensive procedures do not confirm a suspected diagnosis. The yellowish-gray pseudomembranes are densely adherent to the underlying colonic mucosa, interspersed with mucosa that appears normal. Mucosal biopsies may exhibit characteristic findings of epithelial necrosis and micropseudomembranes (so-called volcano lesions), even when pseudomembranes are not grossly visible. Endoscopy should be performed in severely ill patients who present atypically and therefore require a rapid diagnosis.[45]

The enzyme immunoassay (EIA) for toxin A and/or B has been the primary test used in most clinical laboratories, but it is too insensitive and nonspecific to be used as a stand-alone test. In contrast, the use of the polymerase chain reaction (PCR) assay to detect the gene for toxin production (ted B gene) has been increasingly regarded as a superior test that is rapid and sensitive, with a minimum detection limit of 105 bacteria per gram of stool. Although more expensive, it is far more sensitive than EIA. One drawback is that the test will lead to an overdiagnosis of CDI because it does not detect the toxin.[46] This may lead to a two-step algorithmic approach, as has been adopted by the National Health Service laboratories in England as of April 2012.[40]

The offending drug should be discontinued if possible. If symptoms persist, patients who are not seriously ill should receive oral metronidazole, 250 mg tid or qid, for 10 to 14 days. Patients who are seriously ill and those with complicated or fulminant infections should receive oral vancomycin, 125 mg PO qid, for 10 days.[47] If oral intake is not possible, metronidazole, 500 mg IV q6h, is given until oral administration can be accomplished. In patients with ileus, vancomycin enemas can be administered. Metronidazole and vancomycin appear to be therapeutically comparable in non–seriously ill patients, but metronidazole costs less, and there are current concerns about vancomycin-resistant enterococci (VRE).[48] In general, fever resolves within 24 hours, and diarrhea decreases within 4-5 days.

Fidaxomicin is a macrocyclic antimicrobial agent that has little or no systemic absorption after oral administration and which, in in vitro studies, is more active than vancomycin against CDI. It appears to be more effective than vancomycin in patients who require ongoing concomitant systemic antibiotics and also may be associated with a lower incidence of recurrent CDIs.[45]

Relapses average about 20% to 25% following successful treatment with either agent,[49] often involving sporulation, which leads to relapse within 4 weeks after completion of successful treatment. These episodes invariably respond to another course of antibiotic therapy. About 5% to 10% of patients have multiple relapses. In such individuals, vancomycin in conventional doses should be followed by a 3-week course of cholestyramine, 4 g tid and/or Lactinex (a probiotic supplement), 500 mg PO qid, or vancomycin, 125 mg PO every other day. Some have advocated a 6-week schedule consisting of a 2-week course of vancomycin given daily in the standard dose, a 2-week course of the same dose given every other day, followed by a 2-week course at the same dose given every third day. In addition, some have advocated the use of *Saccharomyces boulardii*, a nonpathogenic yeast that inhibits the binding of toxin A to rat ileum, with consequent prevention of enterotoxicity.[50]

Because the pathogenesis of recurrent CDI involves an ongoing disruption of the normal fecal flora and an inadequate host immune response, fecal microbial transplantation (FMT) has become an increasingly popular approach to patients with multiple recurrent infections. This involves infusion of a liquid suspension of intestinal microorganisms from the stool of a healthy donor via intestinal intubation, colonoscopy, or enema. The existing literature indicates that FMT is effective and safe, with no serious adverse effects reported to date, and a response rate of 90% or higher.[51]

Guidelines for prevention of *C. difficile* diarrhea and colitis are based on a few simple practices. See Table 78-2.[52]

TABLE 78-2 Practice Guidelines for Prevention of *Clostridium difficile* Diarrhea

1. Limit the use of antimicrobial drugs.
2. Wash hands between contact with all patients.
3. Use enteric (stool) isolation precautions for patients with C. difficile diarrhea.
4. Wear gloves when contacting patients with C. difficile diarrhea or colitis or their environment.
5. Disinfect objects contaminated with C. difficile with sodium hypochlorite, alkaline glutaraldehyde, or ethylene oxide.
6. Educate the medical, nursing, and other appropriate staff members about the disease and its epidemiology.

Adapted from Fekety R: Guidelines for the diagnosis and treatment of Clostridium difficile-associated diarrhea and colitis. Am J Gastroenterol 92:139-150, 1997, with permission.

Shigella Organisms

These organisms consist of four groups: A (*Shigella dysenteriae*), B (*Shigella flexneri*), C (*Shigella boydii*), and D (*Shigella sonnei*). Group D accounts for most clinical infections in Western countries. In contrast to other enteric pathogens, very few organisms are needed to produce infection, which is spread by fecal-oral transmission between humans and that continues to occur, despite high standards of water purification and sewage disposal. At least 30 gene products are involved in *Shigella* invasion and its intercellular spread. Disease is caused by the invasion of colonic epithelial cells, perhaps in part mediated by cytotoxins produced by *S. dysenteriae* and *S. flexneri*, but enterotoxins may also contribute to early symptoms of nondysenteric diarrhea.[53] Enterotoxins similar to Shiga-like toxins secreted by enterohemorrhagic *E. coli* are believed to mediate the hemolytic-uremic syndrome (HUS) associated with severe colitis caused by *S. dysenteriae* type I.

Symptoms

Colitis is heralded by the passage of bloody mucoid stools associated with urgency, tenesmus, abdominal cramping, fever, and malaise. The frequency of stools is highest during the first 24 hours of illness and gradually diminishes thereafter.

Diagnosis

Stool examination reveals numerous polymorphonuclear cells, and leukocytosis is common. Stool culture grown on selective media is the definitive diagnostic study. Sigmoidoscopy is usually not necessary but, if done, will demonstrate a friable hyperemic mucosa. Barium contrast studies are not indicated.

Treatment

If the illness is mild and self-limited, antibiotics can be withheld. Because resistance to sulfonamides, ampicillin, tetracycline, and even trimethoprim-sulfamethoxazole is now common, treatment with a fluoroquinolone (e.g., ciprofloxacin 500 mg bid for 5 days) is indicated for older or debilitated patients with acute disease to shorten the illness and the duration of fecal excretion of the organism.[54] Antidiarrheal agents prolong the clinical illness and carrying of the organism and should not be administered.[55] The development of a chronic carrier state is rare and difficult to treat.

Pathogenic *Escherichia coli*

These organisms commonly cause disease in developed countries and are a major cause of diarrhea in tourists visiting underdeveloped countries. Because older adults have been increasingly engaging in overseas travel, these organisms can be a major impediment to a successful trip.

Of the five major classes of pathogenic *E. coli*, only enteroinvasive *E. coli* (EIEC) and Shiga toxin–producing *E. coli* (STEC) primarily involve the colon. Both produce a clinical illness similar to that of shigellosis. Once thought to be a pathogen restricted to developing countries, STEC has been shown to produce diarrhea in the United States and is a relatively uncommon cause of traveler's diarrhea. It is more difficult to identify in stool cultures and is not a reportable illness. The clinical illness is generally milder than with shigellosis. A reasonable approach is to treat with a fluoroquinolone, similar to treatment for shigellosis.[53]

Preventive measures include eating cooked food only while it is still hot and avoiding local water, including fruits and vegetables washed with local water. In older tourists, the disease can be shortened by prompt use of a fluoroquinolone.[53]

Shiga Toxin–Producing *Escherichia coli* 0157:H7

This organism has been identified as a major pathogen in the United States and Canada, causing approximately 70,000 U.S. cases annually.[53] In addition to sporadic infections, epidemics have been traced to the consumption of undercooked and raw ground beef, because healthy cattle serve as the primary reservoir for STEC strains. Infections have also been associated with exposure to patients with bloody diarrhea, contaminated water supplies, and nonpreserved apple cider. Clinical manifestations include nonbloody diarrhea, hemorrhagic colitis, and HUS.[56] Unlike most bacterial enteric diseases, *E. coli* O157:H7 is often characterized by low-grade fever or the absence of a fever.[57] The pathogenesis of colitis has been linked to Shiga-like toxins (verocytotoxins 1 and 2), which bind to a glycolipid on the surface of colonocytes, but adherence factors may also play a role. Older age is a risk factor for this infection and increases the risk of HUS and death. It is generally believed that antibiotics are not indicated for active infections and appear to predispose to HUS.[56]

An important emerging group of related pathogens are the non-O157 (STEC), which can produce an illness similar to O157:H7 strains.[58] In Europe, most STEC strains belong to the non-O157 serogroup.

Campylobacter Species

Campylobacter jejuni and *Campylobacter coli* are among the most common bacterial causes of diarrhea and can be manifested by gastroenteritis, pseudoappendicitis, and/or colitis. These organisms are usually transmitted from animals to humans through contaminated food and water and sometimes by direct contact with pets. Constitutional symptoms usually precede diarrhea and abdominal cramps by up to 24 hours, and colitis may be characterized by fever and dysentery lasting for 1 week or more. Diagnosis is made by stool culture. Convalescent carriage up 5 weeks (mean) is common after the onset of illness and is significantly reduced by antimicrobial treatment.

Although the infection is usually self-limited, antibiotics may be given if the illness is severe or if the patient is immunosuppressed.[59] Treatment consists of erythromycin or fluoroquinolones; macrolides such as azithromycin and clarithromycin show excellent in vitro activity. Resistance rates to fluoroquinolones of up to 88% have been reported in Europe and Asia. In areas of high resistance, azithromycin, 500 mg daily for 3 days, is an effective alternative.

Entamoeba histolytica

This organism remains a primary cause of dysentery, which may be complicated by fulminant colitis, toxic megacolon, bleeding, stricture, and perforation. Severe disease is more common in older adults and in patients who are immunosuppressed or debilitated.[60] The disease is typically acquired by ingesting cysts from contaminated water or fresh vegetables but can also be transmitted through sexual practices that promote fecal-oral transmission. Studies on germ-free animals have suggested that intestinal disease does not develop unless bacteria are present. This may partly account for the effectiveness of metronidazole, which is also active against anaerobic bacteria.

The traditional method of diagnosing intestinal *E. histolytica* is by the microscopic inspection of three separate stool specimens. A wet preparation should be obtained within 30 minutes of passage to look for motile trophozoites, which may contain ingested red blood cells. A formalin–ethyl acetate concentration preparation should be examined for cysts. Barium, bismuth, kaolin compounds, magnesium hydroxide, castor oil, and hypertonic enemas all interfere with the ability to detect the parasite in stools.[60] This technique is only 50% to 60% sensitive and can give false-positive results. Antigen detection methods have numerous advantages to microscopy techniques, including higher sensitivity and specificity and good correlation with molecular techniques.[61]

Colonoscopy may reveal erythema, edema, friability of the mucosa, and scattered ulcers 5 to 15 mm in diameter, covered with a yellow exudate. These ulcers may occur anywhere in the colon but are most common in the cecum and ascending colon. Biopsies from the edge of these ulcers may reveal typical hourglass ulcers containing trophozoites. Cathartics and enemas should not be used because they interfere with identification of the parasite.

Because these techniques may miss identifying the parasite, serologic tests for antiamoebic antibody should also be obtained in suspected cases. The indirect hemagglutination assay (IHA) is positive in 75% to 90% of patients with amoebic dysentery and in virtually all patients with amoebic liver abscesses. The IHA remains positive for years after treatment of invasive amoebiasis.[60] An alternative test is the use of the enzyme-linked immunosorbent assay (ELISA) to detect serum IgA antibodies to the organism.[61]

Treatment of acute amoebic dysentery consists of metronidazole, 750 mg tid, for 5 to 10 days or, if not tolerated orally, 500 mg q6h by the intravenous route.[62] This should be followed by phenobarbital (Luminal amebocytes)-acting oral drugs such as paromomycin, 25 to 35 mg/kg tid, for 7 days, or iodoquinol, 650 mg tid daily, for 20 days, to eliminate all cysts and prevent possible relapse.

Cytomegalovirus

Cytomegalovirus (CMV) is a member of the beta herpesvirus group, which transitions to a lifelong latent phase after primary infection in immunocompetent individuals. In patients who are immunocompromised, with diminished T cell function, reactivation may occur and may become persistent, with the reappearance of immunoglobulin M (IgM) anti-CMV antibodies in the serum. Among the GI syndromes associated with CMV are focal and diffuse colitis.

CMV colitis is associated with severe small-volume diarrhea, abdominal pain, and fever. Colonoscopy may reveal variable degrees of focal erythema, petechial hemorrhage, erosions, and, in advanced cases, scattered ulcers. Mucosal biopsy may reveal characteristic intranuclear inclusions (owl's eye lesions) or cytoplasmic inclusions in vascular endothelial cells. In cases in which biopsy is not diagnostic, the PCR assay or in situ hybridization techniques may be helpful, together with serum IgM CMV-specific antibodies.

The treatment of choice is ganciclovir (5 mg/kg IV, q12h, for 21 days) to achieve remission.[63] For patients who relapse after discontinuation of the drug, chronic maintenance therapy (6 mg/kg five times/week) may be instituted. Valganciclovir is as effective as IV ganciclovir because of improved bioavailability over previous oral agents. Because the drug has hematologic side effects such as neutropenia, regular blood counts should be carried out. Human immunodeficiency virus (HIV)-infected patients with CMV colitis should be placed on maintenance therapy indefinitely. Foscarnet (60 mg/kg q8h, adjusted for renal function) is used for patients who do not respond to ganciclovir or who cannot tolerate its toxicity.

INFLAMMATORY BOWEL DISEASE

Both ulcerative colitis and Crohn's disease are more common in early adulthood but are found with increased frequency in older adults. In part, this is because increasing numbers of patients with inflammatory bowel disease (IBD) now live into old age. In addition, ulcerative colitis and Crohn disease exhibit a bimodal age of onset,[64,65] with the peak incidence occurring in the third decade and a minor later peak between the ages of 50 and 80 years. Over 10% of cases have their onset after the age of 60 years. This pattern persists even when other diseases that mimic inflammatory bowel disease, such as ischemic colitis and infectious causes, have been excluded. The reasons for this bimodal pattern are unknown.

Ulcerative Colitis

Ulcerative colitis is a chronic inflammatory process of unknown cause that affects the mucosa and submucosa of the colon in a continuous distribution. Enhanced humoral immunity is more evident in ulcerative colitis than in Crohn disease and probably reflects disturbed immunoregulation, leading to unrestrained T cell activation and cytokine release.[66]

Histopathology

Histologically, there are diffuse ulcerations and epithelial necrosis, depletion of mucin from goblet cells, and polymorphonuclear

TABLE 78-3 Proposed Criteria for Assessment of Disease Activity in Ulcerative Colitis

Parameter	Severity* Severe	Mild
Bowel frequency	>Six daily	<Four daily
Blood in stool	++	+
Temperature	>37.5° C on two of four days	Normal
Pulse rate (beats/min)	>90	Normal
Hemoglobin (allow for transfusion)	<75%	Normal or near normal
Erythrocyte sedimentation rate (mm/hr)	>30	<30

Data from Truelove SC, Witts LJ: Cortisone in ulcerative colitis; final report on a therapeutic trial. Br Med J 2:1041-1048, 1955, with permission.

*Moderate disease is intermediate between severe and mild classifications.

and lymphocytic infiltration involving the superficial layers of the colon to the muscularis mucosa. The finding of crypt microabscesses is characteristic but not pathognomonic. The inflammatory process invariably involves the rectum and extends proximally for variable distances but does not involve the GI tract proximal to the colon. Involvement of the rectum only is designated ulcerative proctitis, whereas disease extending no further than the splenic flexure is known as left-sided disease.

Symptoms and Signs

Symptoms in older patients are similar to those seen in younger persons.[67] The severity of ulcerative colitis may be classified as mild, moderate, and severe and is generally proportional to the extent of colonic inflammation (Table 78-3). Most patients exhibit diarrhea, with or without blood in the stools, although older patients with proctitis only occasionally present with constipation or hematochezia. Systemic manifestations occur during more severe attacks and carry a poorer prognosis. Despite the occurrence of less extensive disease in older patients, older adults more often present with a severe initial attack and have higher mortality and morbidity rates than younger patients.[68]

Toxic megacolon is a feared complication of ulcerative colitis, which occurs more frequently in older patients. Abdominal radiographs show colonic dilation, often to impressive proportions, and patients may exhibit mental confusion, high fever, abdominal distention, and overall deterioration.[69]

Extraintestinal manifestations may occur in ulcerative colitis, including arthralgias, erythema nodosum, pyoderma gangrenosum, uveitis, and migratory polyarthritis. These disorders occur less frequently than in Crohn disease and are generally associated with increased disease activity.

Diagnosis

The diagnosis is made by sigmoidoscopy and rectal mucosal biopsies because the disorder invariably involves the rectum. The extent of the disease is determined by colonoscopy or barium radiography, both of which should be avoided in patients who are severely ill because of the danger of inducing perforation or toxic megacolon. The characteristic findings are diffuse erythema, granularity, and friability of the mucosa, without intervening areas of normal mucosa. Inflammatory pseudopolyps indicate more severe erosion of the mucosa and must be distinguished from true polyps.

Particularly in older adults, it is important to exclude other diseases that may mimic ulcerative colitis, including Crohn colitis (see later), ischemic colitis, radiation proctocolitis, and diverticulitis. In acute presentations, infectious agents should be excluded with appropriate stool cultures, including *Salmonella*, *Campylobacter*, *Shigella*, and *Yersinia* spp., amebiasis, and *E. coli* O157:H7. Finally, *C. difficile*–associated diarrhea and pseudomembranous colitis should be considered in older adults, particularly those who have recently been treated with antibiotics, reside in institutions, or have recently been hospitalized.

TABLE 78-4 Medical Treatment of Ulcerative Colitis

Indication	Drug	Dosage*
Mild to moderate distal disease	Proctofoam HC	as directed, 1-21 d
	VSL#3	1-2 packets/day
	Hydrocortisone enema	hs
	5-ASA enema	hs
	Sulfasalazine	2-4 g
	Mesalamine	2.4-4.8 g
Mild to moderate disease extensive disease	Sulfasalazine	2.4 g
	Mesalamine†	2.4-4.8 g
	Balsalazide†	6.75 g
	Prednisone	40-60 mg
Severe disease (recently receiving steroids)	Prednisolone	60-80 mg IV
	Hydrocortisone	300 mg IV
	Infliximab	5 mg/kg BW at 0, 2, 6 wk
	Vedolizumab	300 mg IV at 0, 2, 6 wk
Severe disease (not recently receiving steroids)	Corticotropin (ACTH)	120 units IV
	Infliximab	5 mg/kg BW IV at 0, 2, 6 wk
	Vedolizumab	300 mg IV at 0, 2, 6 wk
Maintenance	5-ASA (mesalamine) enema (distal disease)	hs to q third night
	Sulfasalazine	2 g
	Mesalamine†	1.2-2.4 g
	Balsalazide†	3 g
	Azathioprine	2-2.5 mg/kgBW
	6-Mercaptopurine	1.5 mg/kg BW
	Infliximab	5-10 mg/kg BW q6-8 wk IV
	Vedolizumab	300 mg IV q8wk

5-ASA, 5-Aminosalicylate; *BW*, body weight; *ACTH*, adrenocorticotropic hormone.

*Daily; PO unless otherwise indicated.

†If patient is intolerant of sulfasalazine.

Treatment

The treatment of ulcerative colitis is based on the extent and the severity of the disease (Table 78-4). Effective medical therapy consists of a number of drugs, which are administered intravenously, orally, or rectally. The major classes of drugs are corticosteroids, 5-aminosalicylate (5-ASA) agents, immunomodulators, anti–tumor necrosis factor-α (TNF-α) agents, and anti-integrin drugs.[70] In older adults, some drugs must be used more carefully than in younger patients. For example, corticosteroids have a higher risk of complications, such as hypertension, hypokalemia, and confusion, whereas sulfasalazine, 5-ASA products, and immunomodulators are generally well tolerated.[68]

Severity of Disease

Severe Disease

Patients with severe or fulminant disease, including toxic megacolon, should be hospitalized for intravenous therapy. This treatment consists of hydrocortisone or adrenocorticotropic hormone

(ACTH) infused in fluids containing sufficient amounts of potassium to avoid hypokalemia. One study has suggested that ACTH is superior for treating patients who have not previously received corticosteroids, whereas hydrocortisone tends to be more effective in those who have.[71] Once improvement is noted, the patient should be converted to oral maintenance therapy (see later).

Anti-TNF agents belong to a class of drugs directed against human TNF-α, an important proinflammatory cytokine that is elevated in ulcerative colitis and Crohn disease. Currently, three anti-TNF agents have been approved by the U.S. Food and Drug Administration (FDA) for the treatment of severe ulcerative colitis.[72]

Infliximab is a chimeric monoclonal antibody that is administered intravenously (5 to 10 mg/kg body weight at 0, 2, and 6 weeks followed by infusions every 8 weeks), whereas adalimumab and golimumab are fully humanized drugs that are given subcutaneously. All three agents appear to have similar safety and efficacy; one meta-analysis has suggested that infliximab may be superior in inducing remission at 8 weeks but was similar to adalimumab at 52 weeks.[73]

In May 2014, the FDA approved vedolizumab, the first selective adhesion molecule inhibitor for use in moderate to severe ulcerative colitis when standard therapy has failed. Vedolizumab is a humanized monoclonal antibody that inhibits the adhesion molecule a4, B7 heterodimer, which blocks leukocyte migration and gut inflammation. The drug appears to be safe and effective when given as 300 mg intravenously at 0, 2, and 6 weeks, followed by once every 8 weeks.[74]

Moderately Severe Disease

Oral corticosteroids are used to achieve or sustain remission after intravenous therapy. Initial therapy should be 40 to 60 mg/day in divided doses, followed by conversion to a single morning dose. Corticosteroids should be viewed as acute-phase drugs and should not be used as long-term maintenance therapy because of significant side effects related to the dose and duration of therapy. Diabetes, congestive heart failure, osteoporosis, cataracts, and hypertension are common in older adults and may be exacerbated by corticosteroids.[68] Corticosteroids should be reduced in a stepwise fashion while monitoring clinical activity and carrying out appropriate laboratory studies.

5-ASAs may be started together with oral corticosteroids. Sulfasalazine is effective and inexpensive but is somewhat limited by side effects, which are often dose-dependent and occur in as many as 30% of patients. Side effects include nausea, anorexia, headache and, less commonly, a generalized rash; in most cases, these conditions are due to the inactive sulfapyridine carrier rather than the 5-ASA moiety. If side effects occur, patients should be switched to the more expensive 5-ASA products, such as mesalamine. Diarrhea is a potential side effect of all 5-ASA drugs.

If patients fail to respond to 5-ASA drugs and cannot be weaned from oral corticosteroids, a trial of azathioprine or 6-mercaptopurine should be considered as an alternative to surgery.[75] These drugs act slowly and have a response time ranging from 3 to 6 months. Complete blood counts should be monitored frequently when these agents are used.

An alternative approach is to use an anti-TNF agent in an induction dose similar to that for severe disease. Prior to starting this therapy, a skin test for tuberculosis should be done because this class of drugs has been associated with reactivation of latent *Mycobacterium tuberculosis*. Another alternative would be vedolizumab, the new selective adhesion molecule inhibitor.

Mild Disease

Patients with mild disease can be treated effectively with 5-ASA drugs, which can be administered orally, by enema in case of left-sided disease, or by suppository in patients with proctitis. Corticosteroid enemas are also effective in left-sided disease but, in general, are not more effective than 5-ASA agents. Because up to 60% of the rectal corticosteroid may be absorbed, they also are less suitable for maintenance therapy. Budesonide is a nonsystemic steroid with a significant first-pass hepatic metabolism that does not affect the adrenal-pituitary-hypothalamic axis. It is available in foam and enema forms for the treatment of mild to moderate proctosigmoiditis or left-sided disease.[76]

In a recent meta-analysis, VSL#3 (bifidobacterium and lactobacillus probiotic) significantly increased remission rates in patients with active ulcerative colitis, with no significant adverse effects.[77]

Treatment

Maintenance Therapy

For patients in remission, long-term maintenance with a 5-ASA agent reduces the frequency of relapses.[78] The usual maintenance dose of sulfasalazine is 1 g bid with little or no long-term adverse effects. For patients who are intolerant to sulfasalazine, mesalamine, 1.2 mg/day, is also effective. For those with ulcerative proctitis or left-sided colitis, 5-ASA suppositories and enemas, respectively, are effective when given every night to every third night. Nonsteroidal anti-inflammatory drugs (NSAIDs) have been reported to activate quiescent inflammatory bowel disease and should be avoided, if possible.[79]

Surgery

Indications for surgery include failure of medical therapy for acute fulminant disease, inability to wean patients from long-term corticosteroid therapy, development of precancerous colonic lesions identified during surveillance studies, and suboptimal response to medical therapy for chronic ulcerative colitis.

The surgical procedure most commonly performed for acute fulminant colitis in all age groups is subtotal colectomy and ileostomy. In the older patient, proctocolectomy and ileostomy also remain the most popular choices for chronic failure of medical treatment or because of the development of premalignant changes. Although procedures that avoid ileostomy, such as the ileoanal pouch, are a viable choice for many younger patients, its increased morbidity makes its use less attractive for older patients who also are at greater risk for fecal incontinence because of age-associated changes in anal sphincter function. Assessment of anorectal function with manometry is mandatory when considering an ileoanal pouch for an older patient.

Risk of Colon Cancer

The risk of developing colorectal cancer in older patients with ulcerative colitis is approximately nine times that of the general population of older adults.[80] The risk in all age groups increases about 8 years after the onset of the disease and is greatest in those with universal colitis. Carcinoma almost always develops many years after quiescent disease has been present and occurs at an earlier age than in the general population. Studies have shown that the risk of patients with ulcerative colitis developing colorectal cancer has decreased steadily over the last 60 years, but the extent and duration of the disease increase the risk.[81] The risk is minimal when the disease is confined to the rectum. Therefore, yearly colonoscopy has been recommended to detect mucosal dysplasia, which is considered a premalignant lesion in ulcerative colitis. Biopsies are obtained randomly throughout the colon and in areas that appear suspicious. Despite some shortcomings in the interpretation of biopsies and in the outcome of surveillance programs, all patients with long-standing ulcerative colitis should undergo periodic colonoscopy and biopsy to look for evidence of mucosal dysplasia. The presence of low-grade dysplasia in the absence of active inflammation is an indication for proctocolectomy.[80]

CROHN DISEASE

Crohn disease is a chronic inflammatory process of unknown cause that usually affects the terminal ileum and/or colon and is characterized by transmural inflammation of the bowel wall, often with linear ulcerations and granulomas.

Histopathology

Histologically, there is transmural inflammation affecting all layers of the bowel, often associated with submucosal fibrosis. Other features that serve to distinguish this disease from ulcerative colitis are linear ulcerations, fissures, fistulas, discrete mucosal ulcers, granulomas, skip areas, and frequent rectal sparing.[82] The disease can involve all areas of the GI tract, from the mouth to the anus, but usually involves the ileum and colon. According to most published series, Crohn disease confined to the colon (Crohn colitis) occurs more frequently in older adults than in younger persons, and left-sided colitis appears to be prevalent in older women.[68] There are also data to support the finding that lower levels of 25(OH) vitamin D increase the risk of incident Crohn disease.[83]

Symptoms and Signs

As with ulcerative colitis, the clinical picture in older patients is similar to that in younger individuals. It includes rectal bleeding, diarrhea, fever, abdominal pain, and weight loss. In patients with colorectal involvement, perianal disease, including fistulas, may be an early manifestation. The prevalence of extraintestinal manifestations such as migratory arthritis, pyoderma gangrenosum, iritis, and erythema nodosum is similar to that in younger patients. Common laboratory abnormalities, such as anemia, leukocytosis, hypoalbuminemia, and an elevated sedimentation rate, vary with the severity of the illness. Rarely, the disease may be manifested by peritonitis due to bowel perforation, but this occurs more commonly with ileal disease. In older patients, peritonitis may occur atypically with mild abdominal pain, often minimal abdominal findings, and mental confusion. Uncommonly, Crohn colitis is characterized by massive lower GI bleeding or bowel obstruction.

Diagnosis

Prolonged delays in diagnosis probably occur more frequently in older patients. It has been speculated that there is a tendency for Crohn colitis to appear in a more indolent fashion than ileal or ileocolonic involvement.[68]

Because the disease may often not involve the rectum, and the distribution in the colon is often not confluent, colonoscopy and CT are the diagnostic tests of choice. Colonoscopy allows superior examination of the mucosa and allows mucosal biopsies to be obtained. Biopsies should also be obtained from grossly normal-appearing mucosa to help distinguish Crohn colitis from other diseases that may mimic it. This is particularly important because of the increased frequency with which diverticula occur in older adults and because of the tendency for ischemic colitis to occur in a discontinuous distribution.

CT provides superior definition of the wall of the colon and can identify extraintestinal abdominal pathology, such as abscesses in patients with fever or palpable masses. CT and ultrasonography can also identify renal lithiasis and ureteral obstruction, which often occur silently.

Perianal involvement is a well-recognized manifestation of Crohn disease and may be characterized by rectal or anal strictures, fissures, fistulas, abscesses, prominent skin tags, and ulcers. MRI is a valuable tool for the evaluation of anorectal disease. For example, it can depict the course of a fistula, its relationship with the anal sphincters, and associated abscesses. Venereal disease (uncommon in older adults) and carcinoma should be excluded, particularly because the latter may complicate long-standing Crohn proctitis. Infectious agents should be excluded by appropriate studies.

Radiologic small bowel follow-through has largely been replaced by MR enterography to assess the extent of small bowel involvement and detect fistulas and strictures.[14] Increasingly, capsule endoscopy is being used in patients without strictures, because it appears to be more sensitive than radiology in the small bowel.[84] Assessment of the small intestine should be done at least once in every patient, usually at the time of diagnosis, to stage the disease.[82]

Treatment

As with ulcerative colitis, treatment of Crohn disease is based on its extent and severity, as well as its distribution. Medical therapy encompasses all the drugs used for treating ulcerative colitis[70]; in addition, selected antibiotics and methotrexate are helpful for some patients (Table 78-5). Recent studies have indicated that patients with Crohn disease and low serum 25(OH) vitamin D levels experience an improved quality of life, less fatigue, and improved social functioning when vitamin D levels are increased to more than 30 ng/mL with supplementation. Normalization of the serum 25(OH) vitamin D level is also associated with a lower risk of Crohn disease–related surgery.[85]

TABLE 78-5 Medical Treatment of Crohn Disease Colitis

Indications	Drug	Dosage*
Ileocolitis or colitis	Mesalamine	2.4-4.8 g
	Metronidazole/ ciprofloxacin	1-1.5 g/0.5-1g
	Prednisone	40-60 mg
	Budesonide	9 mg
Perineal disease	6-Mercaptopurine *or* azathioprine	50-1.5 mg/kg BW *or* 50-2.5 mg/kg BW
	Metronidazone	1-2 g
	Ciprofloxacin	500 mg bid
	Infliximab	5 mg/kg BW IV q8wk
	Certolizumab	400 mg SC q4wk
	Adalimumab	40 mg SC q2wk
Refractory disease or corticosteroid-dependent	6-Mercaptopurine *or* azathioprine	50-1.5 mg/kg BW *or* 50-2.5 mg/kg BW
	Infliximab	5-10 mg/kg BW IV at 0, 2, 6 wk
	Adalimumab	160, 80, 40 mg SC at 0, 2, 6 wk, respectively
	Certilizumab	400 mg SC at 0, 2, 4 wk
	Methotrexate	25 mg SC/wk for 14 wk
Maintenance of remission	6-Mercaptopurine *or* azathioprine	50-1.5 mg/kg BW *or* 50-2.5 mg/kg BW
	Mesalamine	1200-2400 mg
	Methotrexate	15 mg SC/wk
	Infliximab	5-10 mg/kg BW q6-8wk IV
	Adalimumab	40 mg SC q1-2wk
	Certolizumab	400 mg SC q4wk

BW, Body weight.
*Daily; PO unless otherwise indicated.

Ileocolitis and Colitis

Patients with mild to moderate disease often respond to 5-ASA products in doses similar to those used for ulcerative colitis. If the disease remains mild or only moderate in severity but responds inadequately to 5-ASA drugs, metronidazole, 125 to 250 mg bid,[86] ciprofloxacin, 500 mg once or twice daily, or budesonide, 9 mg daily, a steroid with fewer side effects than prednisone, can be tried.

If the disease worsens despite conservative therapy, or if the patient has moderate to severe symptoms, corticosteroids may be started in doses similar to those used for ulcerative colitis. After remission is induced, prednisone is tapered at a rate of 5 to 10 mg/week until a dose of 20 mg/day is achieved. Subsequently, prednisone should be reduced by 5 mg/day every 3 weeks while monitoring clinical activity and laboratory studies.

Increasingly, anti-TNF agents, with or without purine analogues such as azathioprine or 6-mercaptopurine, are being used as first-line therapy in patients with moderate to severe disease or those who have complicated disease.[87] There seem to be no significant differences between intravenous medications such as infliximab and injectable agents such as adalimumab and certolizumab. There is evidence that the combination of infliximab and azathioprine is superior to infliximab or azathioprine alone, both in inducing steroid-free clinical remission and mucosal healing.[88] Thus, purine analogues alone are inferior to anti-TNF agents for the treatment of active Crohn disease.

Similarly, anti-TNF agents have become the dominant strategy for maintenance of remission for Crohn disease and prevention of recurrence after surgery-induced remission. In a cost analysis, the injectable agent (adalimumab) proved to be more effective and less costly than infliximab in the United States, although this strategy might not apply to other health care systems.[89] Alternative agents for maintenance of remission include the folate antagonist methotrexate (MTX, 15 mg/week, intramuscular but not oral)[90] and purine analogues alone.[91] The combination of infliximab and MTX was no more effective than infliximab alone,[90] and budesonide appears to be ineffective for the maintenance of remission beyond 3 months.[92]

Anti-TNF agents are now often used for the treatment of active Crohn disease, which is resistant to mesalamine and antibiotics, and for those who are steroid-dependent.[87,93] They are also used for active fistulizing disease.[94] At all ages, a skin PPD (purified protein derivative) or QuantiFERON gold test should be obtained prior to therapy because of reports of reactivation of latent tuberculosis. In older adults, anti-TNF agents are contraindicated in patients with moderate to severe heart failure and should be used cautiously in patients with mild heart failure.[82] Anti- TNF–treated patients should not receive concomitant immunosuppression with azathioprine, 6-mercaptopurine (6-MP), methotrexate, or corticosteroids chronically because side effects may be increased with no demonstrable benefits.

In contrast to its efficacy in ulcerative colitis, vedolizumab (an a4, B7 integrin antibody) appears to have a somewhat less robust effect in patients with active Crohn disease,[95] with approximately 39% in clinical remission after 52 weeks versus 22% placebo. Unfortunately, vedolizumab was no more effective than placebo in inducing remission at 6 weeks in patients with Crohn disease who had failed anti-TNF agents.[96,97] Some modest improvement was noted in clinical scores at week 10.

Perianal Disease

Perianal fistulas and abscesses can be very debilitating and frustrating to treat. Although perianal disease often improves with standard therapy for bowel inflammation and control of diarrhea, some patients continue to have persistent symptoms. Short-term success has been reported with metronidazole in doses of 1.5 to 2 g/day, but side effects at these doses are not uncommon, and relapses occur when the drug is discontinued or tapered. Ciprofloxacin, 500 mg bid, is a more expensive alternative, albeit one with fewer side effects, but again there is a high relapse rate when the drug is discontinued. If an abscess develops, incision and drainage should be performed.

If perianal disease remains unresponsive to therapy, surgical diversion of the colon may be performed in an attempt to allow healing, but this too may be unsuccessful. Azathioprine or 6-MP may be helpful in some patients with refractory disease.[98] Anti-TNF agents have been reported to be effective in partial fistula closure (>50%) compared to placebo but not for complete closure.[99]

Surgery. Unlike ulcerative colitis, Crohn disease cannot be cured by surgery. Therefore, surgical procedures should be reserved for patients who do not respond to medical therapy.

Protocolectomy with ileostomy is the best surgical option for patients with extensive Crohn colitis. In older patients who are debilitated or malnourished, an initial subtotal colectomy with ileostomy is less debilitating, permits weight gain, and improves physical well-being. If proctectomy is subsequently required, it can be done with a low complication rate but may not be necessary if rectal disease is mild or absent. More limited colonic resections may be appropriate if severe disease is localized or obstructive symptoms are caused by relatively circumscribed bowel involvement.

Surgical treatment for perianal Crohn disease is limited to abscess drainage and noncutting seton placement to prevent reformation of the abscess. A further attempt to treat the fistula is recommended only after endoscopic remission of proctitis has been accomplished.[100] Options for definitive surgical repair include fistulotomy, mucosal advancement flaps, bioprosthetic plugs, and ligation of the intersphincteric fistula tract. The success of any of these procedures cannot be assumed.

LYMPHOCYTIC AND COLLAGENOUS COLITIS (MICROSCOPIC COLITIS)

Lymphocytic and collagenous colitis are uncommon disorders characterized by chronic watery diarrhea and histologic evidence of chronic mucosal inflammation in the absence of endoscopic or radiologic abnormalities of the large bowel. They comprise two histologically distinct disorders that have been grouped under the term *microscopic colitis* and that mainly differ by the presence or absence of a thickened collagen band located in the colonic subepithelium.[101,102] Both lymphocytic and collagenous colitis occur most commonly in those between the ages of 50 and 70 years, with a strong female predominance and a frequent association with arthritis, celiac disease, and autoimmune disorders.

In lymphocytic and collagenous colitis, there is a modest increase in mononuclear cells within the lamina propria and between crypt epithelial cells, primarily consisting of CD8+ T lymphocytes, plasma cells, and macrophages.[103] In collagenous colitis, there is a thickened subepithelial collagen layer, which may be continuous or patchy. Although inflammatory changes occur diffusely throughout the colon, the characteristic collagen band thickening is highly variable, occurring in the cecum and transverse colon in over 80% of cases and less than 30% of the time in the rectum. Although involvement of the left colon appears to be less intense, multiple biopsies of the left colon above the rectosigmoid during flexible sigmoidoscopy is sufficient to make the diagnosis in about 90% of cases.

Patients with collagenous and lymphocytic colitis usually present with chronic watery diarrhea, with an average of eight stools each day, often with nocturnal stools, ranging from 300 to 1700 g/24 hours, occasional fecal incontinence, abdominal cramps, and decreased symptoms when fasting.[104] Nausea, weight loss, and fecal urgency have also been reported but are variable.

Diarrhea is generally long-standing, ranging from months to years, with a fluctuating course of remissions and exacerbations. In one series of 172 patients, the median time from onset of symptoms to diagnosis was 11 months, whereas in another of 31 patients, it was 5.4 years. The physical examination is usually unremarkable, and blood in the stool is absent. Routine laboratory studies are also normal.

Examination of fresh stools has shown fecal leukocytes in 55% of 116 patients with collagenous colitis. Fecal calprotectin may be a more sensitive marker than fecal leukocytes (62%) and is superior to fecal lactoferrin.[105] It is also less time-intensive and less prone to technician error. Mild steatorrhea, mild anemia, low serum vitamin B_{12} levels, and hypoalbuminemia have been reported in variable numbers of patients but are not characteristic. Autoimmune markers that have been identified in patients with collagenous colitis include antinuclear antibodies (up to 50%), perinuclear antineutrophil cytoplasmic antibodies (pANCAs) in 14%, rheumatoid factor, and increased C3 and C4 complement components.

Colonoscopic examinations are usually normal. Infectious agents should be excluded by testing for stool ova and parasites, standard stool cultures, and *C. difficile* toxin assays. Many patients have been diagnosed to have irritable bowel syndrome, a disorder which can be excluded by the abnormal colonic biopsies and the finding of increased stool volume, both of which are not characteristic of irritable bowel syndrome.

Treatment

There have been very few controlled trials for collagenous or lymphocytic colitis and therapy is largely empirical. NSAIDs and other colitis inducing medications should be stopped.[102] About one third of patients respond to antidiarrheal agents such as loperamide or diphenoxylate with atropine, as well as bulk agents such as psyllium or methylcellulose. However, they do not exhibit improvement in inflammation or collagen thickness. In an open-label trial of bismuth subsalicylate in 12 patients,[106] eight chewable tablets/day for 8 weeks resulted in resolution of diarrhea and reduction of stool weight within 2 weeks and, in 9 patients, colitis resolved, including the disappearance of collagen band thickening. Although the basis for its efficacy is unknown, bismuth subsalicylate possesses antidiarrheal, antibacterial, and antiinflammatory properties.

Most other treatment trials for collagenous colitis and lymphocytic colitis have studied 5-ASA compounds and bile acid resins. Alone or in combination, these agents appear to relieve diarrhea and inflammation in some but not all treated patients. Although corticosteroids given via the oral or enema route provide symptomatic improvement and decrease inflammation in over 80% of cases, relapse usually occurs quickly after stopping the drug.[104] Moreover, long-term corticosteroids have undesirable effects, especially in older patients.

Budesonide is a topically acting synthetic corticosteroid with a high receptor-binding affinity and high first-pass effect in the liver. It has fewer significant side effects than prednisone and lower recurrence rates.[107] The recommended dose is 9 mg once daily for 4 weeks, with tapering by 3 mg daily for 2 to 4 weeks.[108,109] Recurrences often occur, and maintenance with 3 mg once daily may be necessary for up to two thirds of patients.[107]

Azathioprine and methotrexate may be considered for steroid-refractory patients.[110] Some studies have suggested that older patients are more likely to be helped with antidiarrheal agents or require no medication in contrast to younger patients.[111]

COLONIC ISCHEMIA

The blood supply to the colon is derived mainly from branches of the superior and inferior mesenteric arteries and is characterized by a rich collateral circulation, except for the potentially susceptible marginal artery of Drummond and the arc of Riolan, located at the peripheral junction of the two mesenteric arteries.[112] Occlusion of a major artery results in immediate opening of collateral vessels to maintain an adequate blood supply to the bowel. Intestinal ischemia may occur as a result of generalized reduction of blood flow (nonocclusive ischemia), redistribution of blood flow (e.g., vessel obstruction with poor collateral circulation), or a combination of the two. Colonic ischemia is the most common vascular disorder of the intestines in older adults, often with multiple comorbidities, and one that is often misdiagnosed unless there is a high index of suspicion and an aggressive diagnostic approach in patients suspected of having this disorder.[113] It is associated with a high in-hospital mortality rate and high rates of surgery, 17% in a recent population-based study.[114]

The clinical spectrum of colonic ischemia includes a vast array of presentations and may be associated with a number of potentiating factors. Ischemia may be classified as reversible and irreversible; the former may present with submucosal or intramural hemorrhage or transient ischemic colitis, which completely resolves within weeks to months, depending on the severity of the process. Irreversible ischemia may be characterized by chronic ulcerations, strictures of varying lengths, colonic gangrene, or fulminant transmural colitis.[115]

In most cases, the cause of colonic ischemia cannot be established with certainty, and no vascular occlusions can be identified. A significant minority of patients is found to have a potentially obstructing process in the colon such as a benign stricture, diverticulitis, or carcinoma. Other contributing factors include hypotension, dehydration, congestive heart failure, use of digitalis, polycythemia, volvulus, and cardiac arrhythmias. One caveat is that it may be the first sign of undiagnosed cardiac disease.[116]

Symptoms and Signs

The most common manifestation is the sudden onset of mild to moderately severe left lower abdominal cramping pain, often accompanied by bloody diarrhea or hematochezia, which may not appear until 24 hours later. Frank hemorrhage is not characteristic of ischemia. The physical examination reveals tenderness at the site of the involved bowel; these sites encompass the distal transverse, splenic flexure, and/or descending colons in about two thirds of patients. Peritoneal signs may last for several hours, but persistence beyond that time suggests a transmural process. Fever, leukocytosis, absence of bowel sounds, and abdominal distention also suggest the possibility of bowel infarction.

Diagnosis

If the diagnosis is suspected on clinical grounds, colonoscopy with minimal insufflation with air is the preferred diagnostic test. When an ischemic segment is encountered, biopsies should be taken from the edge of the ulcerated area and noninvolved tissue and the procedure aborted. Barium studies may reveal thumbprinting in the affected areas of the colon, which represents submucosal or mucosal hemorrhages and edema during the early phase of the process. This corresponds to the hemorrhagic nodules noted on colonoscopic examination. There is no meaningful role for mesenteric angiography in patients with colon ischemia unless there is involvement of the right colon, with suspected mesenteric ischemia of the small intestine. Focal right-sided ischemic colitis has more pain and carries a worse prognosis.[116]

Treatment

Patients should be managed with bowel rest, intravenous fluids, and/or plasma expanders and, in severe cases, systemic antibiotics such as gentamycin and clindamycin.[117] Corticosteroids are of no benefit and should not be administered. In mild disease, symptoms resolve within several days, and radiologic healing occurs within several weeks, although some patients may not heal for up to 6 months.

If the patient continues to have diarrhea, bleeding, or significant obstructive symptoms for more than several weeks, surgical resection is usually indicated. If colonic infarction is suspected, emergency laparotomy with resection of nonviable bowel is needed.[117] With colonic infarction and gangrene, the mortality rate in older adults with multiple comorbid conditions approaches 50% to 75% with surgery, but is universally fatal with nonsurgical treatment.[118]

Prognosis

Recurrent episodes of colonic ischemia occur in less than 10% of patients. Attempts should be made to correct or remove underlying conditions that predispose to this disorder. Peripheral vasculopathy and right colonic involvement are associated with more severe disease.

COLONIC PSEUDO-OBSTRUCTION

Acute colonic pseudo-obstruction, sometimes termed the *Ogilvie syndrome*, is characterized by nonobstructive, nontoxic dilation of the colon.[119] This condition may develop after surgery, especially orthopedic procedures, and also occurs in a setting of serious coexisting illness, including sepsis, pneumonia, acute pancreatitis, spinal cord injury, and administration of anticholinergic, narcotic, or psychotropic drugs. This disorder can compromise respiratory status and cause cecal perforation. The risk of cecal perforation is said to increase when the diameter of the cecum increases beyond 10 cm. A variant of this disorder is the so-called megasigmoid syndrome, often described in psychotic patients but not exclusively seen within this group.

After obstruction has been excluded, treatment includes correction of electrolyte imbalances, discontinuation of offending drugs, treatment of underlying infection or inflammation, nasogastric suction, rectal or colonic decompression tube with positioning of the patient on the right and left sides at intervals of several hours, or medical treatment with intravenous neostigmine.[120] Decompression with colonoscopy may be attempted if there is severe dilation and no response to medical therapy.[121] Surgical decompression under local anesthesia using a stab wound cecostomy can be performed if other measures fail. Postdecompression x-ray films should be obtained for several days to document continued resolution.

Relapses are common after the successful decompression of acute colonic pseudo-obstruction, being as high as 33%. The administration of 29.5 g polyethylene glycol (PEG) daily in two divided doses after successful treatment resulted in no relapses versus a 33% relapse rate for patients receiving placebo.[122]

Chronic colonic pseudo-obstruction, with or without colonic dilation (megacolon), may be associated with amyloidosis, muscular dystrophy, myxedema, dementia, multiple sclerosis, Parkinson disease, quadriplegia, schizophrenia, and idiopathic visceral neuropathy and myopathy. There may be esophageal, gastric, small intestinal, and genitourinary dysfunction. Although most patients have constipation, diarrhea occurs if there is small bowel bacterial overgrowth or overflow around a fecal impaction.[123]

Subtotal colectomy may be necessary in some patients with refractory symptoms and if anorectal function is normal. If anorectal dysfunction is present, proctocolectomy with ileostomy is indicated. Sigmoid resection may be all that is necessary in patients with megasigmoid syndrome. Most patients can be treated conservatively.

VOLVULUS

Factors thought to contribute to colonic volvulus include increasing age, chronic constipation, fecal retention, poor peritoneal fixation during embryologic rotation of the hindgut, and, in some areas of the world, diets very high in fiber. The clinical setting typical of a sigmoid volvulus is an older institutionalized individual with a history of chronic constipation or laxative abuse.[124]

The sigmoid colon, with its copious mesentery, is usually involved, but cecal volvulus can occur when fixation to the posterior parietal wall is incomplete. Volvulus of the transverse colon is the least common. Patients have a sudden onset of severe abdominal pain, followed by rapid and marked abdominal distention. Compromise of blood flow occurs as a result of twisting of the mesentery and marked distention of the loop.

Abdominal x-rays reveal massive distention of a single loop of bowel; the obstructed loop frequently is shaped like a coffee bean, with the concavity marking the point of torsion. The concavity points to the left lower quadrant in patients with sigmoid volvulus and to the right lower quadrant when cecal volvulus is present. Administering contrast through the rectum confirms the diagnosis by the appearance of the pointed twist of the contrast column.

Closely related to a cecal volvulus is a cecal bascule, in which malfixation allows the cecum to fold anteriorly and in a cephalad direction, which can result in a flap valve obstruction with cecal distention. Abdominal x-rays reveal distention of the cecum, but no bird-beak configuration is seen on a barium enema, as in volvulus. However, treatment is identical to that for conventional cecal volvulus.

Attempts to untwist a sigmoid volvulus may be made by gently inserting an endoscope as far as the twisted segment.[125] Successful detorsion must be followed by careful observation should the bowel continue to be ischemic. Nonoperative decompression is more successful with a sigmoid than with a cecal volvulus; attempts to treat a cecal volvulus by nonoperative means can be dangerous and, even if successful, recurrence rates are high. Opinion is divided as to whether the first episode of sigmoid volvulus should be treated with resection. Fixation without resection is not considered a useful option. Certainly, patients with more than one episode of sigmoid volvulus should have resection.

In older frail patients with cecal volvulus, early surgical intervention to untwist the volvulus followed by cecal fixation (cecopexy) is frequently all that is necessary unless bowel necrosis is present. If the latter is present, resection with ileostomy is indicated. In healthy older patients, cecal resection with reanastomosis is the preferred option.

NEOPLASTIC LESIONS

Colonic polyps may be classified into the following groups: neoplastic polyps, which include adenomatous polyps and carcinomas; non-neoplastic polyps, which include hyperplastic, inflammatory, and hamartomatous types; and submucosal tumors, such as lipomas, leiomyomas, hemangiomas, fibromas, lymphoid polyps, and carcinoids.[126]

Most (80% to 90%) colonic polyps are adenomatous or hyperplastic and, of these, about 75% are adenomas. However, when only polyps smaller than 5 mm are considered, 50% are hyperplastic, and most are found in the rectosigmoid colon. A study had suggested that hyperplastic polyps are not of clinical importance.[127] However, this view may be too simplistic. There are sessile serrated polyps that appear to be hyperplastic but with important histologic differences, which do have malignant potential. It is now estimated that the serrated neoplastic pathway accounts for approximately 30% of all colorectal cancers.[128]

Adenomatous polyps

These polyps arise from mucosal glandular epithelium and can be described based on the following characteristic:

1. Size: Approximately 25% of adenomas are larger than 1 cm, and over 80% of large adenomas occur in the left colon and rectum.
2. Architecture: Over 80% of adenomas are tubular, 5% to 15% are villous, and the rest are tubulovillous. Those with a higher proportion of villous elements tend to be larger and carry a higher risk of malignant transformation.
3. Dysplasia: All adenomas are dysplastic, but high-grade dysplasia is strongly associated with malignancy.

In the United States, prevalence rates in men and women are similar. Except in familial syndromes, colonic adenomas are rare before the age of 40 years, increase steadily, and reach a peak after the age of 60 years. Population studies have suggested that the environment strongly contributes to adenoma prevalence and probably to the frequency of colon cancer as well. For example, obesity may be a risk factor, whereas NSAIDs (including aspirin) are associated with decreased risk.[129]

It is logical, although costly, to identify and remove all benign adenomas at an early stage to prevent progression to carcinoma. In one study, screening and polyp removal by rigid sigmoidoscopy during the previous 10 years resulted in a 70% reduction in the risk of fatal cancer of the rectum and distal colon compared to the outcome in nonscreened subjects.[130] In the National Polyp Study, colonoscopic polypectomy reduced the incidence of colorectal cancer by 76% to 90% during a follow-up of almost 6 years.[131] These findings form the basis for current screening recommendations.

There is epidemiologic evidence that aspirin and other NSAIDs may reduce the risk of colorectal cancer.[132] Several large studies, although not all, have found a significant reduction in death rates from colon cancer among men and women who use NSAIDs on a regular basis. Such observations are supported by laboratory studies demonstrating that aspirin and other cyclooxygenase inhibitors have chemopreventive effects in animal models of colon carcinogenesis. There currently are insufficient data supporting the use of NSAIDs as colorectal cancer chemopreventive agents outside appropriately designed trials.

Management

Criteria for the adequacy of colonoscopic polypectomy have been well established for pedunculated malignant polyps.[133,134] In patients with favorable criteria, the risk of residual tumor is 0.3% for pedunculated lesions and 1.5% for sessile lesions, whereas the risk is 8.5% for those with unfavorable criteria. Surgery is therefore strongly considered in the latter situation, although recommendations should be individualized based on patient age and comorbid conditions.

The following are recommendations for treatment after polypectomy[135]:

1. Patients should undergo complete colonoscopy at the time of polypectomy and have removal of all synchronous polyps.
2. Patients at increased risk have three or more adenomas, high-grade dysplasia, villous features, or an adenoma 1 cm or larger. It is recommended that these patients have a 3-year follow-up colonoscopy.
3. Patients at lower risk who have one or two small (<1 cm) tubular adenomas, with no high- grade dysplasia, can have a follow-up examination in 5 to 10 years.
4. Patients with hyperplastic polyps only should have a 10-year follow-up evaluation, as for average-risk individuals.

Screening Strategies

It is generally accepted that colorectal cancer largely can be prevented by the detection and removal of adenomatous polyps. Screening tests may be divided into those that primarily detect cancer early and those that can detect cancer early and detect adenomatous polyps, which can be removed.[136] The sensitivity of Hemoccult II tests for detecting asymptomatic colorectal cancer ranges from 45% to 80% in mass-screened populations but is less than 25% for detecting polyps 1 cm or larger in diameter.[137] Moreover, at least 50% of screened individuals older than 40 years with a positive Hemoccult test are false-positive or have an upper GI source of bleeding. A systematic review of colorectal cancer screening using the fecal occult blood test has indicated that screening is associated with a 16% to 25% reduction in the relative risk of colorectal cancer (CRC) mortality for studies that used biennial screening.[138]

FITs are more sensitive than FOBTs at detecting CRC and adenomas and do not require dietary or medication restrictions, and many tests require only one or two stool samples, making them easier to use.[139] Many countries, including the United States and Europe and Asia, have adopted screening programs using FITs. A systematic review and meta-analysis has concluded that FITs are moderately sensitive, highly specific, and highly accurate for detecting CRC. Diagnostic performance depends on the cutoff value for a positive test result.[140]

In view of the perceived shortcomings of FOBT and FITs, there have been increasing attempts to identify biomarkers for the early detection of CRC and polyps. Thus, sensitivities for CRC detection using fecal DNA markers have ranged from 53% to 87%, and combining fecal DNA markers increases the sensitivity for detecting CRC and adenomas.[141] One panel of serum protein biomarkers has provided a sensitivity and specificity above 85% for all stages of CRC and a PPV (positive predictive value) of 72%. Combinations of fecal and serum biomarkers further improve the early detection of CRC and adenomas.

In a recent study, a multitarget stool DNA test plus a hemoglobin immunoassay detected significantly more CRCs than FIT but had more false-positive test results.[142] It was calculated that the numbers of asymptomatic persons who would need to be screened to detect one cancer were 154 with colonoscopy, 166 with DNA testing, and 208 with FIT. Further research is required to validate biomarkers as a screening technique in population-based studies.

A published consensus document has expressed the strong opinion that colon cancer prevention should be the goal of screening and indicated a preference for tests designed to detect early cancer and adenomatous polyps if resources are available, and patients are willing to undergo an invasive procedure.[136] Testing options under this scenario include flexible sigmoidoscopy or double-contrast barium enema every 5 years, full colonoscopy every 10 years, and CT colonography every 5 years for asymptomatic adults aged 50 years or older. The finding of adenomatous polyps on flexible sigmoidoscopy should be followed by colonoscopy, with removal of all polyps, followed by repeat colonoscopy in 3 to 5 years, depending on the number of polyps and histology. Although somewhat controversial, many think that finding polyps on imaging studies should be confirmed by colonoscopy, with removal of any polyps. Others think that polyps smaller than 1 cm may be followed with repeat studies every 2 years.[12]

Colorectal Cancer

Colorectal cancer is the third most commonly diagnosed cancer and the second most common cause of cancer death in the United States and United Kingdom.[138] Epidemiologic evidence has strongly suggested that colon cancer is an acquired genetic disease produced by chronic exposure to environmental carcinogens. Thus, deaths from colon cancer increase slowly by middle age and rise steeply thereafter. Moreover, immigrants from areas of low incidence acquire, within a single generation, the increased risks of the indigenous population in areas of higher incidence.[143] Except for the increased risk for CRC in individuals with ulcerative colitis and those with a family history of colorectal cancer, no high-risk exposures have consistently been identified in the United States. However, epidemiologic evidence has implicated decreased dietary fiber and increased consumption of animal protein and fat. The fact that CRC is caused by cumulative alterations in the cellular genome, and not by a single genetic alteration, may explain the long latency period between initial exposure to carcinogen(s) and the appearance of cancer.[144]

In about 80% of cases, somatic mutations in the *APC* gene on chromosome 5 are the earliest recognized genetic alterations in sporadic colonic carcinogenesis and are found in the smallest adenomas. These mutations permit unregulated proliferation at the base of the colonic crypt. A multistep genetic model for sporadic colorectal tumorigenesis involves sequential mutations in cellular oncogenes and tumor suppressor genes.[144] Two cellular proteins associated with the *APC* gene have been identified and appear to be involved in cell adhesion, which may provide an important clue about the mechanism of tumor initiation.

In about 15% of sporadic cases, a colon cancer susceptibility gene on the short arm of chromosome 2 has been identified in patients with families with hereditary nonpolyposis colon cancer (HNPCC) and in sporadic colon cancers. Widespread mutations in short repeated DNA sequences due to defective or mutant DNA mismatch repair enzymes have been identified on chromosome 2p. At least six such repair genes have now been identified in the pathogenesis of colon cancer.[145] These tumors appear to have a genetic pathogenesis different from that of the hereditary polyposis syndromes, which results in different clinical features and less aggressive behavior. Microsatellite instability (MSI) is the molecular hallmark of DNA mismatch repair deficiency, and its presence indicates a significantly better overall survival, including disease-free survival.[146,147]

Colon cancers can be classified by gross appearance, histology (well to poorly differentiated, mucinous, signet ring type) or by DNA content. In general, poorly differentiated carcinomas have a somewhat worse prognosis than well-differentiated tumors. More helpful is staging—for example, by the Astler and Coller modified Dukes (Dukes-Turnbull) classification: A, tumor is limited to the muscularis mucosa; B1, tumor extends into the muscularis propria; B2, tumor penetrates through serosa, with no lymph node involvement; C1, four or fewer regional lymph node metastases; C2, more than than four nodes involved; and D, distant metastases. Actuarial 5-year survival rates diminish from 85% to 95% for Dukes A lesions to less than 5% for Dukes D lesions. As expected, prognosis is much poorer when there is vascular or neural invasion.

In an attempt to provide a uniform classification, the American Joint Committee on Cancer introduced the tumor-node-metastasis (TNM) classification for CRC.[148] This system classifies the extent of the primary tumor (T), the status of regional lymph nodes (N), and the presence or absence of a distant metastasis (M). Cases are assigned to one of five stages (0 through IV); it has largely replaced the Dukes classification in therapeutic trials and in clinical practice.

The primary treatment for colorectal cancer is surgical resection. Preoperative studies include a complete evaluation of the colon, preferably by colonoscopy, and chest x-ray. Routine measurement of the carcinoembryonic antigen (CEA) level is often done. Although serial measurements of CEA have been advocated to detect early recurrences after surgery, cancer cures attributable to CEA monitoring appear to be infrequent.[149] In clinical practice, the CEA level is rarely used alone to determine recurrence. Abdominal imaging studies are most useful for detecting advanced disease (e.g., hepatic metastases) but less useful in finding localized extracolonic spread. Moreover, such information can be obtained directly at the time of surgery, and the presence of metastases does not influence the need for surgery or type of surgery that is performed. In contrast, rectal endosonography is superior to CT and MRI in staging rectal cancers.[18]

There is no benefit from adjunctive radiation therapy for colon cancer outside the rectum. However, adjuvant chemotherapy with fluorouracil (5-FU) and levamisole[150] or fluorouracil and leucovorin (5-FU/LV) has been associated with a significant reduction in tumor recurrence and enhanced survival in patients with stage III colon cancer.[151] These data support the use of postoperative adjuvant chemotherapy in stage III colon cancers, including older patients. In contrast, the benefit of adjuvant fluorouracil-based therapy in stage II colon cancer is less clear.[152] The addition of oxaliplatin to 5-FU/LV has shown no benefit in older patients with stage II or III colon cancer, and there may be a trend toward decreased survival.[153]

Treatment of cancer in older patients often requires greater attention because of disabling comorbidities and decline in organ function. Cancer treatment in this population is often associated with more severe toxicities and hospitalizations. The older the patient, the less likely is he or she to receive chemotherapy.[154]

Adjuvant combined radiotherapy and chemotherapy improve postsurgical survival in patients with rectal carcinoma, albeit with increased and often severe toxicity.[155] Some patients with unresectable rectal cancer may become surgical candidates following radiation therapy.

LOWER GASTROINTESTINAL BLEEDING

The two most frequent causes of acute lower GI bleeding in older patients, defined as originating below the ligament of Treitz, are diverticulosis and vascular ectasias (angiodysplasia).[156] These entities account for two thirds of hemodynamically significant lower GI bleeding (Table 78-6). The most common causes of chronic lower GI bleeding are hemorrhoids, angiodysplasia, and colonic neoplasms. Known causes of acute lower GI bleeding other than angiodysplasia and diverticulosis include the following: neoplasm; radiation enterocolitis; ischemic, ulcerative, and Crohn colitis; solitary rectal ulcer syndrome; and internal hemorrhoids. Less frequently reported causes of bleeding include small intestinal and Meckel diverticula, vasculitis, and Dieulafoy lesions of the small intestine and colon.

Causes

Angiodysplasia

Angiodysplasia are small clusters of dilated and tortuous veins that appear in the mucosa of the colon, as well as in the small intestine.[157] They are thought to result from age-associated degeneration of colonic submucosal veins, are often multiple, and are an important cause of lower GI bleeding in older adults; two thirds of patients with angiodysplasia are older than 70 years. The principal theory concerning their development is that repeated episodes of low-grade partial obstruction of submucosal veins occur during muscular contraction or from increased intraluminal pressure, resulting in dilation and tortuosity of the vein.[158] This process may extend to the mucosal veins, which are drained by the submucosal vein. Finally, the precapillary sphincter becomes incompetent, and a small arteriovenous (AV) communication with an ectatic tuft of vessels develops. The tendency of vascular ectasias to occur in the right colon is best explained by the greater tension on the bowel wall, as expressed by the Laplace law relating tension to the diameter of the bowel lumen. A review

TABLE 78-6 Clinical Presentation of Common Causes of Lower Gastrointestinal Bleeding

Symptom	Young Adult	Middle-Aged Adult	Older Adult
Abdominal pain	IBD	IBD	Ischemia, IBD
Painless	Meckel diverticula, polyps	Diverticulosis, polyps, cancer	Angiodysplasia, diverticulosis, polyps, cancer
Diarrhea	IBD, infection	IBD, infection	Ischemia, infection, IBD
Constipation	Hemorrhoids, fissure, rectal ulcer	Hemorrhoids, fissure	Cancer, hemorrhoids, fissure

IBD, Inflammatory bowel disease.

of the literature has cast doubt on a causal association between vascular ectasias and aortic stenosis, also known as Heyde syndrome.[159] Nevertheless, it has been reported that recurrent bleeding from these lesions decreases after replacement of a stenotic aortic valve.[160]

Vascular ectasias remain asymptomatic in most individuals. The usual manifestation is that of painless subacute or recurrent bleeding, which stops spontaneously in most cases. Bleeding may consist of bright red blood, maroon stools or, rarely, melena, or may be occult.[156] About 10% to 15% of patients have episodes of brisk blood loss, and up to 50% exhibit iron deficiency anemia.

Diagnosis may be made by colonoscopy or angiography, but colonoscopy is preferred because it can exclude other causes of bleeding and can be used for therapeutic interventions.[161,162] Because lesions are small, often multiple, and difficult to see, thorough cleansing of the colon is necessary to provide adequate visualization of the mucosa. Colonoscopy is usually performed after bleeding has stopped and within 48 hours to permit identification of other bleeding sources.

Mesenteric angiography is the diagnostic procedure of choice when acute bleeding is brisk. The finding of tortuous, densely opacified clusters of small veins that empty slowly represents the advanced ectatic process. Early filling of the vein, indicative of the presence of an AV communication, is found in most patients who are studied for bleeding. Extravasation of contrast into the bowel lumen is seen when there is active bleeding at a rate of at least 0.5 mL/min; because bleeding is often intermittent, a bleeding site is identified by angiography in only a minority of patients.

Bleeding can be controlled acutely by intraarterial administration of vasopressin in doses ranging from 0.2 to 0.6 units/min. This often permits stabilization of the patient and appears to be more effective when bleeding is from the right colon. When bleeding cannot be controlled, surgery is required. Colonoscopic therapeutic modalities generally involve thermal ablation techniques (e.g., argon plasma coagulation), but rebleeding remains a significant problem.[163] A right hemicolectomy is performed if bleeding from the right colon has been identified by angiography or colonoscopy and if other sources of bleeding have not been identified. The extent of resection should not be influenced by the presence of left colonic diverticulosis. Recurrent bleeding, probably due to undetected ectasias, occurs in up to 20% of patients, who may require more extensive colonic resection or exploratory laparotomy.

Treatment should be conservative whenever possible and consists of blood or iron replacement, as appropriate. For recurrent bleeding, transcolonoscopic electrocoagulation or argon plasma laser coagulation may be attempted; difficulties include identifying the ectatic lesion(s) and excluding other causes of blood loss if bleeding has stopped. Perforation of the right colon with coagulation therapy is a hazard.[164]

The development of capsule endoscopy may reduce the need for diagnostic laparotomy in patients with recurrent bleeding from obscure sites.[165]

Vasculitis

Inflammation and necrosis of blood vessels may lead to ischemia and ulceration, resulting in pain and/or bleeding. Polyarteritis nodosa, Churg-Strauss syndrome, Henoch-Schönlein purpura, systemic lupus erythematosus, rheumatoid vasculitis, Behçet disease, and essential mixed cryoglobulinemia have all been reported to produce GI bleeding. They are best diagnosed with endoscopic procedures in the appropriate clinical setting.

Dieulafoy Lesions

These lesions have been reported to cause bleeding, in several cases massive, in the small intestine and colon.[166] They are characterized by a small mucosal defect with minimal inflammation and a congenitally large, tortuous, thick-walled arteriole at the base, which ruptures into the bowel lumen. The histology of these vessels is normal, and their abnormality is their size relative to their superficial location. Bleeding can be localized with angiography, although occasionally colonoscopy can identify the lesion if bleeding has stopped, and the colon is well prepared. Surgical resection, embolization therapy, thermal coagulation therapy, and endoscopic hemoclipping are the treatments of choice.

Evaluation and Management

The first goal of management is to assess the severity of bleeding and cardiovascular status of the patient rapidly and to resuscitate those with major blood loss (Figure 78-1). Vital signs reflecting orthostatic changes and other signs of hypovolemia should be checked immediately and at frequent intervals thereafter. If signs of shock or hypovolemia are present, one or two large-bore intravenous catheters should be placed to facilitate fluid resuscitation. Initial blood work, including a complete blood count (CBC), platelet count, coagulation profiles, routine blood chemistries, and type and cross-matching should be done immediately. Only after these critical tasks are completed should a more detailed history and physical examination be performed to help determine the site of bleeding and potential causes. Another important step is to distinguish acute bleeding from active bleeding superimposed on chronic blood loss. This is best done by determining the hematocrit and mean corpuscular volume; if the latter is low, chronic bleeding should be suspected.

The third step is to consider the location of the GI bleed based on characteristics of the bleeding and a blood urea nitrogen (BUN)-to-creatinine (Cr) ratio.[167] Although hematochezia, defined as the passage of red blood through the rectum, suggests a lower GI source, up to 20% of patients with upper GI bleeding may present with hematochezia because of the rapid passage of large amounts of blood through the small and large intestines.[168]

These patients always show evidence of severe hemodynamic compromise, and most have a BUN/Cr ratio greater than 25 on initial evaluation.[167] On the other hand, melena is often characteristic of upper GI bleeding but can also be seen in patients with bleeding from the small intestine or right colon when colonic transit is slow. Fresh unclotted blood dripping into the toilet after defecation suggests a very distal anorectal source, whereas blood streaking the stool suggests origin in the left colon.

Exclusion of an upper GI site begins with the passage of a nasogastric tube and examination of gastric contents for red blood, coffee ground material, and bile. The presence of bile and

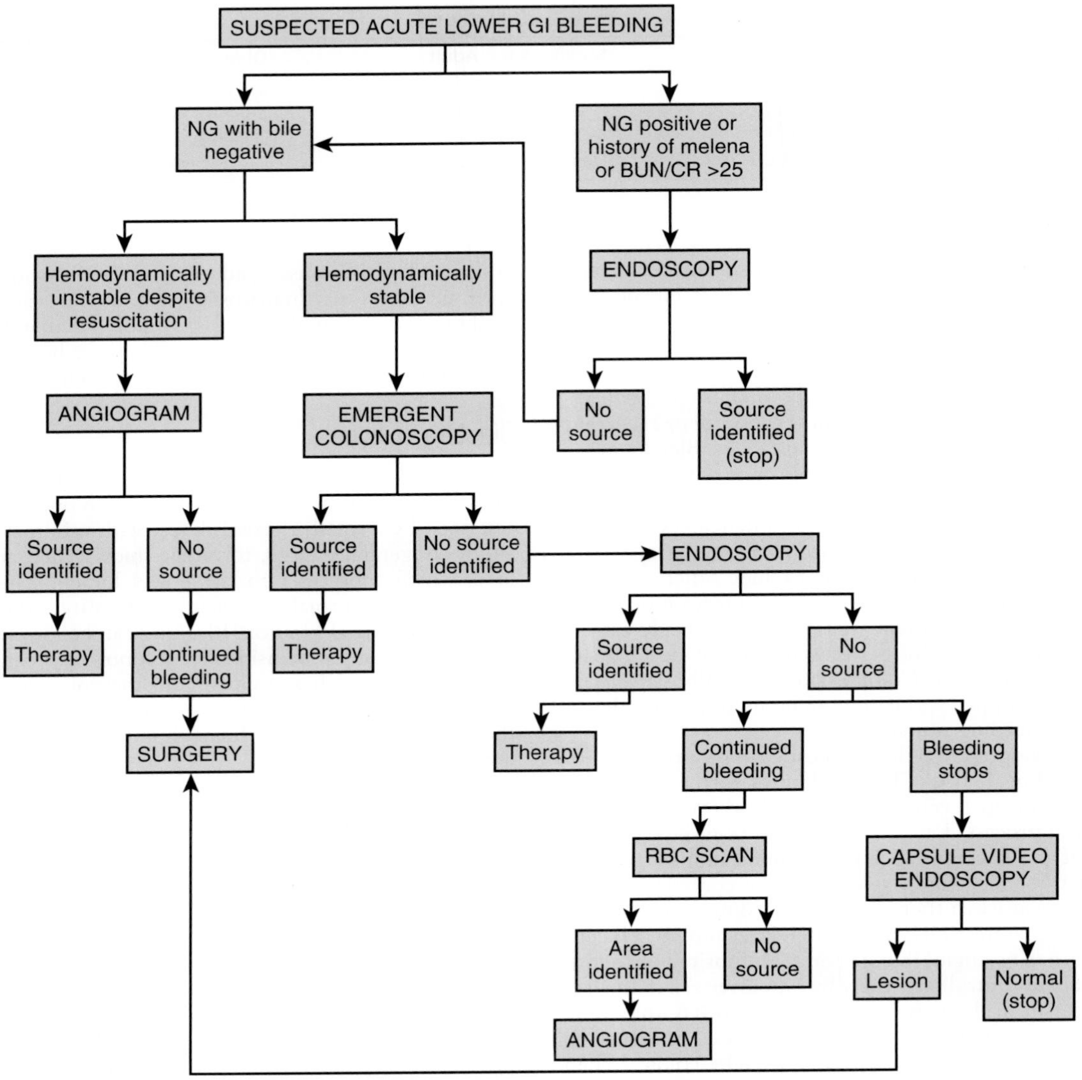

Figure 78-1. Management of suspected acute lower gastrointestinal bleeding. *BUN,* Blood urea nitrogen; *CR,* creatinine; *NG,* nasogastric suction aspiration; *RBC,* red blood cell.

an absence of blood or coffee ground materials significantly diminishes but does not exclude bleeding proximal to the duodenojejunal junction; thus, an upper endoscopy should be performed in a setting compatible with an upper GI source. There is no role for occult blood testing of a nasogastric aspirate in the absence of coffee ground or bloody material. Finally, hemorrhoidal and low rectal bleeding should be excluded by sigmoidoscopy in patients thought to have lower GI hemorrhage.

When evaluating stable patients with acute lower GI hemorrhage, colonoscopy preceded by oral bowel preparation is preferred for identifying and potentially treating a colonic bleeding source. If an emergency colonoscopy is to be considered, the nasogastric tube should be left in place to permit rapid administration of a PEG electrolyte solution to cleanse the colon.

If bleeding is active and bowel preparation cannot be done, scintigraphy with ^{162}Tc-labeled red blood cells can be used in an attempt to locate a bleeding site. This technique detects active bleeding at rates of approximately 0.1 mL/min, and the patient can be serially scanned for up to 36 hours if bleeding is intermittent. Site localization may be impaired if delayed films are taken too infrequently, and the patient must be actively bleeding at the time of the study. Although there were initial enthusiastic reports of an approximately 90% rate of detection of active bleeding, subsequent studies have yielded conflicting results.[169,170] These latter reports have raised serious concerns regarding a rigid policy of routinely performing nuclear scintigraphy prior to mesenteric angiography, particularly in high-risk patients for whom rapid diagnosis is preferred. It may be more accurate if upper GI bleeding has been excluded.[170] If bleeding is active and severe and/or scintigraphy is not diagnostic, selective mesenteric angiography can be used to detect extravasated contrast into the bowel when bleeding rates are 0.5 to 1.0 mL/min or to demonstrate vascular lesions, neovascularity, or tumors in the absence of extravasation.[171] Sensitivity declines when bleeding is recurrent or chronic. Attempts have been made to increase diagnostic sensitivity and accuracy by using systemic heparinization, intraarterial vasodilators, or thrombolytic agents during angiography if the initial study is negative.[172] More extensive experience is needed to determine whether the increased yield justifies the increased risk of bleeding complications.

Angiography also offers the potential for local therapy, provided that selective catheterization can be achieved. These modalities include infusion of vasopressin to control acute arterial bleeding in colonic diverticular disease or angiodysplasia and selective embolization of an identified bleeding site with a gelatin sponge, vascular coils, or polyvinyl alcohol particles.[173] Complications include electrolyte disturbances, cardiovascular complications, and bowel ischemia with vasopressin infusion and bowel infarction following embolization. The latter should be attempted only at centers that have the expertise to perform superselective catheterization. Some investigators have reported that urgent colonoscopy is superior to selective mesenteric angiography in identifying the source of severe lower GI bleeding. If bleeding is massive, emergent surgery with or without intraoperative endoscopy may be the best option. There is little or no place in modern surgical practice for blind colonic resection.

Another approach to detect the site of bleeding is the use of multidetector CT scanning with special angiographic protocols. These are performed without oral contrast to detect intraluminal extravasation of intravenous contrast.[174] In older patients with renal insufficiency, the risk of contrast-induced nephropathy may limit the use of this technique.

If no source of bleeding is detected by colonoscopy and no further bleeding occurs, a small bowel enteroscopy or capsule endoscopy should be performed. Enteroscopes can often be advanced to 60 to 100 cm past the ligament of Treitz if the procedure is done by experienced personnel.[175] The diagnostic yield has varied from 30% to 60%, with arteriovascular malformations accounting for most of the causes of bleeding. Video capsule endoscopy allows visualization of most or all of the small intestine.

Barium radiographic procedures have no role in the evaluation of patients with acute lower GI bleeding. They are unable to demonstrate active bleeding and interfere with attempts to perform colonoscopy or mesenteric angiography. Even if a lesion is detected, there is no proof that it is the source of the bleeding.

KEY POINTS

- Principal functions of the colon are to store fecal wastes and expel them in an appropriate manner. Colonic dysfunction may result in constipation, diarrhea, or fecal incontinence.
- Making a clinical distinction between painful diverticular disease and diverticulitis carries a sizable rate of error in older adults. CT and ultrasonography often help in this important process because treatment approaches are very different.
- Both ulcerative colitis and Crohn disease have been found with increased frequency in older adults. There are more and better drugs to treat these patients, acutely and to maintain remissions.
- Colonic ischemia is often underdiagnosed in older adults, is characterized by the sudden onset of abdominal pain and bleeding, and often is benign and reversible. Colonoscopy is the diagnostic procedure of choice.
- Colon cancers are a frequent but often preventable cause of death in men and women. The aggressive use of colonoscopy to detect premalignant polyps is the gold standard for prevention and should begin at age 50 years in those of normal risk.
- Lower gastrointestinal bleeding in older adults is usually associated with angiodysplasia and diverticulosis. Colonoscopy is the preferred diagnostic test, whereas scintigraphy and angiography are helpful if no source of bleeding is seen or if bleeding is so brisk as to exclude colonoscopy.

For a complete list of references, please visit www.expertconsult.com.

KEY REFERENCES

7. Harari D, Hosk J, Lowe D, et al: National audit of continence care: adherence to National Institute for Health and Clinical Excellence (NICE) Guidance in older versus younger adults. Age Ageing 43: 785–793, 2014.
16. Solan P, Davis B: Anorectal anatomy and imaging techniques. Gastroenterol Clin North Am 42:701–712, 2013.
20. Day LW, Bhuket T, Allison J: FIT testing: an overview. Curr Gastroenterol Rep 15:357, 2013.
24. Templeton AW, Strate LL: Updates in diverticular disease. Curr Gastroenterol Rep 15:339, 2013.
31. Feingold D, Steele SR, Lee S, et al: Practice parameters for the treatment of sigmoid diverticulitis. Dis Colon Rectum 57:284–294, 2014.
40. Oldfield EC, Oldfield EC, III, Johnson DA: Clinical update for the diagnosis and treatment of Clostridium difficile infection. World J Gastrointest Pharmacol Ther 5:1–26, 2014.
45. Khanna S, Pardi DS: Clostridium difficile infection: management strategies for a difficult disease. Therap Adv Gastroenterol 7:72–86, 2014.
72. Neisen OH, Ainsworth MA: Tumor necrosis factor inhibitors for inflammatory bowel disease. N Eng J Med 369:754–762, 2013.
74. Feagan BG, Rutgeerts P, Sands BE, et al, GEMINI 1 Study Group: Vedolizumab as induction and maintenance therapy for ulcerative colitis. N Engl J Med 369:699–710, 2013.
81. Castano-Milla C, Chapano M, Gisbert JP: Systemic review with meta-analysis: the declining risk of colorectal cancer in ulcerative colitis. Aliment Pharmacol Ther 39:645–659, 2014.
85. Ananthakrishnan AN, Cagan A, Gainer VS, et al: Normalization of plasma 25-hydroxy vitamin D is associated with reduced risk of surgery in Crohn's disease. Inflamm Bowel Dis 19:1921–1927, 2013.
87. Antunes O, Filippi J, Hébuterne X, et al: Treatment algorithms in Crohn's—up, down or something else? Best Pract Res Clin Gastroenterol 28:473–483, 2014.
96. Sands BE, Feagan BG, Rutgeerts P, et al: Effects of vedolizumab induction therapy for patients with Crohn's disease in whom tumor necrosis factor antagonist treatment failed. Gastroenterology 147: 618–627, 2014.
107. Gentile NM, Abdalla AA, Khanna S, et al: Outcomes of patients with microscopic colitis treated with corticosteroids: a population-based study. Am J Gastroenterol 108:256–259, 2013.
109. Baert F, Schmidt A, D'Haens G, et al: Budesonide in collagenous colitis: a double-blind, placebo-controlled trial with histological follow-up. Gastroenterology 122:20–25, 2002.
116. Tadros M, Majumder S, Birk JW: A review of ischemic colitis: is our clinical recognition and management adequate? Expert Rev Gastroenterol Hepatol 7:605–613, 2013.
122. Sgouras SN, Vlachogiannakos J, Vassiliadis K, et al: Effect of polyethylene glycol electrolyte-balanced solution on patients with acute colonic pseudo-obstruction after resolution of colonic dilation: a prospective randomized placebo controlled trial. Gut 55:638–642, 2006.
136. Levin B, Lieberman DA, McFarland B, et al: Screening and surveillance for the early detection of colorectal cancer and adenomatous polyps, 2008: a joint guideline from the American Cancer Society, the U.S. Multi-Society Task Force on Colorectal Cancer and the American College of Radiology. Gastroenterology 134:1570–1595, 2008.
140. Lee JK, Liles EG, Bent S, et al: Accuracy of fecal immunochemical tests for colorectal cancer: systematic review and meta-analysis. Ann Intern Med 4;160:171, 2014.
141. Shah R, Jones E, Vidart V, et al: Biomarkers for early detection of colorectal cancer and polyps: systematic review. Cancer Epidemiol Biomarkers Prev 23:1712–1728, 2014.
164. Sami SS, Al-Araji SA, Ragunath K: Review article: gastrointestinal angiodysplasia—pathogenesis, diagnosis and management. Aliment Pharmacol Ther 39:15–34, 2014.

79 Nutrition and Aging

C. Shanthi Johnson, Gordon Sacks

INTRODUCTION

In caring for the older adult population, the nutrition goals are to maintain or even improve their overall health and quality of life as well as to prevent and/or treat age- and nutrition-related problems by improving the nutritional status of individuals and population groups. Whether defined as "the condition of a population's or individual's health as affected by the intake and utilization of nutrients and non-nutrients"[1] or as the degree of balance between nutrient intake and nutrient requirements, nutritional status is extremely important to overall health and to maintaining optimal nutritional status. Not only is optimal nutritional status fundamental to overall health and well-being as people grow older, but it has been shown to influence the aging process, various physiologic systems and functions, body composition, and the onset and management of various chronic conditions. The process of aging also affects nutritional status. Specifically, the aging process has been shown to directly contribute to the changes in nutritional needs with requirements of various nutrients decreasing, increasing, or remaining the same.[2] With aging, changes in economic and social status arise that contribute to decreased access to food, poor food choices, nutrient deficiencies, and poor nutritional status, which in turn lead to increased risk of illness, poor health, and limited mobility and independence, as illustrated in Figure 79-1.[3]

In addition, the nutrition and health status of individuals and populations are influenced by social determinants such as income, educational level, social support, gender, culture, and other factors outlined in the population health framework.[4] These factors partly account for the wide and stubbornly resistant disparities in nutritional and health status that exist in populations. For example, research in the area of food costing shows that seniors living alone are not able to afford nutritious diets.[5] A study investigating supplement use among older adults showed that the consumption of vitamin and mineral supplements was higher among those with higher levels of education.[6] Furthermore, seniors who live alone and lack social support tend to be at greater nutritional risk compared to older individuals with social support.[7]

NUTRITION SCREENING AND ASSESSMENT

There are many physiologic factors that impact the nutritional status and well-being of older adults. An inadequate or excess intake of nutrients is the result of ingestion and utilization of nutrients from a variety of dietary sources, as well as other various elements (e.g., age-related changes, medication intake, socioeconomic factors, and functional and cognitive capacity). These factors facilitate the depletion or storage of tissue stores and changes in plasma nutrient levels, enzymatic activity, and other physiologic functions, which affect anthropometric indicators (e.g., weight, body composition). As a result, anthropometric measures, as well as biochemical, clinical, and dietary factors are critical and must be considered in the assessment of an individual's nutritional status.

Anthropometric measures are used to assess nutritional status through the examination of body proportions and composition, as well as the fluctuations in these indicators over time, and include body weight, weight history, height or other estimates of stature, body mass index (BMI), skinfold thickness, and circumference.[8,9] Self-reported measures are often inaccurate, and standardized measurement protocols should be adopted by trained technicians to reduce measurement error.[10,11] Body weight is a key indicator in nutritional status, and one's weight history serves as an indicator of nutritional risk. Periods of excessive or significant weight loss include 2% body weight in a week, 5% in a month, 7.5% in 3 months, or 10% in 6 months. In addition to weight changes, height changes, which are largely due to compression of the spine, are reliable indicators of an at-risk individual. If unable to stand or stand straight, estimates of stature can be estimated via arm span, demi-span, or knee height. Arm span measurements can determine the maximal height in adulthood rather than one's actual height, while age-, gender-, and race-specific equations are used to estimate stature from knee height measures[12] with supine knee height valued as more reliable than seated knee height. Once height and weight measures are obtained, BMI can be calculated. Body weight (kg) is divided by height squared (m), which evaluates weight independent of height but does not directly measure body fat. For older adults, a BMI of less than 24 is associated with poor nutritional health, a BMI between 24 and 29 is believed to be a healthy weight, and a BMI of over 29 is seen as overweight and may lead to health problems.[13] Skinfold thickness measurements are used to determine body fatness. However, in older adults, skin changes in thickness, elasticity, and compressibility and skinfold thickness measurements are not reliable measurements. Body fat stores can be assessed through circumference measurements (e.g., waist, waist-to-hip ratio, and upper arm circumference), much like measures that are used to estimate skeletal muscle mass (somatic protein stores). Body fat measurement can be used as a quick screening tool to pinpoint high-risk individuals who may be susceptible to under- or over-nutrition and are useful alone or combined with height and weight measurements.

Another useful measure for individuals at risk for nutritional problems is *biochemical markers*, which can be used to find subclinical deficiencies (e.g., through blood or urine specimens). Through such tests, biochemical markers of visceral protein status can be substantiated; these markers include serum albumin, thyroxine-binding prealbumin, serum transferrin, and retinol-binding protein as well as total lymphocyte counts. Although serum albumin is a commonly used marker because it can predict mortality in older adults, it is not always reliable. Values can be elevated as a result of dehydration, or values can decline because of inflammation, infection, and age-related degeneration of muscle mass. Other biochemical measures such as total cholesterol, high-density lipoprotein, low-density lipoprotein, and triglycerides are used to assess lipid status and are also used to measure micronutrient status (e.g., iron status). Low total cholesterol is associated with poor nutritional status and may be a predictor of mortality in older adults. Hematologic assessments can also be used to screen for malnutrition in older adults and include hemoglobin, hematocrit, mean cell volume, mean cell hemoglobin concentration, mean cell hemoglobin, and total iron binding capacity. A combination of these measures is used for a proper clinical diagnosis and can be compared to normative age and gender group values.

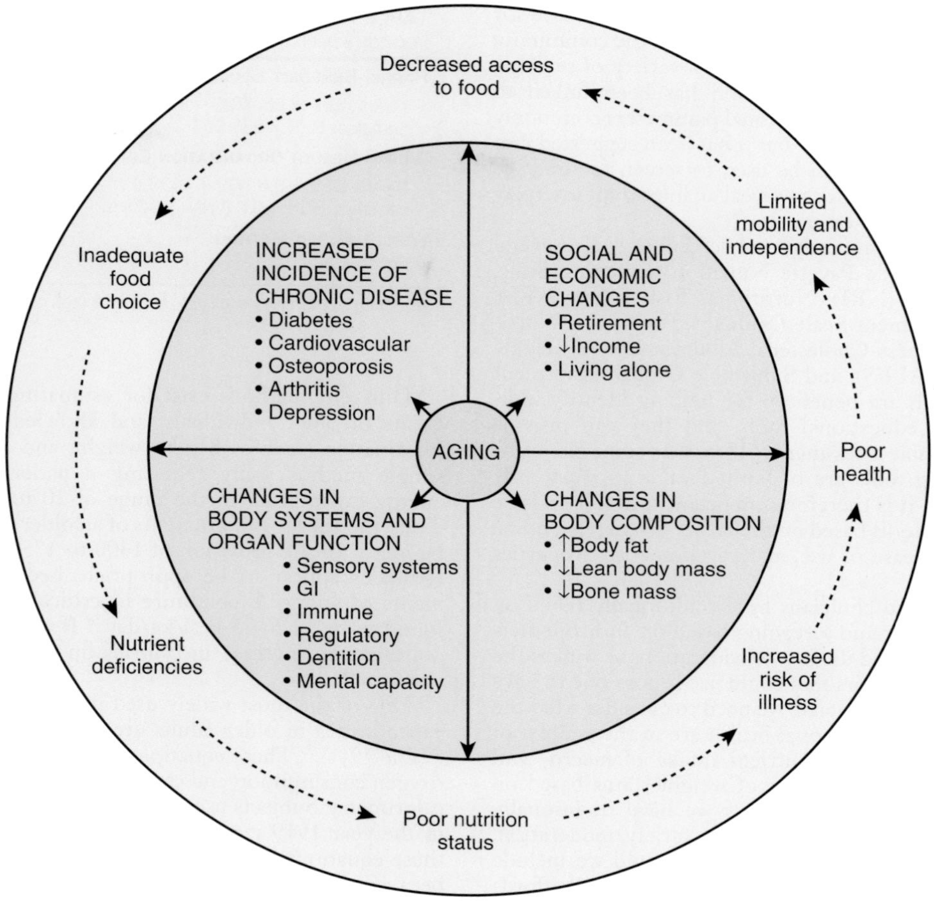

Figure 79-1. Aging cycle showing the changes in economic and social status that contribute to decreased access to food, poor food choices, nutrient deficiencies, and poor nutritional status, which in turn lead to increased risk of illness, poor health, and limited mobility and independence.

Clinical indicators are also used to assess nutritional status. The components of clinical assessment can include medical history and physical signs and symptoms associated with nutritional deficiencies, functional status, and cognitive status. Some clinical signs and symptoms are nonspecific and attributed to the aging process rather than to a particular nutritional deficiency. Functional status can be assessed in several different ways. Most commonly various tools are used to assess the person's abilities to perform basic activities of daily living (ADLs), which include basic self-care such as bathing, grooming, dressing, feeding, and toileting, and instrumental activities of daily living (IADLs), which include cooking, shopping, housekeeping, and managing one's own affairs. These can serve as clinical indicators useful in the assessment of nutritional status. The inability to execute such tasks may indicate a higher risk of poor nutrition, although some clinical signs may be nonspecific and attributed to aging rather than to a specific deficiency. Clinical assessment can include physical signs and symptoms affiliated not only with nutritional deficits but also with functional and cognitive status. Both functional and cognitive status can be assessed in multiple ways.

Dietary assessment is an integral component in the measurement of nutritional status allowing the evaluation of foods consumed and eating patterns. Dietary assessment methods can be categorized as retrospective or prospective. A retrospective assessment involves the recall of all foods and fluids consumed in a particular time frame (often 24 hours). Retrospective assessment can be unreliable if the individual has problems with his or her cognitive status. In this case, a prospective assessment may be favored, as this involves keeping a written record of all foods and fluids consumed in a given period of time (e.g., 3 days [including 2 weekdays and a weekend day] or 7 days). Although this type of assessment aids those with cognitive challenges, it poses a problem for individuals who suffer from a particular functional disability, such as arthritis of the hand or poor vision. A 3-day food record with intakes of 2 weekdays and 1 weekend day recorded is considered to be one of the better dietary assessment methods because it does not depend on memory and can provide detailed intake data, although no single best method exists.

Given that a comprehensive assessment of nutritional status is complex and time consuming, rapid screening is beneficial to identify those who might at risk for poor nutrition and individuals who might need in-depth assessment. Several screening tools exist. The DETERMINE checklist developed as part of the Nutrition Screening Initiative provides public awareness about basic nutrition information and can help identify individuals at risk for poor nutrition in community settings. The checklist is widely used in the United States[14] and is executed in two stages or levels. Level I can include assessments of body weight, eating habits, living environment, and functional status (particularly ADLs and IADLs) and is usually filled out by the individual's primary caregiver.[15] The level II screen can include anthropometric measurements, laboratory data, polypharmacy, and cognitive status assessments. Based on the assessment, a specific nutritional care plan or support is provided. In Canada, a screening tool titled Seniors in the Community: A Risk Evaluation Tool for Eating and Nutrition Version II (SCREEN II) has been developed for assessing nutritional risk among community-dwelling seniors.[16]

The Mini Nutritional Assessment (MNA) is also widely used for initial screening and assessment for individuals in the community as well as in long-term care settings.[17,18] In a variety of settings, using different instruments, malnutrition has been linked to frailty.[19,20] Indeed, not only are nutritional parameters commonly used in frailty assessment tools,[21,22] but it has been suggested that a short version of the MNA can be used to screen for frailty.[23] Still, comprehensive assessment can reveal an important interplay of other factors, including medications.[24]

In addition to these commonly used screening tools, several others exist. These include Payette Nutrition Screening Scale, Nutritional Risk Index (NRI), Nutritional Risk Score (NRS), Nutritional Risk Assessment Scale (NuRAS), Prognostic Nutritional Index (PNI), Sadness-Cholesterol-Albumin-Loss of weight-Eating-Shopping (SCALES), and Subjective Global Assessment (SGA). Screening tools are beneficial for helping identify individuals at risk or as educational tools, and they can provide simple, rapid, and reliable assessment.[25] However, some clinicians suggest that screening tools are of limited value in apparently healthy older adults.[26] It is therefore important to select and use appropriate screening tools based on the target group (e.g., home care, long-term care), ease of use, and psychometric properties (validity/reliability).

While researchers and clinicians have traditionally relied on the nutritional assessment and screening based on anthropometric, biochemical, clinical and dietary considerations as well as the presence of various risk factors that could predispose one to have less than optimal nutritional intake, we need to consider what the appropriate indicators of nutritional health are in the context of the aging population. Is it the nutrient intake of macro- and micronutrients or BMI (an indicator of weight status based on the proportion of weight for height) as we have traditionally measured, or should we pay attention to the variety, moderation, and balance in food group consumption, or should we include indicators of food security such as availability, access, and affordability of nutritious diet? How do we measure availability and access to traditional diet and the quality and safety of traditional foods or cultural foods for minority populations? There is a considerable need for identifying appropriate indicators of nutritional health among the aging population.

NUTRITIONAL REQUIREMENTS

The physiologic, functional, and overall health changes that accompany aging affect the requirements for some nutrients and how nutrient needs should be met. Therefore, determination of a person's nutritional requirements is critical in order to ensure optimal nutrient intake is provided. Reduction in energy requirements is one notable difference between individuals older than 65 years of age and their younger counterparts.[27] For example, it is estimated that total daily energy expenditure decreases approximately by 10 kcal/yr for men and 7 kcal/yr for women aged 30 years and older.[28] Therefore, a man who needs 2200 kcal at age 20 requires only 1700 kcal/day at age 70. In older adults, the decrease in energy needs is largely attributed to the age-related reduction in resting metabolic rate, reduced lean body mass, and decreased physical activity level.[29-31] Yet, other problems, including chewing and swallowing difficulties, living alone, and low income contribute to a decline of energy intake in older adults. Whereas total energy intake significantly increased in the U.S. older adult population from 1977 to 2010, average energy intake decreased with increasing age, with adults older than 75 years having the lowest energy intake for all years.[32] The third National Health and Nutrition Examination Survey (NHANES III, 1988-1991) reported that women and men aged 60 to 69 years and 70 to 79 years consumed an average of 534 kcal/day and 658 kcal/day less than women and men aged 30 to 39 years, respectively.[33]

TABLE 79-1 Formulas for Estimating Energy Requirements of Older Persons (kcal/day)

HARRIS-BENEDICT EQUATIONS	
	Males: BEE = 66.4730 + 13.7516 (Wt) + 5.003 (Ht) − 6.7550 (A)
	Females: BEE = 655.0955 + 9.5634 (Wt) + 1.8496 (Ht) − 4.6756 (A)
WORLD HEALTH ORGANIZATION EQUATIONS	
	Males: BEE = 8.8 (Wt) + 1128 (Ht) − 1071
	Females: BEE = 9.2 (Wt) + 637 (Ht) − 302
WEIGHT-BASED METHOD	
	20-25 (Wt)

A, Age (yr); *Ht*, height (cm); *Wt*, weight (kg).

Different methods exist for estimating the energy requirements of older individuals, and knowledge of patient-specific information (such as height, weight, and age) is required. One simple method, only requiring a patient's weight, estimates energy expenditure in the range of 20 to 25 total kcal/kg/day. Thus, the energy requirements of an older 70-kg individual could be met with the provision of 1400 to 1750 total kcal/day. These estimates appear to be appropriate because indirect measurements of energy expenditure in critically ill older adults were found to be 22 to 25 kcal/kg/day.[34] If weight gain is the desired objective, an increase in calories up to 30 kcal/kg/day may be warranted.

One of the most widely used methods for predicting energy expenditures in older adults are the Harris-Benedict equations (Table 79-1).[35] These equations are based on the measurement of oxygen consumption and carbon dioxide production using direct calorimetry. Subjects used in the development of these equations in the year 1919 ranged in age from 15 to 74 years. However, these equations are often considered inaccurate for older adults because only 9 of the 239 healthy male and female subjects of the population measured were older than 60 years. Some consider equations established by the World Health Organization for people older than 60 years to be more precise than Harris-Benedict equations (see Table 79-1). Recommendations from the National Research Council include multiplying the calculated energy expenditure by coefficients accounting for various levels of physical activity.[36] An activity coefficient 1 to 1.12 times the energy expenditure is used for older adults who are sedentary or fairly inactive. Activity coefficients of 1.27 to 1.45 should be used to account for energy expended by older adults with highly active lifestyles.

Despite the decline of energy requirements with increasing age, it is important that older adults meet intake of protein, fat, and carbohydrate that falls within the acceptable macronutrient distribution range. For protein, this corresponds to between 10% and 35% of total energy intake. Traditionally, guidelines for dietary protein intake have recommended 0.8 g/kg of body weight in order to maintain protein equilibrium and avoid loss of lean body mass for all adults, regardless of age. However, evidence suggests as much as 1.0 to 1.2 g of protein/kg of body weight is required to meet the needs of healthy older adults.[36,37] The increased intake is necessary, in part because of decreased lean body mass, changes in metabolism, changes in body composition, and protein utilization efficiency associated with aging. In addition, protein needs for older adults may reach 1.2 to 1.5 g/kg body weight for those with acute or chronic diseases and as much as 2.0 g/kg body weight for those with severe infections, surgery, or trauma.[36] Geriatric patients generally tolerate moderately high protein intakes without deterioration in renal function. However, those patients with existing renal disease should avoid high-protein diets as they may hasten a greater decline in renal function.[38] Sarcopenia is used to describe the age-associated loss in skeletal muscle and its functional consequences.[39] While the role of dietary protein in the causes and prevention of sarcopenia is unclear, the loss of muscle mass has been linked to sedentary lifestyles, neurogenic processes, and dietary protein deficiencies. There is no consensus on the recommended daily protein intake to enhance muscle protein anabolism and minimize the loss of muscle mass with age. Overall, dietary data from the United States and Canada show protein intakes decline with increasing age. Therefore, intake of high-quality protein sources, such as fish, lean meat, dairy products, eggs, and legumes are recommended at each meal throughout the day.[40,41]

Another key factor in maintaining healthy nutritional status is an appropriate intake of dietary fat. Fats contain twice as many calories per gram as carbohydrates or proteins, and given the fact that higher intakes of dietary fat are associated with an increased risk of developing diabetes, heart disease, and other chronic ailments, it is recommended that lower fat choices such as skim milk, rather than whole milk, are made by older adults. Ideally, total fat intake should fall within 20% to 35% of total daily energy intake; however, if an older adult is unable to consume enough of his or her daily energy requirement, the risks associated with a higher fat intake may be overlooked in favor of meeting the necessary daily energy requirement.

According to the dietary reference intakes (DRI) recommendations developed by the Institute of Medicine, older adults should acquire 45% to 65% of their daily energy intake from complex carbohydrates, such as whole grains, vegetables, and fruits. Dietary fiber requirements decrease for older adults because of overall decreased energy intake. After age 50, 30 g/day for men and 21 g/day for women is needed to improve gastric motility, maintain healthy blood glucose levels, and reduce cholesterol.[28] Along with these fiber requirements, fluid intake must be optimal to ensure regular gastrointestinal motility.

To maintain a healthy nutritional diet and nutritional status, one must maintain an opportune intake of micronutrients, specifically vitamins and minerals, as one ages. Since energy needs decrease, while some vitamin and mineral needs increase, the challenge of maintaining optimal intake for older adults is vital. According to the DRI recommendations, older adults need more calcium, vitamin D, and vitamin B_6 as they age. For example, 1200 mg/day of calcium for women older than 50 years and men older than 70 is essential to protect against decreased absorption of calcium and bone loss. Similarly, the DRI indicates that vitamin D needs increase from 600 IU for individuals aged 19 to 70 to 800 IU for those older than age 70. Hypovitaminosis D is currently a significant problem among older adults. An age-related decline in vitamin D intake is correlated with lower dietary intakes, usually due to limited consumption of milk, which is fortified with vitamin D. Decreased vitamin D intake in older adults is also related to less sun exposure, less efficient skin synthesis of vitamin D, and impaired kidney function, which in turn impairs the conversion of vitamin D from its inactive to active form, thus causing deficiency. Insufficient levels of vitamin B_6, in addition to folate and vitamin B_{12}, are known to contribute higher than normal levels of serum homocysteine, a known risk factor in the development of coronary artery disease, stroke, and depression, as well as a decrease in cognitive function. Individuals older than 50 years need to consume more vitamin B_6 to reduce homocysteine levels and optimize cognitive functioning.[42] Also, older adults may need to rely on supplements to avoid the malabsorption of food-bound B_{12}, since as many as 30% of older adults are deficient in vitamin B_{12} daily.

Water is often overlooked as an essential nutrient, and inadequate hydration poses an additional risk for increased morbidity and mortality in older adults. Age-related decline in intracellular water and fluid reserves, paired with changes in renal function (causing an inability to concentrate urine), can result in difficulty maintaining appropriate fluid levels in older adults. Not only do these physiologic factors impair fluid levels, but altered thirst perception, cognitive impairment, and changes in functional status (such as restricted mobility) can result in reduced fluid intake.[43] External factors, such as adverse effects of medication use, may also contribute to more impediments to balanced fluid intakes. Residents of long-term care facilities are especially at risk for dehydration because of their limited access to oral fluids or underlying conditions (vomiting, diarrhea, colostomy/ileostomy) that increase fluid losses. Institutional issues, including inadequate staffing and a subsequent need for better supervision, places frail older adults at greater risk.[44] Untreated dehydration in hospitalized older adults can result in a mortality rate exceeding 50%.[45] As a result, specific triggers are used by staff at long-term care facilities to detect inadequate hydration (Table 79-2). As such, older adults should make a conscious effort to increase fluid intake and not just rely on thirst perceptions. The adequate intake of fluid is the same for older and younger adults.[46] A water intake of 1 mL/calorie ingested or 30 mL/kg/day with a minimum of 1500 mL/day is generally recommended to meet dietary water requirements and achieve adequate fluid intake in older adults.[47,48]

TABLE 79-2 Risk Factors for Dehydration Among Residents of Long-Term Care Facilities

Deterioration in cognitive status in the last 90 days
Failure to eat or take medication
Diarrhea
Fever
Swallowing problems
Communication problems

Modified from Weinberg AD, Minaker KL, Council on Scientific Affairs, American Medical Association: Dehydration: evaluation and management in older adults. JAMA 274:1552-1556, 1995.

In accordance with Canada's Food Guide to Healthy Eating, dietary guidelines have been created to help avoid energy, vitamin, and mineral deficiencies in the older population by encouraging older adults to meet their needs by choosing from healthy, nutrient-dense dietary sources from all four food groups. The 2010 Dietary Guidelines for Americans and recommendations from MyPlate for Older Adults include limiting foods high in trans and saturated fats, salt, and added sugars and emphasizing whole grains, low-fat dairy products, and bright-colored vegetables and fruit. It also highlights topics such as adequate fluid intake; convenient, affordable, and readily available foods; and physical activity for older adults.

COMMON NUTRITIONAL PROBLEMS AND DEFICIENCIES

Imbalance between nutrient intake and nutrient requirements or less than optimal nutritional status can result from less than optimal dietary intake, age-related changes, disease conditions and their treatment, and/or other contextual factors such as cultural and religious beliefs, practices, and socioeconomic conditions. This imbalance can result in nutrition-related problems and deficiencies among older adults. The most common nutritional deficiencies include malnutrition, which encompasses both under- and overnutrition; micronutrient deficiencies; and dehydration. Malnutrition is very common in older adults and can be divided into protein energy malnutrition and micronutrient deficiency. Whether the imbalance is a result of poor dietary intake, age-related changes, disease conditions and treatments, or other factors such as cultural or religious beliefs, practices, or socioeconomic issues, malnutrition varies in its prevalence.[49] Protein energy undernutrition varies from 1% to 15% in the community to 25% to 85% in long-term care facilities.[50] It is important to recognize that undernutrition is not simply a result of poor dietary intake but is the combination of many factors that interrupt the balance between intake and need. Cognitive decline or dementia, depression, chronic disease, and/or functional deficits are also factors in undernutrition. These are common in individuals suffering from sarcopenia (loss in skeletal muscle and its functional consequences as one ages) and geriatric failure to thrive (GFTT). GFTT is a syndrome in which individuals have involuntary weight loss and fail to maintain functional capacity, social skills, and cognitive skills with no immediately apparent cause. Although the exact prevalence of GFTT is unknown, the incidences increase with age, and it is more common in men and those living in long-term care facilities. In both cases, nutritional interventions and the use of an interdisciplinary team approach have been successful through an increase of energy and protein intake through both dietary sources and oral supplements.[51] Other interventions such as exercise programs have also been beneficial to prevent sarcopenia.

Micronutrient deficiencies among older adults occur when calcium, vitamin D, iron, vitamin B_{12}, and other minerals or vitamins are lacking. Such deficiencies are very common and can be easily remedied through the use of supplements. Vitamin D deficiency is widespread among all age groups but is especially high in older adults.[52,53] Since vitamin D is necessary for calcium absorption, a deficiency contributes to osteoporosis and related fractures among older adults. Recommendations for vitamin D are 600 IU for individuals aged 51 to 70 and 800 IU for those older than 70. These amounts are difficult to obtain from the food alone; therefore, Canada's Food Guide recommends that all adults older than 50 years take a supplement of 400 IU per day. Vitamin D deficiency is also associated with increased risk of certain cancers, such as breast, colon, ovarian, and prostate cancer, particularly among populations living at higher latitudes. Whereas vitamin D has been shown to play a role in maintaining healthy cells and discouraging cancerous cell development, the use of supplements to prevent cancer is unclear. Calcium also plays an important role in maintaining bone health in older adults. The DRI for women 51 years and older and men older than 70 is 1,200 mg/day, with the maximal dose of elemental calcium not to exceed 500 mg at any one time.[54] Similar to vitamin D, adequate intake of calcium is difficult to achieve from food alone; therefore, supplements are often needed. Calcium carbonate is the most cost-effective form of calcium supplement, well absorbed, and tolerated by most individuals when consumed with a meal. Of note, calcium citrate is the preferred form to be used in older adults with intestinal absorption problems, such as achlorhydria or inflammatory bowel disease.[55] Noteworthy changes in B vitamin status occur with advancing age. Vitamin B_{12} deficiency is a concern for older adults; it results from low stomach acid, which limits release of food-bound B_{12} and thus absorption. The Institute of Medicine recommends that individuals older than 50 years meet the DRI by consuming fortified foods or taking a supplement containing vitamin B_{12}. Toxicity of fat-soluble vitamins, such as vitamin A, is a concern in older adults because of increased liver stores and declining renal function associated with increasing age. Osteoporosis and hip fracture are associated with vitamin A intakes that are only twice the current recommended daily intake of 1000 μg retinol equivalents (RE)/day in males and 800 μg RE/day in females.[56] Thus, caregivers of older adults who take vitamin supplements should understand the risks and effects that chronic high intakes of vitamin A may have on bone loss.

The prevalence of obesity has steadily increased over the past three decades. Obesity is generally defined as an unhealthy excess of body fat characterized as a BMI of 30 kg/m^2 or higher. In the United States, nearly 41% of adults 65 to 74 years of age are obese, with incidence dropping to just below 28% for those 75 years of age and older. In 2004, nearly 30% of Canadians aged 55 to 64 were obese, compared to only 20% in 1978.[57,58] This is problematic as higher risks of mortality and other serious medical complications, including type 2 diabetes, hypertension, arthritis, obstructive sleep apnea, urinary incontinence, and cancer, are associated with older men and women who have a BMI of 30 kg/m^2 or higher. The current treatment guidelines for weight management in older persons are lifestyle intervention involving diet, behavior modification with physical activity, and pharmacotherapy.[59] Older adults need to consume a diet rich in nutrient-dense food but not too high in energy. Regular physical activity in the form of stretching, aerobic exercise, and resistance training is important to increase flexibility, strength, and endurance while preventing frailty. Experience with weight-loss medications is limited; however, orlistat appears to be the safest for older individuals. Bariatric surgery is reserved for selected individuals who fail diet and medication therapy and continue to suffer from disabling obesity. The perceived benefits of the procedure in terms of quality of life must be weighed in light of the postoperative morbidity and risk of potential complications.

NUTRITIONAL STRATEGIES

Several strategies can be used to increase dietary intake of the frail older person. High nutrient–dense food can be incorporated into the diet if the individual tolerates traditional solid foods. Peanut butter spread on whole wheat bread, enriched cereal, or powdered instant breakfast products can be substituted at breakfast to increase caloric intake. High-protein and high-calorie snacks, in the form of crackers and cheese, milkshakes, and sandwiches, can be given throughout the day to supplement oral intake.[42] Dietary adjustments and special utensils are often beneficial when physical or neurologic disorders contribute to poor oral consumption. Institutionalized residents often require assistance with eating and drinking.[60] Use of semicircular tables is a simple method to assist understaffed caregivers in feeding several residents at a time in long-term care facilities. Modified spoons have been used to decrease spillage by older adults afflicted with hand tremors. Changes in food texture, such as puréed vegetables or puddings, can prevent intake problems in patients with poor dentition. Patients with swallowing dysfunction should be taught appropriate eating positions and safe swallowing techniques in order to minimize dysphagia.

Enteral nutrition (EN) delivered through a feeding tube is initiated when older patients are unable to maintain adequate nutrient and fluid intake by oral ingestion. Small-bore gastric or duodenal tubes may be placed through the nose to provide short-term (i.e., a few weeks) enteral access to treat older adult patients admitted to a geriatric recuperative care and rehabilitation unit after hip or knee surgery, patients with pressure ulcers, or those with temporary swallowing disorders. Chronic disorders such as head/neck cancer, stroke, head injuries, or neuromuscular disorders impairing the ability to swallow would necessitate placement of a long-term (months to years) enteral access device. Long-term enteral access is achieved with gastric tubes that are inserted directly into the stomach by a surgeon in an operating room or by a gastroenterologist at the bedside. Percutaneous endoscopic gastrostomy (PEG) tubes placed with an endoscope are becoming more common than open surgical gastrostomy tubes since the expense and risks associated with an invasive surgical procedure can be avoided. If gastroparesis or an anatomic defect is present that prevents normal gastric emptying, a feeding tube placed in the jejunum is most appropriate to reduce the risk of aspirating EN into the lungs.

Complications of EN include pulmonary aspiration, diarrhea, and mechanical obstruction of the feeding tube. Aspiration of EN remains one of the most dangerous complications of EN administration. Mortality rates from aspiration of gastric contents range from 40% to 90%.[61] Recommendations for reducing the risk of aspiration in older individuals receiving gastric feedings include elevating the head of the bed higher than 30 degrees and frequent exams for abdominal distention. Among bedridden PEG-fed patients, low-fat elemental diets are associated with more rapid gastric emptying and fewer aspiration occurrences compared with standard EN formulations.[62] EN is often identified as a cause of diarrhea, despite numerous other factors such as medications, hyperosmolar EN formulations, hypoalbuminemia, and infection. Sorbitol is used as a vehicle for many liquid formulations of pharmacologic agents and has been associated with diarrhea. Antibiotics or prokinetic agents such as metoclopramide are examples of concurrent therapies more likely to cause diarrhea than the EN formulation. *Clostridium difficile* is a well-known cause of diarrhea in patients receiving EN and should be ruled out before antidiarrheal agents are initiated.

Geriatric patients who require nutrition support but do not have functional or accessible gastrointestinal tracts are candidates for parenteral nutrition (PN). This may include patients with severe inflammatory bowel disease (e.g., Crohn disease or ulcerative colitis), malabsorption (e.g., celiac sprue), bowel obstruction, a history of extensive bowel surgery (e.g., short bowel syndrome), and severe acute pancreatitis when EN has failed. The primary goal of PN should be to prevent undernutrition from inadequate energy and nutrient intake or to treat undernutrition and its complications. The American Society for Parenteral and Enteral Nutrition (ASPEN) and the European Society for Parenteral and Enteral Nutrition (ESPEN) have published guidelines for appropriate use of PN in older adults.[63,64] Table 79-3 lists some monitoring guidelines for fluid, electrolyte, and micronutrient abnormalities that should be performed in geriatric patients during PN administration.

TABLE 79-3 Complications of Parenteral Nutrition and Management Techniques

Complication	Management
MECHANICAL	
Pneumothorax	Possible chest tube placement; minimize number of catheter insertions; placement by experienced personnel
Air embolism	Placement by experienced personnel
Catheter occlusion	Anticoagulation locally with urokinase or streptokinase; routine line flushing
Venous thrombosis	Anticoagulation; catheter removal
METABOLIC	
Hyperglycemia	Slowly initiate parenteral nutrition (PN); check blood glucose frequently before advancing nutrition; administer insulin if needed
Hypoglycemia	Decrease amount of insulin administered; avoid abrupt discontinuation of PN by tapering rate of infusion; administer 10% dextrose if PN is abruptly discontinued
Hypertriglyceridemia	Decrease lipid volume administered; increase length of infusion time; avoid lipid administration >60% of total calories; assess risk factors for hypertriglyceridemia
Electrolyte disturbance	Monitor fluid intake and output and serum chemistries; replace electrolytes as necessary
Essential fatty acid deficiency	Provide 8% to 10% of total calories as lipid
Prerenal azotemia	Increase fluid intake; decrease protein administered; increase nonprotein calories; analyze nitrogen balance
GASTROINTESTINAL	
Cholestasis	Avoid overfeeding; use gastrointestinal (GI) tract as soon as clinically able
Gastrointestinal atrophy	Use GI tract as soon as clinically able
INFECTIOUS	
Catheter-related sepsis	Remove catheter and place at alternate site; adequately care for catheter site; possible treatment with intravenous antibiotics

NUTRITION PROGRAMS AND SERVICES

Many services are available to support the nutritional and health needs of older adults; these services include meal delivery programs, community meals, grocery delivery service, food banks and food stamps, and nutrition screening and education initiatives. In-home programs such as the Elderly Nutrition Program (ENP) in the United States mandated through the Older Americans Act provides in-home and community-based nutrition services to individuals older than 60 years and targets those at the highest economic and social need.[65] ENP offers meal delivery services, congregate meals, and nutrition screening and assessment. Although a program such as ENP is not available in Canada, a similar array of services are provided for by for-profit and not-for-profit organizations. Despite the benefits of such programs, barriers to achieving optimal outcomes with home-delivered meals still exist; these barriers include inadequate resources, waiting lists, and difficulty with completing food deliveries to rural areas.[66]

Many *meal delivery services* in Canada, such as the Meals on Wheels program, offer meals for older adult Canadians for a nominal fee, and many church groups and for-profit and not-for-profit organizations offer similar programs for those who have difficulty preparing meals for themselves, which places them in a high-risk category. These meal delivery services provide one hot meal, usually lunch, to people's homes at least 5 days a week. Frozen meals are also available to older adults on request. The delivered meal is required to meet one third of the daily nutritional requirement. However, for frail, largely homebound older adults, one meal is insufficient to meet their nutritional needs and prevent nutritional deficiencies. This type of meal delivery service has shown benefit to seniors, who have difficulty preparing meals for themselves and are at risk for poor nutrition. A recent study examining the impact of home-delivered breakfast and lunch showed significant improvement in nutritional intake and quality of life among frail homebound older adults.[67] Targeted nutrition counseling may further extend benefits. After hospital discharge, 12 weeks of follow-up home visits by registered dietitians demonstrated a positive effect on change in weight, energy intake, and protein intake, as well as mobility status in geriatric medical patients.[68]

Congregate and community meals offered by churches and other community-based organizations not only assist older adults by providing them with balanced meals but also function as social events that many seniors would otherwise not experience. The community meals can be served as breakfast, lunch, or dinner, and their frequency ranges from once a week to once a month. Economic need can be offset through the use of *food stamps and/or food banks* on a short-term basis. The selection of foods offered in food banks primarily includes dry goods and nonperishable food items. Some food banks in Canada have facilities for refrigeration and offer selected perishable foods. For accessing these services, a rent receipt, identification, and proof of income may be required. *Community kitchens* allow small groups of individuals to pool resources and cook meals together that are later taken home, thus saving money and creating social time for older individuals. If mobility is an issue, *grocery delivery services* are available for a fee and can be accessed via telephone or the Internet. Lastly, *nutrition screening and education programs* are offered through government agencies such as the ENP, which uses the DETERMINE checklist to aid seniors with nutritional risk assessments. Other lectures and community nutrition education programs are also offered for older adults.

ETHICAL CONSIDERATIONS

A controversial issue that arises with the care of older adults is the withdrawal of nutrition when death is imminent (e.g., within 6 months). Although families may decide to discontinue life-sustaining medical treatment such as mechanical ventilation or dialysis, nutrition and hydration are often considered a basic human right. Most health care professionals agree that the wishes of the individual is the most important factor that should be considered in the development of a nutritional care plan.[69] Thus, most health care teams consider it ethical and acceptable for a competent individual to refuse or halt administration of artificial nutrition. If an individual is considered incompetent, caregivers should provide family members the support needed to facilitate a thoughtful decision with the individual's quality of life taken into consideration. The American Geriatrics Society does not recommend the placement of feeding tubes for EN when eating difficulties arise in older adults with advanced dementia.[70] A common misperception is that EN can increase survival and prevent new episodes of aspiration. On the contrary, a Cochrane review found no evidence of prolonged life or reduced risk of aspiration pneumonia in patients with dementia.[71] Communication among all parties involved (health care personnel, patients, family, friends, guardian) is paramount in making informed decisions concerning the delivery of artificial nutrition and end-of-life issues. Providing hydration solely without EN or PN is an appropriate alternative as patients do not suffer from signs of dehydration. Additional information concerning ethical issues in nutrition support of severely disabled older adults can be found in the cited reference.[72]

KEY POINTS

- Nutritional status influences the aging process and has been linked to frailty.
- Body weight is a key indicator of nutritional status and, especially, of nutritional risk.
- A full nutritional screen overlaps with comprehensive geriatric assessment.
- The total daily energy expenditure decreases approximately by 10 kcal/yr for men and 7 kcal/yr for women older than 30 years.
- Absorption of some nutrients (calcium, iron) and vitamins (D, B_{12}) declines with age, making supplementation often necessary.

For a complete list of references, please visit www.expertconsult.com.

KEY REFERENCES

7. Ramage-Morin PL, Garriguet D: Nutritional risk among older Canadians. Health Rep 24:3–13, 2013.
18. Vellas B, Villars H, Abellan G, et al: Overview of the MNA–its history and challenges. J Nutr Health Aging 10:456–463, 2006.
19. Bollwein J, Diekmann R, Kaiser MJ, et al: Dietary quality is related to frailty in community-dwelling older adults. J Gerontol A Biol Sci Med Sci 68:483–489, 2013.
32. Johnston R, Poti JM, Popkin BM, et al: Eating and aging: trends in dietary intake among older Americans from 1977-2010. J Nutr Health Aging 18:234–242, 2014.
41. Health Canada: Do Canadian adults meet their nutrient requirements through food intake alone? 2012. http://www.hc-sc.gc.ca/fn-an/surveill/nutrition/commun/art-nutr-adult-eng.php. Accessed November 3, 2014.
64. Sobotka L, Schneider SM, Berner YN, et al: ESPEN guidelines on parenteral nutrition: geriatrics. Clin Nutr 28:461–466, 2009.
65. Millen BE, Ohls JC, Ponza M, et al: The Elderly Nutrition Program: an effective national framework for preventive nutrition interventions. J Am Diet Assoc 102:234–240, 2002.
69. Barrocas A, Yarbrough G, Becnel PA: Ethical and legal issues in nutrition support of the geriatric patient: the can, should, and must of nutrition support. Nutr Clin Prac 18:37–47, 2003.
70. American Geriatrics Society Ethics Committee, Clinical Practice and Models of Care Committee: American Geriatrics Society feeding tubes in advanced dementia position statement. J Am Geriatr Soc 62:1590–1593, 2014.
71. Sampson EL, Candy B, Jones L: Enteral tube feeding for older people with advanced dementia. Cochrane Database Syst Rev (2):CD007209, 2009.
72. Monod S, Chiolero R, Büla C, et al: Ethical issues in nutrition support of severely disabled elderly persons: a guide for health professionals. JPEN J Parenter Enteral Nutr 35:295–302, 2011.

80 Obesity

Krupa Shah, Dennis T. Villareal

INTRODUCTION

Obesity is defined as an unhealthy excess of body fat, which enhances the risk of morbidity and untimely mortality. Obesity is a growing epidemic in developed countries and is also becoming increasingly problematic in our aging population. Obesity in older adults is accompanied by an untoward burden of chronic disease, metabolic complications, and a worsening in quality of life. More important, obesity in older adults exacerbates the age-related decline in physical function, which leads to frailty and disability. The current treatment designed for weight loss in older persons includes lifestyle intervention (diet, exercise, and behavior modifications), pharmacotherapy, and surgery. Existing evidence indicates that weight loss therapy in obese older adults prevents or delays functional decline and medical complications and improves quality of life. However, clinicians prescribing weight loss therapy for older adults must consider adverse effects on patients' muscle and bone mass. This chapter describes the clinical importance of obesity in older adults and provides medical professionals with evidence-based guidelines for treating obesity in older adults.

MEASUREMENT

Body mass index (BMI) and waist circumference are widely used and accepted as simple methods to classify overweight and obesity. BMI is calculated as weight (kg)/height squared (m^2). However, the measurement of height is often unreliable and impractical in older adults in nursing homes. In this situation, using alternative measurements such as arm span may be more reliable.[1] Central obesity, as measured by waist circumference, is the excessive accumulation of fat in the abdomen. It is an independent predictor of comorbidities such as diabetes, hypertension, and cardiovascular disease.[2] Table 80-1 incorporates both BMI and waist circumference in the classification of overweight and obesity and estimates relative disease risk.[3]

OBESITY PREVALENCE

The prevalence of obese older adults is rising sharply. According to National Health and Nutrition Examination Survey (NHANES) data from the period 1991 to 2000, the prevalence of obesity increased dramatically for those in the age ranges of 60 to 69 and 70 to 79 years,[2,3] by 56% and 36%, respectively.[4] More recent estimates suggest that 37% of adults 65 years of age or older are obese (BMI $\geq$ 30 kg/m^2), and such prevalence is expected to become even more evident with the aging of baby boomers.[5] The prevalence of obesity in older adults is likely to continue to increase and challenge our health care systems. Moreover, obesity poses an increasing dilemma for long-term care facilities and raises concerns about nursing home preparedness and access.[6] The global growth rate for age-related obesity in developed counties is predicted to be 15% to 20%, and the same trends are being observed in developing countries as they gain more economic affluence.[7]

THE RELATIONSHIP BETWEEN BODY COMPOSITION AND AGING

Aging is associated with significant changes in body composition. After the age of 30 years, individuals tend to show a progressive decrease in fat-free mass (FFM), such as muscle and bone, and an increase in fat mass. Moreover, data from some studies suggest an accelerated loss of FFM in women after they reach age 60 years.[8,9] FFM attains its peak during the third decade of life, whereas fat mass reaches its peak during the seventh decade and is followed by a subsequent decline.[9] In addition, aging is associated with the redistribution of body fat. The intraabdominal fat (central adiposity) increases with aging, whereas the subcutaneous fat and total body fat decrease with aging.[10]

The hormonal changes with aging may explain some of the age-related shifts in proportion of fat and FFM. These age-related changes include a reduced production of the anabolic hormones, growth hormone, insulin-like growth factor 1, testosterone, and dehydroepiandrosterone (DHEA), without a concomitant decline in the catabolic hormone cortisol.[11,12]

CAUSES OF OBESITY IN OLDER ADULTS

Obesity results when total energy intake exceeds the energy output. Energy intake neither changes nor declines with advancing age. Hence, the decrease in total energy output is an important contributor in the gradual accumulation of body fat with aging. Aging is associated with a decrease in all major components of energy output. These components are basal metabolic rate (which explains 70% of energy output), thermal effect of food (10%), and physical activity (20%). The resting metabolic rate decreases with age, largely because of an age-related decline in FFM.[13] The thermic effect of food also declines with aging. The decline in physical activity with aging contributes approximately 50% of the reduction in energy output that occurs with aging.[14]

ADVERSE EFFECTS OF OBESITY

Obesity is associated with several complications that are commonly known to increase mortality and morbidity[15] (Table 80-2). In addition, obesity has a detrimental effect on physical function and quality of life in older adults. These adverse effects of obesity are discussed in this section.

Mortality

Obesity is associated with increased cardiovascular and overall mortality in both younger and older adults.[16] Even though obesity is associated with a higher relative risk of death for younger adults than for older ones, an elevated BMI increases absolute mortality and health risks linearly up to 75 years of age.[17] The relationship of obesity in individuals 75 years or older with total mortality is equivocal. In very old persons, the prevalence of obesity could actually be lower. One explanation for this demographic shift is selective mortality. The underlying diseases can themselves

TABLE 80-1 Classification of Overweight and Obesity by Body Mass Index (BMI), Waist Circumference, and Associated Disease Risk[18]

	BMI (kg/m^2)	Obesity Class	Disease Risk* (Relative to Normal Weight and Waist Circumference) Men <40 Inches; Women <35 Inches	Men >40 Inches; Women >35 Inches
Underweight	<18.5	—	—	—
Normal†	18.5-24.9	—	—	—
Overweight	25.0-29.9	I	Increased	High
Obesity	30.0-34.9	II	High	Very high
	35.0-39.9		Very high	Very high
Extreme obesity	>40	III	Extremely high	Extremely high

*Disease risk for type 2 diabetes, hypertension, and cardiovascular disease.
†Increased waist circumference can be a marker for increased disease risk even in persons of normal weight.

TABLE 80-2 Adverse Effects of Obesity in Older Adults

Disorders Directly Caused by Obesity	Disorders Aggravated by Obesity
Metabolic syndrome	Osteoarthritis
Hypertension	Urinary incontinence
Dyslipidemia	All cardiopulmonary abnormalities
Coronary artery disease	Postoperative complications
Diabetes mellitus	Cataracts
Neoplasia	
Obstructive sleep apnea	

increase the risk of early mortality in obese adults, thus causing an underestimation of the relation between obesity and mortality in older adults. Those who are vulnerable to the adverse effects of obesity die at a younger age. The remaining surviving groups of obese older adults are called the "resistant" survivors.

Comorbid Disease

Obesity and increased abdominal fat are associated with increased morbidity (see Table 80-1), mortality, and poor quality of life.[15] The prevalence of medical conditions commonly associated with obesity (such as hypertension, diabetes, dyslipidemia, and cardiovascular disease) increases with age.[18] Therefore, obesity and weight gain during middle age may contribute to medical complications and the increasing health care expenditures that occur during old age.[19]

The age-related glucose intolerance increases with abdominal obesity and lack of physical activity. Older people who are physically active and do not have increased abdominal girth are much less likely to develop insulin resistance and type 2 diabetes mellitus.[20] In addition, obese older adults have a higher prevalence of dyslipidemia (high triglyceride and low high-density lipoprotein [HDL]) and hypertension.[21,22] In a 15-year longitudinal study, increased BMI in older men was associated with an increase in new cases of coronary heart disease and cardiovascular disease mortality.[23]

Functional Impairment and Quality of Life

Advancing age causes physical dysfunction because of both a progressive decline in muscle mass and strength and an increase in joint immobility and arthritis.[24] These functional limitations adversely affect the activities of daily living (ADLs) and quality of life. Obesity exacerbates this age-related decline in physical function. In addition, medical comorbidities such as diabetes, heart disease, and pulmonary disorders frequently coexist with obesity and contribute to functional decline. Moreover, older adults who are obese (BMI ≥ 30) have a greater rate of nursing home admissions than those who are nonobese (BMI, 18.5-24.9).[25] Both cross-sectional studies and longitudinal studies have consistently demonstrated a strong link between a decline in physical function of older persons and an increase in BMI.[26,27]

Obesity is also associated with frailty syndrome in older adults. In one study, 96% of community-living obese (BMI > 30) older subjects (65 to 80 years old) were frail, as determined by physical performance test scores, peak oxygen consumption, and self-reported ability to perform ADLs.[26] In another study, which was conducted in older women (70 to 79 years old), obesity was linked with a marked increased risk of frailty, determined by weakness, slowness, weight loss, low physical activity, and exhaustion.[28] In a study of community-dwelling older adults, frailty was related to BMI in a U-shaped manner (i.e., increased frailty in people with extremes of low or high BMI). However, in people with large waist circumference (≥35 inches in women and ≥40 inches in men), frailty was shown to exist in all BMI categories.[29]

Despite having higher absolute muscle mass, obese older adults are particularly susceptible to the adverse effects of obesity because not only do they have smaller muscle mass relative to their body weight (relative sarcopenia), but they also have age-related decline in muscle mass leading to sarcopenic obesity.[30,31] With higher fat mass and lower muscle mass, physical activity becomes progressively more difficult. Hence, sarcopenic obesity acts synergistically with aging to augment disability by leading to functional dependence, inactivity, and poor quality of life.

BENEFICIAL EFFECTS OF OBESITY

It should be noted that a potential benefit of obesity with aging is the protection from osteoporosis-related fractures. Higher body weight is associated with greater bone mineral density.[32] This is explained by the bone-stimulating effects of carrying extra body weight as well as hormonal changes (e.g., increased adipose tissue conversion of androstenedione to estrone). Heavier individuals have been found to have higher bone densities even in their non–weight-bearing bones. Furthermore, in the event of a fall, the extra cushioning provided by body fat can serve as protection against fractures, particularly of the hip.

MECHANISMS BY WHICH OBESITY INCREASES MORTALITY AND MORBIDITY

Adipose tissue is recognized as a source of inflammatory mediators by producing cytokines such as tumor necrosis factor-α (TNF-α) and interleukin-6.[33] It appears that the relationship between obesity, insulin resistance, and atherosclerosis may depend partially on the increased production and the release of these inflammatory mediators from adipose tissue. It is postulated that the visceral fat (intraabdominal fat) is most responsible for producing these deleterious cytokines, which in turn leads to diabetes, coronary artery disease, and malignant disease more commonly seen in older adults. Similarly, cytokines and inflammatory mediators produced by adipose tissue may play an important role in the pathophysiology of sarcopenic obesity.[34] A better understanding of the mechanisms that lead from gain in fat mass to muscle loss, or vice versa, seems to be crucial. More research is needed to better characterize this new area of study.

EFFECTS OF INTENTIONAL WEIGHT LOSS IN OLDER ADULTS

Body Composition

Because weight loss results in a decrease in both fat mass (75%) and FFM (25%),[35] it is possible that weight loss in obese older persons could worsen the age-related loss of muscle mass. Nevertheless, adding regular exercise to a weight loss program can attenuate the loss of FFM. This effect was observed in randomized controlled trials (RCTs) conducted on obese older subjects. There was no significant difference in the loss of FFM after regular exercise was added to a diet-induced weight loss program compared to a control group that did not lose weight.[30,36]

Medical Complications

It is well known that weight loss improves or normalizes metabolic abnormalities associated with obesity in young and middle-aged persons.[37] Clinical trials conducted in obese older adults have shown similar results. It was observed that a decrease in multiple coronary artery disease risk factors (including the prevalence of the metabolic syndrome) and insulin resistance, as well as an increase in insulin secretion, resulted from weight loss therapy in obese older adults.[38,39] The results of a recent RCT in obese older subjects showed weight loss improves insulin sensitivity and other cardiometabolic risk factors, but continued improvement in insulin sensitivity is only attained when exercise training is added to weight loss.[40]

Physical Function and Quality of Life

Data from studies conducted in overweight and obese older persons with or without joint disease have shown that the combination of moderate diet-induced weight loss and exercise therapy improves both subjective and objective measures of physical function and health-related quality of life.[30,41] Weight loss in combination with exercise training has also been shown to have beneficial effects on muscle strength and muscle quality (muscle strength/cross-sectional area).[31,42]

Most of the weight loss studies that analyzed physical function as an outcome have included an exercise component. Therefore, data on the effect of weight loss alone on physical function are limited. Nevertheless, one study demonstrated that diet-induced weight loss programs can indeed improve both endurance capacity and exercise tolerance in obese older adults despite the loss of FFM.[43] These findings indicate that obesity is a remediable cause of frailty.

In a 1-year RCT, 107 obese adults aged 65 years and older were recruited for an investigation of the independent and combined effects of weight loss and exercise on physical function, body composition, and quality of life.[36] Participants were randomized into a weight loss program, exercise training program, weight loss plus exercise training program, and a control group. The weight loss program consisted of a balanced diet with an energy deficit of 500 to 750 kcal/day in participants' daily requirements. The exercise intervention included both aerobic and resistance training components. Results demonstrated that although physical function improved in all of the intervention groups compared to the control group, the group with a combined weight loss and exercise training program demonstrated a significantly higher physical function compared to the other interventions. Moreover, the group that received the combined intervention also tended to show increased benefits in terms of reduced loss of lean body mass and bone mineral density, as well as improved aerobic capacity, strength, balance, and gait speed. These findings suggest that the combination of weight loss and exercise programs is more effective at preventing frailty and preserving quality of life for obese older adults compared to interventions focused on a single modality.

In this context, it is important to underline that the combination of weight loss and exercise programs is safe, and the exercise benefits may effectively compensate the reduction of lean mass resulting from the weight loss program.[44] Further studies are needed to determine whether weight loss can be maintained beyond 1 year[45] and how to prevent major health-related outcomes (including mortality and nursing home admissions) in obese older adults. These studies should focus on evaluating whether long-term weight maintenance is likely to produce the most meaningful changes in health outcomes in obese older adults.

Cognition and Mood

A few interventional studies that examined the effect of weight loss on cognition showed mixed findings, but these lacked a rigorous RCT design and focused on middle-aged, not older, adults.[46] A recent RCT conducted in frail, obese older adults demonstrates for the first time that weight loss alone and exercise alone improve cognition and mood, but their combination may provide benefits similar to exercise alone.[47]

Mortality

Epidemiologic studies have shown that older adults who lost weight, or who experienced weight recycling, had an increased relative mortality risk compared to those who were weight stable.[23,48] However, it was not described whether the observed weight changes were intentional or unintentional. Self-reported weight change was used, and in addition, unintentional weight loss is a frequent complication of underlying serious illness, which can confound the explanation of weight loss effects on mortality. Indeed, results from an RCT demonstrated that intentional weight loss was not significantly associated with increased all-cause mortality over 12 years of follow-up in older overweight or obese adults.[49]

Bone Mineral Density

Weight loss can have adverse effects on bone mass. Prospective interventional studies conducted in young and middle-aged adults report that weight loss causes bone loss that may be proportional to the amount of weight loss.[50,51] A clinical trial conducted in young and middle-aged persons showed that diet-induced weight loss, but not exercise-induced weight loss, is associated with reductions in bone mineral density at weight-bearing sites. This suggests that exercise is an important component of a weight loss program designed to offset the adverse effects of diet-induced weight loss on bone.[48] Regular exercise can potentially attenuate weight loss–induced bone loss. Indeed, regular exercise was able to attenuate weight loss–induced bone loss in one study,[44] and this beneficial effect may be specific to sites involved in weight-bearing exercise,[52] mediated by prevention of weight loss–induced increase in sclerostin (a secreted Wnt antagonist that inhibits osteoblastic proliferation and differentiation and thus inhibits bone formation).[53] Therefore, incorporating exercise as part of a weight loss program is particularly important in older persons to reduce bone loss.

TREATMENT

Weight loss in obese persons, regardless of age, can improve obesity-related medical complications, physical function, and quality of life.[15] In older adults, improving physical function and quality of life may be the most important goals of therapy. The current therapeutic options available for weight management in older persons are (1) lifestyle intervention involving diet and exercise therapy, (2) pharmacotherapy, and (3) surgery.

Lifestyle Intervention

Lifestyle intervention is just as effective in older individuals as in younger individuals.[36] The combination of an energy-deficit diet, increased physical activity, and behavior therapy results in moderate weight loss and is associated with a lower risk of treatment-induced complications. Weight loss therapy that reduces muscle and bone losses is recommended for older adults who are obese and who have functional limitations or metabolic complications.

Diet Therapy

A successful diet-induced weight loss program should help patients set a realistic yet clinically meaningful weight loss goal of 8% to 10% reduction in initial body weight by 6 months. Following a calorie-reduced (calorie deficit of approximately 500 to 1000 kcal/day) but balanced diet that provides for as little as 1 or 2 pounds of weight loss a week is recommended for a safe and effective weight loss program[15] (Box 80-1). Because of the increased risk of medical complications, a very-low-calorie diet (<800 kcal/day) should be avoided. The diet should contain 1.0 g/kg high-quality protein/day,[54] a multivitamin, and mineral supplements to ensure that all daily recommended requirements are met. This includes 1500 mg calcium/day and 1000 IU vitamin D/day to prevent bone loss. It is important that health professionals help older adults set personal goals, closely monitor their progress, and use encouragement strategies to improve adherence to the weight loss program. The diet therapy should be consistent with the Therapeutic Lifestyle Changes Diet developed by the National Cholesterol Education Program Expert Panel (Adult Treatment Panel III) (Table 80-3).[55]

Referral to a registered dietitian with experience in weight management is often necessary to ensure that appropriate nutritional counseling is provided. Patients should be educated on food composition, portion control, food preparation, and preferences. Counseling from an exercise specialist or a behavioral therapist who has weight management experience can also facilitate behavior modification. A specific behavioral therapy strategy includes self-monitoring, goal setting, social support, and stimulus control.[56] These techniques can be used to improve compliance.

It is important to realize that changes in the diet and activity habits of older adults may present special challenges because older adults have an increased burden of comorbid conditions, depression, hearing and visual difficulties, and cognitive dysfunction. This increase in chronic disabilities with aging reduces physical activity and functional capacity. Older adults are more likely to have unique psychosocial situations such as dependency on others, cognitive impairment, institutionalization, widowhood, loneliness, isolation, and depression. These situations should be addressed because such factors pose a challenge to weight loss. Because dependency in older age is common, lifestyle-change programs must include participation by family members and caregivers. A successful weight loss and maintenance program should be based on sound scientific rationale. The program must not only be safe and nutritionally adequate, but it must also be practical and applicable to the patient's ethnic and cultural background.

BOX 80-1 Summary of Management Algorithm

INITIAL EVALUATION

- Perform a comprehensive medical history, physical examination, relevant laboratory tests, and medication review to evaluate the patient's current health status and comorbidity risks.
- Gather further information such as the patient's willingness to lose weight, prior attempts at weight loss, and current lifestyle should be gathered before starting weight loss therapy.
- Facilitate the setting of personal goals for the patient and welcome family members and care providers to participate in the management.
- Personalize the weight loss plan after taking into consideration the special needs of this population.
- Advocate a combination of energy-deficit diet, exercise, and behavior modification.

WEIGHT LOSS THERAPY

- Recommend a moderate energy intake (calorie deficit ≈750 kcal/day) containing 1.0 g/kg high-quality protein/day, multivitamin, and mineral supplements (1500 mg Ca and 1000 IU vitamin D/day).
- Recommend referral to a registered dietitian trained in behavior therapy for nutritional education, counseling, and behavior modification techniques.
- Advocate a combination of energy-deficit diet, exercise, and behavior modification.
- Consider bariatric surgery for patients who have failed multiple weight loss attempts.
- Implement weight maintenance efforts after weight loss goals have been achieved.

EXERCISE THERAPY

- Evaluate the need for a stress test before starting the patient on an exercise regimen.
- Recommend an exercise regimen that is gradual, personalized, and monitored.
- Recommend a multicomponent exercise program that includes stretching, aerobic activity, and strength exercises.

Exercise Therapy

The introduction of an exercise component early in the treatment course can improve physical function and ameliorate frailty in older adults.[36] In addition, exercise is a key component in maintaining weight loss. The exercise program should be started

TABLE 80-3 Nutrient Composition of the Therapeutic Lifestyle Changes Diet[51]

Nutrient	Recommended Intake
Saturated fat*	<7% of total calories
Polyunsaturated fat	Up to 10% of total calories
Monounsaturated fat	Up to 20% of total calories
Total fat	25% to 35% of total calories
Carbohydrates†	50% to 60% of total calories
Fiber	20 to 30 g/day
Protein	Approximately 15% of total calories
Cholesterol	<200 mg/day
Total calories‡	Balance energy intake and expenditure to maintain desirable body weight

*Avoid trans fatty acids as well because they increase low-density lipoprotein (LDL) and lower high-density lipoprotein (HDL) cholesterol levels.
†Carbohydrates should be derived from foods rich in complex carbohydrates, including whole grains, fruits, and vegetables.
‡Daily energy expenditure should include at least moderate physical activity.

this is important to exclude in older people who have sustained a stroke or a fall with a prolonged lie.

Multiple myeloma is another condition mostly affecting older adults, of whom approximately 50% will develop renal failure.[43] This is mediated through the direct toxic effects of light chains to renal tubules or intratubular obstruction by their casts. The associated hypercalcemia and hyperuricemia may also give rise to intratubular crystals. Renal failure is reversible in approximately half of these cases, and this is associated with better long-term survival.

About two thirds of cases of acute tubular necrosis are caused by renal ischemia-reperfusion injury,[44] making prerenal AKI and ischemic acute tubular necrosis part of the same continuum. The most common cause is sepsis, particularly with multiple organ failure. There is also increasing evidence suggesting sepsis-associated AKI is an inflammatory event.[45] Postoperative acute tubular necrosis may also occur, often with prerenal causes.

Glomerulonephritis refers to immune-mediated conditions causing inflammation in the kidney, usually classified according to their histologic appearances. Previously thought to be rare in older people, it is now recognized to be a frequent finding as increasing numbers of renal biopsies are performed in this patient group. Rapidly progressive or crescentic glomerulonephritis is more common in older than younger patients.[46] The clinical features depend on the underlying cause, which include antibodies to the glomerular basement membrane, connective tissue diseases, infections, and systemic vasculitides (Table 81-2). Prompt diagnosis and treatment are essential to prevent irreversible loss of renal function. Blood, protein, or red cell casts found on urinalysis are useful clues. A full history and examination will often narrow down the differential diagnosis.

TABLE 81-2 Common Causes of Crescentic Glomerulonephritis and Associated Clinical Features

Causes	Clinical Features
Anti–glomerular basement membrane (GBM) antibody	Goodpasture syndrome—hemoptysis and pulmonary hemorrhage Anti-GBM disease—renal involvement only
Immune complex–mediated disease	Connective tissue diseases Systemic lupus erythematosus—fever, malaise, myalgia, Raynaud phenomenon, hypertension, edema, frothy urine Essential mixed cryoglobulinemia—peripheral neuropathy, arthralgia, skin purpura Henoch-Schönlein purpura—skin purpura, arthritis, abdominal pain, gastrointestinal hemorrhage Infection-associated causes Poststreptococcal infection—edema, hypertension, hematuria Endocarditis—fever, sweats, weight loss Glomerular disease IgA nephropathy—frank hematuria, hypertension Membranoproliferative nephropathy—hypertension, edema
Antineutrophil cytoplasmic antibody (ANCA)–associated systemic vasculitis	Wegener granulomatosis—nasal and upper airway symptoms, pulmonary nodules and infiltrates, c-ANCA positive Microscopic polyangiitis—general malaise, weight loss, cutaneous lesions, p-ANCA positive Churg-Strauss syndrome—late-onset asthma, eosinophilia, gastrointestinal upset, peripheral neuropathy, p-ANCA positive
Others	Malignancies: solid organ carcinomas and lymphoma Drugs: penicillamine, hydralazine

Postrenal Acute Kidney Injury

An obstructive cause must be ruled out in all patients with AKI as prompt relief of the obstruction should result in improvement and recovery of their renal function. The longer this rule-out is delayed, the higher the risk is of irreversible damage. Prostatic disease is a common cause, and a history of hesitancy, poor stream, dribbling, and nocturia is usually present. Other causes include renal calculi, urethral strictures, retroperitoneal fibrosis, renal papillary necrosis, pelvic malignancies, and neurogenic bladder associated with the use of anticholinergic drugs. Examination may reveal a palpable bladder and a large residual volume following catheterization, unless the obstruction is more proximal. Ultrasound scan of the renal tract should show hydronephrosis. A large retrospective study found hydronephrosis in only 5% of patients with AKI, and urinary tract obstruction was the attributable cause in only 2.3%; most cases of hydronephrosis were considered mild and an incidental finding.[47]

Immediate Management

The principal aim is to treat any life-threatening features promptly and stop the decline in renal function before it becomes irreversible. Hypotension, shock, and respiratory failure will be obvious clinically, and sepsis should be treated immediately with appropriate antibiotics and fluid resuscitation, preferably in a high-dependency or intensive care unit. Other life-threatening features associated with AKI are hyperkalemia, pulmonary edema, and severe metabolic acidosis.

Hyperkalemia is dangerous because it precipitates fatal cardiac arrhythmias. Electrocardiogram (ECG) changes include absent or flattened P waves, broadening of the QRS complex, tall tented T waves, and, eventually, ventricular fibrillation or asystole. If any of these ECG changes are present or if the serum potassium level is greater than 6.5 mmol/L, treatment should be started immediately. The myocardium should be stabilized with intravenous calcium, followed by an infusion of insulin and dextrose to increase cellular potassium uptake. Salbutamol has a similar effect to insulin. These measures simply redistribute potassium within the body, and the excess potassium still needs to be excreted, either through restoration of renal function with increased renal potassium excretion or through RRT if the patient remains oliguric or anuric.

Pulmonary edema resulting from volume overload in oliguric or anuric patients is difficult to treat. Respiratory support with oxygen is mandatory, and ventilation may be considered depending on the clinical situation. Opiates and a nitrate infusion may help reduce cardiac workload. Large doses of diuretics may be needed to induce diuresis. However, if these treatments are unsuccessful, then fluid can be removed by RRT.

Severe metabolic acidosis can be treated with intravenous sodium bicarbonate, but there is little evidence that this is beneficial. The acidosis will improve as renal function recovers, but severe acidosis in patients who remain oliguric or anuric will require RRT.

Subsequent Management

AKI is not a disease but a heterogeneous clinical syndrome, often with multiple causes. The cause of AKI should be determined so that treatment is targeted appropriately. Thorough history taking and examination should enable clinicians to establish a differential diagnosis. Several blood tests and radiologic investigations may be helpful (Table 81-3). A renal biopsy may be necessary for accurate histopathologic diagnosis and, although there is a risk of bleeding, it is reasonably safe in older people.[48] In this

TABLE 81-3 Useful Investigations in Acute Kidney Injury

Investigation	Comments
Urea and electrolytes	Identifies renal failure, hyperkalemia, and acidosis
Full blood count	Identifies anemia, infection
Clotting	Coagulopathy may occur
Group and save or cross-match	If acute bleeding suspected
Calcium, phosphate	Hypercalcemia may occur in multiple myeloma
Creatinine kinase, myoglobin	If rhabdomyolysis suspected
Blood cultures, as well as cultures of sputum, urine, wound sites	To identify causative organism in septicemia
Immunoglobulins, protein electrophoresis	If multiple myeloma suspected
Autoantibodies • Antinuclear (ANA) • ANCA • Anti-GBM • Anti–extractable nuclear antigen (ENA) Complement Cryoglobulins Rheumatoid factor	If glomerulonephritis suspected
Antistreptolysin O (ASO) titer, throat swab	If poststreptococcal glomerulonephritis possible
Hepatitis and HIV serology	If urgent hemodialysis considered
Other serology • Cytomegalovirus (CMV) • Epstein-Barr virus (EBV) • Varicella zoster virus (VZV)	If immunosuppressive treatment considered
Urinalysis	Identifies blood, protein, red cell casts
Spot urine albumin-to-creatinine ratio	To quantify proteinuria
Midstream urine	Microscopy, culture, and sensitivities in infection Bence-Jones protein in multiple myeloma
Renal ultrasound scan and/or other radiologic imaging	Identifies urinary obstruction, size of kidneys, renal calculi, other structural abnormalities of renal tract
Electrocardiogram	Changes may occur with hyperkalemia
Renal biopsy	May be required for histopathologic diagnosis

situation, it may be prudent to consider withholding anticoagulants and antiplatelet drugs if it is safe to do so.

Crucial to the management of AKI is accurate assessment of the patient's hemodynamic status and hydration. The majority of patients will be volume deplete and require intravenous fluids. However, bearing in mind the high prevalence of cardiac disease among older people, in particular diastolic dysfunction, this needs to be done cautiously to avoid acute pulmonary edema caused by overzealous fluid resuscitation. Assessment of fluid balance can be difficult in older adults, so a central venous pressure monitor may be useful but is not without its risks.

A urinary catheter should be inserted early, not just because it may relieve obstruction but also to allow accurate measurement of urine output. Relief of upper urinary tract obstruction will require either percutaneous nephrostomy or retrograde cystoscopy with urethral catheterization. Postobstructive diuresis may be up to 20 L/day, and careful management is required to prevent prerenal AKI due to subsequent volume depletion. Hyperkalemic renal tubular acidosis may also occur but generally resolves spontaneously.

All nephrotoxic medications should be stopped as soon as renal failure is identified. Some drugs are removed by dialysis, and this should be considered when elimination is slowed down because of the associated AKI, for example, in toxicity resulting from lithium, salicylates, barbiturates, and inorganic acids. Special considerations and dose adjustments are also necessary when prescribing drugs such as antibiotics and analgesics because patients in renal failure may have altered pharmacokinetics.

Management of AKI is largely supportive, but once a specific cause of AKI is identified, definitive treatment should be commenced as soon as possible. Hypovolemia due to bleeding may need endoscopic or surgical intervention. Uremia itself induces platelet dysfunction and coagulopathies requiring correction with vitamin K and blood products. Glomerulonephritis as suggested by the history, urinalysis, and autoimmune serology requires early involvement of nephrologists. Immunosuppression with corticosteroids or other agents, and occasionally plasma exchange, are necessary treatment measures once the diagnosis is clear. There is no consistent evidence that pharmacologic agents—including diuretics, renal-dose dopamine, fenoldopam, atrial natriuretic peptide, insulin growth factor, statins, *N*-acetylcysteine, calcium channel blockers, and adenosine antagonists—improve renal function in patients with AKI.[31,44]

Renal Replacement Therapy

Life-threatening conditions such as severe metabolic acidosis, pulmonary edema, and hyperkalemia refractory to medical therapy may require urgent RRT. Other indications for initiation of RRT include poisoning with a dialyzable toxin and severe uremia with its complications of pericarditis, encephalopathy, and neuropathy. In the absence of these factors, the optimal timing for initiating RRT for patients with AKI has not been defined.[31] Dialysis tends to be delayed as long as possible, not just because patients may recover on their own but also because of considerable risks associated with RRT, including hypotension, cardiac arrhythmias, complications of vascular access, and need for anticoagulation.

Peritoneal dialysis uses the peritoneum as the semipermeable membrane for dialyzing. Solutes pass from blood into the dialysate along their concentration gradient, and water by an osmotic gradient created by adding glucose or a polymer to the dialysate. This method is less efficient at solute and fluid removal compared to hemodialysis and is rarely used in the acute setting in developed countries. It is still useful where hemodialysis resources are limited and when anticoagulation or vascular access is not possible.

Hemodialysis involves passing blood into a dialyzer, where it interfaces with dialysate across a semipermeable membrane. Molecules diffuse across this membrane, and large volumes of fluid can be removed by ultrafiltration. Good vascular access and anticoagulation with heparin is required. Intermittent hemodialysis is more suitable in severe hyperkalemia, has a lower risk of bleeding, and costs less, but adequacy and hemodynamic control are more difficult. Continuous RRT—for example, continuous venovenous hemofiltration (CVVH) or continuous venovenous hemodiafiltration (CVVHD)—is preferred for patients with cerebral edema and multiple organ failure because it offers better hemodynamic stability and biochemical and fluid volume control. Slowly extended daily dialysis (SLEDD) combines the advantages of both intermittent hemodialysis and continuous RRT by removing fluid more slowly with greater hemodynamic and metabolic control; this type of dialysis may be preferable in older patients. No particular modality has been proven to have better outcomes.[49]

Age alone should not preclude a patient from receiving RRT. Each patient should be assessed individually, taking into account the severity of illness, premorbid functional level and other nonrenal comorbidities, the likelihood of a meaningful physical and cognitive recovery, and the wishes of the patient and the patient's family. A time-limited trial of RRT may be considered, and RRT should be stopped when renal recovery is adequate to meet the patient's needs or when it is no longer compatible with overall goals of care.

Outcome

Although some patients may recover completely, mortality in AKI can be as high as 80%.[34] Prognosis is worse with increasing age and comorbidity and in those with hospital-acquired AKI.[50] Among AKI survivors, 15% to 30% remain dependant on long-term RRT,[51] and many more never fully recover renal function, as AKI is independently associated with an increased risk for CKD and established renal failure (ERF). After a single episode of AKI, the risk for ERF is elevated 2-fold in those with mild AKI and 3-fold to 13-fold in more severe AKI.[52] Close monitoring of post-AKI renal function is therefore vital.

CHRONIC KIDNEY DISEASE

CKD is defined as abnormalities of kidney function or structure for more than 3 months, with implications for health. This includes a decreased GFR of less than 60 mL/min/1.73 m^2 or kidney damage, which may be indicated by persistent proteinuria or hematuria, radiologically demonstrable structural abnormalities, or biopsy-proven chronic glomerulonephritis. Classification of CKD is determined by the level of GFR and albuminuria, regardless of the underlying cause of renal failure (Table 81-4).[2] Category G3 is further subdivided into categories G3a and G3b, in light of evidence that the risk and prevalence of complications accelerate as GFR falls below 45 mL/min/1.73 m^2. Classification now also includes the presence and degree of proteinuria to identify those at higher risk of cardiovascular complications and CKD progression. Urine ACR should be used, as this corrects for urine concentration, and the measurement of albumin offers greater sensitivity and precision for detecting lower levels of proteinuria compared with protein-to-creatinine ratio (PCR). Spot urine samples are sufficient, ideally an early morning sample. ACR of 3 mg/mmol or more is considered clinically significant.

It is well known that GFR declines in parallel with age, and therefore CKD is common in older people. The prevalence of CKD in the United States is estimated to be 13%, with 37% of those older than 70 years in category G3 and above.[54] Prevalence may be even higher in institutionalized care, with over 80% of a residential home population in category G3 or worse and 40% category G3b or worse.[55] A reduced GFR in an older person should not be accepted as normal simply because it is common. However, exactly how much "normal" reduction can be attributable to the aging process and how much is due to pathology remains uncertain. A low GFR implies a reduced reserve and can be used as a guide to risk in that older person, without necessarily labeling the person as chronically diseased.[56]

Causes of CKD

The most common cause of CKD is diabetes mellitus, which accounts for 26% of people commencing RRT in the United Kingdom.[57] In older adults, renovascular disease and hypertension are also important causes, but in the majority of cases the primary renal diagnosis remains unconfirmed. Other causes more common in older patients include obstructive uropathy, myeloma, and systemic vasculitis. Glomerulonephritis, pyelonephritis, and polycystic kidney disease predominantly affect younger patients.

Clinical Manifestations and Complications

CKD is often asymptomatic, even in advanced stages. A large proportion of CKD is found incidentally on blood tests done for other reasons. Clinical features include poor appetite, nausea and vomiting, tiredness, breathlessness, peripheral edema, itch, cramps, and restless legs.

CKD is associated with increased mortality and morbidity, particularly from cardiovascular disease.[58] The cardiovascular risk increases exponentially as CKD progresses, so the risk is increased 2-fold to 4-fold in category G3 and 10-fold to 50-fold in category G5.[59] Hypertension is common in adults with CKD as a result of sodium retention and activation of the renin-angiotensin-aldosterone system. Most CKD patients also have other traditional cardiovascular risk factors such as age, diabetes, dyslipidemia, and smoking. Renal dysfunction itself causes oxidative stress, vascular calcification, increased circulating cytokines due to chronic inflammation and elevated asymmetrical dimethylarginine (ADMA) levels, which inhibit nitric oxide synthesis

TABLE 81-4 Classification of Chronic Kidney Disease

Glomerular Filtration Rate (GFR) and Albumin-to-Creatinine Ratio (ACR) Categories and Risk of Adverse Outcomes		**ACR Categories (mg/mmol), Description and Range**		
		<3 Normal to Mildly Increased	**3-30 Moderately Increased**	**>30 Severely Increased**
		A1	A2	A3
GFR categories (mL/min/1.73 m^2), description and range: G1	≥90 Normal or high	No CKD in the absence of markers of kidney damage		
G2	60-89 Mildly reduced			
G3a	45-59 Mild-moderate reduction			
G3b	30-44 Moderate-severe reduction			
G4	15-29 Severe reduction			
G5	<15 Kidney failure			

Increasing risk (down the rows)

Increasing risk (across the columns)

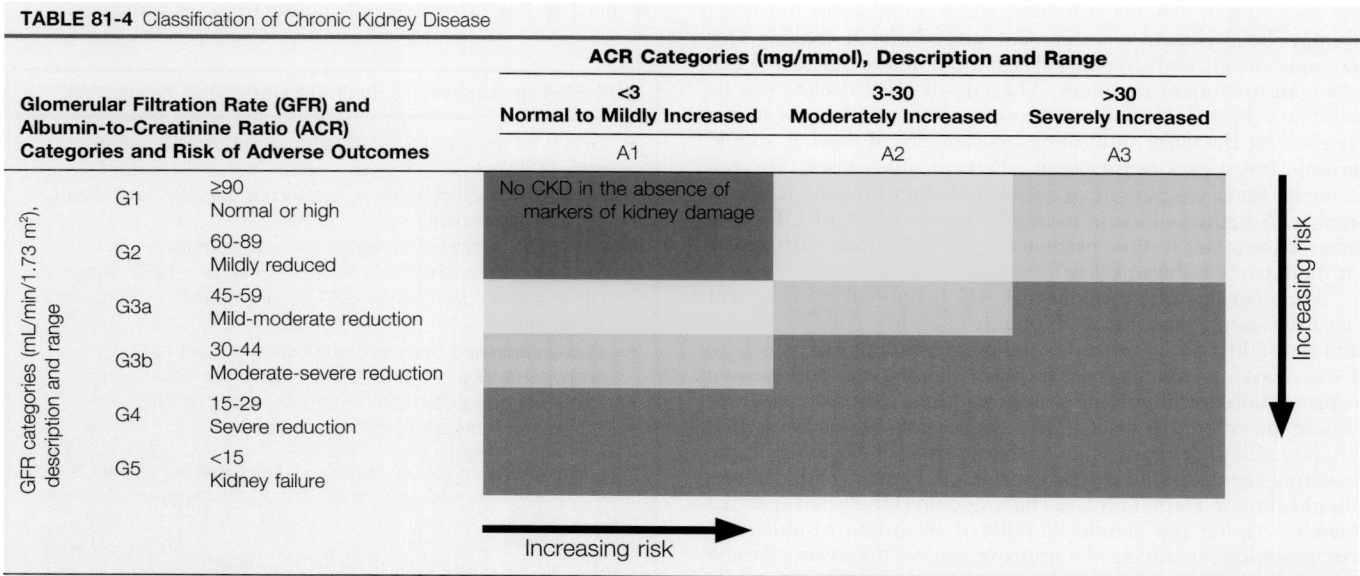

Modified from Kidney Disease: Improving Global Outcomes (KDIGO) CKD Work Group: KDIGO 2012 clinical practice guideline for the evaluation and management of chronic kidney disease. Kidney Int Suppl 3:1–150, 2013.

contributing to endothelial dysfunction and accelerated atherosclerosis. All these mechanisms lead to a higher prevalence of myocardial infarction and ischemic heart disease, cardiac failure, stroke, and peripheral vascular disease.

Other complications of CKD involve the bones, anemia, acidosis, and malnutrition. Renal bone disease and anemia start at category G3. The production of active 1,25-dihydroxyvitamin D is impaired, and secondary hyperparathyroidism occurs as a result of hypocalcemia and hyperphosphatemia. This is particularly significant in older people because of the high incidence of osteoporosis. Anemia results from erythropoietin deficiency, decreased erythrocyte life span and blood loss; if left untreated, it may contribute to cardiac failure, cognitive impairment, and poor quality of life. Metabolic acidosis and malnutrition occur mainly at categories G4 and G5. Acidosis accelerates bone loss, muscle wasting, hypoalbuminemia, and a decline in renal function. Anorexia, dietary restrictions, increased catabolism, and chronic inflammation all contribute to malnutrition in people with CKD, causing muscle weakness, poor exercise tolerance, and increased susceptibility to infection. All of these factors may contribute to an older person's frailty.

Management

The rate of deterioration in renal function can be assessed by reviewing previous biochemistry results. Serum creatinine levels should always be rechecked so that any rapid decline can be identified and treated promptly. Any potentially reversible causes of renal failure should be considered, such as medications and infections. Urinalysis is important to check for hematuria and proteinuria. A urologic malignancy should always be excluded in persistent hematuria. Proteinuria requires confirmation by laboratory confirmation and quantification, as previously discussed. Renal ultrasonography or other radiologic imaging may be indicated, especially in patients with urinary tract obstruction symptoms, hematuria, unexpected or accelerated deterioration in GFR, GFR less than 30 mL/min/1.73 m^2 (category G4 and G5), or in whom a renal biopsy is being considered.[60]

Clinical guidelines[53,60] have been published outlining the management of CKD and indications for referral to nephrologists. Most patients can be managed safely in the community, but disease progression should be monitored with at least annual assessment of GFR and albuminuria. More frequent assessments are indicated in patients at higher risk of progression and when it may help clinical management and decision making, for example, during and after episodes of intercurrent illness or when changing treatment regimens. The rate of GFR decline can be estimated by graphing 1/creatinine over time. Changes in the gradient of the curve, indicating a faster rate of decline, should prompt investigations for potentially reversible causes. There is evidence that a steeper rate of decline in kidney function is associated with higher all-cause mortality, independent of GFR and other known risk factors, particularly for individuals with mildly or moderately reduced GFR.[61,62]

The mainstay of treatment in CKD is optimal management of cardiovascular risk factors. Not only does this reduce mortality and morbidity, but it also slows the progression of early CKD to ERF. Smoking, weight loss, exercise, alcohol use, and sodium consumption are important issues to address. Antiplatelet drugs should be offered for secondary prevention of cardiovascular disease, although there is an increased risk of bleeding. Lipid lowering agents should also be considered. Patients with diabetes should aim for a target glycated hemoglobin (HbA1c) of approximately 7%, but this should be tailored according to individual circumstances, balancing the improvement in microvascular risk with the risk of hypoglycemia.[63] Hypertension should be carefully controlled, aiming for a target blood pressure of either 140/90 or 130/80 if diabetes is present or ACR is 70 mg/mmol or higher. ACE inhibitors or ARBs should be prescribed in patients with an ACR of 70 mg/mmol or higher, diabetics with an ACR of 3 mg/mmol or higher, and hypertensive patients with an ACR of 30mg/mmol or higher. Serum creatinine and potassium levels should be rechecked 2 weeks after commencing or increasing the dose of these drugs. Withdrawal should be considered if serum potassium increases to 6.0 mmol/L or higher and other hyperkalemia-promoting drugs have been stopped, or if creatinine increases by 30% or more or GFR falls by 25% or more. Investigations for renal artery stenosis may be warranted.

Clinicians should take GFR into consideration when prescribing and dosing medications. People in categories G3 through G5 should be advised to temporarily stop potentially nephrotoxic and renally excreted drugs, such as ACE inhibitors, ARBs, diuretics, NSAIDs, metformin, lithium, and digoxin, during an intercurrent illness that increases the risk of AKI. When considering imaging studies, the risk of AKI due to contrast agent should be balanced against the diagnostic and therapeutic value of such a procedure.

All CKD patients should receive dietetic input regarding appropriate sodium, fluid, potassium, and phosphate restrictions. Patients with GFR less than 45 mL/min/1.73 m^2 (category G3b, G4, and G5) should have their hemoglobin (Hb) monitored regularly. Treatment with erythropoiesis-stimulating agents and iron should be considered in anemic patients with Hb 11g/dL or less or if symptomatic, aiming to maintain a stable Hb between 10 and 12 g/dL, depending on their functional needs.[64] Once GFR falls to less than 30 mL/min/1.73 m^2 (category G4 and G5), serum calcium, phosphate, and parathyroid hormone should also be measured. If the parathyroid hormone concentration is raised and serum 25-hydroxyvitamin D is low, treatment with ergocalciferol or cholecalciferol with calcium supplement should be commenced. Alfacalcidol or calcitriol may be offered in categories G4 and G5 if symptoms persist despite correcting vitamin D deficiency. Phosphate binders are also useful in patients with hyperphosphatemia, aiming for a phosphate level of 1.8 mmol/L or less. Supplementary oral sodium bicarbonate can be used to correct acidosis in patients with serum bicarbonate less than 20 mmol/L.

All appropriate patients should be discussed with a nephrologist, taking into consideration the individual's wishes and comorbidities (Box 81-1). This is to ensure that patients are adequately informed about their treatment options as they approach ERF. Most patients need a minimum of 1 year to prepare themselves and their caregivers for RRT,[65] but late referral is significantly more frequent in older patients, contributing to excess mortality.[66]

BOX 81-1 Indications for Referral for Specialist Assessment

- GFR ≤ 30 mL/min/1.73 m^2 (category G4 or G5), with or without diabetes
- ACR ≥ 70 mg/mmol, unless caused by diabetes and already appropriately treated
- ACR ≥ 30 mg/mmol (category A3) with hematuria
- Sustained decrease of ≥25% and a change in GFR category OR sustained decrease in GFR of ≥15 mL/min/1.73 m^2 within 12 months
- Poorly controlled hypertension despite at least four antihypertensive drugs at therapeutic doses
- Known or suspected rare or genetic cause of CKD
- Suspected renal artery stenosis

Data from National Institute for Health and Care Excellence (2014) CG 182 Chronic kidney disease: early identification and management of chronic kidney disease in adults in primary and secondary care. Manchester: NICE. Reproduced with permission. Please visit http://www.nice.org.uk/CG182 for the latest version of the NICE guideline.

ACR, Albumin-to-creatinine ratio; *CKD*, chronic kidney disease; *GFR*, glomerular filtration rate.

ESTABLISHED RENAL FAILURE

The number of older patients on RRT continues to grow, and the median age of patients starting dialysis in the United Kingdom is 64.6 years.[57] Guidelines recommend starting RRT when patients develop symptomatic uremia, difficult fluid balance or blood pressure control, progressive malnutrition, or cognitive impairment. This often occurs when GFR falls to 5 to 10 mL/min/1.73 m^2.[53]

The most common form of RRT in older adults is hemodialysis. Subcutaneous arteriovenous fistula is the preferred vascular access and should be formed at least 6 months before commencing dialysis. In the short to intermediate term, synthetic grafts, central venous catheters, and semipermanent tunneled central catheters may be also be used. Most patients undergo three hemodialysis sessions per week, each lasting 3 to 5 hours, usually in hospital units. Access to home hemodialysis is limited but may be considered for appropriate patients and is associated with good outcomes.[67]

Peritoneal dialysis allows greater independence because it can be carried out in the patient's own home and tailored to the patient's daily routine. However, it is contraindicated in patients with a history of major abdominal surgery or peritoneal adhesions, unrepaired inguinal hernias, or compromised respiratory function, which unfortunately excludes many older people. Common problems include infection and fluid overload as a result of inadequate ultrafiltration, and conversion to hemodialysis may be necessary.

Transplantation can restore renal function completely and is clearly preferable to dialysis. There is no age limit to transplantation. However, scarce donor organs means that many older patients are often not considered for transplantation because of their comorbidity and shorter life expectancy. Despite this, the number of older people receiving renal transplants continues to rise, especially with advances in live kidney donation. In the United Kingdom, adults aged 60 years and older constituted 30% of those who received a deceased donor kidney transplant and 17% of those who received a living donor kidney.[68] Older age at the time of transplantation is a strong risk factor for mortality, and this risk is further increased by presence of comorbid conditions such as cardiac failure, peripheral vascular disease, and cancer.[69] Survival is substantially better for recipients of living donor kidneys; therefore, this should be encouraged as the treatment of choice for all suitable older patients. Renal transplantation has been shown to be worthwhile in older patients with good graft survival rates, provided they are carefully selected and their immunosuppression is tailored sensibly.[70,71] Main complications are graft rejection, infection, and malignancy, but cardiovascular disease remains the leading cause of death.

RRT may not always be in the best interest of older patients. Starting RRT is associated with significant physical and functional decline in the frail.[72] In heavily dependent patients with more comorbidity, survival on RRT is not significantly longer than those treated palliatively.[73] Many older patients on RRT spend a considerable proportion of their time in the hospital with a higher risk of developing multiple complications.[74] Conservative management aims to relieve the symptoms of ERF and maximize health for the remainder of patients' lives. This includes treating anemia with erythropoiesis-stimulating agents and controlling nausea and pruritus with appropriate drugs. Many renal units now have conservative care specialist nurses to facilitate this treatment option for patients. End-of-life care is equally important, not just in patients who choose not to dialyze but also for those who choose to withdraw from dialysis. In the last month of life, patients with ERF have physical and psychological symptom burdens similar or greater than those in patients with advanced cancer.[75] World Health Organization guidelines for pain management should be followed, and close collaboration with palliative care, hospice services, and primary care is essential.

Outcome

Prognosis for CKD and its complications depends on the underlying cause, degree of albuminuria, and other comorbidities. In a large study of community-dwelling older patients with CKD, the majority had minimal or no progression of their disease after a median follow-up of 2 years.[76] Risk factors for CKD progression include proteinuria, cardiovascular disease, AKI, hypertension, diabetes, smoking, untreated urinary tract obstruction, chronic use of , and certain ethnic groups including African, African-Caribbean, and Asian origins. Rapid progression of albuminuria has been associated with worse outcomes. A twofold or greater increase in albuminuria over 2 years has been found to be associated with a 50% higher mortality, whereas a twofold or greater decrease was found to be associated with a 15% lower mortality, independent of baseline albuminuria. Increases in albuminuria were also significantly associated with cardiovascular events, cardiovascular deaths, and renal outcomes, including requirement for dialysis.[77] Mortality increases exponentially with declining GFR, by 17% for category G3 and nearly 600% for G5.[78] Most patients are more likely to die of cardiovascular disease before reaching ERF. The risk of death was 60 times greater than the risk of dialysis in subjects in category G2 and 6 times greater in category G3.[76] In a 5-year observational study in the United States, 3% of patients in categories G2 through G4 eventually required RRT and 24% died.[79] Our efforts should therefore concentrate on early identification and good management of cardiovascular risk factors, which will also delay progression to ERF.

CONCLUSION

The number of people with renal disease will continue to increase as our population ages and the diabetes epidemic grows. Early recognition of risk factors is essential because the disease is often asymptomatic in older people. Age per se should not be a contraindication to good treatment, and appropriate patients should be referred to nephrologists promptly. Bearing in mind the great heterogeneity of older people, each patient should be considered individually. Patients need to be adequately informed about the likely course and prognosis of their disease to guide them in making choices about treatment options.

KEY POINTS

- Renal disease is frequently underdiagnosed and undertreated in older people because they have nonspecific or no symptoms and their serum creatinine may be normal.
- Asymptomatic bacteriuria does not require treatment.
- Iatrogenic renal failure is a growing problem resulting from nephrotoxic drugs and radiocontrast agents.
- Good management of cardiovascular risk factors is important in chronic kidney disease to reduce mortality and morbidity and delay progression to established renal failure.
- Appropriate referral to nephrologists improves outcomes.

For a complete list of references, please visit www.expertconsult.com.

KEY REFERENCES

2. Kidney Disease: Improving Global Outcomes (KDIGO) CKD Work Group: KDIGO 2012 clinical practice guideline for the evaluation and management of chronic kidney disease. Kidney Int Suppl 3:1–150, 2013.
3. National Institute for Health and Care Excellence: Chronic kidney disease, early identification and management of chronic kidney

disease in adults in primary and secondary care (NICE clinical guidelines [CG182]), July 2014.
9. Grabe M, Bjerklund-Johansen TE, Botto H, et al: Guidelines on urological infections. European Association of Urology, 2013.
10. Juthani-Mehta M: Asymptomatic bacteriuria and urinary tract infection in older adults. Clin Geriatr Med 23:585–594, 2007.
17. Scottish Intercollegiate Guidelines Network (SIGN): Management of suspected bacterial urinary tract infection in adults (SIGN publication no. 88), Edinburgh, July 2012.
31. Kidney Disease: Improving Global Outcomes (KDIGO): Acute Kidney Injury Work Group: KDIGO clinical practice guideline for acute kidney injury. Kidney Int Suppl 2:1–138, 2012.
35. Schmitt R, Coca S, Kanbay M, et al: Recovery of kidney function after acute kidney injury in the elderly: a systematic review and meta-analysis. Am J Kidney Dis 52:262–271, 2008.
40. National Institute for Health and Care Excellence: Acute kidney injury: prevention, detection and management up to the point of renal replacement therapy (NICE guidelines [CG169]), August 2013.
58. Van der Velder M, Matsushita K, Coresh J, et al: Lower estimated glomerular filtration rate and higher albuminuria are associated with all-cause and cardiovascular mortality. A collaborative meta-analysis of high-risk population cohorts. Kidney Int 79:1341–1352, 2011.
60. National Institute for Health and Care Excellence: Chronic kidney disease: early identification and management of chronic kidney disease in adults in primary and secondary care (NICE guidelines [CG182]), July 2014.
66. Smart NA, Titus TT: Outcomes of early versus late nephrology referral in chronic kidney disease: a systematic review. Am J Med 124: 1073–1080, 2011.
73. Murtagh FEM, Marsh JE, Donohoe P, et al: Dialysis or not? A comparative survival study of patients over 75 years with chronic kidney disease stage 5. Nephrol Dial Transplant 22:1955–1962, 2007.

82 Disorders of Water and Electrolyte Metabolism

Amanda Miller, Karthik Tennankore, Kenneth Rockwood

INTRODUCTION

With aging, several changes to the regulation of water and electrolyte homeostasis can occur. Total body water (TBW) is commonly reduced. Older adult patients are less responsive to hormonal mediators of water, electrolyte, and mineral balance. Commonly, older adults have impairments in thirst sensation, renal function, and factors that regulate salt and water balance, making them more vulnerable to age-associated diseases and iatrogenic events involving water and electrolytes disturbances.[1] These and other factors make older adults more susceptible to physiologic disturbance and less able to correct or compensate for these metabolic derangements than their younger counterparts. Therefore, with any perturbation in fluid or electrolyte balance, older adult patients are at a significantly increased risk of adverse outcomes. The occurrence and severity of electrolyte abnormalities appear to be increased in older people who are frail. This may result in catastrophic consequences in this population if fluid and electrolyte abnormalities are not promptly recognized and treated. An awareness of this impairment in fluid and electrolyte regulation in aging individuals will help health care providers to better manage these issues.[1]

WATER BALANCE

TBW content is maintained through a number of physiologic responses to changes in fluid status. In middle age, roughly 60% to 65% of body weight is made up of water. With changes in body composition caused by aging (including decreased muscle mass and increased fat mass), the percentage of body water is reduced, such that by 75 years of age TBW comprises only 50% of a person's weight.[1] TBW is reduced by 10% to 15% in older adults,[2] and this reduction is more pronounced in women.[1] In consequence, a given volume of fluid represents a greater relative percentage of TBW, and so older adults may experience more profound derangements in serum electrolyte concentrations as a result of fluid shift compared to younger people.[1] In young adults, TBW is controlled primarily through the thirst and renal responses to either increased or decreased extracellular fluid (ECF) volume and/or serum osmolality. The thirst response is triggered by hypovolemia, often manifested as hypotension, or by an increased serum osmolality. This leads to increased fluid intake, allowing restoration of normal physiologic parameters. Contrarily, thirst is generally suppressed in situations of increased ECF volume or low serum osmolality, a situation in which drinking excess dilute fluid could lead to worsening volume overload and further reduction of serum osmolality.

In addition to less TBW, older adults face challenges in maintaining water homeostasis (and stable ECF volume status) on the basis of a number of impaired physiologic processes (Figure 82-1). Given that frailty results in impaired physiologic reserve, these problems may occur more frequently in frail patients. First, older adult patients have a reduced thirst response with decreased desire for and intake of fluid following a period of water deprivation compared with younger individuals.[3] The mechanism for this is unknown but may be related to the fact that older adults have a higher baseline serum osmolality set point and thus require a greater change in serum osmolality to trigger the thirst center (albeit suboptimally).[4] Additionally, they may have limited access to fluid replacement on the basis of reduced mobility or cognitive deficits.[1] As such, older adults are at higher risk for both dehydration (net water loss) and hypovolemia because of decreased fluid intake. This is especially true after periods of water/fluid deprivation.

As is typical in age-related disorders, the mechanisms behind water homeostasis in older adults are complex: commonly, multiple deficits accumulate to impair function.[5,6] Therefore, it is no surprise that impairment of water homeostasis in older adults is associated with decreased renal mass,[7] reduced cortical blood flow,[8] and a decreased glomerular filtration rate (GFR).[9] The renal response to hypovolemia and increased serum osmolality is reabsorption of free water through stimulation of antidiuretic hormone (ADH). ADH is a peptide hormone secreted by the hypothalamus and stored in the posterior pituitary, which functions to insert water channels (aquaporins) in the renal collecting duct to reabsorb free water and reduce urinary water losses[10] (Figure 82-2, *A*). This results in a more concentrated urine and a decrease in serum osmolality with a concomitant increase in blood volume (Figure 82-2, *B*). Free water retention is valuable in situations where an increase in TBW is required to restore normal physiologic ECF volume status and osmolality, for example, in dehydration. In periods of hypotension, stretch receptors in the aorta and carotid arteries are activated to stimulate ADH secretion so that the body can retain enough fluid to restore blood pressure. Likewise, serum hyperosmolality is detected by osmoreceptors in the hypothalamus, which act to stimulate both ADH secretion and thirst. This leads to free water retention and increased water intake, with reduction of serum osmolality back toward normal level.[9]

Osmoreceptors are much more sensitive at stimulating ADH than are stretch receptors. The body tolerates changes in serum osmolality of only 1% to 2% before stimulating or suppressing ADH secretion. On the contrary, it takes a volume change of 8% to 10% (change in mean arterial pressure by 20% to 30%) before stretch receptors are triggered and ADH secretion is affected.[11] Incomplete coordination of compensatory responses is one manifestation of the impaired repair process associated with frailty,[12] and occasionally there is a mismatch between serum osmolality and ECF volume status. For example, when older adults have solute and volume losses of gastrointestinal (e.g., diarrheal) or renal (e.g., diuretic) cause with access to only solute-poor fluid replacement (e.g., water at the bedside), they can develop progressive hypo-osmolality without full restoration of ECF volume. In this situation, low serum osmolality suppresses ADH, whereas hypovolemia stimulates it. Intuitively, given that preservation of volume status is most essential, ADH will be influenced by ECF volume alone in the face of worsening serum osmolality. In consequence, free water will be reabsorbed and the patient's serum sodium will be further reduced as volume status is corrected.

Further complicating the issue, many older patients have an impaired urinary concentrating ability (see Figure 82-1). As such, in settings where ADH is maximally stimulated (hyperosmolar hypovolemia), the aged kidney is only able to achieve urine osmolalities half that of younger individuals.[1] This submaximal urine osmolality is a result of inappropriate loss of free water in the form of dilute urine, which is maladaptive in the face of reduced TBW and perpetuates the problem of either reduced volume or, in some cases, increased serum osmolality.[1] ADH levels in older

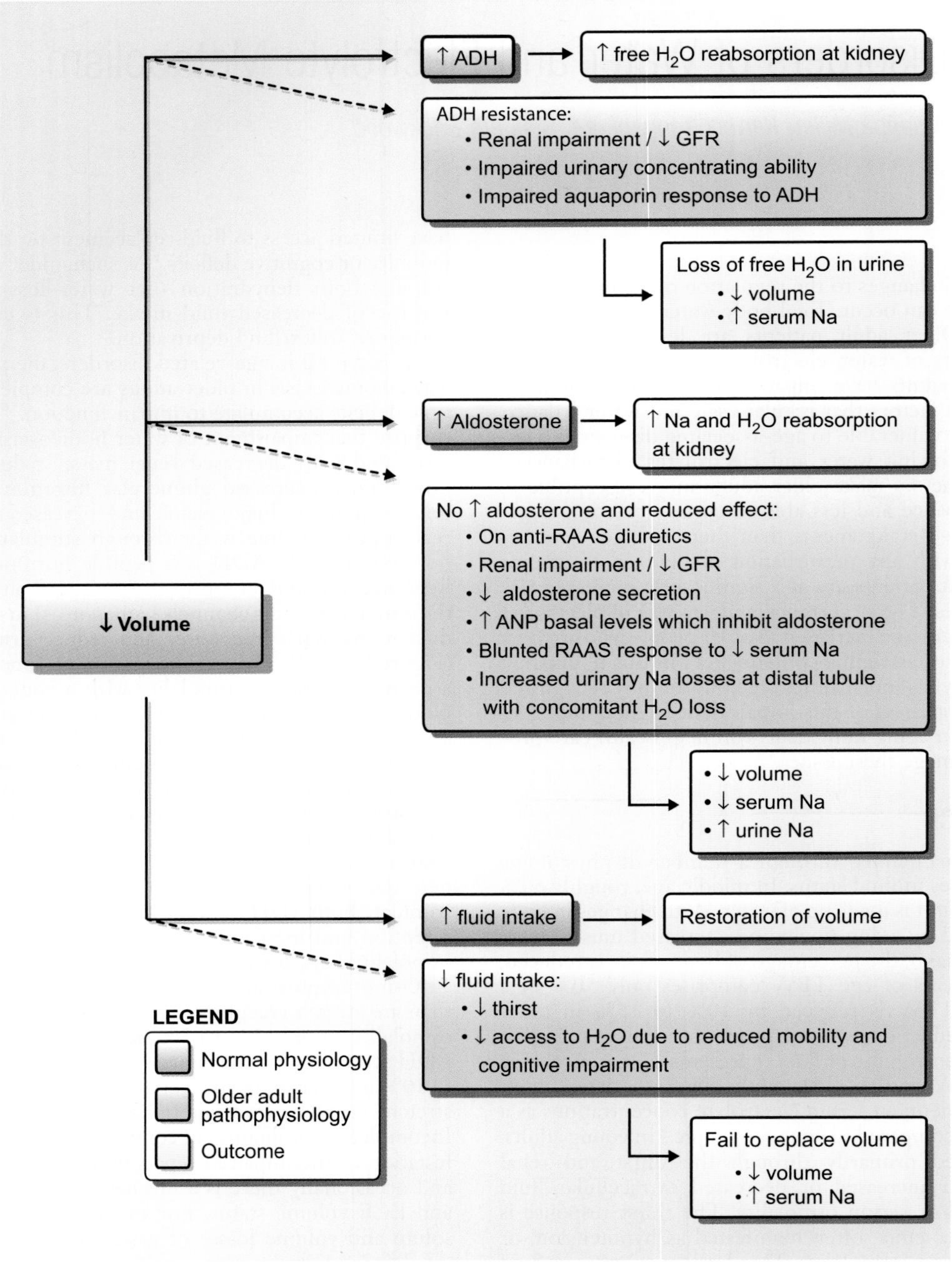

Figure 82-1. Impaired physiologic response to reduced extracellular volume in older individuals. *ADH,* Antidiuretic hormone; *ANP,* atrial natriuretic peptide; *GFR,* glomerular filtration rate; *H_2O,* water; *Na,* sodium; *RAAS,* renin-angiotensin-aldosterone system.

adults are greater than those demonstrated in younger patients, both at baseline and in stimulated states. Thus, inadequate urinary concentrating ability is likely caused by an impaired aquaporin response or a medullary concentrating defect which increases free water excretion in the face of an intact ADH system.[1] It is interesting that in patients with Alzheimer dementia, some studies report a subphysiologic ADH response to dehydration, in comparison to older patients without dementia.[1] The mechanism for this has yet to be elucidated. In combination with functional constraints that may limit a patient's access to water, this inadequate ADH response puts people with Alzheimer disease at an even higher risk for dehydration than other older individuals.[1]

Many other factors can contribute to fluid disturbances in older adults. Those with urinary incontinence often drink less to avoid frequent micturition. Diarrhea, vomiting, and gastrointestinal bleeding can contribute to volume loss in older adult patients, as can decreased intake in the context of anorexia and depression. Poorly controlled diabetes, stroke, draining wounds, fever, rapid breathing, infection, and burns can also impair water and electrolyte balance in aged individuals. In addition to volume loss (with resultant ADH stimulation and increased fluid intake), other conditions such as the syndrome of inappropriate antidiuretic hormone (SIADH) and hypotonic fluid administration can result in hypo-osmolar euvolemia/hypervolemia in older adult

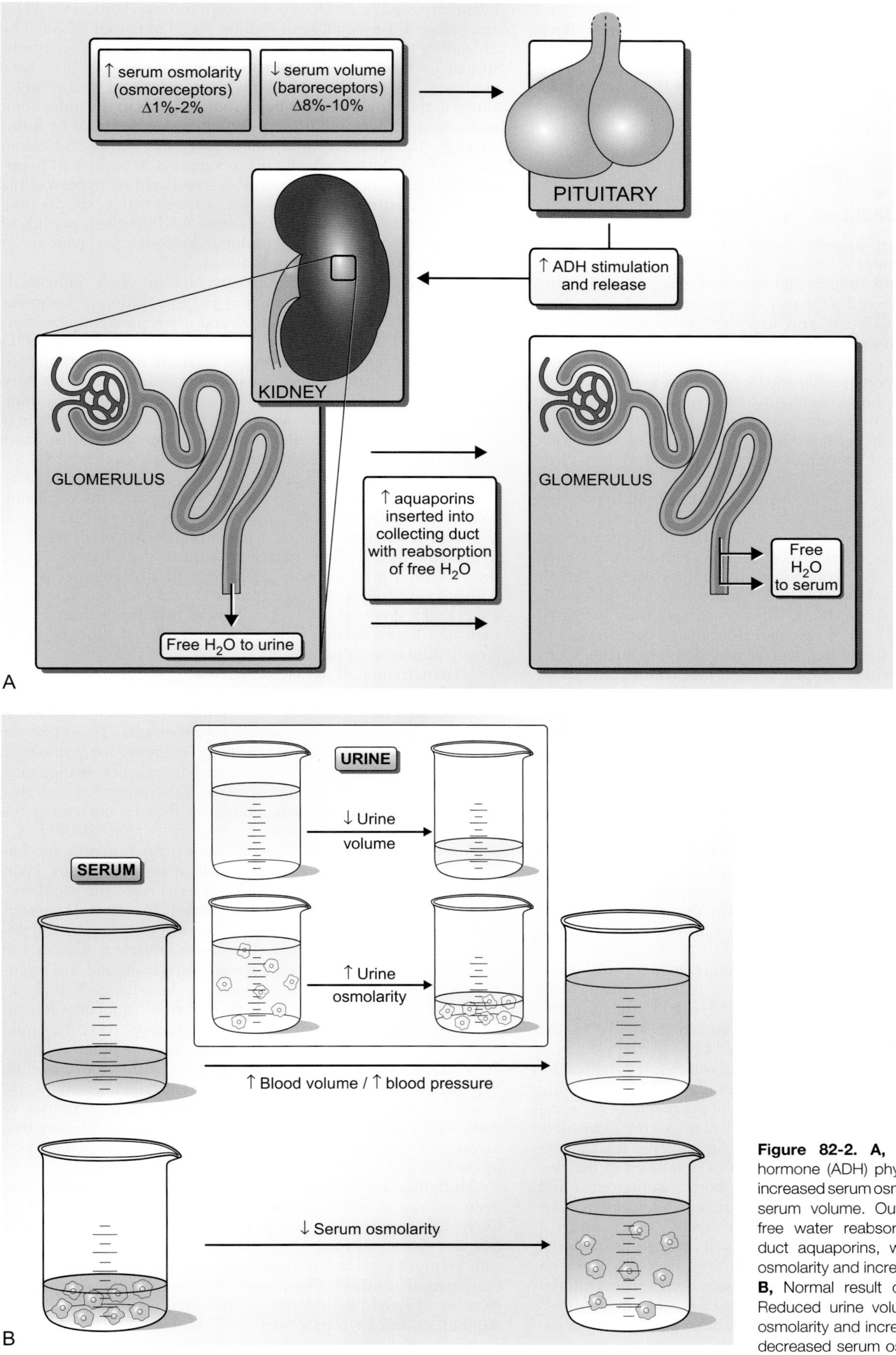

Figure 82-2. A, Normal antidiuretic hormone (ADH) physiology. Stimulus is increased serum osmolarity or decreased serum volume. Outcome is increased free water reabsorption via collecting duct aquaporins, with reduced serum osmolarity and increased serum volume. **B,** Normal result of ADH stimulation. Reduced urine volume/increased urine osmolarity and increased blood volume/ decreased serum osmolarity.

patients. In such cases, compared with younger people, many older adults have a reduced ability to excrete free water, taking 50% longer to return to baseline volume and serum osmolality.[1] This can place them at an increased risk of dilutional hypo-osmolality or volume overload after intake of large volumes of liquids, for example, when receiving hypo-osmolar intravenous fluids during hospitalization.

ELECTROLYTE BALANCE

Sodium Metabolism

The consequences of impaired water homeostasis in older individuals include abnormal volume status and electrolyte abnormalities, most notably hyper- and hyponatremia.[1] Sodium is the major cation in ECF and is the major contributor to serum osmolality in the body. Hyper- and hyponatremia are common in older adults and most evident in hospitalized patients or individuals living in long-term care facilities. Cross-sectional studies have found that hyponatremia may be present in as many as 15% to 18% of nursing home residents.[8] In contrast, approximately 30% of nursing home residents requiring acute hospitalization were shown to be hypernatremic in one study,[13] a result that has been reproduced in studies over a period of almost three decades.[14,15]

Hypovolemia may be a major precipitant of both hyper- and hyponatremia, depending largely on a patient's access to free water. Older patients are at an increased risk of free water loss because of impaired water concentrating abilities in the aged kidney, but they are also prone to urinary sodium losses as a result of dysfunction at the loop of Henle.[16] Taken together, this results in reduced ECF volume status, which is corrected by increased stimulation of ADH and a resultant dilutional hyponatremia in patients with access to water and increased water intake. Conversely, in patients with an impaired thirst mechanism, or in those who don't have access to water because of their impaired mobility or altered cognitive status, the effect on serum sodium is variable. This is because even though ADH is still maximally stimulated in this circumstance, lack of access to water prohibits the development of dilutional hyponatremia. Renal sodium losses are ongoing, if only to a mild degree, and are generally accompanied by some degree of concurrent water loss despite maximal stimulation of ADH. As such, the resulting serum sodium may be either increased or decreased depending on whether relatively more sodium or free water is lost in the urine.

In addition to ADH, sodium status is also influenced by the renin-angiotensin-aldosterone system (RAAS). In periods of low sodium intake, many older patients show an impaired ability to restrict urinary sodium losses compared to their younger counterparts.[1] This may result in hyponatremia and, because water follows sodium along osmotic gradients, in hypovolemia with renal water losses. In addition to loop of Henle dysfunction, the mechanism for reduced sodium concentrating ability in the kidneys of older adults has been proposed to be partially due to a blunted RAAS response to low serum sodium (see Figure 82-1).[17] In younger individuals, hypovolemia stimulates RAAS, resulting in reabsorption of sodium and excretion of potassium in the renal tubules as a means of maintaining euvolemia and electrolyte homeostasis, respectively (Figure 82-3). An impaired RAAS, with less absorption of sodium and excretion of potassium in the face of hypovolemia, may thereby result in both hyponatremia and hyperkalemia in older hypovolemic patients. In addition, in older people, aldosterone is present at lower levels[16] and is under a greater degree of inhibition on the basis of increased basal atrial natriuretic peptide (ANP) levels, which negatively feed back on RAAS, and on aldosterone directly. Furthermore, the renal tubules of older patients are less responsive to the effects of aldosterone.[16] In consequence, in cases of hypovolemia, older adults can develop hyponatremia as a result of both serum sodium dilution via ADH and reduced conservation of sodium via an impaired RAAS. The obligatory renal sodium losses common in older adults is demonstrated by the fact that older people have been shown to have increased 24-hour urinary sodium losses compared with younger adults despite lower renal tubular sodium levels in the older adult population.[17] Increased urinary sodium losses may also be influenced by the fact that older adults have been shown to have an increased ANP level, which fails to suppress in periods of hypovolemia.[1] In younger adults, ANP is stimulated by hypervolemia and serves to stimulate renal sodium wasting with corresponding volume loss. In older patients, elevated ANP levels in periods of hypovolemia can exacerbate volume loss and put patients at increased risk of related complications.

The tendency toward hyponatremia in older individuals appears to reflect a lack of function and integration of a number of physiologic processes. As discussed, there is a frequent tendency toward hypovolemia with resultant stimulation of ADH and dilutional hyponatremia despite a certain degree of impaired urinary concentrating ability. Additionally, older adults often have reduced function of RAAS with concurrent impairment of sodium retention at the loop of Henle, and an increased ANP, which may result in sodium loss.[17] Furthermore, older adults may have impaired sodium homeostasis on the basis of a reduced GFR[17] and are frequently on diuretic therapy and drugs designed to further block the effects of RAAS (angiotensin-converting enzyme [ACE] inhibitors, angiotensin receptor blockers, and aldosterone antagonists). Older patients are particularly sensitive to thiazide-induced hyponatremia because their baseline renal prostaglandin production is lower than that of younger adults. This impairs free water excretion at the level of the kidney, an effect that is counterintuitively enhanced by thiazide diuretics. As such, the hyponatremia induced by thiazides is thought to be largely dilutional in nature.[16,18]

Hyponatremia in older adults may also be attributed to SIADH. In this syndrome, ADH is stimulated in a nonphysiologic manner, such that free water is retained in patients with access to fluid. The eventual outcome is hyponatremia. Treatment for SIADH is removal of the underlying stimulus for pathologic ADH secretion (central nervous system disturbance, malignancy, pneumonia, drugs, etc.) and concurrent fluid restriction such that there is less free water to be absorbed, thereby correcting the hyponatremia. It is important to remember that SIADH is a diagnosis of exclusion: older adults have many potential mechanisms for developing hyponatremia. In many such cases, inappropriate fluid deprivation can further exacerbate the problem.

When hyponatremia is accompanied by central nervous system manifestations or delirium, the morbidity is high. Hyponatremia can cause confusion, drowsiness, muscle weakness, and seizures. A rapid rate of change is most dangerous and will intensify these symptoms, because it does not allow for normal physiologic compensation to the change in serum osmolality. Recent studies have suggested that even in asymptomatic patients, a mild degree of hyponatremia may be detrimental to older adults. A 2011 study reported that older patients with mild-moderate hyponatremia (Na^+ 118 to 131 mM) had significantly worse results in standardized geriatric assessment tests (activities of daily living, Mini-Mental Status Exam, clock completion test, Geriatric Depression Score, Tinetti Mobility Test, the timed get-up-and-go test, and the Mini Nutritional Assessment).[19]

Mild degrees of hyponatremia (Na^+ 131 mM ± 3 mM) have been associated with a greatly increased risk of falls.[20,21] This likely reflects a combination of inattention, postural abnormalities, and gait impairment, demonstrated in patients deemed clinically asymptomatic before assessment and with normal neurologic examination results.[22] These gait abnormalities are comparable to those induced by moderate alcohol intake.[22] In addition, subsequent studies have proposed an additional increased fracture

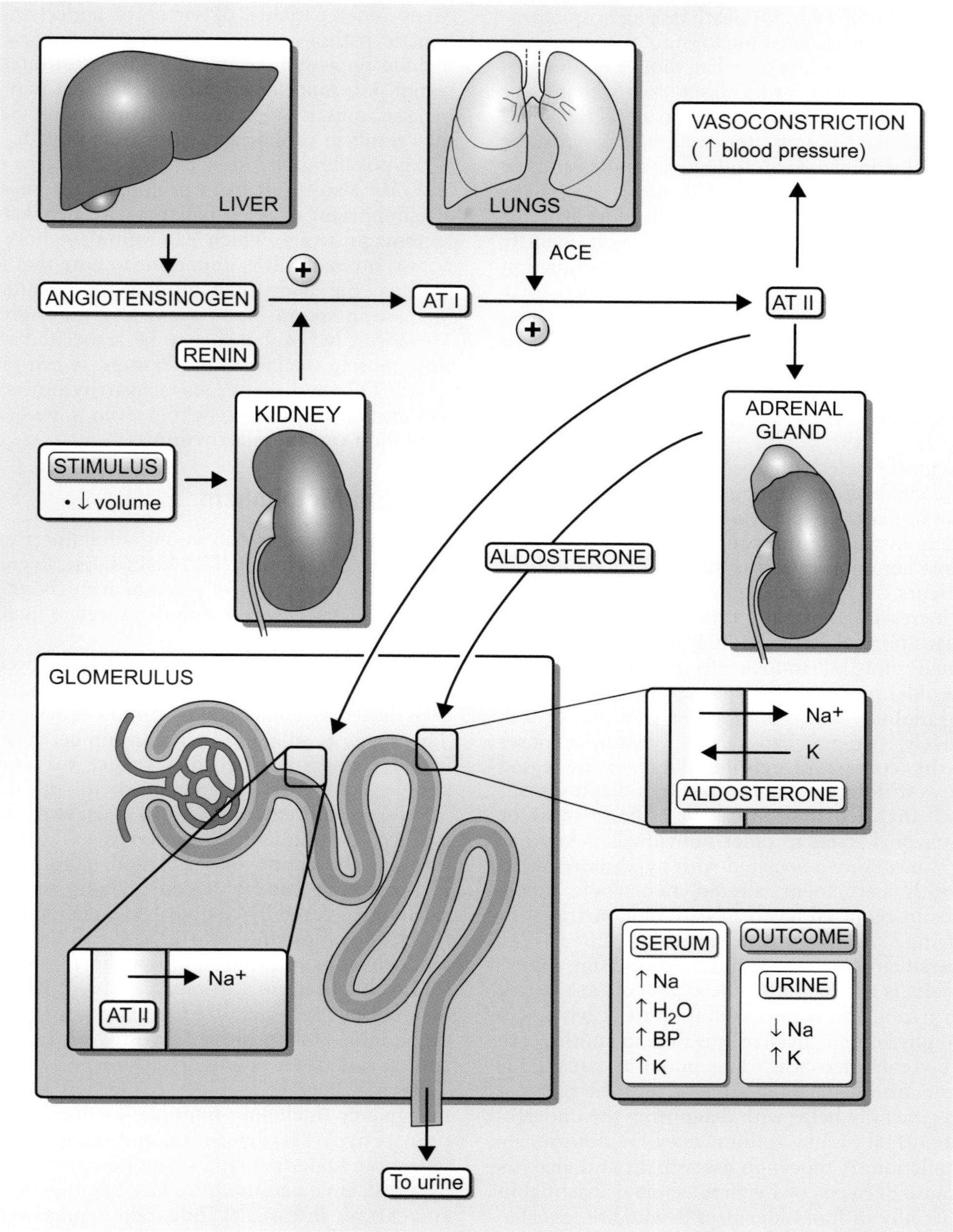

Figure 82-3. Normal renin-angiotensin-aldosterone system physiology. Stimulus is decreased serum volume/blood pressure (aldosterone additionally stimulated by hyponatremia/hyperkalemia). Outcome is increased tubular sodium reabsorption (with concomitant H_2O reabsorption) and urinary loss of potassium. Serum sodium is increased, potassium is decreased, and serum volume/blood pressure is restored. *ACE,* Angiotensin-converting enzyme; *AT,* angiotensin; BP, blood pressure; *H_2O,* water; *K,* potassium; *Na,* sodium.

risk (odds ratio [OR], 2.25) in older individuals with mild hyponatremia, independent of the increased frequency of falls in this population, and taking into consideration age, bone mineral density, presence of chronic kidney disease, and other osteoporotic risk factors.[20] This has been proposed to be on the basis of hyponatremia-induced abnormalities in bone morphology.[22] In addition, the NHANES III study has recently demonstrated a significantly increased risk of osteoporosis in the hip (OR 2.85) in patients with mild chronic hyponatremia (mean Na^+, 133 mM), when accounting for other variables.[21,23] This was confirmed by a subsequent study in 2014, which revealed that in older patients with fragility fractures, hyponatremia was present in 26% of cases.[24] Increased falls and gait abnormalities in the context of weakened bones with reduced density and abnormal bone quality predisposes older patients with mild hyponatremia to orthopedic misadventures. Hyponatremia (Na^+ < 135 mM) is also associated with an increased mortality risk compared with normonatremic patients (Na^+ 135 to 144 mM) during hospitalization as well as at 1 and 5 years after discharge, with adjusted odds ratios of 1.47, 1.38, and 1.25, respectively.[25] Even in mild hyponatremia (Na^+

130 to 134 mM), adjusted odds ratio for death during hospitalization was 1.37 compared with normonatremic patients.[25] At present, there is no clear consensus on what should be done to manage these patients. Recent enthusiasm for vaptans, or V2-receptor antagonists, which block the effects of ADH[23] (and thus correct hyponatremia through free water loss), must be tempered by the need for longer-term follow-up studies and for independent studies that evaluate cost-effectiveness.

The physical examination for volume status in older patients is challenging. The "water offered test" (WOT) aims to identify patients with volume depletion resulting in ADH stimulation and a dilutional hyponatremia. Although older individuals may deny feeling thirsty, they will accept and drink water, when offered, if they are in fact dehydrated or hypovolemic. Any patient with hyponatremia and a positive WOT likely needs frequent encouragement and verbal cuing from caregivers, as well as solute-rich fluid replacement, to remain normovolemic and normonatremic.[26]

Hypernatremia, another electrolyte abnormality common in older patients, is also challenging. Among adults aged 70 years or older, the prevalence of plasma hyperosmolality can be as high as 30%.[27] One study demonstrated surgery (21%) and febrile illness (20%) to be the most common causes of hypernatremia in hospitalized older patients.[28] Hypernatremia has been associated with a sevenfold increased mortality rate compared to age-matched controls with normal serum sodium levels.[28] It is interesting that this may not be influenced by the degree of hypernatremia.[28] In older patients, hypernatremia may be associated with decreased mobility and lack of access to water, or lack of thirst. Alternatively, patients can develop insidious onset hypernatremia in the context of febrile illness or increased ambient temperatures with free water loss through diaphoresis.[29] One study suggested that dehydration can be either a cause or effect of acute confusional states in older individuals.[30] Another demonstrated a 42% mortality associated with hypernatremia in older patients,[29] with permanent altered neurologic status reflected by changes in required levels of care demonstrated in 38% of those surviving.[29]

Overall, the assessment and management of sodium abnormalities in older adults is challenging. These patients are at risk of developing both hypo- and hypernatremia on the basis of a number of impaired physiologic mechanisms that, in youth, serve to maintain electrolyte homeostasis. The potential causes for sodium derangements in older people are vast, and the physical examination, which generally helps with diagnosing the underlying cause of an abnormal serum sodium level, is notoriously difficult in this population. A thorough assessment and analysis of the underlying cause of hypo- or hypernatremia is essential in all patients, but especially in frail older people who are less able to tolerate the consequences of these abnormalities.

Potassium Metabolism

Like sodium, potassium (the chief intracellular ion) needs to be adequately balanced to maintain normal function of the organ systems. Older patients are at risk for developing hyperkalemia due to a number of factors, including decreased GFR, decreased renal blood flow with impaired potassium excretion in the distal secretory sites, and an impaired and blunted RAAS.[1,28] In addition, there is a positive association between increasing age and risk for drug-induced hyperkalemia.[1] Typical offending drugs in the general population include potassium supplements; potassium-sparing diuretics such as spironolactone, triamterene, and amiloride; and ACE inhibitors or angiotensin receptor blockers. Moreover, the use of nonsteroidal antiinflammatory drugs (NSAIDs), cyclosporine or tacrolimus, trimethoprim-sulfamethoxazole, heparin, ketoconazole, and, in rare cases, β-blockers can also lead to the development of hyperkalemia.[1] Many older patients, by virtue of underlying cardiac, renal, or hepatic pathology, may be initiated on low-sodium diets that include potassium-containing salt substitutes that can increase serum potassium levels.[28] Hyperkalemia may present as general malaise, muscle weakness, or palpitations. Severe hyperkalemia may result in cardiac arrhythmias and death.

Hypokalemia is often caused by the use of diuretic therapy and may also result from prolonged diarrhea or vomiting. It is also important to assess patients with hypokalemia for coexistent hypomagnesemia, which can stimulate both urinary and fecal potassium losses. It is important to note that in prolonged hypokalemia, the body may produce less insulin with a resulting increase in serum blood sugar levels and glucose intolerance.[31] Moreover, hypokalemia may be associated with fatigue, confusion, muscle weakness, and cramps. It can predispose to a prolonged QTc and dangerous tachyarrhythmias, especially in those patients on digoxin, in whom even a moderately low level of potassium can cause arrhythmias.

Calcium Metabolism

Calcium homeostasis in young adults is primarily mediated by parathyroid hormone (PTH). In hypocalcemia, increased PTH stimulates resorption of calcium from bone (where more than 99% of body calcium is stored), as well as increased intestinal and renal reabsorption.

In older adults with normal renal function, serum PTH concentrations have been shown to run twofold to threefold higher than those of younger adults with the same serum calcium levels.[28] This suggests an altered relationship between calcium and PTH in older adults,[28] which may reduce the capacity for the older body to compensate for derangements in calcium homeostasis.

Most commonly, older adults are in an overall negative calcium balance, despite normal serum levels (which are maintained through the action of PTH and ongoing bone resorption).[32] Hypocalcemia can be caused by increased urinary excretion of calcium triggered by vitamin D deficiency, a reduced response to PTH, loop diuretics, and glucocorticoid therapy. Additionally, septicemia, pancreatitis, and low dietary calcium intake can also lead to hypocalcemia in older adults. Low serum calcium levels may present as generalized weakness, numbness of the extremities, confusion, a positive Chvostek or Trousseau sign clinically, and, in rare cases, tetany or seizures.

Hypercalcemia in older patients is usually associated with malignancy (including multiple myeloma and bony metastases), primary hyperparathyroidism, and, occasionally, prolonged immobilization. Older patients are at increased risk for immobilization hypercalcemia because of reduced ambulation, general weakness, and chronic disease.[33] While mild hypercalcemia may be asymptomatic, more severe forms (Ca^{2+} persistently > 2.75 mM) can precipitate hypovolemia[34] through a furosemide (Lasix)–like mechanism with concurrent sodium and water loss at the loop of Henle.[35,36] Other consequences of hypercalcemia include loss of appetite, nausea, vomiting, confusion, and even coma.

Phosphate Metabolism

Phosphate homeostasis is maintained by calcium, PTH, activated vitamin D, and the newly identified fibroblast growth factor 23 (FGF-23) phosphatonin and its coreceptor Klotho. FGF-23 promotes renal phosphate wasting at the proximal tubule and is present in increased serum concentrations in chronic kidney disease. In 2012, the Cardiovascular Health Study demonstrated increased all-cause mortality and incident heart failure rates in community-dwelling adults older than 65 years with increased serum FGF-23 levels. This association was independent of renal status but appeared to be further increased in those patients with concurrent chronic kidney disease.[37]

Decreased oral intake (<100 mg of phosphate daily) in older patients may predispose to hypophosphatemia. Additionally, low serum phosphate levels may develop in the context of normal phosphate intake with reduced absorption as a result of chronic diarrhea or the ingestion of magnesium- or aluminum-based antacids, which bind phosphate in the intestinal tract when taken with food.[38] Urinary phosphate wasting on the basis of either renal tubular disease, vitamin D deficiency, or hyperparathyroidism-induced renal phosphate losses can also contribute to hypophosphatemia.[38] Reduced phosphate levels may develop acutely in older patients as a result of intracellular shifts of phosphate precipitated by such driving forces as treatment of diabetic ketoacidosis, refeeding syndrome, and acute respiratory alkalosis.[38] Alcoholic patients may suffer from hypophosphatemia due to a combination of the previously mentioned mechanisms because alcohol can induce a proximal tubular deficiency with urinary phosphate wasting, gastritis with frequent diarrhea and requiring management with antacids, and reduced nutritional intake.[38] Hypophosphatemia may present as a broad spectrum of neurologic abnormalities, including muscle weakness, paresthesias, mental status changes, generalized seizures, and coma. Patients may present with rhabdomyolysis, impaired platelet and white blood cell function, and, infrequently, intravascular red blood cell hemolysis. They also may develop bony abnormalities such as rickets or osteomalacia, impaired diaphragmatic function leading to respiratory failure, or reduced cardiac function and/or cardiac arrest in severe cases.

Renal insufficiency, which increases in prevalence with age, is a risk factor for the development of hyperphosphatemia as a result of decreased phosphate elimination. Alternatively, acute hyperphosphatemia may overwhelm renal excretion abilities, even in patients with apparently normal renal function. This can occur in such circumstances as tumor lysis syndrome, rhabdomyolysis (both cause and effect of increased phosphate), bisphosphonate use, vitamin D toxicity, and ingestion of phosphate-containing laxatives.[38]

Hyperphosphatemia can predispose to vascular calcification with resulting increased risk of ischemic stroke, coronary artery disease, cardiac valvular disease, and peripheral vascular disease. Hyperphosphatemia may also present with nephrocalcinosis or nephrolithiasis and with abnormalities in bone morphology (such as osteitis fibrosis or osteomalacia) due to resultant secondary hyperparathyroidism.[38]

Magnesium Metabolism

Older patients are at an increased risk of hypomagnesemia and reduced tissue magnesium levels. Autopsy studies have reported reduced magnesium in heart and muscle cells in older individuals.[39] In one study, 10% of hospitalized older patients had low serum magnesium levels at admission.[39]

Like other electrolytes, magnesium homeostasis is maintained by a balance between intake, intracellular shifts, and renal excretion.[39] As with other electrolyte abnormalities, many factors can cause hypomagnesemia in older patients. Inadequate magnesium intake in both healthy, older outpatients and hospitalized patients is common.[39] Magnesium loss in the urine is present in diabetic patients because of glucosuria, ketoacidosis, and hypophosphatemia.[16] Magnesium supplementation may improve glucose tolerance and increase insulin sensitivity in peripheral tissues.[40] Hypomagnesemia has also been associated with an increased risk of developing diabetic retinopathy in individuals with type 2 diabetes.[41,42] A number of drugs are associated with the potential for older adults to develop hypomagnesemia; these drugs include proton pump inhibitors, aminoglycosides, digoxin, laxatives, and pamidronate.[39] Loop and thiazide diuretics are particularly common in older individuals who suffer from congestive heart failure and may lead to urinary magnesium wasting.[39] Another common cause of hypomagnesemia in older patients is a history of alcohol abuse, which reduces magnesium levels in a multifactorial manner. Alcohol intake is associated with concurrent metabolic acidosis, hypophosphatemia, and respiratory alkalosis, which reduce serum magnesium levels through cellular shifts, in addition to a direct magnesiuric effect stimulated by acute alcohol consumption.[16] Chronic diarrhea can cause hypomagnesemia because of increased magnesium losses in stool. In addition, previous studies have demonstrated that older patients frequently have inadequate magnesium intake in their diets.[16] In these individuals, any further superimposed magnesium losses may result in hypomagnesemia.[16]

Hypomagnesemia is generally asymptomatic but may present as central nervous system abnormalities such as depression, psychosis, changes in personality, nystagmus, athetoid movements, and seizures. Patients may develop myocardial arrhythmias in settings of severe hypomagnesemia, or they may have nonspecific symptoms such as gastrointestinal complaints, nausea, vomiting, anorexia, or muscle cramps with (in rare cases) progression to tetany.[39] Patients with hypomagnesemia may present with a number of additional electrolyte abnormalities, including hypocalcemia and hypokalemia, both of which are refractory to correction unless magnesium levels are normalized.[39]

Acid-Base Status

The body has two main mechanisms to maintain acid-base status at a stable pH of between 7.35 and 7.45. In acidosis, which is defined as a blood pH less than 7.35, the body compensates by increasing respiratory ventilation to blow off CO_2, and by the renal excretion of H^+ ions in the form of NH_4^+, associated with a concomitant resorption of bicarbonate ions HCO_3^- at the level of the kidney. In alkalosis, respiratory ventilation is reduced, and CO_2 is retained by a slowed respiratory rate. H^+ ions are retained at the level of the kidney with resultant renal loss of HCO_3^-.

With aging, the acid-base regulating ability of the kidney declines dramatically compared with younger individuals. H^+ ions are excreted less efficiently, predisposing patients to exaggerated systemic acidosis as they are less able to compensate.[28] In addition, pulmonary pathology such as obstructive lung disease is much more common in older patients, and this further limits the ability for adequate respiratory compensation in the face of acid-base derangements.[28]

CONCLUSION

Older adults have an impaired ability to regulate body water and electrolyte balance. This is due to multiple factors, including a reduction in thirst sensation and diminished urine concentrating ability, among other issues. Not only are frail older individuals more susceptible to developing abnormalities in salt and water homeostasis, they are also less able to tolerate these derangements compared to younger patients. Thus, scrupulous monitoring of fluid and electrolyte balance is imperative in both community-dwelling and hospital-admitted frail older patients to recognize normal physiologic derangements and to avoid iatrogenic insult.

KEY POINTS

- The occurrence and severity of electrolyte abnormalities appear to be increased in older people who are frail.
- Older adults are at risk of hypovolemia secondary to decreased thirst, gastrointestinal and renal losses, and often limited access to fluid replacement. They are also susceptible to volume overload in settings of large fluid intake (oral or intravenous) because of an impaired ability to excrete free water efficiently.

- Hypovolemia can give rise to both hypernatremia and hyponatremia in older adults, depending on access to free water and/or the tonicity of intravenous fluid replacement and water concentrating ability.
- In older adults, hypovolemia can result in hyponatremia as a result of both continued antidiuretic hormone secretion and an impaired response to activation of the renin-angiotensin-aldosterone system.
- Electrolyte abnormalities are frequent in older adults and may be the direct result of certain medications. In this population, the workup of altered electrolyte concentrations (Na^+, K^+, Ca^{2+}, PO_4^{3-}, Mg^{2+}) should include a thorough medication review and assessment for an offending agent.

For a complete list of references, please visit www.expertconsult.com.

KEY REFERENCES

1. Beck LH: Fluid and electrolyte balance in the elderly. Geriatr Nephrol Urol 9:11–14, 1999.
2. Allison SP, Lobo DN: Fluid and electrolytes in the elderly. Curr Opin Clin Nutr Metab Care 7:27–33, 2004.
4. Kenney WL, Chiu P: Influence of age on thirst and fluid intake. Med Sci Sports Exerc 33:1524–1532, 2001.
8. Beck LH: Changes in renal function with aging. Clin Geriatr Med 14:199–209, 1998.
9. Lindeman RD, Tobin J, Shock NW: Longitudinal studies on the rate of decline in renal function with age. J Am Geriatr Soc 33:278–285, 1985.
16. Elisaf MS, et al: Electrolyte abnormalities in elderly patients admitted to a general medical ward. Geriatr Nephrol Urol 7:73–79, 1991.
17. Refoyo A, Macias-Nufiez JF: The maintenance of plasma sodium in the healthy aged. Geriatr Nephrol Urol 1:65–68, 1991.
20. Renneboog R, et al: Mild chronic hyponatremia is associated with falls, unsteadiness, and attention deficits. Am J Med 119:71.e1–71.e8, 2006.
22. Decaux G: Is asymptomatic hyponatremia really asymptomatic? Am J Med 119(Suppl 1):S79–S82, 2006.
25. Waiker SS, et al: Mortality after hospitalization with mild, moderate, and severe hyponatremia. Am J Med 122:857–865, 2009.
28. Luckey AE, et al: Fluid and electrolytes in the aged. Arch Surg 138:1055–1060, 2003.
29. Arieff AI: Pathogenesis and management of hypernatremia. Curr Opin Crit Care 2:418–423, 1996.
38. Xing XS, et al: A synopsis of phosphate disorders in the nursing home. J Am Med Dir Assoc 11:468–474, 2010.
39. Lowenthal DT, Ruiz JG: Clinical pharmacology-physiology conference: magnesium deficiency in the elderly. Geriatr Nephrol Urol 5:105–111, 1995.

83 The Prostate

William Cross, Stephen Prescott

INTRODUCTION

Prostate gland disorders are extremely common and a frequent reason for medical consultation in older men. The two most prevalent prostate conditions are benign prostatic hyperplasia (BPH) and prostate cancer, both of which increase in incidence with advancing age. Benign prostatic enlargement (BPE) is the fourth most common diagnosed condition, following coronary artery disease/hyperlipidemia, hypertension, and type 2 diabetes, in men older than 65 years.[1] In 2000 in the United States, approximately 4.5 million visits were made to physician offices for a primary diagnosis of BPH, and the estimated direct cost of BPH treatment was $1.1 billion exclusive of outpatient pharmaceuticals.[2] Prostate cancer is the second most frequent cancer diagnosed in American men, with 6 cases in 10 diagnosed in those aged 65 years or older. The estimated cost of prostate cancer care in the United States in 2010 was $11.85 billion (total cost of cancer care $124.57 billion), which is projected to increase to approximately $19 billion by 2020.[3]

As the aging population increases and prostate disorders become more prevalent, the majority of men with prostate conditions will increasingly rely on medical care being delivered by health care professionals other than urologists. It is important that these health care providers are aware of the latest prostate guidelines and care pathways in order to deliver the highest quality of care, improve clinical outcomes, and contain health care costs.

BENIGN PROSTATIC HYPERPLASIA

BPH is a pathologic process that, by definition, can be diagnosed only by histologic assessment and not by physical examination. Historically, many men with lower urinary tract symptoms (LUTS) were labeled as having the symptom complex of "prostatism," which was almost universally attributed to BPH. This clinical assumption has been challenged with the appreciation that male LUTS may be unrelated to the prostate gland and secondary to other pathology or even a side effect of medication (Box 83-1). This greater understanding of the pathophysiology of male LUTS has contributed to an evolution of the clinical terminology, which now offers a more descriptive assessment of the presenting symptoms[4] (Table 83-1). Therefore, although many men present with LUTS suggestive of bladder outflow obstruction (BOO), and on clinical examination have BPE secondary to BPH, it is not uncommon for a man to have significant LUTS without BOO, BPE, or BPH (Figure 83-1). This highlights that the selection of appropriate treatment for male LUTS requires a careful evaluation of symptoms to identify the underlying causative condition(s).

Prevalence of Lower Urinary Tract Symptoms and Benign Prostate Hyperplasia in Men

LUTS are highly prevalent in the male population. The Multinational Survey of the Aging Male (MSAM-7) questioned nearly 13,000 men aged 50 to 80 years in the United States and six European countries.[5] Overall, 31% of respondents reported moderate-to-severe LUTS, which was consistent across the countries. The prevalence was positively related to age, ranging from 22% in men aged 50 to 59 years to 45.3% in men aged 70 to 80 years. One interesting finding is that only 19% of men with LUTS had sought medical help for their urinary symptoms and only 10.2% had been medically treated. The Rancho Bernardo Study, a prospective, community-based study of aging, assessed the prevalence and characteristics of LUTS in community-dwelling men aged 80 years and older.[6] The prevalence of LUTS was 70% in men 80 years and older and 56% in men younger than 80 years ($P = .03$). Compared to the younger men, those aged 80 years or older also reported more severe symptoms.

The prevalence of BPH, similar to that of LUTS, also increases with age. It is important to note that when interpreting and comparing the literature on the prevalence of BPH, caution is needed because epidemiologic studies have used both histologic and clinical definitions to calculate the prevalence. Autopsy studies have revealed that based on histologic criteria, BPH increases from 8% in men aged 31 to 40 years, to 40% to 50% in men aged 51 to 60 years, and over 80% in men older than 80 years.[7] The Baltimore Longitudinal Study of Aging compared the age-specific cumulative prevalence of male LUTS with the autopsy prevalence of BPH and reported a close correlation.[8]

The incidence and prevalence of BPH and LUTS are increasing significantly as the U.S. population ages. Between 1998 and 2007, the age-adjusted prevalence of BPH among hospitalized patients in the United States nearly doubled.[9]

Pathogenesis of Benign Prostatic Hyperplasia

BPH is histologically characterized by an increase in epithelial and stromal cells in the region adjacent to the prostatic urethra. Although the detailed molecular etiology of the hyperplastic process remains to be fully established, it has been shown to be influenced by a combination of androgens, growth factors, estrogens, and epithelial-stromal interactions.[10] Contrary to historical texts, androgens do not directly cause BPH, as there is no direct relationship between the concentration of serum androgens and prostate volume in aging men. However, testicular androgens do have a role, as men castrated before puberty do not develop BPH. In the prostate, testosterone is converted by the enzyme 5α-reductase to dihydrotestosterone, the principal driver of androgen-dependent gene transcription and protein synthesis, resulting in cell proliferation. Inhibition of 5α-reductase is used clinically to induce prostatic involution to treat urinary symptoms secondary to BPH.

BPH causes urethral intrusion and bladder outflow obstruction, resulting in compensatory changes in bladder function. The initial adaptive bladder changes maintain voiding function, but with further deterioration, the bladder muscle can become unstable and/or lose contractility. Men with BPH often experience a complex of symptoms secondary to prostatic obstruction and bladder dysfunction.

Clinical Assessment of Lower Urinary Tract Symptoms

A thorough and comprehensive clinical evaluation of men with LUTS is crucial because it helps render an accurate diagnosis,

BOX 83-1 Causes of Male Lower Urinary Tract Symptoms

Benign prostatic enlargement (secondary to benign prostatic hyperplasia)
Urinary tract infection
Prostatitis
Overactive bladder
Neurogenic bladder dysfunction
Urethral stricture
Bladder neck contracture
Phimosis
Urinary tract stones
Bladder tumor
Advanced prostate cancer
Foreign body in the bladder
Medications, illicit drugs, and dietary factors (including caffeine, alcohol, ketamine, and decongestants)
Diabetes mellitus

TABLE 83-1 International Continence Society Definitions of Lower Urinary Tract Symptoms

Voiding symptoms	*Hesitancy* is difficulty in initiating micturition resulting in a delay in the onset of voiding after being ready to pass urine. *Slow stream* is the perception of reduced urine flow, usually compared to previous performance or in comparison to others. *Splitting or spraying* of the urine stream. *Intermittent stream* (intermittency) is the term used to describe urine flow that stops and starts, on one or more occasions, during micturition. *Straining* to void describes the muscular effort used to initiate, maintain, or improve the urinary stream. *Terminal dribble* is the term used to describe a prolonged final part of micturition, when the flow has slowed to a trickle or dribble.
Storage symptoms	*Increased daytime frequency* is the complaint by the patient who considers that he voids too often during the day. *Nocturia* is the complaint that the man has to wake at night one or more times to void. *Urgency* is the complaint of a sudden compelling desire to pass urine that is difficult to defer. *Urinary incontinence* is the complaint of any involuntary leakage of urine.
Postmicturition symptoms	*Feeling of incomplete emptying* is a self-explanatory term for a feeling experienced by the individual after passing urine. *Postmicturition dribble* is the term used to describe the involuntary loss of urine immediately after finishing passing urine, usually after leaving the toilet.

which, considering the multiple factors contributing to the development of male LUTS, can be difficult. A thorough evaluation also directs therapeutic intervention and treatment. The American Urological Association (AUA) and the European Association of Urology (EAU) have produced evidence-based recommendations to guide and direct clinicians managing men with LUTS.[11,12] These guidelines include recommended tests that should be performed on all men during the initial evaluation and optional tests, usually undertaken in specialist urology clinics (Figure 83-2). If the initial evaluation indicates that a man with LUTS has prostate cancer, hematuria, recurrent urinary tract infection, a palpable bladder, urethral stricture, and/or a neurologic bladder disorder, he should be referred to a urology clinic for appropriate investigation and treatment.

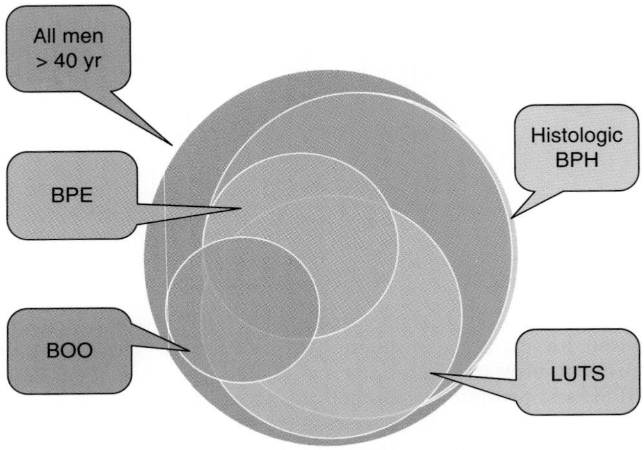

Figure 83-1. Occurance of LUTS with and without BOO, BPE, or BPH. *BOO,* Bladder outflow obstruction; *BPH,* benign prostate hyperplasia; *BPE,* benign prostate enlargement.

All patients should have a focused history taken, addressing urologic and systemic conditions that may cause LUTS. In addition, it is recommended that current medications be reviewed because many drugs commonly prescribed to older people have urinary tract side effects. As part of the history, a self-completed validated symptoms questionnaire can be used to objectively assess and stratify men with LUTS. The questionnaires routinely used in clinical practice were not designed to be used to make a differential diagnosis but were developed to assess the severity of symptoms and to objectively measure the impact of specific therapeutic interventions.

The two most commonly applied questionnaires are the AUA symptom score (Table 83-2) and the International Prostate Symptom Score (IPSS), both of which contain seven symptom questions addressing urinary frequency, nocturia, weak urinary stream, hesitancy, intermittency, incomplete bladder emptying, and urgency. Each symptom is scored on a scale of 0 (not present) to 5 (almost always present) and then summed to stratify the symptom complex as mild (total score 0 to 7), moderate (total score 8 to 19) or severe (total score 20 to 35). The IPSS has an additional disease-specific quality-of-life question: "If you were to spend the rest of your life with your urinary condition the way it is now, how would you feel about that?" A limitation of the AUA score and the IPSS is that they do not address the perception of intrusion on daily life associated with each symptom, unlike other but longer questionnaires such as the International Consultation on Incontinence Questionnaire[13] and the Danish Prostate Symptom Score.[14]

In patients with significant storage LUTS (i.e., frequency, urgency, and nocturia), a frequency volume chart (FVC) is often very useful. The FVC records the volume and time of each void self-recorded by the patient, from which the voiding frequency, total voided volume, and fraction of urine produced during the night can be calculated. To reduce errors, it is recommended that a FVC should be collected over at least 3 days but not too long to cause noncompliance. The FVC will identify 24-hour polyuria (>3 L/24 hr) and nocturnal polyuria (>33% of the 24-hr urine output at night), which can be managed with lifestyle advice and reduced fluid intake.[15]

The physical examination should always include a digital rectal examination (DRE) to assess the shape, symmetry, nodularity, and firmness of the prostate gland, which can be altered in disease states. Normally, the prostate has a consistency similar to that of the contracted thenar eminence muscle of the thumb (opposition of the thumb to the little finger). It is important to note that nodularity within the prostate gland may be secondary

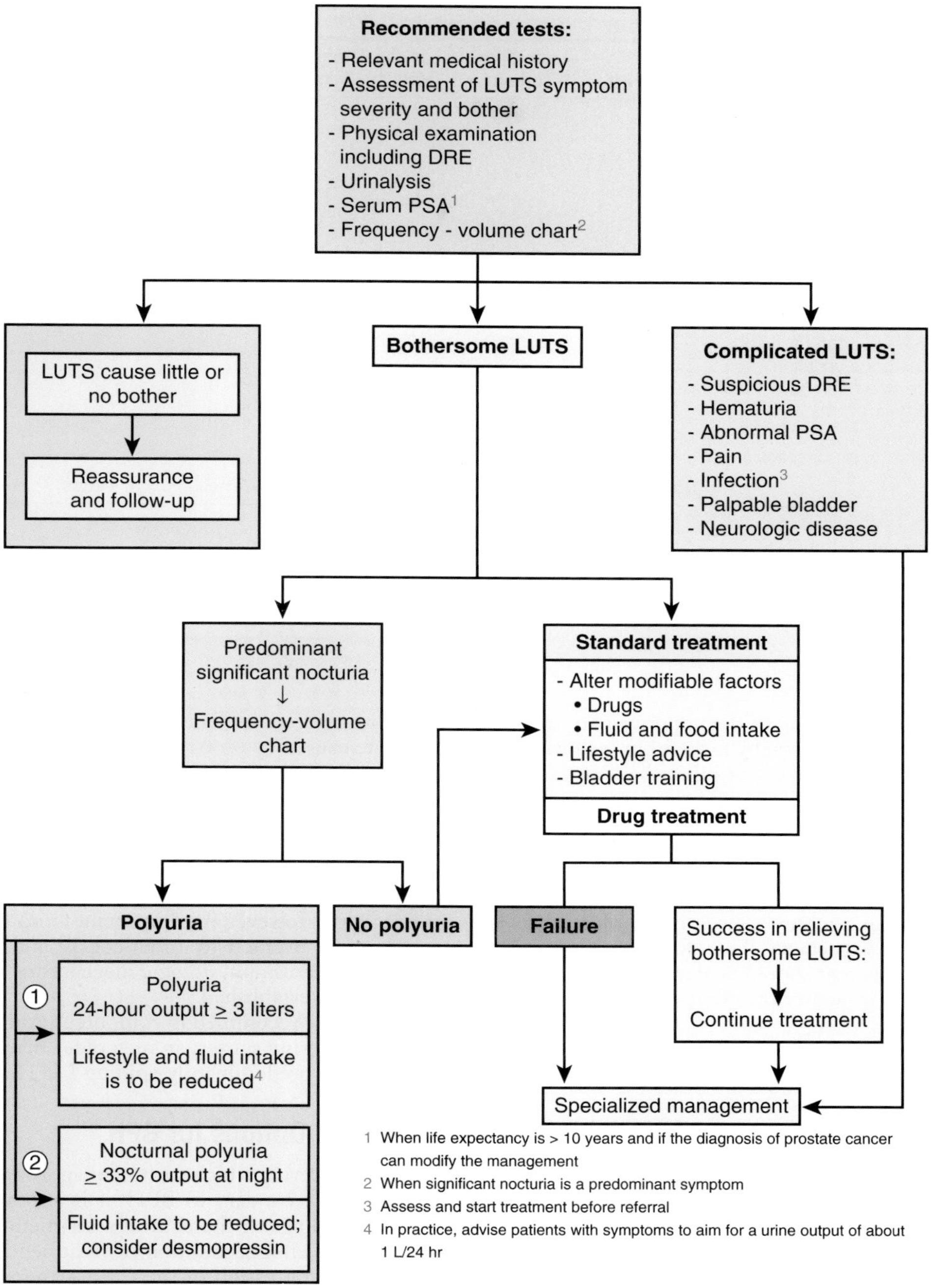

Figure 83-2. Basic management of lower urinary tract symptoms (LUTS) in men. *DRE,* Digital rectal examination; *LUTS,* lower urinary tract symptoms; *PSA,* prostate-specific antigen.

to benign pathology, such as BPH, rather than prostate cancer. Although prostate volume estimation is not crucial in the decision process as to whether a man needs active treatment for his LUTS/BPH, it does have an important role in selecting the most appropriate medical or surgical intervention in those who do need intervention. As assessment of prostate volume by DRE is very unreliable, and often overestimates the volume of small prostates and underestimates the volume in larger glands, prostate size is more accurately measured by ultrasound examination.

Despite the lack of robust evidence, both AUA and EAU guidelines recommend obtaining urinalysis in the routine assessment of men with LUTS. The test is inexpensive and is used to screen for urinary tract infection, diabetes mellitus, and hematuria. If the latter is present, then diagnostic flexible cystoscopy and upper urologic tract imaging should be considered. The role of renal function assessment by serum creatinine or estimated glomerular filtration rate in the investigation of LUTS is controversial. The AUA doesn't recommend obtaining these tests in routine assessment, but the EAU states that "renal function must be performed if renal impairment is suspected, based on history and clinical examination or in the presence of hydronephrosis or when considering surgical treatment for male LUTS." Men with BPH and renal insufficiency have increased risk of postoperative complications, including an increased risk of mortality. Although

TABLE 83-2 American Urological Association Benign Prostatic Hyperplasia Symptom Score

	Not at All	Less Than 1 Time in 5	Less Than Half the Time	About Half the Time	More Than Half the Time	Almost Always
1. Over the past month, how often have you had a sensation of not emptying your bladder completely after you have finished urinating?	0	1	2	3	4	5
2. Over the past month, how often have you had to urinate again less than 2 hours after you have finished?	0	1	2	3	4	5
3. Over the past month, how often have you found you stopped and started again several times when you urinated?	0	1	2	3	4	5
4. Over the past month, how often have you found it difficult to postpone urination?	0	1	2	3	4	5
5. Over the past month, how often have you had a weak urinary stream?						
6. Over the past month, how often have you had to push or strain to begin urination?						
	None	**1 Time**	**2 Times**	**3 Times**	**4 Times**	**5 or More Times**
7. Over the past month, how many times did you most typically get up to urinate from the time when you went to bed at night until the time you got up in the morning?						
Total Symptom Score						

there is no role for routine imaging of the upper urinary tract in men with LUTS, renal ultrasonography is useful in men who are found to have an elevated serum creatinine, hematuria, or a urinary tract infection.

Localized prostate cancer commonly coexists with BPH in older men and can lead to LUTS by producing bladder outflow obstruction. Although the diagnosis of a locally advanced prostate cancer will usually influence the management of LUTS, the detection of small volume prostate cancer in an older man is unlikely to reduce his life expectancy. Therefore, prostate cancer screening by PSA measurement should be done only if a diagnosis of prostate cancer will influence the clinical management of a patient with LUTS.

Optional Test Performed in Specialist Units

In specialist units, assessment of urinary flow rate with a noninvasive flow meter (uroflowmetry) is routinely part of the investigations for men with LUTS. In this test the patient voids into a device that measures the volume of urine voided over time, from which the maximum urinary flow rate (Q_{max}) is calculated. For the results of uroflowmetry to be valid, the patient needs to void more than 150 mL of urine. As a diagnostic test, uroflowmetry has limitations, as it assesses bladder muscle contraction as well as urine flow through the prostate and penile urethra. Therefore, a low urine flow rate may indicate detrusor impairment rather than BOO. Nevertheless, it is a useful and quick test to evaluate male patients for suspected BOO secondary to BPH. A Q_{max} of less than 10 mL/sec is highly suggestive of BOO, whereas very few men with Q_{max} greater than 15 mL/sec have obstruction.

BPH can lead to incomplete bladder emptying and what is often referred to as a postvoid residual (PVR) volume of urine. This volume can be determined by in-out catheterization or, more commonly, by bladder ultrasound scan. Normally the bladder completely empties on voiding.

If BOO due to BPH is clinically suspected and flow rate and PVR are equivocal, then further urodynamic assessment with pressure-flow studies can be considered. Computer pressure-flow studies measure the pressure in the bladder using an electronic transducer passed into the bladder along the urethra. The test is the most accurate method to differentiate men with a low urine flow rate caused by obstruction or impaired bladder muscle contraction. Pressure-flow studies also assess for involuntary bladder muscle contractions (detrusor overactivity) during the bladder-filling phase before voiding. A study of 1271 men with clinical BPH and evaluated by urodynamics found that nearly 61% had detrusor overactivity.[16] Multivariate analysis showed that age and the grade of BOO were independently associated with detrusor overactivity. However, it is important to note that although BOO and detrusor overactivity often coexist and are age-related phenomena, the pathophysiologic mechanisms linking the two have not yet been established.

The EAU recommends computer urodynamic investigation when considering surgery in men older than 80 years of age with bothersome, predominantly voiding LUTS.

Treatment Options for BPH

When considering which treatment approaches to offer a patient with LUTS secondary to BPH, it is important to consider not only the findings of the clinical assessment but also the clinical efficacy, side effects, duration of treatment response, and effect on disease progression of the various therapeutic options. Also, many men have significant comorbidity and/or frailty, which will need to be incorporated into the treatment discussion process.

Conservative Therapy ("Watchful Waiting")

Many men who have symptomatic BPH opt to avoid or at least defer medical intervention, especially if they perceive that their symptoms are not too bothersome, or they are concerned about the potential side effects of medical or surgical intervention, or if significant comorbidity/frailty is present. Once reassured that their symptoms are not secondary to cancer or other serious pathology and that delaying active treatment will not have irreversible consequences, they can be managed with a conservative approach, often referred to as "watchful waiting." Self-management (e.g., fluid restriction, especially in the evening) plays an important role in the conservative management of LUTS/BPH and can reduce both symptoms and progression.

Men with LUTS/BPH and their caring clinicians are often concerned about the potential risks of observation with no active treatment. It is important to emphasize and reassure these men that complications of progressive BPH are rare. Although BOO is associated with increased volumes of residual urine, there is no clear evidence that this predisposes to a significantly increased risk of urinary tract infection. Also, bladder stones due to BOO are rare and there is no indication to screen for their presence, unless clinical symptoms suggest otherwise (e.g., hematuria or urinary tract infection). The development of renal impairment caused by BPH is very uncommon, especially in people with normal renal function at baseline. In the Medical Therapy of Prostatic Symptoms (MTOPS) study, there were no cases of renal insufficiency among more than 3000 men observed for more than 4 years.[17] The most patient-feared risk involved in watchful waiting for BPH is the development of acute urinary retention. In the past, acute urinary retention was an indication for surgical intervention (e.g., transurethral resection of the prostate [TURP]), and today many men go straight to TURP or have surgery if a trial without catheter is unsuccessful. From a patient's perspective, acute urinary retention is often painful and a time-consuming process, necessitating a hospital visit and treatment that, from the health care provider perspective, is costly. A meta-analysis of the placebo arms from three medical therapy trials for BPH reported that the incidence rate of acute urinary retention was 14/1000 patient-years.[18] The risk factors for acute urinary retention include advanced age, symptom severity, increased PSA value, and prostate volume.

The outcomes of watchful waiting in men with LUTS and BPH have been evaluated in a large study comparing conservative therapy and TURP. At 5 years, 36% of men crossed over to surgery, leaving the majority on conservative follow-up.[19] As mentioned, a key component of watchful waiting is patient reassurance and education, which includes the provision of lifestyle advice. Reduction of fluid intake in the evening can reduce nocturia and avoiding or reducing alcohol and/or caffeine consumption can have a positive effect on urinary frequency, urgency, and nocturia. Postmicturition dribbling can be improved with the simple technique of urethral milking.

Drug Therapy

Since the 1980s, there has been a shift in the treatment of LUTS secondary to BPH from surgical intervention to medical therapy. Unless there is an absolute indication for surgery, patients more commonly opt for drug treatment on the basis of efficacy and fewer and less severe side effects.

Medical therapies for LUTS/BPH include α-adrenergic blockers, 5α-reductase inhibitors, antimuscarinic drugs, phosphodiesterase inhibitors, and combinations of these drugs. Despite the absence of clinical trial evidence, many patients also self-medicate with a wide variety of plant extracts that are marketed to have a beneficial effect on LUTS.

α_1-Adrenoceptor Antagonists (α_1-Blockers). It is commonly believed that α_1-blockers mediate their clinical effect by improving bladder outlet obstruction through the reduction of smooth muscle tone in the bladder neck and prostate. However, α_1-blockers have been shown to have very little effect on urodynamically proven BOO, and the mechanisms of action are probably mediated through the bladder and central nervous system as well as in the prostate.

α_1-Blockers are considered the first-line drug therapy for BPH-related symptoms because of their rapid onset of action, good efficacy, and low rates of significant side effects. Five α_1-blockers (alfuzosin, doxazosin, tamsulosin, terazosin, and silodosin) have been approved by the U.S. Food and Drug Administration (FDA) in the United States for the treatment of symptoms related to BPH. Despite the different pharmacokinetic properties of these α_1-blockers, they have similar clinical efficacy in appropriate doses.[20] Symptom improvement may take a few weeks, but most patients notice a benefit in a matter of days. Long-term studies have reported that α_1-blockers appear to have more efficacy in men with smaller prostates (<40 mL) than those with larger glands.[21] Also, α_1-blockers do not prevent BPH progression with the associated risk of acute urinary retention and the need for surgical intervention.[17,21]

The most common side effects of α_1-blockers are dizziness and orthostatic hypotension, with the latter being more common with terazosin and doxazosin than with alfuzosin and tamsulosin. With advancing age, orthostatic hypotension increases in frequency, even in otherwise healthy and unmedicated men. Therefore, care must be taken when prescribing α_1-blockers to older people.[22] Tamsulosin causes ejaculatory dysfunction in up to 10% of men. This side effect is often referred to as retrograde ejaculation, secondary to the passage of seminal fluid through an α_1-blocker–induced open bladder neck. Ejaculatory dysfunction is also possibly related to a decrease in seminal fluid production.

α_1-Blockers, particularly tamsulosin, have been shown to increase the risk of intraoperative floppy iris syndrome in cataract surgery.[23] This syndrome is characterized by a flaccid iris that prolapses toward the incision site and progressive intraoperative miosis. The reported risk of intraoperative floppy iris syndrome among men taking tamsulosin ranges widely (from 43% to 90%), and it remains to be established whether stopping α_1-blocker treatment before surgery reduces the risk of this complication.[11] It is good practice to ask about any planned cataract surgery before prescribing an α_1-blocker and to defer the drug if necessary.

5α-Reductase Inhibitors. 5α-Reductase inhibitors act on the prostate by inhibiting the enzyme (5α-reductase) that converts testosterone to the more potent androgen, dihydrotestosterone. 5α-Reductase exists in two isoforms, 5α-reductase type 1 and 5α-reductase type 2, which is predominantly expressed in the prostate. The FDA has approved two 5α-reductase inhibitors (finasteride and dutasteride) for the treatment of BPH-related LUTS. These agents differ in that finasteride inhibits only 5α-reductase type 1, whereas dutasteride inhibits 5α-reductase types 1 and 2. Whether this difference is clinically relevant is unclear as there are no data from direct comparator trials.

5α-Reductase inhibitors work by causing apoptosis of prostatic epithelial cells, leading to a reduction in prostate volume by 18% to 28% and serum PSA level by 50% after 6 to 12 months. Because of their mechanism of action, 5α-reductase inhibitors are not recommended for the treatment of LUTS in the absence of prostatic enlargement. Although 5α-reductase inhibitors are less effective than α_1-blockers at relieving LUTS in the short term, they significantly reduce the progression of LUTS secondary to BPH, the related risk of acute urinary retention, and the need for surgery.[17,24]

The most commonly experienced side effect of 5α-reductase inhibitors is sexual dysfunction, including reduced libido, ejaculatory dysfunction, and erectile dysfunction. These side effects are reversible.

5α-Reductase inhibitors have been used in two large prostate cancer chemoprevention trials. Both of these studies reported that, in the 5α-reductase inhibitor treatment arm, the incidence of prostate cancer was significantly lower,[25,26] but 5α-reductase inhibitors are not yet FDA approved for prostate cancer prevention.

5α-Reductase inhibitors also have application in the management of refractory hematuria secondary to benign prostatic bleeding. It is important to note that other causes of hematuria (e.g., bladder and renal cancer) need to excluded before a diagnosis of benign prostatic bleeding is made in an older male.

Antimuscarinic Medications. Many men with voiding LUTS secondary to BPH also experience storage symptoms (e.g., urgency, frequency, and nocturia). While voiding symptoms are typically managed with an α_1-blocker, a 5α-reductase inhibitor, or both, storage symptoms are often treated with antimuscarinic drugs. This class of medication reduces smooth muscle contraction in the bladder and may also have a clinical effect by modulating the bladder lining (urothelial cells) and the central nervous system.

The most common reported side effects of the antimuscarinic drugs are dry mouth, constipation and voiding difficulties. It is because of the latter that the AUA recommends that before initiating antimuscarinic therapy, the baseline PVR urine should be assessed and caution should be taken in patients with a PVR volume greater than 250 to 300 mL. If prescribed, it is good practice to monitor the IPSS and PVR urine and warn patients about the risks and symptoms of urinary retention.

Phosphodiesterase 5 Inhibitors. Phosphodiesterase 5 (PDE_5) inhibitors work by reducing smooth muscle contraction and tone in the bladder, prostate, and penile tissues. Three oral PDE_5 inhibitors have been licensed for the treatment of erectile dysfunction, but only one (tadalafil 5 mg once daily) is approved by the FDA for the treatment of male LUTS. A meta-analysis of PDE_5 inhibitor monotherapy reported a significant improvement in erectile function (assessed by the International Index of Erectile Function and the IPSS) but no improvement in the maximum urine flow rate compared with placebo.[27]

PDE_5 inhibitors are contraindicated in patients using nitrates because of the risk of hypotension, myocardial infarction, and stroke. Side effects of PDE_5 inhibitors include headache, flushing, dyspepsia, nasal congestion, and myalgia.

Complementary and Alternative Medicine. A wide variety of products containing plant extracts are marketed to relieve male LUTS. The most commonly used plants include saw palmetto, stinging nettle, South African star grass, pumpkin seeds, and bark of the African plum tree. Because of brand and batch variability, interpretation of the clinical efficacy of these agents in published clinical trials and meta-analyses is extremely difficult. Therefore, the AUA does not recommend any dietary supplement or other nonconventional therapy for the management of LUTS secondary to BPH.

Surgical Treatment

The current gold standard surgical intervention for men with LUTS secondary to BPH is TURP. This procedure involves the removal of inner part of the prostate gland via an endoscopic approach through the urethra. TURP results in a clinically significant improvement in IPSS, maximum urine flow rate, and mean PVR urine. Understandably, many patients are concerned about the morbidity related to surgical intervention, and as such it is important to emphasize that the safety profile of TURP has improved. The mortality following TURP in contemporary series is less than 0.25%.[28,29] Significant complications—including urinary incontinence, urinary tract infection, bladder neck stenosis, urethral stricture, retrograde ejaculation, and erectile dysfunction—are uncommon.[29] A rare complication unique to TURP is the TURP syndrome, which is dilutional hyponatremia resulting from absorption of the irrigant fluid (glycine) used during surgery. Recent technologic advances have allowed saline to be used as the irrigation fluid during TURP, and this has reduced the incidence of TURP syndrome.

An alternative surgical procedure to TURP for men with smaller prostates (<30 mL) is transurethral incision of the prostate gland, a technique in which the bladder neck is incised without removing prostatic tissue to improve voiding symptoms. For men with very large prostates (>100 mL), especially if they have coexisting bladder stones, open prostatectomy via a suprapubic incision is a highly effective but underutilized procedure.

A variety of laser therapies have been developed to treat LUTS secondary to BPH. In these techniques, the laser energy is used to resect, enucleate, or vaporize the prostate tissue. Studies have reported that these laser therapies can reduce length of hospital stay and shorten the period of catheterization, with a similar efficacy to TURP.[30]

KEY POINTS: BENIGN PROSTATIC HYPERPLASIA

- Lower urinary tract symptoms in older men have many causes, including benign prostatic hyperplasia (BPH), and often these coexist.
- BPH can cause bladder dysfunction, expressed as storage lower urinary tract symptoms (LUTS) (urinary frequency, urgency, and nocturia).
- Only consider screening for prostate cancer in men presenting with LUTS/BPH if a diagnosis of prostate cancer is going to influence the treatment decisions.
- In men who are not too bothered by their LUTS, simple reassurance and lifestyle advice (in particular altering fluid intake) is often all that is required.
- α_1-Blockers are first-line medical therapy for LUTS secondary to BPH.
- 5α-Reductase inhibitors reduce clinical progression of BPH, specifically the risk of developing acute urinary retention and the need for surgical intervention.
- A variety of different surgical interventions exist for men with LUTS/BPH who fail medical therapy.

PROSTATE CANCER

Willet Willmore, chief of urology at Memorial Sloan-Kettering Cancer Center (1951-1982), elegantly summarized the dilemma faced by physicians caring for men with prostate cancer: "Is a cure possible in those for whom it is necessary, and is it necessary for those in whom it is possible?"

Prostate cancer is an important health problem in the patient group managed by gerontologists. As the aging population expands, the number of men with a diagnosis of prostate cancer is going to increase, at least until 2030. The majority of prostate cancer diagnoses are made before the age of 75, but most deaths secondary to the disease occur in people older than 75 years. For the general physician, the clinical management of prostate cancer is challenging because of the long and variable clinical course of the disease and the wide range of fitness levels with associated differences in life expectancies. Both EAU (www.uroweb.org) and National Comprehensive Cancer Network (NCCN; www.NCCN.org) guidelines agree that a geriatric assessment of fitness rather than the age of the patient should influence any prostate cancer management plan. This important clinical recommendation has been endorsed by the International Society of Geriatric Oncology Working Group.[31]

Incidence and Natural History

Prostate cancer is the most common solid organ cancer found in U.S. males. According to the National Cancer Institute, in 2011 approximately 2,707,821 men were alive with prostate cancer, and in 2014 there were an estimated 233,000 new cases in the United States (Surveillance, Epidemiology, and End Results Program, http://seer.cancer.gov/statfacts/html/prost.html). Autopsy studies have shown that latent microscopic cancers occur throughout the world, but the incidence of clinical cancers varies by race and geographic region. Currently in the United States, the lifetime risk of being diagnosed with prostate cancer is 16.7%, and the prostate cancer mortality risk is 2.6%. Whereas the median age at diagnosis is 66 years and 80% of cases have been diagnosed by the age of 75 years, the median age at death is 80 years and 70% of deaths occur in men older than 75 years. Incidence rates vary: the incidence among Native Americans, Asians, Pacific Islanders, and Hispanics is below average, whereas in African Americans the rate is approximately 60% higher than average. There is even greater discrepancy in mortality between African Americans and other races whose outcomes are similar. African Americans are more than twice as likely as other ethnic groups to die of prostate cancer.

Overall, the mortality rate has been falling since the peak in 1991. The serum PSA test became available in 1992 and rapidly entered clinical use as an ad hoc prostate cancer screening test. The rapid change in disease-related mortality occurred too soon to be attributed to PSA testing and was more likely the result of more aggressive treatments or more disease being ascribed to prostate cancer through better diagnosis.

Risk Factors

The cause of prostate cancer is not known, but there are multiple risk factors, specifically increasing age, ethnic origin, and heredity.

Heredity

Risk increases with the number of affected first-degree relatives: doubled for one, 5 to 11 times for two, and, if three members are affected, this is defined as hereditary prostate cancer.[32,33] This represents about 9% of prostate cancers; affected individuals usually develop the cancer at a younger age but do not differ in other aspects.

Environment

Whereas the incidence of small-volume latent or incidental disease is similar throughout the world, the incidence of clinical symptomatic disease varies widely from region to region. The geographic variation in incidence—such as the increased incidence of prostate cancer in low-risk Japanese men who have moved to the United States or the increasing risk for Europeans at increasingly northern latitudes—has led to a wide variety of factors being linked to the development of prostate cancer. These include dietary saturated fat and red meat consumption, lifestyle issues, sexual behavior, chronic infection or inflammation, occupation, obesity, and sunlight exposure. From the prevention perspective, a number of supplements—most notably, vitamin E and selenium (Selenium and Vitamin E Cancer Prevention Trial [SELECT]), and vitamin D, lycopene, and aspirin—have been examined. Currently there is no conclusive evidence that chemoprevention of prostate cancer is possible.

Pathology

At autopsy, foci of prostate cancer are present in a large percentage of men without symptoms who died from the disease. This occurs in all parts of the world. The majority of prostatic tumors are *adenocarcinomas*, which arise from the cells lining prostatic acini. Tumors are mainly peripherally sited, most often multifocal, and may be associated with *high-grade prostatic intraepithelial neoplasia* and *intraductal carcinoma* in which cytologically abnormal cells line architecturally normal acini and ducts. The rest of prostatic tumors occur in the periurethral and transition zones. *Ductal carcinomas* arising from the prostatic ducts close to the urethra at the verumontanum are best regarded as high-grade carcinomas. *Small cell carcinomas* with neuroendocrine differentiation similar to those in the lung have a very poor outlook. It is apparent that a multistep process occurs with serial mutations resulting in more aggressive tumors with time. Hence, older men tend to have higher grade tumors at presentation.

The prostate is surrounded by fascial tissues (the capsule), and local spread is typically into periprostatic fat via invasion of intraprostatic blood vessels and nerves that penetrate the fascia. This extension may occur as fine filaments, which are therefore not visible on staging investigations such as magnetic resonance imaging (MRI). Extension may be directly into the ejaculatory ducts and beyond, into the seminal vesicles. Tumor invasion of the seminal vesicles appears to be associated with a step change in the risk of lymphatic spread. This is usually to regional lymph nodes, including the hypogastric and obturator lymph nodes. Hematogenous spread occurs to bone almost always in the axial skeleton (pelvis, spine, ribs, skull). This is possibly related to venous drainage of the prostate through the Batson plexus. It is less common for prostate cancer to invade the liver and lungs.

Clinical Presentation

Currently, most prostate cancers diagnosed are discovered because of formal or opportunistic screening, while others have presenting symptoms that could be related to the tumor. Men with LUTS are more likely to have BPH than prostate cancer because of the relative locations of the conditions in the gland: most cancers are peripherally sited, whereas BPH predominantly affects the periurethral area. In addition to obstructing the bladder outlet, prostate cancer may invade the adjacent neurovascular bundles, resulting in erectile dysfunction. Local disease may also cause epididymitis, hydroceles, hematospermia, and ureteric obstruction with resultant uremia. Nodal involvement may cause lymphedema of the lower limbs. Bony metastasis, especially common in the spine and pelvis, may result in pain, pathologic fracture, paraplegia, or anemia. Approximately 30% of cases of bony metastases of unknown primary site in males are due to prostate cancer. The results of the DRE may raise the suspicion of prostate cancer. However, many tumors are not readily palpable, most often because they lie anteriorly. Nevertheless, the DRE findings are pertinent to the T staging in the TNM system (see "Prostate Cancer Staging," later in this chapter) and to assessment of disease risk in predictive nomograms.

Diagnosis and Staging in the Older Man

The diagnosis of prostate cancer is usually based on results from a needle biopsy or transurethral resection biopsy of the prostate. In some cases, and particularly in the older people who are frail, biopsy may not be appropriate. Investigation of a suspicious DRE and/or marginally raised PSA level in male patients older than 75 years should depend on the exact clinical circumstances. The diagnosis of advanced disease may be made clinically without biopsy on the basis of serum PSA levels (nearly always >20 μg/L) and imaging, especially radionucleotide bone scans.

Blood and Tissue Markers

Prostate-Specific Antigen

The majority of prostate cancers diagnosed today are suspected or diagnosed because of a serum PSA estimation. Prostate-specific antigen is a kallikrein-like serum protease, *specific for prostatic epithelial cells but not for malignancy*. It is a normal component of semen where it acts as an anticoagulant. The amount released into the blood circulation depends on both the amount secreted by the prostate and the permeability of the prostate tissue to the circulation. Therefore, factors such as BPH, prostate cancer, and prostatitis may raise serum levels. For the first two, this may be through the presence of increased numbers of prostate epithelial cells. For inflammatory disorders of the prostate, such as urinary infection (which, in males, inevitably involves the prostate) and bacterial prostatitis, the cause of a serum PSA rise is through increased organ blood flow and tissue permeability. Included in the inflammatory group should be various traumas to the prostate that temporarily increase blood flow; these traumas include prostatic surgery or biopsy, cystoscopy, and urethral catheterization. The serum half-life of PSA is relatively long at 2 to 3 days, and the timing of a PSA test should ideally avoid such events by several weeks. The small effect of DRE is clinically unimportant.

Men may have prostate cancer with a "normal" age-specific serum PSA level. This may be because their background noncancer PSA production is low because they have a small prostate, or because, in certain cases with high-grade disease, the cancer cells fail to secrete PSA.

Based on the natural history of prostate cancer, there is no role for screening asymptomatic people, including older people.

Free-to-Total Prostate-Specific Antigen Ratio

Some PSA in blood is bound to serum proteins and some is free. In the PSA range of 4 to 10 ng/mL, where approximately one third of patients will be diagnosed with prostate cancer, a free-to-total ratio of less than 0.1 is associated with a diagnosis rate of 56%, whereas a ratio of greater than 0.25 is associated with a rate of just 8%.[34]

The Prostate Health Index

The Prostate Health Index (PHI) is a new formula that combines all three forms (total PSA, free PSA, and [-2]proPSA [p2PSA]) into a single score that can be used to aid in clinical decision making.[35] PHI is calculated using the following formula: (p2PSA/free PSA) × $\sqrt{}$PSA. Intuitively, this formula makes sense, in that men with a higher total PSA and p2PSA with a lower free PSA are more likely to have clinically significant prostate cancer.

The Prostate Cancer Gene 3 (PCA3) Test

This test is based on a reverse transcriptase-polymerase chain reaction assay for a prostate-specific gene *(DD3)* and compares the level of this mRNA with the level of PSA-mRNA as a control (ensures that prostate epithelial cells are present). It requires prostate cancer cells, which are obtained by collecting an initial voided urine after an "attentive" DRE. This is too expensive to be used for population screening but may be used to assess the need for repeat prostate biopsy in men with persistently elevated PSA levels.

Prostate Biopsy

The diagnosis of prostate cancer, when indicated, is usually made by prostatic biopsy. The 10 or more core biopsy is usually performed as an office procedure by transrectal ultrasound (TRUS) guidance using a spring-loaded 18-gauge biopsy gun under local anesthesia. Before embarking on this, physicians should be very clear whether or not, in the current clinical context, a tissue diagnosis is required and that the tumor, if confirmed, is likely to be clinically significant. Indeed, the diagnosis of insignificant cancer in an older man should be regarded as an adverse event. Evidence from a systematic review suggests that TRUS-guided biopsy has serious adverse event rates of up to 2% for serious infection (e.g., bacteremia, urosepsis, or abscess), a risk that has been increasing as a result of the emergence of ciprofloxacin-resistant *Escherichia coli*, which can be identified by a prebiopsy rectal swab culture screen. Occasionally, serious bleeding can occur as well as less major adverse events, including hematuria, hematospermia, rectal bleeding, and urinary retention.

Gleason Score

The Gleason scoring system was originally developed using radical prostatectomy specimens and not needle biopsies. It is in universal use today and is the most useful single prognostic factor. It looks at the arrangement of the cells in the tumor and not their individual morphology. The original system graded cases from a sum of 2 (best/lowest grade) to 10 (worst/highest grade) by adding the scores from the dominant and secondary tumor patterns based on a score of 1 (low-grade pattern) to 5 (high-grade pattern).

However, the lower grades (1 and 2) are not relevant today, as they cannot be accurately assessed in needle biopsy specimens. From a clinical standpoint, this renders the older literature on Gleason grading less useful for current-era patients.

Currently, the vast majority of contemporary Gleason grading falls into one of the following scores:

Gleason score 6 (low risk),
Gleason score 7 (intermediate risk), or
Gleason score 8-10 (high risk).

Additionally, tertiary scores for third grades are given especially if they are Grade 5 and contribute more than 5% of the tumor, as these worsen the prognosis.

Molecular Tissue Biomarkers

Molecular biomarkers based on assessment of gene expression profiles in archived paraffin sections of needle biopsies and radical prostatectomies have become commercially available for prostate cancer. The Prolaris test (prostate biopsies and radical prostatectomies) is based on genes within the cell cycle pathway, whereas the Oncotype DX test (needle biopsies only) is based on a number of mechanistic pathways. These have not yet been fully evaluated but may have a role in stratifying risk in both pretreated and posttreated patients.

Prostate Cancer Staging

Clinical staging of prostate cancer is based on a number of factors (Table 83-3). DRE may help to establish local stage with help from radiologic imaging. The PSA level, serum alkaline phosphatase, hemoglobin, and renal function may give clues as to the likely extent of disease.

T Stage

Assessment of local tumor stage, by differentiating whether the cancer has progressed beyond the prostate capsule, is important in terms of treatment planning. Because there is very poor correlation between DRE findings and pathologic stage, imaging is often used to improve accuracy.

Transrectal Ultrasound. Typically a prostate tumor is visible as a hypoechoic peripheral zone lesion, but approximately 40% of tumors are isoechoic and therefore not visible. The main utility of TRUS is to guide systematic prostate biopsies. There is no evidence that TRUS is any more accurate than DRE in establishing risk of extracapsular extension of tumor.

Magnetic Resonance Imaging. The most useful sequence on MRI staging of prostate cancer is the T2-weighted image. Unfortunately MRI is not as sensitive at detecting extracapsular extension of tumor (T3a disease) or seminal vesicle invasion (T3b disease) as has been hoped because extension is usually

TABLE 83-3 Tumor Node Metastasis (TNM) Classification of Prostate Cancer

PRIMARY TUMOR (T)		
TX		Primary tumor cannot be assessed
TO		No evidence of primary tumor
T1		Clinically inapparent tumor not palpable or visible by imaging
	T1a	Tumor incidental histologic finding 5% or less of tissue resected
	T1b	Tumor incidental histologic finding in more than 5% of tissue resected
	T1c	Tumor identified by needle biopsy(e.g., because of elevated prostate-specific antigen[PSA] level)
T2		Tumor confined within the prostate
	T2a	Tumor involves one half of one lobe or less
	T2b	Tumor involves more than half of one lobe but not both lobes
	T2c	Tumor involves both lobes
T3		Tumor extends through the prostatic capsule
	T3a	Extracapsular extension (unilateral or bilateral), including microscopic bladder neck involvement
	T2b	Tumor invades seminal vesicles
T4		Tumor is fixed or invades adjacent structures other than seminal vesicles, e.g., rectum, levator muscles, and/or pelvic wall
REGIONAL LYMPH NODES (N)		
NX		Regional lymph nodes cannot be assessed
NO		No regional lymph node metastasis
N1		Regional lymph node metastasis
DISTANT METASTASIS (M)		
MX		Distant metastasis cannot be assessed
MO		No distant metastasis
M1		Distant metastasis
	M1a	Nonregional lymph node(s)
	M1b	Bone(s)
	M1c	Other site(s)

From Edge S, et al (eds): AJCC cancer staging manual, ed 7, New York, 2010, Springer.

microscopic. However, if these features are seen, then the scan is very accurate.

Multiparametric Magnetic Resonance Imaging. This refers to the addition of functional sequences of diffusion-weighted and dynamic contrast imaging to standard T1- and T2-weighted images to improve sensitivity and specificity of the scan. Multiparametric MRI is particularly useful in identifying larger and more aggressive tumors as well as those in the anterior gland, which may be missed by other techniques. The role of such magnetic resonance scans in both obviating the need for biopsy (if negative) and directing targeted biopsies rather than systematic biopsies is still being evaluated.

Computed Tomography. Computed tomography (CT) does not have a significant role in assessing the T stage. CT is, however, a faster and cheaper alternative to MRI in the assessment of metastatic disease.

N Stage

The assessment of nodal status is of importance because it dictates whether or not the patient will be offered radical local treatment. Conventionally the obturator nodes are those that are assessed by operative lymphadenectomy. At radical prostatectomy, this misses 50% of metastases identified by a more extensive lymphadenectomy. It is more common for nodal status to be decided based on size criteria by CT or MRI. Prediction of rate of node positivity can be assessed by clinical nomograms (e.g., Partin table).

TABLE 83-4 Prostate-Specific Antigen (PSA) Levels

PSA (ng/mL)	Bone Scan Positive (%)[36]
0-9.9	2.5
10-19.9	5.3
20-49.9	16.2
50-99.9	39.2
>100	73.4

M Stage

Among men with detectable bony metastases, 70% will have an elevated serum alkaline phosphatase. Isotope bone scanning is currently the clinical standard for metastatic bone assessment, but other methods (e.g., MRI and positron emission tomography [PET]–CT) are being investigated as alternatives. These newer techniques may be more sensitive and specific for low-volume metastatic disease, but there are cost issues. All patients with bony symptoms or high-grade disease (Gleason sum score 8 or higher) should undergo investigation. Otherwise, only patients with serum PSA levels of higher than 10 ng/mL or possibly 20 ng/mL should be scanned (Table 83-4).

Treatment Modalities

Active Surveillance

Active surveillance is a relatively new term and differs from *watchful waiting*, which means deferring treatment until the patient requires hormonal therapy for symptomatic or metastatic disease. Active surveillance means deferring the decision to carry out radical treatment for localized prostate cancer rather than a deliberate decision to avoid radical treatment. Many men have harmless tumors, and the interventions used to treat them with curative intent carry risks. Observation of tumor evolution over time will more easily help clinicians identify those patients likely to benefit from radical treatment. It makes sense because, despite knowledge of validated parameters used to assign risk to a particular tumor, clinicians are unable to accurately predict outcomes for an individual patient. Although the principles have been used for some time, the protocol for active surveillance is evolving. The NCCN recommends PSA no more than every 6 months, DRE no more than every 12 months, and rebiopsy no sooner than 12 months. The National Institute for Health and Care Excellence (NICE) in the United Kingdom recommends that, in addition, all patients should have an initial MRI assessment, particularly to rule out the presence of a significant anterior tumor that may not have been well biopsied.

Radical Prostatectomy

Radical prostatectomy would be better described as a total prostatectomy with excision of the seminal vesicles and ampullae of the vasa. There is limited scope for wide excision of the gland because of the proximity of important structures (bladder, continence mechanism, and rectum). The terms *nerve sparing* and *non–nerve sparing* relate to the fascial plane that the surgeon uses to dissect around the gland (the nerves important for erections run in the periprostatic tissues). Surgery can be performed retropubically through a lower midline incision; this approach may include pelvic lymph node dissection. During the past decade, there has been a shift to minimally invasive surgery. Robotic-assisted laparoscopic prostatectomy is now the most popular form of radical prostatectomy in the United States.

Radical prostatectomy has the advantages of definitive tumor pathology with confirmation of tumor clearance or otherwise and clarity on PSA follow-up. The serum PSA should have fallen to less than 0.1 ng/mL at 6 weeks after surgery. Adverse pathology or PSA relapse can be identified at an early stage and appropriate steps taken. These factors are more important in younger men. In the SPCG Trial with 22 years of follow-up, men aged younger than 65 years and those with intermediate-risk disease derived the most benefit from undergoing surgery, although it also reduced the risk for metastases from 38.3% to 26.1% (risk ratio [RR], 0.57; $P < .001$) and need for additional treatment such as hormonal therapy (from 67.4% to 42.5%; RR, 0.49; $P < .001$) in older men.[37] The risk of adverse events and complications associated with surgery are increased in the older and less fit patient compared with radiotherapy, after which many of the adverse consequences are delayed for several years. The EAU recommends surgery in selected people older than 70 years.

Radiotherapeutic Options

There are two main methods of radiotherapeutic treatment: external beam radiotherapy (EBRT) and brachytherapy (low and high dose), which is mediated by implanted metallic seeds or needles. Just as there have been technical improvements in surgery, there have also been improvements in radiotherapy techniques and dosimetry. It has been established that the total dose given per course of EBRT was suboptimal at usually around 64 Gy and that increasing the dose to at least 74 Gy improved freedom from biochemical recurrence. So far that has not yet translated into improved overall survival.

For lower risk, localized prostate cancer, EBRT is given in 2-Gy fractions without any androgen deprivation. Treatment is delivered using a conformal three-dimensional planning system and multileaf collimators (known as 3D-CRT) to improve local control while reducing the dose to the rectum. There is increasing use of intensity-modulated radiotherapy in which the radiation source continuously moves relative to the target and monitors the dose given, allowing higher doses to be given to the prostate while reducing scatter to other organs. Most radiotherapy is delivered by photons, although radiotherapy using protons or carbon ions has also been used.

Side effects of EBRT include cystitis, hematuria, urethral stricture, proctitis, chronic diarrhea, and leg edema. There is a significant and rising rate of erectile dysfunction and a low but measurable increased risk of rectal and bladder cancer.

For low-dose brachytherapy, a grid is used to place parallel needles within the prostate to deliver metallic seeds containing a low-energy gamma ray emitter with long half-life. This is most often iodine 125 (half-life 59 days) or palladium 103 (half-life 17 days). If a patient undergoing brachytherapy has bladder outflow obstruction, there is concern for subsequent transurethral prostatectomy because the operative site heals poorly and urinary incontinence is likely. Previous prostatectomy, very large prostate volume (>50 mL), or median lobe enlargement of the prostate similarly make it very difficult to place the seeds. No randomized clinical trials have compared brachytherapy to other radical treatment options. However, because it is a single-treatment method to deliver a radiation dose of greater than 140 Gy to the prostate, brachytherapy is a popular method of treating low-risk localized prostate cancer. The outcomes depend on the ability to deliver an adequate dose. Side effects include urinary retention, and permanent urinary problems may occur in 20% patients. Brachytherapy is given without androgen deprivation therapy unless the initial prostate volume is greater than 50 mL and needs to be reduced for treatment.

High-dose brachytherapy using temporarily inserted radioisotope sources is combined with EBRT to treat higher risk local and locally advanced disease.

Charlson Comorbidities

Aggressive treatment of localized prostate cancer may not be in the best interest of a patient if he has significant comorbidities, frailty, or both. Not only are these a competing cause of death, but also they increase the likelihood of complications from treatment. Using data from the Surveillance, Epidemiology, and End Results–Medicare database, Daskivich and colleagues sampled 140,553 men aged 66 years or older with early-stage prostate cancer who were diagnosed between 1991 and 2007.[38] The risk of cancer-specific mortality between men who received aggressive versus nonaggressive treatment among comorbidity subgroups was then compared. Aggressive treatment was associated with a significantly lower risk of cancer-specific mortality for men who had Charlson comorbidity scores of 0, 1, and 2 but not for men who had Charlson scores of 3 or higher. The absolute reduction in 15-year cancer-specific mortality between men who received aggressive versus nonaggressive treatment was 3.8%, 3%, 1.9%, and −0.5% for men with Charlson scores of 0, 1, 2, and 3 or higher, respectively.

Hormonal Therapy

Hormonal therapy refers to mechanisms to reduce or eliminate circulating androgens in men with prostate cancer, and it has been used since the 1940s. This was originally only used in men with metastatic disease. The original and still underused modality is surgical bilateral orchiectomy, as reported by Huggins and Hodges.[39] This reduces serum testosterone to castrate levels within minutes. For convenience, luteinizing hormone–releasing hormone (LHRH) analogs (e.g., leuprolide and goserelin) have largely replaced surgical castration, but they do have disadvantages. They initially stimulate the production of luteinizing hormone, and thus testosterone, producing what is known as tumor flare. Within a couple of weeks, pituitary gland stimulation is downregulated, levels of gonadotrophins fall, and with them the testosterone level falls. Thus, LHRH analogs have a relatively slow onset of action. It has taken many years to develop an LHRH antagonist (e.g., degarelix). This agent reduces serum testosterone to castrate levels within 3 days and avoids tumor flare. LHRH antagonists or bilateral orchiectomy are therefore particularly useful when rapid response to treatment is required, such as in painful metastatic disease, ureteric obstruction, or spinal compression.

Approximately 10% of testosterone remains after medical or surgical castration because of peripheral metabolism of adrenal androgens. To counteract this, the addition of a nonsteroidal antiandrogen such as bicalutamide to block the androgen receptor produces what is known as combined or total androgen blockade.

The significant change in recent years has been the use of hormonal therapy for earlier disease, particularly in association with radiotherapy where there is a synergism between the two treatments. There is a measurable benefit to starting hormonal therapy before radiotherapy (neoadjuvant hormonal therapy). The synergism is partially due to the tumor volume-reducing effect of neoadjuvant hormone therapy (approximately 30% over 3 to 6 months) and partly due to the sensitizing effects of hormone therapy for radiotherapy-induced cell death.

Treatment by Risk Group

The Geriatric Assessment Tool

The long clinical course of prostate cancer in most men makes management in the older man particularly difficult. A working group was convened in 2010 by the International Society of Geriatric Oncology to examine prostate cancer management in men older than 70 years and again in 2013 to revise recommendations. These recommendations have yet to be widely adopted in routine clinical practice. The key recommendation was that a patient with prostate cancer should be treated on the basis of his individually assessed health status and not his age.[31] The first step is to use the Geriatric 8 assessment tool.

The Geriatric 8 (G8) frailty screening method[40]

A. Has food intake declined over the past 3 months due to loss of appetite, digestive problems, chewing, or swallowing difficulties?
  0 = Severe decrease in food intake
  1 = Moderate decrease in food intake
  2 = No decrease in food intake
B. Weight loss during the last 3 months?
  0 = Weight loss > 3 kg
  1 = Does not know
  2 = Weight loss between 1 and 3 kg
  3 = No weight loss
C. Mobility?
  0 = Bed or chair bound
  1 = Able to get out of bed/chair but does not go out
  2 = Goes out
E. Neuropsychological problems?
  0 = Severe dementia or depression
  1 = Mild dementia
  2 = No psychological problems
F. Body mass index (BMI)? (weight in kg)/(height in m^2)
  0 = BMI < 19
  1 = BMI 19 to < 21
  2 = BMI 21 to < 23
  3 = BMI > 23
H. Takes more than three prescription drugs per day?
  0 = Yes
  1 = No
P. In comparison with other people of the same age, how does the patient consider his/her health status?
  0.0 = Not as good
  0.5 = Does not know
  1.0 = As good
  2.0 = Better

Age
  0: >85
  1: 80-85
  2: <80

If the G8 tool demonstrates impairment, further evaluation should take place that examines the comorbidity status (Cumulative Illness Score Rating Geriatrics [CISR-G]); dependence, using an assessment of the activities of daily living (ADLs) for home independence and instrumental activities of daily living (IADLs) for community independence; and nutritional status by estimating the patient's weight loss over the past 3 months. Using these tools, men can be assigned to one of three groups:

Fit: These patients should be considered for standard treatment.

Vulnerable with a reversible impairment: Grade 3 CISR-G or one Grade 4 CISG-G comorbidity, dependent in one or more IADLs but functionally independent in ADLs, and at risk for malnutrition. After geriatric intervention and management, these patients should be considered for standard treatment.

Frail with irreversible impairment: Patients with Grade 3 CISR-G or one CISR-G comorbidity, dependent in one or more ADLs or severe malnutrition. Treatment should be adjusted to allow for the condition of the patient.

Localized Prostate Cancer

More than 80% of diagnosed cases are localized to the prostate and have widely varying prognoses depending on tumor aggressiveness. The main risk is overtreatment. Data mature enough to provide information on long-term outlook are from an era when pathologic and diagnostic techniques were very different than they are today. There are several risk assessment tools in use for localized prostate cancer. (The most commonly applied is the D'Amico risk stratification.) The NCCN have incorporated these into their risk scoring system. Very low-risk prostate cancer is defined as T1c disease, Gleason score 6 or lower, PSA less than 10 ng/mL, fewer than three cores containing tumor with no more than 50% of any core involved, and a PSA density of less than 0.15 μg/mL/g. Low-risk prostate cancer patients are the remaining D'Amico low-risk group (T1-T2a, Gleason 6 or lower, PSA < 10 ng/mL). The very low-risk group should not immediately be subjected to active treatment if they are over the age of 70 (life expectancy < 20 years). The low-risk group should not be immediately treated if their life expectancy is less than 10 years. If life expectancy is more than 10 years, then radical treatments are an option (radiotherapy more likely than surgery), but there has been a swing toward initial active surveillance.

Intermediate-Risk Localized Prostate Cancer. This group is defined as T2b-T2c disease with a Gleason score of 7 and a PSA of less than 10 ng/mL. Because these patients are more likely to clinically progress, if their life expectancy is considered to be more than 10 years, then they should be offered radical treatment (surgery or radiotherapy). If the life expectancy is limited, most urologists would first offer watchful waiting as a treatment option.

High-Risk Localized and Locally Advanced Prostate Cancer. This includes T3a or Gleason 8-10 or PSA higher than 20 ng/mL. The options here are radical prostatectomy with a pelvic node dissection, EBRT or EBRT with high-dose brachytherapy both with long-course ADT (2 to 3 years). Fit men with a life expectancy of more than 5 years could be considered for this option.

Very High-Risk Localized and Locally Advanced Prostate Cancer. This includes T3b-4, primary Grade 5 disease, or more than four cores Gleason 8-10. A step change occurs when the seminal vesicles are invaded by prostate cancer, when pelvic nodal and systemic disease becomes more likely. Primary therapies alone are much less likely to be curative, but, conversely, treatment is more likely to affect survival. The options are as for high-risk disease: radical prostatectomy with a pelvic node dissection, EBRT or EBRT with high-dose brachytherapy both with long-course ADT (2 to 3 years commencing 3 months prior), but, in addition, those patients unfit for these options may be treated with primary hormonal therapy. Men undergoing surgery who are found to have these adverse features on their postsurgical histology should be considered for adjuvant radiotherapy to the prostate bed with ADT and, if there are pelvic nodes, may be considered for radiotherapy to the pelvic nodes with ADT. For men who have locally advanced tumors with high presenting PSA levels (>40 ng/mL) or high-grade disease and negative metastasis screen, although the likelihood of micrometastasis is high, it has been demonstrated that the addition of radical radiotherapy to ADT improves survival compared with hormonal therapy alone.[41]

Metastatic Disease TXN1M1

There is a wide range of natural history of metastatic prostate cancers. Three prognostic groups can be defined with median survival ranging from 54 to just 21 months[42] (Table 83-5).

The standard therapy for the 4% of men who present with metastatic prostate cancer (usually in bone) has been androgen deprivation therapy. Approximately 50% of these men will achieve a normalized PSA level after 7 months of treatment, most often using an LHRH analog (buserelin, goserelin, leuprolide), and this predicts for survival. If the PSA falls to less than 0.2 ng/mL, the median survival is 75 months; less than 4 ng/mL, 44 months; and more than 4 ng/mL, only 13 months. If a rapid effect is required because symptoms are severe, then surgical castration or an LHRH antagonist should be considered.

In general, it is expected that the PSA nadir will be reached approximately 6 to 8 months after starting treatment. Standard

TABLE 83-5 Prognostic Factors

Prognostic Factors	Good		Intermediate		Poor
Axial bone metastasis and/or nodes	X				
Appendicular bone or visceral metastasis		X	X	X	X
Performance status < 1		X	X		
Performance status > 1				X	X
Gleason score < 8		X			
Gleason score > 8			X		
PSA < 65 ng/mL				X	
PSA > 65 ng/mL					X
Median survival (months)	54		30		21

PSA, Prostate-specific antigen.

therapy is continuous treatment until castrate resistance develops. However, an alternative is intermittent therapy in initial treatment responders (PSA < 4 ng/mL at nadir). The intention is to minimize the side effects of ADT and is based on animal work that suggested consequent prolonged tumor response to castration. These responding patients have treatment holidays until the serum PSA level has risen off treatment to levels most often greater than 20 µg/L or until symptoms develop. It is not certain that these approaches are equivalent, but there is insufficient difference to suggest that intermittent ADT should not be used.[43] The traditional approach has been to step up therapy to combined androgen blockade by the addition of an antiandrogen (e.g., bicalutamide, cyproterone acetate), if the serum PSA starts to rise on treatment. In some patients, initial combined androgen blockade may provide a survival advantage.

Very recently, however, a new approach was suggested by a report of the Eastern Cooperative Oncology Group's randomized trial of 790 patients, which showed that the addition of docetaxel therapy to hormonal therapy improved overall survival by 14 months, and in high-risk patients (those with more bony disease or soft tissue metastases), this increased to 17 months.[44] There was no benefit to those with lower risk disease. The older, less fit patient may not be a candidate for docetaxel.

Castrate-Resistant Prostate Cancer

In the context of a patient receiving androgen ablation for prostate cancer (with a serum testosterone < 50 ng/dL), castrate-resistant prostate cancer (CRPC) is defined as two sequential PSA rises of more than 50% above nadir with a PSA greater than 2 ng/mL, or the appearance of two new bony lesions on an isotope bone scan. It is associated with molecular biologic changes in tumor tissue: increase in bcl-2, p53, and androgen receptor amplification and, in some cases, mutation. Tumors also contain high levels of androgens despite the castrate state. This suggests that there are mechanisms for intracellular production of androgens within castrate-resistant cells with, therefore, the opportunity for self-stimulation.

PSA level is the main, but not the only, measure of response to treatment in this setting, and certainly improvements in quality of life and survival can be achieved without objective PSA responses. Other important measures are performance status, symptoms, hemoglobin, alkaline phosphatase, and radiologic measurements using RECIST criteria.

The management of such patients is in a state of flux as a result of the addition of several new agents to the armamentarium of the oncologist. In general, responses to each will be better the earlier they are given. New agents have dramatically escalated the cost of treatment. In choosing a first-line agent, the previous patient response to hormonal agents and fitness will be taken into account.

If prostate cancer progressed while the patient was on LHRH monotherapy, then there are a number of management options, including the following:

Add an antiandrogen. Bicalutamide 150 mg added to an LHRH analog will reverse the PSA rise in approximately 20% of patients.

Antiandrogen withdrawal. One third of patients on combined androgen blockade will have a PSA response to withdrawal of the antiandrogen of median duration 4 months. The theory is that mutation of the androgen receptor results in the antiandrogen having a stimulatory rather than inhibitory effect.

Low-dose dexamethasone (500 µg daily). Steroids don't significantly increase life expectancy, but they often improve quality of life.

Estrogens orally or as a skin patch. Diethylstilbestrol at a low dose of 1 mg daily is useful with an objective response rate in a retrospective report in this setting of 48%.[45] The feared complication of pulmonary embolus was 3.6% (all nonfatal). An alternative could be to use estriol skin patches, which were shown to be as effective as LHRH analogs in the PATCH trial[46] but carry lower risks because of the avoidance of the effects of first-pass liver metabolism on protein and fat metabolism.

Docetaxel chemotherapy with prednisolone. This single agent paclitaxel (Taxol) is the standard of care, and older people can tolerate it if they are fit (performance status 0-1). The SWOG (formerly the Southwest Oncology Group) 99-16 randomized trial showed a 2- to 2.5-month improvement in median survival compared with mitoxantrone and prednisolone.[47]

Enzalutamide. This new antiandrogen blocks the androgen receptor at a dose of 160 mg daily and improves both overall survival and progression-free survival compared with placebo in the prechemotherapy setting (PREVAIL).[48]

Abiraterone. This inhibitor of 17α-hydroxylase/17,20-lyase (CYP17), a key enzyme in androgen biosynthesis, has the ability to block testicular, adrenal, and intratumoral androgen production. In the placebo controlled, randomized COU-AA-301 trial, abiraterone acetate plus prednisone significantly improved overall survival in men with metastatic CRPC who had progressed after docetaxel chemotherapy by 4.6 months compared with prednisone.[49] Subsequently, abiraterone has been trialed in the prechemotherapy metastatic CRPC setting in the follow-up COU-AA-302 trial.[50] Abiraterone demonstrated significantly prolonged progression-free survival (hazard ratio [HR], 0.53) with a trend toward overall survival (HR, 0.75), which did not reach statistical significance. However, based on these data, the FDA have approved the use of prechemotherapy abiraterone.

Radium 223. This alpha emitter selectively targets bony metastases and was shown to improve median survival of men with metastatic CRPC in the ALSYMPCA trial.[51] Side effects, including marrow toxicity, were not a major problem, and indeed there were less adverse events in the treated than the placebo group. Also, men with CRPC will develop symptomatic problems, which will require consideration of management by other means.

Bone pain. Treatment options include single-fraction palliative radiotherapy, radioisotopes (e.g., radium 223) and intravenous bisphosphonates.

Spinal cord compression. Patient may present acutely with actual or impending paraplegia, which requires urgent investigation and treatment. In practice, after MRI assessment, high-dose steroids and radiotherapy to the affected area is the usual management, although surgery may be required.

Ureteric obstruction. Although this more often occurs in patients with advanced metastatic disease, increasingly, with earlier interventions for prostate cancer, there are patients who develop CRPC that is locally advanced and nonmetastatic. There is often associated distal ureteric obstruction (unilateral or bilateral), and adenocarcinoma may even infiltrate the whole length of the ureter. The increase in availability of treatment for CRPC has shifted the balance from nonintervention in ureteric obstruction to decompression with nephrostomy/antegrade ureteric stenting, but a full and frank discussion should be had with patients (particularly those with symptomatic disease and no further systemic disease treatment options) about the advisability of this before intervention.

Urinary retention. Managed with an indwelling catheter or transurethral resection.

Hematuria. Managed by endoscopic surgical control or palliative EBRT to the prostate gland.

Radiation cystitis. Bladder instillations of hyaluronic acid.

Anemia. Repeated blood transfusions may be necessary.

KEY POINTS

- Prostate cancer is a common cause of mortality and morbidity in older men but because of the long natural history, most localized cancers (which form 80% of diagnoses) do not cause harm.
- The role of prostate cancer population screening is debatable and of no proven value in older men.
- A formal assessment of comorbidities should be made in older men with prostate cancer as life expectancy is the most important determinant of outcome. Complications of treatment may outweigh the benefits for a patient with a high Charlson comorbidity score.
- Low-risk localized prostate cancer should be managed first by observation.
- Options for treatment of intermediate- and high-risk localized prostate cancer might include radical local treatment (surgery or radiotherapy) depending on life expectancy.
- Older men with very high-risk and locally advanced prostate cancer with a life expectancy of more than 5 years are optimally managed by radiotherapy with neoadjuvant and adjuvant androgen deprivation therapy (ADT) or, in selected cases, radical surgery. The optimal duration of ADT remains to be determined.
- ADT (bilateral orchiectomy, luteinizing hormone–releasing hormone [LHRH] agonist or antagonist, or combined androgen blockade with LHRH agonist and antiandrogen) is the mainstay of treatment of metastatic prostate cancer, but recent work suggests that for high-risk metastatic disease, ADT combined with docetaxel chemotherapy may be more effective. Intermittent ADT can be considered to improve quality of life.
- The therapeutic sequence of various new agents (abiraterone, enzalutamide, radium 223) in the management of castrate-resistant prostate cancer remains to be determined, particularly if docetaxel chemotherapy is administered earlier in the treatment pathway.

For a complete list of references, please visit www.expertconsult.com.

KEY REFERENCES

4. Abrams P, Cardozo L, Fall M, et al: The standardisation of terminology of lower urinary tract function: report from the Standardisation Sub-committee of the International Continence Society. Neurourol Urodyn 21:167–178, 2002.
11. McVary KT, Roehrborn CG, Avins AL, et al: Update on AUA guideline on the management of benign prostatic hyperplasia. J Urol 185:1793–1803, 2011.
12. Oelke M, Bachmann A, Descazeaud A, et al: EAU guidelines on the treatment and follow-up of non-neurogenic male lower urinary tract symptoms including benign prostatic obstruction. Eur Urol 64:118–140, 2013.
17. McConnell JD, Roehrborn CG, Bautista OM, et al: The long-term effect of doxazosin, finasteride, and combination therapy on the clinical progression of benign prostatic hyperplasia. N Engl J Med 349:2387–2398, 2003.
21. Roehrborn CG, Siami P, Barkin J, et al: The effects of combination therapy with dutasteride and tamsulosin on clinical outcomes in men with symptomatic benign prostatic hyperplasia: 4-year results from the CombAT study. Eur Urol 57:123–131, 2010.
31. Droz JP, Aapro M, Balducci L, et al: Management of prostate cancer in older patients: updated recommendations of a working group of the International Society of Geriatric Oncology. Lancet Oncol 15:e404–e414, 2014.
37. Bill-Axelson A, Holmberg L, Garmo H, et al: Radical prostatectomy or watchful waiting in early prostate cancer. N Engl J Med 370:932–942, 2014.
38. Daskivich TJ, Lai J, Dick AW, et al: Comparative effectiveness of aggressive versus nonaggressive treatment among men with early-stage prostate cancer and differing comorbid disease burdens at diagnosis. Cancer 120:2432–2439, 2014.
47. Tannock IF, de Wit R, Berry WR, et al: Docetaxel plus prednisone or mitoxantrone plus prednisone for advanced prostate cancer. N Engl J Med 351:1502–1512, 2004.

84 Aging Males and Testosterone

Frederick Wu, Tomas Ahern

INTRODUCTION

As men age, testosterone levels fall, leading to speculation that testosterone supplementation can ameliorate age-related deterioration in physical and psychological functions, health-related quality of life, and life span. Aging and hypogonadism share many clinical features. Age-related decrease in testosterone levels appears to be associated with a combination of the effects of aging on the hypothalamic-pituitary-gonadal (HPG) axis as well as an increasing prevalence of obesity and chronic illness. Testosterone levels fall below the threshold of normality in only a small minority of aging men. The effects of testosterone therapy for older symptomatic men with borderline low testosterone levels are the subject of much debate. Randomized clinical trials (RCTs) of testosterone treatment showed inconsistent benefits, and safety concerns have led to intense scrutiny by the U.S. Food and Drug Administration (FDA). Whether testosterone therapy can improve age-related symptoms and deficits remains unclear, and the conflicting trial data make it challenging to provide a clear explanation of potential risks and benefits of testosterone therapy.

MALE HYPOGONADISM

Male hypogonadism is a clinical syndrome resulting from low testosterone concentrations and deficient spermatogenesis due to pathologic disruption of the HPG axis.[1,2] The condition is usually categorized into primary or secondary hypogonadism caused by testicular or hypothalamic-pituitary disorders, respectively.[3]

Klinefelter syndrome is an example of primary hypogonadism that results from a congenital chromosomal aberration (mostly 47,XXY) and affects approximately 0.2% of male newborns.[4] In addition to low testosterone levels and elevated gonadotropin levels (primary hypogonadism), men with Klinefelter syndrome have small testes and tend to have decreased libido, erectile dysfunction, poor beard growth, infertility (with azoospermia), tall stature, sparse pubic hair, gynecomastia, decreased muscle mass, decreased muscle strength, low bone mineral density (BMD), and anemia.[4] In later life, men with Klinefelter syndrome are more likely to have decreased physical function, diabetes, obesity, bone fracture, and increased mortality.[4]

Hypopituitarism can cause secondary hypogonadism to arise after puberty. Causes include hypothalamic-pituitary tumor (e.g., prolactinoma or nonfunctioning adenoma), hypothalamic-pituitary infiltration (e.g., hemochromatosis), medications (e.g., glucocorticoids, opioid analgesics), brain insult (e.g., traumatic injury, irradiation), and chronic illness (e.g., diabetes and HIV infection).[5] In addition to low testosterone levels and low gonadotropin levels (secondary hypogonadism), men with hypopituitarism after puberty tend to develop similar features to those of men with Klinefelter syndrome, with the exceptions of small penis size, poor beard growth, and abnormal height.[5]

Hypogonadism can result from disruption at more than one level of the HPG axis. Opioids, for example, bind to receptors in the hypothalamus[6] and pituitary[7] glands and inhibit secretion of gonadotropin-releasing hormone[6] and luteinizing hormone (LH).[7] In addition, opioids act directly on the testis to decrease production of sperm and testosterone.[8] Similar to men with primary hypogonadism or secondary hypogonadism, men with hypogonadism caused by multilevel disruption experience adverse effects on multiple organ systems.[6,9]

One of the hallmarks of hypogonadism is an improvement in sexual function and body composition (increased BMD, increased fat mass, and decreased fat mass) in response to testosterone replacement therapy.[10] In cases of pathologic hypogonadism (as described earlier), the efficacy and safety of testosterone replacement has been well established based on long-standing clinical experience.[11,12]

Age-Related Decrease in Testosterone Levels

In the European Male Aging Study (EMAS), a population survey of 3369 community-dwelling men aged older than 40 years, total testosterone concentrations fell by 0.1 nmol/L (0.04%) per year and free (not protein bound) testosterone concentrations fell by 3.83 pmol/L (0.77%) per year.[13] This led to subnormal testosterone levels being detected in a minority of aging men (free testosterone < 220 pmol/L in 12%, total testosterone < 10.5 nmol/L in 8%, and late-onset hypogonadism [see definition later in this chapter] in 1.3%). Both the EMAS and the Boston Area Community Health Survey (BACH) found that the prevalence of a total testosterone concentration below 10.5 nmol/L is between 16% and 26% of men aged 70 to 79 years compared to between 11% and 22% of men younger than 50 years.[3,14]

It is interesting that not all studies have observed lower testosterone levels in older men. Studies of healthy men describe no difference in testosterone concentrations between older and younger men,[15] suggesting that ill health may contribute substantially to the apparent age-related testosterone decline.

Other Factors Related to Decrease in Testosterone Levels

Aging leads to multilevel HPG axis disruption, which is influenced variably by body weight, acute or chronic illness, medications, and lifestyle.

Testicular function declines with aging. Testicular volume of men older than 75 years is 31% smaller than that of men aged 18 to 40 years (20.6 mL vs. 29.7 mL).[16] Leydig cell number is approximately 44% lower in men aged 50 to 76 years than in men aged 20 to 48 years.[17] Congruently, the secretory capacity of the testes, in response to human chorionic gonadotropin or recombinant human LH, is substantially lower in older men than in younger men.[18] Prospective longitudinal studies corroborate these mechanistic data and have found uniformly that LH concentrations rise with aging.[19-22]

Although declining testicular function appears to be the main mechanism underlying the age-related decrease in testosterone, decreased hypothalamic gonadotropin-releasing hormone secretion can also contribute to the dysregulation in the HPG axis in older men.[23] In addition, obesity plays a role in the fall in testosterone levels with aging. Fat mass increases with aging and peaks normally at 65 years.[24] Testosterone concentrations are lower in obese men (BMI > 30 kg/m^2) than in lean men (BMI 20-25 kg/m^2), and obese men's testosterone concentrations decline more quickly.[13] Despite having lower testosterone concentrations than lean men, obese men do not have elevated LH concentrations;

this finding suggests a hypothalamic-pituitary defect,[2] which may be the result of elevated cytokine concentrations[25] and/or insulin resistance.[26]

Chronic illness contributes also to the decline in testosterone levels with aging. Men with chronic illness have lower testosterone levels compared with healthy men.[2] Like men with obesity, LH concentrations are not elevated in those with chronic illness; this finding suggests a hypothalamic-pituitary defect.[2] Chronic illnesses, such as cardiovascular disease and diabetes mellitus type 2 (DM 2), are associated with increased concentrations of proinflammatory cytokines,[27] which, as with obesity, may disrupt the hypothalamus, resulting in lower testosterone levels.[25] Frailty (represented as either a physical syndrome or a health status index) is associated with lower free testosterone and higher LH, suggesting activation of functional reserve in the HPG axis to compensate for impaired testicular function.[28] Statin use[29] and vitamin D deficiency[30] have also been reported to be associated with lower testosterone levels in older men.

Age-Related Low Testosterone Levels and Hypogonadism

In the EMAS, men with low testosterone levels, in the absence of a disease or medication known to affect the HPG axis, had higher BMI, lower muscle mass, lower BMD, higher glucose levels, lower hemoglobin levels, slower walk speeds, and greater illness prevalence compared to men with normal testosterone levels.[31] These features associate only weakly with testosterone levels, however, and are mimicked by chronic illness and the aging process. With the exception of glucose and hemoglobin, no statistically significant relationships persisted after adjustment for age, BMI, and chronic illness.

The Massachusetts Male Aging Study (MMAS) found that the prevalence of loss of libido increased, over the course of 9 years, from 30.6% to 41.1% and that the prevalence of erectile dysfunction increased from 37.4% to 42.3%.[32] Counterintuitively, symptoms of hypogonadism have poor predictive value for low testosterone concentrations and vice versa.[3,14] The BACH study showed that of men older than 50 years, only 20.2% of those with symptoms of hypogonadism had a low total testosterone level (≤10.5 nmol/L) and of men with a low testosterone level, only 20.1% reported low libido and only 29.0% reported erectile dysfunction.[14]

These findings highlight the significant overlap between symptoms of hypogonadism and aging, which have relatively poor specificity for low testosterone levels.

LATE-ONSET HYPOGONADISM

EMAS investigators tried to surmount these issues by defining late-onset hypogonadism (LOH) as the presence of three sexual symptoms (decreased frequency of morning erection, decreased frequency of sexual thoughts, and erectile dysfunction) together with a total testosterone concentration less than 11 nmol/L and a free testosterone concentration less than 220 pmol/L (Figure 84-1).[1] This syndrome affects approximately 3% of men aged 60 to 69 years and approximately 0.1% of men aged 40 to 49 years (Figure 84-2).[1] During the 4.3-year follow-up, nearly 1.5% of eugonadal men developed LOH, and of men with LOH at baseline, nearly 30% recovered. Thus, LOH is not invariably persistent and clinical management strategies need to take this into account.

Adverse Effects of Low Testosterone Levels

International guidelines recommend that a testosterone level that is below the 2.5 percentile in young, healthy adult men be used to define the threshold for a low testosterone level.[11,12] The incidence of depressive illness is greater in men with low testosterone levels.[33] Low testosterone confers also an increased likelihood for the development of poor physical function[34] and frailty,[35] although this relationship becomes nonsignificant after adjustment for chronic illness.[35,36] DM 2 incidence and cardiovascular disease prevalence are also higher in men with low testosterone levels than in men with normal testosterone levels.[37,38] Similarly, men who have undergone androgen deprivation therapy, to effect severe hypogonadism as part of treatment for advanced prostate cancer, have an increased risk of developing diabetes and/or myocardial infarction and have increased mortality.[39]

Mortality and Testosterone Levels

Men with low testosterone levels caused by a disease of the HPG axis usually have testosterone levels that are well below the threshold described previously in this chapter.[40,41] Men with age-related low testosterone levels, however, tend to have testosterone levels that are just below this range.[3] As described earlier, aging, obesity, and chronic illness contribute to the development of age-related low testosterone levels, and these (and perhaps other factors) may be the reason for adverse consequences and not the low testosterone level per se. This is illustrated by prospective studies that found that once the data were adjusted for obesity and chronic illness, age-related low testosterone levels were not associated with increased mortality[42] unless a very low testosterone threshold (<8.36 nmol/L) was used.[43] The situation differs for men at the upper extreme of age (older than 70 years): some studies have shown an association between low testosterone levels with increased mortality and some have not.[44] EMAS data showed an association between sexual symptoms and mortality that was independent of testosterone levels.[43]

TESTOSTERONE THERAPY

Prescription Trends

In the United States, the number of men who received a prescription for testosterone increased from 1.3 million in 2010 to 2.3 million in 2013, with approximately 70% of these aged between 40 and 64 years, approximately 15% aged 65 through 74 years, and approximately 5% older than 75 years.[45] A multinational survey of testosterone prescribing found that between 2000 and 2011, global sales of testosterone sales increased 12-fold from 115 million to 1.4 billion U.S. dollars.[46]

Considerations

Current guidelines of international endocrine societies recommend use of testosterone therapy for men with aging-related hypogonadism provided that testosterone levels are confirmed to be low, the patient has features consistent with hypogonadism, and appropriate screening for disease of the HPG axis is performed.[11,12] These guidelines state also that two consecutive testosterone measurements are required to confirm the presence of low testosterone since the difference between two testosterone measurements on the same person exceeds 20% about half the time.[47] Because of significant diurnal variation in testosterone levels and the considerable effect of food intake on decreasing testosterone levels (by ≈25%), blood for determination of testosterone levels should be taken in the early morning and in the fasting state.[48] It should be noted, however, that the FDA, in contrast to these guidelines, does not consider a low testosterone level due to aging alone an indication for testosterone therapy.[49]

Remediable causes of hypogonadism can be treated specifically by therapies other than testosterone. Dopamine agonist therapy will increase testosterone levels in men with hyperprolactinemia,[50] as will bariatric surgery for men with DM 2, severe

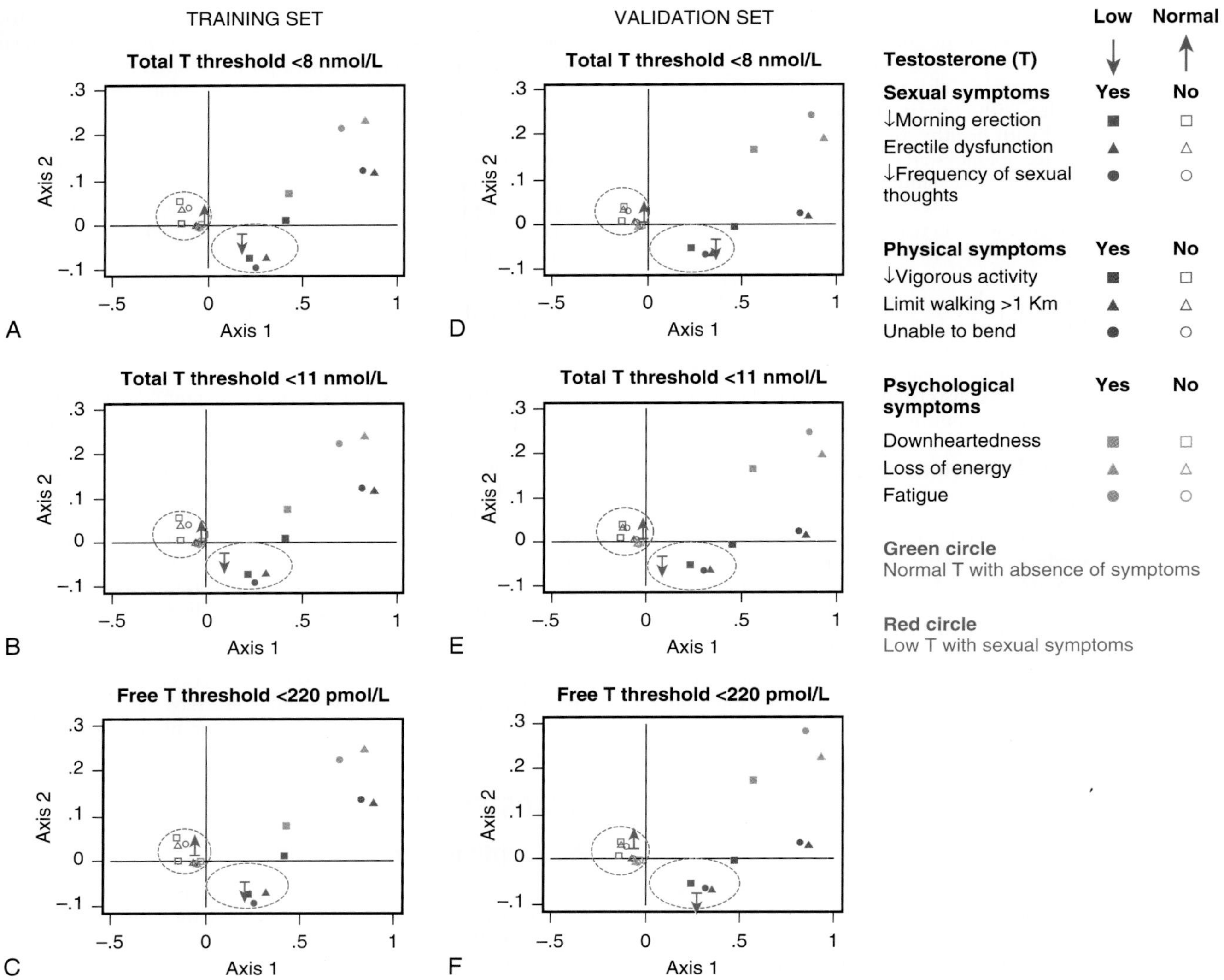

Figure 84-1. Multiple correspondence analysis (MCA) showing associations between symptoms and levels of total testosterone and free testosterone in the training and validation sets. In this MCA plot, variables (including low or normal testosterone levels and the presence or absence of symptoms) are considered to be highly associated if they are at the same distance and in the same direction from the origin where the horizontal axis (axis 1) and the vertical axis (axis 2) cross in the training set and the validation set. Thus, the clustering of the categories of the variables in close proximity to one another is indicative of a syndromic association, which is highlighted by red circles. The values along the axes are indexes of the strength of the association between variables. On axis 1, the presence of symptoms has positive coordinates (to the right of the origin), as compared with the absence of symptoms, with negative coordinates (to the left of the origin). Axis 2 helps identify symptoms that are related to a low testosterone level. The red clusters indicate the presence of the three sexual symptoms, with coordinates similar to those of a low testosterone level. The blue clusters indicate the absence of symptoms, with coordinates similar to those of a normal testosterone level. In contrast, the three psychological symptoms and, to a lesser extent, the three physical symptoms are located far from coordinates for normal and low levels of testosterone, indicating that these symptoms are unrelated or weakly related to the testosterone level. The cluster patterns of symptoms in relation to total or free testosterone levels in the training set are virtually identical to those in the validation set.

obesity, or both.[51] For men with less severe obesity, diet and exercise increases testosterone levels.[52] For men with a low testosterone level and non-elevated LH levels (secondary hypogonadism) who desire fertility, consideration should be given to antiestrogen,[53] aromatase inhibitor,[54] gonadotropin therapy,[55] and/or pulsatile gonadotropin-releasing hormone therapy. The use of aromatase inhibitor therapy, however, is not widely endorsed because long-term safety data are lacking.

An increasing number of preparations are currently available for testosterone replacement therapy.[56] Transdermal and buccal formulations of testosterone therapy require daily administration, whereas intramuscular testosterone ester preparations are given every 3 to 14 weeks. Oral testosterone and 17α-alkylated androgen preparations are not recommended because of potential liver toxicity and variable clinical response. The dose of testosterone therapy should be titrated to maintain a predose

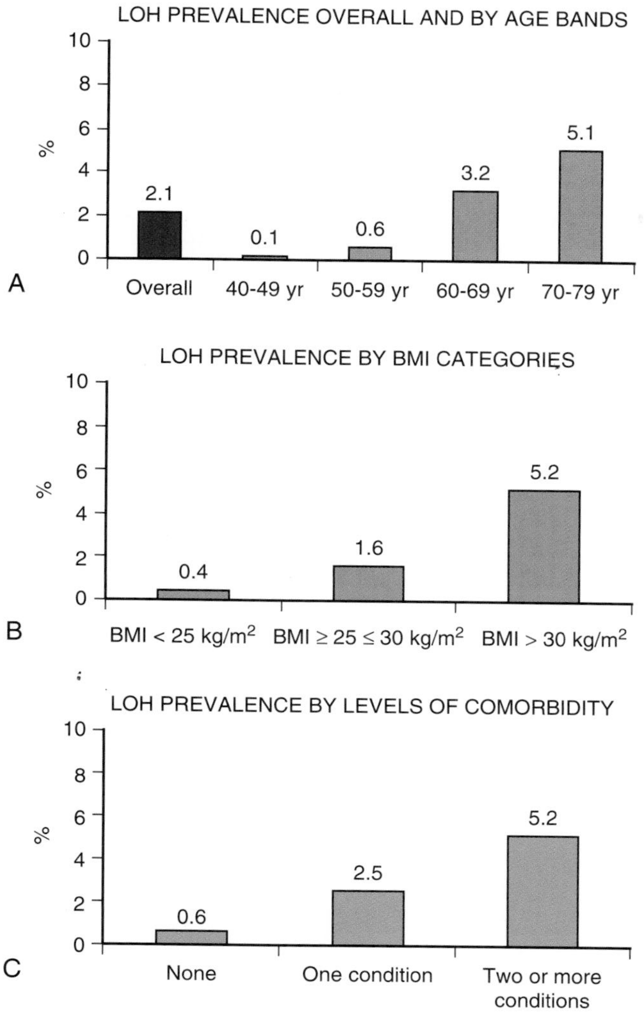

Figure 84-2. The prevalence of the syndrome of late-onset hypogonadism (LOH) in the European Male Aging Study (EMAS), overall and stratified by age, body mass index (BMI), and comorbidity (1). LOH as defined by at least three sexual symptoms associated with total testosterone levels of less than 11 nmol/L and free testosterone of less than 220 pmol/L. A, Overall LOH prevalence and increased prevalence with age. **B,** LOH prevalence increased with BMI. **C,** Prevalence increase with comorbidity (number of coexisting illnesses).

testosterone level in the middle to lower part of the normal reference range. More detailed recommendations on the practical aspects of testosterone therapy are available in published guidelines.[11,12]

Beneficial Effects

Sexual Symptoms

Testosterone supplementation consistently improves sexual interest, spontaneous erections, and, to a lesser extent, erectile dysfunction in hypogonadal men. A meta-analysis of 17 RCTs involving 656 men (mean age 57.5 years) found that testosterone therapy moderately improved sexual symptoms in men with a total testosterone concentration less than 12 nmol/L.[57] Testosterone therapy had no such effect in eugonadal men. Most subsequent studies also have found improvements in sexual symptoms with testosterone therapy in older men with a low testosterone level.[58-60]

Quality of Life and Mood

The effect of testosterone therapy on quality of life in older men with low testosterone levels is unclear, with some studies showing benefit and some not.[58,61] In hypogonadal men with depression, however, testosterone therapy does appear to have a positive impact on mood.[62]

Frailty and Physical Function

In a prospective randomized placebo-controlled trial of 274 men aged 73.8 ± 6.1 years with a low testosterone level (total testosterone < 12 nmol/L), transdermal testosterone therapy, at a dose of 5 mg daily for 6 months (compared to placebo) increased total lean body mass, lower limb muscle strength, and self-reported physical function (SF-36) but did not improve significantly objective physical function except in the subgroups comprising older (aged ≥75 years) and frailer men (≥2 Fried frailty criteria, Figure 84-3).[58] Other RCTs have also not found improvements in physical function with testosterone therapy,[63] suggesting that treatment may benefit only *frail* men with clearly low testosterone levels.

The Testosterone in Older Men with Mobility Limitations trial (TOM) recruited 209 men aged 65 years or older with a total testosterone of 12.0 nmol/L or less. Transdermal testosterone therapy, at double the standard replacement dose (10 mg/day) compared to placebo, improved lower and upper muscle strength but not physical function.[64] This study was terminated early by the safety monitoring board, however, because of a greater incidence of cardiovascular-related events.[65]

Bone Health

Transdermal testosterone therapy for 36 months in men older than 65 years with a low testosterone level (total testosterone < 10.5 nmol/L) increased lumbar spine, but not hip, BMD compared to placebo.[66] Similarly, intramuscular testosterone therapy for 36 months in men aged 65 years and older with a low testosterone level improved lumbar spine BMD (by 9.8 ± 1.4%) and also hip BMD (by 2.5 ± 0.7%).[67] These findings have been confirmed by a meta-analysis of randomized placebo-controlled trials that found also that testosterone therapy improved bone resorption marker concentrations by approximately 17%.[68] Whether these findings translate into a decrease in fracture incidence remains to be determined.

Metabolic Health

Although testosterone levels are lower in men with DM 2, the majority of double-blind, placebo-controlled RCTs involving testosterone therapy for men with DM 2 and/or metabolic syndrome have found no improvement in insulin resistance (as assessed by HOMA2-IR) or in glycemic control (as assessed by hemoglobin A_{1c}).[60,61,69-74]

Risks

Polycythemia

One of the most common adverse effects of testosterone therapy in older men is polycythemia (hematocrit > 52%). Testosterone therapy suppresses hepcidin,[75] leading to an increase in hemoglobin of approximately 1 g/dL, increase in hematocrit of approximately 3%, and a greater than threefold risk of polycythemia.[76]

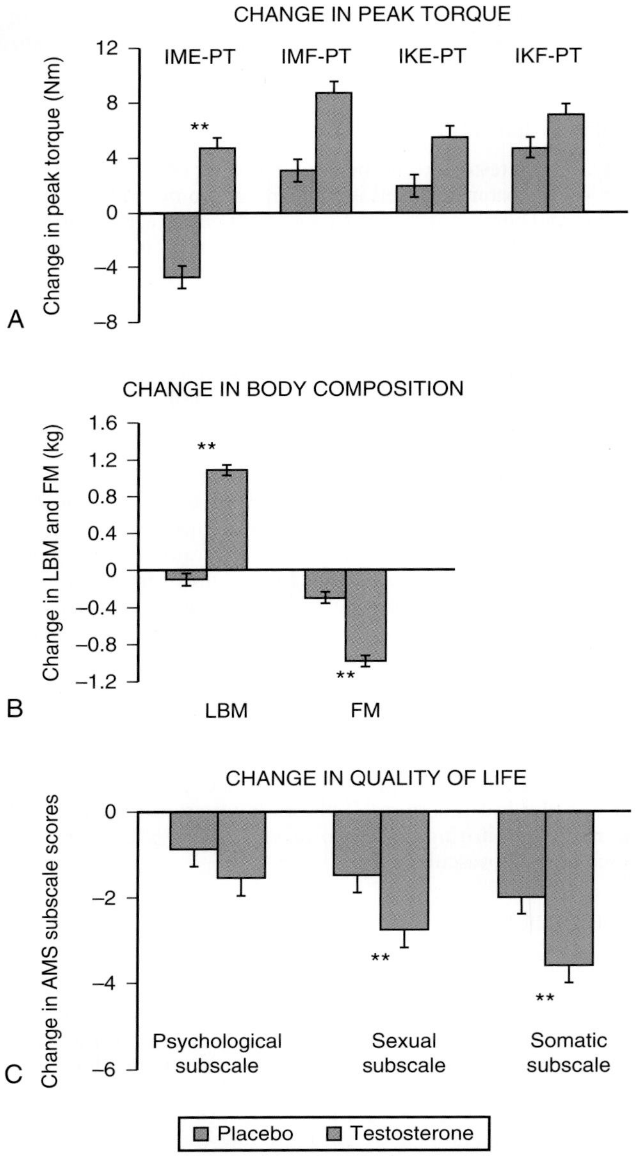

Figure 84-3. Effects of testosterone replacement therapy. A, Change in isometric knee extension peak torque (IME-PT), isometric knee flexion peak torque (IMF-PT), isokinetic knee extension peak torque (IKE-PT), and isokinetic knee flexion peak torque (IKF-PT) in the placebo and T groups at 6 months. **B,** Change in lean body mass (LBM) and fat mass (FM) at 6 months compared with baseline in the placebo and T groups. **C,** change in Aging Males' Symptoms (AMS) scale subscale scores at 6 months compared with baseline in the placebo and T groups. **, Significant difference between groups (ANCOVA, comparing adjusted mean difference between placebo and T groups).

This effect is related to both dose and formulation and can therefore be minimized with careful monitoring and dose titration.[11,12]

Prostate Cancer

The effect of testosterone therapy on prostate cancer incidence is unknown because sufficiently powered RCTs have not been performed (and are unlikely to ever be performed).[77] Although testosterone therapy increases prostate-specific antigen levels,[78] current data suggest no increased risk of prostate cancer.[76]

Cardiovascular Health

Recently, there has been much debate and concern regarding the conflicting data on cardiovascular safety of testosterone treatment in older men.[49] Two retrospective studies found a 39% to 50% reduction in mortality in men with chronic illness who received testosterone therapy.[79,80] These results have been greeted with much caution by experts because of the retrospective, observational nature of the studies and the associated significant limitations.[81] On the other hand, a retrospective case control study of 8709 male veterans with a total testosterone level less than 10.4 nmol/L who underwent coronary angiography observed that testosterone therapy was associated with a 30% increased risk of mortality, myocardial infarction (MI), or stroke over the course of 27.5 months.[82] This was corroborated by another report from a commercial claims database on 55,593 men showing a 36% increase in the rate of MI in men prescribed testosterone.[83] A meta-analysis subsequently found that testosterone therapy did not increase the incidence of new major adverse cardiovascular events (MACE, composite of cardiovascular death, nonfatal acute MI, and stroke) overall, and it decreased MACE incidence in men with DM 2 and/or metabolic syndrome (odds ratio [OR], 0.19 [0.04-0.85]).[84] Baillargeon and colleagues obtained similar findings in their analysis of Medicare beneficiary data.[85]

The widespread concern raised by the previously mentioned publications prompted the FDA to convene an urgent joint advisory committee in September 2014 to investigate the potential for cardiovascular risk associated with testosterone therapy.[49] The committee found significant limitations with all these studies and concluded that available evidence was not sufficient to show an association between testosterone therapy and adverse cardiovascular events. Nevertheless, the committee voted overwhelmingly to (1) limit the indication for testosterone therapy to those with "classical" hypogonadism, and (2) include in the labeling statements regarding the potential for cardiovascular risk, the need for testosterone monitoring and the lack of establishment of safety or efficacy of testosterone therapy in age-related hypogonadism.[49] In March 2015 the FDA issued a drug safety communication stating that "the benefit and safety of these medications (testosterone) have not been established for the treatment of low testosterone levels due to aging." In this statement, the FDA required testosterone manufacturers to change their labeling to clarify that testosterone is FDA approved "only for men who have low testosterone levels due to disorders of the testicles, pituitary gland or brain" and to add information about a "possible increased risk of heart attacks and strokes."[86]

CONCLUSIONS

Testosterone levels fall with aging, leading to LOH in approximately 2% of men aged 40 to 70 years. Aging affects lower testosterone levels directly through deterioration in testicular and hypothalamic function. Aging lowers testosterone levels indirectly also, through an increased prevalence of obesity and chronic illness, which affect pituitary gonadotropin release.

Symptoms associated with age-related low testosterone levels are nonspecific and are highly prevalent among even older men *without* low testosterone levels.

In older men with low testosterone levels, sexual symptoms, mood, and bone health improve with testosterone therapy. In frail older men with low testosterone levels, physical function can improve with testosterone therapy. The effects of testosterone therapy on quality of life and metabolic health are small and/or inconsistent and need to be weighed against the risks of erythrocytosis, prostate disease, and cardiovascular-related events.

These complex issues make the decision to initiate testosterone therapy in older symptomatic men challenging and generate the imperative to establish a formal diagnosis of hypogonadism and to search for an identifiable cause of HPG axis dysfunction. The Testosterone Trials, in which 788 men older than 65 years with a total testosterone concentration less than 9.4 nmol/L will receive transdermal testosterone or placebo for 1 year, will provide important information on the short-term efficacy of testosterone.[77]

It does appear clear, however, that a low testosterone level in an older man should be regarded as a biomarker of chronic illness (overt or occult) and increased mortality and should lead to the use of appropriate interventions with the aim of improving overall health.

KEY POINTS

- Aging and hypogonadism share many clinical features, leading to speculation that testosterone supplementation can ameliorate age-related deterioration.
- Even so, many clinical features of hypogonadism are not related to testosterone levels.
- With aging, most often hypogonadism reflects declining testicular function. Obesity is another important cause and often accompanies a hypothalamic-pituitary defect, indicated by lack of a compensatory elevation of luteinizing hormone. When adjusted for age and obesity, low testosterone levels are not related to mortality.
- Testosterone therapy can improve bone density but, as yet, with no clear impact on fracture incidence.
- Even in men with symptoms of hypogonadism and borderline low testosterone levels, controlled trials of testosterone supplementation have shown inconsistent benefits and risks. Benefit is best established for symptomatic men with low testosterone who are also physically frail, especially if hypothalamic-pituitary compensation is incomplete.

For a complete list of references, please visit www.expertconsult.com.

KEY REFERENCES

1. Wu FC, Tajar A, Beynon JM, et al: Identification of late-onset hypogonadism in middle-aged and elderly men. N Engl J Med 363:123–135, 2010.
2. Wu FC, Tajar A, Pye SR, et al: Hypothalamic-pituitary-testicular axis disruptions in older men are differentially linked to age and modifiable risk factors: the European Male Aging Study. J Clin Endocrinol Metab 93:2737–2745, 2008.
3. Tajar A, Forti G, O'Neill TW, et al: Characteristics of secondary, primary, and compensated hypogonadism in aging men: evidence from the European Male Ageing Study. J Clin Endocrinol Metab 95:1810–1818, 2010.
4. Groth KA, Skakkebaek A, Host C, et al: Clinical review: Klinefelter syndrome–a clinical update. J Clin Endocrinol Metab 98:20–30, 2013.
6. Katz N, Mazer NA: The impact of opioids on the endocrine system. Clin J Pain 25:170–175, 2009.
12. Bhasin S, Cunningham GR, Hayes FJ, et al: Testosterone therapy in men with androgen deficiency syndromes: an Endocrine Society clinical practice guideline. J Clin Endocrinol Metab 95:2536–2559, 2010.
13. Camacho EM, Huhtaniemi IT, O'Neill TW, et al: Age-associated changes in hypothalamic-pituitary-testicular function in middle-aged and older men are modified by weight change and lifestyle factors: longitudinal results from the European Male Ageing Study. Eur J Endocrinol 168:445–455, 2013.
14. Araujo AB, Esche GR, Kupelian V, et al: Prevalence of symptomatic androgen deficiency in men. J Clin Endocrinol Metab 92:4241–4247, 2007.
15. Sartorius G, Spasevska S, Idan A, et al: Serum testosterone, dihydrotestosterone and estradiol concentrations in older men self-reporting very good health: the healthy man study. Clin Endocrinol 77:755–763, 2012.
28. Tajar A, O'Connell MD, Mitnitski AB, et al: Frailty in relation to variations in hormone levels of the hypothalamic-pituitary-testicular axis in older men: results from the European Male Aging Study. J Am Geriatr Soc 59:814–821, 2011.
31. Tajar A, Huhtaniemi IT, O'Neill TW, et al: Characteristics of androgen deficiency in late-onset hypogonadism: results from the European Male Aging Study (EMAS). J Clin Endocrinol Metab 97: 1508–1516, 2012.
36. Krasnoff JB, Basaria S, Pencina MJ, et al: Free testosterone levels are associated with mobility limitation and physical performance in community-dwelling men: the Framingham Offspring Study. J Clin Endocrinol Metab 95:2790–2799, 2010.
37. Ding EL, Song Y, Malik VS, et al: Sex differences of endogenous sex hormones and risk of type 2 diabetes: a systematic review and meta-analysis. JAMA 295:1288–1299, 2006.
40. Citron JT, Ettinger B, Rubinoff H, et al: Prevalence of hypothalamic-pituitary imaging abnormalities in impotent men with secondary hypogonadism. J Urol 155:529–533, 1996.
42. Araujo AB, Kupelian V, Page ST, et al: Sex steroids and all-cause and cause-specific mortality in men. Arch Intern Med 167:1252–1260, 2007.
46. Handelsman DJ: Global trends in testosterone prescribing, 2000-2011: expanding the spectrum of prescription drug misuse. Med J Aust 199:548–551, 2013.
47. Brambilla DJ, O'Donnell AB, Matsumoto AM, et al: Intraindividual variation in levels of serum testosterone and other reproductive and adrenal hormones in men. Clin Endocrinol 67:853–862, 2007.
57. Isidori AM, Giannetta E, Gianfrilli D, et al: Effects of testosterone on sexual function in men: results of a meta-analysis. Clin Endocrinol 63:381–394, 2005.
58. Srinivas-Shankar U, Roberts SA, Connolly MJ, et al: Effects of testosterone on muscle strength, physical function, body composition, and quality of life in intermediate-frail and frail elderly men: a randomized, double-blind, placebo-controlled study. J Clin Endocrinol Metab 95:639–650, 2010.
64. Travison TG, Basaria S, Storer TW, et al: Clinical meaningfulness of the changes in muscle performance and physical function associated with testosterone administration in older men with mobility limitation. J Gerontol A Biol Sci Med Sci 66:1090–1099, 2011.
65. Basaria S, Coviello AD, Travison TG, et al: Adverse events associated with testosterone administration. N Engl J Med 363:109–122, 2010.
66. Snyder PJ, Peachey H, Hannoush P, et al: Effect of testosterone treatment on bone mineral density in men over 65 years of age. J Clin Endocrinol Metab 84:1966–1972, 1999.
68. Tracz MJ, Sideras K, Bolona ER, et al: Testosterone use in men and its effects on bone health. A systematic review and meta-analysis of randomized placebo-controlled trials. J Clin Endocrinol Metab 91:2011–2016, 2006.
86. U.S. Food and Drug Administration: Drug safety communication, 2015. http://www.fda.gov/downloads/Drugs/DrugSafety/UCM436270.pdf. Accessed November 16, 2015.

85 Gynecologic Disorders in Older Women

Tara K. Cooper, Oliver Milling Smith

AGE CHANGES IN THE GENITAL TRACT

The female physiologic aging process accelerates after the menopause, particularly in the genital tract.

Hormone Changes

In perimenopausal women, the ovary becomes less responsive to gonadotropins, which results in a gradual increase in the circulating levels of follicle-stimulating hormone (FSH) and later luteinizing hormone (LH) and a subsequent decrease in estradiol concentrations. FSH levels can fluctuate markedly several years before menses cease, so is an inaccurate diagnostic test, but eventually follicular development fails completely and estradiol production is no longer sufficient to stimulate the endometrium. Amenorrhea then ensues, and FSH and LH levels are persistently elevated, reaching peaks 3 to 5 years after the menopause. Thereafter, there is a gradual decline to premenopausal levels over a 20-year period.[1] A loss of follicles also results in a fall in the production of antimullerian hormone (AMH).

During the reproductive years, the ovary has three components for steroid biosynthesis—the maturing follicle, functioning corpus luteum, and stroma. After menopause, the stroma is the only source of estrogen. Estrone is the major postmenopausal estrogen. It is derived from the conversion of androgens, mainly androstenedione, and produced by the ovaries and adrenal glands. The efficiency of this process increases with age, and estrone levels rise to four times those found in young women. This conversion also relates to body weight because fat has the ability to aromatize androstenedione to estrone.[2] The other postmenopausal estrogens include estriol, which is weak and does not seem to have a significant role, and estradiol, which although secretion is minimal, with blood levels being reduced by 90%, it has 10-fold greater biologic activity than estrone and therefore retains an important role in maintaining hormone-dependent tissues.[3]

Progesterone in the postmenopausal woman is derived mainly from the adrenal glands, and levels fall steadily. Production of testosterone and dehydroepiandrosterone (DHEAS) remains relatively unchanged until later life; surgical oophorectomy will, therefore, result in a decrease of serum testosterone levels of up to 50%.[4]

Anatomic Changes

The major change is atrophy, which results in smaller and smoother structures, flattened epithelial surfaces, and fibrous stroma, with much reduced vascularization and fat content.

Ovary. The postmenopausal ovary is small and sclerotic, with an absence of follicular activity. The cortex involutes, and germinal inclusion cysts are found. Lipid droplets may be seen in the stroma as evidence of continuing steroidogenesis.

Uterus. There is a marked reduction in uterine size so that the uterine body-to-cervix ratio reverts from the 4:1 of reproductive life to the 2:1 of childhood. In the myometrium, there is interstitial fibrosis and thickened blood vessels due to obliterative and subintimal sclerosis. The endometrium becomes a single layer of cuboidal cells with a few inactive glands, which may be dilated due to blocked ducts.

Cervix and Vagina. The cervix becomes more flush with the vaginal vault, and the squamocolumnar junction recedes into the endocervical canal; this can cause stenosis of the external os. The vagina becomes thinner, atrophic, and less elastic, which can make it more vulnerable to trauma. Reduction in estrogen inhibits lactic acid production by the vaginal flora, which raises the vaginal pH and increases the risk of fungal and bacterial infections.[5]

Vulva. Postmenopausal changes are characterized by skin shrinkage, loss of prominent landmarks, and sparse greying hair. The epidermis is thinner, although there is increased keratinization. These features may coincide with a vulvar epithelial disorder (see later).

Pelvic Floor. Aging produces pelvic floor weakness. Damage to the nerve supply starts with parturition,[6] and progressive denervation is found in association with prolapse[7] (see later). An important element of pelvic floor support is collagen, which diminishes after the climacteric. Estrogen receptors are also present in the pelvic organs and decrease after menopause, leading to further weakness of the supporting ligaments and increased risk of prolapse.[8]

MENOPAUSE

Menopause is the permanent cessation of menstruation in nonhysterectomized women. The cessation of ovarian function at menopause has many short- and long-term consequences. The characteristic features of reduced estrogen are systemic, including vasomotor symptoms and localized atrophy of the genital tract.[9] More relevant is the prolonged effect of estrogen deficiency postmenopausally. The average age of menopause has remained around 51 years for centuries. With female life expectancy now reaching over 80 years, there has been a massive increase in the number of postmenopausal women, and the morbidity and mortality secondary to the effects of ovarian failure have become increasingly important. Long-term effects include urogenital atrophy, osteoporosis (see Chapter 70), and effects on cardiovascular function. There is continuing controversy as to whether cognitive performance is adversely affected.

Osteoporosis

In postmenopausal women there is accelerated bone loss, so that by age 70 years, 50% of bone mass is lost, whereas men lose only 25% by 80 years of age.[10] This is due to increased bone resorption by osteoclasts and reduced new bone formation leading to increased turnover. Altered calcium metabolism may be a contributory factor but the primary defect is generalized connective tissue loss, with reduced bone mineral content following breakdown of the organic collagen matrix.[11] The resultant osteoporosis dramatically increases the older woman's fracture rate; 50% of women aged 75 years will have sustained one or more fractures at the most common sites of the wrists, vertebral bodies (resulting in the classic so-called Dowager hump) and neck of the femur. The latter is the most significant consequence of osteoporosis because of its high morbidity and mortality; there is a 20% death rate within the first year, and 50% of survivors will fail to regain their independence.[12]

Two years of hormone replacement therapy (HRT) results in a 66% reduction in hip fracture in the subsequent 2 years and, taken for 10 years, produces a 60% reduction in the overall mortality rate related to osteoporotic fractures.[13] However, studies have highlighted the potential risks of long-term use of HRT (see later, "Hormone Replacement Therapy").

Cardiovascular Disease

Cardiovascular disease (CVD), which includes coronary heart disease and stroke, is five times more common in men than in premenopausal women but, by 70 years, the gender difference is lost. Overall, CVD is the most common cause of death in women. In younger women, estrogen exerts cardioprotective effects through a vasodilatory effect and an alteration in lipid metabolism. Ovarian failure causes increased levels of cholesterol, triglycerides, and low-density lipoprotein (LDL) and a reduction in high-density lipoprotein (HDL). These changes contribute to an increased predisposition to ischemic heart disease.[14] Theoretically, therefore, estrogen therapy should reverse these effects. Observational data have suggested a cardioprotective effect of HRT,[15] but randomized controlled clinical trials have consistently reported that HRT does not reduce, and may slightly increase, the risk of adverse cardiac events after menopause.[16] These studies may have been influenced by the type of HRT investigated and the age range of patients.

Skin and Dentition

Skin changes have been attributed to the aging process but estrogen deficiency and light exposure are significant factors. Skin thickness declines after menopause by 30% in the first 10 years, which is comparable to bone loss over the same time.[17] When HRT is started early, there is maintenance of skin collagen and thickness. Estrogen deficiency also affects teeth; one third of U.S. women older than 65 years are edentulous. HRT may be protective.

Hormone Therapy

Hormone Replacement Therapy

Estrogen therapy has been widely regarded as the appropriate treatment for the consequences of ovarian failure for symptom relief or prevention of long-term effects. However, the Women's Health Initiative (WHI) study and Million Women Study (MWS) results led to considerable uncertainties among health professionals and women about the role of HRT.[18,19]

The British Menopause Society (BMS) published updated recommendations on HRT in 2013.[20] The key recommendation is that all women should be able to obtain advice on how they can optimize their menopause transition and beyond, with particular reference to lifestyle and diet, and an opportunity to discuss the pros and cons of complementary therapies and HRT. Other key points include the following:

- The HRT regimen should be individualized, with an annual review.
- No arbitrary limits on the duration of usage should be established.
- HRT prescribed before the age of 60 years has a favorable benefit-risk profile.
- If HRT is to be used in women older than 60 years, lower starting doses should be used, preferably with a transdermal route.

Currently. most women who request HRT do so for symptom relief, and duration of use is usually less than 5 years.

If HRT is to be used, it should be the lowest dose of estrogen required to relieve symptoms. There is an additional need for progesterone in nonhysterectomized women because unopposed estrogen therapy causes endometrial hyperplasia, which may lead to adenocarcinoma. Progesterone given for 12 to 14 days each month reduces these risks[21] and may be administered orally or transdermally. When HRT is given in this cyclic sequential regimen, there is a withdrawal bleed at the end of each course. In women at least 1 year postmenopausal, progesterone can be given continuously, which prevents endometrial proliferation so there is no bleeding. The levonorgestrel-releasing intrauterine system (Mirena; Bayer) can fulfill this role. Women who start on cyclic HRT can be changed to a continuous combined product when they reach the age of 55 years.

Common adverse effects of estrogen include nausea, headache, and breast tenderness. Unexpected bleeding requires clinical examination, and transvaginal ultrasound with biopsy as required.

Oral Estrogen. Oral administration is the most widely used route and is convenient, relatively inexpensive, and generally well tolerated. Many combinations are available commercially, cyclic and continuous. In perimenopausal women who do not wish frequent withdrawal bleeds, a 3-month bleed preparation can be tried. Tibolone is a synthetic steroid with estrogenic, progestrogenic, and androgenic properties and acts as a continuous combined product. It may also improve libido and may have less effect on breast tissue.[22]

The main disadvantage of the oral route is that estrogen passes directly to the liver, where it is inactivated and partially metabolized to the less effective estrone. This is called the first-pass effect, which means that higher doses are required than with parenteral therapy. It may also result in altered hepatic metabolism, with changes in clotting factors and increased renin substrate, which predisposes to hypertension.

Transdermal Estrogen. Transdermal patches may be matrix or reservoir in type and require changing once or twice weekly. Combination patches with progesterone are also available. Estradiol is delivered at a controlled rate, depending on surface area. The first-pass effect is avoided, and hepatic metabolism is not affected, thus reducing the risk of thrombosis. The main problems are with adhesion, and transient skin reactions can occur in up to 30% of women; the frequency is lower with matrix patches. A transdermal gel may be used instead.

Topical Estrogen. Low-dose vaginal creams, pessaries, tablets, and rings are used primarily for treating symptoms of urogenital atrophy. Systemic absorption and side effects are minimal and, although use may need to be prolonged, progesterone opposition is not required. In general, a short course is adequate; a 14-day course should be followed by two nights' application each week for up to 6 weeks. A problem with this route in older women is reduced acceptability and impaired manual dexterity for self-administration. A low-dose hydrophilic vaginal tablet, which has a fine prelubricated and preloaded applicator (Vagifem; Novo Nordisk) may be acceptable for use in patients with a history of breast cancer after discussion with the oncology team.

Contraindications and Risks With Hormone Replacement Therapy

There are few contraindications to HRT, which provides estrogen replacement at a below-normal premenopausal plasma concentration and that achieved with the high-dose synthetic steroids used in the combined oral contraceptive pill. The main contraindications are estrogen-dependent breast or endometrial cancers, although women with treated breast cancer and debilitating menopausal symptoms may be given HRT under specialist supervision, and there is no evidence of increased recurrence rates.[23]

Oral estrogen is associated with an increased risk of venous thromboembolic disease (VTE), although the absolute risk is low for women younger than 60 years. The risk appears to be lower with transdermal estrogen, so this route is preferable for women with other risk factors, such as smoking and obesity.[24] It is not necessary to stop HRT prior to surgery because most patients will fall into a moderate risk category (in regard to age) and receive antithrombotic prophylaxis.

HRT may be given if there is a preexisting gynecologic condition (e.g., endometriosis, fibroids), but the latter may fail to shrink and cause heavier withdrawal bleeds.

Two large studies (WHI and Million Women Study[18,19]) have suggested a small increase in the risk of breast cancer after 5 years of HRT usage, but current opinion has cast doubt on the ability of these studies to establish a causal association. Similarly, published data on the risk of ovarian cancer are conflicting. The risk of endometrial cancer is largely avoided by the use of combined estrogen-progestogen therapy. Changing to continuous combined HRT as soon as appropriate reduces the endometrial risk to lower than that in an untreated population.[25] There is no association between HRT and cervical cancer. There may be a reduced risk of colorectal cancer.

Despite extensive educational products and improved therapies, such as no bleed continuous HRT, compliance is poor. About 50% of patients do not remain on HRT 12 months after starting treatment, even when at risk of osteoporosis.[26]

Alternatives to Hormone Replacement Therapy

A healthy diet, stopping smoking, and an active lifestyle should be recommended. Symptomatic relief from hot flushes can sometimes be achieved with clonidine, gabapentin, and selective serotonin reuptake inhibitors (SSRIs). There is also a growing trend toward natural products such as black cohosh, red clover, and natural progesterone cream. There are some data on the safety and efficacy of red clover[27] but less so with other products. One study has shown no pharmacologic activity for progesterone cream,[28] and any benefits are likely to be a placebo effect.

As many as 50% to 75% of postmenopausal women will use nonpharmacologic options to treat vasomotor symptoms.[29] It is important to establish what they may be taking because this may affect other medications.

VULVAR DISORDERS

Vulvar epithelial disorders are important because of the severity and chronicity of symptoms—usually itching, soreness, and irritation—and their association with carcinoma. Community-based surveys have demonstrated that round 20% of women have significant vulvar symptoms.[30] There have been conflicting views about the pathogenesis, diagnosis, and terminology of vulvar disorders. Lesions may be infective, inflammatory, localized variants of generalized dermatoses, premalignant or malignant. Management is often difficult, especially because patients may present to a variety of specialists, including gynecologists, dermatologists, geriatricians, and general practitioners. Treatment may therefore be improved by consultation at a dedicated vulvar skin clinic, if available.

Symptoms

Vulvar skin is more sensitive than other epithelium because it is subjected to increased heat, friction, and occlusion. Aging is also a factor, and some chronic vulvar disorders represent an advanced stage of atrophic change. Patients with any of the myriad of diseases of the vulva may complain of symptoms such as dryness, itch, ulceration, and pain.

Management

To diagnose vulvar pathology accurately, a full history and examination are required. The history should explore symptoms at other skin sites and should include a medical and drug history. A family or personal history of autoimmune or atopic conditions should be elicited. Assessment of urinary or fecal incontinence should be made. The examination should extend to other skin and mucosal membranes.

The initial investigation of a woman with vulvar symptoms could include testing for thyroid disease and diabetes if autoimmune-associated conditions are suspected. Swabs for infection should be considered, if appropriate. An initial biopsy is not necessary, especially when the diagnosis can be made on clinical basis. However, if vulvar lesions do not respond to initial treatment or doubt exists as to their cause, they should be biopsied to assist diagnosis and subsequent management.

Specific common vulvar disorders and treatments are discussed below, but general measures such as following should always be discussed to try and improve symptoms:

- Avoid tight, restrictive, or occlusive clothing; cotton underwear is advised.
- Avoid irritants such as soaps, shower gels, scrubs, bubble baths, and fragrances.
- Avoid frequent washing with water; this will dry the skin and worsen symptoms.
- Showering is preferable to bathing.
- Promote the use of emollients and soap substitutes.

Common Vulvar Skin Disorders

As mentioned, the vulvar skin may be affected by a variety of dermatologic conditions, including psoriasis, urticaria, and bullous diseases such as pemphigus. The more common inflammatory conditions found in older adults include dermatitis, lichen planus, premalignant conditions of lichen sclerosus, and vulvar intraepithelial neoplasia. These are described next.

Lichen Simplex Chronic and Vulvar Dermatitis

Women with sensitive skin or eczema can often present with vulvar symptoms and skin changes. Symptoms can include severe intractable itch, especially at night, leading to nonspecific inflammation. Scratching will lead to thickening or lichenification of the skin, termed *lichen simplex*. The cause of this condition may be endogenous (atopic) or exogenous (contact) in nature. In older adults, urine is a common irritant, but a history indicating a change in, for example, soap, fragrances, and underwear, should be sought.

The mainstay of the management of dermatitis and lichen simplex chronic starts with general measures for vulvar care (see earlier section). Moderate or high-potency topical steroids may relieve the itch and can be of value to try and break the itch-scratch cycle. Secondary infection may complicate dermatitis, and swabs should be taken to identify treatable infection. Barrier preparations are valuable in relieving symptoms of contact dermatitis, especially in the presence of urinary or fecal incontinence. However, note that some barrier preparations can cause irritation, worsening the problem.

Lichen Planus

This inflammatory condition may also affect the hair, nails, and mucous membranes. The classic lesions are purple papules, sometimes with a lacy white surface pattern (Wickham striae). The usual complaint is of soreness but itch, dyspareunia, and discharge may be present. If the patient is sexually active and concern exists over vaginal narrowing, vaginal dilators may be of benefit. A more severe presentation of lichen planus may involve an erosive vulvar lesion, leading to profuse discharge and scarring.

Treatment involves general vulvar care. This includes the use of emollients and high-potency topical steroids.

Premalignant Vulvar Disorders

Premalignant conditions of the vulva include a spectrum of disorders, including vulvar intraepithelial neoplasia, lichen sclerosus, and Paget disease of the vulva.

Vulvar Intraepithelial Neoplasia

Vulvar intraepithelial neoplasia (VIN) is divided into usual and differentiated types, depending on histopathologic features. The usual type of VIN is the commoner condition and is found in younger and older women. Although the incidence of this condition is rising in younger women, most cases occur in women older than 50 years.

Usual Type of Vulvar Intraepithelial Neoplasia. This is associated with human papilloma virus (HPV) exposure, in particular subtype 16. Smoking represents an additional strong risk factor, as is chronic immunosuppression. There is no typical appearance of VIN, and the lesions may be unifocal or multifocal.

Differentiated Type of Vulvar Intraepithelial Neoplasia. This is rarer and more common in older women and may arise on the background of conditions such as lichen sclerosus. It has the greatest potential for malignant transformation.[31] Clinically, lesions tend to be unifocal in the form of a plaque or ulcer.

VIN may also be described as VIN type 1, 2, or 3. This classification was revised by the International Society for the Study of Vulvar Disease in 2004 because of a lack of evidence of a disease continuum from VIN 1 to VIN 3 (Box 85-1).[32]

Management. The symptoms of pruritus can be difficult to treat but some benefit may be obtained with the use of emollients or mild steroids. No single ideal therapy for VIN exists. Surgery may be destructive, and medical treatments may be troubled by side effects. Treatment is difficult, and referral to a specialized vulvar skin clinic is advised. Surgical treatment involves local excision and is often mutilating, creates anxiety, affects sexual function, and suffers from high relapse rates. For this reason, a prudent management plan may often involve watching, with repeated biopsies to exclude carcinogenic change.

BOX 85-1 Classification of Vulvar Intraepithelial Neoplasia

Usual type
- Warty
- Basaloid
- Mixed

Differentiated type

Modified from Sideri M, Jones RW, Wilkinson EJ, et al: Squamous vulvar intraepithelial neoplasia: 2004 modified terminology, ISSVD Vulvar Oncology Subcommittee. J Reprod Med 2005; 50:807–810.

Lichen Sclerosis

Lichen sclerosis (LS) is a common problem affecting the aging vulva. The cause is uncertain but there is an association with genetic autoimmune disease factors.[33] The incidence of LS is estimated to be between 1 in 300 to 1000. The vulvar appearance varies but the characteristic lesions are a figure-of-eight configuration around the vulva and anus of white plaques, together with atrophy. The condition does not extend to the vagina. Loss of tissue architecture is common, with fusion of tissue, which may lead to introital stenosis. Chronic scratching complicates the picture, so the skin may be thickened (i.e., lichenified). Although the clinical appearance varies, there are characteristic histologic features, including an atrophic epidermis with hyalinization, areas of thickening (hyperkeratosis), and inflammation.

In older women, management may include investigating for the presence of autoimmune disorders such as pernicious anemia, thyroid disease, and diabetes. General vulvar care advice should be given. However, the mainstay of treatment should include topical use of the potent steroid clobetasol propionate (Dermovate, GlaxoSmithKline UK, Ltd). This should be applied daily at first, reducing the amount as symptoms improve (a 30-g tube is expected to last 3 to 6 months). Response rates are very high but relapse is common, with 84% of women experiencing a relapse within 4 years.[34]

Malignant change may affect from 2% to 9% of older women,[35] and punch biopsies under local anesthetic should be taken of any suspicious areas to exclude atypical change. Punch and incisional biopsies should be targeted at the lesion edge. An excisional biopsy should be avoided because this may complicate subsequent management if cancer is proven (e.g., injection of lesion for sentinel node biopsy).

Squamous carcinoma is more likely when there is a failure to respond to topical steroid use or with the presence of ulceration, raised lesions, or lymph node involvement. These patients should report alteration in symptoms and be checked every 6 to 12 months.

Although the condition is associated with atrophy, topical estrogen is ineffective. It should be considered only for vaginal use.

Extramedullary Paget Disease

This rare condition is a neoplasm of apocrine-bearing skin. It has a peak incidence at 65 years of age. Clinically, it has symptoms to similar to those of other skin conditions of the vulva. Lesions will often appear as white islands, with bridges of hyperkeratinization. A biopsy is required to establish the diagnosis. Treatment is by a specialist and may involve surgery and /or radiotherapy after appropriate discussion with the multidisciplinary team. Prognosis is good if confined to the epidermis, and the challenge is therefore early detection.

Vulvar Discomfort

A complaint of severe pain or discomfort in the vulva for over 3 months is termed *vulvodynia.* Localized pain to light touch at the vaginal vestibule (where the vagina meets the vulva) is termed *localized vulvodynia* (previously known as vestibulitis).

In older women, vulvar pain is more commonly generalized and is characterized by pain, burning, stinging, irritation, and rawness. This is can be termed *dysesthetic vulvodynia* or, more commonly, *generalized vulvodynia.* Unlike localized vulvodynia, which is provoked by touch, women with generalized vulvodynia have a more constant neuropathic pain. The complaint of itch is uncommon, and examination is usually normal. The cause is uncertain but it is recognized that there are both psychological and physical factors involved.[36] Depression is a possible factor because these patients often live alone. Assessment includes neurologic and local examinations with urethral, vaginal, and endocervical swabs to exclude infections. Pathology is rarely found.

Initial treatment should involve explanation of the condition, emphasizing that this is a real condition, although often no physical findings are present. General vulvar care, as previously described, should be given and, in some cases, use of low-strength topical corticosteroids or anesthetics (e.g., 5% lidocaine) may be helpful. The use of pelvic floor exercises to improve muscle tone and blood supply and vaginal retraining dilators can also be used. Some symptoms will respond to low-dose tricyclic antidepressants, such as amitriptyline, 10 mg at night, increasing the dose as side effects permit, to a usual dose of 60 to 150 mg/day. The use of the neuroleptic gabapentin has also been reported as a second-line therapy.[37]

PELVIC ORGAN PROLAPSE

Pelvic organ prolapse (POP) is a common problem, affecting 37% of women older than 80 years.[38] It occurs when there is a weakness in the supporting structures of the pelvic floor, allowing the pelvic viscera to descend and ultimately fall through this anatomic defect. An increase in life expectancy has meant that prolapse has become an increasingly important problem. Although a benign condition, quality of life can be severely affected with bladder, bowel, and sexual dysfunction described. Surgery for POP accounts for approximately 60% of elective major surgery in older women.[38]

Prolapse is most commonly related to childbirth—50% of patients with prolapse are parous[39]—and to postmenopausal hormone deficiency when lack of estrogen causes collagen loss and ligament atrophy.[40] Congenital weakness of sustaining structures and the natural aging process are other factors. Additionally, factors leading to increased abdominal pressure, such as obesity, constipation, and chronic cough, will exacerbate prolapse symptoms.

The main supports of the uterus and upper vagina are the transverse cervical or cardinal ligaments, pubocervical fascia, and uterosacral ligaments. The middle third of the vagina is supported by fascia, and the lower third of the vagina is buttressed by fibers of the pelvic floor. In the erect posture, the anterior vagina rests on the posterior wall, which is strengthened by the rectovaginal fascia and perineal body.

Prolapse of the anterior and posterior vaginal walls occurs independently or together, resulting in any combination of ureterocele, cystocele, rectocele, and enterocele. These are displacements of the underlying urethra, bladder, rectum, and pouch of Douglas (and any contents), respectively.

There are many grading systems to classify POP. The International Urogynaecological Association and International Continence Society (ICS) have recommended the pelvic organ prolapse quantification (POP-Q) system because it has been shown to be reproducible and reliable.[41] The details are beyond the scope of this chapter but, in general, the location of the most distal aspect of the prolapse during straining determines the severity:

- Stage 0: No prolapse
- Stage 1: More than 1 cm above the hymen
- Stage 2: Within 1 cm from the plane of the hymen
- Stage 3: More than 1 cm below the hymen
- Stage 4: Vagina is fully everted

The patient commonly presents with a dragging or bearing down sensation of gradual onset that worsens with activity and settles with rest. A lump may be seen or felt. Urinary symptoms such as frequency, urgency, incontinence, and incomplete or slow emptying result from distortion of the prolapsed bladder and urethra, but they may also be due to atrophy, infection, or detrusor overactivity.[42] Digital replacement of the anterior or posterior vaginal wall is sometimes necessary before micturition or defecation may proceed.

With prolonged uterine descent, edema occurs due to interference with venous and lymphatic drainage, leading to epithelial hyperkeratinization and decubital ulceration. Bleeding may result, but carcinoma rarely develops. With severe prolapse, it is possible to cause ureteric obstruction with subsequent hydronephrosis. In the older woman patient with complete procidentia, a degree of ureteric obstruction is likely, and an ultrasound investigation should be carried out. Further investigation should include pelvic abdominal assessment to exclude a mass. Prolapse is assessed with the patient in the left lateral position, if possible, although standing up may provide good assessment of the degree of prolapse. Asking the patient to cough repeatedly to look for signs of stress incontinence may assess urinary signs. Occult stress incontinence may occur in the older woman patient after correction of prolapse by conservative or surgical methods. It may therefore be advisable to arrange cystometry and uroflowmetry to evaluate potential stress incontinence. If stress incontinence is discovered, this may be addressed at the time of managing the prolapse.

The management of POP depends on how much it affects the quality of life of the woman; if this is minimal, it does not need active intervention. The first line of management is conservative lifestyle modifications, including weight loss, smoking cessation, and correction of constipation. Pelvic floor muscle training (PFMT) has a role in the treatment of prolapse and, if directed by a specialized physiotherapist, has been shown to improve POP objectively.[43]

Surgery offers definitive treatment but suitability of the patient depends on the severity of symptoms, degree of incapacity, and the patient's operative fitness. It includes, as appropriate, anterior and/or posterior pelvic floor repair, vaginal hysterectomy, or vault suspension if hysterectomy has already been carried out. Sacrospinous fixation will reduce the risk of recurrence.

It is now standard practice to give subcutaneous heparin preoperatively and postoperatively to reduce venous thromboembolism risk and to prescribe antibiotics for surgical prophylaxis. Most patients tolerate surgery well because of improved anesthetics and minimal postoperative morbidity. These procedures lead to greater mobility and return to an independent life. Studies have suggested that surgical procedures for prolapse in older women do not entail any increased morbidity as compared to the younger patient.[44]

Recurrence of prolapse will trouble about one third of patients who undergo a surgical corrective procedure.[45] The use of synthetic mesh can reduce the recurrence by up to 30% but has a significantly higher serious complication rate, including exposure or extrusion of the mesh leading to urinary symptoms, vaginal pain, and dyspareunia.

Colpocleisis is the surgical closure of the vagina down to the introitus. It can relieve symptoms of prolapse but precludes sexual intercourse.

When surgery is contraindicated or declined, conservative measures may be used. A variety of pessaries are available, mostly made of polyvinylchloride, which mechanically support the prolapse and relieve pressure on the pelvic organs; these can be as effective as surgery. Women choosing to avoid surgery tend to be older, with less troublesome symptoms.[46] Gellhorn and ring pessaries are equally effective.

The pessary should be inspected and cleaned or renewed every 4 to 6 months to prevent vaginal ulceration. In this case, the ring should be removed for a few weeks to allow epithelial healing.

The use of local estrogen may help healing if hypoestrogenic atrophy is present. If the ring pessary is not effective, usually due to expulsion, a shelf pessary can reduce prolapse. Shelf pessaries lead to a higher degree of vaginal trauma, including the possibility of rectovaginal or vesicovaginal fistulae. However, in older women, particularly if there are comorbidities that prevent surgery or there is a large degree of prolapse, they may be more suitable than the more common ring pessary. They should be inspected in the same way but are more difficult to remove and replace.

URINARY INCONTINENCE

Lower urinary tract symptoms are common in older women and are due to a variety of underlying mechanisms. Diagnosis based on history and examination alone may be correct in only 65% of women who complain of urinary tract symptoms.[47]

Urinary incontinence (UI) is particularly disabling and distressing in older people and can significantly affect quality of life by restricting activities and rendering them housebound but, with current investigative techniques and treatment symptoms may be alleviated, if not cured. UI has been defined by the International Continence Society as "the complaint of any involuntary urinary leakage."[41] The most common types are stress UI and urgency UI, also known as overactive bladder. Continuous leakage is more likely to be associated with neurologic disorders, overflow, urethral diverticulum, or vesicovaginal fistula.

The implementation of assessment and conservative treatment of UI depends on a successful integrated continence service. Most cases of UI can be managed in the community but clearly identified pathways for referral to secondary and tertiary care are vital.[48] UI is discussed in detail in Chapter 106.

GYNECOLOGIC CANCER IN OLDER WOMEN

An association has been noted between aging and cancer development, and there is a tendency for cancer to be at a more advanced stage at presentation. The management of gynecologic cancer patients is now mostly centralized in units staffed by experienced gynecologic oncologists in which the care and outcome is improved. Decisions for care should be undertaken by a multidisciplinary team (MDT), including the gynecologist, medical and radiological oncologists, pathologists, and the patient themselves. Female genital cancer affects four main sites—the vulva, cervix, endometrium, and ovaries.

Vulvar Carcinoma

Vulvar carcinoma is seen most frequently in the 60- to 70-year-old age group and accounts for about 5% of genital neoplasia. Comorbidities are common in older adults, which creates specific challenges in planning management. Early symptoms are pruritus or an asymptomatic lump; however, late presentation is more common because of embarrassment and is usually in the form of bleeding and/or an offensive discharge. The lesion commonly arises in the labium majorum and spreads directly to the urethra, anus, and vagina and by regional lymph glands, the superficial inguinal and prefemoral nodes. Lateral tumors tend to spread to the ipsilateral nodes but centrally placed tumors may involve the contralateral nodes. Hematologic spread is rare and is a late phenomenon leading to metastases to the lung, liver, or bone. The most significant prognostic indicator is nodal status. Overall, groin-negative patients have a 5-year survival rate in excess of 80%.[49]

The aim of management is to carry out the most conservative procedure likely to lead to cure. All cases of suspected vulvar cancer should have the diagnosis confirmed with an incisional biopsy, including an area of epithelium where there is transition from normal to abnormal tissue. Excisional biopsy of suspected cancer should be avoided. The appearance and positioning of lesions should be documented and all findings reviewed by the MDT to plan for specialized management. Factors such as tumor size, location, medical fitness, and patient's wishes will all influence management. Radical vulvectomy with bilateral groin node dissections is no longer the treatment of choice, because morbidity is high, especially in older woman. Morbidity of groin node dissection includes long-term lymphedema and recurrent cellulitis.

Early-Stage Disease

Lesions smaller than 2 cm confined to the vulva or perineum and have a depth of invasion of less than 1 mm (according to the International Federation of Gynecology and Obstetrics [FIGO])—stage 1A—can be managed by wide local excision. In these cases, there is a negligible risk of lymph node metastases.[50] If the depth of invasion is greater than 1 mm or the lesion is larger than 2 cm, dissection of groin nodes is likely to be recommended. This could be unilateral or bilateral, depending on findings; this decision should be determined by the MDT. The aim of surgery on the primary tumor is to achieve a minimal fresh tissue margin of 15 mm because recurrence is inversely related to the margins.[51] More recent evidence has supported the use of sentinel lymph node identification to try and spare the patient more extensive lymph node dissection.[52]

Advanced Disease

Survival rates at 5 years are less than 50%, and the postoperative morbidity can be very high. Resection of advanced disease therefore requires careful planning and will often necessitate a prior examination under anesthetic by a joint surgical team, including the gynecologic oncologist and plastic surgeon. Surgery will aim to achieve adequate margins with wide local or radical excision. Some tumors may require a radical vulvectomy with en bloc groin node dissection. Concern regarding the risk of sphincter damage, risking urinary or fecal incontinence, must always be paramount when planning surgery. If it is a concern, the MDT may consider initial treatment by radiotherapy with curative intent or as an adjunct to delayed surgery after reduction of tumor bulk. Reconstructive surgical techniques should be used to allow for surgical wound closure and to reduce morbidity secondary to scarring.

Radiotherapy is also used to treat recurrence, if not previously used, and is also helpful in the palliative setting. Nursing management may be difficult due to increasing problems with catheterization, poor healing, and discharge, which may be infective or lymphatic in origin.

Cervical Carcinoma

Worldwide, cervical carcinoma is still the most common gynecologic malignancy in all age groups. In developed countries, the incidence has been falling significantly as a result of screening programs. In the United Kingdom, screening programs stop at 60 years of age but if an abnormal smear is found in a woman older than 60 years, it is 16 times more likely to lead to a diagnosis of invasive cancer compared with women younger than 30 years.[53] HPV types 16 and 18 have been incriminated in the pathogenesis of invasive squamous carcinoma and are detectable in over 90% of cases. The introduction of a vaccine against the high-risk HPV subtypes[54] may change the face of cervical cancer in future generations but vigilance is still required.

Older patients will present with symptoms such as offensive vaginal discharge and postmenopausal or postcoital bleeding. Pain is experienced late and is usually related to diffuse pelvic infiltration or bony metastases. The first sign of this cancer may be obstructive renal failure from hydronephrosis due to advanced disease.

As with all cancers, optimal management should be directed by a MDT including the gynecologist, medical and radiological oncologists, pathologists, and the patient. Diagnosis is by biopsy of suspicious areas, preferably under general anesthesia, so that clinical staging according to FIGO criteria can be achieved.[55] Radiologic staging is usually used as the cornerstone of MDT decision making, and magnetic resonance imaging (MRI) of the pelvis should be performed in all patients prior to MDT discussion. Due to the higher sensitivity of detecting lymph node involvement, MDT will often also recommend positron emission tomography (PET) and/or computed tomography (CT) imaging.

Squamous cell cancer accounts for more than 80% of cases. Lymphatic metastases occur quickly. Therefore, up to 50% of early lesions have pelvic spread at presentation. Tumors confined to the cervix may be treated by radical hysterectomy and pelvic node dissection or radiotherapy. Both treatments have similar 5-year survival rates[56] in early stages.

In older adults, radiotherapy may be used more commonly because of the fear of complications from radical surgery or because of the more advanced presentation of disease. However, a fit older woman with early-stage disease will tolerate the procedure well and should not be denied it on the basis of age alone. In advanced disease, the tumor may infiltrate locally, causing fistula formation to the bladder or rectum. As with other squamous carcinomas, the success of chemotherapy alone is limited, but chemotherapy is usually offered concurrently with radiotherapy to potentiate its effect.[57] Patients undergoing chemoradiotherapy with anemia, as indicated by hemoglobin levels of or below 12 g/dL, should have this corrected, because this seems to improve prognosis.[58]

Endometrial Cancer

Endometrial carcinoma is the most common gynecologic malignancy in older women. Postmenopausal bleeding is the most frequent symptom and occurs early. Hence, the prognosis tends to be good, with an overall 5-year survival rate for all stages of around 80%. There are significant associations with nulliparity, late menopause, obesity; diabetes, and hypertension. Unopposed estrogen replacement therapy and tamoxifen use are particularly strong risk factors. The incidence of uterine cancer is increasing in the Western world, and this has much to do with the increasing obesity rates. Of primary endometrial cancers, 80% are adenocarcinomas arising from the glandular endothelium, often on a background of atypical hyperplasia. Hyperplasia is associated with unopposed estrogen action and, when described as atypical, surgical hysterectomy is warranted, because undiagnosed carcinoma may be present. Serous, clear cell, and undifferentiated carcinomas are less common but more aggressive histologic varieties of endometrial malignancies. More rarely, sarcomatous and mixed mesodermal tumors occur and have a poorer prognosis.

Approximately 90% of women with endometrial cancer present with postmenopausal bleeding (PMB), and patients with this complaint have about a 10% chance of being diagnosed with endometrial cancer.[59] The recommended initial assessment of PMB should include transvaginal ultrasound scanning to measure endometrial thickness. A thin endometrium on ultrasound has a high negative predicative value and is reassuring.[60] If a thickening is detected, an endometrial biopsy is required. Thresholds for endometrial thickness will vary between regions but commonly are between 3 and 5 mm, or greater if the woman is currently on HRT. Ultrasound assessment is of little value if the older woman is on tamoxifen due to subendometrial cystic changes. In this situation, the first-line investigation should involve hysteroscopy, with endometrial biopsy. Most cases of PMB are due to benign conditions, including atrophic vaginitis and simple endometrial or cervical polyps.

BOX 85-2 International Federation of Gynecology and Obstetrics (FIGO) Staging for Endometrial Cancer

IA: Tumor confined to the uterus, no or <50% myometrial invasion
IB: Tumor confined to the uterus, >50% myometrial invasion
II: Cervical stromal invasion, but not beyond uterus
IIIA: Tumor invades serosa or adnexa
IIIB: Vaginal and/or parametrial involvement
IIIC1: Pelvic node involvement
IIIC2: Paraaortic involvement
IVA: Tumor invasion bladder and/or bowel mucosa
IVB: Distant metastases including abdominal metastases and/or inguinal lymph nodes

Modified from Mutch DG: The new FIGO staging system for cancers of the vulva, cervix, endometrium, and sarcomas. Gynecol Oncol 115:325–328, 2009.

Endometrial tumors spread directly to the cervix, vagina, and peritoneal cavity via the fallopian tubes. Myometrial invasion is common and may lead to serosal involvement. Lymphatic spread involves the external iliac, internal iliac, obturator, and paraaortic nodes. Hematologic spread may lead to lung metastases. The staging of endometrial cancer relies on surgical assessment of intraabdominal disease combined with pathologic assessment of a hysterectomy specimen (Box 85-2). If the tumor extends to less than 50% of the myometrial depth, there is lymph node spread in less than 5% of cases. If endometrial biopsy suggests high-grade disease or if high malignant histology or MRI suggests deep myometrial involvement, it is recommended that care be provided via a dedicated gynecologic oncologist as part of the MDT.

At a minimum, treatment should involve total hysterectomy, bilateral salpingo-oophrectomy, peritoneal cytology, and upper abdominal inspection. The debate regarding the necessity of lymphadenectomy in these patients led to the Medical Research Council–funded ASTEC (A Study in the Treatment of Endometrial Cancer) trial. One of the study's primary aims was to assess the benefit, or otherwise, of pelvic lymphadenectomy in patients for whom disease was thought to be confined to the corpus. The results suggested that there was no benefit for survival or prevention of recurrence in performing lymphadenectomy for early-stage endometrial cancer. This conclusion remains controversial, and lymph node sampling remains commonplace, especially in older woman with known high-grade histology. It is recommended that optimum management of patients with high-grade histology should be decided preoperatively via the MDT meeting. In much older women, the additional morbidity of lymph node surgery may outweigh any potential benefit, and a simple hysterectomy may be recommended. Radiotherapy may be used if the woman cannot undergo surgery for medical reasons.

Postoperative radiotherapy for stage 1 disease will reduce local recurrence from 14% to 10% but has no effect on overall survival.[61] Radiotherapy is therefore used based on individual risk stratification—myometrial invasion beyond 50%, tumor grade, and age—all influencing this MDT-based decision. Usually, radiotherapy involves vaginal radiotherapy to reduce vault recurrence and, less commonly, additional external beam radiotherapy. Side effects are common, occurring in 25% of older women, and include frequent bowel movements, urinary frequency, pain, and scarring. Patients with advanced disease may be suitable for surgery with adjuvant chemoradiotherapy. Treatment for advanced disease is usually palliative, involving chemotherapy to treat systemic disease and radiotherapy for problems such as vaginal bleeding or bony metastases.

Progestational agents may be used for palliation or when the patient is unfit for other treatment. Tumor deposits may regress for a time. However, high-grade tumors often lack progesterone receptors.

Vaginal vault recurrence can be successfully salvaged with surgery or radiotherapy and a robust patient follow up system is therefore recommended.

Ovarian Cancer

Ovarian cancer remains the most lethal gynecologic malignancy and is currently the fifth leading cause of female cancer deaths. It affects women aged 65 years and older more frequently than younger women, with almost 50% of ovarian tumors occurring in this age group. Early detection of ovarian cancer remains a challenge, and older women are likely to present with advanced disease. Patients with higher stage disease are less likely to be offered radical surgery and chemotherapy. The onset and progress is often insidious, so a high index of suspicion is necessary. The tumor marker CA125 is an indicator of ovarian malignancy but is not elevated in all ovarian carcinomas, particularly in early-stage disease. It can be elevated by nonovarian factors, malignant and benign. In the United Kingdom, women with persistent abdominal distention or feeling full and/or have a loss of appetite or pelvic pain are offered a cancer antigen 125 (CA-125) blood test. Persistent urinary urgency or frequency, especially in postmenopausal women, should also indicate the need for a CA-125 test. If CA-125 levels are elevated, pelvic ultrasound can be performed to look for ovarian pathology. In a postmenopausal woman with ascites, ovarian cancer should be the diagnosis until proven otherwise.

Hereditary ovarian cancers represent around 10% of all ovarian cancers. Currently, there is no satisfactory screening method for ovarian neoplasia that has been shown to offer any reduction in morbidity in the general population or high-risk older women. Screening is therefore not advisable for older women.

The use of CA-125 levels with menopausal status and ultrasound findings provides a useful algorithm, termed the *risk of malignancy index* (RMI). Using the RMI (Table 85-1) provides an 87% sensitivity, 89% specificity, and 75% positive predictive value for detecting ovarian cancer.[62] The greatest utility of the RMI is in facilitating the triage of patients to the care of a gynecologic oncologist or general gynecologist (Table 85-2). Many postmenopausal ovarian cysts are an incidental finding and, if the RMI is low, no action is required. A simple cyst has an RMI of 0, and no intervention is required unless the patient is thought to be symptomatic.

TABLE 85-1 Risk of Malignancy Index (RMI)*

Score		Features†
Ultrasound score	0	No suspicious features
	1	One suspicious feature
	3	Two to five suspicious features
Menopausal score	1	Premenopausal
	3	Postmenopausal

*RMI = ultrasound score × menopausal status × CA-125 (in U/mL).
†Suspicious ultrasound features are multiloculated cyst, solid areas, metastases, bilateral lesions, and ascites.

TABLE 85-2 Triaging According to Risk of Malignancy Index (RMI)

Degree of Risk	RMI	Percentage of Women	Risk of Malignancy (%)
Low	<25	40	<3
Moderate	25-250	30	20
High	>250	30	75

All high-risk patients should be managed by an MDT and have any surgery performed by a trained gynecologic oncologist. In advanced-stage disease, operative mortality is about 1%, and major morbidity is about 5%.

Of ovarian malignancies in older women, 90% are epithelial adenocarcinomas, but other ovarian components may become malignant and give rise to such histologic types as sex cord and germ cell tumors. Up to 10% of ovarian masses are metastases from elsewhere, particularly the upper gastrointestinal and breast. Granulosa cell tumor is the most common sex cord malignancy and may occur after menopause. Hormone production can cause vaginal bleeding due to endometrial hyperplasia.

A complete history is essential to aid diagnosis and assess fitness for surgical and nonsurgical management. Assessment of the Eastern Cooperative Oncology Group (ECOG) performance status is a useful and simple tool in this regard. Investigation includes hematologic and biochemical profiles, chest x-ray, and ultrasound screening of the pelvis, liver, and kidneys. MRI is not routinely indicated, but CT of the abdomen and pelvis may assist in surgical planning and MDT decisions regarding optimal management.

Laparotomy establishes the diagnosis, and examination of the abdominal contents provides accurate staging, which will influence treatment and prognosis. Debulking of the tumor with bilateral salpingo-oophorectomy, total hysterectomy, and infracolic omentectomy is the mainstay of treatment. Peritoneal washings and upper abdominal and diaphragmatic assessment is carried out at the time of laparotomy. Complete cytoreduction is the goal of primary surgery and, if it is thought that this would be difficult to achieve, primary surgery may not be appropriate.[63]

Although cytoreductive surgery is still the gold standard of care for advanced disease, results from trials of primary surgery versus neoadjuvant chemotherapy with interval surgery have suggested a benefit for those with advanced disease.[64] Larger trials on this question are awaited. Postoperative chemotherapy is used in all but stage 1A disease, and many patients will have residual disease after surgery.

The platinum compounds, cisplatin and carboplatin, remain the agents of choice. However, they are toxic, and side effects include myelosuppression, nephrotoxicity, neurotoxicity, and severe emetogenesis. Carboplatin has a better toxicity profile and is usually the first-line agent of choice. Combination therapy of platinum drugs with paclitaxel has been shown to provide some survival benefit over cyclophosphamide-cisplatin (the previous standard of care).[65] Of patients with extensive disease, 40% to 50% will have complete remission with platinum but most relapse within 2 years.

Failure of first-line treatment is ominous because recurrent disease is often resistant to further therapy, but taxanes have been tried in these patients, with some success. Retreatment with platinum-based drugs is appropriate if the tumor was originally sensitive and there has been a disease-free interval of more than 1 year. Recurrent ascites is a major problem and requires repeated paracentesis. Spironolactone may reduce the fluid and limit recurrence. Radiotherapy is limited to unresectable tumors and those with symptomatic recurrence and is used only for palliation. The most common indication for palliative surgery is bowel obstruction; referral to a surgeon should be considered despite a poor prognosis to ensure an optimized quality of life.

Most patients with ovarian cancer present late and die of the disease; although cure is the ultimate goal, it is not often achieved. Surgery and chemotherapy will have a significant impact on a patient's quality of life. Therefore, the informed older woman patient's wishes should always be considered when in planning her care.

KEY POINTS

- The female aging process accelerates after the menopause, particularly in the genital tract, as a consequence of cessation of ovarian estrogen production.
- All women should be able to obtain advice on how they can optimize their menopause transition and beyond, with particular reference to lifestyle and diet and an opportunity to discuss the pros and cons of complementary therapies and HRT.
- Diagnosis of vulvar disorders requires a detailed history, examination, and biopsy, when indicated. Management should be by a dedicated gynecologic skin clinic, where available.
- The implementation of assessment and conservative treatment of urinary incontinence depends on a successful integrated continence service. Most cases of urinary incontinence can be managed in the community but clearly identified pathways for referral to secondary and tertiary care are vital.
- An older woman patient with gynecologic cancer should be offered the same surgical treatment recommended to younger women, but tempered by assessment of comorbidities and frailty status. Management should be by a multidisciplinary team.

For a complete list of references, please visit www.expertconsult.com.

KEY REFERENCES

1. Speroff L, Glass RH, Kase NG: Clinical gynecologic endocrinology, and infertility, ed 5, Baltimore, 1994, Williams and Wilkins, pp 101–111.
12. Cummings SR, Kelsey JL, Nevitt MC, et al: Epidemiology of osteoporosis and osteoporotic fractures. Epidemiol Rev 7:178–208, 1985.
16. Manson JE, Hsia J, Johnson KC, et al: Women's Health Initiative Investigators. Estrogen plus progestin and the risk of coronary heart disease. N Engl J Med 349:523–534, 2003.
19. Whitehead M, Farmer R: The Million Women Study: a critique. Endocrine 24:187–193, 2004.
20. Panay N, Hamoda H, Arya R, et al: The 2013 British Menopause Society & Women's Health Concern recommendations on hormone replacement therapy. Menopause Int 19:59–68, 2013.
24. deVilliers TJ, Pines A, Panay N, et al: Updated 2013 International Menopause Society recommendations on menopausal hormone therapy and preventive strategies for midlife health. Climacteric 16:316–337, 2013.
30. Royal College of Obstetricians and Gynaecologists: Vulval skin disorders, management. https://www.rcog.org.uk/en/guidelines-research-services/guidelines/gtg58. Accessed November 7, 2015.
35. Tidy JA, Soutter WP, Luesley DM, et al: Management of lichen sclerosus and intraepithelial neoplasia of the vulva in the UK. J R Soc Med 89:699–701, 1996.
41. Bump RC, Mattiasson A, Bo K, et al: The standardization of terminology of female pelvic organ prolapse and pelvic floor dysfunction. Am J Obstet Gynecol 175:10–17, 1996.
42. Wyndaele JJ: The overactive bladder. BJU Int 88:135–140, 2001.
44. Gerten KA, Markland AD, Lloyd LK, et al: Prolapse and incontinence surgery in older women. J Urol 179:2111–2118, 2008.
48. National Collaborating Centre for Women's and Children's Health (UK): Urinary incontinence: the management of urinary incontinence in women, London, 2013, RCOG Press.
49. Homesley HD, Bundy BN, Sedlis A, et al: Assessment of current International Federation of Gynecology and Obstetrics staging of vulvar carcinoma relative to prognostic factors for survival (a Gynecologic Oncology Group study). Am J Obstet Gynecol 164:997–1003, 1991.
55. Benedet JL, Bender H, Jones H 3rd, et al: FIGO staging classifications and clinical practice guidelines in the management of gynecologic cancers. FIGO Committee on Gynecologic Oncology. Int J Gynaecol Obstet 70:209–262, 2000.
57. Green J, Kirwan J, Tierney J, et al: Concomitant chemotherapy and radiation therapy for cancer of the uterine cervix. Cochrane Database Syst Rev (3):CD002225, 2005.
59. Ferrazzi E, Torri V, Trio D, et al: Sonographic endometrial thickness: a useful test to predict atrophy in patients with postmenopausal bleeding. An Italian multicentre study. Ultrasound Obstet Gynecol 7:315–321, 1996.
62. Davies AP, Jacobs I, Woolas R, et al: The adnexal mass; benign or malignant? Evaluation of a risk of malignancy index. Br J Obstet Gynaecol 100:927–931, 1993.
65. Scottish Intercollegiate Guidelines Network: Management of epithelial ovarian cancer. http://www.sign.ac.uk/pdf/sign135.pdf. Accessed November 7, 2015.

86 Breast Cancer

Lodovico Balducci, Dawn Dolan, Christina Laronga

Approximately 35% of breast cancers occur in women aged 70 and older, and this percentage is expected to increase with the aging of the population.[1] Age is the most important risk factor for breast cancer.

Breast cancer in the aged is by and large a chronic disease that involves individuals affected by other chronic health conditions, including polymorbidity, polypharmacy, functional dependence, and geriatric syndromes.[2] The primary care provider is pivotal in coordinating the care of these patients, in addressing barriers to treatment, in supporting the home caregiver, and in managing the long-term therapeutic complications. The management of breast cancer in the older woman should be based on individual life expectancy and tolerance of treatment. Personalized treatment plans may require the input of various professionals, including nurses, pharmacist, social worker, and dietician in addition to different medical specialists.

In this chapter we review the basic principles of breast cancer management, the epidemiology of breast cancer in the older women, and the age-specific questions related to the treatment of breast cancer.

PRINCIPLES OF BREAST CANCER MANAGEMENT

Only the management of cancer in the postmenopausal woman is reviewed in this chapter, as the management of the premenopausal woman may involve ovarian suppression that is not pertinent to the older individual. The management is determined by the pathology and the stage of the disease, as well as by the patient's life expectancy and treatment tolerance.

Pathology

The most common histologic forms of breast cancer include ductal carcinoma and lobular carcinoma.[3] Lobular carcinoma is more frequently bilateral than ductal carcinoma. Both forms of cancer may be invasive or in situ. Ductal carcinoma in situ (DCIS) and lobular carcinoma in situ (LCIS) have minimal risk of metastatic disease but may become invasive carcinomas and spread to other organs if left untreated. With the widespread use of mammography, DCIS and LCIS may account for as many as 30% of newly diagnosed breast cancer cases.[4] The value of diagnosing these conditions in individuals with limited life expectancy has been questioned, because the evolution to invasive disease may take several years.

A number of histologic characteristics, including the histologic and nuclear grade and the proliferation rate (commonly assessed by the presence of Ki-67), indicate the aggressiveness of breast cancer and the risk of metastatic spread but have little influence on the treatment choice.[3]

All newly diagnosed breast cancers should be assessed for the presence of estrogen and progesterone receptors and for overexpression of human epidermal growth factor receptor 2 (HER2).[3] In the absence of hormone receptors, hormonal treatment is not effective. Approximately 15% to 25% of breast cancers have HER2 membrane receptor overexpression, which maintains the independent growth of breast cancer. HER2 is part of the family of epidermal growth factor receptors that are present in normal breast. These have an extracellular, a transmembrane, and an intracellular component, consisting of a tyrosine kinase (Figure 86-1). This enzyme, activated by a receptor-generated signal, initiates the transduction cascade that leads to DNA synthesis, cell proliferation, and apoptosis inhibition. A number of monoclonal antibodies and tyrosine kinase inhibitors effectively treat HER2 overexpressing tumors. The so-called triple-negative breast cancers (those in which neither estrogen receptors nor progesterone receptors nor HER2 is expressed) represent the most aggressive forms of breast cancer and those for which the systemic treatment is least effective.

Analysis of the breast cancer genome has allowed clinicians to fine-tune the systemic treatment and, in particular, to identify those patients with hormone receptor–rich tumors for whom chemotherapy may add additional benefit.[5] The genome analysis may also indicate which cytotoxic agents are more promising for treating different types of breast cancer.

Breast Cancer Treatment

The discussion of the staging of breast cancer is very complicated, of limited interest to a primary care or geriatric practitioner, and beyond the scope of this chapter. In describing the management of breast cancer we will refer to localized, locally advanced, and metastatic disease. The management of breast cancer at early stages may involve both local and systemic treatment.[3] Local treatment includes total mastectomy, partial mastectomy with breast preservation, axillary lymph node dissection, and radiation therapy. Nowadays a full axillary lymph node dissection is performed only in individuals who test positive for cancer in the sentinel lymph nodes (SLNs) or those rare cases in which the SLNs may not be identified. SLNs are the first nodes to receive the lymphatic drainage from the breast tumor and may be recognized by mapping of the axilla with radioisotopes or blue dye.

Radiation therapy may be administered to the breast after partial mastectomy to prevent local recurrences and to allow breast preservation. Intraoperative radiation therapy prevents the inconvenience of daily visits to the radiation therapy suite. It may also be administered to the chest walls and to the axilla in patients at high risk of local recurrence after total mastectomy and axillary dissection. These include patients whose primary tumor was larger than 5 cm and those with involvement of four or more axillary lymph nodes. It is debated whether all patients who have had total mastectomy may benefit from postoperative radiation therapy to the chest wall.[6,7] Radiation therapy may also obviate the need for axillary dissection and ameliorate its complications in patients with SLNs involved by the tumor.[8] Radiation therapy is also used for management of metastases in the brain, which may be unreachable by systemic treatment, and for palliation of metastatic disease, such as bone pain.[3]

Systemic therapy of breast cancer involves hormonal, cytotoxic, and biologic agents (Box 86-1). Selective estrogen receptor modulators (SERMs) are currently seldom used in the United States because they may be less effective than the aromatase inhibitors (AIs) and may cause, albeit very rarely, deep vein thrombosis and endometrial cancer.[9] Unlike the AIs, the SERMs prevent osteoporosis and do not cause unfavorable changes in

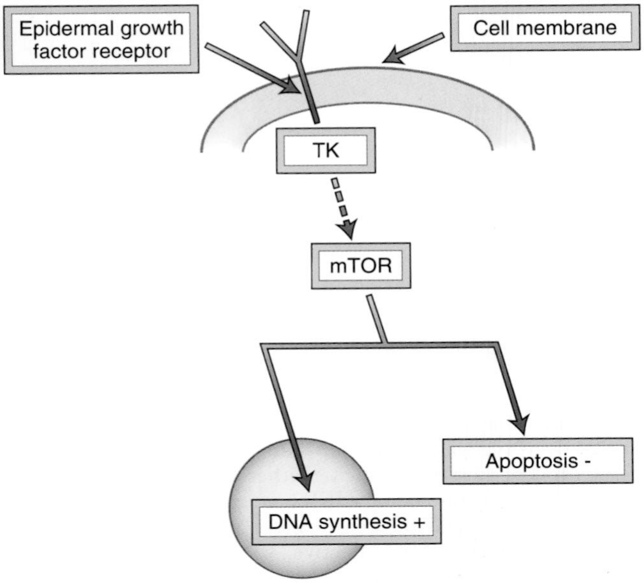

Figure 86-1. Schematic representation of signal transduction. The epidermal growth factor receptors have an extracellular component for the interaction with the growth factors and an intracellular component bound to a tyrosine kinase (TK). The activation of the TK initiates the signal transduction cascade that stimulates tumor growth and prevents apoptosis. The activation of the mammalian target of rapamycin (mTOR) is a key step in signal transduction. The epidermal growth factor receptors may be stimulated by the interaction with the ligand or by polymerization. Polymerization is the only mechanism through which human epidermal growth factor receptor 2 is activated, as it lacks a specific ligand.

lipid profiles. The AIs include steroidal (exemestane) and nonsteroidal (letrozole, anastrozole) drugs.[9] The effectiveness and the risk of complications of various AIs appear the same. The most serious complications include osteopenia and osteoporosis. It is advisable to obtain a baseline dual-energy x-ray absorptiometry (DXA) scan before instituting the treatment and to make sure that older patients are taking calcium and vitamin D supplements even if the DXA scan is normal. In two studies, osteoporosis was prevented by the prophylactic administration of zoledronic acid monthly and every three months,[10,11] but it is not clear whether such intensive regimen is really necessary. Although AIs may cause an increase in cholesterol and low-density lipoprotein (LDL) concentration, it has never been conclusively demonstrated that AIs cause increased risk of coronary artery disease or stroke. Perhaps the most bothersome complication of these compounds is a diffuse arthralgia that may be disabling for older individuals; this complication is the major cause for treatment nonadherence.[9] Before discontinuing the treatment, it is worthwhile to try a compound of a different class (i.e., a steroidal compound if the initial treatment was with a nonsteroidal compound and vice versa).

Unlike the SERMs, which combine antiestrogenic and estrogenic activities, fulvestrant (Faslodex) is a pure antiestrogen.[12] It is administered by intramuscular injection every 4 weeks (after a loading regimen every 2 weeks 3 times). Like the SERMS and the AIs, fulvestrant may cause hot flashes; it can also cause vaginal dryness. The drug is active in patients whose disease has progressed while they were receiving SERMs or AIs. The long-term complications of this compound are poorly known because it has been used only in patients with metastatic disease and the treatment rarely lasted longer than 12 to 24 months. Estrogen in high doses has been the mainstay treatment of hormone-sensitive metastatic breast cancer before the SERMs became widely used and is still active in patients whose cancers progressed with other forms of hormonal treatment. However, high-dose estrogen causes an increased incidence of endometrial bleeding, deep vein thrombosis, fluid retention, and congestive heart failure.[9] Ongoing studies are exploring the possibility of reversing acquired resistance to AIs by using estrogen in patients whose disease progressed after experiencing an initial response. Progestins are rarely used currently, as their activity is marginal after AIs. Likewise, androgens are rarely used because they cause virilization that is burdensome for most patients. Androgens may still have a role in palliating hormone-sensitive breast cancer in patients who are unsuitable for chemotherapy.

A detailed description of the chemotherapy agents used to treat breast cancer is beyond the scope of this chapter.[3,13] They are the mainstay treatment of patients with hormone-unresponsive disease. In patients with metastases, most oncologists prefer to use single agents in sequence (to reduce the risk of complications) and reserve combination chemotherapy for patients with life-threatening metastases, such as lymphangitic lung metastases. All agents may cause neutropenia and thrombocytopenia, whose incidence and seriousness increases with age, and most, albeit not all, agents cause alopecia. The incidence of emetogenic complications used to be particularly high with doxorubicin and platinum derivatives but has been reduced dramatically in recent years

BOX 86-1 Systemic Treatment of Breast Cancer

HORMONAL AGENTS

Selective estrogen receptor modulators (SERMs)
- Tamoxifen
- Toremifene

Aromatase inhibitors
- Anastrozole
- Letrozole
- Exemestane

Pure estrogen antagonists
- Fulvestrant (Faslodex)

Estrogen in high doses
Progestins
Androgens

CYTOTOXIC AGENTS

Alkylating agents (cyclophosphamide, melphalan)
Anthracyclines and anthracenediones (doxorubicin, pegylated liposomal doxorubicin, mitoxantrone)
Antimetabolites (fluorouracil, methotrexate)
Alkaloids (vinblastine, vinorelbine)
Taxanes (paclitaxel, docetaxel, nab-paclitaxel)
Epothilones
Eribulin
Platinum derivatives (cisplatin, carboplatin)
Mitomycin C

BIOLOGIC AGENTS

Monoclonal antibodies directed to human epidermal growth factor receptor 2
- Trastuzumab
- Pertuzumab

Tyrosine kinase inhibitors
- Lapatinib

Mammalian target of rapamycin inhibitors
- Everolimus

BONE-SPARING AGENTS

Bisphosphonates (pamidronate, zoledronate)
Denosumab

thanks to new antinausea medications. The anthracyclines and anthracenediones may cause cardiomyopathy; the risk of this increases with patient age.[14] The risk is reduced but not voided with pegylated liposomal doxorubicin or with the concomitant administration of doxorubicin and dexrazoxane. Peripheral neuropathy, which can be disabling for older individuals, is a common complication of taxanes, epothilones, vinblastine, and cisplatin.[13] Another serious complication is mucositis, which is particularly common with doxorubicin, docetaxel, and fluorouracil.[13] An unusual complication is the so-called hand-foot syndrome, manifested as pain and inflammation of the palms and the soles. This complication may be dose limiting for pegylated liposomal doxorubicin and capecitabine.[15] Preferred single agents in the management of older individuals include capecitabine or weekly intravenous paclitaxel, nab-paclitaxel, or vinorelbine.[16] Capecitabine is an oral prodrug that is activated in the liver and in the cancer itself. Older patients may prefer capecitabine because the dose can be titrated on a daily basis and does not require intravenous infusions.

Trastuzumab and pertuzumab are monoclonal antibodies directed against different domains of the HER2.[17] In this situation, trastuzumab proved very effective in inducing durable complete remissions of breast cancer when combined with chemotherapy. Pertuzumab has limited activity as a single agent, but when used in combination with trastuzumab, it increases both the response rate and the response duration. The main toxicity of trastuzumab includes a reduction in the cardiac ejection fraction, as it may interfere with myocardial trophism and lead to a condition of "frozen myocardium." This complication is more common in older individuals and is reversible in most cases. Recently, an immunoconjugate of trastuzumab with a very active cytotoxic agent, emtansine, was approved for clinical use in patients with breast cancer that progressed while they were receiving trastuzumab.[18] In this case, trastuzumab is used as carrier of the drug to a specific target, the tumor, to enhance its effectiveness and to minimize its systemic complications. Lapatinib is an oral medication that inhibits the tyrosine kinase responsible for transducing the proliferative signals originating from an activated HER2.[19] It is active after progression with trastuzumab, and it enhances the effectiveness of trastuzumab. In patients with a history of heart failure, it may be used in lieu of trastuzumab. Lapatinib penetrates the blood-brain barrier and may represent effective treatment and prevention of brain metastases. Everolimus is an inhibitor of mTOR (mammalian target of rapamycin), a threonine kinase that is a central step in signal transduction.[20] In combination with the AIs, everolimus produces an approximately 20% response rate in patients whose disease has become resistant to hormonal therapy. This oral agent has significant toxicity that includes mucositis, bronchial irritation, and pneumonia, in addition to the financial toxicity. Bisphosphonates (pamidronate and zoledronate) and denosumab (a monoclonal antibody to the RANK ligand) delay the progression of bone metastasis and the occurrence of the so-called skeletal-related events.[21] The bisphosphonates are administered intravenously and denosumab intramuscularly. A serious complication of all these compounds is osteonecrosis of the jaw, which includes failure to heal after oral surgery. Zoledronate has also been used to prevent osteoporosis in patients treated with AIs as adjuvant therapy and may further reduce the risk of systemic recurrence.[10,11]

The management of breast cancer varies with the stage of the disease.[3] When the tumor is resectable, the treatment consists of partial or total mastectomy and SLN sampling. Full axillary dissection or radiation therapy to the axilla may be added in patients who test positive for cancer in the SLN. To ensure breast preservation, partial mastectomy should be followed by radiation therapy of the breast. Local treatment may be followed by systemic adjuvant therapy to reduce the risk of systemic recurrence, which is estimated according to several variables, including the patient's life expectancy.[3] The risk of recurrence increases with the size of the primary tumor, the number of lymph nodes involved, the tumor grade and proliferation rate, the absence of hormone receptors, and the presence of HER2 overexpression.

Adjuvant hormonal therapy is recommended in patients with hormone receptor–rich cancer. The most effective adjuvant hormonal therapy in postmenopausal women includes AIs.[22] These may be used as a single treatment or may be followed by a SERM after 2 to 3 years. The concomitant administration of AIs and SERMs is not recommended, because the drugs may be antagonistic. SERMs alone may be used in patients who do not tolerate AIs. Adjuvant hormonal treatment should be administered for a minimum of 5 years. Recent studies indicate that a more prolonged treatment, up to a lifetime duration, may further reduce the risk of recurrence.[22]

Adjuvant chemotherapy in combination is indicated in patients with hormone receptor–negative tumors and in all patients with involvement of the axillary lymph nodes irrespective of the hormone receptor status.[23] The analysis of the genome allows oncologists to identify a group of patients with negative nodes and hormone receptor–rich tumors that may benefit from adjuvant cytotoxic chemotherapy.[24] In patients with HER2 overexpression, the addition of trastuzumab, for 1 year, to other systemic treatment has further reduced the risk of recurrence by more than 50%.

Sometimes the tumor is locally advanced and unresectable because of involvement of the chest wall or of the skin. In this situation, the primary treatment is systemic to reduce the size of the tumor and to make it amenable to local treatment, which may include both surgery and radiation.[25]

In the case of metastatic disease, the primary treatment is systemic.[26] Chemotherapy is indicated in patients with hormone receptor–poor tumors and in those with hormone receptor–rich tumors that have progressed while receiving all forms of hormonal treatment. Irrespective of the hormone receptor status, combination chemotherapy is indicated in patients with life-threatening metastases, such as lymphangitic lung metastases. In patients with HER2 overexpression, the combination of trastuzumab, pertuzumab, and chemotherapy is the frontline treatment of choice.

Initial Evaluation of the Patient with Newly Diagnosed Breast Cancer

The staging of breast cancer may involve imaging of the chest, abdomen, pelvis, brain, and bone, in addition to symptom history, physical examination, and basic laboratory tests (complete blood count and combined metabolic panel). If there are no contraindications, magnetic resonance imaging (MRI) is the technique of choice for the brain, computed tomography (CT) for the rest of the body, and a radionuclide scan for the bones. Positron emission tomography (PET) may be recommended to confirm the malignancy of CT abnormalities.

The National Cancer Center Network guidelines recommend that in the absence of symptoms or signs of metastases, the full body staging be performed only in patients with a large primary tumor (≥4 cm) or the involvement of three or more axillary lymph nodes.[26] The risks of overstaging include false positive results and cost. When dealing with triple-negative cancer or HER2 overexpressing cancer, full imaging may be indicated even for less advanced disease, given the increased likelihood of metastases. The use of breast cancer–specific tumor markers (cancer antigen [CA] 15-3, CA 15-9, or carcinoembryonic antigen [CEA]) is controversial and is not recommended by many authorities, because they are not specific for breast cancer and are present in normal levels even in patients with metastatic disease. In our experience, these markers, when elevated in metastatic disease, may be useful to follow the effectiveness of treatment without

BOX 86-2 Age-Related Issues in the Management of Breast Cancer

- Assessment of physiologic age (life expectancy and treatment tolerance)
- Postoperative radiation after partial mastectomy
- Axillary lymph node dissection
- Value of adjuvant chemotherapy
- Management of metastatic disease
- Prevention of chemotherapy-related toxicity
- Long-term treatment toxicity

having to repeat the imaging every few months. Before changing systemic treatment, we recommend confirming the presence of progressive disease through imaging.

AGE-RELATED ISSUES IN THE MANAGEMENT OF BREAST CANCER

The breast cancer–related mortality increases with age after age 65.[27,28] The causes of this phenomenon are unknown and mandate careful consideration of current preventive and management strategies of breast cancer in older women. Age may influence each step in the management of breast cancer (Box 86-2).

Prevention

Prevention can include primary and secondary prevention and chemoprevention. Primary prevention refers to the elimination of the causes of the disease. It includes avoidance of radiation, cigarette smoking, and hormone replacement therapy, and some dietary modifications.[3] The combination of estrogens and progesterone is associated with an increased risk of breast cancer and should be avoided.[29] It is not clear whether unopposed estrogens are carcinogenic for the breast.[30] They may be used at the lowest effective dose in women who have undergone a hysterectomy. Alcohol in the amount equivalent to more than two glasses of wine a day is the best known dietary risk factor for breast cancer.[31] Daily folate intake may help prevent breast cancer in the presence of alcohol ingestion. The role of dietary fats in the causation of breast cancer is unclear.

Both SERMs and AIs reduce the risk of hormone receptor–rich breast cancer by approximately 60%, without a reduction in breast cancer–related mortality.[32] Hormone receptor–rich tumors are generally the most indolent forms of breast cancer, and early detection by serial mammograms may also prevent mortality from these neoplasms. Given the risk of complications and the cost of these agents, chemoprevention of breast cancer is controversial and should be individualized, based on individual risk of, and concern for, breast cancer.

Early detection through screening mammogram reduced breast cancer–related mortality in women aged 51 through 69 in three randomized control studies.[33] These results have been debated after the publication of a Canadian study showing that screening mammograms were not superior to serial physical exam of the breast by a health professional.[34] This study has been criticized because the mammogram used was considered inadequate by some authority[35] and at present serial mammographic screening is recommended by the guidelines of major medical organizations. The value of mammogram in women older than 69 years is still controversial. The most common criticisms of screening include the risk of overdiagnosis and unnecessary surgery and the fact that the yield of mammogram may be marginal in patients in whom all prevalence cancers were diagnosed through previous screening. Despite these objections, two retrospective analysis of the data from the Surveillance, Epidemiology, and End Results (SEER) program indicate that the performance of mammogram after age 69 was associated with decreased breast cancer–related mortality, up to age 85, even in women with moderate comorbidity.[36,37] Based on these data, it appears reasonable to recommend serial screening for women 70 and older with a life expectancy of 5 years and longer, as the first benefits of mammogram are seen 5 years after the initiation of screening.

Controversial issues include the frequency of mammograms (whether they should be performed yearly), the role of breast examination by a trained professional (physician, nurse, or advanced practice professional), and the use of new techniques such as MRI of the breast. Digital mammograms are increasingly used and may be considered the standard staging technique.

Once a lesion is detected by mammogram or physical examination of the breast, the nature of the lesion may be further investigated with a sonogram, and biopsy of all suspicious lesions is performed.

Management of Local Disease

Age-related issues in the management of localized disease include the following:

- Primary hormonal treatment of hormone receptor–rich breast cancers in lieu of surgery
- Postoperative radiation after partial mastectomy
- Axillary lymph node dissection
- The value of adjuvant treatment

At least five randomized controlled studies compared primary hormonal treatment of localized breast cancer with surgery followed by adjuvant hormonal treatment. A recent meta-analysis of these studies showed that mastectomy was associated with a better outcome in terms of local progression and breast cancer survival.[38] One may criticize these conclusions because in only one of the five studies hormone receptors were assessed and because the hormonal treatment consisted of tamoxifen instead of a more effective AI. However, considering that mastectomy may be performed even with local anesthesia and that the complications are minimal, it is difficult to justify more studies of this issue that would at most demonstrate the equivalence of surgical and primary hormonal treatment. Primary hormonal treatment of breast cancer should be reserved for patients who refuse mastectomy or for the few cases in which mastectomy is contraindicated.

The risk of local recurrence following partial mastectomy decreases with age, even in the absence of radiation therapy, and some oncologists wonder whether radiation therapy can be omitted in older women. A recent randomized controlled study suggested this may be the case.[39] In women 70 years and older with tumors with the largest diameter of 1 cm, the addition of radiotherapy to surgery reduced the risk of local recurrence at 5 years by 3% and did not affect the cancer-related and overall survival. The main reason to avoid radiation therapy is inconvenience as the toxicity is negligible. When feasible, intraoperative radiation may prevent daily visits to the radiation center.

The issue of axillary dissection is moot since the adoption of SLN mapping, indicating which patients may benefit from dissection. In patients with positive SLN, full axillary dissection may be avoided by administration of radiation to the axilla, unless it is imperative to know the number of positive lymph nodes for the purpose of adjuvant treatment.[40] The risk and severity of lymphedema are less with axillary radiation than they are with dissection.

Adjuvant hormonal therapy with an AI or with an AI for 2 to 3 years followed by a SERM reduces the risk of systemic recurrence in patients with hormone receptor–rich tumors by 40% to

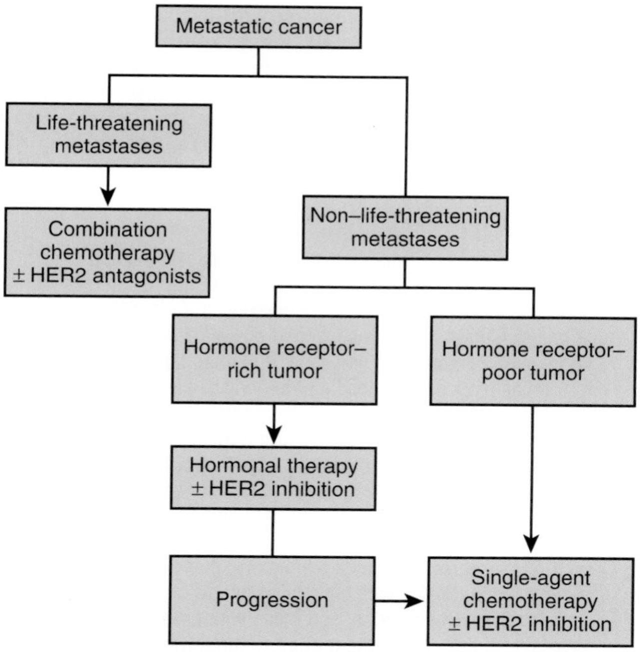

Figure 86-2. Proposed approach to the management of metastatic breast cancer in older women. *HER2,* Human epidermal growth factor receptor 2.

50%.[22] The treatment should last a minimum of 5 years, although a number of studies suggest that more prolonged treatment may be beneficial. In individuals in whom the risk of recurrence is small, the benefits of adjuvant hormonal therapy may be marginal. A number of clinically available genomic analyses identify hormone receptor–rich tumors that may benefit from adjuvant chemotherapy. Currently these assays have been validated only in tumors without involved lymph nodes.

Some form of chemotherapy is considered beneficial in all patients with involved lymph node, at present.[23]

The effectiveness of adjuvant chemotherapy in preventing the systemic recurrence of breast cancer in women 65 and older has been established by a landmark study of the Cancer and Acute Leukemia Group B (CALG-B).[41] Older patients with involvement of the axillary lymph nodes were randomized to receive combination chemotherapy or single-agent capecitabine. Those receiving combination chemotherapy experienced a reduction in recurrence rate and an improved cancer-related survival.

The decision to administer adjuvant chemotherapy to older women may be based on life expectancy and risk of complications in addition to the risk of recurrence of the cancer. A number of instruments modeled on clinical and laboratory evaluation allow the clinician to assess both the risk of cancer-unrelated mortality and of serious complications of chemotherapy.[42-44]

For the management of metastatic disease, we propose the approach shown in Figure 86-2.

Life-threatening metastases are those for which the median survival would be shorter than 3 months, which is the time it may take for the hormonal treatment to work. They include lymphangitic metastases to the lung and diffuse visceral metastases with compromise of organ function.[3]

HER2-inhibiting agents should be added to the management of all tumors that overexpress HER2. Trastuzumab should not be combined with anthracyclines because of the risk of synergistic cardiac toxicity.

Chemotherapy is indicated in hormone receptor–rich tumors once all hormonal treatment options have been exhausted.

Special Considerations in Metastatic Disease

Different metastases are associated with substantially different life expectancies. Metastases limited to the bones are associated with a median life expectancy in excess of 5 years, whereas lymphangitic lung metastases and multiple brain metastases have a mean life expectancy of 3 months if untreated. This difference in life expectancy needs to be kept into consideration when managing the older patients who have breast cancer. Metastatic disease at different sites may also benefit from some special provisions.

Metastases to the Central Nervous System. These include brain and meningeal metastases.[45] Because of the blood-brain barrier, central nervous system metastases are protected from most systemic treatments and require local therapy. There are reports that some agents, including SERMs and lapatinib, may occasionally affect central nervous system metastases. Single brain metastases should be treated with surgery or radiosurgery, whereas multiple metastases require whole brain irradiation. Patient with single metastases may have a prolonged survival following removal. Meningeal metastases have a variable and unpredictable presentation that may include symptoms of increased intracranial pressure or, more often, a peripheral neuropathy involving preferentially cranial nerves. The diagnosis may be suggested by the MRI and is confirmed with the demonstration of tumor cells in the cerebrospinal fluid. The treatment consists of intrathecal chemotherapy with methotrexate or thiotepa.[46] The median survival, even in treated patients, is less than 1 year.

Bone Metastases. These are the most common metastases from breast cancer in postmenopausal women. In addition to the systemic treatment for their breast cancer, these patients receive a bisphosphonate (pamidronate or zoledronate) or denosumab, which delays the development of skeletal complications.[47] If weight-bearing bones are involved, metastases may need surgical stabilization to prevent pathologic fractures. Spinal metastases may need to be evaluated with MRI to rule out impending spinal cord compression, which is a medical emergency and should be treated with high-dose steroids, emergency surgery (if feasible), and radiation therapy.

Hepatic Metastases. Local treatment of hepatic metastases is rarely indicated. In two situations it may be considered. A single metastasis to the liver with no evidence of other systemic disease may benefit from resection, radiosurgery, or thermoablation. Life-threatening liver metastasis may benefit from chemoembolization or radioembolization.[48,49]

Cutaneous Metastases. Although rarely life threatening, cutaneous metastases may be the source of serious complications, including pain, ulceration, and infection. In these cases, local treatment with electron beam or a fluorouracil preparation may be beneficial.[50]

Long-Term Complications of Breast Cancer Treatment

Most breast cancer patients survive 5 and more years and may be susceptible to long-term treatment complications (Box 86-3).

Adjuvant hormonal treatment with AIs may be associated with osteoporosis. This may be prevented with the simultaneous administration of zoledronate irrespective of bone density, with the management of osteopenia when it occurs, or with alternating AIs and SERMs.[9,10,47] As already mentioned, the simultaneous administration of zoledronate may also reduce the risk of systemic recurrence.

BOX 86-3 Long-Term Complications of Breast Cancer Treatment

Aromatase inhibitors ± fulvestrant (Faslodex)
- Osteopenia and osteoporosis
- Abnormal lipid profile
- Hot flushes
- Vaginal dryness and sexual dysfunction

Chemotherapy
- Acute leukemia/myelodysplasia
- Chronic cardiac dysfunction
- Fatigue
- Memory disorders/dementia

The combination of AIs and fulvestrant (Faslodex) is indicated in hormone-sensitive metastatic disease. It is not clear yet whether the combination of these drugs may have an additional deleterious effect on bones and lipid profile.

Age is a risk factor for doxorubicin-induced myelodysplasia[51] and acute leukemia and cardiomyopathy.[52] The genomic analysis will allow the practitioner to limit the number of patients receiving doxorubicin-based chemotherapy and will thus lead to a decreased risk of these long-term complications.

Fatigue is the most common chronic complication of cancer chemotherapy and is associated with increased risk of functional dependence and mortality in older individuals.[53] The management of fatigue is largely unknown and should represent one of the most important areas of future research in cancer survivors.

Although chemotherapy may affect some cognitive domains, it is not clear whether it is associated with an increased risk of dementia.[53] Perhaps the worst symptom is the anxiety patients experience about their own cognitive ability. A normal neuropsychological assessment may be necessary to reassure these individuals.

THE ROLE OF THE PRIMARY CARE PROVIDER

The management of older patients is multidisciplinary in most cases. In our opinion, the primary care provider (PCP), when available, should take the role of team leader. The PCP may fill the unique role of trusted advisor, given her or his awareness of the patient's medical and personal history. As it was highlighted throughout the chapter, the management of breast cancer may involve a number of decision points where the individual balance of risk and benefit needs to be determined. These decision points include mammographic screening, the type of surgical treatment (total vs. partial mastectomy), the administration of adjuvant therapy, and the time to renounce life-prolonging treatment in face of progressive metastatic disease.

In addition to organizing the management of the patient's non–cancer related morbidity, the PCP may have a primary role in estimating the patient's life expectancy and risk of treatment complications, assessing the adequacy of social support, preventing osteoporosis, and managing some of the long-term treatment complications. In addition, the PCP is in the best position to detect unexpected and long-term survivorship issues that are becoming more relevant with the aging of the population and with the improvement of the breast cancer prognosis and outcome.

The cooperation of the PCP and the oncologist may be enhanced with the establishment of patients' home and neighbors and by the ability to communicate electronically through patient charts.

POSTSCRIPT

1. The inhibitor of the cycline-dependent kinases 4 and 6, palbociclib, has been approved for front-line treatment of metastatic disease in combination with letrozol. This combination is considered the most active frontline treatment of metastatic hormone receptor rich breast cancer.
2. A large study reported that denosumab is also effective in preventing osteoporosis and decreasing the risk of breast cancer recurrence when used in combination of an AI in the adjuvant setting letrozol.

KEY POINTS

- In patients aged 65 and older, the risk of cancer-related mortality from breast cancer increases with the patient age. It is not clear whether this excess mortality is a result of more aggressive disease, more advanced presentation, or less aggressive treatment. In any case, it is important to highlight that breast cancer is deadly in older individuals.
- Long-term adjuvant treatment with aromatase inhibitors may be complicated by osteoporosis. This may be prevented by serial administration of zoledronic acid. Bisphosphonates may also reduce the risk of recurrence of breast cancer.
- Adjuvant chemotherapy is beneficial in selected patients, irrespective of age. These may include the majority of patients with hormone-receptor negative tumors; those with hormone receptor–rich tumors who have involvement of more than three axillary lymph nodes; and those with hormone receptor–rich tumors with involvement of up to three lymph nodes, whose genomic profile (Oncotype DX score) suggests a high risk of recurrence.
- Some form of screening for breast cancer is indicated in women with a life expectancy of 5 years or longer. It is not clear whether physical examination of the breast is as sensitive as mammography in older individuals.

For a complete list of references, please visit www.expertconsult.com.

KEY REFERENCES

3. Abeloff MD, Wolff AC, Weber BL, et al: Cancer of the breast. In Abeloff MD, Armitage JO, Niederhuber JE, et al, editors: Clinical oncology, ed 4, Philadelphia, 2008, Churchill Livingstone, pp 1875–1943.
6. Li Y, Moran MS, Huo Q, et al: Post-mastectomy radiation therapy for breast cancer patients with T1-2 and 1-3 positive lymph nodes. A meta-analysis. PLoS One 8:e81765, 2013.
7. Smith BD, Haffly BG, Hurria A, et al: Postmastectomy radiation and survival in older women with breast cancer. J Clin Oncol 24:4901–4907, 2006.
9. Palmieri C, Patten DK, Januszeski A, et al: Breast cancer: current and future endocrine therapy. Mol Cell Endocrinol 382:695–723, 2014.
10. Coleman R, Cameron D, Dodwell D, et al: adjuvant zoledronic acid in patients with early breast cancer: final analysis of the AZURE randomized open label phase III trial. Lancet Oncol 15:997–1006, 2014.
11. Gant M, Mlineritsch B, Stoeger H, et al: adjuvant endocrine therapy plus zoledronic acid in premenopausal women with early stage breast cancer: 62 months follow up from theABCSG-12 randomized study. Lancet Oncol 12:631–641, 2011.
12. Robertson JF: Fulvestrant (Faslodex): how to make a good drug better. Oncologist 12:774–784, 2007.
13. Balducci L: Studying cancer treatment in the elderly patient population. Cancer Control 21:215–220, 2014.
14. Accordino MK, Neugut AI, Hershman DL: Cardiac effect of anticancer therapy in the elderly. J Clin Oncol 32:2654–2661, 2014.
15. Miller KK, Gorcey L, McLellan BN: Chemotherapy-induces hand-foot syndrome and nail changes. A review of clinical presentation, etiology, pathogenesis, and management. J Am Acad Dermatol 4:787–794, 2014.
16. Tew WP, Muss H, Kimmick GG, et al: Breast and ovarian cancer in the older woman. J Clin Oncol 32:2553–2561, 2014.
17. Miles D, Baselga J, Amadori D, et al: Treatment of older patients with HER2-positive metastatic breast cancer with pertuzumab,

trastuzumab, and docetaxel; subset analysis from a randomized double-blind, placebo-controlled phase III trial (CLEOPATRA). Breast Cancer Res Treat 142:89–99, 2013.
18. Peddi PF, Hurvitz SA: Ado-trastuzumab emtansine (T-DM1) in human epidermal growth factor receptor 2 (HER2)-positive metastatic breast cancer: latest evidence and clinical potential. Ther Adv Med Oncol 6:202–209, 2014.
19. Nolting M, Schneider-Merck T, Trepel M: Lapatinib. Recent results. Cancer Res 201:125–143, 2014.
20. Piccart M, Hortobagyi GN, Campone N, et al: Everolimus plus exemestane for hormone-receptor positive, human epidermal growth factor 2 negative metastatic breast cancer: overall survival results from BOLERO-2. Ann Oncol 25:2357–2362, 2014.
21. Clemons M, Gelmon KA, Pritchard KI, et al: Bone-targeted agents and skeletal-related events in breast cancer patients with bone metastases. The state of the art. Curr Oncol 19:259–268, 2012.
30. Roos RK, Paganini-Hill A, Wan PC, et al: Effects of hormone-replacement therapy on breast cancer risk: estrogen vs estrogen plus progestin. J Natl Cancer Inst 92:328–332, 2000.
31. Fagherazzi G, Vilier A, Boutron Rouault MC, et al: Alcohol consumption and breast cancer risk subtypes in the E3N-EPIC cohort. Eur J Cancer Prev 24:209–214, 2014.
32. Advani P, Moreno Aspitia A: Current strategies for the prevention of breast cancer. Breast Cancer 6:59–71, 2014.
33. Gostche PC, Jorgensen KJ: Screening for breast cancer with mammography. Cochrane Database Syst Rev (6):CD001877, 2013.
35. Harris RP: How best to determine mortality benefits from screening mammography: dueling results and methodologies from Canada. J Natl Cancer Inst 106, 2014.
36. McCarthy EP, Burns RB, Freund KM, et al: Mammography use, cancer stage at diagnosis and survival among older women. J Am Cancer Soc 48:1226–1233, 2000.
37. McPherson CP, Swenson KK, Lee MW: The effect of mammography detection and comorbidity on the survival of older women with breast cancer. J Am Geriatr Soc 50:1061–1068, 2002.
38. Morgan JL, Reed MW, Wyld L: Primary endocrine treatment as the treatment of older women with operable breast cancer. A comparison of randomized control trials and cohort study finding. Eur J Surg Oncol 40:676–684, 2014.
39. Hughes KS, Schnaper LA, Bellon JL, et al: Lumpectomy with tamoxifen with and without irradiation in women aged 70 years of older with early breast cancer: long-term follow-up of CALGB 9343. J Clin Oncol 31:2382–2387, 2013.
40. Selton J, Cody H, Tan L, et al: Radiation field design and regional control in sentinel lymph node positive breast cancer patients with omission of axillary dissection. Cancer 118:1994–2003, 2012.
41. Muss HB, Berry DA, Cirrincione CT, et al: Adjuvant chemotherapy in older woman with early stage breast cancer. N Engl J Med 360:2055–2065, 2009.
44. Hurria A, Togawa K, Mohile SG, et al: Predicting chemotherapy toxicity in older adult with cancer: a prospective multicenter study. J Clin Oncol 29:3457–3465, 2011.
45. Liu NU, Amiri-Kordestani L, Palmieri D, et al: CNS metastases in breast cancer: old challenges, new frontiers. Clin Cancer Res 19:6404–6418, 2013.
46. Beauchesne P: Intrathecal chemotherapy for treatment of leptomeningeal dissemination of metastatic tumors. Lancet Oncol 11:871–879, 2010.
47. Rordorf T, Hassan AA, Azim Z, et al: Bone health in breast cancer patients. A comprehensive statement by CECOG/SAKK intergroup. Breast 23:511–525, 2014.
48. Dittman Y, Altendorf-Hoffman A, Schule S, et al: Liver resection in selected patients with metastatic breast cancer. A single center experience and review of the literature. J Cancer Res Clin Oncol 139:1317–1325, 2013.
49. Clark ME, Smith RR: Liver-directed therapy in metastatic colorectal cancer. J Gastrointest Oncol 5:374–387, 2014.
50. Wong CY, Helm MA, Kalb RE: The presentation, pathology, and current management of cutaneous metastases. N Am J Med Sci 5:499–504, 2013.
52. Doyle JJ, Neugut AI, Jacobson JS, et al: Chemotherapy and cardiotoxicity in older breast cancer patients: a population based study. J Clin Oncol 23:8597–8605, 2005.
53. Balducci L, Fossa SD: Rehabilitation of older cancer patients. Acta Oncol 52:233–238, 2013.

87 Adrenal and Pituitary Disorders

Steven R. Peacey

DISORDERS OF THE ADRENAL GLANDS

The need for normal adrenal functioning continues into old age. After decades of speculation, there is now firm evidence that the patterns of basal and stimulated levels of cortisol secretion are substantially unchanged in healthy older adults. Subtle age-related changes have been described related to the metabolism of adrenal hormones, and morphologic features such as nodules appear quite commonly in the aging adrenal glands. Their importance arises from much readier and often serendipitous recognition as advanced imaging techniques are more widely used. It is therefore relevant to open this chapter with a summary of the physiologic and biochemical actions of adrenal steroids, mechanisms controlling their secretion, and techniques available for assessing the function and anatomy of the adrenal glands.

Physiologic Responses to Adrenocortical Steroids

Of the multitude of steroids found in the adrenal cortex, only the secretions of cortisol and aldosterone have undisputed and vital endocrine roles. The distinction between glucocorticoid and mineralocorticoid hormone actions is based on physiologic observations, backed by differential effects on critical enzyme systems in target tissues.

Glucocorticoids

Cortisol (hydrocortisone) is the natural glucocorticoid of humans and most other mammals, but not the rat, which is unable to synthesize cortisol and uses corticosterone instead. It has long been recognized that cortisol, especially in high doses, has mineralocorticoid properties, and this has led to the widespread use of dexamethasone (a synthetic glucocorticoid), effectively without mineralocorticoid properties, as the benchmark glucocorticoid.[1]

This practice has passed from laboratory experiments to clinical investigation, as will be discussed later. There are reasons to question the validity of such assumptions, although the pragmatic clinical tests have proven value. There was previously a tendency to subdivide the actions of glucocorticoids into those seen at low doses and termed *physiologic* and those seen with high doses, typically causing cushingoid side effects, termed *pharmacologic*. There is no sound scientific basis for this differentiation because new effects are not seen with high doses, although the clinical sequelae are striking.

The term *glucocorticoid* derives from the effects on carbohydrate metabolism—antagonism of insulin action, promotion of hepatic glycogen synthesis, and participation in the defenses against hypoglycemia. It may affect resource use by virtue of tissue differences in response to the key glycolytic enzyme, phosphoenolpyruvate carboxykinase.[2] Glucocorticoids have many other actions, often permissive in nature. These include vascular and renal responses affecting control of blood pressure and extracellular water content. Other critical roles include actions on protein and lipid synthesis and complex interactions with the immune system. In addition, there is the well-recognized but poorly characterized function played by enhanced glucocorticoid secretion in combating stress. The stimuli recognized as stressful and capable of evoking enhanced cortisol secretion are numerous; these include fever, trauma, hemorrhage, plasma volume depletion, hypoglycemia, and even psychological disturbance. A unifying hypothesis is thus hard to formulate but, with regard to inflammatory processes, it is now widely believed that the role of glucocorticoids is to curtail the effects of rapidly responding cytokine and acute phase protein production; if protracted, this could be potentially damaging.[3]

Mineralocorticoids

The action of aldosterone is ostensibly simpler, operating primarily via renal mechanisms to control extracellular sodium and potassium levels, with secondary consequences on fluid balance and blood pressure. The effects of mineralocorticoids on other tissues such as the colon, brain, and pituitary have been documented, but their significance is much less certain. The secretion of aldosterone and its circadian rhythm are maintained in older adults, despite a decrease in tonic levels of renin, its principal regulator.[4]

Adrenal Androgens

The adrenal cortex also synthesizes androgens. These include androstenedione and dehydroepiandrosterone; much of the latter is conjugated and secreted as the sulfate. The function of adrenal androgens remains obscure, although much has been made of the phenomenon in childhood of the so-called adrenarche, when enhanced amounts are made from about the age of 7 years. By contrast with cortisol production, there is a well-documented fall in adrenal androgen production in older adults to as little as 5% of young adult levels, with decreased adrenocorticotropic hormone (ACTH) responsiveness, which has been termed the *adrenopause*.[5]

Apart from effects on body hair, it is not at all clear what function the secretion of adrenal androgens serves in normal adults. It has been postulated that the decline in dehydroepiandrosterone levels is partly responsible for the increased atherogenesis and, hence, cardiovascular disease in older adults, but evidence has not supported this hypothesis.[6] It appears more likely that dehydroepiandrosterone has an immunomodulatory and possibly antioncogenic action. Dehydroepiandrosterone replacement in older adults increases natural killer cell cytotoxicity and has been claimed to improve the sense of physical and psychological well-being dramatically.[7]

Biochemical Actions of Steroid Hormones

The effects of hormones on tissues depend on the distribution of specific receptors. Advances in knowledge have simultaneously clarified aspects of steroid hormone action and led to paradoxes that await definitive resolution. Steroids are lipophilic and readily enter cells; steroid receptors are intracellular. The classic model of steroid action is that steroid hormones bind to cytoplasmic receptors, forming activated complexes that are translocated to the nucleus where specific genes are activated, leading eventually to protein products as the end point of hormone influence.[8] A similar pattern was proposed for the structurally dissimilar thyroid hormones. Molecular cloning techniques have not only revealed that all steroid hormone receptors show strong homologies to each other and the proto-oncogene c-*erb*-A, but that the latter actually appears to be a thyroid hormone receptor. All these receptors share homologies in the hormone and the DNA-binding domains and can be regarded as constituting a superfamily of genes whose products are transcriptional regulatory proteins evolved from a common ancestor gene.[9] The steroid hormone receptor is bound to a protein complex containing the heat shock proteins hsp 90, hsp 70, and hsp 65. Exposure to steroid hormone leads to dissociation of the receptor from the complex so that the receptor is able to bind the hormone.[10] Along with the classic genomic mechanisms, the cortisol-glucocorticoid receptor complex can interact with other transcription factors such as nuclear factor-κB and also nongenomic pathways via membrane-associated receptors and second messengers.[11]

The new complex of hormone-plus receptor adopts a different molecular conformation, exposing the DNA-binding domain of the receptor. Thus far, the generalized scheme for steroid hormones applies to glucocorticoids. When it comes to identifying the molecular basis for mineralocorticoid and glucocorticoid actions, difficulties arise. The type 1 receptor—originally considered to bind mineralocorticoids with higher affinity than glucocorticoids—shows no such distinction with more modern techniques. There is a marked relationship shown at the molecular level as well.[12,13] A possible explanation for the failure of the great molar excess of cortisol to swamp the type 1 receptor with regard to aldosterone binding has been suggested for tissues such as kidney, gut, and salivary glands. These tissues possess a potent 11-hydroxysteroid dehydrogenase enzyme system, which rapidly converts cortisol to cortisone, and cortisone does not bind measurably to the receptor.[14]

Acting through the genome, glucocorticoids enhance several key metabolic enzymes, such as hepatic tyrosine aminotransferase[15] and tryptophan oxygenase.[16] In addition to this classic mode of action, it has also been suggested that many of the actions of glucocorticoids on the immune system are mediated by a specific protein product formerly termed *lipocortin*, now termed *annexin A1*, which acts as a second messenger.[17] This has multiple sites of action, especially inhibiting polymorphonuclear leukocyte trafficking, reduction of proinflammatory cytokines, and stimulation of antiinflammatory cytokines.

Regulation of Adrenal Function

Regulation of Glucocorticoid Production

Cortisol secretion is under the immediate control of pituitary ACTH secretion; this acts to promote the conversion of cholesterol to pregnenolone by the removal of the six-carbon fragment from the cholesterol side chain. These steps occur within the mitochondrion. A complex cascade of cytochrome P450 variants has been implicated as steroidogenesis proceeds, shuttling from mitochondrion to endoplasmic reticulum and back. The chronic effects of ACTH affect many more steps in steroidogenesis than just cholesterol side chain cleavage.[18]

Physiologic control of ACTH secretion involves three major areas—circadian rhythms, stress, and negative-feedback inhibition by cortisol. ACTH is synthesized as part of a large 31-kDa precursor polypeptide, pro-opiomelanocortin.[19] This is cleaved and the major fragments, including ACTH and β-endorphin, are usually cosecreted in equimolar proportions. The stimulus to ACTH release is from the hypothalamus via the hypothalamopituitary portal vessels conveying corticotropin-releasing factors.[20]

These are a complex of polypeptides, the major constituent of which is a 41-residue moiety, corticotropin-releasing hormone (CRH). However, this alone has less potent ACTH-releasing properties than crude hypothalamic extracts. It has been shown that vasopressin (AVP) and probably other unidentified compounds act synergistically with CRH.[21] The secretion of these corticotropin-releasing factors appears to be driving pulses of ACTH and cortisol, in turn. The circadian rhythm is composed of pulses of varying amplitudes and frequency, with a nadir reached at midnight, but the onset of activity is at about 3 to 4 AM, reaching a peak at 8 to 9 AM. The pulses of ACTH and cortisol decrease in size and frequency thereafter, although there is often a secondary rise at about lunchtime, which seems to be related to food ingestion.[22]

As mentioned earlier, there is a formidable array of apparently unrelated stressors that can stimulate the release of ACTH and cortisol. There has been preliminary evidence that the relative importance of CRH, AVP, and oxytocin varies according to the stimulus.[23] When inflammation is involved, there is growing evidence for interleukin-1, interleukin-6, and tumor necrosis factor having the capability to stimulate the hypothalamic-pituitary-adrenal axis, thus providing a loop to suppress their own production.[24]

Reports that have suggested extrahypothalamic production of ACTH secretagogues lack confirmation of authenticity or physiologic significance. Negative feedback of cortisol on ACTH production constitutes a sensitive homeostatic regulatory mechanism. The sites of negative feedback include not only the ACTH-producing cells of the anterior pituitary itself, but also higher centers, including the hypothalamus and CA3 field of the hippocampus.[25]

Regulation of Aldosterone Production

Aldosterone is produced by the distinct outer part of the adrenal cortex, the zona glomerulosa. In humans, this is found in cell clusters rather than in a distinct zone. The main regulation of aldosterone is via the renin-angiotensin-aldosterone system (RAAS). The stimuli to renin release from the juxtaglomerular cells of the kidney are low renal perfusion pressure, sodium depletion, and hypokalemia, although hyperkalemia acting directly on the zona glomerulosa is a more potent stimulus for aldosterone release than hypokalemia. Renin acts on renin substrate or angiotensinogen, released into the circulation from the liver, to form angiotensin-I. This decapeptide is converted to the octapeptide angiotensin-II by angiotensin-converting enzyme (ACE), which is of widespread distribution, but is most importantly found in the pulmonary bed.[26]

Angiotensin-II, apart from being a powerful arteriolar vasoconstrictor, stimulates aldosterone secretion from the adrenal cortex. Aldosterone, as noted, acts powerfully to retain salt (and obligatorily water), but promotes kaliuresis, hence closing the homeostatic feedback loop. There are other minor influences recognized as acting on aldosterone secretion, including ACTH, dopamine, and serotonin.

Adrenocortical Function in Normal Aging

Numerous studies indicate that basal, circadian, and stimulated cortisol secretion remains intact well into older age.[27-33] This is particularly important with regard to the ability to withstand stress, and the cortisol response to exogenous ACTH has been shown to be normal in older adults following myocardial infarction.[34] There are well-documented changes in the metabolism of corticosteroids, with an age-related decrease in the catabolism of cortisol.[35,36] Because of the intact negative feedback mechanisms, there is a commensurate reduction in the cortisol production rate. Aldosterone secretion is also normally well preserved in healthy older adults.[37] The recognized decline in adrenal androgen production has been referred to earlier.[30,38-41]

Investigation of Adrenal Function

Tests of adrenal function in older adults are for the reasons noted, mainly those established for the younger adult population. The diminishing reliance on urinary collection is beneficial for practical reasons and also means that some of the physiologically irrelevant changes alluded to earlier will not prove distracting. The key to successful and safe investigation is careful selection.

Glucocorticoid Deficiency

To investigate possible adrenal insufficiency, the basal measurement of greatest value is the plasma cortisol level, measured at the circadian peak at 8 to 9 AM. For most laboratories, a plain clotted sample is required to measure cortisol. Measurement of the midnight cortisol level is uninformative. Random plasma cortisol level measurements at other times of the day are usually worthless, although an undetectable plasma cortisol level (<50 nmol/L)—in the afternoon, for example—might warrant further investigation. If the 9 AM cortisol level is less than 150 nmol/L, the diagnosis of adrenal insufficiency is a strong possibility and, if greater than 450 nmol/L, the patient is normal. For values in between, a formal test of adrenal reserved should be performed. These tests are described here.

Short Synacthen Test. The short Synacthen test (SST) is the simplest and most widely used test. A direct assessment of adrenal reserve can be made by measuring the plasma cortisol level before and 30 minutes after the intramuscular or intravenous administration of 250 μg of tetracosactrin, synthetic ACTH(1-24). Failure of the 30-minute cortisol level to peak above 500 nmol/L may indicate adrenal insufficiency. This test is an excellent choice when primary adrenal insufficiency is suspected, but may also be used to detect secondary adrenal insufficiency due to the fact that chronic ACTH deficiency often leads to adrenal atrophy or adrenal downregulation; thus, rapid cortisol release in response to Synacthen is impaired.[42]

It is important to be aware that false-negative results may occur when using the SST in individuals with secondary adrenal insufficiency. This relates to incomplete downregulation of the adrenals, occurring in some individuals with ACTH deficiency. By performing this test at 9 AM, the possibility of false-negative results can be highlighted when such individuals have a relatively low basal 9 AM cortisol level but have a normal peak cortisol level. However, if an individual fails to achieve a satisfactory peak cortisol (>500 nmol/L), this does not indicate whether this is primary or secondary adrenal insufficiency, and further investigation is required. Traditionally a long Synacthen test was performed to distinguish between these two possibilities.[43] However, given the widely available measurement of ACTH, the distinction is made by measuring ACTH level son two samples approximately 30 minutes apart (due to the pulsatile nature of ACTH) at around 9 AM. A low or normal-range ACTH level indicates secondary adrenal insufficiency, and should prompt further pituitary investigations, whereas a raised ACTH level indicates primary adrenal insufficiency. In malnourished individuals or those with a low protein state (e.g. low albumin level), a falsely low measurement of cortisol can occur related to the reduced level of cortisol-binding globulin (CBG), to which cortisol is mostly bound and that accounts for much of the measured total cortisol—bound and free cortisol.[44]

Insulin Stress Test. If secondary adrenal insufficiency is suspected, a direct assessment of the hypothalamic-pituitary-adrenal axis is required. In those younger than 65 years, the insulin stress test (IST) is still considered the gold standard test (for ACTH and growth hormone [GH] reserve), whereby achieving a peak cortisol of more than 500 nmol/L during insulin-induced hypoglycemia of the IST (<2.2 mmol/L) is considered normal. However, contraindications to the test include a 9 AM plasma cortisol level less than 100 nmol/L, a history of epilepsy, and known ischemic heart disease. Due to the potential for occult ischemic heart disease in older adults, the test is not commonly used, although it has been used successfully.[45]

Glucagon Stimulation Test. The glucagon stimulation test (GST) is an alternative direct test of the pituitary-adrenal axis (as well as a test of GH reserve) and can be used at any age and in patients with epilepsy and ischemic heart disease.[46] Following a basal cortisol measurement in the fasting state, 1 mg of glucagon is given intramuscularly and the cortisol level measured at 150 and 180 minutes. A peak cortisol level of over 500 nmol/L is considered normal[47] and has been closely correlated to cortisol responses during the IST.[48] One disadvantage is the difficulty interpreting unusual results that are sometimes seen with the GST, whereby the basal cortisol is satisfactory but subsequent cortisol levels become reduced during the test, leading to an reputation for unreliability as noted by by some endocrinologists.

Mineralocorticoid Deficiency

Primary but not secondary adrenal insufficiency is associated with reduced aldosterone production. Blood can be sampled at any time of the day for aldosterone and renin, but the exact laboratory requirements should be checked. A plasma sample separated within 30 minutes is often required, implying that such measurements cannot be performed at all facilities. The finding of raised renin and low aldosterone levels confirms mineralocorticoid insufficiency.

Glucocorticoid Excess

Adrenal hyperfunction usually means cortisol excess or Cushing syndrome. Conventional methods of investigation are used first to establish the presence of the syndrome.

24-Hour Urine-Free Cortisol Test. This is a simple and reliable test. Its value derives from the fact that at normal levels of plasma cortisol, most is bound to high-affinity CBG.[49,50] The free cortisol level (thought to be the biologically active fraction) is generally small and is readily excreted in the urine. Because the capacity of CBG is limited and can be saturated with even minor degrees of cortisol hypersecretion, there tends to be a nonlinear and marked rise in urinary-free cortisol when excess cortisol is produced. As always, the cumbersome nature of a 24-hour urine collection may prove a more awkward test for some older patients.

Dexamethasone Suppression Tests. The 1-mg overnight dexamethasone suppression test is widely used as a screen for cortisol excess in an outpatient setting. Dexamethasone, 1 mg, is given orally between 11 PM and midnight, followed by blood sampling for cortisol at 9 AM the following morning. A cortisol level less than 50 nmol/L excludes Cushing syndrome. However, some normal individuals do not suppress to this level (false-positives), and a higher cutoff of less than 140 nmol/L is sometimes used.[51,52] If this higher cutoff value is chosen, there will be a corresponding increase in false- negative results. Further evaluation is often required with a low-dose dexamethasone suppression test, and this must be performed as an inpatient procedure. Dexamethasone, 0.5 mg, is given orally every 6 hours for 48 hours, and the cortisol level should be suppressed below 50 nmol/L at 48 hours. If Cushing syndrome is diagnosed, further evaluation is required to differentiate between adrenal, pituitary, and ectopic ACTH causes. Measurement of the ACTH level at 9 AM is the initial step; an undetectable result indicates an adrenal cause for the excess cortisol level. A normal or raised ACTH level is due to an ACTH-secreting pituitary lesion (Cushing disease) or ectopic ACTH production from another source, commonly a lung tumor.[53] The latter two situations are differentiated using a combination of pituitary and lung imaging, along with the current gold standard test of inferior petrosal sinus sampling for ACTH. Use of the high-dose dexamethasone suppression and corticotropin-releasing hormone (CRH) tests are currently used infrequently.[54]

In cases of adrenal carcinoma, it is not unusual to have mixed patterns of steroid excess. Virilization in women is not uncommon, and plasma testosterone level is raised. A striking rise in the dehydroepiandrosterone sulfate level is characteristic of adrenal carcinoma,[55] and this large production of a weak androgen may greatly increase urinary 17-oxosteroid excretion.[56]

Mineralocorticoid Excess

The mineralocorticoid status can be monitored by measurement of plasma aldosterone level and plasma renin activity, ideally after 30 minutes recumbence. Primary hyperaldosteronism (Conn syndrome) is uncommonly diagnosed in older adults, but may have existed for many years and treated as essential hypertension. Individuals with primary hyperaldosteronism have hypertension and low (or low-normal) potassium levels in association with raised aldosterone and reduced renin levels. Aldosterone may sometimes be within the upper normal range but the aldosterone (pmol/L) to renin (nmol/L/hr) ratio is more than 800 in those with primary hyperaldosteronism. Many antihypertensive drugs interfere with aldosterone and renin levels, and it is important to switch individuals to drugs that interfere less, such as the α-blocker doxazosin. The potassium level should ideally be normalized with supplements prior to the test because hypokalemia can lower the aldosterone concentration. If these tests suggest primary hyperaldosteronism, a confirmatory test is performed—a saline suppression test, whereby 2 L 0.9% saline are given intravenously over 4 hours.[57] The aldosterone level should be suppressed to less than 140 pmol/L to confirm the diagnosis. This test can only be performed if is safe in patients of any age.

Imaging Techniques for Adrenal Disease

Although moderate-sized adrenal abnormalities can be seen with ultrasound, the best initial mode of imaging is computed tomography (CT). In addition, a dedicated adrenal CT with pre- and postcontrast washout calculations can definitively characterize abnormalities as having a benign appearance in many cases.[58] Further characterization can often be made with magnetic resonance imaging (MRI)[59] and positron emission tomography (PET) scanning.[60] Although CT and MRI are very useful in determining whether a lesion has a benign appearance, no indication of the functional nature of adrenal abnormality is provided, and a biochemical evaluation is essential. There remains a small role for isotopic scintigraphy in the diagnosis of adrenal hyperfunction, perhaps more for extra-adrenal or bilateral pheochromocytomas using metaiodobenzylguanidine than using selenocholesterol or its variants in Cushing and Conn syndromes. Adrenal venous sampling is used for the final evaluation of primary hyperaldosteronism when an adenoma is found. However, undertaking this is only of value if surgery is contemplated, and it is more likely that medical therapy would be used (spironolactone or eplerenone) in older adults.

Clinical Patterns of Adrenal Disorders

The patterns of adrenal disease do not differ greatly in older adults from those in younger adults. Because these are well described in standard textbooks of clinical medicine and endocrinology, full descriptions will not be given here in all cases. Instead, emphasis will be placed on issues particularly relevant to older adults.

Adrenal Insufficiency

Primary adrenal failure (usually autoimmune Addison disease) characteristically begins insidiously with nonspecific symptoms, although postural symptoms, nausea, anorexia, and weight loss are often prominent and, in older adults, functional status may be diminished.[61] Although the characteristic ACTH-mediated pigmentation is a useful feature, if present, it is occasionally absent.[62] A large survey has suggested that in older adults, Addison disease is not only more likely to be tuberculous than in younger patients, but likely to prove fatal, and the diagnosis made postmortem.[63] Other rarer causes of adrenal failure, such as hemorrhage, amyloid, and HIV infection, should be borne in mind.[64,65]

Although metastases are commonly found in the adrenal glands, they only compromise cortisol secretion very occasionally.[66] The therapeutic dividend from diagnosing Addison disease is so great that the cortisol response to tetracosactrin (SST) should be assessed at the slightest suspicion. It is certainly not necessary for the electrolytes to be disturbed or random cortisol to be subnormal for significant adrenal insufficiency to be present. Secondary adrenal insufficiency is considered later as part of hypopituitarism.

Treatment. Hydrocortisone replacement therapy is given orally in split doses, between 10 and 30 mg total doses/day—usually 10 mg on waking, 5 mg at lunchtime, and 5 mg around 4 to 6 PM.[67,68] As with patients on long-term corticosteroid therapy, patients needing replacement hydrocortisone should be advised to double or treble the dose of hydrocortisone for 3 days during intercurrent illnesses, and they need parenteral glucocorticoid treatment if oral therapy cannot be tolerated. Mineralocorticoid replacement is given as the synthetic mineralocorticoid, fludrocortisone, 50 to 200 μg once daily, and the dose adjusted to normalize random renin levels.

Cushing Syndrome and Adrenal Carcinomas

Cushing syndrome is rare in older adults. It is usually due to ectopic ACTH production, generally by small cell carcinoma of the lung, but these patients typically have cachexia and profound hypokalemia rather than the characteristic cushingoid appearance. If due to pituitary-dependent disease, trans-sphenoidal surgery may be considered because it causes little systemic disturbance. Nevertheless, in mild cases, medical treatment with metyrapone alone may suffice and be more appropriate. This mode of treatment is certainly helpful for other forms of Cushing syndrome, such as ectopic ACTH secretion. The mixed picture of Cushing syndrome and virilization in adrenal carcinoma may be difficult to recognize; the hirsuteness and thinning of hair on the head may be much more prominent than the features of cortisol excess. Adrenal carcinomas may occasionally secrete estrogen. The main features of Cushing syndrome may be skin atrophy and fragility, with spontaneous bruising. Obesity and plethora may be conspicuously absent. In older adults, certain features are more marked, particularly impaired cognitive function, myopathy, osteoporosis, and diabetes. Hypokalemia is common in all forms of Cushing syndrome other than the pituitary-dependent form. Subclinical Cushing syndrome is increasingly being recognized in cases of adrenal incidentaloma (see later) and may be associated with increased cardiovascular risk.[69,70] Treatment of adrenal Cushings and adrenal carcinoma is primarily surgical unless there are widespread metastases. The use of 1,1 dichloro-2 (*o*-chlorophenyl)-2 (*p*-chlorophenyl) ethane (opDDD) is probably helpful, but may be associated with severe side effects, in which case it should not be used.[71]

Iatrogenic Glucocorticoid Excess

The most common cause of Cushing syndrome in older adults is the exogenous administration of steroids for a variety of medical disorders. The side effects of steroid therapy, often aggravating preexisting problems, are usually more marked in older adults. Particular problems include decreased cognitive function, emotional lability, and dysphoria, osteoporotic fractures, myopathy and muscle wasting with limitation of mobility, skin fragility, and impaired glucose tolerance. Furthermore, patients on maintenance steroids (>5 mg prednisolone daily or equivalent for >2 weeks) are at risk of adrenal insufficiency in the event of intercurrent illness, and the daily steroid dose should be doubled for at least 3 days in these cases.[72]

Adrenal Incidentalomas

The incidental finding of an adrenal nodule or mass during the investigation of nonadrenal symptoms has become increasingly common. It has been estimated from autopsy studies that 7% of individuals older than 70 years have an adrenal nodule.[52,73] The increasing use of CT, MRI, and CT colonography has led to a significant workload for the endocrinologist. A tiny proportion of incidentalomas will represent primary adrenocortical carcinoma but adrenal cancer is rare, with an annual incidence of approximately 2/million.[74] Adrenal masses found in patients with other known malignancy raises the possibility of adrenal metastases, often bilateral.[75,76] Dedicated adrenal CT and MRI can usually characterize adrenal incidentalomas as benign in appearance. The follow-up of such benign appearing lesions is controversial, with some recommending two to three follow-up CT scans,[52] but with others suggesting that no further follow-up imaging is required if the adrenal appearance is are benign.[77,78] The incidence of such lesions developing into adrenal carcinoma is extremely small and estimated to be similar to inducing a new malignancy because of radiation exposure from CT.[78] For adrenal lesions that have an indeterminate appearance, are larger 3 to 4 cm, or have other suspicious features, follow-up imaging is required. Lesions larger than 6 cm have a much greater chance of being malignant and should be surgically removed where appropriate.

Hormonal evaluation should take place at first assessment, particularly in hypertensive individuals. This should include the following: (1) 1-mg overnight dexamethasone suppression test; (2) renin and aldosterone level measurement after 30 minutes recumbence; and (3) urine or plasma metanephrine level measurement. The most common abnormality relates to subclinical cortisol excess—in up to 25% of patients with adrenal tumors incidentally discovered on CT in a number of studies[79,80]—but at present there is no clear guidance on how to manage these individuals.

The late diagnosis of genetic disorders can occur in older adults, including pheochromocytoma in the proband of a family with multiple endocrine neoplasia type 2a (MEN2a), a woman aged 73 years[81] and an 88-year-old woman with congenital adrenal hyperplasia due to 21-hydroxylase deficiency presenting with adrenal insufficiency.[82]

PITUITARY DISORDERS

Pituitary Function

The pituitary gland and normal pituitary function remain important in older adults. In particular, ACTH and thyroid-stimulating hormone (TSH) production remain vital to health, well-being, and sustaining life. Growth hormone production decreases with age (see later). In men, gonadotropin production may decrease with aging, leading to a relative reduction in testosterone levels. In women, gonadotropin levels rise sharply at menopause (physiologic ovarian failure) and thereafter may also decline somewhat during older age. Prolactin has no clear role in the elderly. Maintenance of antidiuretic hormone (ADH) production from the posterior pituitary remains important at all ages.

Testing Pituitary Function

The hormones TSH, free thyroxine (FT_4), luteinizing hormone (LH), follicular-stimulating hormone (FSH), testosterone, prolactin, and insulin-like growth factor 1 (IGF-1), an indirect marker of GH reserve, can all be measured directly in blood (preferably at 9 AM if the testosterone level is measured with the additional measurement of sex hormone-binding globulin (SHBG) to aid in the interpretation of free testosterone levels). However, dynamic tests are required to assess ACTH and GH reserve fully. As described earlier (see section "Investigation of Adrenal Function"), the SST, IST, and GST can be used to check ACTH reserve. GH reserve can be assessed with the IST, GST, and the arginine stimulation test, where appropriate.

Pituitary Tumors

Pituitary tumors are relatively uncommon in older adults, with the exception of nonfunctioning (null cell) adenomas, which increase in incidence in those older than 50 years. Pituitary tumors may present with the following: (1) local complications, usually due to compression of the optic chiasm causing bitemporal hemianopia or, more rarely, due to invasion into surrounding structures, such as the cavernous sinus; (2) clinical or biochemical features of the loss of one or more pituitary hormones; and (3) hormone excess from functioning pituitary tumors, such as in acromegaly and Cushing disease.

As with adrenal incidentalomas, it is increasingly common for older patients to be referred due to the incidental finding of a pituitary mass during the investigation of unrelated conditions with CT and MRI (pituitary incidentaloma). Many of these incidental findings represent small microadenomas (<1 cm), but some are larger pituitary lesions, macroadenomas (>1 cm). All such lesions need dedicated pituitary imaging and biochemical assessment to determine pituitary hormone excess and deficiency.[83]

Primary pituitary carcinoma is exceedingly rare at all ages. However, secondary pituitary lesions due to metastasis from a primary carcinoma may occasionally present with features of local invasion and hypopituitarism, as with pituitary adenomas.[84] Other sella lesions are very uncommon but may include empty sella and infiltrative disorders such as sarcoidosis, Wegener granulomatosis, and tuberculosis.

Trans-sphenoidal pituitary surgery can be considered for larger pituitary adenomas, particularly when the optic apparatus is involved or at risk although, given that glaucoma is common in older adults, visual field assessment may be difficult to interpret when these conditions coexist. Almost all pituitary tumors can be at least debulked by the trans-sphenoidal approach, and the relative simplicity and low morbidity and mortality of this procedure make it the treatment of choice for even the very old patient.[85-90] For inoperable or recurrent adenomas, external beam pituitary radiotherapy and the more recently introduced Gamma Knife radiosurgery offer further treatment options.[91]

Medical therapeutic options are also available for some functioning pituitary adenomas. GH-secreting adenomas often shrink during treatment with long-acting somatostatin analogues such as octreotide and lanreotide.[92] Macroprolactinomas are not infrequently found in older adults and most will shrink following treatment with dopamine agonists such as cabergoline and quinagolide, drugs that have mostly replaced the use of bromocriptine.[93] As with adrenal Cushing disease, ACTH-secreting pituitary adenomas can be treated medically with metyrapone or ketoconazole to reduce the adrenal production of cortisol. Smaller, nonfunctioning pituitary adenomas and larger lesions that pose no threat to surrounding local structures can be followed up with interval MRI scanning, often on an annual basis because most adenomas grow slowly.

Hypopituitarism

Hypopituitarism in older adults may be caused by pituitary adenoma, as in younger age groups, or may be due to any of the above-described lesions of the pituitary, although microadenomas are unlikely to cause hypopituitarism. Pituitary anatomy may show a small shrunken pituitary due to an unknown vascular or inflammatory insult, but may also be completely normal despite clear evidence of pituitary failure. Clinical features of hypopituitarism may be nonspecific, depending on which pituitary axes are affected, and hypopituitarism may remain undiagnosed for a long time. Key features may include weight loss with anorexia, orthostatic hypotension, and hypothyroid features, with inappropriately low TSH levels.[94-97]

Biochemical features of hypopituitarism may include the following: finding inappropriately low gonadotropin levels in an older woman (although it has been reported that these can be depressed in nonspecific illness in the very old)[98]; very low testosterone levels with normal or low gonadotropin levels in men; low FT_4 levels with inappropriately normal or low TSH levels; hyponatremia; low 9 AM cortisol level; and failure of dynamic tests, as described earlier (see "Investigation of Adrenal Function"). Isolated deficiencies of ACTH[99] and TSH[100] are occasionally found. Cranial diabetes insipidus is usually diagnosed by performing a supervised water deprivation test. Suspected hypopituitarism should be investigated with a dedicated pituitary MRI scan.

Growth Hormone Deficiency

GH hormone secretion declines by about 15%/decade from a peak at about 30 years of age,[101] and stimulated GH secretion, using pharmacologic agents and physiologic stimuli (e.g., exercise) is diminished in older adults. This fall in GH secretion is due to a decline in the frequency[102] and amplitude[103] of GH pulses, probably the result of an increase in somatostatinergic tone. Furthermore, there is a decrease in circulating levels of IGF-1, the peripheral mediator of the somatic effects of GH although, in contrast to young adults, IGF-1 levels do not show as strong a correlation with 24-hour GH secretion.

Some of the features of aging are similar to the characteristics of adult GH deficiency, such as the decrease in lean body mass and bone mineral density, increase in fat mass[104] and, possibly, neuropsychological sequelae and increased cardiovascular mortality.[105] The availability of recombinant GH has made the treatment of adult GH deficiency possible.[106]

As with younger patients, the only individuals for whom GH therapy can be recommended are those with pituitary disease requiring at least one form of pituitary hormone replacement therapy, in whom severe GH deficiency has been demonstrated using a pharmacologic stimulation test (peak GH < 3 μg/L) and who have symptoms of GH deficiency, which includes a reduced quality of life.[107-111]

Pituitary Hormone Replacement

Replacement therapy with hydrocortisone (see earlier) is given orally in split doses from 10 to 30 mg total/day. Hydrocortisone replacement should begin at least 2 or 3 days before thyroxine therapy to avoid precipitating an adrenal crisis. As with patients on corticosteroid therapy, those needing replacement hydrocortisone should be advised to double the dose of hydrocortisone for 3 days during intercurrent illnesses, and they need parenteral corticosteroids if they cannot tolerate oral medication while ill. Thyroxine should be commenced in low doses in older adults, gradually increasing every 1 or 2 weeks to a maintenance dose. The aim is to keep the FT_4 level in the normal range, and noting that TSH cannot be used to assess the dose of thyroxine in pituitary failure. Testosterone replacement may still be appropriate in older men, but baseline prostate assessment or a prostate-specific antigen (PSA) test should be carried out, with monitoring of PSA, hematocrit, and blood pressure during follow-up. If GH replacement is considered, it should be given as a small-volume subcutaneous injection each night, and serum IGF-1 levels are used to adjust the dose of GH. Diabetes insipidus is treated with desmopressin (DDAVP) nasal spray or an oral DDAVP preparation.

Acknowledgment

I would like to acknowledge input to this chapter from the seventh edition by the previous authors, Peter Hammond and Paul E. Belchetz.

KEY POINTS

- Patterns of adrenal cortisol secretion are substantially unchanged in healthy older adults.
- The incidental finding of an adrenal nodule during the investigation of nonadrenal symptoms is increasingly common but adrenal cancer is very rare, though more likely with larger larger lesions (>3 to 4 cm).
- Pituitary tumors are uncommon in older adults and may present with local complications (typically compression of the optic chiasm causing bitemporal hemianopia), clinical or biochemical features of the loss of one or more pituitary hormones, and hormone excess from functioning pituitary tumors, such as in acromegaly and Cushing disease.
- Some features of aging are similar to the characteristics of adult growth hormone deficiency (e.g., decrease in lean body mass and bone mineral density, increase in fat mass), but only individuals with well-proven growth hormone deficiency should be treated with growth hormone therapy.

For a complete list of references, please visit www.expertconsult.com.

KEY REFERENCES

11. Rhen T, Cidlowski JA: Antiinflammatory action of glucocorticoids—new mechanisms for old drugs. N Engl J Med 353:1711–1723, 2005.
17. D'Acquisto F, Perretti M, Flower RJ: Annexin-A1: a pivotal regulator of the innate and adaptive immune systems. Br J Pharmacol 155:152–169, 2008.
31. Tourigny-Rivard MF, Raskind M, Rivard D: The dexamethasone suppression test in an elderly population. Biol Psychiatry 16:1177–1184, 1981.
32. Ohashi M, Kato K, Nawata H, et al: Adrenocortical responsiveness to graded ACTH infusions in normal young and elderly human subjects. Gerontology 32:43–51, 1986.
34. Jensen BA, Sanders S, Frolund B, et al: Adrenocortical function in old age as reflected by plasma cortisol and ACTH test during the course of acute myocardial infarction. Arch Gerontol Geriatr 7:289–296, 1988.
52. Grumbach MM, Biller BM, Braunstein GD, et al: Management of the clinically inapparent adrenal mass ("incidentaloma"). Ann Intern Med 138:424–429, 2003.
57. Mulatero P, Milan A, Fallo F, et al: Comparison of confirmatory tests for the diagnosis of primary aldosteronism. J Clin Endocrinol Metab 91:2618–2623, 2006.

71. Luton JP, Cerdas S, Billaud L, et al: Clinical features of adrenocortical carcinoma, prognostic factors, and the effect of mitotane therapy. N Engl J Med 322:1195–1201, 1990.
73. Barzon L, Sonino N, Fallo F, et al: Prevalence and natural history of adrenal incidentalomas. Eur J Endocrinol 149:273–285, 2003.
75. Kasperlik-Zaluska AA, Otto M, Cichocki A, et al: Incidentally discovered adrenal tumors: a lesson from observation of 1,444 patients. Horm Metab Res 40:338–341, 2008.
78. Cawood TJ, Hunt PJ, O'Shea D, et al: Recommended evaluation of adrenal incidentalomas is costly, has high false-positive rates and confers a risk of fatal cancer that is similar to the risk of the adrenal lesion becoming malignant; time for a rethink? Eur J Endocrinol 161:513–527, 2009.
83. Freda PU, Beckers AM, Katznelson L, et al: Endocrine Society: Pituitary incidentaloma: an Endocrine Society clinical practice guideline. J Clin Endocrinol Metab 96:894–904, 2011.
90. Arita K, Hirano H, Yunoue S, et al: Treatment of elderly acromegalics. Endocr J 55:895–903, 2008.
96. Chanson P: Severe hyponatremia as a frequent revealing sign of hypopituitarism after 60 years of age. Eur J Endocrinol 149:177–178, 2003.
97. Kurtulmus N, Yarman S: Hyponatremia as the presenting manifestation of Sheehan's syndrome in elderly patients. Aging Clin Exp Res 18:536–539, 2006.
98. Impallomeni M, Yeo T, Rudd A, et al: Investigation of anterior pituitary function in elderly in-patients over the age of 75. Q J Med 63:505–515, 1987.
109. Feldt-Rasmussen U, Wilton P, Jonsson P: Aspects of growth hormone deficiency and replacement in elderly hypopituitary adults. Growth Horm IGF Res 14(Suppl A):S51–S58, 2004.
111. Gotherstrom G, Bengtsson BA, Sunnerhagen KS, et al: The effects of five-year growth hormone replacement therapy on muscle strength in elderly hypopituitary patients. Clin Endocrinol (Oxf) 62:105–113, 2005.

88 Disorders of the Thyroid

Maria Papaleontiou, Nazanene Helen Esfandiari

As an individual ages, several morphologic and physiologic changes occur in the entire endocrine system, including the thyroid gland. These changes can be explained by the amount of hormones secreted due to changes in target organs or by changes in the rate of metabolism of hormones.[1] Thyroid dysfunction is common in older adults[1] and may be associated with significant morbidity if not treated. Subclinical thyroid disease is the most common thyroid disorder in this population.[2] The classic symptoms of thyroid dysfunction are usually absent or may be overlooked in older patients, making the diagnosis and subsequent management challenging. In addition, interpretation of thyroid function tests in older adults can be challenging due to age-dependent physiologic changes in thyroid function, coexistent chronic illness, and polypharmacy.[1,3-6] Moreover, the risk of harm from treatment in the older adult population further complicates the decision-making process.

In this chapter we will review the epidemiology, clinical presentation, risks and complications, and management of thyroid disorders, including hyperthyroidism, subclinical hyperthyroidism, hypothyroidism, subclinical hypothyroidism, thyroid nodules, and thyroid cancer, in older adults. Unique features in the approach and management of thyroid disorders in older adults are summarized in Table 88-1.

THYROID MORPHOLOGY AND AGING

The normal aging process is associated with changes in the gross and microscopic appearance of the thyroid gland. Several studies have examined the relationship between the size of the thyroid gland and aging. Volumetric analyses performed using ultrasound, computed tomography (CT), or magnetic resonance imaging (MRI) have yielded varying results, with some studies documenting an increase[7] and others no change[8] or a decrease in the size of the thyroid gland occurring with age.[9-11] This discrepancy may be related to diverse dietary iodine intake and because the gland also becomes more nodular with age.[1]

Age-associated histopathologic findings of the thyroid gland have also been documented. These include a reduction in follicle number and size, reduction in colloid content, degeneration and flattening of epithelial cells, increased interfollicular fibrosis of the connective tissue, and varying lymphocytic infiltration.[1,12-16] In addition, the number of parafollicular cells (C cells) in the thyroid gland has been shown to increase with advancing age, with the formation of clusters and micronodular hyperplasia.[15-17]

Thyroid Function and Aging

Several studies have investigated the role of thyroid function in the aging process. Studies have shown increased serum thyroid-stimulating hormone (TSH) levels with increasing age, independent of antithyroid antibody presence[2]; in contrast, others have demonstrated decreased serum TSH levels in older adults.[1,4] Populations in which the dominant thyroid pathology is thyroid deficiency secondary to Hashimoto thyroiditis display a trend for the TSH upper limit to increase with age.[18-20] On the contrary, an inverse relationship between TSH and age is seen in iodine-deficient populations in which the dominant thyroid pathology is nodularity and increasing thyroid autonomy with age.[21] In regard to free triiodothyronine (T_3) levels, most studies have demonstrated an age-dependent decline, whereas free thyroxine (T_4) levels remain relatively unchanged,[1,4] and reverse T_3 (rT_3) levels increase with increasing age. However, interpretation of thyroid function tests in older adults is often complicated by the presence of chronic illness, (in which free T_3 levels can be low and rT_3 levels high), and polypharmacy.[5] Furthermore, differences in iodine intake and the presence of autoimmune thyroid disease make the distinction between age-related and disease-related thyroid function abnormalities even more challenging.[22]

There is convincing evidence that higher levels of TSH are associated with longevity. Serum TSH levels have been shown to be significantly higher in centenarians (mean age, 98 years) as compared to controls ($P < .001$).[23] Increased TSH levels and low to low-normal free T_4 levels have also been shown to be associated with better survival in older adults.[11,12,24,25] It is hypothesized that the association of a higher TSH level with longevity may be due to a correlated lower bioactivity of thyroid hormone, which in turn leads to a lower basal metabolic rate and thus potentially may serve as an adaptive mechanism to prevent catabolism in older adults.[12]

Moreover, the offspring of individuals with longevity were also shown to have higher TSH levels than age-matched controls without familial longevity (mean age, 70 years), indicating a genetic predisposition.[26]

Screening for Thyroid Dysfunction

Thyroid function disorders become increasingly frequent with advancing age. As a consequence, several organizations have issued recommendations regarding screening for thyroid dysfunction in the general population as a means of early detection of altered thyroid function. However, expert panels have continued to disagree about TSH screening of the general population (Table 88-2).

The American College of Physicians (ACP) has recommended that women older than 50 years with one or more general symptoms that could be caused by thyroid disease should be screened with serum TSH testing initially, followed by measurement of free T_4 if the TSH level is undetectable or greater than 10 mIU/L.[27] The American Academy of Family Physicians (AAFP) has recommended routine thyroid function screening in asymptomatic patients older than 60 years.[28] The American Thyroid Association (ATA) has recommended screening in all adults beginning at age 35 years and every 5 years thereafter.[29] The American Association of Clinical Endocrinologists (AACE) has recommended routine measurement of TSH in older patients (age not specified).[29] In contrast, the U.S. Preventive Services Task Force (USPSTF) has not recommended routine screening for thyroid disease in children or adults,[30,31] and the Institute of Medicine has issued a statement that screening is not cost-effective in the Medicare population.[32]

HYPERTHYROIDISM

Hyperthyroidism, or overactive thyroid, is a condition that involves excess synthesis and secretion of the free thyroid hormones, T_3 and/or T_4, by the thyroid gland, leading to the hypermetabolic condition of thyrotoxicosis. It can be primary, indicating thyroid gland pathology, secondary, indicating stimulation of the

TABLE 88-1 Unique Features in Approach and Management of Thyroid Disorders in Older Adults

Thyroid Disorder	Unique Features
HYPERTHYROIDISM	
Overt	• Less symptomatic, with apathetic hyperthyroidism common • Greater likelihood of developing atrial fibrillation or osteoporosis • Antithyroid medications (e.g., propylthiouracil, methimazole)—increased risk of side effects, especially agranulocytosis • Surgery—increased risk of morbidity, but not contraindicated; primarily carried out if large obstructive goiter or suspected malignancy present
Subclinical	• Treat if age > 65 yr, with TSH level persistently < 0.1 mIU/L
HYPOTHYROIDISM	
Overt	• Myxedema coma almost exclusively occurs in older adults • Age > 50 yr—initiate lower dose of levothyroxine, usually 25 μg PO daily and titrate to cardiovascular tolerance • Target a wider TSH range because overtreatment may lead to significant morbidity
Subclinical	• Treat if TSH level > 10 mIU/L or clear symptoms and signs of thyroid failure are present
Thyroid nodules	• Prevalence increases with age
Thyroid cancer	• Greater risk of cancer recurrence and mortality with older age • Age is involved in cancer staging • Greater incidence of poorly differentiated thyroid cancer, including anaplastic, with increasing age • Surgery—higher surgical risk due to comorbidities • Postoperative radioactive iodine ablation—increased risk of empirical dosing exceeding maximum tolerated activity. Consider dosimetry in advanced disease • Thyroxine suppression therapy for some well-differentiated cancers for a limited period—lower doses required

Modified from Papaleontiou M, Haymart MR: Approach to and treatment of thyroid disorders in the elderly. Med Clin North Am 96:297-310, 2012.

TABLE 88-2 Recommendations Regarding Screening for Thyroid Dysfunction in Adults

Organization	Recommendations for Screening
American Academy of Family Physicians (AAFP)	Patients ≥ 60 yr
American Association of Clinical Endocrinologists (AACE)	Older patients, especially women
American College of Physicians (ACP)	Women ≥ 50 yr with incidental finding suggestive of symptomatic thyroid disease
American Thyroid Association (ATA)	Women and men ≥ 35 yr should be screened every 5 yr
U.S. Preventive Services Task Force	Insufficient evidence for or against screening
Institute of Medicine	Screening not cost-effective in Medicare population

thyroid gland from excess TSH, or tertiary, indicating excess thyrotropin-releasing hormone (TRH; rare).

Epidemiology and Pathophysiology

The prevalence of hyperthyroidism in older adults is estimated to be 0.5% to 4%.[32] Even though Graves disease still remains the most common cause, the prevalence of multinodular goiter and toxic nodular adenomas tends to increase with age.[33,34] All can present as apathetic thyrotoxicosis.[35] Graves disease is an autoimmune disorder that results from the stimulatory effects of thyroid receptor antibodies (also known as thyroid-stimulating immunoglobulins) on the thyroid gland. These antibodies stimulate thyroid gland growth and thyroid hormone synthesis and release.[36] Multinodular goiters are common in older adults and may not always be clinically obvious.[37] It has been observed that long-standing euthyroid multinodular goiters can undergo changes and insidiously become toxic, with overproduction of thyroid hormones.[38] A less common cause of hyperthyroidism in older adults is toxic adenoma. This is usually found on thyroid scintigraphy as a solitary hyperfunctioning nodule with suppression of activity in the remaining thyroid gland.[39,40] Toxic multinodular goiter and toxic adenoma are due to focal and/or diffuse hyperplasia of thyroid follicular cells, whose functional capacity is independent of regulation by TSH.

Hyperthyroidism can also rarely occur in a previously euthyroid person following exposure to iodine-containing substances. Ingestion of iodine can lead to hyperthyroidism in areas of iodine deficiency, especially in persons with a nodular goiter.[41,42] Following an increase in iodine supply, underlying areas of autonomy within the thyroid gland produce thyroid hormone independently of normal regulatory mechanisms (Jod Basedow phenomenon), leading to hyperthyroidism.[43] This is usually a self-limiting disorder lasting several weeks to several months.[44] Usually, this occurs following administration of iodinated contrast radiographic agents or exposure to iodine-rich drugs, such as amiodarone.[45] Up to 40% of persons taking amiodarone will have serum T_4 levels above the normal range, but only about 5% will develop clinical hyperthyroidism.[46] Amiodarone is fat-soluble and has a long half-life, so amiodarone-induced hyperthyroidism can last for months and is difficult to treat.[47,48]

Iodine-induced hyperthyroidism is particularly important in the geriatric population because the prevalence of thyroid nodular disease is higher in older than in younger patients, clinical detection of hyperthyroidism is more challenging, and older adults are more likely to have underlying heart disease.[43,49] The risk of iodine-induced hyperthyroidism should always be considered in older patients with known multinodular goiter and/or subclinical hyperthyroidism (see later), and alternatives to imaging with contrast should be pursued when appropriate.

Moreover, the possibility of hyperthyroidism must always be considered in the elderly person who is receiving thyroid hormone, especially if the dosage is greater than 0.15 mg of L-thyroxine daily. Patients who have received such dosages for many years without evidence of hyperthyroidism may insidiously develop features of hyperthyroidism as they age past 60 years because of age-associated slowing in thyroid hormone metabolism.[50]

Rare causes of hyperthyroidism in older adults include TSH-producing pituitary tumors[51,52] and ectopic TSH production by nonpituitary tumors. These can be recognized by the finding of unsuppressed levels of serum TSH in the presence of increased amounts of circulating thyroid hormone. Additional uncommon causes of hyperthyroidism include overproduction of thyroid hormone by metastatic follicular carcinoma and thyroid hormone resistance.

Transient hyperthyroidism may occur in patients with subacute thyroiditis as a result of increased leakage of thyroid hormone into the circulation during the inflammatory phase of the illness.[53] Similarly, radiation injury to the thyroid can be accompanied by a transient increase in circulating thyroid hormone levels with associated symptoms.

Subclinical hyperthyroidism (low or suppressed TSH levels, with normal free T_4 and normal free T_3 levels) is more common than overt hyperthyroidism in older adults. It is estimated to have a prevalence of 3% to 8%.[54-56] It is more common in women than men, especially in patients older than 70 years,[57] smokers, and areas of the world with mild to moderate iodine deficiency.[18,58] In a study of the natural history of subclinical hyperthyroidism in female patients 60 years of age and older ($N = 102$), the progression to overt hyperthyroidism was infrequent, at 1%/year.[59]

Clinical Presentation

Two thirds of older adults with hyperthyroidism present similarly to younger patients.[60] Symptoms are consistent with sympathetic overactivity and include tremors, anxiety, palpitations, weight loss, and heat intolerance. Clinically detectable thyroid gland enlargement (goiter), present in almost all younger patients, is absent in as many as 37% of older patients with Graves disease.[38] Lid lag and lid retraction are frequently seen.[35,38,60-62]

One third of older adults will present with apathetic hyperthyroidism.[35] The paucity of clinical signs and symptoms of hyperthyroidism in older adults has been confirmed by several studies,[60,63-66] with weight loss, apathy, tachycardia, and atrial fibrillation the most commonly occurring symptoms ($P < .001$). However, tachycardia is absent in up to 40% of older hyperthyroid patients, primarily due to coexisting cardiac conduction system disease.[64] Progressive functional decline, muscle weakness with wasting, and depression could also be presenting features in older adults.[38] A large cross-sectional study ($N = 3049$) has shown an increased prevalence of weight loss in older patients (>61 years) and identified shortness of breath as a symptom commonly reported in older adults ($P < .001$). This study also demonstrated a higher proportion of older adults reporting only one or two symptoms, versus five or more in the younger patients.[66] Deep tendon reflexes are often not hyperreflexic. The absence of classic symptoms and signs in older adults presents a diagnostic challenge and may lead to delay in treatment and worse outcomes.[60,66] Often, the initial impression in such patients is that of depression, malignancy, or cardiovascular disease.[35,63]

Patients with subclinical hyperthyroidism have no or very mild clinical features suggestive of hyperthyroidism.[67] However, these patients are at increased risk of developing atrial fibrillation, increased cardiovascular and all-cause mortality, accelerated bone loss, and impaired quality of life.[24,68-72]

Diagnosis

The diagnosis of primary hyperthyroidism is based on thyroid function test results. As in younger patients, the initial diagnostic test for suspected hyperthyroidism in older adults is a serum TSH. Free T_4 and free T_3 levels should also be measured if the TSH level is low or suppressed. However, hospitalized elderly who are acutely ill may demonstrate a depressed TSH without actually being hyperthyroid. A low or suppressed serum TSH level with a high free T_4 and/or high free T_3 level indicates overt primary hyperthyroidism. A low serum TSH level with normal free T_4 and free T_3 levels indicates subclinical hyperthyroidism. Demonstration of anti-TSH receptor antibodies can be helpful in making a diagnosis of Graves disease.[73,74]

In a small proportion of cases of hyperthyroidism, measurement of serum thyroid hormone concentrations results in the expected increase in the serum T_3 level but with the finding that the serum T_4 level is within the normal range, although often at the upper end. This condition has been termed *T_3 toxicosis* and can occur with any type of hyperthyroidism, but is found more commonly in older patients with toxic multinodular goiter or solitary toxic adenoma.[40]

When the clinical presentation of thyrotoxicosis is not diagnostic of Graves disease, a radioactive iodine uptake should be performed to help determine the cause. A thyroid scan should be added if thyroid nodules are also identified.[6]

Risks, Complications, and Sequelae

Atrial Fibrillation

It has been clearly demonstrated that age is independently associated with an increased risk of developing atrial fibrillation. Atrial fibrillation is estimated to be present in up to 20% to 35% of older patients suffering from hyperthyroidism[59-60,75] and is especially common in those with hyperthyroidism secondary to toxic nodule(s).[60] Long-standing low serum TSH concentrations in older patients are associated with a threefold increased risk of developing atrial fibrillation.[69] In a population-based study, euthyroid individuals with a TSH level in the lowest quartile had a higher risk of atrial fibrillation than those in the highest quartile.[76] Because of the greater incidence of underlying cardiac disease, the risk of developing atrial fibrillation is increased in patients older than 60 years. Atrial fibrillation in older adults may sometimes be the only clinical sign of hyperthyroidism. However, the degeneration of the sinus node and fibrotic changes in the cardiac conduction system make the presence of palpitations less likely in this population. In addition, frequent use of β-blockers or amiodarone in these patients can mask the arrhythmia. In contrast, younger hyperthyroid patients often present with sinus tachycardia.[66] Many older adults with hyperthyroidism and atrial fibrillation are at increased risk for thromboembolic events, especially those with a prior history of thromboembolism, hypertension, or congestive heart failure or who have evidence of left atrial enlargement or left ventricular dysfunction.[77]

Cardiovascular Effects and Mortality

Thyroid hormones act on the myocardium to sensitize the heart to β-adrenergic stimulation, with a resultant increase in heart rate, stroke volume, cardiac output, left ventricular mass, ejection fraction, and shortened left ventricular ejection time.[77-79] Overt hyperthyroidism, and less often subclinical hyperthyroidism, can be accompanied by several cardiovascular changes, including widened pulse pressure, increased systolic blood pressure, exercise intolerance, increased risk for atrial fibrillation, exacerbation of angina in patients with preexisting coronary artery disease, increased cardiac mass, and precipitation of congestive heart failure, which responds less readily to digoxin treatment because of increased renal clearance of the drug.[80]

Echocardiographic data further define the cardiac changes in hyperthyroidism. Specifically, it has been demonstrated that diastolic function is enhanced, as evidenced by increased isovolemic relaxation and left ventricular filling in hyperthyroid patients.[81] These alterations in hemodynamic parameters may explain many of the cardiovascular signs and symptoms of hyperthyroidism and many of the cardiac complications associated with hyperthyroidism, including decreased exercise tolerance and increased risk of congestive heart failure.

Several cross-sectional and case-control studies have found that decreased levels of serum TSH are associated with increased cardiovascular mortality in older adults.[82] Collet and colleagues have demonstrated an increased risk of total and ischemic heart disease mortality when the TSH level is lower than 0.10 mIU/L in patients with endogenous subclinical hyperthyroidism.[83] In addition, subclinical hyperthyroidism has been shown to be associated with left ventricular hypertrophy, which is a predictor of cardiovascular mortality.[80]

Osteoporosis and Fracture Risk

Overt hyperthyroidism is a well-recognized risk factor leading to low bone mineral density and osteoporotic fractures, especially in older women.[84] This is critical because hip fracture mortality rates within the year of fracture reach up to 37% in older adults.[85-88] Thyroid hormone acts on osteoblasts and osteoclasts to increase bone turnover, leading to net bone loss.[89] Notably, most studies investigating the relationship between thyroid dysfunction and fracture risk have been specific to women. Bauer and associates, in a large prospective fracture study ($N = 686$), reported that women older than 65 years with a TSH level of 0.1 mIU/L had a threefold increased risk for hip fracture and a fourfold increased risk for vertebral fracture as compared to euthyroid counterparts.[72] In a study of subclinical hyperthyroidism in older adults (mean age, 72.8 years) with gender-specific analyses, men were found to have an increased incidence of hip fractures compared to women (13.8% vs. 12%; $P < .01$).[90]

Ophthalmopathy

There have been contradictory studies regarding the association of symptoms and signs of ophthalmopathy in Graves disease with increasing age. Most studies published on this subject have demonstrated a positive correlation between prevalence and severity of ophthalmopathy with increasing age.[60,91] However, one prospective cohort study has found infiltrative ophthalmopathy with severe proptosis and exophthalmos to be more frequent in younger patients with Graves as compared to older adults (46% vs. 6%; $P < .001$).[66]

Dementia and Cognitive Impairment

Data are also conflicting regarding the link of dementia with hyperthyroidism, but many studies have suggested an association between subclinical hyperthyroidism and increased risk of dementia.[92-94] In a prospective study, women with a mean age of 71 years and a TSH level in the lowest tertile had a twofold increased risk of developing Alzheimer disease compared with those in the middle tertile.[92] In other studies, subclinical hyperthyroidism with a TSH level less than 0.46 mU/L was associated with cognitive dysfunction and increased risk of dementia.[93,95] In addition, it has been shown that a lower serum TSH level within the reference range is independently associated with the risk of cognitive impairment, including mild cognitive impairment and dementia, in older patients.[95] There is a lack of evidence suggesting that antithyroid treatment might ameliorate dementia.[96]

Management

Symptomatic treatment for hyperthyroidism in older adults consists of β-adrenergic blockade. β-Adrenergic blockers act by interfering with some peripheral actions of thyroid hormone but do not correct the hypermetabolic state. They decrease heart rate and systolic blood pressure and can also relieve tremors, irritability, emotional lability, and exercise intolerance. Anticoagulation may be indicated in patients who present with atrial fibrillation. β-Blockers do not interfere with the laboratory assessment of thyroid function and can allow control of symptoms until definitive treatment can be undertaken.

Treatment modalities for overt and subclinical hyperthyroidism are the same. These include radioactive iodine ablation therapy, antithyroid medications, and thyroidectomy.[97]

Radioactive iodine ablation is often used for older adults because of its efficacy, safety, and cost-effectiveness.[98] An appropriate dose is calculated from a thyroid radionuclide uptake and scan obtained prior to radioactive iodine ablation. A drawback to this treatment approach is that hyperthyroidism is reversed gradually over months, and cardiac issues may need to be managed aggressively until the thyrotoxic state is reversed. Over 80% of these patients subsequently develop hypothyroidism and require lifelong thyroid hormone replacement therapy.[99] Periodic monitoring of thyroid function is a necessity for any patient treated with radioactive iodine who has not yet become hypothyroid. Side effects of radioactive iodine treatment include dry mouth (xerostomia), metallic taste, salivary gland swelling, lacrimal duct dysfunction and, rarely, secondary malignancy, such as leukemia. Radiation thyroiditis can also rarely occur.

In regard to antithyroid medications, methimazole is preferred. Propylthiouracil is no longer recommended in this setting unless there is an allergy to methimazole due to its black box warning of severe liver injury and acute liver failure, which may be fatal. Antithyroid medications impair the biosynthesis of thyroid hormone and lead to depletion of intrathyroidal hormone stores and, consequently, to decreased hormone secretion. A decline in the serum T_4 concentration is usually seen by 2 to 4 weeks after initiation of antithyroid drug therapy; the dose can be tapered once thyroid hormone levels reach the normal range to avoid development of hypothyroidism. However, older adults may be at greater risk of recurrence of hyperthyroidism after drug therapy and for medication side effects.[98] Long-term antithyroid drugs are rarely successful in inducing sustained remission in older patients with toxic multinodular goiter. There are data that older adults taking propylthiouracil or high doses of methimazole may be at greater risk for side effects. Agranulocytosis is the major adverse event in this population, occurring in 0.5% of those treated.[99] Routine periodic monitoring of the white blood cell count has not been recommended, but measurement is necessary if the patient experiences the onset of fever, sore throat, or oral ulcerations, and the drug must be discontinued if there is evidence of neutropenia.[99] Rash, arthralgias, and myalgias also occur more frequently.[98]

Depending on comorbidities, surgical approaches are less commonly used in older adults with hyperthyroidism due to the perceived increased risk of morbidity.[100] They are reserved for large goiters with obstructive symptoms or known or suspected malignancy.[101] However, it has been found that thyroid surgery in patients aged 70 years or older is safe, and age alone should not be a consideration factor.[102] Possible complications following thyroid surgery include pain, bleeding, infection, vocal cord paralysis due to recurrent laryngeal nerve damage, and hypocalcemia due to hypoparathyroidism (transient or permanent).

Regarding subclinical hyperthyroidism in older adults, guidelines have recommended periodic clinical and biochemical assessment. Recent ATA/AACE guidelines have recommended that patients older than 65 years be treated if their TSH level is lower than 0.1 mIU/L and that treatment can be considered if their TSH level is 0.1 to 0.5 mIU/L.[55,97] Treatment modalities include antithyroid drugs, radioiodine treatment, and thyroid surgery, as mentioned earlier.

HYPOTHYROIDISM

Hypothyroidism, or underactive thyroid, is a condition in which there is thyroid hormone deficiency (T_4 and T_3) due to decreased synthesis or tissue unresponsiveness to the presence of adequate thyroid hormone levels. Primary hypothyroidism occurs due to dysfunction of the thyroid gland. Secondary hypothyroidism refers to the inadequate release of TSH from the pituitary gland, causing decreased production of T_4 from the thyroid gland. Failure of synthesis or release of hypothalamic TRH leads to rare cases of tertiary hypothyroidism.

Epidemiology and Pathophysiology

Estimates of the prevalence and incidence of hypothyroidism among older adults are variable, depending on the populations studied and criteria used to define the condition.[103] A large screening study (N = 25,000) has revealed that 10% of men and 16% of women aged 65 to 74 years had TSH levels above the upper limit of the reference range.[104] The most recent National Health and Nutrition Examination Survey (NHANES III) has reported that a significantly greater number of women aged 50 to 69 years met criteria for subclinical and clinical hypothyroidism compared to men in the same age range.[18] Moreover, a study evaluating geriatric patients under medical care has demonstrated that 15% of the women and 17% of the men had previously undiagnosed hypothyroidism.[105]

The incidence of hypothyroidism steadily increases with advancing age, predominantly due to a rising incidence of autoimmune thyroiditis.[106-108] In a survey by Reinhardt and Mann, the reported incidence of Hashimoto thyroiditis was 67% in a patient population with a mean age of 73 years (N = 24).[109] A survey of endocrinology clinic patients has revealed that 47% of patients aged 55 years and older presenting with primary hypothyroidism had a diagnosis of autoimmune thyroiditis, whereas 27% had postsurgical hypothyroidism and 10% had postradioiodine hypothyroidism.[110]

Subclinical hypothyroidism is defined as a normal serum free T_4 level in the presence of an elevated serum TSH level. The prevalence of subclinical hypothyroidism rises with age, is higher in women than men, and is lower in blacks than in whites.[18,104,111,112] The prevalence of subclinical hypothyroidism was reported to be 4.3% in 16,533 subjects from NHANES III.[18] In population-based studies, subclinical hypothyroidism prevalence has ranged from 4% to 15%.[104,105,111-114]

Progression of Subclinical Hypothyroidism to Overt Hypothyroidism

Many patients with subclinical hypothyroidism eventually develop overt hypothyroidism, and the cumulative incidence of overt hypothyroidism ranges from 33% to 55% in prospective studies after a 10- to 20-year follow-up.[115-117] In a recent study evaluating 4000 patients older than 65 years, subclinical hypothyroidism persisted in almost 50% of patients at 2- and 4-year follow-up. The highest rates of reversion to euthyroidism were in those patients with lower TSH levels (<7 mIU/L) and a negative thyroid peroxidase antibody titer.[118]

Clinical Presentation

The onset of hypothyroidism in older adults is insidious, and the development of symptoms may take many years, leading to late recognition of the condition in this population. Hypothyroidism can affect several organ systems, including the cardiovascular system, central nervous system (CNS), gastrointestinal tract, and skin.

The most common cardiovascular manifestations are bradycardia and narrow pulse pressure.[77] CNS abnormalities include depression, cognitive impairment, and excessive lethargy. Hypothyroidism has also been studied as a cause of dementia.[119] Constipation is seen in hypothyroidism; however, this is also a common symptom in euthyroid older adults. Integumentary changes are comprised of dry skin, yellowing of the skin, face puffiness, periorbital edema, coarsened and thinned hair, thinning of the outer part of the eyebrows, and brittle nails.[120] Hypothermia and weight gain or loss may also be seen in older adults.

A high index of suspicion is required for the diagnosis of hypothyroidism in older adults because symptoms and signs such as fatigue, weakness, constipation, dry skin, and cold intolerance may be attributed to other diseases common in older patients, medication side effects, or aging itself.[4,121] A prospective study by Doucet and colleagues[122] has compared 24 clinical symptoms and signs of hypothyroidism between older (N = 67; mean age, 79.3 years) and younger patients (N = 54; mean age, 40.8 years). It was concluded that the mean number of clinical symptoms and signs in older adults was 6.6 versus 9.3 in the younger population. Fatigue and weakness were the most common symptoms in older adults, whereas cold intolerance, paresthesiae, weight gain, and abdominal cramps were less common.

Diagnosis

An elevated serum TSH level with a low serum free T_4 level is indicative of overt primary hypothyroidism. There is no diagnostic value in measuring a serum free T_3 level. A low free T_4 level with an inappropriately normal or low TSH level indicates secondary hypothyroidism.

Risks, Complications, and Sequelae

Cognitive Impairment

Hypothyroidism in older adults has been associated with impairment of several cognitive domains, including memory, attention and concentration, language, executive function, and perceptual and visuospatial function.[123,124] Severe hypothyroidism may mimic depression and dementia. Neuropsychiatric symptoms usually improve with treatment and restoration of a euthyroid state.[125] The relationship between subclinical hypothyroidism and cognition is less clear. It has been postulated that older adults may be more vulnerable to the effects of subclinical hypothyroidism, given age-related changes to the hypothalamic-pituitary-thyroid axis. However, several studies in older adults have not shown a significant association between mildly elevated TSH levels and reduced cognitive performance.[126,127]

There have been conflicting data on the role of levothyroxine replacement in subclinical hypothyroidism and improvement in cognition. Several studies have shown improvement in cognition with levothyroxine replacement therapy,[128-130] but others showed no benefit.[126,131]

Cardiovascular Effects

The cardiovascular consequences of hypothyroidism in older adults are thought to be due to a reduction in stroke volume and heart rate, leading to decreased cardiac output.[132,133] Decreased cardiac output contributes to reduced exercise capacity and shortness of breath during exercise. Congestive heart failure and angina can worsen when hypothyroidism develops in patients with preexisting heart disease, which is commonly seen in older adults.

Other cardiovascular effects include increased risk of atherosclerosis, increased arterial stiffness, endothelial dysfunction, and altered coagulation parameters.[134] An increase in peripheral vascular resistance can lead to hypertension. All these abnormalities regress with levothyroxine replacement.

In subclinical hypothyroidism, thyroxine therapy can improve cardiovascular risk factors such as dyslipidemia, markers of inflammation, vascular smooth muscle proliferation, vascular reactivity, ventricular function, endothelial function, and carotid intima media thickness, but the data on decreasing cardiovascular events are limited.[135-145] The Cardiovascular Health Study cohort has shown that in patients aged older than 65 years, subclinical hypothyroidism is not associated with an increased risk of cardiovascular disease, mortality, or heart failure, although the latter was significantly higher in those with serum TSH levels above 10 mIU/L.[68,82] A large prospective cohort of community-dwelling older adults (aged 70 to 79 years) has shown that subclinical hypothyroidism with a TSH level above 10 mIU/L is associated with an increased likelihood of prevalent, not incident, metabolic syndrome.[146]

Mortality

Some studies, but not all, have shown an increased risk of cardiovascular and/or all-cause mortality in patients with subclinical hypothyroidism. In a recent population-based, prospective cohort study (307 participants aged 85 years at baseline), there was no association of TSH or subclinical hypothyroidism with 3-year mortality in the oldest old.[147] Another prospective study of patients older than 65 years with a 7-year follow-up has concluded that alterations in thyroid function test results during hospitalization were associated with long-term mortality in older patients. In particular, low free T4 levels were significantly related to all-cause and cardiovascular mortality.[148] On the contrary, a prospective study of older individuals (>85 years) in the Netherlands with untreated subclinical hypothyroidism has shown that they actually had a lower rate of cardiovascular and all-cause mortality when the TSH level was between 4.8 and 10 mIU/L.[149]

Myxedema Coma

Myxedema coma is defined as severe hypothyroidism leading to decreased mental status, hypothermia, and other symptoms related to slowing function in multiple organs. It occurs almost exclusively in older adults with long-standing untreated primary hypothyroidism and is usually precipitated by a concomitant medical illness. Patients may present with a rapid development of stupor, seizures, or coma, along with respiratory depression. Hallmark signs of myxedema coma include localized neurologic signs, hypothermia, bradycardia, hyponatremia, and hypoglycemia.[132] Myxedema coma is a severe and life-threatening clinical state in older adults, with a mortality rate as high as 40%.[150-152] Early recognition and treatment of myxedema coma are essential. Treatment should be started on the basis of clinical suspicion without waiting for laboratory results.

Serum Lipid and Apolipoprotein Concentrations

Many hypothyroid patients have high serum concentrations of total cholesterol and low-density lipoprotein (LDL) cholesterol, and some have high serum concentrations of triglycerides, intermediate-density lipoproteins, apolipoprotein A1, and apolipoprotein B.[153-157] Subclinical hypothyroidism has also been shown to be associated with an adverse lipid profile.[135,138,158] Several clinical trials investigating the effect of thyroxine therapy in subclinical hypothyroidism on total cholesterol, high-density lipoprotein (HDL), LDL, triglycerides, apolipoproteins A and B, and lipoprotein(a) have shown no significant improvement in these levels.[159] However, some randomized trials of patients with subclinical hypothyroidism who were treated with thyroxine have shown a significant improvement in serum total and LDL cholesterol and apolipoprotein B100 concentrations as compared to placebo.[135,138,158,160-162]

Nonalcoholic Fatty Liver Disease

Because thyroid hormones are known to be involved in the regulation of lipid metabolism and insulin resistance, it has been anticipated that they may play a role in the pathogenesis of nonalcoholic fatty liver disease (NAFLD) and nonalcoholic steatohepatitis (NASH). The prevalence of hypothyroidism has been reported to range from 15% to 36% among patients with NAFLD-NASH.[163] However, studies examining this association have shown inconsistent results. Chung and associates have reported that hypothyroidism is an independent risk factor for increased prevalence of NAFLD.[164] On the contrary, a retrospective study by Mazo and coworkers did not show a direct association between hypothyroidism and NASH.[165] Several other studies have yielded conflicting data. However, no studies have been conducted to date to analyze the association between overt and subclinical hypothyroidism and NAFLD-NASH in older adults.

Effects on Bone and Fracture Risk

Overt hypothyroidism has been linked to osteoporosis in women and men, which can lead to an increased risk of fractures, including hip fractures.[166,167] It is unclear whether subclinical hypothyroidism increases the risk of fractures. The Cardiovascular Health Study has shown no association between subclinical hypothyroidism and hip fracture risk or bone mineral density in men and women aged 65 years and older after a median follow-up of 12 years.[168] Similarly, a retrospective study of 471 patients aged 50 years and older (mean age, 78.5 years), subclinical hypothyroidism was not associated with reduced bone health, including bone mineral density, the level of 25-hydroxy vitamin D, and bone turnover markers.[169] However, a prospective cohort study in community-dwelling adults aged 65 years and older has found that older men with subclinical hypothyroidism are at higher risk for hip fractures. It is unclear if treating subclinical hypothyroidism decreases fracture risk.[170]

Management

Despite the high prevalence of thyroid hormone use in older adults, there are no concrete data on when and at what dose to initiate thyroid hormone replacement. Somwaru and colleagues have collected thyroid hormone medication data from community-dwelling individuals aged 65 years and older (mean age, 72.8 years) enrolled in the Cardiovascular Health Study ($N = 5888$) over the span of 16 years.[171] It was concluded that thyroid hormone use is common in patients older than 65 years, with up to 20% being overtreated with levothyroxine. The incidence of thyroid hormone replacement in adults aged 85 years and older was more than twice as frequent as that in older adults aged 65 to 69 years.[171]

Older patients often have lower levothyroxine dosage requirements. This may be related to several factors, including declining metabolic clearance, slow progression of underlying thyroid failure, declining body mass, and interactions with other medications.[172] On average, older adults with primary hypothyroidism receive initial daily dosages that are 20 μg lower and maintenance daily dosages that are 40 μg lower than those prescribed for younger patients of comparable weight.[173-175] Thyroid hormone increases myocardial oxygen demand, which may induce cardiac arrhythmias, angina pectoris, or myocardial infarction in older patients. Once the cardiovascular tolerance of a starting dose has been assessed, a gradual increase by 12.5 to 25 μg every 4 to 6 weeks is recommended until adequate replacement is confirmed by serum TSH level measurement.[176] In patients with secondary hypothyroidism, the free T_4 level, not TSH, should be assessed to guide treatment.[29]

Physicians treating primary hypothyroidism in older adults should target a normal TSH range.[176] In a survey of ATA members, 39% of them recommended targeting a TSH range of 0.5 to 2.0 mIU/L when treating younger patients, but a comparable number reported being more liberal in their approach to older adults, targeting TSH ranges of 1.0 to 4.0 mIU/L.[176] This avoids overtreatment with excessive doses of levothyroxine, which can be associated with increased risks of atrial fibrillation and progressive loss of bone mineral density in older adults.[177]

Management of subclinical hypothyroidism in older adults is controversial, and guidelines have been published for[178] and against[2,179] routine treatment in older adults. Several placebo-controlled randomized trials have failed to find a reduction in the symptoms of subclinical hypothyroidism with treatment,[128,180] suggesting that there is no benefit to treatment.[129,181] Surks and associates have recommended against routine treatment of patients older than 58 years with TSH levels between 4.5 and 10 mIU/L due to lack of evidence indicating adverse health outcomes in untreated patients in this group, excluding progression to overt hypothyroidism.[2] Chu and Crapo have recommended levothyroxine replacement therapy in patients with a TSH level more than 10 mIU/L on repeated measurements, clear symptoms or signs associated with thyroid failure, family history of thyroid disease, or severe hyperlipidemia not previously diagnosed.[179]

In conclusion, in patients with primary hypothyroidism, the goal of therapy is to keep the TSH concentration in the normal reference range. The mean serum TSH level for the general population is 1.4 mU/L,[18] with 90% having serum TSH levels below 3 mU/L, so a TSH target of 0.5 to 2.5 mU/L in young and middle-aged patients has been recommended by many experts. A TSH target of 3 to 5 mU/L might be more appropriate in patients older than 70 years. Observational studies have shown decreased mortality rates[149] and improved measures of well-being[182] in older adults with TSH levels above the normal range (0.5 to 4.5 mIU/L) for the general population.

THYROID NODULES

A thyroid nodule is a discrete lesion within the thyroid gland that is radiologically distinct from the surrounding thyroid parenchyma. Palpable lesions that do not correspond to distinct radiologic abnormalities do not meet the strict definition of thyroid nodules. Nonpalpable thyroid nodules detected on imaging studies are termed *incidentalomas*.[183]

Epidemiology and Clinical Presentation

Thyroid nodules are usually asymptomatic and are often found incidentally on routine physical examination or during imaging studies evaluating a different condition, such as CT, MRI, or thyroid uptake on a ^{18}F-fludeoxyglucose (FDG) positron emission tomography (PET) scan. High-resolution ultrasound can detect thyroid nodules in up to 67% of randomly selected individuals, with a higher frequency in women and older adults.[184]

It is known that the prevalence of thyroid nodules increases with age.[185] By the age of 65 years, nearly 50% of individuals in iodine-sufficient areas have thyroid nodules when evaluated with ultrasound.[186] Moreover, autopsy studies have demonstrated that thyroid nodules are frequently found in older adults, even when clinical examination of the neck has failed to reveal abnormalities, with a frequency of up to 90% in women and up to 50% in men older than 70 years.[184,187,188] Thyroid nodules may be benign adenomas, cysts, cancer, or inflammation. The clinical importance of detecting thyroid nodules lies with the need to exclude thyroid cancer.[189] Nonpalpable thyroid nodules have the same risk of malignancy as palpable nodules of equal size confirmed by imaging. The risk of malignancy is the same in patients with single thyroid nodules compared to those with multiple thyroid nodules.[190]

The most common presentation in older adults, especially older women, is a large multinodular goiter, often with a substernal component. The finding of a multinodular thyroid gland increases in areas of iodine deficiency. Often, there is a history of goiter dating back to childhood or the young adult years. Very large multinodular goiters, particularly those with a sizable substernal component, may compress the trachea and lead to complaints of dyspnea or the esophagus, causing dysphagia. Sometimes a large substernal goiter is first recognized when the patient has had a chest radiogram and is noted to have compression or deviation of the trachea or a superior mediastinal mass.[191] Occasionally, a thyroid nodule will be associated with an acute onset of neck pain and tenderness, which results from acute or subacute thyroiditis or hemorrhage into a preexisting nodule.

Management

The approach to the management of a solitary thyroid nodule in older adults is the same as that for younger patients (Figure 88-1).

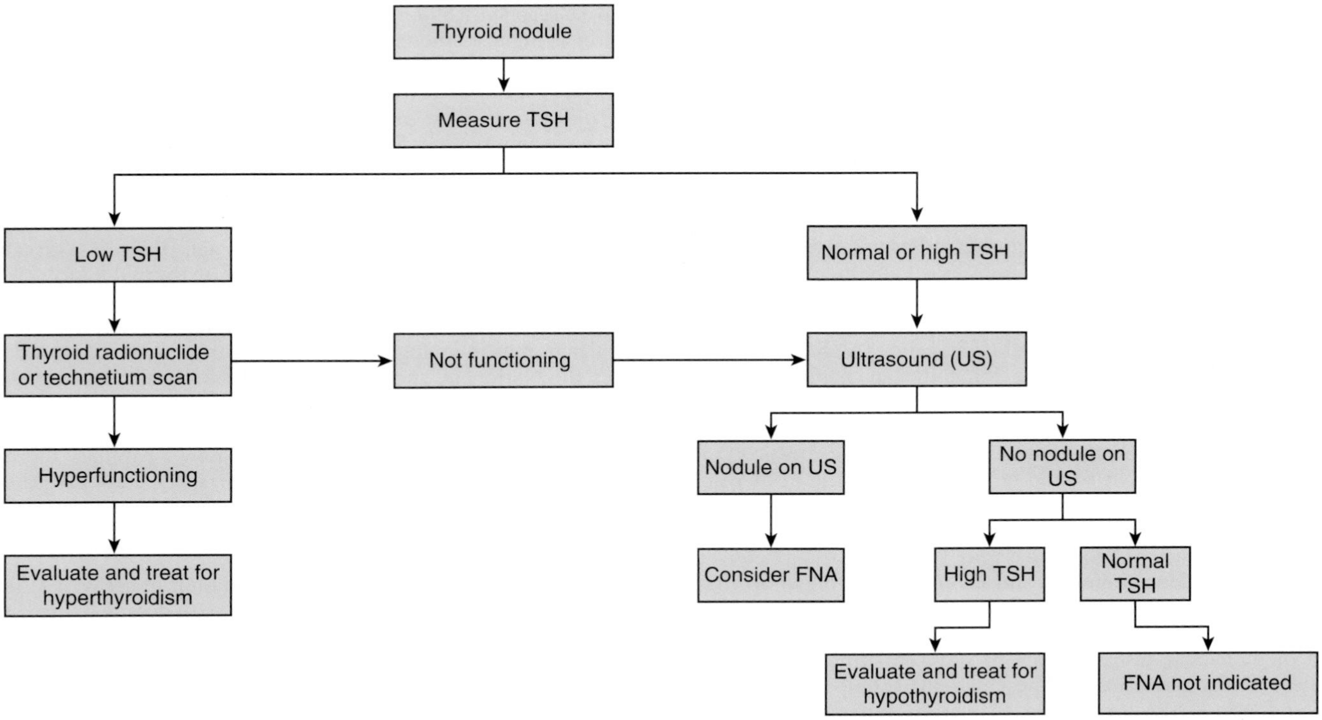

Figure 88-1. Approach to the management of thyroid nodules. *FNA,* Fine-needle aspiration; *TSH,* thyroid-stimulating hormone.

With the discovery of a new thyroid nodule, a complete history and physical examination should be performed. Pertinent questions should include a history of head and neck or whole-body irradiation, exposure to ionizing radiation, and family history of thyroid cancer or syndromes, such as multiple endocrine neoplasia. It is well known that patients who received radiation of the head and neck have a significantly higher risk of developing benign thyroid nodules and thyroid malignancy.[183] Thyroid nodules appear after a latency period of 10 to 20 years, and the incidence of malignant nodules reaches a peak in 20 to 30 years after radiation exposure.[192,193] In the United States, external radiation was used to treat facial acne, tonsillar enlargement, cervical adenitis, and thymic enlargement in the 1950s. Physical findings, such as palpable cervical lymphadenopathy, voice hoarseness, or fixation of the nodule to surrounding tissue, raise suspicion for malignancy.

As per ATA guidelines,[183] the initial evaluation constitutes of measurement of the serum TSH level. If the TSH level is low or suppressed, the next step consists of a radionuclide thyroid scan using technetium pertechnetate or ^{123}I. In a subset of this group of patients for whom the radionuclide thyroid scan suggests nodularity, ultrasound should be performed to evaluate the presence of hyperfunctioning nodules (hot) concordant with the functioning area on the scan. If the nodule is hot the risk of malignancy is very low and does not warrant fine-needle aspiration (FNA) biopsy. If the nodule is cold, then FNA biopsy is usually recommended to rule out malignancy. If the TSH level is found to be normal or high, a radionuclide thyroid scan should not be performed as the initial imaging evaluation. Instead, a diagnostic thyroid ultrasound should be performed in all patients with known or suspected thyroid nodules who have a normal or high TSH level.

Thyroid ultrasound can provide information on the size and location of the nodule, imaging characteristics, such as composition, echotexture, and suspicious cervical lymphadenopathy. If solid thyroid nodules are equal to or larger than 1 cm or smaller than 1 cm with ultrasonographic features associated with a higher likelihood of malignancy, they should be evaluated by ultrasound-guided FNA. Suspicious ultrasound features include hypoechogenicity, increased intranodular vascularity, presence of microcalcifications, absence of a halo, irregular borders, nodule with a height greater than width, and presence of suspicious cervical lymphadenopathy.

Ultrasound-guided FNA biopsy is the procedure of choice for evaluation of thyroid nodules when clinically indicated and is accurate and cost-effective. The Bethesda System for Reporting Thyroid Cytopathology is used to interpret FNA biopsy results.[194] It recognizes six diagnostic categories and provides an estimation of cancer risk, with each category based on literature review and expert opinion. These categories include nondiagnostic and unsatisfactory, benign, atypia of undetermined significance–follicular lesion of undetermined significance (AUS/FLUS), follicular neoplasm or suspicious for follicular neoplasm (FN), Hurthle cell neoplasm or suspicion of Hurthle cell neoplasm, suspicion of malignancy, and malignant (Table 88-3).

As per ATA guidelines,[183] after an initial nondiagnostic cytology result, repeat FNA should be performed. If the FNA result is benign, the patient should be periodically followed on a case by case basis with a physical examination and thyroid ultrasound. Overall, evidence has shown that initial benign cytology conveys an overall excellent prognosis, and a conservative follow-up strategy is reasonable. If cytology is indeterminate (AUS/FLUS, FN, Hurthle cell neoplasm), there has been emerging data about the use of molecular testing to aid in differentiating benign from malignant thyroid nodules. These patients should be referred to an endocrinologist for further evaluation and management. If cytology is suspicious for malignancy or malignant, the patient should be referred for surgery.

TABLE 88-3 Bethesda System for Reporting Thyroid Cytopathology: Implied Risk of Malignancy and Recommended Clinical Management

Diagnostic Category	Risk of Malignancy (%)	Usual Management
Nondiagnostic or unsatisfactory	1-4	Repeat FNA
Benign	0-3	Clinical follow-up
Atypia of undetermined significance or follicular lesion of undetermined significance	~5-15	Repeat FNA
Follicular neoplasm or suspicious for follicular neoplasm	15-30	Surgical lobectomy
Suspicious for malignancy	60-75	Near-total or total thyroidectomy or surgical lobectomy
Malignant	97-99	Near-total or total thyroidectomy

Actual management may depend on other factors (e.g., clinical, sonographic) in addition to the fine-needle aspiration (FNA) interpretation.

Modified from Cibas ES, Ali SZ: The Bethesda System for reporting thyroid cytopathology. Am J Clin Pathol 132:658-665, 2009.

THYROID CANCER

Epidemiology

The incidence of thyroid cancer has been rising[195] and is currently the ninth most common cancer in the United States. Thyroid cancer represents 3.8% of all new U.S. cases of cancer. Approximately 63,000 new cases of thyroid cancer were estimated to have been diagnosed in 2014 in the United States compared with 37,200 cases in 2009.[196] The estimated deaths were reported to have reached 1,890 in 2014. The percentage of thyroid cancer deaths is highest among people aged 75 to 84 years (median age at death, 73 years).[196]

Age is considered to be a risk factor for the development of thyroid cancer. The prevalence of clinically apparent thyroid cancer in adults aged 50 to 70 years has been estimated to be 0.1%.[197] According to the Surveillance, Epidemiology, and End Results (SEER) database, approximately 20% of new cases of thyroid cancer were diagnosed in patients aged 65 years or older between 2007 and 2011.[196] As patients age, there is a greater incidence in poorly differentiated types of thyroid cancer.[198,199] However, well-differentiated papillary thyroid cancer is still the most common thyroid cancer in older adults, with a presentation similar to that in younger patients. A retrospective study of data from the National Cancer Institute's SEER registry has reported that the incidence of papillary thyroid cancer is increasing disproportionally in patients older than 45 years, and the most commonly found tumor in this group is now a papillary thyroid microcarcinoma (<1 cm).[200] It has been speculated that these increased rates are due to the increasing use of imaging studies and subsequent discovery of incidental thyroid nodules in older patients.

Follicular thyroid cancer is more common in areas of iodine deficiency, with the peak incidence in the sixth decade of life.[185,201] Along with Hurthle cell carcinoma, it makes up approximately 23% of thyroid cancers in those older than 60 years.[198,202]

Medullary thyroid carcinoma has a peak incidence in the fifth and sixth decades of life and accounts for 5% of thyroid cancers in older adults.[198] Sporadic forms of medullary thyroid cancer are more common than familial forms in older patients.[203]

Anaplastic thyroid cancer represents only 1% to 3% of all thyroid cancers but is aggressive and has a peak incidence in the seventh decade of life.[185] Based on epidemiologic studies derived from the SEER database, the incidence of anaplastic thyroid cancer held steady in the United States between 1973 and 2002, and the trend has subsequently been decreasing.[196] Risk factors include a prior personal history of goiter and family history of goiter.

Thyroid lymphoma is rare and usually occurs in older women. Virtually all primary thyroid lymphomas are of the mucosa-associated lymphoid tissue (MALT) type arising after 20 to 30 years of lymphocytic thyroiditis in older patients (mean age, 64 years).[204]

Clinical Presentation

In any patient with a thyroid nodule, the initial workup should include history of radiation of the head, neck, and upper thorax, as well as a positive family history, which increase the risk for developing thyroid malignancy.

Well-differentiated thyroid tumors, such as papillary, follicular, and Hurthle cell thyroid cancers, are slow-growing, and most patients are asymptomatic or may present with a painless neck mass. More advanced disease may present with palpable cervical lymphadenopathy,[183,202] usually seen in patients with papillary thyroid cancer as compared to follicular thyroid carcinoma. The most common site of lymph node metastases is the central neck, which is cervical level VI. Cervical lymph node metastases can also occur in the lateral neck compartment, including levels II to V. Other symptoms may include hoarseness, dysphagia, and respiratory distress secondary to local invasion and compression.

Many patients with medullary thyroid cancer present with a palpable neck mass. At the initial presentation, 25% to 63% of these patients have cervical lymph node metastases,[205] and a large number have distant metastases, mainly to the lung and liver.[206] There may be local or systemic symptoms secondary to metastases. Symptoms of hormone hypersecretion include diarrhea, flushing, and bronchospasm. In some cases, medullary thyroid cancer can have an initial presentation of Cushing syndrome due to ectopic adrenocorticotropic hormone (ACTH) hypersecretion.[207]

Anaplastic thyroid cancer often arises within a more differentiated thyroid cancer and usually presents as a rapidly growing neck mass, with metastases at the time of diagnosis. Dysphagia, dysphonia, or voice hoarseness and stridor may also be present. Regional symptoms include a noticeable rocklike mass and neck pain.[208] In a retrospective study, the average anaplastic tumor size at diagnosis was 7.35 cm, with lymph node involvement in 61.5% and distant metastases in 34.5% of cases.[209] Systemic symptoms include anorexia, weight loss, and shortness of breath, with pulmonary metastases.

Thyroid lymphoma typically presents as a rapidly enlarging painless neck mass. It may compress the trachea or larynx.

Risks, Complications, and Sequelae

Thyroid cancer is the only cancer for which age is included in the American Joint Committee on Cancer (AJCC) TNM staging system.[208-210] The mortality rates of patients with thyroid cancer increase starting at age 45 years.[211] A steady decline in survival rates has been reported with increasing age, regardless of the degree of differentiation of the thyroid cancer, suggesting a positive association between age and survival. A large retrospective study ($N = 53,856$) has demonstrated lower 10-year survival rates in patients older than 45 years with papillary (47% to 85% vs. 97%), follicular (57% to 66% vs. 98%), medullary (63% to 80% vs. 88%), and anaplastic (5-year survival rate, 13% vs. 55%) thyroid cancer.[212] Cady and colleagues have documented that women older than 50 years have a 32% risk of thyroid cancer recurrence compared with 10% of those younger than 50 years.[213] Extension of thyroid cancer outside the gland significantly worsened the prognosis in older patients, whereas it did not alter the favorable prognosis in younger patients.[214-216] In a study of the SEER database, the presence of lymph node metastases had no effect on survival in patients younger than 45 years. However, in patients 45 years and older, there was an associated 46% increased risk of death with lymph node positivity ($P < .001$).[217]

Distant metastases are also a serious prognostic sign in older patients with thyroid cancer.[213,214] This may be related to thyroid cancer being less radioactive iodine–avid in older patients than in younger patients.[208,218] Recurrence rates of thyroid cancer have also been shown to be influenced by age.[209]

Management

The modalities used for the treatment of thyroid cancer in older adults are essentially the same as those used in younger patients. Frequently, the surgical approach for a thyroid cancer larger than 1 cm is near-total or total thyroidectomy. Thyroid lobectomy alone may be sufficient for tumors smaller than 1 cm. Central neck dissection should accompany total thyroidectomy in patients with clinically involved central lymph nodes (level VI). If lateral neck lymph nodes are involved, a lateral neck dissection should also be performed.[183] Even though older patients may exhibit a higher surgical risk because of comorbidities, age by itself is not a contraindication to thyroidectomy.[102]

Several studies have shown that thyroid surgery in older patients, including those older than age of 70 years, is safe, with identical operative management and surgical outcomes compared to those in younger patients. The relatively high rate of thyroid carcinoma may justify an aggressive approach in these patients.[102] However, recent studies have found that older patients with thyroid cancer are less likely to receive guideline-concordant care,[219] and older age and Medicare insurance are independently associated with less aggressive management of patients with high-risk thyroid cancer.[220] Even though older patients with thyroid cancer would benefit from referral to high-volume surgical centers,[221] age disparities in referral to a specialist surgical center have been found.[222] Studies have shown that surgical outcomes of thyroid cancer patients, and older patients specifically, are improved with a high-volume thyroid surgeon.[221] However, comorbidities and functional status at the time of thyroid cancer diagnosis may play an important role in determining treatment patterns, especially in older adults. The presence of comorbidities has also been shown to be independently associated with less aggressive treatment in older patients with other malignancies.[223] Possible complications following thyroid surgery include pain, bleeding, infection, vocal cord paralysis due to recurrent laryngeal nerve damage, and hypocalcemia due to hypoparathyroidism (transient or permanent).

Depending on the surgical pathology report, patients are stratified as low risk, intermediate risk, and high risk based on ATA guidelines.[183] If thyroid hormone withdrawal is planned prior to radioactive iodine (RAI) therapy or diagnostic testing, levothyroxine should be stopped for 3 to 4 weeks, with or without T_3 substitution in the initial weeks. Serum TSH levels should be measured prior to radioisotope administration, and a goal TSH higher than 30 mIU/L should be reached in preparation for RAI therapy. Human recombinant TSH stimulation (Thyrogen) can be used as an alternative to thyroxine withdrawal for remnant ablation or adjuvant therapy in patients who have undergone total thyroidectomy. Postoperative RAI ablation is indicated for all patients with known iodine-avid regional and distant metastases, gross extrathyroidal extension of the tumor regardless of tumor size, or primary tumor size larger than 4 cm, even in the absence of other risk factors.[183] RAI ablation is not routinely recommended after lobectomy or total thyroidectomy for patients with unifocal or multifocal papillary microcarcinoma in the absence of other adverse features.[183]

Dosimetry-guided RAI ablation therapy may be preferable to fixed-dose RAI ablation treatment strategies in older patients with advanced thyroid cancer, as evidenced by a study showing that administered activities above 7.4 gigabecquerel (GBq; 200 mCi) will exceed the maximal safe level in a substantial number of patients older than 70 years.[224] Older age, renal failure, and liver failure are associated with a lower clearance of radioiodine.[224] Side effects of RAI treatment include dry mouth (xerostomia), salivary gland swelling, lacrimal duct dysfunction, metallic taste and, rarely, secondary malignancy, such as leukemia.

Serum thyroglobulin measurements are frequently performed as part of the early postoperative evaluation.[183] The predictive value of postoperative thyroglobulin value will be significantly influenced by a wide variety of factors, including the amount of residual thyroid cancer and/or normal thyroid tissue, TSH level at the time of thyroglobulin measurement, functional sensitivity of the thyroglobulin assay, thyroglobulin cutoff used for analysis, time elapsed since thyroidectomy, individual risk of having RAI-avid locoregional or distant metastases, and sensitivity of the post-therapy scanning technique. Postoperative serum thyroglobulin can help in assessing the persistence of disease or thyroid remnant and predicting potential future disease recurrence. Unstimulated thyroglobulin should be periodically assessed. One year after RAI ablation, measurement of thyroglobulin under recombinant human TSH stimulation is useful because it is more sensitive. If the stimulated level is greater than 1 ng/mL, diagnostic imaging studies should be performed for localization of persistent versus recurrent disease.[183]

Thyroxine suppression therapy is used for the treatment of differentiated thyroid cancers. Aggressive thyroid hormone suppression therapy has been shown to be independently associated with longer overall survival in high-risk patients, and moderate thyroid hormone suppression leads to improved overall survival in intermediate-risk patients.[225] Because the outcome is good regardless of intervention, survival is not altered in low-risk patients. The TSH-suppressive doses of 2 to 2.2 µg/kg often required in younger patients with thyroid cancer may be excessive in older adults because thyroxine degradation is reduced with age.[1,226] In the Framingham Heart Study, individuals older than 60 years with TSH levels of 0.1 mIU/L or less had an adjusted relative risk of 3.8 for developing atrial fibrillation during a 10-year follow-up, and those with TSH levels between 0.1 and 0.4 mIU/L had an adjusted relative risk of 1.6.[69] The beneficial effect of TSH suppression is a considerable reduction in recurrence rates of differentiated thyroid cancer, but this should be weighed against potential complications, especially in older adults.

Indications for external beam radiation include the presence of aggressive and unresectable cancer, painful bone metastases, and risk of spinal cord compression.[183]

Cytotoxic chemotherapy has historically produced disappointing results in patients with differentiated thyroid cancers.[227-231] Tyrosine kinase inhibitors, many of which share the common target of the vascular endothelial growth factor (VEGF) receptor, such as sorafenib, vandetanib, cabozantinib, pazopanib, and sunitinib, have emerged as highly promising therapies for metastatic, radioiodine-refractory, differentiated thyroid cancer. Sorafenib has been recently approved by the U.S. Food and Drug Administration (FDA) for use in metastatic radioiodine-refractory differentiated thyroid cancers.[232-238] Tyrosine kinase inhibitors are associated with numerous adverse effects, including diarrhea, fatigue, hypertension, hepatotoxicity, nausea, changes in taste, and skin changes (hand-foot syndrome).[239] Older age may not preclude participation in ongoing clinical trials.

For medullary thyroid carcinoma, the operative procedure of choice is total thyroidectomy because the disease is often multicentric. Routine dissection of the lymph modes is also recommended. Approximately two thirds of patients in their seventh decade will have persistent disease after surgery.[240] The efficacy of surgery can be monitored postoperatively by measurement of the blood calcitonin concentration.[241] Medullary thyroid carcinomas do not respond to ^{131}I therapy, so patients with inoperable residual or recurrent disease are treated palliatively with external irradiation. Recently, tyrosine kinase inhibitors, including vandetanib and cabozantinib, have been FDA approved for the treatment of refractory, metastatic medullary thyroid cancer. The survival rate declines with increase in age at time of initial diagnosis, being substantially lower in patients older than 60 years.[240]

The management of anaplastic carcinoma of the thyroid remains unsatisfactory.[242,243] Relief of symptoms of compression can sometimes be achieved by surgery followed by high-dose (45 to 60 Gy) external irradiation.[242,243] Chemotherapy with doxorubicin may be beneficial in combination with surgery and external irradiation.[208,244]

Patients with thyroid lymphoma should have clinical staging carried out by CT or MRI. The survival rate can approach 100% in response to aggressive external irradiation in combination with chemotherapy (e.g., CHOP—*c*ytoxan, *a*driamycin, *v*incristine, *p*rednisone).[204]

KEY POINTS

- Thyroid disorders are common in older adults. However, the classic symptoms of thyroid dysfunction are usually absent or may be overlooked in older patients, making the diagnosis and subsequent management challenging.
- Expert panels continue to disagree about TSH screening in the general population.
- The serum TSH level has been shown to increase with age and appears to have a survival benefit in older adults. Controversy still exists as to whether asymptomatic older adults with a TSH level above the upper limit of normal but less than 10 mIU/L should be treated.
- Long-standing low serum TSH levels in older adults are associated with an increased incidence of atrial fibrillation, heart failure, osteoporosis, and mortality. Data regarding the link between thyroid dysfunction and cognitive impairment remain conflicting.
- The prevalence of thyroid nodules increases with age. Age is considered to be a risk factor for the development of thyroid cancer, and the prevalence of thyroid cancer in adults older than 50 years is estimated to be 0.1%.

For a complete list of references, please visit www.expertconsult.com.

KEY REFERENCES

2. Surks MI, Ortiz E, Daniels GH, et al: Subclinical thyroid disease: scientific review and guidelines for diagnosis and management. JAMA 291:228–238, 2004.
3. Surks MI, Hollowell JG: Age-specific distribution of serum thyrotropin and antithyroid antibodies in the US population: implications for the prevalence of subclinical hypothyroidism. J Clin Endocrinol Metab 92:4575–4582, 2007.
18. Hollowell JG, Staehling NW, Flanders WD, et al: Serum TSH, T, and thyroid antibodies in the United States population (1988 to 1994): National Health and Nutrition Examination Survey (NHANES III). J Clin Endocrinol Metab 87:489–499, 2002.
20. Papaleontiou M, Haymart MR: Approach to and treatment of thyroid disorders in the elderly. Med Clin North Am 96:297–310, 2012.
23. Atzmon G, Barzilai N, Hollowell JG, et al: Extreme longevity is associated with increased serum thyrotropin. J Clin Endocrinol Metab 94:1251–1254, 2009.

26. Atzmon G, Barzilai N, Surks MI, et al: Genetic predisposition to elevated serum thyrotropin is associated with exceptional longevity. J Clin Endocrinol Metab 94:4768–4775, 2009.
29. Garber JR, Cobin RH, Gharib H, et al: Clinical practice guidelines for hypothyroidism in adults. Endocr Pract 18:998–1028, 2012.
30. Rugge JB, Bougatsos C, Chou R: Screening and treatment of thyroid dysfunction: an evidence review for the U.S. Preventive Services Task Force. Ann Intern Med 162:35–45, 2015.
66. Boelaert K, Torlinska B, Holder RL, et al: Older subjects with hyperthyroidism present with a paucity of symptoms and signs: a large cross-sectional study. J Clin Endocrinol Metab 95:2715–2726, 2010.
68. Cappola AR, Fried LP, Arnold AM, et al: Thyroid status, cardiovascular risk, and mortality in older adults. JAMA 295:1033–1041, 2006.
69. Sawin CT, Geller A, Wolf PA, et al: Low serum thyrotropin concentrations as a risk factor for atrial fibrillation in older persons. N Engl J Med 331:1249–1252, 1994.
75. Cooper DS: Approach to the patient with subclinical hyperthyroidism. J Clin Endocrinol Metab 92:3–9, 2007.
82. Rodondi N, Bauer DC, Cappola AR, et al: Subclinical thyroid dysfunction, cardiac function, and the risk of heart failure. The Cardiovascular Health study. J Am Coll Cardiol 52:1152–1159, 2008.
97. Bahn RS, Burch HB, Cooper DS, et al: American Thyroid Association; American Association of Clinical Endocrinologists: Hyperthyroidism and other causes of thyrotoxicosis: management guidelines of the American Thyroid Association and American Association of Clinical Endocrinologists. Endocr Pract 17:456–520, 2011.
102. Gervasi R, Orlando G, Lerose MA, et al: Thyroid surgery in geriatric patients: a literature review. BMC Surg 12:516–518, 2012.
103. Sawin CT, Castelli WP, Hershman JM, et al: The aging thyroid. Thyroid deficiency in the Framingham Study. Arch Intern Med 145:1386–1388, 1985.
104. Canaris GJ, Manowitz NR, Mayor G, et al: The Colorado thyroid disease prevalence study. Arch Intern Med 160:526–534, 2000.
118. Somwaru LL, Rariy CM, Arnold AM, et al: The natural history of subclinical hypothyroidism in the elderly: the Cardiovascular Health Study. J Clin Endocrinol Metabol 97:1962–1969, 2012.
121. Maselli M, Inelmen EM, Giantin V, et al: Hypothyroidism in the elderly: diagnostic pitfalls illustrated by a case report. Arch Gerontol Geriatr 55:82–84, 2012.
122. Doucet J, Trivalle C, Chassagna P, et al: Does age play a role in clinical presentation of hypothyroidism? J Am Geriatr Soc 42:984–986, 1994.
168. Garin MC, Arnold AM, Lee JS, et al: Subclinical thyroid dysfunction and hip fracture and bone mineral density in older adults: the Cardiovascular Health Study. J Clin Endocrinol Metab 99:2657–2664, 2014.
171. Somwaru LL, Arnold AM, Cappola AR: Predictors of thyroid hormone initiation in older adults: results from the Cardiovascular Health Study. J Gerontol A Biol Sci Med Sci 66:809–814, 2011.
183. Haugen BR, Alexander EK, Bible KC, et al: 2015 American Thyroid Association management guidelines for adult patients with thyroid nodules and differentiated thyroid cancer: the American Thyroid Association guidelines task force on thyroid nodules and differentiated thyroid cancer. Thyroid 26:1–133, 2016.
194. Cibas ES, Ali SZ: The Bethesda System for reporting thyroid cytopathology. Am J Clin Pathol 132:658–665, 2009.
197. Castro MR, Gharib H: Continuing controversies in the management of thyroid nodules. Ann Intern Med 142:926–931, 2005.
200. Hughes DT, Haymart MR, Miller BS, et al: The most commonly occurring papillary thyroid cancer in the United States is now a microcarcinoma in a patient older than 45 years. Thyroid 21:231–236, 2011.
208. Haymart MR: Understanding the relationship between age and thyroid cancer. Oncologist 14:216–221, 2009.
219. Park HS, Roman SA, Sosa JA: Treatment patterns of aging Americans with differentiated thyroid cancer. Cancer 116:20–30, 2011.
221. Ng SH, Wong KP, Lang BH: Thyroid surgery for elderly patients: are they at increased operative risks? J Thyroid Res 2012–946276, 2012.
223. Chen RC, Royce TJ, Extermann M, et al: Impact of age and comorbidity on treatment and outcomes in elderly cancer patients. Semin Radiat Oncol 22:265–271, 2012.

89 Disorders of the Parathyroid Glands

Jane Turton, Michael Stone, Duncan Cole

INTRODUCTION

In most individuals there are just four parathyroid glands, which are usually located at the superior and inferior poles of the thyroid gland and which arise from the third and fourth pharyngeal pouches during the fifth and sixth weeks of fetal development[1] (Figure 89-1).

A parathyroid gland is oval, is yellow in color, measures about 6 mm in a craniocaudal direction, and usually weighs less than 35 mg. Within a gland, there are four cell types: the chief cells, clear cells, oxyphil cells, and adipose cells.[2]

PHYSIOLOGY OF PARATHYROID HORMONE

Parathyroid hormone (PTH) is produced by the chief cells and is an 84–amino acid polypeptide with biologic activity in the N-terminal portion of the molecule. It is synthesized as pre-pro-PTH, and is then sequentially processed to pro-PTH and finally to intact PTH (1-84). PTH is secreted as intact PTH and also in the cleaved C-terminal PTH form (C-PTH). The proportion of C-PTH secreted relative to intact PTH changes in response to circulating free calcium concentration.

Intact PTH has a half-life of less than 5 minutes. It is metabolized by Kupffer cells in the liver, resulting in cleavage of its N-terminal portion and the intracellular degradation of the N-terminal fragment. C-terminal fragments are released back into the circulation from the liver. These fragments are cleared by the kidneys and may be elevated in patients with renal failure. C-terminal fragments have a longer half-life than the intact hormone and constitute the majority of circulating PTH forms.

PTH secretion exhibits both a circadian rhythm, with a peak in the early hours of the morning and nadir in late morning/early afternoon,[3] and a seasonal variation, being highest in the winter and lowest in the summer.[4]

The secretion of PTH occurs predominantly in response to a fall in extracellular free calcium concentration, which is sensed by the calcium sensing receptor (CaSR) on parathyroid chief cells. The CaSR, is a G protein–coupled receptor, found in the intestine, kidney, thyroid C cells, brain, and bone where it is involved in local calcium homeostatic processes.[5] The gene mutation of the CaSR in familial benign hypocalciuric hypercalcemia results in an alteration of the calcium homeostatic set point.[6]

The secretion of PTH is also influenced by circulating levels of 1,25-dihydroxyvitamin D [$1,25(OH)_2D_3$], phosphate, and magnesium. $1,25(OH)_2D_3$ suppresses PTH secretion by inhibiting gene transcription. Hyperphosphatemia increases PTH synthesis and secretion; the converse holds for hypophosphatemia. In states of significant chronic magnesium deficiency, PTH secretion is impaired; however, an acute magnesium deficiency can increase PTH secretion.

In the kidney, PTH stimulates 1α-hydroxylation of 25-hydroxyvitamin D_3 [$25(OH)D_3$] to produce the biologically active $1,25(OH)_2D_3$, promotes calcium reabsorption in the distal convoluted tubule, and inhibits the reabsorption of phosphate from the proximal tubule.

In the small intestine, PTH has a small direct local effect, and circulating $1,25(OH)_2D_3$ produced in the kidney promotes gastrointestinal absorption of calcium and phosphate.[7] PTH increases osteoclastic resorption of bone at cortical surfaces and causes the release of calcium into the extracellular fluid. The net result of PTH action is an increase in extracellular calcium levels and a reduction in phosphate levels.

CALCIUM HOMEOSTASIS AND CHANGES WITH AGE

In older adults, average PTH levels can be up to 35% higher than those measured in a young adult population.[8,9] The cause of this includes the following factors:

- A fall in $1,25(OH)_2D_3$ production by the aging kidney as glomerular filtration rate falls from 125 mL/min at age 20 years to 60 mL/min at age 80[10]
- A reduction in the responsiveness of renal 1α-hydroxylase to circulating PTH[11]
- A reduction in dietary intake and absorption of calcium and vitamin D[12]
- A reduction in vitamin D production in the skin as a result of less frequent and less efficient sunlight exposure. Individuals who are housebound or living in nursing homes are at particular risk of developing abnormal PTH secretion secondary to vitamin D deficiency.[13-16]

(See Box 89-1, Box 89-2.)

SECONDARY HYPERPARATHYROIDISM

Secondary hyperparathyroidism is the most common disorder of calcium homeostasis in older adults and has a prevalence of between 20% and 60% in the population older than 75 years.[17] Secondary hyperparathyroidism occurs when there is vitamin D deficiency or insufficiency, and the resultant decrease in serum calcium causes a reduction in the expression of the CaSR in the parathyroid glands, leading to parathyroid gland hyperplasia, which in turn causes a physiologically appropriate increase in PTH production.

The combination of vitamin D deficiency and secondary hyperparathyroidism is associated with an increased risk of fracture.[17,18] There is an associated increase in mortality from cardiovascular disease[19] independent of bone mass, serum 25(OH)D, and renal function.[20-22]

The first-line treatment for secondary hyperparathyroidism is a combined preparation of elemental calcium 1000 to 1200 mg and vitamin D_3 20 μg (800 IU) daily. Chapuy and colleagues showed that reducing PTH levels and improving serum 25(OH) D_3 levels using this combination could reduce risk of hip fracture by 30% at 18 months and that this efficacy was maintained out to 3 years.[23]

If for any reason a patient cannot or will not adhere to this regime, vitamin D_2 or D_3 alone, 1α-hydroxycholecalciferol, or $1,25(OH)_2D_3$ can be used. $1,25(OH)_2D_3$ is particularly useful for patients with renal failure, although careful monitoring of serum calcium is required.

CASE REPORT 89-1 SECONDARY HYPERPARATHYROIDISM

A female white nonsmoker aged 81 years presented to our clinic with a history of falls and a past history of wrist fracture, osteoarthritis, hypertension, and hypercholesterolemia. She was independent in her activities of daily living and mobile with a walking stick but lacked confidence to go outside alone. Her diet was low in calcium. She was referred for a bone density scan and diagnosed osteoporotic (neck of femur T score, −3.0). She was taking a statin and mild opiate analgesia for arthritic pain. A biochemical screen performed to investigate secondary causes of osteoporosis revealed a profound vitamin D deficiency, secondary hyperparathyroidism, and mild hypocalcemia. She was treated with a combined preparation of 1000 mg calcium and 800 IU ergocalciferol daily, which normalized her biochemistry (see table).

	Baseline	6 Months	12 Months
PTH (pmol/L)	15.5	5	3.3
Vitamin D (μg/L)	5	12.5	27.9
Calcium (mmol/L)	2.21	2.46	2.40

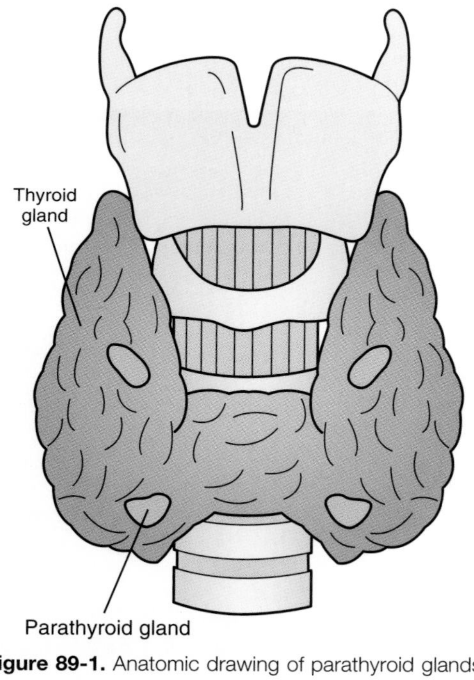

Figure 89-1. Anatomic drawing of parathyroid glands.

BOX 89-1 Clinical Investigation of Parathyroid Disorders

MEASUREMENTS

Bone profile: calcium, phosphate, albumin, alkaline phosphatase
Renal profile: sodium, potassium, urea, creatinine
Plasma parathyroid hormone (PTH)
Serum 25(OH) vitamin D
Magnesium
(Lithium)
24-hr Urinary calcium, phosphate, sodium, and creatinine
Bone density: dual x-ray absorptiometry
X-rays and isotope bone scan
Sestamibi and ultrasound scan for preoperative assessment of primary hyperparathyroidism

BOX 89-2 Parathyroid Hormone Assay

Blood for parathyroid hormone (PTH) assay should be collected into tubes containing ethylenediaminetetraacetic acid (EDTA) because PTH is more stable in EDTA.[12] Intact PTH is measured by noncompetitive immunoassay, which recognizes the C-terminal region. Specificity for the intact PTH is achieved by using a signal antibody that binds to the N-terminal (1-34) region.

CASE REPORT 89-2 PRIMARY HYPERPARATHYROIDISM

A female white patient aged 75 years presented with a history of bone and muscle pain, low mood, indigestion, and a body mass index (BMI) of 18.5. She was referred for bone densitometry, which confirmed severe osteoporosis. Screening for secondary causes of osteoporosis revealed hypercalcemia (corrected calcium, 2.68 mmol/L), normal 25(OH) D_3, a raised parathyroid hormone (PTH) level of 6.8 pmol/L, and raised urinary calcium excretion. She had no vertebral fractures. She was prescribed regular vitamin D_2 and an oral bisphosphonate. She was referred for parathyroidectomy. At surgery she had a solitary right lower parathyroid adenoma measuring 20 × 3 × 2 mm removed. Since her surgery, her PTH and calcium values have remained in the normal range. Her mood has improved, and the muscle and bone pains have eased. Bone mineral densities have increased by 7.5% in the 12 months since her surgery.

PRIMARY HYPERPARATHYROIDISM

The biochemical presentation of primary hyperparathyroidism is a raised plasma PTH and hypercalcemia. The peak incidence occurs between ages 55 and 64 years at 1 : 1000. The prevalence is 2% in persons older than 75 years, and it is three times as common in women as in men.[24] Primary hyperparathyroidism is caused by a single adenoma in 80% of cases, four-gland hyperplasia in 15% of cases, and carcinoma in less than 1% of cases.[25] A rare but notable form of hypercalcemia that can mimic primary hyperparathyroidism is benign familial hypocalciuric hypercalcemia.

Changes in the levels of circulating PTH have been shown to have an effect in bone, increasing the bone remodeling space. In trabecular bone, high levels of PTH increase bone formation. However, in cortical bone, high levels of PTH increase bone loss, cause a fall in bone mineral density (BMD), and increase the risk of fracture independent of 25(OH)D_3 levels.[26-28]

A common presentation of primary hyperparathyroidism follows measurement of serum calcium and the identification of individuals with asymptomatic hypercalcemia. The very old can have an acute disequilibrium hypercalcemia as their renal function progressively declines or if they become acutely dehydrated[29] (Box 89-3).

Although most patients are now identified while asymptomatic, some have presenting symptoms such as lassitude, fatigue, mood swings, muscle pain, generalized weakness, and memory loss.[25] The classical presentation of primary hyperparathyroidism comprising bone cysts, pathologic fractures, and renal calculi, as described by von Recklinghausen in 1891, is very rare.[30]

The treatment of primary hyperparathyroidism can be conservative or surgical. The conservative management involves regular monitoring (serum calcium, BMD, and PTH) and the use of oral or intravenous bisphosphonates. Although the effects on serum calcium are limited and transient,[31] bisphosphonates are effective in treating the associated loss of bone.[32] The use of

BOX 89-3 Differential Diagnosis of Hypercalcemia in Older Adults

Primary hyperparathyroidism
Malignancy
Renal failure
Addison disease
Hyperthyroidism
Immobilization
Medications: thiazide diuretics, calcium supplements, lithium
Milk alkali syndrome
Paget disease (when immobilized)
Sarcoidosis
Tuberculosis
Vitamin D or vitamin A intoxication

SYMPTOMS OF ACUTE HYPERCALCEMIA

Neurologic: drowsiness, confusion, irritability hypotonia, coma
Gastrointestinal: anorexia, nausea, vomiting, acute pancreatitis
Cardiovascular: arrhythmias
Renal: polyuria, polydipsia, dehydration

BOX 89-4 National Institutes of Health 2008 Recommendations for Surgery for Asymptomatic Primary Hyperparathyroidism

Life-threatening hypercalcemia
Reduced creatinine clearance eGFR < 60
Calcium level > 1 mg/dL (0.25 mmol/L) above normal for each laboratory
BMD T score < −2.5 at any site (WHO definition of osteoporosis)
Hypercalcuria

BMD, Bone mineral density; *eGFR,* estimated glomerular filtration rate; *WHO,* World Health Organization.

calcium and vitamin D supplements with bisphosphonates is accepted practice in postmenopausal osteoporosis; however, in primary hyperparathyroidism, calcium supplementation should not be used. It is safe, however, to prescribe regular vitamin D_3 alone to these individuals to ensure that serum vitamin D levels remain normal.

The use of surgery as treatment is becoming more acceptable, even for very old patients, because improvements in imaging have led to successful minimally invasive surgical techniques.[33] The indications for surgery in asymptomatic patients are detailed in Box 89-4. The usual imaging and localization techniques are sestamibi and ultrasound scanning (Figures 89-2 and 89-3). During surgery, PTH[34] is sampled to confirm that the hyperfunctioning tissue has been removed.

After parathyroidectomy, patients can have increases of up to 12% in BMD in the first year, even without further treatment,[35] and the dilemma regarding the use of calcium and vitamin D supplementation is removed.

The mood disturbance, memory loss, and decreased health-related quality of life associated with hyperparathyroidism have been shown to improve after surgery.[36,37]

Calcimimetic medications initially developed for the treatment of hyperparathyroidism related to renal disease and for the treatment of hypercalcemia of malignancy may now be used to treat primary hyperparathyroidism. These medications alter the sensitivity of the CaSR on chief cells of the parathyroid glands to circulating calcium, causing a reduction in the level of circulating PTH and calcium that is maintained up to 12 months of treatment.[38]

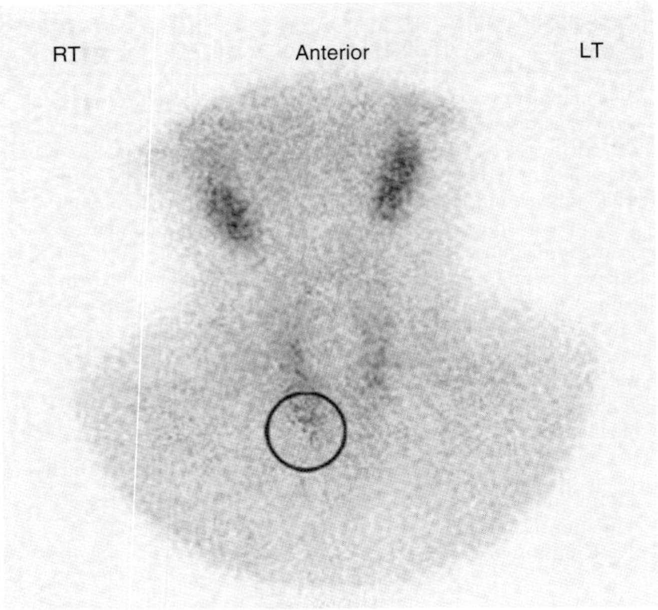

Figure 89-2. Sestamibi scan showing increased uptake at lower right lobe of thyroid.

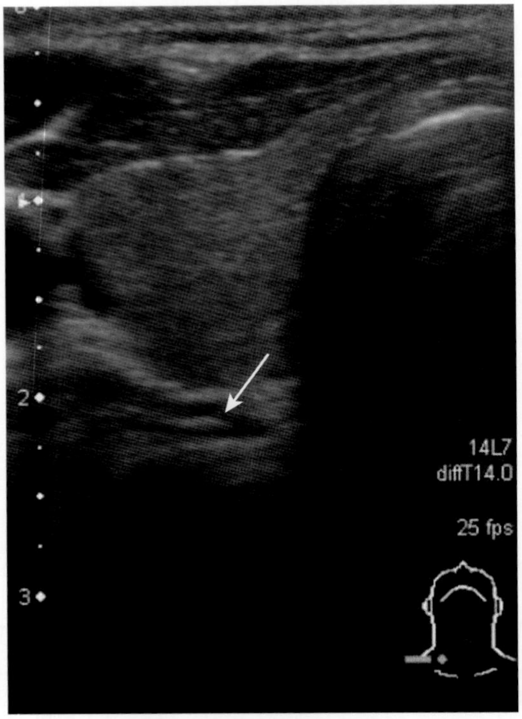

Figure 89-3. Ultrasound showing a hyperechoic region behind right lower lobe of thyroid.

LITHIUM

The combination of hypercalcemia and hyperparathyroidism is common in patients treated with lithium. Lithium-induced

CASE REPORT 89-3 LITHIUM-INDUCED HYPERPARATHYROIDISM

A 65-year-old female presented to clinic with hypercalcemia and osteoporosis identified by our fracture liaison service (corrected serum calcium, 2.78; total spine T score, –4.4). She was being treated for bipolar disorder with oral lithium. She was taking 1000 mg calcium with 400 IU cholecalciferol and oral bisphosphonates as treatment for her osteoporosis at the time of presentation. Her parathyroid hormone (PTH) level was raised, vitamin D level was normal, and her 24-hour urinary calcium value was low (see table). She had preoperative imaging for primary hyperparathyroidism, which did not identify an adenoma, and she was not offered surgery. Her calcium and cholecalciferol combination was replaced with cholecalciferol, and since then serum calcium levels have remained within normal limits.

PTH (0.9-5.4 pmol/L)	Calcium (2.20-2.60 mmol/L)	25(OH)D (8-50 ng/mL)	Phosphate (0.8-1.45 mmol/L)	24-hr Urinary Calcium (<7.0 mmol)
6.6	2.78	25.8	1.34	0.7

hyperparathyroidism has an incidence of 6.3% to 50%, and it can mimic primary hyperparathyroidism.[39,40] However, there are subtle differences between primary hyperparathyroidism and lithium-induced hyperparathyroidism. In lithium-induced disease, there is usually a normal serum phosphate, severe hypercalcemia is rare, 24-hour urinary calcium excretion is low or normal, and there is no adenoma. However, there is a hyperplasia of the parathyroid glands, a condition that is reversible on withdrawing lithium.[41]

Hypercalcemia can occur many years after initiation of lithium therapy, but it is also a recognized effect of a single dosing with lithium, which causes an acute elevation of serum PTH by direct stimulation of the parathyroid gland.[42] Surgical treatment of hypercalcemia with subtotal parathyroidectomy is usually unsuccessful when it is a result of lithium administration, and the hypercalcemia can recur if lithium therapy is continued.[43] The use of calcimimetic medications has been reported in patients with lithium-induced hypercalcemia with good effect.[44]

TERTIARY (REFRACTORY SECONDARY) HYPERPARATHYROIDISM

In individuals who have prolonged secondary hyperparathyroidism as a result of renal failure, there is severe hyperplasia of the parathyroid glands, and the set point for normal inhibition of PTH secretion by calcium is altered. The hyperplastic parathyroid glands show a reduction in CaSR expression, and unlike secondary hyperparathyroidism, patients have high serum calcium and high PTH levels.

Indications for parathyroid surgery in this condition include severe bone pain, fractures, hypercalcemia, heterotopic calcification, and bone cysts; however, if this condition is treated surgically, there is a risk that some patients will subsequently develop adynamic bone disease (Figure 89-4).[45]

HYPOPARATHYROIDISM

Hypoparathyroidism is much less common than hyperparathyroidism. It is very unusual for it to present in the first time in older adults. It presents clinically as hypocalcemia and is a result of insufficiency or resistance to PTH. It can occur after surgery for thyroid or parathyroid disease or reflect autoimmune disease. The reduction in PTH leads to an increase in renal calcium loss and reduced absorption of calcium in the gut because of a fall in $1,25(OH)D_3$ production. Treatment is with hydroxylated products of vitamin D, calcium supplementation, and thiazide diuretics to reduce renal calcium loss.[46]

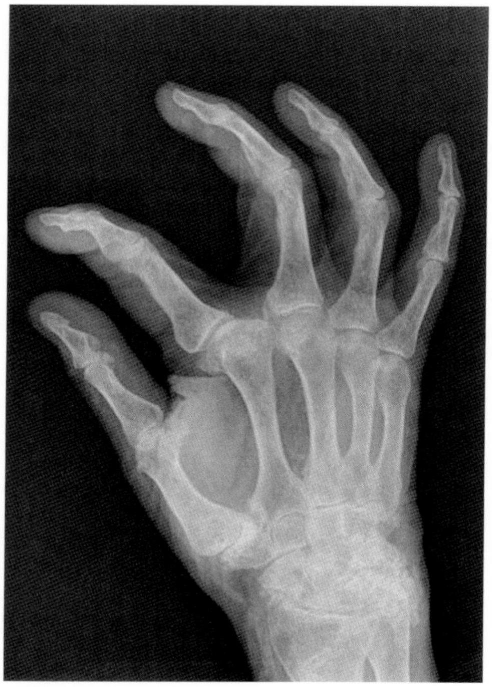

Figure 89-4. Heterotopic tissue calcification in a periarticular distribution.

KEY POINTS

- Vitamin D deficiency and secondary hyperparathyroidism are common in older adults.
- Treatment of frail older adults with simple calcium and vitamin D supplementation significantly reduces the risk of fractures.
- Acute disequilibrium hypercalcemia is an important, life-threatening cause of confusion in older adults.
- The differential diagnosis of raised serum calcium and raised parathyroid hormone includes primary hyperparathyroidism, lithium-induced hyperparathyroidism, familial hypocalciuric hypercalcemia, and tertiary hyperparathyroidism.
- Increasing numbers of older adult patients are now being considered for parathyroid surgery because of improvements in preoperative imaging and the use of minimally invasive surgical techniques.

For a complete list of references, please visit www.expertconsult.com.

KEY REFERENCES

1. Policeni BA, Smoker WRK, Reede DL: Anatomy and embryology of the thyroid and parathyroid glands. Semin Ultrasound CT MR 33:104–114, 2012.
4. Rapuri PB, Kinyamu K, Gallagher JC, et al: Seasonal changes in calciotropic hormones, bone markers, and bone mineral density in elderly women. J Clin Endocrinol Metab 87:2024–2032, 2002.
6. Gunn IR, Gaffney D: Clinical and laboratory features of calcium-sensing receptor disorders: a systematic review. Ann Clin Biochem 41:441–458, 2004.
8. Adami S, Viapiana O, Gatti D, et al: Relationship between serum parathyroid hormone, vitamin D sufficiency, age, and calcium intake. Bone 42:267–270, 2008.
10. Lips P: Vitamin D deficiency and secondary hyperparathyroidism in the elderly: consequences for bone loss and fractures and therapeutic implications. Endocr Rev 22:477–501, 2001.
12. Chapuy MC, Chapuy P, Meunier PJ: Calcium and vitamin D supplements: effects on calcium metabolism in elderly people. Am J Clin Nutr 46:324–328, 1987.
13. Chapuy MC, Schott AM, Garnero P, et al: Healthy elderly French women living at home have secondary hyperparathyroidism and high bone turnover in winter. EPIDOS Study Group. J Clin Endocrinol Metab 81:1129–1133, 1996.
17. Sahota O, Gaynor K, Harwood RH, et al: Hypovitaminosis D and functional hypoparathyroidism the NoNoF (Nottingham Neck of Femur Study). Age Ageing 32:467–472, 2001.
20. Bjorkman MP, Sorva AJ, Tilvis RS: Elevated serum parathyroid hormone predicts impaired survival prognosis in a general aged population. Eur J Endocrinol 158:749–753, 2008.
21. Garnero P, Munoz F, Sornay-Rendu E, et al: Associations of vitamin D status with bone mineral density, bone turnover, bone loss and fracture risk in healthy postmenopausal women. The OFELY study. Bone 40:716–722, 2007.
25. Zarnegar R, Clarke OH: Current indications and decision making leading to parathyroidectomy: a surgical viewpoint. Clin Rev Bone Miner Metab 5:81–89, 2007.
27. Duan Y, De Luca V, Seeman E: Parathyroid hormone deficiency and excess: similar effects on trabecular bone but differing effects on cortical bone. J Clin Endocrinol Metab 84:718–722, 1999.
28. Bargen AE, Repplinger D, Chen H, et al: Can biochemical abnormalities predict symptomatology in patients with primary hyperparathyroidism? J Am Coll Surg 213:410–414, 2011.
29. Mundy GR: Calcium homeostasis: hypercalcaemia and hypocalcaemia, ed 2, London, 1990, Martin Dunitz.
30. von Recklinghausen F: Die Fibrose oder deformierende Ostitis, die Osteomalacie und die osteoplastische Carcinose, in ihren gegenseitigen Beziehungen. Festschr Rudolph Virchow (Berlin) 1–89, 1891.
33. Bilezikian JP, Khan AA, Potts JT Jr: Guidelines for the management of asymptomatic primary hyperparathyroidism: summary statement from the third international workshop. J Clin Endocrinol Metab 94:335–339, 2009.
34. Vignali E, Picone A, Materazzi G, et al: A quick intraoperative parathyroid hormone assay in the surgical management of patients with primary hyperparathyroidism: a study of 206 consecutive cases. Eur J Endocrinol 146:783–788, 2002.
37. Coker LH, Rorie K, Cantley L, et al: Primary hyperparathyroidism, cognition, and health-related quality of life. Ann Surg 242:642–650, 2005.
38. Amgen Ltd 2004 Mimpara: Summary of product characteristics, 1–9, 2013.
40. Livingstone C, Rampes H: Lithium: a review of its metabolic adverse effects. J Psychopharmacol 20:347–355, 2006.
45. Ward BK, Magno AL, Walsh JP, et al: The role of the calcium sensing receptor in human disease. Clin Biochem 45:943–953, 2012.
46. Al-Azem H, Khan AA: Hypoparathyroidism. Best Pract Res Clin Endocrinol Metab 26:517–522, 2012.

90 Diabetes Mellitus

Alan J. Sinclair, Ahmed H. Abdelhafiz, John E. Morley

INTRODUCTION AND BACKGROUND

With increasing aging of the population and urbanization of lifestyle, the prevalence of diabetes has or is likely to reach epidemic levels in most countries, especially in adults older than 75 years.[1] Aging is associated with body composition changes that lead to increased insulin resistance, glucose intolerance, and increased risk of diabetes.[2] As a result, more older adults are developing diabetes. The lifetime risk of developing diabetes is high, reaching 22.4% for women and 18.9% for men from the age of 60 years onward.[3] Older adults with diabetes are exposed to the interplay among metabolic dysfunction, vascular disease, and the aging process in combination with other age-related disorders. Geriatric syndromes and frailty have been emerging as a third category of complications, in addition to the traditional microvascular and macrovascular diseases.[4] Therefore, diabetes in older adults may lead to considerable disability. Unlike other chronic conditions, diabetes care is dependent on self-management, which may be compromised by the presence of comorbidities and geriatric syndromes. Owing to the heterogeneous nature and variations in comorbidity, life expectancy, and functional status, ranging from a fit individual living independently in the community to a fully dependent person living in a nursing home, therapeutic interventions and metabolic targets should be individualized, taking into consideration individual preference while putting quality of life as the basis of care plans. This chapter reviews the phenotype of diabetes in old age and addresses the key areas and special considerations for the care of older adults with diabetes to meet their complex needs.

EPIDEMIOLOGY

The prevalence of diabetes rises with increasing age. Worldwide, the greatest proportional increase in the number of people with diabetes by age group is expected to occur in people aged 60 to 79 years.[3] For example, in France, the prevalence has increased to 14.2% in those aged 65 to 74 years, peaking at 19.7% in men and 14.2% in women aged 75 to 79 years. More than 50% of those with diabetes were older than 65 years.[5] In the United States, 14% of the population is estimated to have diabetes, and the prevalence is highest in those older than 65 years; by 2050, diabetes prevalence could be as high as 33% of the whole population.[6] However, a similar number may remain undiagnosed. In the National Health and Nutrition Examination Survey, the prevalence of diagnosed diabetes in those older than 75 years was 14.9%, and the prevalence of undiagnosed diabetes based on fasting plasma glucose level and 2-hour oral glucose tolerance test was 13.4%. This is a total prevalence of diabetes of 28.3%, with undiagnosed diabetes constituting around 47%. The prevalence of so-called prediabetes, defined as impaired fasting glycemia (IFG) or impaired glucose tolerance (IGT), was 46.7% in those older than 75 years. Therefore, the total prevalence of diabetes and prediabetes was approximately 75% in those older than 75 years.[1] Low- and middle-income countries will have the greatest burden of diabetes, in which the prevalence will increase in adults aged 20 to 79 years by 69% by 2030 compared to only 20% in higher income countries.[7] This is likely driven by the growth and aging of the population and urbanization of lifestyle in these countries.

The prevalence of diabetes among older Chinese in rural Taiwan aged 72.6 years was 16.9% in 2000 and increased to 23.7% in 2005.[8] In minority ethnic groups living in high-income countries, the incidence and prevalence of diabetes are higher than in white populations. For example, the prevalence of diabetes in older Mexican Americans (≥75 years) almost doubled from 1993 to 1994 and 2004 to 2005 from 20.3% to 37.2% in comparison to an increase from 10.4% to 16.4% in the general population of the same age.[9] Diabetes prevalence in nursing homes is also high. Of U.S. nursing home residents in 2004, 24.6% had diabetes; among residents aged 65 to 74, 75 to 84, and 85 years and older, the prevalence of diabetes was 36.1%, 29.5%, and 18.3%, respectively.[10] The prevalence of diabetes steadily increased in U.S. nursing homes between 1995 and 2004—16.9% to 26.4% in men and 16.1% to 22.2% in women. A more recent survey has shown a further increase in the prevalence of diabetes, with 32.8% of residents living with diabetes.[11] Ethnic disparities in diabetes prevalence have also been well documented in care home settings. In U.S. nursing homes, the adjusted odds of diabetes are approximately twofold higher in African American and Hispanic residents relative to white residents, with diabetes present in 22.5% of whites and in 35.6% of those from other ethnic groups.[10]

PATHOLOGIC PROCESS

Glucose homeostasis requires normal insulin secretion by the pancreatic beta cells and normal glucose utilization by the peripheral tissues that are sensitive to insulin. Diabetes in older adults is linked to increased insulin resistance and decreased insulin secretion, with a principal defect of insulin resistance in obese individuals and insulin secretion in lean ones. It is likely that genetic and environmental factors are involved in the pathogenesis of insulin secretory dysfunction and insulin resistance. Because older adults are heterogeneous, the extent and rate of deterioration in glucose homeostasis are variable, leading to insignificant changes in some individuals and diabetes in others (Box 90-1).

Rise in Insulin Resistance

Aging is associated with body composition changes that result in increased insulin resistance.[12] Increased visceral fat is associated with increased rates of lipolysis causing high levels of free fatty acids, which may have a role in reducing peripheral insulin sensitivity.[13] Reduction of muscle mass or sarcopenia occurs with aging through physical inactivity and, because the muscle is the main site of glucose consumption, the loss of muscle mass increases insulin resistance.[12] Accumulation of lipids within the muscles is another factor reducing insulin sensitivity. A reduction in mitochondrial function[14] may also contribute to age-related glucose intolerance by reducing oxidative metabolism, physical fitness, and oxidative capacity. Low concentrations of adiponectin, leptin, and insulin-like growth factor 1 (IGF-1) and high concentrations of tumor necrosis factor-α (TNF-α) are associated with

BOX 90-1 Factors Influencing Glucose Intolerance in Older Adults

- Decreased beta cell function
- Reduced beta cell mass
- Increased visceral fat
- Reduced muscle mass
- Mitochondrial dysfunction
- Low concentrations of adiponectin*
- High concentrations of tumeur necrosis factor-α†
- Reduced insulin-like growth factor-1 concentration‡
- Reduced leptin concentration§
- Physical inactivity
- Altered lipid metabolism

*Secreted by adipose tissue, which improves insulin resistance by increasing fat oxidation.
†Induces anorexia, weight loss, and insulin resistance.
‡A peptide hormone that stimulates glucose uptake.
§Secreted by adipose tissue, which decreases appetite, and its decline may contribute to the increased adiposity and body composition changes seen in older adults.

BOX 90-2 Diabetes Phenotype in Older Adults

- Multiple comorbidities
- Cognitive dysfunction
- Depression
- Physical dysfunction
- Falls and fractures
- Urinary incontinence
- Polypharmacy
- Less muscle mass and poor muscle quality
- Malnutrition
- Frailty
- Nutritional need and hydration
- Irregular eating pattern especially in people with dementia
- Vulnerability to hypoglycemia

aging and have been linked to increased insulin resistance and incident diabetes.[14-16]

Fall in Insulin Secretion

Insulin secretion diminishes by 0.7%/year with increasing age because of reduced function and increased apoptosis of pancreatic beta cells.[17] Beta cell autoimmunity may lead to the activation of an acute-phase response in older adults with diabetes, with hypersecretion of interleukins, C-reactive protein, and TNF-α, which may reduce insulin secretion.[18] Disturbances in the physiology of the gut-derived incretins, gastric inhibitory polypeptide (GIP) and glucagon-like peptide-1 (GLP-1), may be another factor involved in beta cell dysfunction.[19] Both peptides enhance insulin secretion after meals and may have a role in maintaining beta cell growth, proliferation, and inhibition of apoptosis. Aging is associated with reduced levels and function of these peptides.[20]

DIABETES PHENOTYPE IN OLD AGE

Diabetes in older adults is associated with coexistent multiple comorbidity burden, geriatric syndromes, and frailty (Box 90-2).

Comorbidity Impact

Diabetes in older adults is associated with increased atherosclerosis, premature aging, and increased disability. Older adults with diabetes frequently have at least one comorbid chronic disease in addition to diabetes, and as many as 40% have at least three conditions.[21] The comorbidity burden is even higher in nursing home residents with diabetes. For example, those with diabetes have more cardiovascular disease, visual problems, pressure sores, limb amputations, and kidney failure than residents without diabetes.[22] In a retrospective case review of 75 U.K. nursing home residents with diabetes, significant levels of disability were shown in areas of continence, feeding, mobility, and communication. The average number of comorbidities per individual was four (range, one to eight).[23] The mortality rate was 34% after 1 year of follow-up, indicating severe comorbidity.[24] In another study, residents with diabetes had a greater comorbidity burden (hierarchic condition category, 1.90 vs. 1.58), used more prescribed medications, and experienced more hospitalizations than residents without diabetes (37% vs. 18%).[11]

Geriatric Syndromes

Geriatric syndromes, such as cognitive and physical dysfunction, depression, falls, and urinary incontinence, are common in older adults with diabetes and may have subtle presentations.[25] Diabetes is associated with a twofold increased risk of being unable to perform daily physical tasks, such as walking, doing housework, or climbing stairs, and a 1.6-fold greater risk of difficulties performing basic personal care, such as bathing, using the toilet, dressing, and eating. Diabetes complications, such as neuropathy, arthritis, and vascular disease, are contributors to physical disability in older adults with diabetes.[26,27] The Study of Osteoporotic Fractures report[28] has shown that diabetes also increases the risk of falls (odds ratio [OR], 2.78; 95% confidence interval [CI], 1.82 to 4.25). A history of arthritis, musculoskeletal pain, depression, poor vision, and peripheral neuropathy are the main predictors of falling among older adults with diabetes.[28] The risk of developing Alzheimer disease or vascular dementia is twofold higher in older adults with diabetes compared to age-matched adults without diabetes.[29] In the Health, Aging, and Body Composition Study, older adults (70 to 79 years old) with diabetes had an increased incidence of depression compared with persons without diabetes (23.5% vs. 19.0%; hazard ratio [HR], 1.31; 95% CI, 1.07 to 1.61).[30]

Frailty

Frailty is a condition characterized by a reduction in physiologic reserve and the ability to resist physical or psychological stressors.[31] Its definition is largely based on the presence of three or more phenotypes (e.g., weight loss, weakness, decreased physical activity, exhaustion, slow gait speed).[32] Frailty is viewed as a wasting disease, with weight loss being one of its criteria. Undernutrition, which is common in older adults, seems to be a risk factor for frailty. In the United States, about 16% of older adults living in the community are undernourished. These figures rise to 59% in long-term care institutions and to 65% in acute-care hospitals.[33]

Sarcopenia—muscle mass loss—is a component of frailty, which seems to be accelerated when diabetes is present. In a community study of 3153 participants older than 65 years, appendicular lean mass loss in men with diabetes was twice that of men without diabetes (3.0% vs. 1.5%) and, in women with diabetes, was 1.8 times that of those without diabetes (3.4% vs. 1.9%) over 4 years of follow-up. The mechanisms explaining these results may be related to reduced muscle protein synthesis as a result of lower testosterone and IGF-1 levels and increased muscle protein breakdown caused by a higher rate of inflammation.[34] Diabetes also causes sarcopenia through the catabolic effect of insulin deficiency and by increasing intramyocellular lipid accumulation.[35] In another study, older adults with type 2 diabetes had accelerated declines in leg lean mass, muscle strength, and longer sit-to-stand time compared to those with normoglycemia.[36] Another factor related to malnutrition and frailty may be oral health. For example, optimal nutrition may not be maintained because of poor dentition, dry mouth, reduced taste sensation, palatability, and appetite change with increasing age.[37]

CLINICAL MANIFESTATIONS OF DISEASE

Diabetes can be asymptomatic in up to 50% of older adults.[38] However, when symptoms are present, they are mostly nonspecific and may be attributed to aging. Nonspecific symptoms, such as general malaise, fatigue, or lethargy, are common manifestation of diabetes in older adults. Geriatric syndromes, such as falls and urinary incontinence, may be the first manifestation of diabetes. Symptoms may be atypical—for example, anorexia rather than the typical polyphagia. The classic osmotic symptoms are usually less prominent because of the increased renal threshold for glucose, reducing the intensity of polyuria, and impairment of thirst sensation, reducing the intensity of polydipsia. A hyperosmolar hyperglycemic state may be the presenting symptom, or diabetes may first be diagnosed during an acute illness or following a routine blood test (Box 90-3).

DIAGNOSIS

The diagnostic criteria for diabetes are the same, irrespective of age. Clinicians should be aware that the fasting glucose concentration may be normal in the early stages of diabetes and is therefore less sensitive in diagnosing diabetes in older adults; however, the 2-hour glucose tolerance test appears to capture undiagnosed cases.[9]

Since February 2011, glycated hemoglobin (HbA_{1c}) has been used as a diagnostic test for diabetes. However, although HbA_{1c} has high specificity (98.7%), its low sensitivity (46.8%) means that it can miss more than 50%of people with diabetes.[40] There are a number of pitfalls to using HbA_{1c} in older adults. The HbA_{1c} level increases with age after adjustment for glucose, suggesting that nonglycemic factors contribute to this increase. Furthermore, iron deficiency anemia, which is common in older adults, is associated with an increase in the HbA_{1c} level independent of changes in the blood glucose level. Both these factors will lead to an overdiagnosis of diabetes in older adults if the HbA_{1c} level is used instead of the glucose level. The diagnosis should be confirmed by a second laboratory test in the absence of diabetes symptoms, as for younger people.

BOX 90-3 Diagnosis and Assessment Considerations

CLINICAL PRESENTATION AND DIAGNOSIS

- Fasting blood glucose level may be normal in up to one third of cases.
- Postprandial or 2-hour oral glucose tolerance test are more reliable.
- HbA_{1c} is specific but less sensitive as a diagnostic test.
- Symptoms may be absent in up to 50% of patients.
- Osmotic symptoms are less prominent.
- Other symptoms may be nonspecific, such as fatigue or lethargy.

COMPREHENSIVE GERIATRIC ASSESSMENT

A comprehensive geriatric assessment should be performed on initial diagnosis and annually, including assessment of the following:

- Cognitive function
- Screening for depression
- Assessment for frailty
- Falls risk
- Activities of daily living ability
- Presence of urinary incontinence and chronic pain
- Nutritional status
- Medication adherence and polypharmacy
- Social circumstances

TREATMENT AND OTHER MANAGEMENT ASPECTS

The phenotype of diabetes in older adults is highly variable and is affected by comorbidity, geriatric syndromes, and frailty. Therefore, diabetes management should take into account the heterogeneous nature of the diabetes and complex needs of the individual. A comprehensive geriatric assessment should be performed after the initial diagnosis and then annually because age-related comorbidities may impair diabetes control (Figure 90-1) Hyperglycemia should not be treated in isolation but as part of a multifactorial intervention to reduce cardiovascular risk. Cardiovascular complications remain the main cause of mortality, accounting for 50% to 75% of all deaths in people with diabetes.[41] Management includes lifestyle modifications and pharmacologic interventions for hyperglycemia and cardiovascular risk factors (Box 90-4).

Lifestyle Changes

Lifestyle modifications include changes in diet, weight reduction, smoking cessation (the single most effective means of reducing mortality[42]), and regular exercise to reduce visceral obesity and improve insulin sensitivity.

Aging is associated with increased insulin resistance through the loss of skeletal muscle mass.[12] Muscle mass is dependent on a balance between muscle protein synthesis and breakdown; protein intake with exercise training synergistically increases skeletal muscle mass in older adults. In one trial, protein supplementation for frail older adults who were engaged in resistance training resulted in muscle hypertrophy and increases in muscle strength, muscle mass, and performance.[43] A diet that is high in fiber and potassium and low in saturated fats and refined carbohydrates and salt may help achieve an ideal body weight and improve the lipid profile, significantly lowering blood pressure

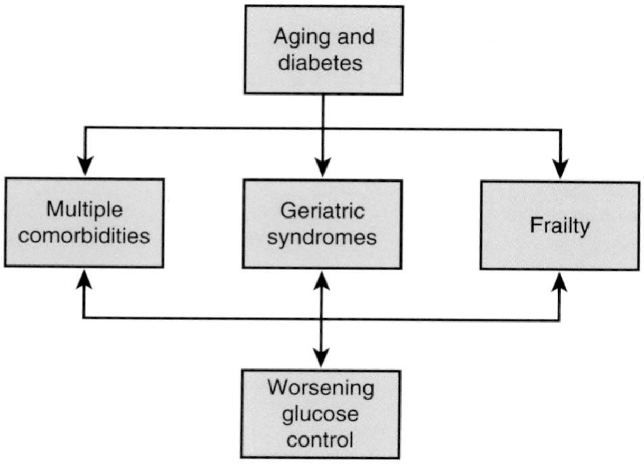

Figure 90-1. Key background conditions affecting glucose control in older people with diabetes.

BOX 90-4 Managing Cardiovascular Risk Factors

LIFESTYLE MODIFICATIONS

- Smoking cessation
- Balanced diet with adequate nutrition, especially in frail individuals
- Regular exercise
- Weight loss in overweight persons

HYPERGLYCEMIA

- Tight control in fit or newly diagnosed people
- Conservative approach in frail persons
- Avoidance of hypoglycemia

HYPERTENSION

- A target systolic blood pressure (BP) of 140 mm Hg is reasonable in fit individuals but a higher target, about 150 to 160 mm Hg, is appropriate in frail or much older (≥85 years) adults.
- Achieving a target BP is more important than the antihypertensive drug class used, and most patients will need more than one drug to achieve the target.

DYSLIPIDEMIA

- Statin therapy in older adults with diabetes is beneficial and should be offered unless specifically contraindicated or life expectancy is limited by frailty and comorbidities.
- The routine use of fibrate or niacin in addition to a statin is not recommended.

ASPIRIN

- Aspirin therapy should be considered selectively for older adults with diabetes and high cardiovascular risk, but after assessment of their bleeding risk.

MULTIPLE INTERVENTIONS

- Hypoglycemia should not be treated in isolation but as part of a multiple cardiovascular risk factors reduction.
- Statins and antihypertensive drugs have the largest effect on reducing cardiovascular events, followed by hypoglycemic agents and aspirin.

REVERSE METABOLISM

- In frail older adults, targets should be relaxed because of the inverse relationship between cardiovascular risk factors and mortality.

and reducing the overall cardiovascular risk.[44] In the Diabetes Prevention Program, lifestyle interventions, including modest weight reduction, healthy low-fat diet, and regular exercise reduced the development of diabetes; this beneficial effect persisted for up to 10 years after the end of the study, especially in older adults (≥60 years).[45] Additional benefits of exercise for older adults may include increased muscle strength and improved walking balance. The Look AHEAD (Action for Health in Diabetes) study in middle-aged and older adults with type 2 diabetes has shown that weight loss and improved fitness lower the risk of loss of mobility.[46]

Hyperglycemia

Although the evidence for reducing microvascular disease by tight glycemic control has been established, there is ongoing debate about whether reducing blood glucose to near-normal levels results in a lower incidence of cardiovascular events (Table 90-1).[47-50] In frail older adults, the benefit of blood glucose control diminishes in the presence of other comorbidities. In a decision analysis to assess the effects of baseline health status on prioritization of therapy, blood pressure control conferred a larger benefit than glucose control for older adults (75 to 79 years), and the expected benefits of both therapies steadily declined as the level of comorbidity and functional impairment increased.[51] Therefore, in older adults who are frail, with multiple comorbidities and functional impairment, tight control may be more harmful by inducing hypoglycemia. It is important to address individual goals of therapy, guided by patient preferences, life expectancy, comorbidities, and influences of therapy on quality of life. The advantages and disadvantages of hypoglycemic medications in older adults with diabetes are detailed in Table 90-2.

Hypertension

A target systolic blood pressure of about 140 mm Hg is reasonable in older adults with diabetes because maintenance of a systolic pressure between 130 and 140 mm Hg is associated with a reduction of adverse cardiovascular outcomes in older adults with hypertension and diabetes. Tighter control, however, is not warranted, because this may be associated with increased adverse events. In the International Verapamil SR-Trandolapril (INVEST) Study, controlling systolic blood pressure to less than 130 mm Hg was not associated with better cardiovascular outcomes than

TABLE 90-1 Summary of Key Studies of Glucose Control in Type 2 Diabetes Mellitus

	Study			
Parameter	*Ukpds Follow-Up*[47]	*Accord*[48]	*Advance*[49]	*Vadt*[50]
Number of participants	3,277	10,251	11,140	1,791
Mean age (yr; SD)	62 (8.0)	62.2 (6.8)	66 (6.0)	60.5 (9.0)
Inclusion criteria	Newly diagnosed type 2 diabetes mellitus (DM)	Age 40-79 yr, with history of CVD Age 55-79 yr, with evidence of atherosclerosis, albuminuria, LVH, or two additional risk factors for CVD	Diagnosis of type 2 DM at ≥30 yr of age *or* age ≥ 55 yr *or* history of macrovascular or microvascular disease	Type 2 DM with inadequate response to maximum dose of an oral agent or insulin therapy
History of cardiovascular disease (CVD)	People with significant CVD excluded	35%	32%	40%
Duration of diabetes on entry (yr)	Newly diagnosed	10.0	8.0	11.5
Cardiovascular outcome	Benefit	Harm	No benefit	No benefit

ACCORD, Action to Control Cardiovascular Risk in Diabetes; *ADVANCE,* Action in Diabetes and Vascular Disease: Preterax and Diamicron MR Controlled Evaluation; *LVH,* left ventricular hypertrophy; *UKPDS,* U.K. Prospective Diabetes Study; *VADT,* Veterans Affairs Diabetes Trial.

TABLE 90-2 Hypoglycemic Medications for Older Adults with Diabetes: Key Messages

Medication	Advantages	Disadvantages
Sulfonylureas	Suitable for those with renal impairment or less risk of hypoglycemia	Increased risk of hypoglycemia and weight gain; long-acting sulfonylureas should be avoided.
Metformin	Less risk of hypoglycemia, cardiovascular benefit, weight neutral	Increased risk of lactic acidosis in those with renal impairment, heart failure, sepsis, and dehydration
Meglitinides	Short-acting, suitable for those with erratic eating pattern	Risk of hypoglycemia and weight gain but less than sulfonylureas
α-Glucosidase inhibitors	Less risk of weight gain and hypoglycemia	Weak hypoglycemic action, gastrointestinal side effects
Pioglitazone	Suitable for those with renal impairment or less risk of hypoglycemia	Fluid retention, worsens heart failure, increases fracture risk, possibly bladder cancer
DPP-4 inhibitors	Low risk of hypoglycemia, weight loss	Gastrointestinal side effects, dose mostly needs to be adjusted with renal impairment
GLP-1 receptor analogues	Low risk of hypoglycemia, weight loss	Injectable, weight loss in frail individuals, not suitable in renal failure, nausea , possible risk of pancreatitis
Sodium glucose cotransporter 2 (SGLT2) inhibitors	Low risk of hypoglycemia, weight loss	Not suitable for frail older adults with weight loss; heavy glucosuria increases risk of urinary tract infections, candidiasis, dehydration, and hypotension
Insulin	Effective, tailored rapidly to changes in need, improves quality of life	High risk of hypoglycemia and weight gain

DPP-4, Dipeptidyl peptidase 4; *GLP-1,* glucagon like peptide-1.

usual control of 130 to 140 mm Hg in individuals 55 years of age and older, and it was associated with a nonsignificant increased risk of mortality (11.0% vs. 10.2%; adjusted hazard ratio [HR], 1.20; 95% confidence interval [CI], 0.99 to 1.45; *P* = .06).[52] Tight blood pressure control (target < 120 mm Hg systolic) was also not beneficial and was associated with adverse outcomes in older adults (40 to 79 years) with diabetes.[53] The Ongoing Telmisartan Alone and in Combination with Ramipril Global Endpoint Trial (ONTARGET) also had similar conclusions for older adults, mean age 66 ± 7 years, of whom 57% were older than 65 years.[54] Two meta-analyses of older adults with diabetes did not show reduced myocardial infarction or mortality rates with a systolic blood blood pressure less than 140 mm Hg.[55,56] In much older adults (>80 years), the targets may be even more relaxed. The Hypertension in the Very Elderly Trial (HYVET), which included older adults older than 80 years, with sustained systolic blood pressure higher than 180 mm Hg, 7% of whom had diabetes, showed a significant 33.7% reduction in cardiovascular events (HR, 0.66; 95% CI, 0.53 to 0.82; *P* < .001), with a target blood pressure control of 150/80 mm Hg. However, the individuals included in the HYVET study were healthier than those in the general population, with a low baseline rate of known cardiovascular disease (CVD; 11.5%), myocardial infarction (3.1%), and heart failure (2.9%). Therefore, the results may not apply to all older adults, especially those with multiple comorbidities or living in nursing homes.[57] In another community study of people older than 85 years, there was a U-shaped relationship, with a systolic blood pressure of 164.2 mm Hg (95% CI, 154.1 to 183.8 mm Hg) being associated with the lowest mortality suggesting that the optimal systolic blood pressure for this age group could be more than 140 mm Hg.[58] Thiazide diuretics, angiotensin receptor blockers, angiotensin-converting enzyme inhibitors, and calcium channel blockers are reasonable first-choice agents although higher doses of diuretics may worsen blood glucose levels and the lipid profile. Most people will require more than one antihypertensive agent.

Dyslipidemia

There have been no large clinical trials of lipid-lowering interventions specifically in older adults with diabetes. Post hoc analysis of the Heart Protection Study, which included participants with diabetes aged between 40 and 80 years, showed a significant 25% risk reductions of cardiovascular events.[59] A meta-analysis of 18,686 people with diabetes in 14 trials of statin therapy for primary prevention showed a similar 20% relative risk reduction in major adverse vascular outcomes in older adults (≥65 years) compared to younger adults (<65 years).[60] In the very old (>80 years), cholesterol targets are unclear. A review of observational studies including 13,622 participants has shown that low total cholesterol (<5.5 mmol/L) is associated with the highest mortality rate in those older than 80 years.[61] The routine use of a fibrate or niacin in addition to a statin therapy failed to reduce cardiovascular events beyond the effects of statins and is not recommended.[62,63] Cardiovascular prevention with statins emerges fairly quickly (within 1 to 2 years), suggesting that statins may be offered to nearly all older adults with diabetes, except those with very limited life expectancy. Chronologic age per se should not exclude people from receiving therapy, but functional or biologic age and the impact of long-term drug therapy on the safety and quality of life should also be considered.

Aspirin Therapy

Aspirin reduces cardiovascular morbidity and mortality in people with a history of cardiovascular disease.[64] However, evidence for aspirin use in primary cardiovascular risk prevention is still unclear. A meta-analysis of aspirin treatment as primary prevention in people with diabetes has demonstrated a trend toward a 10% reduction in cardiovascular events but this needs to be balanced against an increased risk of hemorrhage.[65] The presence of diabetes per se does not justify aspirin use. However, most older adults with diabetes have a high burden of cardiovascular risk factors and are likely to benefit from aspirin therapy. Therefore, aspirin use should be considered selectively in older adults with diabetes and high cardiovascular risk after assessment of the risk of bleeding.

Multiple Risk Intervention

Cardiovascular risk factors tend to cluster in what is known as the metabolic syndrome; age and diabetes increase the prevalence of metabolic syndrome. In a Norwegian study, the prevalence increased from 11.0% in men aged 20 to 29 years to 47.2% in men aged 80 to 89 years and from 9.2% to 64.4% for women in the corresponding age groups.[66] In a population-based study of 5632 white Europeans (65 to 84 years old), the prevalence was 64.9% and 87.1% in men and women with diabetes, respectively, compared to 25.9% and 55.2% in men and women without diabetes.[67] Although metabolic syndrome has been postulated as a risk factor for CVD in a prospective study of 1025 older adults aged 65 to 74 years[68] and an analysis of the outcomes of two prospective studies in people older than 60 years, the metabolic syndrome was shown to be a marker of CVD but did not enhance risk prediction above and beyond the risk associated with its individual components.[69]

Multifactorial interventions are appropriate and have shown that the use of statins and antihypertensive drugs has the largest effect on reducing cardiovascular events, with hypoglycemic agents and aspirin the next most important interventions.[70] More effort is needed to optimize this comprehensive approach; it is still suboptimal because many older adults do not receive this level of care.[71]

Reverse Metabolism

In frail older adults, the power of traditional cardiovascular risk factors, including hypertension, dyslipidemia, and hyperglycemia, to predict the risk of CVD seems to diminish with age, leading to a paradoxic relationship.[72] The more commonly proposed explanations have included the association of low body weight and low cholesterol levels with increased protein energy malnutrition and increased inflammation associated with frailty.[73] In a study of 331 much older adults (mean age, 85 ± 7 years), low body mass index, low blood pressure, low total and high-density lipoprotein (HDL) cholesterol levels, and high insulin sensitivity in individuals without diabetes predicted total mortality, indicating a so-called reverse metabolism, which is probably attributable to malnutrition and chronic disorders that have a negative impact on survival.[74] Low albumin (a marker of malnutrition) and high C-reactive protein (a marker of inflammation) levels were associated with these cardiometabolic factors, limiting their prognostic value for cardiovascular risk in older adults.[74] It is important to recognize that many older adults with diabetes are frail, and the expected benefit of tight metabolic control declines as morbidity and functional impairment increase; thus, functional status and level of comorbidity are important factors when assessing risk.[51]

CONSIDERATIONS IN OLD AGE

Hypoglycemia

Hypoglycemia is more common in older adults with diabetes because of the associated comorbidities, geriatric syndromes, polypharmacy, long duration of diabetes, and increased prevalence of hepatic and renal dysfunction (Box 90-5). Although there is a paucity of data about the incidence of hypoglycemia in older adults, the reported incidence of hypoglycemia varies in the literature owing to differences in the definition used and age of the populations studied. In a U.S. retrospective population-based study of 19,932 Medicaid patients, aged 65 years and older, the incidence of severe hypoglycemia was 1.23 episodes/100 person-years for people treated with sulfonylureas and 2.76 episodes/100 person-years in those treated with insulin.[75] However, the strict definition of severe hypoglycemia—an episode leading to fatal outcome or hospital admission—may have underestimated the true frequency of events. Also, the data were collected before publication of the evidence for the benefit of tight glycemic control in type 2 diabetes in 1998.[76]

The subsequent trends toward tighter glycemic control have resulted in more frequent hypoglycemic episodes, with insulin becoming the second most common medication associated with adverse events reported to the U.S. Food and Drug Administration (FDA) and a threefold increase in reported events from 1998 to 2005.[77] Insulin was the second most frequent medication associated with emergency department visits in older adults older than 65 years; 95.4% of episodes were related to hypoglycemia, 24.1% involved loss of consciousness or seizure, and 25.1% required hospitalization.[78] More recently, in a prospective study from the DiaRegis, a multicenter registry of people with diabetes in Germany involving 3,347 people, median age 66.1 years, the annual incidence of hypoglycemia of any severity was 14.1%.[79] Although hypoglycemia incidence is difficult to estimate accurately, it is likely to be higher in older than younger people. In a prospective observational study of 3,810 people in primary care, 11% of participants reported at least one episode of hypoglycemia of any severity in a 12-month period. Older adults (≥70 years) reported more episodes than younger adults (<60 years; 12.8% vs. 9.0%; $P < .01$). Significant differences were also seen for symptomatic episodes without a need for help (9.2% vs. 5.6%) and symptomatic episodes with a need for medical assistance (0.7% vs. 0.1%).[80] In nursing homes, the incidence of hypoglycemia is likely to be much higher than in a community setting, up to 41.9% in one study over a 1-year period (median, two; range, one to ten episodes/patient-year) because of the higher levels of comorbidity.[81]

BOX 90-5 Hypoglycemia

INCIDENCE

- Increased in older adults due to multiple comorbidities, undernutrition, polypharmacy, long duration of diabetes, and renal or hepatic impairment

DIFFICULT RECOGNITION

- Nonspecific symptoms
- Misdiagnosed as stroke, vertigo, or visual disturbance
- Misinterpreted as dementia-related symptoms, such as agitation or behavior change
- Atypical presentation, such as confusion or passive delirium
- Little warning or unawareness of autonomic symptoms
- Patients with dementia unable to communicate feelings or symptoms

CONSEQUENCES

- Acute events, such as cardiac arrhythmias or stroke
- Chronic consequences, such as mental and physical dysfunction

Recognition

Although hypoglycemia in older adults with diabetes is common, its recognition and diagnosis can be difficult. For example, owing to the predominance of neurologic rather than autonomic symptoms, hypoglycemia may present with symptoms such as dizziness or visual disturbances, resulting in misdiagnosis.[82] Another diagnostic challenge is the similarity in the clinical presentation of hypoglycemia with that of dementia, in which patients may present with agitation, increased confusion, or behavioral changes. Furthermore, symptoms of hypoglycemia tend to be less specific with increasing age. In a survey of hypoglycemia symptom perception by older adults with diabetes (age, 82.3 ± 3.9 years) attending an outpatient clinic, most respondents reported nonspecific symptoms of being generally unwell when their blood glucose level dropped, making the recognition of hypoglycemic episodes more difficult for health care professionals.[83] This was also demonstrated in the Action to Control Cardiovascular Risk in Diabetes (ACCORD) study, with nonspecific fatigue or weakness being the most common symptoms of hypoglycemia experienced by the participants (mean age, 62.2 ± 6.8 years).[84] In older adults, the threshold of autonomic symptoms of hypoglycemia occurs at a lower blood glucose concentration, whereas cognitive dysfunction occurs at a higher level compared with younger adults. Therefore, autonomic and neurologic symptoms occur almost simultaneously, with little warning.[85] This is referred to as impaired awareness of hypoglycemia.[86] Subclinical hypoglycemia or episodes with fewer symptoms may further reduce awareness, leading to a vicious cycle, whereby one episode of hypoglycemia can induce further hypoglycemia.[87] Therefore, many episodes of hypoglycemia may be unrecognized and underreported by those with diabetes and physicians; subsequently, the frequency is likely to be underestimated.

Consequences

Older adults with diabetes are likely to be at a higher risk of the adverse consequences of hypoglycemia because of the increased prevalence of comorbidities, undernutrition, and polypharmacy compared with younger people.[88] Severe hypoglycemia may lead to serious acute vascular events, such as stroke, myocardial infarction, acute cardiac failure, and ventricular arrhythmias.[89,90] The morbidity attributed to recurrent episodes of hypoglycemia is associated with silent and chronic complications, which could lead to significant physical and cognitive dysfunction and eventually to frailty, disability, and increased mortality. In a Taiwanese study of 234 residents aged 77.5 years living in long-term care facilities, of whom 35.5% had diabetes, hypoglycemia was associated with disability and reduced function. Functional status was worse in those who experienced hypoglycemia compared to those with no history of hypoglycemia (mean Barthel Index score, 22.5 vs. 38.2). Complete dependence, defined as a Barthel Index score lower than 30, was also more common in people with hypoglycemia (69.2% vs. 50%).[81] The burden of hypoglycemia leading to hospitalization is higher in older adults and may contribute to increased frailty and reduced quality of life. In a U.S. study of 33,492 people with diabetes, aged about 60 years, accidents resulting in hospital visits occurred in 5.5% of those with hypoglycemia compared to 2.8% of those without. Hypoglycemia was associated with significantly increased hazards for any accident (HR, 1.39; 95% CI, 1.21 to 1.59; $P < .001$), accidental falls (HR, 1.36; 95% CI, 1.13 to 1.65; $P < .001$), and motor vehicle accidents (HR, 1.82; 95% CI, 1.18 to 2.80; $P = .007$) after adjustment for baseline characteristics. In an age-stratified analysis, the risk of falls was twice as high among older adults, 65 years and older, compared with younger individuals, and hypoglycemia was significantly associated with a greater than 50% increase in the hazard of falls (adjusted HR, 1.52; 95% CI, 1.18 to 1.95).[91] Hypoglycemia also increases the risk of fractures, which may lead to disability and frailty. In a retrospective observational study of 361,210 Medicare-covered patients with diabetes older than 65 years, those with hypoglycemic events had a significantly higher proportion of fall-related fractures compared to those without hypoglycemia (5.24% vs. 2.67%; $P < .001$). Hypoglycemic events increased the risk of falls and fractures by 70% (odds ratio [OR], 1.7; 95% CI, 1.58 to 1.83).[92]

Cognitive Decline and Dementia

Progressive decline in cognitive function leading to dementia is common in older adults with diabetes. Persistent hyperglycemia increases the risk of cerebrovascular disease by inducing inflammation, endothelial dysfunction, oxidative stress, and insulin resistance, leading to an increased incidence of vascular dementia.[93] Moreover, accelerated brain aging from altered amyloid metabolism, increased protein glycation, and direct cerebral glucotoxicity may explain the increased incidence of Alzheimer dementia.[94] Structural changes in the brain have been noted in those with with diabetes and dementia. For example, cerebral atrophy and hippocampal atrophy have been reported more frequently in older adults with diabetes and contribute to cognitive dysfunction, especially impairment in immediate memory.[95] It seems that brain insulin resistance increases in Alzheimer disease (AD), suggesting that AD might be caused by a cerebral manifestation of diabetes.

Risk

Among people with diabetes, the relative risk of AD is 1.56 (95% CI, 1.41 to 1.73), whereas vascular dementia is increased 2.27-fold (1.94 to 2.66) and all types of dementia by 1.73-fold (1.65 to 1.82) compared to those without diabetes.[96] In a prospective study of older adults (>60 years) with diabetes, age, microvascular disease, diabetic foot, cerebrovascular disease, cardiovascular disease, acute metabolic events, depression, and level of education were used to develop a risk score for dementia. Over 10 years, the risk of developing dementia was 5.3% (95% CI, 4.2 to 6.3) for the lowest score (−1) and 73.3% (95% CI, 64.8 to 81.8) for the highest (12 to 19) sum scores.[97] The presence of diabetes also accelerates mortality rate in people with dementia. In a retrospective Australian study, the mortality rate for people with diabetes and dementia was almost twice that of those with dementia but without diabetes (HR, 1.9; 95% CI, 1.3 to 2.9).[98]

Implications

Older adults with diabetes and dementia experience difficulties in performing self-care tasks. In a community-based study of 1398 people with diabetes, aged 70 years, adherence to diabetes self-care tasks decreased as cognitive impairment increased, with exercise and diet adherence being the factors most strongly associated with cognitive impairment.[99] The combination of diabetes and dementia is likely to be associated with an increased incidence of treatment adverse events, such as severe hypoglycemia.[100] Due to erratic eating patterns associated with dementia, older adults with diabetes are also at risk of malnutrition, dehydration, and worsening diabetes control. Caregivers of people with diabetes and dementia face extraordinary challenges to care for both conditions, especially in those who develop behavior changes. Their needs should be identified early to allow for greater support from those in the health care system.

Management

Although there is an association between hyperglycemia and cognitive dysfunction, intensive glycemic control does not prevent a decline in mental function.[101] Once dementia develops, diabetes self-care deteriorates, so clinicians need to check for cognitive dysfunction if there is nonadherence to self-care tasks. Clinicians should also be aware that dementia may be associated with language impairment, disorientation, and personality changes, which may mimic the symptoms of hypoglycemia.[102] The Mini-Cog test is a simple screening tool for dementia, with a sensitivity of 86.4% (95% CI, 64.0 to 96.4) and specificity of 91.1% (95% CI, 85.6 to 94.6) and takes only 3 minutes to administer.[103]

Older adults with diabetes and dementia have complex needs because of increased dependency and unpredictable behavioral changes as the decline in cognitive function continues. For example, because of impaired thirst sensation, hydration should be maintained to avoid the risk of volume depletion and hyperglycemic crises. In people treated with insulin, the new class of long-acting insulin analogues may be a good option because they reduce the risk of hypoglycemia and can be conveniently injected once daily.[104] People who have erratic eating patterns and unpredictable caloric intake could be managed with a regimen in which short-acting insulin analogues are administered only after meal consumption, thus reducing the risk of hypoglycemia if a meal is missed or only partly consumed.

Hypoglycemia-Dementia Interaction

The brain is highly dependent on glucose for its metabolism and is particularly vulnerable to hypoglycemia, especially in older adults. After each hypoglycemic episode, major cognitive changes, occur leading to posthypoglycemic encephalopathy. Repeated episodes of hypoglycemia may contribute to cognitive dysfunction, and the relationship appears to be bidirectional. A history of severe hypoglycemia increases risk of cognitive dysfunction,[105] and cognitive dysfunction increases risk of hypoglycemia.[106] Therefore, recurrent hypoglycemia may be associated with impaired cognitive function and development of dementia. In a retrospective study of 16,667 older adults with diabetes, mean age 65 years, the risk of dementia increased by 26% (HR, 1.26; 95% CI, 1.10 to 1.49), 80% (HR,1.80; 95% CI, 1.37 to 2.36), and 94% (HR,1.94; 95% CI, 1.42 to 2.64) in those with a history of one, two, and three or more severe hypoglycemic episodes—defined as hypoglycemia needing hospital admission or an emergency department visit—respectively, independent of glycemic control, medications, and comorbidities. The attributable risk of dementia was 2.39%/year (range, 1.72% to 3.01%/year) in those with a history of hypoglycemia compared to those with no history of hypoglycemia.[105]

In an observational cohort study of 302 participants with diabetes, mean age 75.7 ± 4.6 years, a cross-sectional association between severe hypoglycemia and cognitive function was observed. People with dementia (16% of participants) or cognitive impairment (14%) were significantly more likely to have been hospitalized with hypoglycemia than those with normal cognitive function (3.8%; $P = .004$).[107] A prospective association between a history of hypoglycemia and cognitive decline in a subsample of participants without dementia was not found. However, the prospective phase of this study was limited by the small number of participants ($N = 205$) and short duration of follow-up (18 months), which may have limited the power to detect any association between incident hypoglycemia and cognitive dysfunction.[100]

More recently, in an Edinburgh population-based cross sectional study of 1,066 people with type 2 diabetes, mean age 67.9 ± 4.2 years, self-reported history of severe hypoglycemia was associated with poorer late-life cognitive ability.[108] Those who reported at least one episode of severe hypoglycemia demonstrated poorer performance on tests of verbal fluency (34.5 vs. 37.3; $P = .02$), digit symbol testing (45.9 vs. 49.9; $P = .002$), letter-number sequencing (9.1 vs. 9.8; $P = .005$) and trail making ($P < .001$), independently of diabetes duration, vascular risk factors, or vascular complications. These associations persisted after adjustment for estimated prior cognitive ability, suggesting that the association may be attributable to an effect of hypoglycemia on age-related cognitive decline.[108] A linear relationship was observed between poorer general cognitive ability and increasing frequency of severe hypoglycemia over the year preceding cognitive testing, supporting results of earlier studies.

Glycemic Targets

Glycemic targets should be individualized, taking into consideration overall health and life expectancy.

Targets for Fit Older Adults

For healthier older adults with a low prevalence of cardiovascular risk factors, especially those with a new diagnosis of diabetes, tight glycemic control with an hemoglobin A_{1c} (HbA_{1c}) value of about 53 mmol/mol (7%) is reasonable, because this is likely to reduce complications of diabetes.[47] However, persistent hyperglycemia is associated with an increased risk of falls[109] and mortality,[110] regardless of the associated comorbidities.

Targets for Frail Older Adults

For frail older adults or those with established cardiovascular disease, a safer target, about 58 to 64 mmol/mol (7.5% to 8%) is appropriate. The presence of multiple comorbidities is a potential competitor for the benefit of tight glycemic control in this population. In a decision analysis to assess the effects of comorbid conditions and functional impairment, the expected benefits of tight glycemic control, an HbA_{1c} value of 53 versus 63 mmol/mol (7% vs 7.9%) declined steadily as the level of comorbidities and functional impairment increased. Each comorbidity was allocated one or two points, according to severity, to create a mortality index score. In older adults aged 60 to 64 years with new-onset diabetes, the quality-adjusted days declined from 106 days (95% CI, 97 to 117) to 44 days (range, 38 to 50 days), with three additional points in mortality index score, and to 8 days (range, 5 to 10 days) with seven additional index points.[51]

Targets for Very Frail Older Adults

For very frail older adults and those residents in nursing homes and limited life expectancy, a target HbA_{1c} of 64 to 75 mmol/mol (8% to 9%) is suitable. Tight glycemic control in this population may be harmful by inducing hypoglycemia and reducing quality of life. However, a higher HbA_{1c} value, more than 75 mmol/mol (>9.0%) is associated with increased mortality.[111] Targets in this population should focus on short-term daily blood glucose control, rather than on long-term HbA_{1c}, to avoid hyperglycemia, which may lead to lethargy, dehydration, visual impairment, and infections, and hypoglycemia, which may lead to falls and confusion (Figure 90-2).

Polypharmacy

Clinical guidelines are largely disease-specific, age-neutral, and driven by numeric surrogates, such as HbA_{1c} or blood pressure values, but do not necessarily consider hard end points and outcomes relevant to older adults, such as physical function, disability, and quality of life.[112] The indiscriminate application of guidelines may lead to overtreatment and polypharmacy, with potential harm and increased hospitalization in older adults. For example, older adults are more liable to experience adverse effects to antihypertensive medications, such as renin-angiotensin system blockers, leading to acute kidney injury, hyperkalemia, or hypotension, with further deterioration of renal function, especially in those with existing chronic kidney disease (CKD). Withdrawal of these drugs in older adults (mean age, 73.3 years) with stage 4 or 5 CKD has been shown to improve kidney function.[113] A gradual decrease of blood pressure is an essential strategy in treating older adults with hypertension to avoid an accelerated blood pressure drop, with subsequent falls. Blood pressure should be measured with the patient lying and standing, and patients should be asked about orthostatic symptoms to avoid orthostatic hypotension. It is important to realize that the presence of orthostatic symptoms, such as dizziness, lightheadedness, or faintness, is associated with an increased risk of falls (OR, 8.21; 95% CI, 4.17 to 16.19) rather than orthostatic hypotension per se.[114]

Avoidance of hypoglycemia is essential, especially for those with impaired kidney or liver function, which delay the clearance of hypoglycemic medications.[115] Glycemic goals should be regularly reviewed and hypoglycemic medications adjusted with increasing age, especially in those with the onset of cognitive impairment or frailty. Declining weight, malnutrition, and frailty may lead to a reduced need for hypoglycemic medications while increasing the risk of hypoglycemia. Hypoglycemic medications were safely withdrawn in a cohort of frail nursing home older adults with type 2 diabetes, mean age 84.4 ± 6.8 years,[116] and in another group in the community, mean age, 86.5 ± 3.2 years, who

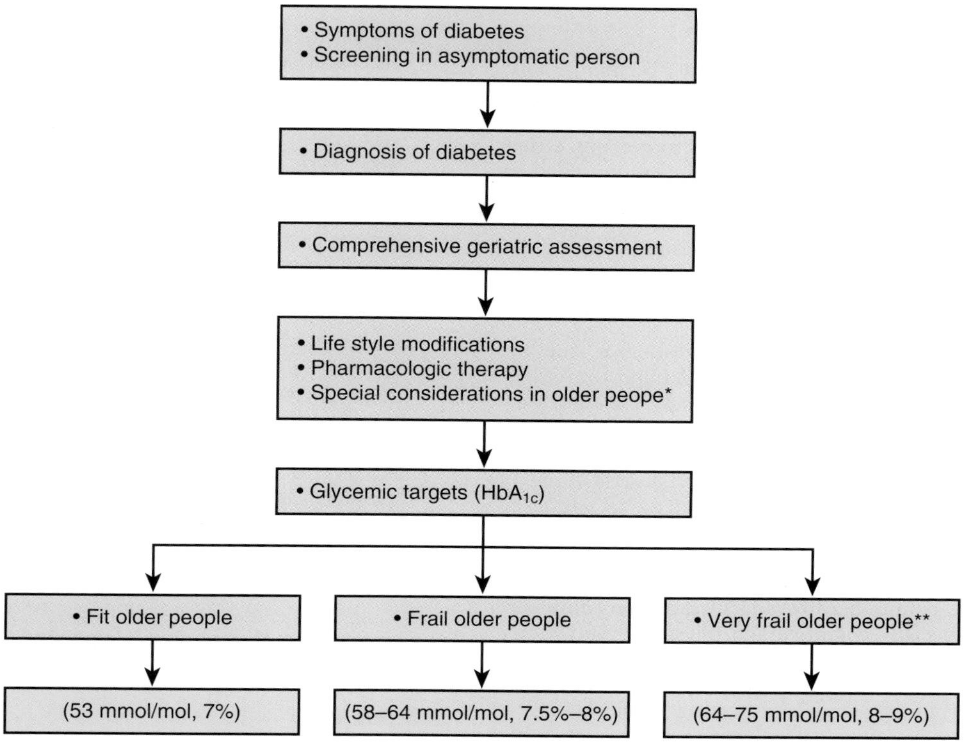

Figure 90-2. Glucose control and functional status categories.

were attending outpatient clinics without deterioration of their glycemic control.[117] Their main features were significant weight loss, increased comorbidities, including dementia, and polypharmacy, with recurrent hypoglycemia.[117] Therefore, people with these criteria appear to be suitable candidates for a trial of hypoglycemic medication withdrawal. Higher doses of statins should be avoided in frail older adults, who may be more susceptible to drug-related myopathy. Nonsteroidal antiinflammatory drugs should be used carefully in older adults with diabetes, especially those with CKD, because of the increased risk of acute kidney injury. Polypharmacy (>4 drugs) is common; in a British nursing home study, 84% of residents with diabetes were taking more than four drugs, with a high proportion of residents (59%) prescribed drugs for CVD prevention. This may be inappropriate in this disabled population with limited life expectancy because polypharmacy leads to an increased risk of drug errors, hypoglycemia, and hospitalization. Therefore, a regular medication review of nursing home residents with diabetes should be undertaken because it has the potential to reduce costs and minimize adverse drug reactions.[118]

Nursing Homes

Nursing home residents with diabetes are likely to be frail, with multiple comorbidities and limited life expectancy. Therefore, short-term glycemic targets with minimal diabetes-related interventions are important to maintain quality of life. Maintaining a random blood glucose level between 4 and 15 mmol/L (70 to 270 mg/dL) is reasonable, because a blood glucose level outside this range is likely to be symptomatic and result in cognitive changes.[119] Maintaining blood glucose in this comfort zone may ensure comfort care, avoiding hyperglycemia and hypoglycemia and thereby reducing malaise and improving mental function and general well-being.[120]

Care Plans

Nursing homes should have a policy for diabetes care, including diabetes screening for residents on admission and individualized care plan for residents. Care plans should be tailored to individual needs and take into consideration patients' values, preferences, life expectancy, comorbidities, and impact of diabetes management (e.g., polypharmacy, glucose monitoring) on quality of life. Medications should be reviewed to switch patients taking longer acting sulfonylureas to shorter acting agents, and polypharmacy should be reviewed regularly. Screening for complications relevant to older adults, such as cognition, physical function, and depression, should be included in the annual review.

Nutrition

Nutritional guidelines should not be too restrictive but tailored to attain optimal health and reflect personal preferences. Individuals are free to exercise personal choices with respect to food selection. Diabetes treatment is then adjusted accordingly. The aims of nutritional intervention include maintenance of healthy body weight and avoidance of malnutrition.

Holistic Approach

An individualized holistic care plan is recommended to address nursing home residents' complex needs.[121] Residents with diabetes should have an annual comprehensive foot examination to identify risk factors for ulcers and amputations. Podiatry input should be available regularly. Residents with diabetes should have an initial comprehensive eye examination and annually thereafter. Optometric services provided in the nursing home may be an option for residents who are not able to travel.

Education

Because older adults are at increased risk of hypoglycemia[82,90] and may tolerate low blood glucose levels with no specific symptoms due to their diminished autonomic response, it is important that residents and nursing home staff be educated to recognize the symptoms and treat hypoglycemia. In a study that provided a diabetes educational program to nursing home staff, staff knowledge improved, was retained at 12 months, and led to improved quality of care for up to 1 year after the intervention.[122]

CONCLUSION

Aging is associated with increased insulin resistance due to decreased muscle mass and increased visceral fat and decreased insulin secretion due to diminished beta cell mass and function, leading to glucose intolerance and diabetes in genetically susceptible individuals. As a result of population aging and increased life expectancy, diabetes has increasingly becoming a disease of older adults. The phenotype of diabetes in older adults is characterized by an increased prevalence of multiple comorbidities, geriatric syndromes, and frailty (see Table 90-2). Therefore, the assessment of older adults with diabetes at diagnosis and annually thereafter should be comprehensive and include screening for these syndromes, especially cognitive and physical dysfunction. Older adults are a highly heterogeneous population, ranging from a fit person living in the community to a frail individual with multiple comorbidities living in a nursing home. Management should therefore be individualized, with variable metabolic targets, from tight control in fit individuals to a conservative approach in frail older adults. More attention should be focused on optimal management of undernutrition in frail older adults by improving nutrition and physical activity to maintain muscle mass and improve overall function. Quality of life should be at the center of the management plan.

FUTURE CARE PROSPECTS

Although tight glycemic control will continue to be the aim for older fit and independent older adults with diabetes, this is not suitable for those who are frail and at a high risk of side effects due to polypharmacy.[123] A new approach to defining glycemic targets based on the level of function has recently been introduced by the International Diabetes Federation and represents the first comprehensive guidance in this area.[124]

There is a need for clinical trials specifically designed for older adults with diabetes to explore the real benefit of glycemic control in this diverse group. Comprehensive geriatric assessment, including physical and mental health assessment, will continue to be essential in view of the epidemiologic shift of diabetes toward older adults. Frailty and geriatric syndromes have been emerging as complications in older adults with diabetes and will need interventions beyond glycemic control. There remains a lack of intervention studies that reduce disability and improve quality of life in older adults with diabetes. A focus on improvements in function may be of greater clinical relevance in frail older adults with diabetes than metabolic targets alone. The MID-Frail study will evaluate the clinical, functional, social, and economic impacts of a multimodal intervention—resistance training exercise, diet, and education—in frail and prefrail participants older than 70 years with type 2 diabetes compared with usual clinical practice.[125] This may have an effect on reducing functional decline, promoting independence and maintaining quality of life.

KEY POINTS

- The phenotype of diabetes in older adults is characterized by an increased prevalence of multiple comorbidities, geriatric syndromes, and frailty.
- A comprehensive functional assessment (physical and cognitive) should be performed at the initial diagnosis of diabetes and annually thereafter.
- Hypoglycemia is common in older adults with diabetes owing to multiple comorbidities and can be less easily recognized or misdiagnosed because of reduced autonomic symptoms.
- A deterioration in glycemic control, unexplained hypoglycemia, or reduced adherence to self-care should alert the clinician to the presence of dementia or depression.
- Tighter glycemic control is reasonable in fit older adults but a relaxed approach is more appropriate in frail older adults at risk of hypoglycemia.
- An individualized and holistic care plan is key for diabetes care in older adults.
- Patient safety and quality of life should always be the focus for individualized care.

For a complete list of references, please visit www.expertconsult.com.

KEY REFERENCES

4. Kirkman MS, Briscoe VJ, Clark N, et al: Diabetes in older adults. Diabetes Care 35:2650–2664, 2012.
27. Volpato S, Blaum C, Resnick H, et al: Comorbidities and impairments explaining the association between diabetes and lower extremities disabilities. Diabetes Care 25:678–683, 2002.
28. Gregg EW, Mangione CM, Cauley JA, et al: Study of Osteoporotic Fractures Research Group: diabetes and incidence of functional disability in older women. Diabetes Care 25:61–67, 2002.
32. Fried LP, Tangen CM, Walston J, et al: Frailty in older adults : Evidence for a phenotype. J Gerontol A Biol Sci Med Sci 56A:M146–M156, 2001.
47. Holman RR, Paul SK, Bethel MA, et al: 10-year follow-up of intensive glucose control in type 2 diabetes. N Engl J Med 359:1577–1589, 2008.
51. Huang ES, Zhang Q, Gandra N, et al: The effect of comorbid illness and functional status on the expected benefits of intensive glucose control in older patients with type 2 diabetes: a decision analysis. Ann Intern Med 149:11–19, 2008.
94. Biessels GJ, Staekenborg S, Brunner E, et al: Risk of dementia in diabetes mellitus: a systematic review. Lancet Neurol 5:64–74, 2006.
111. Huang ES, Liu JY, Moffet HH, et al: Glycemic control, complications, and death in older diabetic patients: the diabetes and aging study. Diabetes Care 34:1329–1336, 2011.
121. Sinclair AJ, Task and Finish Group of Diabetes UK: Good clinical practice guidelines for care home residents with diabetes: an executive summary. Diabet Med 28:772–777, 2011.
123. Sinclair A, Dunning T, Rodriguez-Mañas L: Diabetes in older people: new insights and remaining challenges. Lancet Diabetes Endocrinol. 3:275–285, 2015.
124. Dunning T, Sinclair A, Colagiuri S: New IDF guideline for managing type 2 diabetes in older people. Diabetes Res Clin Pract 103:538–540, 2014.
125. Rodríguez-Mañas L, Bayer AJ, Kelly M, et al: An evaluation of the effectiveness of a multi-modal intervention in frail and pre-frail older adults with type 2 diabetes—the MID-Frail study: study protocol for a randomised controlled trial. Trials 15:34, 2014.

91 Blood Disorders in Older Adults

William B. Ershler

There is an old maxim—"Hematology is the study of blood, and the organs it perfuses." This would seem particularly germane to geriatric medicine. Accordingly, the nuances of the interactions of blood on other organs are outside the scope of this chapter. Instead, we provide broad strokes of key topics in modern hematology while maintaining our focus on geriatric issues of clinical relevance.

Most circulating cells are derived from a single hematopoietic stem cell. The life span of blood cells is genetically predetermined, and the stem cells from which these cells are derived are programmed to survive well in excess of the human life span.[1] Hematopoietic stem cells lack the surface molecules associated with differentiation (maturation), but they do express the $CD34^+$ molecule on their surface, a feature that has important clinical implications. Hematopoietic stem cells give rise to unipotent progenitor cells that then divide and differentiate into recognizable cells of a specific lineage. This differentiation process is considered to be random. Once a specific cell line has been determined (e.g., leukocyte, erythrocyte), the progenitor cells go through further differentiation to manifest their ultimate predestined phenotype. This is accomplished by upregulation of specific receptors under the influence of multiple cytokines and growth factors. Some of these cytokines—for example, erythropoietin and granulocyte colony-stimulating factor—have, in recent years, become important clinical tools.

With aging, there is a notable reduction in the capacity to produce new blood cells. However, unless there is substantial physiologic stress, the number of circulating cells remains fairly constant. Quantitative deficiencies are only apparent when stress produces a demand that exceeds the reserve proliferative capacity. This might occur during an acute infection or after cytotoxic chemotherapy. Significant qualitative deficiencies in blood cell function are not thought to be a consequence of aging, but may be associated with age-associated chronic diseases.[2]

Acknowledging that the discipline of hematology extends well beyond the scope of this chapter, we attempt in this chapter to provide an overview of blood disorders particularly relevant to older adults and common enough to be encountered by the practicing geriatrician. These include anemia, myelodysplasia, myeloproliferative disorders, hematologic malignancies, and disorders of hemostasis.

ANEMIA

Anemia is a significant health problem in older adults due to a high prevalence and significant associated morbidity (Table 91-1).[3] Although there has been a long-established perspective that anemia in older adults is of little consequence, studies have shown that even mild decreases in hemoglobin levels are associated with reduced quality of life, clinical depression, falls, functional impairment, slower walking speed, reduced grip strength, loss of mobility, worsening comorbidities, mortality, and anemia. These therefore require a greater focus on this problem.[4] Currently, screening for anemia is not generally practiced, and thus it is typically discovered during a workup for other conditions, when many of its deleterious effects may have already occurred.

The World Health Organization (WHO) has defined anemia as a hemoglobin level of less than 13 g/dL in adult males and less than 12 g/dL in adult females.[5] In older men and women, anemia by this definition is associated with an increase in mortality.[6-11] It has been noted that the WHO criteria do not take into account inherent racial variations, particularly with respect to African Americans, who may have lower levels of hemoglobin without significant adverse outcomes.[12,13] In a study that analyzed 1018 black and 1583 white older adults aged 71 to 82 years, anemia was associated with increased mortality in whites but not blacks.[12,13]

The issue of defining criteria for the diagnosis of anemia is also relevant in the context of age. Older women, for example, have better physical performance and function at hemoglobin values between 13 and 15 g/dL than from 12 to 12.9 g/dL,[14] suggesting perhaps that a cutoff level of 12 g/dL is too low. Nevertheless the WHO definition remains the current standard used in most current epidemiologic surveys and many clinical laboratories.

Prevalence of Anemia

Guralnik and colleagues have examined the third National Health and Nutrition Examination Survey (NHANES III) database, a nationally representative sample of community-dwelling individuals; they determined age- and gender-specific prevalence rates of anemia in the total U.S. population.[15] For those older than 65 years, by WHO criteria, approximately 11% were anemic (see Table 91-1). The prevalence of anemia was lowest (1.5%) among males from 17 to 49 years of age and highest (26.1%) in men older than 85 years. Among those 65 years of age and older, the prevalence rate was notably higher in African Americans compared to whites and Hispanics. Prevalence rates of anemia in older adults vary in community-dwelling and institutionalized populations. It is also clear that anemia is more common among frail older adults. In nursing homes, for example, anemia prevalence approaches 50% or higher.[16-20]

Pathogenesis

In younger adults with anemia, the cause is usually readily apparent. In older adult patients, however, discerning the cause of anemia can often be challenging (Table 91-2). Inflammation, nutritional deficiencies, and renal insufficiency are commonly observed, but for as many as one third of anemic older adults (and almost 50% for those residing in nursing homes), the anemia cannot be attributed to conventional causes, a condition now termed *unexplained anemia*.[21]

Anemia of Inflammation

Chronic diseases, such as atherosclerosis, diabetes, arthritis, infection, and malignancy, increase in prevalence with age, and each is characterized by inflammatory processes.[22] Although there are several ways in which inflammation can negatively influence erythropoiesis, disordered iron kinetics is a common feature.[23-25] During inflammation, there is reduced iron absorption from the gastrointestinal (GI) tract and defective reutilization of iron

TABLE 91-1 Anemia Prevalence in Older Adults Using the WHO Criteria

Study	Age (yr)	Population	Prevalence (%)
Gurlanik[15]	≥65	Community-dwelling older Americans	10.6
Ferrucci[281]	>70	Community-dwelling older Italians	11
Denny[282]	≥71	Community-dwelling older adults	24
Joosten[283]	≥65	Hospitalized older adults	24 (defined as hemoglobin < 11.5 g/dL)
Artz[16]	Most ≥ 65	Nursing home residents	48
Robinson[19]	Most ≥ 65	Nursing home residents	53
Sahin[20]	Most ≥ 65	Nursing home residents	54

TABLE 91-2 Features of Anemia by Classification

Parameter	MCV	Iron/ TIBC	Ferritin	ESR and CRP	EPO	CrCl
IDA	Small	Low/high	Low	WNL	High	WNL
ACI	Small	Low/low	Low to high	High	High	WNL
CKD	WNL	WNL	WNL	WNL	Low	<30 mL/min
Vitamin B_{12}–folate	LARGE	WNL	WNL	WNL	High	WNL
Hypothyroid	LARGE	WNL	WNL	WNL	High	WNL
MDS	WNL—large	WNL	WNL	WNL	High	WNL
UA	WNL	WNL	WNL	WNL	Low	>30 mL/min

ACI, anemia of chronic inflammation; *CrCl,* creatinine clearance; *CRF,* chronic kidney disease; *CRP,* C-reactive protein; *EPO,* serum erythropoietin; *ESR,* erythrocyte sedimentation rate; *IDA,* iron deficiency anemia; *MCV,* mean corpuscular volume; *MDS,* myelodysplastic syndrome; *TIBC,* total iron-binding capacity; *TSH,* thyroid-stimulating hormone; *UA,* unexplained anemia; WNL, within normal limits.

sequestered in reticuloendothelial cells. Hepcidin, a 25-amino-acid polypeptide produced in the liver in response to inflammatory stimuli, downregulates intestinal iron absorption and macrophage and monocyte iron release, thereby creating functional iron deficiency and resultant hypoproliferative anemia.[26-30] Reduced secretion of erythropoietin due to the action of inflammatory cytokines is also known to play a role in the anemia of chronic inflammation.[31,32]

Iron Deficiency Anemia

The prevalence of iron deficiency in older adults ranges from 2.5% to as high as 30% in some studies. Iron deficiency is usually secondary to iron loss, rather than inadequate intake, and is important to identify because it may be a manifestation of an occult malignancy.[33] For example, in one study of 114 outpatients referred to a gastroenterologist for investigation of iron deficiency, 45 had upper GI bleeding and 18 had colonic sources of bleeding.[34] In an older study of 100 patients in whom the site of bleeding could not be established by any means other than laparotomy, a malignancy was found to be the cause in 10%.[35] In a survey of 1388 patients older than 65 years, 25% were anemic, and approximately one third were iron-deficient. Of those with iron deficiency, GI endoscopy found 57% to have an upper GI lesion and 27% to have colonic lesions. In total, GI malignancy was found in 15% of those with iron deficiency anemia.[36]

Iron deficiency may be the result of GI malabsorption, particularly in patients who have had bowel resection or inflammatory bowel disease or have been on chronic antacid therapy. Furthermore, malabsorption of iron may an early manifestation of celiac disease.[37,38]

For patients who present with anemia and microcytic red blood cell indices, serum levels of iron, ferritin, and transferrin saturation are typically low, and the total iron-binding capacity is elevated. The coexistence of chronic inflammatory disease may complicate analysis. To determine whether patients with chronic inflammation and anemia are iron-deficient, measurement of the soluble transferrin receptor is frequently useful. Under conditions of iron deficiency, the transferrin receptor is upregulated, and increased levels are found in the serum. An index derived by dividing the serum level of soluble transferrin receptor by the log of the ferritin level, has been shown to be helpful.[39] A ratio less than 2 denotes anemia of chronic inflammation, whereas a value greater than 2 identifies patients with uncomplicated iron deficiency anemia or a combination of iron deficiency and inflammation.

In light of the adverse consequences of anemia, older patients with anemia should be treated as possible prior to diagnostic studies to define the cause for the iron deficiency. Parenteral iron is commonly prescribed in current practice,[24] but it is notable that oral replacement can be very effective, even at low doses.[40]

Vitamin B_{12} and Folate

Since the implementation of the U.S. Food and Drug Administration (FDA) policy of folic acid fortification of cereal grain products in 1998, there has been a dramatic reduction in measurable folate deficiency. Just 2 years after implementation, examination of the NHANES cohort IV (1999 to 2000), compared with cohort III (1988 to 1994) revealed the prevalence of low serum folate concentrations (<6.8 nmol/L), decreased from 16% before to 0.5% after fortification.[41] Thus, folic acid deficiency is currently an uncommon cause of anemia. Vitamin B_{12} deficiency, however, remains a problem, particularly in older adults.[42] Most cases of vitamin B_{12} deficiency in older adults is due to food cobalamin malabsorption, with true dietary deficiency or pernicious anemia being significantly less common. An age-associated atrophic gastritis, with or without antacid therapy, is a frequent antecedent. Macrocytic indices, the hallmark of vitamin B_{12} deficiency, may not be apparent because of concomitant inflammatory disease or iron deficiency.

In addition to red cell changes, patients with vitamin B_{12} deficiency may also present with a myriad of hematologic abnormalities, including leukopenia, thrombocytopenia, and pancytopenia, occasionally requiring bone marrow to distinguish it from myelodysplasia or aplastic anemia. Vitamin B_{12} deficiency is usually suspected by the finding of an elevated mean corpuscular volume (MCV) on routine screening or during evaluation of the cause of the anemia. However, other causes for macrocytosis are more common; these include excessive alcohol intake, drug intake (particularly antineoplastic agents), reticulocytosis, myelodysplasia, and hypothyroidism. Levels of vitamin B_{12} below 200 pg/mL reliably indicates vitamin B_{12} deficiency; however, measurement of methylmalonic acid and homocysteine levels, which are elevated, may be necessary to establish the diagnosis for those with higher serum vitamin B_{12} levels. Treatment with intramuscular vitamin B_{12} and crystalline oral vitamin B_{12} are effective in older adults, even in patients with cobalamin food malabsorption.[43]

Renal Insufficiency

Chronic kidney disease (CKD) is an important cause of anemia in older adults.[44,45] Reduced renal erythropoietin (EPO) production is the primary factory leading to anemia in CKD. Serum EPO levels have been shown to be inappropriately low at a creatinine clearance of less than 40 mL/min.[46] The precise degree of renal dysfunction sufficient to cause anemia remains controversial. Mild hemoglobin decreases in adults may be detected at a creatinine clearance of 40 to 60 mL/min.[47,48]

A survey of community-dwelling older adults suggested anemia and low EPO levels independent of age and other factors at a creatinine clearance less than 30 mL/min.[49] Of 6200 residents in a nursing home, 59% were found to be anemic and 43% had calculated creatinine clearances of less than 60 mL/min. This analysis indicated that renal impairment, even at mild levels, increases the risk of anemia.[19]

Unexplained Anemia

Increasingly, it has become recognized that approximately one third of older adults with anemia do not have an obviously discernible cause on routine evaluation (Table 91-3). Typically, this anemia is generally mild (hemoglobin concentration in the 10- to 12-g/dL range), normocytic, and hypoproliferative (low reticulocyte count). It has been postulated that the cause relates to a number of factors, including testosterone level,[50] occult inflammation,[51] reduced hematopoietic reserve with advancing age,[52] inappropriately low serum EPO level,[53,54] and myelodysplastic syndrome (see later). It is clear that this anemia is associated with a low serum EPO level for the degree of anemia. The EPO level usually falls within the normal reference range. However, this is abnormal, because the serum EPO level should increase with falling hemoglobin concentration. The diagnosis of unexplained anemia assumes that the clinician has excluded serious causes. The threshold for performing a bone marrow examination to exclude myelodysplastic syndromes remains unknown. However, we advocate considering a bone marrow examination in all patients requiring red cell transfusion who otherwise have an unexplained anemia. Macrocytosis, thrombocytopenia, neutropenia, splenomegaly, or unexplained constitutional symptoms of fever, chills, early satiety, bone pain, and/or weight loss should prompt consideration of a bone marrow examination.

TABLE 91-3 Features of Unexplained Anemia

Parameter	Value
Hemoglobin	10.5-12 g/dL
Reticulocyte index	Low
MCV	80-95 fL
Serum Iron	Mildly low normal
TIBC	Normal
Iron saturation (%)	Mildly low normal
Vitamin B_{12}, folate, ESR, TSH	Normal
Platelet and white blood counts	Normal
Creatinine clearance	<90 to >30 mL/min

ESR, erythrocyte sedimentation rate; *MCV,* mean corpuscular volume; *TIBC,* total iron-binding capacity; *TSH,* thyroid-stimulating hormone.

MYELODYSPLASIA

The term *myelodysplastic syndrome* (MDS) includes a heterogeneous group of disorders characterized by dysplastic changes within the bone marrow and impaired proliferation in one or more cell lines (e.g., erythroid, myeloid, megakaryocytic).[55] As such, peripheral cytopenias and symptoms related to anemia, leukopenia, or thrombocytopenia are common manifestations of the disease. MDS occurs primarily in older men, with median age of 76 years. Each year, approximately 15,000 patients will be diagnosed with this disorder, although this might be an underestimate.[56] The continues to rise, with the highest incidence found in those older than 80 years (>30 cases/100,000/year).[57-59]

Classification

The long-established French-American-British (FAB) classification[60] has defined five distinct type of MDS—refractory anemia (RA), refractory anemia with ringed sideroblasts (RARS), refractory anemia with excess blasts (RAEB), refractory anemia with excess blasts in transformation (RAEB-T), and chronic myelomonocytic leukemia (CMML). This general classification has been modified by WHO based on salient bone marrow cytogenetic features (e.g., deletion of the short arm of the fifth chromosome [5q-]) and other histopathologic or clinical features (Table 91-4).[61] Thus, RAEB is divided into two groups based on the number of blasts and RA and RARS are divided into those with only anemia or those with multilineage involvement. These modifications have enabled a more accurate estimation of prognosis.[62]

Pathogenesis

Although no distinct cause for MDS can be identified in most cases, there is an association with prior chemotherapy in many cases, particularly with alkylating agents or topoisomerase inhibitors and with prior radiation therapy.[63,64] Treatment-related MDS patients are usually younger and have a worse prognosis than de novo MDS patients.[63] Prolonged exposure to high concentrations of benzene and pesticides appears to increase the risk of MDS, possibly by inducing chromosomal abnormalities.[65] Carcinogens present in cigarette smoke appear to have a similar effect in increasing the risk of MDS, especially of the type associated with deletions of chromosomes 5 and 7.[66] A familial cause for MDS has also been postulated.[65] Chromosomal abnormalities are frequently seen in MDS, very similar to those in acute myelogenous leukemia (AML), including complex karyotypes.[63] Several mechanisms may be involved in the pathogenesis of MDS, including alterations in apoptotic pathways, cytokine regulation, bone marrow microenvironment, mitochondrial enzymes, and immune regulation.[67] Furthermore, there has been evolving evidence that some MDS cases have an autoimmune basis because, clinically, MDS may be associated with other autoimmune disorders, and laboratory evidence has documented oligoclonal T cell patterns in up to 50% of cases.[68]

Clinical and Laboratory Features

Patients with MDS may be asymptomatic or have symptoms and signs related to qualitative or quantitative defects of erythrocytes, leukocytes, and platelets.[69] Fatigue, which significantly affects quality of life,[70] exertional dyspnea, fever, and infections, are some of the reasons for consulting a physician. A complete blood count usually reveals anemia, with normocytic or macrocytic indices. Moderate leukopenia and thrombocytopenia or thrombocytosis may be present. A bone marrow examination may reveal a normal or hypercellular pattern, with dysplastic features identified in erythroid, myeloid, and megakaryocytic cell lines or in all three (trilinear). Commonly seen changes in peripheral blood and bone

TABLE 91-4 WHO Classification and Criteria for the Myelodysplastic Syndromes

Disease	Blood Findings	Bone Marrow Findings
Refractory anemia (RA)	Anemia	Erythroid dysplasia only <5% blasts <15% ringed sideroblasts
Refractory anemia with ringed sideroblasts (RARS)	Anemia	Erythroid dysplasia only <5% blasts ≥15% ringed sideroblasts
Refractory cytopenia with multilineage dysplasia (RCMD)	Cytopenias (bicytopenia or pancytopenia) No or rare blasts No Auer rods <1 × 10^9/L monocytes	Dysplasia in ≥10% of cells in two or more myeloid cell lines <5% blasts in marrow No Auer rods <15% ringed sideroblasts
Refractory cytopenia with multilineage dysplasia and ringed sideroblasts (RCMD-RS)	Cytopenias (bicytopenia or pancytopenia) No or rare blasts No Auer rods <1 × 10^9/L monocytes	Dysplasia in ≥10% of cells in two or more myeloid cell lines ≥15% ringed sideroblasts <5% blasts No Auer rods
Refractory anemia with excess blasts-1 (RAEB-1)	Cytopenias <5% blasts No Auer rods <1 ×10^9/L monocytes	Unilineage or multilineage dysplasia 5% to 9% blasts No Auer rods
Refractory anemia with excess blasts-2 (RAEB-2)	Cytopenias 5% to 19% blasts With or without Auer rods <1 × 109/L monocytes	Unilineage or multilineage dysplasia 10% to 19% blasts With or without Auer rods
Myelodysplastic syndrome, unclassified (MDS-U)	Cytopenias No or rare blasts No Auer rods	Unilineage dysplasia in granulocytes or megakaryocytes <5% blasts No Auer rods
MDS associated with isolated del(5q)	Anemia <5% blasts Platelets normal or increased	Normal to increased megakaryocytes, with hypolobated nuclei <5% blasts No Auer rods Isolated del(5q)

TABLE 91-5 Myelodysplastic Syndrome (MDS): International Prognostic Scoring System (IPSS)—Prognostic Variables

	IPPS Score				
Variable	*0*	*0.5*	*1.0*	*1.5*	*2.0*
Marrow blasts (%)	<5	5-10	—	11-20	21-30
Karyotype	Good	Intermediate	Poor		
Cytopenias	0/1	2/3	—	—	—

Good—normal, -y, del(5q), del(20q); poor—complex (>three abnormalities) or chromosome 7 anomalies; intermediate—any other abnormalities.

marrow include anisocytosis, macrocytosis, basophilic stippling, ringed sideroblasts, pseudo–Pelger-Huet abnormality, blast cells, and hypersegmented neutrophils, micromegakaryocytes, and large platelets.[69]

Prognosis

The International Prognostic Scoring System (IPSS)[71,72] divides patients into low, intermediate-1 (INT-1), intermediate-2 (INT-2), and high categories (Table 91-5). It is based on the number of cytopenias (hemoglobin level < 10 g/dL, absolute neutrophil count < 1,500/μL, platelet count < 100,000/μL), chromosomal abnormalities, and percentage of bone marrow blasts and is used to estimate overall survival and predict progression to AML. Median survival ranges from less than 3 months, regardless of age, in the high-risk groups to almost 12 years in those younger than 60 years in the low-risk group. In the low-risk group, patients older than 70 years seem to have a worse prognosis than younger patients, but age does not seem to change the prognosis significantly in those in the high-risk category. Other factors found to be of prognostic importance include WHO subtypes[73] and transfusion dependence. The IPSS and Revised IPSS (IPSS-R) are used to predict the prognosis of patients with MDS at the time of diagnosis.[71,72] Management recommendations for patients with MDS have largely been based on their IPSS score.[74] Low-risk MDS includes patients with an IPSS score of low/INT-1, and high-risk MDS includes those with an IPSS score of INT-2/high.[74] Older age did not influence prognosis in the refractory anemia group, which is usually associated with good prognosis.[73] Also, MDS associated with a 5q deletion is associated with a good prognosis.[75]

Treatment

Supportive care in the form of transfusions, iron-chelating therapy, and adequate treatment of infection is the backbone of treatment for those with MDS. In the low and INT-1 groups, treatment is deferred unless significant cytopenias are present. Patients with deletion 5q have relatively good prognosis and experience an excellent response to the thalidomide analogue lenalidomide. In one series, 67% of patients became transfusion-independent after treatment with 10 mg of daily lenalidomide and continued to remain so for more than 2 years.[76] Recombinant erythropoietin, with or without granulocyte-stimulating factor, is used to treat symptomatic anemia in those with low serum erythropoietin levels and symptomatic anemia.[77] Older patients in the low INT-1 category but with neutropenia or thrombocytopenia and patients in the INT-2 and high-risk group who are ineligible for transplantation are best treated with DNA methyltransferase inhibitors, such as decitabine[78] or azacytidine[79]; both have been shown to improve quality of life. Although intensive therapy with allogeneic stem cell transplantation has been traditionally reserved for younger patients, reduced-intensity conditioning regimens have extended this therapy to selected older patients, with favorable results. Assessment with the hematopoietic cell transplantation comorbidity index (HCT-CI) has been used in older MDS patients and may help select patients for whom the risk-benefit ratio is favorable for this form of aggressive therapy.[80]

MYELOPROLIFERATIVE DISORDERS

Myeloproliferative disorders (MPDs) are characterized by clonal proliferation of hematopoietic stem cells. They include polycythemia vera (PV), essential thrombocythemia (ET), chronic idiopathic myelofibrosis (CIF), and chronic myelogenous leukemia (CML). CML is identified by the presence of the translocated *bcr-abl* gene and typically has three phases—a chronic phase, seen in more than 80% of patients, blastic phase, and intermediate accelerated phase.

The new 2008 WHO classification has replaced the term *disease* in MPD with *neoplasm* to indicate the possibly malignant nature of these disorders.[61,81] The myeloproliferative neoplasm (MPN) group includes mast cell disease, chronic eosinophilic and neutrophilic leukemia, hypereosinophilic syndrome, and other previously unclassified bone marrow disorders in addition to CML, PV, CIF, and ET. The common feature of these disorders is evident clonal proliferation without dysplasia.

Epidemiology

PV and CIF are more often diagnosed in older adults,[56] equally in both genders, with a median age of 70 years. Incidence rates for all age groups have ranged from 0.7 to 2.6/100,000 for PV and 0.3 to 1.5/100,000 in CIF, but rates as high as 23.5/100,000 have been reported for those from 70 to 79 years of age for PV. An increased incidence among Ashkenazi Jews has been reported. Incidence for ET ranges from 0.59 to 2.53/100,000, with almost twofold higher rates seen in women than in men. Unlike PV, ET is diagnosed at a younger age and is often seen in association with pregnancy. A significant trend toward an increase in ET incidence has been observed, especially among men, although the trends for PV and CIF have not shown any change.[56] Familial studies have shown an almost fivefold increased risk for PV and sevenfold risk for ET in first-degree relatives with MPDs.[82]

Causative Factors

Identification of a specific mutation (*V617F*) in the Janus Kinase-2 gene (*JAK2*) has improved our understanding of the pathogenesis of myeloproliferative disease.[83] *JAK2 V617F* can be identified in almost 95% of PV patients[84] and in more than 50% of ET and CIF patients.[85] Increased activity of this gene enhances the sensitivity of the mutated stem cells to hematopoietic growth factors such as erythropoietin, thrombopoietin, stem cell factor, and granulocyte-stimulating factor, causing clonal trilinear proliferation of myeloid precursors. Also, a mutation in the *mpl* gene, which involves the thrombopoietin receptor, is also thought to play a minor role in the pathogenesis.[86] The *bcr-abl* fusion gene formed as a result of translocation of the *abl* gene from chromosome 9 to the *bcr* region on chromosome 22 causes transcription of proteins with abnormal tyrosine kinase activity, resulting in clonal proliferation usually recognized in CML.[87] Clonal evolution, with additional chromosomal abnormalities frequently involving the 17th, are seen in more than 50% of patients in an accelerated phase of the disease.[88]

Production of growth factors by cytokines secreted from megakaryocytes and monocytes are hypothesized to play a role in the proliferation of fibroblasts, changes in the extracellular matrix, and angiogenesis seen in CIF.[89,90] Abnormal homing of stem cells and endothelial progenitor cells $CD34^+$ to peripheral hematopoietic organs are also known to play a role in the extramedullary hematopiesis of myelofibrosis.[91] Secondary myelofibrosis can result because of the progression of PV and ET, although the progression of true ET has been highly debated.

Clinical Features and Diagnosis

The characteristic clinical features vary by the specific MPD. In ET, they are related to abnormalities in platelet number and function; this is manifest predominantly as thrombotic episodes, although hemorrhagic episodes are also encountered.[92] Thrombotic events can precede the diagnosis of the disease and can involve microvascular and large-vessel arterial circulation, causing ischemic strokes, peripheral vascular disease, and myocardial infarction in addition to venous thrombosis.[93] Erythromelalgia, a specific microvascular condition seen in ET, typically presents with erythremic burning sensations of the extremities and ulceration of the toes.[94] The risk of thrombosis increases with age in PV and ET.[95] A higher incidence of cardiovascular complications is also seen in those older than 65 years who have had a history of thrombosis.[96] It appears that the presence of a *JAK2* mutation[92] and leukocytosis[97] may be additional risk factors for thrombosis in MPN patients. Hemorrhagic complications usually occur in patients with very high platelet counts ($>1500 \times 10^9$/L); the clinical presentation can vary from minor bruising or epistaxis to life-threatening GI bleeding.[95] CIF may be asymptomatic in more than 30% of patients; the diagnosis may be suspected on the basis of a leukoerythroblastic blood picture, presence of classic teardrop cells, or an enlarged spleen, usually in the prefibrotic stage.[98] Presentation in CML is similar to that seen in other MPNs, with constitutional symptoms and hemorrhagic manifestations. A finding of a low leukocyte alkaline phosphatase (LAP) level characterizes CML as compared to the PV, ET, and CIF, which that typically have a normal LAP level.

General signs and symptoms in patients with MPDs include splenomegaly, which can run the spectrum of mild and of little concern to uncomfortable and even life-threatening if rupture occurs. Pruritus may be present in more than 50% of patients. Patients with MPD also have a high incidence of fatigue, which may substantially decrease the quality of life.[99] Weight loss, night sweats, fever, and bone pain are also seen.

Diagnosis

The diagnosis of MPN has undergone a radical change with identification of the *JAK 2* mutation. Previously, standard criteria included physical signs and parameters based on peripheral blood counts, oxygen saturation, bone marrow findings, red cell mass, and presence of splenomegaly. The new WHO criteria, an update of the previous 2001 criteria, include detection of a *JAK2* mutation along with bone marrow biopsy in the diagnosis of *bcr-abl*–negative MPNs. Important changes also include lowering the platelet threshold number for the diagnosis of ET from 600 to 450×10^9/L and establishing a 2-g/dL increase of hemoglobin from normal levels as criteria for PV.[100] Different algorithms using serum EPO levels, morphology of bone marrow megakaryocytes, bone marrow reticulin staining, and use of fluorescence in situ hybridization (FISH) for *bcr-abl* have been proposed to enable differentiation of one MPN from another.[100] It is especially important to differentiate the cause of isolated thrombocytosis, because the prognosis of ET is very different from the thrombocytosis seen in early prefibrotic CIF and that due to CML. The diagnosis of ET also may require exclusion of reactive thrombocytoses such as cancer, iron deficiency anemia, and inflammatory conditions.[101] The diagnosis of CML is straightforward via identifying the Philadelphia chromosome by cytogenetics or the *bcr-abl* gene by the FISH technique.

Prognosis

As noted, survival times vary markedly in each of the MPDs described. One study has shown a 3-year survival rate as high as 92% for ET and 88% for PV. However, older age was associated with lower overall survival for MPDs as a group (90% in those < 50 years and 66% in those > 80 years).[56] ET and PV are associated with reduction in life expectancy, significant morbidity related to thrombosis, hemorrhage, and a small but definite risk for leukemogenic transformation or marrow fibrosis, especially in older adults.[102] Fatigue present in more than 80% of these patients has significant negative effect on the quality of life.[99] It is now recognized that those with the *JAK2* mutation,[92] especially those with higher allelic burden and higher leukocyte counts, have a tendency to higher rates of thrombosis. Age older than 60 years, previous history of thrombosis,[96] and high platelet count ($>1500 \times 10^9$/L) were previously identified as important prognostic factors for thrombosis in these patients. Patients in the prefibrotic stage of CIF have a relatively good prognosis, with a survival of almost 12 years. However, for those with high-risk CIF, life expectancy is significantly reduced.[103] The median length of survival can be as short as 1 year for those at highest risk. AML in patients with primary myelofibrosis carries the worst prognosis, with a dismal median survival of less than 3 months. Numerous scoring systems in CIF using hemoglobin levels, age, and white blood cell count have been described to predict prognosis,[104] and older age appears to be a common negative prognostic factor.[105]

Treatment

Treatment in PV and ET is generally recommended to reduce the morbidity associated with qualitative and quantitative changes in blood cells. Phlebotomy to reduce the hematocrit to less than 45% is the mainstay of treatment in PV because this has reduced the incidence of thrombosis.[106] Low-dose aspirin has been shown to reduce the risk of microvascular and macrovascular complications and is recommended for treatment of all patients with PV.[107] In the European Collaboration on Low-dose Aspirin in Polycythemia Vera (ECLAP) study, which randomized predominantly asymptomatic low-risk PV patients, the incidence of cardiovascular death, nonfatal myocardial infarction, nonfatal stroke, and major venous thromboembolism was lower among those treated with 100 mg aspirin daily as compared to placebo-treated controls (relative risk [RR], 0.4; 95% confidence interval [CI], 0.18 to 0.91]; $P = .0277$).[108] Total and cardiovascular mortality were also reduced by 46% and 59%, respectively. There was no significant increase in the risk of bleeding. In younger low-risk ET patients, treatment is generally not required, although low-dose aspirin can be used to reduce microvascular symptoms.[109] However, in older patients, aspirin may be recommended based on the ECLAP study, especially if other traditional risk factors for vascular disease are also present.[109]

The evidence for benefit with treatment with hydroxyurea (HU) in high-risk ET patients has been clearly demonstrated, particularly with reference to reduced thrombosis (1.6%) compared to no treatment (10.6%).[110-112] Superior benefit was also seen when HU was compared to other cytoreductive agents, including anagrelide.[110] Studies with HU in PV have not been as consistent, and a higher risk of leukemic transformation has been observed in treated patients. However, in high-risk PV and ET patients, HU is considered the standard of care.[106,112]

Primary myelofibrosis is an intractable illness, refractory to standard approaches, and allogeneic hematopoietic stem cell transplantation (HSCT) remains the only potentially curative therapy available. However, age and increasing comorbidity are strong negative prognostic factors for survival, even in these patients, and only 14% of MF transplantation patients older than 45 years survived 5 years after allogeneic HSCT as compared to 62% of younger patients.[113] In that same series, those with a Charlson comorbidity index of 4 to 6 had a greater than twofold risk of mortality. Reduced-intensity conditioning (RIC) regimens have increased response rates and event-free survival (EFS) in older patients but, in most of these studies, patients were considered "old" at the age of 60 years. For patients younger than 70 years, with low comorbidity, an RIC regimen and allogeneic transplantation are reasonable options, worthy of clinical investigation.[114,115] Optimum treatment for those 70 years of age and older remains investigational and, outside of a clinical trial, may be supportive management alone. Control of symptomatic anemia and elevated leukocytes or platelets may require pharmacologic intervention, but treatment is primarily palliative. Splenomegaly is a classic feature of MF, and splenic radiation has provided effective palliation in selected cases.[116]

Erythropoietin and danazol were commonly used to correct anemia, but a recent retrospective study[117] has found an increased risk of transformation to leukemia with the use of these agents in myelofibrosis; thus, enthusiasm for this approach has been tempered. High response rates for patients with anemia and splenomegaly with lenalidomide have been observed in those with the del(5q) group of myelofibrosis.[118] However, patients with del(5q) are exceedingly uncommon.[119]

The management of CML has changed dramatically in the past 2 decades. Survival in CML patients depends on the phase of the disease, with median survival now measured in decades for those presenting in the chronic phase,[120] but still less than 3 months for those in the blastic phase.[121] Prognostic classification incorporating variables such as percentage of blasts, spleen size, platelet count, basophil and eosinophil counts, and age distinguishes three groups—low, intermediate, and high risk—with good correlation with survival.[122] With the introduction of the oral tyrosine kinase inhibitor imatinib and, more recently, with the second-generation tyrosine inhibitors dasatinib[123] and nilotinib,[124] treatment of CML has improved considerably; it appears that response rates and overall survival for CML patients approach that of age-matched individuals without CML.[120] The good news is that older patients respond well to tyrosine kinase therapy, with responses comparable to those observed for younger patients.[125,126]

OTHER HEMATOLOGIC MALIGNANCIES COMMON TO OLDER PATIENTS

Multiple Myeloma

Multiple myeloma (MM), the second most common hematologic malignancy diagnosed in the United States, is a disorder characterized by monoclonal proliferation of plasma cells (>10%) within the bone marrow. Typically, in MM, abnormal amounts of monoclonal immunoglobulin or light chains (kappa or lambda) are present in the serum and/or urine. Manifestations related to involvement of the bone predominate, but symptoms resulting from the extramedullary effects of the circulating abnormal protein or hypercalcemia are also frequently encountered. The median age of myeloma diagnosis is 70 years, and it occurs more frequently in African Americans and in males. The U.S. annual incidence is 4.4/100,000. Curiously, MM incidence and mortality rates are decreasing. However, the 5-year relative survival rates continue to remain less than 20% for patients 65 years and older.[127]

Causative Factors

Lower socioeconomic status, education, and dietary habits seem to account for the differences in incidence between African Americans and whites in the United States.[128,129] Familial studies have shown that the risk of myeloma is higher in patients with a family history of hematologic malignancy, possibly implicating a genetic predisposition.[130] Risk is also known to be higher after radiation or exposure to pesticides, certain chemicals, and asbestos[131] and also in those with a history of inflammatory disease[132] or allergies.[133] High levels of human herpesvirus 8 (HHV-8) virus have been reported in bone marrow stromal cells of myeloma patients, indicating a possible viral cause for the disease in selected cases.[134]

Pathogenesis

Bone pain is the primary symptom in approximately 70% of patients. Radiographs reveal localized punched-out lytic bone lesions or diffuse osteoporosis, usually in bones with active hematopoietic tissue. The discrete lytic lesions are characterized by large and numerous osteoclasts on the bone-reabsorbing surface. An excess of osteoclast-activating factors such as receptor activator of nuclear factor-kappa B ligand (RANKL), macrophage inflammatory protein-1α (MIP-1α), and interleukin-6 (IL-6), coupled with a decrease in osteoblast activity due to the presence of inhibitors such as Dickkopf-related protein 1(DKK-1), contribute to the characteristic osteolytic bone lesions. With bone demineralization and decreased activity because of pain, hypercalcemia may be expected. The symptoms of hypercalcemia (drowsiness, confusion, nausea, thirst) are nonspecific, but their occurrence should alert the physician to investigate this possibility. Cardiac arrhythmias, renal insufficiency, and profound central nervous system (CNS) depression can develop as hypercalcemia progresses.

High levels of circulating monoclonal protein can cause increased whole blood viscosity. This occurs most frequently with immunoglobulin M (IgM; see Waldenstrom disease, later), but may also occur with IgA or even IgG myeloma. Increased viscosity compromises circulation, including that to the brain, kidney, and heart, and symptoms of confusion, light-headedness, and/or chest pain may result. The myeloma protein itself may cause tubular damage in the kidney, and renal insufficiency is a major consequence of uncontrolled myeloma.

Clinical Features

It is important to differentiate myeloma from other plasma cell dyscrasias that occur with increasing frequency with age. Monoclonal gammopathy of undetermined significance (MGUS) once considered a benign disorder secondary to age-associated immune dysregulation,[135] is now thought to be a precursor to myeloma, with a conversion of MGUS to MM of about 1%/year.[136,137] The features of MGUS (Table 91-6) include a marrow with less than 10% plasma cells (and without dysplastic features characteristic of myeloma plasma cells), less than 3-g/dL monoclonal protein in the serum, and no end-organ damage. MGUS patients who have more than 1.5 g/dL of monoclonal protein other than IgG and an abnormal urinary light chain ratio are at a greater risk for earlier progression to MM. Follow-up evaluation, including serum protein electrophoresis and quantitation of the monoclonal protein, is recommended every 3 months so that early conversion to myeloma may be recognized.[138]

TABLE 91-6 Early Myeloma versus Monoclonal Gammopathy of Undetermined Significance (MGUS)

Parameter	Early Multiple Myeloma	MGUS
Pathogenesis	Neoplastic plasma cell disorder (malignant)	Disordered immunoregulation or possibly benign B cell neoplasm
Bone marrow	Frequently > 10% plasma cells with many dysplastic features (myeloma cells)	Usually 10% normal-appearing plasma cells
Bone	Lytic bone lesions or diffuse osteoporosis	Usually no bone disease
Symptoms	Bone pain, constitutional symptoms (e.g., fatigue, weight loss), or those associated with kidney failure or hyperviscosity	Usually no symptoms
Serum spike	Progressively rising	Stable

Smoldering myeloma has the same laboratory features as MM but without end-organ damage. Solitary plasmacytoma is an isolated tumor consisting of plasma cells in bones (solitary myeloma of bone) or soft tissue (extramedullary plasmacytoma), without systemic involvement.[139] In 1% to 2% of patients, MM can progress to plasma cell leukemia, which is more common in younger patients, has more than 20% plasma cells, and is more aggressive than MM.

Renal dysfunction is seen in more than 20% of myeloma patients at the time of diagnosis.[140] The pathogenesis of the renal disease is frequently multifactorial, with contributions from paraproteins, tubular damage, tissue deposition of light chains, amyloidosis, hyperuricemia, and infection.[141-143]

Pathologic fractures are also common. Fatigue related to anemia occurs in 30% to 60% of MM patients and usually occurs in those with a hemoglobin level less than 10g/dL.[144] Signs of amyloidosis (present in up to 30% of myeloma patients) such as macroglossia may also be present. Although constitutional symptoms can occur because of anemia, hyperviscosity, hypercalcemia, renal insufficiency, or infection, it should be remembered that in older adults, these symptoms might be less pronounced. The clinical presentation of MM has changed over the years, with a lower percentage of patients presenting with end-organ damage. MM is usually suspected by the presence of normocytic normochromic anemia and mild renal failure or hypergammaglobulinemia,[145] especially in older adults. Due to the catabolic effects of myeloma-associated cytokines, older patients may present with normocytic anemia and a drop in the serum cholesterol level, even before other signs or symptoms of the disease appear.

Laboratory Data and Diagnosis

Complete blood count, metabolic profile with liver function tests, serum lactic acid dehydrogenase (LDH) level, serum β_2-microglobulin, serum free light chain assay, serum and 24-hour urine protein levels, electrophoresis, immunofixation, skeletal survey, and bone marrow are all important in the initial workup of MM patients.[146] Hypercalcemia, renal insufficiency, anemia, and bony abnormalities, which are the hallmarks of end-organ damage in MM, are usually identified with these evaluations. Other laboratory abnormalities include hypoalbuminemia, elevated LDH level, β_2-microglobulin, platelet, and coagulation abnormalities and rouleaux formation (stacking of red cells) apparent on the peripheral blood smear.[147]

Protein electrophoresis detects a monoclonal protein in approximately 80% of patients in the serum and in 75% of patients in the urine. Immunofixation (or immunoelectrophoresis) allows identification of the isotype, which is usually IgG (60%) or IgA (20%). Of the 20% without detectable monoclonal protein by serum protein electrophoresis, most will have kappa or lambda light chains detected in the urine (light chain myeloma). Only about 1% of myeloma patients will be actual nonsecretors.[147] In the absence of monoclonal protein, the diagnosis of MM is established by the finding of more than 30% plasma cells in the marrow.

Prognosis

Traditionally, the Durie-Salmon staging system—predominantly clinical features and amount of paraprotein—was used to identify patients at higher risk of death because it is a good indicator of tumor burden in MM. However, the International Staging System (ISS) has been shown to provide prognostic information more accurately. This system is based on the levels of serum

β_2-microglobulin and albumin, as well as other measures. In one survey, in stage I or low-risk MM (serum β_2-microglobulin < 3.5 g/dL; serum albumin > 3.5 g/dL), median survival was 62 months. In contrast, for stage III MM (serum β_2-microglobulin > 5.5 g/dL), median survival was 29 months, and for the intermediate stage (stage II), median survival was 44 months.[148] Certain cytogenetic abnormalities, including those detected by FISH, such as deletion of chromosome 13, hypoploidy, t(4;14), t(4;16), 17p–, when combined with a plasma cell labeling index greater than 3% and selected laboratory data (LDH and C-reactive protein [CRP]), have been shown to improve prognostic accuracy.[149]

Although most prior studies did not distinguish significant differences in clinical features of myeloma in younger versus older patients, two reports are notable. The first compared those older and younger than 70 years, and the second compared those older than and younger than 50 years. Both studies showed that older patients presented with more advanced stage, poorer performance, and more adverse clinical features, including lower hemoglobin and higher creatinine levels and, in both reports, the response rates and survival were lower for those in the older group.[127,150,151]

Treatment

Older patients with MGUS and smoldering or asymptomatic myeloma need careful follow-up to detect and intervene if there is evidence for progression to more aggressive disease. In patients with symptomatic myeloma, treatment includes two components—one to manage the disease and the other to provide supportive treatment to control complications or end-organ damage. In older patients, treatment is especially difficult because improvements in progression-free survival and overall survival may lead to adverse effects, such as increased toxicity and poor quality of life. Proper selection of patients using geriatric assessment may reduce the possibility of these adverse outcomes.[127]

Previously, vincristine, doxorubicin, and dexamethasone were used as initial aggressive therapy, although it was difficult to prove that this was more effective than oral melphalan and prednisone (MP) in terms of overall survival. Thalidomide and dexamethasone have become first-line therapy and are even used as induction therapy prior to transplantation. Bortezomib, a reversible inhibitor of 26S proteosome, alone or in combination, has also been used for MM, with excellent results.[152] Retrospective studies have shown similar toxicity profiles and survival outcomes in younger and older patients, despite older adults receiving reduced chemotherapy doses.[153]

Currently, the standard of care in older myeloma patients is treatment with melphalan, prednisone, and thalidomide (MPT). In patients between 65 and 75 years of age, median overall survival was 51.6 months for MPT compared to 33.2 months for MP and 38.3 months for autologous transplantation with a reduced-intensity melphalan conditioning regimen.[154] The complications from MPT include an increased risk of venous thromboembolism, especially when administered with high-dose dexamethasone and erythropoiesis-stimulating agents, as well as peripheral neuropathy, infection, and constipation. Other combinations that have shown benefit in older patients include bortezomib or lenalidomide in combination with dexamethasone. Objective response rates as high as 90% have been seen with both these regimens.[155,156] There have been several new drugs approved for the treatment of myeloma,[157] although the sequence of their use and drug combinations have yet to be established. There remains some controversy with regard to maintenance therapy, although current data would suggest efficacy in terms of progression-free survival.[158]

Treatment with bisphosphonates have benefit with regard to lytic bone disease, bone pain, and osteopenia.[159,160] Radiation is used as a palliative measure to reduce bone pain and, along with dexamethasone, to stabilize tumors of the spine to prevent spinal cord compression and fractures. Newer surgical techniques such as vertebroplasty and kyphoplasty have improved the care of patients with bony complications in MM. Appropriate use of erythropoietic agents for management of anemia, aggressive management of infections, including prophylactic antibiotics, immunoglobulin use, and treatment of hyperviscosity and hypercalcemia are all important for reducing morbidity in MM patients.

LYMPHOMA

Lymphomas are neoplastic disorders of B and T lymphocytes, which predominantly involve lymphoid organs. They comprise a heterogeneous group of disorders, each with a distinct cause, histology, and clinical and prognostic features. Broadly, they can be classified as Hodgkin lymphoma, which make up less than 10% of the lymphoid neoplasms, and non-Hodgkin lymphoma (NHL).[161] Hodgkin lymphoma, characterized by owl eye–like inclusions in the nucleus referred to as Reed-Sternberg cells on histology, usually has a predictable pattern of spread predominantly involving lymphoid organs (lymph nodes, spleen, liver) whereas NHL may involve extranodal tissues and can have widespread systemic involvement at presentation.

Classification of lymphoma has undergone numerous changes. The WHO classification is the currently accepted and widely used classification. B lymphomas, as the name implies primarily arises from lymphocyte of B cell lineage and comprise more than 90% of NHLs as compared to T cell lymphomas.[161] B cell and T cell lymphoma subtypes are further subclassified based on the maturation level of the cells. Categories under mature B and T cell lymphomas include distinct morphologic, immunophenotypic, and clinical subtypes.[162]

Epidemiology

NHL is a disease that affects all age groups, with almost 50% of incident cases occurring in those older than 65 years. Age-adjusted incidence in those older than 65 years for 2001 to 2005 was as high as 88.4/100,000 compared to 9.4/100,000 in those younger than 65 years. Diffuse B cell lymphoma is the most common B cell subtype in all ages, including those older than 75 years. Anaplastic large cell, lymphoblastic cell, and Burkitt lymphoma are less frequently encountered in older adults.[163] White men have the greatest incidence of all lymphomas, with the exception of peripheral T cell lymphoma and mycosis fungoides, which are more common in African Americans. Asians have the lowest incidence of lymphoma.[161] There is an equal male-female distribution of lymphoma subtypes, although a lower incidence of follicular lymphoma and higher incidence of mycosis fungoides have been observed in black females.[161] A decreasing trend in the incidence of lymphomas has been seen in younger but not older age groups. The incidence of mantle cell and Burkett lymphomas has increased in those older than 75 years in recent years.[161] The reason for these trends in older adults, particularly among certain NHL subtypes, is not known, although age-related changes in immune function may be contributing.

Causative Factors

Environmental, infectious, and genetic factors and certain diseases are all known to play a role in the genesis of NHL, mostly by altering or activating immune processes.[164] Immunodeficiency is associated with a greatly increased risk of NHL. It is estimated that HIV patients have an almost 100-fold increased risk for NHL. An increase in NHL has also been reported in association with transplantation, rheumatoid arthritis, Sjögren syndrome, and systemic lupus erythematosus, especially for diffuse follicular and marginal cell lymphomas. NHL has been associated with the use of pesticides, especially in those with the t(14;18) subtype and use of permanent dark hair dyes in women.[165] Obesity and a diet high in animal fat and protein are also known to increase the risk of NHL.[166] Hepatitis C, Epstein-Barr virus, *Helicobacter pylori*, *Campylobacter jejuni*, and *Plasmodium falciparum* are all known to be associated with specific subtypes of NHL.[167] Chromosomal translocations—for example, t(14;18) involving the *bcl-2* proto-oncogene in 85% to 90% of cases of follicular lymphoma[168] and t(8;14) and other translocations involving the c-*myc* proto-oncogene in 100% of Burkett lymphoma cases—can promote lymphoma development.

Diagnosis and Workup

The diagnosis hinges on a tissue diagnosis, usually obtained by lymph node biopsy. A comprehensive evaluation starts with a complete physical examination to document all involved areas, as well as pattern of spread. Further diagnostic procedures include imaging studies to determine occult areas of involvement. These would include computed tomography (CT), magnetic resonance imaging (MRI), and/or positron emission tomography (PET), alone or in combination. A bone marrow biopsy is often recommended to rule out extranodal involvement.

Clinical Features, Prognosis, and Management

Aggressive Lymphomas

Diffuse large B cell lymphoma (DLBCL) is the most common lymphoma subtype seen in older adults.[169] Although characterized by an aggressive course without treatment, DLBCL has a high chance of cure with therapy. It may present as localized disease but this is very unusual. Usually, the disease presents in an advanced stage and with extranodal involvement (e.g., GI tract or bone marrow).[170] Patients may also present with severe systemic systems and sometimes with rapidly progressive organ failure. Immunophenotyping reveals subtypes based on their derivation from a germinal center or activated B cells. Distinct clinical types of diseases, with different presentations and prognoses, also may be recognized based on *bcl-2*, *bcl-6*, *p53*, CD10, and *mum1* expression.

Cytogenetic analysis reveals a deletion of 18q as the most frequent abnormality (20% of cases) as well as a number of other nonrandom alterations. Mantle cell lymphoma, identified by the presence of B cell markers ($CD19^+$, $CD20^+$, $CD22^+$) and a T cell marker (CD5) and lack of $CD23^-$ and $CD10^-$ antigens,[171] is an aggressive type of lymphoma that is seen in more than 75% of cases at an advanced stage.[170] It is a disease of older men, with a median age at presentation of 68 years and a 2 : 1 male-to-female ratio.[170] Despite intensive treatment, the 5-year survival is less than 40%. Lymphadenopathy and bone marrow involvement are common, and splenomegaly is present in more than 60% of cases at diagnosis. Leukemic expression (peripheral blood involvement) is also common in mantle cell lymphoma. Cytogenetic analysis typically reveals t(11;14)(q13;q32) in more than 85% of patients involving the *bcl-1* oncogene and overexpression of cyclin D1.[171]

Treatment. The International Prognostic Index (IPI), which risk-stratifies patients based on age, tumor stage, LDH level, number of extranodal sites, and performance status is useful in determining treatment.[172] Although many studies have shown no definite age differences in clinical presentation,[163] treatment of lymphomas in older adults is associated with significant bias, which may account for some of the observed poorer outcomes.[169,173] More than 60% of older lymphoma patients have at least one comorbidity,[163] and physiologic changes in the key organ reserve may render an older patient more vulnerable to chemotherapy toxicity. As mentioned earlier, a careful and comprehensive assessment of comorbidities, functional status, and social factors are likely to improve outcomes.

Randomized studies have shown that the standard regimen of cyclophosphamide, doxorubicin, vincristine, and prednisone (CHOP) is safe, well tolerated, and comparably effective in younger and older patients.[174] However, a complete response is still seen in only 40% of older patients. The introduction of rituximab, a monoclonal antibody to the lymphocyte cell surface antigen CD20, has greatly improved response rates and survival for patients of all ages with NHL. In previously untreated 60- to 80-year-old patients with DBCL, rituximab CHOP (R-CHOP) resulted in a 76% complete remission rate, with relapse-free survival of 70% at 2 years, a considerable improvement from CHOP alone and without any increase in toxicity.[175] Thus, R-CHOP is currently the standard of care for older patients with DLBCL. The use of granulocyte colony-stimulating factor (G-CSF) has also been recommended for older adults if neutropenia is the only limiting factor to treat patients with a CHOP regimen.[176] Standard treatment for mantle cell lymphoma, such as R-CHOP, results in better remission rates and time to treatment failure but does not significantly improve survival and, for this histology, more aggressive treatment might be required.[177]

In older adults, a hyper-CVAD (hyperfractionated cyclophosphamide, vincristine, doxorubicin, dexamethasone) regimen, alternating with high-dose methotrexate and cytarabine, has shown response rates as high as 90%.[178] However, when rituximab was added to this regimen, a high rate of toxicity and shorter failure-free survival was seen in those older than 65 years (50% vs. 73%).[178] However, rituximab used alone for 2 years as maintenance therapy after a modified hyper-CVAD regimen without methotrexate and cytarabine has shown a complete remission rate of 64%, with acceptable toxicity, and has been recommended for patients older than 65 years.[179] Rituximab in combination with fludarabine, cyclophosphamide, and mitoxantrone in relapsed patients is associated with improved survival in relapsed or recurrent mantle cell lymphoma as compared to standard chemotherapy.[180]

Indolent Lymphomas

Follicular lymphoma (FL) accounts for 20% of lymphomas in older adults. Small painless lymphadenopathy without other symptoms may be the most common presentation.[181] Bone marrow involvement may be present in up to 60% of patients but usually does not signify a poor prognosis unless infiltration is extensive and is associated with peripheral cytopenias.[170] Sometimes, fever and weight loss may be present with lymphadenopathy and warrant immediate investigation. Translocation t(14;18) juxtaposing the *bcl-2* oncogene with the Ig heavy chain promoter may be detected in more than 90% of FLs.[182] FLs are graded from I to III based on the number of large cells in the malignant nodules. Initially, grade III FL was thought to be associated with worse clinical outcomes, but subsequent studies have shown this not to be the case.[183] Historically, FL was considered an indolent lymphoma, with a median survival of 8 to -10 years but generally not curable with standard chemotherapy. The FLIPI, a modification of the IPI,[184] was developed, and five adverse prognostic factors were selected—age older than 60 years, advanced stage, hemoglobin level (<120 g/L), number of nodal areas (>four or ≤four), and serum LDH level (>normal or ≤ normal). Three risk groups were defined as low risk (none or one adverse factor), intermediate risk (two factors), and poor risk (≥three adverse factors), and this system effectively predicts prognosis. Transformation to an aggressive type of lymphoma may occur, especially in those with high-risk FLIPI, and portends poor prognosis.[184,185] In older patients, for whom maintaining quality of life is an important end point, treatment is commonly deferred unless symptomatic or signs of progressive disease develop. Under carefully monitored circumstances, this delay in treatment initiation has been shown not to influence survival significantly.[186] The decision to start radiotherapy, a potentially curative treatment in early-stage disease, is highly individualized, and age older than 60 years is found to be an adverse factor with regard to the effectiveness of localized approaches such as these.[187] No standard chemotherapy regimens are currently available for the treatment of FL. Rituximab-based therapy in combination with traditional chemotherapy regimens, including CHOP[188] and fludarabine,[189] have shown durable response rates as high as 90%.[190] For older patients with comorbidities or functional impairment, rituximab as a single agent is well tolerated and effective.[191]

Marginal cell lymphoma includes three categories—mucosa-associated lymphoid tissue (MALT) lymphoma (typically located in the GI tract), splenic marginal zone lymphoma (SZL), and nodal zone lymphoma (NZL).[192] GI MALT is the most common extranodal presentation of MALT lymphoma, and the stomach is the most common organ involved.[193] Pathogenesis is mainly related to the presence of infection with *H. pylori*,[194] which is seen in almost all cases, and investigation to identify this organism is mandatory in MALT lymphomas.[195] Other commonly involved regions include the salivary gland, ocular adnexa, lung, skin, and Waldeyer ring.[193] Patients with gastric MALT typically present with symptoms of dyspepsia or abdominal pain, and upper endoscopy and biopsy will reveal a tumor with the characteristic histology.[195] Although the prognosis of low-grade MALT (86% 5-year survival) is excellent,[196] those who present with advanced disease and poor IPI scores do not fare well. Eradication of *H. pylori* with antibiotics has been very effective in the treatment of localized gastric MALT and is the standard treatment when *H. pylori* is identified. For those who have *H. pylori*–negative disease or a t(11;18) translocation (associated with resistance to *H. pylori* treatment),[197] initial treatment with radiotherapy or rituximab is generally applied.[198] Treatment of MALT in other sites involves locoregional radiotherapy or surgery, although individualized treatment is the preferred approach NZL zone lymphoma are primarily seen in women. An association with hepatitis C infection is seen in some cases of SZL and NL. The spleen is commonly involved in SZL, as is the bone marrow.[199] M-protein (paraprotein) and immunologic abnormalities may be seen in a high percentage of patients and are associated with a poor prognosis.[200] As with indolent lymphomas, asymptomatic or older patients may be followed frequently for the development of symptoms or progression to aggressive lymphoma. Hepatitis C patients may be successfully treated with appropriate therapy,[193] but splenectomy is the preferred treatment for hepatitis C–negative patients.[200] NZL primarily presents with extensive peripheral and central lymphadenopathy. Survival is lower than for other NZLs, and treatment is not defined, but rituximab-based therapy has been used, with varying success.[193]

Waldenstrom macroglobulinemia (WM; lymphoplasmacytic lymphoma) is a low-grade lymphoma identified by IgM monoclonal protein in serum and presence of characteristic intertrabecular infiltration of bone marrow with plasmacytoid lymphocytes. Immunophenotyping reveals surface IgM^+, $CD10^-$, $CD19^+$, $CD20^+$, $CD22^+$, $CD23^-$, $CD25^+$, $CD27^+$, $FMC7^+$, $CD103^-$, and CD138 cells.[201] The median age at diagnosis is 63 years, and the disease occurs more commonly in whites. Symptoms in WM are primarily related to direct tumor infiltration or the effects of IgM protein. Infiltration can occur in any organ, causing hepatomegaly, splenomegaly, or lymphadenopathy, and the bone marrow is almost always involved.[202] Hypercalcemia secondary to lytic bone lesions may be seen. Hyperviscosity due to the presence of pentameric IgM molecules can give rise to headaches, ocular symptoms, epistaxis, and even altered consciousness.[202] Primary amyloidosis can occur in WM and typically involves the heart and peripheral nerves, leading to cardiac failure and severe peripheral neuropathy. The lungs may also be involved. Cardiomyopathy is more common in older adults and is a primary cause of death in those with WM.[203] Renal dysfunction can be related to glomerulonephritis secondary to tissue infiltration with tumor or cryoglobulin deposition or due to IgM antibody against glomerular basement membrane. Cold agglutinin disease resulting from IgM antibody directed at the red cell antigens can lead to chronic immune hemolytic anemia. Cytopenias may also occur due to bone marrow infiltration of the tumor; 20% of patients may have no symptoms at diagnosis.

Asymptomatic WM patients usually do not require treatment and may be followed by observation alone.[144] A close watch, especially to monitor symptoms of hyperviscosity, is imperative, especially in those with serum monoclonal levels greater than 5g/L.[204] Measurement of serum viscosity is usually not very helpful, although symptoms rarely occur at levels less than 4 centipoises. Plasmapheresis is the treatment of choice for reducing hyperviscosity in these patients.[205] Treatment is usually recommended for symptomatic patients and those with a hemoglobin level less than 10 g/dL and platelet count less than 100×10^9/L.[144] Median survival is about 5 to 10 years for those with WM[204] and older age, high serum β_2-microglobulin, poor performance status, and cytopenias predict a poor prognosis.[206] Especially in older adults, survival may be affected by concomitant comorbidities, because only 50% of deaths in WM patients have been attributed to the disease. When cytoreductive treatment is required, options include single-agent therapy with chlorambucil, fludarabine, or rituximab, with a reported median response duration as long as 60 months,[207] and combination therapy with CHOP and cyclophosphamide and prednisone (CP),207 although their specific activity in those older than 65 years is not known.

T Cell Lymphomas

Peripheral T cell lymphoma (PTCL) and angioimmunoblastic lymphoma (AIBL) are the two most common T cell lymphomas encountered in older adults. Derived from post-thymic lymphocytes, they can be identified by the expression of T cell receptor (TCR) αβ or γδ chains and $CD3^+$, $CD4^+$, or $CD8^+$ cells. The median age of presentation is generally older than 60 years, with a male preponderance. Clinically, they present in advanced stages with a higher rate of B symptoms, worse performance scores, and higher IPI.[208] Involvement of the skin is common in PTCL, and allergic manifestations and symptoms related to proteinuria are typically seen in AIBL, as well as a high seropositivity for Epstein-Barr virus.[209] Molecular cytogenetics has revealed a high rate of chromosomal abnormalities and TCR clonality in β or γ genes. PTCL and AIBL generally have a poor prognosis when compared with B cell lymphomas.[210] IPI is useful in predicting prognosis, with survival less than 1.5 years in the high-risk group and longer than 10 years in the low-risk group,[211] although other molecular findings, such as p53 expression,[212] have also been shown to correlate with poor survival. Treatment with six to eight cycles of standard CHOP or more aggressive regimens for patients with AIBL are all reasonable approaches but should be individualized based on acceptable toxicity and a goal to maintain quality of life in older adults.

Hodgkin Lymphoma

Hodgkin lymphoma (HL) comprises about 8%[161] of total lymphomas in the population. The incidence of HL, at 2.5%, is relatively low and typically demonstrates a bimodal pattern of distribution, with highest rates seen in those to 30 years (4.3%) and 70 to 84 years of age (4.4%). In the younger age groups, HD is more often diagnosed in females than males, whereas the reverse is true in older adults.

The characteristic feature of HL is the presence of lymphadenopathy, which develops in a contiguous fashion and the presence or absence of systemic symptoms that provide useful prognostic information. Of the histologic variants of HL, nodular sclerosing variety is most common, but the mixed cellularity type appears more frequently than in younger patients. Older patients with HL present in more advanced stages and with more constitutional (B) symptoms (fever, weight loss, night sweats) but with less bulky disease than in younger patients.[213] Accurate staging is imperative so that curative therapy can be effectively prescribed. PET-CT has become an excellent method to assist in staging.

Traditionally, stages I and II HL in the absence of B symptoms have been considered to have good outcomes. Additional prognostic factors have been found in early-stage and advanced disease, which further define survival and necessitate treatment modification. In early-stage disease, bulky disease (e.g., mediastinal mass on chest x-ray > one-third the intrathoracic diameter; mass > 35% of the thoracic diameter at T5-T6; any other mass > 10 cm) identifies a subset of patients with less favorable disease especially associated with resistance to radiation. The IPI score,[214] which awards 1 point each for an albumin level lower than 4 g/dL, hemoglobin value lower than 10.5 g/dL, male gender, age older than 45 years, stage IV disease, leukocytosis (white blood cell count at least 15,000/mm, lymphocytopenia [lymphocyte count < 8% of the white blood cell count], and/or lymphocyte count < 600/mm), can predict freedom from disease progression (FFP) and overall survival and has proven to be a useful adjunct to staging in assessing the type of therapy to be undertaken. Those who had none of the above had an 84% rate of FFP compared to 42% for the presence of five or greater.

ABVD (doxorubicin, bleomycin, vinblastine, dacarbazine) has become the standard of care for HL. In early-stage disease, four to six are administered, depending on the presence of bulky disease. In the presence of favorable factors, two cycles may be sufficient. Involved field radiation after completion of chemotherapy and complete response may reduce the relapse rate in these patients,[215] but the long-term risk of a second malignancy is of concern for younger patients. Reports have been inconsistent regarding the outcomes of older patients following chemotherapy. Doxorubicin-based regimens and involved field radiation have been shown to be equally effective in older adults[216] who have been selected appropriately.

Nonetheless, treatment regimens should be chosen with an eye on potential toxicity in older patients. A retrospective analysis of older patients from the German Hodgkin's Study Group[217] has shown that with the exception of minor reactions such as nausea and pain, the frequency of adverse effects was higher in older (>60 years) than younger patients. This excessive toxicity resulted in a reduction of treatment dose and number of cycles and early termination of treatment. As a result, lower response rates and overall survival were observed. Although Hodgkin disease was still the most common cause of death in the older and younger patients, mortality due to treatment-related toxicity and second malignancies was more common in older patients. Appropriate assessment in older adults to individualize treatment programs based on a comprehensive pretreatment evaluation may minimize toxicity, treatment reductions, and less favorable outcomes. Currently, older HL patients are more likely to experience treatment-related cardiovascular disease, second malignancy, and death.[218,219] Age-appropriate cancer screening, annual chest imaging, thyroid function tests, and tests to detect cardiovascular risk factors are essential in all treated patients to identify and prevent late toxicities associated with therapy for HL.

CHRONIC LYMPHOCYTIC LEUKEMIA

Chronic lymphocytic leukemia (CLL)–small lymphocytic leukemia is a disorder classified as a mature (peripheral) B cell neoplasm according to the WHO classification.[220] There have been almost no reported cases in those younger than 30 years, and only about 10% of the cases occur in those younger than 55 years. Although not significant, there has been a trend toward a slight decrease in the incidence rates of CLL, including in those aged 75 years and older.[161] It is a disease predominantly seen in whites, occurring slightly more frequently in males, and the incidence is very low among Asians and Pacific Islanders.[161] An increased risk of CLL has been observed in patients with pernicious anemia,[221] chronic sinusitis, recurrent pneumonia, and herpes simplex and zoster viral infections.[222,223] Interestingly, there is a decreased incidence of CLL in patients with chronic rheumatic and nonrheumatic valvular heart disease. Population and family studies have highlighted the importance of genetic factors in the cause of B cell CLL (B-CLL). The relative risk of CLL in first-degree family members can be eightfold higher than in controls.[224,225] Some have suggested that the risk increases with the degree of relationship between the affected member and family members,[224] and it is apparent that the age at onset of disease occurs earlier in successive generations, a phenomenon termed *anticipation*.[226]

Clinical Features and Diagnosis

A rapid proliferation in the use of automated systems to evaluate peripheral blood counts have led to an increase in the diagnosis of asymptomatic individuals with elevated lymphocyte counts and those in early-stage CLL.[227,228] The median age of patients diagnosed in early-stage CLL has also been increasing. Lymphadenopathy is the most common feature in symptomatic patients, and the lymph nodes are usually painless and mobile on examination.[229] Inguinal lymphadenopathy is uncommon. Nonspecific symptoms such as malaise, fatigue, and weight loss also predominate in symptomatic CLL patients. Other findings include anemia, hepatomegaly, and splenomegaly.[230] Bruising secondary to thrombocytopenia may also occur in these patients. Cytopenia seen in CLL may result from bone marrow failure (more common) or secondary to autoimmune disease.[231] Clinical features are very similar in younger and older patients,[232] except that younger patients (<50 years) usually present with a higher hemoglobin level.[233]

Autoimmune hemolytic anemia can occur in CLL as a presenting feature or during the course of the disease, with a prevalence of approximately 4%. Older men appear to have a higher rate of autoimmune hemolytic anemia.[234] Treatment with steroids for this condition is frequently successful[234] but can significantly increase the morbidity and mortality if older patients require prolonged treatment. Other autoimmune disorders such as immune thrombocytopenic purpura and pure red cell aplasia occur but are uncommon. Infections secondary to hypogammaglobulinemia may precede the diagnosis of CLL but usually occur during the course of the disease, especially following CLL treatment. Although bacterial infections with encapsulated organisms are the most common, fungal and viral infections are also fairly frequent.[235] Transformation to diffuse B cell lymphoma (Richter syndrome) also occurs in CLL patients, with a 10-year incidence of 16.5%,[236] and older adults appear to be at an increased risk.[237] This can occur even in early-stage disease and is heralded by the development of systemic symptoms and rapidly growing lymphadenopathy.

CLL cells contain unmutated or mutated immunoglobulin heavy chain variable (IGHV) genes. ZAP-70 (zeta chain–associated protein) is a 70-kDa intracellular tyrosine kinase involved in TCR signaling.[238] By gene expression analyses, it has been discovered that CLL cells with unmutated IGHV differ from CLL cells with mutated IGHV in the expression levels of a small subset of genes, one of which encodes ZAP-70. It has been established that patients with CLL cells that have unmutated

IGHV have more aggressive disease, and measurement of ZAP-70 may be used as a surrogate marker for the expression of unmutated IGHV.[239] Furthermore, the expression of the cell surface marker CD38⁺ on CLL cells also defines those with more aggressive disease,[240] but the two markers (ZAP-70 and CD38⁺) do not always coincide.[241] Using both markers, clinicians are now better prepared to determine which patients at presentation are likely to be best served by aggressive treatment—those positive for ZAP-70 or CD38⁺—and those for whom specific therapy can be delayed.

Diagnosis and Management

The International Working Group has updated CLL guidelines[242] for diagnosis and management. CLL is usually diagnosed by the presence of lymphocytosis in the peripheral blood (>5 × 10^9/L present at least for 3 months), with less than 55% being atypical cells (prolymphocytes or lymphoblasts). Flow cytometry is essential in the diagnosis of CLL and reveals the characteristic immunophenotype, with CD5⁺, CD23⁺, FMC7⁻, weak expression of surface Ig (sIg), and weak or absent expression of membrane CD22⁺ and CD79b⁺.[243] Bone marrow usually has 30% or more lymphocytes, although bone marrow examination is not required for diagnosis.

Clinical staging using the Rai[244] or Binet[245,246] classification is used to determine prognosis and guide therapy. It is well known that CLL is a heterogeneous disease, with survival for some only 2 years, and for others, 2 decades. However it is also appreciated that more than 30% of patients show progression from an early stage to a more advanced stage within 3 years of diagnosis.[242] Numerous prognostic indicators have been identified that can detect those individuals at high risk of progression and also correlate with survival.

Features associated with poor prognosis include older age,[247] absolute lymphocyte count more than 50 × 10^9/L, diffuse bone marrow involvement, low platelet count, lymphadenopathy, low hemoglobin level, and presence of fever.[248,249] A diagnosis of CLL has significant effects psychologically on quality of life more, more so in older adults, and this aspect should be considered in decision making.[250]

Currently, the guidelines do not recommend treatment for early asymptomatic disease (stage 0 Rai and stage A Binet)[242] because more than 50% of these patients are alive at 10 years, and treatment for indolent disease did not improve outcome. For all stages, more than 65% of patients older than 80 years did not receive treatment at the time of initial diagnosis as compared to less than 45% in those younger than 40 years. However, analysis of relative survival from the National Cancer Database[251] has revealed that older patients succumb to CLL more often than from existing comorbid diseases.

Treatment

Treatment in the early and intermediate stages is offered only for those with CLL-attributable symptoms. Chlorambucil, with or without prednisone, was initially the drug of choice but this has been largely replaced by fludarabine, alone or in combination with cyclophosphamide or rituximab.[252] However, the incidence of autoimmune hemolytic anemias is increased in patients treated with fludarabine, and hematologic toxicity appears to increase in those older than 70 years. Pentostatin, cyclophosphamide, and rituximab have also been found to be effective treatment of CLL, with no significant differences in overall response (83% vs 93%) or complete response rate (39% vs. 41%) when older patients (≥70 years) were compared with younger patients (<70 years).[253] In patients with 17p deletion, associated with p53 mutations and poor prognosis, alemtuzumab, a humanized anti-CD52 monoclonal antibody, has achieved objective response rates as high as 40%.[254] Curiously, older patients appeared to do better than younger patients, and currently this agent is recommended as front-line therapy for those older than 70 years with 17p deletion or refractory CLL. There is an increased risk of infection with alemtuzumab, and appropriate prophylaxis should be administered. Reduced-intensity allogeneic stem cell transplantation may be considered for younger patients (<65 years) with good performance status after first remission or refractory disease, but supportive care and observation may be best for older patients in this setting.

ACUTE MYELOGENOUS LEUKEMIA

AML is primarily a disease of older adults. The median age at diagnosis is 67 years and, according to the National Cancer Institute Surveillance, Epidemiology and End Results (SEER) registry, the age-adjusted incidence rates for people aged 65 years and older is 16.4/100,000 as compared to 1.7/100,000 for those younger than 65 years.[255] Furthermore, there has been a progressive increase in the incidence of AML in older adults 85 years of age, with the highest incidence and mortality in those 74 to 85 years old. Although in earlier years the incidence of AML was shown to increase with each year, the annual percentage change in the age groups 65 to 74 years and older than 75 years has shown a significant downward trend for the years 2001 to 2005. However, mortality rates have continue to increase in those older than 75 years. There is a slight gender difference, with males being more affected, and this difference becomes more pronounced with age.

Diagnosis and Classification

AML is diagnosed by the demonstration by a minimum of 20% myeloblasts in a bone marrow sample. Environmental, genetic, and iatrogenic factors have been implicated in its cause.[256] AML may arise or, as is generally the case with older patients, as a progression of MDS or after treatment for a primary malignancy (secondary or treatment-related AML).[257] In people older than 60 years cigarette smoking (number of cigarettes and duration of smoking) is associated with an increased risk, particularly of the M2 subtype of the FAB AML classification.[258] A higher carrier rate of human T cell lymphotropic virus-1 (HTLV-1) has been observed in patients with acute promyelocytic (FAB M3) leukemia.[259]

As with most of the hematologic malignancies, classification schemes have been revised in consideration of new molecular and genetic understandings of disease pathogenesis. Thus, the classic French-American-British (FAB) system has been replaced by the WHO classification of acute leukemia (Table 91-7).

Clinical Features

Clinical features in AML are related to the uncontrolled proliferation of leukemic blasts in the bone marrow and infiltration into body tissues. Anemia and thrombocytopenia are frequently seen. CNS infiltration, which is more often noted in those with an initial white blood cell count more than 100,000/mm^3 and in those with monocytic leukemia, may present as meningeal involvement, bleeding, or a distinct mass (chloromas). Lumbar puncture should be considered in patients with neurologic features if imaging studies do not reveal pathology. Chloromas may also present as a space-occupying mass when present on the spine. In older adults, more subtle symptoms such as weakness, fatigue, or generalized malaise may be initial presenting features. Acute promyelocytic leukemia may present with disseminated intravascular coagulation (DIC) and bleeding manifestations. Older patients with AML typically present with a worse performance status and greater percentage of complex and high-risk

TABLE 91-7 WHO and French-American-British (FAB) AML Classification

WHO	Description	FAB
I	AML with recurrent genetic abnormalities	
	t(8;21)(q22;q22);(AML1/ETO)	
	inv(16)(p13;q22) or t(16;16)(p13;q22);(CBFβ/MYH11)	
	t(15;17)(q22;q12)(PML/RARα)	
	11q23 (MLL) abnormalities	
II	AML and MDS, therapy-related	
	Alkylating agent–related	
	Topoisomerase type II inhibitor–related	
III	AML with multilineage dysplasia	
	Following MDS	
	Without antecedent MDS	
IV	AML not otherwise categorized	
	AML without maturation	M1
	AML, minimally differentiated	M2
	AML with maturation	M3
	Acute monocytic leukemia	M4
	Acute myelomonocytic leukemia (AMMoL)	M5
	Acute monoblastic leukemia, AMMoL with eosinophilia	M5e
	Acute erythroid leukemia	M6
	Acute megakaryoblastic leukemia	M7
V	Acute leukemia of ambiguous lineage	

AML, Acute myelogenous leukemia; *MDS*, myelodysplastic syndrome; *MLL*, mixed-lineage leukemia.

karyotypic abnormalities but lower numbers of peripheral and bone marrow blasts.[260]

Treatment and Prognosis

Cytogenetic evaluation and immunophenotyping are absolutely essential in the initial workup of leukemia to classify subtypes and determine prognosis.[261] Although age itself is a poor prognostic factor in AML, the demonstration of high-risk karyotypes or immunophenotypes might portend an even greater risk of standard therapy failure.[262] Treatment of AML in otherwise fit older adults remains an anthracycline (e.g., daunorubicin, idarubicin) and cytosine arabinoside. For more frail older patients, alternative regimens or supportive care alone have been recommended.[263]

Outcomes

Outcomes for older patients with AML remain unsatisfactory, although there has been some improvement in survival over the past 3 decades.[264] Standard induction therapy, although not as effective as in young adults, is associated with better outcomes for those older than 60 years, particularly those with low-risk features.[265] Although the rate and duration of hospitalization are greater in older patients, treatment is often gratifying, with a return to a baseline level of functioning after discharge. For those younger than 75 years, with good performance status and favorable cytogenetics,[266] cytosine arabinoside combined with an anthracycline and followed by consolidation therapy is still considered the standard of care. Reduced-intensity conditioning regimens followed by stem cell transplantation can be effective curative therapy for older patients, with excellent performance status once in remission. However, this approach is still considered investigational and should be performed in the setting of a clinical trial.

Newer treatment approaches may also be relevant for older patients. For example, treatment with gemtuzumab, an ozogamicin calicheamicin conjugated to monoclonal antibody specific for the CD33+ receptor, was found to be associated with improved median survival in older patients with relapsed disease.[63] For patients with significant comorbidities, or those older than 75 years and with unfavorable cytogenetics or other high-risk factors, the standard induction therapy (cytosine arabinoside and an anthracycline, such as daunorubicin) often results in very poor outcomes, and these patients may best be managed by low-intensity therapy or supportive care. However, involvement of the patient in decision making and consideration of available psychosocial support are important in all decisions regarding AML management. Support with G-CSF after chemotherapy may be considered for older patients because it has been shown to improve remission rates and reduce hospitalizations.[267]

Older adults are susceptible to tumor lysis syndrome, which should be considered in all patients, particularly those who present with a very high white count. Also, older adults are particularly susceptible to the cerebellar toxicity of certain drugs, most notably cytosine arabinoside. When this drug is used in higher doses, such as during remission consolidation, careful neurologic checks should be performed before each dose of drug is administered.

DISORDERS OF HEMOSTASIS

Hemostasis is maintained by intricate and complex interactions involving vascular, platelet, and coagulation components. With advancing age, alterations in function of at least one of these components is likely, and there is a tendency for bleeding or clotting to result. This may be a consequence of aging, but it is equally likely to be associated with the use of one or many prescription drugs that can influence coagulation or platelet function. However, as a general rule, coagulation defects in older adults may be treated just as they are for those in other age groups.

Senile Purpura

Senile purpura occurs mainly on the extensor surfaces of the forearms and hands and may be seen in many otherwise normal older adults. Loss of subcutaneous fat and changes in aging connective tissue permit undue mobility of older skin, and shearing forces result in rupture of small vessels. Platelets are typically normal qualitatively and quantitatively in patients with senile purpura, and no correlation has been shown with ascorbic acid deficiency.

Purpura Due to Platelet Defects

Thrombocytopenia may occur as a primary (idiopathic) disorder or as a secondary phenomenon (e.g., drug-induced or associated with other blood diseases, infections, neoplasia, or other conditions). Occasionally, thrombocythemia, thrombasthenia, or combined defects may be present.

Autoimmune (Idiopathic) Thrombocytopenic Purpura

Autoimmune (idiopathic) thrombocytopenic purpura (ITP)is usually secondary to IgG autoantibodies against platelets, which sensitizes the platelets for destruction[268] and has a higher incidence in older adults as compared to younger adults.[269] Antibody to platelet antigens may be observed in a number of medical conditions, including systemic lupus erythematosus, HIV, immunodeficiency disorders, or a B cell lymphoproliferative syndrome (e.g. CLL). In older adults, the onset is usually insidious and is not clearly related to another illness. More than two thirds of patients may present with signs of mucosal or visceral bleeding, such as hematuria. The course is usually chronic and intermittent. An association of chronic ITP with current or past *H. pylori* infection has suggested an association that might be very relevant in older patients.[270]

Few platelets are seen in the peripheral blood smear, and those present are large (so-called megathrombocytes). The bone marrow typically reveals an increase in megakaryocytes. There is usually no splenomegaly. Diagnosis is primarily clinical; however, testing for the presence of antibodies on platelet surfaces has been associated with many false-positive results, and the assay has not been proven to be of great value in most situations.[271] Treatment is usually initiated if bleeding occurs or prophylactically in the setting of a very low platelet count (usually <10,000/μL) or prior to surgery. Therapy usually involves corticosteroids (prednisone, 1 to 2 mg/kg/day), which results in improvement in about 80% of patients but sometimes only after 2 or more weeks of treatment.[272] Other approved treatment options include intravenous immunoglobulin and danazol. Anti-CD20 antibody (rituximab)[273] and the thrombopoietin (TPO) receptor agonist eltrombopag[274] have undergone investigative trials. Splenectomy is usually considered only for refractory cases but provides excellent cure rates, with complete remission in more than 60% of cases.[275]

Secondary Thrombocytopenia

Drugs are a very important cause of thrombocytopenia. They may be direct marrow toxins or cause idiosyncratic hypersensitivity reactions or immune-mediated platelet destruction. Some drugs are known to cause selective thrombocytopenia only by decreasing megakaryocytes. Commonly used drugs associated with thrombocytopenia include sulfonamides, penicillin, tetracycline, desipramine, chlorothiazide, digitoxin, insulin, cimetidine, and myelosuppressive drugs used as chemotherapeutic agents.[276] Secondary thrombocytopenia is seen with acute and chronic leukemia, lymphoma, infection, myelodysplastic syndrome, MPD, chemotherapy treatment, collagen vascular diseases, splenomegaly, paraproteinemia, cirrhosis of the liver, and hypersensitivity reactions.

Heparin-induced thrombocytopenia results from antibodies against heparin that bind to and activate platelet Fc receptors.[277] Patients are at risk of severe bleeding from the thrombocytopenia, as well as arterial thrombosis, and one or the other can be lethal. Management includes immediate discontinuation all heparin-related products, including low-molecular-weight heparin and warfarin and the use of alternative antithrombotics, such as argatroban and hirudin before restarting warfarin.[277] Although the incidence of this complication is low, the widespread use of heparin in clinical practice makes it a familiar problem.

Thrombotic Thrombocytopenic Purpura

Thrombotic thrombocytopenia purpura (TTP) is a disseminated thrombotic microangiopathy that can be triggered by infection, drugs (e.g., clopidogrel), autoimmune disease, or an unknown risk factor. The syndrome is due to deficiency of ADAMTS-13 protein. ADAMTS-13 is a protease discovered in normal plasma that cleaves von Willebrand factor (vWF) and prevents platelet aggregation and clot formation.[278] TTP has a rapid onset, with widespread manifestations appearing over the course of 1 or 2 days. In the classic case, fever, thrombocytopenia with bleeding, microvascular hemolytic anemia, acute renal failure, and CNS disturbances are seen. Elevated LDH, bilirubin, and low haptoglobin levels are often present, and schistocytes or fragmented red cells may be seen on the peripheral blood smear. Other clotting studies are usually normal, fibrinogen levels are normal or increased, and split products are usually absent.

TTP is usually treated by large-volume plasma exchange. Cryodepleted (vWF-poor) plasma can be used in combination with steroids. This form of therapy has decreased the mortality rate of TTP from 90% to less than 50%. In patients with TTP who do not respond to plasma exchange, a combination of steroids, antiplatelet agents, and emergency splenectomy has been used, with some success.

COAGULATION DEFECTS

Survival with congenital coagulation disorders in later life is possible, especially von Willebrand disease. Acquired disorders include vitamin K deficiency, which leads to a reduction in prothrombin (factor II) and in factors VII, IX, and X. This condition may occur in malabsorption syndromes, liver disease, prolonged obstructive jaundice, and biliary fistula and with oral broad-spectrum antibiotic therapy. Renal failure, extracorporeal circuits, and acquired inhibitors may result in significant blood coagulation defects.

Anticoagulant therapy with warfarin reduces hepatic synthesis of the same four factors. Although warfarin has been associated with an increased risk of hemorrhagic complications, particularly intracranial hemorrhage,[279] maintaining international normalized ratio (INR) values between 2.0 and 3.0 remains appropriate in older adults[279] to derive adequate benefit. Levels of D-dimer, fibrinogen, factor VIII, and thrombin are known to increase with age and may be an explanation for the high incidence of vascular disorders in older adults. These have also been shown to predict adverse outcomes, including hospitalization, mortality, and poor functional outcomes.

Disseminated Intravascular Coagulation

A syndrome of diffuse intravascular coagulation (DIC) may be seen in older adults people in an acute, subacute, or chronic form. There is typically a serious underlying disease process leading to thromboplastic substances entering the circulation or injuring endothelial cells directly. Liver disease, acute pancreatitis, incompatible transfusions, cancer, and nonbacterial thrombotic endocarditis have also been associated with the occurrence of DIC.[280] DIC may also complicate the clinical course in acute promyelocytic leukemia in older adults. Criteria for diagnosis are not well defined; the most useful are a low platelet count, prolonged prothrombin time, positive plasma protamine test for fibrin, monomer-fibrinogen complexes, D dimers, and levels of fibrinogen and fibrin degradation products related to the clinical condition. Primary treatment should include control of underlying disease.

Therapy may include restoration of depleted blood components with platelet and fresh-frozen plasma infusions in bleeding patients. The use of heparin in the treatment of DIC remains controversial. Most studies have found heparin to be of little or no value and may in fact result in exaggerated thrombocytopenia or thrombosis. Even in complex situations, such as promyelocytic leukemia, the routine use of heparin remains controversial.

KEY POINTS

- Anemia is common in older adults but is not normal and affects quality of life, function, and outcomes. Causes should be sought.
- The incidence of myelodysplasia, myeloproliferative disorders, myelofibrosis. and multiple myeloma increases with age. This requires careful diagnostic evaluation in older adults and generally can now be more successfully treated, especially multiple myeloma.
- Almost 50% of non-Hodgkin lymphomas occur in those older than 65 years. Diffuse B cell lymphoma is the most common B cell subtype in all age groups, including those older than 75 years. Anaplastic large cell, lymphoblastic cell, and Burkitt lymphomas are less frequently encountered in older adults.
- With advancing age, alterations in hemostasis are likely, and there is a tendency for bleeding or clotting to result. This may be a consequence of aging but is equally likely to be associated with the use of one or many prescription drugs, which can influence coagulation and platelet function.

For a complete list of references, please visit www.expertconsult.com.

KEY REFERENCES

2. Geiger H, Denkinger M, Schirmbeck R: Hematopoietic stem cell aging. Curr Opin Immunol 29:86–92, 2014.
20. Sahin S, Tasar PT, Simsek H, et al: Prevalence of anemia and malnutrition and their association in elderly nursing home residents. Aging Clin Exp Res 2015.
22. Fraenkel PG: Understanding anemia of chronic disease. Hematology Am Soc Hematol Educ Program 2015:14–18, 2015.
24. Camaschella C: Iron-deficiency anemia. N Engl J Med 372:1832–1843, 2015.
25. Ganz T, Nemeth E: Hepcidin and iron homeostasis. Biochim Biophys Acta 1823:1434–1443, 2012.
32. Nemeth E, Ganz T: Anemia of inflammation. Hematol Oncol Clin North Am 28:671–681, 2014.
40. Lindblad AJ, Cotton C, Allan GM: Iron deficiency anemia in the elderly. Can Fam Physician 61:159, 2015.
43. Couderc AL, Camalet J, Schneider S, et al: Cobalamin deficiency in the elderly: aetiology and management: a study of 125 patients in a geriatric hospital. J Nutr Health Aging 19:234–239, 2015.
54. Sriram S, Xenocostas A, Lazo-Langner A: Erythropoietin in anemia of unknown etiology: a systematic review and meta-analysis. Hematology 2016.
57. Dinmohamed AG, Visser O, van Norden Y, et al: Trends in incidence, initial treatment and survival of myelodysplastic syndromes: a population-based study of 5144 patients diagnosed in the Netherlands from 2001 to 2010. Eur J Cancer 50:1004–1012, 2014.
74. Killick SB, Carter C, Culligan D, et al: Guidelines for the diagnosis and management of adult myelodysplastic syndromes. Br J Haematol 164:503–525, 2014.
90. Hoermann G, Greiner G, Valent P: Cytokine regulation of microenvironmental cells in myeloproliferative neoplasms. Mediators Inflamm 2015:869242, 2015.
112. Tefferi A, Barbui T: Essential thrombocythemia and polycythemia vera: focus on clinical practice. Mayo Clin Proc 90:1283–1293, 2015.
115. Deeg HJ, Bredeson C, Farnia S, et al: Hematopoietic cell transplantation as curative therapy for patients with myelofibrosis: long-term success in all age groups. Biol Blood Marrow Transplant 21:1883–1887, 2015.
116. Kitanaka A, Takenaka K, Shide K, et al: Splenic irradiation provides transient palliation for symptomatic splenomegaly associated with primary myelofibrosis: a report on 14 patients. Int J Hematol 2016.
120. Thompson PA, Kantarjian HM, Cortes JE: Diagnosis and treatment of chronic myeloid leukemia in 2015. Mayo Clin Proc 90:1440–1454, 2015.
127. Tuchman SA, Shapiro GR, Ershler WB, et al: Multiple myeloma in the very old: an IASIA conference report. J Natl Cancer Inst 106:5, 2014.
157. Ria R, Reale A, Vacca A: Novel agents and new therapeutic approaches for treatment of multiple myeloma. World J Methodol 4:73–90, 2014.
158. Stewart AK, Jacobus S, Fonseca R, et al: Melphalan, prednisone, and thalidomide vs melphalan, prednisone, and lenalidomide (ECOG E1A06) in untreated multiple myeloma. Blood 126:1294–1301, 2015.
263. Minakata D, Fujiwara SI, Ito S, et al: A low-dose cytarabine, aclarubicin and granulocyte colony-stimulating factor priming regimen versus a daunorubicin plus cytarabine regimen as induction therapy for older patients with acute myeloid leukemia: a propensity score analysis. Leuk Res 2016.

92 Geriatric Oncology

Margot A. Gosney

Cancer is a major cause of death and morbidity in older adults. In England and Wales, more than 331,000 people were diagnosed with cancer in 2011, and there were over 162,000 cancer deaths in 2012; of these, 52% were 75 years of age or older.[1] Female death rates from lung cancer have increased, whereas female mortality for breast and bowel cancer are the lowest they have been in 40 years. Unlike women, male mortality rates for lung cancer have fallen to their lowest levels in 40 years, and this has also been seen in bowel cancer. Men are 36% more likely than women to die from cancer, and mortality rates in the United Kingdom have decreased by more 24% since the mid-1980s. Improvements in treatment, early diagnosis, and public awareness are the main reasons for this progress. In the United Kingdom, it has been estimated that cancer costs over £15 billion/year; this figure includes £17.6 billion in economic costs, £5.6 billion for health, and £21.6 billion for unpaid care.[2] In 2011, it was announced that an excess of 14,000 cancer deaths/year is seen in the U.K. population aged 70 years and older.[3,4]

The full impact of cancer in older people is unclear if poor histologic verification occurs. Although this was a common occurrence 20 years ago, now only 6% men and 7% of women die of an unknown primary.[1] In the United States and in Europe, specialized groups have been formed to focus attention on geriatric oncology, such as the International Society for Geriatric Oncology (SIOG; http://siog.org) and European Society of Medical Oncology (ESMO; http://www.esmo.org).

CANCER AND AGING

Older adults are more likely to develop cancer, and differences in tumor growth and spread occur as a result of aging. The relationship between cancer and aging is complex, and various factors, including changes in host tumor defenses and exposure to carcinogens, have roles to play in the autology of tumors.[5] Current theories of cancer causation in older adults include decreased ability to repair DNA, oncogene activation or amplification, tumor suppressor gene loss, decreased immune surveillance, prolonged duration of carcinogenic exposure, and increased susceptibility of aged cells to carcinogens.

There is debate as to whether carcinogenesis and aging are related phenomena. Many state that such a relationship exists,[6,7] with some postulating that cancer develops as a consequence of normal aging processes, although others favor common causative factors for cancer and aging.[8] There is a relationship between chromosomal alterations and malignancy.[9] Several inherited disorders featuring chromosomal breakage and an increased frequency of malignant disease show abnormalities of DNA repair or recombination,[10] and many genetically determined syndromes have an accelerated progression of biologic aging and high frequency of malignant disease.

The increased incidence of cancer with age can be interpreted by the two major theories of aging. The first, the damage, or error, theory holds that over time, there is an accumulation of damage to vital areas of cellular or organ function, which culminates in the manifestations of the aging process. Mutations may occur in certain key genes or in many individual genes on a random basis. The multistep model of carcinogenesis fits with this theory because successive cancer-causing mutations accumulate during the aging process. The alternative, or program, theory considers aging as a later stage of a program that proceeds throughout embryogenesis to growth development and maturation. During aging, certain genes become expressed, and others are shut down.

The response of the body to a cancer is not a unique mechanism. There has been much interest in circulating concentrations of insulin-like growth factor 1 (IGF-1) and IGF-binding protein 3 (IGFBP-3) and their association with an increased risk of common cancers. Although these associations are modest, and vary among sites, further clarification is required,[11-13]

There is conflicting opinion regarding the growth and spread of cancer in older patients. Although some evidence shows death to be earlier in older subjects, coexisting diseases have obvious effects on morbidity and mortality. Some experimental work has demonstrated slower tumor growth, fewer metastases, and longer survival in older rodents, and others have shown decreased tumor growth associated with impaired T cell function.[14] Cultures from melanoma cell lines have demonstrated that T cells from young but not old donors stimulate the growth of tumor cells, and T cells from young but not old mice produce angiogenic factors, resulting in a richer vascular supply that may be responsible for increased growth and metastases.

Many older adults have been exposed to carcinogenic agents as a result of their occupation (e.g., working with asbestos, inorganic chemicals such as arsenic or nickel, and plant products such as aflatoxin, polycyclic hydrocarbons, and dyes). The key lifestyle environmental factors in older adults are tobacco consumption and atmospheric pollution. Studies have shown an increased incidence of cancer of the endometrium and breast associated with diet, and other dietary factors such as fiber protect against the development of carcinoma of the bowel.[15]

The relationship between cancer and aging is clearly complex. Various factors, including exposure to carcinogens and changes in the host defense, have roles to play in the development of tumors.

PREVENTION

Prevention may be classified into three types.[16] Primary prevention aims to prevent the onset of a disease, and secondary prevention aims to halt progression of a disease once it has been established. By identifying the disease early, often while the patient is still asymptomatic, prompt and effective treatment may be given to stop progression of the disease. Tertiary prevention aims to rehabilitate people with an established disease to minimize residual disabilities and complications. The focus of many cancer studies is primary and secondary prevention. Approximately 80% of all cancers are potentially preventable, and many public health strategies have been aimed at behavior modification.

For screening to be applicable, a disease must be common and curable if diagnosed early, and the test involved must be highly sensitive. Screening in the United Kingdom is almost exclusively for tumors of the breast, cervix, and colon. Older adults are less likely than those from younger age groups to participate in screening and cancer detection programs, which may be due to inadequate knowledge about cancer,[17,18] lower educational level,[19] perceived susceptibility,[20] and ethnic background.[21] Other factors, such as fear of cancer[22] and its treatment, difficulty differentiating between normal physiologic changes and early symptoms or signs of cancer, and fatalism[23] have also been implicated. Men participate less than women in screening procedures,[24] although the role of ethnicity, marital status, availability of screening test, and physician attitude are all known to have effects on this gender inequality. Older adults who scored higher in a health perception questionnaire that measured current health, prior health, health outlook, health worries and concerns, resistance or susceptibility to illness, and rejection of the sick role were also more likely to have participated in cancer screening programs.[25]

Older adults involved in health promotion have been found to have significant improvement in their quality of life, and therefore this should be advocated.[26] If the screening of older adults is to increase, the involvement of health care providers will be important.[27] Many exploratory studies have found that individuals who fail to undergo cancer screening tests have cited a lack of involvement with their health care provider in the previous year; also, in some countries, there are financial implications of taking such screening tests. Agist attitudes must not prevent physicians from recommending screening, nurses must not remove a patient's autonomy, and screening services must not exclude those most at risk. Educating health care practitioners, instilling confidence in their ability to teach certain self-examination techniques to patients and increasing the education of patients, is essential.

U.S. citizens show high enthusiasm for cancer screening,[28] although participation by certain subgroups (e.g., Hispanics) is reduced.[24] In the United Kingdom, many older adults have reported that they wish to continue to be actively invited for cancer screening, even though they may not all take up the offer.[29]

To improve the early detection of cancer, several questions, including the attitudes of older people toward screening and the barriers perceived by the patient, especially for skin, breast, and cervical cancers, need to be asked.[30] The comprehensive geriatric assessment (CGA) process can be used to identify suitable candidates for cancer screening in older adults.[31] The presence of a comorbid illness may reduce[32] or increase[33] the participation rate in cancer screening.

Breast Cancer Screening

First-line screening is through teaching breast self-examination. Studies have suggested that nurses do not view teaching breast health as part of their role in patient intervention, particularly in the acute care setting.[27] A clinical breast examination does not increase the accuracy of breast screening when combined with mammography.[34] Despite there being a number of clear guidelines for breast cancer screening, those most at risk still reject screening.[35]

The information on mammographic screening presented on various websites is not necessarily balanced. Some provide advice that is not in accord with AMA and General Medical Council guideline recommendations for informed consent. In one study, all the advocacy groups involved were receiving industry funding, apparently without restrictions, and the major harms of screening were mentioned in only a small proportion of websites.[36] A number of groups, including older, low-income, and African American women, are less likely to be screened,[17,23,37] as well as those with long-term limitations in their activities of daily living due to disability.[38-40] Other factors may reduce a patient's likelihood of attending screening, including male radiographers; younger women were more likely to describe embarrassment than older women, but there was a universal view that male radiographers result in a poor return for future screening appointments.[41]

The American Cancer Society (ACS) considers that screening decisions should be individualized and, as long as the woman is in reasonably good health and fit enough to be a candidate for treatment, she should continue to be screened with mammography. However, if the individual has a life expectancy of less than 3 to 5 years, severe functional limitations, or multiple or severe comorbidities likely to limit life expectancy, it may be appropriate to consider cessation of screening.[35] Data obtained from the Surveillance, Epidemiology, and End Results (SEER) program has shown a life extension of 178 days for those older than 85 years and 617 days for those aged 65 to 69 years[42] if screening was extended.

Colorectal Cancer Screening

Unfortunately, despite well-documented evidence of the benefits of screening for colorectal cancer (CRC), there is a relatively low participation rate, particularly when comparing the screening programs that exist for breast or cervical cancer.[43] In 1996, Hardcastle and colleagues published the results of a 10-year U.K. study that collected fecal occult blood from over 152,000 people aged 45 to 72 years. They found that 360 people had died from colorectal cancer in the screened group compared with 420 in the control group, a 15% reduction in cumulative mortality in the screened group.[44] At 2002 prices, the cost was £5,290/cancer detected, and the incremental cost per life year gained as a result of the screening was £1,584.[45] A similar French study invited participants up to 94 years of age and found that of the 206 adenocarcinomas detected, 47.6% were stage 1 and 23.8% were stage 2.[46] There are, however, a variety of time- and priority-related reasons why individuals fail to undergo fecal occult blood testing; these include the following: "did not notice test in mailbox" or "forgot," as well as more health-related issues such as "severe illness" and "family circumstances."[47] Although much of the evidence was from younger people, a Dutch study screened individuals up to 80 years of age, when colonoscopy capacity was unlimited, and up to 75 years of age, when colonoscopy capacity was decreased. They found that increasing the colonoscopy capacity substantially increased health benefits.[48] Worldwide, the age for screening is variable (lower age limit, 50 years, to upper age limit, 74 years). Although improved adherence with fecal occult blood testing is associated with being female, younger, and more educated, recommendation by a physician increases compliance,[19] as does the design of instructions.[49]

The U.K. National Screening Committee (UKNSC) currently offers screening every 2 years to all men and women aged 60 to 74 years. Although individuals older than 74 years can request a kit, they are not sent one automatically. In certain areas of the United Kingdom, starting in December 2016, all men and women 55 years of age will be asked to undergo sigmoidoscopy; this will affect older groups in the future. Controversy exists over the previous upper age limit of 69 years, but the suggestion by Hardcastle and associates[44] and Kronborg[50] of an upper age limit of 74 years has been accepted. It is expected that for every 100 patients screened, 98% will receive a normal result and be returned to routine screening, and the remaining 2% will be offered a colonoscopy. For every 20 individuals offered colonoscopy, 16 will accept the invitation and, of them, 50% are likely to have nothing abnormal detected, 38% are likely to have one or more polyps detected, and 12% are likely to have colorectal cancer detected.[51]

The 5-year risk of colorectal cancer after a negative screening colonoscopy is extremely low—1.3% of advanced adenomas detected approximately 5 years after a negative colonoscopy,[52] although higher in some series.[53] The role of screening colonoscopy in very old patients is a balance between increased prevalence of neoplasia (26.5% in the 75- to 79-year-old group vs. 28.6% in those aged 80 years or older) versus life expectancy in the two different age groups. Screening colonoscopy in those aged 80 years and older results in only 15% of the expected gain in life expectancy seen in younger patients; this should therefore only be performed after careful consideration of potential benefits, risks, and patient preferences.[54]

Although colonoscopy is relatively safe in older adults, the process is not without morbidity and, in rare cases, mortality. Increasing age increases the risks of poor bowel preparation and failed procedures. However, older patients can prove to be more tolerant than younger patients during the procedure and can undergo colonoscopy without sedation because the individual's pain threshold is not exceeded. With an entire bowel-cleansing preparation, there can be a 71.5% completion rate in older people.[55] Older adults who have not had a previous colonoscopy have higher baseline anxiety scores, but informational videos can reduce anxiety, as can more education about the purpose of the procedure, procedural details, and knowledge of potential complications.[56] Local data from several countries have demonstrated that colonoscopy in the very old can be safe and worthwhile.[57] The U.K. flexible sigmoidoscopy screening trial investigators found that a one-time flexible sigmoidoscopy was an acceptable, feasible, and safe screening regimen. This relatively simple procedure was carried out on almost 50 people/week, with two or three colonoscopy referrals being generated per center. The control group was not screened, and therefore comparisons could not be undertaken.[58] The limitations of bowel preparation and depth of insertion of the sigmoidoscope clearly affects the yield.[59]

Computed tomography (CT) colonography takes approximately 10 to 15 minutes, and the accuracy is similar to that of conventional colonoscopy.[60] It is, however, more expensive,[61] and is influenced by the experience of those reporting the scan.[62] It is good for identifying polyps that may be missed on colonoscopy,[63] may identify extracolonic abnormalities,[64] and requires minimal preparation, which may be of particular benefit for older adults.[65]

Investigating the older frail patient with lower bowel symptoms is difficult. It may result in up to 25% of flexible sigmoidoscopies being unsatisfactory due to poor bowel preparation.

Prostate Cancer Screening

There has been much controversy about the benefits of prostate cancer screening. The American Cancer Society and American Urological Association recommend annual prostate-specific antigen (PSA) screening for average-risk men aged 50 years and older if they have more than a 10-year life expectancy.[66] However, there is not yet evidence of overall mortality benefit from PSA screening.[67]

Lung Cancer Screening

The use of a baseline radiograph for lung cancer detection was investigated in the U.S. Prostate, Lung, Colorectal, and Ovarian (PLCO) Cancer Screening Trial. This study, of almost 155,000 participants, included individuals up to the age of 74 years. In the initial screening, approximately 9% of radiographs were suspicious for lung cancer, and these rates were highest for older age groups and for smokers.[68] The U.S. National Lung Cancer Screening trial found that cancer mortality was reduced by 20%. In an Italian study of older patients (mean age, 58 years), some of whom were up to the age of 84 years, there was little evidence of benefit for the routine use of screening.[69] Other lung screening trials have adopted low-dose CT (LDCT) and included individuals up to the age of 74 years who had a smoking history or were current smokers.[69,70]

CANCER INCIDENCE

De Rijke and colleagues have used high-quality data from the Netherlands and reported that total cancer incidence rates in men and women were highest in the 85- to 94-year-old age group.[71] In middle-aged groups, there was a stable rate of the most common tumors, but increasing rates in the oldest age groups. Although it was speculated that this might be due to an increase as a result of a decrease in mortality from other diseases, they also suggested that it might be related to an artifactual increase resulting from increased cancer detection rates in those in the very old group. With increasing interest in older patients with malignant disease, the latter rather than the former seems more likely.

Although age-specific rates and age-adjusted rates can be calculated for major cancers using incidence data at different cancer registries, there is a disconnect between cancer mortality in Europe and the US. However, trends are favorable although not consistent across all age groups.[72,73]

ASSESSMENT

The CGA is widely used internationally, and the results are used to modify treatment based on the extent of frailty.[74-79] A 2015 Cochrane systematic review of a mixed population of patients has reported that although there were limitations within the meta-analysis, there was evidence that patients who had undergone a CGA were more likely to be alive and in their own home following admission to hospital.[80]

CGA is essential in the management of older patients with cancer. There are, however, different views on whether a complete CGA is required. Overcash and colleagues, in 2005 and 2006, reported that a 15-item abbreviated CGA could be used to identify older adults presenting with cancer who would benefit from the entire CGA process.[81,82] They identified that four domains—functional status, instrumental activities of daily living, depression (using the geriatric depression scale), and cognition (using the Mini Mental State Examination [MMSE])—should be scored separately. Any score suggestive of deficits in these areas should be a marker for an in-depth assessment. In a pilot study, a mini geriatric assessment (MGA) administered by a gastroenterologist was used during decision making by a multidisciplinary cancer team. They found that the concordance between the MGA and CGA was good for the assessment of cognitive function, psychological status, and functional status but less accurate for nutritional status and comorbidity.

The Vulnerable Elders Survey-13 (VES-13) is an instrument to identify vulnerable older people in the community.[83] It has been used to predict functional decline and survival in different cancer types.[84] In older patients with cancer, the VES is highly predictive of impaired functional status and is a preliminary means of assessing older adults before undertaking a full CGA.[85] Higher VES-13 scores are linked with an increased probability of not completing radiotherapy for a variety of different tumor types.[86] The VES-13 has performed almost as well as a conventional CGA in detecting geriatric impairments in populations of older men with prostate cancer receiving androgen ablation[87] and, in other patients with several different tumor types, VES-13 is a useful predictor for survival.

Postal screening questionnaires (surveys) have been used in geriatric medicine since the 1980s,[88] and there has been interest in postal questionnaires and computer-based, self-administered questionnaires for older patients with cancer.[89-91] Although this screening identifies some potential issues, patients probably benefit from broader, more in-depth clinical assessment, and the high support needs of patients were often identified only in follow-up telephone calls.

For patients with cancer admitted for surgery, there is some evidence for embedding a CGA geriatric assessment service.[92] However, only one third of geriatricians responding to a British Geriatrics Society survey identified that their hospital provided some geriatric medicine input to older general surgical patients. Only 20% delivered care postoperatively; barriers to input were work force issues, lack of interspecialty collaboration, and funding.[93]

Comorbidity is particularly prevalent in older patients with cancer. However, cancer may be more likely to be diagnosed in healthier older patients due to primary care professionals being more reluctant to refer patients with cancer and poor general health.[94] Older adults with cancer experience a high number of concurrent symptoms (3 to 18), and there is a growing body of literature that describes specific symptom clusters in such patients. Unfortunately many symptoms may be attributed to the cancer and the so-called giants of geriatric medicine, such as urinary and fecal incontinence, fatigue, and frailty.[95] In 1987, Charleson and associates developed a method of classifying prognostic comorbidity using longitudinal studies. This index has been widely implemented into daily practice.[96] Predictably, increasing age and comorbidity are prognostic factors,[97] but comorbidity and functional status are independent prognostic factors in older cancer patients.[98] In the year following diagnosis, functional status in patients with all tumors, especially lung and colon, and with the exception of prostate, decline. The decrease in functional status is independent of cancer diagnosis but comorbidities, as well as age, smoking, and obesity, are clear predictors.[99,100] Age is associated with increasing comorbidity in older cancer patients,[101] and age-matched patients without cancer have fewer comorbidities.[102] Many comorbidity indexes use retrospective financial data,[103] but it is important that comorbidity be assessed prospectively, especially if it is being used during treatment decisions in multidisciplinary cancer team meetings.[104] Comorbidity indices may predict short-term outcomes,[104] patients who can undergo curative treatment, and overall survival rates.[105]

Although there are clear roles for a GGA in most cancer types, it is unclear from the many reports as to which intervention occurred following the assessment. It may, therefore, be the intervention that affects outcomes rather than the underlying issues that are identified through the CGA process. However, a CGA is strongly predictive of hospital readmission in older adults with cancer,[106] survival,[107,108] and treatment-related toxicity.[109-111] The CGA may be used to tailor therapy to optimize patients prior to surgical management[112-115] and help make a final therapeutic decision.[116]

In breast cancer patients, a CGA has been used to measure comorbidity retrospectively using Medicare claims.[117] CGA used prospectively has identified an average of six initial problems, with a further three problems identified during follow-up.[118] The most important questions that the CGA might be able to answer include the following[119]:

- Which older women should be screened for breast cancer?
- What is the best first-line treatment?
- Which older women require adjuvant radiotherapy?
- Which older women should receive adjuvant chemotherapy, if indicated by tumor?
- Which chemotherapy is appropriate for older women using a palliative approach?

Although the CGA is associated with improved outcome in older patients, the data so far have suggested that further work, including a randomized controlled trial, may be necessary to answer many of these questions. It must be used to support and improve therapy decisions rather than simply to prevent older women from receiving definitive treatment. Patients with more comorbidity identified by CGA at diagnosis were significantly less likely to have had surgical treatment 6 weeks later, but this may be appropriate.[120]

The primary care process should ensure that frailty and/or comorbidity are reliable detected in older patients.[121] Systematic reviews have identified the high prevalence of frailty in older adults with cancer and its effect on outcomes.[122,123] Therefore, quantitative and qualitative outcome measures cannot be considered without appropriate adjustment for frailty.[124-127] Some frailty tools identify frailty more accurately, so only well-validated tools should be selected.[128] Identification of frailty may help predict a higher risk of hospitalization or primary care usage, although this has yet to be proven definitively.[129]

DIAGNOSIS AND STAGE OF DISEASE

Diagnosis

For many patients, early diagnosis is the key to improved survival. There is evidence that the stage of disease varies in older adults at presentation. For those with breast cancer, it has been found to be an earlier stage when screening is used. The proportion of cancer cases diagnosed and confirmed by mammography in older women appears to be increasing.[130] However, many older patients delay seeking medical advice, which may result in cancer being diagnosed at a more advanced stage.

There is controversy as to whether the patient's age alone influences the method and thoroughness of a diagnostic investigation. Significantly more older patients with colorectal cancer present as emergency cases with advanced disease when compared with younger patients. These emergency cases are often not referred to surgical units, which may be partly explained by an atypical presentation, general frailty, or the patient being unsuitable for surgery. Geriatricians are experienced in assessing preexisting disability and concurrent disease and understanding functional status, level of dependency, and psychological adjustment. This enables joint decisions to be made with regard to further therapy before rehabilitation and, it is hoped, recovery of the older patient with cancer.[131]

With improved screening and diagnostic tests, older patients should present with an earlier stage of cancer. The knowledge of and ability to treat comorbidity should ensure that older patients are just as likely to be investigated as their younger counterparts. This should be particularly encouraged in patients with tumors for whom low-risk elective surgery can be undertaken and has been found to have similar morbidity and mortality in all age groups.[132]

Stage of Disease

Cancer staging is an important component of management, and histology and clinical stage of the cancer are independent predictors of survival.[133] There is a clear relationship between age and stage at diagnosis and between age at diagnosis and treatment received by the patient with cancer, although this difference is diminishing.[134]

TREATMENT

Older patients should now be receiving therapy comparable to that of their younger counterparts, although historically this may not always have been the case. In the 1980s and 1990s, older adults with cancer were less likely to receive definitive treatment than younger patients. Currently, there are few patients who, following assessment of comorbidity, should not be considered for active curative treatment. There is, however, an issue regarding the inclusion of older adults in clinical trials. U.S. data comparing 1996 to 1998 with 2000 to 2002 showed an increase in the total number of trial participants, with only 1.3% of 65- to-74-year-old patients and 0.5% of patients older than 75 years being represented. With increasing age, study participation becomes reduced.[135] There has been an underrepresentation of women and black and ethnic minority groups in clinical trials; the underrepresentation of patients older than 65 years was documented even in 1999.[136] At this time, many trials explicitly excluded older adults but, even in studies in which recruitment of older individuals was attempted, there was still underrepresentation in regard to breast cancer treatment and, to a lesser extent, for other tumor types.[136] White patients in suburban areas, and those who were uninsured, had better, although not representative, recruitment in older age groups.[137] These findings are not exclusive to the United States or United Kingdom.[138,139] The reasons given by newly diagnosed patients were "feeling too anxious" (40%), "not interested" (25%), "no time" (12.5%), "too sick" (5%), or "too healthy" (5%) to be included in clinical trials.[140]

Some have argued that older patients are more likely to suffer from toxicity with chemotherapy, although newer drugs have reduced toxicity and allow good palliation for most cancers.[141] Younger patients often report more nausea, fatigue, and vomiting than their older counterparts and therefore these side effects should not overtly restrict the recruitment of older adults.[142] Other reasons given for the nontreatment of older adults with cancer have included advanced disease at presentation. Although there is some evidence that patients older than 55 years have more advanced disease at presentation, this is not a universal finding.[134,143,144]

Some physicians responsible for older patients with cancer believe that they are less likely to want treatment than their younger counterparts.[144a] This was not the finding of Yellen and colleagues, who used structured scenarios to assess patients' willingness to accept toxic chemotherapy to enhance survival. They reported that older patients were as willing to choose chemotherapy as younger patients, although the former required a greater survival advantage before they would choose a toxic regimen over a less toxic alternative.

Myths about cancer may affect treatment. If older patients believe that a cancer treatment is worse than the disease itself, or if they have a greater fear of cancer than younger patients,[145] they may decline treatment. If adequate information is given to older patients, they are likely to accept treatment in a similar fashion to younger patients[146,147] and may experience less emotional distress following the diagnosis of cancer. Bilodeau and Degner have found that older women with breast cancer prefer to assume a passive role in treatment decision making.[148] Whereas most younger women thought that the stage of disease, likelihood of cure, and treatment options were the most important aspects of the information they received, older women considered that self-care issues were more important.[148,149]

The attitudes of physicians with regard to informing older adults about a cancer diagnosis may also influence the treatment that they receive. Although there is a widely held view that older adults do not wish to be informed about a new cancer diagnosis, 80% of respondents aged 65 to 94 years wanted to be informed of a cancer diagnosis, with 70% of respondents also wanting their relatives to be informed when the diagnosis was made.[150] This is in contrast to how relatives of cancer patients feel, for whom 6% did not want the diagnosis to be disclosed.[151] It must, however, be remembered that collusion with relatives and nondisclosure to patients have a negative effect on those caring for the patient.[152]

There are three categories of decision making roles about treatment—preferred, actual, and perceived roles. There is often a mismatch between patients' preferred and actual roles and, although this occurs in patients of all ages, it must be carefully avoided when dealing with older patients about to begin cancer treatment.[153] The communication skills required to deliver cancer care have been defined following a number of consensus meetings.[154]

The need for information and support when viewed through the eyes of patients, relatives, and professionals is often different. Patient education should therefore be tailored to reflect older patients' information support needs and abilities, rather than using generic materials.[155] Patient preferences can be assessed using a patient-driven questionnaire,[156] and their satisfaction can be measured through questionnaires administered via paper or the Internet.[157] Although why older adults with cancer accept or decline prime treatment varies considerably when systematically studied,[158] this is also consistent with other evidence on nonadherence.[159] Overall, many older cancer patients prefer to receive less information about their illness and treatment and assume a less active role in making treatment decisions.[160] Therefore, communication to patients about cancer must improve.[161] At the end of treatment, if decisions to limit treatment are made, many relatives support patients in voicing their preferences, but one third may act against the known or presumed wishes of the patient.[162] Therefore, although relatives play some role in end-of-life decision making and treatment decisions, physicians must guard against relatives voicing different decisions than those expressed by the patient.

Surgery

Surgery is considered to be the treatment of choice for most cancers, and patients should not be denied surgery on the basis of chronologic age. Nonetheless, mortality and morbidity rates are often increased in older patients who undergo cancer surgery. Multidisciplinary care and teamwork can, however, minimize mortality and morbidity.[163]

Advanced age per se is often used by the patient's family or health care professional to justify not proceeding with surgery. However, this agist attitude has fortunately been declining. Surgery for octogenarians now results in better clinical outcomes for cancer and noncancer patients. Even octogenarians can undergo high-risk cancer surgery, such as pancreatectomy, esophagectomy, and lung cancer resection, for which survival is again associated with preoperative comorbidities.[164] A number of guidelines exist for the management of perioperative patients undergoing noncardiac surgery,[165] and even older patients should be considered for surgical resection of metastatic cancer.[166] The POSSUM score (Physiological and Operative Severity Score for the enUmeration of Mortality and morbidity) was devised from retrospective and prospective data.[167] Both APACHE II and POSSUM scores reliably predict perioperative complications and mortality in patients with different types of cancers who undergo surgery.[168,169] Preoperative assessment of any older surgical patient is essential, particularly to identify those most at risk of postoperative cognitive dysfunction (POCD).[170]

Drug Therapy

The normal physiologic changes of aging affect drug absorption, distribution, metabolism, and elimination. Older patients with cancer may receive a wide range of drugs, including chemotherapeutic agents, analgesics, antiemetics, and antibiotics in addition to drug therapy that had been previously prescribed for coexisting medical disorders.

Some normal changes of aging can affect drug absorption. Oral drugs are modified by gastric motility and emptying time, whereas the absorption of parenterally administered drugs is dependent on local blood flow in muscles and fatty tissue. Drug distribution is affected by the decrease in total body water and albumin and change in the ratio of lean body weight to fat. The reduction in the albumin level results in a greater concentration of unbound, highly lipophilic drugs in the circulation that can exert their effects.

Drug metabolism is affected by decreased liver mass and hepatic blood flow, as well as decreased microsomal enzymatic activity in the liver. Elimination is affected by a reduction in the glomerular filtration rate, decreased renal blood flow, and renal tubular function and is particularly important with cyclophosphamide and methotrexate, which are both excreted renally.

Unfortunately, as with younger patients with cancer, many older adults with cancer may be taking multiple medications, which will increase the risk of adverse drug reactions, drug-drug interactions, and nonadherence. Many clinical trials do little to include typical older patients with frailty. As a result, progress in the understanding of many of the pharmacologic issues when treating older individuals with cancer has yet to be fully addressed.[171]

Chemotherapy

Older patients are less likely to receive chemotherapy and, if treated, it is more likely to be outside a clinical trial, although this is gradually improving. All drug therapy in older adults is affected by their altered pharmacokinetics and pharmacodynamics, and some chemotherapeutic agents pose special problems.[172] Reduction of chemotherapeutic drug dosages may reduce toxicity at the expense of response rates, lower response rates without any effect on toxicity, or result in better tolerance, but provide no survival advantage. Reducing dosages on the basis of age alone is not justified.

A prospective pilot study by Chen and coworkers has found that although older patients undergoing chemotherapy experience some toxicity, they could generally tolerate it with limited impact on their independence, other comorbidities, and quality of life.[173] This, however, is in contrast to the views of Repetto,[174] who considered that age was such a clear risk factor for chemotherapy-induced neutropenia and its complications, particularly in the treatment of lymphoma or solid tumors, that without the use of colony-stimulating factors better outcomes would not be achieved.

The use of erythropoietin to treat anemia[175] may not be without risks.[176] Chemotherapy- induced anemia may also be treated with darbepoetin alfa.[177] The pharmacology and polypharmacy associated with the older cancer patient has been extensively reviewed by Lichtman and Boparai,[178,179] and others have highlighted the risks of concomitant medication and potential drug interactions.[180-182] Complications such as renal insufficiency,[183] febrile neutropenia,[184] and chemotherapy-induced alopecia[185] are similar to those seen in the younger population. Anticancer therapy must be targeted using evidence from older and younger individuals[186] and, when new drugs are developed, they must be evaluated in older adults, who are now becoming the main recipients of oncology drugs.[187] ESMO, in 2013, presented a position paper on the current and future roles of medical oncologists but failed to mention their role in the older cancer patient.[188] There is clear evidence of a disparity in race, gender, and age when considering recruitment to clinical trials,[135] and evidence has suggested that education may reduce this barrier.[189] Although evidence is essential for the treatment of older patients, the ACTION trial attempted to randomize woman older than 70 years to investigate the effects of adjuvant chemotherapy.[190] The trial was terminated after 10 months when only four patients had been randomized. Despite widespread support, including input from patient groups, the trial failed to recruit due to the inability to convince older patients to accept randomization.[190]

It may be appropriate for frail patients to receive chemotherapy dose reductions, so-called older adult–friendly chemotherapy regimens, but higher rates of premature withdrawal and early deaths may still occur compared to nonfrail patients. Patients with frailty may have a shorter survival, but this may be related to frailty rather than to chemotherapy or other treatments; therefore, clinical trials that recruit frail older cancer patients are urgently needed.[191]

Hormone Therapy

Hormone therapy may provide benefit to older patients with advanced cancer of the breast, prostate, and endometrium. In the management of metastatic breast cancer, the beneficial effects of estrogen therapy increase steadily with age in all postmenopausal women, probably because of the increased incidence of receptor-positive tumors in older women that result in an increased response rate to this type of therapy.

Radiotherapy

If a tumor is radiosensitive, radiotherapy may be appropriate and have positive results, particularly for older patients in good health.[192-194] Organ-specific tolerance to radiation is related to aging. Lymphocytes from older experimental animals and humans are more susceptible to damage induced by ionizing radiation. When radiotherapy in older patients is palliative in intent, it is important that minimal toxicity be experienced. However, radiotherapy can be highly effective, with many older patients completing treatment with no serious complications. Radiotherapy may be used at times with curative intent, particularly in early-stage, non–small cell lung cancer (NSCLC), which is inoperable. In such cases, a large fraction size can be given safely, even to older adults.[195] Zachariah and colleagues have found that 94% of patients aged 80 years or older diagnosed with cancer of the head and neck, lung, pelvis, or breast tolerated and completed the planned course of radiotherapy, curative or palliative, without serious complications.[196] Side effects are often few and usually mild, with most older patients tolerating delivery of their radiotherapy over 1 week.[197] Unless the patient is severely debilitated, there is no reason to modify a potentially curative approach.[198] When radiotherapy is being used for the treatment of cancer pain, there is no evidence that age influences the efficacy of such treatment and factors such as the pain score before the onset of radiotherapy or the presence of radiating pain are much better predictors of who will benefit from the treatment. Follow-up of such patients is often difficult, and use of the Edmonton Symptom Assessment System (ESAS) by telephone follow-up may be more appropriate for older adults.

Myelosuppression may be problematic because older patients have less functional bone marrow and a slowed recovery of normal tissue. Fatigue may result in compliance problems, and radiation may result in dry skin that is more susceptible to infection. The normal aging of the gastrointestinal (GI) tract may result in increased susceptibility to anorexia and stomatitis following radiotherapy.

The more commonly seen radiation side effects that occur in older adults are predicated on preexisting conditions. Thus, radiation to emphysematous lungs will increase dyspnea, and irradiation of the mediastinum will impair declining left ventricular function. Compliance with radiotherapy in older adults is additionally hampered by multiple visits and traveling. The use of split fractions does, however, reduce toxicity and is essential for the treatment of many tumors in older patients.

Treatment of the Three Most Common Cancers

The three most common cancers that geriatricians will encounter are colon, lung, and breast cancers.

Colon Cancer

Frailty is an independent predictor of survival in older patients with colorectal cancer.[199]

Surgery. The preoperative bowel cleansing that has rendered many older adults fecally incontinent, with severe electrolyte disturbances, is now considered to be no longer required.[200,201] Preoperative carbohydrate administration, as well as barring the use of nasogastric tubes, which increase pulmonary morbidity and slow the recovery of GI function, are both part of fast-track surgery, which may benefit the older patient.[202] The MRC CLASICC trial in 2005 has shown that laparoscopic surgery for cancer of the colon is as effective as open surgery.[203] Laparoscopic rectal surgery can preserve the pelvic autonomic nerves in selected patients when performed by appropriately trained surgeons.[204] Older patients often present as an emergency, which is associated with poor outcome,[205] although there is little difference in outcomes between patients who present with perforated or obstructed lesions.[206] Postoperative mortality features in patients older than 80 years have illustrated that age, American Society of Anesthesiologists (ASA) grade, operative urgency (emergency vs. elective), no cancer excision, and metastatic disease are poor prognostic indicators.[207] Age, presence of another site of recurrence, and time of diagnosis are all independent factors associated with resection of curative intent.[208] Even patients older than 70 years can have good outcomes following surgical treatment of liver metastases and age per se should not preclude consideration.[209]

The impact of surgery on the older frail cancer patient has been reviewed.[210] Some investigators have found that frailty indicators do not necessarily predict a decline in physical function after colorectal cancer surgery.[211] However, there is evidence that screening for frailty among older patients with cancer who may be candidates for abdominal surgery is clinically important and eminently justified[212] because frailty is an independent predictor of surgical outcomes.[213,214]

Chemotherapy. Adjuvant chemotherapy with fluorouracil and levamisole for 1 year after surgical resection of node-positive colon cancer was developed in 1990.[215] A variety of different drugs have been investigated since then, some in association with radiation therapy. Age, gender, comorbidity, and socioeconomic status often influence treatment decisions,[216] despite older patients being able to tolerate adjuvant chemotherapy alone or in combination with radiation therapy.[217,218] Although outcomes may be worse among the older population,[219-221] a number of chemotherapy regimens have been used for metastatic colorectal cancer and, despite small numbers of patients older than 75, such treatment should not be discounted in older adults.[222,223] In a trial that included a small number of individuals in their 70s, preoperative chemotherapy improved the outcome of resection of liver metastases.[224]

Lung Cancer

The European Organisation for Research and Treatment of Cancer (EORTC) and International Society of Geriatric Oncology (SIOG) recently published an updated review on the management of older patients with NSCLC. They recommended the use of a multidimensional, multidisciplinary CGA, which leads to better individualized treatment after taking into account of the patient's life expectancy, functional cognitive and emotional status, and presence of comorbidities. Clearly, patient preference is also incorporated into such treatment decisions.[225] Other reviews have yielded consistent advice and highlighted the barriers to the recruitment of older patients to clinical trials.[226,227] In the United Kingdom, the online audit tool (LUCADA database) collects data on treatment rates and survival and separates patients into age bands (<70, 70 to 74, 75 to 79, 80 to 84, and >85 years). In 2009, 7,593 of 32,068 diagnoses of lung cancer (23.7%) were made in those 80 years of age or older.[228]

Although lung cancer incidence has been falling in men, there are more women being diagnosed in the United Kingdom due to increased cigarette smoking.[229] Noninvasive investigations such as positron emission tomography (PET) scanning may reduce the number of invasive staging procedures and be useful to select older adults who may have curable lung cancer.[230,231]

Mesothelioma

Mesothelioma is a universally fatal disease, with an increasing incidence. The mean survival from presentation is 9 to 12 months. Its association with industrialized countries has resulted in a large excess of men being diagnosed with the condition; therefore, an accurate occupational history must be taken in all older adults presenting with breathlessness and a pleural effusion.[232] Of all new diagnoses, 50% are in those aged older than 70 years because of the long latency period between exposure and development of mesothelioma.[233] The addition of chemotherapy to active symptom control offers no significant benefits in terms of overall survival or quality of life, although the use of vinorelbine may be promising.[234] Weekly paclitaxel gives a median progression-free survival of 9.7 months,[235] and bevacizumab may also have a place in this group of patients.[236] Unfortunately, some drugs, such as oral idarubicin, have shown lack of efficacy and unacceptably high toxicity in those older than 70 years.[237]

Radiotherapy. Patients with stage 1 NSCLC who are not medically fit for surgery may be offered conventionally fractionated radiotherapy. Hypofractionated schedules, with three fractions during week 1, may be appropriate in patients up to the age of 84 years.[238] Two-year local control and cancer-specific survival rates have been shown to be 94.7% and 77.6%, respectively, in a small series representing all age groups.[195] Radiotherapy plus chemotherapy may be used prior to resection in selected patients with stage 3A NSCLC, although most of the studies have been done in patients younger than 80 years.[239]

Chemotherapy. The feasibility of delivering chemotherapy to older NSCLC patients has been determined in a number of studies.[240] There is a significant association between cardiac dysfunction and the use of chemotherapy or radiation therapy, although this may be an option for older adults.[241] The use of carboplatin, gemcitabine, and paclitaxel has varying effects on quality of life and toxicity[242,243] and, for some patients with advanced NSCLC and poor performance status, a single oral drug agent may be more appropriate.[244] Older patients with small cell lung cancer may be too frail for treatment, and a CGA must guide decision making, especially in these patients.[245]

Surgery. Surgery provides the best opportunity for cure at all ages. Although postoperative mortality after surgery for lung cancer increases with age (1.7% for patients < 60 years and up to 9.4% for those >80 years).[246] Previous cigarette smoking, as well as age, may increase cardiac comorbidity, although is not necessarily a risk factor for mortality and morbidity following surgery for primary NSCLC. Cardiac function should be rigorously assessed and not used as the only factor for final decision making.[247] Less extensive surgery in the form of lobectomy is now often superseded by sublobar resection, with no reduction in survival.[248]

Breast Cancer

Radiotherapy. A study of more than 8,700 women aged 70 years or older who were treated with conservative surgery for small lymph node–negative, estrogen receptor–positive breast cancer has shown positive benefits. The radiation therapy was associated with an absolute risk reduction of four events/100 women at 5 years and was most likely to benefit those women 70 to 79 years without comorbidity. Although those who derived least benefit were those 80 years of age or older with moderate to severe comorbidity, the number needed to treat to prevent one event was 61 to 125 patients, illustrating some benefit, albeit reduced compared to the younger group.[249] In a study including women of all ages, those who received adjuvant radiotherapy were younger, had fewer comorbidities, and were more likely to be white, married, from an urban area, and diagnosed in the later years of the study compared to those who did not receive adjuvant therapy. However, it is of note that they were more likely to have a surgeon who was female, had a Doctor of Medicine (MD) degree, and was caring for more than 15 patients, adding support to the multifactorial nature of patient selection.[250]

Chemotherapy. A CGA is essential prior to adjuvant chemotherapy and is often insufficiently taken into account in routine practice.[251,252] Not all patients require systemic adjuvant therapy,[253,254] but in those for whom chemotherapy is appropriate, the most common reasons for not offering it were "other treatments more appropriate" or "benefits too small" (in 63% and 54% of patients, respectively). Comorbidities and frailty were less commonly used as reasons for not administering chemotherapy, although they became more frequent with increasing age.[255] Much of the data presented included individuals up to the age of 69 years at entry into trials.[256] However, studies comparing small numbers of individuals older than 70 years have found that age alone should not be a contraindication to the use of optimal chemotherapy regimens in older women who are in good health.[257]

Surgery. Martelli and colleagues[258] have found that older patients with early breast cancer and no palpable axillary lymph nodes could be safely treated with conservative surgery and adjuvant tamoxifen, without the need for axillary dissection or postoperative radiotherapy. During prolonged follow-up (median, 15 years), they found that 83% of the deaths were unrelated to breast cancer. This provides data that may enable some older women to choose more limited surgery and adjuvant tamoxifen over extensive surgery and postoperative radiotherapy. In 2008, the results of two large trials that investigated extending tamoxifen treatment beyond 5 years were reported. On the basis of these studies, it is now suggested that following 5 years of adjuvant tamoxifen, an aromatase inhibitor (AI) may be used for a further 4 years in postmenopausal women.[259-261]

Endocrine Therapy. A Cochrane review of surgery versus primary endocrine therapy for women older than 70 years with operable primary breast cancer has summarized the findings of seven studies. It was concluded that primary endocrine therapy should be offered only to women with estrogen receptor–positive tumors who are unfit for or who have refused surgery. If a woman has significant comorbid disease, and estrogen receptor–positive tumors, it is possible that primary endocrine therapy may be a superior option to surgery, although this requires further evidence.[262] AIs are considered to be clinically effective compared with standard tamoxifen treatment, but their long-term effects still remain unclear. Tamoxifen is responsible for a small but statistically significant increase in endometrial cancer, thromboembolic events, and stroke. However, AIs are associated with an increased risk for osteoporosis.[259] Older patients who are healthy, are older than 70 years, and have completed 5 years of tamoxifen should be considered for extending adjuvant therapy with letrozole.[263]

NURSING AND CAREGIVERS

Patients with cancer will have a variety of symptoms, and many report fatigue, which may be particularly difficult to treat in older patients with comorbidity.[264] It is important that fatigue be measured and managed following surgery and chemotherapy.[264-267] Practical advice is essential, as well as the identification of common reversible causes.[268]

In the community, much of the physical and psychological care of the patient is placed on the family, with the attendant risk of caregiver strain. Many patients with cancer have depressive symptoms, and there is a positive correlation between a patient's self-care needs and mood. A brief intervention delivered by nonspecialists may promote adjustment in newly diagnosed cancer patients at high risk of developing anxiety or depressive disorders.[269] Although androgen deprivation therapy is consider by some to result in more depressive symptoms in men with nonmetastatic prostate cancer, this has not been substantiated.[270] The older cancer patient may have treatment goals that focus on pain relief and comfort, but they receive fewer prescriptions for opioids.[271] This finding was confirmed by Kurtz and associates,[272] who assessed the mental health of patients and family members and found that of the 208 patients in the study, 83 of whom were aged 65 years or older, the most common five symptoms were fatigue, pain, nausea, poor appetite, and constipation. In this study, there was no relationship between age and the level of symptoms, although older adults tended to underreport, which may counteract a genuine age-related increase in symptoms.

Caregivers are more likely to be wives than husbands and to perform care single-handedly. Wives provide twice the hours of care than husbands, although this is compensated by female patients having more outside care than males.[273] Unfortunately, when illness or treatment results in restricted activity, finance is limited, or caregivers are not spouses, patients with cancer are more likely to report unmet needs.[274,275] Using data from noninstitutionalized older adults without cancer, there is further evidence of married disabled women receiving fewer hours per week of informal home care than married disabled men, again stressing the need to target resources, particularly to married disabled women who, without the input of their children, may be deficient in necessary care.[276] In 82% of cases, the caregivers were spouses of the patients, and it is likely, therefore, that older spouses will be solitary caregivers and have little support from other friends and relatives.[277] Although caregivers provide essential support for older cancer patients, they may misunderstand the informational needs of the patient. Therefore, talking to relatives to determine an older patient's information preferences may not accurately predict what the patient wants.[278] Although the burden of caregiving is high, it must be remembered that even caregivers with chronic health problems have a lower mortality risk than noncaregivers, even those providing 50 or more hours of caregiving per week.[279] Worldwide, counseling in relation to depression and anxiety, as well supportive care and advice on diet, exercise, and weight control, are unmet needs for people of all ages with cancer.[280]

PREHABILITATION AND REHABILITATION

Where data are available on older patients following treatment for cancer, functional status assessment is usually via oncology-specific measures, which ignore many of the more important activities of daily living that are included in the well-validated rating scores frequently used in geriatric medicine. Without accurate clinical assessment of older adults with cancer, rehabilitation cannot be targeted. The role of comorbidity scores is limited, and therefore there is a need for a more overarching comprehensive assessment.[281]

The role of a structured exercise training program has been investigated in older patients undergoing rectal[282] and prostate[283] cancer surgery. Both studies have confirmed the feasibility of such regimens. In the rectal cancer study, patients up to the age of 84 years were included. Prehabilitation improved the return of fitness to baselines at 6 weeks.

There is randomized controlled trial evidence that postacute care delivered in small community hospitals is associated with improved independence outcomes.[284] Further evidence for improving independence in noncancer patients has been provided in a review of 774 inpatient medical rehabilitation hospitals (148,807 patient records), and a substantial reduction in mean length of stay was observed.[285] A systematic review of 16 effectiveness and six cost-effectiveness studies of rehabilitation in cancer survivors was published in 2012.[286] Although it was concluded that the evidence for multidimensional interventions and economic impact of rehabilitation studies is scarce, the findings were positive, with most notable improvements in fatigue and physical functioning.[286] Regular exercise can also improve psychological well-being during cancer treatment.[287]

SURVIVAL

Relative survival is lower among older adults with cancer than among their younger counterparts. There are many possible explanations for these differences, including the tendency for cancer to be diagnosed at a later stage in older adults and differences in treatment received by older patients. Other age-related factors, such as frailty and comorbidity, obviously influence outcomes.[288]

The development of cancer-specific brief questionnaires for patients will also facilitate the identification of symptoms that require palliation.[289] Patients wish to know the mode of disease progression, mode of death, and prognosis and are more content with realistic versus unrealistic time scales. In addition, a prognosis does not in itself cause depression; therefore, collusion and physician anxiety must not detract from information giving, particularly with older patients.[290] Novel delivery of specialized care may be more appropriate for older patients, many of whom wish to remain at home. This not only improves quality of life but also improves survival.[291] In addition, patients close to death are often prepared to undergo chemotherapy, even for small gains, and this may be particularly true in older cancer patients.

SUMMARY

The SIOG[292] and ESMO[293,294] have provided clinical practice guidelines. The challenge for clinicians is the rapidly changing clinical environment, particularly for those treating patients aged 70 years and older.[295,296]

Frailty has been well described in the geriatric medicine literature since 1990.[297] It is now a major issue in geriatric oncology, with much agreement that the CGA should become more widely used.[298,299] Cancer trials in the future will need to consider the frail older patient as a target population to ensure that realistic results from intervention trials are obtained.[300] Geriatricians have a major role in pretreatment assessment, identification of frailty, advice on how to optimize patient, and liaison with surgical and oncologic colleagues.

KEY POINTS

- Cancer is a major cause of death and morbidity in older adults.
- The relationship between cancer and aging is complex and several factors, including lifetime exposure to carcinogens and changes in host defense, are influential.
- Improving outcomes for older adults with frailty is now a major issue in geriatric oncology, with an understanding that the comprehensive geriatric assessment should be more widely used.
- The International Society of Geriatric Oncology and European Society for Medical Oncology have provided clinical practice guidelines
- Cancer trials in the future will need to consider older adults with frailty as a target population to ensure that realistic results from intervention trials are obtained.
- Geriatricians have a major role in pretreatment assessment, identification of frailty, advice on how to optimize patient, and liaison with surgical and oncologic colleagues.

For a complete list of references, please visit www.expertconsult.com.

KEY REFERENCES

85. Luciani A, Ascione G, Bertuzzi C, et al: Detecting disabilities in older patients with cancer: comparison between comprehensive geriatric assessment and vulnerable elders survey-13. J Clin Oncol 28:2046–2050, 2010.
89. Kalsi T, Babic-Illman G, Hughes S, et al: Validity and reliability of a comprehensive geriatric assessment screening questionnaire (CGA-GOLD) in older people with cancer. Age Ageing 43(Suppl 1):i30, 2014.
92. Harari D, Hopper A, Dhesi J, et al: Proactive care of older people undergoing surgery ('POPS'): designing, embedding, evaluating and funding a comprehensive geriatric assessment service for older elective surgical patients. Age Ageing 36:190–196, 2007.
104. Stairmand J, Signal L, Sarfati D, et al: Consideration of comorbidity in treatment decision making in multidisciplinary cancer team meetings: a systematic review. Ann Oncol 26:1325–1332, 2015.
106. Chiang LY, Liu J, Flood KL, et al: Geriatric assessment as predictors of hospital readmission in older adults with cancer. J Geriatr Oncol 6:254–261, 2015.
109. Versteeg KS, Konings IR, Lagaay AM, et al: Prediction of treatment-related toxicity and outcome with geriatric assessment in elderly patients with solid malignancies treated with chemotherapy: a systematic review. Ann Oncol 25:1914–1918, 2014.
110. Hamaker ME, Vos AG, Smorenburg CH, et al: The value of geriatric assessments in predicting treatment tolerance and all-cause mortality in older patients with cancer. Oncologist 17:1439–1449, 2012.
111. Baitar A, Van Fraeyenhove F, Vandebroek A, et al: Geriatric screening results and the association with severe treatment toxicity after the first cycle of (radio)chemotherapy. J Geriatr Oncol 5:179–184, 2014.
116. Chaibi P, Magne N, Breton S, et al: Influence of geriatric consultation with comprehensive geriatric assessment on final therapeutic decision in elderly cancer patients. Crit Rev Oncol Hematol 79:302–307, 2011.
120. Parks RM, Hall L, Tang SW, et al: The potential value of comprehensive geriatric assessment in evaluating older women with primary operable breast cancer undergoing surgery or non-operative treatment—a pilot study. J Geriatr Oncol 6:46–51, 2015.
121. Pal SK, Katheria V, Hurria A: Evaluating the older patient with cancer: understanding frailty and the geriatric assessment. CA Cancer J Clin 60:120–132, 2010.
122. Handforth C, Clegg A, Young C, et al: The prevalence and outcomes of frailty in older cancer patients: a systematic review. Ann Oncol 26:1091–1101, 2015.
123. Hamaker ME, Jonker JM, de Rooij SE, et al: elderly patients with cancer: a systematic review. Lancet Oncol 13:e437–e444, 2012.
158. Puts MT, Tapscott B, Fitch M, et al: A systematic review of factors influencing older adults' decision to accept or decline cancer treatment. Cancer Treat Rev 41:2197–2215, 2015.
188. Popescu RA, Schafer R, Califano R, et al: The current and future role of the medical oncologist in the professional care for cancer patients: a position paper by the European Society for Medical Oncology (ESMO). Ann Oncol 25:9–15, 2014.
279. O'Reilly D, Rosato M, Maguire A, et al: Caregiving reduces mortality risk for most caregivers: a census-based record linkage study. Int J Epidemiol 44(6):1959–1969, 2015.

93 Clinical Immunology: Immune Senescence and the Acquired Immunodeficiency of Aging

Mohan K. Tummala, Dennis D. Taub, William B. Ershler

CHANGES IN THE HUMAN IMMUNE SYSTEM WITH AGING

As a fundamental organ necessary for the maintenance of life, the immune system first appeared in primitive organisms about 480 million years ago.[1] The intricate relationship between acquired immunity and infection was apparent early in recorded history. Observing an epidemic of plague in 430 BC, Thucydides reported that anyone who had recovered from the disease was spared during future outbreaks. The era of modern immunology was launched with Jenner's report in 1798 of an effective vaccine using cowpox pustules to prevent smallpox in humans. Improved understanding of immunity and infection continued throughout the nineteenth and twentieth centuries. For example, identification of bacterial organisms ultimately resulted in the discovery of antibodies that could neutralize these microbes and/or their toxins, eventually leading to endorsement of the concept of vaccination. The discovery of antibody structure during the 1960s finally began the era of modern immunochemistry. With regard to cellular immunity, despite the early work of Metchnikoff and his followers, the role of cells in acquired immunity was not truly appreciated until the 1950s. Although theories of self-recognition and autoimmunity appeared early in the twentieth century, autoimmune diseases remain incompletely understood.

As a concept, immunogerontology is a relatively recent focus of interest. In 1969, Walford proposed that declining immune function contributes to the biologic processes of aging.[2] He speculated that disorders in the immune system that occur with aging account for three major causes of disease in older adults—increased autoimmunity, failing surveillance, allowing the expression of cancers, and increased susceptibility to infectious diseases. Current evidence supports the notion that the decline in immune function with aging may be viewed as a form of acquired immunodeficiency of modest dimension. Complicating the assessment of aging on immune function, older people are more likely to have diseases, conditions, or exposures that contribute to declining immune function.[3]

CHANGES IN THE HUMAN IMMUNE SYSTEM WITH AGING

Nonspecific Host Defense

Primary (innate) immunity is the first line of defense against invading pathogens. It differs from secondary (acquired) immunity in that it does not require sensitization or prior exposure to offer protection. Primary immunity involves tissues (e.g., mucocutaneous barriers), cells (e.g., monocytes, neutrophils, natural killer [NK] cells) and soluble factors (e.g., cytokines, chemokines, complement) coordinated to mediate the nonspecific lysis of foreign cells.

A feature of innate immunity is the detection of pathogens using pattern recognition receptors such as Toll-like receptors (TLRs), which recognize specific molecular patterns present on the surface of pathogens that trigger a variety of signaling pathways. After processing of antigen by the antigen-presenting cells (APCs), the peptide fragments are presented along with major histocompatibility (MHC) class II molecules to $CD4^+$ T cells or with MHC class I molecules to $CD8^+$ T cells to generate efficient T cell responses. The APCs also provide additional costimulatory stimulus (e.g., ligation of B7.1 or CD80 on APCs with CD28 on T cells) to lower the threshold of T cell activation and survival following the recognition of antigens. The ligation of TLRs on APCs enhances the phagocytosis of the pathogen through the release of chemokines and other peptides, which then result in the activation and recruitment of immune cells to the sites of infection.

Phagocytosis

Phagocytosis involves the engulfment, lysis, and/or digestion of foreign substances. The capacity of neutrophils, macrophages, and monocytes for phagocytosis is determined by their number and ability to reach the relevant site, adhere to endothelial surfaces, respond to chemical signals (chemotaxis), and complete the process of phagocytosis.[4] The study of alterations in phagocytosis with age must then involve examinations of each of these steps, which is inherently more difficult in human populations than in disease-free, inbred animals. Extrapolation of studies of senescent mice to humans suggests that age itself does not attenuate the response to bacterial capsular antigens in a well-vascularized area such as the lung.[5,6] Niwa and colleagues have reported a deterioration in neutrophil chemotaxis and increase in serum lipid peroxidase levels in the nonsurviving cohort of a 7-year longitudinal study, suggesting a preterminal but not necessarily normal aging alteration in these factors.[7] However, age-related effectiveness in chemotaxis may be reduced in less vascular tissues in vivo, such as in the skin, which also has a number of other changes that may impair the ability of cells in the vascular compartment to reach a site of infection.[8] Although older adults preserve the number and overall phagocytic capacity, in vitro neutrophil functions (e.g., endothelial adherence, migration, granule secretory behavior such as superoxide production, nitric oxide, and apoptosis) appear to be reduced with age,[9-11] and significantly fewer neutrophils arrive at the skin abrasion sites studied in older adults.[12] How this translates to immune response and immune-mediated repair in infected or otherwise physiologically stressed older adults remains unknown. Although the expression of TLRs and granulocyte macrophage colony-stimulating factor (GM-CSF) receptors are not diminished, ligation of these receptors results in altered signal transduction. With aging, alterations in signal transduction of these receptors may be involved in the defective function of neutrophils, with decreased response to stimuli such as infection with gram-positive bacteria.[13,14] These changes in older adults, unlike in younger persons, could be the result of changes in the recruitment of TLR4 into lipid rafts and no-raft fractions (the domains on plasma membrane that play an important role in cell signaling) with lipopolysaccharide (LPS) stimulation.[15] Similarly, the activation through GM-CSF on the surface of these cells is also altered in older adults because of an age-related presence of a phosphatase in the lipid raft, blocking cell activation and contributing to a decreased response to GM-CSF in neutrophils from older adults.[16]

Macrophage activation also appears to change with age; this may be partially attributable to a reduced interferon-γ (IFN-γ) signal from T lymphocytes.[17,18] A decrease in the number of macrophage precursors and macrophages is observed in bone marrow.[19] Although it is not clear if there is an age-associated decrease of TLR on the surface of aged macrophages, defective production of cytokines has been observed after TLR stimulation, possibly due to altered signal transduction.[20,21] With aging, there is diminished expression of MHC class II molecules in humans and mice, resulting in diminished antigen recognition and processing by these APCs.[19,22] In addition, activated macrophages from humans and mice produce higher levels of prostaglandin E2, which may negatively influence antigen presentation.[19] Fewer signals at the site of infection may be a consequence of reduced numbers of activated T cells locally due to the reduced antigen-processing capacity of macrophages. Fewer T cells and the defective expression of homing markers to attract T cells from peripheral blood into inflamed tissues[23] suggests that increased susceptibility of old mic—for example, to tuberculosis—reflects an impaired capacity to focus mediator cells and the additional cytokine they may express at sites of infection (see more on T cell changes with age in later discussion). These observations may help explain why late-life tuberculosis or reactivation tuberculosis occurs and remains clinically important in geriatric populations. The change in function of antigen-presenting dendritic cells (DCs) with aging is less well defined. A decrease in the number and migration of Langerhans cells in skin has been described in older adults,[24] but their function remains sufficient for antigen presentation.[25] In contrast, DCs from older adults who are considered frail have been demonstrated to have reduced expression of costimulatory molecules, secrete less interleukin12 (IL-12), and stimulate a less robust T cell proliferative response when compared with those who are not frail.[26]

Cell Lysis

Cell lysis is mediated through a variety of pathways, including the complement system, NK cell, macrophage-monocyte, and neutrophil activity. Complement activity does not appear to decline significantly with age, and neutrophil function also appears intact. However, in longitudinal studies of nonhuman primates, NK cell activity does appear to be affected by age[27] and acute stressors such as illness.[28] The functioning status of NK cells is dependent on a balance of activating and inhibitory signals delivered to membrane receptors.[29] A well-preserved NK cell activity is observed in healthy older adults,[30] explaining, in part, a lower incidence of respiratory tract infections and higher antibody titers after influenza vaccination.[31] However, older adults with chronic diseases and frailty are characterized by lower NK cell cytotoxicity and a greater predisposition to infection and other medical disorders.[32,33]

Although little is known about any changes in expression of activating and inhibitory receptors in older adults, NK activation and cytotoxic granule release remain intact.[30,34] Secretion of IFN-γ after stimulation of purified NK cells with IL-2 shows an early decrease, which can be overcome with prolonged incubation.[35] IL-12 or IL-2 can upregulate chemokine production, although to a lesser extent than that observed in younger subjects.[36] These observations suggest that NK cells have an age-associated defect in their response to cytokines, with a subsequent detriment in their capacity to kill target cells and synthesize cytokines and chemokines.

Specific Host Defense

There are well-defined alterations in cellular and humoral immunity with advancing age. In the cellular immune system, most studies have shown no significant changes with human aging in the total number of peripheral blood cells, including total lymphocytes, monocytes, NK cells, or polymorphonuclear leukocytes.[35,37-41] The appearance of lymphocytopenia is associated with mortality in older adults, but is not an age-related finding.[42-44] Most studies have shown no changes in the percentages of B and T lymphocyte populations in the peripheral blood,[45,46] although chronically ill older adults may, in particular, have a decline in total T cell numbers. Equivocal changes in the ratio of helper cells to suppressor cells (T4/T8) occur in normal aging.[39,40,45,47,48] These findings are in contrast to human immunodeficiency virus (HIV)–induced acquired immunodeficiency syndrome (AIDS) associated with a decreased T4/T8 ratio. Finally, there is a specific age-related increase in memory cells, cells that express the CD45 surface marker.[49-52]

Qualitative Changes in Cell Function

Changes in T Cell Function

The function of lymphocytes is altered with aging. This may be a consequence of decreased thymic function, an important factor for age-related changes in thymus-dependent immunity and adaptive T cell immunity. Declines in serum thymic hormone levels precede the decline in thymic tissue. By the age of 60 years, few of the thymic peptides are measurable in human peripheral blood,[53] and the thymus undergoes progressive reduction in size associated with the loss of thymic epithelial cells and a decrease in thymopoiesis. Thymic hormone replacement may improve immune function in older adults,[54,55] but there are no current clinical indications in this regard.

T cells may be considered naïve or memory on the basis of prior antigen exposure and, with advancing age, there has been noted a relative expansion of the memory T cell pool. The competency of adaptive immune function declines with age primarily because of a dramatic decline in the production of naïve lymphocytes due to a decline in thymic output and an increase in inert memory lymphocytes (see later discussion). Naïve $CD4^+$ T cells isolated from older adults and animals display decreased in vitro responsiveness and altered profiles of cytokine secretion to mitogen stimulation, expand poorly, and give rise to fewer effector cells when compared with naïve $CD4^+$ T cells isolated from younger hosts. Naïve $CD4^+$ T cells from aged animals produce about half the IL-2 as younger cells on initial stimulation with APCs. Also, the helper function of naïve $CD4^+$ T cells for antibody production is also decreased.[56] However, newly generated $CD4^+$ cells in aged mice respond well to antigens and are able to expand with adequate IL-2 production, with good cognate helper function. Thus, these age-related defects in naïve $CD4^+$ T cells appear to be a result of the chronologic age of naïve $CD4^+$ T cells rather than the chronologic age of the individual. These aged naïve $CD4^+$ T cells proliferate less and produce less IL-2 in response to antigenic stimulation than naïve $CD4^+$ T cells that have not undergone homeostatic divisions in the peripheral blood. The mechanism underlying homeostasis-associated dysfunction of naïve CD4 T cells is not known. In contrast to naïve cells, however, memory $CD4^+$ T cells are long-lived, maintained by homeostatic cytokines, and are relatively competent with age. Isolated $CD4^+$ T cells from healthy older adults and old mice are normal in regard to antigen proliferation in vitro.[57] Memory $CD4^+$ T cells generated from a young age respond well to antigens over time, whereas memory $CD4^+$ T cells derived from older age respond poorly.[58] Memory T cells generated from aged naïve T cells, on stimulation, survive and persist well, but are markedly defective in proliferation and cytokine secretion during recall responses, with impaired cognate help for humoral immunity. Healthy older adults can mount a $CD4^+$ T cell response comparable to that observed in younger individuals when vaccinated with influenza vaccine, but they exhibit an impaired long-term $CD4^+$ T cell immune response to the influenza vaccine.[59] Vaccination with influenza results in increased IL-2 secretion in response to viral antigen in vitro.[60,61] However, the number of influenza-specific cytotoxic T cells declines with age, with no increase after vaccination.[62]

Alteration in cell surface receptor expression (e.g., the loss of costimulatory receptor CD28 on the surface of $CD8^+$ T cells) is one of the most prominent changes that occurs with aging. $CD28^-CD8^+$ T cells are absent in newborns but become the majority (80% to 90%) of circulating $CD8^+$ T cells in older adults. Functionally, these $CD28^-CD8^+$ T cells are relatively inert and have a reduced proliferative response to TCR cross-linking, but maintain their capacity for cytotoxicity and are resistant to apoptosis.[63] This loss of CD28 expression is associated with a gain of expression of stimulatory NK cell receptors in $CD28^-CD8^+$ memory T cells, enabling their effector function as a compensation for impaired proliferation.[64]

There is a reduction of naïve $CD8^+$ T cells with some degree of oligoclonal expansion of $CD8^+$ T cells with age observed in healthy older adults.[65] This expansion may reflect a compensatory phenomenon to control a latent viral infection or fill available T cell space as a result of diminished output of naïve T cells from the thymus. When this clonal expansion reaches a critical level, the diversity of the T cell repertoire is reduced, and its ability to protect against new infections is compromised, as seen when older adults are exposed to new antigens. For example, the effect of host age was studied in the severe acute respiratory syndrome (SARS) outbreak, and it was discovered that the antigen recognition repertoire of T cells was approximately 10^8 in younger adults but only 10^6 in older adults.[66] Notably, most of the SARS mortality was observed in infected persons older than 50 years. The accumulation of $CD28^-CD8^+$ T cells is also found in viral infections, such as cytomegalovirus (CMV), Epstein-Barr virus (EBV), and hepatitis C virus, so $CD28^-CD8^+$ T cells may be derived from $CD28^-CD8^+$ T cells after repeated antigenic stimulation.[67] This clonal expansion of $CD28^-CD8^+$ T cells appears to be associated with increased infections and failed response to vaccines in older adults. As a result of the combination of thymic involution, repeated antigen exposure, and alteration in susceptibility to apoptosis (increased for CD4 and decreased for CD8), the thymic and lymphoid tissue in the aged host becomes populated with anergic (nonresponsive) memory $CD28^-CD8^+$ T cells, resulting in impaired cell-mediated immunity. The potential for far-reaching effects of the presence of senescent T cells is illustrated by the correlation between poor humoral response to vaccination in older adults and an increase in the proportion of CD8 T cells that lack expression of CD28.[68,69]

There is also a decline in delayed-type skin hypersensitivity (DTH),[70-73] and the assessment of this has become a useful measure of cell-mediated immunity. Generally, a battery of skin test antigens (usually four to six antigens) is required to assess DTH adequately. The number of skin test positive reactions declines with age, from more than 80% in younger individuals to less than 20% in older adults.[73] As with most functional measures in geriatric populations, there is remarkable heterogeneity. In one study,[72] 17.9% of subjects older than 66 years and living at home were anergic compared with 41% living in a nursing home but able to care for themselves and 60% who were functionally impaired and living in a nursing home. Although skin testing is a good indicator of cell-mediated immunologic health, it is heavily influenced by acute and chronic illnesses and the component of anergy because of aging is difficult to discern. Furthermore, concomitant in vitro testing has suggested that not all anergic patients have impaired in vitro responses,[37,74] suggesting that some of the observed skin test anergy may be technical (i.e., due to difficulty in intradermal injection in the skin of older adults) or be caused by a deficit in antigen presentation, as described earlier. Thus, both in vivo cutaneous DTH assessment and in vitro lymphocyte testing may be necessary to identify more adequately those who are truly anergic and presumably immunodeficient. The relevance of this type of determination is apparent by the repeated demonstrations of an association between anergy and mortality.[43,72,73,75-77]

The issue of an age-associated decline in DTH has particular relevance for the testing of past or current tuberculosis exposure.[78-82] Acknowledging the high incidence of anergy in older adult patients, care must be given to assess response to control antigens, such as *Candida*, mumps, or streptokinase-streptodornase (SKSD) before concluding that a negative tuberculin reaction indicates the absence of tuberculosis exposure. Furthermore, for healthy older adults, false-positive skin test results may be observed in those who have had repeated testing (the so-called booster effect).[82]

Changes in B Cell Function

In the humoral immune system, there are no consistent changes in the number of peripheral blood B cells with age. The decline in antibody production following vaccination in older adults is the result of reduced antigen-specific B cell expansion and differentiation, leading to the production of low titers of antigen-specific immunoglobulin (IgG). Most studies have indicated a mild to moderate increase in total serum IgG and IgA levels, with no change in IgM levels.[83,84] Declines in antibody titers to specific foreign antigens have been noted, including naturally occurring antibodies to the isoagglutinins[85] and titers of antibody to foreign antigens such as microbial antigens.[86-90] Both the primary[91] and secondary immune responses to vaccination are impaired. Older patients tend to have lower peak titers of antibody and more rapid declines in titers after immunization,[92,93] with the peak titer occurring slightly later than in younger people (2 to 6 weeks, rather than 2 to 3 weeks postvaccination).[94] In contrast, serum autoantibodies may have organ specificity, such as antiparietal cell, antithyroglobulin, and antineuronal antibodies.[46,95-101] With aging, there is a decreased generation of early progenitor B cells, resulting in a low output of new naïve B cells, with clonal expansion of antigen-experienced B cells. This results in a limited repertoire in immunoglobulin generation (through class switch) in B cells as observed in older adults and old mice,[102] with limited antigen-specific B cell expansion and differentiation leading to the production of reduced titers of antigen-specific IgG. The antibodies produced by older B cells are commonly of low affinity due to reduced class switching and somatic recombination in the variable region of the immunoglobulin gene necessary for antibody production and diversity. The generation of memory B cells is highly dependent on germinal centers, the formation of which is known to decline with age. The formation of germinal centers is dependent to some extent on interactions of B cells with $CD4^+$ T helper cells, and the age-related quantitative and qualitative changes in T and B cells may account, in large part, for the clinically observed diminished response to vaccines. For example, although 70% to 90% of individuals younger than 65 years are effectively protected after influenza vaccination, only 10% to 30% of frail older adults are protected.[105]

Organ-nonspecific autoantibodies, such as antibodies to DNA and rheumatoid factors, also increase with age. Circulating immune complexes may also increase with advancing age.[95,106] The reason why autoantibodies increase with age is not known. Several explanations are possible, including alterations in immune regulation and an increase in stimulation of B cell clones because of recurrent or chronic infections or increased tissue degradation.

Cytokine Dysregulation and Aging

There has been an increased awareness of alterations in the production and degradation of cytokines with age (Table 93-1). In vitro studies to assess functional aspects of lymphocytes after stimulation with mitogens have shown a decline in proliferative responses, possibly as a result of decreased T cell lymphokine production and regulation, particularly IL-2.[44,48,107,108] Decreases in the percentage of IL-2 receptor–positive cells, IL-2 receptor density, and expression of IL-2 and IL-2 receptor–specific mRNA in older adults have been reported.[48,109] IL-2 production in response to specific antigens also declines. There is a profound decline in the proliferative capacity of T lymphocytes to nonspecific mitogens.[46,48,73,110] In addition, antigen-specific declines in the proliferative potential of T cells have been demonstrated.[70,111] The number and affinity of mitogen receptors on T lymphocytes do not change with age.[112] However, the number of T lymphocytes capable of dividing in response to mitogen exposure is reduced, and the activated T cells do not undergo as many divisions.[80] Superimposed on the accumulation of a relatively inert naïve T cell fraction observed with advancing age, there appears also to be a shift in predominance of helper T cell responses from type 1 (Th1) to type 2 (Th2). Cells of the Th1 type produce IL-2, IFN-γ, and tumor necrosis factor-α (TNF-α) and predominantly mediate cell-mediated immune and inflammatory responses, whereas cells of the TH2 type produce IL-4, IL-5, IL-6, and IL-10, factors that enhance humoral immunity (Figure 93-1).[56] Whereas the decline in IL-2 and IL-12 may contribute to the observed decline in cellular immune function, the increase in proinflammatory cytokines (particularly IL-6) may contribute to the metabolic changes associated with frailty. It has been proposed that a chronic exposure to such proinflammatory signals contributes to the phenotype of frailty.[113] In fact, elevated IL-6 levels have been shown to correlate well with functional decline and mortality in a population of community-dwelling older adults.[114] Thus the inflammation-related biomarkers are powerful predictors of frailty and mortality[115,116] in older adults, a phenomenon termed *inflammaging*.[49]

In the steady state (i.e., in the absence of stress, trauma, infection, or disease), IL-6 is tightly controlled, and serum levels are typically measured in the very low picogram range. Among the regulators of IL-6 are sex steroids (estrogen, testosterone) and, at menopause, detectable IL-6 levels appear in the blood in apparently healthy older women. This inappropriate presence of a circulating proinflammatory molecule has garnered great interest among biogerontologists because it provides a rational explanation for many of the phenotypic features of frailty and levels associated with a number of age-associated disorders, including atherosclerosis, diabetes, Alzheimer disease, and osteoporosis.[117-120]

TABLE 93-1 Immunologic Markers of Aging

Decreased	Increased
Thymic output	Memory T and B cells
Naïve peripheral T cells	Oligoclonal expansion of memory lymphocytes
Diversity of T and B cell repertoire	CMV specific $CD8^+/CD4^+$ T cells
Costimulatory stimuli to T cells	CD45 RO^+ T cells
$CD28^+$ T cells	$CD28^-$ T cells
$CD45^+$ T cells	IL-6, SCF,* LIF†
IL-2, INF-γ, IL-12, IL-10, IL-13	Anergic T cells
Proliferation with mitogens	
Delayed-type hypersensitivity	
Response to vaccination	

*Stem cell factor.
†Leukemia inhibitory factor.

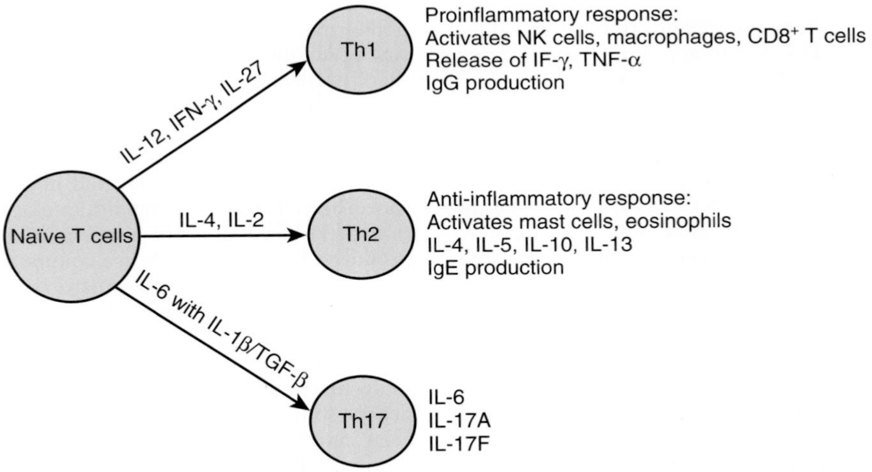

Figure 93-1. Differentiation of a naïve T helper cell (Th cell) into effector T cells. The differentiation of naïve T cells into various effector T cell subsets occurs in response to stimulation by distinct antigen-presenting cells and cytokine exposure. These functional subsets include Th1, Th2, Th17, and regulatory T (Treg) cells. These subsets play distinct roles in the genesis and control of cell-mediated immunity and inflammation. Traditionally, the Th1 cell responses have been implicated in many autoimmune and inflammatory disease states and cytokines produced by these cells, primarily IL-2, IFN-γ, and TNF-α, induce mononuclear and polymorphonuclear cell infiltration and activation in the target tissues. In this fashion, deregulated expression of proinflammatory cytokines is thought to play a central role in the development of autoimmune diseases and chronic inflammatory responses. In contrast, Th2 cells secrete IL-4 and IL-10 that promote humoral immunity and inhibit Th1 cell responses and have been implicated in the amelioration and remission of autoimmune and inflammatory diseases. A third Th cell subset, named Th17, has been described that depends on IL-23 for survival and expansion and has been identified as a major mediator of pathogenic inflammatory responses associated with autoimmunity, allergy, organ transplantation, and tumor development. Treg cells of several types have been identified and been shown to play an active role to suppress autoreactive T cells. However, these cells are also capable of suppressing the host's ability to mount an optimal cell-mediated immune response to antigens and tumor cells if their numbers and activity are not controlled.

CLINICAL CONSEQUENCES OF IMMUNE SENESCENCE

Autoimmunity

Waldorf and coworkers[91] have speculated that autoimmunity plays an important role in the aging process. Cohen has alternatively proposed that autoimmunity may play an important physiologic role in the regenerative and reparative process that is ongoing during aging.[121] Certain autoimmune diseases have their highest incidence in older adults, such as pernicious anemia, thyroiditis, bullous pemphigoid, rheumatoid arthritis, and temporal arteritis, suggesting that the age-related increase in autoantibodies may have clinical relevance,[122-127] although this latter point remains unproven.

Autoimmunity may also play a role in vascular disease in older adults.[128] Giant T cell arteritis is a common disease in older adults[124,129] and is associated with degenerative vascular disease. Immune mechanisms may cause atherosclerosis, a final common pathway of pathology secondary to a variety of vascular insults.[130] A number of antivascular antibodies have been described in humans[131-134] that are associated with diseases of the vasculature. Antiphospholipid antibodies are associated with a variety of pathologic states of the vasculature, including stroke and vascular dementia, temporal arteritis, and ischemic heart disease.[135-138] However, the exact mechanism whereby antiphospholipid antibodies cause vascular injury remains unknown.[139] The increased occurrence of antiphospholipid antibodies with age[140-142] and the association of these autoantibodies with vascular disease may represent a predisposing immunologic factor for immune-mediated vascular disease in older adults. Autoantibodies to vascular heparan sulfate proteoglycan (vHSPG) may also be important in vascular injury in older adults[133] because vHSPG play an important role in normal anticoagulation and cholesterol metabolism.[143]

Immune Senescence

Immune Senescence and Cancer

Age is the single greatest risk for cancer.[144] It has long been postulated that immune mechanisms play an important role in recognizing and destroying tumor cells; thus, an age-associated decline in immune function might be invoked to explain the increased rate of cancer in older adults. The problem with this hypothesis is that as rational as it sounds, it has been very difficult to prove (see later discussion). Furthermore, there are other explanations for the observed increased malignant disease in older adults, not the least of which is the estimated prolonged time (measured in decades for many epithelial tumors) that it takes to sustain the multiple genetic and epigenetic events required for malignant transformation and tumor growth to the point of clinical detection. An alternative explanation suggests that the host and host factors change over time, favoring progression and expression in later life. These two hypotheses to explain the increase in late-life malignancy have aptly been described as "seed versus soil."[145]

From an immunologic and soil standpoint, there are two principal observations that relate to malignancies and age—deregulation of proliferation of cells directly controlled by the immune system and evidence of increased malignancies in later life that could be hypothetically restrained by nonsenescent immunity. These will be discussed sequentially.

Proliferative disorders of the lymphocyte are common in older adults. Although bimodal in incidence, the peak in late-life lymphoma includes a disproportionate incidence of nodular B cell types.[146] Both older adults and mice commonly exhibit a monoclonal gammopathy (paraprotein) in the last quartile of their life span.[147-150] Monoclonal gammopathies increase with age and may occur in 79% of sera from subjects older than 95 years.[151-153] Radl and colleagues[151] have defined four categories of age-associated monoclonal gammopathy—myeloma or related disorders, benign B cell neoplasia, immunodeficiency, with T cell greater than B cell loss, and chronic antigenic stimulation. They speculated that the third category is the most common and that this is what occurs with immune senescence. It is possible that age-associated immune dysfunction is initially associated with markers of aberrant immune regulation, such as increased levels of paraproteinemia and/or autoantibodies, which may later contribute to the pathogenesis of lymphoma. Monoclonal gammopathies may cause morbidity, particularly renal disease, in the absence of overt multiple myeloma.[154] In a minority of cases of monoclonal gammopathies, a malignant evolution may occur.[154-156] Multiple myeloma also demonstrates an age-related increase in incidence.[157] Although treatment is not generally indicated for monoclonal gammopathies,[152] treatment of myeloma is often useful. Another common malignant transformation of the lymphocyte in older adults is chronic lymphocytic leukemia.[158] Non-Hodgkin lymphoma also increases in incidence with age, whereas Hodgkin lymphoma has a bimodal distribution.[159]

Finally, a discussion of cancer development and aging would not be complete without considering the importance of the decline in immunity and associated failure of immune surveillance.[160-163] It has long been proposed that the decline in immune function contributes to the increased incidence of malignancy. However, despite the appeal of such a hypothesis, scientific support has been limited, and the topic remains controversial.[164] Proponents of an immune explanation point to experiments in which outbred strains of mice with heterogeneous immune function were followed for their life span.[165,166] Those that demonstrated better function early in life, as determined by a limited panel of assays available at the time on a small sample of blood, were found to have fewer spontaneous malignancies and a longer life than those estimated to be less immunologically competent. Furthermore, it is difficult to deny that profoundly immunodeficient animals or humans are subject to a more frequent occurrence of malignant disease. Thus, it would stand to reason that others with less severe immunodeficiency would also be subject to malignancy, but perhaps less dramatically. However, the malignancies associated with profound immunodeficiency (e.g., with AIDS or after organ transplantation) are usually lymphomas, Kaposi sarcoma, or leukemia and are not the more common malignancies of geriatric populations (e.g., lung, breast, colon, prostate cancers). Accordingly, it is fair to say that the question of the influence of age-acquired immunodeficiency on the incidence of cancer in older adults is unresolved. There is much greater consensus on the importance of immune senescence in the clinical management of cancer, including the problems associated with infection and disease progression.

Immune Senescence and Infections in Older Adults

An aging immune system is less capable of mounting an effective immune response after infectious challenge; thus, infection in older adults is associated with greater morbidity and mortality.[167,168] Most notable in this regard are infections with influenza virus, pneumococcal pneumonia, and various urinary tract pathogens. However, older adults are also more susceptible to skin infections, gastroenteritis (including *Clostridium difficile* infection), tuberculosis, and herpes zoster (shingles). There is also an increase in hospital- and nursing home–acquired infections in older adults. These susceptibilities to infection are due to immune senescence and other changes more common among older adults, such as the following: reduced ciliary escalator efficiency and cough reflex predisposing to aspiration pneumonia; urinary and fecal incontinence predisposing to urinary tract and perineal skin infections; and immobility predisposing to pressure sores and wound infections.

Infections in older adults frequently present atypically.[74,144,169] Older adults may not have typical hard signs of infection, such as spiking fever, leukocytosis, prominent inflammatory infiltrates on chest x-rays, or rebound tenderness for those with an acute abdomen. Thus, a change in mental status or mild malaise might be the only clinical indication of urinary tract infection or even pneumonia. Lower baseline temperatures may require the need for monitoring the change in temperature, rather than the absolute temperature. This is particularly true in frail older adults, for whom infections caused by unusual organisms, recurrent infections with the same pathogen, or reactivation of quiescent diseases such as tuberculosis or herpes zoster virus can be counted on to present atypically and also to be resistant to standard therapy.

Influenza

Most of the significant morbidity and excess mortality during influenza epidemics occurs in older adults.[170] Age itself, in addition to and separate from the many comorbid conditions of older adults, is a significant risk factor for severe complications of influenza.[171] It is widely believed that much of the increased susceptibility of older adults to influenza and its complications are attributable to immunologic factors, including reduced antibody responsiveness and influenza-specific cell-mediated immunity (see earlier). The role of humoral immunity, especially in the form of neutralizing antibodies, is perhaps most important for preventing and limiting the initial infection[172] rather than promoting recovery. T cell–mediated responses appear to be more important and are primarily involved in postinfection viral clearance and recovery; influenza-specific cytotoxic T lymphocyte (CTL) activity correlates with rapid clearance of virus in infected human volunteers, even in the absence of detectable serum antibody.[173] This has been experimentally confirmed in several studies through the adoptive transfer of influenza-specific CTLs in mouse models.[174,175] Influenza-specific antibody declines with age, whether because of natural infection or vaccination,[176-178] and this presumably translates to an increased risk of influenza infection. However, and perhaps equally important, CTL,[62,179] human leukocyte antigen (HLA) restriction by influenza-specific T cell clones, and lymphocyte proliferative responses also decline with age. T cell–mediated cytokine responses, most notably IL-2, also decrease with age, although this has not been as clearly established for healthy older adults[61] as it has been for frail older adults.[60] Together these observations account for much of the age-related increase in influenza susceptibility and morbidity. Furthermore, although influenza in otherwise healthy unvaccinated older adults leads to an illness that lasts nearly twice as long as that in their younger counterparts, influenza illness duration in older adults previously vaccinated (i.e., vaccine failures) is comparable to the illness duration in vaccinated, healthy, younger adults. This observation remains true when the vaccine to circulating strain match is poor, negating poor vaccine match as a reason not to vaccinate older adults annually.

In the long-term care setting, influenza vaccination was found to be effective in reducing influenza-like illness and preventing pneumonia, hospitalization, and deaths (both infectious and all-cause mortality). Among older adults residing in the community setting, the benefits of annual vaccination have been demonstrably modest in some studies[180] but found to be more effective in others.[181,182] Among many efforts to increase the immune response and hence protection from influenza vaccination in older adults, a component hemagglutinin dose within the vaccine and higher doses were found to be more immunogenic.[183] It is important to note that despite all the changes occurring with age and comorbid conditions in older adults, influenza vaccine is still highly cost-effective in reducing influenza-related infections and complications, especially in the high-risk older adult population.[171,182,184]

Pneumococcal Disease

Reduced immune competence, whether due to age, disease, or drug therapy, introduces risk for complications from pneumococcal disease. For example, one study has found the incidence of pneumococcal disease to be 70 cases/100,000 in individuals older than 70 years compared with 5 cases/100,000 in younger adults.[185] *Streptococcus pneumoniae* is a gram-positive, lancet-shaped diplococcus that normally colonizes the nasopharynx and was present in up to 70% of individuals in the preantibiotic era. The pathogenic form is encapsulated, and antigenic variants of the polysaccharide capsule are sufficiently immunogenic to be useful as vaccine targets. The rising prevalence of penicillin-resistant *Pneumococcus*[186] renders infection treatment more difficult and reinforces the need for prevention as a primary management strategy for pneumococcal disease.

Pneumonia is the most prevalent expression of infection with *S. pneumoniae*, but other sites of infection are also clinically important. These include otitis media, sinusitis, meningitis, septic arthritis, pericarditis, endocarditis, peritonitis, cellulitis, glomerulonephritis, and sepsis (especially postsplenectomy). Chronic obstructive pulmonary disease is an independent risk factor for the occurrence of and complications from pneumococcal infection, which might relate to the altered mechanics of clearing secretions and altered immunity within the lung itself. Risk factors for pneumococcal infections also include conditions that predispose an individual to aspirate pneumococci, such as swallowing disorders, a feature not uncommon in stroke survivors.

Prevention is the best form of defense, and the polysaccharide antigens of the pneumococcal vaccine have been used to generate T cell independent responses, a theoretical advantage for older adults because immune senescence is thought primarily to perturb T cell more than B cell responses (see previous discussion). However, studies on pneumococcal vaccine efficacy in disease prevention often have been disappointing or inconclusive,[178,187] with other studies suggesting efficacy and cost-effectiveness.[188-191] Consequently, underuse of pneumococcal vaccine has been held accountable for the development of outbreaks in nursing facilities in which vaccination rates were low.[192,193] Currently, revaccination is recommended for persons aged 65 years and older if they received vaccine 5 or more years prior and were younger than 65 years at the time of vaccination. Meanwhile, new vaccine designs aim to stimulate the immune response better in older adults by recruiting T cell help through polysaccharide conjugation with a peptide combined with cytokine[194] or by using a peptide target.[195] Whether these approaches are superior for an immune senescent patient remains to be defined.

Varicella Zoster Virus

Herpes zoster (shingles) is caused by varicella zoster virus (VZV) and is increasingly prevalent with advancing age, as are its severity and complications.[196-200] Most cases occur after the age of 60 years[201] and, by 80 years, the annual attack rate is 0.8%. Two major complications of herpes zoster, postherpetic neuralgia and cranial nerve zoster (often of the ophthalmic nerve, and not infrequently resulting in lower motor neuron paresis), are the most disabling. Postherpetic neuralgia occurs in more than 25% of patients 60 years of age and older and is strongly associated with sleep disturbance and depression.[202-206] Bell palsy[207] and Meniere[208] disease, both conditions associated with advanced age, have also been linked to herpes zoster. VZV-specific cell-mediated immunity correlates closely with susceptibility to herpes zoster in large populations, such as patients with lymphomas, bone marrow transplant recipients, and immunocompetent older adults.[209-216] Whereas a decline in VZV-specific cell-mediated immunity is a major precipitant for VZV reactivation,[217] demonstrable VZV immunity limits the viral replication and spread.[218]

In a randomized clinical trial with a live attenuated VZV vaccine among adults aged 60 years and older, vaccination reduced the incidence of herpes zoster and postherpetic neuralgia compared with those who received a placebo.[219] The magnitude of benefit with a reduction in postherpetic neuralgia was more pronounced in those 70 years of age or older. This study led to the approval of a vaccine for those older than 60 years in the United States and in Europe and Australia.

SECONDARY CAUSES OF ACQUIRED IMMUNODEFICIENCY IN OLDER ADULTS

In contrast to the normative changes that may result in a mild idiopathic-acquired immunodeficiency with aging, a variety of secondary causes of acquired immunodeficiency occurs in older adults that may be severe yet reversible. The distinction between secondary causes of immune deficiency from so-called normal age-related changes is an important clinical distinction. The clinician needs a high index of suspicion for acquired immunodeficiency in older adults, because many causes are reversible and can be the primary reason for infection risk, altered presentation of infection, or inadequate response to usual therapy.

Malnutrition

The effects of malnutrition on the immune system may be profound and clearly increase the risk of infection in older adults.[220,221] Immune deficits in undernourished ambulatory older adults may be reversed by nutritional supplementation. Malnutrition affects up to 50% of hospitalized older adults and is highly associated with poor acute care outcomes, including death.[222-224] Severe protein, calorie, vitamin, and micronutrient deficiencies may cause immune impairment, resulting in poor outcomes in response to infection.[225,226] An absolute lymphocyte count below 1500 cells/mm^3 often indicates some degree of malnutrition, and a count below 900 cells/mm^3 is a frequent correlate of severe malnutrition and immunodeficiency.

Comorbidity

Chronic illnesses such as congestive heart failure[227] and Alzheimer disease may be associated with progressive cachexia, despite adequate food intake, and may be mediated by tumor necrosis factor or other inflammatory mediators.[94,102] In older patients with dementia, despite adequate food intake, malnutrition is common and is associated with a fourfold increase in infection.[102] Diabetes mellitus, common in geriatric populations, is frequently associated with diminished immune function.

Polypharmacy

Because older adults frequently consume a number of prescription or over-the-counter medications, drug-induced acquired immunodeficiency is probably far more common than has generally been appreciated. Numerous commonly prescribed drugs cause neutropenia and lymphocytopenia. Analgesics, nonsteroidal antiinflammatory drugs, steroids, antithyroids, antibiotics, antiarthritic drugs, antipsychotics, antidepressants, hypnotics-sedatives, anticonvulsants, antihypertensives, diuretics, histamine type 2 (H2) blockers, and hypoglycemics are among a long list of commonly prescribed medications that may suppress inflammatory and/or immune responses.[228-230] T lymphocytes also have calcium channels along with cholinergic, histaminic, and adrenergic receptors, and drugs that work on these targets may have unappreciated effects on immune function.[227] Hypogammaglobulinemia may also be induced by medications.[231] Other studies have also demonstrated that medications may also be associated with an impaired or enhanced response to vaccination.[232,233]

HIV and Other Infections

HIV infection may be a cause of acquired immunodeficiency in older adults and should always be considered part of the differential diagnosis of acquired immunodeficiency in older patients with lymphopenia and appropriate risk factors.[234-238] The most common source of AIDS in older adults was until recently transfusion, but now is acquired through sexual activity.[239-241] Dementia is often a common presenting feature of AIDS,[242] and AIDS should be considered part of the differential diagnosis of dementia in older patients with appropriate risk factors. The possibility that many cases of AIDS will go undetected in older adults has considerable implications for geriatric health care workers. In the United States, approximately 11% of patients with AIDS are older than 50 years of age—a recognized health issue in the geriatric population—and age could be an independent risk factor in rapid progression of the disease.[240,243]

Stress

Psychosocial isolation, depression, and stress are probable causes of immune dysfunction in older adults.[244,245] There is an increased incidence of cancer during periods of psychosocial stress and depression related to bereavement.[246,247] Social isolation and marital discord may impair immune function.[248] Chronic stress in the form of caregiving for a demented spouse also reduces the influenza vaccine response.[249] Interventions to enhance social contact demonstrably improve immune function, as determined by a variety of laboratory measures.[250] Immobility may also cause immune dysfunction, and exercise may maintain function in older animals and older adults.[251] These aspects of psychoneuroimmunology obviously have particular relevance in the interdisciplinary practice of geriatrics, given the high prevalence of psychosocial problems in older adults.

IMMUNE FUNCTION ASSESSMENT AND IMMUNE ENHANCEMENT

Immune Function Assessment

The tests necessary to perform an immunologic evaluation to establish the diagnosis of acquired immunodeficiency in older adults are readily available to the clinician.[252] The humoral immune system is readily tested by measuring total serum protein and quantitative immunoglobulin (IgG, IgA, and IgM) levels. Serum protein electrophoresis and immunoelectrophoresis are useful to rule out monoclonal gammopathy, myeloma, and some forms of lymphoma, and may also provide clues to chronic inflammatory disease (polyclonal gammopathy, reduced albumin levels). Specific antibody titers such as isoagglutinins also provide additional information regarding B cell function. The integrity of the cellular immune system is tested by blood leukocyte counts (including absolute lymphocyte counts), delayed skin test hypersensitivity using a panel of at least six antigens, and in vitro testing, such as measurement of lymphocyte subsets, proliferative capacity of lymphocytes in response to a mitogen or specific antigens, and cytokine production. The latter tests are often performed in a standard clinical immunology laboratory. Other more sophisticated immune tests are also available from the clinical immunology consultant and research laboratory.

Specific potentially reversible causes of acquired immunodeficiency, such as malnutrition or medications, should be sought in older patients with recurrent or unusual infections, particularly those with lymphocytopenia and/or anergy. At a minimum, a medication review and nutritional assessment should be performed, with monitoring of neutrophil or lymphocyte counts during nutritional supplementation or medication withdrawal. HIV infection should always be considered in high-risk patients, including the very old, particularly because of the risk for spread of HIV among health care workers and family members caring for frail older adults.

Immune Enhancement and Other Clinical Strategies

Numerous interventions have been used in an attempt to enhance immune function in older adults. The use of thymic and other hormones, medications, and cytokines have been proposed as immunoenhancing agents, but none of these has gained clinical acceptance.[253] In animals, caloric restriction without undernutrition clearly prolongs life and is associated with immune competence into late life; however, the benefits of caloric restriction in people remain unknown.[254] Supplemental zinc and other trace metals may also have benefit in some older patients in restoring lymphocyte proliferation in vitro and in enhancing delayed-type skin hypersensitivity reactions, but their effects in preventing or reducing the morbidity of infections or other problems potentially related to immunodeficiency in older adults have not been demonstrated.[255-258] Vitamin C and other antioxidants may also have beneficial effects on immune function.[259,260] However, megadose dietary supplementation does not significantly improve immune function in the normal-aged animal.[261]

Vaccinations are critically important in maintaining the health of older adults in the face of declining immunity and are effective in preventing pneumococcal pneumonia, influenza, and tetanus and in reducing mortality from these illnesses.[251,262-264] Although older adults achieve lower peak titers and more rapid declines of serum antibody levels, most healthy older adults reach achieve titers that are generally presumed protective.[89,92,265,266] However, chronically ill, frail older adults, particularly institutionalized malnourished individuals, may not achieve adequate protective peak antibody titers against pneumococcal pneumonia or influenza when immunized with a single dose of vaccine; Therefore, supplemental doses have been recommended by some experts.[267-269] Older adults may require revaccination with tetanus toxoid more frequently than every 10 years (as currently recommended) to maintain protective levels of antibodies in the serum.[88,270] The use of protein conjugate and immunoconjugate vaccines may improve the response in older adults.[271-273]

CONCLUSIONS

There are mild to moderate changes in the immune system with normal aging; these render an individual susceptible to certain infections and may also affect the clinical presentation. A more profound deficit in immune function is commonly observed in geriatric populations but, when this occurs, the clinician should be highly suspicious that secondary causes (i.e., causes other than just aging) are involved. Reversible causes of acquired immunodeficiency in this age group include comorbid diseases, malnutrition, medications, stress, and possibly infections, including HIV. Newer therapeutic approaches may ultimately be useful in the treatment of acquired immunodeficiency in older adults, particularly in high-risk individuals who are substantially impaired by the effects of aging and diseases of old age on the immune system.

KEY POINTS

- The immune system changes with age, primarily affecting T cell and B cell functions.
- Changes in the immune system are relevant to the changing clinical presentation and expression of disease.
- Immune senescence affects vaccine effectiveness.

For a complete list of references, please visit www.expertconsult.com.

KEY REFERENCES

13. Fortin CF, Larbi A, Dupuis G, et al: GM-CSF activates the Jak/STAT pathway to rescue polymorphonuclear neutrophils from spontaneous apoptosis in young but not elderly individuals. Biogerontology 8:173–187, 2007.
14. Tortorella C, Simone O, Piazzolla G, et al: Age-related impairment of GM-CSF-induced signalling in neutrophils: role of SHP-1 and SOCS proteins. Ageing Res Rev 6:81–93, 2007.
26. Agrawal A, Agrawal S, Cao JN, et al: Altered innate immune functioning of dendritic cells in elderly humans: a role of phosphoinositide 3-kinase-signaling pathway. J Immunol 178:6912–6922, 2007.
161. Koebel CM, Vermi W, Swann JB, et al: Adaptive immunity maintains occult cancer in an equilibrium state. Nature 450:903–907, 2007.
162. Swann JB, Smyth MJ: Immune surveillance of tumors. J Clin Invest 117:1137–1146, 2007.
167. Larbi A, Franceschi C, Mazzatti D, et al: Aging of the immune system as a prognostic factor for human longevity. Physiology (Bethesda) 23:64–74, 2008.
190. Johnstone J, Marrie TJ, Eurich DT, et al: Effect of pneumococcal vaccination in hospitalized adults with community-acquired pneumonia. Arch Intern Med 167:1938–1943, 2007.
211. Hovens MM, Vaessen N, Sijpkens YW, et al: Unusual presentation of central nervous system manifestations of varicella zoster virus vasculopathy in renal transplant recipients. Transpl Infect Dis 9: 237–240, 2007.
212. Miller GG, Dummer JS: Herpes simplex and varicella zoster viruses: forgotten but not gone. Am J Transplant 7:741–747, 2007.
227. Gelinck LB, Teng YK, Rimmelzwaan GF, et al: Poor serological responses upon influenza vaccination in patients with rheumatoid arthritis treated with rituximab. Ann Rheum Dis 66:1402–1403, 2007.
228. Gelinck LB, van der Bijl AE, Beyer WE, et al: The effect of anti-tumour necrosis factor alpha treatment on the antibody response to influenza vaccination. Ann Rheum Dis 67:713–716, 2008.
229. Gelinck LB, van der Bijl AE, Visser LG, et al: Synergistic immunosuppressive effect of anti-TNF combined with methotrexate on antibody responses to the 23-valent pneumococcal polysaccharide vaccine. Vaccine 26:3528–3533, 2008.

94 Skin Disease and Old Age

Kacper K. Pierwola, Gopal A. Patel, W. Clark Lambert, Robert A. Schwartz

INTRODUCTION

Aging affects all organ systems, including the integument. Cell replacement, sensory perception, thermal regulatory function, and immune defense systems are among the many components that are compromised. The skin appearance changes, depending on environmental and genetic factors. The psychosocial impact, including cosmetic disfigurement and social stigma, in addition to vulnerability to skin disease, must be addressed in older patients. The role of the physician is to diagnose, treat, and guide patients through this visible component of aging while preventing avoidable disease.

EPIDEMIOLOGY

The U.S. population older than 65 years has been greatly expanding. Skin complaints constitute a significant and growing portion of geriatric ambulatory patient visits. A 2005 U.S. study demonstrated that 21% of all patients seen by family practitioners had a skin problem. It was their primary complaint 72% of the time.[1] Also in 2005, the National Ambulatory Medical Care Survey (NAMCS) showed that the number of outpatient visits was highest in the 45- to 64-year-old age group, a shift up from the 1995 survey, suggesting increasing medical use by the baby boomer population, which is now entering the 65 years and older bracket.[2] A more recent 2012 NAMCS survey has further supported this shift in demographics.[3] Among all patient age groups, 1 in 20 visits to an outpatient office are of skin, hair, or nail concern.[2] Diseases such as cutaneous melanoma are on the rise, with lifetime risks shifting from 1 in 250 in 1980 to 1 in 65 in 2002 based on a U.S. population study.[4] These data emphasize the importance of skin disease recognition in older adults.[5] Skin cancer, for example, is often preventable and, with early diagnosis, can be 100% curable. Also, the role of cosmetic services and the impact on psychosocial well-being that can be traced to skin disease is of added concern.

APPROACH TO THE PATIENT

A complete medical history is desirable for the skin disease patient, regardless of age. One should pay attention to medicines or chemicals used, including topical, systemic, cosmetic, or complementary and alternative agents. The duration of a complaint, previous therapy, close contacts, and patient opinion on cause may assist or obfuscate diagnosis and treatment. Hygiene, including bathing and laundering habits, should be assessed. Geriatric patients should undergo a thorough skin evaluation under good lighting.

Older patients often have trouble with medication compliance. Dermatologic treatments are further challenging because of their frequent topical nature. Patients may need to apply creams on difficult to reach areas (e.g., feet, back) or may be immobilized. Shampooing, showering, or complicated treatment regimens can confuse and challenge geriatric patients. The clinician needs to be aware of all these barriers and accommodate accordingly.

SELECTED SKIN CONDITIONS

Eczematous Disorders

The older patient population's chief complaint is often of a pruritic (itchy) rash or lesion that turns out to be an eczematous disease. The prevalence of eczema is between 2.4% and 4.1% in the U.S. population.[6] In older adults, natural aging of the skin predisposes patients to eczematous diseases. In a Turkish study of more than 4000 patients, eczematous disorders constituted nearly 22% of diagnoses in the 65- to 74-year-old age group.[7]

Xerosis (Eczema Craquelé, Asteatotic Eczema)

Xerosis describes rough or dry skin, which is seen in almost all older adults. Conditions of low humidity, such as artificially heated rooms, especially forced hot air heating, exacerbate this condition. Xerosis is actually a misnomer, because water is not absent throughout the entire thickness of the skin. There is only diminished hydration in the superficial corneum.[8,9] Xerosis has also been misclassified as a sebaceous gland disorder. Although sebaceous gland activity decreases with age and thus depletes the skin's moisture, it only plays a partial role in xerosis development.[10] Other factors include an irregular epidermal surface caused by maturation abnormalities. Deficits in skin hydration and lipid content impair normal desquamation, leading to the formation of the skin scales that characterize xerosis. Furthermore, old age results in altered lipid profiles and decreased production of filaggrin, which are filament-associated proteins that bind keratinocytes. Both factors contribute to xerosis.[9]

Xerosis may appear scaly, with accentuated skin lines, often occurring on the anterior legs, back, arms, abdomen, and waist. The scales are a result of epidermal water loss, and focal dryness may be deep enough to cause bleeding fissures. Superimposed pruritus is possible, leading to secondary excoriations, inflammation, and lichen simplex chronicus.[9] Allergic and irritant contact dermatitis may also complicate xerosis. Secondary infection may follow a break in the skin barrier.[11] Xerosis is also a secondary feature of many of the conditions discussed in this chapter.

Untreated xerosis progresses to flaking, fissuring, inflammation, dermatitis, and infection. Topical emollients make dry skin more comfortable and avoid such complications. Alpha-hydroxy acids (e.g., 12% ammonium lactate) are helpful because of their keratolytic nature, although some patients report stinging and irritation.[12] Formulations containing ammonium lactate or other alpha-hydroxy acids help restore barrier function and improve xerosis.[13] Liberal use of moisturizers throughout the day is recommended. Topical steroids (classes III and VI) are recommended in moderate to severe cases, along with antipruritics for symptomatic itching. Further recommendations include decreasing hot water baths, reducing use of soap or harsh skin cleansers, avoiding rough clothes on the skin, using a humidifier in a dry environment, and adding emollient substances, such as oatmeal, to bathwater.

Simple xerosis is a common cause of pruritus in older adults. Asteatotic eczema is a dermatitis superimposed on xerosis that often flares in the winter. It is dry scaly skin, sometimes in extreme cases resembling cracked porcelain, with bleeding from damaged dermal capillaries. The cracked porcelain, or so-called crazy paving, pattern is best termed *eczema craquelé*.[14] Asteatotic eczema is a common condition on the shins of geriatric patients, although it is also seen on other regions of the body. There are several associations of asteatotic eczema—one related to hard soaps, one to corticosteroid therapy, one to neurologic disorders, and an idiopathic form often located on the shins of older patients. Prevention is the key to controlling this problem. Contributing factors include cleansers used, frequency of showers, diet, medications, and temperature exposure. Specifically, patients should reduce the use of hot showers and irritant detergents. Creams, humidifiers, and topical steroids can improve the effects of asteatotic dermatitis.[14] Alcohol-based lotions feel good just after application but eventually cause increased dryness and should be avoided.

Seborrheic Dermatitis

Seborrheic dermatitis is a chronic condition that typically manifests as an erythematous and greasy scaling eruption, usually affecting areas with abundant sebaceous glands, including the scalp, ears, central face, central chest, and intertriginous spaces.[15] When present in the scalp, it tends to cause flaking known as dandruff. It may also appear as marked erythema over the nasolabial fold during times of stress or sleep deprivation. Although the prevalence of seborrheic dermatitis is approximately 5% in the general adult population, estimates in those aged 65 years and older report a range from 7% to as high as 67% in institutionalized patients.[16-18] Seborrheic dermatitis is also found in greater frequency with neurologic conditions such as Parkinson disease, a concern in the geriatric population.[19] Facial nerve injury, spinal cord injury, syringomyelia, and neuroleptic treatment are also associated with seborrheic dermatitis.

The pathogenesis of seborrheic dermatitis, although controversial, has been attributed to the yeast *Malassezia* species (e.g., *Malassezia furfur, Malassezia ovalis*; formerly known as *Pityrosporum*).[20] This yeast is a normal resident in more than 90% of healthy adults, but when overgrown it can be proportionally related to the severity of seborrheic dermatitis. Treatment options against *Malassezia* spp. have been effective for seborrheic dermatitis, supporting a causal relationship. Antifungals along with topical steroids are used, such as ketoconazole cream or shampoo and hydrocortisone valerate cream.[15] Furthermore, topical ketoconazole has inherent antiinflammatory properties. One classic study comparing these two agents determined that 2% ketoconazole cream was 80.5% effective in resolving seborrheic dermatitis, as opposed to 94.4% efficacy with 1% hydrocortisone cream.[21] Although not as effective as hydrocortisone, ketoconazole serves as an effective steroid-sparing agent. The calcineurin inhibitors tacrolimus and pimecrolimus are macrolide immunosuppressants that are alternative agents for use on the face, again to reduce the use of steroids in this sensitive area. A 2008 randomized prospective controlled study comparing 1% pimecrolimus cream and 2% ketoconazole cream showed equal efficacy between the two, but there were greater side effects with pimecrolimus.[22] Side effects included burning, itching, and redness. Both tacrolimus and pimecrolimus have a black box label by the U.S. Food and Drug Administration (FDA) warning of skin cancer or lymphoma formation in some patients using this drug, although an established link remains controversial.[23] Shampoos with ketoconazole, selenium sulfide, salicylic acid, zinc pyrithione, or tar are also effective for relieving seborrheic dermatitis in hair-bearing regions.[24]

Pruritus

Older patients often experience localized or generalized pruritus, which can be severe. The cause of itching in older patients is often difficult to determine. Renal, hematologic, endocrine, cholestatic, allergic, infectious, and malignant causes all potentially contribute to the older patient's itch. Entities causing pruritus include the following[25,26]:

- Uremia
- Cholestasis
- Pregnancy
- Cancers (e.g., lymphoma, leukemia, multiple myeloma)
- Polycythemia vera
- Thyroid disease
- Iron deficiency anemia
- Diabetes mellitus
- HIV infection
- Multiple sclerosis
- Drug hypersensitivity
- Psychogenic causes
- Senile pruritus
- Sjögren syndrome
- Carcinoid syndrome
- Dumping syndrome

Some of these are addressed here.

Physiologically, specific C-fiber neurons that terminate at the dermoepidermal junction transmit the itch sensation to the brain. These fibers possess receptors sensitive to histamine, neuropeptide substance P, serotonin, bradykinin, proteases, and endothelin. Rubbing or scratching further stimulates these receptors.[27] As the itch and scratch cycle progresses, the skin is driven to a point of barrier function compromise, which is worrisome in older patients with limited means of self-care.

Pruritus is one of the most distressing concerns of a patient suffering from cholestasis. The exact cause of pruritus in this disease is unknown, although an altered role of opioid receptor function has been suggested.[28] Treatment of the underlying disease process often resolves itching. However, some diseases, such as primary biliary cirrhosis (PBC), cannot easily be cured. Ursodeoxycholic acid (UDCA) treatment for PBC often does not resolve the patient's pruritus.[29] Cholestyramine, rifampin, naloxone, and phenobarbital are other agents used for pruritus, all of which have substantial side effects in older adults.[30]

Generalized pruritus is recognized as a key marker of underlying malignancy, particularly lymphomas and leukemias.[31] Generalized pruritus is noted in up to 30% of patients with Hodgkin disease and may be the only presenting symptom.[32,33] Pruritus is also a key feature of multiple myeloma, polycythemia rubra vera, Waldenström macroglobulinemia, and malignant carcinoid.[34]

Pruritus is best resolved by identifying and treating the underlying systemic cause. Unfortunately, nonspecific therapies must often be used for older patients with an atypical disease presentation. Emollients are valuable interventions, regardless of suspected cause, because some level of pruritus exacerbating xerosis is present in most older patients. Topical use of alcohol, hot water, or harsh soaps and scrubbing must be discouraged. Proper humidity, cool compresses, nail trimming, and behavior therapy may all improve the itch and scratch cycle.[27] Topical anesthetics such as benzocaine and dibucaine have been used for relief. A trial of oilated soap and antihistamines may also be helpful before an invasive workup, including hematologic studies, imaging for malignancy, skin biopsy, skin scrapings, skin culture, and HIV testing.[34] Antihistamines should be used with caution because they are not universally effective and may cause sedation in the vulnerable and often highly medicated older patient.

Vascular-Related Disease

Stasis Dermatitis

Stasis dermatitis is a common condition affecting 15 to 20 million patients older than 50 years in the United States.[35] It often presents as a circumscribing dermatitis around the calf and ankle in patients with chronic venous insufficiency and venous hypertension. However, any body area constantly under pressure against a hard surface may be affected. Pitting edema may be present, in addition to loss of hair, waxy appearance, and yellow-brown pigmentation.[36] If untreated, stasis dermatitis may progress to a chronic nonhealing wound, with erythema and oozing. Stasis dermatitis results from poor function of the deep venous system in the legs, which leads to backflow and hypertension in the superficial venous system.[37] Often, both lower legs show stasis dermatitis. An associated self-perpetuating cutaneous inflammatory response follows.[37] The workup includes venous Doppler studies to identify flow in the involved venous plexus.

Several treatment approaches are useful in resolving stasis dermatitis. Compression of the legs to control superficial venous hypertension is critical. This can be achieved by the use of Unna boots, compression stockings, or elastic wraps. In one study of more than 3000 patients, those with stasis dermatitis had a compliance of 46% for the use of compression stockings.[38] Leg elevation 6 inches above the level of the heart during sleep also improves blood flow. Topical treatments include corticosteroids and the calcineurin inhibitors, pimecrolimus and tacrolimus. Corticosteroids have an associated risk of tachyphylaxis and must be used carefully because of the high risk of infection in these patients.[39,40] Topical antibiotics such as bacitracin, neomycin, or polymyxin B may be added if there is evidence of skin barrier compromise and infection.

For more information on stasis ulcers, see Chapter 37.

Elephantiasis Nostras Verrucosa

Patients with a long history of stasis dermatitis with chronic lymphedema due to nonfilarial causes such as infection, surgery, radiation, neoplastic obstruction, obesity, portal hypertension, or chronic congestive heart failure may develop a condition known as elephantiasis nostras verrucosa (ENV).[41] Physical examination may show dependent edema with hyperkeratosis and lichenification, papillomatous plaques, crusting, cobblestone-like nodules, and erythema of the affected area (Figure 94-1).[42,43] Management of ENV is similar to that of stasis dermatitis because it relies on treating the underlying condition of lymphedema using limb elevation, skin hygiene, lymphatic drainage, compression bandages, support stockings, and lymphatic pumping as well as weight loss and infection control.[44]

Cherry Angiomas

Cherry angiomas, also known as cherry hemangiomas or Campbell de Morgan spots, are the most common vascular proliferations of the skin and are nearly ubiquitous after the age of 30 years. They appear as firm, smooth, red papules ranging in size from 0.5 to 5 mm. They may also appear as a myriad of tiny spots resembling petechiae. Although patients may be concerned with a new cherry angioma, the condition is benign. Cosmetic concern may merit electrocautery or laser coagulation treatment.[45]

Venous Lakes

Venous lakes are dark blue to violet-colored papules that occur on sun-exposed areas of older patients. They are compressible lesions common on the face, lips, and ears. The differential diagnosis includes blue nevus and malignant melanoma. Venous lakes are benign lesions and treatment is for cosmetic purposes or bleeding. Electrodesiccation, excision, or lasers may be used to remove venous lakes.[46]

Infectious Diseases

Herpes Zoster (Shingles)

Herpes zoster (shingles) is a reactivation of the varicella zoster virus, the causative agent of varicella. It is a significant ailment of older adults, ranging from 690 to 1600 cases/100,000 person-years in those 60 years and older.[47-49] The varicella zoster virus remains latent in the dorsal root ganglia of the nervous system after its initial infection usually resolves in childhood.[50,51] A weakened or impaired immune system is thought to precede reactivation, so underlying conditions such as lymphoma, leukemia, and possible HIV infection should be considered. Local steroid injection has also been associated with a herpes zoster flare.[52] Herpes zoster begins as a prodromal sharp pain localized to a dermatomal region, followed by a rash and vesicular eruption (Figure 94-2). Itching, burning, and weakness of muscles associated with the involved nerve may be noted. More than 20 vesicles outside of the primary dermatome suggest disseminated zoster,

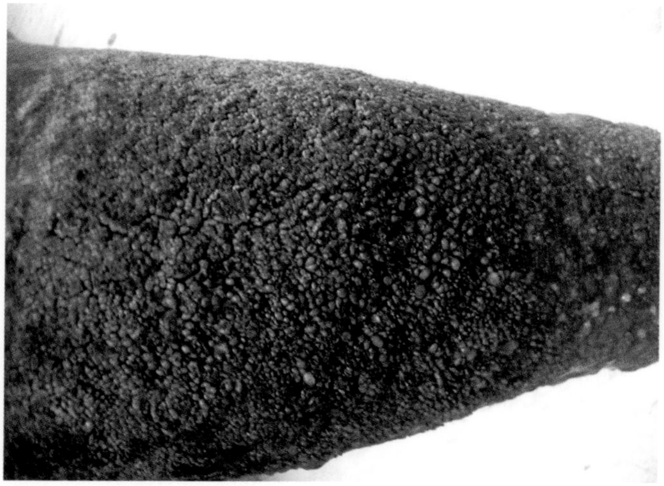

Figure 94-1. Typical papillomatous projections and cobblestone-like nodular appearance of elephantiasis nostras verrucosa.

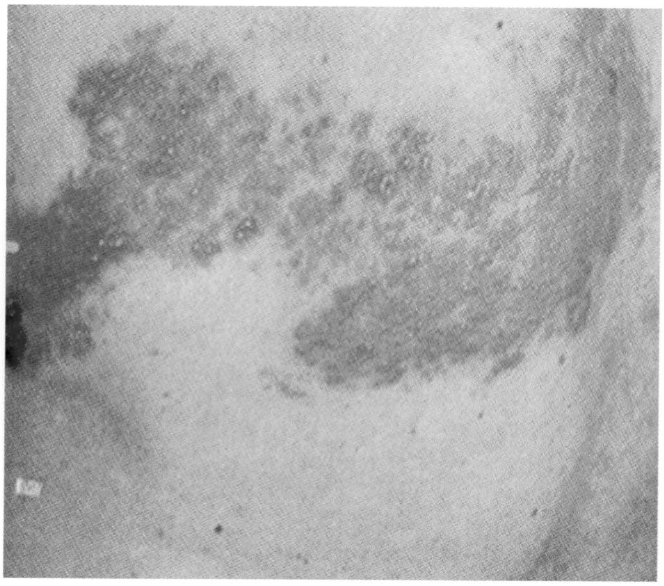

Figure 94-2. Vesicular lesions from herpes zoster on the back of an older man in a typical dermatomal distribution.

as may be seen in immunocompromised patients[53] or patients with granulocytic lesions. The long-lasting pain of zoster may be mistaken for gallbladder, kidney, or cardiac pain, depending on location. Chronic pain or chronic pruritus localized to the dermatome may follow. This is known as postherpetic neuralgia (PHN) or postherpetic itch, respectively.[54]

Herpes zoster is diagnosed by a Tzanck smear of a sample scraped from the base of an intact vesicle. The appearance of multinucleated giant cells may indicate a herpetic infection.

Treatment of herpes zoster includes early antiviral therapy, within 72 hours of onset. Acyclovir is a safe but variably efficacious agent, although famciclovir is also used. In one double-blind, randomized group study of 55 patients, it was found that famciclovir was well tolerated and had a more favorable adverse event profile than acyclovir.[55] Valacyclovir is an L-valine ester form of acyclovir and is converted to acyclovir in vivo. It provides three to five times the oral bioavailability of acyclovir and has been shown in clinical trials to reduce pain severity better.[56] In 2006, the FDA approved the use of a live zoster vaccine (Zostavax) for the prevention of shingles in immunocompetent patients older than 60 years. According to the multicenter Shingles Prevention Study, vaccine administration reduces the incidence, burden, and PHN complications in older patients.[57] Oral antibiotics covering staphylococci and streptococci are used to control secondary infection.[50]

PHN is most evident in older adults, and 10% to 18% of zoster patients develop this neuralgia, according to a community-based U.S. study.[58] Treatment is more challenging for PHN and requires the concomitant use of pain medication, such as topical capsaicin. The prompt prescription of analgesia, recommended when zoster is still active, often reduces long-term negative outcomes for PHN.[59]

Scabies

Scabies is among the oldest recognized infections to occur in humans, with more than 300 million yearly cases detected worldwide.[60,61] A U.K.-based study showed an incidence of 788/100,000 person-years of scabies.[62] Risk factors include nursing home residence, especially older (>30 years) and poorly staffed (>10:1 bed–to–health care provider ratio) institutions.

The causative agent for scabies is the mite, *Sarcoptes scabiei*, whose life span is about 1 month. Transmission requires direct skin contact or indirect contact with bedding or clothing. Once the pregnant female mite is on a new host, she digs into the skin to lay eggs. The eggs, saliva, feces, and the mites themselves lead to a delayed type IV hypersensitivity reaction from 2 to 6 weeks after contact so that at onset, multiple lesions are typically seen. These immune reactions lead to intense pruritus. In previously infected patients, the immune system response may present in 1 to 4 days after contact.[63]

Scabies manifests as papules, pustules, burrows, nodules, and urticarial plaques. Severe pruritus affects most patients unless they are immunocompromised.[64] In the latter case, scabies may resemble psoriasis or a hyperkeratotic dermatosis. The infection is not life-threatening but is often debilitating and depressing. Common areas infected include the finger webs, wrists, waistline, axillary folds, genitalia, buttocks, and nipples.[65] Any area of concern should be scraped and microscopically examined for mites. Early confirmation is imperative to avoid secondary infection and rapid spread in the susceptible nursing home environment.[66] Treatment includes permethrin cream or rinse, which should be applied to all areas of the body for an 8- to 14-hour period. Mild burning, stinging, and rash may develop. Lindane cream, crotamiton, and sulfur were used previously but with less efficacy. Ivermectin is an alternative agent with the benefit of oral administration, but the FDA has not officially approved its use for scabetic infection.[64] It is particularly helpful in cases of scabetic resistance to permethrin, although cases of ivermectin resistance have also been documented.[67,68] Pruritus and inflammation may be treated with steroids and antihistamines.[69]

Pediculosis

Parasitic lice are known to infest hair-bearing areas of the human body. Louse infection, or pediculosis, affects up to 12 million Americans each year. The offending human agents include *Pediculosis humanus humanus*, *Pediculosis humanus capitis* (larger body louse), and *Phthirus pubis* (pubic louse).[70] Similar to scabies, transmission may be direct or indirect through brushes, clothing, or bedding. Higher levels of crowding increase transmission rates, as seen in some nursing homes. Pathogenesis involves deposition of eggs (nits) on hair shafts and subsequent hatching under conditions of 70% humidity and temperatures of 28° C (82° F) or higher.[69]

The main symptom of lice infestation is pruritus.[25] Bite reactions, excoriations, lymphadenopathy, and conjunctivitis are other possible manifestations. Hair combing may be associated with a "singing" sound because of the interaction of the tines with the nits. Red bumps on the scalp that progress to crusting and oozing are noted in *P. humanus capitis*. Pediculosis is further complicated by the potential of co-transported infections. Diagnosis is established by visualization of the lice or nits. This often requires a good light source and use of a comb to expose the hair. The difficult to remove nits on the hair shafts appear as white specks on examination.[70] Prevention is the best way to address lice infestations, such as avoiding continued contact with an infested individual. Chemical pediculicides, including permethrin, malathion, lindane, and pyrethrin, are the main treatment modalities. These treatments should be repeated every 7 to 10 days and, because of increasing resistance, must often be rotated.[71] So-called bug busting with a wet comb and conditioner has limited efficacy. Dimethicone has been shown to treat pediculosis in a randomized controlled study in which 69% of patients were cured, and only 2% had irritant reactions.[72] More studies are necessary for widespread recommendation of this treatment. All family members and contact persons should be included in therapy and prevention measures during patient treatment.

Onychomycosis

Fungal infections are among the most prevalent integumentary concerns in older adults, and onychomycosis is a leading entity. Defined as a fungal infection involving the nail and nail plate, over 90% of onychomycosis is attributable to dermatophytes known as tinea unguium, and 10% to nondermatophytic molds, or *Candida*. The prevalence of onychomycosis has been estimated at almost 6.5% overall in the Canadian population.[73] Studies have shown that onychomycosis increases with age, possibly because of poor circulation, diabetes, trauma, weakened immunity, poor hygiene, and inactivity.[74] Some studies have shown the prevalence of onychomycosis in patients older than 60 years to be 20%.[75]

There are several classifications of onychomycosis, including distal-lateral subungual, superficial white, candidal, and proximal subungual. Distal-lateral subungual onychomycosis is the most common clinical type, often caused by *Trichophyton rubrum* invasion of the hyponychium, the white area at the distal edge of the nail plate. The nails become yellow and thick, with parakeratosis and hyperkeratosis leading to subungual thickening and onycholysis. Superficial white onychomycosis is often associated with HIV infection and appears as a chalklike white plaque on the dorsum of the nail.[76] The proximal subungual type is also relatively uncommon and may present in immunocompetent or immunocompromised patients. In this case, the infection penetrates near the cuticle and migrates distally, resulting in hyperkeratosis, leukonychia, and onycholysis. *T. rubrum* is again the most frequent causative agent. Candidal onychomycosis is seen in patients with chronic mucocutaneous candidiasis.[74]

A patient history, physical examination, microscopy, and culture are all critical to diagnosis. Onychomycosis is best diagnosed by clipping the toenail very proximally and scraping the newly exposed subungual debris for laboratory evaluation. Toenails are 25 times more likely to be infected than fingernails.[74] Typical presentation involves two feet and one hand (the dominant hand of a patient).

Treatment options include topical and systemic medications, along with surgical approaches. A surgical trimming and débridement may be effective initially. Systemic therapy includes griseofulvin, fluconazole, itraconazole, and terbinafine.[77] Multiple double-blind controlled studies have shown terbinafine to be more effective than fluconazole or itraconazole for dermatophyte infections.[78-83] Systemic antifungals may have significant contraindications in patients on other medications. Topical treatments using amorolfine, ciclopirox, efinaconazole, or tavaborole have shown significant efficacy in the treatment of mild to moderate onychomycosis.[84,85]

Cutaneous Cancer

Skin cancer is an increasingly important public health issue for the geriatric population. Current rates indicate that one in five people in the United States develops skin cancer at some point in their lifetime, with melanoma incidence increasing faster than any other cancer worldwide.[86] The economic burden of skin cancer is substantial in the United States.[86] The risk of skin cancer has been related to ultraviolet (UV) exposure, which has varying roles in basal cell carcinoma, squamous cell carcinoma, and melanoma pathogenesis. The use of sunblock, avoidance of peak hours of sunlight, and proper clothing are simple preventive measures that can be followed by all patients, young and old. Early detection is critical in older patients because a 100% cure rate is possible.[87]

Actinic Keratosis

Actinic keratosis (AK), or solar keratosis, may be defined as a premalignant precursor of squamous cell carcinoma or an incipient cutaneous squamous cell carcinoma.[88] There are about 5.2 million physician visits annually for AK in the United States, 60% by the Medicare population.[89] These precancers are most common in light-skinned populations with year-round sun exposure who have not used appropriate sunscreens. Areas most affected include the forehead, scalp, ears, lower lip, forearms, and dorsal aspect of the hands.[90]

AK development is attributable to UV radiation–induced DNA mutation in select keratinocyte genes. With time, AKs may develop into invasive squamous cell carcinomas. They appear as small, skin-colored to yellowish-brown macules or papules, often with a dry adherent scale. They may feel rough to palpation, reminiscent of sandpaper, although they are asymptomatic in most patients.[91] If an AK becomes painful, indurated, eroded, or greatly erythematous, squamous cell carcinoma transformation must be highly suspect. AKs may also proliferate and become exophytic so as to constitute a so-called cutaneous horn. This is particularly evident on the ear.[92] Treatment for few and discrete AKs is best performed with cryosurgery (liquid nitrogen), which approaches almost 100% effectiveness and is convenient and economical. Topical treatment includes 5-fluorouracil, imiquimod, diclofenac, and photodynamic therapy with a light-sensitizing compound.[90] Sun safety practice is helpful for prevention, such as proper coverage and limited outdoor activity between 10 AM and 4 PM.

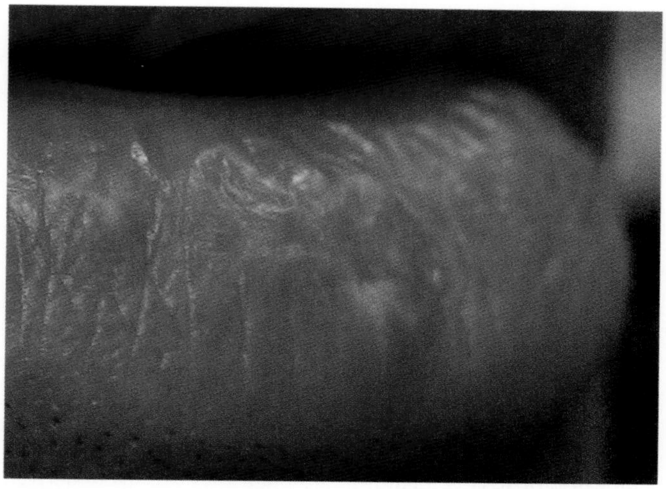

Figure 94-3. Older man with a white plaque identified as solar cheilosis (actinic cheilitis) on his lower lip, likely due to chronic exposure to ultraviolet radiation.

Solar Cheilosis

Solar cheilosis (SC), also known as actinic cheilitis or cheilosis, is a subset of AK confined to the mucosa of the lips. It has a high risk of progression to squamous cell carcinoma; risk factors include chronic exposure to UV radiation, Fitzpatrick skin phototypes I and II, advanced age, occupational and leisure activities that involve sun exposure, geographic latitude of residence, male gender, genetic predisposition, and immunosuppressive therapy.[93] It presents as a white scaly plaque that has a rough sandpaper feel usually limited to the lower lip (Figure 94-3). Histologically, hyperkeratosis, acanthosis, perivascular inflammation, and solar elastosis may be present.[93] Treatment of mild and moderate SC includes topical agents such as imiquimod, 5-fluorouracil, and diclofenac gel. These drugs can also be used as adjuncts to surgical intervention, which remains the definitive treatment but is usually not preferred because of scarring, prolonged healing, and cosmetic disfigurement.[94]

Squamous Cell Carcinoma

Squamous cell carcinoma (SCC) is a cancer arising from the epithelium, with an estimated 200,000 cases diagnosed each year.[95] SCC is often separated into two groups based on malignant potential. The more common type develops from sun-damaged skin and AKs and is less likely to metastasize. For people in this group, the lifetime risk of having SCC after developing a single AK is between 6% and 10%.[96] The more aggressive type arises from areas of prior radiation or thermal exposure, chronic drains, chronic ulcers (Marjolin ulcer), and mucosal surfaces. In general, prolonged UV radiation exposure induces DNA damage and subsequent carcinogenesis in select keratinocyte, leading to SCC formation.[90]

SCCs arising from AKs often appear with a thick adherent scale. The tumor is soft to hard, locally movable, and has an erythematous inflamed base. SCCs are frequently found on the same areas as noted for AKs. If a SCC is diagnosed on a mucous membrane or on non–sun-damaged skin, it may be aggressive and can rapidly metastasize to regional lymph nodes. An SCC described as firm, movable, and elevated, with minimal scale and a sharp border, is usually derived from actinically damaged skin but not typically from a precursor AK. The differential diagnosis for SCC is wide and includes seborrheic keratosis, melanocytic nevus, AK, and chromomycosis. Diagnosis is established by skin biopsy. When SCC is in situ, it is commonly known as Bowen disease.[90] However, what Bowen originally described is slightly different and includes the presence of large atypical cells (Bowen cells) within the lesion.[97] Smaller SCCs are treated with electrodesiccation and curettage, whereas larger tumors in sensitive locations such as the face are often best handled with Mohs micrographic surgery. Other treatment options include radiation therapy, carbon dioxide laser, and oral 5-fluorouracil for refractory lesions.[98]

Keratoacanthoma

Keratoacanthomas (KAs) are a common and distinct neoplasm with a histologic pattern resembling SCC, thus challenging the diagnosis. They are often found in sun-exposed areas of light-skinned older patients, peaking at ages 50 to 70 years and increasing in incidence with advancing age.[99,100] The face, forearms, and hands are frequently afflicted sites, although any area is possible. The cause of KAs is unknown, although they are likely derived from hair follicles, with UV light, chemical carcinogens, immunocompromised status, and viruses contributory to their incidence and progression. KAs are usually solitary and appear as firm, round, skin-colored or erythematous dome-shaped papules. They often have a central umbilication with a keratin plug. Diagnosis is best established by incorporating affected tissue with normal lateral tissue in a biopsy specimen to help distinguish SCC from KA. KAs grow rapidly in a period of 2 weeks but may slowly involute over a period as long as 1 year if no intervention is implemented.[101] Although the regression rate of KA may reach 98.1%, surgical excision is still recommended as the primary therapy.[102]

Basal Cell Carcinoma

Basal cell carcinomas (BCCs) are the most common type of cancer in pale-skinned individuals. It is estimated that more than 1 million new diagnoses are made each year in the United States, comprising 25% of all cancers diagnosed.[103] People who burn easily and severely in the sun without tanning are those at greatest risk for BCC. Fortunately, BCCs only rarely metastasize and are better described as a local infiltrator, with the potential of destroying underlying structures if unattended. However, our group and others have described a rare variant of facial BCC that is extremely aggressive and rapidly involves deep tissue, especially bone. UV light exposure is the main causative agent, but x-rays, thermal injury, and scars may all contribute to BCC formation.[104]

There are five major subtypes of BCCs:

- Noduloulcerative BCC is the most common, with a pearly dome-shaped nodule, central umbilication, and telangiectatic border. This type enlarges slowly, with a 4-mm-sized tumor taking years to develop.
- Pigmented BCCs may display a uniform dark pigment and can resemble melanoma.
- Cystic BCCs are uncommon and are described as bluish gray cystic nodules.
- Superficial BCCs are flat plaques with pearly translucency and thin borders. This subtype is most common on the trunk, unlike the high occurrence on the face of other subtypes.
- Sclerosing BCCs appear as fibrosing and infiltrating plaques. When these resemble a scar, it is often an ominous sign of deep invasiveness.[104] Such morpheiform BCCs must be excised with wide margins.

After biopsy-proven diagnosis, several treatment options are available. These include cryotherapy, curettage and electrodesiccation, radiotherapy, and excisional or Mohs micrographic surgery. For carefully selected thin and small BCCs, topical treatment options include imiquimod and 5-fluorouracil. A 2004 study of 5% imiquimod cream for superficial BCCs showed clearance rates of almost 75% based on clinical and histologic examination.[105]

Melanoma

Melanoma, a malignancy of melanocytes, comprises 4% of all skin cancers but is the leading cause of skin cancer deaths worldwide.[106] According to the American Cancer Society, cutaneous melanoma accounts for 60,000 cases but about 9,000 deaths annually. The annual melanoma incidence peaks at 30 to 50 years of age. The median age of diagnosis is 59 years, with 19.5% of cases diagnosed in those between 55 and 64 years, 17.8% diagnosed between 65 and 74 years, 16.4% diagnosed between 75 and 84 years; and 5.5% diagnosed in those older than 85 years. The median age for death is 68 years, with 15% dying between 45 and 54 years, 18.8% dying between 55 and 64 years, 21.3% dying between 65 and 74 years, 23.6% dying between 75 and 84 years, and 11.0% dying when older than 85 years of age. The incidence is 18.5 to 28.5/100,000 for whites and 0.9 to 1.1/100,000 for blacks for all types of melanoma.[107] Malignant melanoma formation is a multistep process of mutations, with risk factors including blistering tendencies in the sun, high number of dysplastic moles, actively changing mole, family history of melanoma, previous history of melanoma, and older age.[108]

There are several subtypes of melanoma:

- Superficial spreading melanoma is characterized as a flat or slightly elevated dark brown lesion, with variegate colors.
- Nodular melanoma manifests as a rapidly growing dark brown or black papule or nodule that is at risk for ulceration and bleeding. Both are common on the trunk and legs.[108]
- Lentigo maligna (Figure 94-4) is a slower growing subtype on the rise in the United States, which when invasive is called lentigo maligna melanoma.[109] It is found on chronically sun-damaged areas of the head and on the neck and arms, with a peak incidence at 65 years of age. It is characterized as a brown to tan-colored macule with possible areas of

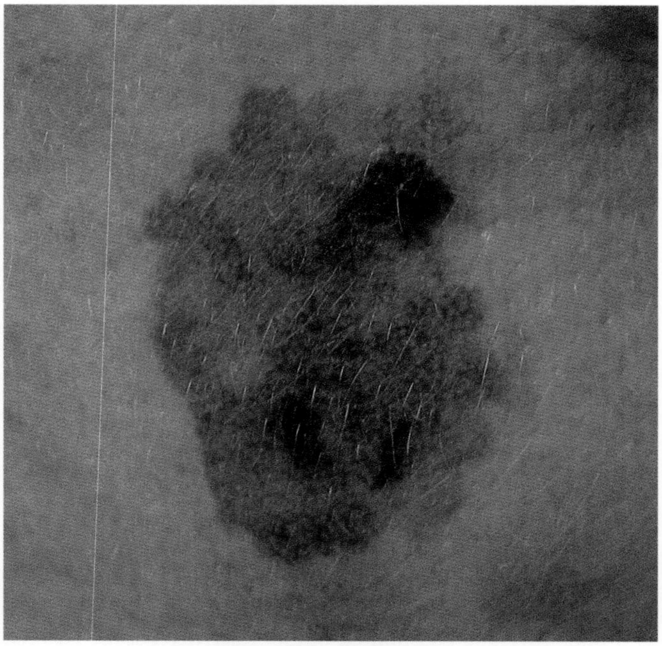

Figure 94-4. Older woman with lentigo maligna on her right cheek.

hypopigmentation and later raised blue-black nodules with dermal invasion.

- The last major subtype, acral melanoma, is the least common, comprising 2% to 8% of all melanomas in lightly pigmented people and 29% to 72% in darkly pigmented people. Although the proportion is higher in dark-skinned individuals, the incidence is similar across all skin types.[110] Acral melanomas are noted on the palms, soles, and subungual areas and thus are more difficult to identify, with late diagnosis leading to poor outcome. They usually appear dark brown to black, with irregular borders.

The subungual type may show the Hutchinson sign, or proximal nail fold dark pigmentation.[111] Of all melanomas, 2% to 8% are amelanotic, showing no pigmentation.[108]

Diagnosis involves a proper history and physical examination, along with lymph node evaluation. The ABCDE criteria (***a***symmetry, ***b***order irregularity, ***c***olor variegation, ***d***iameter, ***e***volution of lesion or change over time) frequently mentioned is a useful tool during the initial examination, and all components must be used in concert to establish a level of suspicion. A biopsy with pathologic confirmation is essential to rule out mimicking lesions such as pyogenic granuloma and pigmented basal cell carcinoma. After biopsy-confirmed diagnosis and evaluation for metastasis, the primary mode of treatment is surgery.[108]

Angiosarcoma

Angiosarcomas are rare and malignant neoplasms of endothelial origin. The age-adjusted incidence for soft tissue sarcoma was 3.1/100,000 men and women/year in the 2000 to 2004 period, with angiosarcomas constituting 4.1% of such sarcomas.[112,113] Angiosarcomas have a peak incidence in the seventh decade, although any age group may be affected. Cutaneous angiosarcoma of the scalp and face is the most common form and appears as an enlarging bruise, dark blue to black nodule, or unhealed ulceration. After biopsy and staging, treatment remains challenging, with a combination of surgery and radiation therapy being most successful. Studies have demonstrated beneficial activity of paclitaxel and liposomal doxorubicin against angiosarcoma of the scalp and face.[114]

Kaposi Sarcoma

Kaposi sarcoma (KS) is a tumor of endothelial origin in which the classic form is usually found in men in their 60s. Human herpesvirus-8 is linked to the pathogenesis of all types of KS, including the classic form. Classic KS is found as a rare and indolent lesion in older men of Jewish and Mediterranean descent. Specifically, it represents about 0.2% of cancers in older U.S. men of Mediterranean and Central-Eastern European (Ashkenazi) Jewish lineage in the United States.[115] In Israel, rates of classic KS of 2.07/100,000 in men and 0.75/100,000 in women have been calculated.[116]

Clinically, it is often apparent on the distal extremities as a bluish-red hematoma resembling a macule. It can develop into plaques and nodules and may become hyperkeratotic and ulcerate. The disease progresses slowly, and patients may live for decades with the tumor. Therefore, death in these patients may be from other causes of aging.[116] In localized disease, treatment can involve radiotherapy and intralesional chemotherapy. Systemwide chemotherapy, including agents such as doxorubicin, vincristine, and etoposide, are helpful in metastasized or aggressive KS. Immunotherapy, including imiquimod, interferon-α, and sirolimus have been used, but specific health concerns of each older patient need to be carefully addressed.[117,118] Other types of KS, including those in immunocompromised and AIDS patients, do not occur preferentially in older adults.

Bullous Pemphigoid

Bullous pemphigoid is an autoimmune blistering disease primarily of older adults. The average age of affected patients is 65 years, and incidence reports vary by region.[119,120] Rates of 0.7 cases/100,000 were reported in Germany in 1995 and up to 4.3 cases/100,000 in the United Kingdom in 2008.[120,121] The disease is characterized by large tense bullae on an erythematous base on flexor areas of the extremities, axillae, groin, and abdomen. Clear or sanguineous exudates exist in these bullae. The size can range from 0.5 to 7 cm. Postinflammatory pigmentary changes may follow rupture of these bullae. Mucosal lesions are rare but heal quickly, if present. There have been associations of bullous pemphigoid with other autoimmune conditions such as psoriasis, diabetes mellitus, and rheumatoid arthritis.[122]

Consistent with its autoimmune cause, immunoglobulin G (IgG) and C3 have been demonstrated in the epidermal basement membrane of bullous pemphigoid. IgG autoantibodies specifically bind to hemidesmosome adhesion complexes (components BP180 and BP230) of the basement membrane.[123] A subepidermal blister forms, with eosinophils, and possible lymphocytes, histiocytes, and neutrophils. Diagnosis is established on clinical and histologic findings. A fresh blister biopsy shows eosinophils in a subepidermal cleft, whereas direct immunofluorescence demonstrates IgG or C3 linearly deposited at the basement membrane zone.[122]

Topical or systemic corticosteroids are used for treatment, with systemic therapy most effective for multiple lesion disease.[124] Before starting systemic corticosteroids, tetracyclines, with possible niacinamide, may be explored for mild to moderate disease.[124]

The use of steroids in older patients should be coupled with calcium and vitamin D to help prevent osteoporosis complications. Supplemental antiinflammatory agents such as dapsone are useful for tapering steroid doses. Dapsone therapy requires close evaluation of liver and bone marrow function, as well as ruling out glucose-6-phosphate dehydrogenase deficiency, and the adverse effect profile is severe. Other ancillary treatments include azathioprine, methotrexate,[125] chlorambucil, cyclosporine, cyclophosphamide, plasmapheresis, and mycophenolate mofetil.[124,126] The effectiveness of plasma exchange or azathioprine as adjuncts has not been conclusively determined.[124] According to a 2008 Swedish study of 138 patients comparing methotrexate, prednisone, methotrexate plus prednisone, and topical steroid groups, methotrexate was found to be an excellent option for patients.[127]

Bullous pemphigoid may be fatal if appropriate treatment is not administered. The main predictors of poor prognosis include old age, female gender, associated chronic morbidities, and poor hygiene.[128,129] Mortality rates from 19% to 43% were reported in some studies, and death may be related to chronic high-dose steroid use.[128,130-132]

Erythema Multiforme

Erythema multiforme (EM) is a skin disorder believed to be the result of a hypersensitivity reaction causing well-demarcated plaques, with characteristic target or iris lesions that have a red or pink border with central clearing[133] (Figure 94-5). It is usually a self-limiting condition that begins distally on the extremities and progresses proximally. The most common causes of EM include infection by herpes simplex virus (HSV) and *Mycoplasma pneumoniae* and drug reactions, with the latter most commonly associated with severe forms of EM. The severe forms of EM are mostly linked with barbiturates, hydantoins, nonsteroidal antiinflammatory drugs, penicillins, phenothiazines, and sulfonamides.[134] Diagnosis is usually made clinically after identifying characteristic lesions, and treatment depends on the severity of symptoms. Mild EM can be treated with oral antihistamines and topical steroids. Oral acyclovir is used for patients with

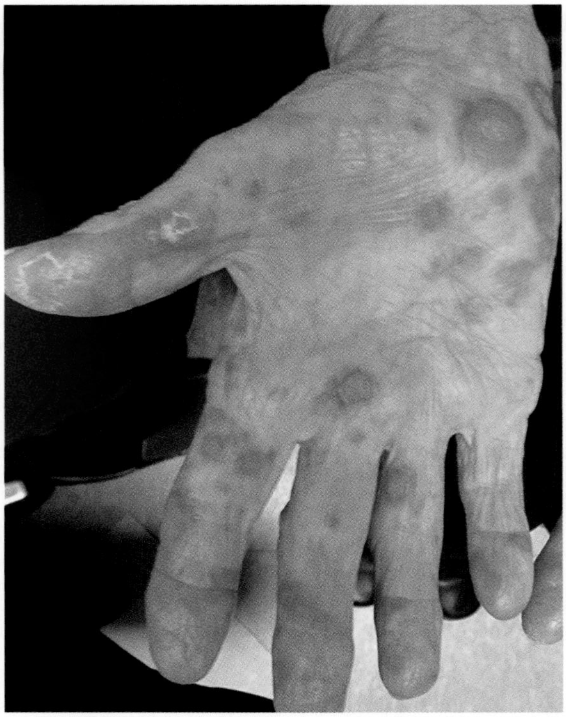

Figure 94-5. Older women with bullous erythema multiforme, cause uncertain.

coexisting HSV infection and recurrent EM. However, EM may be severe and life-threatening, to the extent that it may be classified as EM major, Stevens-Johnson syndrome, or toxic epidermolysis, with the latter producing widespread sloughing of skin involving the gut, liver, and lungs. Prednisone and rituximab have been used for severe cases of EM, but their use remains controversial.[134,135]

Systemic Concerns of Older Adults with Cutaneous Complications

Diabetes Mellitus

Diabetes mellitus (DM) is an endocrine disease of epidemic proportions in the United States. The Centers for Disease Control and Prevention in a 2005 study showed that those older than 60 years had a diabetes prevalence of 20.9%.[136] Diabetes manifests in many organ systems, including the nervous, renal, ocular, integumentary, and cardiovascular systems. Older patients suffer greatly from complications such as functional disability, depression, cognitive impairment, injury, and urinary incontinence.

Diabetic dermopathy, also known as shin spots, is found in 9% to 55% of diabetics.[137-141] It appears as round, slightly indented patches of brown to purplish skin. Diabetic dermopathy is the most common cutaneous complication of DM and suggests advanced internal disease of the heart, liver, or kidney.[138]

DM is the cause of the greatest number of nontraumatic amputations in the United States. This is a result of nonhealing ulcers in diabetics with long-standing neuropathy and reduced pain sensation. Up to 25% of diabetics suffer from leg ulcers in their lifetime.[142] Proper and frequent examination of the feet and immediate treatment of ulcers is a critical component of diabetic patient care.

Perforating dermatosis is a condition found in diabetics who suffer from severe renal disease or in patients with chronic renal failure alone. This condition presents as hyperkeratotic, pruritic, and umbilicated papules and nodules on the extensor surfaces of the legs, trunk, and face.[143]

Acanthosis nigricans is probably the most recognized dermatologic sign of diabetes. It reflects insulin resistance and is common among the obese. This diffuse, darkened, and velvet-like thickening is seen on the skin of the neck, axilla, groin, umbilicus, hands, submammary area, and areola. In exuberant form, this condition can also be a signal of internal malignancy; thus, a thorough examination is critical.[31]

Necrobiosis lipoidica diabeticorum presents as a red papule that grows peripherally, becomes atrophic in the center, assuming an apple jelly–like coloration, and eventually appears telangiectatic and porcelain like. Although rare, a striking 75% of patients with necrobiosis lipoidica have or will be diagnosed with diabetes.[144] Patients may respond to topical or intralesional corticosteroids, among other medications, but strict diabetes management does not improve the papules of necrobiosis lipoidica.

Thyroid Disease

Thyroid disease, including hypothyroidism and hyperthyroidism, affects up to 20% of older patients.[145] Cutaneous manifestations of thyroid disease also depend on overproduction or underproduction of thyroid hormones. There is an increased incidence of alopecia areata and vitiligo associated with autoimmune thyroid disease.

Characteristic features of hyperthyroidism include palmar erythema, warm and moist skin, and fragile scalp hair, or alopecia. These signs are often useful for diagnosis. Pretibial myxedema is a specific dermopathy of hyperthyroidism in Graves' disease (an antibody-mediated autoimmune thyroid reaction). Firm nonpitting nodules or plaques form on both legs in an asymmetric pattern. The color may be pink, purple, or fleshlike.[146] An accumulation of mucopolysaccharides in the dermis is suspected to lead to this appearance. These signature features of hyperthyroidism should trigger appropriate diagnosis and treatment of the underlying disease process. Hypothyroidism is a condition occurring in about 10% of women and 2% of men older than 60 years.[147] It manifests with a cutaneous feature of myxedema that is more prolonged and diffuse. In advanced cases, the overall appearance of the skin becomes dry, scaly, and yellowish, with sparse hair.[148] With progressing myxedema, the face may also appear flat and expressionless. Palmoplantar keratoderma, or hyperkeratosis on the palms and soles, is possible in severe cases. Hair and fingernails are prone to break as well.[145] Onycholysis, or separation of the nail plate from the nail bed, is found in patients with thyrotoxicosis and hypothyroidism but decreases in incidence in patients older than 60 years.[146]

Renal and Adrenal Disease

Cushing syndrome and Addison disease are two conditions of the adrenal gland with cutaneous manifestations. In Cushing disease, the main cause of Cushing syndrome, there is hypersecretion of adrenocorticotropic hormone (ACTH).[148] ACTH levels may rise from neoplasms of the pituitary gland or from ectopic neoplasms such as oat cell lung cancer.[149] The primary clinical features include hypertension and weight gain. A buffalo hump or redistribution of fat to the upper back is evident, along with purple striae on the torso. Hypertrichosis, excessive bruising, poor wound healing, and hirsutism are additional complications.[148] In Addison disease, autoimmune destruction of the adrenals leads to adrenocortical insufficiency. The main dermatologic feature is hyperpigmentation of skin creases, new scars, vermilion border, nipple, and areas of constant pressure.[149] The mechanism is attributable to the stimulation of melanocytes by ACTH or the closely related melanocyte-stimulating hormone (MSH). This darkening of the skin may be the presenting feature.[150]

Chronic kidney disease (CKD) is a life-threatening condition affecting more than one third of patients 70 years of age and older according to the National Health and Nutrition Examination Survey.[151] Cutaneous examination of patients has shown that 50% to 100% have at least one dermatologic symptom.[152] The list of cutaneous sequelae is extensive, including pruritus, xerosis, ischemic ulcerations, prurigo nodularis, calcinosis cutis, calciphylaxis, Kyrle disease, bullous disease of dialysis, nephrogenic fibrosing dermopathy, and uremic frost. Most of these improve with appropriate renal management.

Pruritus and xerosis have been attributed to uremia in CKD patients.[153-155] Pruritus may be local or generalized, mild or severe, or episodic or constant. Evidently, it is highly patient-specific, with no demographic biases.[152] Both xerosis and pruritus may improve with kidney disease management, with xerosis specifically responding to emollients.[155] Calcinosis cutis is the result of insoluble calcium deposition in the skin, appearing as multiple, firm, whitish papules, plaques, or nodules. They may ulcerate, extruding a chalky white substance.[156] Calciphylaxis refers to vascular calcification with skin necrosis. Patients have firm painful lesions with central necrosis along a vascular track. These may begin initially as violaceous mottling.[157] Kyrle disease is the occurrence of widespread papules with central keratin and cellular debris plugs that usually begins as a silvery scaled papule.[158] Bullous disease of dialysis resembles porphyria cutanea tarda, with blistering and mechanical fragility of the skin in sun-exposed areas. The incidence is 1.2% to 9% in patients with CKD on hemodialysis.[159-162]

Nephrogenic fibrosing dermopathy is a condition with fibrosis of the skin and internal organs that is distinct but reminiscent of scleroderma. Large areas of indurated skin, brawny discoloration, and tightening occur. Nephrogenic fibrosing dermopathy occurs almost exclusively in patients with end-stage renal disease who have had imaging studies with gadolinium.[163] Uremic frost is the aggregation of fine, white to off-white, friable urea crystal deposits on the skin. This condition is usually observed on skin containing pilosebaceous units such as the neck, scalp, forearms, and chest and occurs at blood urea nitrogen levels of approximately 200 mg/dL.[164]

Nutrition

Proper nutrition, including daily recommended levels of essential vitamins and minerals, is critical in older adults to prevent disease with cutaneous manifestations, such as scurvy and pellagra. More information on these topics is presented in Chapter 74.

Menopause

Menopause leads to significant changes in skin biology. On physical examination, the skin is thinner and less lubricated than premenopausal skin. The risk of infection is higher, and atrophy, pruritus, stiffness, alopecia, and dryness result.[165] Topical estrogen-based creams have been shown to result in some improvement in elasticity and moisturization. Specifically, collagen content and dermal thickness are improved with estrogen use after menopause.[166,167] The risks and benefits for each individual patient must be assessed before initiating therapy for moderate improvement.

Tobacco Use

Tobacco use is a leading cause of preventable morbidity and mortality in the United States. In addition to risks of lung cancer, chronic obstructive pulmonary disease, and cardiac disease, the skin suffers significant damage from smoking. Early skin aging, SCC, melanoma, oral cancer, acne, and hair loss are some problems faced by long-term smokers. One study of 63 volunteers has noted that a 35–pack-year smoking history leads to a significantly greater skin furrow depth of the volar forearm when compared to that of nonsmokers ($P < .05$).[168] A few specific signs of tobacco smoking include harlequin nail, which is a demarcation between the yellow and pink on the nail of someone who has recently quit smoking. The term *smoker's face* refers to a constellation of deep lines and furrows at right angles from the lips and corners of the eye, prominence of bony structures, and general graying of the skin. In vitro and epidemiologic evidence strongly support premature aging of the skin from tobacco smoke.[169]

KEY POINTS

Skin Cancer

- Current incidence rates suggest that one in five people in the United States will develop skin cancer in his or her lifetime.
- Basal cell carcinoma is the most common type of skin cancer and the one least likely to metastasize.
- Melanoma comprises 4% of skin cancers, and suspicion is guided by ABCDE criteria (***a***symmetry, ***b***order irregularity, ***c***olor variegation, ***d***iameter, ***e***volution of lesion).
- Actinic keratosis is considered to be a precancerous form of squamous cell carcinoma, although its classification as a malignant neoplasm is debated.
- All patients should use a dermatologist-recommended sunscreen appropriate for their skin type and should avoid sun exposure during the peak hours of sunlight.

Skin Disease and Old Age

- Skin diseases are common in older adults and, although rarely deadly, may degrade quality of life.
- Skin cancer is increasing in incidence in the light-skinned U.S. population and is curable if diagnosed early.
- Xerosis and pruritus are the most common complaints of older adults and may be manifestations of many systemic diseases.
- Early treatment, within 3 days of onset, is most effective for herpes zoster patients.
- Tobacco use and unregulated sun exposure are major preventable factors in skin cancer predisposition and skin aging.

For a complete list of references, please visit www.expertconsult.com.

KEY REFERENCES

9. Norman RA: Xerosis and pruritus in the elderly: recognition and management. Dermatol Ther 16:254–259, 2003.
15. Schwartz RA, Janusz CA, Janniger CK: Seborrheic dermatitis: an overview. Am Fam Physician 74:125–130, 2006.
25. Klecz RJ, Schwartz RA: Pruritus. Am Fam Physician 45:2681–2686, 1992.
26. Schwartz RA: Superficial fungal infections. Lancet 364:1173–1182, 2004.
37. Pascarella L, Schonbein GW, Bergan JJ: Microcirculation and venous ulcers: a review. Ann Vasc Surg 19:921–927, 2005.
41. Schissel DJ, Hivnor C, Elston DM: Elephantiasis nostras verrucosa. Cutis 62:77–80, 1998.
50. Janniger CK, Droana AN Herpes zoster. http://emedicine.medscape.com/article/1132465-overview. Accessed October 6, 2009.
58. Yawn BP, Saddier P, Wollan PC, et al: A population-based study of the incidence and complication rates of herpes zoster before zoster vaccine introduction. Mayo Clin Proc 82:1341–1349, 2007.
60. Steen CJ, Carbonaro PA, Schwartz RA: Arthropods in dermatology. J Am Acad Dermatol 50:819–842, 2004.
64. Janniger CK, Micali G, Hengge U, et al: Scabies. http://author.emedicine.com/ped/topic2047.htm. Accessed October 6, 2009.
73. Vender RB, Lynde CW, Poulin Y: Prevalence and epidemiology of onychomycosis. J Cutan Med Surg 10(Suppl 2):S28–S33, 2006.

90. Butani AK, Arbesfeld DM, Schwartz RA: Premalignant and early squamous cell carcinoma. Clin Plast Surg 32:223–235, 2005.
93. Jadotte YT, Schwartz RA: Solar cheilosis: an ominous precursor. Part I. Diagnostic insights. J Am Acad Dermatol 66:173–183, 2012.
94. Jadotte YT, Schwartz RA: Solar cheilosis: an ominous precursor. Part II. Therapeutic perspectivs. J Am Acad Dermatol 66:187–198, 2012.
100. Schwartz RA: Keratoacanthoma. In Schwartz RA, editor: Skin cancer: recognition and management, ed 2, Oxford, England, 2008, Blackwell, pp 66–80.
102. Takai T, Misago N, Murata Y: Natural course of keratoacanthoma and related lesions after partial biopsy: Clinical analysis of 66 lesions. J Dermatol 42:353–362, 2015.
104. Schwartz RA: Basal cell carcinoma. In Schwartz RA, editor: Skin cancer: recognition and management, ed 2, Oxford, England, 2008, Blackwell, pp 87–99.
108. Cohen PJ, Hofmann MA, Sterry W, et al: Melanoma. In Schwartz RA, editor: Skin cancer: recognition and management, ed 2, Oxford, England, 2008, Blackwell, pp 152–199.
112. Toro JR, Travis LB, Wu HJ, et al: Incidence patterns of soft tissue sarcomas, regardless of primary site, in the surveillance, epidemiology and end results program, 1978-2001: an analysis of 26,758 cases. Int J Cancer 119:2922–2930, 2006.
117. Schwartz RA, Micali G, Nasca MR, et al: Kaposi sarcoma: a continuing conundrum. J Am Acad Dermatol 59:179–206, quizzes 207-178, 2008.
122. Di Zenzo G, Marazza G, Borradori L: Bullous pemphigoid: physiopathology, clinical features and management. Adv Dermatol 23:257–288, 2007.
133. Stampien TM, Schwartz RA: Erythema multiforme. Am Fam Physician 46:1171–1176, 1992.
138. Morgan AJ, Schwartz RA: Diabetic dermopathy: a subtle sign with grave implications. J Am Acad Dermatol 58:447–451, 2008.
154. Schwartz IF, Iaina A: Management of uremic pruritus. Semin Dial 13:177–180, 2000.
164. Saardi KM, Schwartz RA: Uremic frost: a harbinger of impending renal failure. Int J Dermatol 55:17–20, 2016.

95 Aging and Disorders of the Eye

Scott E. Brodie, Jasmine H. Francis

Loss of vision, one of the most feared forms of medical disability, falls disproportionately on older adults. Unfortunately, the damage to the delicate tissues of the eye from the various metabolic insults that may occur throughout life is generally cumulative. Consequently, most forms of ocular pathology occur ever more frequently, and in more debilitating forms, with increasing age.

Estimates of the prevalence of blindness from all causes vary by perhaps a factor of 13 between industrialized and Third World countries.[1] Nevertheless, regardless of the degree of economic development, the prevalence rate for blindness in any society is typically 100-fold greater among individuals older than 65 years than among children in the same country.[2] In developed countries, the major causes of blindness (Box 95-1) are primarily cataract, glaucoma, and retinal disease (mostly macular degeneration and diabetic retinopathy), all of which are strongly related to advancing age.[3] In the Third World, the major causes of blindness are cataract, corneal scarring, glaucoma, and retinal disease.[4]

Delivery of adequate eye care to older adults remains an unsolved problem, even in wealthy countries. Recent surveys in the United States have identified significant rates of untreated eye disease among older adults. The nursing home population appears to be notably underserved.[5,6]

Discussion of age-related ocular problems is organized in this chapter by considering the visual apparatus in anatomic order, from anterior to posterior.

EYELIDS

The eyelids are vital for the proper circulation of tears and maintenance of the smooth ocular surface necessary for clear image formation by the eye. With increasing age, the skin of the eyelids, as elsewhere, loses elasticity, and the lids become more loosely apposed to the globe. Atrophy of the fascial planes within the eyelids may lead to herniation of the orbital fat into the lid tissue, producing the bags under the eyes frequently seen in older adults (Figure 95-1). Atrophy or disinsertion of the aponeurosis of the levator palpebrae muscle, which ordinarily supports the upper eyelid, may cause the opened lid to fail to uncover the pupil, as seen in senile ptosis, despite normal levator muscle function (Figure 95-2). Senile ptosis must be differentiated from ptosis due to mechanical and neuromuscular causes, such as oculomotor nerve palsies and myasthenia gravis.[7]

Laxity of the lower lid may allow the free lid margin to rotate away from the eyeball, a condition known as ectropion (Figure 95-3). If severe, the lacrimal punctum may fail to make contact with the pool of tears adjacent to the lower lid. This prevents the normal conduction of tears into the lacrimal sac, which may result in persistent tearing (epiphora), even in the absence of lacrimal duct obstruction. More dangerous is entropion, in which a loosening of the adhesions between tissue planes in the lid allows the muscle tone of the orbicularis oculi to rotate the lid margin inward (Figure 95-4).[8] Frequently, the lashes come to rub directly against the cornea or conjunctiva, producing irritation or scarring.

The treatment of eyelid malpositions is generally surgical. For senile ptosis, resection of the levator aponeurosis is generally performed.[9] Ectropion and entropion are generally treated by resection of redundant lid tissue.[10]

Of the tumors of the eyelid skin, basal cell carcinomas are the most common; squamous cell carcinomas are also possible. Both these tumors are frequently a consequence of lifetime exposure to sunlight. If the lesions are detected early, a curative local resection is often possible. In advanced cases, the tumor may cause massive destruction of facial structures by local extension. Metastases are very rare.[11]

LACRIMAL APPARATUS

The lacrimal apparatus consists of the lacrimal glands, which secrete the tears, and lacrimal sac and ducts, which convey the tears into the nasal cavity. Secretory function of the lacrimal glands declines with age, and many older adults develop dry eye syndrome. This nonspecific reduction in tear production is much more common than the full-fledged Sjögren syndrome, which is an autoimmune disease process affecting salivary and lacrimal secretion.[12] Paradoxically, many tear-deficient patients complain of excess tearing because the chronically irritated eyes may stimulate reflex tear production. Dry eyes are treated with artificial tear eye drops, as often as needed. Some patients respond well to topical treatment with cyclosporin A.[13] In patients whose eyes dry out overnight, lubricant ointment at bedtime may be helpful. In severe cases, small silicone plugs may be placed to obstruct the lacrimal puncta,[14] or surgical occlusion of the lacrimal puncta may be performed to conserve the available tears.

Obstruction of the lacrimal ducts also leads to epiphora. Uncomplicated mechanical stenosis may occasionally be relieved with simple probing, but severe cases (often following bacterial infection of the lacrimal sac) are treated surgically. A dacryocystorhinostomy is performed to anastomose the mucosa of the nasal cavity to the lacrimal sac through an osteotomy made in the lacrimal bone.[15]

CONJUNCTIVA

Subconjunctival hemorrhage, a localized accumulation of blood seen between the conjunctiva and globe, is frequently encountered in older adults, either following minor trauma or occurring spontaneously (Figure 95-5). The Valsalva maneuver may be a precipitating event. Such hemorrhages are rarely of any consequence, but they are often alarming in appearance. They resolve spontaneously without treatment over a period of several days. Occasionally, recurrent hemorrhages may suggest an underlying disease such as hypertension or a coagulation disorder, or perhaps an occult tumor.

Chronic exposure to sunlight, particularly at tropical latitudes, may cause a degeneration of the connective tissue in the exposed sector of the conjunctiva between the eyelids, leading to thickening of the conjunctiva (pinguecula), which may grow over the cornea from the periphery toward the pupil (pterygium). If the growth threatens to cover the visual axis, surgical excision may be indicated. Recurrence after surgery is, unfortunately, not uncommon.[16]

Tumors such as squamous cell carcinoma and melanoma may arise from the conjunctiva. Primary acquired melanosis and squamous dysplasia must be distinguished from malignant tumors. Local excision and cryoablation may be adequate in early cases, but advanced cases may require other interventions (e.g., radiation

BOX 95-1 Major Causes of Blindness in Older Adults

IN DEVELOPED COUNTRIES

- Cataract
- Glaucoma
- Diabetic retinopathy
- Macular degeneration

IN DEVELOPING COUNTRIES

- Cataract
- Corneal scarring
- Glaucoma
- Diabetic retinopathy
- Macular degeneration

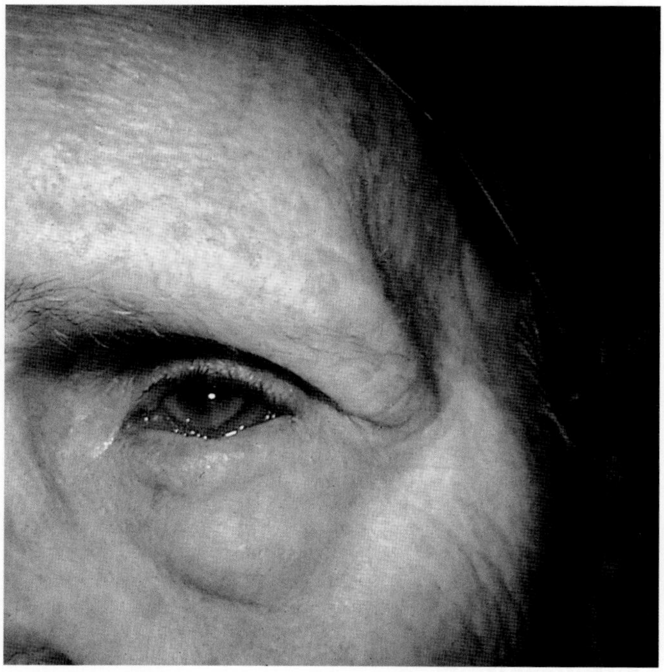

Figure 95-1. Prolapse of orbital fat through atrophic fascial planes in the eyelid produces bags under the eyes. *(Courtesy Dr. Murray Meltzer.)*

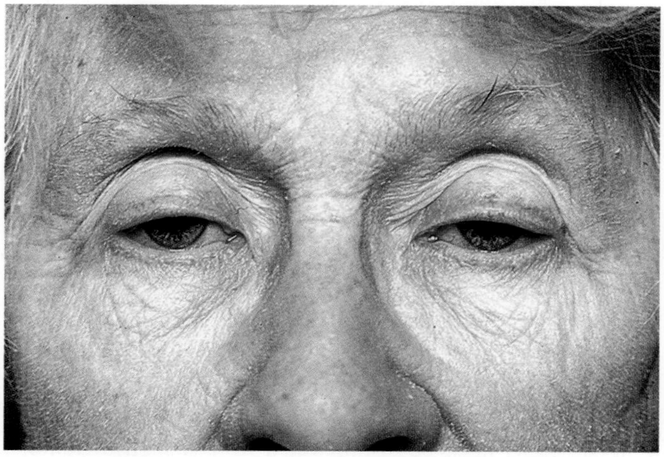

Figure 95-2. Senile ptosis. Note the low lid level and loss of the normal lid folds. *(Courtesy Dr. Murray Meltzer.)*

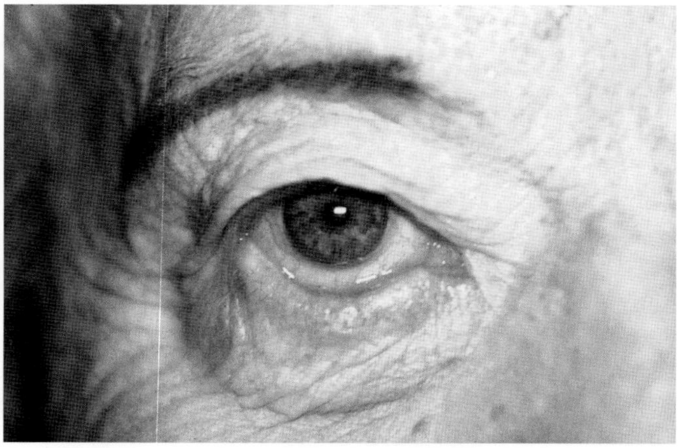

Figure 95-3. Ectropion. Laxity of the lower eyelid allows the lid margin to rotate away from the eyeball. *(Courtesy Dr. Murray Meltzer.)*

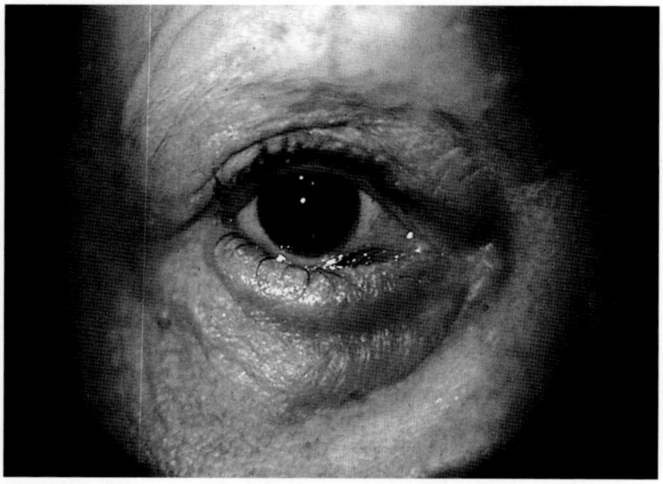

Figure 95-4. Entropion. Breakdown of the adhesion between the tissue planes in the eyelid allows the muscle tone of the orbicularis oculi muscle to rotate the lid margin inward. The eyelashes may chronically irritate the surface of the eyeball. *(Courtesy Dr. Murray Meltzer.)*

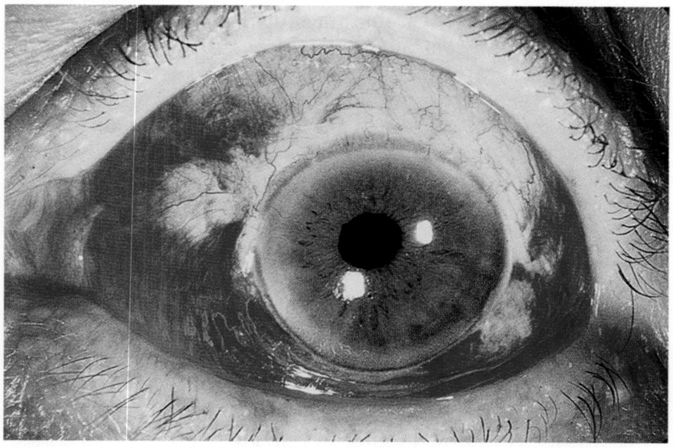

Figure 95-5. Subconjunctival hemorrhage. This small hematoma, seen through the transparent conjunctiva, is benign unless recurrent.

therapy, systemic treatment with chemotherapy or potentially with targeted molecules) or even orbital exenteration.[17,18]

CORNEA

The eye is unique in its requirement for transparent tissues, including the cornea and crystalline lens. The need for transparency places many constraints on the architecture and metabolism of these ocular structures. In particular, the eye must nourish these tissues with a cell-free fluid, because red blood cells preclude transparency. Similarly, the transparent tissues must rely primarily on anaerobic glycolytic metabolism because the enzyme systems required for oxidative phosphorylation (aptly named *cytochromes*) strongly absorb visible light. Even in the absence of these absorbent components, the tissues must be constructed in a highly compact and regular manner so that light scattering from tissue organelles does not cause a white opaque appearance. This requirement is met in the case of the cornea by a highly regular arrangement of collagen fibrils and an active metabolic pump in the corneal endothelial cell layer, which dehydrates the corneal stroma. Absence of these tissue features explains why the sclera, which is otherwise histologically similar to the cornea, is opaque.[19]

The corneal endothelial cells, on which the dehydration critical for corneal transparency depends, do not divide during adulthood. Endothelial cell density declines slowly with age.[20] If the number of endothelial cells falls below a critical level, the cornea imbibes fluid, swells, and becomes cloudy (Figure 95-6). Edema fluid percolates to the epithelial surface and may coalesce into subepithelial bullae. Mild cases may be managed with the use of hypertonic saline eye drops and ointment to withdraw fluid from the cornea osmotically. If these measures fail, a corneal graft, which replaces the deficient endothelium, is necessary to restore vision.[21] In addition to full-thickness corneal transplants, there are now options for partial-thickness procedures (Descemet stripping and automated endothelial keratoplasty [DSAEK] and Descemet membrane endothelial keratoplasty [DMEK]),which replace only the diseased back layer of the cornea. These procedures have the advantage of being sutureless and offer quicker recovery times.

Bacterial ulcers of the cornea (Figure 95-7) seem to occur with greater frequency in older adults, perhaps reflecting impairments of tear secretion, epithelial integrity, and cellular and humoral immunity, and are associated with a poorer prognosis in older adults.[22] Intensive antibiotic therapy is generally required. Fourth-generation fluoroquinolones have been shown to be as effective as fortified antibiotics[23,24] and may be easier to obtain.

The ring-shaped deposition of lipid in the far periphery of the cornea, termed the *arcus senilis*, is completely benign.

UVEAL TRACT

The uveal tract (uvea) is comprised of the iris, ciliary body, and choroid, which form a continuous, highly vascular layer inside the sclera. Inflammation of the uvea occurs frequently as a primary disease process in response to infections, in many patients with rheumatic disease, and as a sequela to accidental or surgical trauma. Clinically, inflammatory cells are seen in the aqueous or vitreous humor. These inflammatory reactions can cause ocular injury by many mechanisms. They may occlude the trabecular meshwork, causing glaucoma. They may accumulate on the inner surface of the cornea as keratic precipitates, where they may injure or destroy the corneal endothelial cells and cause corneal edema. Inflamed tissues often develop pathologic adhesions, which may derange normal ocular function. Adhesions between the anterior surface of the peripheral iris and anterior chamber angle (peripheral anterior synechiae) may occlude the trabecular meshwork, leading to chronic angle-closure glaucoma. Adhesions between the posterior surface of the iris and anterior surface of the crystalline lens can seal off access of the aqueous humor to the anterior chamber (pupillary block), forcing the iris to bow forward (iris bombé). In cases in which the peripheral iris becomes apposed to the trabecular meshwork, the egress of aqueous humor from the eye is blocked, resulting in angle-closure glaucoma. In the posterior segment, inflammatory cells in the vitreous humor may obscure vision and lead to fibrovascular proliferation, which may distort the retina or even cause a retinal detachment.

Treatment in most cases of uveitis is generally empirical. Dilation of the pupil with cycloplegic eye drops is generally advisable to prevent posterior synechiae and pupillary block and relieve the discomfort (photophobia) caused by light-induced miosis of the inflamed iris. If the inflammation is confined to the anterior segment, topical corticosteroid eye drops are usually sufficient. In cases involving the posterior segment, periocular corticosteroid injections or systemic administration of corticosteroids are frequently required.[25] In the most severe cases, systemic administration of immunomodulators or biologics has proven to be useful.[26] Typically, a workup for associated systemic disease is appropriate. If a treatable condition is discovered, such as syphilis

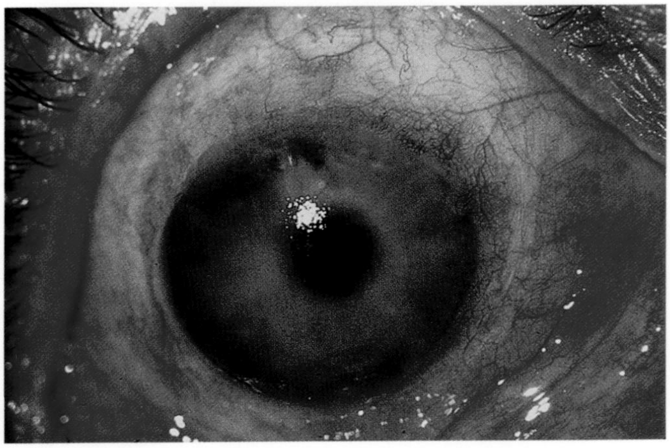

Figure 95-6. Corneal edema. The cornea is thickened and cloudy because of failure of the corneal endothelium to dehydrate the tissue adequately. *(Courtesy Dr. Calvin Roberts.)*

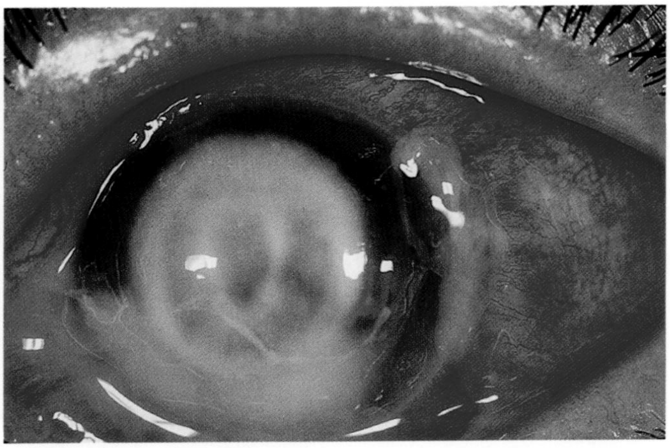

Figure 95-7. Corneal ulcer. A localized infection causes an epithelial defect and attracts an infiltrate of white blood cells. *(Courtesy Dr. Michael Newton.)*

or tuberculosis, specific treatment for the underlying condition may simultaneously cure the uveitis.

Intraocular tumors in older adults usually occur within the uveal tract. Melanomas are the most common primary tumor. Although prompt enucleation (surgical removal of the eyeball) was long the traditional management, many authorities now recommend that eyes containing small uveal melanomas be followed closely, rather than enucleated, because they have only a low propensity for metastasis.[27] Medium-sized tumors have been successfully treated in many cases with irradiation by temporary implantation of a radioactive plaque applied to the overlying sclera[28] or administered by external beam x-ray or proton beam.[29] A large prospective clinical trial found no difference in 5-year survival between groups of patients randomized to treatment by radioactive plaque or by enucleation.[30] Primary enucleation is often recommended for large tumors. Metastatic melanoma is usually detected initially in the liver. Annual magnetic resonance imaging (MRI) of the abdomen and monitoring of hepatic enzyme activity in the serum are advisable for patients at risk.[31] Traditionally, estimates of the risk of metastatic disease have been based on the clinical features and histologic architecture of the primary tumor. Recent studies have suggested that better estimates of metastatic risk may be obtained via determination of the genetic underpinnings of the intraocular tumor. This can be achieved by using DNA- and RNA-based assays.[32,33] For example, a somatic mutation in *BAP1* (BRCA-associated protein 1) has been implicated in tumors at high risk for metastases.[34] Furthermore, a germline mutation in *BAP1* has been associated with a hereditary cancer syndrome that includes uveal melanoma, lung mesothelioma, renal cell carcinoma, and gastric cancer.[35] Genetic mutations within the metastatic tumor may qualify the patient for novel systemic treatments that target the aberrant molecular pathway.[36]

Tumors metastatic to the choroid are actually more frequent than primary intraocular tumors. Lung primaries predominate in men and breast primaries in women.[37] Because the eye is seldom the sole site of metastasis, these patients generally require systemic chemotherapy. Additional treatments often used for sight-threatening lesions include radiation, anti–vascular endothelial growth factor (VEGF) injections, and lasers.[38]

GLAUCOMA

Glaucoma is a form of progressive atrophy of the optic nerve, frequently associated with increased intraocular pressure (IOP; Figures 95-8 and 95-9).

Open-Angle Glaucoma

In many cases, the primary pathology is presumed to lie in the trabecular meshwork, the ring of porous tissue located in the anterior chamber angle through which aqueous humor drains from the eye. Impaired facility of aqueous outflow through the trabecular meshwork is generally idiopathic (so-called primary open-angle glaucoma). This condition is generally reported to increase in prevalence with increasing age, at least in most Western populations.[39] Loss of outflow facility may also arise from various insults to the trabecular meshwork, including trauma, uveitis, hemorrhage, and dispersion of intraocular pigment.

Visual impairment from open-angle glaucoma is generally insidious and chronic, with visual field damage occurring initially in the far periphery, where it is rarely noticeable except by formal testing. The ability to diagnose this condition in its early stages is imperfect. The actual risk of visual field loss in untreated individuals with modestly elevated IOP is only 1% to 2%/year[40]; conversely, histologic studies have shown that as many as 40% of the optic nerve fibers must be destroyed before any abnormality of the visual field is detectable by standard techniques.[41]

Initial treatment is usually medical. The goal of therapy is to lower the IOP with topical (or, rarely, systemic) medications to a level that is tolerated by the optic nerve, as demonstrated by arrest of the progressive visual field loss. Available medications include parasympathomimetic miotics (rarely used), anticholinesterase miotics (rarely used), sympathomimetics, β-adrenergic blockers, carbonic anhydrase inhibitors, and prostaglandin analogues. The potential side effects of the various topical and systemic pressure-lowering drugs are occasionally serious, particularly in older patients (see later, "Systemic Complications of Ophthalmic Medications").

If medical treatment is unsuccessful or poorly tolerated, the IOP may be further lowered by laser treatments to the trabecular meshwork or by so-called filtering surgery, which creates a fistula between the anterior chamber and subconjunctival space, allowing easier egress of aqueous humor. Complications of filtering surgery may include hypotony, choroidal effusion, and cataract. Supplementary medical treatment after filtering surgery may also be required. The optimal stage in the disease process for surgical intervention is unclear. Some authors have reported better long-term visual results with earlier surgery.[42] One large study has suggested that laser treatment to the trabecular meshwork may also be suitable as initial therapy.[43]

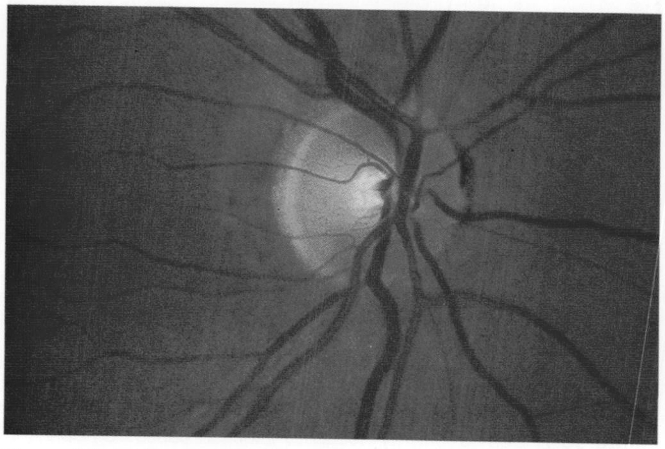

Figure 95-8. Normal optic nerve head. The cup-to-disc ratio is about 0.3.

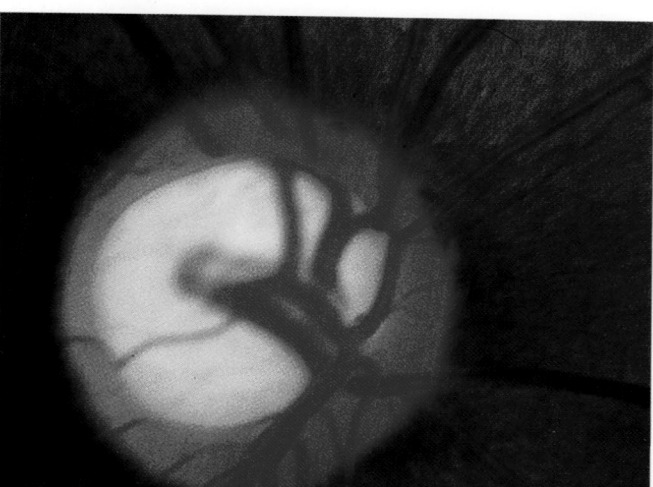

Figure 95-9. Glaucomatous optic nerve head cupping. Loss of neural tissue is seen as a narrowing of the neural rim of the optic disc and enlargement of the central cup. (Compare with Figure 95-8.)

Angle-Closure Glaucoma

Occasionally, alterations in the intraocular anatomy may predispose the iris to cover the trabecular meshwork, suddenly preventing aqueous outflow and causing an acute elevation of the IOP. Common scenarios include adhesions between the iris and lens (pupillary block), which may cause the iris to bow forward so as to occlude the trabecular meshwork, and dilation of the pupil, which may occur spontaneously in the dark or following pharmacologic mydriasis. Gradual enlargement of the lens with increasing age or cataract formation is an important factor that predisposes the eye to this process in older adults. Acute angle-closure glaucoma is generally a dramatic event, with symptoms that include severe pain, blurring of vision, perception of colored haloes around lights, nausea, and vomiting. Diagnosis of acute angle-closure glaucoma is easy once attention is directed to the eye, but may be missed if attention is diverted to the gastrointestinal symptoms. Cases have been reported from the emergency departments of general hospitals where concentration on the nausea and vomiting of a patient with acute angle-closure glaucoma actually led to exploratory laparotomy.

The massive elevation of IOP following acute angle-closure glaucoma (often to triple the normal upper limit of 21 mm Hg) may cause permanent optic nerve damage within a matter of weeks. Acute angle-closure glaucoma is initially treated by lowering the IOP with systemic and topical medications, including miotic eye drops and systemic osmotic agents. In cases of pupillary block, a small hole (peripheral iridotomy) is made in the iris by laser or invasive surgery to bypass the pupillary block and allow passage of aqueous humor from the posterior segment into the anterior chamber. This prevents subsequent angle-closure glaucoma attacks. Because the anatomic factors that predispose an eye to acute angle-closure glaucoma are generally found bilaterally, it is usually considered prudent to perform a peripheral iridotomy prophylactically in the fellow eye after an attack of angle closure. However, recent evidence suggests that cataract extraction may be the optimal means of controlling IOP in eyes with primary angle-closure glaucoma.[44]

Prolonged episodes of angle-closure glaucoma may result in permanent damage to the trabecular meshwork or even adhesions between the iris and sectors of the trabecular meshwork, leading to chronic angle-closure glaucoma. If the angle is sufficiently compromised, filtering surgery may be necessary.

Normal-Tension Glaucoma

Although an elevated IOP has historically been the hallmark of the diagnosis of glaucoma, it has become clear in recent decades that many patients with otherwise typical glaucomatous optic atrophy and visual field loss seldom, if ever, are found to have elevated IOP. Identification and treatment of this so-called low-tension glaucoma (more accurately termed *normal-tension glaucoma*) remains problematic although, even in this cohort, reduction of IOP is thought to convey some benefit. This entity is probably more common than previously thought—population-based surveys have demonstrated a substantial incidence of otherwise typical glaucomatous field loss in patients with normal IOP.[45]

CRYSTALLINE LENS

The crystalline lens of the eye is a unique ectodermal structure that develops entirely within the primordial lens vesicle. Only the cells on the extreme periphery of the lens divide, adding cells to the outer surface of the growing lens. Thus, the center of the adult lens represents the earliest tissue laid down during embryonic development. There is no mechanism whereby these cells can turn over, unlike the situation in typical ectodermal structures, such as the skin. The metabolism of the lens is largely confined to anaerobic glycolysis because neither hemoglobin-mediated oxygen transport nor cytochrome-mediated oxidative phosphorylation is available because of the need for transparency. The lens is at a further metabolic disadvantage because of the need to maintain a state of great disequilibrium with its surroundings—the lens must maintain the highest protein concentration and one of the lowest water concentrations of any tissue in the body. Thus, relatively modest metabolic insults or osmotic stresses may overwhelm the lens metabolism, resulting in protein denaturation and cataract formation.[21]

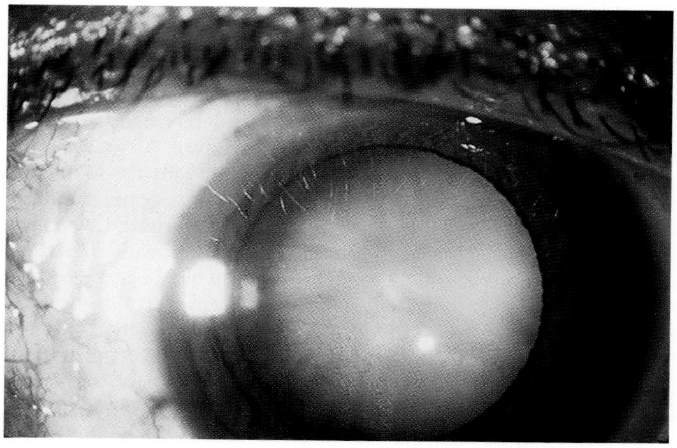

Figure 95-10. Cataract. Loss of transparency of the crystalline lens impairs visual acuity. *(Courtesy Dr. Calvin Roberts.)*

The lens of the eye continues to grow and mature throughout life. As the lens ages, it becomes more rigid and responds less effectively to changes in ciliary muscle tone, decreasing the effectiveness of accommodation, the eye's mechanism for focusing from distant to near objects. This loss of accommodation (presbyopia) is managed with reading glasses, bifocals, or other refractive strategies.

The lens responds to virtually any mechanical or metabolic insult by loss of optical clarity, resulting in the formation of a cataract (Figure 95-10). Several patterns of opacities are commonly encountered:

Oxidation (browning reactions) of lens proteins, particularly in the older, central portions of the lens, is termed *nuclear sclerosis*, which may result in alterations in the refractive index of the lens, as well as frank opacity. The most common refractive change is in the direction of an increase in myopia or decrease in hyperopia. In some cases, this refractive shift will allow the patient to read without reading glasses (so-called second sight). This improvement in visual performance is usually only temporary and often heralds the development of a more debilitating lens opacity. Refractive changes in the lens need not be uniform. Patients will occasionally report monocular diplopia from inhomogeneous refraction by distinct portions of the lens, resulting in two distinct images being formed on the retina. The notion that monocular diplopia is generally indicative of hysteria is incorrect.

Denaturation of lens proteins in a sector of adjacent cortical lens fibers results in wedge-shaped or cuneiform cortical opacities. These are often found in the far periphery of the lens but frequently spare the optical zone near the center.

Aberrant proliferation of lens fibers on the posterior lens capsule produces a posterior subcapsular cataract. This is often induced by topical or systemic corticosteroid treatment and is frequently seen in other disease states, such as retinitis pigmentosa.

Treatment of cataract is generally surgical. With rare exceptions, the lens proteins that constitute the opacity are irreversibly denatured, precluding medical treatment.[46] Surgical strategies for removal of the lens material have evolved greatly. In all cases, an incision must be made in the eyeball. A cataract cannot be removed—even with a laser—without an ocular incision. The simplest operation is to remove the entire lens intact within its lens capsule, a so-called intracapsular procedure. At present, the extracapsular procedure, in which the opaque lens tissue is carefully aspirated from within the lens capsule, has become standard, because retention of the capsule to serve as a barrier between the anterior and posterior segments of the eye appears to reduce the rate of complications. Greater emphasis has been placed on the development of minimally invasive surgical methods for cataract extraction. Often, the cataract can be liquefied by the mechanical action of a rapidly vibrating needle (phacoemulsification) and aspirated from the eye through an incision only 3 to 4 mm in length.[47] Frequently, such wounds can be constructed to be self-sealing, eliminating the need for sutures.[48] The femtosecond laser has been used to assist in some of the key steps in cataract surgery, including corneal incision, opening of the lens capsule, and fragmentation of the lens material.[49]

Indications for cataract surgery should be determined in relation to the visual needs of each individual patient. Occasionally, cataract extraction is recommended for technical reasons, such as those rare cases when the lens itself is causing injury to the eye (as in phacolytic glaucoma, when lens proteins leak from a cataractous lens and occlude the trabecular meshwork) or when a cataractous lens prevents adequate visualization or treatment of disease of the posterior segment of the eye, such as diabetic retinopathy. Otherwise, cataract surgery is appropriate whenever the anticipated improvement in visual function would be of benefit to the patient. In general, a visual result of 6/12 (20/40) or better may be anticipated in 90% to 95% of cases without other known concurrent ocular disease; thus, surgery is generally recommended only when the acuity has fallen to the level of 6/15 (20/50) or worse. In some patients, difficulties with glare, contrast sensitivity, diplopia, or specific occupational demands may justify cataract extraction, even with less severe loss of visual acuity.

Optical rehabilitation of the aphakic eye requires replacement of the focusing power of the cataractous lens that was removed. Where economic conditions permit, this is usually provided by means of a plastic intraocular lens prosthesis, which is generally implanted at the time of the primary cataract operation. Intraocular lenses were once thought to be an inaccessible expense and an option limited to those in developed nations. However, India is now tackling its burden of cataract blindness and is able to implant 90% of its cataract patients with intraocular lenses due to low-cost, indigenous lens manufacturing.[50] Recent intraocular lens designs can even restore a degree of accommodation, reducing the need for reading glasses or bifocals in many cases, and these so-called premium intraocular lenses have favorable outcomes for some patients.[51,52] Alternatives include contact lenses (often worn on an extended-wear basis) and thick aphakic spectacles, which subject the patient to substantial optical distortions and, if the aphakia is unilateral, may cause substantial difficulties because of unequal perceived image size in the two eyes. Indeed, the difficulties with spectacle correction of unilateral aphakia are sufficiently severe that if spectacle correction is the only modality of optical rehabilitation available, most surgeons recommend deferral of surgery until visual acuity in the better eye falls to 6/18 (20/60) or worse. In some developing countries, local custom may discourage the use of spectacles after cataract surgery. In these situations, the attitude and customs of the patient must be taken into account in the decision about whether to perform a cataract extraction.

Some yellowing of the lens proteins is nearly universal with aging. Sufficient opacity to impair visual acuity results in more than 3.5 million cataract extractions each year in the United States, the vast majority in individuals older than 65 years. In developing countries, the rate of cataract formation appears to be even higher, so that untreated cataract is typically the largest single cause of acquired blindness.[3] In India, as recently as 8 years ago, the rate of procedures each year was finally able to surpass the rate of new cataract formation in the general population.[50] This feat has been attributed to a number of factors, including low procedural costs and internal manufacturing of eye care goods.

Cataract formation may occasionally reflect an underlying metabolic abnormality, such as galactosemia or renal failure. Cataract onset is accelerated in diabetic patients and may be triggered by various drugs (particularly topical or systemic corticosteroids). In addition to these specific associations, several studies have shown a nonspecific excess mortality among cataract patients compared with age-matched control patients undergoing other elective surgical procedures.[53,54]

RETINA AND VITREOUS

Diseases of the retina, particularly diabetic retinopathy and so-called age-related macular degeneration (formerly referred to as *senile macular degeneration*) constitute the most frequent cause of acquired blindness, at least in developed countries.

Diabetic Retinopathy

Diabetic retinopathy shows a steady increase in incidence and severity with increasing duration of diabetes mellitus, with significant visual complications rarely occurring before 10 to 15 years after the onset of the disease.[55] Thus, although juvenile-onset (type 1) diabetic patients may develop severe retinopathy as early as the third decade of life, the retinal burden of adult-onset (type 2) patients is borne largely by older adults. The disease seems to attack primarily the retinal capillary circulation. Initially, small innocuous microaneurysms are noted ophthalmoscopically. With time, the retinal capillaries begin to leak fluid into the surrounding tissue, causing retinal edema and precipitation of exudates into the retina, with a concomitant reduction in visual acuity (Figure 95-11). At this stage of the disease, the preferred treatment is the intraocular injection of anti-VEGF medications, which block the effects of VEGF secreted by ischemic

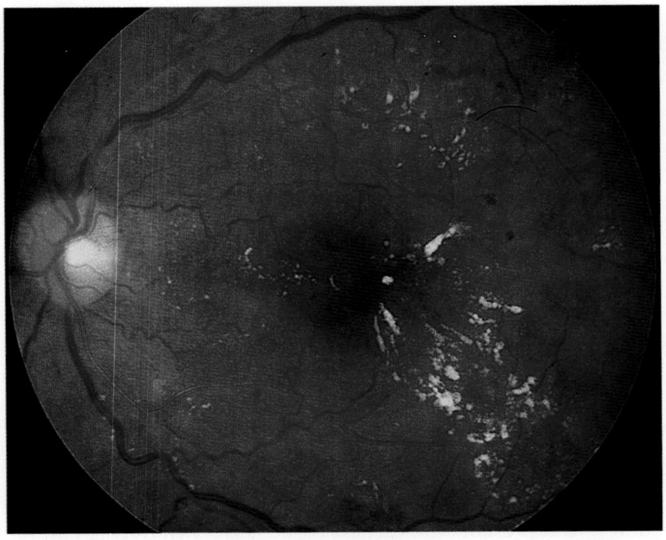

Figure 95-11. Background diabetic retinopathy. Microaneurysms (dot hemorrhages), intraretinal hemorrhages (blot hemorrhages), and hard exudates indicate deterioration of the retinal microcirculation.

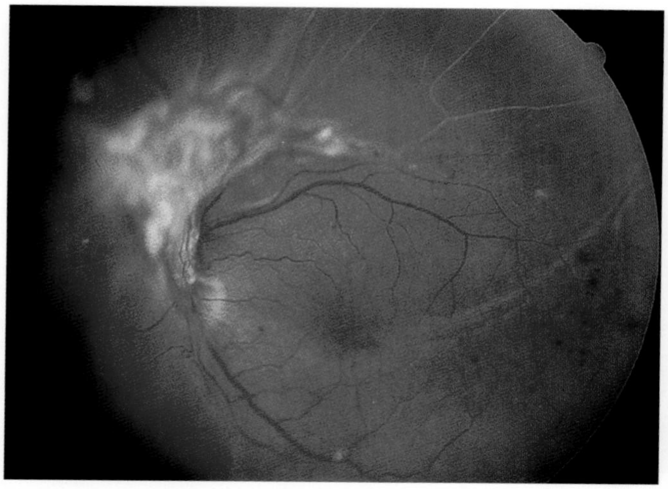

Figure 95-12. Proliferative diabetic retinopathy. A membrane of fibrovascular tissue has sprouted from the optic disc in response to prolonged retinal ischemia.

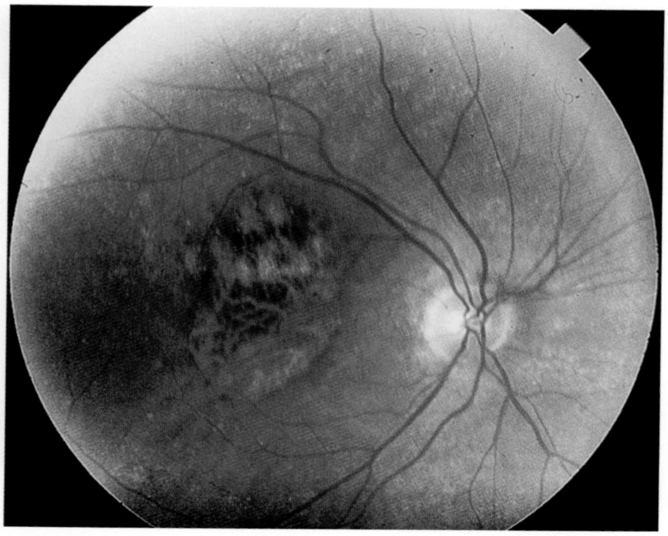

Figure 95-13. Atrophic (dry) age-related macular degeneration. Geographic atrophy of the retinal pigment epithelium causes loss of central vision.

retinal tissue.[56] Loss of visual acuity may be reduced through the use of laser treatments, either directed at leaking microaneurysms or, if the leakage is diffuse, placed in a grid pattern over the leaky sectors of the retinal capillary bed.[57] In contrast to anti-VEGF injections, which frequently result in recovery of visual acuity, laser treatment has been shown only to reduce the likelihood of future visual loss.

In later stages, perfusion of small regions of the retinal capillary bed fails (capillary dropout), leading to localized retinal infarctions, which may be seen ophthalmoscopically as cotton wool spots. The remaining capillaries are often seen to become dilated, irregular, and leaky. Ultimately, in many patients, the ischemic retina develops a neovascular proliferative response, sprouting new blood vessels that may grow along the retinal surface or along the posterior surface of the vitreous body. These aberrant blood vessels are prone to leaking and hemorrhages. Vision may also be lost through traction exerted on the retina by fibroblastic membranes that accompany the neovascular proliferation (Figure 95-12). In severe cases, the neovascular response may extend to the anterior segment, producing neovascularization on the surface of the iris (rubeosis iridis). If the fibrovascular membrane extends over the anterior chamber angle, it obstructs the filtration of aqueous humor through the trabecular meshwork, producing a refractory neovascular glaucoma.

Proliferative retinopathy may often be arrested through the ablation of a large fraction of the peripheral retina with laser photocoagulation.[58] In severe cases, blood in the vitreous cavity and fibrovascular membranes may be removed surgically by introducing mechanized suction cutter instruments through small scleral incisions over the ciliary body (pars plana vitrectomy). Intraocular injection of anti-VEGF medications is often very effective at suppressing neovascularization in the retina or the anterior segment, but the effects are not permanent,[59] and combined treatment with panretinal photocoagulation and/or vitrectomy is often necessary.

The benefit of tight control of the blood glucose level in the management of diabetic retinopathy depends on the stage of the disease. Many attempts to retard the progression of established retinopathy by improving the degree of glucose control have been disappointing.[60] In some studies, tight control has been associated with a worsening of retinopathy. Similarly, in one study, successful pancreatic transplantation, with near-perfect normalization of blood glucose levels, failed to improve diabetic retinopathy compared to the retinal disease in fellow pancreatic transplant patients whose allografts failed, requiring resumption of daily insulin injections, with the usual deficiencies in control of blood glucose levels.[61] However, it has been demonstrated in types 1 and 2 patients that better glucose control in recent-onset diabetic patients helps retard the onset of diabetic retinal disease.[62,63]

Age-Related Macular Degeneration

Age-related macular degeneration is a common cause of impaired vision, although not of total blindness, in older adults. In the atrophic form, the retinal pigment epithelium and choriocapillaris underlying the macula appear to degenerate, resulting in dysfunction of the overlying photoreceptors (Figure 95-13). There is no known treatment. In the exudative form, a neovascular net emanates under the macular region of the central retina from the choroidal circulation, proliferating between the retina and underlying retinal pigment epithelium or underneath the pigment epithelium.[64] Leakage of plasma components and frank subretinal hemorrhage or scarring cause loss of vision (Figure 95-14).

Treatment of exudative macular degeneration has been revolutionized with the introduction of injectable drugs directed against the tissue factor, VEGF, which is elaborated by ischemic retina, stimulating increased vascular permeability and the sprouting and growth of new retinal blood vessels from adjacent vascular beds.[65] The anti-VEGF drugs currently in widespread use (ranibizumab [Lucentis], bevacizumab [Avastin], and aflibercept [Eylea]) appear to be equally effective, preventing visual loss in up to 90% of patients and inducing improvement in visual acuity in up to 40% of cases (Figure 95-15).[66,67] Bevacizumab, which is used for this purpose on an off-label basis, can be dispensed and injected at considerable savings compared with the other drugs.

These anti-VEGF treatments are demanding of the patient and physician. The drugs are administered under sterile conditions—iodophor skin preparation, sterile drape and lid speculum, sterile gloves—by injection into the vitreous compartment of the eye through the sclera and pars plana of the ciliary body. After injection, the eye must be checked for elevation of the IOP. Injections must be repeated every 4 to 8 weeks, potentially indefinitely. Alternatively, patients can be treated on an as-needed basis, but regular monthly eye examinations are still required. Each eye

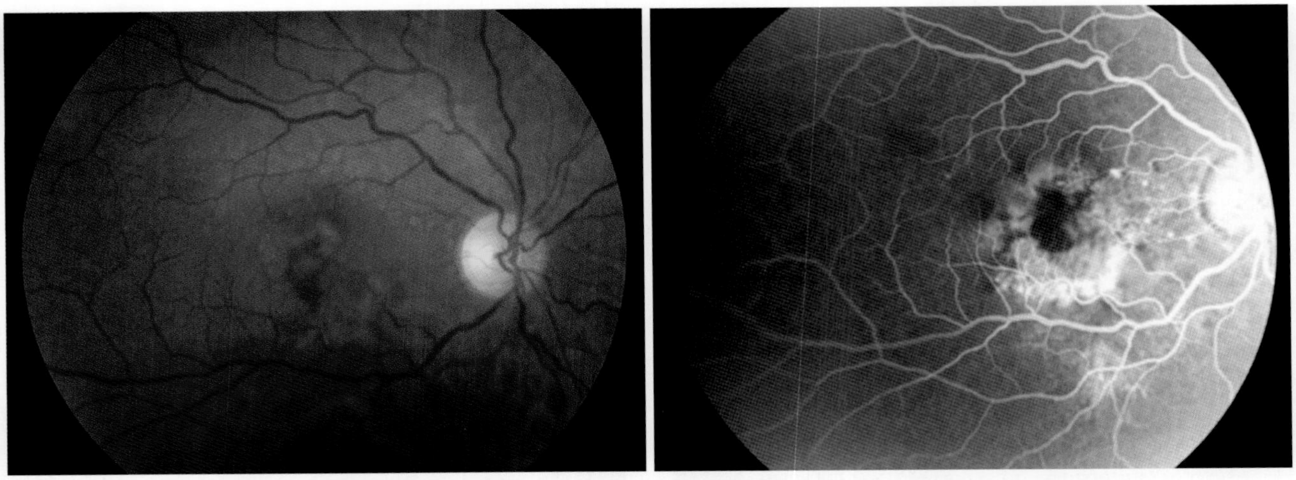

Figure 95-14. Exudative (wet) age-related macular degeneration. Leakage and scarring from a subretinal neovascular membrane impairs central retinal function. Note the subretinal hemorrhage in the color photograph *(left)*, confirmed in silhouette in the fluorescein angiogram *(right)*.

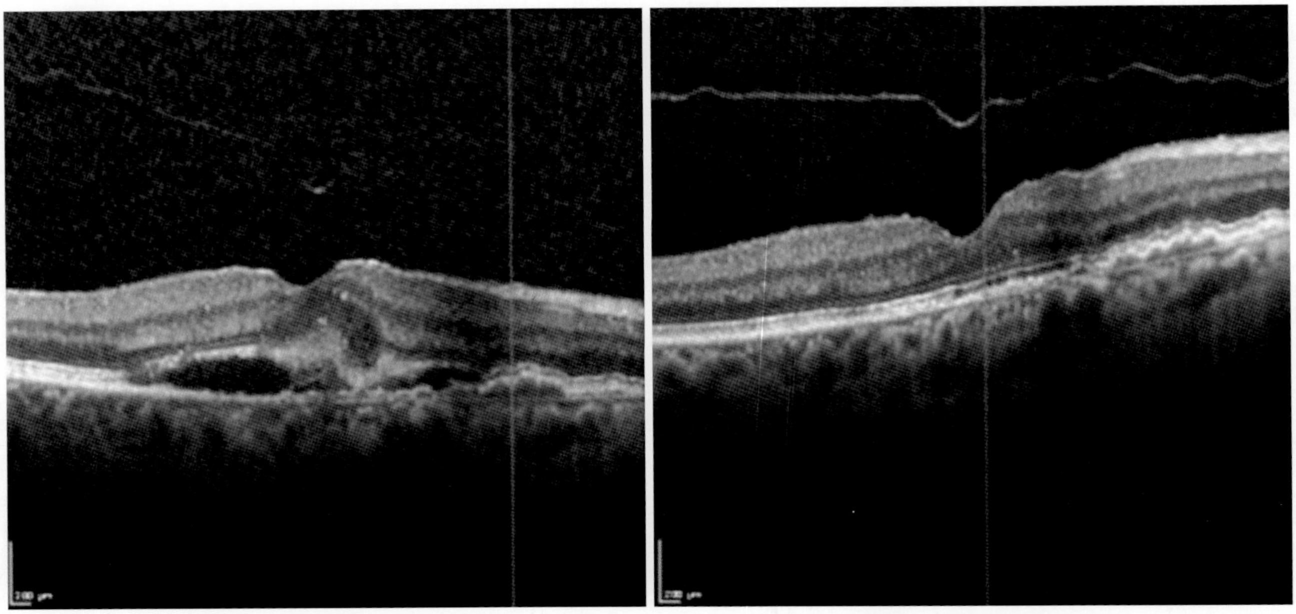

Figure 95-15. Treatment of wet age-related macular degeneration in a 68-year-old man with intravitreal bevacizumab injections, demonstrated by spectral-mode optical coherence tomography (OCT) cross-sectional images through the foveal center (same eye as shown in Figure 95-14). Note subretinal fluid and shallowing of foveal depression prior to treatment *(left)*. After two intravitreal bevacizumab injections *(right)*, subretinal fluid has resolved, and normal foveal contour is restored. Visual acuity improved from 20/60 to 20/20.

must be treated separately. Complications are rare, with an infection rate below 1 per 1000 injections in competent hands and rare incidents of cataract and retinal detachment.

Where available, anti-VEGF treatment has largely supplanted thermal laser and photodynamic therapy and corticosteroid medication for the treatment of exudative macular degeneration.

It should be emphasized that these various modalities of treatment for age-related macular degeneration have significant limitations. Anti-VEGF agents may be very expensive and require frequent injection—in principle, indefinitely. Many patients fail to recover visual acuity. Few patients with advanced visual loss are restored to normal or near-normal visual function.

In the atrophic and exudative types of macular degeneration, the pathologic process appears to be confined to the posterior pole. These diseases thus spare the peripheral retina in nearly all cases, so that most affected patients retain sufficient vision indefinitely for independent ambulation and may be reassured that they are not going to go completely blind.

Pale white dots, known as drusen, frequently seen in the retinas of older patients, are usually benign. They correspond to small deposits of amorphous hyaline material seen histologically between the Bruch membrane and retinal pigment epithelium. However, these lesions appear to serve as a predisposing factor in the evolution of exudative macular degeneration.[68] Older patients with drusen or who have lost vision in one eye because of age-related macular degeneration may be advised to check their vision every day by examination of an Amsler grid, a 10-cm square of ruled graph paper. Any abnormality or distortion of the central vision should prompt immediate examination of the retina. This will maximize the chance that a subretinal neovascular net will be discovered before it undermines the fovea, when treatment is most effective.

Studies have suggested that nutrition may play a role in the development of macular degeneration. In one large prospective randomized study, patients at risk for age-related macular degeneration were randomized to dietary supplementation with a combination of antioxidant vitamins (C, E, β-carotene, and zinc) or to placebo. Treated patients at high risk for exudative macular degeneration, as indicated by the presence of large or confluent drusen, extensive geographic atrophy, or advanced macular degeneration in the fellow eye, experienced a 27% reduction in risk compared with controls.[69] There was no benefit to patients at lesser risk. The antioxidant plus zinc regimen was also of no value in preventing the development of cataracts. A follow-up study has shown that the carotenoids lutein and zeaxanthin may be substituted for the β-carotene in the vitamin cocktail. This has been considered contraindicated in smokers for whom it entails an increased risk of lung cancer, but found no benefit from adding omega-3 fatty acids.[70]

Retinovascular Occlusive Disease

The retinal arteries and retinal veins are subject to sudden occlusive events, particularly in older adults. Retinal artery occlusions are usually embolic or arteritic in nature. Embolic occlusions are due to the occlusion of a retinal artery by a small particle derived from the more proximal circulation, usually a cholesterol fragment from an ulcerated atherosclerotic plaque. A small refractile cholesterol crystal may often be visualized within a retinal artery (Hollenhorst plaque). Acutely, the affected sector of the retina appears pale and cloudy. Various measures to encourage migration of the occlusive plaque toward the retinal periphery have been recommended, including lowering of the IOP by medical means, withdrawal of a small amount of fluid from the anterior chamber with a fine needle, or dilation of the retinal arterial tree by having the patient breathe an elevated concentration of carbon dioxide. However, no convincing benefit of these maneuvers has been demonstrated.[71]

Transient obscurations of vision, typically lasting less than 10 minutes (amaurosis fugax), are generally believed to represent embolic arterial occlusions that are quickly dislodged into the far retinal periphery.[72] These attacks indicate an elevated risk of occlusive stroke.[73]

Arteritic disease (e.g., temporal arteritis) may also cause occlusion of the arteries of the retina or optic nerve head. An elevated erythrocyte sedimentation rate is commonly, but not invariably, observed. The diagnosis is usually confirmed by temporal artery biopsy. Prompt treatment with systemic corticosteroids is indicated and may prevent visual loss in the fellow eye.[74] If the diagnosis of temporal arteritis is suspected, most authorities recommend immediate initiation of systemic corticosteroid treatment; it is unwise to wait until the erythrocyte sedimentation rate and the results of a temporal artery biopsy can be obtained because the fellow eye may lose vision in the interim. If the tests are negative, the steroid treatment can usually be stopped promptly, without a period of tapering doses.

Retinal vein occlusions result in a pattern of vascular tortuosity and intraretinal hemorrhage in the affected sector of the retina. Most retinal vein occlusions seem to be due to compression of a retinal vein by an adjacent retinal artery, frequently exacerbated by hypertension, arteriosclerosis, or glaucoma. Although there is no treatment for the occlusion itself, retinal vein occlusion carries a significant risk of subsequent neovascular complications, particularly glaucoma. In those in whom retinal ischemia can be demonstrated, typically by fluorescein angiography or electroretinography, retinal ablation by laser photocoagulation can substantially reduce the risk of subsequent neovascularization.[75] Treatment by injection of anti-VEGF agents is very effective at reducing retinal edema, with frequent recovery of visual acuity.[76] In some cases, after recanalization of the occluded vein, anti-VEGF injections may be discontinued.

OPTIC NERVE

Older adults are particularly susceptible to ischemic injury to the optic nerve. Infarctions of the entire optic nerve head cause sudden obscuration of vision in one eye and present ophthalmoscopically with optic nerve head swelling and hemorrhages. Many patients present with infarction of only a portion of the optic nerve head, resulting in the sudden onset of a monocular visual field defect. As with retinal artery occlusions, it is important to distinguish between arteritic and nonarteritic occlusions,[77] because only the former respond well to systemic corticosteroids.

Ischemic optic neuropathy is also occasionally seen in the period following otherwise uncomplicated cataract extraction. Visual recovery is rare, and the benefit of corticosteroids in this setting is unproved.[78]

The term *papilledema* is reserved in ophthalmic usage for optic disc swelling as a result of increased intracranial pressure. In these patients, visual acuity is rarely impaired, at least initially; the only visual field abnormality is typically an enlarged blind spot. In chronic papilledema, optic atrophy may ensue, with progressive visual impairment. Treatment is directed at the underlying intracranial cause of the increased pressure. In occasional cases of idiopathic intracranial pressure elevation (pseudotumor cerebri), medical treatment with carbonic anhydrase inhibitors or surgical decompression of the central nervous system (CNS) via a shunt or fenestration of the optic nerve sheath may be of value.[79] Other causes of optic disc swelling that must be distinguished from papilledema include ischemic optic neuropathy, malignant hypertension, and severe uveitis.

OCULOMOTOR NERVES AND POSTERIOR VISUAL PATHWAYS

The oculomotor nerves and posterior visual pathways are targets in older adults for ischemic injury and for compressive injuries caused by intracranial mass lesions, typically tumors or aneurysms, and shifts of the intracranial contents. Sudden loss of function of a single isolated cranial nerve is common. An isolated trochlear or abducens nerve palsy in a patient otherwise susceptible to atherosclerotic disease is usually a benign event, and spontaneous recovery is frequently seen.[80] Ischemic insults to the oculomotor nerve typically spare the pupillary fibers.[81] In older patients at risk for ischemic disease, an atraumatic pupil-sparing (but otherwise complete) third nerve palsy may be attributed to an ischemic event and the patient monitored for recovery over the next several weeks. However, if extraocular motor function is only incompletely impaired (e.g., if the patient presents with normal levator function), or if the pupil is involved, the risk of compression of the nerve by aneurysm or tumor is sufficient that CNS imaging is recommended.[82] Patients with multiple cranial nerve deficits or in whom pupillary dilation has occurred require a thorough neurologic evaluation, preferably including CT or MRI, if available. The differential diagnosis can be broadly defined as including infectious, neoplastic, autoimmune, traumatic, and vascular causes. Given that neoplasms account for 25% of cases, a prompt workup to determine the underlying diagnosis should be undertaken.[83]

Abnormalities of the visual field should be thoroughly investigated. Scotomas that affect only one eye or that respect the horizontal meridian are generally the result of injury to the retina, optic disc, or optic nerve or to glaucoma. Injuries at or posterior to the level of the optic chiasm will impair vision in both eyes. Of particular importance are bitemporal hemianopsias, which suggest compression of the optic chiasm, typically by a pituitary tumor, and highly congruous homonymous field defects, which suggest an injury of the occipital cerebral cortex.

ORBIT

Tumors of the orbit generally present with horizontal, vertical, or anterior displacement of the globe (proptosis). In older adults, the most frequently diagnosed entities include orbital pseudotumor (idiopathic inflammation of one or more orbital tissues, typically the extraocular muscles, lacrimal gland, or infiltration of the orbital fat), hemangiomas, and lymphangiomas, lymphomas, and primary tumors of the lacrimal gland. Management frequently requires orbital exploration for histopathologic diagnosis as well as for anatomic correction.[84]

Thyroid ophthalmopathy (Graves disease) is a well-known orbital problem. The impairment of ocular motility, lid retraction, and exophthalmos are largely due to infiltration of the extraocular muscles. The orbital fat is rarely, if ever, involved.[85] Progression of the orbital disease is poorly correlated with the actual thyroid hormone levels, and restoration of the euthyroid state, although desirable for many reasons, is not particularly effective as a tool in the management of the ocular complications. Early cases respond well to systemic corticosteroids, but the benefits are often only temporary. In long-standing cases, patients should be monitored closely for signs of optic nerve compression and be promptly offered surgical decompression, generally achieved by fracturing the orbital bones to provide more room for the swollen orbital contents, if the optic nerve is at risk.[86]

FURTHER CONSIDERATIONS

Ophthalmic Complications

Systemic Diseases

The vision of older patients is at risk, not only from primary ocular diseases, but also from the effects of systemic diseases. In addition to the effects of diabetes mellitus and thyroid disease mentioned earlier, a few of the more prominent disease entities with serious ophthalmic sequelae include hematologic disorders (e.g., leukemia, polycythemia), rheumatic diseases (e.g., rheumatoid arthritis, ankylosing spondylitis, systemic lupus erythematosus), Marfan syndrome, and renal failure. Treatment is usually directed at the primary disease process, but topical or systemic corticosteroids or other immunomodulators may be needed to control ocular inflammation.

In addition to the local mechanical effects of metastasis to the eye or orbit, systemic malignancy may also exert a deleterious remote effect on retinal function, greatly impairing vision.[87,88] Paraneoplastic syndromes can affect vision and result from an immune response that is directed against shared antigens on both the tumor and normal tissue. Chemotherapy directed at the primary malignancy has occasionally led to visual improvement. The role of immunomodulatory therapy remains unclear, however, although some favorable results have been reported.

Systemic Medications

Many older patients receive several concurrent medications, some of which may frequently cause ocular symptoms. A few of the more common problems are described here.[89]

Tricyclic antidepressants have a mild parasympatholytic action, which may cause mydriasis and paralysis of accommodation. Major tranquilizers, such as chlorpromazine, may also cause mydriasis and interfere with accommodation and may cause a pigmentary retinopathy. Significant visual impairment has generally been reported only with protracted chronic use. Chloroquine may also cause a bull's-eye maculopathy, with impairment of central vision, particularly after prolonged use with a total dosage exceeding 100 g of the chloroquine base. Hydroxychloroquine appears to be less retinotoxic than chloroquine, but the risk of retinal toxicity increases with cumulative dosage and prolonged use, especially beyond 1000 g or 10 years.[90]

Systemic corticosteroids may precipitate an open-angle glaucoma, which frequently does not abate until several weeks after cessation of the drug, as well as accelerate the formation of cataracts. Digitalis derivatives may produce various visual disturbances in addition to the classic yellow vision (xanthopsia). Ethambutol is also reported to produce dyschromatopsia, as well as optic atrophy and visual field defects. Anti-impotence drugs such as sildenafil may cross-react slightly with the retinal isoform of phosphodiesterase and cause transient perception of a bluish haze or increased light sensitivity.[91]

Precipitation of an acute angle-closure attack by the mydriatic action of systemic medications is extremely rare.

Molecularly targeted agents are increasingly being used in oncology and, because many of the targets are expressed in ocular tissues, some agents are associated with ophthalmic toxicities. These include surface abnormalities (e.g., dryness, inflammation of the eyelid, aberrant eyelashes) from epithelial growth factor receptor (EGFR) inhibitors and subretinal fluid (akin to central serous chorioretinopathy) from MEK inhibitors, which affect the mitogen-activated protein kinase (MAPK) pathway.[92,93]

Ophthalmic Medications. Because the dosages of topical eye medications are generally much smaller than the dosages used for systemic treatment, systemic complications from the use of eye drops are rare. However, these drugs are rapidly absorbed across the conjunctiva and nasal mucous membranes and occasionally cause systemic complications. Also, it is also sometimes necessary to treat localized eye disease with systemic medications, which may cause further systemic problems.[89]

The topical anticholinergics used as mydriatics or cycloplegics may occasionally cause the full spectrum of systemic atropinic toxicity. Of the drugs in common use, cyclopentolate appears to cause these problems most frequently. Conversely, the parasympathomimetics, such as pilocarpine and carbachol, and the anticholinesterases, such as echothiophate, may cause side effects such as abdominal cramps, diarrhea, and nausea.

Topical adrenergic agents, such as phenylephrine (Neo-Synephrine), may cause tachycardia, hypertension, and even frank arrhythmias. Conversely, topical β-blockers, such as timolol maleate, may cause the full spectrum of side effects of β-blockade, including bradycardia, asthma, and hypotension. The use of cardioselective β-blockers, such as betaxolol, has not completely eliminated these problems.

The topical use of chloramphenicol has resulted in a few reported cases of aplastic anemia, generally after prolonged treatment. There have also been rare reports of Stevens-Johnson syndrome following topical administration of sulfa antibiotics. Otherwise, there have been few reports of serious systemic toxicity from topical antibiotics other than local ocular hypersensitivity reactions.

Mannitol and glycerin are administered as osmotic agents to lower IOP in those with acute glaucoma. The fluid shifts that result may also cause congestive heart failure, renal shutdown, and altered mentation. Patients undergoing repeated treatments should be closely monitored for electrolyte imbalances and signs of renal decompensation.

Systemic carbonic anhydrase inhibitors, such as acetazolamide and methazolamide, are occasionally used to treat glaucoma. These are difficult drugs for many patients, frequently causing anorexia, depression, impotence, and paresthesias, in addition to such rare complications as bone marrow depression, gout, and acidosis. Carbonic anhydrase inhibitors are now available in topical formulations, which have largely eliminated many of these complications. Patients whose quality of life is intolerable on these medications should be offered medical or surgical alternatives.

Low-Vision Rehabilitation

The rehabilitation of individuals who have sustained an irremediable loss of vision is an important component of effective medical care, particularly among older adults. In the United States, more than two thirds of individuals with acuity less than 6/18 are older than 65 years. Conversely, of individuals older than 65 years, 7.8% are reported to have acuity worse than 6/18, a fraction that increases to 25% among individuals older than 85 years. Loss of vision has been ranked as the third most common chronic condition, after arthritis and heart disease, for which individuals older than 70 YEARS require assistance with the activities of daily living (ADLs).[94]

Low-vision rehabilitation attempts to allow vision-impaired individuals to make the most effective use of whatever vision they retain to facilitate their ADLs, prolong independence, and enhance self-confidence. Successful rehabilitation frequently requires the coordinated efforts of a team of care providers, including the ophthalmologist, optometrist, and occupational therapist, as well as the assistance and understanding of the patient's family, friends, and caregivers. Rehabilitation is generally most successful if it begins as soon as permanent visual disability has been diagnosed. Critical to the functional outcome is acceptance by the patient of the need to adopt compensatory visual strategies to cope with the loss of vision, rather than to continue vain attempts to reverse the visual loss.

Rehabilitation programs should center on the needs of the patient. A thorough functional history should be obtained. Emphasis should include the patient's perceptions of the impact of the visual disability on accustomed activities and on goals for the future. Every attempt should be made to identify specific tasks that the patient's visual limitations have curtailed and whose recovery would be particularly valued. Typical problems include inability to read, mend, or pay bills; loss of independent mobility; and difficulty with distance vision, such as watching television or reading signs.

The severity of the visual deficit should be determined, including measurements of visual acuity, visual fields, and contrast sensitivity. It is often helpful to be more specific in identifying the level of visual acuity than is usual in general ophthalmic practice. Placement of eye charts as close as 1 yard (≈1 m) may be used to expand the range of acuity testing. It is frequently essential to allow a substantially greater amount of time than usual for visual assessment in low-vision patients, especially older adults.

Rehabilitation may then proceed.[95] A comprehensive program frequently entails the dispensing and instruction in the use of optical aids (e.g., spectacles, telescopes, magnifiers) and nonoptical aids (e.g., improved lighting, large-print reading materials, high-contrast guides for reading and writing, closed-circuit television magnifiers). Training in the use of residual vision, such as eccentric viewing for individuals who have lost central macular function, may be attempted but may require many hours of practice over many months to obtain optimal performance. Training in adaptations for ADLs and the introduction of suitable equipment, such as needle threaders or large-print playing cards, can help the individual recapture self-confidence and facilitate independence. Professional counseling, often in a group setting, can play an important role in helping patients deal with the emotional impact of their visual disability.

It is important that the patient adopt reasonable goals for low-vision rehabilitation. In nearly every case, it is impossible to recover the level enjoyed before the loss of visual function. Each patient must individually decide whether the results achieved are worth the extra effort that will remain necessary to perform most visual tasks. The best results are achieved when specific tasks are targeted.

KEY POINTS: TREATMENTS FOR MAJOR CAUSES OF BLINDNESS

CATARACT

- Surgical extraction, ideally with intraocular lens implant

GLAUCOMA

- Initial—lower intraocular pressure with topical, systemic medications
- Additional options—laser treatment to trabecular meshwork; filtering surgery

DIABETIC RETINOPATHY

- Tight control prevents or delays retinopathy in early stages
- Intravitreal injection of anti-VEGF drugs, focal or grid laser treatment for macular edema
- Panretinal laser treatment or anti-VEGF injections for proliferative retinopathy
- Pars plana vitrectomy for persistent vitreous hemorrhage or traction retinal detachment

MACULAR DEGENERATION

- Atrophic (dry)—no treatment available
- Exudative (wet)
  - Intravitreal injection of anti-VEGF agents
  - Photodynamic therapy
  - Thermal laser ablation of neovascular membranes
  - Dietary supplementation with antioxidant vitamins and zinc may reduce risk of progression from dry to wet macular degeneration.

For a complete list of references, please visit www.expertconsult.com.

KEY REFERENCES

1. Pascolini D, Mariotti SP: Global estimates of visual impairment: 2010. Br J Ophthalmol 96:614–618, 2012.
6. Dev MK, Paudel N, Joshi ND, et al: Psycho-social impact of visual impairment on health-related quality of life among nursing home residents. BMC Health Serv Res 14:345, 2014.
11. Mohs FE: Micrographic surgery for the microscopically controlled excision of eyelid cancers. Arch Ophthalmol 104:901–909, 1986.
18. Griewank KG, Westekemper H, Murali R, et al: Conjunctival melanomas harbor BRAF and NRAS mutations and copy number changes similar to cutaneous and mucosal melanomas. Clin Cancer Res 19:3143–3152, 2013.
24. Hanet M-S, Jamart J, Chaves AP: Fluoroquinolones or fortified antibiotics for treating bacterial keratitis: systematic review and meta-analysis of comparative studies. Can J Ophthalmol 47:493–499, 2012.
25. Jabs DA, Akpek EK: Immunosuppression for posterior uveitis. Retina 25:1–18, 2005.
30. Diener-West M, Earle JD, Fine SL, et al: The COMS randomized trial of iodine 125 brachytherapy for choroidal melanoma, III: initial mortality findings. COMS Report No. 18. Arch Ophthalmol 119:969–982, 2001.
32. Harbour JW: A prognostic test to predict the risk of metastasis in uveal melanoma based on a 15-gene expression profile. Methods Mol Biol 1102:427–440, 2014.
40. Gordon MO, Beiser JA, Brandt JD, et al: The Ocular Hypertension Treatment Study: baseline factors that predict the onset of primary open-angle glaucoma. Arch Ophthalmol 120:714–720, 2002.

42. Jay JL, Murray SB: Early trabeculectomy versus conventional management in primary open angle glaucoma. Br J Ophthalmol 72:881–889, 1988.
47. Kelman CD: Phaco-emulsification and aspiration of senile cataracts: a comparative study with intra-capsular extraction. Can J Ophthalmol 8:24–32, 1973.
50. Aravind S, Haripriya A, Sumara Taranum BS: Cataract surgery and intraocular lens manufacturing in India. Curr Opin Ophthalmol 19:60–65, 2008.
54. Xu L, Cui TT, Wang YX, et al: Cataract and mortality. The Beijing eye study. Graefes Arch Clin Exp Ophthalmol 246:615–617, 2008.
56. Rajendram R, Fraser-Bell S, Kaines A, et al: A 2-year prospective randomized controlled trial of intravitreal bevacizumab or laser therapy (BOLT) in the management of diabetic macular edema: 24-month data: report 3. Arch Ophthalmol 130:972–979, 2012.
58. The Diabetic Retinopathy Study Research Group: Indications for photocoagulation treatment of diabetic retinopathy: Diabetic Retinopathy Study Report no. 14. Int Ophthalmol Clin 27:239–253, 1987.
59. Osaadon P, Fagan XJ, Lifshitz T, et al: A review of anti-VEGF agents for proliferative diabetic retinopathy. Eye (Lond) 28:510–520, 2014.
66. CATT Research Group, Martin DF, Maguire MG, et al: Ranibizumab and bevacizumab for neovascular age-related macular degeneration. N Engl J Med 364:1897–1908, 2011.
70. Aronow ME, Chew EY: Age-related Eye Disease Study 2: perspectives, recommendations, and unanswered questions. Curr Opin Ophthalmol 25:186–190, 2014.
71. Augsburger JJ, Magargal LE: Visual prognosis following treatment of acute central retinal artery obstruction. Br J Ophthalmol 64:913–917, 1980.
73. Poole CJ, Ross Russell RW: Mortality and stroke after amaurosis fugax. J Neurol Neurosurg Psychiatry 48:902–905, 1985.
78. Hayreh SS: Anterior ischemic optic neuropathy. IV. Occurrence after cataract extraction. Arch Ophthalmol 98:1410–1416, 1980.
80. Rush JA, Younge BR: Paralysis of cranial nerves III, IV, and VI. Cause and prognosis in 1,000 cases. Arch Ophthalmol 99:76–79, 1981.
90. Melles RB, Marmor MF: The risk of toxic retinopathy in patients on long-term hydroxychloroquine therapy. JAMA Ophthalmol 132:1453–1460, 2014.
93. Liu CY, Francis JH, Brodie SE, et al: Retinal toxicities of cancer therapy drugs: biologics, small molecule inhibitors, and chemotherapies. Retina 34:1261–1280, 2014.
94. Eaglestein A, Rapaport S: Prediction of low vision aid usage. J Vis Impair Blindness 85:31–33, 1991.

96 Disorders of Hearing

Barbara Weinstein

A guiding principle for the care of older adults is the delivery of person-centered care (PCC), with patient preferences elicited and incorporated into medical decision making. A cornerstone of PCC is communication wherein individuals can make themselves understood and understand what others are saying. When older adults are unable to communicate because of untreated or unrecognized hearing loss (HL), the health consequences are dramatic, especially among those with multimorbidity. Ironically, HL is considered a little recognized consequence of aging, despite the physical, psychosocial, and cognitive correlates of this unavoidable aspect of aging. With Americans living longer and functional status and remaining life expectancy emerging as important prognostic indicators, an understanding of HL and its prevalence, cause, consequences, and treatment are crucial to optimization of therapies and care planning.

Life expectancies at ages 65 and 85 years have increased dramatically, bringing with it an increase in the amount of time spent in all major activities, including work and retirement. Older adults are spending an increasing proportion of their life in retirement, so the ability to communicate effectively takes on even greater importance with these retirement and work force trends. As people age, the likelihood of experiencing one or more chronic conditions increases. Over 50% of older adults have three or more chronic diseases, typically referred to as multimorbidity. Coincident with increases in life expectancy, the number of older adults with multimorbidity has been increasing dramatically. Communicating with the patient about clinical management options within the context of risks, burdens, benefits, time horizon to benefit, import of adherence, and prognosis (e.g., functional status, quality of life) is key to the delivery of quality care.

Considered a geriatric syndrome, age-related hearing loss (ARHL) is a major public health problem and a contributor to the global burden of disease.[1] Hearing impairment is one physical disability that is increasing in prevalence in society in general and in older adults in particular. Globally, adult-onset HL is the second leading cause of years living with disability (YLD) behind depression and is a larger nonfatal burden than alcohol use, osteoarthritis, and schizophrenia.[2] Over the last generation, the HL population has grown at a rate 1.6 times that of U.S. population growth, with 36 million Americans self-reporting hearing impairment. By the year 2030, at least 21 million Americans older than 65 years are projected to have a hearing impairment. HL prevalence ranges from 30% to 47% among persons older than 65 years, doubling with each age decade, so that nearly two thirds of persons 70 years of age and older and 80% of persons older than 85 years having a HL that affects their communication ability.[3] The risk of experiencing a HL increases dramatically with each additional decade, with rates of decline more accelerated for the oldest old cohort and with 50% having at least a moderate HL.[1] Mean hearing levels of persons 95 years of age and older are consistent with moderately severe to profound HL, significantly poorer than the cohort between 80 and 94 years. The high prevalence and severity of hearing impairment among the oldest old has will affect transitions in care, palliative care, and home care.

Hearing impairment, increasing age, and male gender are the most relevant risk factors for tinnitus, with 11% of adults suffering from ARHL experiencing permanent and persistent tinnitus.[4,5] Because the inner ear subserves the sense of hearing and balance, age and high-frequency HL are risk factors for vestibular dysfunction, which is highly prevalent among older adults. Prevalence ranges from 69% among 70- to 79-year-olds to 85% among those older than 80 years.[6] The sensation of dizziness is highly prevalent among people older than 65 years, accounting for 8 million primary care physician visits in the United States. Among those 70 years of age and older, high-frequency HL is associated with reduced saccular function, with age and noise exposure significantly associated with cochlear and saccular dysfunction.[7] Older adults with chronic dizziness or imbalance are two to three times more likely to fall in comparison with older adults who do not experience these problems. Finally, population-based studies of persons older than 50 years have revealed a prevalence of between 5% to 10% of persons with objectively measured concurrent hearing and visual problems; this is termed *dual sensory impairment* (DSI).[8] DSI increases in prevalence with age, so that the oldest old are at greatest risk for DSI, with woman having a slightly greater prevalence than men. The likelihood of comorbid and secondary conditions is greater in persons with DSI than in those with a hearing or vision problem.[9] DSI is associated with mortality, especially among older adults with concurrent moderate to severe HL and any presenting or best-corrected vision loss.[10]

MODIFIABLE AND NONMODIFIABLE RISK FACTORS FOR HEARING LOSS

ARHL is a multifactorial condition with a number of modifiable and nonmodifiable risk factors.[11] Nonmodifiable factors include increasing age, genetic predisposition, race (decreased risk in African Americans), and gender (males, increased risk).[11] Modifiable risk factors include environmental exposure (e.g., noise, ototoxicity), smoking, and multiple health comorbidities, including cerebrovascular disease, cardiovascular disease (CVD), and diabetes. Cognitive decline increases the risk for hearing impairment, and kidney disease, metabolic conditions such as lupus, thyroid dysfunction, and head trauma are also medical conditions associated with HL. Alcohol consumption in moderation appears to be a buffer against developing HL. When present in older adults with chronic conditions ranging from CVD to diabetes and falls, HL is likely to increase the burden of these problems. Data from the Health ABC Study, a population-based prospective cohort study, has revealed that history of smoking is associated with poorer high-frequency hearing levels in men.[12] Similarly, data from the NHANES cross-sectional survey has confirmed that heavy smoking increases the odds of HL nearly twofold.[13] Exposure to loud noise accelerates age-related HL, and noise exposure and history of CVD appear to have a synergistic effect, elevating hearing threshold levels.[13]

CVD risk factors, including higher levels of triglycerides and poorer resting heart rate, are related to poorer hearing.[12] This association is likely linked to the fact that an insufficient cochlear blood supply can disrupt the chemical balance of the fluids within the inner ear, influencing the activity of the hair cells and activation of the auditory nerve.[12] Similarly, a history of diabetes mellitus is linked to poorer hearing sensitivity, most likely due to the effect on the cochlear vascular system, with a prevalence higher among persons with diabetes as compared to those without.[13,14]

Adverse drug reactions (ADRs) in the form of auditory or vestibular symptoms are prevalent and severe among older adults.

ADRs occur for a variety of reasons, including lack of compliance due to compromised understanding of the prescription. This could be attributable to hearing or visual problems or possibly because of confusion between two medications that might sound alike (e.g., Plavix or Paxil) to a hearing-impaired person or may look alike to a visually impaired older adult. Some of the auditory or vestibular side effects of medications include dizziness, ear discomfort, lightheadedness, vertigo, bilateral HL that is often profound and delayed in onset, and tinnitus. The severity and time of onset of is dose-dependent and typically rapid in onset, occurring soon after the drug is administered. Although symptoms may appear months after the medication has been administered, the effects often progress for several months after cessation of the medication, especially in the case of chemotherapeutic agents. Older adults with HL prior to chemotherapy with cisplatin are more likely to experience a threshold shift following administration of the drug, and close monitoring and counseling are recommended. Otoprotective medications should be considered as well. When aminoglycoside antibiotics are administered with loop diuretics, the ototoxic effect is synergistic and powerful. Symptoms of ototoxicity include development or intensification of tinnitus in one or both ears, appearance of a new sound in the ear different from already existing tinnitus, fullness or pressure in the ears (i.e., different from that caused by infection), progression of an already existing HL, and development of a spinning sensation aggravated by motion, which might be accompanied by nausea. Ototoxic medications include but are not limited to the following: aminoglycoside antibiotics, chemotherapeutic agents, including cyclophosphamide, carboplatin, cisplatin, loop diuretics, and aspirin or salicylate-containing medications.

Cognitive impairment increases the risk for HL, and HL increases the risk of developing cognitive impairment.[1] Predictors of rate of change in hearing levels over an 11-year time frame include baseline age, gender, and probable cognitive impairment. Probable cognitive impairment (Mini Mental State Examination [MMSE] score ≤ 23) at baseline is associated with faster rates of change in hearing levels and poorer initial hearing levels at baseline.[1] Greater rates of change in hearing levels take place in persons with clinically diagnosed hypertension at baseline. The incidence of cognitive impairment is also associated with poorer hearing levels.[1] HL is independently associated with all-cause dementia, and the risk of all-cause dementia increases linearly with HL severity.[15] The mechanisms for the observed association have not yet been determined, but researchers have speculated about a possible common neuropathologic process or via the pathway of reduced social network size, diminished quality interpersonal relations, and social isolation, which is linked to hearing impairment.

THE AGING AUDITORY MECHANISM

The auditory system is an integrated system involving an interplay among its many components, including the outer, middle, and inner ears (peripheral auditory system) and the brain (central auditory system).[16] An impoverished output from the peripheral auditory system due in part to age-related changes affects the integrity of the input to the central auditory system and ultimately the communication challenges associated with ARHL. The lack of uniformity in pathologic and physiologic changes across individuals may help explain e individual differences in speech understanding in a challenging acoustic environment, which is the hallmark of ARHL.

Age-related changes in the outer and middle ears have few implications for communication ability. Increased activity of cerumen glands in the cartilaginous portion, physical obstruction due to a hearing aid, frequent use of cotton-tipped swabs, or production of drier and less viscous cerumen contribute to the excessive accumulation of wax to which older adults are susceptible. One of the most common reasons for physician visits is accumulation of cerumen because of failure of the self-cleaning mechanism. Accumulation of excessive cerumen (cerumen impaction) is present in approximately one third of older adults, with estimates ranging from 19% to 65%. It is more common in older adults, nursing home residents, and persons with cognitive impairment. The primary sequela of impacted cerumen is HL, which typically produces noticeable improvements in hearing and understanding following treatment. Curettage and irrigation are the two approaches to removing cerumen in primary care, and each is associated with risks and benefits. In diabetics or immunocompromised patients, for example, management can pose problems for primary care physicians.

The middle ear is susceptible to minor age-related changes that have little impact on hearing, whereas the site of conversion of mechanical energy to an electrophysiologic signal, the inner ear, is composed of several functional components vulnerable to the effects of aging. The organ of Corti is the structure most susceptible to age-related changes that ultimately interfere with the transduction process integral to the reception of sound. Historically ARHL has been classified into three types—sensory, neuronal, or metabolic.[11]

The primary histopathologic changes in the organ of Corti include loss of hair cells beginning in the extreme basal end, greatest in persons older than 70 years and most pronounced for outer hair cells (OHCs). It is now well accepted that changes in OHCs are due in large part to noise trauma rather than age. The resulting HL is primarily for high-frequency sounds (e.g., *s*, *sh*, *th*), which are processed in the basal end of the cochlea. Neuronal pathology tends to manifest as loss of spiral ganglion neurons and is diffuse, involving all three turns of the cochlea and resulting in considerable difficulty understanding speech. The deleterious effects of aging are typically first seen in highly metabolic tissues in the body, and the most prominent feature of age-related HL of the metabolic variety is atrophy of the stria vascularis, an area very high in metabolic activity.[17] The most common feature of ARHL in the periphery is degeneration of the stria vascularis. Loss of function of the cells in the stria vascularis and/or spiral ligament appears to result in disruption of inner ear ion homeostasis, thereby causing a decline in endocochlear potential (EP).[11] When strial degeneration exceeds 50%, EP values drop rather substantially.[18]

A hallmark of ARHL is neuronal loss in the periphery, which may begin at any age. The neuronal changes which tend to impact processing of speech sounds include the following: (1) disrupted neural synchrony, which is associated with reduced amplitude of the action potential; (2) decreased neural inhibition; (3) longer neural recovery time; (4) a decrease in the number of neurons in the auditory nuclei; (5) changes in synapses between inner hair cells and the auditory nerve; and (6) age-related changes in the level of inhibitory neurotransmitters.[19,20] The overall loss of neurons and loss of acoustic nerve activity interfere with temporal resolving abilities, which contributes in large part to the auditory processing and speech understanding problems experienced by many older adults.[21] Impoverished auditory signals and reduced stimulation from the impaired cochlea disrupt the tonotopic organization throughout the central auditory system, including the cochlear nucleus, inferior colliculus, and midbrain, precipitating changes in cortical reorganization and brain morphometry.[22] Specifically, decreased acoustic input associated with age-related changes in the auditory periphery is associated with a selective downregulation of normal adult inhibitory γ-aminobutyric acid (GABA)–ergic function in the inferior colliculus (IC). Decreased acoustic input from the auditory periphery is associated with significant changes in GABA neurotransmission in the normal adult IC. Central auditory reorganization due to plasticity does take place, so that intact regions of the tonotopic map adjacent to the impaired regions tend to become responsive, confirming an auditory reorganization.

Age-related changes also take place in the temporal lobe of the aging brain. Recent neuuroimaging studies have demonstrated an independent association of hearing impairment with reduced cortical volumes in the auditory cortex, as well as accelerated rates of atrophy in the lateral temporal lobe and whole brain.[22,23] Regarding the latter, magnetic resonance imaging (MRI) studies have revealed that persons with hearing impairment have significantly more shrinkage (i.e., specific volume declines) in the structures responsible for processing speech information—namely, the superior, middle and inferior temporal gyri.[22] The temporal region of the auditory cortex is involved in processing spoken language and is integral to linguistic, cognitive, and speech processing in challenging situations, such as semantic memory and sensory integration.[23]

BEHAVIORAL IMPLICATIONS OF ANATOMIC AND PHYSIOLOGIC CHANGES

The classic complaint of older adults with ARHL—"I can hear people talking but cannot understand what they are saying, especially in noisy situations"—aptly describes the problems resulting from the reduction in transmission, reception, and perception of the speech signal attributable to sensorineural HL. ARHL (presbycusis) is sensorineural, characterized by a loss of acuity and loss of clarity (distortions). The attenuation or loss of audibility for low- and high-frequency sounds interferes with the detection of warning signals and with speech understanding. The distortion component of sensorineural HL is associated with reductions in spectral and frequency resolution, which further compromise speech understanding. Specifically, older adults have difficulty comprehending the following: (1) speech in quiet and noisy situations; (2) speech when the rate of speaking is fast; (3) accented speech; (4) speech spoken from a distance; and (5) when multiple talkers are speaking. Characteristics of the speaker's voice, complexity of the message, listener's knowledge of the language, use of gestures, and availability of contextual information also influence speech understanding. Speech understanding is compromised when presented without the benefit of contextual information, when multiple speakers are talking, and when the speaker is not nearby. Communicating in challenging situations demands the expenditure of mental effort. making it an effortful and fatiguing process.[24] Cognitive processing (e.g., working memory, speed of information processing, divided attention), which also declines with age, is crucial to the functions of listening and comprehending, further compromising communication ability.[24] Finally, the advantages of binaural listening, including directional hearing, are reduced in older listeners, potentially compromising their safety. Brain plasticity enables compensation when older adults can use knowledge and context to advantage during listening. Although many aspects of cognitive processing that are important to speech understanding decline with age, knowledge and use of context are well preserved and can enhance recall, comprehension, and communication.

Consequences of Age-Related Hearing Impairment

The behavioral implications of hearing and speech understanding difficulties that characterize older adults are considerable. The myth that HL is harmless has been debunked, and it is becoming increasingly clear that when untreated, HL can be costly to the individual and family members. The unique features of ARHL can be summarized using the four Is, as shown in Figure 96-1. Considered an invisible handicap, ARHL is (1) insidious, developing gradually so that the individual does not notice or admit to HL until 7 to 10 years after it typically begins to set in; as the HL progressively worsens, the individual's personality, behaviors, and outlook toward life may change; (2) interfering, notably with communication and performance of many of the instrumental and routine activities of daily living; (3) impacting on self-esteem, sociability, and quality of life, if left untreated; and (4) invisible, so people adapt by using avoidance behaviors that enable them to get by in many situations.

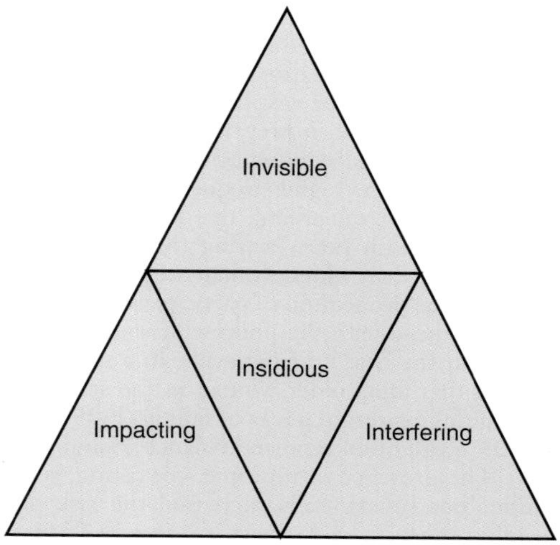

Figure 96-1. The four "I's" of hearing loss.

Given the insidious and invisible nature of ARHL, it is not surprising that its consequences interfere with many facets of daily life, posing a threat to healthy and active aging. The incidence of depressive symptoms is higher among persons self-reporting a hearing handicap as compared to those without, and self-reported hearing handicap is an independent predictor of depressive symptoms.[25,26] Furthermore, the prevalence of moderate to severe depression (Patient Health Questionnaire [PHQ-9] score = 10) is dose-dependent, with 4.9% of individuals reporting excellent hearing, 7.1% good hearing, and 11.4% reporting a little trouble, or greater HL.[27] HL and a self-reported hearing handicap are associated with perceived social isolation for those with moderately severe to severe HL, and a person with a significant self-reported hearing handicap is at greatest risk for being subjectively and objectively socially isolated.

HL may be mechanistically associated with cognitive decline through social isolation.[28] HL is independently associated with accelerated cognitive decline and incident cognitive impairment in community-dwelling older adults. Individuals having HL were found to have a 30% to 40% accelerated rate of cognitive decline and a 24% increased risk for incident cognitive impairment over a 6-year time period as compared with individuals having normal hearing.[28] Compared to individuals with normal hearing, individuals with a mild, moderate, or severe hearing impairment, respectively, have a twofold, threefold, or fivefold increased risk of incident all-cause dementia over more than 10 years of follow-up.[29]

Additionally, increased severity of HL is associated with impaired activities of daily living (ADLs) and instrumental ADLs; those with moderate to severe HL have higher odds of having difficulty with ADLs as compared to those without HL.[26] Older adults with HL have increased use of community support and informal support networks. Use patterns are related to HL severity, with those with moderate to severe HL at the greatest risk of developing reliance on community support systems.[30] The link between HL and independence is highlighted by the fact that persons with baseline HL were found to have a higher likelihood of relying on support systems than those with normal hearing at 5-year follow-up.[30] The prevalence of falls increases with age and is highest among those in poor health, those with two or more functional limitations, and those with HL, visual loss, and depression.[31] Persons with hip fractures have a higher prevalence of hearing impairment, followed by vision impairments and dual sensory impairment.[32] The latter findings are not surprising, given the fact that age-related vestibular abnormalities appear to be bilateral and to increase in prevalence with advancing age.[33] There is a decline in saccular function with age, which has been correlated with HL in the higher frequencies.[7] The more severe the high-frequency HL, the greater the decline in saccular function. Older women with poor hearing threshold levels had an higher risk for falls than older woman with essentially normal hearing acuity.[34] The proportion of participants with two or more falls was 30% in those with the poorest hearing levels and 17% in the group with the best hearing levels. In a subsequent study, it was reported that most older woman in the sample reporting walking difficulties expressed a fear of falling (FOF), and persons reporting FOF more often reported balance, vision, and hearing difficulties.[35] The presence of multiple, coexisting, self-reported sensory difficulties substantially increased the risk of mobility decline, leading the authors to speculate that FOF may serve as an exacerbating behavioral factor, increasing mobility decline in persons with sensory impairments.

Anatomically, the link between HL, mobility limitations, and falls makes sense because the hearing and vestibular organs share fluid-filled bony compartments and blood circulation and have similar mechanosensory receptor hair cells, which detect sound, head movements, and orientation in space.[34] An additional explanation may be related to cognitive load. Older adults with impaired hearing must allocate a greater proportion of their attention to maintaining their balance during daily activities, including walking and talking. Impaired hearing may "place additional demands on attention sharing and thus further increase fall risk." [34] Among persons 60 years of age and older, ambulation and hearing were predictive of mortality.[35] Disability in hearing showed a stepwise and strong impact on mortality, and disability in ambulation was associated with a stepwise increase in mortality. There exists a link between hearing impairment and mortality risk which was mediated by falls, poor self-rated health, and poor cognitive status (MMSE score ≤ 24).[36] Compared with participants having normal hearing, those with HL at baseline were more likely to be male, older, cognitively impaired, diabetic, and underweight and more likely to have a self-reported history of angina, myocardial infarction, stroke, low self-rated health, and observed difficulty in walking or use of walking aids. Using a structural equation modeling (SEM) pathway analysis to model the relationship over a period of 5 years between hearing impairment, mortality, and covariables, a significant association emerged between hearing impairment and mortality after adjusting for confounders such as age and gender. There was no gradient effect from the severity of HL and mortality risk.

Another possible explanation for the link among falls, mobility restrictions, and HL is that FOF or a history of falls may decrease participation in various activities, which in turn may accelerate the disablement process, thereby increasing risk of falling.[34] There is a connection between self-reported and objectively measured physical activity levels and HL.[37] Participants with moderate HL or greater had a greater odds of reduced self-reported physical activity and less accelerometer-measured activity than individuals with normal hearing. Reduced physical activity levels is one of the criteria that characterizes frailty or low physiologic reserve and vulnerability to stressors.[38] Unintentional weight loss, slow walking speed, weakness and exhaustion are also classic signs of frailty. Using data on individuals 70 years of age and older, the 1999 to 2002 cycle of the National Health and Nutrition Examination Survey (NHANES) self-reported HL was independently associated with frailty in women.[39] Because frailty is associated with hospitalization, it is of interest that HL is also associated with burden of disease and odds of hospitalization, health care use, and health care expenditures. The literature linking mortality risk, mobility limitations, reduced physical activity levels, and HL underscores the need to screen the hearing of patients at risk for falls or those having a history of falls; perhaps treating hearing impairment via one of the interventions along the continuum can be effective in reducing mortality risk.[32,36]

HL is independently associated with increased burden of disease, poorer self-reported health, history of CVD, and increased rates of hospitalization and health care use.[40,41] Longitudinal studies have demonstrated that the physical composite score and mean scores for seven of the eight SF-36 domains were significantly lower at the 10-year follow-up among participants with self-reported hearing handicap at baseline. Furthermore, the greater the degree of HL, the higher the likelihood of experiencing functional disability, with those with moderate to severe HL at greatest risk. This finding is not surprising because communication is integral to performing routine instrumental ADL tasks, such as talking on the telephone and shopping. The presence of distracters is in part responsible for the latter associations. Similarly, driving performance **is** affected by HL, especially in the presence of visual and auditory distractions.[42] Older drivers with moderate to severe hearing impairment demonstrate worse driving performance in the presence of distracters as compared to those with normal to mild hearing impairment. Hence, the use of GPS systems, speaking on the telephone, conversing with other passengers, or listening to the radio could create in-car distractions, which may diminish driving performance. This finding is consistent with the so-called effortfulness hypothesis, which holds that the extra effort associated with listening to and understanding a degraded auditory signal consistent with ARHL takes resources from other cognitive processes. Because the typical HL characterizing the oldest old tends to be moderate to severe, these individuals are at greatest risk for many of the negative consequences of HL (Box 96-1). Based on a data set of over 600,000 Australians, it appears that at each stage of advancing HL and resultant disability, there was a change in health status.[43] Notably, at the point of severe and profound self-reported hearing disability, the decline in health status is most pronounced. When asked to rate the disability that caused the most disability, respondents rated HL as the third most problematic condition after chronic pain and restrictions in physical activity.

Finally, declines in vision and hearing are associated with decreased quality of life, increased physical disability, falls, hip fractures, and increased mortality risk. Persons reporting hearing and visual impairments report lower rates of excellent health and higher rates of poor health.[9] Interestingly, having a dual sensory impairment had higher rates of comorbid conditions than those

BOX 96-1 Negative Consequences of Hearing Loss: Difficulty Understanding Words and the Meaning of Everyday Language

- Accelerated cognitive decline
- Depression
- Incident cognitive impairment
- Higher rates of comorbid conditions
- Increased mortality risk, burden of illness, functional disability, health care expenditures, and social isolation
- Increased reliance on community and family support
- Increased risk of institutionalization, falls, hospitalization, and motor vehicle accidents
- Poorer health-related quality of life and self-rated health
- Reduced functional independence and physical activity levels (self-reported and objectively measured)
- Self-reported hearing handicap
- Slower gait speed

with a visual or hearing impairment. As compared to older adults without vision impairment and HL, persons with vision and hearing problems were more likely to have additional chronic conditions, including hypertension and heart disease. Regarding activity limitations and participation restrictions, older adults with dual sensory impairment were more likely to report difficulty walking and to experience falls and hip fractures. In light of the threat to social engagement, focusing on strategies to promote participation in community activities is essential for those with sensory impairment(s). With most older adults choosing to age in place, there will be an increase in older adults with significant HL who are homebound and receiving palliative care and who will have an increased need to communicate with health care professionals, caregivers, and family members. Finally, it is important to note that limited social activity and lack of physical activity are considered risks or threats to brain health and, given their link to untreated hearing impairment, the contribution of hearing to brain health is an area of great importance.

MANAGEMENT STRATEGIES

Gains in communication function are associated with timely and appropriately administered audiologic rehabilitation (AR), including the use of sound amplification systems. Sound amplification systems can be considered as a social technology, and AR can be considered as an intervention that promotes health relationships among support patients and providers. AR is a person-centered management process designed to reduce activity limitations, decrease participation restrictions, promote communication efficiency, improve quality of life, and improve the quality of interpersonal interactions. Using a person-centered approach, audiologists strive to collaborate with the patient and caregiver to develop a solution designed to overcome challenges posed by hearing impairment. AR is a highly variable process with several components, including the following: (1) sensory management to optimize auditory function using a continuum of devices ranging from personal sound amplifiers (PSAPs) to hearing aids, assistive listening devices, or implantable devices; (2) instruction in the use of technology and control of the listening environment; (3) perceptual training to improve speech perception and communication; and (4) counseling designed to increase participation in activities and promote the use of communication strategies and realistic expectations and that addresses emotional and practical limitations. Cost-utility analyses have confirmed that the most favorable outcomes are achieved when hearing aids are dispensed in the context of a comprehensive rehabilitation program. Furthermore, of the various approaches to AR, group programs that focus on counseling, communication strategy training, and computer-assisted techniques to enhance perceptual learning are of proven cost-utility and effectiveness.[44] There is reasonably good evidence that hearing-related quality of life improves when adults participate in counseling-based group AR programs.

Of the components of AR, sensory management, or the provision of some form of amplification ranging from a hearing enhancement device to a hearing aid and hearing assistive technology (HAT) to medical technologies, such as a cochlear implant (CI) or bone-anchored hearing aid, is the treatment of choice. Despite advances in hearing aid technologies, most older adults with HL do not use hearing aids. Given the negative health outcomes associated with moderate to severe HL and the variety of available interventions, older adults should be encouraged to purchase hearing aids and AR services before HL becomes an intolerable burden and less responsive to intervention. Stakeholders must also understand that the length of time needed to achieve a clinically meaningful reduction in negative health outcomes associated with hearing aid use (e.g., reduction in depression, social isolation, improved quality of life) is relatively brief (6 weeks to 3 months) and, with CIs, is about 6 months.

Because hearing problems are diverse, there is no "one size fits all" solution, and communication accessibility must be fostered via a universal design of the environment conducive to communication and through technologies that can improve audibility of the signal relative to background noise. Technologic interventions, which address four sets of receptive communication needs, including face to face interactions in quiet and noisy settings, media, telecommunication, and alerting devices for home office and public places, fall along a continuum consistent with the severity of HL and communication challenges,

Sensory Management to Optimize Auditory Function: Hearing Aids and Implants

Hearing Aids

Hearing aids improve the audibility of the sounds of speech in a wide range of settings while also preserving comfort and sound quality for persons with HL. They do not restore hearing to normal but do reduce speech understanding difficulties, especially in a noisy setting, in a large and reverberant room, and they make communication less effortful for the person with HL and his or her communication partners. Hearing aids are available in many shapes and sizes. The introduction of miniature behind the ear hearing aids has led to their resurgence as the style of choice, given their small size and features including comfortable fit, better sound quality, feedback reduction, directionality, noise reduction, less occlusion of the ear, and elimination of the need for a custom ear mold. Directional and remote microphone technology and the ability to control the hearing aid using smartphone software are innovations that have affected functionality and end user experience. Inclusion of a telecoil switch on the hearing aid or CI expands options for their use in public settings equipped with induction loop systems. Using a telecoil and hearing loop together is seamless, cost-effective, and unobtrusive, in that it obviates the need for persons with HL to seek out and obtain special equipment to facilitate their understanding.

Despite technologic advances, prevalence of hearing aid use is consistently low among persons with HL, yet penetration does increase with age and HL severity. Drivers of hearing aid use include difficulty understanding friends and relatives, when someone speaks in a whisper, watching television, self-perception of the handicapping effects of HL, readiness, and self-efficacy. Stigma and financial considerations are deterrents to hearing aid use. Third-party reimbursement for hearing aids is limited, with the exception of veterans, who are all eligible for hearing aids through the Veterans Administration; they recognize that veterans must be able to hear and understand their physicians so they can "participate and be partners in their care."

Although most older adults with mild to severe sensorineural HL are candidates for hearing aids, the U.S. Food and Drug Administration (FDA) lists a number of conditions for the sale of hearing aids and mandates a medical evaluation prior to purchase. The conditions that are considered red flag signs and symptoms, which preclude hearing aid fitting and require immediate referral to a physician, include the following: (1) visible congenital or traumatic deformity of the ear; (2) history of active drainage from the ear within the previous 90 days; (3) history of sudden or rapidly progressive HL within the previous 90 days (according to clinical practice guidelines, sudden HL is typically idiopathic at presentation and is defined as a rapid onset, occurring over a 72-hour period, of a subjective sensation of hearing impairment in one or both ears; a presenting symptom is a stuffed ear); (4) acute or chronic dizziness; (5) unilateral HL of sudden or recent onset within the previous 90 days; (6) audiometric air-bone gap equal to or greater than 15-dB HL at 500, 1000, and 2000 Hz; and (7) visible evidence of significant cerumen accumulation or a foreign body in the ear canal.

A body of evidence has begun to accumulate demonstrating that gains in communication function using hearing aids are associated with improved social and emotional function, reduced depressive symptoms and social isolation, and improved quality of life and cognitive ability. They are considered to be a relatively cost-effective strategy to rehabilitate hearing-impaired older adults.[45] According to one report, the greatest mean functional improvements after 3 months of hearing aid use include the following: (1) feeling less frustrated when talking to the family; (2) experiencing fewer difficulties in hearing the television and radio; (3) having less difficulty understanding at a party; (4) having fewer difficulties while visiting family and friends; and (5) not feeling as left out in a group.[46] Significant others (SOs) have also reported fewer communication challenges with their family member or spouse following hearing aid use. Notably, the SOs felt less frustrated because the volume of the television was significantly reduced, reported less difficulty when communicating in noisy settings, and reported feeling more relaxed because of improved ease of communicating. Persons with more significant HL demonstrated the greatest improvements with hearing aids, as did those wearing the units more hours each day. Persons using hearing aids have reported better health-related quality of life (HRQL) than those not using hearing aids.[43] Notably, however, hearing aid users still reported poorer HRQL as compared to that of the general population, underscoring the burden of HL.

In light of the connection between loneliness, subjective social isolation, and HL, we explored whether hearing aid use could serve as a buffer against feelings of loneliness.[47] Participants had predominantly mild to severe sensorineural HL, normal cognitive function, and large social networks. A subset of the population considered to be among the oldest old (mean age, 87 years) had moderately severe HL, typical of that age cohort. Social and emotional loneliness were measured using the De Jong Gierveld Loneliness Scale. Results were dramatic in that prior to hearing aid use, 60% of participants were not lonely, whereas 40% were lonely. Following hearing aid use, 80% of participants were not lonely, and 20% were reportedly lonely. The changes in categorization of loneliness were statistically significant. Also, hearing aid use was associated with a statistically and clinically significant improvement in loneliness scores. Among the oldest old, a similar pattern emerged in that the proportion of hearing aid users considered to be lonely decreased. Thus, the evidence is clear that the impact of HL on communication function can be mitigated through the use of hearing aids in older adults with mild to moderately severe HL. Gains in communication function are also associated with reversal of depressive symptoms and subjective social isolation.[48]

Cochlear Implants

More than 300,000 older adults suffer from severe to profound HL and, for these individuals, CIs may be a more viable and sustainable option than hearing aids. Surgically implanted devices, CIs consist of an internally placed receiver-stimulator connected to an electrode array coiled within the cochlea of the inner ear, which delivers the unique electrical representation of each speech sound to the auditory nerve. Age and duration of deafness have a negligible effect on postsurgical outcomes among persons 65 years and older. CIs improve the user's access to verbal communication and environmental sounds, enhance telephone communication and enjoyment of music, increase confidence and participation in social activities, improve self-reported communication performance and HRQL, and provide significant gains in HRQL (e.g., cost-utility estimate of $9,530/quality-adjusted life-year in older adults using CIs).[49] CIs narrow the functional gap between older adults with profound HL and older adults with less severe HL who were using hearing aids in that for older deaf adults, scores on physical, psychological, and social evaluations were closer to scores enjoyed by hearing aid users with less severe loss.[50] The positive outcomes associated with CI use in combination with the numerous negative health outcomes associated with severe to profound HL and poor speech understanding underscore the importance of earlier intervention with CI once hearing aids no longer prove to be beneficial. Earlier intervention with a CI may help forestall the downstream effects of HL.[49] It is important to note that a recent indication for CI is single-sided deafness accompanied by severe tinnitus. Long-term results have shown that implantation provides durable tinnitus relief in these patients.

Bone-Anchored Hearing Aids

Older adults with single-sided deafness (unilateral severe to profound HL) may benefit from a surgically implanted, contralateral, bone-anchored hearing aid (BAHA), wherein sound is delivered into the skull via sound vibration. The sound vibrations transfer sound from the bad ear side to the good ear side through the skull. The BAHA can be used in persons with conductive HL, particularly those with chronically discharging ears, or in persons with complete or near-complete single-sided deafness (SSD) or deafness in one ear. Persons with SSD may be quite handicapped because of difficulty localizing sound and understanding speech in noisy environments, especially when the speaker is on the side of the bad ear. Wireless CROS hearing aids, which do not require surgical intervention, provide significant benefits to persons with SSD. Before proceeding with the surgical procedure, individuals can try the BAHA to gain a feel for the experience of hearing via bone conduction and might consider the wireless CROS hearing aid because anecdotal reports have suggested that the benefits are impressive.

Middle Ear Implants

Middle ear implants (MEIs) are a relatively new class of technology available for partial restoration of hearing for those with moderate to severe sensorineural HL. Unlike cochlear implants, the success of an MEI rests on the health of the cochlea; the amplified vibratory signal is delivered to the inner ear via a normally functioning middle ear structure. They are similar to CIs in that the internal processor is surgically attached to the skull behind the ear, and an external processor delivers sound to the internal processor.

Hearing Assistance Technologies

Hearing aids are ideal in small group and quiet situations, but many users continue to have difficulty understanding in noisy situations and in reverberant environments. Their disadvantage lies in the fact that in many listening situations, the hearing aid microphone, which is worn at the listener's ear, is typically some distance from the sound source, making speech difficult to understand. Designed to be used as a complement to or in lieu of hearing aids or CIs, HAT enhances or helps maintain the functional communication capacities of the hearing-impaired by enhancing the level of the signal relative to the noise. By making the signal louder, HAT is akin to binoculars for the ears. In essence, placing a microphone close to the talker's mouth catches the desired speech before it travels across the room, loses energy, and becomes degraded by noise and reverberation, preserving the intensity level and clarity of the speech. HAT improves the reception of face to face, small- and large-group communication, enhances reception of media, and facilitates understanding of telecommunication devices. HAT is effective in a variety of settings, including home, work, private practice, theater, and hospital. In addition to setting specific uses, HAT can be classified according to portability; it can be personal or private, portable versus stationary, or hard-wired rather than wireless.[51] Alerting devices inform persons of warning signals, including the sound of the doorbell, telephone, smoke alarm, or alarm clock. Collectively, these devices rely on auditory, visual, or tactile information to help the user monitor environmental sounds. Added value of HATs include their simplicity, low cost, and commercial availability.

Hearing Aids, Hearing Assistance Technology, and Counseling-Based Audiologic Rehabilitation Leading to Improved Function

Following device selection, goal setting, communication training, device-related and personal adjustment, positive disconfirmation counseling, perceptual and listening retraining, and familiarity with effective communication strategies will help debunk many of the myths surrounding hearing aid use and provide realistic expectations critical to success. To ensure maximal benefit, older adults must have realistic expectations, patience, and the understanding that hearing aids are not very smart in that they do not automatically do a good job of helping the user to discriminate between the sounds the person wants to hear (i.e., speech) and those the person wants to ignore (i.e., background noise). New hearing aid users should not expect suddenly to hear normally. Users must understand that it takes time to realize the potential benefit from hearing aids, and thus they should not become discouraged early. Their ears and brains must become reeducated to hear selected patterns of sounds that have been made louder by the hearing aid. In a sense, new hearing aid users are suddenly being exposed to or bombarded with a world of sounds that they forgot existed, such as the blare of street noises in the city, and they must become reoriented to or acquainted with the location and source of these “new” sounds.

If patients complain that some intense sounds produce an uncomfortably loud hearing sensation, they should alert the dispensing audiologist at the follow-up visit because a simple adjustment can usually be made. Many hearing aid users report that although at first they prefer natural-sounding louder sounds as their ears and mind adjust, they tend to prefer a boost in the high-frequency response of the hearing aid that makes the consonants of speech crisper and easier to understand. It is of utmost importance that new hearing aid users schedule and keep all follow-up appointments (a minimum of 2 to 4 weeks following receipt of the hearing aid) so that the audiologist can make the necessary adjustments to ensure that sounds are comfortable, audible, tolerable, and understandable. At these visits, the audiologist and new hearing aid user work together to modify the response of the hearing aid for optimal speech understanding and user comfort. Finally, new hearing aid users should accept their HL and not continue to consider it as a disgrace or a stigma. They should not cover their hearing aids as a way of hiding the HL, because hearing aids signal others that a HL exists and that they should speak clearly. If the hearing aid user accepts the HL and hearing aid, so will persons to whom they are speaking. In short, acceptance of HL and motivation to overcome its consequences are conditions for hearing aid satisfaction and success. Finally, hearing aids may not solve all communication challenges, so persons with HL should be encouraged supplement hearing aids with technologies to promote better understanding in noisy settings, over the telephone, and in large listening situations.

Role of Physicians in Managing Age-Related Hearing Loss

It is well accepted that HL disrupts social behavior and has significant functional, behavioral, and physical consequences. Although physicians have numerous opportunities to identify HL and provide appropriate referrals, there appear to be relatively few cases in which HL is identified opportunistically.[52] Mounting evidence has suggested that at least 25% of persons between 65 and 75 years of age have undiagnosed HL that could be detectable via routine, inexpensive hearing screening activities. Despite the high prevalence of hearing and balance problems among persons of Medicare age, most physicians do not screen older adults. Acknowledging the importance of wellness and preventive care, Medicare covers an Annual Wellness Visit (AWV), which provides Personalized Prevention Plan Services (PPPS) at no cost to the beneficiary (not subject to a co-payment; the physician can bill Medicare for the visit). Key elements of the first AWV providing PPPS include detection of any cognitive impairment, review of potential risk factors for depression, review of functional ability based on direct observation or appropriate screening questions, and a screening questionnaire. This includes a minimum assessment of the following: (1) hearing impairment; (2) ability to perform ADLs successfully; (3) risk of falls; and (4) home safety.

Hearing screening is an important condition to target for screening because people are living longer and want to remain socially engaged; adequate hearing is central to engagement. Additionally, the horizon to benefit tends to be brief ranging, from 3 to 6 weeks for hearing aids and 3 to 6 months for CIs. Another reason to screen is that older adults underreport or fail to report hearing deficits, and hearing deficits are one of the few geriatric syndromes missed during the traditional medical examination.[16] Physicians should consider screening an older adult in the following situations: (1) if a family member reports a concern about hearing or understanding; (2) if the patient presents with chronic conditions or multimorbidity, which places them at risk for HL, including mild cognitive impairment; (3) if the patient takes ototoxic medications; and (4) if the patient suffers from tinnitus. Furthermore, if a patient has a recent history of depression, it would behoove the physician to conduct a hearing screen because it may be that untreated HL is a contributing factor. It is well accepted that if a physician recommends a hearing test and possible treatment, it increases the likelihood that the patient will take action, because physicians have considerable influence over actions pertaining to health matters, which is why it is so important.

In conclusion, the ability of the patient to understand the physician during medical encounters and during transitions is integral to achieving PCC and is a guiding principle of care of older adults with multiple geriatric syndromes.[53] An important conclusion from the American Geriatrics Society Expert Panel on the Care of Older Adults with Multi-morbidity is as follows: “inadequate communication skills and educational materials are also barriers to the care of older adults with multi-morbidity. Because conversations about prognosis and preferences can often be difficult for clinicians, training of all health care team members must address communication skills.”[53]

CONCLUDING REMARKS

Nearly two thirds of persons 70 years of age and older and 80% of persons older than 85 years have a HL. Although adults older than 55 years make up 81% of all hearing aid users, most do not use hearing aids, HAT, or CIs. The stigma associated with hearing aid use, coupled with persistent complaints from experienced users about difficulty understanding in public places, especially noisy environments, has kept penetration rates stable but low over time. Technologically sophisticated hearing aids, in combination with some form of audiologic rehabilitation and cochlear implantation, are more effective than ever before and are a boon to older adults, who are living longer and must remain socially engaged, given the link to healthy aging. There is much evidence regarding the negative outcomes associated with untreated hearing loss and the contribution of hearing aids and cochlear implants to improved quality of life. The availability of situation-specific assistive technologies that can be used in isolation or as a supplement to hearing aids and cochlear implants is an important avenue for persons with hearing impairment to pursue. The physician has reliable, valid, and inexpensive tools at her or his disposal to identify persons with hearing problems who require and can benefit from the expertise of audiologists. Working together, physicians and audiologists can reduce the burden of hearing loss and promote the quality of life of the increasing population of older adults suffering from a handicapping hearing impairment.

KEY POINTS

- Age-related hearing loss is a public health problem.
- Untreated age-related hearing loss is associated with increased burdens of health and health care expenditure.
- Untreated hearing loss places individuals at risk for cognitive decline; people with self-reported hearing loss report poorer physician patient communication than those who do not report hearing loss.
- Hearing aid use is associated with reductions in perceived social and emotional loneliness and depression.

For a complete list of references, please visit www.expertconsult.com.

KEY REFERENCES

1. Kiely K, Gopinath B, Mitchell P, et al: Cognitive, health, and sociodemographic predictors of longitudinal decline in hearing acuity among older adults. J Gerontol A Biol Sci Med Sci 67:997–1003, 2012.
3. Lin F, Niparko J, Ferrucci L: Hearing loss prevalence in the United States. JAMA Intern Med 171:1851–1853, 2011.
5. Gopinath B, McMahon C, Rochtchina E, et al: Incidence, persistence, and progression of tinnitus symptoms in older adults: the Blue Mountains Hearing Study. Ear Hear 31:407–412, 2010.
12. Helzner E, Patel A, Pratt S, et al: Hearing sensitivity in older adults: Associations with cardiovascular risk factors in the health, aging and body composition study. J Am Geriatr Soc 59:972–979, 2011.
16. Weinstein BE: Geriatric audiology, ed 2, New York, 2012, Thieme.
22. Lin F, Ferrucci L, An Y, et al: Association of hearing impairment with brain volume changes in older adults. Neuroimage 90:84–92, 2014.
26. Gopinath B, Hickson L, Schneider J, et al: Hearing-impaired adults are at increased risk of experiencing emotional distress and social engagement restrictions five years later. Age Ageing 41:618–623, 2012.
27. Li CM, Zhang X, Hoffman HJ, et al: Hearing impairment associated with depression in US adults, National Health and Nutrition Examination Survey 2005-2010. JAMA Otolaryngol Head Neck Surg 140:293–302, 2014.
28. Lin F, Yaffe K, Xia J, et al: Hearing loss and cognitive decline in older adults. JAMA Intern Med 173: 293-299, 2013.
29. Lin F: Hearing loss and cognition among older adults in the United States. J Gerontol A Biol Sci Med Sci 66:1131–1136, 2011.
30. Schneider J, Gopinath B, Karpa M, et al: Hearing loss impacts on the use of community and informal supports. Age Ageing 39:458–464, 2010.
35. Feeny D, Huguet N, McFarland B, et al: Hearing, mobility, and pain predict mortality: a longitudinal population-based study. J Clin Epidemiol 65:764–777, 2012.
36. Karpa M, Gopinath B, Beath K, et al: Associations between hearing impairment and mortality risk in older persons: the Blue Mountains Hearing Study. Ann Epidemiol 20:452–459, 2010.
37. Gispen F, Chen D, Genther D, et al: Association between hearing impairment and lower levels of physical activity in older adults. J Am Geriatr Soc 62:1427–1433, 2014.
38. Lin F: Associations between hearing impairment and mortality risk in older persons: the Blue Mountains Hearing Study. Ann Epidemiol 62:1186–1187, 2014.
39. Kamil R, Li L, Lin FR: Association between hearing impairment and frailty in older adults. J Am Geriatr Soc 62:1186–1188, 2014.
40. Genther D, Frick K, Chen D, et al: Association of hearing loss with hospitalization and burden of disease in older adults. JAMA 309:2322–2324, 2013.
41. Gopinath B, Schneider J, McMahon C, et al: Severity of age-related hearing loss is associated with impaired activities of daily living. Age Ageing 41:95–200, 2012.
49. Clark J, Yeagle J, Arbaje A, et al: Cochlear implant rehabilitation in older adults: literature review and proposal of a conceptual framework. J Am Geriatr Soc 60:1936–1945, 2012.
52. Schneider J, Gopinath B, McMahon C, et al: Role of general practitioners in managing age-related hearing loss. Med J Aust 192:20–22, 2010.

PART III Problem-Based Geriatric Medicine

SECTION A Prevention and Health Promotion

97 Health Promotion for Community-Living Older Adults

Maureen F. Markle-Reid, Heather H. Keller, Gina Browne

INTRODUCTION

The older adult population (older than 65 years) is growing worldwide[1] as a result of economic prosperity and improved health care, sanitation, and education. In Canada, as the baby boom generation reaches the age of 65, seniors will make up a substantial part of the population: about 23% of Canadians by 2030 will be old by today's standards. The fastest-growing segment is people 80 years and older; this reality has implications for how we provide health care.[2]

Increasingly, as in many countries, Canada's older citizens are aging in place, a change attributable to technologic advances, investments in affordable and social housing, age-friendly communities, support for caregivers, programs to combat homelessness, and changes in options for care. In 2011 in Canada, 92% of seniors lived in a private home.[2] Rates of institutionalization for older people have decreased and formal community-based care has expanded, such that the proportion of older people receiving community care now outweighs that receiving services through an institution.[3] Over the past two decades, hospital beds have been reduced by 30%, nursing home beds by 11%, and ambulatory care has increased. The result is increasing pressure on community-based services to maintain accessible, high-quality, and comprehensive health care despite economic constraints.[3-5]

The benefits associated with aging in place are well documented. Residing at home optimizes older persons' health,[6,7] independence, control, sense of well-being,[8] and social connectedness.[7,9] Managers and policy makers face questions about the most efficient mix of service strategies for health promotion in this more community-based system.

As the population of older adults increases and medical advances continue to convert previously acute life-threatening diseases into chronic illnesses, there is an associated increase in the prevalence of chronic conditions and frailty.[10-12] More than 90% of older adults live with at least one chronic disease requiring daily self-care and management[13] and 65% to 85% have two or more chronic diseases.[14] Approximately 33% of community-living older adults have multiple chronic conditions (three or more).[15] Seniors with three or more chronic conditions report poorer health status, take five or more medications, have higher rates of health care utilization, and are at high risk for adverse events (e.g., death, hospitalization, and falls).[15,16] They account for 40% of health care use among seniors in Canada, with the intensity of use increasing as the number of chronic conditions increases.[15] Left unchecked, these conditions may overwhelm the health care system and threaten its sustainability.[17] The long-term solution must involve health promotion to prevent or better manage these conditions to improve quality of life and reduce demand for health care services.[18]

Approximately 15% of community-living seniors fall into the category of *frail*, defined as the accumulation of multiple interacting illnesses, impairments, and disabilities.[12,19,20] Of those considered frail, 17% are at high risk of experiencing functional decline that will jeopardize their ability to live independently.[21] These people are typically 75 years of age or older, living with multiple acute and chronic health conditions and functional disabilities.[22] They may also have cognitive impairment or unstable social support networks.[22,23] These characteristics put frail older adults at increased risk for morbidity, disability, health service use, and death.[24]

However, chronic disease and frailty should not be considered an inevitable or irreversible consequence of aging.[25] As individuals age, they are at greater risk of developing chronic health problems, but these conditions are not inherent in the aging process.[26] A majority of the most costly health conditions are preventable, treatable, or manageable.[18] At least one third of the total economic and social burden of disease in developed countries is caused by a handful of largely avoidable risks: tobacco, alcohol, high blood pressure, high cholesterol, and obesity.[27-29]

Evidence suggests that chronic disease is preventable and can be better managed to reduce its health and economic effects on older adults. Many chronic disease risk factors, such as physical inactivity and poor nutrition, are modifiable. The negative effects of many risk factors can be reversed, with even modest reductions in risk factor levels producing large improvements in health.[30] For example, with healthy eating, regular exercise, not smoking, and effective stress management, over 90% of cases of type 2 diabetes and 80% of cases of coronary heart disease could be avoided.[27,28] Even a 5% reduction in preventable illnesses could lead to substantial savings in medical and other costs.[18] Consequently, identifying modifiable factors that can reduce or delay health service use and increase quality of life in older adults is a priority.

Family caregivers, particularly women, provide up to 80% of the care for community-living older adults with chronic conditions or disabilities. These caregivers provide vital help with activities of daily living, such as personal hygiene, toileting, eating, and moving about inside the home. Family caregivers also help with meal preparation, housework, medication management, shopping, and transportation and provide emotional support.[31] In 2012, an estimated 8.1 million Canadians provided care to a family member or friend with a long-term health condition or aging-related needs.[32] Although many caregivers find this to be a rewarding role, it is often carried out at the expense of their own health and well-being. The level of caregiver strain increases with the number of chronic conditions the older adult has, resulting in negative health outcomes and more health service use in caregivers.[33] Despite this evidence, little is known about the best way to support family caregivers.

A growing body of research suggests that older community-living adults can benefit considerably from proactive health promotion interventions.[34-41] The ultimate goal of these programs is to proactively identify and address factors influencing health and to promote positive health behaviors and autonomy of older people living in the community to prevent or delay institutionalization, reduce health care costs, and improve health-related quality of life and function.[42]

The purpose of this chapter is to summarize this research and identify how health promotion and disease prevention for community-living older adults can be improved. The specific objectives of this chapter are (1) to describe three groups of older adults and their need for health promotion and disease prevention, (2) to describe a conceptual framework for health promotion and disease prevention for frail older adults, (3) to describe a framework for economic evaluation of health care programs, (4) to argue in favor of the importance of screening to identify older adults who could benefit from health promotion and disease prevention efforts, (5) to describe successful health promotion and prevention efforts among community-living older adults, (6) to discuss the barriers to implementing effective health promotion programs, and (7) to demonstrate the need for further policy and research on health promotion and disease prevention for community-living older adults.

THE HETEROGENEITY OF OLDER ADULTS AND THE NEED FOR HEALTH PROMOTION

Older adults are a very heterogeneous group, with aging occurring at different rates in different people. Chronological age does not tell the full story of functional ability or quality of life, and most disabilities of old age are not inevitable.[25] The trajectories of aging after age 65 have been described as "successful," "usual," and "accelerated."[43-45]

Those who are *successfully aging* continue to experience good health for an extended period of time. "This is the 65-year old who plans to take a cycling tour of France, the 75-year old who plays tennis twice a week, or the 80-year old who walks two miles each day."[43] Successfully aging adults have minimal health problems; they may visit their primary health care provider for preventive checks, such as blood pressure, and may have a few risk factors (e.g., family history of heart disease), but they are quite healthy, with no modifiable risk factors. These older adults are likely to be on no medications. They watch what they eat and try to exercise. They develop signs of chronic disease only late in life, thus spending less time dealing with chronic disease.[43]

Usually aging older adults have some signs of chronic disease. They take a few medications to manage hypertension or cholesterol levels, may be bothered by the occasional bout of arthritis pain, and see their doctor routinely to monitor their conditions. These conditions do not drastically affect their quality of life, because they still travel and do most of their normal activities, such as driving, babysitting grandchildren, and taking cruises.[43] Approximately 80% of seniors are experiencing successful or usual aging.[46]

Older adults experiencing *accelerated aging* appear frailer and more functionally dependent for their age. These people, who represent between 15% and 20% of seniors, are typically older than 75 years and have co-occurring physical health problems, both acute and chronic.[20,47] They are highly vulnerable, living with supports that are prone to breakdown with any shift in their health and well-being.[21-23] Many live in isolation and are cut off from community services because of a lack of information or transportation or the will to initiate action.[48] Many single seniors live in poverty or near-poverty, without the benefit of the two pensions that married older adults get.[49] The prevalence of depression among those with accelerated aging is between 26% and 44%, at least twice that among older people in general.[50] These characteristics lead to a greater risk for loss of functional independence, institutionalization, and death.[12] Long-term care facilities take care of approximately 25% of seniors with accelerated aging and the remainder reside at home.[20] These frail older adults pose a challenge to health care systems, because they are frequent users of acute hospitalization and home care services.[23,38] Frail seniors living at home are particularly difficult to reach and are at high risk for loss of functional independence and institutionalization.[12] These facts underline the need for health promotion efforts in this group.

Before discussing health promotion and disease prevention in relation to frail older adults, it is important to clarify what is meant by "frailty" (see also Chapter 14). Despite the recent increase in the use of this term, there is a lack of consensus about frailty and its meaning, beyond agreement that people who are frail are at an increased risk of adverse outcomes compared with others their own age.[24] What does frailty look like? How is it defined, framed, and understood? Exactly how frail is frail?[51,52] A first step in addressing the problem of frailty is to understand better how to identify those who are frail.[53] However, the components of frailty have not been sufficiently defined to identify populations at risk or in need of proactive interventions.[24]

A literature review of definitions and conceptual models of frailty in relation to older adults suggests that frailty is a multiple-determined state of vulnerability in which an individual is at risk of becoming more or less frail over time.[24] The implication of this definition is that the process of frailty can be modified or reversed,[24] highlighting the need for rational, theoretically based interventions directed toward health promotion and disease prevention for this population. This chapter gives guidelines for a taking a new theoretical approach to the concept of frailty in older adults. This new approach to the concept of frailty (1) is multidimensional and considers the complex interplay among behavioral, biological, social, and environmental determinants of health rather than a single influence[12,54,55]; (2) is not age-related; (3) is subjectively defined; and (4) considers both individual and environmental factors that influence health (Table 97-1).[24]

Despite the differences in the three types of aging groups, each could benefit from health promotion and disease prevention efforts targeted to its specific needs.[28,38] Programs and services that promote the health of older adults, focused on keeping them healthy rather than solely being reactive to symptoms, are underdeveloped in North America.[45,56] The lack of such programs may reflect the narrow viewpoint that older adults cannot change behaviors such as smoking, eating, and exercising.[57] However, seniors are interested and can change behaviors when given the support to do so. Calls have been made for the development of more public health interventions for older adults[58] that target motivation to acquire or maintain important health behaviors. The goal of any health promotion program should be to optimize the individual's current health, even if minimal change in quality of life is achieved.[1] Given the heterogeneity of older adults, it is essential to consider differences in health trajectories and quality of life when making decisions about the type and number of health promotion activities required. As the population ages and the number of people aging in place increases, there is an urgent need to identify effective and efficient ways of promoting the health of community-living older adults.

CONCEPTUAL FRAMEWORK FOR HEALTH PROMOTION AND DISEASE PREVENTION FOR FRAIL OLDER ADULTS

Empirical evidence alone is insufficient to direct the design and evaluation of interventions. Theory is essential for program development, implementation, and evaluation, as it provides explanation and can predict outcomes. Theory enhances the

TABLE 97-1 Dimensions of Frailty

Dimensions	Supporting Evidence
The concept must be multidimensional and consider the complex interplay among behavioral, biologic, social, and environmental determinants on health rather than a single influence.	This view is consistent with the observation that many social, socioeconomic, and lifestyle factors are associated with health and that determinants of health are often highly inter-related.[12,54,55] Theoretical models need to address the complexity of problems rather than focusing on a single problem, since older people typically have co-existing physical, emotional, and social problems interrelated with one another and with external factors.[24,192]
The concept must not suggest a negative and stereotypical view of aging.	Theoretical models should reflect a positive view of aging that emphasizes the capacity for autonomy and independence and maximizes a person's strengths[193] as well as deficits.[24]
The concept must take into account an individual's context and incorporate subjective perceptions.	The trajectory of frailty is unique for each individual.[194] The emphasis is on the individual's perception of health rather than the person's objective circumstances. Research supports the hypothesis that an individual's poor adjustment to chronic illness or affective state is not related to the specific physical disease or level of disability but rather to the negative meaning the individual attributes to it.[195] Theoretical models need to incorporate subjective measures and allow for individual variability.[24]
The concept must take into account the contribution of both individual and environmental factors that influence health.	Frailty can originate from within an individual or from conditions in the environment. Theoretical models need to address the constellation of individual and environmental factors that influence health.[24]

generalizability of the results by providing the basis for the systematic development and implementation of intervention strategies, as well as evaluation indicators.[59] Furthermore, there is evidence to support higher effectiveness of theory-based versus non–theory-informed interventions.[60]

An adapted version of the model of vulnerability[61] incorporates the key concepts of frailty (discussed earlier) to guide the development, implementation, and evaluation of health promotion and disease prevention interventions. Vulnerability is a net result of the interaction between a person's personal resources (cognitive, emotional, intellectual, and behavioral) and environmental supports (social, material, and cultural), both of which, along with biologic characteristics (age, gender, and genetic endowment), are determinants of health. Within an individual, personal resources and environmental supports intersect, as shown in Figure 97-1, and can be synergistic and cumulative.[39] The base of the triangle represents the degree of vulnerability[61] and thus also health status and quality of life. Use of health services increases with the level of vulnerability.[34]

Even if personal resources hold constant, changes in the individual's environmental supports can alter his or her degree of vulnerability and thus his or her use of health and social services.[39] What is needed is "a 'fit' between the needs and resources of the person and the demands and resources of the environment" (p. 68).[61] This vulnerability model provides a schema of the basic

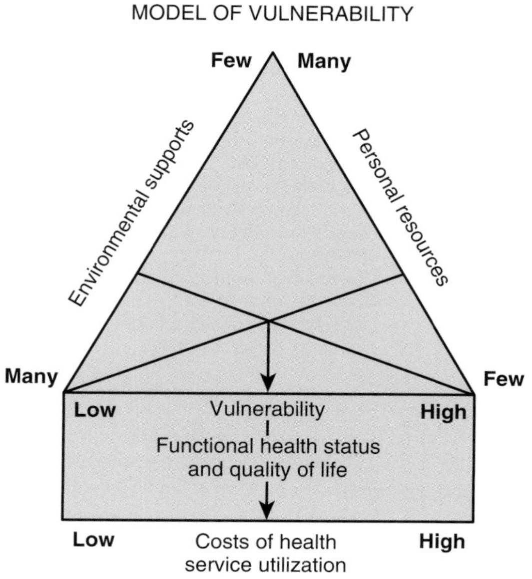

Figure 97-1. Model of vulnerability. *(Modified from Rogers AC: Vulnerability, health and health care. J Adv Nurs 26:65–72, 1997.)*

components of a multidimensional health promotion and disease prevention intervention. Such interventions, targeted at either the individual or the environment, can identify and strengthen available resources, thereby reducing vulnerability and the on-demand use of expensive health services, while enhancing quality of life. Hence, strategies for optimizing health in the model of vulnerability are multilevel.[61]

Personal resources can be defined as either inborn or acquired characteristics, which interact with the environment to influence health.[61] Inborn characteristics include nonmodifiable factors such as age, gender, race, temperament, genetic predisposition to disease, susceptibility to illness, sensitivity to drugs, and chemical imbalances. Acquired characteristics are modifiable factors known to increase risk for functional decline in older adults. *Environmental supports* are factors that interact with personal resources to influence health[61] (Table 97-2).

FRAMEWORK FOR ECONOMIC EVALUATION

Although the literature contains many evaluations of programs seeking to achieve improved outcomes for vulnerable populations, such as frail older community-dwelling adults, few of them evaluated the efficiency of these programs. In economic terms, efficiency involves maximizing outcomes for a given cost or minimizing costs for a given level of outcome.[62] As depicted in Figure 97-2, the economic evaluation of health care programs[63] yields nine possible outcomes (the more favorable ones are within the triangle). In outcome 1, increased effects or health benefits are achieved with increased expenditure or additional resources consumed—this is called *cost-effective*. Outcome 4 is also favorable, because increased effects are achieved at equivalent costs. Outcome 7 represents the "win/win" situation, whereby more effect is produced at lower costs. Outcome 8 represents the situation where different health programs produce the same effect, but some approaches are associated with lower costs. Options 7 and 8 are superior to the often-implemented option 9, in which funding for a program is cut because of reduced effects, releasing resources for other purposes.[63]

This approach can be used to classify the main effects and expenses of comparative community health interventions. In addition, it can be used to determine who benefits most and at

TABLE 97-2 Model of Vulnerability

Dimensions	Factors	Supporting Evidence (Reference)
PERSONAL RESOURCES		
Inborn	Age, gender, race, temperament, genetic predisposition to disease, susceptibility to illness, sensitivity to drugs, and chemical imbalances	61,196
Acquired	Recently moved	22
	Recently discharged from hospital	197
	Poor self-perceived health	109
	Depression and anxiety	108,109
	Falling	39,198
	Taking multiple medications	54
	Cognitive impairment	109
	Using assistance for activities of daily living	40,140
	Impaired vision or hearing	109
	Social isolation	109
	Comorbid health conditions	109,199
	Nutritional risk	156
	Low level of physical activity	163
	Excessive consumption of alcohol, smoking	109
ENVIRONMENTAL SUPPORTS		
	Societal attitudes and stereotypes of aging	61
	Living alone, social isolation	109
	Low income	200
	Low levels of education	196,201

Modified from Rogers AC: Vulnerability, health and health care. J Adv Nurs 26:65–72, 1997.

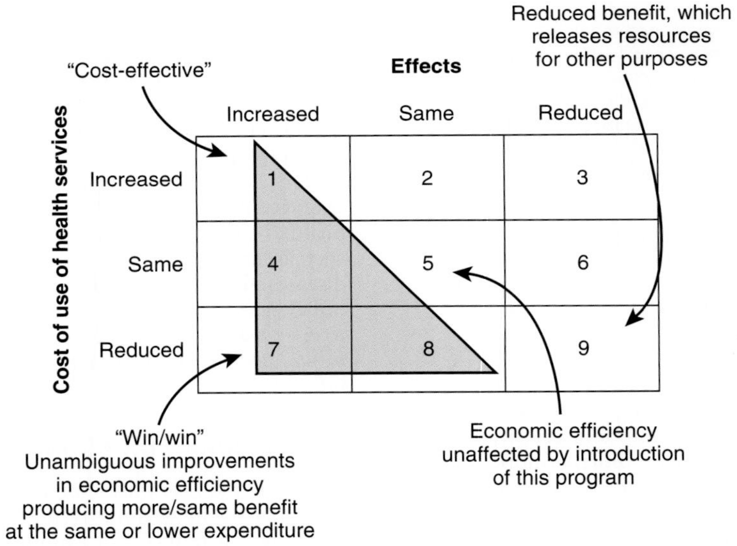

Figure 97-2. Framework for evaluating possible outcomes of economic evaluation of health care programs. *(From Birch S, Gafni A: Cost-effectiveness and cost utility analyses: methods for the non-economic evaluation of health care programs and how we can do better. In Geisler E, Heller O, editors: Managing technology in healthcare, Norwell, MA, 1996, Kluwer Academic.)*

what expense when various interventions are available. This is of concern especially in systems of government health insurance, in which some people may use services inappropriately.[64]

SCREENING AND ASSESSMENT: IDENTIFYING OLDER ADULTS WHO COULD BENEFIT FROM HEALTH PROMOTION AND DISEASE PREVENTION EFFORTS

A growing body of international evidence suggests that early detection of older people at risk for functional decline or loss of autonomy is beneficial. Several studies of screening and case finding have been conducted to proactively identify and address unmet needs of older adults, to reduce the on-demand use of costly resources. These will be reviewed here.

Many older adults living the community have unrecognized risk factors. Health concerns or risk occur in almost all older adults, with up to 83% having at least one unreported or unrecognized risk.[65-67] Many of these risk factors are social problems[67] that can affect a senior's support network and have the potential to increase health care expenditures if left undetected. Unsolicited home visits by a health visitor can be a means of recognizing these unmet needs. Using this service, Harrison and colleagues[68] found that 35% of patients older than 70 years of age had unidentified risks and could benefit from preventive programs. Brown and coworkers,[69] in an audit of 40 general practices in the United Kingdom, reported that 44% of patients older than 75 years had at least one health problem that was previously undetected. Ramsdell and associates[70] found that compared with an office-based assessment, a home-based assessment of older adults resulted in the detection of up to four new problems. Stuck and colleagues[71] identified several key advantages of in-home visits versus office-based visits. A home-based assessment allows for appraisal of the physical environment to identify risk factors and equipment needs, review of medications, contact with family members, and convenience for clients with mobility problems. Furthermore, an office-based visit often has a specific focus and limited time to solicit additional risks.

Browne and coworkers,[34] in a review of 12 randomized controlled trials evaluating a community-based approach to care in a Canadian setting, found that for clients with multiple problems (such as the frail older adult), it is more expensive to *not* provide proactive and comprehensive disease prevention and health promotion. Similarly, Caulfield and associates[65] (p. 87), in a review of the literature on geriatric screening programs, concluded that "home based, comprehensive screening of the older adult for undetected physical, mental and socioeconomic problems by nursing or other trained personnel may be able to prolong survival, improve quality of life, and perhaps even postpone dependency or institutionalization." Screening eliminates a barrier between the need for help and gaining access to that help.

Screening and assessment in three areas—falls, nutrition, and depression—are advocated for community-dwelling older adults, because these conditions are readily preventable through health promotion efforts. The term *screening* refers to the process of detecting or identifying a health condition or risk factor among a specific population. The term *assessment* refers to the process that follows a positive screen and involves evaluating older adults in a more specific way to confirm the problem or establish the diagnosis and develop a treatment plan.[72]

Risk of Falls

As detailed in the chapter on mobility and its assessment (see Chapter 102), falls and fall-related injuries negatively affect older adults' quality of life and health care resources. Thirty percent of community-living adults older than 65 years fall at least once a year, increasing to 50% for those older than 80 years.[73] Fall-related injuries often trigger a downward spiral in health that is associated with activity restriction,[74] high health care costs,[75] long-term care admissions,[76] and death.[77] The costs of health care associated with fall-related injuries are staggering. The 2004 cost of fall injuries to seniors in Canada was $4.5 billion. With an aging population and an associated increase in fall-related injuries, these cost estimates are projected to rise as high as $240 billion by 2040.[75]

Aside from the cost, the negative effect of a fall on health and quality of life should not be underestimated. Fall injuries often result in fear of falling,[78,79] leading to self-imposed restriction of activity and loss of confidence,[80] low self-esteem, depression,[79] chronic pain, and functional deterioration.[81] Falls and fall-related injuries and complications are the leading cause of death among seniors.[82] Frail seniors are at increased risk of falls,[83] are more likely to sustain serious injury, and take longer to recover after falling.[75] Falls are caused by multiple interacting factors, some of which are modifiable. Factors such as postural hypotension; the use of multiple medications; and impairments in cognition, vision, balance, gait, and strength increase the risk of falling.[84] Although no single factor causes all falls, the risk of falling increases with the number of risk factors present.[85]

Evidence suggests that most falls are predictable and preventable. Intervention studies showed that 30% to 40% of falls can be avoided.[86-88] A 10% reduction in the number of nonfatal falls would mean 7931 fewer falls and health care savings of $138.6 million.[18] Categorizing individuals into different levels of risk through screening is important from both clinical and economic perspectives; it is the seniors with the highest risk of falling who will benefit most from preventive efforts.[87] Preventing falls in any group of older persons requires knowledge of where that group sits on the risk spectrum, because this will determine the type and amount of services required, as well as the effectiveness of the program.[81] Fall risk screening is a means of targeting limited home and community care resources.

Home and community care providers are well positioned to play a major role in preventing falls in older people through screening and intervention. Because of the rising concern for fall-related injuries, several fall risk screening instruments for community-living older adults have been developed.[89] The most effective fall reduction programs involve routine and systematic fall risk assessments, followed by targeting of interventions to an individual's risk profile.[83,90] This conclusion has been substantiated by meta-analyses of many randomized controlled trials[90,91] and by consensus panels of experts who have developed evidence-based practice guidelines for the detection and management of fall risk.[83,92,93,87] The importance of this direction cannot be overstated. Reducing just one fall risk factor can have a great effect on the frequency and morbidity of falls.[88]

Risk of Nutritional Problems

Nutrition problems in older adults are common, because of the diverse determinants of food intake in this age group[44] (see also Chapters 79 and 109). Low intakes of various food groups, energy, protein, and micronutrients in the older adult population have been reported.[38,94] Poor-quality, energy-dense food, and lack of exercise lead to obesity.[94] Obesity, coupled with poor function, results in a precarious state for older adults. Those who are frail, exhibiting accelerated aging, are also highly susceptible to malnutrition.[38,94,95]

Several nutrition screening indices have been developed[96] in response to concerns for the nutritional health of older adults.[38,57] Nutrition screening is a means of targeting limited nutrition resources, especially dietitian services.[97] Unfortunately, most research to date has focused on describing "at-risk" populations or identifying linkages between nutrition risk and negative health outcomes, without demonstrating that nutrition screening can change practice and prevent these outcomes. Prevalence of risk varies, depending on the index used and the subgroup of older adults screened; estimates range from 34% in "usually aging" seniors to 69% in those who are frail.[98-101] Risk factors associated with poor food intake or nutrition risk include poor self-rated health,[100,102] functional limitations,[44,102,103] education, income, social support, dentition, smoking, vision,[98,102,103] stress,[99] lack of transportation, poor social networks, and living alone.[38,98] Food intake is very complex because of its multifactorial determinants. Interventions to promote food intake need to be comprehensive and multisectoral.

In the United States, the Elderly Nutrition Program provides nutritious meals and other nutrition services to older adults who are especially vulnerable.[94] Although not mandatory, screening, assessment, and interventions, such as counseling and basic nutrition education, can be provided within individual communities. Screening within the program is meant to target interventions,[94] but no research on the effectiveness of the screening process has been documented. Only 20% of older adults who could benefit from this program are reached,[104] and targeting of services to those most in need is required.[105]

A 2008 article described a nutrition screening program with the Nutrition Risk Screening 2002 in 26 European hospital departments in 12 countries.[106] The average age of the 5051 patients screened was 60 years, and 33% were considered to be "at risk." These patients were more likely to have complications, death, and a longer length of hospital stay than those without risk. Subsequent interventions, if any, were not described. Regardless of setting, screening needs to be followed with assessment and efficacious treatment.

There is only one known evaluation of a nutrition screening program focused on older adults in the community, limited to describing and assessing the process of screening.[43] The Bringing Nutrition Screening to Seniors in Canada project[43] involved developing, implementing, and process evaluating screening programs in five diverse communities in Canada. Approximately 1200 seniors were screened. Those who were found to be at risk were provided with referrals to community services. An ethical screening process, which included follow-up, helped to identify the effect of the program. Seniors indicated that screening helped them recognize their problem areas and become aware of the programs and services available in their community. Some individuals reported improving their food intake as a result of the screening, although objective data were not collected.[43] Now that nutrition screening tools are available, researchers need to focus on determining the effectiveness of screening and early nutrition interventions in this population.

Risk of Depression

Depression is one of the most common treatable causes of mortality, morbidity, functional decline, and increased health care use among community-living older adults.[107-109] Despite the high prevalence of depression in this population, its incidence is often missed or suboptimally managed.[110] Depression affects 5% to 10% of individuals in primary care but is recognized in only about 50% of cases.[111] In a recent study of older adults receiving home care services, only 12% of those with depression received adequate treatment.[110]

Many challenges to the diagnosis and management of depression in older adults have been identified, including difficulties disentangling coexisting medical, psychiatric, and social morbidity[112]; transportation and access difficulties; social isolation[113]; health care provider attitudes toward mental health disorders and treatment; and reluctance of older adults to accept the diagnosis of depression.[114,115] Thus, seniors may be particularly vulnerable to suboptimal depression care. The magnitude of the problem has potential to increase as a result of the rising number of seniors[46] and the associated increase in the prevalence of depressive symptoms.[72]

Clinician and health care system factors also impede the recognition and treatment of depression. Older people at risk of, suffering from, or recovering from depression have limited access to professional services promoting mental health, especially nursing.[116] Other barriers to optimal depression care include inadequate collaboration among home and community care providers, primary health care providers, and specialized mental health care providers; no continuity among providers; difficulties accessing specialized mental health care services; lack of knowledge among home care providers in recognizing and managing depression[113,116-118]; and underuse of depression screening tools. A final barrier is the lack of evidence-based practice standards specific to the assessment and management of depression in home care for older adults.[116]

Unrecognized, untreated, and undertreated mood disorders generate enormous personal, economic, and societal costs.[110,119] Depression in older people often coexists with other chronic illnesses, and untreated depression is a significant risk factor for functional decline, diminished quality of life, mortality from comorbid medical conditions or suicide, dementia, social isolation, poor adherence to treatment, increased demands on family caregivers, and increased use of expensive health services.[120,121] In 1998, depression cost Canadians approximately $14.4 billion dollars.[122,123] These costs are compounded by indirect costs, such as those to family caregivers, who are more prone that noncaregivers to experience symptoms of depression.[124] Depression is also associated with unhealthy lifestyles and noncompliance with medical treatment.[125,126]

Frail seniors are at increased risk of depression.[19,127] The prevalence of depression among frail older persons receiving home care services is 26% to 44%, at least twice that among older persons in general.[110,128,129] They also suffer from a fourfold increase in more severe forms of depression than the general population.[130] Clearly, recognition is key to referral and subsequent treatment for depression in this population.[115]

Multiple interacting physical, psychological, and social factors increase the risk of depression in old age. These include comorbid health condition(s); functional limitations; taking medications such as centrally acting antihypertensive drugs, analgesics, steroids, and antiparkinsonian agents; social factors; and history of depression.[131]

Routine depression screening and assessment have been shown to improve the recognition and management of depression in community-living older adults.[115,117,132-137] Several instruments have been developed to reflect the differences in presentation of depression in older adults and to address such issues as the presence of concurrent medical disorders (e.g., dementia).[138]

Community providers can play a pivotal role in screening for depression in older adults. An understanding of the risk factors for depression will increase clinicians' ability to effectively target the use of screening, because screening is most effective when targeted to higher risk groups.[72] Current Canadian recommendations suggest that screening for depression in primary care settings should only be carried out if effective follow-up and treatment can be provided.[139] Although access to specialized geriatric mental health services remains limited in some settings, primary health care practitioners are able to provide appropriate follow-up and treatment.[72]

Importance and Implementation of Screening

Awareness of the importance of screening is required at several levels: older adults, their families, their home care providers, and the community.[38] Although older adults seem to be interested in health promotion, they often do not think they are at risk for falls, poor nutrition, or depression. Screening may increase their attentiveness or self-awareness. Assessment of risk can be used to guide the allocation of limited community resources to those most likely to benefit from preventive efforts.

Home and community care providers play an important role in the early identification and management of risk factors for functional decline. This is best accomplished by performing a multifactorial assessment using validated screening instruments, followed by targeting of interventions to an individual's risk profile.[90] There is a need for greater standardization and multidisciplinarity of assessments, which was identified as one of four factors that influence the "margin" between institutional and community-based care for community-living seniors.[140]

Screening in the community is complex and providers need support to build capacity.[38] Tools used for assessment of risk may not be standardized and often lack rigorous reliability and validity testing.[48,141] To be acceptable to practice and relevant for a diverse group of older adults, risk screening instruments need to be reliable, valid, brief, and easy to use. They need to be acceptable to both the individual being assessed and the provider performing the assessment.[89] Different instruments may be required for different segments of the heterogeneous older population.[142]

In addition to an appropriate screening instrument, capacity for screening in the community is based on the development of an ethical screening process.[143,144] The ethical screening process has three steps: (1) targeting people in need of resources or education through consistent administration of a valid and reliable screening tool; (2) providing those identified to be "at risk" with feasible options for assessment and treatment through resources, services, or education; and (3) following up with these individuals to ensure that their identified needs are met.[144] Development of an ethical screening process is complex and requires time, resources, and effort.[144] Research and best practice guidelines should be translated into practice, so that risk assessment is implemented and appropriate interventions are tailored to individual needs.

PROMOTING HEALTH IN COMMUNITY-LIVING OLDER ADULTS: LESSONS FROM FIVE INTERVENTION STUDIES

Health promotion is the process of enabling people to take control over the determinants of health and thereby improve their health.[145] Health promotion strategies are based on a participatory model of health,[146] which seeks to expand an individual's positive potential for health. This is in contrast to disease prevention, which is grounded in the traditional biomedical model of health,[146] which seeks to avoid or decrease risks to health and well-being.[147]

A participatory approach to health involves activities that empower individuals and promote positive attitudes, knowledge, and skills to maintain and enhance health.[148,149] Health promotion strategies involve goals such as autonomy, empowerment, and independent decision making.[39] Health promotion interventions are developed, implemented, and evaluated together with individuals, families, and stakeholders from different organizations.[150] Empowerment for health goes beyond illness and the management of a single disease. Its success is seen in enhanced health, well-being, quality of life, and sense of self-esteem and self-worth.[151]

According to the World Health Organization, health promotion strategies include developing personal health skills, creating supportive environments, strengthening community action, reorienting health services, and building healthy public policy.[151] Thus, health promotion strategies are multilevel, focusing on family, community, and society, as well as individuals. Health promotion is concerned not only with facilitating the development of life skills, self-concept, and social skills but also with environmental intervention through a broad range of political, legislative, fiscal, and administrative means.[146]

Whereas health promotion is approach-motivated, disease prevention is avoidance-motivated.[147] The aim of disease prevention is to reduce premature morbidity and mortality.[146,147,152] Health promotion and disease prevention efforts are categorized as primary, secondary, or tertiary. *Primary prevention* is focused on removal of risk factors for disease or functional decline from the individual or the environment. Activities of this type are implemented for successfully or usually aging older adults who are asymptomatic and free of clinical evidence of the targeted disease or health condition. *Secondary prevention* activities focus on early identification and prompt treatment of risk factors before they lead to functional decline.[144] In essence, secondary prevention is the way to add "life to years."[1] Secondary prevention can slow progression through the stages of functional decline for successfully or usually aging older adults. *Tertiary prevention* is typically provided to older adults with accelerated aging, focused on those who exhibit some signs of functional decline. These interventions aim to limit the progression of disease, functional decline, and loss of independence[26] and to maximize function.

Our knowledge base concerning the potential role for health promotion and secondary prevention in older people is relatively small.[26,38] The current health care system was created to respond to acute, episodic care provided in hospitals by individual physicians.[153] Most community-based interventions for older adults occur at a tertiary prevention level, focusing on illness and the treatment of disease, largely ignoring health promotion, secondary prevention, and partnering approaches between and among all professionals and older people with chronic diseases.[39,154] In the United States, less than 4 cents of every health care dollar is spent on prevention and public health.[18] The health care system has been criticized for narrowly focusing "downstream," diverting scarce resources away from primary and secondary prevention. Functional disabilities and illnesses in older people often are managed as acute medical problems, not as ongoing life challenges.[41] Older people need both health promotion and disease prevention, so it is essential that health professionals become engaged in all areas of activity.[155]

This section describes five examples of Canadian health promotion and disease prevention interventions designed for community-living older adults, in which either falls, nutrition, or depression were areas of focus:

I. Evergreen action nutrition: an example of a secondary prevention program[144,156,157]
II. Home support exercise intervention for frail older adults using home care services[158]
III. Nursing health promotion for frail older adults using home care services[40]
IV. Interprofessional nurse-led fall prevention for older home care clients at risk of falling[159]
V. Interprofessional nurse-led mental health promotion for older home care clients with depressive symptoms[160,161]

Studies I and II are prospective cohort studies of older adults living in the community with comparable types and severity of illnesses and disabilities, who self-select to one community-based approach over another. Studies III and IV are randomized controlled trials that control for the methodological problem of self-selection that confound Studies I and II. Measures of well-being and the costs of use of health services provided to older adults randomly assigned to health-oriented, proactive care were compared with those of similar clients receiving reactive, unplanned, and disease-oriented approaches to care. Study V is a one-group pretest-posttest study. The interventions in all studies were delivered using existing home and community services, with the goal of integrating the intervention into practice once the studies ended. The major findings from each study are described, and lessons, as they relate to using results to inform practice, policy, and future research, are summarized.

Study I. Evergreen Action Nutrition: An Example of a Secondary Prevention Program

Evergreen Action Nutrition is a nutrition education program provided, since 1999, in a seniors recreation center in southern Ontario. Using a community-based approach, this program was developed, implemented, and evaluated by an advisory committee that included senior members of the center.[162] Nutrition screening was used to identify needs, raise awareness, and evaluate activities. The program was voluntary. Seniors could participate solely through reading education materials or they could be involved in hands-on activities such as cooking groups. The program included stocking the center library with quality nutrition books, a nutrition column in the monthly newsletter, monthly nutrition and nutrition displays, cooking groups for men, support groups for persons managing their weight or diabetes, food demonstrations that included hands-on activities and food consumption, celebrity chefs, and monthly deliveries of a fresh vegetable and fruit box. Process evaluation showed that the program was effective.[144] The program had a large reach, with approximately two thirds of members (approximately 2000 seniors) having participated in some way during a 3-year period. Respondents to a randomly mailed follow-up survey were less likely to be at nutrition risk than those surveyed at baseline (39% vs. 57%). Participants in the program had better fruit and vegetable intake than nonparticipants. Food demonstrations and cooking groups helped overcome barriers to trying new foods and recipes.[156,157] Participants reported intention to change cooking and eating behaviors. This program was funded from a research grant for the first three years and has continued with minimal funding from the seniors association that runs the center and from monies collected from participants. Lessons learned from this program are that diverse education activities are needed to reach a wide audience; no single intervention will appeal to all seniors. Seniors are interested and motivated to improve their nutrition knowledge and behaviors. A recreation center is an ideal setting for this activity because it is a nonthreatening environment that provides consistent educators and other staff important for building trust and program continuity. Finally, a participatory approach that involves the target group is essential for developing and implementing meaningful education activities.

Study II. Home Support Exercise Intervention for Frail Older Adults Using Home Care Services

This prospective cohort study was designed to determine the effectiveness of a home support exercise program (HSEP) for frail older adults receiving home care services.[158] Home exercise is an effective means to prevent falls, maintain functional independence, and promote rehabilitation following injury or illness.[163] The study sample consisted of 98 frail older adults (65 years or older) using home support services in a home care program in southern Ontario. Sixty subjects self-selected to receive the HSEP, and 38 matched controls were allocated to receive standard home care without the HSEP. A total of 77 subjects (79%) completed the 4-month follow-up. The HSEP is a 4-month in-home physical activity intervention provided by a trained personal support worker (PSW). It consists of 10 simple, functional, and progressive exercises that are to be done daily. Once the exercises have been introduced, the PSW continues to monitor the client's progress and offer motivational support. Participants who received the HSEP reported general improvement, such as feeling better, being less stiff and stronger, and being able to walk more easily. The control group reported that they felt worse than they did 4 months previously. Between groups, significant differences in mobility and walking scores were observed, with an average improvement of 14% to 34% in the HSEP group compared with only minor improvement or functional decline in the control group. Significant improvements for balance confidence were also observed in the HSEP group, whereas the control group experienced little or no change. The findings support the effectiveness of the HSEP, as well as the importance of proactive and regular exercise interventions and support in this population.[158]

Study III. Nursing Health Promotion for Frail Older Adults Using Home Care Services

This single-blind, randomized controlled trial with a 6-month follow-up, conducted in a home care program in southern Ontario, was designed to determine the effects and costs of adding nursing health promotion and disease prevention to usual home care services.[40] The study sample consisted of 288 older adults (75 years or older) using personal support services who were randomized to intervention or control groups. A total of 242 (84%) subjects completed the 6-month follow-up. In addition to usual home care, the nursing group received monthly in-home visits by a registered nurse (RN) over 6 months. The primary outcome was health-related quality of life. Secondary outcomes were depression, perceived social support, coping ability, and cost of use of health services, from a societal perspective. Results showed that providing older adults with proactive nursing health promotion and disease prevention, compared with providing nursing services on a reactive and episodic basis, results in better mental health functioning and a reduction in depression, at no additional cost. The overall conclusion of this study is that home-based nursing health promotion proactively provided to frail older people with chronic health needs enhances quality of life at no additional expense. The results underscore the need to reinvest in nursing services for health promotion for frail older adults receiving home care services.[40]

Study IV. Interprofessional Nurse-Led Fall Prevention for Older Home Care Clients at Risk of Falling

This single-blind, randomized controlled trial with a 6-month follow-up, conducted in a home care program in southern Ontario, was designed to determine the effects and costs of an interprofessional, nurse-led team approach to fall prevention, compared with usual home care for older home care clients at risk of falling.[159] The study sample consisted of 109 older adults (75 years or older) who were randomized to intervention or control groups. A total of 92 subjects (84%) completed the 6-month follow-up. The intervention was a 6-month multifactorial and evidence-based prevention strategy involving an interprofessional team. In addition to usual home care, the intervention group received monthly in-home visits by members of the interprofessional team (RN, home care case manager, physiotherapist, and occupational therapist) over 6 months. Each participant's treatment regimen was discussed by the interprofessional team at monthly case conferences. The primary outcome was the change in the number of falls. Secondary outcomes were changes in fall risk factors and costs of use of health services, from a societal perspective. Results showed no difference between groups in the mean number of falls at 6 months. However, subgroup analyses showed that the intervention was effective in reducing falls in men aged 75 to 84 years who had a fear of falling or a negative history of falls. The intervention group had a greater reduction in number of slips and trips and a greater improvement in role functioning related to emotional health. These improvements were achieved at no additional cost. The overall conclusion of this study is that a multifactorial, interprofessional team approach was more effective and no more expensive than usual home care in improving quality of life, reducing the incidence of slips and trips, and reducing falls among males (75 to 84 years) with a fear of falling or a negative history of falls.[159] This study is important because of the high prevalence of falls among older adults receiving home support services. The baseline fall rate of 72% in the sample greatly exceeded the fall rate of 30% typically reported for community-dwelling older adults.[83] Home care policy makers, agencies, and funders should work together to ensure that an interprofessional team approach is available to the subgroups of seniors who could benefit from it most to reduce future falls, enhance quality of life, and reduce on-demand use of health services.

Study V. Interprofessional Nurse-Led Mental Health Promotion for Older Home Care Clients with Depressive Symptoms

This one-group pretest-posttest study with a 1-year follow-up, conducted in a home care program in southern Ontario, was designed to determine the feasibility and acceptability of a new 6-month interprofessional, nurse-led mental health promotion intervention and to explore the effects of the intervention on reducing depressive symptoms in older home care clients (older than 70 years) using personal support services.[161] Of 142 participants, 98 (69%) completed the 6-month and 87 (61%) completed the 1-year follow-up. In addition to usual home care, the intervention group received monthly in-home visits by an RN and a PSW over 6 months. Each participant's treatment regimen was discussed by the RN/PSW dyad at monthly case conferences. The primary outcome was the change in severity of depressive symptoms immediately following the intervention. Secondary outcomes were changes in the prevalence of clinically significant depressive symptoms, severity of anxiety, health-related quality of life, and costs of use of health services, from a societal perspective. Results showed that the intervention was feasible and acceptable to older home care clients with depressive symptoms. It was effective in reducing depressive symptoms and improving quality of life at 6 months, with small additional improvements at 1 year. The intervention also reduced anxiety at 1 year. Significant reductions were observed in the use of hospitalization, ambulance services, and emergency room visits. The findings provide initial evidence for the feasibility, acceptability, and sustained effects of the nurse-led mental health promotion intervention in improving client outcomes, reducing use of expensive health services, and improving clinical practice behaviors of home care providers.[161]

Lessons Learned

Collectively, these studies of health promotion and disease prevention interventions suggest that, in a system of government health insurance such as in Canada, proactive, comprehensive, and integrated interventions for older adults with varying characteristics can result in better health outcomes for the same or sometimes lower cost compared with providing services on a limited, reactive, and piecemeal basis. Across these studies, subjects were assessed with different outcome measures appropriate to their circumstances, yet the same approach to economic evaluation was employed.[164] Studies III and IV of frail older home care populations illustrate that interprofessional nurse-led health promotion and disease prevention interventions, compared with on-demand care, result in improved outcomes at no more expense to society (see outcome 4, Figure 97-2). Study V provided initial evidence for the feasibility, acceptability, and sustained effects of an interprofessional nurse-led mental health promotion intervention in improving client outcomes and reducing use of expensive health services (see outcome 7, Figure 97-2). Expenditure data in these studies include the cost of the health promotion and disease prevention intervention. The studies illustrate the different kinds of economic efficiencies that are achieved with populations with more or less initial access to services.

As a whole, the results of these studies provide empirical support for the positive synergistic and cumulative effects of bolstering personal resources and environmental supports on health status and related quality of life[61] to considerable economic effect (no additional or lower expense). Health care providers need to be able to assess older adults' areas of strength and vulnerability. Awareness of the sources of vulnerability and barriers to health care may assist health care providers to provide more holistic, comprehensive care to their clients.[61]

These five studies illustrate several features of successful community-based health promotion programs for community-living older adults. First, the results show that comprehensive and coordinated services aimed at all the broad determinants of health are superior to individual, fragmented, and disease-oriented approaches to care.[34] Because health is determined by many more things than physical needs, such approaches must extend beyond the care of medical problems to address other nonmedical determinants of health.[4] This approach represents a shift away from a "replacement function" focused solely on physical needs to an "empowerment function" to enhance seniors' independence, autonomy, and problem-solving skills.[165] The results of these studies suggest that interventions that address single problems or single risk or protective factors are less effective in reducing health problems or enhancing competencies in people with synergistic risks than proactive, health-oriented, and comprehensive interventions.[35,39] In particular, there is a need for multiple health behavior interventions for older adults. Optimizing health service delivery for older adults requires a shift away from single-disease models of care.[166] It also requires access to a comprehensive range of services provided in the right amount, by the right care provider, in the right place, and at the right time.[140] There is a need for more research on complex interventions that consist of a range of interacting activities.[167,168]

Second, successful health promotion interventions need to be tailored to individual needs. The most expensive services are those that are not tailored to people's needs (or vulnerabilities).[35] No single intervention or mix of community services will meet the health promotion needs of all seniors. Hence, there is a need to classify who (with what characteristics) most benefits, and at what expense, from various interventions. Screening plays a part in targeting those who are most likely to benefit. Seniors are interested and motivated to change their behavior to enhance health. Successful behavior change is associated with the empowerment of individuals through the provision of appropriate communication, information, and support. Interventions need to respond appropriately to an individual's readiness to change through various strategies tailored to an individual's needs. Models of care should be flexible and contextualized, taking into account individual needs and comorbidities and paying particular attention to vulnerable, at-risk populations. This information can be used to target scarce resources to those most likely to benefit from preventive efforts.

Third, health promotion needs to focus on increasing self-management of long-term conditions. Self-management has been defined as "the care taken by individuals towards their own health and well-being: it comprises the actions they take to lead a healthy lifestyle; to meet their social, emotional and psychological needs; to care for their long-term condition; and to prevent further illness or accidents," and can include responding to symptoms, managing acute episodes, employing relaxation techniques, exercising, stopping smoking, managing the emotional effect of conditions, and working effectively with health professionals and other community resources.[169] Self-management may include patient education, support for decision making, self-monitoring, and psychological and social support. Self-management has the potential to make an important contribution to efficient health care delivery, by increasing client engagement in care, improving uptake of preventive activities, and reducing reliance on formal health care services by better management of existing conditions. The evidence suggests that self-management support interventions can improve health outcomes and reduce health service utilization.[169,170] Nutri-eSCREEN, a self-management Internet site based on nutrition screening and educational messages based on individualized screening results was developed to meet this need (www.nutritionscreen.ca/escreen).

Fourth, to be successful, health promotion needs to occur across multiple settings and sectors. In these studies, the interventions involved a wide range of actions operating at three levels: the individual clinician (e.g., promoting changes in practice behavior), interprofessional team (e.g., fostering interdisciplinary collaboration), and health care system (e.g., influencing the financing, management, and delivery of services). When health problems are chronic, care must be organized and coordinated over time, among providers, and across settings.[165] There is a need for a shift away from isolated, solo professionals to team-based nonconventional and conventional providers. Multisector work requires good communication and a close affiliation so that individual home and community-based services do not operate in isolation but are part of a broader, integrated approach to a comprehensive and coordinated system of services.

Fifth, models of care need to be functionally based (from the client's perspective) rather than disease based. The emphasis is on the individual's perception of health, rather than that individual's objective circumstances, and on determining his or her decision to take action. Studies focusing on patient-relevant outcomes have less emphasis on managing particular diseases and greater focus on optimizing function, reducing symptoms, and preserving independence. However, unanimity does not exist regarding which outcomes are most appropriate in different groups of older adults. Given the variability of individual preferences, it is unlikely that a single intervention or care pathway would prove feasible. There is an urgent need to develop patient-reported outcome measures in this population.[171]

Sixth, there is a need for new approaches to determining scopes of practice of individual providers. A recent report suggests that this approach needs to be (1) supportive of innovative models of care, (2) flexible so that it can respond to the varying needs of older adults, and (3) accountable to the public and funder. It should also recognize the importance of collaboration among providers as a central feature of the delivery of community-based care.[153] This aspect is particularly important for older adults with multiple chronic conditions, because no single discipline can identify and address all the factors involved in the early identification, prevention, and management of chronic health problems. Specifically, there is a need for an accountability model embedded within a collaborative community-based practice that ensures that all team members are working optimally to meet the needs of older adults and their family caregivers. Indeed, because the purpose of collaboration is to address clients' needs, clients and their caregivers should be considered true members of the team.[172] It is unrealistic to think that simply bringing providers together in teams will lead to collaboration.[173] Providers need to be motivated to start collaborating with each other.[172] Other key elements to optimizing collaborative practice include (1) a common vision, values, and philosophy; (2) mutual trust and respect; (3) effective communication; (4) education and professional development to facilitate effective collaboration; (5) clear understanding of team members' roles and responsibilities; (6) flexibility to allow each provider to practice to the full extent of his or her scope of practice; (7) adequate resources; and (8) accountability for provision of care.[153]

Finally, it is important to take a comprehensive approach to examining expenditures associated with different approaches to home and community-based care.[34] In addition to savings within the health care sector, a program might expect to see a return on its investment in other sectors.[18] Economists argue that the effect of a publicly funded home and community-based service on society as a whole should be considered when making decisions about the use of that service.[174] This comprehensive societal viewpoint is often ignored in economic analyses of health care services.[34]

BARRIERS TO IMPLEMENTATION OF SUCCESSFUL HEALTH PROMOTION PROGRAMS

There are several evidence-based recommendations on the delivery of effective health promotion programs, but numerous challenges hamper their implementation in community-based settings. Many of these challenges result from a need for considerable reorganization of the delivery of community-based health care for community-dwelling older adults with comorbid chronic conditions. Examples include physical limitations, minimal transportation services, episodic use of community-based and primary care services, limited access to services for health promotion and prevention, heavy workloads and limited time, limited follow-up care, poor coordination of existing services, insufficient provider training, lack of evidence-based treatment guidelines for older persons with comorbid chronic conditions, and poor collaboration and communication among various providers.[175] Further complicating matters, most clinical guidelines are disease-specific and do not explicitly account for the role of chronic disease (either single or multiple) or take into account clients' goals and preferences for health care.[176]

THE NEED FOR LEGISLATION AND POLICY

Despite the important role of home and community-based services in health promotion and disease prevention for older adults, several realities continue to impede this direction. Within the persistently biomedically and institutionally focused health care arena, in-home and community-based care still suffer from underfunding of services, underfunding of research to inform policy and practice, and limited consideration of the broader determinants of health.[154] Over the past couple of decades, Canada's health care system has been challenged to provide more home and community care services to older, more vulnerable, and frail individuals while limiting the growth of health care expenditures.[177-179] Between 1995 and 2000, the demand for home and community care grew by 140%,[179] attributable to several factors, namely, technologic advancements, changing demographics, patient preference, and the presumed cost-effectiveness of home care.[177] With the increasing life expectancy of Canadians, an 80% increase in home care expenditures is expected by 2026.[180]

Yet, the allocation of funding for home care has not kept pace with the increased demand for services.[179] Home care programs have been growing at an annual rate of 9.0%, compared with an annual increase of only 2.2% in average health care spending.[177] The result has been a shift in the allocation of scarce home care services away from prevention and health promotion to meet the more pressing need for post–acute care substitution.[181] This emphasis, coupled with the sustained biomedical orientation of services, has meant that the focus on prevention and health promotion for seniors with chronic needs is minimal at best.[154] The allocation of home and community services has been largely based on physical needs or medical services, suggesting that nonmedical services are unrelated to health outcomes despite evidence to the contrary.[18]

A growing body of research, done mostly within a system of government health insurance, suggests that, for older people with chronic health needs, these trends combine to create a fragmented system of health care delivery, characterized by providing health services on a reactive, episodic, and piecemeal basis, rather than a comprehensive and proactive system of care.[23,35] Delays or errors in detecting and responding to chronically ill older people's changing health needs can contribute to more complications, functional decline, negative changes in quality of life,[182] and an increased demand for expensive institutional-based care such as acute hospitalization.[35] Furthermore, experience with the acute care system often undermines chronically ill seniors' self-confidence and interest and ability to participate in their own care. The result is a vicious circle of reliance on institutionalized care.[149]

This review highlights the need for increased emphasis on health promotion and disease prevention for this population. Raphael and colleagues[183] reported that Canada was one of the few industrialized nations not to have a formal plan at various government levels to meet the evolving and complex health promotion needs of older adults. Legislation and policy at national and provincial levels are needed to move forward with this agenda. A 2008 scan of government websites revealed that policy specific to nutrition is lacking in Canada.[56] There have been recent calls for health promotion for the general population; in its December 2007 report, the Health Council of Canada presented a case for immediate, comprehensive, and sustained action to promote healthy living, prevent long-term health problems, and improve chronic illness care. Changing how the health care system works can change health outcomes.[29] Specifically, there is a need for primary prevention targeting modifiable risk factors in older adults. To address effectively the growing burden of chronic disease and frailty in older people living in the community, healthy home and community care policies are needed to provide vision, set priorities, and establish standards. Such policies and standards should support the development of basic competencies for health promotion and disease prevention among providers, as well as systemic changes within home and community care organizations to allow the allocation of adequate resources for assessment of risk and delivery of health promotion and prevention strategies. There is a need to move away from a "find it and fix it" episodic orientation that does not match the ongoing care needs of older people with chronic conditions, who need a "find it, manage it, and prevent it" approach.[29]

Despite the crucial role of family caregivers in managing the health of older adults, support for them is lacking, is inconsistently available, or does not completely meet their needs. This lack of support can have a negative effect on the physical and mental health of caregivers and on their personal and professional lives, as well as on the quality of care that they provide.[184] As reported by a forum of Canada's leading cancer, mental health, and caregiver groups, "Failure to recognize, acknowledge and support family caregivers heightens their risk of becoming 'collateral casualties' of the illness, compromises their health, reduces the efficacy of the help they can provide to their relatives, and increases costs to the health and social service systems."[184] Including older adults and their caregivers in the development of health care plans is beneficial (e.g., improved self-esteem for patients, updated and improved patient-information resources, and organizational attitudes that are supportive to patient involvement).[185] Community-based health promotion programs need to shift from a patient-focused approach to a combined patient- and caregiver-focused approach that addresses the needs of family caregivers. Ongoing support for family caregivers of community-living older adults with chronic conditions should be an essential component of a publicly funded health care system.

Home and community-based programs need to provide a continuum of services, including health promotion, prevention, and post–acute care substitution services.[177] Enhanced funding and focused health promotion and disease prevention activities should be applied to mitigate the risk factors for functional decline and loss of independence, so that living at home, even with significant challenges, can become a true reality for older persons. Without this legislation and resource provision, improvements in the health of older adults will continue to be an ad hoc affair with limited effect.[38]

THE NEED FOR MORE RESEARCH

With the increasing demand for home and community-based services for older people, there is increasing pressure for evidence to show that community-based health promotion and disease prevention for older people is an efficient use of health care resources in developed countries.[186] A report for policy makers by the World Health Organization[28] on the future direction of health promotion evaluation emphasized the need for evidence about effective and efficient health promotion and disease prevention strategies. This evidence is needed to ensure that the most appropriate services are available to people who most need them so that the best health outcomes can be attained.[179] However, our knowledge base concerning the role for health promotion and secondary prevention in older people remains small.[26,38] Further investigation is needed regarding the most efficacious ways of providing health promotion and disease prevention to the different groups with successful, usual, or accelerated aging. These groups have different needs, risks factors, and health conditions, and they experience different barriers and facilitators to health promotion.[187]

Older adults experiencing accelerated aging have been identified as being at increased risk for functional decline, institutionalization, and death,[12] but these individuals are often excluded in community-based trials.[188] There is a need to establish a knowledge base about the needs of this vulnerable group. Understanding which factors in the individual and the environment are most predictive of morbidity and use of health services is essential to move forward with health promotion efforts in this group.

Large randomized trials are required to test new and innovative approaches to health promotion and secondary prevention strategies for community-living older adults. Such studies should provide information on client-important outcomes, such as functional health status and related quality of life, mental health, and social support. They should also address more process-oriented outcomes associated with health promotion, such as autonomy, empowerment, and decision making.[146] Such studies should also compare outcomes achieved with different providers and different combinations of providers to inform how best to meet the needs of this client group. Future research also needs to incorporate a full economic evaluation and identify the subgroups of clients that will benefit most.

A major gap in the research on home-based health promotion is the lack of a theoretical framework.[39] As a result, it is difficult to assess the appropriateness of the intervention to the outcomes being measured or to formulate hypotheses regarding why or how a particular intervention should be expected to result in a particular outcome.[37,150] Future research should use a theoretical framework and provide descriptive and contextual details about the health promotion strategies and measures of process to enable their replication and provide information about why an intervention was or was not found to be effective.[189] Further testing of the vulnerability model is needed to provide a knowledge base for designing and evaluating health promotion strategies.

Finally, research is needed on older adults' awareness and perceived need for health promotion. Despite being identified as at risk and having an awareness of the benefits associated with certain health behaviors, not all older adults decide to make positive behavioral changes.[187] Furthermore, some people, such as the oldest cohorts and women, may be less likely to change health behaviors,[190] and it may be necessary to target strategies to these groups. Qualitative studies would help identify the processes involved in the decision to change behavior, including the factors that influence compliance with recommendations. This information could be used to identify the most effective ways of supporting health promotion behavioral change to ultimately improve older adults' quality of life.

Overall, future research should assist with targeting limited home and community resources and improving the effectiveness of efforts. A 2006 discussion paper titled *Healthy Aging in Canada* identifies the need for a home and community care research and knowledge development agenda and the transfer of what is learned in ways that policy makers, practitioners, seniors, and their families can understand and use.[191]

KEY POINTS

- Prevention of chronic disease and frailty needs to be a focus of health and community services to meet the challenges of the growing older adult population; policy and legislation are currently lacking to support this investment in prevention.
- Many chronic diseases and their accumulated deficits that lead to frailty have a common basis that is potentially preventable; smoking, obesity, poor-quality diets, sedentary behaviors, and stress are key targets for preventive efforts.
- Community providers can screen for risk (e.g., nutrition risk/malnutrition, depression, falls) in older adults to identify those who need and should receive preventive programs and services.
- Successful health promotion programs that address various risk factors have been developed and evaluated and can be used as models for future program development and evaluation.
- Segmenting the older adult population into groups of successful, usual, and accelerated aging can help to develop and target health promotion services; further tailoring to the individual's needs and risks is paramount for successful health promotion.

Acknowledgments

Dr. Maureen Markle-Reid holds a Tier 2 Canada Research Chair in Aging, Chronic Disease and Health Promotion Interventions from the Canadian Institutes of Health Research (CIHR) (2012-2017). She is the co-founder and director of the Aging, Community and Health Research Unit, funded by the Ontario Ministry of Health and Long-Term Care and CIHR. She received a Career Scientist Award (2004–2009) from the Ontario Ministry of Health and Long-Term Care, Health Research Personnel Development Fund, which allowed her to complete much of her work on health promotion interventions cited in this chapter.

Dr. Heather Keller is a research chair with the Schlegel-UW Research Institute for Aging (2012-2017). She received a New Investigator Research Award (2000-2006) from CIHR, which allowed her to complete much of her work on screening and community nutrition education interventions cited in this chapter.

Dr. Gina Browne is the founder and director of the System-Linked Research Unit, funded by the Ontario Ministry of Health and Long-Term Care, which supported many of the studies cited in this chapter.

For a complete list of references, please visit www.expertconsult.com.

KEY REFERENCES

24. Markle-Reid M, Browne G: Conceptualizations of frailty in relation to older adults. J Adv Nurs 44:58–68, 2003.
35. Browne G, Roberts J, Byrne C, et al: The costs and effects of addressing the needs of vulnerable populations: results of 10 years of research. Can J Nurs Res 33:65–76, 2001.
38. Keller HH: Promoting food intake in older adults living in the community: a review. Appl Physiol Nutr Metab 32:991–1000, 2007.
39. Markle-Reid M, Weir R, Browne G, et al: The effectiveness and efficiency of home-based nursing health promotion for older people: a review of the literature. Med Care Res Rev 63:531–569, 2006a.
40. Markle-Reid M, Weir R, Browne G, et al: Health promotion for frail older home care clients. J Adv Nurs 54:381–395, 2006b.
44. Payette H, Shatenstein B: Determinants of healthy eating in community-dwelling elderly people. Can J Public Health 96(Suppl): S27–S31, 2005.
87. Gillespie LD, Robertson MC, Gillespie WJ, et al: Interventions for preventing falls in older people living in the community. Cochrane Database Syst Rev (9):CD007146, 2012.
92. Federal/Provincial/Territorial Committee of Officials (Seniors) for the Minister Responsible for Seniors: A best practices guide for the prevention of falls among seniors living in the community, Ottawa, Ontario, 2001, Minister of Public Works and Government Services Canada.
94. American Dietetic Association: Position paper of the American Dietetic Association: Nutrition across the spectrum of aging. J Am Diet Assoc 105:616–633, 2005.
96. Green SM, Watson R: Nutritional screening and assessment tools for older adults: literature review. J Adv Nurs 54:477–490, 2006.
98. Ramage-Morin PL, Garriguet D: Nutritional risk among older Canadians. Health Rep 24:3–13, 2013.
100. Roberts KC, Wolfson C, Payette H: Predictors of nutritional risk in community-dwelling seniors. Can J Public Health 98:331–336, 2007.
106. Sorensen J, Kondrup J, Prokopowica J, et al: EuroOOPS: an international, multicentre study to implement nutritional risk screening and evaluate clinical outcome. Clin Nutr 27:340–349, 2008.
113. Ayalon L, Fialova D, Arean PA, et al: Challenges associated with the recognition and treatment of depression in older recipients of home care services. Int Psychogeriatr 22:514–522, 2010.
114. Ell K: Depression care for the elderly: reducing barriers to evidence-based practice. Home Health Care Serv Q 25:115–148, 2006.
133. Brown EL, Bruce ML, McAvay GJ, et al: Recognition of late-life depression in home care: accuracy of the outcome and assessment information set. J Am Geriatr Soc 52:995–999, 2004.
139. MacMillan HL, Patterson CL, Wathen CN: Screening for depression in primary care: recommendation statement from the Canadian Task Force on Preventive Health Care. CMAJ 172:33–35, 2005.
143. Keller HH, Goy R, Kane SL: Validity and reliability of SCREEN II (seniors in the community: risk evaluation for eating and nutrition—version II). Eur J Clin Nutr 59:1149–1157, 2005a.
153. Nelson S, Turnbull J, Bainbridge L, et al: Optimizing scopes of practice: new models for a new health care system, Ottawa, Ontario, 2014, Canadian Academy of Health Sciences.
157. Keller HH, Hedley M, Hadley T, et al: Food workshops, nutrition education and older adults: a process evaluation. J Nutr Elder 24:5–23, 2005b.
159. Markle-Reid M, Browne G, Gafni A, et al: The effects and costs of a multifactorial and interdisciplinary team approach to falls prevention for older home care clients "at risk" for falling: a randomized controlled trial. Can J Aging 29:139–161, 2010.
160. Markle-Reid M, Browne G, Gafni A: Nurse-led health promotion interventions improve quality of life in frail older home care clients: lessons learned from three randomized trials in Ontario, Canada. J Eval Clin Pract 19:118–131, 2011.
161. Markle-Reid M, McAiney C, Forbes D, et al: An interprofessional nurse-led mental health promotion intervention for older home care clients with depressive symptoms. BMC Geriatr 14:62, 2014.
169. Panagioti M, Richardson G, Small N, et al: Self-management support interventions to reduce health care utilization without compromising outcomes: a systematic review and meta-analysis. BMC Health Serv Res 14:356, 2014.
191. Federal/ Provincial/Territorial Committee of Officials (Seniors) for the Minister Responsible for Seniors. Healthy aging in Canada: a new vision, a vital investment from evidence to action. 2006. http://www.swsd.gov.nl.ca/publications/pdf/seniors/vision_rpt_e.pdf. Accessed November 30, 2015.

98 Sexuality in Old Age

Carien G. Hartmans

INTRODUCTION

Sexuality, sexual behavior, and intimacy are considered aspects of quality of life and remain important throughout all phases of life. Sexuality is also associated with physical health, which makes it even more important to understand and address sexual function in late life.[1] However, knowledge and attitudes about sexuality in older adults is still limited.[2,3] Most studies focus on frequency of sexual activity and report a decrease in older adults.[4] Furthermore, there is no unified definition of sexuality in later life, making it difficult to interpret or compare the available data. Studies that use a broad definition of sexuality and sexual behavior indicate how a percentage of older adults report continuance of sexual activity, feelings of desire, and intimate relationships throughout their lives.[5-8]

During a medical examination, the sexuality of older patients is often not discussed by physicians, and older patients are reluctant to bring up the subject themselves.[9] Personal beliefs, stereotyped views, and lack of professional medical education are the main reasons for neglecting late-life sexuality during a medical examination. As a result, physicians may fail to diagnose sexual dysfunction and recommend treatment possibilities. Discussing sexuality in later life can offer older patients reassurance about the normal changes in sexuality that may be troubling them. Furthermore, patients should be informed about the possible side effects of medications that can affect sexual behavior negatively.[10]

The psychological effect of a sexual problem usually affects both patient and partner. For example, in heart patients, fear of another heart attack or even death during intercourse may interfere with the patient's and partner's ability to perform and enjoy having sex.[11] Involvement of the partner is an important indicator for therapy to be successful or effective. Psychosexual treatments can vary, ranging from basic sex education through improved partner communication to cognitive behavioral therapy.[12]

SEXUALITY IN OLDER MEN AND WOMEN

The World Health Organization (WHO) defines sexuality as follows[13]:

> *Sexuality is a central aspect of being human throughout life and encompasses sex, gender identities and roles, sexual orientation, eroticism, pleasure, intimacy and reproduction. Sexuality is experienced and expressed in thoughts, fantasies, desires, beliefs, attitudes, values, behaviors, practices, roles and relationships. While sexuality can include all of these dimensions, not all of them are always experienced or expressed. Sexuality is influenced by the interaction of biological, psychological, social, economic, political, cultural, ethical, legal, historical, religious and spiritual factors.*

This broad definition underlines the various aspects of how sexuality can be expressed and the variety of difficulties that may occur. However, it also clarifies how asking about the frequency of sexual activity alone is not enough. A study on the perception of sexuality among older adults (mean age, 71 years; 54% women) showed that 42% of respondents agreed that sexuality was still important, and almost 70% reported a continued need for touch and intimacy.[8] The phases of the sexual response cycle—desire, excitement, and orgasm—remain the same throughout life, although it may take longer to become aroused and more stimulation may be needed.[14] Intimacy also remains important in later life; studies have shown that infrequent sexual touching can be associated with arousal and orgasm difficulties in men and women.[15]

Physical problems associated with acute and chronic diseases are more prevalent in older adults. In addition to the physical effects of a medical condition, patients often regard the sexual loss or inability to engage in sexual activity to be the most devastating aspect of their condition.[16] As such, awareness of psychological effects during treatment of a medical condition is essential and requires a holistic approach.

Male Sexuality

With aging, the male orgasm may last a shorter time, with a decreased force of ejaculation and the volume of ejaculate. Increased blood flow through the paired cavernosal arteries is the main mechanism for obtaining an erection.[17] Erectile dysfunction (ED) is characterized as the inability to maintain an erection during intercourse. Studies on prevalence data have reported that 10% of men in their 60s, 15% of men in their 70s, and 30% to 40% of men in their 80s suffer from ED.[18]

ED may be an early warning sign of a medical condition, such as diabetes, heart disease, and hypertension.[19] Most ED cases have physical causes, including vascular, neurologic, and endocrine disorders (Table 98-1).[10,20] Structural abnormalities such as Peyronie disease (incidence, 0.39% to 3.2%) also affect sexual activity.[21]

Surgical procedures and the use of medication and substances may also lead to sexual problems (Tables 98-2 and 98-3).[10,20,22]

Finally, psychological causes, such as performance anxiety, can also adversely affect sexuality and lead to ED. As described earlier, cardiovascular patients may experience performance anxiety, which interferes with one's ability to perform and enjoy having sex.[11]

Sildenafil, tadalafil, and vardenafil are three potent selective phosphodiesterase type 5 (PDE5) inhibitors approved by the U.S. Food and Drug Administration (FDA) and the European Medicines Agency (EMA) with proven efficacy and safety in treating ED. Avanafil was recently approved by the FDA and EMA and works similarly to sildenafil, tadalafil, and vardenafil. Alternative treatments for ED include vacuum devices, intracavernosal drugs, and penile prosthetic implants.[12] Penile revascularization surgery is also a treatment possibility but is mainly effective in men who younger than 50 years.[17]

Although several natural preparations claim to treat sexual problems, including erectile problems, research about effectiveness and possible side effects is still limited. Use of over-the-counter preparations such as yohimbine should be determined by physicians because of possible interaction with prescription medications. The studies on yohimbine have reported several side effects, such as increased blood pressure and tachycardia.[23]

Female Sexuality

Research shows that a lack of interest in sex and inability to reach orgasm are frequent in women, but are not so dependent on aging.[24] In general, healthy older women report feelings of desire and can continue their earlier patterns of sexual behavior,

TABLE 98-1 Effects of Medical Conditions on Sexuality

Medical Condition	Effect on Sexuality	Treatment
Arthritis	Sexual desire is usually unaffected, but disability due to osteoarthritis and rheumatoid arthritis may interfere with performance.	Trying sexual positions that do not aggravate joint pain; planning sexual activity for times of day when pain and stiffness are diminished
Chronic emphysema and bronchitis	Shortness of breath hinders physical activity, including sex.	Rest, supplemental oxygen
Chronic prostatitis	Pain may diminish sexual desire.	Antibiotics, warm sitz baths, prostatic massage, Kegel exercises
Chronic renal disease	Impotence, possibly with anxiety and depression	Dialysis, psychotherapy for underlying emotional problems, kidney transplantation may restore sexual capacity
Diabetes mellitus	Impotence is common.	Very tight control of diabetes may restore potency
Heart and vascular disease		
Myocardial infarction	8- to 14-wk recuperation period recommended before resuming sexual intercourse; depression and antidepressant drugs may reduce libido and capacity; fear of bringing on another heart attack if patient resumes sexual activity.	Reassurance from the physician about safety of sexual activity, exercise programs to improve cardiac function
Heart failure	Sexual dysfunction resulting from physical symptoms or medications; a 2- to 3-wk week recovery period is advised before resuming sex in cases of pulmonary edema.	Reassurance from the physician about safety of sexual activity for patients with effectively managed heart failure, exercise programs to improve cardiac function
Coronary bypass surgery	Abstinence for at least 4 wk is recommended before resuming sexual intercourse.	Alternatives such as self-stimulation or masturbation can usually be started earlier in recovery period, exercise programs to improve cardiac function
Pelvic steal syndrome	Example of vascular impotence—male loses erection as soon as he enters his partner and begins pelvic thrusting due to gravity's redirecting blood supply away from the pelvis.	Changing position may help (man should lie on his back or side)
Hypertension	Incidence of impotence in untreated male hypertensive patients is about 15%; effects on women have not been established.	Choose hypertensive drugs that do not impair sexual response.
Parkinson disease	Lack of sexual desire in men and women; impotence in men	Levodopa can improve sex drive and performance in some men for a limited period.
Peyronie disease	Intercourse is painful for many men with the disease; penetration may be difficult or impossible when penis is angled too sharply.	Psychotherapy to help patient adjust to changes in the penis; symptoms occasionally disappear spontaneously; surgery helps in some cases.
Stress incontinence	Sexual dysfunction has been reported in up to 50% of women with this condition.	Solving the underlying problem may help. Kegel exercises to strengthen muscles supporting bladder. estrogen taken orally or locally to firm up vaginal lining. biofeedback training
Stroke	Sexual desire may not be impaired, but sexual performance is likely to be affected (e.g., male erectile dysfunction because of physical or psychological reasons, anesthetic areas, or physical limitations due to paralysis).	Mechanical adjustments to assist positioning necessary for sexual activities. treatments for impotence

TABLE 98-2 Effects of Surgery on Sexuality

Surgical Procedure	Effect on Sexuality
Hysterectomy	Need to refrain from sexual activity during healing (6-8 wk after surgery), depression, possible reduction in sensation during orgasm
Mastectomy	Emotional reactions such as depression, loss of sexual desire because of emotional reactions of patient and partner
Prostatectomy	Need to refrain from sexual activity during healing (6 wk), possible impotence because of surgery (nerve-sparing techniques help avoid this effect in some cases), possible psychogenic impotence
Orchiectomy	Impotence common
Colostomy and ileostomy	Emotional reactions that can affect desire and potency (participation in ostomy clubs recommended)
Rectal cancer surgery	Impotence common

Modified from Butler RN, Lewis MI: Sexuality. In In Beers M, editor: Merck manual of geriatrics, ed 3, Whitehouse Station, NJ, 2000, Merck, pp 1156-1164; and Butler RN, Lewis MI: The new love and sex after 60, New York, 2000, Ballantine Books.

including maintaining orgasmic capacity. However, with aging, there is less vasocongestion. A decline of sexual hormone levels influences sexuality after menopause. Although some women report an increased sexual interest, for most women menopause negatively interacts with aging, resulting in emotional and physical problems (e.g., mood swings, sleep deprivation, changed sexual desire, poor arousal and lubrication, dyspareunia, lack of satisfaction).[25] As such, a multidisciplinary approach is essential in managing female sexual dysfunction. Health care providers can contribute significantly to healthy aging and partnership by enhancing coping strategies in women facing sexual changes in midlife.

Hormone replacement therapy (HRT) can help relieve some of the menopausal symptoms. The long-term effects of hormone therapy have been studied by the National Institutes of Health's Women's Health Initiative (WHI), which ended early because results indicated an increased risk of stroke, breast cancer, thromboembolic complications, and coronary heart disease in women who received both estrogen and progestin compared to placebo. However, further WHI subanalyses and other recent studies have shown how the use of HRT can be considered, but this needs to be carefully assessed by analyzing risks and benefits of the therapy for each individual woman.[26,27]

TABLE 98-3 Selected Medications and Substances That May Adversely Affect Sexual Functioning

Psychotropics	β-Blockers
• Tricyclic antidepressants	• Propranolol
• Clomipramine	• Atenolol
• Amitriptyline	• Metoprolol
• Doxepin	• Bisoprolol
• Imipramine	• Timolol
• Nortriptyline*	• Betaxolol
• Desipramine*	α_1-Blockers
Monoamine oxidase inhibitors	• Prazosin*
• Isocarboxazid	• Doxazosin*
• Phenelzine	α_2-Agonists
• Tranylcypromine*	• Clonidine
Serotonin reuptake inhibitors	• Guanfacine
• Fluoxetine	ACE inhibitors‡
• Paroxetine	• Captopril*
• Sertraline	• Enalapril
• Fluvoxamine	Calcium channel blockers
• Venlafaxine	• Amlodipine
Mood stabilizers and anticonvulsants	• Verapamil
	• Diltiazem
• Lithium†	Anticancer drugs
• Valproate*	• Vinblastine
• Carbamazepine	• 5-Fluorouracil
• Phenytoin	• Tamoxifen
• Phenobarbital	Cold and allergy medications
Antipsychotics and neuroleptics	• Chlorpheniramine
	• Diphenhydramine hydrochloride
• Phenothiazines	• Pseudoephedrine
• Chlorpromazine	Antiulcer medications
• Fluphenazine*	• Cimetidine
• Perphenazine	• Famotidine*
• Thioridazine	• Nizatidine*
Other	• Ranitidine*
• Haloperidol	Stimulants and anorectics
• Thiothixene	• Phentermine
• Risperidone	• Fenfluramine
Antianxiety agents and tranquilizers	• Phenylpropanolamine
	• Diethylpropion
• Benzodiazepines	• Mazindol
Diuretics	Commonly abused substances
• Thiazide-type	• Alcohol
• Chlorthalidone	• Barbiturates
• Hydrochlorothiazide	• Cannabis
• Indapamide*	• Cocaine
Loop diuretics	• Opioids
Potassium-sparing	• Methylphenidate
• Spironolactone	• Amphetamine
Antihypertensives	• Nicotine
• Reserpine	Hormones
• Methyldopa	• Progesterone
• Guanethidine	• Cortisol

Modified from Crenshaw TL, Goldberg JP: Sexual pharmacology: drugs that affect sexual functioning, New York, 1996, WW Norton.

*Studies indicate that these drugs may have fewer sexual side effects than others in their class.

†Direct sexual side effects of lithium are confirmed only when it is taken in conjunction with benzodiazepines.

‡ACE inhibitors have fewer sexual side effects than other classes of antihypertensives.

Alternative interventions may include exercise, diet, and nonhormonal drugs, such as bisphosphonates. Off-prescription, water-based vaginal lubricants can relief vaginal dryness, irritation, and pain during intercourse. Prescription drugs for cholesterol and blood pressure can lower the risk of heart disease.[4,28,29]

As in men, surgery in women can also result in impaired sexual functioning and capacity. Embarrassment after surgical procedures such as a mastectomy can negatively affect sexual interest and sexual functioning (see Table 98-2).[10,20] Substance abuse (e.g., alcohol, tobacco) and medications can also lead to sexual problems (see Table 98-3).[22]

Another factor that might influence female sexual behavior in later life is longevity. In comparison to men, women live longer and, in general, outlive their partners and may not get romantically involved in the remaining years.

MEDICAL EXAMINATION

Sexual problems reported by the older patient should not be considered a mere consequence of aging, but as a response to stressors in multiple life domains. This in turn affects both patient and partner.[12,30]

A medical evaluation of older patients should include questions about sexual history, current sexual function, and desires. The physician should initiate the conversation about sexual behavior and sexual concerns because older patients may not volunteer information about their sex life themselves. Physicians need to familiarize themselves with the effects of neurologic, circulatory, and endocrine disorders on sexuality. A discussion of sexual functioning in later life should inform the older patient on how sexual problems are not automatically considered to be a result of aging, but may be a possible indicator of underlying physical problems.[31]

The physician should also be aware that age itself does not protect patients from sexually transmitted diseases (STDs). Almost 25% percent of all AIDS patients in the United States are older than 50 years, and not all of them contracted HIV through blood transfusions.[32]

Sexual dysfunction in men and women can also be caused by emotional or relational problems. When identified, these patients should be referred for psychological or psychosexual treatment. Also, asking about marital status alone is not enough, because one can be involved in a romantic relationship or practice solo sex (self-gratification).

Finally, physicians need to be aware of alternative sexual expression.[4] A recent survey has found that 1.9% of older adults (≥65 years) identify themselves as lesbian, gay, bisexual, or transgender (LGBT).[33] Many LGBT individuals are involved in long-term relationships. Sexual problems reported by LGBT couples involve many of the same interpersonal, physical, social, and psychological problems as those faced by heterosexual couples.[31]

EFFECTS OF MEDICAL PROBLEMS, SURGERY, AND MEDICATIONS

Sexuality and Illness

Several diseases and mental illnesses can have a huge impact on sexual desire, sexuality, and sexual functioning. For example, loss of libido is often reported by patients diagnosed with depression either because of the condition itself or as a side effect of using antidepressants. Some of the most common disorders that can adversely affect sexual functioning are heart failure, stroke, and diabetes. Cardiovascular patients and their partners often report fear of renewed sexual activity. With the increased heart rate during intercourse, they may fear inducing another heart attack. So, they may refrain from expressing sexual behavior in ways prior to the condition, which in turn might lead to feelings of depression in patient and partner. Physicians should inform patients and their partners how sexual activity is not contraindicated because the highest energy expenditure during sexual activity does not exceed oxygen usage compared to climbing three flights of stairs or performing general housework activities.[19]

Other medical conditions known to affect sexuality significantly are osteoarthritis and rheumatoid arthritis, back pain, Parkinson disease, dementia, chronic emphysema and bronchitis, chronic prostatitis in men, and stress incontinence in women (see Table 98-1).[10,20]

Sexuality and Medication

Medications can affect sexual functioning and sexual desire and cause sexual dysfunction. Whenever possible, physicians should consider prescribing a lower dosage, which may avoid or limit the negative side effects on sexual functioning.[22] For example, wellbutrin is one of the least problematic antidepressant drugs. In case of hypertension, angiotensin-converting enzyme (ACE) inhibitors are less apt to cause sexual dysfunction than methyldopa. Widely used prescribed medications that adversely affect sexuality are listed in Table 98-3.[22]

Sexuality and Cognitive Functioning

Early human experiments measured pleasurable feelings through deep brain stimulation of the amygdala, and later studies reported how neurologic disease can alter the sexual response. The amygdala has a central role in emotional processing, learning, and memory. While engaging in sexual activity, other brain regions and structures are also activated. For example, the parietal lobes and other higher cortical regions are associated with cognitive, emotional, and sensorimotor aspects of central control of sexual behavior, whereas the hypothalamus coordinates activation of the autonomic aspects of sexual drive.[16]

The aging process is strongly associated with cognitive functioning and with increasing age, a certain decline in cognitive functioning is inevitable. Understanding the extent of cognitive decline of older patients is essential because sexual behavior, like any type of behavior, is initiated by the brain. Two studies have shown how sexual activity is associated with better overall cognitive functioning.[5,34]

The role of cognitive functioning is important throughout the entire sexual response cycle—desire, excitement, and orgasm. Interpretation of genital sensations and sensory stimulation is necessary for sexual arousal (Figure 98-1).[35]

Complex executive functions such as decision making and memory are essential to perform in all stages of the sexual response cycle. Simply being aroused is not enough to reach the orgasmic phase. Decisions making processes involve judgment, the capacity to consent to sex, and a sense of self and others. These processes may then lead to the motor responses necessary for further engagement and finally reaching the orgasmic phase. Memory is also important, because the person has to remember previous actions, experiences, and nature of the current relationship.[35]

In neurodegenerative disorders such as dementia, all areas of life are affected due to progressive declines in social, behavioral, and cognitive functioning, which in turn are associated with sexual functioning. Although discussing sexuality with older patients is often neglected, discussing this topic in case of dementia seems to be even more controversial. Data on the frequency of sexual activity in those with dementia are limited, but the results have shown a continuance of sexual activity in a percentage of dementia patients and their spouses.[36-38]

Dementia disrupts the equality and reciprocity in a relationship because partners also have to become caregivers. The stage of dementia, quality of the past sexual relationship, and perceived impact of the diagnosis are some of the aspects that interact with one's sexual capacities or need for sexual expression and activity in patient and partner. A study on sexual satisfaction in mild to moderately demented outpatients and their spouses has reported sexual activity by 64% of the patients and 56% of the spouses. One third of the female and male patients reported dissatisfaction with the sexual activity.[38]

Demented patients may experience a decrease or increase in libido. Before prescribing medication for sexual problems in demented patients, the physician should evaluate the current sexual relationship with patient and partner because patients may have different needs than their partners. Inappropriate sexual behavior is also reported, which may be a direct result of impaired cognitive functioning expressed as the inability to take into account the contextual environment or feelings of others or as disinhibition.[39]

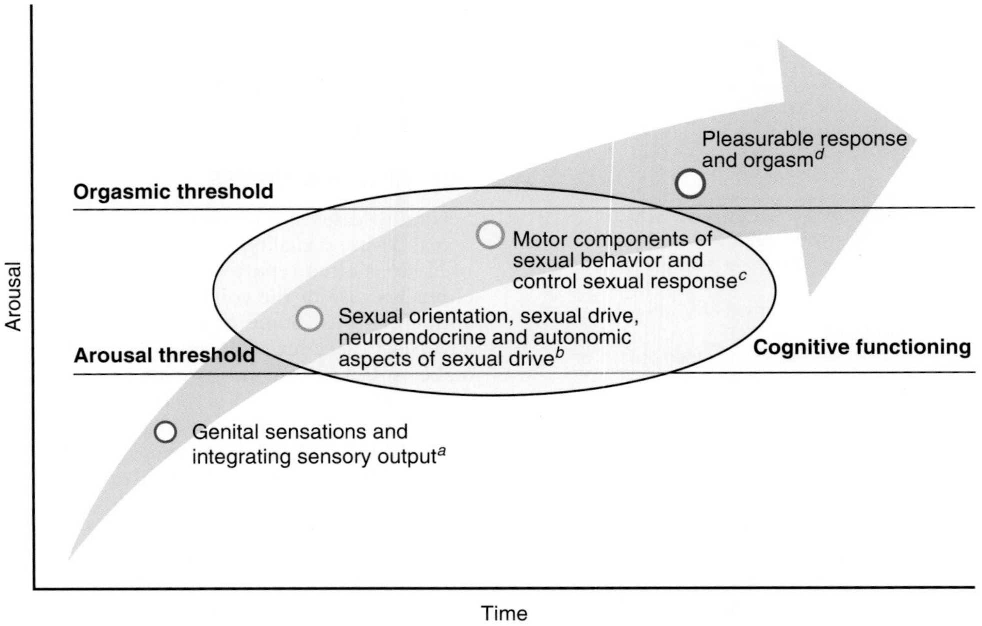

a: Parietal lobes; *b*: Amygdala, ansa lenticularis, globus pallidus, and hypothalamus; *c*: Frontal lobes; *d*: Septal region.

Figure 98-1. Cognitive functioning in the process of sexual functioning.

LET'S TALK ABOUT SEX

Sexuality is one of the indicators of quality of life and, as such, sexuality remains important throughout life. Research has shown how a percentage of older adults report sexual activity in late life. In general, those older patients who value their earlier sexual relationships as satisfying can continue to do so in later life but it may take longer to become aroused, and more stimulation is needed to reach a climax. Health care workers and physicians need to be aware of the continued need for intimacy, sexual expression, and sexual activity in older patients. When older patients are informed about sexuality and the normal changes due to aging and changes due to a medical condition, they are offered an opportunity to redefine what sexuality means to them. The information can further enable older patients to maintain a meaningful form of physical intimacy.[40] Knowledge about sexual feelings and desires should also provide the physician with information on which medical treatment can be based. Patients with an active sexual life should, to some extent, be able to decide with their physician about taking prescription medication with the least side effects. For those who report no longer being sexually active, higher dosages or other medications may be considered. Furthermore, whenever possible, partners should also be involved during treatment and informed about the influence of the medical condition or medication on sexual functioning. In addition to discussing physical limitations and side effects, physicians should also inquire about psychological functioning because a medical condition may cause feelings of depression or anxiety in patient and partner. If necessary, they can be referred for psychological treatment.

Finally, sexual functioning is also associated with cognitive functioning. The extent of impaired cognitive functioning, as seen in case of neurologic damage or dementia, may negatively influence one's capability for sexual performance in all stages of the sexual response cycle.

CONCLUSION

Physicians should acknowledge their personal values and attitudes regarding sex and sexuality in later life, as well as the values and attitudes of older patients. They should integrate sexual functioning (history and current) during a medical examination or treatment because medical conditions can adversely affect sexuality. Sexual problems such as erectile dysfunction can also be an early warning sign of a medical condition. Most older patients are willing to talk about their sexual concerns but are reluctant to start the discussion. They should therefore be invited by the physician, who in turn needs to be able to talk about sex freely and in a comforting manner. Older patients are usually unaware of how sexual difficulties can be related to a medical condition and are often not informed about treatment possibilities or side effects of medications.

KEY POINTS

- Research has shown continued sexual functioning in older adults. Physicians should initiate questions about sexual history, current functioning, and desire during a medical examination.
- Sexual functioning can be adversely affected by medical conditions, surgery, and medications. The physician should provide basic management including explanation, suggestions, and, if necessary, drugs.
- The phases of the sexual response cycle (desire, excitement, and orgasm) remain the same throughout life, although it may take longer to become aroused, and more stimulation is needed.
- Sexual problems may have a physical cause, but can also be psychologically induced. Patients and their partners should then be referred to a psychologist for treatment.
- Medical conditions that often influence sexuality are cardiovascular disease, diabetes, osteoarthritis and rheumatoid arthritis, Parkinson disease, chronic emphysema and bronchitis, chronic prostatitis in men, and stress incontinence in women.
- Sexual functioning and expression in later life may be influenced by impaired cognitive functioning or dementia.

For a complete list of references, please visit www.expertconsult.com.

KEY REFERENCES

3. Snyder RJ, Zweig RA: Medical and psychology students' knowledge and attitudes regarding aging and sexuality. Gerontol Geriatr Educ 31:235–255, 2010.
4. Lindau ST, Schumm P, Laumann EO, et al: A study of sexuality and health among older adults in the United States. N Engl J Med 357:762–774, 2007.
5. Padoani W, Dello Buono M, Marietta P, et al: Influence of cognitive status on the sexual life of 352 elderly Italians aged 65-105 years. Gerontology 46:258–265, 2000.
8. Hartmans C, Comijs H, Jonker C: The perception of sexuality in older adults and its relationship with cognitive functioning. Am J Geriatr Psychiatry 23:243–252, 2015.
10. Butler RN, Lewis MI: Sexuality. In Beers M, editor: Merck manual of geriatrics, ed 3, Whitehouse Station, NJ, 2000, Merck, pp 1156–1164.
11. Mandras SA, Uber PA, Mehra MR: Sexual activity and chronic heart failure. Mayo Clin Proc 82:1203–1210, 2007.
12. McMahon CG: Erectile dysfunction. Intern Med J 44:18–26, 2014.
16. Rees PM, Fowler CJ, Maas CP: Sexual dysfunction in men and women with neurological disorders. Lancet 369:512–525, 2007.
17. Dabaja AA, Teloken P, Mulhall JP: A critical analysis of candidacy for penile revascularization. J Sex Med 11:2327–2332, 2014.
19. Jaarsma T, Fridlund B, Mårtensson J: Sexual dysfunction in heart failure patients. Curr Heart Fail Rep 11:330–336, 2014.
20. Butler RN, Lewis MI: The new love after 60, New York, 2000, Ballantine Books.
22. Crenshaw TL, Goldberg JP: Sexual pharmacology: drugs that affect sexual functioning, New York, 1996, WW Norton.
31. Butler RN, Lewis MI: Sexuality in old age. In Fillit HM, Rockwood K, Woodhouse K, editors: Brocklehurst's textbook of geriatric medicine and gerontology, ed 7, Philadelphia, 2010, Saunders, pp 854–858.
35. Hartmans C, Comijs H, Jonker C: Cognitive functioning and its influence on sexual behavior in normal aging and dementia. Int J Geriatr Psychiatry 29:441–446, 2014.
38. Dourado M, Finamore C, Barrosa MF, et al: Sexual satisfaction in dementia: perspectives of patients and spouses. Sex Disabil 28:195–203, 2010.
39. Eloniemi-Sulkava U, Notkola IL, Hämäläinen K, et al: Spouse caregiver's perceptions of influence of dementia on marriage. Int Psychogeriatr 14:47–58, 2002.

99 Physical Activity for Successful Aging

Olga Theou, Debra J. Rose

INTRODUCTION

Regular participation in physical activity is associated with positive and meaningful outcomes in older adults.[1-4] Physical inactivity has been linked to all-cause mortality, functional decline, nursing home admissions, health care spending, and increased risk for common chronic diseases and conditions such as coronary heart disease, hypertension, stroke, metabolic syndrome, type 2 diabetes, breast and colon cancer, cognitive disorders, depression, falls, obesity, osteoporosis, and sarcopenia. Increased physical activity is associated with reduced pain, decreased risk of injury, and improved emotional health, confidence level, and quality of life. Virtually every system in the human body is affected in some way by physical activity. The World Health Organization has identified physical inactivity as the fourth leading risk factor for global mortality, after high blood pressure, tobacco use, and high blood glucose levels.[5] Worldwide, 5.3 million deaths annually are attributed to inactivity, and eliminating inactivity is expected to increase the world's population lifespan by 0.68 years. If inactivity were reduced by 25%, more than 1.3 million deaths could be averted per year.[6]

In relation to the burden of noncommunicable diseases, the impact of physical inactivity is similar to that of established risk factors such as smoking and obesity.[6] Far more Americans are inactive compared to those with elevated cholesterol levels or those who smoke. In fact, since 1990, the American Heart Association (AHA) has stated that physical inactivity is a primary risk factor for cardiovascular disease.[7-9] In a 2013 report, the AHA suggested that a physical activity assessment be considered a vital health measure and, similar to all other major modifiable cardiovascular risk factors (e.g., diabetes mellitus, hypertension, hypercholesterolemia, obesity, smoking) that are assessed routinely, should be tracked regularly over time.[10] In this chapter, we will describe current and recommended levels of physical activity among older adults, discuss ways in which physical activity can be incorporated within clinical settings, and describe the physiologic adaptations to exercise.

TYPES OF PHYSICAL ACTIVITY

Physical activity is defined as "any bodily movement produced by skeletal muscles that requires energy expenditure."[5] Exercise is a type of physical activity that is planned or structured with the objective of increasing or maintaining physical fitness.[11] Other types of physical activity include leisure, transportation, occupational, and household and domestic activities. Exercise encompasses a broad range of activities and can be categorized as endurance (aerobic), resistance (strength), balance, and flexibility training. Endurance training refers to exercises in which the body's large muscles move in a rhythmic manner for prolonged periods. Popular aerobic activities for older adults include walking, stationary cycling, treadmill walking, dancing, and swimming. Resistance training is defined as exercises that cause muscles to work or hold against an applied force or weight. Resistance training is distinctly different from aerobic or endurance exercise, in which muscles contract against little or no resistance. Balance training refers to a combination of activities designed to improve postural control and stability in static and dynamic environments, enhance neuromotor coordination, and reduce the likelihood of falling. Flexibility training refers to activities designed to preserve or extend joint range of motion.

Exercise can also be differentiated by intensity, based on the energy expenditure measured in metabolic equivalents (METs), from light-intensity activity, in which the individual exercises at an intensity level ranging from 1.5 to 3 METs, to moderate-intensity activity in which the individual exercises at an intensity ranging from 3 to 6 METs, and finally to vigorous-intensity activity, in which the individual exercises at an intensity of 6 METs or more. One MET is defined as the amount of energy burned while an individual is at rest. During waking hours, when individuals are not physically active, they are engaging in sedentary behaviors. Sedentary behavior has been defined as any waking activity characterized by an energy expenditure of less than 1.5 METs in a sitting or reclining position.[12] Common sedentary behaviors include screen time (e.g., watching TV, playing video games, using computers), driving, and reading—essentially, any waking activity that is performed while sitting or lying down. Even though engaging in moderate or vigorous activity reduces the time spent in sedentary behavior, high levels of physical activity can still be offset by high levels of sedentary time. The "active couch potato" phenomenon describes people who exercise and meet the current recommendations for physical activity but nevertheless spend large amounts of time being sedentary.

PHYSICAL ACTIVITY GUIDELINES FOR OLDER ADULTS

The adaptive responses to regularly performed physical activities, and especially exercise, have been repeatedly demonstrated to have remarkably beneficial effects on overall health and can slow the age-related decline by 10 to 15 years. The list of these adaptive responses is extensive. Currently the Lifestyle Interventions and Independence for Elders (LIFE) study is the largest and longest duration randomized trial of physical activity in older adults. This study enrolled 1635 sedentary adults older than 70 years who were at risk for mobility disability into a health education program or a multicomponent, structured physical activity program of moderate intensity. The LIFE physical activity program was a feasible and effective way to reduce the burden of disability, especially among those with lower physical function at baseline.[13]

Some countries such as the United States, Canada, United Kingdom, and Australia have developed national physical activity guidelines for older adults (>65 years) that outline how much physical activity is generally recommended to realize health benefits.[14-16] These national guidelines are based on the most current scientific evidence, and considerable overlap in the type of recommendations is evident. The guidelines suggest that older adults should accumulate at least 2.5 hours of moderate-intensity physical activity each week, in single bouts of at least 10 minutes. In addition, resistance training is recommended at least 2 days/wk. The American College of Sports Medicine (ACSM) recommends that balance training (neuromotor exercises) should also be included in the exercise program of older adults; however, more research is needed before definitive recommendations are made regarding the frequency, duration, and intensity of balance training.[17] The guidelines also state that some physical activity is better than none, and that older adults who participate in any amount of physical activity will gain some health benefits.

The physical activity guidelines can be applied to older adults across all levels of frailty. Engaging in physical activities that require moderate effort is safe for most people[18,19]; however, adjustments may be needed based on fitness level and individual health risks or limitations. The ACSM[16] has recommended that resistance and/or balance training should precede aerobic training for frail older adults. In addition, they stated that exercise is more beneficial for frail older adults than any other intervention and that the contraindications to exercise for this segment of the population are the same as those for younger and healthier people. Multicomponent exercise seems to be the most effective physical activity intervention for frail older adults; however, the optimal design of the exercise protocol for this segment of the population is not clear.[20]

The physical activity guidelines suggest that to stay healthy, people need to engage in activities that are strenuous enough to burn at least three times more energy than expended when sitting quietly. The ACSM recommends that older adults should do at least 150 minutes of moderate-intensity activity or at least 75 minutes of vigorous-intensity activity, or an equivalent combination of moderate and vigorous activity.[16] This is based on research evidence showing that greater health benefits can be obtained if physical activity is performed at a more vigorous intensity level.[21,22] For example, brisk walking is considered to be better than slow walking.

Health benefits can still be derived from engaging in low-intensity physical activities such as slow walking[23]; however, there is currently insufficient evidence on the health benefits of light-intensity activities and/or the consequences of sedentary behaviors in older adults. Despite the lack of any published guidelines related to sedentary behavior, there is enough evidence to suggest that regardless of participation in physical activity, including exercise, sedentary behaviors can still increase the risk of adverse outcomes, such as mortality and the incidence of cardiovascular disease, cancer, and type 2 diabetes.[24] Reducing sitting time to less than 3 hours/day has the potential to increase life expectancy by 2 years, and reducing television viewing to less than 2 hours/day will increase life expectancy by almost 1.5 years.[25] In short, it appears all hours of the day have an impact on health—not just those spent in moderate- or vigorous-intensity physical activity. Therefore, older adults should not only exercise regularly, but should also try to limit the number of hours/day that they are engaged in sedentary behavior.

Some important principles that must be considered when designing physical activity programs for older adults are heterogeneity, challenge, adaptation and tailoring, and functional relevance.[26] Older adults are very heterogeneous and, when trying to increase their physical activity level, we need to consider the number and type of medical conditions that they have, medications they are taking, and range of their physical function. Not all older patients age in the same way or at the same rate. Although the exercise prescription for the healthy older adult might look similar to that designed for a younger adult, a more tailored approach will be needed for older adults who are more frail. For example, the frequency, duration, type, and intensity of exercise prescribed for a frail older adult will be very different from that prescribed for their healthier peers. They will likely need a longer duration program that includes shorter and less frequent training sessions to allow for sufficient rest and recovery. Exercises will also need to be performed at a lower intensity and emphasize balance training during the early stage of the program.[20] The selected exercises also need to challenge the participants to perform to the best of their ability, while still keeping activities enjoyable. However, participants should not exceed their intrinsic abilities and should not reach a point of pain or overexertion. The health and physical function of older adults can fluctuate, especially in the frailest people, and these changes need to be recognized by designing exercise programs that are tailored to their individual needs and can be adapted during periods of fluctuating health. For example, after a prolonged hospitalization or acute illness, the older adult may feel weak and fatigue easily, so it will be important to modify the exercise prescription by lowering the exercise intensity until they have returned to their usual levels of activity. Finally, exercise programs need to be functionally relevant to older adults and simulate movements of daily activities. For example, during the resistance training component, incorporate movements such as squats to improve transfer abilities, chest press and seated row exercises to simulate pushing and pulling actions, and bicep curls to improve lifting capabilities.

PATTERNS OF PHYSICAL ACTIVITY

Overall, levels of physical activity seem to have decreased in the past decades in most countries due to urbanization, which has resulted in an increase in motorized travel, sedentary desk-bound jobs, and the use of labor-saving technology in the home.[27,28] However, participation in sports and leisure physical activities has remained stable or increased slightly, with the number of fitness memberships increasing from 120 millions in 2009 to 144.7 millions in 2014.[29] Even though the number of younger people exercising may have increased, most of the population is still very inactive.

Children aged 6 to 11 years are the least sedentary group in the United States (6.1 hours/day) whereas young adults between the ages 20 and 29 years are, on average, sedentary for 7.5 hours/day. Thereafter, sedentary time increases approximately 1 hour/day (8.4 hours/day) by the age of 60 years and 2 hours/day by the age of 70 years (9.3 hours/day).[30] Similarly, in Canada, only 17.5% of young adults (20 to 29 years) and 13% of adults older than 60 years are meeting the physical activity guidelines of 150 min/wk of moderate to vigorous activity.[31] The frailest individuals are the most sedentary group of the population, with only 1% of Canadian frail people meeting the physical activity guidelines.[32] Older Canadians spend the highest mean hours per day viewing television: 47% of those aged 65 to 74 years and 52% of those older than 75 years spend 15 or more hours watching television per week. Computer screen use, although currently low in the 65 years and older age groups (11.2% of 65- to 74-year-olds and 6% of those older than 75 years report 11 or more hours/wk), is expected to increase.

Egerton and Brauer[33] have found that older adults living in the community spend 7.2 hours/day upright (standing or moving), whereas those living in a long-term care facility spend only 2.3 hours/day upright, of which less than 1 hour includes walking. Levels of inactivity are even greater in acutely ill older patients during hospitalization. Even when these patients can walk independently, they spend much of their time lying in bed, with less than 1 hour spent upright and only 7 minutes spent walking per day.[34,35] Although this finding could be related to their poor health, it may also be due to the prevailing environments of long-term care facilities and hospitals, which usually do not promote physical activity.

PROMOTING PHYSICAL ACTIVITY IN CLINICAL SETTINGS

The effectiveness of exercise in treating chronic debilitating disease remains largely unexplored. For example, fatigue is the most common complaint of patients with cancer, and increased rest is commonly advised by oncologists. However, just as cardiac rehabilitation has been demonstrated to provide an important mechanism for patients with a post–myocardial infarction to improve fitness and reduce the risk of a second event, exercise can greatly improve fitness and reduce much of the fatigue associated with cancer and its treatment.[36] Furthermore, the proven effects of resistance training in enhancing nitrogen retention and increasing muscle size and strength can provide positive benefits for patients with wasting diseases (e.g., HIV infection). Resistance exercise may also prove to be effective for patients with chronic renal failure, who must consume low-protein diets to slow the progression of their disease.[37] Exercise therapy for patients experiencing extended periods of inactivity during dialysis could also improve their functional status and decrease the fatigue associated with disuse. The potential value of a well-designed exercise program is great and warrants further investigation. A thoughtful and appropriate exercise prescription for any older adult patient has been recommended as the standard of care.[38]

Most older adults visit a primary care physician multiple times per year and consider health care professionals to be the primary source of advice for lifestyle changes, including physical activity. Therefore, clinical settings, and especially primary care, are ideal for identifying inactive people and promoting physical activity. Previous studies have shown that counselling middle-aged and older adults on increasing physical activity in primary care can be effective and improve patients' quality of life.[39] Similarly, physical activity counselling done by primary care physicians or nurses with follow-up to exercise specialists has been shown to increase physical activity levels and quality of life while lowering the number of hospitalizations for older adult patients.[40] We need to take advantage of the interactions between patients and health care professionals in the clinical setting to promote physical activity in all adults, and especially older adults, who are the most inactive, have the highest proportion of chronic diseases, and use the most health care resources.[41]

An objective of the Department of Health and Human Services' Healthy People 2020 agenda is to "increase the proportion of physician office visits that include counseling or education related to physical activity."[42] Likewise, the American College of Preventive Medicine has recommended that primary care health professionals incorporate physical activity counselling into routine patient visits.[43] Exercise is Medicine is a global health initiative that was launched in 2007 by the American Medical Association and the ACSM. This initiative focuses on encouraging primary care physicians and other health care professionals to assess and record physical activity as a vital sign regularly during patient visits, include physical activity when designing patient treatment plans, and conclude each visit with an exercise recommendation and/or referral to a certified health fitness or allied health care professional for further counselling and support.

In addition, all eligible Medicare recipients are entitled to receive an annual wellness visit under the U.S. Affordable Care Act. Physical activity is listed as a component of that visit, which should focus on prevention versus illness. Despite these efforts, health care professionals have not widely taken up the recommendations. In 2010, only 30% to 40% of older Americans received advice from their physician or other health care professional to increase their physical activity level.[44] In the near future, we hope to see an even greater proportion of the medical community recommending participation in physical activity. Given that health care professionals are more likely to encourage patients to increase their physical activity levels if they are active themselves,[45] it will be important that strategies also be developed to promote physical activity among health care providers.

A systematic review[45] has shown that health care professionals, especially those working in primary care settings, believe that physical activity is important and that they have a role to play in its promotion. Even so, they also recognize barriers to integrating physical activity into clinical settings. Two key barriers are lack of reimbursement and time constraints.[45] Medicare reimburses U.S. health care professionals for physical activity counseling as part of the annual wellness visit; however, this is not a common practice worldwide. Although in some cases effective intervention can be as brief as 3 to 5 minutes, longer counseling sessions may be needed to ensure that the exercise prescription is appropriate for some patients.[46] To address this problem, patients could fill out a physical activity questionnaire while they are in the waiting room, and a shorter counseling session could be supplemented with written material and/or referral to an exercise specialist. Also, innovative strategies such as Internet-based counseling and phone and text reminders could be incorporated into the treatment plan.

Many primary care health professionals are not comfortable providing detailed advice about physical activity and are not certain whether their counseling will result in their patients becoming more active.[45] Behavioral counseling techniques should be included in medical school curricula, and training should be offered to members of professional organizations on how to promote physical activity. In addition, educational material related to physical activity can be provided though Internet-based courses and grand rounds.[45] Using structured counseling protocols that have been shown to be effective could overcome some of the barriers that health care professionals are experiencing. Some examples of these are the green prescription intervention,[39] the Patient-centered Assessment and Counseling on Exercise plus nutrition (PACE+) intervention,[47] and the 5As (***a***sk, ***a***dvise, ***a***gree, ***a***ssist, ***a***rrange) approach[48] to physical activity counseling.[49]

Many physical assessment tools are available to track an individual's physical activity level. No one instrument will work for every situation. The two main categories are subjective (e.g., questionnaire, diary) and objective methods (e.g., pedometer, accelerometer). Choosing among the many options available can be confusing to health care professionals. For this reason, the AHA has developed a decision matrix based on the primary outcomes of interest (e.g., total physical activity, exercise) and other factors such as feasibility, resources, and administration considerations that can assist health care professionals in choosing the most appropriate assessment method.[10]

PHYSIOLOGIC ADAPTATIONS IN RESPONSE TO EXERCISE

Aerobic Exercise

Maximal aerobic exercise capacity is termed VO_{2max}. VO_2 (volume of oxygen consumed during maximal aerobic exercise) is defined using the Fick equation (VO_2 = cardiac output × arteriovenous oxygen difference). This equation demonstrates two important determinants of VO_{2max}—central factors, which control the delivery of oxygen to skeletal muscle, and the capacity of skeletal muscle to extract and use oxygen for adenosine triphosphate (ATP) during exercise. Regularly performed aerobic exercise increases VO_{2max} through the following mechanisms: increased cardiac output resulting from an expansion of plasma volume (≈15%) and from an increase in stroke volume as a result of cardiac hypertrophy and improved capacity to extract and use oxygen by skeletal muscle. This enhanced oxidative capacity of muscle is due to increased capillarization, mitochondrial density, and myoglobin content.

VO_{2max} declines with advancing age. This age-associated decrease in VO_{2max} has been shown to be approximately 10%/decade after the age of 25 to 30 years.[50] This decline is likely to be due to a number of factors, including changing cardiac function (e.g., decreased maximum cardiac output) and reduced muscle mass. The decline in maximal aerobic capacity with age accelerates after the age of 70 years.[51] Because a decline in maximal heart rate with advancing age is linear, this accelerated decline in late life is ascribed to factors related to skeletal muscle, such as capillary density and muscle oxidative capacity. Short and colleagues[52] have shown that most of the age-related decline in maximal aerobic capacity can be explained by a decrease in muscle mass and muscle mitochondrial function (oxidative capacity). Earlier studies demonstrated that the age-related decline in VO_{2max} may be ameliorated by physical activity.[53-55] Bortz and Bortz,[55] reviewing world records of master athletes up to age 85 years for endurance events, noted that the decline in performance occurred at a rate of 0.5%/year. They concluded that this decline of 0.5%/year may represent the effects of age (or biologic aging) on VO_{2max}, and the remainder of the decline may be the result of an increasingly sedentary lifestyle. However, more recent studies[50,51,56] have concluded that VO_{2max} declines at the same rate in athletic and sedentary men, and that 35% of this decline is due to sarcopenia.[55]

The responses of initially sedentary younger men (20 to 30 years) and older (60 to 70 years) men and women to 3 months of aerobic conditioning (70% of maximal heart rate, 45 min/day, 3 days/wk) were examined by Meredith and associates.[57] They found that the absolute gains in aerobic capacity were similar between the two age groups. However, the mechanism for adaptation to regular submaximal exercise appears to be different between older and younger adults. Muscle biopsy specimens taken before and after training showed a more than twofold increase in oxidative capacity in older adults, whereas that in the younger subjects showed smaller improvements. In addition, skeletal muscle glycogen stores in the older adults, significantly lower than those in the young men and women initially, increased greatly. Spina and coworkers[58] have observed that older men increased maximal cardiac output, whereas healthy older women demonstrated no change in response to endurance exercise training.

Aerobic Exercise and Carbohydrate Metabolism

Aerobic exercise is generally prescribed as an important adjunct to weight loss programs. Aerobic exercise combined with weight loss intervention has been demonstrated to increase insulin action to a greater extent than weight loss through diet restriction alone. Also, regularly performed aerobic exercise is an important way for older adults to improve their glucose tolerance. The fact that aerobic exercise has significant effects on skeletal muscle may help explain its importance in the treatment of glucose intolerance and type 2 diabetes. Kirwan and colleagues[59] have found that 9 months of endurance training at 80% of the maximal heart rate (4 days/wk) resulted in reduced glucose stimulated insulin levels. Coker and associates[60] examined the effects of intensity of aerobic exercise (50% vs. 75% VO_{2max}) on insulin-stimulated glucose uptake in older overweight men and women. They demonstrated that after 4 months, only those in the high-intensity group demonstrated a significant improvement in insulin sensitivity. These findings demonstrate that higher intensity exercise (without weight loss) may be necessary to reduce the risk of insulin resistance and type 2 diabetes significantly.

Endurance training and dietary modifications are generally recommended as the primary treatment in the non–insulin-dependent diabetic. Hughes and coworkers[61] compared the effects of a high-carbohydrate (60% carbohydrate and 20% fat), high-fiber (25 g dietary fiber/1000 kcal) diet with and without 3 months of high-intensity (75% maximum heart rate reserve, 50 min/day, 4 days/wk) endurance exercise in older glucose-intolerant men and women. No improvement was seen in glucose tolerance or insulin-stimulated glucose uptake in the diet or diet plus exercise group. However, the exercise plus high carbohydrate diet group demonstrated a significant and substantial increase in skeletal muscle glycogen content and, at the end of the training, the muscle glycogen stores were considered saturated. Because the primary site of glucose disposal is skeletal muscle glycogen, the extremely high muscle glycogen content associated with exercise and a high-carbohydrate diet likely limited the rate of glucose disposal. Thus, when combined with exercise and weight maintenance diet, a high-carbohydrate diet had a counterregulatory effect.

Resistance Training

Although endurance exercise has been the more traditional means of increasing cardiovascular fitness, strength or resistance training is an important component of an overall fitness program. Resistance training can be accomplished by virtually anyone and is particularly important for older adults due to age-associated declines in muscle mass and increased weakness. In the past, some health care professionals directed their patients away from resistance training in the mistaken belief that it can cause undesirable elevations in blood pressure. This can be avoided by instructing the patient in the correct technique while performing resistance exercises. Because muscle weakness is a primary deficit in many older adults, increased strength may stimulate participation in more aerobic activities, such as walking and cycling. Campbell and colleagues[62] have demonstrated that through increases in the resting metabolic rate and physical activity, resistance training results in an approximately 15% increase in energy expenditure in older men and women. As clinicians recognize that patients need higher levels of strength and endurance for many activities of daily living, muscle-strengthening exercises are rapidly becoming a critical component of cardiac rehabilitation programs. Churchward-Venne and associates[63] have found that all older adults responded to resistance training and concluded that this type of training "should be promoted without restriction to support healthy aging in the older population."

Strength conditioning or progressive resistance training is generally defined as training in which the resistance against which a muscle generates force is progressively increased over time. Progressive resistance training involves few contractions against a heavy load. The metabolic and morphologic adaptations resulting from resistance and endurance exercise are quite different, however. Muscle strength has been shown to increase in response to training at intensities between 60% and 100% of the one-repetition maximum (1RM).[64] An 1RM is the maximum amount of weight that can be lifted in a single contraction. Strength conditioning will result in an increase in muscle size, which is largely the result of increased contractile proteins. Lifting weight requires that a muscle shorten as it produces force, which is termed a *concentric muscle contraction*. Lowering the weight, on the other hand, forces the muscle to lengthen as it produces force, termed an *eccentric muscle contraction*. These lengthening muscle contractions have been shown to produce ultrastructural damage (microscopic tears in contractile protein muscle cells) that results in an acute-phase response and increase in muscle protein turnover.[65-69]

Muscle power may be a more important determinant for functional capacity in older adults than strength. Bassey and coworkers[70] have demonstrated that power (force production × time) is more closely related to functional capacity than strength in frail nursing home residents. It is therefore possible to design resistance exercise programs that increase strength and power.[71] Increasing muscle power should, perhaps, be the most important goal when designing the resistance training component for older adults.[72]

Effects of Resistance Exercise on Insulin and Protein Metabolism

Studies of insulin secretion after resistance but not endurance exercise have provided evidence for insulin's role in maintaining muscle mass. Arginine-stimulated insulin secretion is decreased with endurance training.[73,74] In contrast, acute resistance exercise in rats has been shown to increase insulin secretion.[75] A single bout of concentric exercise is a recognized enhancer of insulin action, whereas eccentric exercise transiently impairs whole-body insulin action for at least 2 days after the bout.[76] The decreased insulin action and delayed glycogen synthetic rate have been shown to result from a decreased rate of glucose transport rather than decreased glycogen synthase activity.[77] This transient resistance to insulin and impaired resynthesis of glycogen can result in a systemic hyperinsulinemia, which in turn may result in an increase in the rate of muscle protein synthesis. Another study[78] has demonstrated age-related differences in the insulin response to hyperglycemia following a single bout of eccentric exercise. Two days following upper and lower body eccentric exercise, younger subjects demonstrated a pronounced pancreatic insulin response during a hyperglycemic clamp, whereas this response was blunted in healthy older men.

The effects of resistance exercise on insulin availability appear to be opposite those of endurance exercise, thus stimulating net protein accretion. Insulin has been demonstrated to have profoundly anabolic effects on skeletal muscle. In the resting state, insulin has been demonstrated to decrease the rate of muscle protein degradation. Fluckey and colleagues[75,79] have argued that insulin is not likely to stimulate muscle protein synthesis in quiescent muscle. An insulin infusion may not increase the rate of protein synthesis in nonexercised muscle. However, using a resistance exercise model, investigators have demonstrated that resistance exercise alone does not stimulate an increase in the rate of protein synthesis. It was only with the addition of insulin that an exercise-induced increase in the rate of soleus and gastrocnemius protein synthesis was seen. This effect of insulin stimulation of the rate of protein synthesis was preserved with advancing age.

High-intensity resistance training is clearly anabolic in younger and older individuals. A 10% to 15% decrease in nitrogen excretion is observed at the initiation of training that persists for 12 weeks. That is, progressive resistance training improved nitrogen balance, so older subjects performing resistance training have a lower mean protein requirement than sedentary subjects.[80] Strawford and associates[81] have also demonstrated similar effects of resistance exercise training on nitrogen balance in patients with HIV-related weight loss. These studies, taken as a whole, demonstrate the powerful effects of resistance exercise training on protein nutriture. The anabolic effects have important implications in the treatment of many wasting diseases and conditions such as cancer, HIV infection, aging, chronic renal failure, and undernutrition seen in many very old men and women. By effectively lowering dietary protein needs, resistance exercise can limit further losses of skeletal muscle mass while simultaneously increasing muscle strength and functional capacity.

Resistance Exercise and Aging

High-intensity resistance training of the knee extensors and flexors (80% of 1RM, 3 days/wk) in older men (age, 60 to 72 years) increased knee flexor and extensor strength by 227% and 107%, respectively. Total muscle area by computed tomography analysis increased by 11.4%, and the muscle tissue showed an increase of 33.5% in type I fiber area and 27.5% increase in type II fiber area. In addition, lower body VO_{2max} increased significantly, whereas upper body VO_{2max} did not, indicating that increased muscle mass can increase maximal aerobic power. Improving muscle strength can enhance the capacity of many older men and women to perform many activities, such as climbing stairs, carrying packages, and even walking.

This same training program was conducted with a group of frail, institutionalized older men and women (mean age, 90 ± 3 years; range, 87 to 96 years).[82] After 8 weeks of training, the 10 subjects in this study increased muscle strength by almost 180% and muscle size by 11%. A similar intervention in frail nursing home residents demonstrated not only increases in muscle strength and size, but increased gait speed, stair-climbing power, and balance. In addition, spontaneous activity levels increased significantly, whereas the activity of a nonexercised control group was unchanged.[83] In this study, the effects of a protein-calorie supplement combined with exercise were also examined. The men and women who consumed the supplement and exercised gained weight compared with those in the three other groups examined (exercise control, non–exercise-supplemented, and non–exercise control). In addition, investigators[84] demonstrated that the combined weight lifting and nutritional supplementation increased strength by 257% and type II fiber area by 10.1%, with a similar trend for type I fiber area (12.8%). Exercise was associated with a 2.5-fold increase in neonatal myosin (a form of myosin found in growing muscle) staining and an increase of 491% in insulin-like growth factor-1 (IGF-1) staining. Ultrastructural damage increased by 141% after exercise training. Strength increases were largest in those with the greatest increases in myosin, IGF-1, damage, and caloric intake during the trial. Very old frail adults respond robustly to resistance training with musculoskeletal remodeling, and significant increases in muscle area are possible with resistance training in combination with adequate energy intakes. It should be pointed out that this was a very old, very frail population with diagnoses of multiple chronic diseases.

OTHER EFFECTS OF EXERCISE

Balance and Falls

Three different exercise approaches have been shown to reduce fall risk and/or fall rates significantly among community-dwelling older adults—multicomponent group exercise programs (i.e., at least two or more exercise components), group-based tai chi programs, and individually tailored exercise programs conducted in the home.[85] Combining the components of balance and resistance exercise can be particularly effective in reducing fall rates. Based on a systematic review of 54 randomized controlled trials investigating the effects of different types of exercise interventions on fall incidence rates, Sherrington and coworkers developed a set of best practice recommendations to guide practitioners in the development of exercise programs designed to reduce falls.[86,87] Effective programs were characterized by the inclusion of balance exercises that became progressively more challenging over time, provided a sufficient amount of exercise (at least 50 hours of supervised exercise), and were tailored to the level of fall risk identified. Whether the exercise was delivered in a group- or home-based setting did not affect the outcomes.

Bone Health

Nelson and colleagues[88] have examined the interaction of dietary calcium and exercise in a study that included 41 postmenopausal women consuming a high-calcium (1462 mg/day) or moderate-calcium (761 mg) diet. Half of these women participated in a year-long walking program (45 min/day, 4 days/wk, 75% of heart rate reserve). Independent effects of the exercise program and dietary calcium were seen. Compared with those in the moderate-calcium group, the women consuming a high-calcium diet displayed reduced bone loss in the femoral neck, independently of whether the women exercised. The walking prevented a loss of trabecular bone mineral density seen in the nonexercising women after 1 year. Thus, it appears that calcium intake and aerobic exercise are both independently beneficial to bone mineral density at different sites.

The effects of 52 weeks of high-intensity resistance exercise training were examined in a group of 39 postmenopausal women.[89] In this group, 20 were randomly assigned to the strength training group (2 days/wk, 80% of 1RM for upper and lower body muscle groups). At the end of the year, significant differences were evident in lumbar spine and femoral bone density between the strength-trained and sedentary women. However, unlike other pharmacologic and nutritional strategies for preventing bone loss and osteoporosis, resistance exercise affected more than just bone density. The women who underwent strength training improved their muscle mass, strength, balance, and overall levels of physical activity. Thus, resistance training can be an important way to decrease the risk for an osteoporotic bone fracture in postmenopausal women.

Giangregorio and associates have critically reviewed and graded the quality of the research evidence related to exercise and osteoporosis, with the goal being to develop exercise recommendations for individuals with osteoporosis or vertebral fractures.[90] Using a follow-up Delphi consensus process, they recommended that individuals with osteoporosis participate in multicomponent exercise programs that emphasize resistance training, balance, and postural alignment.[91] Providing patients with guidance on protective spine-sparing techniques during the performance of activities of daily activities and leisure activities was also recommended by the expert panel. For older adults with a history of vertebral fractures, consultation with a physical therapist prior to development of the exercise prescription was recommended.

Cognitive Function

Leisure activities (e.g., reading, playing board games, playing musical instruments, dancing) have been associated with a decreased risk of developing dementia in men and women older than 75.[92] A recent systematic review[93] has shown that 88% of the cohort studies and 100% of the cross-sectional studies that examined the relationship between physical activity and various cognitive health outcomes found a significant association. This review also demonstrated that the estimated population-attributable risk was particularly high for physical activity (31.9%; 95% confidence interval [CI], 22.7 to 41.2) compared to other modifiable risk factors. Middleton and colleagues[94] used double-labeled water, the gold standard measure of total physical activity, and showed that greater activity energy expenditure was protective against cognitive impairment in a dose-response manner. A randomized controlled trial of a 24-week physical activity intervention in 170 older adults with memory problems, but not diagnosed dementia, showed a persistent effect of the exercise on memory over an 18-month period after cessation of the exercise intervention.[95]

A growing body of literature[96,97] has suggested that aerobic exercise is better than other types of exercises for improving cognitive function in older adults and will reduce the risk of dementia and Alzheimer disease (AD). Resistance exercise has also been demonstrated to have a significant and positive effect on select components of executive function (e.g., memory, selective attention, sensory conflict resolution) in older adults.[98,99] Therefore, combining exercise types may be more beneficial for the cognitive function of older adults. Even though there are no clear guidelines for the optimal duration and intensity of an exercise program, longer interventions are likely to lead to better cognitive outcomes.

The mechanisms that underlie the potentially protective effects of increased physical activity on cognitive function are likely multifactorial. Physical activity has been shown to enhance cerebral blood flow and cerebral nutrient supply, as well as improve neuroplasticity by modifying the brain-derived neurotropic factor. In animal studies,[100-102] voluntary exercise results in direct effects on brain function through an increase in hippocampal brain-derived neurotrophic factor expression and decrease in inflammation. Physical activity is also associated with greater gray matter volume in the prefrontal cortex and hippocampus.[103]

Finally, studies have suggested that physical activity improves aerobic capacity and reduces the risk of many cardiovascular conditions (e.g., hypertension), obesity, and type 2 diabetes, which have been shown to be associated with an increased risk of cognitive decline.

CONCLUSION

Physical activity exerts powerful acute and chronic effects on virtually every system in the human body. In assessing these effects and prescribing exercise, it is important to keep in mind the very different effects of the different types of physical activity and their collective role in disease prevention and health promotion. Older adults, in particular, can benefit from regularly engaging in physical activity because they are the most sedentary group. Increasing physical activity in this group can be a realistic strategy for maintaining functional status and independence. Clinicians should regularly assess and record physical activity as a vital sign during older patients' visits and provide physical activity counselling as a routine part of their practice.

KEY POINTS

- Physical activity exerts a powerful acute and chronic effect on virtually every system in the human body and delays age-related decline.
- Older adults in particular can benefit from regularly performed physical activity.
- Older adults should accumulate at least 2.5 hours of moderate intensity physical activity each week and should do resistance training at least twice per week.
- Balance training is beneficial for older adults to enhance neuromotor coordination and reduce the likelihood of falling.
- An individualized and targeted prescription of exercise should be the standard of care within clinical settings for any older adult.

For a complete list of references, please visit www.expertconsult.com.

KEY REFERENCES

1. Garatachea N, Pareja-Galeano H, Sanchis-Gomar F, et al: Exercise attenuates the major hallmarks of aging. Rejuvenation Res 18:57–89, 2015.
4. Jones CJ, Rose DJ: Physical activity instruction of older adults, Champaign, IL, 2005, Human Kinetics.
6. Lee IM, Shiroma EJ, Lobelo F, et al: Lancet Physical Activity Series Working Group. Effect of physical inactivity on major non-communicable diseases worldwide: an analysis of burden of disease and life expectancy. Lancet 380:219–229, 2012.
10. Strath SJ, Kaminsky LA, Ainsworth BE, et al: American Heart Association Physical Activity Committee of the Council on Lifestyle and Cardiometabolic Health and Cardiovascular, Exercise, Cardiac Rehabilitation and Prevention Committee of the Council on Clinical Cardiology, and Council. Guide to the assessment of physical activity: clinical and research applications: a scientific statement from the American Heart Association. Circulation 128:2259–2279, 2013.
13. Pahor M, Guralnik JM, Ambrosius WT, et al: LIFE study investigators. Effect of structured physical activity on prevention of major mobility disability in older adults: the LIFE study randomized clinical trial. JAMA 311:2387–2396, 2014.
14. Tremblay MS, Warburton DE, Janssen I, et al: New Canadian physical activity guidelines. Appl Physiol Nutr Metab 36:36–46, 47–58, 2011.
15. Department of Health, Physical Activity, Health Improvement and Protection: Start active, stay active: a report on physical activity for health from the four home countries' Chief Medical Officers. https://www.gov.uk/government/uploads/system/uploads/

attachment _data/file/216370/dh_128210.pdf. Accessed November 10, 2015.

16. American College of Sports Medicine; Chodzko-Zajko WJ, Proctor DN, et al: American College of Sports Medicine position stand. Exercise and physical activity for older adults. Med Sci Sports Exerc 41:1510–1530, 2009.
17. Garber CE, Blissmer B, Deschenes MR, et al: American College of Sports Medicine: American College of Sports Medicine position stand. Quantity and quality of exercise for developing and maintaining cardiorespiratory, musculoskeletal, and neuromotor fitness in apparently healthy adults: guidance for prescribing exercise. Med Sci Sports Exerc 43:1334–1359, 2011.
20. Theou O, Stathokostas L, Roland K, et al: The effectiveness of exercise interventions for the management of frailty: a systematic review. J Aging Res 2011:569194, 2011.
33. Egerton T, Brauer SG: Temporal characteristics of habitual physical activity periods among older adults. J Phys Act Health 6:644–650, 2009.
39. Elley CR, Kerse N, Arroll B, et al: Effectiveness of counselling patients on physical activity in general practice: cluster randomised controlled trial. BMJ 326:793, 2003.
43. Jacobson DM, Strohecker L, Compton MT, et al: Physical activity counseling in the adult primary care setting: position statement of the American College of Preventive Medicine. Am J Prev Med 29:158–162, 2005.
45. Hébert ET, Caughy MO, Shuval K: Primary care providers' perceptions of physical activity counselling in a clinical setting: a systematic review. Br J Sports Med 46:625–631, 2012.
47. Calfas KJ, Sallis JF, Zabinski MF, et al: Preliminary evaluation of a multicomponent program for nutrition and physical activity change in primary care: PACE+ for adults. Prev Med 34:153–161, 2002.
48. Whitlock EP, Orleans CT, Pender N, et al: Evaluating primary care behavioral counseling interventions: an evidence-based approach. Am J Prev Med 22:267–284, 2002.
49. Carroll JK, Fiscella K, Epstein RM, et al: A 5A's communication intervention to promote physical activity in underserved populations. BMC Health Serv Res 12:374, 2012.
52. Short KR, Bigelow ML, Kahl J, et al: Decline in skeletal muscle mitochondrial function with aging in humans. Proc Natl Acad Sci U S A 102:5618–5623, 2005.
60. Coker RH, Hays NP, Williams RH, et al: Exercise-induced changes in insulin action and glycogen metabolism in elderly adults. Med Sci Sports Exerc 38:433–438, 2006.
63. Churchward-Venne TA, Tieland M, Verdijk LB, et al: There are no nonresponders to resistance-type exercise training in older men and women. J Am Med Dir Assoc 16:400–411, 2015.
87. Sherrington C, Tiedemann A, Fairhall N, et al: Exercise to prevent falls in older adults: an updated meta-analysis and best practice recommendations. N S W Public Health Bull 22:78–83, 2011.
90. Giangregorio LM, Papaioannou A, Macintyre NJ, et al: Too Fit To Fracture: exercise recommendations for individuals with osteoporosis or osteoporotic vertebral fracture. Osteoporos Int 25:821–835, 2014.
93. Beydoun MA, Beydoun HA, Gamaldo AA, et al: Epidemiologic studies of modifiable factors associated with cognition and dementia: systematic review and meta-analysis. BMC Public Health 14:643, 2014.
94. Middleton LE, Manini TM, Simonsick EM, et al: Activity energy expenditure and incident cognitive impairment in older adults. Arch Intern Med 171:1251–1257, 2011.
103. Erickson KI, Leckie RL, Weinstein AM: Physical activity, fitness, and gray matter volume. Neurobiol Aging 35(Suppl 2):S20–S28, 2014.

100 Rehabilitation: Evidence-Based Physical and Occupational Therapy Techniques for Stroke and Parkinson Disease

Geert Verheyden, Annick Van Gils, Alice Nieuwboer

INTRODUCTION

Rehabilitation services are typically provided by a group of health care professionals, each of whom has a different health education background. Interdisciplinary rehabilitation—the collaboration and interaction between these professionals with regard to patient care—is believed to be of benefit for the patient. This chapter will present the work of physical and occupational therapists within the rehabilitation process and discuss general therapy techniques for treating the older geriatric patient, as well as specific, evidence-based therapy techniques for people with stroke and Parkinson disease.

PHYSICAL THERAPY

The World Confederation for Physical Therapy (WCPT) defines physical therapy as follows[1]:

> *Physical therapy provides services to individuals and populations to develop, maintain and restore maximum movement and functional ability throughout the lifespan. This includes providing services in circumstances where movement and function are threatened by ageing, injury, pain, diseases, disorders, conditions or environmental factors. Functional movement is central to what it means to be healthy. Physical therapy is concerned with identifying and maximizing quality of life and movement potential within the spheres of promotion, prevention, treatment/intervention, habilitation and rehabilitation. This encompasses physical, psychological, emotional, and social well-being. Physical therapy involves the interaction between the physical therapist, patients/clients, other health professionals, families, caregivers and communities in a process where movement potential is assessed and goals are agreed upon, using knowledge and skills unique to physical therapists.*

The physical therapy process entails a series of steps[1]: (1) assessment of the patient and evaluation of the assessment within a process of clinical reasoning; (2) diagnosis and prognosis, not in terms of the underlying health condition or disease but in terms of the mainly physical consequences of the health condition of the patient; (3) intervention and treatment; and (4) reassessment in terms of the predefined outcomes.

Both physical and occupational therapists work within the framework of the International Classification of Functioning, Disability and Health. This framework is based on the biopsychosocial model and considers a person with a health condition as having problems on three different levels[2]: (1) the body functions and structure level, (2) activity level, and (3) participation level. Additionally, contextual factors, including environmental and personal factors, affect the relationship among the three different levels. For example, a person with stroke (health condition) can have a variety of impairments (problems in body functions and structure), such as muscle weakness, sensory deficits, cognitive problems, and emotional disorders. These impairments will result in activity limitations—difficulties an individual may have in executing activities—such as the inability to walk over uneven ground and, consequently, leave the house and use public transport. Finally, the activity limitations will result in participation restrictions, which are problems that an individual may experience in life situations, such as the inability to go out with friends to a museum, movie, or theater. Contextual factors can positively or negatively influence this interaction; for example, a restrictive environmental factor would be living on the third floor without an elevator for a hemiparetic person with stroke, whereas a stimulating personal factor would be a patient having a wide network of social support.

General Physical Therapy Techniques

Motor rehabilitation in the field of physical and occupational therapy is underpinned by motor learning principles because motor recovery is based on motor (re)learning.

Key Principles

The key principles of motor learning are as follows.[3]

Intensity. Repetition is a key aspect of motor learning. Patients should be stimulated to perform exercises in subsequent series, with adequate rest breaks. This regimen should not only be applied in the face to face therapeutic setting, but also in group sessions and self-training programs.

Progression. Based on a high number of repetitions, motor skills will be (re)learned and, to continue motor learning, exercises should be made more difficult and more challenging for the patient, yet still be within her or his capabilities. An exercise that is too difficult can lead to demotivation.

Variation. Performing the same exercise over and over again might also lead to reduced motivation. Thus, it is important in a therapeutic setting to incorporate a variety of similar exercises to train one specific motor skill. This is a different aspect than progression in that variation of an exercise does not mean that the difficulty of the exercise increases.

Task Specificity. Exercises performed in a therapeutic setting will lead to improvement in that specific exercise. For example, if balance has to be improved, therapy should primarily be focused on performing balance exercises. There is little to no evidence in the rehabilitation literature that exercises have what is called a carryover effect. For example, this would mean that a muscle-strengthening exercise on its own will improve walking. This implies that therapy should mainly consist of performing functional exercises to improve functional activities.

Goal-Oriented. Conducting exercises without a clear goal or aim are meaningless for patients and, again, can reduce motivation. Thus, therapists should incorporate specific goals for all the exercises conducted in a therapeutic session.

Feedback. The patient should be provided with feedback about the performance of the exercise—how the movement was conducted—and the actual result, if the goal was achieved. This is called knowledge of performance and knowledge of result, respectively.

Incorporation of Motor Learning Principles

This example is presented to clarify the incorporation of these motor learning principles for an older adult who has difficulty standing up from a chair. Based on the visual movement analysis and assessment, it appears that the trunk is not moving sufficiently far forward to bring the body weight forward to transfer the body weight (center of mass) over the feet (base of support). The therapist can use a standardized measurement, which includes a sit-to-stand movement to assess the current state and subsequently to evaluate progress during and after treatment. A measurement that could be used is the five times sit-to-stand test (timed test) or, if the person is still able to walk, the timed get-up-and-go (TGUG) test. An exercise for this patient could be to perform sit-to-stand movements with a little knee-high box in front of him or her. The person should, while standing up, bring the hands in front and touch the box with the hands. Touching the box with the hands is a goal-oriented movement; the exercise is also task-specific because sit-to-stand is specifically designed for this person. It can be varied by performing the same exercise from a different chair (with and without an arm rest or back rest) or sofa, as is necessary in daily life. Progression is incorporated by moving the box further forward; this would require a greater forward leaning posture when touching the box before being able to stand up. Alternatively, the seat height could also be lowered systematically, because this would make the overall sit-to-stand more difficult. The person has to perform these sit-to-stands eight to ten times, if possible, after he or she rests for 30 to 60 seconds, with a total of three to five series conducted before variation or progression is incorporated. Finally, feedback is provided by the therapist (orally) about the performance and result. The person also receives feedback when touching the box, knowing that there was an adequate forward lean and knowing performance, and when standing up, knowing that a successful sit-to-stand was conducted and knowing the result.

Evidence-Based Physical Therapy Techniques

For Stroke

Veerbeek and colleagues have recently published a systematic review and meta-analysis of the evidence for physical therapy poststroke.[4] This was an update of the 2004 study of Van Peppen and associates,[5] which included 123 randomized controlled trials in the field of physical therapy poststroke. The updated review included 467 randomized controlled trials involving 25,373 patients. More importantly, the quality (risk of bias) of physical therapy trials improved over the last decade; the median PEDro score (http://www.pedro.org.au) improved from 5 of 10 in 2004 to 6 of 10 in 2014.

Evidence-based therapy techniques will be discussed based on the recent review[4] for the following domains: gait and mobility-related function and activity, arm-hand activities, and physical fitness. Only (positive or negative) results from meta-analyses or phase III randomized controlled trials will be presented. For more information, the reader is directed to Verbeek and coworkers' report.[4]

Gait and Mobility-Related Function and Activity. Reaching activities in sitting beyond arm's length have a significant positive effect on sitting balance. Practicing standing balance with biofeedback has a significant positive effect on postural sway. Balance training has a significant positive effect on balance and activities of daily living (ADLs). Body weight supported treadmill training demonstrates a significant positive effect on comfortable gait speed and walking distance. Electromechanical gait training leads to a significant positive effect on maximum gait speed, walking distance, peak heart rate, and ADLs. Incorporating functional electrical stimulation with electromechanical gait training has a significant positive effect on balance and walking capacity, but only in the early rehabilitation phase (<3 months poststroke). Treadmill training has a significant positive effect on maximum gait speed and step width. Walking overground (as frequently done in regular face to face physical therapy sessions) demonstrates only a significant positive effect on fear. It has a significant negative effect on aerobic capacity in people unable to walk. Circuit class training has a significant positive effect on walking distance, balance, walking capacity, and physical activity. Training of the caregiver by the physical therapist demonstrates a significant positive effect on ADLs and caregiver strain. Hydrotherapy has a significant positive effect on muscle force. Neuromuscular electrostimulation has a significant positive effect on motor function, muscle force, and muscle tone. Finally, transcutaneous electrical nerve stimulation (TENS) shows a significant positive effect on muscle force and walking capacity.

Arm-Hand Activities. Positioning of the arm shows a significant positive effect on passive range of motion for outward rotation of the shoulder. The use of inflatable splints has a significant negative effect on muscle tone in the early rehabilitation phase (<3 months poststroke). The original constraint-induced movement therapy (CIMT) concept demonstrates a significant positive effect on arm-hand activities and self-reported use and quality of the arm and hand. In the original CIMT concept, therapy is provided for 2 weeks, with the patient wearing a padded mitt over the unaffected hand for 90% of her or his waking hours to stimulate use of the affected hand. Additionally, during these 2 weeks, 6 hours of therapy is given daily.

High-intensity CIMT (therapy provided from 3 to 6 hours daily) has a significant positive effect on arm-hand activities and self-reported use and quality of the arm and hand. Low-intensity CIMT (wearing the padded mitt between zero and 90% of the waking day and receiving from 0 to 3 hours of therapy daily) also has a significant positive effect on motor function, ADLs, arm-hand activities, and self-reported use and quality of the arm and hand. Robot-assisted training focusing on the shoulder and elbow demonstrates a significant positive effect on proximal motor function, muscle force, and pain. Robot-assisted training focusing on the elbow and wrist has a significant positive effect on proximal motor function and muscle force. Interestingly, a meta-analysis of trials investigating robot-assisted training focusing on the shoulder, elbow, wrist, and hand did not show any significant effect.

Mental practice has a significant positive effect on arm-hand activities. Virtual reality training demonstrates a significant positive effect on ADLs, but a significant negative effect on muscle tone—the meta-analysis showed an increase in muscle tone. Neuromuscular stimulation for the flexors and extensors of the wrist and fingers has a significant positive effect on motor function and muscle force. Neuromuscular stimulation of the shoulder has a significant positive effect on a subluxation. Electromyography (EMG)–triggered neuromuscular stimulation of the extensors of the wrist and fingers demonstrates a significant positive effect on motor function, arm-hand activities, and active range of motion. The use of trunk restriction to promote upper limb movement has a significant negative effect on self-reported arm and hand use. Finally, somatosensory stimulation demonstrates a significant positive effect on somatosensory function and muscle tone.

Physical Fitness. Fitness training focusing on the lower limb has a significant positive effect on muscle force, muscle tone, and spatiotemporal gait parameters. Interestingly, a meta-analysis of fitness training focusing on the upper limb did not show significant effects. Training of aerobic capacity demonstrates a significant positive effect on aerobic capacity and respiratory function. A mixed fitness approach (muscle force and aerobic training) has a significant positive effect on lower limb motor function, lower limb muscle force, comfortable and maximum gait speed, walking distance, aerobic capacity, heart rate at training, balance, physical activity, and quality of life.

The review[4] also reported that a statistically significant effect on outcome can be seen if an increase in therapy time of, on average 17 hours over a number of weeks, was included. The effect size ranged from 5% to 15%; with a typical measurement error for clinical outcomes of around 10%, several statistically significant results are in the measurement error interval. As a result, this was not a true reflection of change in the patient's performance. Future research should therefore focus on combining effective therapy approaches and evaluating whether effect size improves due to the combination of approaches.

For Parkinson Disease

Parkinson disease (PD) is a highly prevalent condition in those older than 60 years.[6,7] Age-specific prevalent rates indicate that PD is present in 1% of those older than 60 years, rising to 4% in the oldest age groups.[6] Although mortality is significantly increased versus age-matched controls (by ≈1.5) and disease progression varies greatly, mean disease duration is estimated to be from 6.9 to 14.3 years.[8] The basal ganglia are the central nervous system structures affected by PD, so patients lose the ability to move automatically. This overarching automaticity deficit can be defined as the ability to perform a motor task while at the same time focusing on executing an additional task.[9] Loss of automaticity implies that patients find it difficult to maintain movement amplitude, rhythm, balance, and postural tone without consciously attending to movement activity. As a consequence, dual task interference is exacerbated in PD, over and above that seen as a result of aging.[10] Another correlate of dual task interference, constituting a particularly bothersome problem of PD, is freezing of gait (FOG). FOG is defined as a brief episodic absence or marked reduction of forward progression of the feet, despite the intention to walk.[11] FOG often occurs during starting to walk, when almost reaching the intended destination, and during turning. FOG is a very disabling symptom and severely curtails functional independence.[12] Other debilitating symptoms of PD include rigidity, bradykinesia, and postural instability. The varied ways in which these symptoms present themselves in different patients determines the heterogeneity of the gross motor dysfunction, gait impairment, and fine motor deficits inherent to PD.[13] PD symptoms can only partially be relieved by medical treatment and, with disease progression, induce a significant loss of functional activity.[14]

Patients with PD have a lower level of physical activity than healthy older adults, not only resulting from motor[15,16] but also from cognitive decline,[17] including executive dysfunction,[18] mood disturbance, depression, and fatigue.[19] A sedentary lifestyle threatens overall physical capacity, exaggerates signs of frailty, and increases the risk of comorbidity.[15] Secondary changes associated with PD include cardiovascular and respiratory problems but also osteoporosis in early to mid-stage disease,[20] as well as contractures, bed sores, and pneumonia in later stages of the disease.[21] Falls in people with PD occur frequently and recurrently[22] and are particularly common with increasing disease duration, age, and cognitive impairment.[23,24] The basal ganglia are also crucially involved in motor learning, particularly during the consolidation phase.[25] Therefore, the most important challenge that physiotherapists face is to use the most optimal strategies to deal with PD patients' lack of movement automaticity and inherent difficulty with motor learning retention.

Effects of Physical Therapy. Physical therapy has the potential to modify the risk factors of inactivity and falling in PD.[15,26] Tomlinson and colleagues[27] have published a systematic review and meta-analysis based on randomized controlled trials that included 39 trials with 1827 patients. This high-quality evidence demonstrated overall efficacy of physical therapy in the short term (mean follow-up, 3 months). More specifically, significant benefits of exercise interventions were found for gait speed, 6-minute walk test, FOG score, and TGUG test. In addition, positive effects of physical therapy were demonstrated on the functional reach test, Berg balance scale, and unified Parkinson disease ratings scale (UPDRS) motor scores. Most of the observed between-group changes were small, but three outcomes (gait speed, Berg balance, and UPDRS) showed clinically meaningful improvements, approaching or beyond the minimal detectable change threshold. No effects of physical therapy were found on patient-rated quality of life or on fall frequency. This comprehensive review also did not show differential treatment effects among various types of physical therapy interventions. Current thinking about which components of a physical therapy program are most optimal for PD point to exercise on the one hand and goal-directed motor learning on the other, despite the known learning limitations.[28,29] Because patients with PD are particularly sensitive to external motor drive due to their loss of automaticity, various methods of external pacing (or cueing), visual targets, and visual feedback are recommended to enhance practice and learning.[28]

Exercise for PD usually incorporates a mixture of repetitive practice to optimize physical activity, increase strength, and prevent secondary consequences, such as loss of flexibility and fitness. Usually, exercise is embedded in functionally relevant movements to optimize transfer to ADLs. For example, PD patients in all disease stages exhibit difficulties in rising from a chair.[30] The inability to stand up from a seated position prohibits engaging in upright activities such as walking, thus reinforcing the vicious circle of physical deconditioning and functional deterioration. The sit-to-stand task involves large muscle work from the trunk and lower limbs and is therefore a valuable exercise to increase fitness, postural control, and leg muscle strength. Sit-to-stand has proved as trainable for those with PD as for age-matched controls by using repetitive muscle work and biofeedback.[31]

Most recent publications indicate that there is an important role for progressive resistance training in PD.[32,33] These studies have shown that twice-weekly, supervised, progressive strength training continued for 2 years induce strength increases and functional improvements, overruling the deterioration predicted by disease progression.

Generally, evidence is lacking about what the optimal dose and intensity of exercise intervention should be, particularly in a geriatric setting. Currently, clinical advice on exercise is guided by age, health status, disease stage, and general World Health Organization's guidelines for exercise.[34] As was demonstrated by the progressive resistance training studies,[32,33] it is as important in PD as in other populations that the intensity of exercise be appropriately set and progressed to achieve physiologic adaptations. Furthermore, maximizing the intensity of exercise in a PD-specific way can be achieved by prompting patients to move with large amplitude and optimal speed.[35]

PD patients' needs vary according to the different stages of the disease. In the early stages, interventions can still aim at motor learning, stimulating consolidation and automaticity. A review of 11 motor learning studies[36] has shown that the capacity for motor learning of novel tasks remains relatively preserved in PD. This applied to well-defined discrete movements of upper and lower limbs as well as balance maneuvers, postural sequences, and obstacle stepping performed in a laboratory-based environment. Interestingly, most acquisition slopes were similar in PD to those in healthy age-matched controls, although final performance never reached healthy control levels. However, retention of learning, although sometimes preserved in PD for up to 2 months, was also impaired and appeared more dependent on the learning condition. The close relationship between practice context and retention effects emphasizes the importance of training functionally relevant tasks if the goal is to implement the learned tasks in daily life. In the later stages, and in some specific patient subgroups in which motor and cognitive deterioration is more advanced, the generalization of learning will be affected even more, and the use of compensation strategies will become more crucial.

Most patients experience symptom fluctuations. Motor learning and exercise are best applied during the "on" phase of the medication cycle—when medication works best. Strategies to tackle FOG or bed transfers need to be practiced during the off phase as well, when medication is working suboptimally.

Cueing and Feedback. Given the chronic character of the disease, physical therapy needs to be adapted over time, and exercise needs to be offered in an attractive and challenging fashion to ensure sustained adherence. Technology-aided rehabilitation methods—for example, computerized balance boards or exergames—are important tools for PD rehabilitation because of their ability to provide online performance information and combine motor and cognitive training. PD patients rely more than healthy controls on attention, external cueing, and feedback for movement, implying a change from a habitual to goal-directed mode of motor control.[28] Cueing is defined as providing discrete external sensory information, usually via rhythmic auditory or visual stimuli, which serve as a reference, target, or trigger for movement generation.[37] Feedback refers to the continuous online provision of external information, which supplements sensory (proprioceptive) pathways to guide motor performance. In contrast, cognitive strategies, often referred to as internal cueing, is a method of self-generated cognitive prompting and monitoring to improve specific movement components.[38] All these compensatory methods are critical in guiding PD patients toward better motor performance. Focusing attention on taking big steps, for example, has been shown to improve gait strongly in PD.[34,38] However, attentional focus rapidly declines with time and during prolonged dual tasking. To a lesser extent than with cognitive strategies, cueing and feedback also call on the ability to allocate attention and executive function flexibly, an ability that is crucially dependent on the patient's cognitive reserve.[18]

Many studies have shown that visual and auditory cueing modalities enhance spatiotemporal gait features, effects that remain for short retention periods (<24 hours) after cue removal.[38,39] In general, visual cues are used to improve spatial gait characteristics (e.g., step amplitude), whereas auditory cues influence temporal factors such as cadence or step time variability. In addition to immediate cueing effects, sustained cued training with a continuous rhythm of a metronome was shown to enhance motor learning and retention compared to training without cues.[40,41]

FOG is best tackled using a combined training approach, with external cueing to train maintenance of rhythm and amplitude and cognitive strategies to alleviate FOG flexibly.[42,43] FOG is often accompanied by high-frequency trembling movements in the legs, which generate incomplete weight displacements from one leg to the other.[11] Gait training to improve rhythmic continuity and reduce hastening using auditory and visual pacing has been found to be effective to reduce FOG.[43] Patients with FOG also benefit from cognitive strategies that encourage voluntary stopping during FOG, which alleviates the involuntary trembling and allows the decoupling of the movement intent from the inability to generate stepping. This permits resetting the freezing behavior, after which gait can be re-initiated. Conscious facilitation of alternating weight displacement before or during FOG is another useful cognitive strategy to restore weight shifting so that an appropriate swing phase can be resumed. Equally, lifting the feet high in confined spaces, or initiating weight shifts by shoulder or head movements, are strategies that need to be taught during daily situations to facilitate generalization of learning. In patients with cognitive deficits, it is recommended to keep strategies very simple and just focus on the repetitive practice of simple strategies in various settings to encourage learning transfer. Surprisingly, a pilot study has shown that providing auditory rhythmic cueing prompts better gait as effectively as in cognitively intact patients.[44]

Balance and Risk of Falls. A recent review on fall predictors in PD and the potential of rehabilitation to remediate these factors identified the following most important predictors: (1) freezing of gait; (2) impaired balance; and (3) cognitive impairment.[26] Less consistently reported fall risk factors include poor mobility, reduced leg muscle strength, difficulty performing daily activities, depression, fear of falling, and impulsivity. Strength training, balance exercises, and strategies to reduce FOG were found to improve these factors but a reduction in fall risk was not demonstrated.[45] Beneficial effects of balance training in PD have so far only been shown in small studies with considerable methodologic weakness.[46] A recent meta-analysis has shown that the level of balance challenge is crucially related to the effect size achieved.[47] In addition, balance training using augmented feedback showed better retention than traditional lower limb strength training for balance.[48] So far, one study has shown that balance training could reduce actual fall frequency in PD.[49] The approach on whether and how to train dual tasking crucially depends on the individual's fall risk and cognitive reserve. Optimally dividing attention over multiple tasks while deciding what to prioritize to ensure safety can be trained during physical therapy and has been shown to be effective in PD in a pilot study.[50] Depending on the severity of the dual-task problem, integrated dual-task training (training two or more tasks simultaneously) or consecutive training of each task separately is recommended.[51] Training effects of cognitive exercises have been shown in PD and can be combined with gait and balance work, especially in the early to mid stages.[52]

In the late stages of the disease, many patients need to be advised regarding the use of walking aids to maintain independence and safety. A walking stick is recommended mainly for patients with well-preserved cognitive functioning because, in some patients, using a stick is experienced as performing a dual task and makes walking more complex. A standard walking frame without wheels is not effective for PD patients, particularly not those with gait initiation problems, which requires continuous starting and stopping. Most PD patients benefit from a wheeled walking frame with compression breaks.[53]

In conclusion, physical therapy is an important tool to address the motor problems occurring in older adults with PD. Patients with PD particularly benefit from exercise and motor learning when supported with feedback and cueing modes. The five key targets for exercise are increasing strength, improving walking, maintaining balance, getting up from sitting, and freezing of gait. To date, no studies have shown the long-term effects of physical therapy. Given the long disease course, rehabilitation methods are needed that promote long-term adherence to exercise, not necessarily with hands-on professional input.

OCCUPATIONAL THERAPY

Occupational therapy has been defined by the World Federation of Occupational Therapists (WFOT)[54] as follows:

> *... a client-centered health profession concerned with promoting health and well-being through occupation. The primary goal of occupational therapy is to enable people to participate in the*

activities of everyday life. Occupational therapists achieve this outcome by working with people and communities to enhance their ability to engage in the occupations they want to, need to or are expected to do, or by modifying the occupation or the environment to better support their occupational engagement.

This definition of occupational therapy reflects the current paradigm of occupation as well as the initial occupational therapy paradigm known as the roots of the profession as stated by Meyer early in the twentieth century.[55] Occupational therapy is grounded in the Arts and Crafts movement of the nineteenth century and the paradigm of occupation that emerged at the beginning of the twentieth century.[56,57] At this time, it was assumed that participation and involvement in purposeful activities had a key role in the health and well-being of the individual.[55] In the mid–twentieth century, a paradigm shift occurred in occupational therapy reasoning, driven by a more biomedical approach, whereby the focus on activity and occupation had to give way to a more restricted approach with limited occupational therapy goals, such as ameliorating functions such as amplitude and strength rather than activity, participation, and occupation.[56-58] During the last decades of the twentieth century, occupational therapy reasoning and practice returned to the previous views of participation and involvement in meaningful occupation[56-58] These views have persisted and are therefore incorporated in the definition of occupational therapy as formulated by the WFOT.[54]

Process

Occupational therapy in geriatric rehabilitation usually is implemented in a multidisciplinary rehabilitation approach. The primary target of occupational therapy is to enable people to perform meaningful occupations by enhancing their ability or modifying the environment or occupation.[54,59] In geriatric rehabilitation, occupational therapy intervention will focus on the consequences of a condition such as stroke or PD, principally by increasing an older adult's ability to perform self-care activities using a range of rehabilitation techniques. This requires a twofold approach, whereby the restoration of the functional capacity of the individual is considered together with modification of the activity to address the individual's ability. Moreover, in addition to the attention given to patient and activity, the environment is targeted to facilitate participation where restricted by physical and sociocultural barriers.[59] This holistic approach, in which the older adult, occupation, and environment are involved, leads to greater independence in ADLs and less deterioration in stroke patients, who receive occupational therapy as part of their multidisciplinary rehabilitation.[60] Furthermore, the client-centered practice is an even more crucial construct in occupational therapy, which implies a dynamic process between patient and therapist, with active involvement of the patient in the rehabilitation process. Clinical reasoning in occupational therapy entails a cyclic process of assessment, therapy planning, and implementation and evaluation.

Assessment

Occupational therapy assessment comprises two major objectives:

1. To identify the patient's needs, and in particular to determine the occupations that are meaningful and important to the patient
2. To explore why these occupations present limitations to the patient and to define the underlying deficits that restrict the performance of purposeful activities[61,62]

The Canadian Occupational Performance Measure (COPM) is a commonly used assessment that addresses the first objective of occupational therapy assessment, specifically to identify an individual's concerns in everyday life performance and hence provides the basis for setting intervention goals and intervention priorities in occupational therapy.[62] In geriatric rehabilitation, a wide range of assessments targeting measures of motor and cognitive skills, as well as specific occupational therapy measures such as the Assessment of Motor and Process Skills (AMPS)[63] or the Perceive, Recall, Plan, and Perform System of Task Analysis (PRPP),[64] are available. These relate to the second objective of occupational therapy. Both assessments (AMPS and PRPP) are based on the observation of task performance and subsequently task analysis to determine the underlying processes that affect task performance.[63,64] AMPS and as PRPP both provide the benefits of a standardized assessment while allowing observation of task performance in a naturalistic context,[62] and results of both lead to more specific goal setting and guide the occupational therapist to individualized therapy interventions.[63,65]

Planning

Regardless of the rehabilitation setting or rehabilitation stage, the use of purposeful and meaningful occupations in occupational therapy interventions is considered to be beneficial, whether the purpose is remediation or compensation of the deficits that the patient is facing.[66] Most common occupational therapy objectives in geriatric stroke rehabilitation include increasing independence and participation in daily living, improving posture and positioning, and providing training and education to caregivers.[59] This is in line with the definition of occupational therapy by the WFOT, which also emphasizes that participation in everyday life activities is the key objective in occupational therapy; this is achieved by two main therapeutic interventions, enhancement of the patient's capacities through restoration of functions and adjustments of the environment or activity to the patient's abilities.[54]

Evaluation

The evaluation of occupational therapy intervention at an individual patient level involves ongoing reassessment of the patient's needs and meaningful occupations, as informed by the restrictions experienced in occupational performance.

Evidence-Based Measures

Occupational Therapy Techniques for Stroke

Multidisciplinary team care is the basis for stroke rehabilitation. Improved outcomes with regards to mortality, institutionalization, and independence for ADLs in stroke survivors who received multidisciplinary care have been demonstrated in several systematic reviews.[67,68] Although the benefits of multidisciplinary stroke care are evident, because of the complex package of treatment, which is usually individualized, it is difficult to determine the responsible components.[69] In the literature, inpatient organized stroke unit care and therapy-based, in-home rehabilitation are described as multidisciplinary care systems improving outcome after stroke.[67,68]

Furthermore, a good rehabilitation outcome seems to be associated with high patient motivation and engagement.[69] It is therefore recommended that rehabilitation goals be determined in collaboration with the patient and caregivers[62] through standardized assessments such as COPM (see earlier) or by interview.[62] Setting goals relevant to the needs of the patient might improve rehabilitation outcome.[69] In occupational therapy, the ultimate goal in stroke rehabilitation is engagement in a range of meaningful occupations, achieved by a collaborative process between the occupational therapist and patient.[62] During the acute stage after stroke, major concerns in occupational therapy intervention are preventing the development of secondary impairments and maximizing recovery.[62] Subsequently, the rehabilitation focus is on improvement in activities within recovery patterns, as well as the restoration of independent occupational performance.[62,70] Finally, in the long-term stage, when recovery is tempered, occupation and environment are targeted, and adjustments or adaptations are made to overcome barriers to optimum independence.[62]

However, overall, occupational therapy interventions increase independence in the ability of performing personal ADLs and instrumental ADLs and improve participation after stroke.[60,66,69] Everyday life occupations should be embedded in stroke rehabilitation by the occupational therapist. The thoughtful use of purposeful occupations applied as a therapeutic measure to remediate impairments, or adjusted to the individual's capability to improve occupational performance, is considered to be highly valuable in stroke rehabilitation.[66] This occupational approach enriches the rehabilitation intervention and is in line with well-accepted principles in stroke rehabilitation, such as task-specific and context-specific training.[69] Occupational therapy services at home, provided within 1 year after stroke, has been shown to improve performance in ADLs,[71] suggesting that occupational therapy should be preferentially provided in the patient's home environment.

Occupational Therapy Techniques for Parkinson Disease

Although PD is a progressive neurologic condition that affects ADLs and social participation, occupational therapy involvement is not very common in the management of PD, perhaps because of the limited evidence of the efficacy of occupational therapy in the management of PD.[72] However, multidisciplinary guidelines do include recommendations for occupational therapy in the management of PD.[73] Because of the complex nature of PD, a patient-centered approach is recommended, whereby the occupational therapy intervention is supporting participation in daily life through the engagement in purposeful occupations. According to multidisciplinary and occupational therapy guidelines in PD,[73,74] occupational therapy intervention should target the following aspects: (1) maintenance of family roles, home care, and leisure activities; (2) improvement and maintenance of transfers and mobility; (3) improvement of self-care activities—eating, drinking, washing, and dressing; (4) consideration of environmental issues; (5) improvement in safety and motor functions; and (6) cognitive assessment and appropriate intervention.[73,74] Recent research has suggested the effectiveness of occupational therapy intervention for patients with PD with home-based, individualized occupational therapy resulting in improvements in self-perceived performance in daily activities.[72]

Practice and Research in Occupational Therapy

Evidence-based practice in occupational therapy is described as a dynamic process based on the best scientific research, knowledge and experience of the occupational therapist, and patient's knowledge and experiences.[75] Although research in occupational therapy has attracted increased interest over the last several decades, it is not yet routinely evidence-based.[59] However, the increase in research-aware occupational therapists is resulting in a more critical approach and a better evidence base for clinical practice.

SUMMARY

Results of occupational therapy research were scarce until the second half of the twentieth century.[76] Although the initial research publications, influenced by the contemporary dominant biomedical approach, reported mainly quantitative research, since the 1980s occupational therapy literature has reported a diverse range of qualitative research, including phenomenologic, narrative, and participatory approaches.[76] In 2007, a study conducted to explore the quality and quantity of occupational therapy research demonstrated huge variations, although some topics were more frequently studied. Research designs of higher quality evidence, such as randomized controlled trials or well-conducted systematic reviews, have been limited.[77] However with the increasing number of research-active therapists and the publication of higher quality research in peer-reviewed journals, this situation is likely to change.

KEY POINTS

- Motor rehabilitation should consist of task-specific and goal-oriented exercises, including a high number of repetitions as well as progression, variation, and adequate feedback.
- Optimal rehabilitation for Parkinson disease involves allocating attention for movement, with or without external feedback and cues.
- Cognitive impairment is the most important barrier to achieving retention of motor learning.
- Effective occupational therapy interventions in neuromotor rehabilitation encompass the use of everyday life occupations.

For a complete list of references, please visit www.expertconsult.com.

KEY REFERENCES

2. World Health Organization: Towards a common language for functioning, disability and health. http://www.who.int/classifications/icf/en. Accessed October 11, 2014.
3. Carr J, Shepherd R: Neurological rehabilitation. Optimizing motor performance, 2010, Elsevier Churchill Livingstone.
4. Veerbeek JM, van Wegen E, van Peppen R, et al: What is the evidence for physical therapy poststroke? A systematic review and meta-analysis. PLoS One 9:e87987, 2014.
25. Nackaerts E, Vervoort G, Heremans E, et al: Relearning of writing skills in Parkinson's disease: a literature review on influential factors and optimal strategies. Neurosci Biobehav Rev 37:349–357, 2013.
26. Canning C, Paul S, Nieuwboer A: Prevention of falls in Parkinson's disease: a review of fall risk factors and the role of physical interventions. Neurodegen Dis Manage 4:203–221, 2014.
27. Tomlinson CL, Patel S, Meek C, et al: Physical therapy versus placebo or no intervention in Parkinson's disease. Cochrane Database System Rev (8):CD002817, 2012.
28. Rochester L, Nieuwboer A, Lord S: Physical therapy for Parkinson's disease: defining evidence within a framework of intervention. Neurodegen Dis Manage 1:57–65, 2011.
29. Petzinger G, Fisher B, Van Leeuwen J-E, et al: Enhancing neuroplasticity in the basal ganglia: the role of exercise in Parkinson's disease. Mov Disord 25(Suppl 1):S141–S145, 2010.
32. Corcos DM, Robichaud JA, David FJ, et al: A two-year randomized controlled trial of progressive resistance exercise for Parkinson's disease. Mov Disord 28:1230–1240, 2013.
37. Nieuwboer A, Kwakkel G, Rochester L, et al: Cueing training in the home improves gait-related mobility in Parkinson's disease: the RESCUE trial. J Neurol Neurosurg Psychiatry 78:134–140, 2007.
60. Legg L, Drummond A, Langhorne P: Occupational therapy for patients with problems in activities of daily living after stroke. Cochrane Database System Rev (4):CD003585, 2006.
62. Sabari J, Lieberman D: American Occupational Therapy Association: Occupational therapy practice guidelines for adults with stroke, Bethesda, MD, 2008, American Occupational Therapy Association.
70. Steultjens E, Dekker J, Bouter L, et al: Evidence of the efficacy of occupational therapy in different conditions: an overview of systematic reviews. Clin Rehabil 19:247–254, 2005.
72. Sturkenboom I, Graff M, Hendriks J, et al: Efficacy of occupational therapy for patients with Parkinson's disease: a randomised controlled trial. Lancet Neurol 13:557–566, 2014.

101 Geriatric Pharmacotherapy and Polypharmacy

Jennifer Greene Naples, Steven M. Handler, Robert L. Maher, Jr., Kenneth E. Schmader, Joseph T. Hanlon

INTRODUCTION

Medications are the most frequently used and misused therapy for the medical problems of the aged. Geriatric health care professionals and their patients rely heavily on pharmacotherapy to cure or manage diseases, palliate symptoms, improve functional status and quality of life, and potentially prolong survival. In the past several decades, knowledge about the epidemiology and clinical pharmacology of drugs in older adults has increased dramatically. The purpose of this chapter is to identify issues related to the efficacy and safety (including medication-related problems) of pharmacotherapy in older populations, to examine approaches to reduce these problems, and to discuss principles of optimal geriatric pharmacotherapy.

EFFICACY AND SAFETY OF PHARMACOTHERAPY FOR OLDER PATIENTS

Historically, older adults have been excluded from clinical drug trials, thereby limiting knowledge regarding the efficacy and safety of geriatric pharmacotherapy.[1] There are, however, encouraging signs that this pattern is changing. For example, evidence for the efficacy of medications in older patients has been bolstered in recent years by a number of seminal randomized controlled clinical trials (RCTs) for geriatric conditions (e.g., behavioral complications with dementia) and diseases (e.g., hypertension).[2,3] The advent of linked administrative databases for pharmacy, laboratory, hospital, and outpatient visits should allow the execution of studies large enough to detect differences in effectiveness and safety of currently marketed drugs in older adults.[4] In addition, the future seems bright for medication discoveries that may benefit older people, as nearly 435 new medicines in the United States are currently in phase I to phase III testing.[5] Organizations responsible for safe medication use have also formally endorsed this shift in clinical research. In 2011, the European Medicines Agency published a document stating it "will ensure that the assessment process gives adequate consideration to the information available to ensure safety and effective use of products in older adults."[6] A similar supportive call to improve the inclusion of older adults in clinical drug trials was published by the U.S. Food and Drug Administration.[7]

Currently, however, there is a paucity of information about the efficacy and effectiveness of available drugs, especially in the frail oldest-old (i.e., those individuals aged 85 years or older). Thus, it is difficult for prescribers to use evidence-based medicine to choose the most appropriate drug therapy for frail older patients while avoiding medication-related problems.

MEDICATION-RELATED PROBLEMS IN OLDER PATIENTS

Information about medication-related problems is derived from postmarketing observational studies of specific therapeutic classes or conditions. Issues commonly associated with medication use include medication errors and adverse drug events (ADEs) (Figure 101-1).[8] A medication error can be defined as "an event that may cause or lead to inappropriate medication use or patient harm while the medication is in the control of the health care professional, patient, or consumer."[8-10] These errors may occur at the prescribing, order communication, dispensing, administration/taking, or monitoring stages of the medication use process and are considered preventable.

Medication errors may result in an ADE, defined as "an injury due to a medication."[9] Of the three different types of ADEs, the most common is an adverse drug reaction (ADR), classified as "a response to a drug that is noxious and unintended and occurs at doses normally used for the prophylaxis, diagnosis, or therapy of disease, or for modification of physiological function."[11] The second type of ADE is an adverse drug withdrawal event (ADWE), characterized as "a clinical set of symptoms or signs that are related to the discontinuation of a drug."[11,12] Lastly, a therapeutic failure (TF) is defined as "a failure to accomplish the goals of treatment resulting from inadequate drug therapy and not related to the natural progression of disease (e.g., omission of necessary medication therapy, inadequate medication dose or duration, and medication non-adherence)."[11] Recent studies of medication errors and ADEs in older adults have been described in annual summaries.[13-18] The following sections describe some of the most pertinent studies pertaining to the epidemiology of these three distinct types of ADEs.

EPIDEMIOLOGY OF ADVERSE DRUG REACTIONS

Emergency department evaluation and hospitalization are some of the worst adverse consequences of pharmacotherapy. A meta-analysis of older studies found that 16% of all hospitalizations in older adults were because of ADRs.[19] A more recent systematic review identified seven additional studies between 2000 and 2013 in which hospitalization rates ranged from 5.0% to 30.4%.[20] This review, however, did not include two important studies from the United States. In the first, Budnitz and colleagues identified 5077 cases of ADRs over a 2-year time period, which extrapolated to 98,628 hospitalizations of adults older than 65 years; nearly half involved patients aged 80 and older.[21] In the second study of 678 veterans who were at least 65 years old, 10% of unplanned hospitalizations over 2 years were determined to be related to an ADR according to the Naranjo ADR causality algorithm.[22,23] Of these, only 36.8% were deemed preventable, with suboptimal prescribing identified as the primary precipitator. Extrapolation to the U.S. population of older veterans receiving primary care suggests that approximately 8000 would have been hospitalized secondary to an ADR.

Few investigators have studied ADRs in older outpatients or nursing home residents. In a large cohort study of 27,617 older ambulatory adults, 5.5% experienced an ADR over the 12-month study period, of which 27.6% (421) were considered preventable.[24] Another prospective cohort study of 626 Medicare beneficiaries aged 65 and older with mobility limitations found that 38 (22%) self-reported an ADR.[25] Finally, a retrospective cohort study used a causality algorithm to examine the prevalence of type

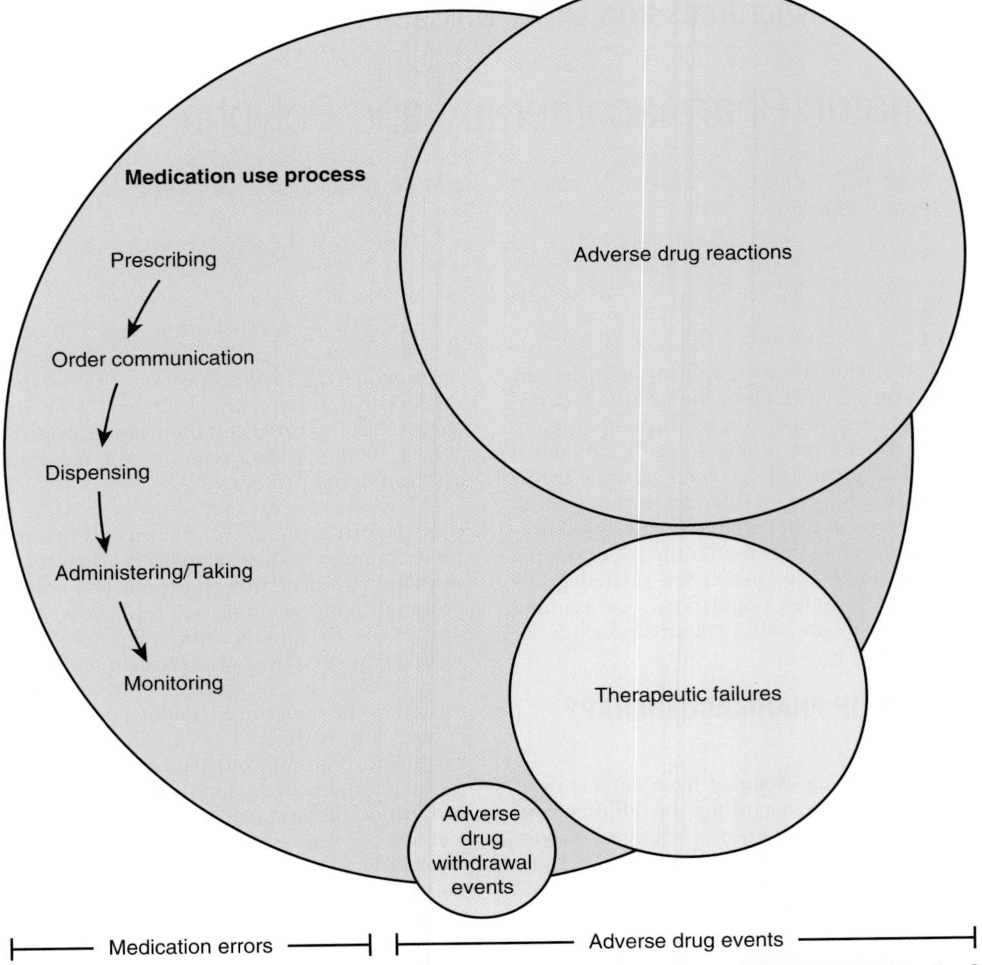

Figure 101-1. Conceptual model for medication-related problems in older adults. *Modified from Handler SM, Wright RM, Ruby CM, et al: Epidemiology of medication-related adverse events in nursing homes. Am J Geriatr Pharmacother 4:264–272, 2006.*

A ADRs (i.e., ADRs due to an exaggeration of the expected pharmacologic effect of a drug) in ambulatory adults.[26] Among 359 frail older veterans transitioning from hospital to community and prescribed a high-risk medication, 31.8% were found to have one or more type A ADRs rated at least "possible" on the Naranjo ADR algorithm scale.[22,26]

Gurwitz and colleagues studied the occurrence of ADRs in 18 nursing homes in the U.S. state of Massachusetts.[27] Over a 1-year period, 2916 nursing home residents had 546 ADRs, an incidence rate of 1.89 ADRs per 100 resident-months. Overall, nearly 44% of ADRs were fatal, life-threatening, or serious, and 51% were preventable. Subsequently, Gurwitz and colleagues also examined the combined incidence of ADRs in two academic nursing homes.[28] In this 9-month prospective observational study, 815 ADRs were detected among 1247 nursing home residents, an incidence rate of 9.8 ADRs per 100 resident-months. The majority (80%) of ADRs occurred at the monitoring stage of the medication use process and, as in the previous study, a large proportion (42%) was considered preventable. Collectively, these studies from a variety of settings demonstrate that ADRs are common phenomena in older patients.

In published studies discussing ADRs in older adults, only polypharmacy has been consistently identified as a risk factor, although some have suggested that ADRs may be attributed to a select few medication classes (e.g., antithrombotics, antidiabetics, and opioids).[21,29,30] Reducing the number of medications in older patients with multiple comorbidities may be challenging, however, because these concomitant diseases often require pharmacotherapy. It is also difficult to avoid drug classes most associated with ADRs because they are essential to the management of older persons. There is some evidence that specific types of medication errors (e.g., inappropriate prescribing, suboptimal lab monitoring, and medication nonadherence) increase the risk of ADRs.

Inappropriate prescribing refers to the selection of a medication where either the risks associated with its use outweigh the benefits or utilization does not agree with accepted medical standards.[31,32] Whether using explicit or implicit criteria, potentially inappropriate prescribing is common regardless of care setting, affecting 25% to 92% of older patients.[33-35] Since the last edition of this book, four studies have been published that found inappropriate prescribing increases the risk of ADRs as measured by explicit criteria such as the Screening Tool of Older Persons (STOPP) and American Geriatric Society Beers criteria.[25,36-38] Similar results were seen in five studies using a reliable and valid implicit measure, the Medication Appropriateness Index (MAI).[26,37,39-41] Drug-drug and drug-disease interactions may be the most important types of potentially inappropriate prescribing that increases the risk of ADRs.[25,26] This is clinically sensible given that aging is associated with decreases in organ function and hemostatic reserve, changes in drug pharmacokinetics and pharmacodynamics, and increases in the number of comorbidities requiring drug therapy.

Suboptimal monitoring may also increase the risk of ADRs in older adults.[42,43] In the ambulatory care setting, a substantial proportion of older adults does not receive appropriate laboratory monitoring while taking chronic prescription medications.[44,45] Indeed, as many as 70% of the ADRs in nursing homes are related to a failure to appropriately monitor medications.[27,28]

The most common medication adherence problem is underuse.[46,47] However, the contribution of medication nonadherence to ADRs is likely minor, as older patients may be adherent with up to 75% of their total number of medications.[48]

EPIDEMIOLOGY OF ADVERSE DRUG WITHDRAWAL EVENTS

Because ADWEs are not formally examined in clinical trials, practitioners must rely on clinical experience and published data in the postmarketing period to glean information about these problems.[12,49] ADWEs may manifest either as a physiologic withdrawal reaction (e.g., β-blocker withdrawal syndrome) or as an exacerbation of the underlying disease.[12,49] A 2008 review summarized data from clinical trials about the benefits and risk of discontinuing specific drugs/classes.[50]

Few studies have examined ADWEs when multiple different drug classes are discontinued in older patients. Of those presented here, all used causality algorithms such as the Naranjo scale. Overall, ADWEs were much less common than ADRs or TFs, rarely severe, and almost always preventable. Gerety and coworkers investigated ADWEs in a single nursing home in the U.S. state of Texas over an 18-month time period and found that 62 nursing home patients experienced a total of 94 ADWEs (mean 0.54 per patient), corresponding to an incidence of 0.32 reactions per patient-month.[51] Cardiovascular (37%), central nervous system (22%), and gastrointestinal (21%) drug classes were most frequently associated with an ADWE. A study of ambulatory older patients by Graves and associates in the U.S. examined ADWEs in 124 patients. Of 238 drugs discontinued, 62 (26%) resulted in 72 ADWEs in 38 patients.[52] Again, cardiovascular (42%) and central nervous system (18%) drug classes were the most frequently implicated. Only 26 drugs (36%) discontinued led to ADWEs that required hospitalization, emergency department evaluations, or urgent care clinic visits. Most of these ADWEs were exacerbations of an underlying disease, and some withdrawal events occurred up to 4 months after the medication was discontinued. In a study by Kennedy and colleagues, ADWEs were investigated in the postoperative period at a single hospital.[53] Of 1025 patients studied, 50% were older than 60 years. Thirty-four patients suffered postsurgical complications resulting from drug therapy withdrawal. Specific drug classes involved included antihypertensives (especially angiotensin-converting enzyme inhibitors), antiparkinson medications (notably levodopa/carbidopa), benzodiazepines, and antidepressants. A retrospective chart review of 627 older patients in Japan evaluated the incidence of ADWEs for the first three months after admission to a long-term care facility. Of the 230 patients with medication reduction, only 5 (2.2%) experienced an ADWE. Discontinuation of antipsychotics resulted in confusion in three cases. Relapse in depression and hyperglycemia were seen in the other two cases after stopping antidepressants and sulfonylureas, respectively.[54]

Recently, case reports suggest that the abrupt cessation of donepezil may also be associated with ADWEs, including agitation and delirium, beginning approximately 3 to 5 days after discontinuation. In two cases where donepezil was restarted, symptoms resolved entirely.[55,56] When donepezil rechallenge was not employed, symptoms fluctuated, disappearing by day 10 after cessation.[55] No causality algorithm was used in these studies. Finally, a study in the U.S. examining medication changes between bidirectional nursing home and hospital transfers illustrated that half of the ADEs attributed to medication changes were the result of drug discontinuation.[57]

Little is known about the risk factors for ADWEs. In the study by Gerety and colleagues ADWEs were associated with multiple diagnoses, multiple medications, longer nursing home stays, and hospitalization.[51] The number of medications stopped has also been shown to significantly predict ADWEs.[52] Additionally, the risk of ADWEs may rise as the length of time off a medication increases.[53]

EPIDEMIOLOGY OF THERAPEUTIC FAILURE

There are very few published trials examining TF in older patients. In a U.S. study of TF leading to hospitalization, investigators used the reliable Therapeutic Failure Questionnaire (TFQ) to measure causality in 106 frail older adults admitted to 11 Veterans Affairs hospitals.[58] Eleven percent of these individuals had probable TF leading to hospitalization, with congestive heart failure and chronic obstructive pulmonary disease representing the most commonly-associated comorbidities. Italian investigators found that 6.8% of patients in the emergency department had evidence of TF, with nearly two-thirds occurring in patients older than 65 years.[59] A U.S. investigation of drug-related emergency department visits in older patients found that 28% of drug-related visits were due to TF.[60] Using an implicit Likert scale, researchers on a geriatric hospital ward in Belgium noted that 9 of 110 (8.2%) admissions were due to TF, specifically resulting from nonadherence and subtherapeutic dosing.[61] Marcum and associates also reported that, based on the TFQ causality algorithm, 34 of 678 (5%) veterans with unplanned hospitalizations had evidence of TF. Thirty-two instances were deemed preventable, as medication nonadherence and suboptimal prescribing were the most common reasons for TF.[62]

Risk factors for TF have not been clearly delineated. The most recently published study found that African American veterans were significantly more likely to experience TF-related hospital admissions than were white veterans.[62] This may be because of lower medication adherence rates in African American versus white older adults.[63] Other reasons for TF may include low prescribed doses, hepatic metabolism enzyme induction, drug interactions, drug resistance or nonresponse, inadequate therapeutic monitoring, or underprescribing of necessary drug therapies.

Nonadherence was the most common reason for TF in two U.S. TFQ hospitalization studies (46% and 58%) and in the U.S. emergency department visit study (66%).[50,58,62] Older patients may fail to fill or take their prescriptions, skip doses, take the drug erratically, or take reduced doses. These behaviors may be intentional (e.g., adverse effects, health beliefs, concerns about taking too many drugs) or unintentional (e.g., cognitive impairment, poor vision or dexterity, lack of transportation).[42] Cost-related nonadherence is a particularly important and prevalent subtype of intentional nonadherence among older adults with limited means.[63,64]

Another major factor related to TF is the underprescribing of medications, defined as the omission of drug therapy indicated for the treatment or prevention of a disease or condition.[65] A study that applied the explicit Assessing Care of Vulnerable Elders criteria found that 50% of 372 vulnerable adults were not prescribed an indicated medication.[66] The most common omissions were gastroprotective agents for high-risk users of nonsteroidal inflammatory drugs, angiotensin-converting enzyme inhibitors in diabetics with proteinuria, and calcium and/or vitamin D for those with osteoporosis. Studies using the explicit START (Screening Tool to Alert doctors to the Right Treatment) criteria have reported rates of underprescribing of 22% to 74% in older patients.[31,67-69] A group of U.S. investigators using the Assessment of Underutilization of Medication measure found evidence of medication underuse in 62% of 384 frail older patients at hospital discharge.[70] The necessary drug classes most likely to be absent were cardiovascular agents (e.g., antianginals), blood modifiers (e.g., antiplatelets), vitamins (e.g., multivitamins), and central nervous system medications (e.g., antidepressants). Patients with greater comorbidity and limited ability to perform basic activities of daily living were at higher risk for undertreatment.

APPROACHES TO REDUCE MEDICATION-RELATED PROBLEMS IN OLDER PATIENTS

Given that medication-related problems are common, costly, and clinically important, how can they be reduced? Finding a specific answer to this question is surprisingly difficult because there are few health services intervention clinical trials in older patients that examine approaches to reduce ADRs, ADWEs, or TF. Therefore, health policy makers and clinicians must look to reasonable, empirical approaches based on existing epidemiologic and clinical information. These approaches include better health systems design, improved health services, and patient and caregiver education. (Professional education is discussed in the section "Principles of Optimal Geriatric Pharmacotherapy.")

Health Systems Design

Medication-related problems can be reduced by designing health care systems that make it difficult for individuals to do the "wrong" thing and easy to do the "right" thing.[71] In an Institute of Medicine report, the authors provide a number of specific recommendations to improve medication safety.[9] One suggestion proposes that all health care organizations immediately make complete patient-information and decision-support tools available to clinicians and patients. Another recommendation encourages health care systems to capture information about medication-related issues and use this information to improve overall safety. Health care organizations should also implement the appropriate systems to enable providers to (1) have access to comprehensive reference information concerning medications and related health data; (2) assess the safety of medication use through active monitoring and use these monitoring data to inform the implementation of prevention strategies; (3) write prescriptions electronically; and (4) subject prescriptions to evidence-based, current clinical decision support. Systematic reviews of studies have found that computerized physician order entry and clinical decision support systems improve the quality, efficiency, and cost of health care for elders.[72-75] Few have explicitly examined the effect of computerized order entry and clinical decision support systems on ADEs, but it is likely that continued development and refinement will lead to a reduction in medication errors and medication-related adverse events in a variety of care settings.[76] For example, a cluster RCT found when patient-specific risk estimates of the likelihood of falls secondary to central nervous system medications were provided in the electronic health record, the risk of injury was reduced for vulnerable older outpatients.[77] Another RCT in nursing homes used pharmacist drug regimen review supported by computer software to identify patients taking medications that put them at risk for geriatric syndromes and health services use.[78] This study demonstrated a significantly decreased risk of delirium and a nonsignificant decrease in ADE-related hospitalizations.[78]

Health Services Approaches

A number of reviews and book chapters have discussed health services approaches designed to improve suboptimal prescribing, including academic detailing, clinical pharmacist consultation, and geriatric medicine services.[79-85] However, only four RCTs to date have demonstrated the ability of these strategies to actually decrease ADEs in older adults. One such successful health services strategy is the provision of geriatric medicine services, also known as geriatric evaluation and management (GEM). In this model, a multidisciplinary team of specialists, including a geriatrician physician, nurse, social worker, and pharmacist, collaborate to provide comprehensive patient care. An important component of GEM is the assessment and optimization of medications. One study by Schmader and colleagues showed that GEM care reduced underuse of medications and decreased the risk of serious ADRs in frail outpatients.[86] Another RCT found that clinical pharmacist activities improved suboptimal prescribing in older hospitalized patients and reduced subsequent ADE readmissions.[37,87] Finally, a multidisciplinary education intervention was shown in a RCT to both improve medication appropriateness and reduce drug-related readmissions.[40] Additional large, multicenter controlled trials are needed to determine the effectiveness of these and other approaches for optimizing medication use on medication-related ADEs in older adults.

Patient and Caregiver Education

Providing systematic education to patients and caregivers about potentially inappropriate medications and possible ADEs may have multidimensional benefits. Use of high-risk medications may be reduced and, if ADEs do occur, patients or caregivers may be able to recognize and report issues earlier, allowing clinicians to adjust medications sooner. A novel recent RCT initiated at 30 community pharmacies tested the impact of patient education booklets describing the risks of benzodiazepine use and the importance of tapering schedules in 3303 older outpatients.[88] Under the supervision of the physician or pharmacist, more patients receiving booklets discontinued benzodiazepines (25%) or reduced the dose (16%) than those not receiving education. It is conceivable that a larger study might have also found a reduction in falls or fractures associated with benzodiazepine reduction. Although not measured in this study, it is also possible that education regarding the necessity of a slow benzodiazepine taper instead of abrupt cessation may have helped prevent ADWEs. Another study examining the effects of pharmacist medication counseling for patients and caregivers at hospital discharge showed reduction in the rate of ADRs.[89] Finally, a recent review summarizing RCTs designed to enhance medication adherence in older adults found that patient education and adherence aids improved medication adherence, thereby reducing potential TF-related hospitalizations resulting from a patient or caregiver's decision to stop a beneficial medication.[90]

PRINCIPLES OF OPTIMAL GERIATRIC PHARMACOTHERAPY

Clinicians who care for older patients must know and be able to apply principles of optimal geriatric pharmacotherapy in order to maximize the benefits of medications and minimize medication-related problems (Box 101-1). The first step in prescribing is to decide whether drug therapy is truly necessary, as many medical problems in older patients do not require a pharmacologic solution. This assessment should take into account life expectancy and the time to benefit required for medications.[91] If a medication is indicated and its benefits outweigh its risks, then selection of an agent should be based on the medication's pharmacokinetics, possible adverse effects, potential drug interactions, and the patient's disease states, including renal and hepatic function.[92] In older patients, starting at lower doses and/or extending the dosing interval before modifying the dosage may be necessary. Evaluating cost, establishing clear therapeutic end points, and incorporating patient preference in pharmacotherapy decisions

BOX 101-1 Principles of Optimal Geriatric Pharmacotherapy

1. Consider whether medication therapy is necessary.
2. Understand the pharmacology of the medication in relation to age.
3. Know the adverse effect profile of the medication in relation to the patient's other medication(s) and disease(s).
4. Choose initial dose, and adjust it carefully (doses will often need to be lower in older people).
5. Select the least costly alternative.
6. Establish clear, feasible therapeutic end points.
7. Monitor for adverse drug reactions, an important cause of illness in older adults.
8. Slowly taper medications to prevent or minimize adverse drug withdrawal events (if possible).
9. Regularly review the need for chronic medications and discontinue unnecessary ones.
10. Assess whether there is omission of needed medication for an established diagnosis or condition.
11. Review adherence, simplify the medication regimen, if possible, and consider use of aids.

are also important, especially when considering the use of a medication in patients with multiple comorbidities in which actual risks and benefits have not been established.

As part of continuous care management, clinicians should monitor for potential ADRs via patient history, physical examination, and, where appropriate, laboratory data.[85] Identifying ADRs can be challenging in older patients because ADRs may present in a vague or atypical fashion, and the causal link can be difficult to establish. ADRs should be included in the differential diagnosis of most geriatric syndromes. If the adverse event is a known side effect of one or more of the patient's medications, confidence in establishing ADR causality can be increased by determining the temporal relationship between medication initiation and event onset, evaluating competing causes, and assessing the effects of rechallenge or dechallenge among other factors.[22] Nonetheless, in some cases it may be difficult or impossible to establish the causal link between a medication and subsequent adverse event in an older patient.

In patients who have recently stopped a medication, it is important to consider the possibility of an ADWE. In older patients, ADWEs can be overlooked when the withdrawal reaction is mistaken for a patient's disease state. Everyday events that can lead to an ADWE include discontinuation of unwanted therapies, intentional nonadherence, medication cessation before surgical procedures, and managed care practices of therapeutic interchange within classes of medications. Table 101-1 lists medications commonly used by older patients that may be associated with withdrawal syndromes or exacerbation of the underlying disease.[51,52,93,94] To prevent ADWEs, clinicians should consider the dose, duration, and pharmacokinetics of medications.[49] Risk can be minimized or eliminated by slow, careful tapering of the medication over a prolonged period of time. This approach is similar to that taken in the initiation and titration of a new medication. Unfortunately, precise tapering schedules have not been established for most medications.

At each visit it is necessary to review and, if possible, simplify the patient's medication regimen. This may be achieved by altering the dosing schedule and/or discontinuing medicines that are no longer warranted. Measures such as the MAI may be used to facilitate medication reviews when providers are evaluating older patients taking multiple medications (Box 101-2).[32,95] Standardized tools can also be used to evaluate possible omissions of necessary therapies. For example, the Assessment of Underutilization of Medication requires a health professional to match a patient's complete list of chronic medical conditions to the prescribed medications after reviewing the medical record.[70] In this manner, omissions of evidence-based medications for a given disease state based on scientific literature may be identified. For each condition, one of three ratings can be made: omission, marginal omission (e.g., have used an appropriate nonpharmacologic approach), or no omission.

Once suboptimal prescribing is addressed, it is important to assess how a patient takes his or her medications and to identify risk factors for poor adherence (e.g., impaired hearing, vision, and cognition) so that an individualized plan may be developed.[46] Health care professionals may consider providing adherence aids to their older patients and should follow up on adherence recommendations with regular monitoring. General methods to enhance

TABLE 101-1 Medications Associated With Adverse Drug Withdrawal Events in Older Adults

Medications	Type of Withdrawal	Withdrawal Syndrome
α-Antagonist antihypertensives	P, D	Hypertension, palpitations, headache, agitation
Angiotensin-converting enzyme inhibitors	P, D	Hypertension, heart failure
Antianginal agents	D	Myocardial ischemia
Anticholinesterase inhibitors	D	Delirium, agitation, anxiety, insomnia, difficulty concentrating, rapidly changing mood
Anticonvulsants	P, D	Seizures, anxiety, depression
Antidepressants	P, D	Akathisia, anxiety, irritability, gastrointestinal distress, malaise, myalgia, headache, coryza, chills, insomnia, recurrence of depression
Antiparkinson agents	P, D	Rigidity, tremor, pulmonary embolism, psychosis, hypotension
Antipsychotics	P	Nausea, restlessness, insomnia, dyskinesia
Baclofen	P	Hallucinations, paranoia, insomnia, nightmares, mania, depression, anxiety, agitation, confusion, seizures, hypertonia
Benzodiazepines	P	Agitation, confusion, delirium, seizures, insomnia
β-Blockers	P	Angina, myocardial infarction, anxiety, tachycardia, hypertension
Corticosteroids	P	Weakness, anorexia, nausea, hypotension
Digoxin	D	Heart failure, palpitations
Diuretics	D	Hypertension, heart failure
Histamine-2 blockers	D	Recurrence of esophagitis and indigestion symptoms
Opioids	P	Restlessness, anxiety, anger, insomnia, chills, abdominal cramping, diarrhea, diaphoresis
Nonsteroidal antiinflammatory drugs	P	Recurrence of arthritis and gout inflammatory drugs
Sedative/hypnotics (e.g., barbiturates)	P	Anxiety, muscle twitches, tremor, dizziness
Statins		Early neurological deterioration, heart failure, myocardial infarction, ventricular arrhythmia, cardiogenic shock

D, Exacerbation of underlying disease; *P*, physiologic withdrawal.

BOX 101-2 Medication Appropriateness Index

QUESTIONS TO ASK ABOUT EACH MEDICATION

1. Is there an indication for the medication?
2. Is the medication effective for the condition?
3. Is the dosage correct?
4. Are the directions correct?
5. Are the directions practical?
6. Are there clinically significant drug-drug interactions?
7. Are there clinically significant drug-disease/condition interactions?
8. Is there unnecessary duplication with other medication(s)?
9. Is the duration of therapy acceptable?
10. Is this medication the least expensive alternative compared to others of equal utility?

adherence in older patients include simplifying regimens, providing written instructions, and considering generic formulations to reduce costs. Pill boxes, larger font size on prescription labels, calendars, easy-to-swallow dosage forms, pill cutters, oral dosing syringes, insulin syringe magnification, tube spacers for inhalers, and easy-open caps may be specific strategies to improve adherence in this population. Electronic adherence aids (e.g., alarm watches with messages, automated pill delivery systems, medication bottles with alarms) may also prove beneficial. Finally, active patient and family involvement should be encouraged.

SUMMARY

Pharmacotherapy may greatly enhance the quality of life of geriatric patients by effectively palliating, preventing, or treating many conditions in late life. The clinical trial evidence for the efficacy of medications in older patients has significantly increased in past decades, and many more potentially beneficial medications are in development. However, clinical trial data may be limited by underrepresentation of older patients, exclusion of frail older or oldest-old patients, and lack of postmarketing studies designed to assess the effectiveness of competing medications. In addition, the benefits of medication therapy can be offset by ADRs, ADWEs, and TF. Although frequency estimations vary, many epidemiologic studies agree that these medication-related problems are common, costly, and clinically important in older patients. Potential solutions include designing better health systems, implementing health services approaches, and educating patients and caregivers, but more research is needed to determine the feasibility and effectiveness of these approaches. Clinicians who care for older patients must know and apply principles of optimal geriatric pharmacotherapy in order to maximize the benefits of medications and minimize medication-related problems.

KEY POINTS

- Knowledge about the efficacy and safety of medications in older adults is limited.
- Medication-related adverse patient events, such as adverse drug reactions, adverse drug withdrawal events, and therapeutic failure, are common and result in considerable morbidity in older adults.
- Strategies to modify or reduce medication-related problems, including polypharmacy, will require health systems to design and institute new approaches to delivering health care to older adults.
- Clinicians should strive to conduct periodic systematic reviews of older patients' medication regimens as well as adhere to other principles to optimize geriatric pharmacotherapy.

For a complete list of references, please visit www.expertconsult.com.

KEY REFERENCES

4. Hilmer SN, Gnjidic D, Abernethy DR: Pharmacoepidemiology in the postmarketing assessment of the safety and efficacy of drugs in older adults. J Gerontol Med Sci 67:181–188, 2012.
11. Edwards IR, Aronson JK: Adverse drug reactions: definitions, diagnosis, and management. Lancet 356:1255–1259, 2000.
19. Beijer HJ, de Blaey CJ: Hospitalisations caused by adverse drug reactions: a meta-analysis of observational studies. Pharm World Sci 24:46–54, 2002.
23. Marcum ZA, Amuan ME, Hanlon JT, et al: Prevalence of unplanned hospitalizations caused by adverse drug reactions in older veterans. J Am Geriatr Soc 60:34–41, 2012.
29. Maher R, Hanlon JT, Hajjar ER: Clinical consequences of polypharmacy in elderly. Expert Opin Drug Saf 13:57–65, 2014.
31. American Geriatrics Society: 2015 Beers Criteria Update Expert Panel: AGS updated Beers criteria for potentially inappropriate medication use in older adults. J Am Geriatr Soc 63:2227–2246, 2015.
32. Hanlon JT, Schmader KE: The Medication Appropriateness Index at 20: where it started, where it has been and where it may be going. Drugs Aging 30:893–900, 2013.
34. O'Mahony D, O'Sullivan D, Byrne S, et al: STOPP/START criteria for potentially inappropriate prescribing in older people: version 2. Age Ageing 44:213–218, 2015.
42. Steinman MA, Handler SM, Gurwitz JH, et al: Beyond the prescription: medication monitoring and adverse drug events in older adults. J Am Geriatr Soc 59:1513–1520, 2011.
46. Hughes CM: Medication non-adherence in the elderly. Drugs Aging 21:793–811, 2004.
49. Bains K, Holmes H, Beers M, et al: Discontinuing medications: a novel approach for revising the prescribing stage of the medication use process. J Am Geriatr Soc 56:1946–1952, 2008.
62. Marcum ZA, Pugh MV, Amuan ME, et al: Prevalence of potentially preventable unplanned hospitalizations caused by therapeutic failures and adverse drug withdrawal events among older veterans. J Gerontol Med Sci 67:867–874, 2012.
65. Cherubini A, Corsonello A, Lattanzio F: Underprescription of beneficial medicines in older people: causes, consequences and prevention. Drugs Aging 29:463–475, 2012.
80. Spinewine A, Schmader KE, Barber N, et al: Appropriate prescribing in elderly people: how can it be measured and optimized? Lancet 370:173–184, 2007.
81. Tjia J, Velten SJ, Parsons C, et al: Studies to reduce unnecessary medication use in frail older adults: a systematic review. Drugs Aging 30:285–307, 2013.
82. Patterson SM, Cadogan CA, Kerse N, et al: Interventions to improve the appropriate use of polypharmacy for older people. Cochrane Database Syst Rev (10):CD008165, 2014.
83. Alldred DP, Raynor DK, Hughes C, et al: Interventions to optimise prescribing for older people in care homes. Cochrane Database Syst Rev (2):CD009095, 2013.
85. Hajjar ER, Hanlon JT, Maher RM: Drug-related problems in older adults. In Hutchison L, Sleeper R, editors: Fundamentals of geriatric pharmacotherapy: an evidence-based approach, ed 2, Bethesda, MD, 2015, American Society of Health-System Pharmacists.
91. Holmes HM, Min LC, Yee M, et al: Rationalizing prescribing for older patients with multimorbidity: considering time to benefit. Drugs Aging 30:655–666, 2013.

102 Impaired Mobility

Nancy L. Low Choy, Eamonn Eeles, Ruth E. Hubbard

INTRODUCTION

Impaired mobility and balance dysfunction each become more common with aging. Acute changes in each ("off legs," falls) remain among the "geriatric giants" or now, as they increasingly are called, acute geriatric syndromes. Whether slower changes in mobility and balance are physiologic (and inevitable) or pathologic (and potentially mutable) remains unclear. The accumulation of deficits, including those that affect motor performance, may be inevitable at an advanced age. However, factors such as sedentary behavior, emergence of chronic diseases, and low levels of physical activity, which all make significant negative contributions to mobility integrity, can be mitigated.

This chapter addresses impaired mobility and the integral relationship with balance, but does not focus on the issue of falls, the theme of Chapter 103. We briefly review some essential features of how mobility changes with age. This is approached from a hierarchical perspective that includes higher order, executive function through gait speed to gait initiation, transitions from sitting to standing and, finally, from lying to sitting. Next, we describe some common gait disorders and how a structured approach to assessment can facilitate their classification. The clinical assessment of balance and mobility for older adults is reviewed to highlight strengths of specific tools for management in community and hospital settings. Finally, we explore the relationship between impaired mobility and frailty and appraise current interventions for impaired mobility across the frailty spectrum.

AGE-RELATED CHANGES IN MOBILITY

Mobility is the term used to refer to a number of fundamental daily activities that range from walking to sitting and standing tasks to in-bed mobility. In this section, we explore the age-related changes that occur with each of these activities, providing a foundation for the assessment and management of balance and mobility.

Executive Function

Walking was traditionally seen as an automatic task requiring little input from higher mental functions. However, an intricate interaction between gait and executive function is now recognized.[1] Older healthy adults with the greatest declines in executive function, relative to cognition, exhibit impaired functional mobility[2] and experience more falls.[3] As executive function declines, an increase in the double support phase and step time of the gait pattern occurs.[4]

Studies investigating dual tasks, which are dependent on intact executive function, have demonstrated that older adults are less able to maintain normal walking while performing an additional task, particularly talking.[5] Even in physically fit older adults, dual tasks influence balance during walking through a direct effect on body sway and stride variability and an indirect effect on gait velocity.[6] Task shifting when multitasking is also impaired with aging, with inhibitory control, mental set shifting, and attentional flexibility predictive of functional mobility in older adults.[7]

The pathophysiology of these changes may originate in the prefrontal cortex, which plays a crucial role in executive functioning and is particularly vulnerable to microvascular damage.[8] Hypoactivation of the medial frontal gyrus, a region involved in motor planning, is linked with falls in older adults[7] although, intriguingly, frontal executive network disruption does not appear to be predictive of fallers.[9] Pilot studies have shown that targeted executive function training is feasible and may improve gait parameters, including balance.[10]

Gait Speed

Older adults tend to walk more slowly than young adults. In a nationally representative sample of community dwellers in Ireland, usual walking speed declined after the age of 50 years, with the most pronounced drop after age 65.[11] Although this sample excluded patients with severe cognitive impairment, dementia, and Parkinson disease (PD) and those living in residential care facilities, individuals with chronic disease were included. This raises the question of whether declines in gait speed are secondary to pathologic processes rather than being age-related changes. Studies of the fittest older adults support the latter hypothesis. Cross-sectional investigations of elite athletes have shown reductions in speed and endurance of approximately 3.4%/year between 50 and 74 years, with notable acceleration after older adults 75 years.[12] However, although some slowing of gait speed is to be expected with increasing age, there is a growing body of evidence to suggest that this may not be benign.

Generally speaking, gait speed is reflective of overall health status. The mean walking speed of older community dwellers is significantly faster than their age-matched peers in the hospital[13] or in residential care facilities.[14] Slow gait speed is also associated with adverse outcomes. A systematic review of 27 different studies has concluded that slowness (measured by walking at a usual pace over 4 m) identified autonomous older adults at risk of future disability, cognitive impairment, and institutionalization.[15] Similarly, in pooled data from 34,485 people older than 65 years followed for between 6 and 21 years, survival increased across the full range of gait speeds, with significant increments per 0.1 m/sec.[16] Gait speed has therefore been advocated as a marker of frailty, either exclusively[17] or in combination with other markers of strength and vitality.[18] Indeed, in a study of seven potential frailty criteria, including weakness, weight loss, and exhaustion, slow gait speed was the strongest predictor of chronic disability and the only significant predictor of falls.[19] The dynamic nature of frailty has also been explored and supported by the measurement of mobility changes in older adults.[20]

The cause of slow gait speed has not yet been fully elucidated, but cerebrovascular disease is likely to be the key pathophysiologic factor. Slow walking has been linked to white matter hyperdensities and with gray matter changes in the medial temporal area.[9,21] A smaller volume of the prefrontal area seems to contribute to slow gait through slower information processing and motor planning.[22] Similarly, the association between faster gait speed and larger cerebellar gray matter volume is significantly influenced by information-processing ability.[23] Hypertension may also be a critical contributor. In the Cardiovascular Health Study, hypertension accelerated slowing of gait speed[24] and mediated the association between the degree of white matter hyperintensities and mobility impairments.[25]

Gait Initiation

Gait initiation requires the integrated control of limb movement and posture and is achieved with purposeful postural shifts at toe off, including relaxation of the triceps surae for swing and synergistic contraction of ventral, hip abductor and quadriceps muscles for support, modulated by controlled knee flexion mid stance. These culminate in a forward step, with steady-state velocity being achieved in less than two steps.[26] Gait initiation is well preserved in healthy older adults.[27] Abnormalities of gait initiation are a sensitive but not specific sign of disease processes in older adults, such as those with PD, multiple cerebral infarcts, normal-pressure hydrocephalus, progressive supranuclear palsy, and cervical myelopathy.

Transitions Into Standing from Sitting

The ability to stand from a bed or chair is a critical aspect of mobility, independently predicting mobility disability and activities of daily living disability in community-dwelling older adults.[28] The activity of standing up involves a number of phases, including the following: (1) a preparatory phase that positions the feet for weight acceptance, along with forward inclination of the trunk to shift the center of mass forward over the feet; (2) a peak force phase, enabling weight acceptance onto the feet to commence standing up; (3) a phase of controlled extension enabling attainment of upright stance; and (4) a stabilization phase in stance that enables the individual to remain steady.[29] Inefficient preparatory patterns may occur when people are obese[30] or present with chronic obstructive airway disease,[31] along with PD or some other neurologic gait disturbance.[27] Reduced range of motion in the hips, pelvis, knees, and spine is common with aging and impedes the initial shift of the total body center of mass over the feet. Weakness of the hip girdle muscles is also a frequent finding in older adults and is a manifestation of general deconditioning, and those affected may need to use their arms to help themselves up. Chair stands are sensitive to changes in postural control, strength, and coordination and thus are useful as a physical performance measure[32] for frail and high-function older adults.

Transitions from Lying to Sitting Over the Bed Edge

One study of older adults has shown the importance of the start position in bed and strength in the upper limbs when weak trunk musculature makes it difficult for older adults to sit up over the bed edge.[33] Preparatory positioning of the person (rolling the person onto his or her side or elevating the bed head), in conjunction with use of the upper limbs, can provide effective assistance during sitting over the bed edge when trunk muscles are weak.[34] In addition, the lower limbs can be used for added momentum if well-timed with upper limb and trunk components. When trunk muscles are weak, ongoing reliance on the upper limbs for support during sitting up and sitting will be required.[34] Thus, for an older adult to be independent in getting out of bed, muscles of the trunk and upper and lower limbs need to be targeted in intervention programs.

COMMON DISORDERS OF GAIT

Gait disturbances associated with aging are often multifactorial, a combination of sensory, neurodegenerative, and negative mental-cognitive biofeedback.[35] Pragmatically, disorders of gait may be divided into those that are clinically obvious and others that are less apparent. The following gait patterns would be evident to experienced clinicians and are classified according to level of impairment and interaction with the nervous system[36]:

Middle-level disorders include the following:

- The slow and shuffling gait of parkinsonism
- The stiff limb with clumsy circumduction and scuffing of footwear due to hemiparesis, usually observed in a stroke victim
- Sensory cerebellar ataxia and vestibular pathology—share unsteadiness as a core feature but can be discriminated clinically by isolating and unmasking the affected organ

Lowest level disorders include the following:

- Antalgic gait pattern with a shortened phase on the injured side to alleviate pain experienced when bearing weight on that side, often secondary to disease in the ankle, hip, or knee
- A combination of problems (frequently secondary to arthritis or arthrodesis of the ankle) that cause alterations in load bearing and secondary stress in adjacent joints (antalgic gait), muscle weakness of the tibialis anterior (foot slap or toe drag gait), and compensatory gait patterns (steppage gait) involving recruitment of the long toe extensors, with hammer toe deformity a consequence

Because these disorders are covered in other chapters, here we shall concentrate on gait disorders that may present more of a diagnostic challenge. The term *gait apraxia* has largely been superseded by the term *higher level gait disorder*. This is based on abnormalities of the highest sensorimotor systems and assumes integrity in basic sensorimotor circuitry.[36] Gait pattern in higher level disorders is attributed to a motor programming failure comparable to the problems encountered in PD. These abnormalities can be classified according to their functional or neuroanatomic associations. Even so, their exact nature is still debated, and the present uncertainty is reflected by the many classification systems that have been proposed (Table 102-1).[36-38]

For locomotion, interrelated higher level structures (the corticobasal ganglia–thalamocortical loop) meet the demands of the personal desire to move and the maintenance of posture within the confines of environmental limitations.[38] Pathology in any of these regions or their connections therefore results in an array of gait disorders, such as the following:

- Suppression of conversion of personal will into task execution manifesting as hesitation or freezing and problems initiating

TABLE 102-1 Classification of Higher Gait Disorders*

Parameter	Location Classification[36]			
	Frontal Gait Disorder	*Frontal Dysequilibrium*	*Subcortical Dysequilibrium*	*Speculative*
Phenomenology classification[36]				Isolated gait ignition failure
Clinical findings	Extrapyramidal features, some postural imbalance	Bizarre ineffective gait	Loss of postural balance reflexes	Inability to initiate a continue movement
Liston classification[37]	Mixed gait apraxia	←------------------Equilibrium apraxia------------------→		Ignition apraxia
		←-----------------------------------Mixed gait apraxia----------------------------------→		
Elble classification[38]	←-------Dysfunctional or absent postural righting------→		Gait ignition failure	

*Cautious gait, psychogenic gait, and extrapyramidal overactivity probably retain their separate identities and have been omitted from the table.

gait or making turns (particularly affected by abnormalities of the supplementary motor area and its connections)[38]
- Dysfunctional processing with gait adversely influenced by emotional and environmental information
- Dysfunctional or absent postural righting reflexes, resulting in injurious falls
- In contrast to hypokinesis implicit in basal ganglia underactivity, disturbance in basal ganglia function may also lead to excessive, involuntary and uncontrolled limb movements.[39]

Classifications of gait have been criticized for their lack of consistency.[37] The Nutt classification, for example, includes frontal gait disorder, cautious gait, frontal disequilibrium, and cortical disequilibrium as distinct entities.[36] The older adult, with accumulation and overlap of pathology, may exhibit problems of higher gait that are not reducible to such discrete categories. Distinct gait parameters have been identified by Liston and colleagues according to their own clinically proposed subtypes.[37] This allows for the theoretical inclusion of mixed pathology and gait subtypes. The amalgamation of disordered balance in conjunction with ineffective gait by Elble[38] seems a sensible if not altogether precise way to overcome the lack of connection between the site of pathology and physical characteristics of the gait disturbance.

The phenomenologic entanglement of cautious gait is worthy of consideration.[40] Frequently multifactorial, a cautious gait may be more classically considered as a sensory disorder across locomotor afferent axes—vestibular, visual, or peripheral nervous system.[41,42] The slower gait speed associated with loss of balance confidence and fear of falling implicates a compensatory consolidation of remaining locomotor sensorimotor processing. Cautious gait may be entirely appropriate in the setting of a recent fall, with loss of confidence or a perceived fear of falling.[40] Cross-sectional studies have suggested that a cautious gait is common and is associated with poor standing balance, depression, anxiety, fear of falling, and reduced strength.[41,43] It is these features that indicate a cautious gait as a marker of high risk but one potentially amenable to targeted interventions. The distinction between dysfunctional and excessive compensatory mechanisms and a primary disturbance of gait is important.[44] Identification and attempted correction of underlying factors contributing to the syndrome of cautious gait should precede attribution of a primary gait disorder.[43]

In direct contrast to cautious gait, those with careless gait[15-17] exhibit disinhibition of movement, with an inability to match their judgment to their physical limitations or the hazards posed by the external environment. Although many studies have reported that older adults with dementia walk slowly,[45] if their overall degree of physical impairment is taken into account (e.g., use of walking aids, functional impairment), they may actually walk too quickly.[46] Such recklessness implicates frontal lobe disturbance, as noted, and may account for the high incidence of injurious falls observed in those with dementia. Similarly, in hospitalized older adults, those with delirium are at increased risk of falls because of excessive ambulation and lack of insight into mobility problems.[47] Conceivably a motor expression of dysexecutive syndrome, and therefore measurable, the development of tools to test ambulatory impulsivity would have clinical utility and the potential to predict risk.

Drug burden exponentially challenges the vertical and multiple pathways involved. This may be less of a direct effect on the locomotor system, except in the case of extrapyramidal consequences of neuroleptics, and more an impact on the executive-cognitive hierarchy. Any drug or combination that impinges on sentient capability can affect mobility adversely and will make a preexisting mobility impairment even more precarious.[48] Conversely, treating cognitive impairment may improve gait characteristics, showing that assessment and thoughtful pharmacologic management of cognition is the prerequisite of a holistic approach to the optimization of mobility.[49,50]

CLINICAL ASSESSMENT OF BALANCE AND MOBILITY

Community ambulation imposes challenges to mobility and balance through the demands of speed, distance, surface (e.g., cement, gravel, sand), terrain (e.g., slope, curb, and road challenges) and stairs that is further challenged by dual tasks (e.g., talking, carrying objects), objects in the environment (e.g., people, animals, physical structures), different lighting (e.g., dark, dim, shade, sunlight), and weather conditions.[51] Balance is integral to mobility and may be associated with stabilizing activities (e.g., preserving upright posture while standing), more dynamic and adaptive responses to internal perturbations, or reactive responses to external perturbations.[52]

Balance and gait impairments can be quantified using different tests. These measure varying balance parameters, gait speed, and impact of other graded challenges, including secondary tasks that require attention and higher order executive function. A range of balance and mobility tools[32,53-76] is summarized in Table 102-2 in relation to reliability, validity, performance norms for older adults, sensitivity to change across short (e.g., acute hospital stay) or longer time periods (e.g., subacute rehabilitation, community-based care), and ability to predict adverse health or fall outcomes. The functional gait assessment,[72-77] BEST test and mini–BEST test,[69-72] and timed up-and-go (TUG) test, with or without dual task components,[60-64] have emerged as the stronger tools to consider in relation to outcomes and for predicting risk of falls in rehabilitation and community contexts. Evidence has also suggested that monitoring backward walking[78] and stair climbing in conjunction with gender and fear of falling[79] are critical elements indicating the risk of falls in home and community settings.

A broader functional approach to balance and mobility assessments, with the inclusion of bed mobility, sitting and standing balance, transfers, and walking, appears to be better suited to the acute ward setting when frail older adults are hospitalized. Some tools (Table 102-3) have been mainly investigated in subacute rehabilitation settings (e.g., Clinical Outcome Variables Scale [COVS],[80] modified elderly mobility scale [MEMS][81]) and residential care settings (PMS),[82-84] whereas the de Morton mobility index (DEMMI)[85-89] and hierarchical assessment of balance and mobility (HABAM)[90-93] have been more thoroughly examined in the acute ward setting. The assessment of balance and mobility across a range of motor tasks offers several clinical benefits, such as the following:

- Risk stratification of health—using mobility and balance as a noninvasive tool to identify physiologic decline before conventional means of evaluation register such concerns
- Exploration of relationships between mobility and balance and specific diagnoses and/or geriatric syndromes
- Identification of objective thresholds of improvement to determine suitability and timing of more intensive rehabilitation programs
- Visual demonstration of progress to inform patients and caregivers, facilitate teaching and learning opportunities, and enable multidisciplinary understanding
- Assessment of mobility and balance to provide a culture of clinically meaningful patient contact without redress to expensive technologies

Given the importance of mobility and balance as an overall correlate of an individual's state of health, selection of a mobility tool with the capacity to track daily changes in a patient's health, such as the HABAM (Figure 102-1),[93] is an important criterion to consider when managing an acutely unwell patient. This has

TABLE 102-2 Measures of Balance and Gait for the Hospital, Rehabilitation, or Community Settings

Clinical Balance and Gait Measures	Items Rated or Measured by Scale or Test	Reliability and Validity for Older Adults	Normative Data for Older Adults	Predictive of Adverse Health or Falls and Fall Risk	Floor and Ceiling Effects
Clinical Test for Sensory Integration of Balance (CTSIB)[53,54]	Feet apart—firm EO/EC, foam EO/EC Feet together—firm EO/EC, foam EO/EC	Well established[53]	Pass-fail; 30-sec trials[53]	Failed trials on foam EO/EC linked to adverse health and fallers[54]	Ceiling effect with higher functioning older adults
Five times sit to stand (5×STS)[32,55,56]	Time to complete standing up and sitting down five times	Well-established acute and rehabilitation settings[32,55]	60-69 yr = 11.4 sec; 70-79 yr = 12.6 sec; 80-89 yr = 14.8 sec[55]	>13.6 sec (older adults with disability) >15 sec linked to recurrent fallers	No ceiling effect; real change = 2.5 sec[56]
Berg Balance Scale (BBS): 0-56 points[57-59]	14 items rated 0-4—sitting, standing, transfers, stepping, 360-degree turn, pick up object on floor	Well established across settings	>56 MDC= 4-7 points[58]	41-56: low fall risk 21-40: moderate fall risk 0-20: high fall risk[59]	Ceiling effect with higher functioning older adults
Timed up-and-go (TUG) test—TUG manual; TUG cognitive[60-64]	Time to stand, walk, turn at 3 m, return to chair and sit down[60,61]	Well established across acute, rehabilitation, and community settings	60-69 yr < 8.5 sec; 70-79 yr < 9.5 sec[63]	>13.5 sec moderate predictor of falls Faller-nonfaller 3.69 sec difference >13.5 sec Predictive of 83% of prospective fallers in 6-mo[60,64]	No ceiling effect MDC = 2.5 sec[60]
10-m walk test (10MWT)[65]	10-m timed (sec) over 14-m walkway	Well established	Age-matched healthy adults = 1.36 m/sec	Not established	No ceiling effect
6-m walk test (6MWT)[66]	Distance walked over 30-m walkway	Well established	Older men > 550 m Older women > 450 m	Fallers walk < 250 m MDC varies between clinical groups by ≈90 m	No ceiling effect defined
Dynamic Gait Index (DGI)—score 0-24; eight walking items rated 0-3[67,68]	Standard—change walk speed; walk + head movements, pivot turn, step over and around obstacles, walk up and down stairs	Well established	Healthy older adults score = 21 ± 3[67,68]	Moderate risk for fall < 19[68] Fallers = 11 ± 4 Predictive of 67% of prospective fallers across 6 mo	Ceiling effect with higher functioning older adults
BEST test—score 0-108; 36 items rated 0-3 (six categories of balance and gait tested)[69-73]	Biomechanical, stability, transitions anticipatory control, reactive control, sensory orientation, walking tasks and gait	Well established	Healthy older adults score >69%[71]	Predictive of fallers[73]	No ceiling effect established in older adults
Functional gait assessment—score 0-30; 10 items rated 0-3[73-77]	Standard—change walk speed, walk + head movements, pivot turn, step over obstacles, heel-toe walk, walk with EC, backward walking, walk up and down stairs	Well established[86,88]	Healthy older adults score > 22 MDC = 5[77]	<22/30—high fall risk up to 80 yr of age <20—high fall risk if >80 yr Predictive of 100% of fallers across 6 mo[73,76,77]	No ceiling effect established in older adults

EC, Eyes closed; *EO,* eyes open; *MDC,* minimal detectable change.

particular utility in frail older adult patients, in whom traditional signs of illness may not be present.

IMPAIRED MOBILITY AND FRAILTY

Falls are frequently pivotal events in the life of a frail individual. Trauma aside, the loss of confidence, mobility decline, deconditioning, social withdrawal, and fear of falling can become overwhelming. The most consistent independent predictors of future falls in older adults are gait or balance deficits.[94] This is consistent with the paradigm of frailty in older adults as the failure of a complex system.[95]

Normal ambulation requires the coordination of many different muscles acting on multiple joints; it is accomplished by the integration of activity in spinal neuronal circuitries with sensory feedback signals and descending commands from the motor cortex.[96] The central nervous system coordinates this activity, adjusts it to fit environmental conditions, and refines it when required, all while maintaining a remarkable degree of precision. This is evident when foot position is considered during normal walking, in which multiple joints and muscles act to ensure that the foot is elevated by 1 to 2 cm above the ground and the position varies by less than 4 mm.[97,98] The computational task solved by the human brain to accomplish this feat is extraordinary, given the infinite number of combinations of joint and muscle positions that have to be attained relative to each other to arrive at the desired outcome. Bipedalism is a higher order function that requires a significant degree of connectivity and coordination among several interdependent components (muscular, skeletal, and nervous) of the complex system that is the human body. Consequently, it is not surprising that frail individuals who have gait and balance deficits and who have lost the ability to integrate multiple inputs in the face of stress often present with impaired mobility and falls.[99]

There is a direct relationship between frailty and mobility; impairment in balance and mobility is universal at a high frailty

TABLE 102-3 Functional Mobility Measures for Acute Wards, Residential Care, and Rehabilitation Units*

Functional Mobility Measures	Items Rated or Measured by Scale or Tool	Reliability and Validity for Older Frail Adults	Predictive for Falls and Fall Risk	Minimal Detectable Change	Floor and Ceiling Effects
Clinical Outcome Variables Scale (COVS)—0-91 points; 13 items rated 1-7[80]	Bed mobility, horizontal and vertical transfers, wheelchair mobility; upper limb function; walking ability—speed, distance, external challenges	Established in subacute rehabilitation settings	Not established	7 points[7]	Ceiling effect with higher functioning adults
Modified elderly mobility scale—0-23 items rated 0-3[81]	Lying down and sitting up, sit to stand, standing balance, gait speed, gait independence, stairs, functional reach	Established in subacute rehabilitation settings	Not established[81]	Not defined	Ceiling effect with higher functioning adults
Physical mobility scale (PMS)—0-46[82-84]	Bed mobility, sitting, transfers, walking[82,83]	Established in residential care settings	Inverse relationship between level of mobility and risk of falls[94]	5 points[82,83]	None reported in aged care context
De Morton mobility index (DEMMI)—converted score, 0%-100%[85-89]	15 items of graded challenge—bed mobility, sitting, standing, gait, advanced gait activities	Established in acute ward, rehabilitation, and community settings[86-88]	Not established	9 points[89]	None reported with older adults
Hierarchal assessment balance and mobility (HABAM)—0-65[90-93]	Three broad categories of graded challenge mobility (bed, sitting, standing)—walking, 0-26; transfers, 0-18; balance, 0-21 (no aid)	Established for acute hospital settings[90-93]	Not established	Sensitivity to change in health status reported in acute setting[93]	None reported with older adults

*Functional mobility includes a range of motor tasks from bed mobility to walking.

burden[100] and leads to functional decline, with physical activity a critical element in the prevention of this deterioration. Although mobility and balance impairment are sensitive if nonspecific indicators of acuity in frail patients, these elements may be insufficient to define frailty fully in keeping with the tenet that multiple systems, not just mobility, are implicated. Thus, holistic management is required that is best informed through a comprehensive geriatric assessment.[101]

Through a comprehensive assessment, targeted interventions can be implemented. Several groups have emphasized the need to understand osteoporosis and sarcopenia (the reduction of muscle mass and function) in the pathogenesis of frailty,[102-104] as well as the negative impact of chronic diseases (e.g., degenerative arthritis, obesity) on the progression to frailty.[105] Because immobility and lack of exercise are major factors responsible for the emergence of chronic diseases and development of sarcopenia, objective evaluation of physical performance has been advocated as an indicator of frailty in older adults.[85,93] Poor performance on selected tests characterize those who may benefit from targeted and multifactorial interventions.[106-108]

Some components of frailty may be more predictive of adverse outcomes. Women with lower limb osteoarthritis or rheumatoid arthritis have a mild to moderate risk of falls and balance impairments in comparison to age-matched older women.[105] Among very frail older adults, those with mobility disability had a higher risk of mortality and nursing home placement than those without disability.[109] The effects of osteoporosis and sarcopenia have been implicated in more severe presentations of frailty in community-dwelling older women.[103,104] In participants in the MacArthur Study of Successful Aging, six frailty subdimensions were identified, involving different combinations of four or more of ten criteria: weight loss, weak grip, exhaustion, slow gait, low physical activity, cognitive impairment, high interleukin-6 level, high C-reactive protein level, subjective weakness, and anorexia. Each had a different predictive validity for disability and mortality, suggesting "that pathways to frailty differ and that sub-dimension-adapted care might enhance care of frail seniors."[110]

Although some researchers in the aging field have emphasized the conceptualization of frailty as a risk state and others have aimed to clarify components of the risk state, the importance of mobility impairment is universally recognized. Both approaches to frailty are motivated by the need to increase our understanding of the pathways to poor health in older adults, and they are not irreconcilable. Inouye and associates,[111] for example, have identified impaired mobility as one of four shared risk factors—along with older age, baseline cognitive impairment, and baseline functional impairment—for five common geriatric syndromes (delirium, pressure ulcers, incontinence, falls, and functional decline) and for the overarching geriatric syndrome of frailty. It is certainly feasible to unite the two different approaches to frailty, recognizing and investigating the importance of components of frailty, yet managing it as a complex condition.

INTERVENTIONS FOR IMPAIRED MOBILITY

The prevalence of impaired mobility and frailty requires a continuing emphasis on interventions within the community, residential care, and hospital settings.

Community-Dwelling Older Adults

Exercise programs of varying design have diverse positive effects in community-dwelling older adults, including improved muscle strength and gait speed,[112] reduction in falls,[113] and improved balance.[114] In longitudinal cohort studies, physical activity is protective of impaired physical function.[115] Participation in frequent and intense training can result in even greater improvements in reactive balance performance; for example, older athletes undertaking long-term, high-intensity training demonstrate better and more rapid stabilization of posture following perturbation than healthy older adults under challenging conditions.[116] A systematic review and meta-analyses of intervention programs involving older adults[117] has revealed stronger effects in programs that included exercises that challenged balance, used a higher dose of

Hierarchical Assessment of Balance and Mobility

Completed By: ______________________ Date Completed: ______________

Date Assessed																		
Instrument Day	-14	01	02	03	05	06	07	08	09	10	11	12	13	14	15	16	17	18
BALANCE																		
21. Stable ambulation	21								21	21	21	21						
14. Stable dynamic standing								14										
10. Stable static standing							10											
7. Stable dynamic sitting						7												
5. Stable static sitting		5	5	5	5													
0. Impaired static sitting																		
TRANSFERS																		
18. Independent and vigorous	18									18	18	18						
16. Independent									16									
14 Independent but slow								14										
12. One-person standby							12											
11. One-person minimal assist						11												
7. One-person assist			7	7	7													
3. Two-person assist		3																
0. Total lift																		
MOBILITY																		
28. Unlimited, vigorous																		
26. Unlimited																		
25. Limited >50 m, no aid																		
21. Unlimited, with aid																		
19. Unlimited with aid, slow																		
18. With aid >50 m	18											18						
16. No aid, limited 8-50 m										16	16							
15. With aid 8-50 m									15									
14. With aid <8 m+								14										
12. 1 person standby/+/-aid						12	12											
9. 1 person hands-on/+/-aid				9	9													
7. Lying-sitting independently		7	7															
4. Positions self in bed																		
0. Needs positioning in bed																		

Notes for scoring the HABAM.

- Baseline (-14) is taken as 2 weeks prior to the current assessment.
- Each domain (balance, transfers, mobility) is scored at the highest level attained.
- In balance, "**dynamic**" refers to withstanding a force, either administered externally (e.g., a sternal nudge) or internally (e.g., reaching forward).
- In transfers, **standby assist** refers to no hands-on assistance but presence of an aide for security; **minimal assist** refers to hands on with little force, chiefly for guidance.
- In mobility, **<8 m** corresponds to not being able to walk outside the room; **8-50 m** mobility is being able to get to the nursing station and back; **>50 m** is more than one trip around the ward.
- The HABAM should be scored using the patient's usual walking aid.

A

Figure 102-1. Hierarchical assessment of balance and mobility form. **A,** The patient's mobility and balance had deteriorated considerably from baseline. The patient could only move from side to side in bed and required the assistance of two people to transfer and to walk. By the second hospital day, however, recovery had begun and accelerated after day 5.

HIERARCHICAL ASSESSMENT OF BALANCE AND MOBILITY

Completed By: ______________________ Date Completed: ______________

Date Assessed																		
Instrument Day	-14	01	02	03	05	06	07	08	09	10	11	12	13	14	15	16	17	18
BALANCE																		
21. Stable ambulation	21																	
14. Stable dynamic standing																		
10. Stable static standing																		
7. Stable dynamic sitting																		
5. Stable static sitting		5																
0. Impaired static sitting			0	0	0	0												
TRANSFERS																		
18. Independent and vigorous	18																	
16. Independent																		
14 Independent but slow																		
12. One-person standby																		
11. One-person minimal assist																		
7. One-person assist																		
3. Two-person assist		3	3															
0. Total lift				0	0	0												
MOBILITY																		
28. Unlimited, vigorous																		
26. Unlimited																		
25. Limited >50 m, no aid																		
21. Unlimited, with aid																		
19. Unlimited with aid, slow																		
18. With aid >50 m	18																	
16. No aid, limited 8-50 m																		
15. With aid 8-50 m																		
14. With aid <8 m+																		
12. One-person standby/+/-aid																		
9. One-person hands-on/+/-aid																		
7. Lying-sitting independently		7																
4. Positions self in bed			4															
0. Needs positioning in bed				0	0	0												

Notes for scoring the HABAM.

- Baseline (-14) is taken as 2 weeks prior to the current assessment.
- Each domain (balance, transfers, mobility) is scored at the highest level attained.
- In balance, "**dynamic**" refers to withstanding a force, either administered externally (e.g., a sternal nudge) or internally (e.g., reaching forward).
- In transfers, **standby assist** refers to no hands-on assistance but presence of an aide for security; **minimal assist** refers to hands on with little force, chiefly for guidance.
- In mobility, **<8 m** corresponds to not being able to walk outside the room; **8-50 m** mobility is being able to get to the nursing station and back; **>50 m** is more than one trip around the ward.
- The HABAM should be scored using the patient's usual walking aid.

B

Figure 102-1, cont'd. B, Another patient with a similar level of decline continued worsening on the second and third hospital days; this signaled a rapidly fatal course that ended in death by day 6. *(Modified from MacKnight C, Rockwood K: Rasch analysis of the hierarchical assessment of balance and mobility [HABAM]. J Clin Epidemiol 53:1242-1247, 2000; and Rockwood K, Rockwood MR, Andrew MK, et al: Reliability of the hierarchical assessment of balance and mobility in frail older adults. J Am Geriatr Soc 56:1213-1217, 2008.)*

exercise, and did not include a walking program. These elements are integrated into the balance strategy training program,[118] Otago Exercise Program,[119] and tai chi[120,121] to promote healthier aging of sedentary and active older adults. Intervention programs involving frail older adults may need to be modified to accommodate problems such as degenerative arthritis,[105] osteoporosis and sarcopenia,[103,104] and the age-related decline in sensorimotor systems.[122]

Because the benefits of exercise are rapidly lost when exercise is ceased, the issue of adherence to interventions and exercise continues to need attention.[123] Although adherence to exercise is a multifactorial issue, follow-up of older adults participating in an exercise-based intervention after discharge to home has revealed that being female, with a low self-efficacy[124] for falls, as well as concern regarding pain during exercise, are critical factors to consider.[125] Other studies have emphasized the need to screen for cognitive impairment before commencing interventions.[126] Limited but fairly consistent findings in trials of higher methodologic quality have shown that home-based exercise and fall-related multifactorial programs,[106-108] along with community-based tai chi programs delivered in a group format,[120,121] have been effective in reducing fear of falling in community-living older adults. Of note, frail older females positively engaged in a home-based intervention program when provided with supportive phone follow-up across the intervention period,[125] supporting one strategy for future delivery of home-based programs for frail older adults. It is thus important to monitor physical capacity and balance, along with cognition and self-efficacy, when individuals enroll in intervention programs in home or community contexts. Physical capacity along with self-efficacy will help inform goal setting and the type of instruction and support that individual participants may require to maximize community ambulation.

Older Adults in Residential Care Facilities

Exercise programs for frail older adults in long-term care have yielded conflicting results. A systematic review of physical training in institutionalized older adults has indicated positive effects on muscle strength, but effects on gait, disability, balance, and endurance were inconclusive.[109] In some studies, exercise programs involving very frail older people resulted in no improvements in physical health or function,[127] with an increase in musculoskeletal injury and falls[128] reported. In contrast, other studies have concluded that exercise improves physical performance scores,[129] slows further functional decline, and reduces falls.[100,130] Given these discrepancies in reported adverse events, it is likely that the status of an individual needs to be understood so that the benefits of exercise can be attained while the potential for adverse outcomes, such as falls, can be reduced through appropriate selection of the delivery mode. Tools with predictive capacity for falls in the residential care setting, such as the Physical Mobility Scale,[84] could be instructive in this context, enabling clinicians to meet the needs of residents to participate safely in exercise programs for improved health.

Older Adults in Hospital

Impaired mobility in the hospital should be considered a negative prognostic sign. Mobility decline in hospital is an important determinant of poor functional recovery,[131] as well as a predictor of mortality.[132] Measured through accelerometry, lower mean daily step count is associated with readmission to hospital,[133] and an inability to engage with performance-related tasks is linked to failure to achieve premorbid mobility.[132] Note also that many acutely ill people cannot walk, decline in bed mobility which can be tracked by the HABAM, is also a herald of death.[93] Hence, if physicians only think about walking before they concern themselves with mobility, they will miss informative clinical signs.

What can be done to mitigate these adverse outcomes? Even in ambulatory hospitalized patients, the time spent standing or walking is only of the order of 1 hour/day.[132] Interestingly, the risk-averse culture within health profession may contribute to the restriction of mobility activities in an effort to provide "care and keep them safe."[134]

Avoidance of nosocomial disability requires identification of frail inpatients with interventions to address the multifactorial nature of mobility disturbance. Again, interventions to improve outcomes in hospitalized older adults have centered on exercise. A Cochrane systematic review[135] has determined the effect of exercise interventions for acutely hospitalized older medical patients on functional status, adverse events, and hospital outcomes. Of 3138 potentially relevant articles screened, seven randomized controlled trials and two controlled clinical trials were included. Although the effects of exercise on functional outcome measures were unclear, there was level 2 evidence that multidisciplinary intervention that includes exercise may increase the proportion of patients discharged to home, and reduce the length and cost of the hospital stay for acutely hospitalized older medical patients.

Nutritional support also improves outcomes of hospitalized older adults.[136] Although mobility outcomes were not explicitly reported, attention to nutrition significantly reduced patients' risk of dying after hip fracture.[137] Anabolic agents are theoretically attractive as therapeutic agents in hospitalized older adults, reducing the negative nitrogen balance and improving body composition, but small randomized controlled trials have shown no effects on mobility or function, and further studies with longer follow-up periods are needed.[138]

Embedding nutritional support, early mobilization and cognitive stimulation in an Eat, Walk, Engage model has shown promising effects on outcomes such as length of hospital stay.[139] This holistic approach is congruent with informing interventions through a comprehensive geriatric assessment (CGA),[101,140] with subsequent optimal outcomes for older adults.

CONCLUSION

Mobility impairment is integral to frailty, however it is defined. The need to quantify mobility performance during the acute care period is compelling, with selection of tools that are sensitive to changes in health status. Measures of balance and gait that include a graded challenge are more instructive for rehabilitation and community contexts. Assessment tools deliver a number of functions—for inpatients, they can provide clinicians with valuable information on which to make decisions regarding readiness for discharge from the acute hospital environment; for community dwellers, they provide predictive indicators for falls so that preemptive prevention interventions can be implemented.

Multifactorial and multidisciplinary interventions are essential to manage impaired mobility in older adults at the frailer end of the health spectrum. Exercise modes that include balance training, functional strength, and endurance training seem to be most effective to manage the demands of community ambulation and promote healthier aging. Knowledge of the factors limiting engagement and adherence to exercise modes is another challenge that requires the attention of health professionals with physical capacity, cognition, and self-efficacy emerging as issues to be considered when planning intervention programs for older adults.

KEY POINTS

- In general, gait speed reflects overall health status.
- Impaired mobility and balance should be investigated as signs of pathophysiology and/or illness and not accepted as inevitable with aging.
- Assessment tools that capture representative levels of mobility impairment and are sensitive to change in health status may provide valuable clinical information during acute care management.
- Management of frail, older adults should be accompanied by a comprehensive geriatric assessment as impaired mobility and balance are common.
- Assessment tools that offer a graded challenge to mobility are required for optimal management of older adults who are completing rehabilitation and/or participating in community contexts.
- Exercise programs that include a focus on balance training, in addition to strength and walking, have a particular role in the treatment of impaired balance and mobility in older adults across the frailty spectrum.
- Planning for optimal patient engagement of older adults in exercise programs needs to consider physical capacity, cognition, and self-efficacy of participants.

For a complete list of references, please visit www.expertconsult.com.

KEY REFERENCES

9. Hsu CL, Voss MW, Handy TC, et al: Disruptions in brain networks of older fallers are associated with subsequent cognitive decline: a 12-month prospective exploratory study. PLoS ONE 9:e93673, 2014.
13. Peel NM, Kuys SS, Klein K: Gait speed as a measure in geriatric assessment in clinical settings: a systematic review. J Gerontol A Biol Sci Med Sci 68:39–46, 2013.
14. Kuys SS, Peel NM, Klein K, et al: Gait speed in ambulant older people in long term care: a systematic review and meta-analysis. J Am Med Dir Assoc 15:194–200, 2014.
18. Fried LP, Tangen CM, Walston J, et al: Frailty in older adults: evidence for a phenotype. J Gerontol A Biol Sci Med Sci 56:M146–M156, 2001.
36. Nutt JG, Marsden CD, Thompson PD: Human walking and higher-level gait disorders, particularly in the elderly. Neurology 43:268–279, 1993.
37. Liston R, Mickelborough J, Bene J, et al: A new classification of higher level gait disorders in patients with cerebral multi-infarct states. Age Ageing 32:252–258, 2003.
38. Elble RJ: Gait and dementia: moving beyond the notion of gait apraxia. J Neural Transm (Vienna) 114:1253–1258, 2007.
54. Low Choy NL, Brauer S, Nitz J: Timed stance performances reflect differences in age, prevalence of co-morbidities, medication use, fall's history and activity level: early screening for balance loss is indicated. Australas J Ageing 26:29–34, 2007.
57. Berg KO, Wood-Dauphinee SL, Williams JI, et al: Measuring balance in the elderly: validation of an instrument. Can J Public Health 83:S7–S11, 1992.
60. Podsiadlo D, Richardson S: Timed "Up & Go": a test of basic functional mobility for frail elderly persons. J Am Geriatr Soc 39:142–148, 1991.
61. Muir-Hunter SW, Clark J, McLean S, et al: Identifying balance and fall risk in community-dwelling older women: the effect of executive function on postural control. Physiother Can 66:179–186, 2014.
81. Kuys S, Brauer S: Validation and reliability of the modified elderly mobility scale. Australas J Ageing 25:140–144, 2006.
82. Nitz JC, Hourigan SR: Measuring mobility in frail older people: reliability and validity of the physical mobility scale. Australas J Ageing 25:31–35, 2006.
84. Barker AL, Nitz JC, Low Choy NL, et al: Mobility has a non-linear association with falls risk among people in residential aged care: an observational study. J Physiol 58:117–125, 2012.
85. de Morton NA, Davidson M, Keating JL: The de Morton mobility index (DEMMI): an essential health index for an ageing world. Health Qual Life Outcomes 6:63, 2008.
90. MacKnight C, Rockwood K: A hierarchical assessment of balance and mobility. Age Ageing 24:126–130, 1995.
93. Hubbard RE, Eeles EM, Rockwood MR, et al: Assessing balance and mobility to track illness and recovery in older inpatients. J Gen Intern Med 26:1471–1478, 2011.
95. Clegg A1, Young J, Iliffe S, et al: Frailty in elderly people. Lancet 381:752–762, 2013.
99. Nowak A, Hubbard RE: Falls and frailty: lessons from complex systems. J R Soc Med 102:98–102, 2009.
100. Davis DH, Rockwood MR, Mitnitski AB, et al: Impairments in mobility and balance in relation to frailty. Arch Gerontol Geriatr 53:79–83, 2011.
107. Fairhall N, Sherrington C, Lord SR, et al: Effect of a multifactorial, interdisciplinary intervention on risk factors for falls and fall rate in frail older people: a randomised controlled trial. Age Ageing 43:616–622, 2014.
115. Lang IA, Guralnik JM, Melzer D: Physical activity in middle-aged adults reduces risks of functional impairment independent of its effect on weight. J Am Geriatr Soc 55:1836–1841, 2007.
119. Yang XJ, Hill K, Moore K, et al: Effectiveness of a targeted exercise intervention in reversing older peoples mild balance dysfunction: a randomised controlled trail. Phys Ther 92:24–37, 2012.
122. Low Choy NL, Brauer S, Nitz J: Age-related changes in strength and somato-sensation during mid-life support rationale for targeted preventive intervention programs. Ann N Y Acad Sci 1114:180–193, 2007.
135. de Morton NA, Keating JL, Jeffs K: Exercise for acutely hospitalised older medical patients. Cochrane Database Syst Rev (1):CD005955, 2007.

103 Falls

Stephanie Studenski, Jessie Van Swearingen

INTRODUCTION

Falls are a major focus of geriatric medicine because they are common among older adults, have complex interacting causes and serious consequences, and require multiple disciplines for effective management. The goals of this chapter are to present the scope and impact of the problem, explore various perspectives on causation, provide guidance about clinical evaluation and treatment, and examine opportunities to implement programs across health care settings and communities.

EPIDEMIOLOGY

Falls are common among older adults. Up to one third of community-dwelling persons older than 65 years fall annually, and about 20% to 25% of them will fall repeatedly.[1] Falling is more common among women than men and increases in prevalence with advancing age. In acute care settings, falls are the most commonly reported adverse incident, with rates varying from 3 to 13 falls/1000 bed days.[2] In chronic care settings, falls are so common that typically over 50% of residents are fallers; average rates can run from 1.5 to two to six falls/resident/year.[3] The most obvious adverse consequence of falls are injuries, which develop in about 10% of community fallers and 30% of fallers in acute and chronic care.[1,2,4] Injuries are more likely in recurrent fallers.[1]

Falls can be fatal; they are the fifth leading cause of death among older adults.[1] Falls are a major contributor to serious injuries, including not only hip fractures but also other fractures, cervical spine injuries, and severe head trauma.[5,6] Falls are a common precipitator of hospitalization and contribute to the need for long-term institutionalization.[1,7] In acute and chronic care institutions, falls are also a source of complaints from families and even may lead to litigation.[8] Although injuries and health care use are serious concerns, falling also creates other serious problems for the older adult, including functional limitations, fear of falling, restricted activity, and social isolation.[1,8] Falling can be a precipitator of a vicious cycle of failing health and function, leading to death.

In the past, there was no widely agreed on definition of falls. More recently, ProFaNE (Prevention of Falls Network Europe,www.profane.eu.org), a multinational work group dedicated to reducing falls and injuries through research and implementation of evidence-based interventions, has proposed the following as the most reliable and valid definition: "A fall is an unexpected event in which the participant comes to rest on the ground, floor or lower level."[9]

Although this definition provides some consistency for reporting, there are still areas of confusion. It is not clear if it is appropriate to include in the definition of falls those events associated with loss of consciousness or overwhelming external forces, such as being hit by a moving vehicle. Similarly, it may or may not be important to include events such as a near-fall, in which the individual barely avoids a fall to the floor by suddenly grabbing for furniture or wall or is caught by another person. Frequent near-falls, such as stumbling and tripping, are risk factors for future falls. There are also problems with fall reporting. Fall events may not be remembered retrospectively, especially if there were no injuries. Prospective monitoring improves accuracy but can be burdensome. Although falls in general are important, it is possible that the most clinically relevant concern is the recurrent faller or a fall injury. There are also serious health-related concerns for those who does not actually fall because they have restricted their own activity. This group may also be at high risk for future falls, injuries, and social isolation. Another area of recent discussion has encompassed the role of exposure intensity in estimates of fall risk. Just as in estimates of automobile accidents, for which rates are adjusted for the exposure to miles driven, adjusting for physical activity intensity has been proposed as a more appropriate indicator of fall risk.[10]

CAUSATION

Falling is considered a classic geriatric syndrome because it is often due to multiple interacting conditions that create an organism with reduced tolerance to any type of external stress. The evidence base that has been used to define the causes of falls is highly dependent on the perspective and priorities of the researchers, definitions of falling and fallers, time frame and approach to monitoring for falls, characteristics of the population under study, factors that were measured, and how interactions between factors were assessed in the analyses. Whatever the focus of the research, it is clear that many fallers demonstrate multiple abnormalities and that interactions among these abnormalities influence fall risk.

Epidemiologic Perspective

Epidemiologic observational studies of older adults in the community and in acute and chronic care institutions have identified risk factors for falls; all suggest that risk increases as the number of risk factors increases. Table 103-1 summarizes risk factor profiles by the setting in which older adults were studied. Across settings, altered mobility and cognition are major risk factors for falls. Interestingly, it is possible to be too immobile to fall.[11] For example, in one chronic care setting, residents with fair standing balance had the highest fall rates, those with good standing balance had intermediate fall rates, and persons with poor standing balance had the lowest fall rates.[12] Risk factor patterns and appropriate preventive interventions may differ substantially by overall mobility capacity; active older adults may experience falls and injuries for reasons very different than those for persons who stand and walk with difficulty, who in turn may fall for very different reasons than those who cannot stand.

Risk factors for injurious falls may differ from risk factors for all falls. In a study of older adults in residential care facilities, fracture risk among fallers was higher in those with better balance and no history of falls, perhaps suggesting that in some persons, activity increases the risk of producing sufficient force to fracture.[13] Risk factor profiles are also limited in that they generally only identify chronic and stable risk factors, sometimes called predisposing risk factors. Many falls might occur because an individual with a predisposing risk has additional acute precipitating factors.[14] For example, an older adult with limited mobility and cognition might not become a faller until he or she develops diarrhea, becomes dehydrated and dizzy, and tries to rush to the bathroom. Because risk factor studies have rarely accounted for these more transient and dynamic precipitating contributors, much less is known about them.

TABLE 103-1 Predisposing Risk Factors for Falls in Older Person in Three Settings*

Community Dweller	Acute Care	Chronic Care
Fall history Weakness Balance problem Gait problem Visual problem Mobility limitation Cognitive impairment Decreased functional status Postural hypotension	Gait instability Agitated confusion Urinary incontinence and frequency Fall history High-risk medications	Cognitive impairment Visual impairment Weakness Neurologic problems Gait and balance problems Cardiovascular problem

*Based on observational studies.

BOX 103-1 Components of Postural Control

SENSORY SYSTEMS
Vision
Vestibular functions
Somatosensation

CENTRAL NERVOUS SYSTEM
Perfusion
Speed, attention
Postural reflexes

EFFECTOR SYSTEMS
Strength
Flexibility

TABLE 103-2 Environmental Risk Factors for Falls

Indoor Falls	Outdoor Falls
Poor lighting	Uneven and broken sidewalks
Loose or absent railings	Wet surfaces
Throw rugs	Poor lighting
Trailing cords and wires	Irregular steps
Uneven transitions (e.g., level change between rooms)	Unpredictable level changes
Lack of bars in the bathroom	
Slippery floors	
Cluttered walkways	

Risk factors for falls overlap substantially with risk factors for other geriatric syndromes.[15] Older age and impairments in cognition, mobility, and function are risk factors for falls, incontinence, delirium, and frailty.[15] Thus, there is a population of older adults with multiple impairments who are at risk for numerous geriatric syndromes, including falls and injuries. There may be other populations of older adults who are at risk for different types of falls; active older adults may fall and injure themselves during demanding activities, whereas very immobile older adults may fall out of bed and chairs or even be dropped by caregivers. In the future, more distinct risk factor profiles might be defined based on overall mobility status.

Epidemiologic studies have also identified environmental risk factors for falls. Virtually all falls can be considered the result of interactions between a person and her or his environment. The individual has some level of ability to move, and the environment has some level of challenge. The issue is the context in which the person and environment interact. The risk factors identified in Table 103-1 are sometime called intrinsic factors because they relate to the individual, and risk factors associated with the environment are sometimes called extrinsic factors. The typical older faller experiences a fall in an environment and while performing tasks that would not cause a healthy young person to fall. This phenomenon of falling under a low challenge is the rationale for believing that many falls in older people are due largely to intrinsic factors. If an older adult has many intrinsic risk factors, it is possible that only modest problems with the environment or modest degrees of challenge in a task will precipitate a fall.

Table 103-2 lists environmental risk factors for falls. Commonly reported indoor environmental factors are uneven walkways, loose rugs, absence of grab bars in the bathroom, and poor lighting.[16,17] Outdoor hazards are less frequently assessed but might be important, especially for more active older adults. Other extrinsic elements, such as the availability of help, may be an important factor in falls among persons living in the community and are even more likely to contribute to falls in an institutional setting.[10] Additional risk factors for falls include psychological and attitudinal characteristics such as risk preference.[11,18] Other risk factors for injury include osteoporosis, low body weight, and fall direction.[19]

Physiologic Perspective

Contributors to falls can be examined from the perspective of physiologic systems that affect balance. The rationale for using a framework of organ-based physiologic systems that affect balance is based on models of disablement. These models draw links between pathologic processes and altered organ system performance (termed *impairments*), which combine to affect body movements (termed *functional* or *performance limitations*), then affect functional abilities and disability, and ultimately interfere with social roles such as being a homemaker or volunteer (termed *handicap*). There are several disablement models. When assessing causation of problems of aging, these multisystem physiologic approaches are helpful for several reasons. First, such approaches can address interactions between systems. Second, they can include mild or subclinical impairments that might affect function without being clinically obvious for an individual. Third, well-functioning systems might actually serve to compensate for problems with other systems. Thus, individual organ systems and even overall functions such as balance are on a continuum; they might be obviously abnormal, subclinically abnormal under usual conditions, abnormal only under stressful conditions, normal, or even have backup or reserve excess capacity.

From a physiologic perspective, balance dysfunction results from impairment in one or more of the following systems: peripheral sensory receptors for input, central nervous system (CNS) structures for processing sensory input and planning motor output, and effector organs to carry out the movement plan (Box 103-1). In many situations, it is the combination of deficits across these systems that produces instability and falls.

There are three main sensory systems used for balance—vision, somatosensation, and vestibular function. Visual functions such as acuity, depth perception, dark adaptation, contrast sensitivity, and peripheral vision help determine body position and trajectory in space and monitor the environment.[20] Because bifocal glasses prioritize two focal lengths, one in the lower field at about 20 inches for reading and one in the upper visual field at about 20 feet for distance, bifocals can limit acuity in the critical zone in front of the feet while walking.[21] Diseases of the aging eye that affect multiple visual functions are common; these include glaucoma, macular degeneration, and cataracts. Medications that cause miosis, or constriction of the pupil, can reduce dark adaptation.

Peripheral sensation is important for balance. These sensors provide information about the position of the body relative to the support surface and gravity and reflect the relationship of one body part to another during rest and movement. Peripheral sensation is the most important system for monitoring the characteristics of the weight-bearing surface and distribution of body weight onto the feet. Peripheral sensory loss is common in older adults due to diabetes and peripheral vascular disease. In case of peripheral sensory loss, visual systems can compensate by supplementing information about body position. Thus, a combination of vision loss and peripheral sensory loss can create serious problems with the ability to monitor body position.

The vestibular system detects the position of the head with respect to gravity, monitors linear and angular acceleration of the head, and coordinates head and eye movements to maintain gaze and visual field stability while moving. Vestibular system impairments can occur with usual aging and are affected by ischemia or head trauma.[22] Several widely recognized vestibular conditions, such as benign paroxysmal vertigo and perhaps Meniere disease, are common in older adults. Others are also common but less well recognized, such as chronic bilateral vestibular hypofunction.[23]

The CNS has numerous structures that contribute to balance. Structures in the brainstem and spinal cord are considered central pattern generators that produce stepping behaviors. Balance is further controlled by higher level brain structures, including the frontal cortex, basal ganglia, cerebellum, and motor cortex. Degeneration of brain regions can affect balance, as in the basal ganglia in Parkinson disease and in cerebellar degeneration. All brain processes depend on adequate levels of brain perfusion, so any threats to perfusion affect central processes of gait and balance. Thus, many of the conditions that produce syncope or presyncope can cause transient cerebral hypoperfusion and falls, such as orthostatic hypotension, tachyarrhythmias, bradyarrhythmias, and critical aortic stenosis.[24]

There has been increased awareness of the role of more diffuse microvascular brain disease as a contributor to balance disorders and falls.[25] This mechanism is posited to involve ischemia in vulnerable brain areas, especially the frontal lobes, and in important white matter tracts connecting the frontal lobes to critical subcortical areas. Radiologically, this ischemia is manifested as leukoaraiosis (white matter disease) on magnetic resonance imaging scans. White matter disease has been associated with specific patterns of cognitive dysfunction involving psychomotor slowing and altered attention and executive functions, such as sequencing and visual spatial organization.[25-27] These cognitive abnormalities have been associated with alterations in gait, especially excessively variable length and timing of stepping, and with falls.[28,29] Thus, there is an emerging concept of altered balance and gait due to abnormal nonamnestic cognitive functions and movement planning produced by regional microvascular brain disease. This condition may be manifest by irregular walking patterns and exacerbated by placing stress on cognition and movement. Tasks that simultaneously stress cognition and movement are part of an emerging conceptual approach to balance assessment termed *dual tasking*.[30,31] Older adults whose performance worsens substantially when asked to walk and solve cognitive problems simultaneously may be at increased risk for falls.[32]

The CNS also operates a multisynaptic righting reflex that produces automatic correcting movements when balance is lost. Typically appearing as a stepping response that occurs much more quickly than what can be done voluntarily, this righting reflex is lost in many CNS disorders, including extrapyramidal diseases and other forms of multisystem atrophy. Sedation, clinical or subclinical, may further reduce alertness and attention. Thus, both sleepiness and sedative medications have been found to increase fall risk.[33,34] Less specific but potentially important are psychological factors, such as fear of falling and risk preferences.[11,35]

Muscles and joints are effector organs critical for balance and mobility. Muscle weakness is widespread in older adults and can be due to primary muscle mass loss (sarcopenia), disorders of peripheral nerves or neuromuscular junctions, or inactivity. Specific muscle diseases such as inflammatory myositis or steroid myopathy can produce proximal muscle and trunk weakness that presents with falls. Lower motor neuron conditions, radicular nerve deficits due to spinal stenosis, or peripheral nerve damage can result in localizing strength deficits that affect specific muscle groups and more distinct functional movements. For example, a foot drop due to damage to the peroneal nerve prevents the forefoot from lifting to clear obstacles and can induce trips and stumbles. Evidence has suggested that low vitamin D levels may contribute to muscle weakness and falls.[36] Low testosterone levels have been found to be associated with falls in men younger than 80 years.[37] Other common conditions such as arthritis can reduce range of motion and produce pain that alters stepping and weight bearing.[38] Deformities distort the weight-bearing surfaces of the foot and cause pain. Fatigue, generalized or localized to muscle, can contribute to loss of balance. Thus, acute conditions such as overworked muscles or chronic conditions associated with fatigue such as anemia[39] or congestive heart failure might increase risk for falls. Although traditional assessments of strength have focused on the extremities, more recent thinking has emphasized the role of trunk or core strength involving the abdomen and pelvis as critical to postural control, which is a novel avenue to pursue interventions.[40]

When fall onset is abrupt or there is a major change in balance, the likelihood is higher that there is a medical event that has affected the CNS. Any illness or episode that reduces cerebral perfusion through hypoxia, decreased oxygen-carrying capacity, or hypotension could present as dizziness, lightheadedness, unsteadiness, and falls. Toxic or metabolic abnormalities due to medications, infection, or electrolyte disorders could present as unsteadiness and falls through effects on attention. New focal neurologic deficits due to stroke can also present as unsteadiness. Older adults with predisposing subclinical balance disorders could be more vulnerable to such precipitating factors. These types of physiologic acute, and sometimes transient, changes are harder to include in research studies because stable chronic effects are usually the focus of an investigation.

Biomechanical Perspective

A biomechanical approach to fall risk is based on the concepts of mass, force, momentum, and acceleration of the body as a whole, as well as of body segments. The standing human body is a long tall column that rests over a small base of support. The main task of movement is to displace and recover this column while the base of support changes. Therefore, the assessment of balance includes two main conditions: (1) static balance, defined as steadiness of the fixed column over a constant base of support; and (2) dynamic balance, defined as control of the column and supporting structures during movement. The most essential and classic dynamic balance task is walking. Walking involves alternating the use of one leg to support the body while the other swings from behind to in front of the body. There is an extensive knowledge base about normal and abnormal walking based on a set of biomechanical characteristics; it uses a specialized terminology. Walking can be characterized by the pattern of steps using spatial factors such as step length, stride length (distance between two heel contacts from the same foot), and step width (Figure 103-1). Walking can also be characterized by temporal factors such as double support time (the duration of the stride when both feet are on the ground at the same time) and cadence (step frequency). Walking has been described as controlled falling because the body column moves forward past the base of support, and the feet must be timed to contact the support surface at the right location and time in anticipation of the moving location of the trunk.[41] When this timing is altered by disease, gait becomes irregular, and trunk movement can be altered. Walking can also

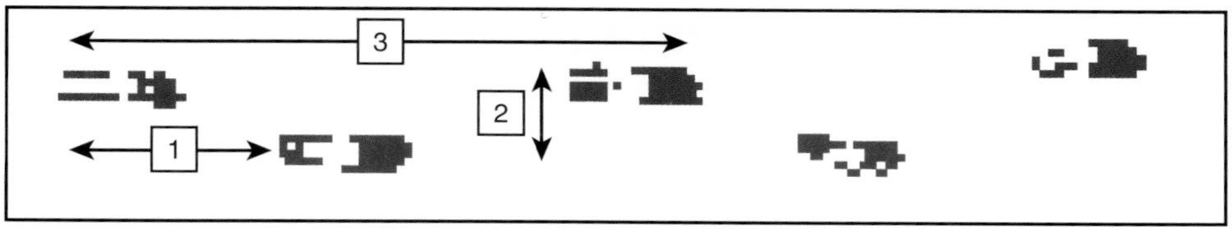

Figure 103-1. Terms used to describe normal walking: (1) step length; (2) step width; (3) stride length.

be characterized by changes in other body segments and joints. During normal walking, the foot begins a step with a push-off from the toe, lifts the foot to swing through, and ends with a heel strike and forward rolling foot contact to initiate the next push-off. The knee is in full extension at the time of toe push off, swings forward with slight flexion to aid foot clearance and then returns to full extension at the point of heel contact. The hip is in extension behind the trunk at push off and swings into flexion at heel contact. The arms swing alternately and in a sequence opposite to the step sequence of the legs. Biomechanical factors that have been found to be abnormal in fallers encompass both static and dynamic balance. Abnormal static balance associated with falling is manifested as increased sway during quiet standing. Some studies have suggested that increased sway to the side, or mediolateral plane, is especially associated with falls.[42] Alterations in dynamic balance among fallers are diverse, depending on the underlying cause. Frequently observed abnormalities include prolonged double support time during walking, increased step width, increased trunk sway during movement, increased or decreased toe clearance, reduced hip extension, abnormal lateral stepping, and delayed correcting movements at the hip or ankle when the trunk is displaced.[43,44]

SCREENING

Screening for fall risk has two main goals, to identify persons at high risk and identify remediable factors for intervention. Screening for risk alone can be more efficient than assessment for modifiable factors, so screening sequences that first identify risk and then assess remediable factors may make the best use of scarce resources. Because fall risk varies by population and type of fall, there is unlikely to be a single screening approach that works well in all settings. Certainly in diverse community populations, it makes sense to identify groups who are at low risk and who therefore can be spared more detailed, time-consuming assessments. The American Geriatrics Society and British Geriatrics Society have recommended fall screens that identify risk as the following: (1) more than one fall in the last year; (2) one or more falls with injury; (3) self-report of unsteadiness; or (4) unsteadiness on performance testing.[45] Many older adults do not complain about falling to health care providers, so it is important to ask about falls explicitly. Some older adults fail to report falls because they have forgotten them, and some may actively hide the fact that they are falling because they worry that the family or health care provider will insist on relocation or activity restrictions.

Screening in chronic care settings differs from screening in primary care. In chronic care settings, fall rates are often high, and screening tool are more likely to have high false-negative rates. If prevalence is very high, it may be sensible to consider almost everyone as high risk and act accordingly. Fall risk screening in acute care is a high priority, but some have argued that no screening tool is accurate enough to justify the current investment in detailed admission fall screening because it consumes much nursing staff time, with little real benefit.[46] In addition, general screens for functional problems in acutely ill, hospitalized older adults may do as well at predicting falls as more specific fall screens, and general screens can be used for a number of nursing issues.[47] There is some evidence that nursing global judgment is comparable in accuracy to formal screening tests in some chronic care settings.[48]

There are two main types of screening tools—those based on professional assessment of various historical and health factors and those based on observed performance of mobility and balance tasks. Some of the more common tools are described in Table 103-3. There are no clearly superior tools that have been shown to have high accuracy in multiple settings, so the optimal tool must be tailored to the population, goals of screening, and time and other resources available.

EVALUATION AND MANAGEMENT

Evaluation

When an individual has been identified as being at high risk for falls, a more detailed evaluation is needed. The goals of evaluation are as follows: (1) identify impairments that contribute to the problem; (2) gain an overall sense of mobility and balance capacity; and (3) consider special risk factors for injury. Because falling is multifactorial in regard to cause, multidisciplinary teams can provide a range of expertise. Disciplines that can make valuable contributions include physicians, nurses, physical therapists, occupational therapists, social workers, pharmacists, and others. Although the older adult should always be interviewed, other informants may be helpful. Table 103-4 illustrates elements of the history and physical examination that can be used to evaluate potential impairments. It is important to recall that older adults often have more than one impairment, so finding one problem does not mean that others are not present. The history should include circumstances of one or more recent falls, history of injuries from falls, course of the problem over time, associated symptoms, and effect on overall mobility and activity. A fall description should include location, time of day, activity, symptoms, use of assistive devices, and ability to get up again.

It is sometimes helpful to explore potential relationships to medication dosing schedules. Various patterns may suggest differing clusters of contributors. Recurrent backward falls tend to be associated with degenerative brain diseases. Acute onset is more likely to be due to a toxic or metabolic effect or perhaps an acute cerebrovascular or cardiac condition. Fear of falling can develop with or without a history of falling and can lead to severe activity restriction. Falls associated with dizziness may suggest some specific diagnoses (Table 103-5). Dizziness is common and nonspecific, so the interviewer must probe more deeply to distinguish potential contributors. True vertigo is defined as a hallucination of rotatory motion and is generally due to vestibular problems. Lightheadedness sometimes implies a sense of imminent loss of consciousness or presyncope. In this case, consider contributors to decreased cerebral perfusion. A third type of dizziness is perceived as not in the head and only occurs when the person upright. It may be an indicator of multisensory disequilibrium, when more than one sensory impairment reduce the ability to monitor body position.

Medications are sometimes implicated in falls and can be among the most treatable contributors, so a thorough medication

TABLE 103-3 Scales Used for Fall Risk Screening and Balance Assessment

Instrument	Items	Setting: Community	Setting: Acute	Setting: Chronic
Multifactorial Reports				
STRATIFY[71]	Five items—history of falls, agitation, visual impairment, frequent toileting, able to stand but needs assistance with moving		X	X
Morse Fall Scale[72]	Six items—history of falls, secondary diagnoses, parenteral therapy, use of ambulation aids, gait, mental status		X	X
FROP-Com[73]	13 risk factors in 26 items—fall and fall injury history, medications, medical conditions, sensory loss, feet, cognitive status, toileting, nutrition, environment, function, behavior, balance, gait; total score, 0 to 60; fall risk high with score > 24	X		
Fall risk for residential care[74]	Among persons who can stand without assistance—poor balance or two of three the following: fall history, nursing home residence, urinary incontinence Among persons who cannot stand without assistance—one of three of the following: fall history, hostel residence, use of nine or more medications			X
Functional Mobility				
Berg Balance test[50,75]	14 tasks scored 0 to 4; total range 0 to 56; fall risk increases as score decreases	X	X	X
Functional reach[76]	Distance reached in inches without moving the feet; fall risk < 7 inches	X	X	X
Performance-oriented mobility and balance[77]	Balance subscale score 0 to 16, gait subscale 0 to 12, summary score 0 to 28; summary score < 19 indicates high fall risk	X		X
Timed up and go[78]	Time in seconds to rise from a chair, walk 3 m, turn, walk back, and sit down; <10 sec normal; fall risk increases with time > 13.5 sec	X		X
Dynamic gait index[51]	Eight walking tasks scored 0 to 3, total score 0 to 24; <18 or 19 indicates fall risk	X		
Functional mobility tests[79]	Time to complete eight step ups (alternate step test) > 10 sec, timed sit to stand five times > 12 sec, 6-m walk time > 6 sec increased fall risk	X		
Physiologic profile assessment[80]	Performance in five domains: sway, reaction time, strength, proprioception, contrast sensitivity; total score 0 to > 3; fall risk increased with score ≥ 2	X		

TABLE 103-4 Clinical Assessment Based on Components of Postural Control

Organ System	Impairment	Clinical Evaluation	Potential Cause
Eye	Decreased acuity	Vision chart	Presbyopia, macular degeneration, cataracts
	Reduced visual fields	Confrontation, perimetry	Glaucoma, posterior circulation stroke
	Decreased depth perception	Stereo or depth testing	Monocular vision
	Decreased dark adaptation	Self-report—inability to dilate pupil in low light	Aging, miotic agents for glaucoma
Vestibular apparatus	Otoliths	Ability to detect true vertical, Hallpike maneuver	Benign positional vertigo
	Semicircular canals	Ability to detect position during rotation with eyes closed, nystagmus, visual acuity during head motion	Meniere disease, vestibular hypofunction
Peripheral nerve	Peripheral neuropathy	Light touch, filaments, two-point discrimination, vibratory sense	Diabetes, peripheral vascular disease, vitamin B_{12} deficiency
Circulation	Reduced cerebral perfusion	Low blood pressure, altered level of consciousness, lightheadedness	Medications, arrhythmias, postprandial hypotension
	Orthostatic hypotension	Positional change in blood pressure	Medications, autonomic dysfunction, dehydration
Brain	Reduced attention	Ability to perform dual tasks like timed up and go with cup of water, executive function tasks	Mild cognitive impairment, dementia, medications
	Psychomotor slowing	Timed tapping, timed finger to nose test, trails A test (connect the dots)	Medications, degenerative and vascular brain diseases
	Altered postural reflexes	Absent or slowed righting reflexes	Parkinson disease, other extrapyramidal and degenerative brain diseases
Muscle	Reduced strength	Manual muscle testing, strength-based functional performance (chair rise, squat)	Generalized—inactivity, sarcopenia, vitamin D deficiency, myopathies Focal deficits, spinal cord and peripheral motor nerve conditions
Musculoskeletal pain	Loss of flexibility	Contractures, decreased range of motion	Arthritis, inactivity
	Bone and joint deficits	Weight-bearing pain	Arthritis, fractures, periarticular conditions, foot problems
	Disturbance of spinal cord, roots, nerves	Leg and back pain with activity	Spinal stenosis, radiculopathies, peripheral neuropathies

history is essential. Although there are long lists of medications with adverse effects on balance, there are just a handful of major mechanisms whereby they cause falls. Common mechanisms include sedation, orthostatic hypotension, extrapyramidal effects, myopathy, and altered dark adaptation of vision. See Table 103-6 for examples of medications listed by potential mechanism. Those who take multiple medications that alter balance are especially vulnerable.

Functional status should be assessed because mobility and balance are central to the ability to care for oneself and live independently. Many older adults use assistive devices for walking, so it is important to explore when and how they were obtained,

TABLE 103-5 Differential Diagnosis and Management of Dizziness

Condition	Symptoms	Evaluation	Management
Orthostatic hypotension	Lightheadedness with change in position	Measure blood pressure in multiple positions, both immediately after change and then again after several minutes. Clinically important systolic drop is not well defined but is more likely to be significant if >20 mm Hg or drops <100 mm Hg	Taper or eliminate medications, fluorinated corticosteroids, salt loading, lower extremity muscle contractions prior to arising, compression hose
Arrhythmia, especially tachy arrhythmia or bradyarrhythmia	Lightheadedness or syncope not associated with position, occasionally with palpitations	Rhythm monitoring—important to capture symptomatic episode so monitoring may be prolonged.	Antiarrhythmic agents, medications for heart rate control, pacemakers
Benign paroxysmal positional vertigo (BPPV)	Short periods of true vertigo with head movement, even without upright body movement such as rolling over in bed or looking up	Dix-Hallpike maneuver reproduces symptoms when in head-down position and precipitates rotatory nystagmus in direction of involved ear	Epley maneuver to reposition otolith debris; Brandt Daroff exercises
Meniere disease	Severe episodes of vertigo with perceived ear pressure, decreased hearing, nausea and vomiting	Usually diagnosed based on classic presentation, often incorrectly diagnosed when true cause is not known	Diuretics, dietary modifications to reduce salt intake
Uncompensated vestibular hypofunction	Unsteadiness that worsens when vision is reduced; blurred vision with head motion	Rotational chair testing, caloric testing, dynamic visual acuity testing	Vestibular rehabilitation, optokinetic stimulation
Multisensory dysequilibrium	Sensation of lack of confidence in body position that only occurs when upright	Decreased sensory function in more than one sensory system (e.g., vision, vestibular, and peripheral sensations)	Treat sensory disorders; carry out rehabilitation for use of sensory aids.

TABLE 103-6 Medications That Affect Components of Postural Control

System Affected	Examples
CNS—attention and psychomotor speed	Benzodiazepines, sedating antihistamines, narcotic analgesics, tricyclic antidepressants, SSRIs, antipsychotics, anticonvulsants, ethanol
Basal ganglia and extrapyramidal system in general	Antipsychotics, metoclopramide, phenothiazines, SSRIs
Blood pressure regulation	Antihypertensives, antianginals, Parkinson drugs, tricyclic antidepressants, antipsychotics
Muscle—myopathy	Corticosteroids, colchicine, statins, ethanol, interferon
Pupil—miosis	Some glaucoma medications, especially pilocarpine

SSRI, Selective serotonin reuptake inhibitor.

TABLE 103-7 Modifications for the Physical Environment

Area	Modifications
Lighting	• Nightlights in the bedroom, bathroom, and hallways leading to the bathroom • Flashlight kept next to the bed • Timer or motion-activated lighting systems • Light switches located near all doors and both ends of stairways
Flooring	• Nonglare, nonskid flooring • Avoidance of loose area rugs or use of nonskid backing • Nonskid strips on steps • Bevel or ramp—uneven transitions between rooms • Increased contrast at level changes
Stairwells	• Sturdy handrails, sometimes on both sides of steps • Chair lift (stair glide) • Rearrange rooms for single-floor living arrangement
Bathroom	• Elevated toilet seat • Grab bars • Nonskid strips or mat on floor of shower or bathtub • Shower chairs • Tub bench
Kitchen	• Commonly used items placed at easily accessible height • Countertop clutter cleared to maximize working space
Walkways	• Clear and straight as possible • Increased width by removing obstacles and furniture to accommodate walkers • Elimination of e tripping hazards such as cords and tubing

where they are used and not used, and if there are areas of problem or concern. Because balance and mobility problems can limit function, it is important to determine if able and willing helpers are available. Older adults without access to helpers may be at special risk when they attempt to perform tasks that have become difficult.

Because the environment influences mobility and safety, a home assessment is an important element of fall risk evaluation. Although some aspects of the environment can be explored through an interview, a direct home assessment by professionals from a home visit agency can be invaluable. Key aspects of home assessment are described in Table 103-7.

The physical examination is useful to detect impairments that contribute to poor balance and assess overall functional performance. Table 103-4 describes maneuvers that can be performed during the physical examination to detect impairments. Most of these assessments are familiar to health care providers, but a few are somewhat unique to balance assessment. Peripheral sensory testing is important because neuropathy is common among older adults. Although proprioception (joint position sense) is important for balance, testing is insensitive. Because proprioception and vibratory sensation use similar nerve fibers, testing vibratory sense may be more sensitive. A common strategy is to evaluate vibration sense using a 128-Hz tuning fork applied over a bony prominence such as the medial malleolus. The Romberg test, in which standing balance is compared with eyes open and closed, is a useful strategy for detecting visual dependence. An abnormal result suggests a peripheral nerve or vestibular disorder. Abnormal muscle tone can indicate a variety of conditions. Increased tone implies upper motor neuron disease whereas decreased tone suggests lower motor neuron dysfunction. Increased tone can exist throughout the range of motion (lead pipe rigidity) or intermittently (cogwheeling rigidity). Coordination should be assessed in the upper and lower extremities using tests of rapid alternating movements. Soft neurologic signs suggestive of a Parkinson disease–like condition, with rigidity and loss of balance, has been reported to be common among older fallers.[49] Every balance assessment should include a test of righting reflexes. To perform the assessment, the examiner stands behind the patient and asks the patient to prepare to respond to a push or pull with any reaction they prefer. The examiner pulls the patient's pelvis backward sufficiently to displace the body outside the base of support. A normal response is a brisk step backward. An abnormal response is a complete lack of stepping, called a timber reaction. The patient can also be displaced to the side.

The evaluation is also used to determine functional mobility and balance capacity. Physical performance measures can serve as a guide, but it is important to target the performance assessment to the mobility capacity of the individual. Thus, an older adult who is wheelchair-bound needs detailed assessment of bed mobility, transfers, and standing balance, whereas an active older adult may need more of a focus on high-level skills such as obstacle avoidance, dual tasks, and stair climbing. Table 103-3 includes commonly used functional performance assessment tools for mobility and balance. The Berg balance scale has been used to predict fall risk[50] but does not assess balance during walking. The Dynamic Gait Index is especially helpful for detecting subtle, higher level problems because it includes challenging conditions.[51] The Performance-Oriented Mobility Assessment (POMA) assesses static balance and gait and is widely used, but does not assess higher level functions.[52] Balance assessments have added dual-task tests that combine mobility assessment with distraction or a cognitive task. These divided attention tasks can sometimes uncover abnormal gait or balance not seen under usual simple conditions. Being unable to walk and talk at the same time is a risk factor for falls.[53] Reduced endurance during walking can create a sense of fatigue and leg weakness, so a long walk might be a useful element of the examination.

The third element of evaluation is to determine special risk factors for injury. Because fractures are a major cause of morbidity in fallers, every unsteady person should be assessed for osteoporosis. Another special concern is the risk of bleeding in persons who take anticoagulants. Loss of protective reflexes also increases the risk of injury. Normal protective responses involve use of the upper extremity to moderate impact force and protect the head, so injuries to the head, face, and orbit are especially worrisome. An absent righting reflex on physical examination is a significant indicator of increased risk of injury.

Management

The goals of management are as follows: (1) treat impairments, where possible; (2) build on systems that work well to compensate for deficits; and (3) provide physical and human resources to assist when necessary. Table 103-8 provides suggestions for management strategies based on impairments detected during the evaluation. As always, it is important to engage the older adult and family in the discussion of management options and incorporate patient preferences into the plan.

Assistive devices can promote mobility in persons with balance problems through several mechanisms. In general, they all increase the base of support, thus increasing stability. Assistive devices can also provide sensory information about the walking surface directly to the upper extremity and therefore are especially helpful to people with sensory loss in the feet. This ability to use sensory information from any part of the body to promote awareness of body position is termed *haptic sensation*. Assistive devices should be professionally assessed, and patients need training in their proper use. Older adults notoriously acquire poorly fitting devices from family and friends. Canes increase the base of support and take up much less space than walkers. Walkers provide much more stability than canes but are bulkier and difficult to maneuver in tight spaces. Newer four-wheeled walkers are lightweight and have hand-activated wheel locks, seats, and baskets that make them an attractive option for older adults. The larger wheels also make them more maneuverable on uneven sidewalks, grass, and gravel than the small wheels found on traditional walkers. Wheeled walkers also are easier to learn to use than traditional pick-up walkers.

Inappropriate footwear can be modified, but there is no clear evidence to guide optimal characteristics of the shoe for fall reduction. Shoes with low wide heels promote stability. Shoes should fit comfortably but snugly so that the foot and shoe move together. There is controversy about the optimal characteristics of the bottom of the shoe. Rubber-soled shoes reduce pressure areas in persons with insensitive feet but also decrease sensory information about the walking surface. Hard, leather-soled shoes provide better sensory information and reduce tripping because they don't catch on surfaces, but do increase the risk of slipping.

It is important to attend to the needs of the caregiver as well. Caregivers should receive training in body mechanics and transfer assists. They can also be educated about how to help get the older adult up after a fall.

Injury prevention is an important element of falls care. If a faller has had a fracture or is found to have osteoporosis, serious consideration should be given to prescribing appropriate medications. Hip protectors have been found to reduce injury in some studies, but other studies have shown less benefit.[54,55]

There is now a body of clinical trial evidence that supports the effectiveness of interventions to prevent falls.[56,57] Interventions that have been found to reduce falls include multiple risk factor reduction, professionally directed group and individualized rehabilitation, professionally led home hazard assessment and remediation, psychotropic medication withdrawal, and cardiac pacemakers for fallers with cardioinhibitory carotid sinus hypersensitivity. Overall interventions yield about a 20% relative risk reduction and 10% absolute risk reduction, so there is certainly room for further improvement.

Emerging evidence from exercise intervention studies has suggested that multiple types of exercise, dose, and targeting of exercise for functional abilities are important factors. Effective fall reduction exercise programs include some type of balance exercises combined with a range of strengthening, endurance, walking, stepping, movement control, and dual-task exercises and have been found to be more effective than any single exercise–type training.[57-60] Exercise for 12 weeks or longer for approximately 2 hours/week is the effective minimum dose to reduce falls.[59] Among older adults who are frail or have multiple comorbidities, group and home-based exercise programs have been less effective and may not be appropriate for fall reduction.[57,60] Alternatively, individualized physical therapy exercise programs are often underdosed. In the future, linking individualized rehabilitation exercise intervention with transition to community group or home-based exercise and health promotion physical activity appears key to reduce and prevent falls.[58,60,61]

SYSTEM-WIDE IMPLEMENTATION

There has been sufficient evidence from formal clinical trials to suggest that interventions to reduce falls may be effective in some settings.[8,62-64] Despite the evidence, these programs have not yet translated into system-wide changes in practice. It has been suggested that translation to practice may be feasible and effective. A large nonrandomized study that compared fall injury rates and medical service use between two comparable geographic regions before and after a system-wide intervention was implemented in one of the regions.[65] The intervention consisted of recommendations for medication reduction, management of postural hypotension and vision and foot problems, hazard reduction, and training for balance, gait, and strength. Using multiple media, seminars, opinion leaders, and site visits, the intervention was targeted at

TABLE 103-8 Management of Impairments That Contribute to Instability and Falls

Organ System	Impairment	Medical Management	Restorative Services	Environmental Modifications
Eye	Decreased acuity	Corrective lenses	Low vision rehabilitation	Lighting
	Reduced visual fields	Prisms in spectacles	Low vision rehabilitation, teach to scan using head rotation	
	Loss of depth perception	Cataract removal, if indicated	Teach to use shadows to detect depth	Lighting to accent shadows, contrast
	Poor dark adaptation	Switching to glaucoma medications that do not cause miosis		Lighting
Vestibular system	Benign paroxysmal positional vertigo (BPPV)	Epley maneuver	Vestibular rehabilitation	
	Meniere disease	Cautious use of meclizine, diuretics; rarely, surgery	Vestibular rehabilitation	
Peripheral nerve	Neuropathy	Footwear to protect foot and maximize sensation	Assistive devices for haptic enhancement	Hand holds, railings
Central circulation	Reduced brain perfusion	Treatment varies by cause Arrhythmias—medications to control rate and rhythm, pacemakers Postprandial hypotension—frequent small meals		
	Orthostatic hypotension	Treatment varies by cause Adjust offending medications Autonomic neuropathy—salt loading, fluorinated corticosteroids Dehydration—hydration, reduce diuretic dose	Compression hose, calf muscle contractions	
Brain	Reduced attention	Medication adjustment	Practice dual tasks	
	Psychomotor slowing	Medication adjustment	Practice movement speed	
	Abnormal righting reflexes	Antiparkinsonian medication helps bradykinesia more than balance.	Assistive devices, practice getting up after a fall	Protective clothing
Effector muscle	Weakness	Reduced activity—treat contributing causes (e.g., CHF, anemia, COPD, arthritis)	Strength-training exercises	Raise chair height
		Focal motor deficit due to spinal stenosis—sometimes surgery	Orthotics, exercise, assistive devices	
		Myopathy—adjust offending medications, possibly steroids for myositis		
Musculoskeletal	Decreased range of motion		Active and passive range of motion exercise, orthotics	
Pain	Bone and joint	Analgesics, injections	Physical modalities (e.g., heat, massage, assistive devices, orthoses, adaptive equipment)	Place items within easy reach
	Spinal cord, roots, nerves	Injections, surgery, analgesics	Orthoses, assistive devices	Place items within easy reach

CHF, Congestive heart failure; *COPD*, chronic obstructive pulmonary disease.

primary care physicians, home health agencies, and emergency departments. Injury rates were lower in the intervention region, and medical use increased less than in the usual care region. Other system interventions have been effective in emergency departments[66] but not nursing homes[67,68] or public health departments.[69] Keys to widespread implementation require that system barriers such as provider time limits, lack of knowledge, care fragmentation, and lack of reimbursement be addressed.[1] A major new fall prevention trial embedded in multiple U.S. health care systems has been funded by the Patient-Centered Outcomes Research Institute (PCORI) through a research partnership with NIH.[70]

SUMMARY

Falling is common and has serious consequences for older adults. Fallers often have multiple contributing impairments that interact to affect balance. Multidisciplinary interventions have been effective in some settings, but evidence from research has not yet translated into usual clinical practice.

KEY POINTS
- This chapter presents the scope and impact of falls in older adults.
- Causes of falls are discussed.
- Guidelines for clinical evaluation and treatment are provided.
- Opportunities to implement programs across health care settings and communities are described.

For a complete list of references, please visit www.expertconsult.com.

KEY REFERENCES

1. Tinetti ME, Gordon C, Sogolow E, et al: Fall-risk evaluation and management: challenges in adopting geriatric care practices. Gerontologist 46:717–725, 2006.
9. Lamb SE, Jorstad-Stein EC, Hauer K, et al: Development of a common outcome data set for fall injury prevention trials: the Prevention of Falls Network Europe consensus. J Am Geriatr Soc 53:1618–1622, 2005.
10. Etman A, Wijlhuizen GJ, van Heuvelen MJ, et al: Falls incidence underestimates the risk of fall-related injuries in older age groups: a comparison with the FARE (Falls risk by Exposure). Age Ageing 41:190–195, 2012.
15. Inouye SK, Studenski S, Tinetti ME, et al: Geriatric syndromes: clinical, research, and policy implications of a core geriatric concept. J Am Geriatr Soc 55:780–791, 2007.
18. Feldman F, Chaudhury H: Falls and the physical environment: a review and a new multifactorial falls-risk conceptual framework. Can J Occup Ther 75:82–95, 2008.
19. Lord SR: Aging and falls: causes and prevention. J Musculoskelet Neuronal Interact 7:347, 2007.
20. Reed-Jones RJ, Solis GR, Lawson KA, et al: Vision and falls: a multidisciplinary review of the contributions of visual impairment to falls among older adults. Maturitas 75:22–28, 2013.
23. Ward BK, Agrawal Y, Hoffman HJ, et al: Prevalence and impact of bilateral vestibular hypofunction: results from the 2008 US National Health Interview Survey. JAMA Otolaryngol Head Neck Surg 139:803–810, 2013.
25. Kuo HK, Lipsitz LA: Cerebral white matter changes and geriatric syndromes: is there a link? J Gerontol A Biol Sci Med Sci 59:818–826, 2004.
27. Liu Y, Chan JS, Yan JH: Neuropsychological mechanisms of falls in older adults. Front Aging Neurosci 6:64, 2014.
30. Montero-Odasso M, Verghese J, Beauchet O, et al: Gait and cognition: a complementary approach to understanding brain function and the risk of falling. J Am Geriatr Soc 60:2127–2136, 2012.
31. Amboni M, Barone P, Hausdorff JM: Cognitive contributions to gait and falls: evidence and implications. Mov Disord 28:1520–1533, 2013.
33. Stone KL, Ewing SK, Lui LY, et al: Self-reported sleep and nap habits and risk of falls and fractures in older women: the study of osteoporotic fractures. J Am Geriatr Soc 54:1177–1183, 2006.
45. American Geriatrics Society, British Geriatrics Society, and American Academy of Orthopaedic Surgeons Panel on Falls Prevention: Guideline for the prevention of falls in older persons. J Am Geriatr Soc 49:664–672, 2001.
46. Oliver D: Falls risk-prediction tools for hospital inpatients. Time to put them to bed? Age Ageing 37:248–250, 2008.
49. Fasano A, Plotnik M, Bove F, et al: The neurobiology of falls. Neurol Sci 33:1215–1223, 2012.
57. Gillespie L, Robertson M, Gillespie W, et al: Interventions for preventing falls in older people living in the community. Cochrane Database Syst Rev (9):CD007146, 2012.
58. Maetzler W, Nieuwhof F, Hasmann S, et al: Emerging therapies for gait disability and balance impairment: promises and pitfalls. Mov Disord 28:1576–1586, 2013.
59. Sherrington C, Whitney J, Lord S, et al: Effective exercise for the prevention of falls: a systematic review and meta-analysis. J Am Geriatr Soc 54:2234–2243, 2008.
60. Shubert T: Evidence-based exercise prescription for balance and falls prevention: a current review of the literature. J Geriatr Phys Ther 34:100–108, 2011.
61. Cameron I, Gillespie L, Robertson M, et al: Interventions for preventing falls in older people living in care facilities and hospitals. Cochrane Database Syst Rev (12):CD005465, 2012.
63. Coussement J, De Paepe L, Schwendimann R, et al: Interventions for preventing falls in acute- and chronic-care hospitals: a systematic review and meta-analysis. J Am Geriatr Soc 56:29–36, 2008.
64. Gates S, Fisher JD, Cooke MW, et al: Multifactorial assessment and targeted intervention for preventing falls and injuries among older people in community and emergency care settings: systematic review and meta-analysis. BMJ 336:130–133, 2008.
71. Oliver D, Papaioannou A, Giangregorio L, et al: A systematic review and meta-analysis of studies using the STRATIFY tool for prediction of falls in hospital patients: how well does it work? Age Ageing 37:621–627, 2008.
80. Lord SR, Menz HB, Tiedemann A: A physiologic profile approach to falls risk assessment and prevention. Phys Ther 83:237–252, 2003.

104 Podiatry

Hylton B. Menz

INTRODUCTION

The foot plays an important role in all weight-bearing tasks. When walking, the foot contributes to shock absorption, adapts to irregular surfaces, and provides a rigid lever for forward momentum. Aging is associated with significant alterations to the cutaneous, vascular, neurologic, and musculoskeletal characteristics of the foot, all of which may impair this important weight-bearing function.[1] As a consequence of these age-related changes, foot pain and deformity are a common accompaniment of advancing age. This chapter briefly outlines the prevalence and consequences of foot problems in older people and provides an overview of the management of some common conditions affecting the feet of older people.

EPIDEMIOLOGY OF FOOT PAIN IN OLDER PEOPLE

Foot pain has long been recognized as a common problem in older people. A recent systematic review and meta-analysis of 31 studies estimated the population prevalence of foot pain to be 24% in people aged 65 years and over, with approximately two thirds reporting at least moderate disability.[2] Women report a higher prevalence of foot pain compared to men, possibly because of the detrimental influence of wearing fashion footwear.[3] Other identified risk factors for the development of foot pain include obesity, chronic conditions such osteoarthritis, psychological factors such as anxiety and depression, and socioeconomic disadvantage.[4-6]

There is strong evidence that foot pain and deformity have a significant impact on mobility and health status. Several studies of older people have demonstrated that foot pain is associated with decreased ability to undertake activities of daily living,[7] problems with balance and gait,[8] an increased risk of falls,[9] and poorer health-related quality of life.[10] Approximately 20% of older people who are unable to leave their home specifically attribute this to foot pain.[11]

CLINICAL ASSESSMENT OF THE FOOT IN OLDER PEOPLE

Physical examination is the basis for diagnosing foot disorders. Observation and palpation, in conjunction with detailed history taking, are generally sufficient to diagnose most common conditions.[12] Physical examination of the older person with foot problems involves assessment of skin and appendages, vascular status (including pulse palpation and ankle-brachial index measurement), neurologic status (including sensory testing with graded monofilaments and reflex testing), orthopaedic examination (including foot posture and range-of-motion measurement of the ankle, subtalar, midtarsal, and metatarsophalangeal joints), manual muscle testing, footwear assessment, and observational gait analysis.[13]

Many interventions for foot problems require some degree of self-management in the home environment. For this reason, an essential component of clinical assessment of older persons with foot problems is evaluating their ability to undertake basic foot care tasks such as cutting and filing nails, applying creams, washing and drying feet, putting on shoes and socks, changing wound dressings, and examining the foot for lesions. To perform these tasks appropriately, the older person requires adequate cognition, grip strength, flexibility, visual acuity, and manual dexterity.[14]

COMMON FOOT DISORDERS IN OLDER PEOPLE AND THEIR MANAGEMENT

Nail Disorders

Onychauxis

Onychauxis refers to hypertrophy of the nail plate, which may result from injury, chronic low-grade trauma from ill-fitting shoes, infection, peripheral vascular disease, diabetes, or nutritional deficiency (Figure 104-1, *A*). Onychauxis is often accompanied by onychophosis, the formation of hyperkeratosis in the nail grooves. If left untreated, hematomas may form under the nail, creating a potential site for infection. Regular maintenance of basic foot hygiene and selection of appropriate footwear may prevent excessive thickening of the nail. However, advanced cases may require treatment by a podiatrist, who will use a special drill to reduce the thickness of the nail. Surgical removal is occasionally indicated, particularly in cases of long-term neglect where the nail may become grossly thickened, curved, and elongated.

Onychocryptosis

The term *onychocryptosis* refers to "ingrown" toenail, where a spicule of nail penetrates the skin, leading to pain, inflammation, and risk of secondary infection. People with abnormally curved nails or overriding toes are more likely to develop onychocryptosis; however, in many cases, the condition is simply caused by inappropriate nail cutting or tightly fitting footwear. Toenails should be cut straight across, and shoes should have sufficient room in the toe box to prevent constriction. Applying topical antiseptics and allowing the nail to grow out normally can successfully manage most cases, but recurrent cases may require removal of the offending portion of nail under local anesthetic. Partial nail avulsion combined with phenolization to destroy nail matrix cells is more effective at preventing recurrence compared to surgical excision, although healing times may be slower.[15]

Onychomycosis

Onychomycosis (fungal nail infection) is usually caused by dermatophyte, saprophyte, or yeast organisms and results in yellow-brown discoloration, thickening, and crumbling of the nail plate. Conscientious management of foot hygiene, including washing the feet with soap and water and changing socks daily may prevent many fungal nail infections. Once the condition has developed, it may take some time to achieve a complete cure. A wide range of treatments have been used to treat the condition. However, the gold standard treatment is terbinafine, an oral medication that has been shown to cure the condition in 3 to 6 months.[16] In the presence of contraindications to oral medication, topical treatments may be used; however, relief of symptoms

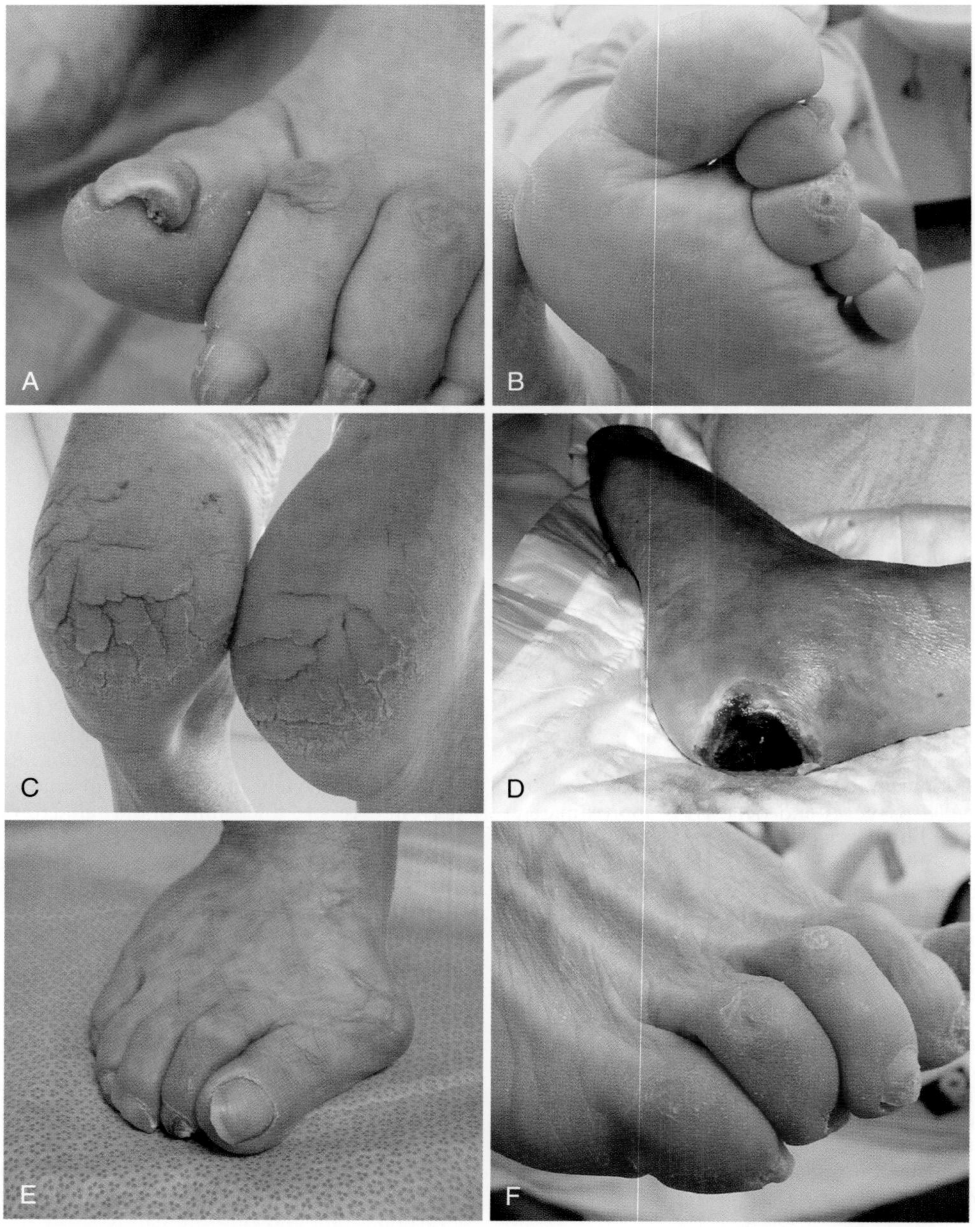

Figure 104-1. Common foot problems in older people. **A,** Onychauxis. **B,** Corns. **C,** Heel fissures. **D,** Decubitus heel ulcer. **E,** Hallux valgus. **F,** Claw toes.

takes much longer and cure rates are significantly lower.[17] Modest improvements in cure rates can be achieved by combining oral and topical treatments, although achieving adequate compliance may be difficult.[18] To prevent recurrence, infected footwear and socks should be discarded or sterilized.

Skin Disorders

Hyperkeratosis

Hyperkeratosis is a normal physiologic response to friction applied to the skin, and it develops as a protective mechanism to prevent damage to deeper tissues. However, when the friction applied to the skin becomes excessive, the resultant focal thickening can become extremely painful, increasing the pressure on the underlying dermis. The foot is a common site for the development of hyperkeratosis because of its load-bearing function[19] and compression from footwear.[3] Broadly, there are two types of hyperkeratosis: *calluses*, which generally develop on the plantar surface of the foot and appear as a diffuse thickening, and *corns (heloma)*, which are more common on the toes and can be differentiated from a callus by the presence of a sharply demarcated central core (Figure 104-1, *B*). Corns may also develop underneath the nail bed (*subungual heloma*)[20] or in between the toes (*interdigital heloma*). Because of the associated moisture, interdigital corns are often soft and macerated.[21]

Calluses and corns are caused by a range of factors, including ill-fitting footwear, bony prominences, short or long metatarsals, and abnormal plantar loading patterns. In addition to the selection of more appropriate footwear, calluses and corns should be débrided and enucleated by a podiatrist. Simple foam and silicon pads available over the counter at pharmacies can offer effective temporary relief.[22] Medicated corn plasters containing salicylic acid are more effective at reducing pain and recurrence of corns than is regular scalpel débridement.[23] However, because the application of salicylic acid–containing corn plasters can lead to ulceration in older people with frail skin and/or impaired peripheral vascular supply, they should be used with considerable caution, particularly in people with diabetes.[24] Long-term management includes foot orthoses to redistribute excessive plantar loads and surgery to correct any underlying osseous deformity.

Xerosis

Xerosis, or dehydration of the skin, is particularly prevalent in older people with diabetes or peripheral vascular disease. Dry skin around the heels often leads to the development of fissures that may extend to the dermis, resulting in pain and risk of infection (Figure 104-1, *C*). A wide range of emollient preparations (including urea, α-hydroxy acids, lactic acid, lanolin, and ammonium lactate) have been shown to be similarly effective in rehydrating the skin,[25,26] with the frequency of application likely to be as important as the active ingredient in the preparation. Deep heel fissures may require débridement of the callused edges and application of an adhesive bandage to limit lateral expansion of the heel when weight bearing, or the application of cyanoacrylate adhesive to seal the fissures until they heal.

Foot Ulceration

Aging is associated with several changes to the structure and function of the skin, including a marked loss of collagen and elastin fibers, resulting in increased skin fragility, and a reduction in Langerhans and mast cells, which reduces the inflammatory response to infection. These changes, combined with reduced peripheral blood flow, increase the likelihood of tissue damage and impair the ability of the skin to heal.[27] Consequently, chronic and recurrent foot ulceration is a common problem in older people, particularly those in residential care facilities.

Foot ulcers tend to have a characteristic appearance depending on their primary cause. *Arterial* ulcers resulting from peripheral arterial disease most commonly affect the dorsum of the toes or the heel and typically have well-defined edges with a dry base. Limb elevation exacerbates symptoms as a result of reduced peripheral blood flow. *Venous* ulcers resulting from venous insufficiency most commonly affect the region between the ankle and calf and are generally shallow, with irregular borders and substantial exudate. The surrounding tissue is often edematous and hyperpigmented. *Diabetic* ulcers most commonly form in weight-bearing areas such as the metatarsal heads and heel. They are usually deep with undermined edges and surrounded by hyperkeratosis. Pressure ulcers (also known as *decubitus* ulcers) result from long-term compression of the skin and most commonly affect the posterior heel in older people who are confined to bed (Figure 104-1, *D*).[28]

Effective treatment of foot ulceration involves addressing the underlying cause (e.g., surgical revascularization for arterial ulcers and reduction of venous stasis using compression therapy for venous ulcers) in addition to débridement, management of infection, and the application of appropriate wound dressings. Alleviation of pressure is particularly important for ulcers affecting the foot and can be achieved using padded stockings, orthoses, custom footwear, and casting techniques.

Musculoskeletal Foot Disorders

Hallux Valgus

Hallux valgus is a condition affecting approximately 36% of people older than 65 years in which the first metatarsophalangeal joint is progressively subluxed as a result of the lateral deviation of the hallux and medial deviation of the first metatarsal (Figure 104-1, *E*).[29] Factors thought to be associated with the development of hallux valgus include constrictive footwear, an overly long first metatarsal, and a rounded first metatarsal head.[30] The condition has also been shown to be highly heritable.[31] The enlarged first metatarsal head creates problems with finding suitable footwear, and the friction created by the shoe often leads to the formation of a bursa. Treatment of hallux valgus includes changing footwear to that with a broader toe box, the application of foam or silicon pads over the joint, foot orthoses, and surgery. Surgery has been shown to provide better long-term results than have foot orthoses.[32]

Lesser Toe Deformity

Long-term wearing of ill-fitting footwear, in association with abnormal foot mechanics and intrinsic muscle atrophy, can lead to the development of clawing, hammering, and retraction of the lesser toes (Figure 104-1, *F*).[33] Hammer toes and claw toes often lead to the development of corns on the dorsum of the interphalangeal joints and calluses under the metatarsal heads. There is also evidence to suggest that toe deformity may impair balance and increase the risk of falls in older people.[34] Treatment involves footwear modification, various splinting devices, and management of secondary lesions. Severe cases often require surgery to realign and stabilize the affected metatarsophalangeal or interphalangeal joints and/or lengthen the long flexor or extensor tendons.

Tibialis Posterior Dysfunction

With advancing age, there is a tendency toward a lowering of the medial longitudinal arch of the foot, which may be the result of a gradual weakening and elongation of the tibialis posterior tendon.[1] An advanced form of this process is known as *tibialis posterior dysfunction*, in which the tibialis posterior tendon weakens and may partially rupture, leading to a progressive and disabling acquired flatfoot deformity.[35] Although the exact cause is unknown, tendon degeneration as a result of reduced blood supply has been implicated, and the condition is more common in people with obesity, hypertension, diabetes, or previous trauma. Treatment selection depends on the degree of severity. Early stages may be effectively managed with nonsteroidal antiinflammatory medications, foot orthoses, braces, and footwear modifications, whereas more advanced stages require tendon reconstruction or surgical fixation of joints in the rearfoot.

Plantar Heel Pain Syndrome

Pain in the region of the heel has been estimated to affect 15% of older people.[36] There is a range of causes of heel pain, including proximal plantar fasciitis, nerve entrapment, calcaneal stress fracture, and plantar calcaneal bursitis. Systemic conditions can also lead to heel pain, including Paget disease, rheumatoid arthritis, psoriatic arthritis, gout, Reiter syndrome, and ankylosing spondylitis. Older people may be more likely to develop heel pain because of the effects of aging on the structure and function of the plantar heel pad. Compared to younger people, older people have thicker but more compressible heel pads that dissipate more energy, which may result in greater impact being applied to the musculoskeletal and neural structures in the heel region.[1] Interventions shown to be effective for the treatment of plantar heel pain include taping, foot orthoses, night splints, and, for short-term pain relief, corticosteroid injection.[37] Full-length foot orthoses may be more effective in older people than simple cushioning heel pads, as they prevent the heel from spreading and redistribute loads from the heel to the midfoot.[38]

THE ROLE OF FOOTWEAR AND FOOT ORTHOSES

Footwear advice and modification are essential in the management of foot problems in older people. Wearing shoes narrower than the foot is associated with corns, hallux valgus, and foot pain, while wearing shoes that are too short is associated with hammer toes and claw toes.[3] However, a recent randomized trial demonstrated that the provision of extra-depth footwear with a broad, pliable upper to accommodate toe deformity was effective at reducing foot pain and recurrence of hyperkeratotic lesions in older people.[39] This suggests that ill-fitting footwear is a modifiable risk factor and that, in many cases, changing footwear may be the only intervention required to alleviate foot pain in people of this age group.

Footwear modification (*pedorthics*) is also a useful conservative management strategy for older people with foot problems. The aim of footwear modification is to relieve excessive pressure from sensitive or painful areas; to accommodate, correct, and support deformities; and to control or limit painful motion of joints. This may be achieved by the prescription of shoes with extra depth in the forefoot, addition of balloon patches to the upper of the shoe to accommodate bony prominences, insertion of a wedge of soft material into the heel region to improve shock absorption, and/or addition of an external "rocker bar" to the sole of the shoe to enhance propulsion.[40]

Foot orthoses are devices placed within the shoe that aim to decrease pain and improve function by altering the biomechanical function of the lower limb. Foot orthoses can be divided into two broad functional categories: those that aim to improve function by redistributing pressure beneath the foot (*pressure-redistributing orthoses*) and those that improve function by limiting excessive motion of tarsal joints (*motion-controlling orthoses*). Pressure-redistributing orthoses are generally made from compressible materials and are commonly used to offload sites of high pressure, whereas motion-controlling orthoses are made from firmer materials and are most commonly used to manage conditions related to flat foot. Several studies have shown that various types of orthoses can redistribute plantar pressures away from high-pressure areas to reduce pathologic loading on specific regions of the foot,[38,41] and preliminary evidence indicates that these approaches are effective at reducing foot pain in older people.[42]

KEY POINTS

- Normal aging results in significant alterations to the cutaneous, vascular, neurologic, and musculoskeletal characteristics of the foot.
- Foot pain affects 1 in 4 older people and is associated with impaired mobility and an increased risk of falls.
- The most common foot problems in older people are nail disorders, keratotic disorders (corns and calluses), and toe deformities.
- Many foot problems can be successfully managed with conservative interventions such as regular podiatry treatment, selection of appropriate footwear, and foot orthoses.

For a complete list of references, please visit www.expertconsult.com.

KEY REFERENCES

1. Menz HB: Biomechanics of the ageing foot and ankle: a mini review. Gerontology 61:381–388, 2015.
2. Thomas M, Roddy E, Zhang W, et al: The population prevalence of foot and ankle pain in middle and old age: a systematic review. Pain 152:2870–2880, 2011.
3. Menz HB, Morris ME: Footwear characteristics and foot problems in older people. Gerontology 51:346–351, 2005.
9. Menz HB, Morris ME, Lord SR: Foot and ankle risk factors for falls in older people: a prospective study. J Gerontol A Biol Sci Med Sci 61:M866–M870, 2006.
23. Farndon LJ, Vernon W, Walters SJ, et al: The effectiveness of salicylic acid plasters compared with "usual" scalpel debridement of corns: a randomised controlled trial. J Foot Ankle Res 6:40, 2013.
29. Nix SE, Smith M, Vicenzino BT: Prevalence of hallux valgus in the general population: a systematic review and meta-analysis. J Foot Ankle Res 3:21, 2010.
31. Hannan MT, Menz HB, Jordan JM, et al: Hallux valgus and lesser toe deformities are highly heritable in adult men and women: the Framingham Foot Study. Arthritis Care Res 65:1515–1521, 2013.
32. Torkki M, Malmivaara A, Seitsalo S, et al: Surgery vs orthosis vs watchful waiting for hallux valgus: a randomized controlled trial. JAMA 285:2474–2480, 2001.
36. Hill CL, Gill T, Menz HB, et al: Prevalence and correlates of foot pain in a population-based study: the North West Adelaide Health Study. J Foot Ankle Res 1:2, 2008.
39. Menz HB, Auhl M, Ristevski S, et al: Effectiveness of off-the-shelf, extra-depth footwear in reducing foot pain in older people: a randomized controlled trial. J Gerontol A Biol Sci Med Sci 70:511–517, 2015.

105 Constipation and Fecal Incontinence in Old Age

Danielle Harari

INTRODUCTION

Fecal incontinence (FI) in older people is a distressing and socially isolating symptom and increases the risk of morbidity,[1,2] mortality,[3,4] and dependency.[2,4] Many older individuals with FI will not volunteer the problem to their general practitioner or nurse. Regrettably, health care providers do not routinely inquire about the symptom, which is why it is a routine prompt in a standard comprehensive geriatric assessment. This "hidden problem" can lead to a downward spiral of psychological distress, dependency, and poor health. The condition can especially take its toll on informal caregivers of home-dwelling patients,[5] with FI being a leading reason for requesting nursing home placement.[6,7] Even when older people are noted by health care professionals to have FI, the condition is often managed passively (e.g., pads provision without assessment). Current surveys show limited awareness of appropriate assessment and treatment options among primary care physicians.[8] The importance of identifying treatable causes of FI in frail older people is strongly emphasized in national and international guidance,[7,9-12] but successive audit shows that adherence to such guidance is generally poor, with nonintegrated services, and suboptimal delivery by professionals of even basic assessment and care.[13-15]

Constipation is a common concern for adults as they age beyond 60 years, reflected by a notable increase in primary care consultations and burgeoning laxative use. Older people reporting constipation are more likely to have anxiety, depression, and poor health perception. Qualitative studies show older adults feel doctors can be dismissive about the problem and that useful and empathic professional advice is hard to find,[16] and this is confirmed in primary care studies that reveal that general practitioners view constipation as less important than other conditions (such as diabetes).[17] Clinical constipation in frail individuals can lead to significant complications such as fecal impaction, FI, and urinary retention precipitating hospital admission. Constipation and FI are costly conditions, with high expenditure, including laxative spending and nursing time.[5] For instance, it is estimated that 80% of community nurses working with older people in the United Kingdom are managing constipation (particularly fecal impaction) as part of their caseload. A 2014 health care utilization study of patients with chronic constipation (mean age 64) in Sweden documented an average of 2.4 constipation-related health care contacts per year at an annual cost of 951 Euros per patient.[18]

DEFINITIONS

The World Health Organization (WHO) International Consultation on Incontinence defines FI as "involuntary loss of liquid or solid stool that is a social or hygienic problem."[10] There is, however, a lack of standardization in defining FI in published prevalence studies, hindering cross-study comparisons. Most community-based studies examine prevalence of FI occurring at least once over the previous year, which may overestimate prevalence but also provide the upper limit for FI occurrence. Nursing home studies mostly measure weekly or monthly occurrence. Systematic reviews examining FI prevalence have highlighted the need for consensus on definitions.[19,20] A study of women mostly aged 60 years and older with FI looked at patient-preferred terminology for FI symptoms: important outcomes were predictability, awareness, ability to wipe, and burning discomfort, in addition to the usual primary outcomes of frequency, amount of leakage, and "bother."[21]

Definitions of constipation in older people in medical and nursing literature have also been inconsistent. Studies of older people have defined constipation by subjective self-report, specific bowel-related symptoms, or by daily laxative use. Self-reported constipation (e.g., "Do you have recurrent constipation?") often means different things to different individuals.[14] It is now increasingly required in both clinical practice and research to use standardized definitions for constipation based on specific symptoms (Rome III criteria)[22-25] (Table 105-1). Important constipation subtypes affecting older people, such as rectal outlet delay and constipation-predominant irritable bowel syndrome (IBS-C), are easier to identify by using standard definitions.[22,24,25] Rome criteria are symptom-based: objective assessment relies on finding fecal loading in the rectum, colon, or both. Such objective assessment is particularly important in frail older people in whom constipation can be underestimated (Table 105-2).

PREVALENCE OF CONSTIPATION AND CONSTIPATION-RELATED SYMPTOMS

Constipation is a hugely prevalent problem in older people. Approximately 63 million people in North America meet the Rome III criteria for constipation, with a disproportionate number being older than 65 years.[26] Age is strongly associated with nonspecific self-reporting of constipation.[27-29] It is therefore striking that the report of infrequent bowel movements (two or fewer per week) is no more prevalent in older than younger people in community-based studies.

- Only 1% to 7% of both younger and older people report two or fewer bowel movements a week.[27,29,30]
- This consistent bowel pattern across age groups persists even after statistical adjustment for greater laxative use among older people.[27]
- Of older people complaining of constipation, less than 10% report two or fewer weekly bowel movements, and more than 50% move their bowels daily.[29,31]
- In contrast, two thirds of older people have persistent straining, and 39% report passage of hard stools.[31]

The symptoms predominantly underlying self-reported constipation in older people tend not to be infrequent bowel movements but straining and passing hard stools. Difficult rectal evacuation is a primary cause of constipation in older people. Among community-dwelling people aged 65 and older, 21% have rectal outlet delay (see Table 105-1),[32] and many describe the need to self-evacuate.[16,32] Two thirds of nursing home residents taking laxatives still report frequent straining.[33] Among these frailer individuals, difficult evacuation can lead to recurrent rectal impaction and overflow. Fecal impaction was a primary diagnosis in 27% of acutely hospitalized geriatric patients admitted over the course of 1 year in the United Kingdom,[34] and a survey of patients with FI found that fecal loading was present in 57% of older acute hospital inpatients and 70% of care home residents.[35]

TABLE 105-1 Definitions of Constipation

CONSTIPATION (ROME III CRITERIA)
Symptoms for longer than 6 months and two or more of the following symptoms on more than 25% of defecations during the past 3 months:
Straining
Lumpy or hard stools
Two or fewer bowel movements per week
Sense of incomplete evacuation
Loose stools not present and insufficient criteria for irritable bowel syndrome (abdominal distention or pain relieved by defecation, passage of mucus)
RECTAL OUTLET DELAY OR DIFFICULT EVACUATION
Sensation of anorectal blockage
Need for manual maneuvers (e.g., pressing in or around the anus) to facilitate defecations
CLINICAL CONSTIPATION
Large amount of feces (hard or soft) in rectum on digital examination and/or
Fecal loading on abdominal radiograph

TABLE 105-2 Factors Potentially Leading to Underestimation of Constipation and Fecal Incontinence in Frail Older People

Frail older people may:

- Be unable to report bowel-related symptoms because of communication or cognitive difficulties
- Have regular bowel movements despite having rectal or colonic fecal impaction
- Have impaired rectal sensation and inhibited urge to go and so be unaware of rectal stool impaction
- Have nonspecific symptoms associated with colonic fecal impaction (e.g., delirium, anorexia, functional decline)
- Be less likely to have symptoms of urgency associated with fecal incontinence and more likely to have passive leakage

Frail older people have a higher prevalence of two or fewer weekly bowel movements, affecting one third of care home residents reporting constipation.[36] Up to 80% of care home residents are constipated according to Rome III criteria,[37] a surprising figure considering that 50% to 74% of long-term care residents use daily laxatives.[36,37] A recent nationwide care home study in Spain similarly found a 71% prevalence of chronic constipation, of whom only 43% had the condition controlled with 8% rectally impacted on digital examination.[38] Acute hospital admission is in itself a risk factor for constipation—43% of adult patients acutely admitted to medical wards developed constipation during the first 3 days of hospital stay (incidence rate 143/1000 patient days), with older people being more severely affected.[39]

PREVALENCE OF FECAL INCONTINENCE IN OLDER PEOPLE

Table 105-3 summarizes data on prevalence and risk factors in FI. Meta-regression analysis of prevalence studies in community-dwelling people shows that age has a significant influence on rates of solid and liquid FI.[20] Prevalence is equal between genders in older people, except in the care home setting, where it is greater in men.[40-43] A prospective U.S. population-based study in community-dwelling men and women aged 65 and older showed a high incidence rate for new FI of 17% over 4 years, strengthening the case for screening of older patients in primary care.[44] In U.K. primary care, the rates of first diagnosis for FI in patients older than 60 years was 11% in people with dementia and 3% in those without dementia.[45] There is equal reason to screen care home residents. A prospective study in French nursing home residents[3] found a baseline FI prevalence of 54% and a 10-month incidence in those continent at a baseline of 20%. New-onset FI was transient (less than 5 days) in 62% and long standing in 38%. In the latter group, 1-year mortality was 26% compared with 7% in those who remained continent.

The prevalence of FI varies according to the general health of the study population and therefore by proxy to the study setting.

- Community: 6% to 12% in adults older than 65 years and 18% to 29% in those older than 80 years[4,5,40,46-54]
- Acute hospital: 14% to 33% in adults older than 65 years[55,56]
- Long-term care: 37% to 54%[3,36,42,43,55,57]

Of note, U.K. care home studies have shown wide variations in prevalence between individual homes,[42,50] which may well be more reflective of different standards of care rather than of different patient characteristics. A national study of care home in Norway found an overall prevalence for FI of 47% with similar risk factors of diarrhea, dementia, and longer residential stay, but the risk was reduced in residents needing help to transfer between bed and chair as compared to those transferring independently; it is important that increased risk of FI (and indeed falls) should not promote less assistance with toilet mobility in care settings.[57]

These prevalence data represent case-finding statistics within epidemiologic studies, but in real clinical settings, FI is often overlooked. Reasons for this include that older people do not seek help ("it is embarrassing" and "nothing that can be done") and that providers do not find cases and do not follow through when the problem is identified. In British primary care surveys, less than 50% of home-dwelling older people with FI (or their caregivers) reported discussing the problem with a health care professional.[58] Recent U.S. surveys of consultation and screening in older women with FI show that more than two thirds do not seek help,[59] they have little knowledge about availability and effectiveness of treatments, and most would prefer physicians to ask them directly about the symptom.[60] Younger women are more likely to seek help for less severe FI symptoms than older women,[60,61] yet even in younger cohorts, most cases of FI are still not recognized by general practitioners.[62] Primary care studies showing incidence of FI in home-dwelling people with dementia highlight the opportunity to build early intervention and support pathways to avoid incontinence being a factor for insitituionalization.[63]

Poor provider awareness of FI is just as prevalent among older adults in institutions as it is in home-dwelling adults despite greater opportunity for patient observation. In the acute hospital setting, only one in six patients reporting FI have the symptom documented by ward nursing staff,[64] and care home nursing staff are aware of FI in only half of those residents self-reporting the condition.[36] Professional ignorance about how to treat FI may, in part, underlie this poor provider awareness of the condition. A U.K. care home survey found that trained staff cited advanced age as the main cause of both urinary and fecal incontinence.[65] Auditing bowel care in care homes to improve quality of care may seem like a solution, but this proved challenging in a recent high-profile nationwide audit of urinary and fecal incontinence care in older people in the United Kingdom.[14,15] Many care homes declined participation, and those who did partake generally reported hampered data collection (because of limited access to clinical records and information technology) and staff shortages. The audit showed that patients admitted to these care homes with preexisting FI tended to be placed on a containment management plan rather than being assessed for causes and possible treatment, and this was despite having good access to continence specialist care. On a similar theme, a U.S. National Institutes of Health State-of-the-Science Statement commented that health care provider education alone is not enough to improve the identification of adults with FI and recommended key requirements to improve detection in the practice setting (see Table 105-3).[7]

TABLE 105-3 Epidemiology of Fecal Incontinence in Older People and Recommendations for Identifying Cases

EPIDEMIOLOGIC DATA SUMMARY

- Fecal incontinence (FI) affects 1 in 5 older people (aged 65 and older) living in the community and half of all residents living in care homes.[93]
- Prevalence of FI increases with age alone, particularly in the eighth decade and beyond.[93]
- The prevalence of FI is higher in acute hospital and nursing home settings than in the community[93]; thus, the group most affected is frail older people.
- The prevalence of FI in frail older people is equal to or greater in men than women.[1] This predominance of older men over women with FI is most striking among nursing home residents.[1]
- The prevalence of FI varies dramatically between institutions in nursing home studies.[1]
- FI coexists with urinary incontinence in the majority of frail older people.[93]
- Aside from age, the following are primary risk factors for FI in older people[1]:
  - Loose stool/chronic diarrhea
  - Impaired mobility
  - Dementia (up to 27% of people with dementia living at home are affected)
  - Stroke (and any neurologic disease)
  - Urinary incontinence
  - Higher parity (women)
  - Diabetes
  - Depression
  - Higher body mass index
  - Cigarette smoking
  - Chronic medical conditions and/or poor general health
- Fecal loading and constipation are clinically linked to FI, but there is little epidemiologic work assessing this association.
- Physicians and nurses in primary care, acute hospital, and long-term health care settings do not have a high awareness of FI in older people.[1]
- Within nursing homes, there is a low rate of referral by nursing staff of residents to either primary care physicians or continence nurse specialists for further assessment of FI,[1] and there is a tendency toward passive management (e.g., use of pads only without further evaluation).[1] Fecal loading is often present in older care home residents with FI.[1]
- Older people may be reluctant to volunteer the symptoms of FI to their health care provider[1] for social or cultural reasons or because of a popular misperception that the condition is part of the aging process and therefore "nothing can be done about it."
- FI is associated with reduced quality of life and poor health perception.[1]

RECOMMENDATIONS: IDENTIFYING FI IN OLDER PEOPLE

- Bowel continence status should be established by direct questioning and/or direct observation in:
  - All nursing and residential home residents
  - Hospital inpatients aged 65 and older
  - People aged 80 and older living at home
  - Older adults with impaired mobility
  - Older adults with impaired cognition
  - Older adults with neurologic disease
  - Older adults with chronic disease
- Primary care staff, hospital ward staff, and long-term care staff should routinely inquire about FI in frail older patients.
- Inquiry about FI should be systematic and include stool consistency, severity of FI, and impact on activities of daily living and quality of life.
- Health care providers should be sensitive to cultural and social barriers discouraging patients from talking about the condition.
- Frail older patients with restricted ability to access primary care, such as nursing home residents, and those with mobility, chronic illness, or cognitive impairments should be screened for FI through systematic case-finding methods.
- Systematic outreach programs that make it easier for frail older people and those who care for them to voluntarily report the problem to their primary care provider should be implemented.
- There are significant geographic variations in provision of specialist expertise in bowel care (both medical and nursing) nationally and globally, which may affect case finding in older people.
- Further examination of underlying reasons for the variations in prevalence of FI between nursing homes (standards of care, patient case mix, reporting) is needed.
- Urinary and fecal incontinence often coexist; continence care workers (e.g., nurse specialists) should be trained in identification and management of fecal and urinary incontinence in older people.
- Key requirements to improving detection in the practice setting should be implemented:
  - Education of health care workers to embed both a sense of value in identifying FI and confidence that the condition can be treated
  - Protocols clarifying all details of screening inquiry (who will ask, how to ask, when to ask, and who to ask)
  - Patients and caregivers should have access to educational materials at the point of inquiry

RISK FACTORS FOR FECAL INCONTINENCE AND CONSTIPATION IN OLDER PEOPLE

Urinary incontinence is strongly linked to FI, with 50% to 70% coexistence in community-based studies.[1,41,48,66] Perhaps unsurprisingly, diarrhea or loose stool is a strong predictor for FI in all settings, but what is striking is the prevalence of chronic diarrhea in frail older people.[1,5,43,50] Medical comorbidity and physical disability are equivalent or greater than age in strength of assocation.[1,2,5,41,66] A cohort study of community-dwelling patients aged 65 and older found that severe FI (at least once weekly) was associated with increased mortality after 42 months, independent of age, gender, and poor general health.[4] Depression is repeatedly linked in cross-sectional studies, probably as both cause and effect.[1,48,41] A 15-year study showed a strong association between self-reported depression and persistent constipation in community-dwelling older women.[67] Independent factors for FI in acutely hospitalized patients (in order of strength of association) are loose/liquid stool consistency, illness severity, and older age.[56] In older hospital inpatients, contributing factors are fecal loading (57%), functional disability (83%), loose stools (67%), and cognitive impairment (43%)[35]; those with loose stools and less comorbidity are more likely to have transient FI with resolution after 3 months.

Most risk factor studies for constipation are cross-sectional, but one prospective study examined baseline characteristics predictive of new-onset constipation (two or fewer bowel movements per week or persistent straining) in older U.S. nursing home patients.[68] Seven percent (n = 1291) developed constipation over a 3-month period. Independent predictors were poor consumption of fluids, pneumonia, Parkinson disease, decreased bed mobility, more than five medications, dementia, hypothyroidism, white race, allergies, arthritis, and hypertension (the latter three conditions were postulated to be associated primarily because of the constipating effect of drugs used to treat them). What is evident is that many of these factors are potentially modifiable. Table 105-4 summarizes practice guidance in constipation based on the epidemiologic data described in this section.

Reduced Mobility

Greater physical activity (including regular walking) is associated with less constipation in older people living at home.[28,69] Reduced mobility is the strongest independent correlate (following adjustment for age and comorbidities) of heavy laxative use among nursing home residents,[70] and gut transit time in bedridden older subjects can be as long as 3 weeks.[71] Exercise increases colonic propulsive activity ("joggers diarrhea"), especially when measured postprandially.[72] In a survey of younger women (36 to 61 years), daily physical activity was associated with less constipation (constipation measured as two or fewer bowel movements per week), and the association strengthened with increased frequency of physical activity.[73] This leads to speculation that increasing physical activity in adulthood may reduce the likelihood of constipation problems in older age. Epidemiologic studies in older people have repeatedly shown that poor mobility is also a strong risk factor for FI after adjustment for other variables.[2,3,5,41,43]

Polypharmacy and Drug Side Effects

Polypharmacy itself increases the risk of constipation in older patients, particularly in nursing homes where each individual takes an average of six prescribed medications per day.[71] Certain drug classes are particularly implicated. Anticholinergic medications reduce contractility of the smooth muscle of the gut via an antimuscarinic effect at acetylcholine receptor sites, and in some cases (e.g., patients with schizophrenia taking neuroleptics), long-term use may result in chronic megacolon. Anticholinergic medications have been independently associated with daily laxative use in nursing home studies,[74] symptomatic constipation in community-dwelling older U.S. veterans,[55] and FI in older stroke survivors.[75] Although older people are certainly susceptible to the constipating effects of opiate analgesia, a study of nursing home residents with persistent nonmalignant pain showed equivalent constipation rates in chronic opiate users and nonusers over a 6-month period; those taking opiates showed improved function and social engagement.[76] Chronic pain is often undertreated in frailer older people, possibly through fear of adverse effects of analgesic drugs, so it is important to note that constipation in this context can be effectively managed by laxative and suppository coprescribing. Transdermal patches (e.g., fentanyl) are associated with lower constipation risk than sustained-release oral morphine.[77] All types of iron supplements (sulfate, fumarate, and gluconate) cause constipation in adults, the constipating factor being the amount of elemental iron absorbed.[78] Slow-release preparations have a lesser impact on the bowel because they carry the iron past the first part of the duodenum into an area of the gut where elemental iron absorption is poorer. Intravenous iron does not cause constipation and can be an alternative in patients with chronic anemia (e.g., chronic kidney disease) who become constipated on oral iron. Constipation was the main side effect in a 5-year study of calcium supplementation in older women (treatment 13.4% versus placebo 9.1%).[79] Calcium supplementation reduced bone turnover and fracture rates in women who took it, but long-term compliance was poor, and constipation may have contributed to this. Calcium channel antagonists impair lower gut motility, particularly in the rectosigmoid.[80] Severe

TABLE 105-4 Practice Guidance for Constipation Based on Epidemiologic Evidence

SCREENING

- Constipation symptoms should be routinely asked about in patients aged 65 and older in view of the high prevalence of the condition in this population.
- Men and women in their eighth decade and beyond should be regularly screened for constipation symptoms, because prevalence increases with advancing age.
- Periodic objective assessment for constipation in older nursing home residents should be incorporated into routine nursing and medical care. Patients unable to report symptoms because of cognitive or communication difficulties should be especially targeted. Such an assessment should occur at minimum every 3 months (3-month incidence rate of new-onset constipation is 7% in nursing home residents), and optimally monthly.

IDENTIFYING RISK FACTORS

- The identification of risk factors for constipation in older people is critical to effectively managing the condition.
- The following are risk factors for constipation in older people:
  - Polypharmacy (five or more medications)[1]
  - Anticholinergic drugs (tricyclics, antipsychotics, antihistamines, antiemetics, drugs for detrusor hyperactivity)[93]
  - Opiates[1]
  - Iron supplements[2]
  - Calcium channel antagonists (nifedipine and verapamil)[1]
  - Calcium supplements[1]
  - Nonsteroidal antiinflammatory drugs[1]
  - Impaired mobility[1]
  - Nursing home residency[1]
  - Dementia[1]
  - Parkinson disease[93]
  - Diabetes mellitus[93]
  - Autonomic neuropathy[1]
  - Stroke[2]
  - Spinal cord injury or disease[93]
  - Depression[2]
  - Dehydration[1]
  - Low dietary fiber[2]
  - Hypothyroidism
  - Hypercalcemia
  - Hypokalemia
  - Uremia
  - Renal dialysis[2]
  - Mechanical obstruction (e.g., tumor, rectocele)
  - Lack of privacy or comfort
  - Poor toilet access[2]
- Systematic identification of multiple risk factors in vulnerable older people with constipation should be incorporated into good practice guidelines in all health care settings.
- Patients at increased risk of constipation from recognized comorbidities (e.g., Parkinson disease, diabetes) should be regularly assessed for the condition.

ASSESSMENT

- Identifying specific bowel symptoms in older individuals reporting constipation is important to guide appropriate management of this common complaint.
- Reduced bowel movement frequency, although specific, is not a sensitive symptom indicator for constipation in community-dwelling older people.
- Difficulty with evacuation and rectal outlet delay are primary symptoms in older individuals.
- An objective assessment should be undertaken in frail older people with constipation because these patients are at increased risk of developing complications.
- Increased wandering and agitation in patients unable to communicate because of dementia should prompt an assessment for constipation.
- Older patients being prescribed laxatives on a daily basis should be regularly reviewed for symptoms of constipation and rectal outlet delay, and treatment should be appropriately adjusted.

constipation has been reported in older patients taking calcium channel antagonists, with nifedipine and verapamil being the most potent inhibitors of gut motility within this class. Nonsteroidal antiinflammatory drugs (NSAIDs) increase the risk of constipation in older people, most likely through prostaglandin inhibition. In a large primary care study, constipation and straining were more prevalent reasons for stopping NSAIDs than was dyspepsia.[81] NSAIDs have also been implicated in increasing the risk of fecal impaction[82] and stercoral perforation in patients with chronic constipation. Aluminium antacids have been associated with constipation in both nursing home[70] and community settings.[83]

Dietary Factors

Low consumption of fiber in the form of wheat bran, vegetables, and fruit predisposes toward constipation, and in the United Kingdom, consumption of all of these decreases with advancing age. Community studies of older Europeans who eat a Mediterranean diet rich in fruit, vegetables, and olive oil show lower rates of constipation (4.4% in people aged 50 and older).[84] A study of nutritional factors within all the nursing homes in Helsinki found an association between malnutrition and constipation.[85] This may be two-way in that marked constipation can cause anorexia, whereas low calorie intake can promote constipation. Constipation is a recognized problem in patients receiving enteral nutrition. A prospective survey of older hospitalized patients receiving nasogastric tube feeding identified constipation as a complication of treatment in 30% of patients.[86] Enteric feeding products containing fiber are available, although there are no data on whether constipation is any less of a problem with their use.

Low fluid intake in older adults has been related to symptomatic and slow-transit constipation.[68,87] Withholding fluids over a 1-week period in young male volunteers significantly reduced stool output.[88] Older people are generally at risk of dehydration because of the following factors:

- Impaired thirst sensation
- Less effective hormonal responses to hypertonicity
- Limited access to drinks because of coexisting physical or cognitive impairments
- Voluntary fluid restriction in an attempt to control urinary incontinence

Population studies have suggested that alcohol consumption is a preventive factor for constipation symptoms in both men and women.[69,73]

Diabetes Mellitus

Over half of diabetic outpatients report constipation symptoms, with neuropathy symptom scores correlating with laxative usage and straining.[89] Diabetic autonomic neuropathy can result in slow colonic transit and impairment of the gastrocolic reflex.[90] However, one third of diabetic patients with constipation do not have neuropathic symptoms,[89] so unrelated reversible factors (e.g., drugs, mobility, fluids) should be considered, particularly in older people. Colonic transit time in frail older people with diabetes and constipation is extremely prolonged at a mean of 200 hours.[91] Administering acarbose, an alpha-glucosidase inhibitor with a potential adverse effect of causing diarrhea significantly reduced transit in these patients.[91] Diabetes is a risk factor for the development of FI, especially in men.[92] FI may occur through mechanisms of[93] bacterial overgrowth resulting from prolonged gut transit causing characteristic nocturnal diarrhea and[1] multifactorial anorectal dysfunction (reduced basal and squeeze pressures, spontaneous relaxation of the internal anal sphincter, reduced rectal compliance, abnormal rectal sensation).[90,94] Acute hyperglycemia can further inhibit anorectal function and colonic peristalsis. It should be noted that a number of oral diabetic medications such acarbose, metformin, thiazolidinediones (e.g., pioglitazone), and the gliptins can cause loose stools (and other gastrointestinal side effects), increasing the risk of FI.

Neurologic Diseases

Patients with Parkinson disease (PD) suffer from multiple primary pathologies that lead to constipation[93]: dopaminergic neuron degeneration and increased presence of Lewy bodies in the myenteric plexus, prolonging colonic transit (independent of age, physical activity, medications)[1,95]; pelvic dyssynergia, causing rectal outlet delay and prolonged straining[95]; and small increases in intraabdominal pressures on straining. Constipation can become prominent early in the course of the disease, even before motor symptoms develop. In a 24-year longitudinal study, less than one bowel movement a day was associated with a threefold risk of future PD in men.[96] Constipation, delayed gastric emptying, and dysphagia are increasingly being recognized as early features of PD that can frequently precede the neurologic manifestations.[97] Fifty-nine percent of PD patients report constipation according to Rome criteria, with 33% being very concerned about their bowel problem.[98] Antiparkinsonian drugs may further exacerbate constipation. Pelvic dyssynergia affects 60% of people with PD and may be hard to treat. Botulinum toxin injected into the puborectalis muscle has been used to improve rectal emptying in PD patients with good effect, although repeated injections every 3 months are required to maintain clinical benefit.[99] Constipation in patients with PD is often associated with other nonmotor symptoms, all of which may adversely impact quality of life and should be managed symptomatically.[100]

Dementia predisposes individuals to rectal dysmotility,[34] partly through ignoring the urge to defecate. Epidemiologic studies show a significant association between cognitive impairment and nurse-documented constipation in nursing home residents. Patients with non-Alzheimer dementias (PD, Lewy body, vascular dementia), compared with those with Alzheimer dementia, are more likely to suffer from constipation as part of autonomic symptoms.[101] Constipation in long-term care residents unable to communicate because of dementia has been linked to physically aggressive behavior[102] and development of wandering behavior[103] by independent association.

Depression, psychological distress, and anxiety are all associated with increased self-reporting of constipation and with FI in older persons. The symptom of constipation can also be a somatic manifestation of psychiatric illness. A careful assessment is required to differentiate subjective complaints from clinical constipation in depressed or anxious patients.

Constipation affects 60% of those recovering from stroke on rehabilitation wards,[104] and a high number of these have combined rectal outlet delay and slow transit constipation.[105] Major FI is 4½ times more prevalent in stroke survivors than in the nonstroke population.[106] FI may develop months after acute stroke and can be transient, consistent with constipation with overflow as one possible cause.[75] Epidemiologic data suggest that FI is associated more with disability-related factors (particularly functional difficulties in using the toilet, and anticholinergic medications) than stroke-related factors (e.g., severity and lesion location).[75,106,107] Weak abdominal and pelvic muscles following stroke also contribute to problems with evacuation.

Metabolic Disorders

Hypokalemia and hypomagnesemia produce neuronal dysfunction that minimizes acetylcholine stimulation of gut smooth muscle and so prolongs transit through the gut. This should especially be looked for and corrected in patients who have acute colonic pseudo-obstruction. Hypercalcemia causes conduction delay within the extrinsic and intrinsic gut innervation of the gut neuromuscular bowel dysfunction (which may be reversed following parathyroidectomy). Constipation is not an unusual presenting symptom for clinical hypothyroidism, particularly in older women. Patients on long-term renal hemodialysis have prolonged age-adjusted transit time[108]; 63% to 72% complain of constipation, with important contributors being diabetes, high (49%) use of resin to prevent hyperkalemia, suppression of the defecation urge while undergoing dialysis, and low fiber intake.[109,110] In addition, resin administration can increase the risk of impaction in frail older patients.

Colorectal Cancer

There is controversy as to whether constipation as a sole symptom should prompt colonoscopy. Following adjustment for age and potential confounders, two or fewer reported bowel movements a week was associated with a greater than twofold risk of colon cancer in a U.S. study, with the association being stronger in women than men; no association was seen with laxatives.[111] Another study conducted colonoscopy in 700 patients with constipation and found polyps in 6% (more so in older patients) but no cancer; their conclusion was that colonoscopy for constipation should only be warranted in older people.[112] Comparing underlying causes for FI in younger and older men shows colon and prostate cancer to be significantly more common in the older group,[113] so the index of suspicion for colorectal cancer should be higher in older adults with bowel symptoms.[114]

Constipation-Predominant Irritable Bowel Syndrome

Constipation-predominant irritable bowel syndrome (IBS-C) is a prevalent subtype of IBS that most commonly affects older people, with a preponderance of women.[115] Although clinically, IBS-C shares some of the Rome III diagnostic criteria for constipation, it is even more multifactorial, being consistently associated with lower socioeconomic status, anxiety, depression, and somatization.[116] It also has a different disease pathophysiology to chronic constipation, so patients respond less well to conventional laxatives and better to newer prokinetic and prosecretory agents. Although available, these newer agents have not been sufficiently tested in older people.

Diverticular Disease

A case control study of patients (mean age 68) with acute uncomplicated diverticulitis showed 74% to have prolonged transit.[117] Left-sided diverticulosis coli affects 30% to 60% of people older than age 60 in developed countries. High intraluminal pressures while straining at stool in people who have a low fiber diet contributes to the cause of the condition. Uncomplicated diverticular disease may not cause colonic symptoms,[118] but symptomatic diverticular disease needs to be correctly diagnosed because the condition shares characteristics with IBS-C of recurrent episodes of abdominal pain and erratic bowel habit with diarrhea sometimes alternating with constipation.[116] Distinguishing features are that symptomatic diverticular disease affects an older population and both sexes equally, and patients are likely to have a fever with prolonged episodes of abdominal pain.

PATHOPHYSIOLOGY OF CONSTIPATION AND FECAL INCONTINENCE IN OLDER PEOPLE

Physiologic studies suggest that changes in the lower bowel predisposing toward constipation in older people are not primarily age-related. This is compatible with the epidemiology showing that bowel movement frequency alters with aging and that constipation symptoms are more prevalent in older people with comorbidities. Extrinsic causes such as reduced mobility, decreased fluid intake, reduced dietary fiber, comorbidities, and medication impact colonic motility and transit and influence the pathophysiology of constipation. Studies of anorectal function, however, show age-related changes predisposing to FI.

Colonic Function

Colonic motility depends on the integrity of the central and autonomic nervous systems, gut wall innervation and receptors, circular smooth muscle, and gastrointestinal hormones. Propagating motor complexes in the colon are stimulated by increased intraluminal pressure generated by bulky fecal content. Studies of total gut transit time (passage of radiopaque markers from mouth to anus, normally 80% passed within 5 days), colonic motor activity, and postprandial gastrocolic reflex show no differences between healthy older and younger people.[118-120] Conversely, older people with chronic constipation have prolonged transit of up to 9 days.[118,121] Transit time can be diagnostically measured by the newer wireless motility capsules technique.[122] Markers pass especially slowly through the left colon with striking delay in the rectosigmoid, suggesting that total transit time is prolonged because of segmental dysmotility in the hindgut.[123] The prolongation is even greater in institutionalized or bedridden older patients with constipation, with transit time ranging from 6 to more than 14 days.[71] Slow transit results in a cycle of worsening constipation by reducing stool water content (normally 75%) and shrinking fecal bulk, which then diminishes intraluminal pressures and hence the generation of propagating motor complexes and propulsive activity. Aging is associated with some intrinsic physiologic mechanisms that may alter colonic function, predisposing older people to this "constipation cycle"[124]:

- Reduced number of neurons in the myenteric plexus and impaired response to direct stimulation,[123,125] leading to intrinsic myenteric dysfunction
- Progressive loss of interstitial cells of Cajal in the colon[124]
- Increased collagen deposit in left colon, leading to altered compliance and motility[125]
- Reduced amplitude of inhibitory junction potentials and hence inhibitory nerve input to circular colonic muscle, causing segmental motor incoordination[126]
- Increased binding of plasma endorphins to gut receptors in adults older than 60 years[127]

Anorectal Function

In normal defecation, colonic activity propels stool into the rectal ampulla, causing distention and reflexic intrinsically mediated relaxation of the smooth muscle of the internal anal sphincter (or anal canal). This is followed promptly by reflex contraction of the external anal sphincter and pelvic floor muscles, which are skeletal muscles innervated by the pudendal nerve. The brain registers a desire to defecate, the external sphincter is voluntarily relaxed, and the rectum is evacuated with assistance from abdominal wall muscle contraction. There is a tendency toward an age-related decline in internal sphincter tone and thickness, particularly beyond the eighth decade.[120,128-130] This reduction in internal anal sphincter pressure lowers the threshold for balloon (stimulated stool) expulsion and is much more notable in frail older people with FI.[131,132] The clear age-related decline (greater in women than men) in external anal sphincter and pelvic muscle strength[128,129] may contribute to both incontinence and evacuation difficulties. Rectal motility appears to be unaffected by healthy aging,[120] but an age-related increase in anorectal sensitivity thresholds and reduced rectal compliance have been observed, starting at an earlier age in women than men.[133] Patients with dementia and FI tend to exhibit multiple uninhibited rectal

TABLE 105-5 Types of Anorectal Dysfunction Causing Rectal Outlet Delay in Older People

	Pathophysiology	Clinical Picture
Rectal dysmotility	Reduced rectal motility and contractions Increased rectal compliance Variable degree of rectal dilation Impaired rectal sensation with blunting of urge to pass stool Over time, increasing rectal distention required to reflexively trigger the defecation mechanism	Rectal hard or soft stool retention on digital examination of which patient may be unaware Chronic rectal distention leads to relaxation of the internal sphincter and fecal soiling One postulated cause is diminished parasympathetic outflow as a result of impaired sacral cord function (e.g., from ischemia or spinal stenosis). May also develop through persistent disregard or suppression of the urge to defecate as a result of dementia, depression, immobility, or painful anorectal conditions
Pelvic floor dyssynergia	Paradoxical contraction or failure to relax the pelvic floor and external anal sphincter muscles during defecation Manometric studies show paradoxical increases in anal canal pressure on straining	Severe and long-standing symptoms of rectal outlet delay Parkinson disease More common in younger women
Irritable bowel syndrome	Increased rectal tone and reduced compliance Lower pain threshold on distending the rectum during anorectal function tests	Usually constipation-predominant in older people Rome criteria symptoms: abdominal distention or pain relieved by defecation, passage of mucus, and feeling of incomplete emptying

contractions in response to rectal distention.[131] Younger women with FI are more likely to have isolated anal sphincter defects (often related to child-bearing),[134] whereas the anorectal pathology is more multifactorial in older women, including pudendal neuropathy, hemorrhoidectomy, diabetes, and rectal and vaginal prolapse.[135] Failure of the anorectal angle to open and excessive perineal descent in older women can also lead to constipation,[125] and consequent prolonged straining may compress the pudendal nerve further, exacerbating any preexisting neuropathy. Table 105-5 describes the three main types of anorectal dysfunction that predispose older people to rectal outlet delay.

CLINICAL EVALUATION

The causes of FI and constipation in older people are usually multifactorial. Comprehensive geriatric assessment (evaluating medical, functional, and psychosocial factors in addition to the bowel) is key to identifying all contributing causes and developing a goal-focused management plan. There is much room for improving standards of bowel assessment in older people in current routine practice; surveys indicate a lack of thoroughness by doctors and nurses in all settings, with failure to obtain an accurate symptom history or to perform rectal examinations.[12,15,136] A recent U.K. national audit comparing care in older (65 years and older) and younger patients with FI against National Institute for Health and Care Excellence (NICE) standards in primary care, acute hospital, and care home settings showed that bowel history was not documented in 41% older versus 24% younger patients in the hospital and 27% versus 19% in primary care. In older people, there was no documented focused examination in one third of hospital patients, one half of patients in primary care and three quarters of patients in care homes. Overall less than half had documented treatment for an indentified bowel-related cause of FI. FI was frequently attributed to comorbidity. Few patients received copies of the treatment plan, and quality-of-life impact was poorly documented, especially in hospitals. Organizationally it highlighted the fact that assessments of FI in older people were done by geriatricians in only 19% of cases, with low general practitioner involvement also, and concluded that clinicians need to lead on improving care in this area.[12,15] It is important for health care providers services and organizations to buy into continence care. Table 105-6 provides an example of a tool (based on U.K. NICE guidance)[12,13] that can promote continuous audit with real-time quality improvement in FI management.

Clinical History

It is helpful to have patients or caregivers keep a stool chart for 1 week to document bowel pattern and episodes of FI. Self-report of bowel symptoms are generally reliable and reproducible in older cohorts, including those in long-term care.[137-139] Proxy responses by informal caregivers for questions concerning FI have also been shown to concord well with index responses given by older patients.[140]

Documentation of stool consistency is diagnostically critical[7] for both FI and constipation, and the pictorial Bristol Stool Chart (Figure 105-1) is commonly used to aid patients in describing their stool. Overflow FI typically presents as frequent passive leakage of watery stool, sometimes confusing patients and caregivers (and occasionally health care providers) into thinking they have "diarrhea" rather than constipation. Patients with anal sphincter dysfunction tend to leak small amounts of stool, with urgency before leaking where external anal sphincter weakness predominates and more passive (unconscious) leakage when internal sphincter dysfunction is the main cause.[141] Fecal urgency and/or loose stool should prompt investigation for diarrheal disease (see "Treatment of Fecal Incontinence in Older Adults"). Patients with dementia-related incontinence tend to pass complete formed bowel movements, usually after meals. A recent history of altered bowel habit should prompt an exploration of precipitants (e.g., medications, stroke) and, where unexplained, an evaluation for colorectal cancer (colonoscopy, or in frailer patients a computed tomography [CT] enema; see Table 105-6 for bowel preparation).

Abdominal pain, rectal bleeding, and any systemic features such as weight loss or anemia should prompt further investigation for an underlying neoplasm. IBS-C should be a diagnosis of exclusion in older people and should be made only in those with a long history of IBS symptoms (Table 105-7). Abdominal pain is a warning symptom for constipation complications such as impaction with obstruction, stercoral perforation, sigmoid volvulus, or urinary retention and requires further radiologic imaging, ideally with a CT scan. Abdominal pain with fever is characteristic of diverticulitis, especially in the context of more prolonged episodes of pain; prompt diagnosis and antibiotic treatment may prevent the further complication of diverticulitis of intraabdominal sepsis and fistula formation. Rectal pain associated with defecation in older people may be caused by rectal ischemia and

TABLE 105-6 Example of Continuous Quality Improvement and Audit Tool for Adults with Fecal Incontinence

Goal Name	Improving Fecal Incontinence Care According to NICE Quality Standard 54 and NICE Clinical Guideline 49
Description of indicator	QS **Statement 2**. Adults reporting or identified as having bowel control problems are offered a full baseline assessment, which is carried out by health care professionals who do not assume that symptoms are caused by any existing conditions or disabilities. **Statement 3**. Adults with fecal incontinence and their caregivers are offered practical support, advice, and a choice of appropriate products for coping with symptoms during the period of assessment and for as long as they experience episodes of fecal incontinence. **Statement 4**. Adults with fecal incontinence have an initial management plan that covers any specific conditions causing the incontinence, as well as diet, bowel habit, toilet access, and medication.
Numerator	1. Percentage of patients with fecal incontinence who have baseline assessment, which includes medical history, physical examination (including anorectal examination), and medication review [adapted from NICE clinical guideline 49, recommendation 1.2.2], and questions about diet and how the bowel problems affect their day-to-day life. Examples of specific questions to ask as part of a baseline assessment are available in Table 1 of NICE clinical guideline 49. 2. Percentage of patients with fecal incontinence who are offered advice, support, and a choice of products (such as pads, plugs, skin care products, and disposable gloves) to help them deal with bowel control problems [NICE clinical guideline 49 recommendations 1.1.5,1.3.11, 1.3.12, and 1.3.13]. 3. Percentage of patients with fecal incontinence who have an initial management plan that covers any specific conditions causing the incontinence, as well as diet, bowel habit, toilet access, and medication. Interventions may include addressing specific conditions causing the incontinence and addressing diet, bowel habit, toilet access, and medication needs [adapted from NICE clinical guideline 49 recommendations 1.3.1 to 1.3.15]. Specific conditions that might cause fecal incontinence and require condition-specific interventions include the following: • Fecal loading • Potentially treatable causes of diarrhea (e.g., infective, inflammatory bowel disease, and irritable bowel syndrome) • Warning signs for lower gastrointestinal cancer, such as rectal bleeding and change in bowel habit, as defined in recommendations 1.5.4 to 1.5.10 of referral guidelines for suspected cancer [NICE clinical guideline 27] • Rectal prolapse or third-degree hemorrhoids • Acute anal sphincter injury, including obstetric and other trauma • Acute disc prolapse/cauda equina syndrome [NICE clinical guideline 49 recommendation 1.2.3]
Denominator	Number of hospital inpatients and/or primary care patients who report or who are identified as having fecal incontinence. A minimum of 25 patients with FI will be surveyed quarterly.
Rationale for inclusion	Fecal incontinence may have different underlying causes and contributing factors. There is a risk that health care professionals could make assumptions that fecal incontinence is related to a preexisting condition or disability (such as a neurologic condition or cognitive impairment) without carrying out a full assessment. Fecal incontinence may have different contributing factors in people with the same long-term condition. A baseline assessment that takes account of the individual person, rather than assuming incontinence is related to a preexisting condition, is therefore essential. Correct identification of contributing factors will promote better access to care and ensure that appropriate management can be planned. Fecal incontinence can be depressing, demoralizing, and detrimental to everyday life, and it is important that people are able to cope with symptoms. Because some interventions may take time to be effective, people have to cope with symptoms while undergoing baseline assessment and sometimes during the period of initial management, while waiting for specialist referral, or while undergoing specialist assessment or management. People for whom specialist management has not been effective and people who do not wish to pursue active treatment also have to cope with symptoms. Access to support, advice, and appropriate coping strategies, including a choice of appropriate products, can allow people with fecal incontinence to lead active lives with as much independence as possible. Most symptoms of fecal incontinence can be improved, and many resolved, with initial management. Considering simple management options that may improve or resolve symptoms, in addition to providing support and advice on coping, should lead to the biggest improvements in quality of life for people with fecal incontinence. Effective initial management may reduce the risk of skin conditions and falls and reduce the number of referrals to some specialist services. It can also help caregivers to cope, preventing caregiver breakdown and potentially delaying the need for domiciliary or residential care. People for whom early specialist referral is indicated should also be offered initial management during any period of waiting.
Data source	Patient records (including electronic) for inpatients and/or primary care patients. Data can be collected on a quarterly basis examining a minimum of 25 patients with fecal incontinence.
Final indicator value (payment threshold)	80% of patients with fecal incontinence with all three elements: Baseline assessment Advice and support Management plan Evidence: Provider reports showing number of patients with fecal continence, number of patients whose fecal incontinence problems have been assessed and managed References and sources of information: • Fecal incontinence. NICE quality standard 54 (2014) • Patient experience in adult NHS services. NICE quality standard 15 (2012) • Lower urinary tract symptoms in men. NICE quality standard 45 (2013) • Fecal incontinence. NICE clinical guideline 49 (2007) • Irritable bowel syndrome. NICE clinical guideline 61 (2008) • Lower urinary tract symptoms in men. NICE clinical guideline 97 (2010) • Urinary incontinence in neurologic disease. NICE clinical guideline 148 (2012) • Urinary incontinence in women. NICE clinical guideline 171 (2013)

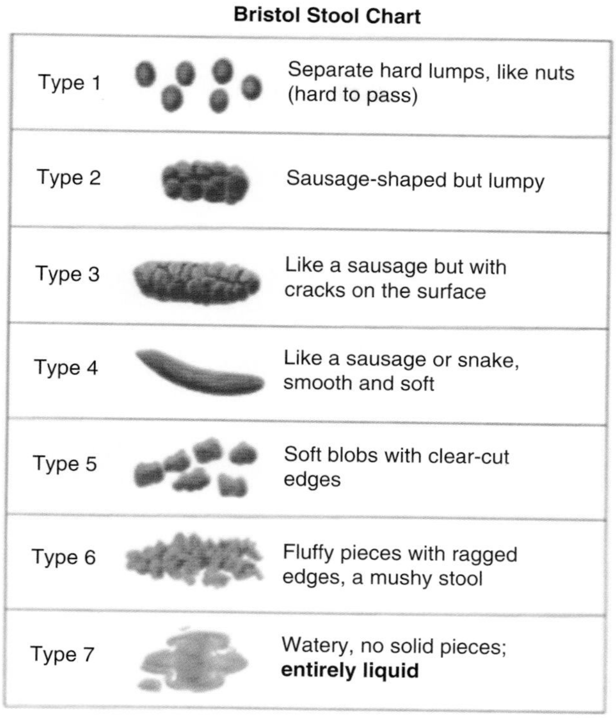
Bristol Stool Chart
Type 1
Separate hard lumps, like nuts (hard to pass)
Type 2
Sausage-shaped but lumpy
Type 3
Like a sausage but with cracks on the surface
Type 4
Like a sausage or snake, smooth and soft
Type 5
Soft blobs with clear-cut edges
Type 6
Fluffy pieces with ragged edges, a mushy stool
Type 7
Watery, no solid pieces; entirely liquid

Figure 105-1. Bristol Stool Scale Chart. *Modified from Lewis SJ, Heaton KW: Stool form scale as a useful guide to intestinal transit time. Scand J Gastroenterol 32:920–924, 1997.*

TABLE 105-7 Diagnosis of Constipation and Fecal Incontinence in Older People

Bowel History
Number of bowel movements per week
Stool consistency
Straining/symptoms of rectal outlet delay
Fecal incontinence/soiling (frequency)
Duration of constipation symptoms or fecal incontinence
Irritable bowel syndrome symptoms (abdominal pain, bloating, passage of mucus)
Diverticulitis symptoms (intermittent prolonged bouts of abdominal pain, associated fever, PR bleeding)
Rectal pain or bleeding
Laxative use, prior and current
Psychological and quality-of-life impact of bowel problem
Urinary incontinence/lower urinary tract symptoms
Pad use and laundry changes
General History
Mood/cognition
Symptoms of systemic illness (weight loss, anemia)
Relevant comorbidities (e.g., diabetes, neurologic disease)
Mobility
Diet
Medications
Toilet access (location of bathroom, manual dexterity, vision)
Specific Physical Examination
Digital rectal examination, including external and internal sphincter tone
Perianal sensation/cutaneous anal reflex
Rectal prolapse/hemorrhoids
Pelvic floor descent/rectocele
Abdominal palpation, auscultation
Postvoid residual volume
Neurologic, cognitive, and functional examination
Tests
Indications for Plain Abdominal Radiograph
Empty rectum with clinical suspicion of fecal impaction
Persistent fecal incontinence despite clearing of any rectal impaction
Evaluation of abdominal distention, pain, or acute discomfort
Persisting complaints of constipation with increasing laxative usage
Indications for Colonoscopy/CT Enema
Systemic illness (weight loss, anemia, etc.)
Bleeding per rectum
Recent change in bowel habit without obvious risk factors
Prolonged abdominal pain
Indications for Anorectal Function Tests
Severe or persistent symptoms of rectal outlet delay, suggesting pelvic dyssynergia
Persistent fecal incontinence with preserved anorectal sensation and clinically weak anal sphincter

other more common anorectal conditions. Urinary incontinence and lower urinary tract symptoms (frequency, urgency, straining and hesitancy, dysuria, nocturia) frequently coexist with FI and constipation[135,142] and should be characterized. Urinalysis and postvoid bladder residual volume measurement (preferably by handheld scan) should also be undertaken if present.

Fecal Impaction

In frail patients, fecal impaction may present as a nonspecific clinical deterioration; more specific symptoms are anorexia, vomiting, and abdominal pain. Findings on physical examination may include fever, delirium, abdominal distention, reduced bowel sounds, arrhythmias, and tachypnea secondary to splinting of the diaphragm. The mechanism for the fever and leucocytosis response is thought to be microscopic stercoral ulcerations of the colon. A plain abdominal radiograph will show colonic or rectal fecal retention associated with lower bowel dilation (Figure 105-2). Presence of fluid levels in the large or small bowel suggests advanced obstruction; the closer the fecal impaction is to the ileocecal valve, the greater the number of fluid levels seen in the small bowel.

Rectal and Pelvic Examination

Stool impaction on digital rectal examination does not have to be hard; soft stool retention is commonly seen in older people taking laxatives who have problems with rectal outlet delay. Absence of stool on rectal examination does not exclude the diagnosis of constipation.[28] A dilated rectum with diminished sensation and retained stool suggests rectal dysmotility. Digital assessment of squeeze and basal tone has been shown to be as sensitive and specific as manometry in discriminating sphincter function between continent and incontinent patients older than 50 years.[143] Easy finger insertion with gaping of the anus on finger removal indicates poor internal sphincter tone, whereas reduced squeeze pressure around the finger when asking the patient to "squeeze and pull up" suggests external sphincter weakness. Preserved sensation (urge to stool, awareness of wind) improves likelihood of response to anal strengthening maneuvers. Absent cutaneous-anal reflex (gentle scratching of the anal margin should normally induce a visible contraction of the external sphincter) and, in particular, perianal anesthesia points to sacral cord dysfunction with possible related gut neuropathy. Proctoscopy is a simple, quick, and useful test for diagnosing internal hemorrhoids (engorged fibrovascular cushions lining the anal canal, symptomatically affecting almost 50% of people aged 50 years and older),[144] anal fissure (a painful condition strongly associated with chronic constipation),[145] and abnormalities of the rectal wall.

Perineal examination is relevant in view of the association between urogenital prolapse (particularly rectocele) and FI in

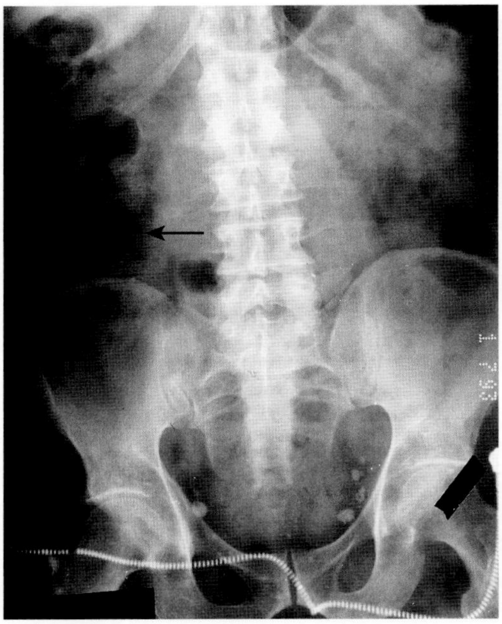

Figure 105-2. Abdominal radiograph of a 73-year-old man with chronic schizophrenia who has taken anticholinergic neuroleptics for many years. This was his third hospital admission for colonic impaction. The arrow points to the cecum, which is full of stool, indicative of slow transit. Fecaliths are visible in the pelvic region.

older women.[135] An examination for posterior vaginal prolapse (bearing down in the gynecologic position) is appropriate in all women with constipation, especially those reporting incomplete rectal emptying. Excessive perineal descent is observed by asking the patient to bear down while lying in the lateral position. Normal perineal descent is less than 4 cm (can be eye-balled by drawing an imaginary line between the ischial prominences). Rectal prolapse is associated with both constipation and FI and may also be observed in this manner, although lesser degrees of prolapse may be only identified by having the patient strain while sitting or squatting.[146] FI is a primary independent risk factor for pressure sores in older people,[5,147] so evaluation of skin integrity (with pressure ulcer risk assessment) is important.

Rectosigmoid fecal loading may impinge on the bladder neck, causing a degree of urinary retention.[148,149] Constipation increased the risk of urinary retention fourfold (other predictors being urinary tract infection and previous urinary retention) in hospitalized women aged 65 and older.[149] Urinary symptoms of difficult voiding are unreliable in diagnosing retention in older people, so it is good practice to check postvoid residual volumes in older patients with constipation or FI.

Plain Abdominal X-ray

Incontinent patients without evidence of rectal stool impaction should ideally undergo a plain abdominal radiograph to establish or rule out the diagnosis of overflow. Abdominal x-ray is required in the presence of abdominal pain or dilation to identify impaction with obstruction and more severe complications, such as sigmoid volvulus, colonic pseudo-obstruction, and stercoral perforation.[121] Acute colonic pseudo-obstruction (Ogilvie syndrome) is most likely to occur in hospitalized frail older people with a history of chronic constipation who are acutely medically ill or postoperative. It occurs with abdominal distention and colonic dilation on x-ray, with a cecal diameter of 10 cm or larger. Abdominal x-ray can be helpful in evaluating constipation.[150]

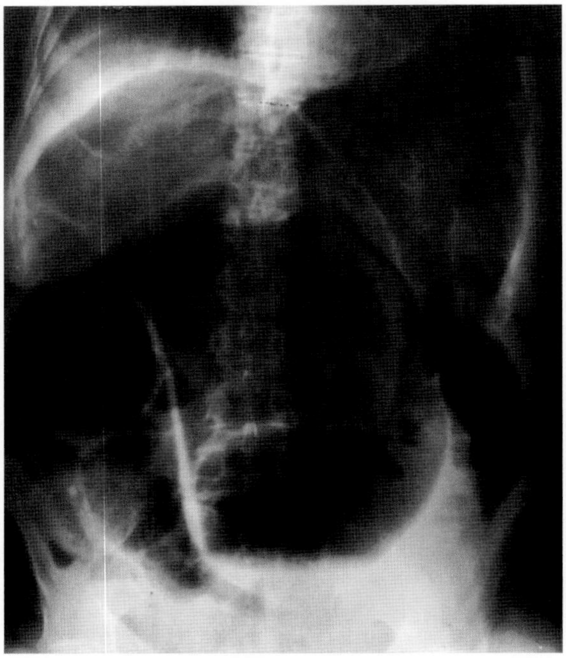

Figure 105-3. Abdominal radiograph of an 83-year-old man with Parkinson disease and long-standing symptoms of continuous fecal leakage. As his caregiver at home, his wife was changing his clothing up to six times a day. The rectosigmoid colon is completely impacted, and the dilated bowel loop implies obstruction. He was briefly hospitalized for disimpaction with enemas and laxatives, resulting in complete resolution of incontinence. He and his wife were educated in regular use of laxatives and suppositories and in lifestyle measures.

Marked fecal loading in the descending and sigmoid colon correlates well with prolonged transit time, as does the presence of feces rather than air in the cecum (Figure 105-3). Dilation of the colon (>6.5 cm maximum diameter) in the absence of acute obstruction points to a neurogenic component to bowel dysfunction and thus identifies patients at risk of recurrent colonic impaction. Rectal dilation (>4 cm) implies dysmotility and evacuation problems.

Colonoscopy and Bowel Preparation

Chronic constipation alone is generally not considered an appropriate indication for colonoscopy; the range of neoplasia found is similar to that in asymptomatic patients undergoing primary colorectal cancer screening.[151] A review of 400 colonoscopies in people aged 80 and older showed a good safety profile but low cancer detection rate for symptoms (e.g., constipation, abdominal pain) other than bleeding (2% vs. 12%).[152] Further investigation is warranted in the context of rectal bleeding (even if hemorrhoids are present), systemic illness, or laboratory abnormalities. Inadequate colonoscopies because of poor bowel preparation are common in older people, especially those with chronic constipation (and other risk factors), so, whenever possible, a personalized approach to bowel preparation should be adopted (Table 105-8).[153]

Anorectal Function Tests

Anorectal physiology tests are not generally required in older people with constipation or FI because they do not tend to alter the clinical examination conclusions or the management plan.[154] These tests have a role in confirming pelvic dyssynergia in people

TABLE 105-8 Bowel Preparation in Older People

- Older age, constipation, reported laxative use, tricyclic antidepressants, stroke, diabetes, and dementia are associated with inadequate preparation and thus taking longer to instrument the cecum.
- Even in those who take 75% to 100% of their prescribed treatment, bowel preparation is satisfactory in only 50%.

GUIDANCE

- Give regular laxatives (e.g., Movicol 2 sachets daily) and enemas or suppositories for at least 1 week before the procedure, with a longer run-up period in patients known to have constipation and in those with comorbidities such as diabetes.
- Individualize the cathartic regimen (e.g., 1 to 2 L of GoLYTELY daily over 2 to 3 days in those unable to drink 4 L, or use of alternative preparations such as sodium picosulfate).
- Identify potential nonadherence. ("Can the patient drink 4 L of GoLYTELY in 24 hours?")
- Preempt unpleasant side effects. ("Will the patient be able to reach the toilet in time to avoid fecal leakage?")
- Use oral phospho soda with caution as administration in older people increases serum phosphate, even in patients with normal creatinine clearance.
- Consider preprocedure plain abdominal x-ray for evaluation of persisting fecal loading.
- Where possible, give clear fluid diet before administration of bowel preparation.

with persistent rectal outlet delay, a condition amenable to biofeedback. Endoanal ultrasound or magnetic resonance imaging (MRI) measures the integrity of the anal sphincters and thus guides management of incontinence toward biofeedback therapy or surgical intervention (sphincter reconstruction). This investigation is appropriate in those patients with clinically weak sphincters and preserved sensation whose FI persists after conservative measures (e.g., pelvic floor exercises, loperamide) have been taken.

Physical Function and Toilet Access

Functional FI can occur in individuals who are unable to access the toilet in time because of impairments in mobility, dexterity, or vision but who may have normal lower gut function. Withholding evacuation because of access problems can lead to constipation. Evaluation of toilet access should ideally be multidisciplinary and include assessment of function (e.g., Barthel Index), mobility (e.g., timed get-up-and-go test), visual acuity, upper limb dexterity (e.g., undoing buttons), and cognition. A practical assessment is to watch someone transfer and manage clothing on the toilet or commode. Toilet or commode design should be adapted to each individual (e.g., trunk support, adaptability, mobility, foot support).[155] For patients with functional difficulties, the physical layout of their home in relation to the bathroom should be assessed (location, distance from main living area, width of doorway for accommodating walking aids, presence of grab rails or raised toilet seat, lighting levels).

Psychological Impact and Quality of Life

Constipation and FI affect quality of life, daily living, and morale in older people, even following adjustment for other chronic illnesses.[49,156] A 15-year study of community-dwelling older women showed that those with persistent constipation had significantly lower quality-of-life scores and higher levels of self-reported depression.[157] In routine practice, patients' attitude toward their bowel problem (positive, acceptance, denial, distress, apathy) and its impact on their quality of life (changes in usual family, social, physical, and work-related activities) should be included when taking a history.

TREATMENT OF CONSTIPATION IN OLDER PEOPLE

Nonpharmacologic Treatment

The consultation between a general practitioner and an older person reporting constipation will more often than not result in a laxative being prescribed. Nursing home studies show high rates of self-reported constipation, despite very substantial levels of laxative prescribing. These observations suggest that nonpharmacologic treatments for constipation are underused. They should be first-line treatment in nonsevere constipation and combined with laxative treatment. A 1997 systematic review of nonpharmacologic treatment of chronic constipation in older people found no studies evaluating the effect of exercise therapy and only a few nonrandomized trials examining fiber and fluid supplementation,[158] and there has been little further robust research in this area since then. Available data, expert opinion, and practical recommendations are summarized here.

Education of Patients and Caregivers

Educating patients as to what constitutes normal bowel habit is helpful, and those with no or mild symptoms of constipation should be encouraged to discontinue laxative therapy. Patients who require laxative treatment for constipation should be advised to aim for regular, comfortable evacuation rather than daily evacuation, which is often their preconceived norm.

Educational interventions promoting lifestyle changes should include written educational materials (ideally produced with input from users). A single nurse assessment and education session, including provision of booklet in older stroke patients with constipation and FI, showed that 1 year later they were still more likely to be altering their diet and fluid intake to control their bowel problem.[105] Table 105-9 illustrates some of the patient-centered instructions from this study booklet, which are relevant to all older people with constipation and FI.

Other randomized controlled trials (RCTs) have sought to influence fiber intake at a population level. Nutrition newsletters sent to older Americans in their homes significantly improved their dietary fiber intake. Another community intervention used media and social marketing in educational targeting of small retirement communities under the theme "Bread: It's a Great Way to Go" and reported a 49% decrease in laxative sales and 58% increase in sales of whole meal bread.

Diet

Evidence for the effectiveness of fiber in treating constipation in older people is somewhat equivocal. In one community study, higher fiber intake was associated with lower laxative use among older women,[162] but in another study, higher intake of bran was associated with no reduction in constipation symptoms and greater fecal loading in the colon, as found on an abdominal radiograph.[28] There have been several "before and after" studies in nursing home residents reporting that addition of dietary fiber (ranging from bran to processed pea hull) or fruit mixtures (apple purée to fruit porridge) to the daily diet improved bowel movement frequency and consistency and reduced laxative intake and need for nursing intervention; despite the possibility of bias, these observational studies demonstrate the usefulness of increasing dietary fiber, fluid, and fruit in older people at high risk of constipation. In practical terms, at least 10 g of fiber with additional fluids should be recommended to patients. Although coarse bran rather than more refined fiber is more effective in increasing stool fluid weight, it is far less palatable and is more likely to cause initial symptoms of increased bloating, flatulence, and irregular bowel movements. Fiber should therefore be recommended in the form of food, such as whole meal bread, porridge, fresh fruit

TABLE 105-9 Patient Education

Toilet Habits and Positioning

- Do not delay having a bowel movement when you feel the urge.
- Put aside a particular time each day (we would advise after breakfast) when you can sit on the toilet without being in a hurry.
- A relaxed attitude to bowel evacuation will help, especially if you have problems with straining or a feeling of anal blockage.
- If straining is a problem, place a footstool under your feet while sitting on the toilet because this increases the ability of your abdominal muscles to help evacuation of stool.

Abdominal Massage

- Lie on the bed with pillows under your head and shoulders.
- Bend your knees, and place a pillow underneath them for support.
- Cover your abdomen with a light sheet.
- Massage your abdomen with firm but gentle circular movements, starting at the right side and working across to the left side.
- Continue the massage for about 10 minutes.
- This massage should be a pleasant experience; if you feel any discomfort, then stop.

Diet

- To help prevent constipation, you should eat more of the food from list A and less of the food from list B. Food in list A tends to make the stool softer and easier to pass because it is high in fiber. Food in list B tend to make the stool harder because it binds together the contents of the bowel.
  - List A: Fresh fruit, prunes and other dried fruit, whole meal bread, bran cereals and porridge, salad, cooked vegetables (with skin where possible), beans, lentils
  - List B: Milk, hard cheese, yogurt, white bread or crackers, refined cereals, cakes, pancakes, noodles, white rice, chocolate, creamed soups
- You should increase your fiber intake gradually because sudden change in fiber content may cause temporary bloating and irregularity. It is important to eat the food that contains fiber all through the day and not just at one meal such as breakfast.
- Increase the amount of fluid that you drink gradually up to 8 to 10 glasses a day. Try to drink more water, fruit juices, and carbonated drinks.

Sphincter Strengthening

Learning to Do Your Exercises

- Sit in a comfortable position with your knees slightly apart. Now imagine that you are trying to stop yourself passing wind from the bowel. To do this, you must squeeze the muscle around the back passage. Try squeezing and lifting that muscle as tightly as you can. You should be able to feel the muscle move. Your buttocks, abdomen, and legs should not move at all. You should be aware of the skin around the back passage tightening and being pulled up and away from your chair. Really try to feel this. You are now exercising your anal sphincter muscles. (You do not need to hold your breath when you tighten the muscles!)

Practicing Your Exercises

- Tighten and pull up the anal sphincter muscles as tightly as you can. Hold tightened for at least 5 seconds, then relax for at least 10 seconds.
- Repeat this exercise at least 5 times. This will work on the strength of your muscles.
- Next, pull the muscles to about half of their maximum squeeze. See how long you can hold this for. Then relax for at least 10 seconds.
- Repeat at least 5 times. This will work on the endurance, or staying power, of your muscles.
- Pull up the muscles as quickly and tightly as you can and then relax and then pull up again. See how many times you can do this before you get tired. Try for at least 5 quick pull-ups. Try this quick pull-up exercise at least 10 times each day.
- Do all these exercises as hard as you can and at least 5 times a day. As the muscles get stronger, you will find that you can do more pull-ups each time without the muscle getting tired.
- It takes time for exercises to make muscle stronger. You may need to exercise regularly for several months before the muscles gain their full strength.

Instructions for Using Suppositories

- These may be inserted into your rectum (back passage) by your nurse or caregiver or yourself if you are physically able to do it.
- If necessary, go to the toilet and empty your bowels if you can.
- Wash your hands.
- Remove any foil or wrapping from the suppository.
- Either lie on your side with your lower leg straight and your upper leg bent toward your waist or squat.
- Gently but firmly insert the suppository, narrow end first, into the rectum using a finger. Push far enough (about 1 inch) so that it does not come out again.
- You may find your body wanting to push out the suppository. Close your legs and keep still for a few minutes.
- Try not to empty your bowels for at least 10 to 20 minutes.

(preferably unpeeled), seeded berries, kiwi,[163] raw or cooked vegetables, beans, and lentils.

Fluids

An RCT of chronic constipation in adults showed that the beneficial effect of increased dietary fiber was significantly enhanced by increasing fluid intake to 1.5 to 2 L daily.[164] Adding two 8-oz beverages a day for 5 weeks to the fluid intake of dependent nursing home residents significantly increased bowel movement frequency and reduced laxative use.[165] This "hydration program" used a colorful beverage cart and four beverage choices to stimulate residents' interest in drinking. An RCT found that drinking carbonated versus tap water significantly improved constipation scores, along with benefiting functional dyspepsia and gallbladder emptying.[166] Probiotic supplementation (particularly *Bifidobacterium lactis*) decreases intestinal time, with greatest clinical effects in constipated and older people,[167] and increases defecation frequency in older people.[168]

Physical Activity

An RCT in middle-aged inactive patients with chronic constipation showed that daily physical activity (30-minute brisk walk and 11-minute home exercises) decreased transit time and improved constipation measured according to Rome II criteria.[169] Physical activity interventions in older adults are generally most effective if incorporated naturally into their daily routine. Exercise interventions in older nursing home patients have shown a disappointingly modest impact on constipation,[170,171] but existing evidence would support exercise programs (e.g., prompting to walk to toilet, bed exercises for chairbound[172] within the context of addressing other risk factors as well).

Abdominal Massage

There is some evidence to support abdominal massage in alleviating chronic constipation in patients with spinal cord injuries and in older people.[172] A vibrating device that applied kneading force to the abdomen daily for 20 minutes in older constipated nursing home residents resulted in softening of stool, increased bowel movement frequency, and a 47% reduction in transit time after 3 months.[173] Patients can self-administer after receiving training (see Table 105-9).

Toileting Habits

Small nonrandomized studies show that regular scheduled toileting habits restore comfortable evacuation in stroke survivors[174] and in older postoperative inpatients. The preservation of the gastrocolic reflex with aging supports the rationale for postprandial toilet visits. Voluntary increase in intraabdominal pressure during defecation can compensate for rectal dysmotility to produce enough of an increase in rectal pressure for evacuation to occur, but older people are often limited by weakened abdominal musculature. A straight-backed sitting position and raising the knees above bottom level (feet on footstool or toilet block) are useful bowel management techniques[175] that can also optimize the Valsalva maneuver.[10]

Toileting Access—Privacy and Dignity

A U.K. study asked frail older patients with FI about privacy during defecation.[176] Adequate privacy was reported by 23% of nursing home residents and 50% of hospital inpatients. Lack of privacy, particularly in dependent older people in institutions, is a major care issue. Reluctance to use the toilet in institutional settings has been linked to residents developing severe fecal impaction in case reports. Table 105-10 summarizes basic but important recommendations relating to toileting and maintaining privacy and dignity.

TABLE 105-10 Toilets and Toileting: Maintaining Privacy and Dignity

A multidisciplinary assessment should be made of older persons' ability to access and use the toilet.[2]
Commodes/sani-chairs/shower chairs:
Should be available to residents in institutional settings.[2]
Should provide a safe seated position for prolonged use by older people with skin vulnerability and trunk support problems (e.g., padded seat, footstool if feet are unsupported, back and arm support, grab rails, etc.).[2]
Older people should be given the opportunity to use the toilet (either directly or by using a sani-chair or shower chair) rather than a bedside commode.[2]
Bedpans should be avoided for defecation purposes.
Transportation to the toilet and use of the toilet or commode should be carried out with due regard to privacy and dignity.
A direct method of calling for assistance should be provided when an older person is left on the toilet/commode.
When using a commode:
Methods to reduce noise and odor should be offered.
Methods to facilitate bottom wiping should be available.
If in living area and cannot be emptied immediately, a chemical toilet should be offered instead.[2]

Modified from Potter J, Norton C, Cottenden A: Bowel care in older people: research and practice. London, 2002, Royal College of Physicians.

Pharmacologic Treatment

Many reported trials of laxative treatment in older people have generally been of low quality and limited by unclear definitions for constipation, inconsistent outcome measurement, and underreporting of potential confounding factors during the trial period (e.g., fiber intake). The absence of good level evidence specific to older people may in part underlie the somewhat empirical way in which laxatives are prescribed.[158,177] However, efficacy (compared with placebo) and safety, in adults with chronic constipation, have been shown for osmotic salts, sugars and sugar alcohols, polyethylene glycol (PEG), anthraquinones, diphenolic laxatives, and diphenylmethanes (bisacodyl and sodium picosulfate).[158,178-180] In trials that have been conducted in older people, significant improvements in bowel movement frequency were observed with a stimulant laxative (cascara)[2] and lactulose,[1] and psyllium[1] and lactulose[1] were individually reported to improve stool consistency and related symptoms in placebo-controlled trials. Level 1 evidence supports the use of PEG in adults, and level 2 evidence supports the use of lactulose and psyllium in adults.

Newer agents such as prucalopride, lubiprostone, and linaclotide have been tested against placebo, but, because comparative RCTS are lacking, it is unclear whether these newer agents offer advantages over the older agents.[179] In addition, there has been little testing of these agents in older people. Because of concerns regarding cardiac side effects of prokinetic agents, these are not to be recommended in older people at present. Secretagogues may have a future role in treating older people, particularly those with IBS-C, but there are no data on this population at this time (Table 105-11).

In the few trials conducted in older adults (older than 55 years), there is little evidence of differences in effectiveness between categories of laxatives, and so a stepped approach to laxative treatment in older people is recommended (Table 105-12), starting with the milder and cheaper forms. However, patterns of general practitioner prescribing have been changing in the United Kingdom, and possibly elsewhere, with PEG rather than lactulose and senna now being the most commonly prescribed[181]; this can present problems in older people with constipation in whom first-line PEG may cause overlaxation and FI. Individual risk assessment is key; in patients with low risk, milder laxatives are often appropriate first-line treatment using the stepped approach. In patients with higher risk (either short-term, such as post neck-of-femur fracture in patients on opioids,[182] or long-term, as in neuropathic bowel), use of PEG as first-line treatment (combined, if necessary, with enemas) would be appropriate.

Table 105-11 lists the indications, efficacy, and safety of laxatives, and Table 105-12 provides guidance to pharmacologic treatment of constipation in older people based on available evidence and best practice. Ineffective patterns of prescribing, such as giving docusate to care home residents,[183,184] may partly explain the reports of high constipation rates despite heavy laxative use. A U.K. study of laxative use in older people in care homes concluded that the laxative used varied between homes and that use may not be based on rational criteria.[185]

Another factor may be undertreatment of rectal outlet delay by enemas and suppositories. Enemas have a role in acute disimpaction and in prevention of recurrent impactions in susceptible patients.[186,187] Enemas induce evacuation as a response to colonic distention and by plain lavage; the most common reason for a poor result from an enema is inadequate administration. Frail older patients with recurrent episodes of overflow FI despite regular laxative and suppository use can benefit from weekly enemas. In one study of nursing home residents with overflow incontinence associated with fecal impaction found on rectal examination, daily phosphate enemas continued until no further result was effective in completely resolving incontinence in 94% of patients.[187] Regular use of phosphate enemas should be avoided

TABLE 105-11 Summary of Laxatives

Type and Agent	Indication, Action, Administration, Side Effects
Stimulant Senna (alternate is bisacodyl)	Cheap, safe, and effective for use in chronic constipation. Improves propulsive action (direct stimulation of myenteric plexus) and softens stool (prostaglandin E–like effect). Onset 8-12 hr. Give at bedtime. Long-term use associated with melanosis coli (mucosal pigmentation with no clinical significance) does not cause "cathartic colon."
Bulk Psyllium Ispaghula husk Methyl cellulose Calcium polycarbophil	First-line laxative in ambulant older people with mild-moderate constipation, safe long-term, underprescribed in older people. First-line in diverticular disease (limits flare-ups of diverticulitis), facilitates painful defecation with hemorrhoids, reduces abdominal pain in IBS. Reduces incontinent episodes in FI associated with loose stool. Psyllium lowers cholesterol (binds bile acids in intestine). Hydrophilic fibers resistant to bacterial degradation, leads to bulkier and softer stool and peristaltic stimulation. Onset 12-72 hr. May initially cause bloating and unpredictable bowel habit, increased risk of impaction with poor fluid intake.
Magnesium hydroxide (Milk of Magnesia)	Unsuitable for treatment of chronic constipation. Rapid onset, so commonly prescribed to older hospital inpatients. Stimulates release of cholecystokinin, increases secretion of electrolytes and water into gut lumen. May cause watery stool, dehydration, FI, hypermagnesemia in renal insufficiency.
Hyperosmolar Lactulose	Second-line laxative for chronic constipation, relatively expensive. Nonabsorbable disaccharide degraded into low-molecular-weight acids, which osmotically draws water into the colon causing reflex prolonged tonic gut contractions. Shortens transit time and softens stool. Onset 24-48 hr. May cause abdominal cramps and flatulence, especially with fruit diet.
Hyperosmolar Polyethylene glycol (PEG) Movicol, GoLYTELY	Useful for acute disimpaction (effective in care home residents and hospitalized patients) and rapid clear-out for bowel preparation. Reduces recurrence of acute pseudo-obstruction if administered after initial resolution of colonic dilation. Long-term use only in patients with neuropathic bowel or resistant constipation. Potent hyperosmotic action, shortens transit time. Onset 30-60 min, low starting dose and titrate against effect. May cause nausea, abdominal cramps, FI, and loose stool.
Stool softener Docusate	Ineffective in treating constipation although commonly prescribed. Reduces surface tension and promotes penetration of water into stool. No effect on colonic motility or bowel movement frequency. Increases risk of FI in care home residents. Can cause perianal dermatitis in incontinent patients.
Enterokinetic agents 5-HT_4 receptor agonists (e.g., prucalopride)	Effective but insufficient safety data to recommend use in older people. Altered serotonin (5-HT) signaling may predispose to chronic constipation. 5-HT_4 receptor agonists (e.g., prucalopride) stimulate gastrointestinal motility and increase stool water content. Meta-analysis of 13 placebo RCTs showed 5-HT_4 receptor agonists superior for mean spontaneous complete bowel movements/week. Two of these studies were done in an older population and prucalopride was superior to placebo. 5-HT_4 receptor agonists have a high risk of cardiac events and currently are not approved in the United States. Currently there are insufficient safety data related to older people.
Secretagogues (lubiprostone, linaclotide)	Lubiprostone: effective in older people in small substudies but no demonstrated advantage over older laxatives so not recommended for routine use without further comparative trials. May be helpful with IBS-C symptoms but further trials needed in older people. Linaclotide: potential use in older people with IBS-C or refractory constipation but cannot be recommended as no studies have been performed in the older population. Lubiprostone is a bicyclic fatty acid compound derived from a metabolite of prostaglandin E_1, which acts locally in the small intestinal mucosa, inducing secretion of fluid and electrolytes through the activation of the type-2 chloride channels in the intestinal apical cell membrane. Two studies were published in older population extrapolated from a larger RCT. A substudy in 57 adults 65 years and older showed that 24 μg bid lubiprostone significantly improved number of spontaneous bowel movements, consistency, and straining rate compared to placebo in a 4-week trial and was well tolerated. Substudy of 163 older adults showed significant improvement in constipation severity, abdominal bloating, and discomfort compared with placebo. Meta-analysis of seven RCTs of linaclotide in patients with IBS-C or chronic constipation showed that linaclotide increases the number of complete spontaneous bowel movements per week, improved stool form, and reduced abdominal pain, bloating, and overall symptom severity in both groups.

FI, Fecal incontinence; *IBS*, irritable bowel syndrome; *IBS-C*, constipation-predominant irritable bowel syndrome; *RCTs*, randomized controlled trials.

in patients with renal impairment because dangerous hyperphosphatemia may occur.[188] Tap water enemas are the safest type for regular use, although they take more nursing administration time and are not available in certain countries. Peanut oil retention enemas (checking first for peanut allergy) are particularly useful in loosening colonic impactions. In patients who have a firm and large rectal impaction, manual evacuation should be performed before inserting enemas or suppositories, using local anesthetic gel if needed to reduce discomfort.

The predominance of rectal outlet delay (including manual evacuation) in older people, many of whom take regular laxatives, is likely to be linked to underuse of suppositories. Although research data are lacking, in clinical practice, suppositories are useful in symptoms of prolonged straining and incomplete rectal emptying. Regular suppository administration (usually three times a week, ideally after breakfast) may be needed. With appropriate education, many older people can learn to use suppositories (see Table 105-9 for patient instructions). People with

TABLE 105-12 Guidance for Pharmacologic Treatment of Constipation in Older People

CHRONIC CONSTIPATION
In ambulant older people:
Bulk laxative 1-3 times daily with fluids as required
If symptoms persist, add senna 1-3 tablets at bedtime
In individuals with questionable fluid intake or those intolerant of bulk laxatives:
Start with senna 1-2 tablets at bedtime
If symptoms persist, add sorbitol or lactulose 15 mL daily as needed, titrating the dose to achieve regular (three or more times a week) and comfortable evacuation
In high-risk patients (bed- or chair-ridden individuals, patients with neurologic disease, patients with history of fecal impaction):
Senna 2-3 tablets at bedtime and sorbitol or lactulose 30 mL daily, titrating upward as needed
If symptoms persist, give polyethylene glycol (PEG) (½-2 sachets of Movicol daily)
COLONIC FECAL IMPACTION
Clinical or radiologic obstruction:
Daily retention enemas (e.g., peanut oil) until obstruction resolves, before starting oral laxatives
Colonic disimpaction:
Daily enemas (preferably tap water) until no further washout result
PEG (½-2 L daily or 2-3 sachets of Movicol) with fluids
Ensure that patient has easy access to toilet to avoid fecal incontinence
When impaction resolves, give laxative regimen for chronic constipation in high-risk patients long-term to avoid recurrence
RECTAL OUTLET DELAY
Rectal disimpaction:
Manual disimpaction where necessary, followed by phosphate enema(s) for initial complete clearance of rectal impaction
Regular treatment:
Glycerin suppositories at least once a week and as required to relieve symptoms
For persistent symptoms, use bisacodyl suppositories instead of glycerin suppositories
In patients at high risk of rectal impaction (rectal dysmotility, neurologic disease), give regular enemas (usually once weekly) and daily suppositories
If stool is hard or infrequent, add daily laxative as for chronic constipation

impaired dexterity can be helped with suppository inserters designed for patients with spinal cord injuries. Glycerin, a hyperosmolar laxative used solely in suppository form, should be used as a first-line treatment. If glycerin is ineffective, bisacodyl suppositories in PEG base (effective in patients with spinal cord injuries)[189] should be substituted. Suppository onset of action varies on an individual basis from 5 to 45 minutes (most likely influenced by the neurogenicity of the rectum), so patients should be advised to set aside a quiet time for effective evacuation.

TREATMENT OF FECAL INCONTINENCE IN OLDER ADULTS

Table 105-13 summarizes the clinical evaluation and management of FI in older adults, emphasizing the structured comprehensive clinical approach, which can be undertaken by doctor or nurse specialist.[10]

Multicomponent Treatment of Fecal Incontinence in Frail Older People

Although a multidimensional approach to FI treatment would clearly be indicated in view of the multifactorial causation in older people, there are few published studies of multicomponent interventions. An RCT in older stroke survivors living in the community with constipation and/or FI evaluated a one-off assessment according to the algorithm in Figure 105-4, leading to patient/caregiver education and treatment recommendations to routine health care providers,[105] showed a benefit at 6 months in percentage of "normal" defecations. A U.S. evaluation of the impact of wound, ostomy, and continence nurses as additions to home health care services showed a benefit in rates of FI and associated pressure sores and urinary tract infections.[190] The continence nurse specialist is a valuable resource for education, training, and clinical care, but such services are subject to health care policy and commissioning, and currently in the United Kingdom, numbers of continence nurse specialists are on the decline.

A nursing home RCT found that a structured daily exercise program, combined with increased fluid intake and regular toileting opportunities, significantly improved FI and increased appropriate toilet use.[191] These types of evaluations do not identify any specific action to have a particular benefit; rather, they test a multicomponent approach that nonspecialist doctors and nurses

TABLE 105-13 Treatment of Fecal Incompetence in Older People: Evidence-Based Summary and Recommendations

OVERFLOW FI
• Stimulant laxatives, osmolar laxatives (polyethylene glycol [PEG] and lactulose), suppositories, and enemas can be effective in treating fecal impaction in older people at risk of overflow.[1]
• Complete rectal clearance is required to reduce overflow fecal incontinence (FI),[1] but this may be hard to achieve in frail older patients.[1] Weekly digital rectal examination and prolonged treatment are helpful in increasing effectiveness of a bowel clearance program.[1]
FRAIL OLDER PEOPLE AND DEMENTIA-RELATED FI
• Structured approaches to bowel care can reduce the frequency of FI in the nursing home setting.[1]
• Prompted toileting can be effective in reducing FI in patients with dementia within a structured bowel care plan.[1]
• Multicomponent structured nurse-led assessment and intervention can improve bowel symptoms and alter bowel-related habits in older stroke patients.[1]
FI ASSOCIATED WITH LOOSE STOOL
• Treatable causes of loose stool (e.g., infection) must first be identified.
• Dietary fiber supplementation can reduce episodes of FI associated with loose stool.[93]
• Caffeine reduction can reduce FI and urgency.[2]
• Some patients with FI benefit from limiting dietary dairy products, fiber (e.g., unpeeled fruit, vegetable, whole meal, etc.), sorbitol, and alcohol.
• Loperamide can reduce frequency of FI, particularly when associated with loose stool.[1]
FI ASSOCIATED WITH WEAK ANAL SPHINCTERS
• Older people with FI associated with weak sphincters and preserved sensation can benefit from sphincter strengthening exercises[2] and biofeedback.[1]
LIFESTYLE AND EDUCATION
• Self-care practices are prevalent in older people with FI.[1] Women are more likely to alter their diet than men.
• Patient and caregiver education (using verbal and written materials) should be undertaken to promote self-efficacy, other coping mechanisms, and, where appropriate, self-management (e.g., reducing risk of constipation and impaction through dietary and lifestyle measures, advice on how to take loperamide). Advice on skin care, odor control, and continence aids is also important.
PRIVACY AND DIGNITY
• Dependent older people with FI in care homes and hospitals often lack privacy during defecation.[2]
• Privacy and dignity of care during defecation should be afforded to all older people in institutionalized settings. Particular attention should be paid to this in patients with FI because privacy may be relatively overlooked in their care.

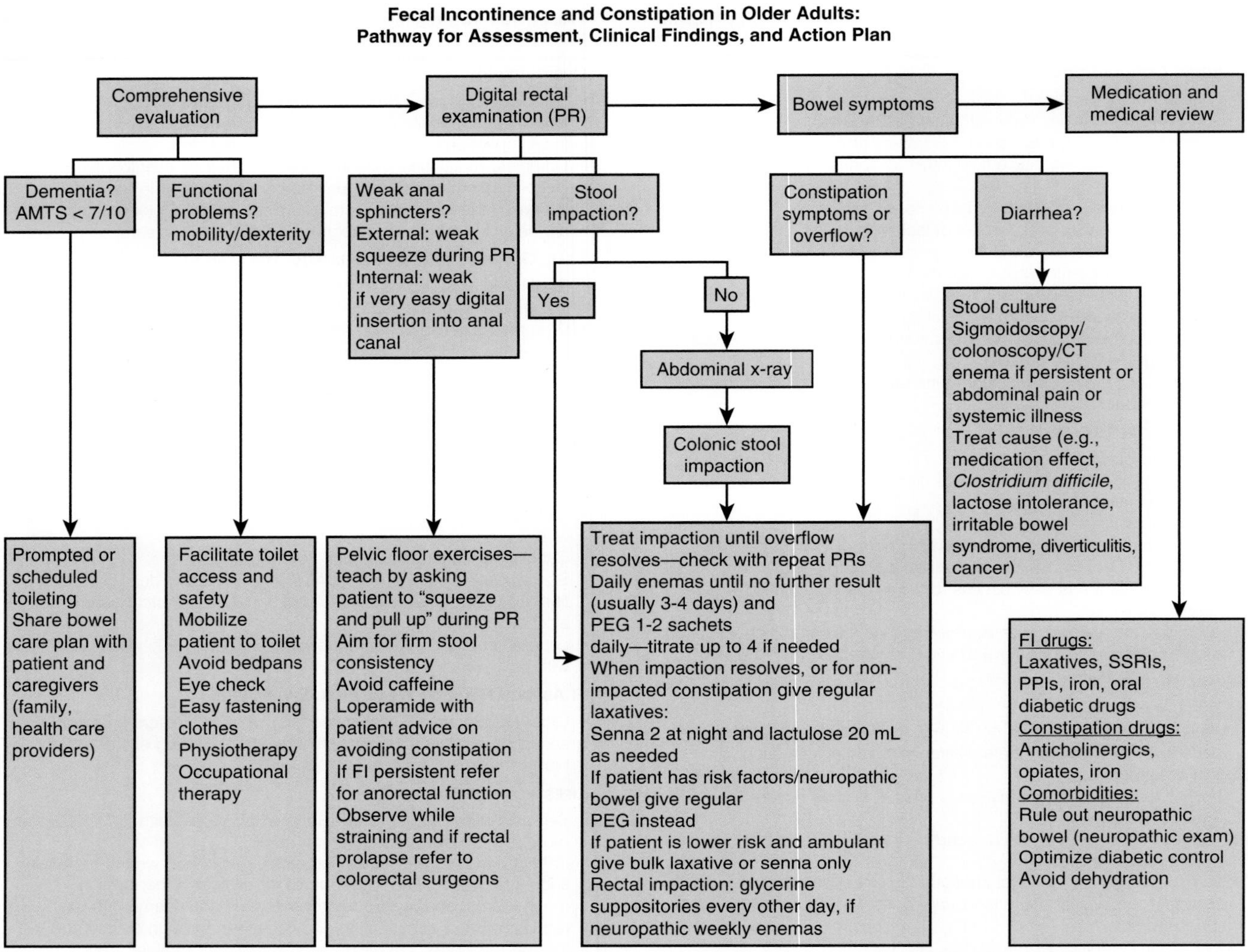

Figure 105-4. An algorithmic approach to assessment and treatment of constipation in older people. *AMTS,* Abbreviated Mental Test Score; *FI,* fecal incontinence; *PEG,* polyethylene glycol.

could feasibly apply in various settings. In reality, staff implementing an intervention such prompted voiding in people with dementia may feel concerned about their patient's autonomy, and so reflective support on an individual case basis is important especially, where this can be embedded in existing ways of working.[192] An example of this is a recent U.K. study that tested a clinical benchmarking tool working with district nurses and care home staff to individualize bowel care. The study showed that in one care home, there was a reduction in episodes of avoidable FI and overall evidence of improved person-centered care and staff awareness.[6,193]

Lifestyle and Diet

A U.S. study of self-care practices among home-dwelling older people with FI found that the most commonly used strategies for managing FI were changing the diet, wearing pads, and limiting activity.[194] Women, more so than men, altered their diet and missed meals to prevent FI. Reducing intake of fiber foods (whole grain bread, fruits, etc.) can limit FI in some people. Likewise, some individuals may benefit from limiting dairy products and sorbitol sweeteners. In the context of FI associated specifically with loose stool, an RCT of dietary fiber supplementation (psyllium or gum agar) significantly reduced incontinent episodes.[195]

Caffeine reduction can also help—black coffee increased rectosigmoid motility within 4 minutes of ingestion in young healthy volunteers (a reaction not observed with ingestion of hot water), implying that caffeine triggers the gastrocolic reflex.[196] Caffeine has also been shown to stimulate defecation urgency in some patients with FI.[10]

TREATMENT OF OVERFLOW FECAL INCONTINENCE IN OLDER PEOPLE

An effective therapeutic program for overflow incontinence depends on the following elements:

- Regular toileting (ideally every 2 hours, which also promotes mobility)
- Monitoring of treatment effect by rectal examination and bowel chart
- Responsive stepwise drug and dosage changes
- Prolonged treatment (at least 2 weeks)
- Subsequent maintenance regimen to prevent recurrences

Two trials evaluated treatment of overflow FI in frail older care home residents. The first, a U.K. trial, evaluated an intervention based on treatment recommendations to general practitioners.[187] Patients with rectal impaction and continuous fecal soiling were classed as having overflow. The recommended treatment was giving enemas until no further response, followed by lactulose. Complete resolution of incontinence was achieved in 94% of those who were fully treated, but general practitioner and care home staff compliance with the recommended treatment was obtained in only 67% of patients. The second, a French study, found that treatment of constipation was only effective in improving overflow FI (incontinence at least once weekly associated with impaired rectal emptying) when long-lasting and complete rectal emptying (monitored by weekly rectal examinations) was achieved using daily lactulose plus daily suppositories, plus weekly tap water enemas.[186] The number of FI episodes was reduced by 35% and staff workload (based on soiled laundry counts) fell by 42% in those with complete rectal emptying; complete clearance, however, was achieved in only 40% of study subjects. These trials demonstrate the challenges of treating overflow FI in care homes where it is highly prevalent, both in terms of delivering the right care and of needing to persevere with treatment to achieve good clear-out and restoration of continence. They also emphasize the need for combined laxative and enema or suppositories and for treatment persistence (lasting weeks rather than days) to achieve effective bowel clearance.

TREATMENT OF LOOSE STOOL

Treatable conditions affecting older people include the following:

- Excessive laxative use. Stool softeners in particular have been linked to FI in frail older people.[42]
- Drug side effects. Loose stool can be caused by proton-pump inhibitors (which also increase risk of *Clostridium difficile*),[197] selective serotonin reuptake inhibitors, magnesium-containing antacids, cholinesterase inhibitors, or oral diabetic agents.
- Lactose intolerance. Lactose malabsorption affects 50% of healthy women aged 60 and older, compared with 15% in women aged 40 to 59 years.[198] Only certain individuals will develop a clinical intolerance to dairy products.
- Antibiotic-related diarrhea. Among hospitalized patients, age, female gender, and nursing home residency significantly increases the risk for antibiotic-related *C. difficile* diarrhea.[199] The diarrhea also takes longer to resolve following treatment of *C. difficile* in more frail older patients.[199] Infective causes of loose stool should always be ruled out before settling on a chronic FI management plan (e.g., with loperamide or fiber).
- Diabetes. Treatment with erythromycin and metoclopramide is indicated where slow-transit with bacterial overgrowth is diagnosed. Acarbose may also be beneficial.[91]
- Crohn disease. This condition has a second incidence peak in the sixth decade and beyond.

TREATMENT OF DEMENTIA-RELATED FECAL INCONTINENCE

It is important to look for all other causes of FI (e.g., constipation, drugs, reduced function) in patients with cognitive impairment because only those with severe cortical deficit will have FI related primarily to dementia. Prompted toileting (by reminder or by accompaniment, depending on cognition) is the mainstay approach in these patients and has been evaluated in two care home resident RCTs. One significantly increased the number of continent bowel movements but had no impact on FI frequency,[200] whereas the other significantly reduced the frequency of FI and increased the rate of appropriate toilet use but interestingly did not impact the primary outcome measure of pressure ulcers.[191] Prompted toileting is also an appropriate intervention in the hospital and at home, although it has not been evaluated in those settings. Pharmacologic control of disinhibited bowels in patients with dementia was demonstrated in a small care home study using daily codeine phosphate and twice-weekly enemas; continence was achieved in 75% of those treated.[187] This approach can be effective in practice but requires careful bowel planning and monitoring to prevent impaction.

Educating home caregivers on maintaining fecal continence in patients with dementia (focusing on constipation and other contributors) increases knowledge levels,[159] although impact on FI is unknown. Interventions for urinary incontinence in people with dementia living at home, in which caregivers were advised to follow prompted voiding and individualized toileting schedules, revealed difficulties and barriers to caregivers following through on this advice.[160] One study interviewed caregivers for patients with incontinence and dementia living at home and found that although they used problem-solving strategies, these strategies were often not acceptable or understood by the person with dementia.[161] Most caregivers reported protecting the person's dignity by not seeking health professional help until a point of crisis. Once help was sought, it was sometimes less than helpful, including inconsistencies related to provision of continence products. So, although home caregiver involvement in bowel care plans is crucial in treating patients with FI, it should include specific awareness of caregiver needs and challenges with ongoing practical support including the right type of pads, bed sheets, odor control, cleansing products, and other items.

TREATMENT OF ANORECTAL FECAL INCONTINENCE IN OLDER ADULTS

Older patients with an FI pattern suggestive of anorectal incontinence (small amounts of leakage, weak anal sphincters) should be taught sphincter strengthening exercises (see Table 105-9). These are similar to pelvic floor exercises, a treatment shown to be effective in older women with urinary incontinence.[201] It is helpful to teach the exercises while placing the examining hand resting on the posterior vaginal wall, so that verbal feedback can be given as the patient contracts the pelvic floor; an RCT in older women with urge urinary incontinence showed that this teaching method was just as effective as formal biofeedback.[201] Similar verbal feedback can be given to men during digital examination of the anal sphincter. There is no evidence to suggest that frail older people without severe cognitive problems are any less able to adhere to such programs. Combined with the exercises should be advice to reduce caffeine intake and to increase fiber (psyllium can be prescribed).[202] If FI persists after several months of this approach, other nonsurgical treatments should be considered through specialist referral. A study of biofeedback in older patients with no cognitive impairment, good motivation, and intact anorectal sensation showed a 75% reduction in incontinent episodes in the short term.[203] Transcutaneous posterior nerve stimulation has been shown to be feasible in care home residents with some improvements in fecal urgency and incontinence.[204] Sphincter reconstructive surgery improves quality of life, although older versus younger people are more likely to have a deterioration in FI in long-term follow-up.[205]

Loperamide

The most extensively tested drug treatment for FI associated with loose stools is loperamide. In one adult study, loperamide significantly reduced FI, with no additional benefit when combined with fiber supplementation.[206] A small placebo-drug crossover trial in older adults showed that loperamide significantly reduced visual analogue scores for incontinence and urgency, prolonged colonic transit, and increased basal tone.[158] It is appropriate to start at low doses in older people (1 mg available in liquid form or 2-mg tablets), with monitoring for impaction and instruction on titration. Self-administration of loperamide can greatly restore confidence in older people whose social activities have been restricted because of FI.

KEY POINTS

- Constipation is a common problem as people age; the definition of constipation includes symptoms of evacuation difficulty, fewer bowel movements, or both.
- Fecal incontinence (FI) is common among older people who are frail but can be missed if not inquired about routinely. Such inquiry properly forms part of a comprehensive geriatric assessment.
- A wide range of problems can give rise to FI in older adults, including problems in cognition, mobility, gastrointestinal motility, and anorectal dysfunction. A systematic approach is therefore essential.
- Interinstitutional differences in patterns of bowel function are associated more with differences in standards of care than with different patient characteristics.
- Common precipitants of constipation include low fluid volume intake, neurologic disorders, anticholinergic medications, iron supplementation, and dysautonomia.
- Fecal impaction can result in overflow diarrhea, so that the presenting complaint can be entirely at odds with the diagnosis. Note, too, that stool impaction on digital rectal examination does not have to be hard.
- Evidence supports various nonpharmacologic ways to treat constipation, including increased fluid intake, dietary fiber, physical exercise, and abdominal massage, although more research is needed, especially in relation to older people who are frail.
- A stepped approach to laxative treatment in older people is justified, starting with cheaper laxatives before proceeding to more expensive alternatives.
- Treatment of FI starts with understanding the type (overflow, diarrheal, anorectal, functional, neurogenic).
- Many frail older adults will have more than one cause of FI, and although a multidimensional approach would be indicated, there are few published studies of multicomponent interventions.

For a complete list of references, please visit www.expertconsult.com.

KEY REFERENCES

3. Chassagne P, Landrin I, Neveu C, et al: Fecal incontinence in the institutionalized elderly: incidence, risk factors, and prognosis. Am J Med 106:185–190, 1999.
7. Landefeld CS, Bowers BJ, Feld AD: National Institutes of Health state-of-the-science statement: prevention of fecal and urinary incontinence in adults. Ann Intern Med 148:449–458, 2008.
12. National Institute of Health and Care Excellence: Faecal incontinence in adults (NICE quality standard [QS54]), February 2014. http://www.nice.org.uk/guidance/qs549. Accessed December 10, 2015.
15. Harari D, Husk J, Lowe D, et al: National audit of continence care: adherence to National Institute for Health and Clinical Excellence (NICE) guidance in older versus younger adults with faecal incontinence. Age Ageing 43:785–793, 2014.
20. Pretlove SJ, Radley S, Toozs-Hobson P, et al: Prevalence of anal incontinence according to age and gender: a systematic review and meta-regression analysis. Int Urogynecol J Pelvic Floor Dysfunct 17:407–417, 2006.
35. Akpan A, Gosney MA, Barrett JA: Factors contributing to fecal incontinence in older people and outcome of routine management in home, hospital and nursing home settings. Clin Interv Aging 2:139–145, 2007.
44. Markland AD, Goode PS, Burgio KL, et al: Incidence and risk factors for fecal incontinence in black and white older adults: a population-based study. J Am Geriatr Soc 58:1341–1346, 2010.
60. Kunduru L, Kim SM, Heyman S, et al: Factors that affect consultation and screening for fecal incontinence. Clin Gastroenterol Hepatol 13:709–716, 2015.
68. Robson KM, Kiely DK, Lembo T: Development of constipation in nursing home residents. Dis Colon Rectum 43:940–943, 2000.
96. Abbott RD, Petrovitch H, White LR, et al: Frequency of bowel movements and the future risk of Parkinson's disease. Neurology 57:456–462, 2001.
97. Rayner CK, Horowitz M: Physiology of the ageing gut. Curr Opin Clin Nutr Metab Care 16:33–38, 2013.
105. Harari D, Norton C, Lockwood L, et al: Treatment of constipation and faecal incontinence in stroke patients: randomised controlled trial. Stroke 35:2549–2555, 2004.
125. Camilleri M, Lee JS, Viramontes B, et al: Insights into the pathophysiology and mechanisms of constipation, irritable bowel syndrome and diverticulosis in older people. J Am Geriatr Soc 48: 1142–1150, 2000.
170. Simmons SF, Schnelle JF: Effects of an exercise and scheduled toileting intervention on appetite and constipation in nursing home residents. J Nutr Health Aging 8:116–121, 2004.
179. Muller-Lissner S: Pharmacokinetic and pharmacodynamic considerations for the current constipation treatments. Expert Opin Drug Metab Toxicol 4:391–401, 2013.
186. Chassagne P, Jego A, Gloc P, et al: Does treatment of constipation improve fecal incontinence in institutionalized elderly patients? Age Ageing 29:159–164, 2000.
191. Bates-Jensen BM, Alessi C, Al-Samarrai NR, et al: The effects of an exercise and incontinence intervention on skin health outcomes in nursing home residents. J Am Geriatr Soc 51:348–355, 2003.
193. Goodman C, Davies S, Norton C, et al: Can district nurses and care home staff improve bowel care for older people using a clinical benchmarking tool? Br J Community Nurs 18:580–587, 2013.
196. Bliss DZ, Jung H, Savik K, et al: Supplementation with dietary fiber improves fecal incontinence. Nurs Res 50:203–213, 2001.
200. Schnelle JF, Alessi C, Simmons SF, et al: Translating clinical research into practice: a randomized controlled trial of exercise and incontinence care with nursing home residents. J Am Geriatr Soc 50:1476–1483, 2002.

106 Urinary Incontinence

Adrian S. Wagg

INTRODUCTION

There is an often used quote stating that the bladder is an unreliable witness and the symptoms a patient describes do not point to the true pathology.[1] This belief has arisen from the assumption that patients can be fitted into clearly separate diagnostic categories, in which a set of unique symptoms leads to distinct diagnoses. Given that there is likely to be a spectrum of disease, reflecting the variability inherent in any biologic system, diagnostic categories most likely form intersecting continua that share symptoms. Epidemiologic surveys have revealed this complex coexistence of lower urinary tract symptoms. The bladder detrusor muscle has a relatively limited repertoire with which to respond to any number of insults (e.g., ischemia, obstruction, diabetes mellitus, aging). Essentially, it can become overactive or fail. There is mounting evidence from human studies that there is a transition from one state to the other over time, which also accounts for the occurrence of bladder overactivity and impaired emptying in the same individual.[2] The great majority of symptoms can be explained by the physiologic and mechanical principles that govern the lower urinary tract and its interplay with the central nervous system—what patients say usually makes sense. Experimental data have supported this thesis,[3] but there is a continual search for classification, discrimination, and scoring of disease variables, which largely leads to greater understanding of disease or advances in treatment.

This chapter examines the prevalence, assessment, and management of urinary incontinence (UI) and troublesome lower urinary tract symptoms in older adults, both robust and frail. For frail older adults, this take into account their remaining life expectancy and expectations, as well as those of their caregivers, for the treatment and amelioration of UI.

Impact of Incontinence

Although incontinence is a common symptom of later life, it is not an inevitable consequence of aging. UI has a demonstrable negative impact on quality of life, leading to social isolation and deconditioning.[4-7] Incontinence is also associated with various adverse consequences, including falls and fractures, skin infections, functional impairment, and depression.[8-11] UI is also an independent predictor of institutionalization.[12,13] The per capita cost of incontinence increases with age, with many of the expenses attributable to the costs of absorbent products and nursing home care.[14,15]

Urinary Urgency and Urgency Incontinence

Urinary urgency is the hallmark symptom of overactive bladder (OAB), which for approximately one third of the population is associated with UI.[5] The prevalence and incidence of urgency and urgency incontinence increase in association with aging. In the EPIC (European Prospective Investigation into Cancer and Nutrition) study of adults older than 40 years (based on structured telephone interviews of over 19,000 people from four European countries and Canada), 19.1% of community-dwelling men (95% confidence index [CI], 17.5 to 20.7) and 18.3% of women older than 60 years (95% CI, 16.9 to 19.6) indicated that they had urinary urgency and 2.5% of men (95% CI, 1.9 to 3.1) and 2.5% of women (95% CI, 1.9 to 3.0) indicated that they had urgency incontinence.[4]

Similarly, in the NOBLE study, a population-based U.S. survey of 5,204 adults, the overall prevalence of OAB was 16% in men and 16.9% in women, increasing in association with age.[6] More recently, reports from longitudinal studies in cohorts of men and women have illustrated the age-related increase in lower urinary tract symptoms, including urgency and urgency incontinence over time. In one study of women, 2,911 responded to a self-administered questionnaire in 1991; of these women, 1,408 replied to the same questionnaire in 2007. Over that time, the prevalence of UI, OAB, and nocturia increased by 13%, 9%, and 20% respectively. The proportion of women with OAB and urgency incontinence increased from 6% to 16%.[16] In a similar study of men,[17] 7,763 responded to a self-completed questionnaire in 1992, and 3,257 responded again in 2009. In a similar fashion as in women, the prevalence of UI and OAB increased in the men assessed in 1992 and 2003 (overall UI, from 4.5% to 10.5%; OAB, from 15.6% to 44.4%). The prevalence of nocturia, urgency, slow stream, hesitancy, incomplete emptying, postmicturition dribble, and daytime frequency also increased. Only a minority of men, as opposed to a considerable proportion of women, reported any regression of symptoms, although the limitations of regression in the context of epidemiologic survey time frames need to be taken into account.

UNDERLYING CAUSES OF URINARY INCONTINENCE

Stress Urinary Incontinence

Stress urinary incontinence (SUI), urinary loss that occurs on exertion or effort, appears to have its peak incidence in women in midlife. In the EPIC study,[4] 3.7% of women younger than 39 years (95% CI, 3.1 to 4.3) and 8.0% of women older than 60 years (95% CI, 8.1 to 9.0) had the condition. In men, most SUI occurs following prostate surgery, with rates varying depending on the type of operation. Transurethral resection of the prostate is associated with rates of approximately 1%,[18] whereas retropubic radical prostatectomy is associated with higher rates, from 2% to 57%.[19,20] Some of this variation, however, is explained by differences in the definition used, date of the report, time of ascertainment of SUI following surgery, and population surveyed; however, the proportion of men with SUI is generally most prevalent in the oldest groups. The EPIC study has revealed a prevalence of 0.1% (95% CI, 0.0 to 0.2) in those younger than 39 years and 5.2% (95% CI, 4.2 to 6.1) in those older than 60 years.

According to current evidence, if a woman describes stress incontinence, there is a 78% probability that sphincter dysfunction exists. Although there is a reduction in the maximum closing pressure that can be generated in the urethra in association with increasing age, this closing pressure must exceed the pressure of urine at the bladder neck for continence to be maintained. As the bladder fills, a pressure will develop equal to the hydrostatic pressure of urine in the bladder plus the weight of any viscera pressing on it. If the maximum urethral closure pressure is reduced below this, the woman will develop a sense of impending incontinence, because the hydrostatic pressure rises with positional changes, which typically exacerbates this. The woman will thus be forced to maintain a bladder capacity below the threshold. Frequency, urgency, and urgency incontinence may all therefore be induced by an incompetent urethral sphincter. Additionally, rising during or at the end of the night, with a full bladder and suddenly applying an increased hydrostatic pressure to the bladder neck and faulty sphincter will lead to very severe urgency and precipitancy.

Mixed Urinary Incontinence

Mixed symptoms—that is, urinary incontinence with symptoms of urinary urgency incontinence and exertional incontinence—are highly prevalent in primary care.[21] Urodynamic studies of women with mixed symptoms have predominantly identified only urodynamic stress incontinence, although to what extent this reflects the imprecision of urodynamic testing is unclear. Some epidemiologic data have suggested that mixed incontinence accounts for approximately one third of all cases of incontinence in women, but age in the EPIC study of mixed UI only accounted for 4.1% of incontinence in women older than 60 years, probably highlighting the difficulty with the operational definition.[4,22]

Voiding Inefficiency

It is not uncommon to find a postvoid residual volume of urine in older adults. In one survey of community-dwelling men and women older than 75 years, more than 10 mL of residual urine was found in 91 of the 92 men (median, 90 mL; range 10 to 1502 mL) and in 44 of the 48 women (median, 45 mL; range 0 to 180 mL).[23] In a study of men undergoing a urologic workup, a postvoid residual volume more than 50 mL was 2.5 times greater for men with a prostate volume greater than 30 mL than in men with smaller prostates. The postvoid residual was not associated with the American Urological Association symptom index score (now International Prostate Symptom Score), age, or peak urinary flow rate. Men with a postvoid residual greater than 50 mL were about three times as likely to have subsequent acute urinary retention with catheterization during the subsequent 3 to 4 years and, in another study, a residual volume more than 300 mL predicted the need for invasive therapy over a similar time period.[24,25] Another study in older women found a residual volume of 100 mL or more in up to 10% of older women, many of whom were asymptomatic. It appeared that the residual volume remitted over a 2-year period.[26] The clinical irrelevance of a small residual volume is clear, but the extent to which residuals may vary from void to void, and the natural history of ineffective voiding in older persons, are less clear, although what constitutes a normal or acceptable postvoid residual urine in older adults is still widely debated. The widely held concerns about recurrent urinary tract infection, incontinence, and upper renal tract damage are not well substantiated in otherwise normal older adults.

Nocturnal Enuresis

Whereas nocturia is extremely common in older adults, nocturnal enuresis (NE) is less so in community-dwelling older adults. In a study of 3884 community-dwelling men and women 65 to 79 years of age, it was reported by 2.1% and was significantly higher among women (2.9%) compared with men.[27] NE occurred in 35% (495 of 1429) residents older than 65 years in nursing homes sampled as part of a national audit of continence care from England and Wales. In 2010, the reported prevalence in the same setting was 43% (477 of 1097).[28-30] It is often accompanied by other associated lower urinary tract symptoms (LUTS) and is complicated by comorbid conditions or the effects of medications affecting sleep. Congestive heart failure, functional disability, depression, use of hypnotics at least once weekly, and nocturnal polyuria have been associated with the condition, and the persistence of childhood nocturnal enuresis into adulthood has been well described. Adult-onset NE without daytime symptoms in an older person without significant comorbidity is a serious symptom that usually signifies significant urologic pathology and should be thoroughly investigated.[31,32] Unfortunately, there is little available evidence on which to guide the management of older adults in any setting, from acute care to nursing home resident. Older studies that have addressed the problem describe punitive interventions, which would by today's standards never be ethically approved.[33]

Functional Incontinence

Urinary incontinence in older adults may be wholly unrelated to lower urinary tract dysfunction. Successful toileting requires sufficient cognition and physical function, including manual dexterity, to reach the toilet, undress, and void in a timely and socially appropriate fashion. For many frail older adults, the burden of physical or cognitive impairment renders this less likely. Incontinence in these situations is termed *functional incontinence*. There is little systematic evaluation or assessment of the prevalence or management of this clinical entity; much of what is practiced is a result of received wisdom involving behavioral and conservative techniques used for the general management of incontinence in frail older adults (see later).

PHYSIOLOGIC CHANGES IN LOWER URINARY TRACT FUNCTION ASSOCIATED WITH AGING

Much data are derived from older men and women with LUTS, often without comparative controls. In more recent studies, people with LUTS have been compared across all age groups.[34-37] Of the potential subtypes of urinary incontinence, urgency incontinence appears to be the most common cause in older adults. Among outpatients presenting with lower urinary tract symptoms, between 75% and 85% of women and 85% to 95% of men aged 75 years and older will be found to have detrusor overactivity.[38] The observed changes associated with older age in men and women with LUTS undergoing cystometry are listed in Box 106-1.

In men, the influence of the enlarging prostate on the outflow tract appears to dominate the evolution of bladder physiology. In older men and women, detrusor overactivity is associated with lower bladder capacities than in those with normal bladders.

BOX 106-1 Observed Changes in Lower Urinary Tract Physiology Associated With Older Age

DECREASED

- Urinary flow rate
- Speed of contraction of detrusor
- Collagen—detrusor ratio (women only)
- Maximum bladder capacity
- "Functional" bladder capacity (usual bladder capacity at normal voiding)
- Sensation of filling

INCREASED

- Postvoid residual volume of urine
- Urinary frequency
- Outflow tract obstruction (men only)

Older adults void less successfully in late life, and voiding is associated with higher residual urine volumes. The explanations for this are probably complex. There is evidence for a reduced speed of detrusor shortening as well as problems in sustaining adequate voiding contractions.[36,39] The transmission of force from the detrusor is dampened by the accumulation of collagen and connective tissue, giving the impression of impaired contractility, a common misnomer.

The combination of detrusor overactivity and incomplete bladder emptying in older adults is commonly found in combination. Detrusor hyperactivity and impaired contractile function (DHIC) were described as involuntary detrusor contractions, postmicturition residual urine volume, and reduced speed and amplitude of isometric detrusor contractions.[40] Elbadawi and colleagues[41] performed electron microscopy studies of bladder biopsy specimens from older men (n = 11) and older women (n = 24); they reported four structural patterns precisely matching four urodynamic groups, with no overlap. However, these findings have not been corroborated; Carey and associates[42] reported finding some of the defining histologic characteristics described by Elbadawi's group evenly distributed between normal women (n = 15) and women with detrusor overactivity (n = 22).

In vitro studies of detrusor muscle contraction have revealed a lower level of acetylcholine release in association with increasing age.[43] There are also data showing a reduction in the number of acetylcholinesterase-containing nerves within the muscle.[44] There are also changes in urethral function. Older age is associated with lower values of the pressures at which urine begins and stops flowing, even in the presence of detrusor overactivity. Data from studies measuring the maximum urethral closure pressure have also shown a similar decline in association with increasing age. Histologically, there is evidence of an age-related apoptosis of striated muscle cells of the urethral sphincter.[45,46] The combination of reduced bladder capacity, increased urinary frequency, impaired bladder sensation, and the central mechanisms discussed next means that an older person has less time than a younger person to respond to a full bladder, explaining the commonly expressed complaint of older adults that "when they have to go, they have to go."

Central Mechanisms of Urinary Urgency

There is a known association between vascular risk factors and LUTS.[47] The presence of white matter hyperdensities within periventricular and subcortical regions of the brain are associated with functional and cognitive impairment, increased incidence of urinary urgency and detrusor overactivity on cystometry, and difficulty in maintaining continence.[48,49] There is also accumulating evidence that the frontal regions of the older person's brain "work harder" to suppress urinary urgency than that of a younger person. This in turn suggests that the micturition center in the pons might be normally "on" but continually suppressed, rather than a simple "on-off" switch, as has hitherto been thought.

Associated Factors

Multimorbidity

Many people with UI will have at least one coexisting chronic medical condition; many of these are associated with the development or worsening of UI, or their presence may make successful continent toileting more difficult. In a large population-based observation study, UI (defined as the use of pads) was increasingly associated with the existence of other geriatric conditions (e.g., cognitive impairment, injurious falls, dizziness, vision impairment, hearing impairment)—one condition in 60% of those studied, two or more conditions in 29%, and three or more in 13%.[50] The impact of other chronic diseases has not been as well evaluated, but conditions such as peripheral vascular disease, Parkinson disease (PD), diabetes mellitus, congestive heart failure, venous insufficiency and chronic lung disease, falls and contractures, recurrent infection, and constipation have all been implicated as exacerbating factors. Similarly, hypertension, congestive heart failure, arthritis, depression, and anxiety have all been associated with a higher prevalence of UI. In one study, a linear relationship was demonstrated between the prevalence of UI and number of comorbid conditions. (correlation coefficient = 0.81).[51]

Comorbid conditions can affect incontinence through a number of mechanisms. For example, diabetes mellitus, present in approximately 15% to 20% of older adults, may cause UI by diabetes-associated LUT dysfunction (e.g., DO, OAB, cystopathy, incomplete bladder emptying), or by poor diabetic control (e.g., hyperglycemia causing osmotic diuresis and polyuria). The Nurses Health Studies has shown an increase in weekly urgency incontinence (odds ratio [OR], 1.4) in women with type 2 diabetes compared to those without. Findings from the National Health and Nutrition Examination Survey (NHANES) 2001-2002 survey showed that the prevalence of UI is significantly higher in women with impaired fasting glucose levels and diabetes mellitus compared to those with normal fasting glucose levels. Two microvascular complications caused by diabetes, peripheral neuropathic pain and microalbuminuria, were associated with weekly UI.[52] Table 106-1 lists common conditions associated with UI in older adults. There are studies on interventions only for PD, obstructive sleep apnea, and obesity. Data from nursing home residents have suggested that older adults with incontinence are more significantly burdened by multimorbidity than those without.[53]

Dementia

The likelihood of incontinence increases in association with the severity of dementia but older longitudinal studies did not identify an association with incident cases.[54,55] Another more recent longitudinal study of 6,349 community-dwelling women has found that a decrease in mental functioning, as measured by a modified Mini Mental State Examination (MMSE) score, was not associated with increased frequency of urinary incontinence over 6 years, but did predict a greater impact of the condition.[56] Despite strong associations with baseline incontinence in the Canadian Study of Health and Aging, moderate or severe cognitive impairment measured using the modified MMSE was not associated with incident UI over 10 years.[57] However, in a longitudinal study of 12,432 women aged 70 to 75 years, with a 3-year follow-up, there was a strong association with a dementia diagnosis (OR, 2.34).[58] Similarly, over a 9-year follow-up of 1,453 women aged 65 years, dementia was strongly associated with incident UI (relative risk [RR], 3.0).[13]

Likewise, in a Scottish study, the prevalence of UI increased with decreasing MMSE scores and was notably more common in those with impairments of attention and orientation, verbal fluency, agitation, and disinhibition.[59] Incontinence in dementia adds to caregiver burden[60] and influences decisions to relocate people to nursing homes.[13] It is unknown whether successful management **of** incontinence can reduce this associated burden or alter nursing home decisions, because the evidence is limited to case reports and anecdotes. Incontinence is associated with a reduced quality of life and impaired nutrition and mobility in older adults with dementia,[61,62] but is sadly neglected in terms of the amount of attention paid to it, despite the acknowledged adverse effects on quality of life and associated costs of management.[63] In England and Wales, the National Institute for Health and Care Excellence (NICE) quality standard for UI has noted that active treatment is better than containment.[64] A dementia diagnosis should not preclude an attempt to manage incontinence with behavioral methods, but for those with a compromised

TABLE 106-1 Comorbid Conditions That Can Cause or Contribute to Urinary Incontinence in Frail Older Adults

Conditions	Comments	Implications for Management
COMORBID MEDICAL ILLNESSES		
Diabetes mellitus	Poor control can cause polyuria and precipitate or exacerbate incontinence; also associated with increased likelihood of urgency incontinence and diabetic neuropathic bladder	Better control of diabetes can reduce osmotic diuresis and associated polyuria, improve incontinence
Degenerative joint disease	Can impair mobility and precipitate urgency UI	Optimal pharmacologic and nonpharmacologic pain management can improve mobility, toileting ability
Chronic pulmonary disease	Associated cough can worsen stress UI	Cough suppression can reduce stress incontinence and cough-induced urgency UI
Congestive heart failure Lower extremity venous insufficiency	Increased nighttime urine production at night can contribute to nocturia and UI	Optimizing pharmacologic management of congestive heart failure, sodium restriction, support stockings, leg elevation, and late afternoon dose of rapid-acting diuretic may reduce nocturnal polyuria, associated nocturia, nighttime UI
Sleep apnea	May increase nighttime urine production by increasing production of atrial natriuretic peptide	Diagnosis and treatment of sleep apnea, usually with continuous positive airway pressure devices, may relieve UI, reduce nocturnal polyuria and associated nocturia
Severe constipation and fecal impaction	Associated with "double" incontinence (urine and fecal)	Appropriate use of stool softeners Adequate fluid intake and exercise Disimpaction if necessary
NEUROLOGIC AND PSYCHIATRIC CONDITIONS		
Stroke	Can precipitate urgency UI and, less often, urinary retention; also impairs mobility	UI after acute stroke often resolves with rehabilitation; persistent UI should be further evaluated. Regular toileting assistance essential for those with persistent mobility impairment
Parkinson disease	Associated with urgency UI; also causes impaired mobility and cognition in late stages	Optimizing management may improve mobility, improve UI Regular toileting assistance essential for those with mobility and cognitive impairment in late stages
Normal-pressure hydrocephalus	Presents with UI, along with gait and cognitive impairments	Patients presenting with all three symptoms should be considered for brain imaging to rule out this condition; may improve with a ventricular-peritoneal shunt
Dementia (Alzheimer, multi-infarct, others)	Associated with urgency UI; impaired cognition and apraxia interfere with toileting and hygiene	Regular toileting assistance essential for those with mobility and cognitive impairment in late stages
Depression	May impair motivation to be continent; may also be a consequence of incontinence	Optimizing pharmacologic and non-pharmacologic management of depression may improve UI
MEDICATIONS	See Table 106-3.	Discontinuation or modification of drug regimen
FUNCTIONAL IMPAIRMENTS		
Impaired mobility, impaired cognition	Impaired cognition and/or mobility due to a variety of conditions (listed above) and others can interfere with ability to toilet independently and can precipitate UI	Regular toileting assistance essential for those with severe mobility and/or cognitive impairment
ENVIRONMENTAL FACTORS		
Inaccessible toilets Unsafe toilet facilities No contrasting color between toilet and seat Caregivers unavailable for toileting assistance	Frail, functionally impaired persons require accessible and safe toilet facilities and, in many cases, human assistance to be continent	Environmental alterations may be helpful; supportive measures such as pads may be necessary if caregiver assistance not regularly available.

UI, Urinary incontinence.

ability to learn behavioral change, this is clearly inappropriate. A stepwise approach to initiating interventions and assessing the results seems like a reasonable first step in management.

Medications

Some medications may predispose older adults to incontinence. Wherever possible, they should be reviewed and, if possible, any offending drugs should be removed or the dose reduced. Evidence exists for diuretics, calcium channel blockers, prostaglandin inhibitors, α-blockers, selective serotonin reuptake inhibitors, cholinesterase inhibitors, and systemic hormone replacement therapy,[65-72] but the list is more extensive due to the potential of adverse effects of some drug classes to affect continence status (Table 106-2). Cholinesterase inhibitors for dementia are of particular relevance because their use appears to be associated with an increased risk of urinary urgency and urgency incontinence.[73] Older nursing home residents with dementia newly treated with cholinesterase inhibitors are more likely to be prescribed a bladder antimuscarinic than those with dementia.[74] Treatment with bladder antimuscarinics in addition to cholinesterase inhibitors has not been associated with delirium but, in one study, a decrease in the ability to carry out the activities of daily living (ADLs) in the most functionally independent people at baseline was noted.[75]

In a study of trospium and galantamine co-prescription, no effect on cognition or ADLs and some benefits on continence-related outcomes were found.[76,77] The current weight of evidence, albeit of low quality, appears to be that a positive outcome in terms of bladder control can be achieved without a significant detriment in cognition or ADLs. Currently, there are no data on quality of life outcomes for this group of older adults who are treated with this combination of agents. Obviously, there needs to be due consideration about the risks and benefits of treatment with either agent before taking any action.

TABLE 106-2 Medications That Can Cause or Contribute to Urinary Incontinence in Frail Older Adults

Medications	Effects on Continence
α-Adrenergic agonists	Increase smooth muscle tone in urethra and prostatic capsule may precipitate obstruction, urinary retention, related symptoms
α-Adrenergic antagonists	Decrease smooth muscle tone in urethra may precipitate stress urinary incontinence in women
Angiotensin-converting enzyme inhibitors	Cause cough that can exacerbate UI
Anticholinergics	May cause impaired emptying, urinary retention, and constipation, which can contribute to UI; may cause cognitive impairment, reduce effective toileting ability
Calcium channel blockers	May cause impaired emptying, urinary retention, and constipation, which can contribute to UI; may cause dependent edema, which can contribute to nocturnal polyuria
Cholinesterase inhibitors	Increase bladder contractility, may precipitate urgency UI
Diuretics	Cause diuresis and precipitate UI
Lithium	Polyuria due to diabetes insipidus
Opioid analgesics	May cause urinary retention, constipation, confusion, immobility, all of which can contribute to UI
Psychotropic drugs Sedatives Hypnotics Antipsychotics Histamine1 receptor antagonists	May cause confusion and impaired mobility and precipitate UI; anticholinergic effects; confusion
Selective serotonin reuptake inhibitors	Increase cholinergic transmission, may lead to urinary UI
Others—gabapentin, glitazones, nonsteroidal antiinflammatory drugs	Can cause edema, which can lead to nocturnal polyuria and cause nocturia and nighttime UI

UI, Urinary incontinence.

EVALUATION OF THE OLDER ADULT WITH INCONTINENCE

In line with current recommendations, a screening question about bladder and bowel problems should be asked as part of all health care interactions between an older person and clinician.[78] A simple question such as "Do you have any problems with bladder or bowel function?" is usually recommended. If the answer to that question is positive, an assessment should be offered.

There has been little systematic evaluation of the utility of components of the clinical assessment in older adults. Generally, the traditional biomedical model of history taking and examination has been applied. In England and Wales, the national guidelines for LUTS in men suggest that the following be carried out: (1) general medical history to identify possible causes and comorbidities; (2) review of medications that may be contributing to the problem; (3) physical examination guided by symptoms and other medical conditions; (4) examination of the abdomen and external genitalia; and (5) digital rectal examination and urine dipstick test to detect blood, glucose, protein, leukocytes, and nitrites. The guidelines for women are a variation on these.[79,80]

In the United States, data have suggested that primary care practitioners fail to follow the U.S. Agency for Healthcare Research and Quality UI guidelines (now obsolete), and nursing home practitioners rarely follow federal guidelines for UI care regarding recommended physical examination, postvoid residual volume (PVR) testing, urinalysis, and identification of potentially reversible causes.[81] Okamura and colleagues have investigated the diagnosis and treatment of LUTS by general practitioners and found adherence to the guidelines, reinforced by educational and promotional activities, resulted in better treatment outcomes.[82,83] Although it is unusual for guidelines to consider multimorbidity, the International Consultation on Incontinence does include guidance on the assessment and management of fecal and urinary incontinence in frail older adults.[78]

Assessing Cognitive Function

Older cognitively impaired people are less able to cooperate in lifestyle interventions for their incontinence and may also be at risk of developing further impaired cognition in response to high-dose antimuscarinic therapy or high preexisting antimuscarinic burden.[84] However, the actual occurrence of this is rare in community-dwelling older adults, and studies have suggested that it is only those at the highest levels of exposure who might be affected. The modified MMSE does not appear to be sensitive enough to detect the magnitude of change associated with the bladder antimuscarinics and the results of other tests, such as the Montreal Cognitive Assessment, are not known. The best that might be achieved is an overall assessment of global thought processes and everyday decision making by the older adult or family member or caregiver.

Bladder Diaries

Obtaining a reliable completion of a bladder diary requires considerable effort and observation, particularly if there are a considerable number of incontinent voids. This may not be possible for people with more advanced frailty or cognitive impairment. The process might therefore involve caregiver observations with regular wet checks to determine a pattern of voiding. The utility of a bladder diary in adding to the assessment must be weighed against the burden of achieving it, because an incomplete diary may represent a considerable burden but may not be helpful to clinical decision making.

Physical Examination

A physical examination should be performed for all people complaining of new or worsening UI. At a minimum, this should consist of a rectal examination to exclude fecal loading as a precipitating factor for the incontinence and assessment of the prostate in men; there are no data on the clinical utility of a digital rectal assessment in women. Palpation of the abdomen will detect large volumes of urine in the bladder but a transabdominal ultrasound assessment of postmicturition residual volume may be useful in selected cases. As noted, there are no studies evaluating the utility of PVR measurement on clinical diagnosis and treatment outcomes. A urogenital examination is important to exclude contributing or complicating pathologies, such as urogenital atrophy or prolapse, which can cause urinary symptoms. Visual inspection of the skin will also help in the planning of treatment to maintain skin integrity if this is threatened. A clinical assessment incorporating the cough test in older women may have some utility. In one study of older women, a test with leakage symptoms was 78% accurate, with only 6% false-negatives for SUI, but was only 44% accurate, with 45% false-negatives for urgency UI.[85] A urinalysis to exclude acute symptomatic infection and the presence of hematuria should also be performed and a specimen sent for more detailed analysis, according to the results of the test.

Urodynamic Testing

Urodynamic testing is feasible and safe, even in frail nursing home residents.[86] There is no evidence, however, that a cystometric diagnosis changes the clinical outcome following treatment. Expert guidelines have recommended urodynamic testing before surgical or minimally invasive UI treatment in frail older adults, but there have been no studies that assess whether its use changes outcomes following treatment. Whereas multichannel subtracted cystometry is not required in women with symptoms of stress UI only,[87] this is a rare occurrence in older women, and cystometry before surgery is probably still warranted to assess voiding function prior to a potentially obstructive surgical procedure. Cystometry in frail older adults should be used with consideration of the likely benefits, harms, and feasibility of its use.

TREATMENT STRATEGIES

Interventions

Lifestyle Interventions

Several lifestyle interventions have been evaluated in healthier older women, including dieting and medication to help with weight loss, fluid selection (caffeine, alcohol, and volume), and constipation management. There are much fewer data in healthier older men and almost no data on frail older adults.[88] The recent International Consultation on Incontinence suggested that should there be evidence of efficacy for any intervention in a general population of older adults, it would seem unreasonable not to offer that intervention to frail older adults, with the proviso that the intervention is feasible and congruent with the aims of management and expectations of that person.[78] A trial of caffeine restriction, for example, may superficially result in little harm, but may adversely affect the hydration status of an older person for little perceived benefit.

Behavioral Interventions

Behavioral interventions have been especially designed for frail older adults with cognitive and physical impairments. Because they have no side effects, they have been the mainstay of UI treatment in frail older adults.[89] The technique with the most evidence of benefit is prompted voiding. Individuals are prompted to use the lavatory and encouraged with social reward when successfully toileted. This technique increases patient requests for toileting and self-initiated toileting and decreases the number of UI episodes.[90] A 3-day trial during which the number of incontinent episodes should be reduced by 20% should be considered successful.

The second commonly used technique, habit retraining, requires identification of the incontinent person's individual toileting pattern and UI episodes, usually by means of a bladder diary. A toileting schedule is then devised to preempt them.[91,92] Timed voiding involves toileting at fixed intervals, such as every 3 hours. There is no patient education, reinforcement of desirable behaviors, or attempt to reestablish normal voiding patterns.[93]

Functional Intervention Training

This incorporates musculoskeletal strengthening exercises into toileting routines by nursing home care aides (nursing assistants).[94] There has been increasing evidence for the effectiveness of physical exercise as an intervention for UI in populations in diverse settings. In a U.S. veterans nursing home population, the combination of individualized prompted voiding, functionally oriented endurance, and strength-training exercises offered four times/day, 5 days/week, for 8 weeks delivered by trained research staff was effective in significantly reducing UI.[95] An intervention that provided exercise and incontinence care every 2 hours from 8 AM to 4:30 PM (total of four daily care episodes) for 5 days/week over 32 weeks in a nursing home population was also found to be effective in significantly reducing incontinence.[96] Similarly, a study of walking exercise for 30 minutes/day in a small group of cognitively impaired residents over 4 weeks resulted in a significant reduction in daytime incontinence episodes and an increase in gait speed and stamina.[97] In community-dwelling older adults, a 30-minute evening walk proved effective in reducing nocturia while also improving daytime urinary frequency, blood pressure, body weight, body fat ratio, triglyceride levels, total cholesterol, and sleep quality.[98] Cognitive and functional impairment, common in frail older adults, may preclude the use of some of these interventions. Additionally, the context in which care is provided needs to be considered.[99-101] Many of these interventions are time-consuming and need effective staff engagement to deliver them effectively.[102]

Although pelvic floor muscle rehabilitation has not been studied extensively in frail older adults, age and frailty alone should not preclude their use in appropriate patients with sufficient cognition to participate.

Pharmacologic Therapy

Overactive Bladder/Urgency-Frequency Syndrome

The main target for pharmacologic therapy of UI associated with storage symptoms is for OAB and urgency-frequency syndrome. Here, antimuscarinic drugs are the current mainstay of treatment. There has been accumulating evidence that older adults are more dependent on antimuscarinic drug therapy to control their OAB symptoms[103] and are more likely to need higher doses of drug to achieve most benefit, particularly in the oldest old (>75 years).[104,105] This might be because of the increased severity of UI in older adults or because behavioral or lifestyle measures have been less successful. There is evidence of the efficacy of antimuscarinic agents in community-dwelling older adults from post hoc pooled analyses from registration trials of antimuscarinic agents and, increasingly, from trials specifically designed to assess the efficacy of newer agents in older adults. There are fewer data about the use of these agents in older men and in older frail individuals; one study of extended-release oxybutynin examined the cognitive effects in nursing home residents with dementia and urgency UI.[106] Published trials of the efficacy of transdermal oxybutynin included subjects up to the age of 100 years and in institutional care settings, but did not stratify results by age or comorbidity.[107] Fesoterodine has been studied in older people identified as frail in a survey of vulnerable older adults.[108,109]

Briefly, meta-analyses have suggested that the efficacy of each of the antimuscarinic drugs in relieving the symptoms of OAB and improving quality of life is essentially comparable. However, high-dose oxybutynin is associated with an increased incidence of unwanted effects.[109a] Also, the side effect profile of immediate-acting oral oxybutynin, and its potential for subclinical cognitive impairment in those cognitively at risk, particularly at high doses, mitigates against its use in older adults.

Responses to commonly used antimuscarinics from post hoc analyses of older adults and from other studies are shown in Table 106-3. The common side effects of antimuscarinics are dry mouth and constipation, which may limit their use in some older adults. A recent network meta-analysis has illustrated the relative incidence of side effects in a comparative study.[110] The newer antimuscarinics have a place in management, and physicians should be confident in using them (increasing the dose where necessary) and swapping them if they are found not to be efficacious. There are specific data on the cognitive effects of the bladder antimuscarinics (e.g., darifenacin, fesoterodine, solifenacin, tolterodine, transdermal oxybutynin gel, trospium chloride) in cognitively intact older adults and for solifenacin in older adults with mild cognitive impairment.[84,111-116] The quaternary

TABLE 106-3 Resolution of Symptoms and Incontinence

Trial	Reduction (vs. Comparator, *P*) in:				Proportion With Resolution of Incontinence (vs. Comparator, *P*)
	Mean Urgency of Episodes	*Micturition Frequency*	*Nocturia Episodes*	*Incontinence Episodes*	
Chapple[146] (12 wk, darifenacin vs. placebo)	−88.6% vs. −77.9%, *P* = NS	−25.3% vs. −18.5%, *P* < .01			70% vs. 58%, *P* = .021*
Malone-Lee[147] (12 wk tolterodine vs. oxybutynin, patients > 50 yr)		−1.7 vs. −1.7, *P* = NS		−1.3 (−54%) vs. −1.7 (−62%), *P* not reported	
Wagg[148] (12 wk, solifenacin, pooled analysis vs. placebo)	−3.2 (5 mg) −3.2 (10 mg) vs. −1.1, *P* < .05	−2.0 (5 mg) −2.5 (10 mg) vs. −1.1, *P* < .05		−1.5 (5 mg), −1.9 (10 mg) vs. −1.0, *P* < .005	49.1% (5 mg), 47.3% (10 mg) vs. 28.9%, *P* < .001
Kraus[104] (pooled analysis, fesoterodine vs. placebo >65 to <75 yr and ≥75 yr vs. placebo	>65 to <75 yr, −2.04 (4 mg), −2.19 (8 mg) vs. −0.77, *P* < .05; ≥75 yr, −1.13 (4 mg), −2.01 (8 mg) vs. −0.31, *P* < .05 (8 mg)	>65 to <75 yr, −1.83 (4 mg), −1.68 (8 mg) vs. −1.08, *P* <0.05; ≥75 yr, −0.69 (4 mg), −1.90 (8 mg) vs. −0.36, *P* < .05 for 4 mg (>65 yr) and 8 mg (≥75 yr)		>65 to <75 yr, −2.38 (4 mg), −2.41 (8 mg) vs. −0.98, *P* < .05; ≥75 yr, − 87 (4 mg), −2.44 (8 mg) vs. −0.91, *P* < .05 for 8 mg	
Szonyi[149] (6 wk oxybutynin combined with bladder retraining vs. placebo; results expressed as difference in change)		W = 577, 95% CI, −27.0 to −6.0, *P* = .0025	−6 (95% CI, −5 to 7),† *P* = NS	−9.5 (95% CI, −11.0 to 3.0),† *P* = NS	
Wagg[150] (12 wk fesoterodine vs. placebo)	−3.47 vs. −1.92, *P* < .001‡	−1.91 vs. −0.93, *P* < .001‡	−1.0 vs. −0.7, *P* = .003‡	−1.0 vs. −0.7, *P* = .729‡	53% vs. 45%, *P* = 0.11§
Sand[151] (pooled analysis 12 wk trospium vs. placebo)	−2.53 vs. −0.61, *P* = .004	−2.15 vs. −0.37, *P* < .008	−0.76 vs. −0.08, *P* = .01	−1.77 vs. −0.54, *P* = .003	
DuBeau[152] (12 wk, fesoterodine vs. placebo)	−4.14 vs. −2.75, *P* = .001	−1.5 vs. −2.34, *P* < .01	−2.2 vs. −2.84, *P* =.002		36% vs. 50%, *P* = .002
Wagg[117] (12 wk pooled analysis, efficacy, plus 1-yr safety		>65 yr, −0.02 (95% CI, −0.69 to 0.30); >75 yr, 0.83 (95% CI, −0.26 to 1.93); no comparative e-statistics vs. placebo		>65 yr,§ −0.66 (95% CI, −0.95 to −0.37) >75 yr,§ −0.65 (95% CI, −1.17 to −0.13); no comparative e-statistics vs. placebo	

As reported from clinical trials of overactive bladder medications in older adults.
NS, Not significant.
*>50% reduction.
†Totaled over final 14 days and compared to first 14 days of run-in.
‡Change from baseline to wk 12.
§Wet at baseline, dry at wk 8 and 12.

ammonium compound, trospium chloride, does not cross the blood-brain barrier in older adults in the absence of significant disease and has a low potential for drug-drug interactions. Darifenacin, trospium, and 5-hydroxymethyl tolterodine penetrate the blood-brain barrier but are substrates for permeability glycoproteins and are actively transported from the central nervous system. Transdermal preparations of oxybutynin are associated with low levels of antimuscarinic side effects.

There are data on the comparative pharmacokinetics of mirabegron in older adults but not specifically frail older adults. In available studies, there were no statistically significant differences in mirabegron exposure between older volunteers aged 55 years and older and younger volunteers (18 to 45 years). The area under the curve was predicted to be 11% higher in a subject aged 90 years. Pooled analyses of phase 3 registration trials have shown efficacy of mirabegron in those older than 65 and 75 years, with evidence of safety over a year-long extension period.[117] Unfortunately, many geriatricians reject antimuscarinics for OAB out of hand, despite evidence for their efficacy and tolerability and despite evidence showing that treatment with the newer antimuscarinics is not associated with an excess of falls, precipitation of delirium, or widespread cognitive impairment. This is unfortunate and leads to the undertreatment of many older adults whose life is adversely affected by their incontinence. For most older adults, if pharmacologic therapy is required, a newer antimuscarinic agent, started at a low dose for tolerability, should be recommended. High-dose, immediate-release oxybutynin should be avoided in older adults. For frail older adults at more than moderate risk of cognitive impairment (e.g., with Parkinson disease), mirabegron may be a sensible first choice if there is no uncontrolled hypertension. For older men with storage and voiding symptoms, prescription of an α-adrenoreceptor blocker (e.g., tamsulosin) should precede antimuscarinic prescription by 4 to 6 weeks.

Nocturia

Nocturia is highly prevalent among older adults. Typically, nocturia of two or more nightly episodes is associated with a significant impact on quality of life. Also, some studies have associated nocturia with falls, increased mortality, and early development of coronary vascular disease. Although nocturia may also be associated with bladder outflow tract obstruction and OAB, most patients with nocturia do not have overactive bladder. Most patients with OAB do, however, have nocturia. Antimuscarinics are not usually effective for nocturia but may be effective for nocturnal voids due to urgency.[118] Other associated conditions include obstructive sleep apnea, subclinical heart failure, and loss of circadian variation in antidiuretic hormone (ADH; vasopressin) levels and other fluid-retaining states. Once a non–lower urinary tract underlying cause has been elucidated and, where possible, treated, nocturia may be classified into nocturnal polyuria (>33% of total 24-hour urinary output overnight) or nocturnal frequency. Afternoon doses of loop diuretics (e.g., furosemide,[119] bumetanide[120]) have some evidence supporting their use for this condition. The use of synthetic ADH (deamino-8-D-arginine vasopressin [DDAVP]) is also effective in reducing nighttime urine output and increasing the mean amount of sleep.[121-123] The drug is not licensed for use in those older than 65 years due to the risk of developing significant hyponatremia, which occurs in up to 20% of adults within the first 3 days of treatment.[124] If a baseline serum sodium level is determined, followed by 3 days of therapy, and another estimation of the serum sodium level is made—the patient having been instructed to stop the drug until notified otherwise—DDAVP may be used safely in selected older adults. Evidence has suggested that the serum sodium level remains relatively stable for up to 1 year on therapy but needs to be measured if medication that might affect sodium balance (e.g., antidepressants) is started or the patient develops an intercurrent illness.[125] Preparations of DDAVP with evidence for a difference in dose sensitivity according to gender are available but these have not yet been evaluated in frail older adults. Studies have supported their use in robust, community-dwelling older adults, with fewer adverse events.[126,127]

Nocturnal Enuresis

Nighttime sleep in older adults is often fragmented and disrupted. In nursing homes, much of this fragmentation and disruption is caused by noise, light, and the care routines. When older adults are dependent on caregivers for going to bed, either in their own home or care facility, they may spend long periods of time in bed overnight, which in itself may predispose them to enuresis. Interventions that have been investigated to enhance the quality and duration of sleep for residents with UI include daytime physical activity programs, alone or combined with a night staff behavior program aimed at reducing noise, light, and sleep disruptive care practices.[128] Congestive heart failure, functional disability, depression, use of hypnotics, and nocturnal polyuria are all amenable to interventions to reduce the occurrence of enuresis.

Surgery

There are data that support the use of anti-incontinence surgery in selected older adults, but there have been few studies on frail older adults. Both botulinum toxin for urgency incontinence and midurethral tapes for stress urinary incontinence are effective, and there have been some studies in frail older adults.[129-133] Hellberg and coworkers have shown that at 3 months, women 75 years old had a cure rate of 81.6% compared with a rate of 92.8% in women younger than 75 years.[133a] At later follow-up, regardless of length of time since the tension-free vaginal tape (TVT) procedure, the proportion of women with cure for any incontinence decreased with increasing age. In a randomized controlled trial of TVT versus 6-month wait list control, the intervention group at 6 months had a statistically significantly greater improvement in mean incontinence–quality of life, patient satisfaction, and urinary problem scores.[134]

On botulinum toxin, therapy is effective, albeit less so than in younger women, but is associated with a higher rate of increased risk of large postvoid residual urine volume.[133] Older women experience more adverse events than younger women, and the proportion reporting improvement or cure (however defined) may not be as high as in a younger group. There are fewer data, other than those for deobstructing operative intervention, on surgery for incontinence in older men. Some case series for clam ileocystoplasty include men up to the age of 90 years, but they were undoubtedly carefully selected. Nevertheless, with appropriate selection and precautions, optimizing premorbid conditions, use of measures to reduce delirium, adequate hydration, nutrition, and analgesia, early proactive rehabilitation, treatment of postoperative delirium, treatment of functional impairment, and use of specialized care units for older adults, excellent operative outcomes for older adults are achievable. As with all surgery, due regard should be given to potential benefits and harms, and the potential patient should be appropriately counseled, taking note to include input from relevant caregivers, if necessary. In Australia, but not in the United Kingdom, older women appear to have benefited from the less invasive options available for the treatment of stress incontinence.[135,136]

Pads, Catheters, and Appliances

A huge variety of handheld urinals, bedpans, and collection devices are available for those with UI and for those whose incontinence is complicated by physical impairment. The International Consultation on Incontinence, in collaboration with the International Continence Society, has produced a comprehensive product directory for use by patients, families, and caregivers, which enables them to obtain advice on the suitability of different products (http://www.continence productadvisor.org). A comprehensive review is available.[137] Older adults should be seen by specially trained health care professionals with a view to providing appropriate products for their type and severity of incontinence. Ideally, a range of products should be made available to address varying situations. Unfortunately, where products are made available by some health care services (e.g., in the United Kingdom), rationing maintenance products because of financial constraints commonly occurs. There is also evidence of the use of arbitrary local eligibility criteria that people have to fulfill to be given free pads.[138] The most expensive product may not be the best and, likewise, the least expensive product does not necessarily may not be the worst.[139-141]

Attention should be paid to the type of pad, frequency of changing, ease of application and removal and, overall, the personal preference of the intended user. However, the first step in assessment should not be the provision of free pads. These should only be offered as part of a planned assessment and management plan, again in accordance with current guidance. The use of intermittent catheterization for voiding inefficiency in older adults should not be neglected. There are aids to assist with difficult catheterization, and some home care service aides will do this two or three times a day if the older person or willing and able caregiver is unable to do so. The use of a single catheterization before bed—for example, to ensure an empty bladder before sleep—can transform the life of the patient with ineffective voiding and nocturnal frequency. If intermittent catheters cannot be used, long-term catheterization can offer a practical solution to an intractable problem. Guidelines have suggested the use of suprapubic catheters for long-term use, chiefly for the avoidance of urethral complications and relative ease of replacement.[142]

Attention should be paid to the type and required function of collection bags to minimize the inhibiting influence of traditional collection bags and stands on mobility. If the generation of high pressures is not a major problem, the use of a flip flow valve should be considered, ensuring that the older person has the dexterity to open and close the tap. A sheath catheter may also form a practical solution to dribbling incontinence but these present their own challenges to men in terms of application and remaining in situ. Generally they are preferred to indwelling catheter use for incontinence without urinary retention and will not be affected by bypassing due to detrusor overactivity.[143] Attention should be paid to skin health because these devices are not without complications.[144]

Environmental Adaptations

The environment in which the older person lives has a significant role in his or her ability to toilet successfully; this is particularly true in institutions. The provision of a bedside commode or handheld urinal for those with difficulty in transferring or with mobility may be a practical solution to the problem. However, many commodes are of poor design with regard to stability and present challenges to privacy and dignity, particularly in a shared living space. The cleaning and maintenance of such equipment may also prove challenging in the home setting. The provision of hand rails, low-level lighting, adequate seating, and adapted clothing may similarly make a great difference to an older person's ability to toilet successfully, and the role of the occupational therapist in the assessment and provision of appropriate aids should be taken into consideration. at all times.

CONCLUSIONS

Evidence for the efficacy of interventions for incontinence in older adults and increasingly in frail older adults continues to accumulate. Older adults should not be denied treatments simply on the basis of age, but sometimes proactive advocacy is required to ensure that appropriate treatment is considered.[145] For most people, taking into account the remaining life expectancy, their wishes for treatment, and likely expectations, incontinence can be treated with a reasonable expectation of a positive outcome.

KEY POINTS

- Urinary incontinence is a common symptom in older adults and has a profound negative impact on quality of life.
- There is increasing evidence for effective management of urinary incontinence in robust and frail older adults.
- There is probably no reason to assume that interventions that work for community-dwelling older adults should not also be effective in frail older adults. This assumption should guide practice when there is a dearth of direct evidence, but consideration should be made of potential benefits, harm, and feasibility.
- Incontinence in older adults, in common with other geriatric syndromes, requires a multicomponent, often multidisciplinary, approach to obtain the optimal outcomes from treatment.

For a complete list of references, please visit www.expertconsult.com.

KEY REFERENCES

2. Chancellor MB: The overactive bladder progression to underactive bladder hypothesis. Int Urol Nephrol 46(Suppl 1):S23–S27, 2014.
4. Irwin DE, Milsom I, Hunskaar S, et al: Population-based survey of urinary incontinence, overactive bladder, and other lower urinary tract symptoms in five countries: results of the EPIC study. Eur Urol 50:1306–1314, 2006.
36. Malone-Lee J, Wahedna I: Characterisation of detrusor contractile function in relation to old-age. Br J Urol 72:873–880, 1993.
37. Collas D, Malone-Lee JG: Age associated changes in detrusor sensory function in patients with lower urinary tract symptoms. Int Urogynecol J Pelvic Floor Dysfunct 7:24–29, 1996.
48. Kuchel GA, Moscufo N, Guttmann CR, et al: Localization of brain white matter hyperintensities and urinary incontinence in community-dwelling older adults. J Gerontol A Biol Sci Med Sci 64:902–909, 2009.
49. Kuo HK, Lipsitz LA: Cerebral white matter changes and geriatric syndromes: is there a link? J Gerontol A Biol Sci Med Sci 59:818–826, 2004.
74. Gill SS, Mamdani M, Naglie G, et al: A prescribing cascade involving cholinesterase inhibitors and anticholinergic drugs. Arch Intern Med 165:808–813, 2005.
78. Wagg A, Gibson W, Ostaszkiewicz J, et al: Urinary incontinence in frail elderly persons: report from the 5th International Consultation on Incontinence. Neurourol Urodyn 34:398–406, 2015.
84. Wagg A: The cognitive burden of anticholinergics in the elderly—implications for the treatment of overactive bladder. Eur Urol Rev 7:42–49, 2012.
88. Landefeld CS, Bowers BJ, Feld AD, et al: l. National Institutes of Health state-of-the-science conference statement: prevention of fecal and urinary incontinence in adults. Ann Intern Med 148:449–458, 2008.
89. Roe B, Ostaszkiewicz J, Milne J, et al: Systematic reviews of bladder training and voiding programmes in adults: a synopsis of findings from data analysis and outcomes using metastudy techniques. J Adv Nurs 57:15–31, 2007.
97. Jirovec MM: The impact of daily exercise on the mobility, balance and urine control of cognitively impaired nursing home residents. Int J Nurs Stud 28:145–151, 1991.
108. DuBeau CE, Kraus SR, Griebling TL, et al: Effect of fesoterodine in vulnerable elderly subjects with urgency incontinence: a double-blind, placebo-controlled trial. J Urol 191:395–404, 2014.
117. Wagg A, Cardozo L, Nitti VW, et al: The efficacy and tolerability of the β3 adrenoreceptor agonist mirabegron for the treatment of symptoms of overactive bladder in older patients. Age Ageing 43:666–675, 2014.
125. Cornu JN, Abrams P, Chapple CR, et al: A contemporary assessment of nocturia: definition, epidemiology, pathophysiology, and management—a systematic review and meta-analysis. Eur Urol 62:877–890, 2012.
152. Dubeau CE, Kraus SR, Griebling TL, et al: Effect of fesoterodine in vulnerable elderly subjects with urgency incontinence: a double-blind, placebo controlled trial. J Urol 1:395–404, 2014.

107 Pressure Ulcers

Bryan D. Struck

Five centuries ago, French physician Ambroise Paré described one of the earliest pressure ulcers in the medical literature, noting that "the bedsore on the buttock has come from having been too long a time lying on it, without moving himself."[1] Today, pressure ulcers continue to be a significant problem. costing billions of dollars annually.[2,3] The United States, the United Kingdom, and the European medical community spent significant time and effort creating staging guidelines, identifying risk factors, and outlining prevention strategies.[4-6] Even with these guidelines, pressure ulcers continue to haunt medicine in the twenty-first century. The older adult population is especially at risk. Incidence rates of pressure ulcer in the United States approach 38% in acute care, 40% in critical care units, and 24% in long-term care facilities.[4] Average cost to treat a pressure ulcer in the United States is $40,381, which results in $11 billion annually.[7] Prevalence rates in the United Kingdom range from 8% to 20% for hospitalized patients.[8,9] The cost in the United Kingdom to treat varies from 1,214 to 14,108 pounds, resulting in GBP 1.4 to 2.1 billion annually.[10,11] In 2008 the Centers for Medicare and Medicaid implemented policy to limit reimbursement to hospitals for certain hospital-acquired conditions. Pressure ulcers are one of the most common hospital-acquired conditions, diagnosed at 30.38/1000 Medicare discharges. The limits are set to begin in fiscal year 2015.[10] This chapter describes how normal aging affects the known risk factors for pressure ulcer development, reviews the pathophysiology of pressure ulcers, describes new staging classification, and discusses prevention and treatment options.

NORMAL AGING

With increasing age, several changes occur throughout the skin, resulting in increased risk of pressure ulcer development. Epidermal turnover rates decrease by 30% to 50% by the age of 70, resulting in rougher skin with decreased barrier function.[12] Theoretically, this change plays a role in decreased healing of epidermal wounds. The dermal-epidermal junction flattens, resulting in decreased contact between the two layers. As a result, the two layers may separate easily, making older skin more likely to tear and blister.

The dermis provides the basic structure of the skin between the epidermis and the deeper structures (muscle and bone). The dermis is a complex connective tissue matrix consisting of collagenous, elastic, and reticular fibers, which provide strength and elasticity. The blood vessels, lymphatics, nerves, and deeper portions of the hair follicles are located in the dermis. Normal aging changes the structure and function of the dermis. Basal and peak levels of cutaneous blood flow are reduced by about 60%, resulting in compromised vascular responsiveness during injury or infection.[12] This change may be mediated by endothelial dysfunction.[13] With age, collagen synthesis decreases and degradation increases, resulting in a loss of the connective tissue matrix and impaired wound healing.[12] Elastic fibers decrease in number and size, resulting in decreased skin elasticity. Photo aging may worsen these normal changes.

Subcutaneous fat decreases with age, decreasing its ability to protect deeper structures from injury. Distribution of subcutaneous fat changes (decreasing in face and hands, increasing in thighs and abdomen), which decreases pressure diffusion over bony prominences.

PATHOPHYSIOLOGY OF PRESSURE ULCERS

Pressure that disrupts normal circulation to the skin and deep structures is the primary factor in the development of pressure ulcers. A complex vascular system, consisting of large vessels and a network of capillaries, courses through the dermis to supply the skin with oxygen and nutrition and remove waste. Motor nerves monitor arterioles and excretion production.[14] Blood flow through the macrocirculatory system is controlled by the microcirculatory system. Small conductance vessels in between these two systems conduct blood and resist flow.[15,16] Dermis capillary blood flow pressures range from 11 mm Hg at the venule side to 32 mm Hg on the arterial side. If capillary pressures rises above 32 mm Hg, blood flow will be disrupted, causing ischemia within hours.[17,18] An older adult patient, supine on a bed, generates pressure between 50 and 90 mm Hg at the location of the heel and greater trochanter, well above the capillary filling pressure. Animal skin studies suggest damage can begin in 2 hours in the presence of only 100 mm Hg pressure.[19]

In addition to pressure, friction and shear also are extrinsic factors contributing to ulcer development. Friction causes epidermal injury, which can increase damage already present by pressure. This often occurs when objects such as bed linen or clothes are allowed to rub on the skin, removing the epidermis. The age-associated decrease in epidermal turnover rate may delay repair. Moisturizer use can decrease effects of friction.

Shear is the internal force that is generated when a body shifts or moves in a direction parallel to the plane of contact.[20] As an older person slides down in the bed, the skin adheres to the bed surface but the underlying structures move with the body. This causes tearing of capillaries and disruption in blood flow. Now less pressure is needed to occlude blood flow. These phenomena may be worsened by the loss of subcutaneous fat seen with normal aging. Using a draw sheet and keeping a low head of bed elevation can minimize shear.

The final extrinsic factor contributing to pressure ulcer development is excessive moisture. Moisture from urinary or fecal incontinence or profuse sweating can lead to skin maceration and perhaps increased friction and sheer forces when left the skin is left sticky and wet. Absorbent pads can improve moisture.

Aside from extrinsic forces, several intrinsic forces also impact the development of pressure ulcers. These factors include immobility, poor nutrition, decreased sensory perception, and low body mass.[18] Older adults are at increased risk for immobility because of increased rates of cerebral vascular disease, hip fracture, and increased recovery time from acute illness or surgery. If these comorbidities are present, physical therapy and occupational therapy consults may minimize the effects of immobility. Decreased sensory perception may be the result of diabetic neuropathy or cerebral vascular disease, which may prevent an older adult from feeling the pain associated with damage from extrinsic forces. Inadequate nutrition increases risk for ulcer development and impairs healing.[21] Large wounds may require twice the normal protein intake to heal.[22] Tube feeding has not been associated with preventing or healing pressure ulcers in advanced dementia.[23]

Although the extrinsic and intrinsic factors previously discussed may initiate pressure ulcer formation, cell death results from ischemia-reperfusion injury.[20] The initial ischemic injury occurs when blood flow ceases. Deeper structures such as skeletal muscle can tolerate only short periods of ischemia, compared to the epidermis, which can tolerate longer periods. Initially, the microcirculation dilates and releases histamine (blanchable erythema). Next, the capillaries and venules engorge with red blood cells and then hemorrhage (nonblanchable erythema). Necrosis of all skin structures is seen by stage III.[24] Reperfusion begins with removal of pressure. Damage seen with blanchable and nonblanchable erythema may be reversible. Nitrous oxide production decreases during ischemic periods, causing blood vessel constriction. During reperfusion, blood vessels dilate as nitrous oxide production increases. If damage is extensive, the reperfusion spreads toxic metabolites and oxygen free radicals, destroying surrounding tissue.[20]

RISK ASSESSMENT

Prevention remains the mainstay of pressure ulcer treatment. The health care provider should carefully examine high-risk areas for pressure ulcer development, such as the occiput, spine, sacrum, ischium, heels, trochanter, knee, and ankle. Several scales, including the Norton, Braden, and Waterlow scales, exist to assess patients at risk for pressure ulcer development. The Norton scale assesses five areas on a 4-point scale; these areas are physical condition, mental condition, activity, mobility, and incontinence. A modified scale deducts 1 point for each of the following: comorbidities (diabetes, hypertension), low hemoglobin, low hematocrit, low albumin (<3.3 mg/dL), fever higher than 99.6° F, polypharmacy, and mental status changes/lethargy in the past 24 hours. A score of 10 is high risk.[25] The Braden scale is used in both research and clinical settings. This 3-point scale assesses risks in six categories: sensory perception, activity, mobility, nutrition, moisture level, and friction/shear. The maximum score is 23. A score of 18 indicates increased risk for older patients.[26,27] The Waterlow scale is a modification of the Norton scale and assesses eight factors: build, sex, age, continence, mobility, appetite, medication, and special risk factors.[28] The higher the score on this complex scale indicates an increased risk. A 2007 review and study using the three scales in an inpatient geriatric setting showed that sensitivity and specificity of all scales depended on selected cutoff points sample changes.[29] The positive predictive value of the Braden and Norton scales is approximately 37%.[30] As a result, it is recommended that the scales be used in conjugation with a good physical examination by a nurse or physician.[7,29] In a 2014 update, the *Cochrane Database of Systemic Reviews* found two studies (one randomized controlled) that showed no statistical significance between assessment and pressure ulcer incidence; the authors concluded assessment does not reduce pressure ulcer development.[31]

PRESSURE ULCER CLASSIFICATION

The National Pressure Ulcer Advisory Panel (NPUAP) defines a pressure ulcer as localized injury to the skin and/or underlying tissue usually over a bony prominence as a result of pressure or pressure in combination with shear and/or friction. Blanchable erythema or reactive hyperemia often precede pressure ulcer development and can resolve in 24 hours if treatment starts. However, once the skin changes go beyond the initial stage, pressure ulcer formation has started. The NPUAP uses a four-stage system of pressure ulcer classification.[32] In 2007, two new stages were added: suspected deep tissue injury and unstageable.[33]

Suspected deep tissue injury is a purple or maroon localized area of discolored intact skin or blood-filled blister caused by damage of underlying soft tissue. The skin may be painful and may be a different temperature compared with surrounding skin. Deep tissue injury may progress rapidly to a pressure ulcer, despite treatment. Stage I is intact skin with nonblanchable erythema of a localized area usually over a bony prominence. The skin may be painful and may be a different temperature compared with surrounding skin. This indicates that there is inadequate perfusion to the cutaneous microcirculation. Stage II is a partial thickness loss of dermis presenting as a shallow open ulcer with a red-pink wound bed, without slough or bruising. An open or ruptured blister may also be present. At this stage, tissue anoxia has progressed to such an extent that the epidermis starts to necrose. Stage III is full-thickness tissue loss associated with undermining and tunneling. Subcutaneous fat may be visible, but bone, tendon, or muscle is not exposed. Ulcers on areas with no subcutaneous tissue (nose, ear, malleolus) may be very shallow compared with areas with significant subcutaneous tissue such as the sacrum. Stage IV is full thickness tissue loss with exposed bone, tendon, or muscle. It is often associated with slough or eschar, undermining and tunneling, and osteomyelitis. An unstageable ulcer is full thickness tissue loss in which the base of the ulcer is covered by slough (yellow, tan, gray, green, or brown) and/or eschar (tan, brown, or black) in the wound bed. The slough and/or eschar must be removed before the true stage can be determined. However, an eschar on the heels is considered stable if it is dry, adherent, and intact without erythema and should not be removed.

Once staging of the ulcer is completed, ulcer progression must be documented. One method of documenting a wound is as follows[34]: (1) stage the ulcer, time present, setting where occurred; (2) describe the location anatomically; (3) measure ulcer in centimeters (length × width × base); (4) describe percentage of ulcer covered by granulation tissue versus yellow slough versus necrotic tissue/eschar; (5) note any odor; (6) describe the surrounding tissue; and (7) document undermining or tunneling (use clock as reference point).

MANAGEMENT AND TREATMENT

As described earlier, pressure ulcer development occurs from a combination of extrinsic and intrinsic factors. Pressure ulcers are chronic wounds, and amount of time to heal is very variable.[35] Management and treatment should focus on (1) pressure relief, (2) wound care, and (3) complications. In 2006, *Wound Repair and Regeneration* published *Guidelines for the Treatment of Pressure Ulcers (GTPU)*, which were evidence and consensus based.[31] Evidence level (EL) were classified as I (multiple clinical trials supporting use), II (at least one trial), or III (suggestive but lacking sufficient data).

Pressure relief is the first line of treatment. According to the NPUAP, patients should be turned every 2 hours while in bed or every 1 hour while seated. Patients should be positioned or padded to minimize pressure on at-risk areas or minimize pressure on existing ulcers (GTPU EL II). Support surfaces can reduce pressure but not eliminate pressure, so repositioning is still important. Static support surfaces are usually foam, air, or water overlays and can reduce pressure, especially for stage I and stage II ulcers and if the patient can move[36,37] (GTPU EL I). These surfaces lie over the existing mattress or replace the existing mattress and can be used in the home.

Dynamic support surfaces are low air loss beds, alternating pressure beds, and air-fluidized beds. These devices are usually reserved for stage III and stage IV ulcers (GTPU EL I). The low air loss beds and air-fluidized beds reduce pressure by keeping the person floating on a bed of air or fluidized beads. By contrast, alternating pressure beds reduce pressure by reproducing the alternation of high and low pressure in the weight-bearing areas, which occurs in normal people as a result of postural changes in response to pressure pain. They consist of two alternating systems of air cells powered by a pump, which causes them to inflate and deflate reciprocally over a 5- to 10-minute cycle, thus continually changing the supporting areas of pressure on the body. These beds are expensive and large and thus difficult to use in the home setting; in addition, they may increase immobility for older patients. One dynamic surface has not been shown to be superior to another one in treatment of pressure ulcers.[38]

Pressure ulcers require consistent wound care, which includes débridement, cleansing, and dressing. Necrotic tissue or slough may require débridement to promote healing (GTPU EL I). Sharp débridement requires a scalpel and scissors, removing only the dead tissue. Mechanical débridement is performed with wet to dry dressings, whirlpool, and irrigation; this is a nonselective method and may remove healthy tissue. Enzymatic débridement uses enzymes to slowly break down the fibrin and collagen in the necrotic tissue. The enzymatic ointments are expensive. Autolytic débridement uses the wound's own enzymes to slowly remove the necrotic tissue through use of an occlusive dressing.

Wound cleansing should be done with tap water or saline. Antiseptics should be avoided because they will destroy healthy tissue (GTPU EL III).

The purpose of the dressing is to manage fluid balance in the ulcer by adding moisture or absorbing excess moisture (GTPU EL I). Films are semiocclusive or occlusive, are usually transparent, promote autolytic débridement, and are often used on stage II ulcers. Hydrogels provide moisture to the ulcer and are best used for ulcers that have adequate granulation tissue and minimal necrotic tissue. Hydrocolloid dressings are occlusive, adhere to the wound, and promote autolytic débridement. Alginate dressings are derived from seaweed and, because they can absorb 20 times their weight in fluid, they are good for draining ulcers. Silver impregnated dressings are used to decrease microbial count and improve healing. Although they have been used in infection-prone wounds, such as burns and leg vein graft sites, their use in chronic wounds such as pressure ulcers is unclear; however, data suggest that dressings may be changed less frequently, saving clinician time, which offsets their expense. If stage III or IV pressure ulcers fail to improve after these therapies, consider using a negative pressure wound therapy such as V.A.C. therapy (GTPU EL I). However, hyperbaric oxygen therapy has not been shown to improve healing (GTPU EL I).

The primary complication of pressure ulcers is infection, resulting in poor healing, sepsis, or osteomyelitis. All ulcers are colonized and do not require antibiotics. However, if an ulcer does not improve in 14 days, infection should be considered (GTPU EL II). To prevent contamination with colonizing organisms, a culture should be obtained by deep aspiration or biopsy. Initiate treatment if greater than 10^5 colonies are present.[39]

QUALITY INIDICATOR AND LITIGATION

Google "pressure ulcer" and the search will return a list of law firm websites. Because pressure ulcers are considered preventable, their development is used as a quality indicator for long-term care facilities, hospitals, and effectiveness of a physician's care. It is argued that some pressure ulcers are unavoidable if the facility assessed the risk and implemented interventions or if the patient's medical condition (cachexia, metastatic cancer, severe peripheral vascular disease, or terminal illness) impedes healing or promotes development of ulcers.[40] In 2014, the NPUAP reached consensus that unavoidable pressure ulcers do occur.[41] Yet litigation over pressure ulcers in the United States continues to grow. Pressure ulcer cases account for 13% to 15% of litigation against long-term care facilities and are second only to fall claims (25% to 26%).[42,43] A review of pressure ulcer cases against long-term care facilities showed that the number of cases increased 2.6 times from 1984 to 2002, with 87% of the plaintiffs receiving some type of recovery from the facility.[44] The mean recovery for the period 1984 to 1999 was $3,359,259 compared to a mean of $13,554,168 for the period 1999 to 2002.[44] In Great Britain, there is usually little to be gained in litigation as there would be little payable compensation. However, the National Health Service has a statutory procedure for handling pressure ulcer complaints in coordination with the Patient Advocacy and Liaison Service.[45]

When a family appears with a digital camera to photograph a pressure ulcer, one can conclude that the photo will be used in future litigation. When it appears that a family is contemplating legal action, the entire health care team should work with the patient and family. Table 107-1 summarizes risk management measures for pressure ulcers.[46] Pressure ulcer prevention programs also appear to limit litigation.[44] Other ways to minimize litigation include giving clear documentation of the skin exam at admission and discharge, aligning care plans with patient's care goals (curative vs. palliative), carefully documenting interventions and response, and discussing the factors for "unavoidable" pressure ulcers.[47] If the patient is receiving palliative care or is on hospice, the underlying illness may prevent the healing of the pressure ulcer. In this situation, discussion with a palliative care specialist may be required to address issues of pain, the need for fewer dressing changes, and the need for control of odor and infection.

TABLE 107-1 Minimizing Litigation from Pressure Ulcers

Principle	Action
Avoid defensiveness, anger, and confrontation.	If family members request help in documenting the pressure ulcer, immediately ask administration for assistance.
Involve the entire team, even administration.	Maintain professionalism and avoid blame and finger pointing.
Attempt to reestablish trust with the family and patient.	Meet frequently with the family; try new interventions.
Educate the family and provide realistic goals.	Notify family as soon as pressure ulcer is noted; inform them that end-stage diseases will affect healing.
Review the history and reassess the patient.	Prepare a time line of events leading up to the pressure ulcer; discuss alternative pressure relief devices.
Reevaluate the care plan.	The best care plans are individualized. Clearly state the role of each discipline in treatment.
Obtain proper studies and consultations.	Obtain Doppler scan for evaluation of peripheral vascular disease for leg ulcers, and conduct swallow study for patients with poor nutrition.
Document problem behaviors and provide appropriate interventions.	Be specific in the record with date and time. When describing behaviors, be objective, consistent with terms, and nonjudgmental (e.g., family interfered with care, patient had a leave of absence during care).
Establish a feedback loop for quality improvement.	When pressure ulcer occurs, review policy and procedures.

Modified from Levine JM, Savino F, Peterson M, et al: Risk management for pressure ulcers: when a family shows up with a camera. J Am Med Dir Assoc 9:360–363, 2008.

CONCLUSION

The best plan for pressure ulcer prevention and treatment continues to be informed health care providers that are always vigilant in their examination of the older patient's skin and assessment of risk factors. Older adults have decreased epithelial cell turnover, decreased dermal blood flow, impaired collagen synthesis, and loss of subcutaneous fat. These changes make the skin more susceptible to pressure ulcers from extrinsic factors, such as pressure, friction, shear, and moisture. Because impaired mobility often accompanies illness in older people who are frail, the clinical index for suspicion for pressure ulcers must be high and require pressure-reducing protocols immediately.

KEY POINTS

- As skin ages, there is decreased epithelial cell turnover, decreased dermal blood flow, impaired collagen synthesis, and loss of subcutaneous fat. These changes make the skin more susceptible to pressure ulcers.
- Extrinsic factors that cause pressure ulcers are pressure, friction, shear, and moisture.
- An older patient, supine on a bed, generates pressure between 50 to 90 mm Hg at the heel and greater trochanter, well above the 32 mm Hg arterial capillary filling pressure.
- Intrinsic factors that cause pressure ulcers are poor nutrition, decreased sensory perception, low body mass, impaired mobility, and endothelial dysfunction.
- Impaired mobility often accompanies illness in older people who are frail; the clinical index for suspicion for pressure ulcers must be high.
- Pressure ulcers can be reliably staged using the National Pressure Ulcer Advisory Panel classification (from nonblanchable erythema to full-thickness tissue loss with exposed bone, tendon, or muscle).
- Management relies on relieving pressure and a variety of treatments; no one treatment has yet been reliably shown to be superior.
- Pressure ulcer development can be considered an indication of negligent care and lead to litigation.

For a complete list of references, please visit www.expertconsult.com.

KEY REFERENCES

4. National Pressure Ulcer Advisory Panel: Pressure ulcers in America: prevalence, incidence, and implications for the future. An executive summary of the National Pressure Ulcer Advisory Panel monograph. Adv Skin Wound Care 14:208–215, 2001.
6. European Pressure Ulcer Advisory Panel: Pressure ulcer prevention and treatment guidelines. http://www.epuap.org/glprevention.html. Accessed September 4, 2015.
17. Bansal C, Scott R, Stewart D, et al: Decubitus ulcers: a review of the literature. Int J Dermatol 44:805–810, 2005.
23. Finucane TE, Christmas C, Travis K: Tube feeding in patients with advanced dementia. JAMA 282:1365–1370, 1999.
24. Witkowski JA, Parish LC: Histopathology of the decubitus ulcer. Am Acad Dermatol 6:1014–1021, 1982.
34. Garcia AD, Thomas DR: Assessment and management of chronic pressure ulcers in the elderly. Med Clin North Am 90:925–944, 2006.
40. American Medical Directors Association: Pressure ulcers in long-term care setting: clinical practice guideline, Columbia, MD, 2008, AMDA.
44. Voss CA, Bender SA, Ferguson ML, et al: Long-term care liability for pressure ulcers. J Am Geriatr Soc 53:1587–1592, 2005.
46. Levine JM, Savino F, Peterson M, et al: Risk management for pressure ulcers: when a family shows up with a camera. J Am Med Dir Assoc 9:360–363, 2008.
43. Studdert D, Spittal M, Mellow M, et al: Relationship between quality of care and negligence litigation in nursing homes. New Engl J Med 364(13):1243–1250, 2011.
41. Eisberg LE, Langemo D, Baharestani MM, et al: Unavoidable pressure injury: state of the science and consensus outcomes. J Wound Ostomy Continence Nurs 41:313–334, 2014.

108 Sleep in Relation to Aging, Frailty, and Cognition

Roxanne Sterniczuk, Benjamin Rusak

SLEEP AND HEALTH

Getting adequate sleep and maintaining normal daily sleep-wake rhythms are important to sustaining good lifelong physical and mental health and reducing the risk of disease development. Acute sleep loss leads, for example, to disruption of endocrine function and glucose metabolism.[1-3] Chronic sleep loss and daily rhythm disruption also lead to numerous negative long-term health consequences,[4] including increased risk for obesity,[5] cardiovascular disease,[6] and type 2 diabetes.[7] In addition, disrupted sleep-wake and circadian rhythms (e.g., as a result of chronic shift or night work) have been linked to an increased risk for developing cancer[8-10] and for resistance to cancer treatments.[11]

Some of the negative consequences of sleep loss may be related to its impact on immune system function. Disturbed or short sleep weakens immune system function,[12,13] which can lead to impaired healing and recovery,[14-16] as well as inadequate immune system responses to vaccinations.[17] Increased risk of metabolic diseases, weakened immune responses, and inadequate tissue repair are in turn associated with accelerated health deficit accumulation and increasing frailty in older adults.[18,19]

Sleep has also been shown to be involved in brain plasticity and consolidation of newly acquired information, so disrupted sleep can interfere with learning and memory.[20,21] Sleep has also been proposed to play an important role in facilitating clearance of the metabolic products of neuronal metabolism, including the substance most closely linked to the development of Alzheimer disease, β-amyloid.[22,23] These physiologic effects of sleep loss may be the basis for findings of increased risk for cognitive decline and ultimately for the development of Alzheimer disease in those with sleep problems.[24,25]

SLEEP AND CIRCADIAN RHYTHM DISTURBANCES IN OLDER ADULTS

Several changes in sleep patterns have been associated with aging, including an advance in the timing of sleep onset and waking to earlier clock times, more disrupted sleep, reduced slow-wave sleep with more light sleep, and increased daytime napping.[26-28] As a result, more than 80% of those older than 65 years report some degree of disrupted sleep.[29] Older adults also have more difficulty adjusting to changes in daily rhythms resulting from travel or shift work schedules.[30] Although the types of sleep shown, degree of sleep continuity (i.e., sleep maintenance or lack of interruption by wake episodes), and distribution of sleep across the 24-hour cycle change with age, total daily sleep time remains relatively stable in healthy aging, with those 60 years of age and older sleeping an average of 6.5 to 7 hours a day.[31,32]

Sleep changes during aging may be related to the disruption of sleep regulatory mechanisms in the brain.[33,34] However, it is important to bear in mind that many medical conditions that disrupt nocturnal sleep, and consequently can provoke daytime sleepiness, also increase in frequency with age. These include sleep-related breathing disorders (e.g., sleep apnea), pain syndromes (e.g., arthritis), prostatism in men, and menopause-related hot flashes in women. In addition, sleep may be disrupted early in the prodromal stages of neurologic diseases (e.g., Parkinson and Alzheimer diseases).[25,35] These and other potential contributors to sleep disruption in older adults should be ruled out before considering whether changes intrinsic to sleep regulatory or circadian mechanisms are implicated in these features.[36]

One impact of the circadian system on sleep is to promote sustained waking during the day and sleep at night; a reduction in the strength of this circadian impact can contribute to increased sleep disruption and redistribution of sleep during the 24-hour day. There is evidence from animal models and human studies that the amplitude of oscillation of the circadian pacemaker in the hypothalamic suprachiasmatic nucleus is reduced during aging.[37-39] In addition, the molecular mechanisms responsible for generating these daily rhythms may be disrupted with age.[40] Aging also affects various physiologic rhythms that influence sleep, such as body temperature, melatonin secretion, and fluctuations in other neuroendocrine systems (e.g., declining secretion of luteinizing, growth, and thyroid-stimulating hormones; lower serotonin levels).

CHANGES IN SLEEP ARCHITECTURE DURING AGING

Non–Rapid Eye Movement Sleep

Although older adults spend more time in bed than younger adults, they experience pronounced deterioration in the quality of sleep, as measured by changes to sleep architecture[41] (Figure 108-1). Sleep tends to become shallower and lighter with advancing age, and there are fewer sleep spindles and smaller amplitude K complexes observable during non–rapid eye movement (REM) stage 2 sleep (N2), as measured by electroencephalography (EEG). One of the most profound changes observed in older adults is a reduction in the number and amplitude of electroencephalographic delta waves, which corresponds to a significant decrease in the percentage of time spent in slow-wave sleep or non-REM stage 3 sleep (N3, formerly divided into stages 3 and 4[42]), or even the virtual absence of this sleep stage in the oldest cohorts.[43,28] A meta-analysis of 65 studies has demonstrated that there is a significant decrease in total sleep time, sleep efficiency (time spent asleep as a proportion of the time spent in bed), percentage of slow-wave sleep, and REM sleep latency, from young adulthood to about age 60 years, after which only sleep efficiency appears to continue to decrease. These changes are accompanied by an increase in the percentage of non-REM stage 1 sleep (N1), the lightest stage of sleep characterized by low-voltage, mixed-frequency waves, as well as N2. An increase in sleep latency and time spent awake after sleep onset also occurs.[28]

Rapid Eye Movement Sleep

Many reports have suggested as much as a 50% reduction in REM sleep in older as compared to younger adults.[28,44] However, when the effects of mental and physical illnesses are taken into consideration,[36] the percentage of REM sleep is relatively well preserved from age 60 years onward.[28]

SLEEP DISORDERS IN AGING

Late-Life Insomnia

Insomnia is usually defined as inadequate or unrefreshing sleep and is characterized by self-reports of difficulty falling or staying

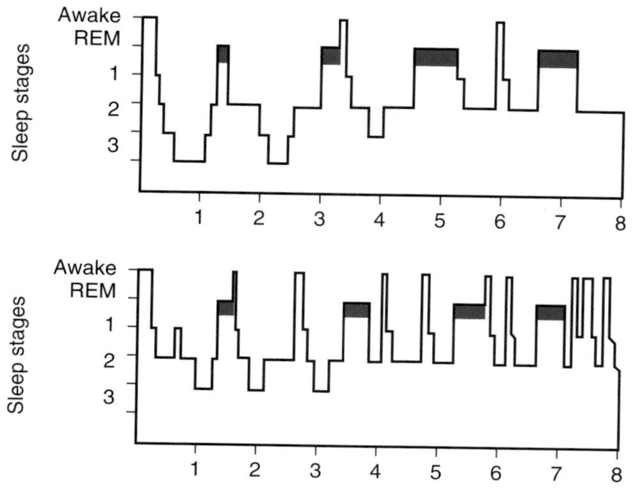

Figure 108-1. Typical distribution of sleep architecture across an 8-hour sleep cycle in a young adult *(top)* and an older adult *(bottom)*. *REM,* Rapid eye movement.

TABLE 108-1 Common Sleep Disorders in Older Adults

Sleep Disorder	Prevalence	Characteristic Features
Late-life insomnia	Up to 50% in those > 65 yr	Difficulty falling or staying asleep Early-morning awakenings Disrupted sleep continuity at night
Obstructive sleep apnea	Up to 62% in those > 65 yr	Five or more episodes/hr of reduction or complete cessation of airflow
Periodic limb movements	Up to 45% in those > 65 yr	Involuntary repetitive leg jerks that occur at 20- to 40-sec intervals Occurs during non-REM sleep
Restless legs syndrome	Up to 35% in those > 65 yr	Irresistible urge to move one's legs due to a restless crawling sensation or pain Associated with sleep onset
REM sleep behavior disorder	0.5% of those in the general population	Acting out elaborate movements during sleep (e.g., punching, kicking, yelling) Occurs during REM sleep

REM, Rapid eye movement.

asleep, typically accompanied by increases in sleepiness and functional impairment during the day. It is the most common sleep complaint in most age groups, including older adults[45] (Table 108-1). Complaints of insomnia are often,[29,46,47] but not always,[48,49] reported to increase with age. Women are more likely to complain of insomnia, especially during and after menopause, and this gender difference appears to increase after the age of 65 years. Insomnia symptoms tend to persist over time,[31,32,50] with early-morning awakenings and disrupted sleep continuity during the night being highly associated with older age groups; younger adults tend to exhibit greater difficulty initiating sleep.

Sleep-Disordered Breathing

Sleep-related respiratory disorders encompass those conditions that cause abnormal respiratory events during sleep, ranging from mild snoring to a reduction (hypopnea) or complete cessation of airflow (apnea).[51] Obstructive sleep apnea is one of the most common sleep disorders. It is caused by relaxation and subsequent collapse of muscles in the back of the throat, causing obstruction of the upper airway. The increased prevalence of sleep apnea in older adults, which has been reported to be as high as 62% in those older than 60 years,[52] may be due to the increased occurrence of obesity, age-related decline in muscle tone, or impaired pharyngeal sensory detection thresholds. Sleep apnea often goes unrecognized in older adults because the overt symptoms that are reported—fatigue, daytime sleepiness, morning headache, mood changes, poor concentration, or memory loss—tend to be attributed to other comorbidities or to the aging process.

Peaking at age 50 to 60 years, snoring is also a frequent complaint of older adults. Interestingly, the prevalence of snoring has been shown to decrease after the age of 75 years, possibly reflecting a survivorship effect. Snoring may be related to various comorbidities, especially obesity and sleep-disordered breathing, that ultimately contribute to premature death in this age group. Narrowing of the upper airway, which contributes to snoring, is also associated with the many health consequences of sleep-disordered breathing, including hypertension, heart disease, and stroke.[53-55]

Periodic Limb Movements in Sleep and Restless Legs Syndrome

Periodic limb movements are repetitive leg jerks or kicks that occur specifically during sleep. They can range from subtle contractions of the ankle or toe muscles to dramatic flailing of the limbs. These movements often occur during N2, resulting in sleep disruption and excessive daytime sleepiness. Its prevalence increases with age and can be found in as many as 45% of community-dwelling older adults.[56]

Restless legs syndrome is commonly comorbid, and often confused, with period leg movement disorder. It is characterized by uncomfortable, restless, crawling sensations in the legs, creating an irresistible urge to move or walk, typically when one first goes to bed. These sensations can contribute to sleep-onset insomnia as well as disrupted sleep. The condition is also more prevalent in older adults, occurring in up to 35% of those older than 65 years, with about twice as many women being affected. Restless legs syndrome has been associated with iron deficiency and abnormal dopaminergic signaling; it can be treated with interventions aimed at these features.[57]

Rapid Eye Movement Sleep Behavior Disorder

REM sleep behavior disorder involves movement during dreams due to the absence of muscle atonia, which normally occurs during REM sleep.[58] Individuals may engage in punching, kicking, yelling, or even more elaborate behaviors during REM sleep; the behaviors are often aggressive in nature and can injure the sleeper or bed partner. This condition is relatively rare in the general population (0.5%) and occurs almost exclusively in men older than 60 years.[59,60] The cause of REM sleep behavior disorder is unclear, but has been strongly linked to the subsequent development of neurodegenerative diseases known as synucleinopathies, including Parkinson disease, Lewy body dementia, and multiple system atrophy.[61]

Sleep Disturbance and Comorbidity

Despite the characteristic sleep changes that are experienced by older adults, these typically age-associated sleep disturbances may not be an inevitable part of the healthy aging process, but rather a consequence of other changes that accompany aging. Insomnia, in particular, appears to be a major factor contributing to the increase in age-associated sleep complaints.[62-64] However, the decreased ability to fall asleep or maintain sleep once initiated is frequently linked to a comorbid health condition. There is an increased risk for various medical and psychiatric conditions (e.g., depression, diabetes, arthritis, chronic pain, loss of bladder elasticity) during aging, which may indirectly disturb sleep.[41] In addition, pharmacologic treatments for these conditions (e.g., antidepressants, β-blockers, diuretics, corticosteroids) are often not recognized as factors that may contribute to sleep disturbances. Although one study has reported that an extensive health assessment can identify medical conditions that account for most sleep complaints in older adults,[36] an estimated 10% to 16% of community-dwelling adults older than 65 years still report chronic (primary) insomnia in the absence of an obvious precipitant.[65,66]

Sleep and Frailty

Frailty can be conceptualized as an increasing vulnerability to poor health outcomes (i.e., disability, institutionalization, mortality) as a result of accumulating age-associated declines in physiologic systems; because health deficits increase with age, so does frailty.[67,68] Little is known about the relationship between frailty and sleep or about the consequences of sleep disturbances in frail populations.[69,70] In addition, the sparse literature on this topic has focused primarily on community-dwelling older adults.[25,71-74]

Daytime drowsiness is associated with a higher level of frailty,[74] and older adults who exhibit poor subjective sleep quality, increased nighttime waking, and greater nighttime hypoxemia have been found to be at higher risk for increasing frailty about 3 years later.[73] Those with excessive daytime sleepiness, frequent nighttime awakenings, and sleep apnea may also be at greater risk for mortality up to about 3 years later, whereas short sleep duration and prolonged sleep-onset latency are not clearly associated with increased frailty or risk of early death.[73] Given that sleep disturbances are associated with poorer health, frail individuals, who are already more vulnerable to the accumulation of stressors, may also be affected by the consequences of sleep impairment to a greater extent than healthy older adults (e.g., responses to sleep medication, impact of insomnia or other sleep disorders). Alterations to the sleep-wake cycle may have prognostic utility in predicting future decline in health and increasing frailty. If so, then treating specific sleep disorders in frail adults may reduce the rate of acquisition of deficits and development of dependency.

Sleep in Critically Ill Older Adults

Patients who are especially susceptible to the adverse effects of accumulating deficits are those in the intensive care unit (ICU). Sleep disturbance and insomnia are common in ICU patients,[75,76] in particular in older adults.[77] Sleep disruption in the ICU has also been linked to impaired healing and recovery, and even to increased mortality.[78,79] In addition, up to 41% and 96% of older patients in the general and surgical wards, respectively, are prescribed sedative-hypnotic drugs. As discussed later, these drugs tend to have greater negative effects in older adults and may interact adversely with other medications that may also be prescribed for them. Several analyses have concluded that the risk of adverse health outcomes from sedative agents does not justify the small benefit achieved.[80,81] It remains unclear how age and premorbid frailty levels affect sleep quality in older adults who are treated in the ICU.[82] Determining how sleep quality in this environment affects health outcomes, such as cognitive decline and mortality, will help provide guidance about appropriate treatments for vulnerable older patients in this high-risk situation.

SLEEP AND COGNITION

Sleep deprivation has long been known to have negative consequences for subsequent cognitive performance, including impaired attention, working memory, decision making, and logical reasoning.[83] There is mounting evidence that sleep disturbance, particularly reduced sleep duration, sleep fragmentation, and sleep-disordered breathing (e.g., obstructive sleep apnea), may play a significant role in the future development of cognitive impairment. Less consistent evidence has been found for a relationship between impaired cognition and insomnia or circadian rhythm dysfunction.[84]

In addition to the disruption of cognitive functions following acute or chronic sleep loss, there is also a large body of evidence demonstrating that sleep loss after new learning may impair retention of the learned material or skill, or so-called offline improvement. This refers to the improvement in later performance that occurs during sleep after learning in the absence of any additional practice or waking experience of the task.[85-87] There is considerable controversy about which sleep stages are important for enhancing performance and which categories of learning (e.g., semantic, motor, sensory, emotional) may be most influenced by each of these sleep stages.

Enhancement of later performance following sleep has generally been modeled as involving the enhancement or stabilization of neural connections that have been newly formed or strengthened during a waking learning experience. There is evidence at a cellular level in animal models that such strengthening of neural connectivity occurs during sleep.[88] One view is that the neurochemical profile of the waking brain is especially suited to acquiring new information, whereas that of the sleeping brain is biased toward stabilization of already acquired information.[87] Depending on the type of learning involved, this strengthening process has been attributed to processes occurring during slow-wave sleep, REM sleep, or N2.

An alternative view is that waking results in a global strengthening of synaptic connections throughout active areas of cortex, and that sleep downregulates synaptic strength globally. This process is hypothesized to strengthen memories by making synapses that have been most strongly enhanced more salient, and also to make subsequent learning possible by preventing everyday experiences from saturating the capacity for synaptic potentiation.[89]

NEURODEGENERATIVE DISORDERS AND SLEEP

With age, there is an increased risk of neurodegenerative disease, which often includes a lengthy prodromal period that can include impaired sleep. Alterations to the sleep-wake cycle and circadian rhythms have been observed prior to the onset of Parkinson disease (PD)–related motor symptoms and appear to signal an increased risk of mild cognitive impairment and dementia, including Alzheimer disease (AD),[24,25,90] Lewy body dementia,[91] and possibly frontotemporal dementia.[92] For example, early-stage AD has been characterized by more nocturnal awakenings, sleep-wake fragmentation, and daytime sleepiness, whereas excessive daytime sleepiness and REM sleep behavior disorder tend to be more prominent in those with Lewy body dementia or PD.[35,91,93]

Sleep loss has been implicated in the mechanisms giving rise to AD in several ways (Figure 108-2). β-Amyloid levels and the formation of cortical plaques, a key neuropathologic feature of the disease, are increased by sleep loss,[22] and clearance of β-amyloid from the brain is enhanced during sleep.[23] In addition, aggregation of β-amyloid has been shown to disrupt sleep-wake cycles, suggesting that there is a detrimental reciprocal feedback relation between sleep loss and amyloid levels.[94] In addition, better sleep quality has been reported to attenuate the risk of AD in those carrying the apolipoprotein (Apo) e4 allele, which confers an elevated risk of developing AD by decreasing neurofibrillary tangle density.[95] These findings suggest that enhancement of sleep quality in older adults and those otherwise at an increased risk of developing AD may be a useful therapeutic strategy for delaying progression to AD.

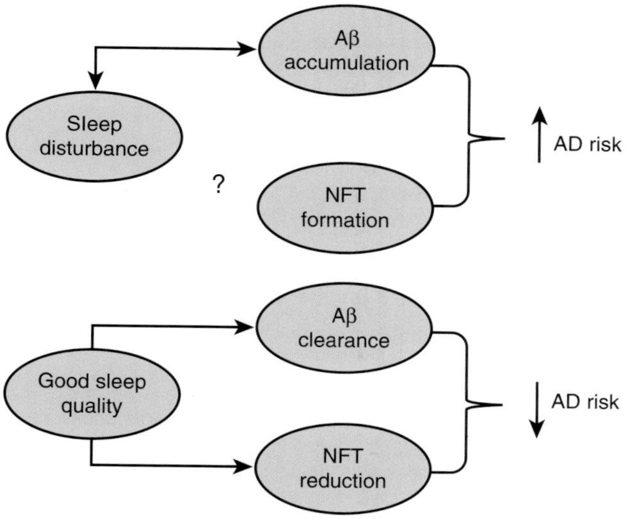

Figure 108-2. Potential mechanisms mediating effects of sleep loss on the development of Alzheimer disease (AD) neuropathology. *Aβ,* β-Amyloid-beta plaques; *NFT,* neurofibrillary tangles; *?,* further work is still needed to establish a relationship.

Interpreting changes in sleep quality and patterns during aging requires caution. Some changes may be characteristic of healthy aging and may not predict disease development. Other sleep changes may be secondary consequences of disease processes, such as the neurodegenerative damage to sleep regulatory systems that occurs during the development of PD. Other sleep changes may actually contribute to the development of disease because of the loss of some of the beneficial effects of sleep for brain health and function, such as clearance of β-amyloid. It is not yet clear which of the changes in sleep patterns observed in older adults fall into each of these categories—normal changes unrelated to health status, changes secondary to brain disease, and changes contributing to brain disease development. Detecting connections between altered sleep patterns or sleep disorders and disease is made more difficult by the lengthy periods over which neurodegenerative disease symptoms may emerge. Thus, there may be years or even decades between the onset of REM sleep behavior disorder symptoms and later development of PD.[96]

TREATMENT OF SLEEP DISORDERS IN OLDER ADULTS

Behavioral Treatments

Although older adults often receive pharmacologic agents for sleep problems, including insomnia, accumulating evidence has suggested that behavioral approaches may be more effective than medications and should be considered as first-line treatment for this population (Table 108-2). The most effective behavioral approach to treating sleep disturbance is the use of cognitive behavioral therapy for insomnia (CBT-I). This technique involves addressing unrealistic expectations or misconceptions related to sleep and promoting behaviors consistent with good sleep quality while avoiding environmental and internal conditions that tend to disrupt sleep (sleep hygiene). Recommendations for improving sleep hygiene include, but are not limited to the following: limiting heavy food and drink, especially caffeine and alcohol, near bedtime; exercising no closer than 4 to 8 hours before bedtime; maintaining a routine schedule for sleep and wake times; avoiding or limiting daytime napping; and creating a comfortable sleep environment (e.g., good ventilation and temperature, no noise, minimal light exposure, no direct access to a clock).[97] Other educational components include reviewing the influence that medical comorbidities, drugs, and environmental conditions may have on achieving a good night's sleep.

TABLE 108-2 Evidence-Based Treatment Options for Treatment of Insomnia

Nonpharmacologic Treatments: Cognitive Behavioral Therapy	Pharmacologic Treatments
Cognitive intervention • Modification of maladaptive or unrealistic thoughts and attitudes related to sleep Behavioral interventions • Improvement of sleep hygiene • Stimulus control therapy • Sleep restriction therapy • Relaxation techniques	Benzodiazepines Nonbenzodiazepines (Z-drugs) Melatonin or agonist (e.g., ramelteon) Orexin (hypocretin) receptor antagonists (e.g., suvorexant)

Behavioral approaches, such as stimulus control therapy, sleep restriction therapy, and relaxation techniques, are the approaches most often used in addition to the promotion of good sleep hygiene.[98,99] Stimulus control therapy is based on the idea that poor sleep can result from maladaptive classic conditioning—that is, the association of being in bed with a variety of non–sleep-related behaviors. This treatment involves instructing clients to use their beds strictly for sleep or sex and not for reading, watching television, using electronic devices, eating, or working. In addition, they must get out of bed if they fail to fall sleep after 20 minutes and only return when they are sufficiently sleepy; this process continues for 20 minutes at a time until they are able to fall asleep.

Sleep restriction therapy is based on enhancing sleep efficiency (e.g., reducing time spent in bed awake, often ruminating about the impact of lack of sleep or other problems) by limiting the time spent in bed to no more than 15 minutes beyond the actual time spent asleep. Once sleep has lengthened to fill the extended period, the allowed time in bed is again increased by 15 minutes until an adequate sleep duration has been achieved. Limiting time in bed may sound counterintuitive for someone complaining of insomnia; however, this approach is effective because if often switches the individual's perspective from being reluctant to go to bed because of anxiety about falling asleep to looking forward to being permitted to spend a little more time in bed. This attitude change, in combination with an already significant sleep debt, can have excellent effects on sleep quality.[100,101]

The components of CBT are typically used together; however, each may stand alone depending on the individual's sleep habits and concerns. Treatment typically takes 6 to 8 sessions, but clinical improvements may not be evident for several weeks.[102] Not only are these methods simple to use, but there is a large body of evidence demonstrating the effectiveness and long-lasting benefits, of CBT-I,[100] including among older patients.[101]

Pharmacologic Treatment

Because of the number of medical and psychiatric issues that develop in older adults and are treated with pharmacologic agents, polypharmacy is very common in this age group. There is typically little consideration given to the effects of individual drugs or combinations of drugs on sleep in older adults. Thus, some sleep symptoms that appear in older adults may be secondary to drug treatments for other conditions; they may be relieved by a careful assessment of drug effects on sleep and identification of alternative treatments that may have less of an impact on sleep. Whenever possible, older adults should take sedating medications near bedtime, and stimulating medications or others that may cause disruption of sleep at night (e.g., diuretics) should be taken during the day.

Several classes of medications are available to treat insomnia and decrease sleep disturbance, including sedative-hypnotics, antidepressants, antipsychotics, antihistamines, and anticonvulsants. Of the sedative-hypnotics, benzodiazepines (BZDs) are the most commonly prescribed medications for sleeping problems. Relative to barbiturates, which are now rarely used as sleep aids, they have a lower risk of toxicity and development of tolerance, but may have harmful effects when taken in conjunction with other sedatives or alcohol.

Different BZDs have different durations of action. Those with intermediate or long half-lives are more effective in maintaining sleep throughout the night, but may also cause residual hangover effects during the following day. These may include daytime sleepiness, confusion, memory problems, and motor problems, which may increase the risk of falls, especially in older adults. Discontinuation after prolonged use may trigger rebound insomnia. Thus, these sleep aids are generally recommended only for acute use (up to 4 weeks).

A newer class of short-acting non-BZD drugs, so-called Z-drugs (e.g., zopiclone, zolpidem, zaleplon) have been promoted as having fewer side effects than BZDs, but they actually act on part of the same γ-aminobutyric acid A ($GABA_A$) receptors on which BZDs act. There have also been reports of amnestic effects and dissociative disorders related to use of these drugs, generally when combined with other nervous system depressants (e.g., alcohol), and they appear to offer few, if any, clinical advantages in efficacy or tolerability in older adults.[103] Like BZDs, they are reported to increase the risk of falls and cognitive side effects, so there is little support for their long-term use in this population.[104]

Neurohormones

Many studies have evaluated the use of the neurohormone melatonin as a sleep aid. Melatonin is secreted from the pineal gland with a pronounced daily rhythm, rising in the evening about 1 hour before usual sleep onset and remaining elevated for much of the night phase. There has been good experimental evidence that melatonin level elevation is a component of the circadian system's transition to the night phase and helps promote sleep onset under appropriate conditions. Although the clinical findings have been mixed in the different populations that have been studied, most studies have indicated that nightly melatonin supplementation, alone or combined with magnesium (which also improve measures of insomnia[105]), can reduce sleep onset latency, promote sleep in older adults,[106-108] and diminish symptoms of REM sleep behavior disorder.[109]

Melatonin levels have been reported to decrease in old age (and, in some studies, much earlier in life),[110,111] and some medications also suppress melatonin secretion (e.g., β-blockers, antiinflammatories). Although melatonin itself is not a patentable drug, pharmaceutical companies have developed melatonin receptor agonists that are available for the treatment of sleep-onset insomnia, such as ramelteon, which has shown promise of clinical effectiveness in older adults.[112] Another drug recently approved by the U.S. Food and Drug Administration (FDA) for the treatment of insomnia, suvorexant, is an antagonist that blocks receptors for the alertness-promoting neurotransmitter orexin, also called hypocretin.

SUMMARY

Adequate sleep is an integral component of good physical and mental health. Sleep disruptions are more common in older adults, who often show profound changes in sleep architecture, efficiency, and distribution across the 24-hour day. Although there are changes in sleep architecture and patterns in older adults, many sleep disturbances can actually be attributed to medical or psychiatric conditions or the drugs used to treat them. The relationship between sleep and frailty is not well understood, but excessive daytime sleepiness, frequent nighttime awakenings, and sleep apnea appear to contribute to increasing frailty and have been shown to increase the risk of death within a few years. In addition, sleep disturbance may contribute to increased vulnerability for a wide variety of age-associated neurodegenerative disorders. Depending on the disorder, treatment may include pharmacologic and/or cognitive behavioral strategies; however, the latter is recommended as a first-line treatment in older adults.

KEY POINTS

- Sleep disturbances are commonly reported in older adults, but are not an inevitable part of healthy aging.
- The most profound changes to sleep architecture in older adults include decreased sleep efficiency, increases in N1 and N2, and reduction in N3.
- Comorbid medical or psychiatric conditions, as well as medications and primary sleep disorders, can account for most sleep problems in older adults.
- Frail older adults may be more vulnerable to the effects of sleep disturbances.
- Disturbed sleep is not only a marker of several neuropsychiatric conditions, but may also contribute to degenerative changes in the brain.
- Sleep is an important factor in the enhancement of cognitive performance, such as learning and memory, but the underlying mechanisms are still not well understood.
- Behavioral interventions should be the first line of treatment when managing sleep disturbances in older adults.

For a complete list of references, please visit www.expertconsult.com.

KEY REFERENCES

4. Knutsson A: Health disorders of shift workers. Occup Med (Lond) 53:103–108, 2003.
9. Megdal SP, Kroenke CH, Laden F, et al: Night work and breast cancer risk: a systematic review and meta-analysis. Eur J Cancer 41:2023–2032, 2005.
12. Gamaldo CE, Shaikh AK, McArthur JC: The sleep-immunity relationship. Neurol Clin 30:1313–1343, 2012.
18. Clegg A, Young J, Iliffe S, et al: Frailty in elderly people. Lancet 381:752–762, 2013.
19. Mitnitski A, Song X, Rockwood K: Assessing biological aging: the origin of deficit accumulation. Biogerontology 14:709–717, 2013.
21. Walker MP: Cognitive consequences of sleep and sleep loss. Sleep Med 9(Suppl 1):S29–S34, 2008.
22. Kang JE, Lim MM, Bateman RJ, et al: Amyloid-beta dynamics are regulated by orexin and the sleep-wake cycle. Science 5:146–148, 2009.
28. Ohayon MM, Carskadon MA, Guilleminault C, et al: Meta-analysis of quantitative sleep parameters from childhood to old age in healthy individuals: developing normative sleep values across the human lifespan. Sleep 27:1255–1273, 2004.
30. Monk TH: Aging human circadian rhythms: conventional wisdom may not always be right. J Biol Rhythms 20:366–374, 2005.
33. Simic G, Stanic G, Miadinov M, et al: Does Alzheimer's disease begin in the brainstem? Neuropathol Appl Neurobiol 35:532–554, 2009.
34. Sterniczuk R, Dyck RH, Laferla FM, et al: Characterization of the 3xTg-AD mouse model of Alzheimer's disease: part 1. Circadian changes. Brain Res 12(1348):139–148, 2010.
37. Hofman MA, Swaab DF: Living by the clock: the circadian pacemaker in older people. Ageing Res Rev 3:33–51, 2006.

39. Wu YH, Swaab DF: Disturbance and strategies for reactivation of the circadian rhythm system in aging and Alzheimer's disease. Sleep Med 8:623–636, 2007.
41. Ancoli-Israel S, Ayalon L, Salzman C: Sleep in the elderly: normal variations and common sleep disorders. Harv Rev Psychiatry 16:279–286, 2008.
63. Wolkove N, Elkholy O, Baltzan M, et al: Sleep and aging: 1. Sleep disorders commonly found in older people. CMAJ 176:1299–1304, 2007.
64. Wolkove N, Elkholy O, Baltzan M, et al: Sleep and aging: 2. Management of sleep disorders in older people. CMAJ 176:1449–1454, 2007.
68. Rockwood K, Mitnitski A: Frailty in relation to the accumulation of deficits. J Gerontol A Biol Sci Med Sci 62:722–727, 2007.
69. Cochen V, Arbus C, Soto ME, et al: Sleep disorders and their impacts on healthy, dependent, and frail older adults. J Nutr Health Aging 13:322–329, 2009.
84. Yaffe K, Falvey CM, Hoang T: Connections between sleep and cognition in older adults. Lancet Neurol 13:1017–1028, 2014.
87. Rasch B, Born J: About sleep's role in memory. Physiol Rev 93:681–766, 2013.
94. Roh JH, Huang Y, Bero AW, et al: Disruption of the sleep-wake cycle and diurnal fluctuation of β-amyloid in mice with Alzheimer's disease pathology. Sci Transl Med 4:150ra122, 2012.
100. Morin CM, Bootzin RR, Buysse DJ, et al: Psychological and behavioral treatment of insomnia: update of the recent evidence (1998–2004). Sleep 29:1398–1414, 2006.
103. Bain KT: Management of chronic insomnia in elderly persons. Am J Geriatr Pharmacother 4:168–192, 2006.
111. Karasek M: Melatonin, human aging, and age-related diseases. Exp Gerontol 39:1723–1729, 2004.

109 Malnutrition in Older Adults

Larry E. Johnson, Dennis H. Sullivan

Malnutrition is a global term representing any condition resulting from insufficient, excessive, or imbalanced consumption, absorption, or utilization of nutrients. With increasing severity and duration, malnutrition can lead to a decline in health, including deterioration in physical and cognitive function, loss of vitality, and reduced overall quality of life and longevity. This chapter will focus on one of the most common forms of malnutrition in older adults—protein-energy undernutrition (PEU)—including its assessment and treatment. Optimal nutrition, including vitamin use, is covered in Chapter 79; sarcopenia, a protein deficiency state, is covered in Chapter 72; and obesity, including overnutrition, is covered in Chapter 80.

PEU is a common, frequently unrecognized, and often inadequately treated condition in older adults.[1,2] Its prevalence is reported to range from 5% to 10% among community-dwelling older adults, between 30% and 61% among hospitalized older adults, and between 12% and 85% among older adults in long-term and subacute care facilities.[3-8] Because there is no uniformly accepted criteria for defining PEU in older adults, the accuracy of these estimates is unknown. Many of the putative diagnostic criteria used in prevalence studies, such as serum secretory protein levels, anthropometric measurements, and muscle strength, lack adequate sensitivity and specificity as nutritional indices. However, they are reasonably good indicators of overall health status and nutritional risk; the more abnormal each of these measures, the greater the individual's risk of experiencing subsequent adverse clinical outcomes and failure to maintain an adequate nutrient intake. For example, older hospitalized patients categorized as protein-energy undernourished based on these criteria have longer lengths of stays, higher costs, and increased mortality.[9] And, their nutrient intakes are often dangerously low. In one study of 700 older hospitalized men, 21% had an average daily nutrient intake of less than 50% of their estimated maintenance requirements. Those in this low nutrient intake group had an eightfold higher risk of mortality, even after adjusting for baseline health status and other indicators of disease severity.[10] Although acute illness may produce profound anorexia, the study indicated that there is often a nosocomial component contributing to the nutritional deficiencies; hospitalized patients are sometimes not fed for extended periods of time in preparation for various procedures. As is true within hospitals, health care providers in other clinical settings also frequently fail to recognize PEU and fail to prioritize its importance correctly among the many other coexisting health problems.[11,12]

Weight loss is a cardinal manifestation of PEU and can develop in association with many disorders, including cancer, heart failure, pulmonary disease, diabetes mellitus, and thyroid disease. Detection of weight loss is important in the care of older adults because it often represents the development of PEU and portends a bad prognosis. However, when evaluating a weight history, it is important to recognize that many older adults experience significant fluctuations in total body water as a result of disease progression or treatment (including dialysis and diuretics), especially those with a history of ascites, edema, or anasarca. Such fluid fluctuations can mask or mimic serious protein-energy nutritional deficiencies and should prompt a careful nutritional assessment. Unassessed weight loss is associated with a high risk of adverse outcomes. In a study of older community-residing men, those who lost more than 3 kg/year over 5 years had a 3.5 times greater mortality risk than those who had no weight change.[13] In a large multisite study, long-term care residents who experienced a 5% weight loss in any one month had a tenfold higher risk for death compared to those who gained weight during the same interval.[14] Even a slow loss of weight, such as 5% over 1 year or 10% over several decades, is associated with an increased mortality risk.[15,16] Weight loss may also precede the diagnosis of Alzheimer disease by many years and may be the consequence of pre-Alzheimer brain pathology.[17] In addition, it is important to be wary of trying to distinguish voluntary from involuntary weight loss, particularly in older adults[18]; any weight loss in this population, even in the obese, should be considered potentially serious. On the other hand, stable weight or weight gain in physically inactive older adults who are obese may mask muscle loss, leading to the condition of sarcopenic obesity.[19,20]

The cause of PEU has important implications in terms of its assessment, treatment, and prognostic implications. It has long been recognized that PEU can present in different ways, and that some forms of PEU are much more resistant to nutritional interventions than others. Based on studies conducted decades ago of children in famine-stricken, third-world countries, it was recognized that some had primarily weight loss and general wasting, whereas other children were developing edema and abdominal distention along with loss of muscle and fat. These conditions were labeled marasmus and kwashiorkor, respectively. Although these terms are sometimes used to describe adult PEU, there is considerable controversy as to which nutritional and pathophysiologic mechanisms distinguish these two conditions in children and whether these same factors are relevant to older adults. For these reasons, the utility of these terms in clinical care is questioned. Alternatively, it has been proposed that the cause(s) of PEU represent a spectrum from inadequate nutrient intake, absent any other pathology, to a serious systemic disorder characterized by abnormal nutrient metabolism, insulin resistance, general protein catabolism, and profound anorexia. The former has been termed *simple starvation*, implying that careful refeeding would be adequate to prevent further nutritional deterioration and reverse established deficits. This condition could result from self-deprivation (e.g., hunger strike), lack of access to food, or other situations in which physical or psychological barriers to adequate food consumption exist.

The metabolic disarray that characterizes the other end of the PEU spectrum is often referred to as cachexia. Although far more needs to be learned about the metabolic basis of cachexia, there is growing evidence that disease-induced inflammation triggers the nutrition-resistant catabolic response that characterizes this disorder. Even when protein and energy intakes are adequate to meet estimated requirements, there is continued catabolism of fat and lean body mass, particularly skeletal muscle. Anorexia and weakness are also major components of the cachexia syndrome; as weakness becomes more pronounced, the individual's level of physical activity declines, which can result in further muscle atrophy.[21] The combination of low nutrient intake, disuse muscle atrophy, and inflammation-induced catabolism often leads to rapid and profound loss of body mass and death if the underlying condition(s) triggering the cachexia cannot be controlled. Certain forms of cancer, uncontrolled infections, and other chronic inflammatory disorders can produce cachexia. However, this is usually a diagnosis of exclusion. Older adults with low nutrient intake or other signs of PEU can fall anywhere along the spectrum from pure starvation to nutrition-resistant cachexia. As discussed later, it is important that clinicians evaluating such individuals conduct a careful search for potentially treatable conditions that could be contributing to the anorexia and weight loss, develop and implement an appropriate intervention plan to treat the underlying conditions and improve nutrient intake, and then closely monitor and modify the plan, as needed, based on treatment effectiveness.

ANOREXIA OF AGING

With advancing age, appetite and food intake often decline, even in the absence of overt serious acute or chronic disease. Paralleling the change in appetite, there is usually an associated decline in total energy expenditure, which results from a loss of lean body mass (producing a drop in basic metabolic rate) and a reduction in the level of physical activity (i.e., energy expenditure of activity).[22,23] Whether the declines in energy intake and expenditure are causally related to each other or to the progressive weight loss seen in many older adults after about 60 to 70 years of age is not known with certainty. The magnitude of this problem is indicated by population-based studies that show a progressive decline in the prevalence of overweight and obesity and an increase in the prevalence of those who are underweight (body mass index [BMI] < 18.5 kg/m^2) with each decade of life after 60 years of age.[24] It is known that with advancing age, the physiologic processes that regulate body weight and link nutrient intake and energy expenditure apparently lose their compensatory responsiveness to changes in energy demands.[25] This was demonstrated in one study of younger and older adults who were placed on energy-restricted diets. Both groups lost weight. However, at the end of the fast, the older adults regained their lost weight more slowly and less completely than the younger subjects.[26] These findings suggest that a reduced ability to regulate appetite and food intake may contribute to the progressive loss of weight that many older individuals experience as they age. They are also consistent with some clinical observations.

Investigators have conducted thorough assessments of older adults who had lost weight to determine if there were potentially reversible causes and to assess the severity of the anorexia.[27] In some cases, the extensive evaluation failed to find any contributing causes for the anorexia and weight loss. The term *anorexia of aging* is often used to describe such older adults with isolated anorexia. It is hypothesized that this age-associated anorexia may result from any number of physiologic changes seen in older adults, including impaired gastric motility, exaggerated adiposity signals from leptin and insulin, and/or postprandial anorexigenic signals from cholecystokinin (CCK) and peptide YY (PYY).[28] As noted, it may also entail a cytokine-dependent process because many older adults have elevated blood levels of inflammation-associated cytokines such as interleukin-6 (IL-6).[29,30] Given the high prevalence and potential seriousness of involuntary weight loss in older adults, more needs to be learned about the causes and prevention of the apparent anorexia in this population.

DIAGNOSIS AND ASSESSMENT OF PROTEIN-ENERGY UNDERNUTRITION

There is no gold standard laboratory test for PEU. The so-called nutritional biochemical markers (e.g., serum albumin, prealbumin [transthyretin], α_1-acid glycoprotein, or transferrin) have low specificity as indicators of protein-energy nutritional status. The synthesis and distribution of all these serum proteins are probably more strongly affected by cytokine-associated inflammation (as negative acute-phase reactants) than nutrient intake. The sensitivity of these markers is also low. This is particularly true of serum albumin. The serum concentration of albumin may remain normal during uncomplicated slow starvation, often dropping only when secondary complications develop as a premorbid event. However, because of their responsiveness to physiologic stress, serum albumin and some of the other serum secretory proteins are important health status indicators; low levels are associated with increased morbidity and mortality, independent of nutritional status.[31] No biomarker is readily available to distinguish simple starvation from cachexia; the diagnostic utility of measuring nonspecific markers of inflammation, such as erythrocyte sedimentation rate or C-reactive protein, has not been established.

Nutritional Screening

Recognition of nutritional problems is not a priority for many health care providers and institutions.[32] Thus, malnutrition is commonly not considered, not recognized, or minimized as to its importance. Although provider recognition of patients at nutritional risk can be improved through nutritional screening, the impact on patient outcomes is less uncertain.[33] This may relate to a lack of proper follow-through on the part of clinicians. Nevertheless, screening is an important first step in addressing the problem. A number of nutrition screening instruments are available (see later). These instruments can be used in various clinical settings to identify individuals who are at risk for having protein-energy nutritional deficiencies. They do not necessarily confirm that an individual is malnourished; these at-risk patients need to be more thoroughly evaluated to confirm the diagnosis of PEU and to identify potentially reversible contributors to the patient's nutritional deterioration. However, such an evaluation requires considerable provider skill and knowledge. Because there is no gold standard whereby nutrition status can be defined or measured, the clinician must rely on a wide array of surrogate measures and know how each can best be used. The sensitivity and specificity of these measures as indicators of protein-energy deficits vary dramatically within the clinical context of a careful history and thorough physical examination. For example, the nutritional implications of weight or weight change can be impossible to determine in a patient with significant dependent edema, poorly controlled heart failure, or other conditions that can produce large fluctuations in total body water. On the other hand, for appropriately selected patients, serial weights can be a powerful tool for assessing protein-energy nutritional status. Weight stability over time, however, does not exclude a clinically significant change in body composition. Muscle mass often declines with advancing age, but weight remains stable or increases as a result of increases in total body fat.

Weight measurement accuracy is highly dependent on the skill of the examiner; weights obtained by trained persons maintaining strict adherence to protocol are more reliable and can differ substantially from those obtained routinely by nursing staff.[34] Establishment of protocols that define proper weighing techniques and ongoing training of clinical staff in the use of these protocols can have a dramatic impact on improving the reliability and accuracy of weight measurements obtained in clinical settings.[34,35]

Calculation of the BMI requires measurement of height. Direct measurement of height may not be valid due to the presence of spine curvature. An older patient's memory of current or maximal adult height is frequently inaccurate. Formulas to estimate height using demispan (half the total arm span), ulnar length, or knee height (using special calipers) are available, but they may not be any more accurate than the patient's own estimate.[36]

Several recent reviews have evaluated nutrition screening tools.[37-40] In one review of 10 well-studied and commonly used screening instruments, the Malnutrition Screening Tool (MST) was ranked highest in terms of validity and reliability.[41] This instrument uses unintentional weight loss and reduced appetite as the basis for gauging nutritional risk. The Mini Nutritional Assessment (MNA) is another well-studied instrument that consists of a six-question screening test.[42] If an older adult scores at nutritional risk, there are 12 more questions (including estimates of consumption, self-assessment, and anthropometric measures of midarm and calf circumference) to aid in assessing the probability of malnutrition. The Malnutrition Universal Screening Tool (MUST) has also been validated for older adults and has alternative measurements for patients whose height cannot be measured or who cannot be weighed (for detailed information, go to www.BAPEN.org.uk).[43,44] In the United States, nursing home residents are required to have a Minimum Data Set (MDS) completed within 14 days of admission, with any major change in condition, and at yearly intervals.[45] This document includes the following: an assessment for nutritional risk, including chewing or swallowing problems or pain; IV or parenteral feeding; feeding tube use, or mechanically altered or therapeutic diets; planned weight change programs; an estimate of percentage of calories or fluid amounts received by artificial feeding over the previous 7 days; height and weight over the previous 30 days; and weight loss or gain over the past 30 and 180 days. The MDS regulations for nursing home residents require a thorough evaluation for any resident who loses (or gains) 5% of weight in 1 month or 10% in 6 months.[45]

In addition to weight, other surrogate measures have been promoted for use in assessing the adequacy of an individual's nutrition status. Clinicians need to recognize the limitations of all such measures. Some, such as many of the biochemical measures, are now thought to have little utility as nutritional markers. As noted, this is particularly true of the serum secretory proteins (e.g., albumin, prealbumin [transthyretin]), which are now recognized to be influenced more by inflammation and hydration than by nutrition. Other measures may be too invasive, costly, or inadequately validated for use in all patients or clinical settings. This includes imaging modalities (e.g., dual-energy x-ray absorptiometry [DXA], magnetic resonance imaging [MRI], computed tomography [CT]), strength or performance tests (e.g., hand grip strength),[46] anthropometric measurements, and tests of immune function. It is also important to remember that endocrine factors, nervous system integrity, immune function and inflammation, and level of physical activity are equally important as determinants of body composition and physiologic function as nutrition. For these reasons, nutritional status should never be assessed in isolation; the assessment needs to involve a multicomponent evaluation that is comprehensive enough to allow the assessing clinician to interpret each measure in context. The goal of nutrition assessment is to determine whether nutrient intake has been and continues to be adequate to maintain or attain optimal body composition and physiologic function for the health and long-term survival of the individual. For this reason, an assessment of nutrient needs and nutrient intake is a very important component of the nutritional assessment.

Unfortunately, obtaining an accurate estimate of actual nutrient intake is almost always a challenge. It is probably the most error-prone component of the nutritional assessment. Having appropriately trained staff to perform accurate nutrient intake assessments on patients in acute, intermediate, and long-term care settings is vital to patient welfare. Obtaining a good diet history from outpatients can also be valuable.

Identifying Barriers to Adequate Nutrient Intake

In addition to assessing the severity of nutritional deficits and nutritional requirements, it is important to identify all potential barriers to volitional nutrient intake. Strategies to improve nutrition should be individualized to reduce or eliminate as many of these barriers as possible (Box 109-1); the most successful strategies entail using a multidisciplinary team approach.

Appetite may improve when depression, pain, and constipation are treated, so these common disorders should be searched for whenever appetite is poor. Many medications (e.g., psychotropics, anticholinergics, cardiac medications) cause confusion and anorexia. For institutionalized older adults, appropriate social stimulation, one on one feeding support, increasing the variety of choices at and between meals, and a liberal food substitution policy are associated with increased caloric intake.[47] Nursing home residents who are physically unable to feed themselves are at particularly high risk for weight loss if adequate care is not provided. This risk can be reduced by the provision of feeding assistance by appropriately trained personnel, including volunteers. Less well recognized, many nursing home residents assessed by the nursing staff to be physically independent are also at high risk for weight loss. Recent studies have indicated that these individuals can also benefit from close supervision, verbal cueing, and other forms of staff support at mealtime.[48,49] Using non-nursing staff to transport patients to the dining room, deliver meals and provide substitute foods, document intake, and increase social stimulation may allow nursing staff to spend more time with mealtime feeding assistance.[48]

The onset of eating problems in persons with dementia is associated with poor survival.[50] Weight loss in patients with dementia is often due to many interacting factors: self-feeding, chewing, and/or swallowing difficulties; loss of hunger drive; and, occasionally, higher energy expenditure due to pacing coupled with failure of intrinsic regulatory systems for maintaining body weight.[51] Unless other diseases are present, there is no consistent evidence that patients with dementia have higher resting energy expenditure or other evidence of hypermetabolism. Obstinacy and feeding aversions—turning the head away when food is offered, keeping the mouth shut, pushing the spoon or hand away, and spitting out food—are common in those with dementia and often require individualized and creative and persistent approaches to maintain an adequate nutrient intake.[51-54] Education and involvement of the family and caregiver at this stage will help them understand that weight loss and clinical deterioration are not due to staff neglect.

Artificial (tube) feeding has many negative consequences in patients with advanced dementia, and patients with early dementia and their families and caregivers should plan ahead to avoid artificial feeding and to use comfort feeding (assisted oral feeding), if required.[55-58]

Chewing and Swallowing

Healthy aging is generally associated with little clinical change in chewing and swallowing. Many medications (particularly anticholinergic and antimuscarinic drugs), Sjögren syndrome, and radiation therapy for head and neck cancers decrease salivation, causing xerostomia, which increases the risk of dental caries and hampers chewing and swallowing.[59] Poor dental hygiene, missing teeth, and poorly fitting or missing dentures are common and cause reduced food intake, requiring the evaluation of a dentist.[60] Leaving dentures in the mouth of frail older adults overnight may increase pneumonia risk, which can lead to a rapid deterioration in nutritional status.[61] Proper routine dental care for the uncooperative patient requires training for the family, caregiver, nursing staff, and dentist. *Mouth Care Without a Battle* (www.mouthcarewithoutabattle.unc.edu), available as a DVD set, provides evidence-based approaches to mouth care for persons with cognitive and physical impairments. Finding a dentist specially trained in examining and treating resistive patients can be challenging if a gerodentist is not available.

Dyspraxia and Dysphagia

Chewing dyspraxia and dysphagia (difficulty swallowing) can arise as a consequence of problems in any phase of eating,

BOX 109-1 Causes and Feeding Options for Patients Who Are Not Eating Enough*

ALL PATIENTS

Liberalize diet; offer variety of snacks between meals; offer food substitutions at meals.
Offer high-calorie supplements (between meals to avoid food substitution).
Reduce or eliminate so-called therapeutic diets (e.g., low cholesterol, low fat, low salt).
Treat pain, constipation, and depression.
Have a dental evaluation performed.
Give medications with high-calorie liquid protein drinks.
Reduce or eliminate sedating and other medications that often reduce appetite, if possible (e.g., anticholinergics, nonsteroidal antiinflammatory drugs [NSAIDs], some antidepressants and other psychotropic medications, dementia medications)
Train volunteers to feed patients and encourage family and caregiver participation.

PHYSICALLY CAPABLE PATIENTS

Educate and provide preferred and varied beverages, buffets, social stimulation, and encouragement.
Assess for depression.
Encourage exercise.

DEMENTIA PATIENTS

Offer foods and a variety of high-energy, high-protein snacks frequently between meals; integrate fluids into activities, happy hours; have roving beverage and snack carts available.
Provide intensive dietitian involvement and staff education and awareness.
Have the patient eat out of bed, in a chair and at a table, if possible.
Use nonverbal and verbal cueing to encourage self-feeding, physical guidance; hand-over-hand technique to initiate and guide self-feeding; demonstrate eating movements for patient to imitate; show how to use utensils.
Reduce distraction; turn off television.
The patient should have dentures in and eyeglasses on.
Simplify: give one food or plate at a time.
Observe for pocketing ("cheeking") foods.
Have less emphasis on healthy eating and more on food preferences.

PATIENTS WHO CANNOT OR WILL NOT EAT OR DRINK

Dysphagia

Speech-language therapist evaluation (see text)
Assess for mouth and throat infections.

Physically Dependent

Provide adequate assistance.
Allow sufficient time to eat a meal.

Who Will Not Eat or Drink

Note: *Patients who are apathetic to eating or drinking may have frontal lobe dysfunction.*
Sippers, those with eating disorders—the patient should have a geropsychiatry evaluation.
Fears incontinence—adjust timing of diuretics and consider alternatives.

END-OF LIFE-CARE

Review advance directives; discuss natural dying with patient, family, and caregiver and the risks of artificial nutrition and hydration.
Treat pain, constipation, and depression.
Avoid medication side effects.
Provide adequate hand feeding and assistance.

*Most recommendations are based on consensus (more suggestions are available at www.Consult GeriRN.org).[47,51,109,178] Persons with coexisting inflammation and cachexia may respond poorly to efforts at increasing nutritional intake.

including the anticipatory, preparatory, mastication (oral), and swallowing (pharyngeal) phases and/or passage of food or fluids down the esophagus (esophageal phase).[62] Details of the neurophysiology of swallowing can be found elsewhere.[63] Signs and symptoms of difficulty chewing or swallowing include the sensation of food getting stuck in the throat or chest and/or coughing or choking with swallowing. Patients with these symptoms require a thorough history and physical examination, especially of the head and neck regions, to identify possible causes. The reported prevalence of dysphagia ranges from 7% to 28% among community-dwelling older adults and up to 33% among those in independent living centers.[64,65] In all settings, the prevalence increases with frailty and the number and severity of comorbid pathologies, especially neurodegenerative disease, stroke, and head and neck cancers.[64,66]

The type of dysphagia varies by disease. Oropharyngeal dysphagia occurs commonly after strokes and during the course of many neurodegenerative diseases, such as dementia and Parkinson disease. Dysphagia following a stroke is associated with decreased survival in the 3 months after a stroke and with increased risk of nursing home placement.[67] Dysphagia is an expected complication of head, neck, and esophageal cancers, as well as many of the therapies directed at these conditions; pretreatment swallowing exercises may benefit some of these patients.[68] Esophageal stage disorders (e.g., esophageal cancer, candidiasis, reflux esophagitis, Zenker diverticulum, hiatal hernia, varices, Barrett esophagus, Schatzki ring) will need assessment by a gastroenterologist with esophagogastroduodenoscopy (EGD) or other specialized evaluations. Persons with degenerative neurologic disorders such as Alzheimer disease and other dementias may also have a tonic bite or other aversive feeding behaviors (refusing to open their mouths when fed) or may hold food in the mouth for a prolonged period (swallowing apraxia, oral phase dysphagia). However, dysphagia may be present with fewer or no obvious symptoms and should be considered whenever there is weight loss, decreased appetite, prolonged eating time, food falling from the mouth, food debris staying in the mouth, nasal or oral regurgitation, wet voice, or hoarseness after eating.[69] Any symptoms suggestive of oral or pharyngeal dysphagia that do not quickly resolve should be assessed by a speech-language pathologist (SLP) or ENT (ears, nose, and throat) specialist.

Assessment and Treatment

SLP assessment can be very useful in assessing persons who are not chewing or swallowing normally, who cough with eating, or who are losing weight for unknown reasons. These experts can assess chewing and swallowing using many modalities and often provide valuable treatment suggestions, although evidence of the effectiveness of many of these strategies is limited. The most accurate diagnostic test for dysphagia is considered to be videofluoroscopy (or the modified barium swallow), but this requires radiation exposure. Fiberoptic endoscopic evaluation of swallowing (FEES) also appears to be accurate and can be performed at bedside. As part of this test, an observable swallow is triggered by blowing air through the endoscope in the nose down onto the soft palate or by the application of slight pressure to the pharyngeal muscles.[70,71] In the absence of these resources, certain bedside tests may be useful, although they generally have only low to moderate sensitivity and specificity for dysphagia (and aspiration risk).[72] The Gugging swallow screen (GUSS) is an example of such a test. It involves observing patients during a saliva swallow, then after they swallow semisolid thickened liquids, thin liquids, and finally dry toast.[73] Other evidence-based tools include the 3-ounce (84-mL) water test (observing for coughing during and for up to 1 minute after the subject swallows the water),[74] V-VST (volume-viscosity swallowing test), and TOR-BSST (Toronto bedside swallowing screening test).[72] A comprehensive nursing protocol to assess and manage swallowing problems in frail older adults is also available.[75]

A variety of treatment options are used by SLP experts to try to restore a normal swallow, including electrical stimulation, thermal stimulation, muscle exercises, and acupuncture.[76] However, there is no evidence-based algorithm for dysphagia rehabilitation, and more invasive interventions (e.g., cricopharyngeal muscle myotomy, botulinum toxin injections) have an uncertain role.[77,78] A modified diet can improve the safety of swallowing; SLPs and dietitians can provide guidance to patients, families, caregivers, and staff on the use of such diets. For patients with difficulty swallowing thin liquids, adding thickening agents to provide nectar-thick, pudding-thick, and honey-thick fluids is an option.[79,80] However, thickened liquids are often less palatable and may increase the risk for dehydration.[81] Sitting patients upright when eating (and for some time afterward), chin tucking when swallowing, eating more slowly, and use of various swallowing maneuvers are additional techniques (Box 109-2). Methods that are successful in persons with a particular cause for dysphagia may not work as well for another cause (see later, "Aspiration and Aspiration Pneumonia").[82,83]

Nutrition and the Aging Gastrointestinal Tract

The gastrointestinal tract generally shows little dramatic change with aging, although the accumulation of multiple small changes may contribute to the development of the anorexia of aging (see earlier) and swallowing problems.[84] Esophageal motility may be impaired (presbyesophagus), with less efficient peristalsis. Medication transit and absorption may be affected by this change, and pills may remain for a prolonged period in the esophagus of supine older adults. It is therefore recommended that older adults take more fluids with medications and then remain upright for at least 30 minutes, rather than lying down immediately. This is a particularly important issue for older adults taking medications known to cause esophageal irritation. Gastroesophageal reflux and hiatal hernia increase with aging, with associated dyspepsia. In most cases, symptoms are managed with dietary avoidance of foods that increase symptoms; universal avoidance of hot and spicy foods is not necessary. Many older adults take antacids, histamine 2 (H2) blockers, or proton pump inhibitors for dyspepsia; these medications reduce gastric symptoms but can increase the risk of pneumonia—stomach acid is valuable in killing bacteria that are swallowed—and may reduce absorption of some vitamins and minerals (e.g., vitamin B_{12} and iron) in very frail older adults.[85-87] Further workup of uncomplicated dyspepsia (e.g., endoscopy, *Helicobacter pylori* testing) is necessary only if alarm symptoms or signs appear such as weight loss, fall in hemoglobin level, or gastrointestinal bleeding. Constipation is a common cause of poor food intake in the frail or bedridden older adult, and proper monitoring of bowel movements can be very useful in assessing reasons for reduced dietary intake of these patients. The older adult is prone to constipation for many reasons (e.g., anticholinergic and opioid medications, poor fluid intake, poor fiber intake, little physical exercise, laxative dependence, neurologic disorders [such as Parkinson disease]).

BOX 109-2 Reducing Risk of Aspiration and Aspiration Pneumonia in Older Adults*

HAND FEEDING

Provide a rest period (>30 minutes) prior to feeding time.
Have the patient sit upright at 90 degrees or highest position allowed by medical condition.
Avoid rushed or forced feeding; feeding by syringe is risky.
Alternate liquids with solids.
Recognize the high risks of sedatives, hypnotics, and other psychotropic medications, and try to wean or reduce dosages.
Speech-language therapist referral: Evaluate patient for possible benefit of chin-down position when swallowing or of adjusting liquid viscosity; thickened liquids of varying types may improve swallowing in some patients (ice cream and Jello are considered thin liquids).

TUBE FEEDING

Note: Both nasogastric and gastrostomy tube feeding may increase aspiration risks.
Consider continuous feedings rather than intermittent (bolus) feedings.
Keep back rest elevated at least 30 degrees during feedings, if possible.
Consider pump-assisted feedings rather than gravity-controlled feedings.
A gastric residual volume > 200 mL during continuous feeding or before intermittent feedings may increase risk (but this remains controversial).[179]
Prokinetic agents such as metoclopramide or erythromycin may improve feeding tolerance, but are associated with their own serious potential side effects.
Placing the feeding tube tip beyond the pylorus (jejunostomy, gastrojejunostomy) may reduce aspiration in some patients.
Using colored dye in tube feeding is contraindicated (it was originally thought that adding coloring to liquid tube feeding formulas would help identify probable feeding aspiration if the dye was found after throat and pulmonary suctioning).[180]

*Most of these suggestions are consensus and expert opinions rather than evidence-based.[181-184]

Aspiration and Aspiration Pneumonia

Aspiration pneumonia is common in older frail adults, particularly those who are hospitalized or institutionalized and those with acute or chronic neurologic disease. It may also make up 5% to 15% of all community-acquired pneumonias.[88] The highest predictors of aspiration pneumonia, which vary among differing patient populations, include the need for suctioning, chronic obstructive pulmonary disease (COPD) and congestive heart failure (CHF) diagnoses, presence of a feeding tube, feeding or oral care dependency, and being bedridden.[89,90] Risk factors for pneumonia following a stroke include COPD, failure to cough when aspirating (silent aspirators), and decreased consciousness.[91] Patients on respirators are also at very high risk. Aspiration pneumonia in frail older adults (as well as all pneumonias in this population) frequently presents with few typical symptoms; delirium (confusion with agitation or lethargy), an unexplained elevated white blood cell count, or tachypnea may be the only early indicators. Aspiration itself may occur without any obvious clinical signs (silent aspiration) or with only episodic fever or reduced oxygen saturation.[92-94] Approaches to reducing the risk of aspiration and aspiration pneumonia are outlined in Box 109-2.

Although controversial, formal dysphagia rehabilitation programs may reduce aspiration pneumonia risk.[95] For this reason, patients who have dysphagia should be evaluated to assess their aspiration risk and to determine whether this risk is influenced by the texture of the foods consumed. In some of these patients, thin liquids present a particular problem. For these individuals, dietary modifications and adoption of specialized swallowing techniques may be of help in reducing risk (see earlier, "Chewing and Swallowing"). A recent study of patients with dementia or Parkinson disease (PD) did not find any clear difference in aspiration pneumonia risk between drinking thin liquids in a chin-down posture or thicker liquids in a normal posture.[96] However, follow-up was limited to 3 months, and care providers were not blinded. Furthermore, the study did not address the issue of whether these techniques were more effective than no intervention as a no-treatment control group was not included. A videofluorographic swallow study (VFSS) currently appears to be the best test to document the extent of aspiration and is recommended prior to restricting intake of thin liquids.[70] In patients with dementia or PD, honey-thickened liquids appeared to work better at reducing aspiration than nectar-thickened liquids or chin-down posture.[82] However, 50% of patients in this study received no benefit from these maneuvers, particularly those with the most severe dementia. It is also important to recognize that despite SLP interventions or recommendations, debilitated patients will continue to aspirate oral secretions and refluxed gastric contents, and this is at least as important as prandial aspiration.[97] Many patients and their families and caregivers refuse to accept thickened liquids and prefer to accept the aspiration risk of thin liquids. It is critically important to document that they have been provided education regarding the relationship between diet modification and aspiration risk and that they were provided the opportunity to share in all evaluation and treatment decisions.[98,99]

Several medications have been proposed to reduce the risk of aspiration pneumonia, most notably the angiotensin-converting enzyme (ACE) inhibitors, but the evidence in support these interventions remains inadequate.[88,100] Improved oral hygiene and regular tooth brushing may also reduce the risk of aspiration pneumonia.[101-103] Treatment of aspiration pneumonia should include coverage for gram-positive and gram-negative organisms, including anaerobic mouth organisms.

Thirst and Hydration

Inadequate fluid intake and dehydration are associated with an increased risk of falls, constipation and laxative use, poor rehabilitation outcomes, and postprandial orthostatic hypotension.[104,105] Risk for dehydration increases with advanced age, use of certain medications (e.g., diuretics, laxatives, psychotropics, general polypharmacy), physical dependency, dementia, delirium, and chronic disease.[104,105] Healthy older adults have an age-associated decrease in thirst sensation (hypodipsia) and consume less fluid in response to the same degree of dehydration than younger adults.[106-108] Hypodipsia can be even more pronounced in older adults suffering from chronic disease; perhaps 30% of nursing home residents are dehydrated at any point in time.[109] Urine color (very dark amber), blood urea nitrogen-to-creatinine ratio (>25 : 1 mg/dL), serum osmolality (>300 mmol/kg), serum sodium level (>150 mEq/L), urine specific gravity (>1.029), and urine output (<800 mL/day) may aid in the detection of dehydration.[110-112] Skin turgor is not a reliable indicator of hydration status in older adults. Older adults at highest risk of dehydration include those who have a diminished thirst drive due to neurodegenerative conditions, those who cannot access or safely consume fluids due to physical or cognitive impairments or dysphagia, those who will not drink enough because of fears of urinary incontinence or have never consumed many fluids, and those at the end of life.[109] Distinguishing patients in this manner may aid in selecting the optimal prevention and treatment strategies.

Water requirements are not well defined for adults, let alone older adults. In healthy adults, hydration status remains normal, despite large individual differences in intake. Fluid goals should be tailored to each individual; for example, there may be competing goals with fluid overload (as found with congestive heart failure), with hyponatremia in the syndrome of inappropriate antidiuretic hormone (SIADH), and with changing activity level or environmental temperature. A daily water intake (including water in beverages and food) of 3.7 L for men and 2.7 L for women meets the needs of most healthy persons, including those of advanced age.[113] This should not be considered a minimum intake. It may be reasonable for sedentary older adults to begin with 30 mL/kg/day (1500 to 2000 mL/day) of fluids; this goal can then be adjusted based on blood urea nitrogen levels, serum sodium levels, urinary output, and clinical status. Possible intervention strategies are presented in Box 109-3. The poorer palatability of thickened liquids may reduce intake, making it more difficult to meet patients' fluid requirements.[81] For residents of long-term care institutions who experience a temporary decline in oral fluid intake—for example, due to an acute infection—subcutaneous infusion of fluids (hypodermoclysis) for 1 or 2 days until oral fluid intake is again adequate, is easy to accomplish and may avoid the need for intravenous (IV) lines or hospitalization.[114]

NUTRITIONAL SUPPORT

Refeeding Syndrome

Nutritional requirements are discussed in Chapter 82. When determining dietary recommendations or developing enteral feeding orders, there are several formulas that can be used for calculating estimated caloric needs; the Harris-Benedict equations (Box 109-4) are the most extensively validated and can serve as a starting point for average individuals.[115] However, caution must be exercised when caring for patients with severe undernutrition such as that which can develop after prolonged starvation. Because these patients often have profound depletion of total body nutrients, rapid refeeding can result in the refeeding syndrome, characterized by the following: a rapid fall in blood

BOX 109-3 Strategies to Reduce Dehydration in Older Adults

- Prepare for dehydration in older adults in high-risk situations (e.g., summer heat without air conditioning, acute illness, delirium).
- Evaluate patient for possible benefit to drink using a straw.
- Offer a variety of fluids during recreational and social activities—"happy hours," "tea time."
- Consider offering options to water [juices, soups, water-rich fruits [watermelon, grapes, peaches] and vegetables [tomatoes, lettuce, squash]).[185]
- Discuss side effects and timing of diuretics to anticipate voluntary dehydration.
- Offer a choice of fluid options, rather than only one or two.

BOX 109-4 Harris-Benedict Equations for Estimating Caloric Requirements

MEN

66.4 + (13.75 × weight [kg]) + (5.0 × height [cm]) − (6.8 × age)

WOMEN

655.1 + (9.6 × weight [kg]) + (1.85 × height [cm]) − (4.7 × age)

phosphorus, potassium, and magnesium levels; sodium and water retention (leading to fluid overload, resulting in heart failure and pulmonary edema); hypoglycemia; and other metabolic complications.[116-120] Altered mental status, cardiac decompensation, cardiac arrhythmias, and death can occur within hours. High carbohydrate intake increases thiamine requirements and can precipitate acute Wernicke encephalopathy in any individual (e.g., alcoholics) deficient in this vitamin.

Individuals at high risk for refeeding complications require thiamine and other micronutrient supplements at the initiation of any nutrition repletion strategy. For those at risk for the refeeding syndrome, it is prudent to provide only about 25% of the estimated daily caloric needs within the first 24 hours (permissive underfeeding). Glucose and electrolytes should be assessed prior to refeeding and then monitored every 4 to 6 hours for the first several days. Initial fluid intake should be restricted to less than 1000 mL/day and weights accurately measured daily. A weight gain of more than 1 kg/week should prompt a careful assessment for fluid overload. As tolerated, intake can be increased slowly, with the goal of reaching targeted daily intake after 3 to 5 days.[116,117]

Appetite Stimulation

Although the appetite-stimulating properties of many pharmaceutical agents have been investigated, none have been proven very effective in improving lean body mass or clinical outcomes in older adults. Relatively few studies of appetite stimulants have targeted the frail older adult, and studies of cancer patients or those with AIDS should not be presumed translatable to the aging patient. Many of the putative appetite stimulants have considerable side effects or costs. Corticosteroids, cyproheptadine, thalidomide, and human growth hormone lack proven effectiveness as appetite stimulants and are not recommended for appetite stimulation in older adults.

Relatively weak evidence has indicated that the cannabinoid dronabinol is effective in promoting weight gain in patients with Alzheimer disease.[121,122] However, this medication is very expensive, and many frail patients do not tolerate the dysphoria that is a common side effect. If careful monitoring can be provided, a trial of use in patients with anorexia can be considered. Megestrol acetate (MA, a progestagenic corticosteroid) is another appetite stimulant that may be prescribed for frail older adults who are losing weight. Studies have indicated that it is occasionally effective in increasing nutrient intake, inducing weight gain, and decreasing serum inflammation-associated cytokine levels.[123] However, the physiologic significance of this latter effect is not known, the weight gain is primarily fat and/or water, and MA often produces several potentially serious side effects. Many of these side effects are thought to be the result of its known corticosteroid agonist and antagonist properties. It has been clearly established that MA can induce profound pituitary-adrenal axis suppression, leading to acute Addison crisis and a Cushing syndrome, especially in older adults. Its use is also associated with muscle loss, insulin resistance, salt and water retention, suppression of testosterone to castrate levels, and increased risk of venous thromboembolism and death.[124-126] In one randomized study of older men in a rehabilitation program, MA negated the beneficial effects of muscle-strengthening exercises.[127]

Appetite stimulation and weight gain are potential side effects of certain antipsychotics and antidepressants, which fact may have relevance when choosing therapies. Depression is common in older adults with anorexia, and the clinician should actively and repeatedly screen for it in these patients (see Chapter 56). If depression is identified, a trial of antidepressant therapy is justified. Because certain antidepressants, such as mirtazapine (up to its maximum dose), are associated with weight gain as a potential side effect, they would be a reasonable choice as initial therapy. It is also reasonable to initiate a trial of antidepressant therapy with one of these agents in any older adult who has unexplained anorexia and weight loss, even when the diagnosis of depression is uncertain. Whenever starting such therapies, close monitoring is indicated because any of the antidepressants may increase or decrease appetite in any patient. Assessment by geropsychiatry should be considered for patients who do not respond to initial therapy.

As discussed, systemic inflammation may induce catabolism, which when severe can lead to a state of nutrition-resistant cachexia.[28,128,129] Inflammation-associated cytokines, such as IL-6, are recognized to play a central role in the inflammatory process. There is some evidence that blocking the production or action of these cytokines or other mediators of inflammation may improve appetite and prevent or reverse the catabolism.[130] However, far more research in this area is needed. To date, no biologic antiinflammatory agent has received U.S. Food and Drug Administration (FDA) approval to be used for this purpose. The antiinflammatory properties of a number of nutrients, such as omega-3 polyunsaturated fatty acids and various vitamins and minerals, are also being investigated. However, their clinical benefit in reversing inflammation-induced catabolism, reducing heart disease or cancer, or improving clinical outcomes of patients with these conditions has yet to be demonstrated. Any role for ghrelin is unknown. The benefits of anabolic steroids, including testosterone and its derivatives (e.g., nandrolone), have also been intensively studied. All these agents can produce potentially serious side effects, and their use in persons who are anorexic and losing weight cannot be recommended currently. The risks and benefits of testosterone replacement or supplementation in older men are highly controversial, even when hypogonadism is documented (see Chapter 13). Selective androgen receptor modulators (SARMS) have not yet been fully investigated but may play a future role.[131]

Enteral Nutrition and Tube Feeding

When oral intake is inadequate and is likely to remain so for an extended period, artificial nutritional support should be considered. The nutritional assessment should consider several factors, including the urgency of the need, prognosis of the underlying condition, whether the individual has a functioning gastrointestinal (GI) tract, and personal preferences. If the GI tract is not functioning properly, peripheral or total parenteral nutritional support should be considered. If it is functioning and tube feeding is appropriate, it is then necessary to choose the type of tube and formula to be used, as well as the rate, schedule, and method of formula delivery. The many risks of tube feeding, including aspiration, should be thoroughly reviewed with the patient, family, and caregiver to allow informed consent.[132,133] Although feeding tubes are frequently placed in persons who are at high risk for aspiration, studies have suggested that such tubes further increase (not decrease) the risk of aspiration pneumonia in these individuals.[134-136]

The patient's overall prognosis is a critical consideration before beginning enteral (i.e., tube) feedings. If the underlying condition contributing to the older adult's loss of desire or ability to eat can be treated, and the individual has a reasonable expectation of recovering independent function, it is often advisable to provide nutritional support during the recovery period.[137] This might be the case when the decline in nutrient intake occurs in association with major surgery, acute medical or psychiatric illness, or as an acute and likely reversible exacerbation of a chronic medical condition. If the patient's BMI is greater than 18 kg/m^2, the individual does not have a condition associated with exceptional metabolic demands, and volitional nutrient intake is expected to return to adequate levels within 5 days, nutritional support is probably not necessary.[137-139] In these cases, efforts should focus on identifying and eliminating any possible contributor to the patient's low intake (as discussed earlier). Older patients who have not had any appreciable nutrient intake for more than 5 days, or who are unlikely to resume oral feedings within a comparable amount of time, nutritional support is warranted.[137-139] For patients with very little nutritional reserve (e.g., BMI < 18 kg/m^2), or high metabolic demands (e.g., extensive burns), beginning nutritional support should be strongly considered if volitional intake cannot be restored within 2 or 3 days.[137-139]

If it is anticipated that tube feedings will be needed for less than 6 weeks, a soft (e.g., silicone or polyurethane), small-bore, nasoenteric feeding tube can be used. These tubes can be inserted at the bedside, and their use avoids the need for an invasive procedure. The disadvantages of nasoenteric feeding tubes include increased risk of aspiration, sinusitis, and local nasal irritation; need for x-ray confirmation of correct placement prior to use; possibility of the tube being dislodged with coughing or vomiting; and poor patient tolerance. Although gastric paresis is common in older, acutely ill patients, the benefits of passing a nasoenteric feeding tube beyond the stomach are not clearly established.

For patients requiring long-term enteral nutritional support (i.e., >6 weeks), a tube enterostomy is preferable. Tubes can be placed endoscopically, radiologically, or surgically. Surgical placement is usually used only when there is a contraindication to less invasive procedures or the patient will be undergoing to surgery for another reason. Tubes placed radiologically or endoscopically can be used within hours, and the procedure is often done on an outpatient basis. Tubes that are long enough to be passed into the duodenum or jejunum can be considered when there is significant gastroparesis or other pathology preventing gastric feedings or when there is intractable intolerance to gastric feeding. Placement distal to the ligament of Treitz may also lower the risk of large volume aspiration, but these tubes are easily obstructed or displaced, and their benefits are not proven.[140] Use of percutaneous jejunostomy tubes is usually limited to hospitalized patients with complex GI problems. Major complications of percutaneous endoscopic or radiologic gastrostomy occur in approximately 3% of patients; these include hemorrhage, bowel perforation, fistula, aspiration, and erosion of the internal tube bumper into the abdominal wall.[137-139]

The type of formula to be used should be determined based on the needs of the patient. In most cases, a nutritionally complete, polymeric, lactose-free formula is the best option. The polymeric formulas differ in terms of the ratio of fat, protein, and carbohydrates; caloric density; and fiber content. Although some patients, such as those whose medical condition cannot tolerate high fluid intake, may benefit from high-calorie or high-nitrogen formulas, other patients do not tolerate the higher osmolality of such formulas, which may contribute to the development of diarrhea. With very narrow tubes, it is important to avoid the use of formulas of high viscosity and not to insert crushed medications into the tube.

Partially digested and elemental (e.g., amino acid) formulas are available for patients who have difficulty digesting whole nutrients. However, these formulas are rarely required and are expensive. If the infusion rate of the formula is increased slowly or pancreatic enzymes are provided when needed, standard polymeric formulas can usually be used.

For patients who are severely undernourished, tube feedings should be started slowly to avoid metabolic complications (see earlier, "Refeeding Syndrome").[116,117,141] Diarrhea, abdominal pain, and vomiting may also occur when tube feedings are increased too rapidly. The use of tube feeding protocols to increase feeding rates to desired amounts and closely monitoring laboratory values are recommended. Measuring gastric residual volumes in tube-fed patients and adjusting feeding rates based on these amounts does not reduce aspiration, even in patients on a ventilator.[142,143] Staff estimations of daily caloric intake in patients who are being fed enterally are frequently inaccurate because the feedings are frequently held for procedures, emesis, and other reasons.

The method of delivering enteral nutritional support is an important consideration, whether using a nasoenteral or gastrostomy tube. Some patients are eventually able to tolerate multiple, intragastric bolus feedings per day. This approach may be more physiologic and offers the advantage of allowing the patient to be disconnected intermittently from the feeding apparatus to enjoy more freedom of movement. This approach may also allow volitional oral feedings to be slowly introduced. Cyclic or nightly feedings may provide a similar advantage. For patients who do not tolerate bolus feedings or who need to be fed distally to the stomach, slow formula infusion by a pump is the preferred method. To minimize the risk of aspiration, the patient should be sitting upright at more than 30 degrees during feedings, whether fed by bolus or slow infusion.[144] Unless there is an absolute contraindication, patients receiving enteral nutritional support should always be allowed, and even encouraged, to resume volitional oral intake if tolerated. "Recreational" oral feeding, even in small amounts, may be offered to patients with low aspiration risk to allow some of the hedonic sensations of eating.

NUTRITION AND HYDRATION AT THE END OF LIFE

There are significant emotional, cultural, and religious aspects to providing nutrition and hydration to someone nearing the end of life and, in some cases, legal constraints as well (see Chapter 114).[145-147] It is often difficult to determine when aggressive nutritional support should be pursued and when someone should be allowed to die naturally. Ideally, an ongoing dialogue among the patient, family members, caregivers, and health care team regarding the use of nonvolitional methods of hydration and feeding should begin earlier in adulthood, when the patient is healthy. Such advanced care planning should include a discussion of the potential benefits and risk of these interventions, how the individual defines quality of life, medical futility, dying naturally, unrealistic expectations, and medically prolonged death.[136,148] As age advances and health changes, these directives should be reconsidered, taking into consideration any newer evidence and the patient's changing preferences. Encouraging the participation of nurses and nursing aides in the hospital or nursing home, and also providing them with the latest clinical evidence, may allow the health care team to present a unified, consistent, and supportive message and maximize the chances for a peaceful death.[149] Early involvement by a palliative care team is often of benefit to the patient, family, caregivers, and health care team, particularly in helping guide decision making on important matters such as hospice referral, which is otherwise often needlessly delayed or avoided until shortly before death.[150]

The role of nutrition in end-of-life care is complex and controversial. Estimating life expectancy in patients with incurable disease is imperfect.[150,151] Average life expectancy after diagnosis differs significantly from one disease to another, and there is considerable controversy as to how best to define the terminal stage of most conditions, whether it is metastatic cancer, heart failure, or end-stage dementia. The issue is further complicated by the fact that the type of care provided may have a significant impact on the duration of life, but not necessarily the quality of life. This is particularly true of nutritional support. As noted, certain cancers and other forms of inflammation-associated cachexia are generally resistant to increasing nutrient intake and nutritional support is usually not effective in prolonging life. In contrast, some patients with Alzheimer disease and other dementias can be kept alive for many years if provided with adequate oral or enteral nutritional support (and excellent nursing care).

However, there is no evidence that nutritional support slows the progression of the cognitive deficits or lowers the risk of aspiration, pressure sores, or infections, and it does not lead to improvement in physical function.[56,136,152-156] Several observational studies have failed to identify a survival advantage for patients with advanced dementia who received a new feeding tube, and some found an association between feeding tube placement and increased mortality.[157-161] Whereas eating is associated with pleasure, enteral feedings are not thought to add to the quality of life. Thus, artificial nutrition and hydration are considered appropriate for reversible diseases, but decisions may become more complicated with irreversible illness and when the patient does not have an advance directive and cannot make informed decisions (see Chapter 115).

Complicating the issue further, clinicians' attitudes toward the role of nutritional support at the end of life differ significantly by specialty, region of the world, and personal beliefs.[162] Many health care providers, including oncologists and SLPs, encourage artificial nutrition and hydration and may cause confusion for patients and families (as well as other staff) by using terms such as *life-sustaining* and *starvation*.[97,163,164] Dietitians and SLPs are more likely to recommend artificial nutrition and hydration than other health care professionals.[165,166] Diverse ethnic and religious backgrounds (of both patients and clinicians) may result in different goals and values, and different attitudes toward end-of-life care that are often poorly appreciated or anticipated.[167] Encouraging "comfort feeding" (offering food by mouth as long as possible) helps relieve fears about neglect and abandonment by the family, while family members observe the disease progression, and is a goal-directed alternative to tube feeding.[55,168,169] If the family still insists on artificial feeding and hydration, a therapeutic and finite trial of tube feeding can be instituted and can then be discontinued if the patient's condition has not improved, or if the patient continues to be unable to consume enough food or fluids by mouth. This often allows family members to witness the futility of the purpose of the feeding and to come to terms with their depression and grief. An excellent education resource is *Making Choices: Feeding Options for Patients with Dementia* (www.med.unc.edu/pcare).

The dying process is often extremely stressful for families and caregivers to observe. There are often many fears and unasked questions. Proactively discussing the natural dying process with patients, families, and caregivers can be very beneficial, including education regarding the dying patient's naturally slow cessation of food and fluid intake and the evidence that there is no apparent suffering from this decline in intake.[170,171] Families need to be educated that IV hydration is unlikely to provide comfort and may actually increase secretions and respiratory difficulty in the dying patient. Patients receiving IV hydration at the end of life often require diuretics for edema and/or respiratory distress.[172] Families, patients, and caregivers need reassurance that pain management and treatment side effects (e.g., constipation, lethargy, confusion) will be anticipated and effectively treated.

Two clinical practice guidelines from France and Canada have addressed artificial nutrition in terminally ill cancer patients.[173,174] Parenteral nutrition is recommended only in selected persons with GI obstruction due to cancer, a life expectancy of more than 6 to 12 weeks, and good functional status (Karnofsky score > 50%). These guidelines can improve decision making and reduce the inappropriate use of these interventions.[175] Educating patients, families, caregivers, and staff that artificial feeding and nutrition in persons who are terminally ill may increase suffering and may not improve outcome is recommended.[176,177]

KEY POINTS

- Protein energy undernutrition is common in older adults and is a marker of their overall state of health.
- It is also common in older adults in hospital. There, even adjusting for illness severity, it remains an independent risk of death.
- The causes of protein-energy undernutrition range from inadequate nutrient intake to a serious systemic disorder characterized by abnormal nutrient metabolism, insulin resistance, general protein catabolism, and profound anorexia.
- In those with severe undernutrition, rapid refeeding can result in the refeeding syndrome, requiring prophylaxis by permissive underfeeding and careful monitoring of glucose and electrolyte levels, including phosphorus and magnesium.
- Initiation of enteral feeding needs to consider the metabolic demand, nutrient reserve, volitional nutrient intake, and timing in relation to the overall goals of care.

For a complete list of references, please visit www.expertconsult.com.

KEY REFERENCES

2. Jensen GL, Compher C, Sullivan DH, et al: Recognizing malnutrition in adults: definitions and characteristics, screening, assessment, and team approach. JPEN J Parenter Enteral Nutr 37:802–807, 2013.
7. Bell CL, Tamura BK, Masaki KH, et al: Prevalence and measures of nutritional compromise among nursing home patients: weight loss, low body mass index, malnutrition, and feeding dependency, a systematic review of the literature. J Am Med Dir Assoc 14:94–100, 2013.
8. White JV, Stotts N, Jones SW, et al: Managing postacute malnutrition (undernutrition) risk. JPEN J Parenter Enteral Nutr 37:816–823, 2013.
21. Kortebein P, Ferrando A, Lombeida J, et al: Effect of 10 days of bed rest on skeletal muscle in healthy older adults. JAMA 297:1772–1774, 2007.
48. Simmons SF, Schnelle JF: Feeding assistance needs of long-stay nursing home residents and staff time to provide care. J Am Geriatr Soc 54:919–924, 2006.
55. Palecek EJ, Teno JM, Casarett DJ, et al: Comfort feeding only: a proposal to bring clarity to decision-making regarding difficulty with eating for persons with advanced dementia. J Am Geriatr Soc 58:580–584, 2010.
58. Teno JM, Gozalo PL, Mitchell SL, et al: Does feeding tube insertion and its timing improve survival? J Am Geriatr Soc 60:1918–1921, 2012.
114. Remington R, Hultman T: Hypodermoclysis to treat dehydration: a review of the evidence. J Am Geriatr Soc 55:2051–2055, 2007.
119. Palesty JA, Dudrick SJ: Cachexia, malnutrition, the refeeding syndrome, and lessons from Goldilocks. Surg Clin North Am 91:653–673, 2011.
136. American Geriatrics Society Ethics Committee and Clinical Practice and Models of Care Committee: American Geriatrics Society feeding tubes in advanced dementia position statement. J Am Geriatr Soc 62:1590–1593, 2014.
147. Brody H, Hermer LD, Scott LD, et al: Artificial nutrition and hydration: the evolution of ethics, evidence, and policy. J Gen Intern Med 26:1053–1058, 2011.
158. Schwartz DB, Barrocas A, Wesley JR, et al: Gastrostomy tube placement in patients with advanced dementia or near end of life. Nutr Clin Pract 29:829–840, 2014.
168. Hanson LC, Ersek M, Gilliam R, et al: Oral feeding options for people with dementia: a systematic review. J Am Geriatr Soc 59:463–472, 2011.
169. Hanson LC: Tube feeding versus assisted oral feeding for persons with dementia: using evidence to support decision-making. Ann Longterm Care 21:36–39, 2013.

110 Geriatric Dentistry: Maintaining Oral Health in the Geriatric Population

Andrea Schreiber, Lena Alsabban, Terry Fulmer, Robert Glickman

INTRODUCTION

Whereas dental textbooks address the management of medically compromised older patients—generally including a review of the basic pathophysiology of a disease, clinical signs and symptoms of the condition, common therapeutic interventions, and how the disease itself or the medications for it might affect planned dental care—in general, medical textbooks, even those on geriatric medicine, do not address the impact of oral health on the overall systemic health of a patient. Physicians are uniquely situated to screen older patients for common oral diseases.

Older adults tend to have low use rates of dental services, due perhaps to a lack of insurance coverage for these services or limited access to care secondary to infirmity. Although more than 90% of adults older than 75 years seek medical care on a regular basis, only approximately one third of them seek dental care.[1]

In a pilot study[2] investigating the physician's role in the diagnosis and management of oral disease in a geriatric population, four primary care physicians and four geriatricians were asked to identify oral conditions on 30 color slides. The rate of correct diagnosis was 55%, and appropriate treatment decisions were made 70% of the time.

In another study[3] performed to assess hospital physician knowledge and views concerning oral health in older patients, 70 respondents completed a survey and were asked to diagnose 12 different oral conditions demonstrated on clinical slides. Although 84% of respondents thought that it was important to examine the oral cavity, only 19% reported that they did so. Of the responding physicians, 56% did not feel confident in examining the oral cavity and 77% thought that that they had insufficient training to do so. Of the 70 physicians, only 2 (3%) were able to identify all 12 oral conditions depicted in the slides correctly.

The focus of this chapter will be on the maintenance of oral health for the geriatric patient and how physicians and dentists can ensure that this goal is attained. Topics to be discussed include the definition of oral health, how oral health is measured, changing dental needs of the geriatric population due to advances in medicine and dentistry, impact of oral health on systemic health, recognition and management of common oral conditions in older adults, and access to care issues for community-dwelling older adults and residents of long-term care facilities. Prevention and management of oral disease will improve systemic and oral health.[4]

Definition of Oral Health

Any discussion concerning the maintenance of oral health as a goal must start with a definition of the term.[5] Mouradian[6] defined it as "…encompassing all of the immunologic, sensory, neuromuscular and structural functions of the mouth and craniofacial complex. Oral health influences and is related to nutrition and growth, pulmonary health, speech production, communication, self-image and societal functioning." Although Mouradian was addressing the oral health needs of the pediatric population, this definition of oral health seems to apply to the population in general and to the geriatric population in particular. Conditions that adversely affect the oral and maxillofacial complex are common and pervasive in older adults and can affect an individual's general health and quality of life.

Measures of Oral Health and Function

Common measures of oral health include the number of teeth present in the mouth, presence of caries (Figure 110-1) and restorations, and presence or absence of periodontal disease (infection of the gingiva and tooth-supporting structures; Figure 110-2) and oral mucosal lesions (Figures 110-3 through 110-6). Many attempts have been made to quantify the effect of these parameters on oral function and relationship of adequate oral function to an individual's quality of life. In a literature review[7] focused on determining the relationship between dentition and oral function, four specific areas were investigated—overall masticatory function, aesthetics and psychosocial ability, posterior dental occlusal stability and support, and other functions, including taste and phonetics. In this study, 83 articles met inclusion criteria for review. Satisfactory masticatory function was linked to the total number of teeth present—specifically, 20 teeth with 9 or 10 dental contacts (upper and lower teeth in occlusion). Patients with fewer teeth and/or fewer contacts demonstrated limited masticatory function. Dental aesthetics and psychosocial satisfaction were linked to the loss of anterior teeth with variations in satisfaction noted among age groups, cultures, and socioeconomic status.

Occlusal stability was noted with three to four posterior units in individuals with a symmetric pattern of tooth loss and five to six posterior units in those with a nonsymmetric pattern of bone loss. Patients did not attribute a high value to phonetics or taste. The conclusion of the authors was that the World Health Organization's goal of maintaining 20 natural teeth throughout life as a means of ensuring an acceptable level of oral function is supported by current literature.

Measures of oral health-related quality of life (OH-QoL) assume functional and psychosocial impacts on the quality of life but exactly what is being measured by a variety of instruments designed for this purpose still remains to be clearly elucidated.[8] Many efforts have been underway to verify the validity of the QoL assessment tools used to measure the impact of oral health on QoL or to add subscales to current tools to aid in quantifying a qualitative question.[9,10] In a survey investigating the association among tooth loss, chewing ability, and association with oral and general health-related QoL issues, two survey instruments were used, the Oral Health Impact Profile and EuroQoL Visual Analogue Scale. In addition to the patient survey, functional tooth units were assessed by calibrated dentists on more than 700 Australians older than 50 years. The number of functional tooth units was positively related to chewing ability and general health, thereby reflecting the importance of oral health to general well-being.[11]

The aim of the Ontario Study of Oral Health of Older Adults (OSOHOA) was to document the natural history of oral diseases and disorders in older adults and to document the impact on physical, functional, and psychological well-being.[12] This was an

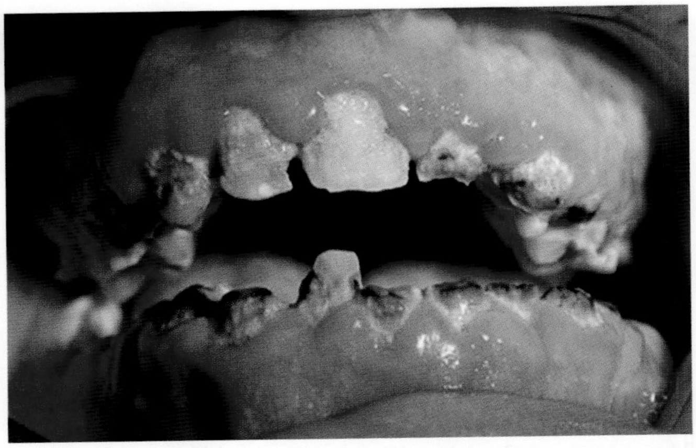

Figure 110-1. Rampant dental caries. *(From Dr. Miriam Robbins, New York University College of Dentistry, New York.)*

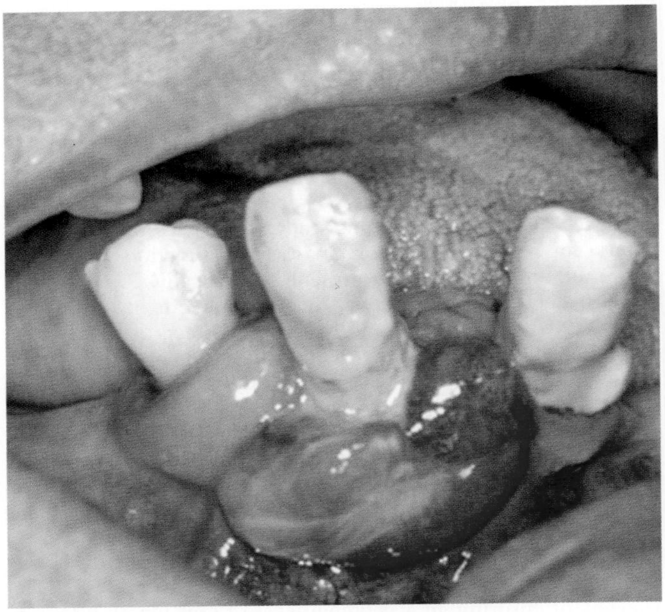

Figure 110-2. Periodontal abscess associated with bone loss around root of the tooth. *(From Dr. Miriam Robbins, New York University College of Dentistry, New York.)*

observational cohort study of a random sample of adults who were older than 50 years when recruited. The study consisted of a baseline phase and 3- and 7-year follow-ups. The ability to chew was assessed using an index of six different foods. Descriptive statistics were used to measure changes in chewing ability over time. The proportion of individuals experiencing increased chewing problems rose from 24% at baseline to 33.8% over the 7-year period. An increased prevalence and severity of chewing dysfunction was most notable for edentulous patients.

Other studies have noted that approximately one third of older adults have trouble biting some foods and that this percentage increases with advancing age and number of teeth missing.[13] Chewing ability or lack thereof can influence food choices and result in malnutrition in community dwelling and long-term care residents (Figure 110-7). Weight loss and poor nutrition in long-term care facilities have been linked to chewing problems.[14,15]

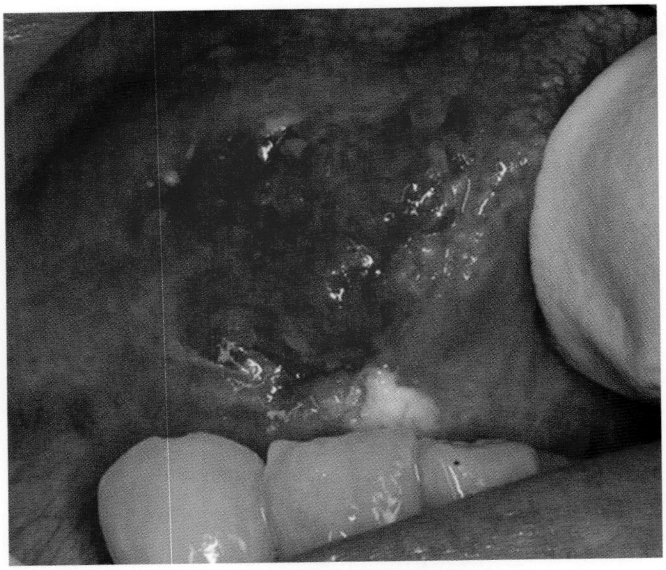

Figure 110-3. Oral dysplasias—right lateral border of the tongue. *(From Dr. Miriam Robbins, New York University College of Dentistry, New York.)*

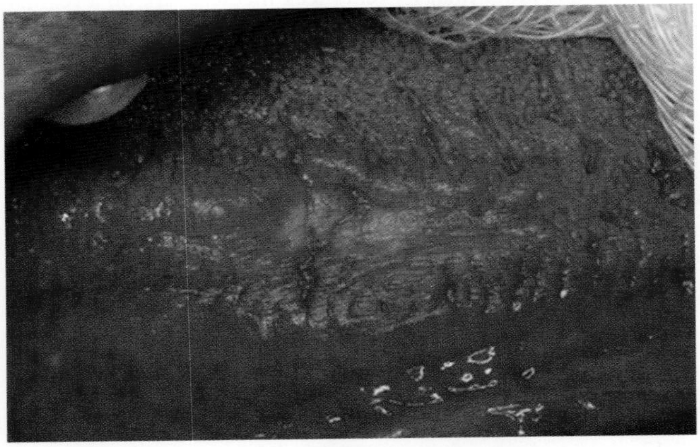

Figure 110-4. Leukoplakia or white lesion—left lateral border of the tongue. *(From Dr. Miriam Robbins, New York University College of Dentistry, New York.)*

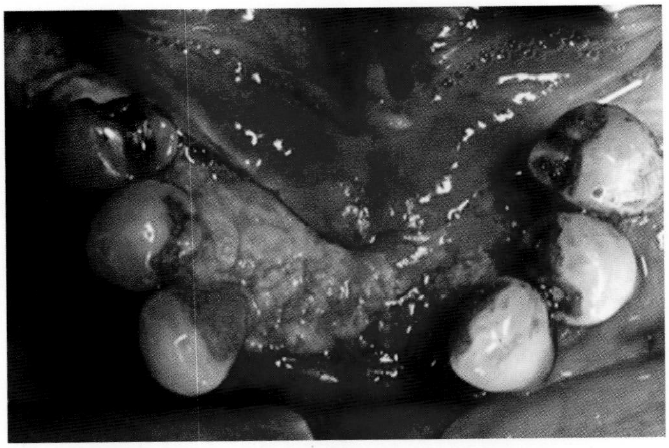

Figure 110-5. Squamous cell carcinoma—floor of the mouth. *(From Dr. Miriam Robbins, New York University College of Dentistry, New York.)*

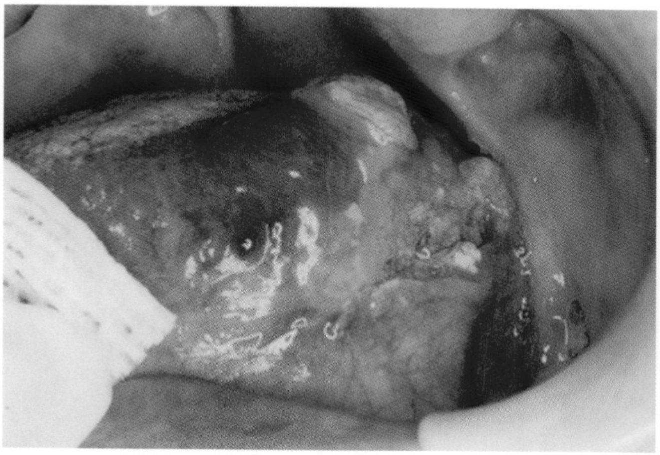

Figure 110-6. Squamous cell carcinoma—left lateral border of the tongue. *(From Dr. Miriam Robbins, New York University College of Dentistry, New York.)*

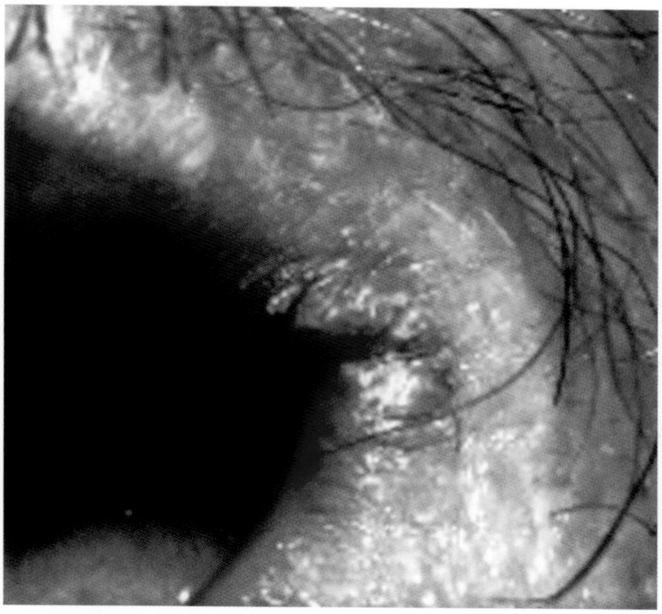

Figure 110-7. Angular cheilitis caused by loss of dentition, poor diet, and candidiasis. *(From Dr. Miriam Robbins, New York University College of Dentistry, New York.)*

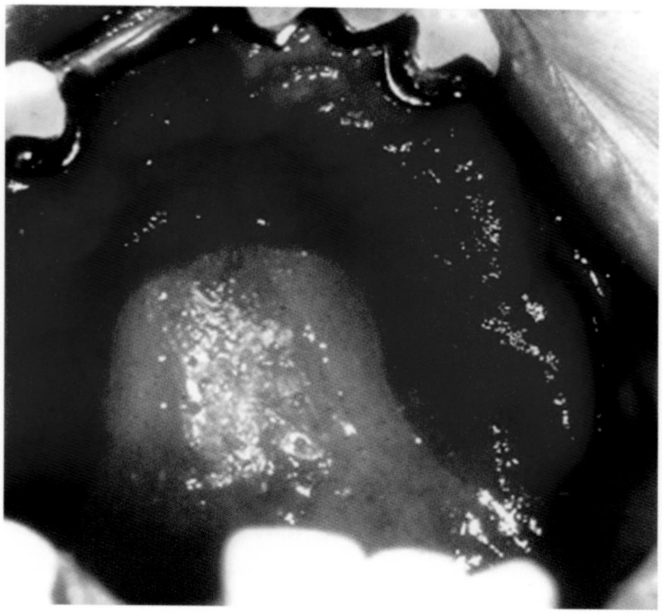

Figure 110-8. Denture stomatitis—ill-fitting denture and candidiasis. *(From Dr. Miriam Robbins, New York University College of Dentistry, New York.)*

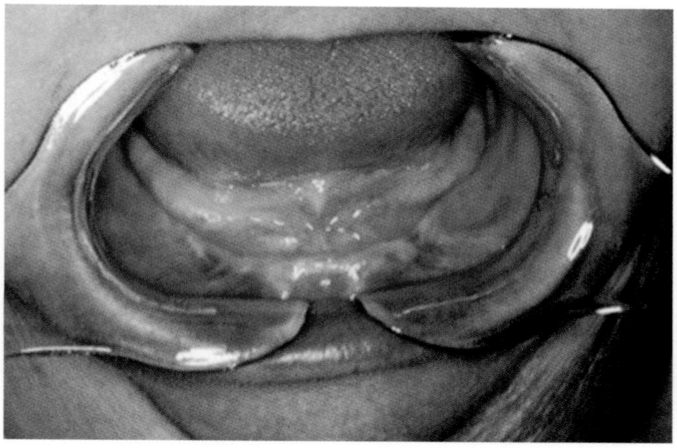

Figure 110-9. Atrophic mandible—early loss of dentition and long-term denture wear. *(From Dr. Kenneth Fleisher, New York University College of Dentistry, New York.)*

Changing Need for Dental Care in Geriatric Patients

Advances in dental research have resulted in a lower incidence of tooth loss and caries in the general population as a result of the widespread use of fluoride, patient education, and dental hygiene programs.[16] Simply put, people are living longer with more teeth. The fully edentulous octogenarian is and will continue to be less frequently encountered in the twenty-first century. However, edentulous patients, despite the absence of teeth, may have a host of problems that can adversely affect oral and systemic health, including denture or non–denture-related soft tissue lesions, oral candidiasis, malnutrition from ill-fitting dentures (Figure 110-8) or lack of thereof, resorption under existing dentures (Figure 110-9), gastrointestinal problems, masticatory insufficiency, swallowing disorders, and aspiration pneumonia. They are still susceptible to mucosal diseases (see Figures 110-3 and 110-4) and oral cancers (see Figures 110-5 and 110-6), despite the absence of teeth. The Surgeon General's Report on Oral Health in America in 2000 cited 30,000 new diagnoses of oral cancer each year, mainly in individuals with a median age in the sixth decade of life.[17]

The types of problems encountered by a dentate or partially edentulous geriatric patient may include dental caries, chronic facial pain and/or temporomandibular dysfunction, and benign or malignant lesions of the oral mucosa or jaws. Periodontal disease, an inflammatory disorder that results in alveolar bone loss and chronic tissue inflammation (Figure 110-10), is a primary cause of tooth loss in older adults, which has been shown to have a strong association with the pathophysiology of certain systemic diseases, including cardiovascular disease, cerebrovascular disease (CVD), and diabetes mellitus.[18] Patients with periodontal disease are up to twice as likely to develop cardiovascular disease.[19] Medications taken for comorbid conditions may result in decreased salivary flow, which in turn affects the ability to chew, swallow,

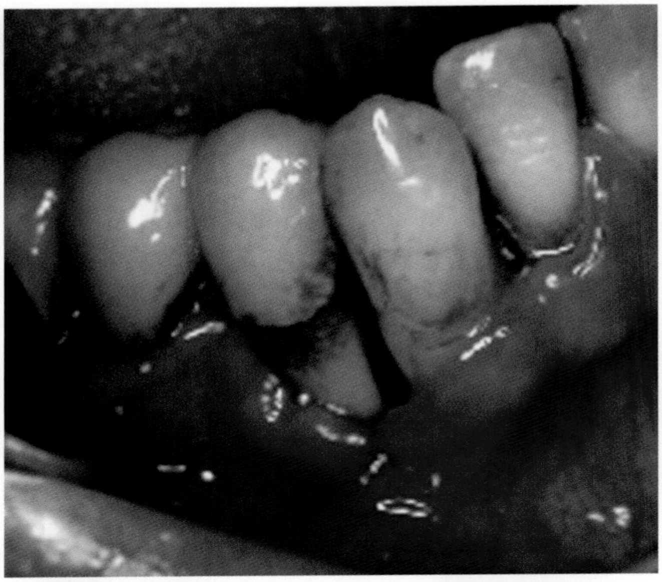

Figure 110-10. Severe periodontal bone loss. *(From Dr. Miriam Robbins, New York University College of Dentistry, New York.)*

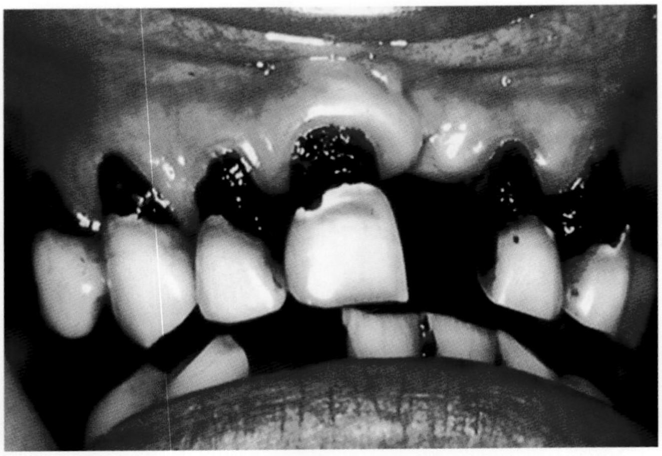

Figure 110-11. Severe cervical decay. *(From Dr. Miriam Robbins, New York University College of Dentistry, New York.)*

and cleanse the oral cavity. Additionally, xerostomia may be accompanied by painful or burning sensations. Finally, maxillofacial trauma as a result of gait disturbance, neuromuscular disease or, in some cases, elder abuse, is another factor affecting the oral health of the geriatric population.[5]

As advances in medical research result in increasing patient life span, older adults have become the fastest growing portion of the population. In the United States, population projections indicate that by the year 2030 more than 20% of the population will be 65 years of age or older.[20] Because concurrent advances in dental research have resulted in less tooth loss in older adults, these patients will require an increased need for dental care in the future, most especially with the advent of dental implants leading to less reliance on conventional dentures as a primary form of treatment. Although the trend is toward less tooth loss in older adults, there are still regional demographic variations, with higher levels of edentulism in areas of lower socioeconomic status. With increased tooth retention comes the continued risk of recurrent and cervical caries. The pattern of caries differs in the geriatric versus the general population in that coronal (chewing surface) caries are less frequent than root caries. Root or cervical caries (Figure 110-11) are characterized by rapid progression and increased difficulty in restoration, often necessitating extraction (see Figure 110-1).[20,21]

Dentists are now challenged with treating an increasing number of community-dwelling older adults with chronic but stable systemic diseases, along with caring for the dental needs of more debilitated and frail older adults, with physiologic and cognitive impairments. According to the Surgeon General's report in 2000, more than 20% of home-bound or institutionalized older adults require emergency dental care annually. As this population increases, so too will the need for care.[17]

Oral Health Impact on Systemic Health

The well-established links between oral and systemic diseases have served as a wake-up call to improve oral hygiene and access to dental care for older patients in long-term care facilities.[22,23] One such risk is aspiration pneumonia, which has long been recognized as a common cause of death in infirm homebound and long-term care facility residents. Bacterial pneumonia is directly linked to aspiration as a result of dysphagia and/or poor oral hygiene and the elevated numbers of respiratory pathogens in oropharyngeal secretions. Attention to improved oral hygiene is a method or strategy to decrease the incidence of bacterial pneumonia in susceptible populations.[24]

The main causes of community-acquired pneumonia are *Streptococcus pneumoniae* and *Haemophilus influenzae*. The organisms usually associated with hospital-acquired pneumonia are *Staphylococcus aureus* and *Pseudomonas aeruginosa*. Hospital-acquired pneumonia commonly occurs in frail older adults with a compromised immune system.

Aspiration is most likely to occur in patients with functional dependence on oral care and feeding.[25,26] Studies have demonstrated increased levels of bacteria in the oral secretions of institutionalized versus home-dwelling older adults.[27] Aspiration usually occurs with feeding or during sleep. The risk of developing an infection subsequent to aspiration depends on the state of the individual's host defenses—cough reflex, mucociliary adequacy, and cellular immunity—and on the type and volume of aspirate. The higher the bacterial load of the aspirate and the lower the host defenses, the greater the risk.[28]

Oral care for functionally dependent older patients in long-term care facilities has been documented as being sorely lacking in numerous studies.[29,30] Poor oral hygiene leads to the proliferation of dental plaque, which is a biofilm responsible for dental and periodontal disease (see Figure 110-2). As the biofilm matures, organism shedding is facilitated. Reduced salivary flow in older adults as a consequence of medications, aging, or disease may also enhance microbial growth in the oral cavity. Similarly, long-term use of broad-spectrum antibiotics may contribute to the overgrowth of certain organisms in the oral cavity.

A study by Adachi and colleagues[31] investigated the incidence of fever higher than 37.8° C and aspiration pneumonia in the residents of two nursing homes for 2 years. Patients who received professional oral health care were compared with patients who did not. The prevalence of fevers and rate of aspiration pneumonia were significantly lower in the patient group that received professional oral health care than in the group that did not. It has been demonstrated that improved oral hygiene efforts in long-term care facilities result in a decreased incidence of fevers and pneumonia deaths. Effects of improved oral health care on other systemic diseases, such as cerebrovascular accident, diabetes mellitus, and myocardial infarction, have yet to be fully investigated.

Desvarieux and associates[32] have investigated the relationship between periodontal disease and tooth loss with subclinical atherosclerosis. Subjects received comprehensive periodontal examination, a carotid scan, and evaluation of cardiovascular disease risk factors. A significant association was noted between observed prevalence of carotid plaque formation and the number of teeth missing. Approximately 60% of individuals missing more than 10 teeth demonstrated carotid artery plaque, and this association was greatest among patients older than 65 years. The mechanisms underlying the relationship between periodontal disease and cardiovascular disease are not well understood but are likely due to chronic bacteremia and elevated inflammatory markers. Interestingly, in a follow-up study, gender variations were noted in the relationship between periodontal disease, tooth loss, and subclinical atherosclerosis, with men being affected more frequently than women.[33]

The relationship between cardiovascular disease and stroke and periodontal disease has been the object of numerous studies in the last decade, with most focusing on the role of inflammatory markers, such as C-reactive protein (CRP), interleukin, and tumor necrosis factor. Periodontal disease results in elevations of CRP and interleukin levels, but a clear link between periodontal disease and the pathogenesis has yet to be elucidated. Studies have been conducted to explore the possible link between periodontal health and cardiovascular disease. Bartova and coworkers have concluded that circulating microorganisms or their products may promote pathogenesis and enhance local inflammatory changes in vessel walls leading to clotting and clot formation, a potential risk factor for atherosclerosis development.[34]

Kalburgi and colleagues noted that periodontitis may cause systemic changes in plasma levels of CRP and numbers of circulating leukocytes and neutrophils. CRP, leukocyte, and neutrophil levels have been positively correlated with the severity of periodontitis. Thus, periodontitis, a common chronic condition, may predispose affected patients to CVD by increasing the levels of systemic markers of inflammation, which may contribute to the development of atherosclerosis.[35]

The therapeutic implications for such an association are significant, given the prevalence of periodontal disease in the general population and the relative ease with which oral hygiene improvement can be accomplished. Other risk factors for the development of CVD, such as gender, hypertension, obesity, hyperlipidemia, and smoking, are less readily addressed and modified. Animal studies have indicated that chronic infections lead to increased systemic inflammation and the accelerated development of atherosclerotic plaque.[36]

The results of the meta-analysis of five prospective cohort studies involving more than 85,000 patients have indicated that patients with periodontal disease had a 1.14 times higher risk of developing cardiovascular disease than patients without periodontal disease. The highest risk (1.24) was assigned to individuals with fewer than 10 remaining teeth. A meta-analysis of five case-control studies involving more than 1400 individuals demonstrated an even higher risk of individuals with periodontal disease developing CVD.[37]

Several studies have been conducted to determine whether there is a relationship among periodontal disease, treatment, and diabetic control. Although some results were optimistic, Engebretson and associates found that nonsurgical periodontal therapy did not improve glycemic control in patients with type 2 diabetes and moderate to advanced chronic periodontitis. Thus, nonsurgical periodontal treatment in patients with diabetes for the purpose of lowering levels of hemoglobin A_{1c} (HbA_{1c}) cannot be supported at this time.[38]

Issues Facing Community Dwelling Versus Long-Term Care Facility Residents

Ohrui and colleagues[39] have studied more than 400 Japanese nursing home residents and have evaluated the relationship between dental status and mortality. Participants were divided into three groups—individuals with adequate dentition, edentulous individuals who wore full dentures, and individuals without adequate dentition and without a dental prosthesis. All groups were followed for 5 years. The 2- and 5-year risks for mortality were greater for the functionally edentulous individuals than for the other groups. It was concluded that the dental status of institutionalized older adults should be systematically evaluated and optimized.

Older patients with dementia may demonstrate difficulty with activities of daily life, including oral care and, as such, they pose unique challenges to caregivers in the community and in institutions. Connell and coworkers[40] have evaluated changes in the nursing home environment that could foster improved oral health care. These changes included modification of the physical environment to compensate for cognitive defects and physical incapacity and staff instruction on cues to overcome cognitive and noncognitive deficits. Improved visual cues, single step cues, and closing doors to decrease distractions all resulted in improved oral hygiene status. Improved wheelchair access to sinks, access to mirrors, and change from conventional toothbrushes to those designed with better-grip handles also resulted in improved oral hygiene.

A study of 192 nursing home residents investigating oral health status, cognitive function, and the need for dental treatment, as assessed by dental professionals and nursing staff, was performed by Nordenram and Ljunggren.[41] The results indicated that dentate status coupled with a loss of cognitive function were predictive for the need for oral treatment. Patients with the best cognitive function were found to have better chewing ability; 30% of patients were found to have a functional chewing deficit based on lack of dentures, ill-fitting dentures, or poor dental status. Assessment of need by staff versus dental practitioners was compared; clinical dental function and oral hygiene were assessed by both groups. The two groups varied widely in their assessment of the oral health status of the nursing home residents—the dentists found that 93% of residents required oral hygiene assistance, whereas the nursing assessment was that only 11% of the population required such aid. Such disparity in findings between nursing home staff and dentists clearly indicates the need for improved training in the recognition of oral hygiene neglect and related oral health conditions.

Physical disability, cognitive impairment, or a combination of the two can result in making nursing home residents who are no longer functionally independent vulnerable to poor oral health. Numerous studies have documented the need for improved oral health care for long-term care residents and homebound older adults. Reports of severe periodontal disease, untreated root caries, and poor oral hygiene on remaining teeth and on dentures abound in the literature. Frenkel and colleagues[75] have reported that more than 70% of nursing home residents had not seen a dentist in 5 years and that more than 20% reported untreated dental problems.

Murray and associates[42] have observed soft tissue lesions and dry mouth in 6% of the nursing home population that they studied. Oral hygiene, as measured by the amount of calculus on crowns of teeth or on dentures, increased with patient age and length of time of denture wear. Less than 25% of nursing home patients had minimal or no calculus.

In an article reviewing the prevalence and consequences of poor oral health care or lack of care in geriatric patients in long-term care facilities, Pino and coworkers[43] have concluded that the effects on the general health and well-being of these patients were far-reaching. Poor oral hygiene or oral health neglect may result in problems that range from socially embarrassing to life-threatening. Systemic complications, including deep fascial space infections, endocarditis, cavernous sinus thrombosis, and brain abscesses, are well documented in dental and medical literature.

Nutritional status, conversing, smiling, and eating are all dependent on adequate oral health.

Institutionalized older adults are not the only ones at risk. Studies of oral health status in the United States and Europe have documented the need for attention to oral health care in older adults. Tooth loss results in masticatory insufficiency, which can result in swallowing and digestive disorders in addition to poor diet due to the need to alter food choices. Periodontal disease may present clinically with erythematous, edematous gingival tissue associated with bleeding, tooth mobility, and fetid oris locally (see Figure 110-2) and aspiration pneumonia and local and distant spread of infection systemically.[43]

In a study evaluating functional tooth number (≥10) and overall mortality in more than 500 individuals older than 40 years who were followed for 15 years, Fukai and colleagues[44] found that adults older than 80 years demonstrated increased mortality and decreased functional tooth number in comparison to the other groups. An increased risk of malnutrition was assessed in 130 community-dwelling older adults in Japan using the Mini Nutritional Assessment (MNA) tool. Factors affecting an increasing risk of malnutrition included cognitive impairment, physical disability, poor oral health status, and difficulty with meal preparation, resulting in an unbalanced diet. Of the participants, 12% were found to be at risk for malnutrition.[45]

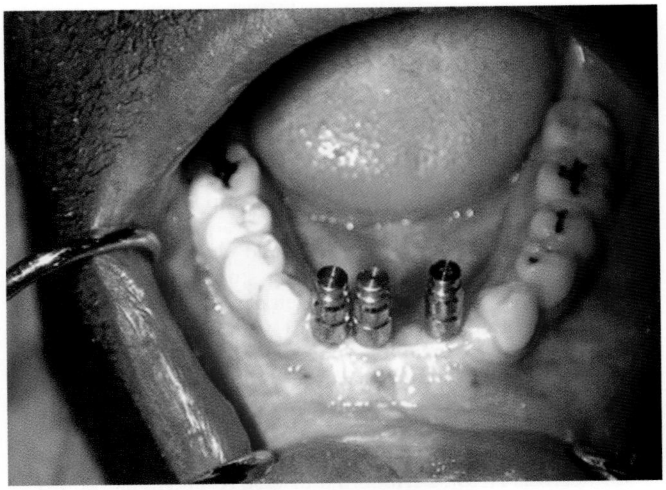

Figure 110-12. Dental implants before fabrication of prosthesis and/or bridge. *(From Dr. Miriam Robbins, New York University College of Dentistry, New York.)*

RECOGNITION AND MANAGEMENT OF COMMON ORAL CONDITIONS IN OLDER ADULTS

Caries and Periodontal Disease

Although the incidence of caries (tooth decay) is highest in children and young adults, dentate geriatric patients are not immune from the development of these lesions. To the contrary, cervical or root caries and recurrent caries under existing restorations are common in older dentate patients. Cervical caries tend to progress more rapidly than caries on occlusal surfaces, and restoration of teeth with cervical caries is often more difficult, ultimately leading to extraction. Partially edentulous older adults often alter their diets to softer consistency foods, which are high in carbohydrates and increase the chance of caries formation, especially when coupled with inadequate home care. The Centers for Disease Control and Prevention (CDC) has estimated that 30% of adults older than 65 years have untreated caries and that 94% of adults with one or more natural teeth have experienced caries.[46]

Periodontal disease is a chronic inflammatory process involving the gingiva and alveolar bone, which ultimately results in gingival erythema, edema, bleeding, recession, and loss of alveolar bone resulting in tooth mobility and, ultimately, tooth loss. In a study of more than 300 patients aged 65 to 95 years, Stabholz and associates[47] found that caries accounted for 30% of extractions and periodontal disease accounted for 65% of extractions. In another study, which followed 179 geriatric patients at three long-term care facilities over a period of 30 months, a logistic regression demonstrated that the relative risk of a worsening periodontal condition or loss of teeth was twice as high for patients not enrolled in a preventive program than for those that were.[48] The benefit of an oral health preventive program for severely frail older adults or terminal patients appears to demonstrate no significant improvement.[49]

Edentulism, Partial Edentulism, Dentures, and Implants

Caries and periodontal disease, left untreated, are the primary causes of tooth loss. Although the number of teeth present is a common tool used in evaluating oral health and masticatory function, evaluation of functional tooth units, which involves description of the arrangement and number of remaining teeth, is perhaps a more reliable tool to evaluate masticatory function in older adults. Hildebrandt and coworkers[50] have found that a low number of functional tooth units results in food avoidance patterns and swallowing of coarser boluses of incompletely chewed food.

The fabrication of full or partial dentures has long been the primary method of ensuring masticatory sufficiency in adults with missing teeth. Long-term use of these prostheses often leads to resorption of alveolar bone and associated soft tissue changes, including ulcerations and hypertrophic areas. This ultimately results in the need for dentures to be refitted continuously. In some cases, resorption may be so severe as to obviate the fabrication of stable prostheses. The advent of dental implants (Figure 110-12) and the ability to provide implant-supported bridges and dentures have improved the masticatory capabilities, diet, and nutrition of countless adults in the last 2 decades. The greatest benefit appears to be for patients with the most ridge resorption.[51] Implant-supported prostheses may demonstrate secondary benefits, such as improvements in facial aesthetics and lip support, which complement improvements in masticatory function.[52] In a survey of 125 patients, loss of function was the most common complaint of wearers of full dentures, whereas patients with fixed prostheses had fewer complaints.[53]

Before the advent of implants for the treatment of full or partial edentulism, removable dental prostheses were the primary means of oral rehabilitative care. Full and partial dentures did and do provide for improvements in mastication, swallowing, speech, and facial aesthetics. Implant-supported prostheses provide a more comfortable, functional, and stable alternative to conventional dentures. A study[54] was conducted of 15 patients older than 60 years who were treated with implant-supported lower dentures and then evaluated for impact of this treatment on their QoL. The reported benefits of this treatment included improvements in eating, speaking, and social interactions.

Dental implants to treat full or partially edentulous conditions have become a common treatment option, with more than a 90% success rate reported at 10 years. Neither advanced age nor systemic disease are absolute contraindications to implant placement.[55] Some studies appear to have demonstrated an increased risk of implant failure associated with diabetes mellitus, smoking, oncologic treatment (e.g., chemotherapy, head and neck radiation), and postmenopausal hormone therapy.[56] Patients should be evaluated as candidates for implants based on the level of control of their systemic disease, ability to withstand surgical stress, life expectancy, and QoL.[57] Evidence of implant failure due to systemic disease is not prevalent.[58]

Grant and Kraut[59] placed 160 implants in the maxillas and mandibles of 47 patients older than 79 years, with a median age of 89 years. All but one of the implants healed successfully. The authors concluded that geriatric patients in stable medical condition are suitable implant patients. It appears that concerns about the success of osseointegration in older patients in regard to bone remodeling and resorption and decreased soft tissue response may not be entirely warranted. There is no strong body of evidence to support an increased failure rate of implants based on advanced patient age. A review of the literature regarding the success of implants in older patients has revealed that old age, in and of itself, is not a significant concern.[60] Al Jabbari and associates[61] concluded that even limitation in oral hygiene capacity in older adults is not a contraindication to implant placement. Treating dentists need to first consider whether the patient is in optimal condition to withstand the procedure and be less concerned about whether osseointegration is likely to occur in the older patient.

Saliva and Salivary Glands

Xerostomia may occur with medication use, chemotherapy, radiation therapy for head and neck cancer, or as a symptom of Sjögren syndrome. Common sequelae include an inability to tolerate a dental prosthesis, difficulty swallowing, alteration of nutritional status, and increased incidence of dental caries because of changes in the dental plaque biofilm. The decreased ability to chew comfortably can result in malnutrition and decreased enjoyment of food and the social interaction of meals.[62] Dry mouth is a common complaint in older adults, possibly secondary to polypharmacy for multiple comorbid conditions. It is more common among patients who take several medications, especially if antipsychotics are included.[63]

Dry mouth or xerostomia has a number of possible causes, including smoking, use of alcohol or caffeinated beverages, mouth breathing, and a host of medications. Some drugs may cause the sensation of dry mouth, whereas others may result in measurable hyposalivation.[64] The drugs that are most commonly implicated in dry mouth are antipsychotics, tricyclic antidepressants, β-blockers, antihistamines, and atropine.[65] Advancing age and medication use were shown to be related to objective evidence of hyposalivation, whereas female gender and psychiatric issues were strongly correlated to subjective complaints of oral dryness.[66]

No specific medication has been singled out as being more xerogenic, but polypharmacy does increase the likelihood of dryness. The severity of a dryness complaint appears to be increased with female gender and antianginal, antiasthma, and antidepressant medications.[67]

Drugs can affect salivary flow rate or composition by antagonizing or mimicking any of the regulatory aspects of salivation. The mechanism of action of xerogenic drugs may be the result of an anticholinergic action mediated by parasympathetic (M3 muscarinic receptor) neurotransmission to the salivary glands.[62] Tricyclic antidepressants have been shown to reduce salivary flow, whereas selective serotonin release inhibitors do not. This lower incidence of dry mouth complaint is thought to be related to the lower anticholinergic effects of this group of medications. Approximately 25% of patients on tricyclics develop a complaint of dry mouth. Muscarinic receptor antagonists, such as oxybutynin, which are used to treat the overactive bladder symptoms of frequency and urgency, with or without incontinence, are nonspecific for the bladder and also cause dry mouth. Tolterodine demonstrates in vivo selectivity for the bladder over the salivary glands and may be a good choice for older patients who are taking other xerogenic medications.

Anticholinesterase inhibitors such as donepezil, used in the treatment of Alzheimer disease, may also induce dry mouth. Many antihypertensive agents, including β-blockers, angiotensin-converting enzyme (ACE) inhibitors, and α-methyldopa, have been associated with complaints of dry mouth.

A study of 175 home-dwelling older patients[63] who were hospitalized for an acute change in health status were compared with 252 outpatients. The parameters evaluated included medical diagnosis, prescribed medications, oral examinations, and analysis of saliva samples. Of these older patients, 63% of hospitalized patients and 57% of outpatients complained of dry mouth, whereas 13% of hospitalized patients and 18% of outpatients complained of burning mouth. There were no differences in the biochemical analysis of the saliva between the two groups. The complaint of dry mouth was associated with polypharmacy, whereas this was not the case for the complaint of burning mouth. Dry mouth and burning mouth were rarely reported simultaneously.

The management of dry mouth is challenging, and saliva substitutes have been the mainstay of treatment for many years, along with alcohol-free mouth rinses, increased water intake, lubricating gels, and alteration of food consistency (blenderized diet). Because dentate patients diagnosed with xerostomia are prone to an increased incidence of caries, a comprehensive and aggressive caries monitoring protocol should be instituted, including fluoride treatments, sealants, and use of sugar-free lubricating gum. Stimulation of salivary secretion with yohimbine, an α_2-adrenoreceptor antagonist, has been somewhat effective in patients being treated with psychotropic drugs. Another strategy for patients on multiple medications is for physicians to evaluate the xerogenic potential of each medication prescribed and to alter the medication regimen, if possible. A persistent dry mouth may necessitate alteration of drug dose or prescription.[63]

Oral Lesions

Oral mucosa possesses an essential protective function, which is presumed to diminish with age as the tissue becomes more permeable. This theory appears to be supported by the reported increased incidence of oral lesions with advancing age.[68] However, Wolff and coworkers[69] have found that the incidence of oral mucosal lesions in healthy older adults was not significantly higher than that of the general population. Other factors contributing to the development of oral mucosal lesions include general health and nutrition status, medication usage, and presence of ill-fitting dentures.

Common oral mucosal conditions of older denture wearers include candidiasis (Figure 110-13), epulis fissuratum (soft tissue hyperplasia), traumatic ulcers, angular cheilitis (see Figure 110-7), and coated tongue. Although most oral mucosal lesions appear to be benign, premalignant and malignant lesions are also present, usually in the form of leukoplakias (see Figure 110-4), erythroplakias, and squamous cell carcinomas (see Figure 110-6).

Denture stomatitis is a generally asymptomatic inflammatory process found on mucosal surfaces underlying full or partial removable dentures (see Figure 110-8), with a commonly reported prevalence of 10% to 75% of denture wearers.[70] Causative factors for the development of denture-related stomatitis include trauma from ill-fitting dentures, poor oral hygiene, reduced vertical dimension (atrophy), continuous use of prosthesis, unstable occlusion, hyposalivation, and nutritional deficiency. The increased incidence of lesions was found to be associated with a greater number of years of denture use. Interestingly, advanced age and high alcohol consumption did not correlate with incidence of these lesions.[71]

A retrospective study of 4098 adults investigating the prevalence of oral lesions and association of those lesions with age,

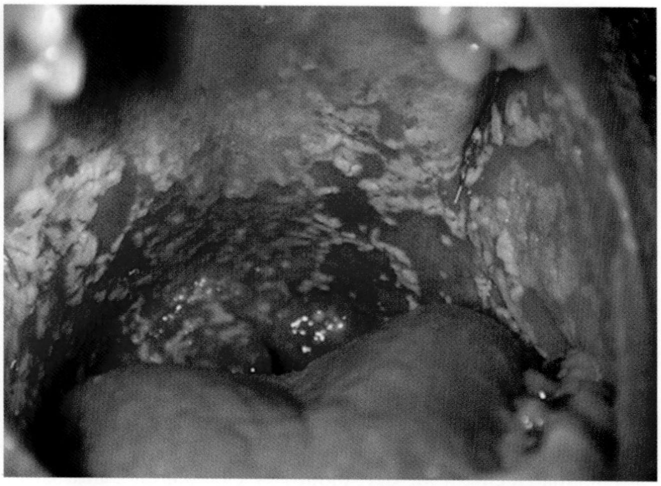

Figure 110-13. Oral candidiasis. Note the striae throughout, indicative of fungal infection. *(From Dr. Miriam Robbins, New York University College of Dentistry, New York.)*

dentures, tobacco, or alcohol use, found that the overall prevalence of oral mucosal lesions appears to be linked to risk behaviors and age. More than 27% of the men and 22% of the women were noted to have a mucosal lesion. The use of alcohol and tobacco appeared to be linked to the incidence of leukoplakia, nicotinic stomatitis, and frictional lesions. Denture-related lesions, in the form of candidiasis and traumatic and frictional lesions, appeared to be the most prevalent.[72]

The incidence of oral mucosal lesions[73] in a Thai population of 500 adults older than 60 years was investigated in relation to the type of lesion, age, gender, and presence or absence of dentures. The incidence of oral mucosal lesions in this study population was 83.6%, with no significant gender difference. The incidence of oral mucosal lesions appeared to increase with advancing age and denture use. The three most prevalent oral mucosal conditions were traumatic ulcers, fissured tongue, and lingual varices. Premalignant lesions were detected in 5% of subjects, and squamous cell carcinoma was detected in less than 1% of subjects.

In one study,[74] older patients, especially women, appeared to be at increased risk of developing malignant lesions and, curiously, those who never smoked appeared to be at greater risk. Oral squamous cell carcinoma usually occurred on the ventral and lateral tongue, floor of the mouth, and retromolar regions. Angular cheilitis is characterized by cracking fissures at the commissures of the lips, which may be caused by saliva accumulation in this region secondary to ill-fitting dentures, candida infections, or vitamin deficiencies (vitamin B; see Figure 110-7). Discomfort with eating and speaking are often attendant complaints. Treatment is aimed at the cause and may include topical antifungal ointments, vitamin supplements, dietary changes, and denture adjustments or, in some cases, the fabrication of new dentures or implant-supported prostheses.

Poor oral hygiene, immune compromise, or both can lead to an overgrowth of candida on dentures, resulting in denture stomatitis and oral-pharyngeal candidiasis (see Figure 110-13). It is frequently asymptomatic and may be found on routine examination. On occasion, complaints of a painful or burning sensation may be elicited. Common clinical characteristics include erythema or pinpoint hyperemic areas in denture-bearing locations. Frank fungal colonies are also sometimes observed. If the affected region is limited to the denture-bearing areas, dentures should be routinely brushed and may be soaked in chlorhexidine or a dilute hypochlorite solution. In more extensive areas, oral antifungal troches are administered. Denture stomatitis may occur in up to 50% of edentulous patients who wear full dentures.[75]

Oral cancer occurs most frequently in older adults, usually in or after the sixth decade of life, with more than 95% of cases occurring in individuals older than 45 years.[20,76] These cancers account for approximately 3% of all cancers in the United States. The National Institute of Dental and Craniofacial Research has estimated that more than 28,000 Americans will be diagnosed with oral cancer and that 7,000 individuals will die from it this year. Oral cancer affects men more frequently than women by a ratio of approximately 2 : 1. Tobacco and alcohol use remain primary risk factors for the development of oral cancers, with the risks increasing with increased usage of either or both substances. The 5-year survival rate remains at 59%.[77]

Early detection remains the key to an improved prognosis. Common clinical signs and symptoms include nonhealing ulcers and areas of leukoplakia, erythroplakia, or mixed lesions. Lesions that do not resolve on removal of a suspected irritant or within a few weeks of detection should be biopsied because histologic evaluation is necessary to determine if any dysplastic or malignant changes are evident. If a malignancy is detected, treatment is then predicated on the staging of such lesions and may involve surgical ablation, chemotherapy, radiation therapy, reconstruction with vascularized grafts, and oral rehabilitation.

Medication Related Osteonecrosis of the Jaw

Recently there has been a growing number of osteonecrosis cases involving the maxilla and mandible associated with medications prescribed for older patients (e.g., antiresorptive medications, bisphosphonates, antiangiogenic agents), known as medication-related osteonecrosis of the jaw (MRONJ). The America Association of Oral and Maxillofacial Surgeons Special Committee on MRONJ has supported a multidisciplinary approach to the treatment of patients who benefit from antiresorptive or antiangiogenic medications. This approach would include consultation with an appropriate dental professional when it is determined that a patient would benefit from an antiresorptive or antiangiogenic drug. There is considerable support for early screening and initiation of appropriate dental care, which would not only decrease the incidence of MRONJ but also accrue the benefits that all patients enjoy with optimum oral health.[78]

CONCLUSION

Compromised oral health may result in a variety of illnesses and conditions that can adversely impact an individual's quality of life or life span. Engaging in conversation, enjoying a good meal, kissing a loved one, smiling, and laughing—many of life's little pleasures—require a functioning and aesthetically acceptable dentition. The ability to engage in these activities improves socialization, self-esteem, and quality of life for all but the most infirm and cognitively impaired individuals. Additional benefits of good oral health on an individual's systemic health include improved diet and nutrition and decreased frequency of aspiration pneumonia in frail older adults. The association between periodontal disease and CVD, stroke, diabetes, and myocardial infarction may prove to have the most far-reaching health benefit.

The key to maintaining oral health in older adults remains timely access to care. Community-dwelling dependent older adults, homebound frail older adults, and long-term care facility residents face many more obstacles to receiving dental care than healthy, independent older adults. Therefore, physicians play a primary and crucial role in ensuring adequate oral health for these individuals. Familiarity with common oral conditions afflicting dentate and edentulous older adults is the first and most basic step in ensuring their improved oral health.

KEY POINTS

- Impact on quality of life: Conditions that adversely affect the oral and maxillofacial complex are common and pervasive in older adults and can affect an individual's general health and quality of life.
- Oral health impact on systemic health: Poor oral health and loss of teeth adversely affect nutritional status and gastrointestinal health by limiting food choices secondary to masticatory insufficiency.
- Recognition and management of common oral diseases of older adults: The link between oral and systemic disease has been reinforced, specifically in relationship to cardiovascular disease. The risk of aspiration pneumonia in nursing home residents has been demonstrated to be decreased with improvements in oral hygiene care.
- The America Association of Oral and Maxillofacial Surgeons Special Committee on Medication-Related Osteonecrosis of the Jaw (MRONJ) supports a multidisciplinary approach to the treatment of patients who benefit from antiresorptive or antiangiogenic medications, including consultation with an appropriate dental professional.
- Early screening and initiation of appropriate dental care: This would not only decrease the incidence of ONJ, but also accrue the benefits that all patients enjoy with optimum oral health.

For a complete list of references, please visit www.expertconsult.com.

KEY REFERENCES

1. Pyle MA, Terezhalmy GT: Oral disease in the geriatric patient: the physician's role. Cleve Clin J Med 62:218–226, 1995.
2. Jones T, Siegel MJ, Schneider JR: Recognition and management of oral health problems in older adults by physicians: a pilot study. J Am Board Fam Pract 11:474–477, 1998.
3. Morgan R, Tsang J, Harrington N, et al: Survey of hospital doctors' attitudes and knowledge of oral conditions in older patients. Postgrad Med J 77:392–394, 2001.
11. Brennan D, Spencer A, Roberts-Thomson KF: Tooth loss, chewing ability and quality of life. Qual Life Res 17:227–235, 2008.
22. Shay K: Infectious complications of dental and periodontal diseases in the elderly population. Clin Infect Dis 34:1215–1223, 2002.
23. Loesche WJ, Lopatin DE: Interactions between periodontal disease, medical diseases and immunity in the older individual. Periodontol 1998:80–105, 2000.
26. Terpenning MS, Taylor GW, Lopatin DE, et al: Aspiration pneumonia: dental and oral risk factors in an older veteran population. J Am Geriatr Soc 49:557–563, 2001.
27. Terpenning MS, Bretz W, Lopatin D, et al: Bacterial colonization of saliva and plaque in the elderly. Clin Infect Dis 16(Suppl 4):5314–5316, 1993.
33. Desvarieux M, Schwahn C, Volzke H, et al: Gender differences in the relationship between periodontal disease, tooth loss and atherosclerosis. Stroke 35:2029–2035, 2004.
34. Bartova J, Sommerova P, Lyuya-Mi Y, et al: Periodontitis as a risk factor of atherosclerosis. J Immunol Res 2014:636893, 2014.
35. Kalburgi V, Sravya L, Warad S, et al: Role of systemic markers in periodontal diseases: a possible inflammatory burden and risk factor for cardiovascular diseases. Ann Med Health Sci Res 388–392, 2014.
36. Dave S, Van Dyke TE: The link between periodontal disease and cardiovascular disease is probably inflammation. Oral Dis 14:95–101, 2008.
37. Bahekar A, Singh S, Saha S, et al: The prevalence and incidence of coronary heart disease is significantly increased in periodontitis: a meta-analysis. Am Heart J 154:830–837, 2007.
38. Engebretson SP, Hyman LG, Michalowicz BS, et al: The effect of nonsurgical periodontal therapy on hemoglobin a1c levels in persons with type 2 diabetes and chronic periodontitis: a randomized clinical trial. JAMA 310:2523–2532, 2013.
40. Connell B, McConnell E, Francis T, et al: Tailoring the environment of oral health care to the needs and abilities of nursing home residents with dementia. Alzheimers Care Q 3:19–23, 2002.
41. Nordenram G, Ljunggren G: Oral status, cognitive and functional capacity versus oral treatment need in nursing home residents: a comparison between assessments by dental and ward staff. Oral Dis 8:296–302, 2002.
44. Fukai K, Takiguchi T, Ando Y, et al: Functional tooth number and 15 year mortality in a cohort of community-residing older people. Geriatr Gerontol Int 7:341–347, 2007.
45. Itzaka S, Tadaka E, Sanada H: Comprehensive assessment of nutritional status and associated factors in the healthy, community-dwelling elderly. Geriatr Gerontol Int 8:24–31, 2008.
63. Pajukoski H, Meurman JH, Halonen P, et al: Prevalence of subjective dry mouth and burning mouth in hospitalized elderly patients and outpatients in relation to saliva, medication and systemic diseases. Oral Surg Oral Med Oral Pathol Oral Radiol Endod 92:641–649, 2001.
66. Bergdahl M, Bergdahl J: Low unstimulated salivary flow and subjective oral dryness: association with medication, anxiety, depression and stress. J Dent Res 79:1652–1658, 2000.
67. Thomson WM, Chalmers JM, Spencer AJ, et al: Medication and dry mouth: findings from a cohort study of older people. J Public Health Dent 60:12–20, 2000.
71. Figueiral MH, Azul A, Pinto E, et al: Denture-related stomatitis: identification of aetiological and predisposing factors-a large cohort. J Oral Rehabil 34:448–455, 2007.
73. Jainkittivong A, Aneksulk V, Langlais RP: Oral mucosal conditions in elderly dental patients. Oral Dis 8:218–223, 2002.
78. Ruggiero S, Dodson T, Fantasia J, et al: American Association of Oral and Maxillofacial Surgeons position paper on medication-related osteonecrosis of the jaw—2014 update. J Oral Maxillofac Surg 72:1938–1956, 2014.

111 Pain in the Older Adult

Patricia Bruckenthal

Despite its increased prevalence in older adults, pain should not be considered a normal consequence of aging. Pain is always due to pathology, even if not easily identified or fully appreciated by the clinician. An understanding of the complex cellular, molecular, and genetic contributions to the experience of pain are beginning to emerge, along with their relationship to physical, psychological, and environmental factors. Persistent pain interferes with enjoyment of life and has deleterious effects on mood, social interaction, function, mobility, and independence. For many reasons, pain remains undertreated in this population. This chapter examines age-related changes in the prevalence and perception of pain and approaches to assessment and treatment. The focus is on pain and suffering, rather than the underlying causes of pain. The management of specific painful conditions is not discussed.

COMPONENTS OF PAIN

The pain experience is best understood by considering the influence of four determinants—nociception, pain perception, suffering, and pain behaviors.[1] Nociception is the detection of tissue damage by specialized transducers on primary afferent A delta and C nerve fibers in response to noxious stimuli. The subsequent perception of pain by the individual is affected by central processing of nociceptive input from the periphery or from lesions in the peripheral and central nervous systems. Pain consequent to nerve damage can occur with or without somatic nociceptive input. In the former case, the perception of pain is altered from what is usually reported following nociception. The intensity of pain under these circumstances bears little relationship to the extent and severity of observable pathology and tends to be less responsive to traditional analgesic medications. Adjuvant medications, or those formerly not used to treat pain, have demonstrated efficacy in treating pain that results from changes in the central and peripheral nervous systems.

Suffering is a negative emotional response induced by pain and also by fear, anxiety, loss, and other psychological states. Patients often use the language of pain to describe suffering, such as "heartache," although not all suffering is caused by pain. Pain behaviors, such as grimacing, lying down, limping, and avoidance of physical activity may result from pain perception and suffering. The clinician infers the existence of nociception, pain, and suffering from the patient's history, physical examination, and observation of pain behaviors.[1] Recognition of the multiple components of the pain experience will guide the clinician in assessing and planning age-appropriate pain management.

TYPES OF PAIN

A simple classification differentiates pain as acute or chronic. Acute pain can be of visceral or somatic origin. It usually has an identifiable temporal relationship with an injury or disease. Autonomic overactivity, such as diaphoresis and tachycardia, may be present. In this setting, pain may be seen to serve a useful role in drawing attention to injured tissues, altering behavior, and hence preventing further tissue damage. Acute pain often leads the individual to seek medical attention. Pain often resolves before healing is complete. As people age, there may be a blunting of protective warning signals. Age-related dysfunction along pain pathways may account for age-related differences in pain perception.[2-4] Pain associated with visceral causes are prevalent and may present atypically in older adults. Visceral pain associated with cardiac, pulmonary, and abdominal disease is associated with morbidity and mortality and can be difficult to diagnose in older adults. Clinicians need to be especially vigilant in their pain assessment technique in this population.

Chronic pain persists beyond the normal duration of injury or tissue damage or is associated with progressive disease. The time frame for the transition from acute to chronic pain is somewhat arbitrary, often determined by the underlying pathology, and not necessarily characterized by a change in quality or severity of symptoms. Thus, chronic pain is often defined as pain persisting for longer than 3 to 6 months or beyond the expected time of healing. There may be no identifiable pathology to account for the pain. Psychological and functional features are often associated with chronic pain, and autonomic overactivity is not usually present. Chronic pain may be persistent (always present) or intermittent, such as migraine headache. Pain intensity may vary during the day or be related to activity level. Musculoskeletal disease, arthritis, orofacial, and neuropathic pain conditions are common in older adults. Once reversible factors have been excluded, the pain rather than the pathology is considered the major problem. At this stage, the goal of treatment shifts from a disease focus to reduction of pain, suffering, and disability.

Prevalence Studies

Pain in older adults is common and has a tremendous impact on quality of life in this age group. Pain is an important health deficit, and its presence adds to the risk associated with health deficit accumulation, particularly in relation to this risk, it is greater in men than in women.[5] There is great variability in the reported prevalence, likely due to differences in the reporting period for pain, intensity of pain reported, and composition of the older population studies. Crook and colleagues[6] have reported age-specific rates of 29% for those between 71 and 80 years of age when asked "how often are you troubled by pain during the past 2 weeks…?" Brattberg and associates[7] have reported a 12-month prevalence of mild to severe pain in 75% of those older than 75 years. Persistent pain ranges from 26% to 30% in the population, with those between the ages of 60 to 69 years reporting the most pain.[8] Persistent pain has been reported in approximately half of community-dwelling older adults,[9,10] and older adults at the end of life report an even higher incidence of pain.[11] The fact that prevalence data has not changed significantly in the past 30 years illustrates the complexity of pain management in older adults.

Pain affecting the joints, feet, legs, and back is increased with age but pain in the head, abdomen, and chest is reduced. The high prevalence of degenerative joint disease overwhelms any contribution from other causes in all surveys. Osteoarthritis (OA) is reported in 12% of adults, with the incidence increasing with age. Painful OA is present in 26% of women and 13% of men older than 71 years, whereas OA of the knee is present in 17% of adults older than 45 years. These rates are significantly higher than those reported in younger adults.[12] Persistent intermittent back pain ranges from 13% to 49% in persons 65 years of age and older.[13,14]

Other musculoskeletal noncancerous conditions contribute to pain in older adults. Bone demineralization leading to osteoporosis and vertebral compression fractures are common in postmenopausal women[15]and can contribute to traumatic long bone fractures.[16] Vitamin D deficiency can predict osteoporosis and OA and is associated with a significantly higher prevalence of chronic back pain in women.[17] Postherpetic neuralgia (PHN) and painful diabetic neuropathy (PDN) are common in older adults. In persons older than 60 years who develop acute herpes zoster, approximately 12.5% will develop PHN,[18,19] and PDN affects 15% of older patients with diabetes.[20] Persistent and inadequately treated pain can lead to decreased quality of life, including impaired sleep, mobility, and function and decreased socialization and independence, among other consequences. Efforts by clinicians to understand, assess, and treat pain in this population are imperative.

Age-Related Changes in Pain Perception

Pain may not be the cardinal symptom of disease in older adults. Silent myocardial infarction is more common with age.[21,22] Similarly, in a retrospective study of older patients with peritonitis, abdominal pain was absent in nearly 50% of cases.[4] The physiologic basis of these observations is uncertain. Clinicians should not underestimate the potential seriousness of underlying pathology in an older person because of the absence of severe pain.

There are widespread morphologic, electrophysiologic, neurochemical, and functional changes within the nociceptive pathways, and psychological factors may alter pain experience in older adults.[23] Most studies of experimental pain have supported the view that pain thresholds to short-duration noxious stimuli are increased in older adults.[24,25] There is controversy regarding the effect of age on pain thresholds; pain thresholds to thermal, ischemic, and mechanical stimuli have been shown to increase with age, but aging does not predict decreasing sensitivity to pain.[26] However, a decrease in the function of the descending inhibitory pain control pathway as a person ages[23] suggests greater sensitivity to noxious experimental pain. In other studies, reticence, self-doubt, and reluctance to label a stimulus as painful underlie the perception that stoicism to pain increases with age. However, when pain is perceived, the experience is the same or, under some circumstances, enhanced or prolonged.[27,28] Tolerance to severe pain may even be reduced in older adults.

Age-related loss of neurochemicals, such as serotonin,[29] glutamate, γ-aminobutyric acid GABA),[30] and opioid receptors,[31] implicated in pain modulation, may contribute to altered pain processing in older adults. Changes in the aging brain[32,33] have been associated with older adults processing and response to pain. Taken together, these studies suggest that pain is dependent on a complex neuroprocessing system that is affected by aging and has implications for the pain experience in older adults.

PATHOPHYSIOLOGIC PERSPECTIVE

Inferences about the underlying pathophysiology of a painful condition assist the clinician in the selection of therapy and determining prognosis. Clinicians must keep in mind that older adults often have more than one source of pain. Pain may be subdivided into three pathophysiologic subtypes—nociceptive, neuropathic, and psychogenic. Pain that arises from noxious stimulation of specific peripheral or visceral nociceptors is termed *nociceptive pain*. Examples include pain arising from OA, soft tissue injuries, and visceral pathology. Pain arising from pathology of the peripheral nerves or within the central nervous system leading to aberrant somatosensory processing is termed *neuropathic pain*. This term encompasses a diverse range of conditions, including painful peripheral neuropathies, phantom limb pain, postherpetic neuralgia, trigeminal neuralgia, and central poststroke pain. Pain of neuropathic origin is often associated with abnormal and unpleasant sensations (dysesthesia) and may have a burning or shooting quality. Mild, normally non-noxious stimuli in the affected region may cause pain (allodynia), normally noxious stimuli may result in a heightened sensitivity response (hyperalgesia), or repetitive stimulation can result in summation and pain persisting longer than the stimulus (hyperpathia). There may be a delay between the precipitating injury and onset of pain. The onset of central poststroke pain syndrome occurs commonly between 1 and 3 months following a stroke, but may occur more than 1 year later.[34] Pain often persists in the absence of ongoing tissue damage. Pain associated with psychological factors is termed *psychogenic pain*. It is probably more useful to consider the impact of psychological influences on the pain presentation, choice of treatment, and response to treatment than the potential influence that the label of psychogenic pain may convey.

The multidimensionality of chronic pain has long been recognized to include sensory-discriminative, affective-motivational, and cognitive-interpretative dimensions. These are influenced by biologic, psychological, and social factors. The ability of the individual to adapt to biopsychosocial changes in response to stress may be diminished with age. The term *pain homeostenosis* has been introduced to describe an organism's diminished ability to respond effectively to the stress of persistent pain.[5,33] Clinicians should be aware of factors that contribute to these phenomena, such as cognitive function, decreased density of opioid receptors, medical comorbidity, polypharmacy, and effect of aging on pharmacokinetics and pharmacodynamics, social isolation, depression, and altered activities of daily living. There are specific assessment techniques and tools to assist in assessing these factors.

Depression is common in people with chronic pain. Patients who are depressed may exhibit decreased energy, decreased engagement in treatment modalities, or avoidance of pleasant diversional activities. Anxiety has also been closely associated with pain[35,36] and often coexists with depression in this population. Anxiety may play a part in fear-related behavior that might inhibit participation in physical rehabilitation efforts. Social networks and economic resources are important assessment parameters. Involvement with family and friends can provide pleasurable experiences and diversion away from a constant focus on pain. In addition to the availability of social support, the type of relationship should be assessed. Negative social reinforcement may present in the form of overly solicitous family members who encourage sedentary behavior. Other negative effects are likely if long-term caregivers become resentful of their support role. Economic resources have a great impact on access to potential treatment options and must to be identified.[37] Finally, beliefs and attitudes about pain can affect the overall pain management plan. Pain can signify loss of independence, debilitating illness, or be regarded as a general consequence of the aging process and therefore underreported. If older patients have a good understanding of the underlying cause of pain, what it means in terms of function, and possible treatment options, it is likely that they will participate in the plan of care and obtain more satisfactory outcomes.

EVALUATION

Pain is inherently subjective; the individual's self-report is the gold standard for assessment. The history should focus on the onset and temporal pattern of the symptoms, site, and quality of the pain, severity, aggravating and relieving factors, and impact of the pain on the patient's lifestyle. The assessment of a patient with a complex pain problem may need to take place over several consultations. The reliability of the history can be affected by the chronicity of the pain, past interventions, and age-related conditions that affect cognition. A collaborative history from a family member is often helpful. Special emphasis should be placed on musculoskeletal and neurologic examinations because of their importance in the genesis of pain in older adults. The assessment should include functional and psychological aspects and, where possible the individual should be assessed within his or her own environment. The open-ended question, "What would you do if you no longer had pain?" often reveals valuable information regarding mood state, attitudes, and disability. Part of the assessment needs to focus on the patient's comorbidities, how these affect function, their contribution to altered mood state their propensity to affect management with medications, and physical or psychological interventions.

Back pain is illustrative. An estimated two thirds of adults will experience back pain at some stage of their lives. Experimental studies have revealed that pain may originate from any one of many structures. However, after clinical evaluation, no precise pathoanatomic diagnosis can be established in 85% of cases.[38] Investigations are used to confirm a diagnosis and exclude more serious pathology. The diagnostic probabilities change with increasing age, with cancer, compression fractures, and spinal stenosis becoming more common. Plain radiology is not highly sensitive but findings on computed tomography (CT) and magnetic resonance imaging (MRI) are nonspecific and thus may be misleading. CT and MRI studies of asymptomatic individuals older than 60 years have shown that about 80% have abnormal findings, such as disc prolapse and spinal canal stenosis. Therefore, the identification of pathology on diagnostic investigation does not necessarily indicate causality. Deyo and Weinstein[38] have suggested that it is more helpful to address three questions during the assessment of a patient with low back pain:

1. Is a systemic disease causing the pain?
2. Is there social or psychological distress that may amplify or prolong pain?
3. Is there neurologic compromise that may require surgical evaluation?

Under most circumstances, these questions can be answered from a careful history and physical examination. without the need for further tests.

Although these scales only assess unidimensional pain intensity, older adults with mild to moderate cognitive impairment have demonstrated successful use of numeric rating scales[39,40] and verbal descriptor scales.[37,41] Several validated psychometric instruments can help quantify and communicate the patient's pain experience. The widely used McGill Pain Questionnaire[42,43] consists of 78 adjectives describing emotional, sensory, and evaluative dimensions of the pain experience. Words such as throbbing, sharp, cramping, burning, and aching describe a sensory dimension, whereas tiring, exhausting, cruel, punishing, fearful, and sickening describe an affective component. There is no shortage of geriatric assessment instruments available to clinicians. A recommendation from a comprehensive review of assessment of pain in older adults[44] has suggested the Brief Pain Inventory[45] combined with the Short Form-McGill Pain Questionnaire[43] as an appropriate 10-minute battery for cognitively intact older adults.

Modification to accommodate sensory, motor, perceptual, and cognitive changes in older adults may be necessary. Proper lighting, attention to tone, speed, and pacing of voice, reduction of extraneous noise, and using tools with large bold print is helpful. The Mini-Cog is a brief (3-minute) cognitive screen that includes a clock drawing and three-item recall,[46] which can establish the ability to obtain a self-report of pain.[47]

Psychological Assessment

A comprehensive psychological assessment is not usually required in the setting of acute pain. However, chronic pain may have profound effects on mood, interpersonal relationships, and activity level, and it may be difficult to ascertain which is cause and which is effect. A psychological evaluation is indicated when contributing factors are discovered on history taking or medical evaluation fails to explain the severity of pain behaviors adequately. Psychological evaluation can also be valuable when the pain results in excessive health service use or interference with normal activities or interpersonal relationships. Chronic pain patients are often resistant to psychological evaluation, considering this an inference that the pain is "in the head," rather than being a physical problem. Patients often require careful explanation regarding the complex interaction between mind and body, which often influences pain, suffering, and disability.[48] Acknowledging that the pain is real preserves the patient's sense of legitimacy and allows for a more complete evaluation of the psychological factors contributing to the maintenance of pain. Moreover, pain is commonly accompanied by depression, and this relationship persists, even for people who are frail, for whom it can affect disease expression.[49]

It is important to evaluate how the patient, family, and caregiver(s) conceptualize the pain and goals of treatment. They may believe that the pain has persisted because the medical assessment has been inadequate or specific interventions denied. Each time a new intervention is tried and fails, the psychological distress is reinforced. Psychological strategies are not likely to be effective in teaching the patient how to manage ongoing pain while the patient remains focused on seeking a cure. Pain behaviors such as limping, grimacing, inactivity, and verbalizing of pain complaints may be reinforced by social influences such as gaining attention, sympathy, or the ability to avoid unpleasant responsibilities. Fear of causing further pain or injury may lead to avoidance of activity. Attempts at management with medications and physical therapies, without addressing psychological factors, are often unsuccessful.

Assessment of Pain in the Presence of Cognitive Impairment

Cognitive impairment represents a major impediment to the evaluation and management of pain. A hierarchical approach is recommended as a guide to assess pain in persons not able to self-report pain.[50] Interpretation of a pain stimulus may be altered in persons with dementia.[51] Additional evidence has suggested that cognitive impairment does not necessarily change the pain intensity experienced.[52-54]

When assessing pain in severely cognitively impaired patients, the clinician must rely on behavioral indicators. These include nonverbal cues such as restlessness and guarding, verbal cues such as crying, moaning, and groaning, and facial expressions such as grimacing.[55-57] Changes in usual activity may also indicate pain. There is tremendous variability in pain behavior, and certified nursing assistants will often be the first to notice behavioral changes, including combativeness, resisting care, a decrease in social interactions, increased wandering, difficulty sleeping, and refusing to eat.[58] Behavioral indicators for pain in this population and pain assessment tools have been developed for cognitively impaired persons. The assessment instruments vary greatly on their reliability, validity, and applicability for easy clinical use.[59-61] Because pain behaviors may be absent during rest, observations should take place during movement such as bathing, dressing, or transferring.

Defining the Goals of Therapy

Before embarking on a treatment program, the patient and clinician should agree on the goals of therapy, particularly when pain eradication is not feasible. An essential outcome should include improvement in physical an psychosocial functioning.

Involvement of family members and caregivers often assists with enhanced compliance to treatment and successful outcomes. A frank discussion about the prognosis and therapeutic options is important, particularly for individuals who have had unsatisfactory experiences and expectations in the past. Even if the sensory component of pain cannot be eliminated, improved outcomes can be achieved by addressing factors such as disability and mood disturbance. Management of severe pain often requires establishing a balance between the severity of sensory symptoms, level of disability, and medication side effects. Disability may be more important to the patient than the pain. An improvement in the distance that an individual can walk before being stopped by pain may be considered a positive outcome, although the intensity of maximum pain remains unaltered. Medication side effects may be more troublesome than the condition for which they were prescribed. Pain management programs that combine cognitive and rehabilitative approaches to enhance coping strategies and minimize the impact of persistent pain on the individual can be helpful.

MANAGEMENT

Medications

The management of pain can be tricky. Pain medications can be less well tolerated in frail older adults, so attention to whatever other medications they are on is needed.[62] Selection of appropriate drug therapy for older patients requires an understanding of age-related pharmacokinetic and pharmacodynamic changes and needs to take into account any coexisting diseases and other medications, including those obtained without prescription. Selection of therapy needs to balance the potential efficacy with the potential for harm from the intervention. Physiologic changes associated with aging, such as intestinal motility, secretions, and blood flow, can alter drug absorption, bioavailability, and transit time, Hepatic and renal functions are diminished and alter the metabolism and excretion of water-soluble drugs. Guidelines are available to mitigate the potential risks of adverse effects and medication toxicity due to the age-related changes,[63] as summarized in Box 111-1.

The timing of drug administration is important. Analgesics may be prescribed on an "as required" basis for occasional pain or prophylactically for induced pain. However, for continuous pain, analgesics are best prescribed on a regular basis. Additional doses may be required before an activity known to exacerbate pain or for breakthrough pain. Medications with long half-lives may be used to reduce the frequency of dosing. In general, medications should be started at low doses, titrating upward and stopping at the lowest dose that achieves the desired outcome. Finding the appropriate medication and dose may take a long of time due to tolerability and efficacy and should be explained to the patient to reduce the potential for prematurely abandoning treatment.

BOX 111-1 Treatment Options

MEDICATIONS

Paracetamol

- First-line analgesic for older patients with chronic pain
- Often as effective as NSAIDs
- Best given regularly for persistent pain, rather than as required

NSAIDs

- Increased risk of GI and renal complications in older adults
- Avoid if possible

Selective COX-2 Inhibitors

- Preferable to nonselective NSAIDs
- Similar nongastrointestinal side effects to nonselective NSAIDs

Adjuvant Analgesics

These include antidepressants and anticonvulsants.

- Proven role in neuropathic pain states
- Total pain eradication is unlikely
- Selection of medication based on side effect profile rather than comparative efficacy
- Started at low dose, increased slowly

Opioid Analgesics

- Have a role in chronic noncancer pain
- Treat constipation preemptively
- Drug dependence uncommon in older adults

NONPHARMACOLOGIC APPROACHES

These include physical and psychological therapies.

- Will reduce reliance on medications
- Failure to use these strategies often accounts for treatment failure.

Simple Analgesics

Acetaminophen (APAP, paracetamol) 500 mg qid is the preferred analgesic for older adults.[64-66] A trial of acetaminophen is warranted as initial therapy on the basis of cost, efficacy, and toxicity profile. Dosages should be limited to 4000 mg/day, with lower doses used for persons with diminished renal or hepatic function or for those requiring chronic use. It is absorbed rapidly and metabolized by the liver. Because of the risk of hepatoxicity, acetaminophen should be used with caution in patients with liver disease, chronic alcoholism, malnutrition, and dehydration.

As a class, nonsteroidal antiinflammatory drugs (NSAIDs) have been among the most frequently prescribed medications, particularly for pain associated with OA and inflammatory arthropathies. However, they should not be used as first-line analgesics for persistent pain. The side effect and drug interaction profile of NSAIDs is of particular concern. Dose-related and prolonged exposure to NSAIDs contribute to gastric mucosal adverse events, which are significantly increased in those older than 75 years.[67-69] Renal toxicity is another concern. Risk factors for renal failure in patients with intrinsic renal disease treated with NSAIDs include age older than 65 years, history of hypertension, congestive cardiac failure, and concomitant use of diuretics or angiotensin-converting enzyme (ACE) inhibitors. Most NSAIDs have a dose-response relationship, with a ceiling effect. Increasing the dose above the recommended level or adding a second NSAID does not impart any greater analgesia, but increases the likelihood of drug toxicity.

The rate of NSAID-related gastrointestinal (GI) complications has decreased in recent years, in part due to extensive medical education campaigns and a move away from NSAIDs as first-line management of OA.[70] Patients with inflammatory arthritides should preferentially be treated with disease-modifying drugs. The options for management of patients with NSAIDs who are at high risk of serious upper GI events are the use of a nonselective NSAID with gastroprotective therapy or the use of a cyclooxygenase-2 (COX-2) specific inhibitor. Coadministration of misoprostol has been demonstrated to reduce the upper GI complication rate of nonselective NSAIDs but is not well tolerated. Proton pump inhibitors are an acceptable alternative. Histamine H2 receptor antagonists have been shown to prevent duodenal ulceration only and cannot be recommended.[71] Celecoxib is the only COX-2 selective NSAID currently available in the United States.[4] The primary short-term advantage of this class of agents is its lack of effect on platelet function. Because these drugs are frequently prescribed for pain control in rheumatoid arthritis and OA, their usefulness for long-term therapy is limited. In addition, COX-2 inhibitors appear to affect renal function in a similar fashion as nonselective NSAIDs, and particular care is required in patients with renal impairment or those taking diuretics and ACE inhibitors. COX-2 inhibitors may diminish the antihypertensive effects of ACE inhibitors and diuretic effects of furosemide and thiazides. Celecoxib inhibits the cytochrome P450 (CYP450) enzyme (CYP2C9) and thus may cause elevation of plasma concentrations of drugs metabolized by this enzyme, such as some β-blockers, antidepressants, and antipsychotics.[72] Topical NSAIDs are an effective and safe alternative for some patients, especially for the management of pain associated with OA[73] and acute musculoskeletal and soft tissue inflammatory pain.[74,75] Diclofenac gel and patch formulations are currently available, with several other NSAID formulations under development. Although GI side effects are less common than with oral preparations, there is still a risk, especially in those who have previously experienced previous side effects from NSAIDs.[76]

Opioid Analgesics

Opioid analgesic medications are considered second- or third-line pharmacologic therapy for persistent moderate to severe pain.[65,77,78] Older patients tend to be more sensitive to equivalent doses and blood levels of opioids due to physiologic changes associated with aging and the effects of polypharmacy. For example, the analgesic effects of codeine (methylmorphine) are mediated by its conversion to morphine via the CYP450 D6 (CYP2D6) system. About 8% of whites and 2% of Asians are genetically deficient in CYP2D6 and obtain little pain relief with codeine. A number of medications frequently prescribed for older patients are capable of inhibiting CYP2D6, including cimetidine, quinidine, amitriptyline, and the selective serotonin reuptake inhibitors (SSRIs; e.g., fluoxetine, paroxetine, fluvoxamine). Starting doses should be 25% to 50% lower than standard adult doses, and titration should be done cautiously and slowly.[66] For patients requiring round the clock dosing, a steady state is generally reached through five half-lives of repeated dose administration.[78,79] Effectiveness of the drug therapy can then be evaluated. Clinicians, therefore, need to be familiar with specific opioid pharmacology, starting doses, titration schedules, and monitoring of effectiveness, side effects, and potential for abuse and diversion.

All opioid analgesic medications carry the side effect profile of potential nausea, constipation, sedation, respiratory depression, and cognitive alterations. Older adults should be placed on a prophylactic bowel regimen. They may be at greater risk for accident-related injuries when starting therapy.[80] Methadone should only be prescribed by those familiar with the drug. An initial electrocardiogram (ECG) with periodic reassessments are necessary due to the potential for prolonged QTc intervals, especially with doses above 100 mg/day.[65,81,82] Older adults without a prior history of substance abuse disorder are at low risk for developing an addiction to opioid analgesics, but opioid misuse is a public health concern. Strategies to assess for misuse and diversion need to be in place for all older adults receiving opioid therapy. These include periodic pill counts, urine drug screening, use of a prescription drug monitoring program, and securing medications in a locked container.[78,83] Newer abuse-deterrent formulations have the potential to mitigate abuse and diversion of opioid analgesic medications.

Weak opioids include tramadol, tapentadol, and buprenorphine and may be better tolerated by older adults. Tramadol is a centrally acting synthetic analgesic with opioid-like effects. Its mode of action is through binding to the μ-opioid receptor and inhibition of noradrenaline and serotonin reuptake. The efficacy of tramadol is comparable to that of ibuprofen in patients with hip and knee OA. Dose reduction may be required in older patients, Tapentadol is a centrally acting analgesic and acts as a μ-opioid receptor agonist and noradrenaline reuptake inhibitor.[84] Buprenorphine is a semisynthetic opioid analgesic that acts primarily as a partial agonist at the μ-opioid receptor. The transdermal formulation provides continuous delivery of buprenorphine, resulting in a relatively consistent plasma drug concentration throughout a 7-day dosing interval.[85] The more traditional weak opioids may be effective but have a ceiling effect for analgesia due to the combination and limits of acetaminophen. If adequate pain relief is not obtained at optimal doses, change to a strong opioid should be considered.

Morphine is the prototypic opioid. Its analgesic properties are not limited by a ceiling effect, but side effects are common. Tolerance to side effects develops more rapidly than tolerance to analgesic effects, although constipation tends to persist. Once the daily opioid requirements have been established through the administration of a short-acting opioid on a regular basis, the use of delayed-release opioid agents should be considered. Delayed-release morphine and oxycodone preparations may be used in older patients but care must be taken to prevent drug accumulation. Other strong opioids include methadone, hydromorphone, and fentanyl. Methadone must be used with caution because it has a long half-life of up to 2 or 3 days, resulting in accumulation in older patients.

When carefully monitored, opioid analgesics can be very effective in treating pain in older adults. However, achieving efficacy and tolerability is sometimes compromised by two related clinical manifestations of this treatment approach, opioid tolerance and opioid-induced hyperalgesia (OIH). Tolerance may develop with repeated administration of all opioids whereby higher doses are required to maintain equivalent analgesic effects. The rate of development of tolerance varies greatly, but is not as common as once believed. OIH is described as a paradoxic response in which prolonged opioid administration results in an atypical increase rather than a decrease in pain that appears unrelated to the original nociceptive stimuli.[86,87] Clinical differences between the two conditions have been described. Opioid tolerance is characterized by a decrease in the efficacy of the drug, which can be overcome by increasing the drug dosage. Conversely, OIH is not overcome by increasing the drug dosage and will worsen the pain. In this scenario, pain is improved by reducing or eliminating the drug.[88] Clinical recognition and management is a challenge for clinicians.

Before tolerance is suspected in a patient with a previously established opioid dose, evidence of advancing disease, new-onset disease or injury, or psychosocial cause should be investigated. If these are negative, the dose or frequency of dosing may be increased. Cross-tolerance with other opioids is not complete because they often act through different combinations of receptors. The problem may be overcome by changing to another oral opioid, commencing at 50% of the equianalgesic dose. When a patient is unable to tolerate oral opioids or has refractory pain, parenteral analgesia by the transdermal, subcutaneous, venous, epidural, or intrathecal route should be considered. A transdermal fentanyl patch offers the advantage of one application every 72 hours. It has a similar side effect profile to other opioids, although some patients report less constipation than with other preparations. Fentanyl accumulates in skeletal muscle and fat and then is slowly released into the blood. Minimum effective concentrations are reached approximately 6 hours after application. Serum fentanyl concentrations decrease by 50% approximately 17 hours after removing the patch. The clearance of fentanyl is delayed in older, cachectic, and debilitated patients. The 25-μg/hr transdermal fentanyl patch is equivalent to about 90 mg of morphine/day. It is not recommended for opioid-naive patients.

Clinical criteria for diagnosing OIH have been proposed, including the following: (1) increased pain intensity during ongoing opioid treatment; (2) no evidence of underlying disease progression; (3) no evidence of opioid withdrawal; (4) no evidence of opioid tolerance (tested by decreased pain in response to added dose); (5) decrease in pain intensity in response to dose reduction; and (6) no evidence of addictive behavior.[87] Several mechanisms for neural changes in response to exposure to μ-opioid agonists that lead to OIH have been proposed. Although not fully understood, management approaches are related to the sensitization of glutamenergic systems, *N*-methyl-D-aspartate (NMDA) receptor activation, and enhanced descending descending facilitation to the dorsal horn of the spinal cord.[86,87] Opioid-sparing strategies with adjuvant drug therapies, such as anticonvulsants and antidepressants, and heat, cold, and exercise programs have been used to treat OIH. Opioid rotation has demonstrated effectiveness in treating opioid tolerance and increased opioid sensitivity.[89-91] NMDA receptor blockade studies have had mixed results. Ketamine, methadone, dextromethorphan, and COX-2 inhibitors all have a theoretical rational in OIH treatment[87] but should be used cautiously in older adults.

Clinical strategies to manage these potential opioid administration–related conditions as well as other potential opioid side effects begins with vigilant monitoring and early problem identification. Treatment can be time-consuming and may require multiple office visits. Rational polypharmacy, including nonopioid medications and nonpharmacologic approaches in conjunction with opioid analgesics, can be very effective in older adults.

Adjuvant Analgesics

Adjuvant analgesics are drugs that have a primary indication other than pain, are analgesic in many pain syndromes, but have been most studied in neuropathic pain syndromes. They include medications from heterogeneous therapeutic classes, including selected antidepressants, anticonvulsants, topical lidocaine, and herbal remedies. Antidepressants act by modulating pain through direct pathophysiologic mechanisms or by treating underlying depression that might augment pain perception. Tertiary amines (e.g., amitriptyline, imipramine, doxepin) should be avoided in older adults because of anticholinergic side effects, including sedation, constipation, urinary retention, delirium, and dizziness. Amitriptyline entails the risk of cardiac arrhythmia. Secondary amines (e.g., nortriptyline, desipramine) tend to have a more favorable adverse event profile in older adults.[92] Serotonin norepinephrine reuptake inhibitors (SNRIs), such as duloxetine and venlafaxine, have been approved for the treatment of diabetic peripheral neuropathic pain, but SSRIs do not appear to be effective for pain management. Among the anticonvulsant drug class, the calcium channel alpha-2/delta-1 ligands (gabapentin and pregabalin) are associated with a more favorable adverse event profile and with fewer drug-drug interactions.[92]

Neuropathic pain (NeP) has been defined as pain arising as a direct consequence of a lesion or disease affecting the somatosensory nervous system.[93] Toth and Au[94] have reported a prevalence rate for NeP of 45% for patients presenting with polyneuropathy from a variety of causes. Treatment based on clinician and patient preference, usually gabapentin, pregabalin, topiramate, and amitriptyline, suggests an average number needed to treat (NNT) of 2 to 3 for more than 30% relief. The average NNT was 5 to 7 for more than 50% relief. Average NeP pain relief was 31% to 42% on a visual analogue scale (VAS) after 6 months, and amitriptyline had a slightly greater intolerable side effect profile.[94]

The selection of an adjuvant analgesic agent for the management of neuropathic pain should be based on the side effect profile and the potential for drug interaction rather than on the relative efficacy of different agents. There is considerable individual variation in the response to these agents. Failure to respond to one agent is not predictive of the response to another agent in the same therapeutic class.

Topical lidocaine patches have been licensed for use in PHN in the United States[95] and are an effective treatment for diabetic neuropathy.[96] In addition, herbal products and dietary supplements are used by many Americans. Marinac and coworkers have found that 21% of persons older than 60 years were using at least one herbal or dietary supplement, with 19% at risk for a potential adverse drug reaction.[97]

Nonpharmacologic Therapies

Nonpharmacologic approaches, alone or in combination with pharmacologic treatment, should be an integral part of the care plan for older adults with chronic pain. These approaches encompass a broad range of physical, psychological, and other treatment modalities. They are widely used by patients, often without the knowledge of their health care provider. Nonpharmacologic interventions can also refer to invasive approaches such as epidural steroid injections and spinal cord stimulators. This section will focus on noninvasive approaches.

Psychological Approaches

Psychological factors may contribute to the maintenance of pain or be causally related to the pain. Regardless of the pathophysiologic basis of chronic pain, psychological strategies have a role in management. The essence of management is to establish appropriate pain-coping strategies and discourage behaviors that may perpetuate the pain syndrome. Generally, a combination of behavioral and cognitive strategies is used. Cognitive strategies are aimed at modifying belief structures, attitudes, and thoughts to modify the experience of pain and suffering. This approach also includes distraction therapy, relaxation, biofeedback, and hypnosis. The patient is encouraged to take an active role and accept responsibility for pain management, rather than being a passive victim. These strategies have been demonstrated to be effective for managing pain in older adults.[98] Although difficulties in accessing treatment have been cited, models to mitigate the access barrier have been emerging.[99-101]

Other self-management strategies such as yoga, tai chi, and music therapy, have shown promise for reducing pain and increasing function in older adults.[100,102-104] The use of telephone- and Internet-delivered interventions may increase access to these therapies for older adults.

Physical Therapies

Simple adjustments in posture and daily routines, such as preparing meals in a seated position, breaking up the housework, or providing a walking aid can reduce the impact of pain on daily life. The use of a walking frame, which causes a mild degree of lumbar flexion, will often ease the pain of lumbar canal stenosis.

Exercise is a major component of most pain management programs, alone or in conjunction with pharmacologic and other nonpharmacologic approaches. Even frail and institutionalized older adults may benefit. Exercise can lead to decrease in pain, improvements in function, and elevation of mood.[105,106] Low-impact exercises, such as walking and water aerobics, may be helpful in reducing pain and improving function.[107,108] Hydrotherapy should be considered when weight-bearing exercises aggravate pain.[105,109] The buoyancy effect of water reduces the weight of the body, allowing joints to be moved with minimal friction through a full range of movements. The warmth of the water decreases pain and muscle spasm. Transcutaneous electrical nerve stimulation (TENS) is a popular method of symptom relief for a wide range of painful conditions in older adults, such as low back pain, OA, and PHN.[105,110] Other physical therapies used for a wide range of painful conditions include massage, cold and heat treatments, acupuncture, and electrotherapies such as ultrasound, low-level laser therapy, and biofeedback. Combined with drug therapies, nonpharmacologic interventions may have an additive or synergistic effect on the management of pain and improved function in older adults.

Pain and Cancer

Half of all cancers occur in those older than 60 years.[111] In the advanced stages of cancer, 64% experience pain, and the pooled prevalence of pain in all types of cancer at all stages is more than 50%. Many patients (>33%) report moderate to severe and persistent pain.[112] Despite clear guidelines, pain associated with cancer persists in older adults.[113]

The World Health Organization (WHO) method for relief of cancer pain is based on a three-step approach to the use of analgesia. The first step of the WHO analgesic ladder is nonopioid analgesics, including acetaminophen and NSAIDs. The second step is weak opioids, and the third step is the strong opioid group. Nonopioid analgesics are usually combined with an opioid in steps 2 and 3 to give additive analgesia.[114] The relevance of this approach has come into question due to newer pharmacologic delivery systems (e.g., rapid-onset opioid analgesics) and the need to bypass earlier steps in many cases.[115-118] The use of strong opioids as first-line therapy compared to the WHO analgesic ladder has demonstrated better pain control, with fewer changes in therapy.[119] A more recent guideline has supported the role of opioid analgesics as first-line therapy for patients with pain associated with cancer.[120]

CONCLUDING REMARKS

Advancing age is associated with an increased incidence of painful pathology. Anyone who has persistent pain, despite what appears to be conventional treatment, should be carefully reassessed to determine why there has been a failure of response to therapy. One should never conclude that it is the patient who has failed to respond to treatment; it is the treatment that has failed to achieve the desired result. Severe unrelieved pain has a profound impact on an individual. Various factors may preclude the older patient from the benefit of definitive therapy to eradicate pain and, under these circumstances, symptom management is indicated. This must take into consideration the effect of comorbidities on the expression, assessment, diagnosis, and treatment of the painful condition. Overemphasis on pharmacologic approaches ignores the potential benefits of physical and cognitive-behavioral strategies. The persistence of pain despite apparently appropriate therapy raises the possibility of unrecognized mood disturbance, pain of neurogenic origin, or advancing pathology. Under these circumstances, a multidisciplinary pain management approach involving medical, physical, and psychological therapeutic modalities is often more effective than a single disciplinary approach.[121] Multidisciplinary pain management clinics have emerged over the past 30 years, but are limited geographically and by expertise in geriatric medicine. Age should not, however, be regarded as a barrier to successful outcomes from the multidisciplinary management of pain problems. Even if pain cannot be eradicated, worthwhile improvements can often be achieved by addressing pain as a problem in a broader sense, not simply as a sensory symptom.

KEY POINTS

ASSESSMENTS

- Contribution of nociceptive and neuropathic factors
- Impact of pain on function and mood state
- Comorbidities affect assessment, function, and treatment selection.

INVESTIGATIONS

- Presence of radiologic abnormalities does not prove causality.
- Unexplained change in symptoms warrants reassessment to exclude serious pathology.

For a complete list of references, please visit www.expertconsult.com.

KEY REFERENCES

10. Patel KV, et al: Prevalence and impact of pain among older adults in the United States: findings from the 2011 National Health and Aging Trends Study. Pain 154:2649–2657, 2013.
23. Lariviere M, et al: Changes in pain perception and descending inhibitory controls start at middle age in healthy adults. Clin J Pain 23:506–510, 2007.
33. Karp JF, et al: Advances in understanding the mechanisms and management of persistent pain in older adults. Br J Anaesth 101:111–120, 2008.
44. Hadjistavropoulos T, et al: An interdisciplinary expert consensus statement on assessment of pain in older persons. Clin J Pain 23(Suppl):S1–S43, 2007.
50. Herr K, et al: Pain assessment in the patient unable to self-report: position statement with clinical practice recommendations. Pain Manag Nurs 12:230–250, 2011.
61. Hadjistavropoulos T, et al: Pain assessment in elderly adults with dementia. Lancet Neurol 13:1216–1227, 2014.
63. American Geriatrics Society 2012 Beers Criteria Update Expert Panel: American Geriatrics Society updated Beers Criteria for potentially inappropriate medication use in older adults. J Am Geriatr Soc 60:616–631, 2012.
65. American Geriatrics Society Panel on Pharmacological Management of Persistent Pain in Older Persons: Pharmacological management of persistent pain in older persons. J Am Geriatr Soc 57:1331–1346, 2009.
66. Gloth FM 3rd: Pharmacological management of persistent pain in older persons: focus on opioids and nonopioids. J Pain 12(Suppl 1):S14–S20, 2011.
99. Broderick JE, et al: Nurse practitioners can effectively deliver pain coping skills training to osteoarthritis patients with chronic pain: a randomized, controlled trial. Pain 155:1743–1754, 2014.
103. Reid MC, et al: Self-management strategies to reduce pain and improve function among older adults in community settings: a review of the evidence. Pain Med 9:409–424, 2008.
110. Park J, Hughes AK: Nonpharmacological approaches to the management of chronic pain in community-dwelling older adults: a review of empirical evidence. J Am Geriatr Soc 60:555–568, 2012.

112 The Mistreatment and Neglect of Frail Older People*

Anthea Tinker, Simon Biggs, Jill Manthorpe

Evidence about the abuse, mistreatment, and neglect of frail older people has been emerging over the past decades. In this chapter, we first examine the development of concern, definitions, prevalence rates, and risk factors. We then discuss ways in which the risks of elder abuse may be identified in clinical practice as well as in public health strategies and consider prevention and responses. We write from the perspective of developments in the United Kingdom and draw mainly on studies in the wider European and North American context. However, the publication of "Hidden Voices" by the World Health Organization (WHO) in 2002[1] followed by the WHO European report on preventing elder mistreatment in 2011[2] has revealed widespread recognition of this problem internationally. There is scope for continuing to draw lessons from cross-national perspectives, while recognizing differences in service and legal provisions as well as cultural interpretations of abuse between countries. Although there are lessons to be learned from child abuse, simplistic parallels should not be drawn. For example, there are dangers in interventions narrowly focused on the *protection* of older people (although *safeguarding their rights* is of growing importance) if they are ageist in philosophy or undermine autonomy and rights in civil and criminal law. The European Convention on Human Rights, now incorporated into U.K. domestic law, offers an important counter to these dangers, as does the growing emphasis on empowerment. This suggests the importance of being aware of overlaps with cases of domestic violence[3] and the acknowledged difficulty of working within long-standing family conflict. Elder abuse, however, is not confined to family or domestic settings, and clinicians have responsibilities for the well-being of their patients in hospitals and in long-term care facilities.

HISTORICAL DEVELOPMENT

Early concerns about mistreatment of older people were raised by doctors who detected a parallel with child abuse and placed the issue in the wider context of the care of older people both in their own homes and in long-term care facilities, emphasizing the importance of good geriatric practice.[4,5] However, an evidence base was slow to develop despite notable exceptions.[6,7] In its absence, abuse was linked to concerns about the stress placed on family caregivers supporting older people, particularly those with dementia. Policy in many countries has drawn on developments from the United States, which advocates the creation of local protocols when abuse is suspected or revealed. In the United Kingdom, policy developments have also responded to professional and pressure group concerns that elder abuse has been insufficiently resourced and prioritized.[8]

DEFINITIONS

The WHO[9] defines elder mistreatment as "a single or repeated act or lack of appropriate action occurring within any relationship where there is an expectation of trust, which causes harm or distress to an older person" (p. 6). The U.S. National Research Council[10] supplies an operational definition that includes "intentional actions that cause harm or create a serious risk of harm (whether or not harm is intended) to a vulnerable elder by a caregiver or other person who stands in a trust relationship to the elder" and "failure by a caregiver to satisfy the elder's basic needs or to protect the elder from harm" (p. 40).

Box 112-1 provides definitions of types of mistreatment, including both behavior and effect. The terms *elder abuse, mistreatment*, and *neglect* refer to the ill-treatment of an older person (usually defined as older than 60 years) by acts of commission or omission. They may occur in domestic settings (the older person's own home, a relative's home, or supported housing), in long-term care facilities (assisted living, nursing homes, and hospitals), or in the community. Some kinds of behavior are criminal acts, such as assault and theft; other forms, such as verbal abuse, the restraint of someone who is aggressive, or apparent overmedication, may be more contingent on particular circumstances. Definitions are important, but multiple terms are used and sometimes overlap. For example, abuse and neglect generally refer to behavior within a relationship connoting trust. This distinguishes actions by those closely linked to the older person (such as family members) or others in positions of responsibility for their care (such as nursing staff or family physicians) from actions by strangers. These boundaries are not always clear; for example, electronic fraud is a growing crime that may also fall under the definition of abuse when the older person is vulnerable because he or she has dementia. A recent trend has been to broaden understanding of abuse to include resident-on-resident abuse in long-term care facilities,[11] the characteristics of abusive environments,[12] contextual factors permitting abuse,[13] and the relationship of abuse to caregiver stress or characteristics.[14]

Different Types of Abuse and Neglect

There is now widespread agreement about five categories of abuse: physical violence; psychological abuse, often measured by persistent verbal aggression; financial abuse; sexual abuse; and neglect.[15] However, there remains very limited information on how often these types of abuse occur together and whether they are separate phenomena, but the research suggests that they both occur singly *and* in combination and that explanations for the abuse, and therefore the factors relevant to risk, may vary accordingly. The U.K. prevalence study[16,17] distinguished between forms of abuse that are interpersonal and of an intimate nature, financial forms, and neglect. Whether or not a common label and tendency to a common response are useful requires further research. The U.K. study used a series of behavioral definitions of abuse to take frequency and severity into account, and these definitions may be of greater use to professionals than those intended for policy makers. Prevalence studies are now available from a number of countries in Europe, North America, and East Asia, but comparisons should be made with caution. For example, social abuse and isolation were identified as an additional category by some East Asian studies.[18]

Vulnerability of Frail Older People

In the context of elder abuse, vulnerability may be related to physical and mental frailty, as well as disability. Socioeconomic factors such as low income, minority ethnic background, and poor housing have been associated with enhanced risks.[17] The majority

*With acknowledgments to Claudine McCreadie, who coauthored the original chapter with Anthea Tinker.

BOX 112-1 Definitions of Types of Abuse, with Examples of Behavior and Effects

Physical abuse: Nonaccidental infliction of physical force that results in bodily injury, pain, or impairment
- *Examples of behavior:* hitting, slapping, pushing, burning, physical restraint
- *Examples of effects:* bruises, fractures, burns, broken teeth, sprains, cuts, hair loss, bleeding from scalp, fear, anxiety, depression

Psychological abuse: The persistent use of threats, humiliation, bullying, swearing and other verbal conduct, and/or of any other form of mental cruelty that results in mental or physical distress
- *Examples of behavior:* treating an older person as a child, blaming, swearing, intimidating, name-calling, threatening violence, isolating older person
- *Examples of effects:* fear, depression, confusion, loss of sleep, loss of appetite

Financial abuse: Unauthorized and improper use of funds, property, or any resources of an older person
- *Examples of behavior:* misappropriating money, valuables, or property; forcing changes to will; denying access to personal funds
- *Examples of effects:* loss of money, etc., inability to pay bills, deterioration in health or standard of living, lack of amenities, unusual activity in bank accounts, signatures on documents uncertain, lack of solid arrangements for financial management, eviction or house sale notices

Sexual abuse: Direct or indirect involvement in sexual activity without consent
- *Examples of behavior:*
  Noncontact: looking, photography, indecent exposure, harassment, serious teasing or innuendo, pornography
  Contact: touching breast, genitals, anus, mouth; masturbation of either or both persons; penetration or attempted penetration of vagina, anus, mouth, with or by penis, fingers, other objects
- *Examples of effects:* difficulty in walking or sitting, bruises, bleeding, venereal disease, psychological trauma

Neglect: Repeated deprivation of assistance needed by the older person for important activities of daily living
- *Examples of behavior:* failure to provide food, shelter, clothing, medical care, hygiene, personal care; inappropriate use of medication or overmedication
- *Examples of effects:* malnutrition, pressure ulcers, oversedation, untreated medical problems, depression, confusion

of prevalence studies have collected data from older people living in community settings. Evidence from other locations about abuse and neglect tends to arise from public inquiries, inspection reports, and case studies, for example, the major U.K. inquiry into events at Mid Staffordshire NHS hospital where hundreds of older patients' care was poor, abusive, and neglectful.[19]

Residents of nursing homes or other long-term care facilities may be deemed vulnerable or at risk by virtue of their increased disability or their living situations. Professionals are particularly likely to have contact with these groups of older people, who, because of their physical and/or mental impairments, are least able to protect themselves. However, while there are various discussions about individual risks, it may also be worth thinking about vulnerable situations. This means analyzing the context rather than personal vulnerability. For example, not all people with dementia are at risk, but those who are may have few people to safeguard their best interests and may be easy prey for the unscrupulous.[20]

PREVALENCE AND INCIDENCE

Table 112-1 shows prevalence (in percentages) of elder mistreatment in North America, Canada,[21] the United Kingdom, Ireland, Amsterdam (the Netherlands), and Spain.[22] Studies have also taken place in Spain, the Czech Republic, Finland, Sweden, and Germany. The Spanish study[22] is one of national community prevalence, indicating a figure of 0.8% reported by older people but 4.5% by caregivers. Some studies of community prevalence in North America were based on telephone interviews.[6] The U.K. survey was based on individual face-to-face interviews with people aged 66 and older.[16] Overall in this survey, 2.6% of people aged 66 and older living in private households reported that they had experienced mistreatment involving a family member, close friend, or care worker (i.e., those in a traditional expectation of trust or trust relationship) during the past year. When this 1-year prevalence of mistreatment was widened to include incidents involving neighbors and acquaintances, the overall prevalence increased to 4.0%. The Irish study[23] found less neglect but more psychological abuse than the U.K. study. Data from Hong Kong[24] and mainland China[25] are also available, reporting higher instances of mistreatment than other studies. Variation between national studies cannot be taken to indicate ethnic or cultural differences in prevalence because standardized measurements were not used.

One particular difficulty for studies using the general population is that people who are highly reliant on another person for activities of daily living, and particularly people who have severe cognitive impairment, are unable to participate, except by proxy. In the U.K. and Spanish studies, people with severe dementia or otherwise unable to take part were excluded from the research. In the Dutch study, nonresponse was relatively high for those with mental and physical incapacity (although all were living independently).[26] Yet it is precisely these people whom practitioners might identify as most vulnerable or at risk.

TABLE 112-1 Prevalence of Elder Abuse

Type of Abuse	Boston (United States), 1986[6] (%)	Canada, 1990[22] (%)	United Kingdom, 2006[16,17] (%)	Amsterdam (Netherlands), 1994[26] (%)	Spain, 2006[22] (%)	Ireland, 2010[23] (%)
Physical	2	0.5	0.4	1.2	0.3	0.5
Psychological*	1.1	1.1	0.4	3.2	0.6	1.2
Financial	Not in study	2.5	0.7	1.4	0.9	1.3
Neglect	0.4	0.4	1.1	0.2	0.6	0.3
Sexual	Not in study	?	0.2	?	0.1	0.05
Multiple	Not in study	0.8	Any 2.6	Not in study	0.8†	Any 2.2

*Persistent verbal abuse.
†Any type of abuse.

RISK FACTORS

There seems to be no single risk factor for mistreatment and abuse but rather "many risk and protective factors on five different levels: factors relevant for the victim, offenders, family system, institutions and society"[27] (p. 9). WHO has pointed to the lack of high-quality studies of risk and prevention.[2] Clinical and forensic markers indicating abuse and neglect point to the importance of dementia, depression, psychosis, and alcohol abuse as risk factors among older people but also among those in contact with them. Declining health, loneliness, and depression have been associated with enhanced risk factors, but these may also affect resilience.[16]

Physical Abuse

The most thoroughly researched area of physical abuse is that taking place in domestic settings, although the following risks may also apply to people living in long-term care facilities and hospital patients.

1. Risk is higher for older people who live with someone.[6,14,22,26] Older people may be abused by their partners or by other relations, including their adult children. Living in congregate accommodation may also be a risk[2] (p. 29).
2. Some research links abuse with sociodemographic variables such as marital status and occupation.[16] Ethnic background has been the subject of more debate,[17] and it is not clear if minority status increases risks or whether it may be protective.
3. Some abuse is long-standing—Homer and Gilleard[28] referred to the "elderly graduates of domestic violence." However, the predominance of women as victims of domestic violence at younger age groups is not so marked in the case of elder abuse.[6,16,22] Lachs and colleagues[29] concluded, "Clinicians should be particularly aware of high-risk situations in which functional and/or cognitive impairment are present, especially in circumstances where violent behavior has been known to exist previously."
4. Lachs and colleagues[29] found that the number of activities of daily living impairments approximately doubled the chance of reported abuse or neglect. The researchers did not, however, consider that reporting bias substantially influenced this finding.
5. There is little evidence that the stress of caring for an older person is, on its own, a cause of abuse. Large numbers of caregivers are under stress but do not abuse their relative. How caregivers react to the stresses associated with caring, however, may be important.[23]
6. Risk appears to depend more on problematic characteristics associated with the abuser, particularly their physical and mental health and notably, according to many studies, their heavy consumption of alcohol or drug substances.[30] Research with general practitioners (family physicians) linked identification of abuse with knowledge of these factors in patients' households. Those general practitioners who identified 5 or more of 15 risk situations were seven times more likely (all other variables held constant) to have identified a case of abuse.[31]
7. The role of dementia as a risk factor is complex, but abusive behavior by family caregivers toward people with dementia is reported to be common. Among a sample of caregivers accessing specialist mental health services in England, one third reported important levels of abuse and one half reported some abusive behavior.[32] Lachs and colleagues[29] observed that cognitive impairment, particularly if it was new, was highly significant. Early research with people with dementia and their caregivers found that the factors distinguishing abusive situations related to caregivers.[28] Behavioral and psychological symptoms of dementia, such as aggression or apathy, may be associated with aggression on the part of the person caring for a person with dementia.[28]

Long-Term Care Settings

Knowledge about abuse and neglect in long-term care facilities is also growing.[33] The WHO identified risk factors, including being a woman, having a physical or mental disability, being cognitively impaired, having few or no family members, and having few visitors.[2] In the United Kingdom, the Department of Health and the charity Comic Relief commissioned a number of studies (but not a national prevalence study) and summarized their findings under the title of "Respect and Protect."[34] These studies investigated the experiences of older people and staff in care homes and hospitals (studies also undertook data analyses and engaged with definitional debates). Methods of caring and cultures of care in both settings assumed significance, particularly as the prevalence of physical and mental frailty is generally high among older people in long-term care facilities. Numerous inquiries in Britain into grave deficiencies of care found abuse flourishes within a culture that allows it to be acceptable.[19] Reasons may include poor training of and lack of support for staff, tolerance of violence, inadequate support for activities of daily living of residents or patients, and lack of both respect and autonomy for older people.[2] The ability to report abuse to authorities anonymously may be necessary.[35] The leadership role of clinicians in such settings should include attention to complaints, staff turnover and its reasons, and risk management, as well as direct patient care. It is the worst of all possible worlds, as older people themselves are only too aware, to move an older person to a long-term care facility for safety only for them to be abused there.

Sexual Abuse

This type of abuse has been little researched, but a groundbreaking study from Australia[36] offered details of some older women's experiences. Those affected relied on others for their care, but others were also at risk. Abusers may have problems themselves and need help. Attention should be paid to the potential for sexual abuse in long-term care facilities and to the risk of sexual abuse by other residents or visitors. During physical examinations, health care professionals should be alert to possible indicators of abuse, such as unexplained trauma in the genital area or bites.

Financial Abuse

Nearly all definitions of elder abuse include financial abuse (theft, undue influence, and exploitation), but this is sometimes not included in research studies. The U.K. prevalence study found this to be the most common form of abuse (after neglect) with a rate of 0.7%.[16] On the one hand, the financial affairs of older people, with dementia in particular, appear often to be complex or confusing for them, thus increasing the risk of financial abuse. On the other hand, people with dementia may be vulnerable to financial abuse and specifically targeted. Some evidence shows that financial abuse is more likely to be perpetrated by the extended family than by partners or paid care workers.[15] When allied with physical and psychological abuse, the offender or perpetrator may be a close adult relation (usually an adult child) with problems of his or her own, particularly relating to alcohol or drug misuse.[10] In England and Wales, the Mental Capacity Act 2005 has strengthened the ability of people to make arrangements for their finances in the event of losing capacity to manage their money. A system of legal safeguards was set up to reduce the likelihood of financial abuse, but it has not eradicated the risk. The implications for clinicians are that when an older person is in unexplained financial trouble, that where there seems to be a sudden drop in their living standards so that they seem unable to afford previously affordable items, that when they appear under pressure, then professionals should report concerns to adult protective services.[37]

Neglect

Neglect is generally interpreted as omission. However, opinion is divided about the appropriateness of classifying self-neglect as mistreatment in the context of adult protective systems, and local procedures will assist in determining the clinical and care pathways. People whose needs are insufficiently met or ignored may be mentally frail and, unsurprisingly, in poor health.[17] Neglect may occur in care facilities, including hospitals, with pressure ulcers giving cause for concern but also lack of personal care and lack of hydration.[19] Moreover, family members may be unwilling or unable to provide necessary care, which may lead to a situation of neglect; such is the seriousness of deliberate or willful neglect that, in some jurisdictions, it may be a criminal offense for both practitioners and family caregivers.[38]

IDENTIFICATION

Elder abuse is often hidden. The U.K. prevalence study,[16] for example, indicated that only approximately 3% of mistreated older people were in touch with adult protective services (in England termed *adult safeguarding*). It estimated that approximately 1 in 40 older people visiting their family physician would, statistically speaking, be suffering some form of mistreatment but that contact with adult protection services was far less than might be expected. The majority of cases, whether in domestic or other settings, may be likely to arise in either primary or secondary care as part of some other presenting problem. People who are abused are unlikely to volunteer information and may fear retribution, not trust formal authorities, or not wish to criminalize significant others. Identification often depends on a high index of suspicion. An early survey in England showed that many family physicians might not recognize abuse and would welcome training in both identification and management.[31] Physical symptoms, such as bruising, may be common to frail older people and may be unreliable indicators alone.[26] As prevalence is relatively low, assessment assumes great importance. Incorrect diagnosis of abuse, followed by misplaced interventions, can damage all those concerned. Apart from increased sensitivity and awareness of the possibility of abuse, the first general principle, common to all good practice in geriatric medicine, family medicine, and psychiatry, is that assessment must be person centered, holistic, and interdisciplinary.[39] Although there is no definitive list of "red flags," it has recently been stated that "doctors should be aware of the various "red flags" that initiate suspicions of abuse. Unexplained injuries may be discovered on examination or reported by a third party"[40] (p. 30). Assessment may be time-consuming and some doctors may, under pressure of time and shortage of resources, be particularly unwilling to address issues of family violence, family conflict, or financial complexities. The logic of current research is that criminal justice and helping professionals should work together. Clinicians may be asked for opinions about possible abuse, and their testimony may be vital in safeguarding an older person from further abuse or in exonerating an innocent relative or careworker.

In the United States, where, in some states, the law requires mandatory reporting of suspected abuse cases, it is recommended that routine questioning should be built into daily practice and that in every clinical setting there should be a protocol for the detection and assessment of elder abuse. Knowing what to look for is key, but so too is listening. There are benefits of a protocol or framework for questioning,[11,14] and this can be useful in the context of possible financial abuse as well as physical and psychological abuse. Consultation with the older person alone may be difficult but is advisable.[40]

Financial abuse is an issue that doctors may encounter in various ways.[14] They may be approached to advise on the mental capacity of people to make financial and other decisions. For example, they may be asked whether a person has the mental capacity to make a will, appoint a proxy decision maker (attorney), or dispose of assets. They need to know to whom to refer people for appropriate guidance, to know the professional and legal requirements and procedures in their national context, to be aware of protocols around data sharing and evidence collection, and to ensure that the person understands what is happening and that, if not, the person is not left unsupported.

Clinicians may also come across possible abuse in the course of other patient contact where it is equally necessary to know about local safeguarding or adult protective systems. A small study of the views of U.S. geriatricians found that the average number of cases of elder abuse diagnosed per year was about eight per geriatrician.[40] Their diagnostic work rested on a combination of history taking and physical examination.

PREVENTION, TREATMENT, AND MANAGEMENT

The key objectives remain the prevention of abuse and the promotion of the older person's human rights.[10,41,25] At the level of policy and guidance, it is essential that the medical profession is represented where any professional or local initiatives are taking place to develop responses to abuse. The use of excessive or inappropriate medication as a form of abuse highlights the need for clinicians themselves to be careful of their own practices and those of their colleagues.

Two additional general principles are meticulous documentation and liaison with other professionals, both within and outside health services. The taking of photos, video footage, or drawings and the careful recording of suspected injuries and conversations are important evidence of abuse. The difficulty and time involved in collecting this information need to be taken into account when arranging consultations. The need to work interprofessionally raises difficult ethical questions in terms of confidentiality of the doctor-patient relationship, should the older person request the doctor to "do nothing." Older people's rights to autonomy have to be balanced with decisions that may need to be made in their best interests should they not have the capacity to consent to or refuse information sharing. The need for police intervention and other data sharing may arise if a crime is suspected in order to address possible dangers to others. The assessment of mental capacity, therefore, is of crucial importance and helps direct physicians to the options for intervention if an older patient is unwilling to accept any help. Advocacy can be a particularly valuable service for the older person at the center of this concern, and in England and Wales this is now available by right for some people who are lacking mental capacity and are in situations of suspected abuse.

Figure 112-1 should be interpreted in relation to the type of abuse and to the legal and service provision context in which medical practitioners are working. In most countries, the number of laws that potentially bear on abuse is considerable, and advice may be needed from adult protective services. In the event of an emergency, the medical practitioner should make immediate contact with other responsible agencies and act to protect the older person from harm. Doctors and other health professionals "need to familiarise themselves with the policies and procedures concerning safeguarding"[40] (p. 33), although a systematic review of knowledge, detection, and reporting of abuse by health and social care professionals suggests that practice is variable.[42] Although safety of the alleged victim is the first priority, it is also essential to pay attention to the physical and psychological health of the other party, who also may be frail.

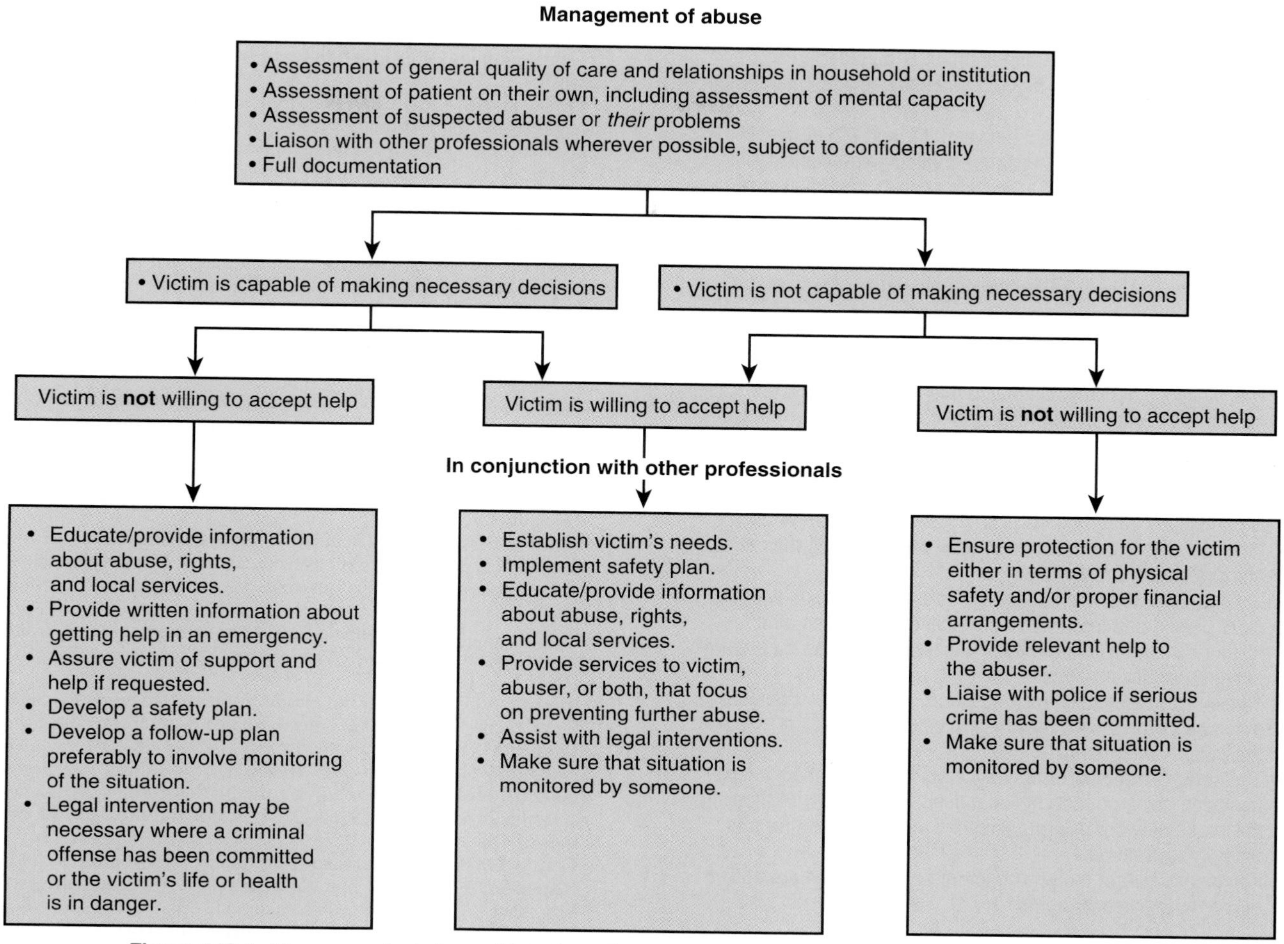

Figure 112-1. Management of abuse. *(Data from Fisk J: Abuse of the elderly. In Jacoby R, Oppenheimer C, editors: Psychiatry in the elderly, ed 2, Oxford, England, 1997, Oxford University Press, pp 736–748; Lachs MS, Pillemer KA: Abuse and neglect of elderly persons. N Engl J Med 332:437–443, 1995; Kurrle S: Elder abuse: a hidden problem. Mod Med Aust 9:58–72, 1993; and American Medical Association.)*

SUMMARY AND CONCLUSION

Elder abuse can be divided into four forms—physical, psychological/emotional, sexual, and financial—as well as neglect, which together are often referred to as *elder mistreatment*. It may be a one-time incident or be part of a long-term pattern.[37] The development of behavioral definitions, better understanding of risk factors, and more knowledge of the characteristics of the parties involved are leading to greater understandings of the circumstances associated with each form of elder abuse. Across all settings, the principal aim is to prevent abuse and neglect from occurring through building safe and responsive systems, regular monitoring, and interprofessional collaboration. Medical practitioners have key roles in ensuring that systems are safe and in responding to suspicions and allegations by providing expert medical intervention and testimony. They are often trusted and accessible. Their responsibilities for the treatment of physical harm are evident, but they may also arrange or offer support to people in risky situations. Elder abuse or neglect is similar to domestic violence but is wider in scope and form. Abuse and neglect may best be currently understood within human rights frameworks.

This means that the primary aim should be to prevent abuse from occurring. There are at least four planks in prevention. The first is the provision of effective health and welfare services for older people, including income and medical provision, resilience building, and social support.[41] The second is awareness among all professions that abuse exists and requires a response, which may be most effective when it is multidisciplinary and reflective of what older people want to happen. This may involve criminal justice interventions, skills development,[11,39] and agreement to follow guidelines but, above all, listening to the older person. It may also involve working with people who have mistreated older people or neglected them in order to prevent harm from reoccurring. However, there is limited evidence about whether interventions work.[2] Third, in the context of a policy emphasis on care in people's own homes is the need for support for caregivers and care providers, who may be both abuser and/or abused, older or younger, and have physical and/or mental health problems, including stress.[32,43] Finally, in the context of long-term care facilities,[43] monitoring and regulation of the quality of care and care cultures are essential, and clinicians have important roles here since they generally have access to the frailest patients and residents.

KEY POINTS

- Elder abuse refers to the mistreatment of an older person (usually defined as older than 65 years) by acts of commission or omission.
- It has been shown to affect between 2% and 6% of people older than 65 years depending on definition and context.
- It is generally understood to include physical, psychological/emotional, sexual, and financial forms, as well as neglect.
- Risk of physical or verbal abuse appears to depend more on problematic characteristics associated with the abuser—particularly their physical and mental health and, notably, alchohol and drug misuse.
- There is little evidence that the stress of caring for an older person is, on its own, a cause of such abuse.
- The likelihood of being mistreated may vary depending on gender, separation or divorce, socioeconomic position, declining health, and depression. Frailty may affect a person's ability to raise concerns, report incidents, and recover from harm.
- Identification may be enhanced by a high index of suspicion and is particularly important because of relatively low prevalence.
- Physicians need to be aware of local protocols and their legal and professional responsibilities.
- Holistic assessment is necessary, through discussion with the older person and informants, physical examinations, and history taking, including mental capacity. The wider care team may be usefully involved.
- Those involved in suspected abuse as offenders or suspects may need support and may have health care needs of their own.
- The severity of effect of the abuse, its frequency, how long it has been going on, and the intentions and capacity of those in the social network help practitioners judge the case for and type of intervention.
- Key objectives are the prevention of abuse and the promotion of the older person's rights.

For a complete list of references, please visit www.expertconsult.com.

KEY REFERENCES

1. World Health Organization, International Network for the Prevention of Elder Abuse: Missing voices: the views of older persons on elder abuse. Geneva, Switzerland, 2002, WHO.
2. World Health Organization: European report on preventing elder maltreatment, Geneva, Switzerland, 2011, WHO.
4. Baker AA: Granny-battering. Mod Geriatrics 8:20–24, 1975.
6. Pillemer KA, Finkelhor D: The prevalence of elder abuse: a random sample survey. Gerontologist 28:51–57, 1988.
7. Ogg J, Bennett GCJ: Elder abuse in Britain. Br Med J 305:998–999, 1992.
9. World Health Organization. A global response to elder abuse and neglect: building primary health care capacity to deal with the problem worldwide: main report. Geneva, Swtizerland, WHO, 2008.
10. Bonnie RJ, Wallace RB, editors: Elder mistreatment, abuse, neglect, and exploitation in an aging America. National Research Council, Panel to Review Risk and Prevalence of Elder Abuse and Neglect, Washington DC, 2003, National Academies Press.
12. Stevens M, Biggs S, Dixon J, et al: Interactional perspectives on the mistreatment of older and vulnerable people in long-term care settings. Br J Sociol 64:267–286, 2013.
16. O'Keefe M, Hills A, Doyle M, et al: UK study of abuse and neglect of older people: prevalence survey report. London, National Centre for Social Research, 2007.
17. Biggs S, McCreadie C, Manthorpe J, et al: Mistreatment of older people in the United Kingdom: findings from the first national prevalence study. J Elder Abuse Negl 21:1–14, 2009.
19. Francis R, chair: Mid Staffordshire NHS Foundation Trust Public Inquiry. 2013. www.midstaffspublicinquiry.com/report. Accessed December 3, 2015.
20. Samsi K, Manthorpe J, Chandaria K: Risks of financial abuse of older people with dementia: findings from a survey of UK voluntary sector dementia community services staff. J Adult Protection 16:180–192, 2014.
21. Podnieks E, Biggs S, Penhale B: Elder mistreatment an international report: learning through comparison. J Elder Abuse Negl 21:14, 2008.
22. Iborra I: Elder abuse in the family in Spain. Documentos Series no 3, Valencia, Spain, 2008, Queen Sophia Center for the Study of Violence.
23. Naughton C, Drenman MP, Treacy A, et al: Abuse and neglect of older people in Ireland: report on the National Study of Elder Abuse and Neglect. Dublin, Ireland, 2010, National Centre for the Protection of Older People.
26. Comijs H: Elder mistreatment: prevalence, risk indicators and consequences, Amsterdam, The Netherlands, 1999, Vrije Universiteit.
27. Van Bavel M, Janssens K, Schakenraad W, et al: Elder abuse in Europe (Background and position paper 01062010). Utrecht, The Netherlands, 2010, European Reference Framework Online for the Prevention of Elder Abuse and Neglect (EuROPEAN).
30. Manthorpe J: Elder abuse. In Crome I, Wu L, Rao T, et al, editors: Substance abuse and older people, Chichester, NY, 2014, Wiley.
34. Lupton C, Croft-White C: The experience of older people and staff in care homes and hospitals, London, 2013, Department of Health, Comic Relief.
37. British Medical Association: Safeguarding vulnerable adults – a tool kit for general practitioners, London, 2011, BMA.
43. Manthorpe J, Stevens M: Adult safeguarding policy and law: a thematic chronology, relevant to care homes and hospitals, social policy and society. Soc Policy Soc 14:203–216, 2014.

113 HIV and Aging: Current Status and Evolving Perspectives

Julian Falutz

INTRODUCTION

The HIV/AIDS epidemic continues to affect millions of people throughout the world more than 30 years after it was first described.[1] Acquired immunodeficiency syndrome (AIDS) refers to a complex of often fatal infectious and malignant conditions occurring as a result of the severe and progressive immunodeficiency caused by infection with a novel retrovirus, human immunodeficiency virus (HIV). The median time from HIV infection to the development of AIDS is 10 years. Most people are relatively asymptomatic during this clinically latent phase and, unless specifically tested for HIV, are unaware of being infected. During the first 10 to 15 years of the epidemic, effective anti-HIV therapy was unavailable, and most patients died within 2 to 3 years after their first AIDS-defining illness.[2] During this early period, rapid advances occurred in understanding the biology of HIV infection. This led to the development of effective antiretroviral (ARV) drugs. Their use has transformed AIDS into a mostly manageable chronic disease, so that now few effectively treated patients develop AIDS-related complications.[3] However, for various sociopolitical and economic reasons, these benefits are only available to a minority of infected persons worldwide.

Treated patients are living longer, and overall survival has increased.[4] This has had a significant impact on the age distribution of the infected population. Most people were infected as young adults during the early phase of the disease. Currently, about 50% of infected persons in high-income countries are older than 50 years,[5] and similar proportionate increases have occurred in low- and middle-income countries. At present, older HIV patients are generally not considered as being elderly, because this term is understood by most health care providers working within the traditional confines of geriatric medicine.

This chapter will summarize the biologic and clinical principles relevant to the effective management of older HIV patients. It will focus on the evolving clinical parameters related to the complex interrelationship between the current paradigm of HIV infection and those aging with HIV. The underlying biologic and psychosocial similarities between the traditional older adult population and aging HIV population will be considered.

HIV INFECTION: EVOLUTION OF CLINICAL PROFILE AND MANAGEMENT

In 1981, reports appeared of usually rare and severe opportunistic infections and malignancies occurring in previously healthy gay men living in high-income countries. All patients had a significant loss of cellular immunity, denoted by very low levels of CD4$^+$ T-helper cells (normal level > 600 to 800/μL) and disruption of normal immune homeostasis parameters. By 1983, it was shown that AIDS was caused by infection with HIV,[6] which caused immunodeficiency by specifically targeting CD4$^+$ cells.

HIV originated as a benign chimpanzee virus (simian immunodeficiency virus [SIV]) within a localized area of sub-Saharan Africa, the Congo River Basin. SIV crossed species barriers early during the twentieth century because of increased rates of hunting and eating chimpanzee meat. SIV mutated to the much more pathogenic HIV, which then spread slowly but efficiently via sexual, bloodborne, and perinatal transmission through the increasingly urban population. Clinical disease was not recognized as a distinct entity because of its generally nonspecific manifestations. Dissemination then occurred progressively from sub-Saharan Africa to industrialized countries in the late 1960s and 1970s.[6]

Approximately 75 million people have been infected worldwide, and more than 50% of them have died. Since HIV has been identified as the cause of AIDS, effective HIV risk prevention and education programs have significantly reduced new infection rates, although new infections clearly occur. Older adults remain at particular risk for exposure to HIV and other sexually transmitted infections. Health care workers infrequently discuss sexual issues, including HIV, with older patients.[7] This is associated with a perception of low personal HIV risk among older adults.

Soon after the cause of AIDS was discovered, the HIV life cycle and pathogenesis of the ensuing immunodeficiency were characterized.[8] This facilitated the development of effective ARVs, which disrupt HIV replication by acting at multiple points in its life cycle.[9] Zidovudine, a nucleoside reverse transcriptase inhibitor, the first ARV, was approved in 1987. Since then, drugs of different classes continue to be produced; more than 30 ARV drugs are now licensed. Since 1996, these drugs have been used in various combinations, referred to by the acronym HAART (***h****ighly* ***a****ctive* ***a****nti****r****etroviral* ***t****herapy*). Currently available ARVs have minimal toxicity, resulting in improved adherence compared to that associated with the large number of drugs required to be taken in the 1990s. Several ARVs are now co-formulated, allowing for the daily use of a single pill.[10] This allows the drug's potent and durable antiviral effects to be exerted fully. These regimens are increasingly available to many people worldwide through innovative programs involving close collaboration among the pharmaceutical industry, government and public organizations, and affected communities. At present, there is no consensus that specific HAART regimens are better tolerated and more effective in older compared to younger patients.

Untreated HIV infection results in very high plasma HIV viral loads (HIV-VL), often greater than 1 million copies/mL. There is an inverse relationship between the concentration of HIV-VL and extent of CD4$^+$ cell reduction. All HAART regimens effectively reduce HIV viral replication to below the level of detection of current assays (<40 copies/mL) resulting in a slow and variable but progressive immune recovery.[6] This reduces the risk of AIDS-related complications; the higher the CD4$^+$ recovery, particularly to levels more than 500/mL, the lower the risk of AIDS. This relationship informs the clinical scenarios faced by aging HIV patients.

AIDS-related morbidity and mortality in treated patients declined dramatically following the introduction of HAART. Overall long-term survival has improved significantly in adherent patients with reliable access to ARVs but remains at only 75% to 85% of that of the general population.[11] Importantly, patients who maintain an undetectable HIV-VL and CD4$^+$ count more than 500/mcL for over 5 years are predicted to achieve normal long-term survival.[12] The major burden associated with taking HAART is the need for strict adherence to prescribed regimens. Poor adherence leads to the rapid emergence of drug resistance, with resulting recurrence of viral replication.[13] The main predictor of the extent of immune recovery is the nadir CD4$^+$ count, referring to the lowest CD4$^+$ count that a patient had prior to starting HAART. Counts less than 200 CD4$^+$cells/mL are associated with poor immune recovery,[14] which is especially relevant to understanding older patients' ability to respond to treatment.

The age of 50 years has been used in HIV infection as a transition point separating older from younger patients, recognizing that there is no specific biologic rationale for this age to represent older patients. Its use likely stems from the fact that during the first decade of the epidemic, only 10% of affected patients in industrialized countries were older than 50 years,[15] a proportion that has progressively increased to 50%.

The term *long-term survivors* refers to patients infected early in the epidemic who did not develop AIDS or who survived those complications to benefit from the first HAART regimens. Their survival is the main explanation for the overall increasing age of infected persons.[5] In addition, the mean age at the time of HIV seroconversion has also increased.[16] Older adults are more likely to have become exposed to HIV heterosexually than younger people; this is partially related to increased divorce rates and longevity, maintaining an active functional status, including sexual activity,[17] availability of effective drugs for erectile dysfunction, and infrequent use of condoms between nonmonogamous partners.[18]

As AIDS-related complications have decreased, the spectrum of illness occurring in treated patients has evolved and now consists generally of otherwise common medical conditions. These include cardiovascular disease, bone demineralization, metabolic disorders and associated body composition changes, several malignancies, certain hepatorenal diseases, and nondementing cognitive dysfunction.[19] In general, their clinical presentation, course, and response to treatment are broadly similar to that occurring in non-HIV infected persons. However, the risk of developing these complications, referred to by various acronyms, such as serious non-AIDS related events (SNAREs), is variable and related to a post-HAART plateau CD4$^+$ count less than 500 copies/mL.[20] This immune outcome is more likely to occur in older HIV patients.[5]

Older HIV patients are more likely to present initially with advanced immunosuppression or AIDS-related complications, likely because HIV is less often considered in the differential diagnosis of otherwise common HIV-related symptoms. Older patients' baseline CD4$^+$ counts are often lower at the initial clinical presentation, possibly because age-related immunosenescence may be accelerated in HIV patients, leading to a lower CD4$^+$ count.[21]

Although consensus remains elusive, older patients are generally less likely to attain the same degree of post-HAART immune recovery than younger patients, and their plateau CD4$^+$ counts are also lower.[22] They therefore remain at a higher risk of developing AIDS-related complications. Older patients' survival after developing AIDS is also less than that of younger patients.[23] However, plausible data has suggested that after starting HAART, older patients achieve an undetectable HIV-VL as often as younger patients.[22] Furthermore, they are more likely than younger patients to maintain an undetectable HIV-VL, likely due to better adherence to drug therapy.[24]

IMMUNE ACTIVATION AND CHRONIC INFLAMMATION

Patients with untreated HIV infection have laboratory features consistent with an activated immune state, even in the absence of concurrent infectious or malignant complications.[6] This refers to processes involving immune cell activation and proliferation, as demonstrated by increased levels of inflammatory cytokines, monocytes, activated T cells, and coagulation parameters.[25] HAART reduces increased activation markers but generally not to pre-HIV infection levels.[26] Several factors predispose to chronic immune activation. Treated patients with undetectable HIV-VL continue to have ongoing low-level HIV replication,[25] itself a strong stimulus to chronic immune activation. Other contributors include thymic dysfunction leading to impaired T cell maturation[27] and co-infection with specific viruses, including hepatitis B and C virus, human papillomavirus (HPV), and cytomegalovirus (CMV).[25] Immune activation is also related to microbial translocation, which refers to the passage of intestinal microbial products to the systemic circulation. This occurs because of incomplete HAART-associated restoration of the severe initial HIV-related disruption of gut-associated lymphatic tissue (GALT), which causes epithelial injury and loss of CD4$^+$ cells. Incomplete restoration of GALT allows passage of biologically active products, including lipopolysaccharide (LPS), to the bloodstream, which activate monocytes and macrophages, B and T cells, plus coagulation factors, and contribute to immune activation.[28] Microbial translocation occurs in normal aging,[29] also considered to be a state of chronic immune activation, although to a much more limited extent than HIV. Persistent immune activation contributes to incomplete CD4$^+$ recovery,[30] a risk factor for developing SNAREs. Although older HIV patients generally have lower nadir and plateau CD4$^+$ cell counts, it is unknown if they have an increased risk of developing SNAREs compared to younger patients with a similar CD4$^+$ count.

Markers of chronic inflammation include cytokines such as interleukin-6 (IL-6), tumor necrosis factor-α (TNF-α), IL-1β, and acute-phase reactants, which attract further immune system components. Physiologic aging itself is accompanied by such a state of low-grade inflammation, leading to a chronic increase in inflammatory mediators.[31] These may contribute to an increase in age-related diseases such as atherosclerosis, dementia, diabetes, cancer, and sarcopenia. This proinflammatory state may also occur if the normal mechanisms that turn off the otherwise effective immune response are defective or inefficient. In treated HIV infection, ongoing low-grade HIV viremia and the resulting chronic immune response plays an important pathogenic role in the development of the major non-AIDS complications. These include atherosclerosis, osteoporosis, neurocognitive decline, and the increasingly recognized geriatric frailty syndrome.[32]

The term *inflamm-ageing* was coined almost 15 years ago to describe the tripartite interaction among the upregulated inflammatory response, subsequent low-grade chronic inflammation, and increase in inflammation-driven chronic illnesses that are seen in older adults.[33] This process incorporates neuroendocrine activation via a chronically stimulated hypothalamic-pituitary-adrenal axis, so that glucocorticoid hypersecretion functions as the major counteractive response; this has its own long-term toxicities.[34] A similar scenario may be active in treated HIV disease.[35]

IMMUNOSENESCENCE AND HIV

Chronic immune activation and related chronic inflammation also contribute to the development of *immunosenescence*, a term describing the quantitative and functional changes in immune parameters that occur in normal aging.[36] These have been mostly studied in persons older than 80 years who have an increased vulnerability to infections, decreased effectiveness in responding to recommended vaccines, and increased risk of disorders in which chronic inflammation plays a pathogenic role.[37] Genetic signals also affect several factors, including gender, diet, and age-related thymic involution, which affect immune parameters.[36]

Immunosenescence affects all aspects of immune function, including innate immunity components such as neutrophils, natural killer (NK) cells, monocytes and macrophages, dendritic cells, and T cell and B cell lymphocyte senescence markers.[37-39] These are described in the chapter on the clinical immunology of aging (see Chapter 93). Many of the immune dysfunction changes occurring in response to chronic untreated HIV infection and, to a lesser extent, in those on HAART, are similar to those occurring in normal aging. Treated HIV has therefore been described as a state of accelerated immunosenescence.[40]

Age-related changes in immune parameters are related to chronic simulation of the immune system and genetically determined rates of telomere shortening,[39] possibly modifiable by lifestyle factors. Chronic immune stimulation is associated with lifelong exposure to environmental antigenic stresses, persistence of noncurable infections (e.g., CMV, herpesviruses), increase in age-related microbial translocation via the gut, and thymic atrophy resulting in decreased thymic hormone levels. These stimuli cause the following: (1) expansion of the pool of terminally differentiated senescent memory $CD28^-$ T cells, which then release the proinflammatory cytokines IL-6 and TNF-α, further contributing to chronic inflammation; (2) reduction of the pool of naive T cells capable of responding to new antigenic stimuli; and (3) an inverted T helper–to–T suppressor cell ratio, which is normally greater than 1 to 1.5.[37,39] The inverted T cell ratio is a key feature that was shown to predict short-term morbidity and mortality in the Swedish OCTO and NONA studies of community-dwelling octogenarians and nonagenarians.[41] These studies have also shown that CMV seropositivity contributes to expansion of the $CD8^+$ and $CD28^-$ T cells.[42]

Similar immune changes occur to a variable degree in untreated and treated HIV patients, including a low $CD4^+/CD8^+$ ratio, low numbers of naive T cells, low T cell proliferation potential, expanded $CD8^+/CD28^-$ numbers, reduced T cell repertoire, increased IL-6 production, reduced thymus function, reduced T cell telomere lengths, expanded CMV-specific $CD8^+$ T cells, and reduced vaccine responses.[43-45] This similarity between immunosenescence-related changes in people with HIV and in older adults is further supported by the finding that young HIV patients with severe immunosuppression have naive T cell numbers comparable to those of healthy seronegative persons older than 80 years.[41] Rates of telomere shortening in terminally differentiated $CD8^+$ and $CD28^-$ cells of young HIV patients are also comparable to those in healthy seronegative centenarians.[46] Levels of a known biomarker of aging, CDKN2A, a cell senescence mediator, are increased in treated younger patients, suggesting that increased biologic aging may occur in these patients.[47]

Chronic CMV infection also contributes to overall immune dysfunction in HIV and older patients. In the very old, CMV seropositivity contributes to expansion of the $CD8^+$ and $CD28^-$ T cells and to an inverted $CD4^+/CD8^+$ T cell ratio, referred to as the immune risk phenotype (IRP), which is associated with poor health-related outcomes.[48] The overall T cell response to latent herpesvirus infections in older adults is important and represents up to 20% of the total memory T cell compartment.[49] Treated HIV patients with good immune recovery have a strong anti-CMV response.[50] They also have an inverse association between strong anti-CMV T cell responses and lower total and naive $CD4^+$ T cell numbers.[51] Treated CMV-negative HIV patients have higher $CD4^+/CD8^+$ T cell ratios, are more likely to achieve normalization of their $CD4^+/CD8^+$ T cell ratios (>1.0), and are less likely to have immunosenescence-related markers.[52] Although CMV seropositivity in treated HIV patients represents a latent infection, the anti-CMV drug valganciclovir may decrease $CD8^+$ T cell activation markers in treated patients.[53]

HIV, AGING, AND SELECTED AGE-RELATED COMORBIDITIES

Treated HIV patients develop age-related, non-AIDS complications at a younger age compared to controls (Box 113-1), which is one of the reasons proposed for why HIV represents a state of accelerated aging. Careful epidemiologic comparisons do not, however, consistently support the conclusion that HIV and HAART increase a true aging phenotype.[54] The increase in comorbidities may alternatively represent a state of accentuated aging, in which HIV and HAART increase the risk of chronic conditions occurring at all ages.[55] Nevertheless, of treated HIV patients 50 to 60 years old, 35% have at least two non-HIV related comorbidities, and 20% have three, whereas in patients older than 60 years, 15% have three comorbidities, and 5% have four. This age-controlled prevalence is higher than in controls.[56]

BOX 113-1 Age-Related Conditions That May Occur at a Younger Age in HIV-Infected Persons

- Immunosenescence
- Cardiovascular disease
- Body composition changes
- Non–AIDS-defining cancers
- Hepatorenal disease
- Bone demineralization

Cardiovascular Disease

Treated HIV patients have a higher risk of typical cardiovascular disease (CVD) compared to seronegative controls, and this increases with age.[57] Many elements are in play, but common CVD factors account for most of the risk; tobacco smoking in particular is more prevalent in affected populations.[58] HIV viral components increase endothelial tissue factor levels, augmenting proatherosclerotic signals.[59] HIV also interferes with reverse cholesterol transport, decreasing high-density lipoprotein (HDL) cholesterol levels.[60]

Metabolic complications contribute to the increased CVD risk. Untreated, severely immunosuppressed patients develop an inflammatory lipid profile with increased triglycerides, and low HDL and low low-density lipoprotein (LDL) cholesterol levels.[61] After HAART initiation, specific ARVs further increase triglycerides. LDL levels increase, although this might represent a return to health effect phenomenon rather than a specific ARV effect; HDL levels infrequently increase, however. These lipid changes occur much less frequently with current ARVs.[62] Insulin resistance and type 2 diabetes are increased in HIV and are associated with specific ARVs and lifestyle factors.[63] The prevalence of obesity has increased, both in untreated and treated HIV patients.[64] This likely reflects the increase in obesity occurring in the general population and will contribute to obesity-related complications in treated patients, just as in seronegative individuals. The prevalence of the metabolic syndrome has been increasing,[65] but it is unknown whether older HIV patients are affected more often. Body composition changes, particularly increased visceral adipose tissue (VAT), may occur and affects CVD risk.[66] Increased VAT also occurs normally with aging and may therefore be more common in older HIV patients.[67]

Coronary artery and epicardial vessel calcium levels are increased,[68,69] and the absolute amount of carotid intima-medial thickness (cIMT) and its rate of progression are also increased.[70] A proatherosclerotic effect of the chronic inflammatory state also occurs. This was clearly demonstrated in a prospective ARV study, the SMART study, whose primary goal was to determine whether comparing episodic HAART with continuous therapy limits ARV toxicities. Patients on episodic HAART had an increased risk of SNAREs, and CVD events in particular.[71] The inflammatory marker IL-6 and D-dimer, a coagulation marker, were increased in patients on episodic HAART.[72] The impact of chronic inflammation is further supported by the finding that after controlling for traditional CVD risks, cIMT and CRP levels are increased in a group of unique HIV patients, referred to as elite controllers, compared to uninfected persons.[73] These patients represent a very small and much-investigated group of HIV patients who maintain a normal immune profile and undetectable HIV-VL without HAART.[74]

The clinical presentation, atherosclerotic burden, and response to standard management are similar to those seen in HIV-negative controls. An aggressive approach to risk assessment is advocated. However, the standard CVD risk assessment tool, the Framingham Risk Score, may underestimate HIV patients' risk by about 10% compared to controls.[75] Ongoing investigations will determine the most accurate tools to assess CVD risk and determine the best treatment strategies.

Body Composition Changes

Soon after the general introduction of HAART in 1996, significant changes in body composition were seen in patients who were responding well. These consisted of the diffuse loss of subcutaneous fat, termed *lipoatrophy* (LA), often occurring concurrently with abdominal obesity, termed *lipohypertrophy* (LH), which is due to increased VAT.[76] LA is related to specific ARVs—thymidine nucleoside reverse transcriptase inhibitors (tnRTIs)—which cause mitochondrial toxicity and apoptosis of peripheral adipocytes. The incidence of LA has decreased because these drugs are used less often today and current ARVs rarely cause LA. However, HIV itself can cause mitochondrial toxicity and may contribute to the persistence of LA.[77] In normal aging, physiologic loss of subcutaneous fat occurs.[67] Thus, in chronically treated older HIV patients, LA persists or may develop to a lesser degree. The cause of LH is more complex and includes pre-HIV exposure body composition and both HIV-related and specific ARV effects on intermediary metabolism. Overall, LH still develops in some treated patients. The clinical consequences of these fat mass alterations, in addition to their metabolic effects, include decreased self-esteem and quality of life and risk of poor adherence to otherwise effective HAART.

Treating peripheral LA by stopping the offending ARV or switching to a newer drug that is less associated with LA only partially reverses the fat loss. The treatment of LH is more complicated, because switching away from an associated ARV is ineffective. Exercise and diet are only as effective in HIV patients as in the general population. Recently, a multinational study of a synthetic human growth hormone–releasing agent, tesamorelin, has confirmed its ability to reduce VAT in HIV patients with increased VAT.[66] This drug is licensed in the United States and Canada.

Malignancies

The use of HAART has caused a significant decrease in the incidence of AIDS-defining cancers (ADCs), such as Kaposi sarcoma, primary central nervous system (CNS) lymphoma, and invasive endometrial cancer. However, as with the increase in CVD and other SNAREs, there is an increased risk of other non–AIDS-defining cancers (NADCs), which are now a leading cause of death in treated HIV patients. These include certain head and neck tumors, anal carcinoma, hepatocellular carcinoma in patients with hepatitis B or C (HBV or HCV) co-infection, and non-Hodgkin lymphoma.[78] Increasing age is a major risk for NADCs, as is duration of HIV, a low $CD4^+$ T cell count (<200/μL), and possibly the use of HAART, although this may be a surrogate for increased survival.[79] Other contributing causes of NADCs include a decrease in competitive causes of death, a possible oncogenic effect of the HIV tat gene,[80] and impaired tumor surveillance related to HIV immunosuppression in treated patients. A common thread among these malignancies is their confirmed or strongly supported association with an underlying infectious cause—HPV with head and neck, endometrial, and anal cancers, Epstein-Barr virus with lymphomas, HBV and HCV with hepatocellular carcinoma.

The incidence of cancers not associated with an infectious cause, such as lung cancer (the higher incidence is more than can be attributed to the expected tobacco-associated risk[81]) and melanoma,[82] has also increased in the post-HAART era. The risk of other age-related, non–infection-associated cancers, including colon, breast, and prostate cancers (whose risk may actually be decreased in HIV[83]) has not increased.

HIV-associated immunosuppression, by causing impaired T cell immunity and chronic inflammation, even if reduced by effective HAART, may increase cancer risk via interaction with the oncogenic effects of the concurrently present infectious agents. These represent chronic co-infections capable of inducing host responses, with potentially deleterious immune consequences. This has been shown particularly for CMV. MicroRNAs, particularly MiR-155, may serve as an intermediate between chronic inflammation and the associated cancer risk by causing a mutagenic effect.[84] The $CD4^+$ T cell response to HAART has also been associated with virus-related NADCs.[85] Increasing age is the most consistently documented risk factor for ADCs and NADCs, and thus aging HIV patients are a particularly vulnerable population. Inconsistent evidence has suggested that NADCs, and lung cancer in particular, may present more aggressively and at more advanced stages in HIV patients.

Limiting the increased rates of certain cancers may be achieved by encouraging the timely diagnosis of HIV in older patients and the early initiation of HAART when substantial immune recovery is more likely. Aggressive cancer screening, based on accepted algorithms for the specific cancers, is indicated. Optimal screening strategies may differ in HIV patients, and further research is needed to determine how best to proceed.[86]

Renal Complications

Renal dysfunction is common in older HIV patients and has many causes. Older age is clearly a strong risk, as are other conditions more common in HIV disease, such as type 2 diabetes, hypertension, and HCV co-infection.[87] HIV-associated nephropathy (HAN) is due to a specific histologic entity and is the leading cause of end-stage renal disease (ESRD), especially in HIV patients of African ethnicity.[88] Microalbuminuria occurs more frequently in HIV disease, suggesting premature endothelial dysfunction, which increases CVD risk.[89] ESRD occurs more frequently but at a similar age among HIV patients compared to controls.[90] ARVs may also contribute to renal dysfunction. The highly effective and widely used nucleotide reverse transcriptase inhibitor tenofovir causes the low prevalence of a minimal, and mostly reversible, nephrotoxicity.[87]

Bone-Related Disorders

Sporadic reports of low bone mineral density (BMD) in the pre-HAART era were reinforced following the introduction of HAART by the use of dual energy x-ray absorptiometry (DXA) scans to assess body composition. Osteoporosis may be three times more common in untreated patients. In treated patients, osteopenia and osteoporosis are, respectively, about ten- and threefold higher than in controls.[91] This low BMD is clearly associated with an increased fracture risk in males and females at all ages and is estimated to be between three and five times higher than in controls.[92] In addition to age, smoking, white ethnicity, and the number of comorbidities also contribute to fragility fractures.

The pathogenesis of low BMD in HIV is multifactorial and includes common risk factors such as low weight, alcohol and tobacco use, hypogonadism, and vitamin D deficiency (VDD), in addition to HIV-specific and ARV-related factors. Specific HIV viral proteins stimulate osteoclast activity and decrease osteoblast function, leading to uncoupling of the carefully regulated interactions between bone resorption and formation. In untreated and treated patients, immune activation, inflammation, and immunodeficiency, signaled by low CD4+ cell counts and increased HIV-VL, also lead to disordered osteoclastic and osteoblastic activity.[93]

Initiation of all HAART regimens cause an early decrease in BMD of about 2% to 6%, which then stabilizes and may be related to increases in bone turnover. Specific ARV effects on BMD have been identified. Protease inhibitors (PIs) are associated with an increased fracture risk through uncertain mechanisms. Tenofovir, in addition to its renal toxicity, causes a greater loss of BMD at HAART initiation than other ARVs, which is associated with a small but significantly increased fracture risk.[94] Tenofovir nephrotoxicity leads to osteomalacia, which may be worsened by concurrent VDD. VDD is very common in HIV patients, as it is in the general population, and is also associated with inflammation and increased abdominal obesity in treated patients.[95] The commonly used ARVs ritonavir and efavirenz may also independently increase the risk of VDD.

Because of the increased prevalence of low BMD and fracture risk, suggested recommendations include a screening DXA scan for HIV-positive postmenopausal women and all men older than 50 years, although the cost-effectiveness of this has not been studied. It has been suggested that HIV be considered as a secondary cause of osteoporosis.[96] Common secondary causes of low BMD should be vigorously determined. The decision to treat should be based on confirming osteoporosis at the femoral neck or spine or on a 10-year risk of hip fracture more than 3% or a major related fracture of more than 20% using the computer-based fracture risk assessment tool (FRAX). Treatment with biphosphonates is as effective as in the general population.[97]

Common Geriatric Syndromes

The focus of clinical geriatrics is to assess and guide an older adult to maintain a safe and functional status, as appropriate in their particular environment. Challenges to maintaining functional status are often due to complex geriatric syndromes, which cannot be easily defined using traditional medical paradigms and that represent the clinical consequence of interactions between multiple age-related morbidities and their impact on integrative, high-order functions. These typically include cognitive decline, impaired mobility and related falls, polypharmacy, sensorimotor dysfunction, social isolation, genitourinary problems, and frailty.[98] Treated aging HIV patients remain at risk of developing multiple, often concurrent, conditions, which resemble profiles seen in older adults (Box 113-2).

Social Isolation

In the general population, a variety of social factors have been associated with poor health status and a range of adverse health and social outcomes.[99] Older adults, especially those living in high-income countries, often have limited social support networks, including family and friends, and frequently require social, nursing, home care, and community services to maintain functional independence. They frequently have fixed incomes, with limited flexibility to increase health care expenditures.

HIV patients often come from socially and financially disenfranchised communities with higher rates of substance abuse, alternative lifestyles, social discrimination, and stigmatization. They are less likely to access community support networks effectively, which are often limited and ill prepared to deal with the multiple issues that HIV patients deal with regularly. Unemployment and financial restraints are common, further limiting access to support structures.[100] The increasing incidence of affective and nondementing cognitive impairment that can occur in treated patients further contributes to these problems.

These multiple interacting factors are compounded in older HIV individuals. Being both HIV-positive and older places them under a significant double stigma.[101] Older HIV patients are more socially isolated, which increases the risk of frailty, hospitalization, and mortality.[102] Because HIV is now a highly treatable, chronic disease, models of care increasingly take on an approach usually associated more with geriatric patients than with acutely ill adults.[103] However, there is limited information regarding the particular needs of these patients on which to base recommendations. Caregivers involved with older adults, although generally aware of HIV/AIDS and are open to caring for these patients, still lack fundamental information about their particular medical and psychosocial needs.[104] Community support networks and long-term care facilities are also mostly unprepared to look after these older patients. More fundamental research, across different chronic care models, is urgently needed, as are active interdisciplinary exchanges among the affected communities, funding agencies, and care providers.[105]

BOX 113-2 Clinical States in Treated HIV Patients*

- Social isolation
- Polypharmacy
- Disability and falls
- Cognitive dysfunction
- Frailty

*With features similar to those of common geriatric syndromes.

Polypharmacy

Polypharmacy occurs more often in treated older HIV patients than in controls and is an important contributor to morbidity and mortality because of the well-known increased risk of adverse drug events, use of inappropriate drugs, and poor adherence to required medications.[106] HAART currently consists of at least three separate ARVs. HIV patients often take nonprescription drugs, as well as drugs used to treat comorbidities. The median number of drugs being taken by all patients is from five to nine,[107] a level that has been associated with an increased risk of falls, frailty, and mortality in the general population.[108] From 15% to 75% of HIV patients in their 60s meet criteria for polypharmacy and take four or more non-ARV drugs, most of which are either vitamins and supplements or drugs for cardiovascular or neurologic disorders[109]; 15% may take drugs with potential anticholinergic toxicity.[106]

The large number of drugs taken by older treated HIV patients also increases the chances of important pharmacokinetic interactions with ARVs. Many treated HIV patients develop dyslipidemia and require statins. There is a well-known risk of statin-induced myopathy and rhabdomyolysis in patients on certain PI drugs that inhibit CYP3A4 and increase statin levels normally metabolized via cytochrome P450. Proton pump inhibitors, some of which are available over the counter, are also used by HIV patients but may lower serum levels of the important PI atazanavir, potentially leading to therapeutic failure and drug resistance.[110] One third of treated patients with chronically suppressed HIV-VL do not achieve immune recovery to more than 500 CD4+ cells/mL and remain at risk for specific AIDS-related infections. These can be prevented using low doses of specific antibiotics as primary prophylaxis but add to the pill burden, risk of drug interactions, and toxicity. HIV-knowledgeable pharmacists are essential members of the HIV treatment team.

Disability and Falls

Treated HIV patients are at particular risk for conditions contributing to disability. Visual impairment has been emerging as an important comorbidity in treated patients. In the pre-HAART era, CMV retinitis occurred frequently and was a debilitating AIDS-defining illness. Treated patients with a plateau $CD4^+$ cell count less than 200/mL have a higher risk of increased ocular lens density[111] and cataracts.[112] Visual acuity may also be impaired in patients with poor immune recovery.[113] These deficits contribute to social isolation, falls, and decreased quality of life.

The severe loss of fat and muscle that occurred in the early pre-HAART era, known as the AIDS wasting syndrome, rarely occurs today, but ongoing, low-level weight loss persists in some treated patients.[114] Muscle mass is lower overall in treated men than in controls, and increasing age is a risk factor for sarcopenia in the general population. Hypogonadism contributes to sarcopenia and remains a problem, especially in older treated patients.[115] Decreased limb muscle mass puts patients at risk for disability and predicts 5-year mortality in treated HIV patients.[116]

Objectively determined excessive or severe chronic fatigue has been reported in 50% and 28% of treated patients, respectively. This may contribute to disability by increasing the risk for impaired locomotor function.[117]

Assessment of physical impairment has been studied in HIV patients using locomotor function tests adapted from geriatric assessment measures. These include the Berg balance scale, 6-minute walk test (6MWT), timed get-up-and-go (TGUG) test, functional reach test, one-leg standing test, and five times sit-to-stand test (5STS).[118] Of middle-aged HIV patients, 60% have at least one abnormal result, and 50% have poor lower extremity function based on the 5STS.[119] A validated and easily constructed scale comprised of both HIV-related and routinely determined laboratory parameters, the Veterans Aging Cohort Study Index (VACS-I), predicts mortality and hospitalization in HIV patients and is inversely correlated with routine tests of quadriceps function, grip strength, and 6MWT, suggesting that it may identify patients at risk for disability.[120] A functional assessment tool devised for HIV patients, the Veterans Aging Cohort Study Function Scale, which includes questions about activities of daily living (IADLs), instrumental activities of daily living (IADLs), mobility, and vigorous activity performance, correlates with the standard SF-12 physical subscale and predicts survival. HIV patients in their 50s with comorbidities such as chronic lung disease have functional status scores similar to those of controls more than 18 years older.[121] The association of inflammatory markers in patients with impaired function, determined using the short physical performance battery (SSPB), 400-m walk distance (400MWD), and presence of frailty supports the early diagnosis and treatment of older patients.[122]

Risk factors for falls in the community include multiple comorbidities, physical impairments, and polypharmacy. These conditions occur at increased rates in older treated HIV patients and, not surprisingly, falls are common in these patients. Nearly 30% of HIV-positive men in their early 50s reported a fall in the previous year, a rate occurring in controls 15 years older.[123] Standard metrics to evaluate sensorimotor function should be evaluated and adapted for routine use in older HIV patients. Impaired function may be amenable to targeted interventions aimed at improving performance status.

Cognition

In the pre-HAART era, impaired cognition with severe functional impairment developed in about 20% of patients and was due to a form of subcortical dementia referred to as the AIDS dementia complex.[124] This typically caused severe loss of attention and concentration, frequently accompanied by motor slowing and behavioral changes. It was often the initial manifestation of AIDS in older patients,[125] in whom it occurred more often (23%) than in younger patients (14%).[126] In the post-HAART era, the prevalence of the AIDS dementia complex has decreased significantly, to about 5%. However, milder forms of cognitive decline still occur.[127] Currently, the spectrum of cognitive impairment is known as HIV-associated neurocognitive disorders (HANDs). Formal diagnostic criteria for these disorders, occurring in 35% to 55% of all patients, have been adopted. HANDs includes the following: (1) asymptomatic neurocognitive impairment (ANI) in about 20% to 25% of all patients; (2) mild neurocognitive disorder (mNCD) in about 25% to 30%; and (3) HIV-associated dementia (HAD) in 3% to 5%. mNCD is distinguished from ANI by the presence of impaired IADLs.[128] A reliable assessment of prevalence remains tentative because of limitations related to the selection of appropriate controls, need for extensive formal neuropsychologic testing, and challenges of reliably determining functional status in a younger population.[129]

Several factors contribute to ongoing HIV-associated cognitive decline. Mood disorders, also increased in HIV patients, must be carefully considered. Opportunistic CNS infections may present initially with subtle cognitive manifestations in untreated older patients. HIV is a neurotropic virus and crosses the blood-brain barrier early after HIV infection but does not directly infect neurons. Penetration into the brain is associated with CNS immune activation and increased cerebrospinal fluid (CSF) cytokine levels characteristic of inflammation. Neuronal dysfunction occurs secondarily to activation of CNS macrophages, microglia, and astrocytes.[130] Chronically treated patients with an undetectable serum HIV-VL may have increased CSF HIV-VL and activation markers.[131] An association between immune activation and cognitive decline also occurs in the general population.[132,133] Brain imaging shows atrophy, reduced cerebral blood flow, and impaired neuronal networks.[134] Other factors predicting cognitive dysfunction include a low nadir and current serum $CD4^+$ cell count, high HIV-VL, and HCV co-infection.[127] Concomitant lifestyle-related disorders affecting neurobehavioral status are common in many patients, complicating assessment and treatment options.

Concern has been raised that HANDs may predispose to Alzheimer disease (AD). CSF biomarkers suggestive of AD may be more prevalent in HIV patients than in controls. HIV patients homozygous for apolipoprotein E4 (ApoE4) perform worse on HIV-related cognitive tests than those without the allele.[135] The contribution of HIV-related metabolic cofactors to cognition is being investigated. In the general population, hypertension, dyslipidemia, abdominal obesity, and diabetes increase the risk of vascular dementia and AD.[136,137] In treated HIV patients, older age, hypertension, proteinuria, abdominal obesity, and both insulin resistance and type 2 diabetes impair performance on standard cognitive function tests.[138-140]

Although screening for cognitive dysfunction is recommended, there is no consensus at present regarding which tool most accurately diagnoses ANI and mCND. Given the subcortical nature of functional abnormalities and evidence of executive dysfunction, the Mini-Mental Status Exam is ineffective. The recently developed HIV Dementia Scale (HDS) and standard Montreal Cognitive Assessment (MoCA) have only moderate performance features to diagnose HAND, with particular limitations for diagnosing mild impairment.[141-143]

Individual ARVs have variable CSF penetration but, overall, all current HAART regimens significantly reduce CNS inflammation, resulting in less neurocognitive impairment.[131] Detectable CSF HIV-VL reflects this variable CNS penetration by ARVs. The correlation between variable CNS penetration by ARVs and ongoing neurocognitive symptoms has been strategized using a pharmacologic-based, CNS-penetrating effectiveness (CPE) score.[144,145] Most[146] but not all studies[147] have suggested that HAART regimens with higher CPE scores improve neuropsychological outcomes. However, some ARVs may be neurotoxic; efavirenz, an effective and commonly used drug, causes neuropsychiatric toxicity in a minority of patients.[131] Diagnosing HIV early in older patients and initiating a well-tolerated HAART regimen with the lowest pill burden and toxicity is likely to be the cornerstone of preventing long-term cognitive impairment.

Frailty

Frailty refers to a state of impaired homeostatic response of interrelated physiologic systems resulting in an increase vulnerability to biologic and environmental stressors. Frailty increases the risk of falls, delirium, hospitalization, loss of independence, and mortality. Frailty has been operationalized in the general population using various tools, most commonly with the frailty index (FI) and the frailty phenotype (FFP).[148] The FI represents accumulated, nonspecific, aging-related health problems and is determined by calculating the proportion of confirmed deficits present out of the total number counted. The specific deficits counted are not fixed as long as at least 30 distinct deficits are used.[149] The FI has been evaluated in diverse settings, and the ability to predict impaired outcomes are consistent. In contrast, the FFP is considered as a syndrome encompassing five deficits, including unintentional weight loss, impaired grip strength, slow walking speed, subjective fatigue, and decreased activity levels. Having at least three deficits is said to constitute frailty.[150] The FP also reliably predicts morbidity and mortality. There is no consensus as to which metric captures all elements of frailty, predicts outcomes, and can be most easily applied in a clinical setting.

Frailty has been assessed with the modified FFP in untreated and treated HIV patients and in uninfected controls in several large cohort studies. The Multicenter AIDS Cohort Study (MACS) has been a prospective multicenter study of HIV-positive and seronegative urban gay men who have undergone extensive biannual evaluation. HIV-positive subjects are more likely to be frail if they had a history of AIDS, a $CD4^+$ count less than 350/mL or HIV-VL more than 100,000 copies, longer duration of HIV, or were older. The prevalence of being FFP-positive was increased in those with or without AIDS in the pre-HAART era compared, respectively, to the post-HAART era—24% versus 10% and 3.3% versus 2.9%. HIV-positive men were more likely to be FFP-positive at consecutive visits compared to uninfected subjects, and the risk of developing AIDS or death was higher in those who had a sustained FFP-positive diagnosis at follow-up visits.[151-154] The Women's Interagency HIV Study (WIHS) has shown that subjects are more likely to be FFP-positive if they were HIV-positive with a $CD4^+$ cell count less than 100/mL (20%), had a prior diagnosis of AIDS (12%) compared to HIV-positive women with $CD4^+$ cells more than 500/mL (6%), or were seronegative (8%).[155] The AIDS Linked to the IntraVenous Experience (ALIVE) Cohort has shown that 14.5% of HIV-positive subjects were frail compared to 11.4% of seronegatives, and that being both HIV-positive and frail predicted mortality.[156] Higher scores on the VACS-I, described earlier, are associated with inflammatory markers and predict mortality, hospitalization, fragility fractures, and neurocognitive impairment. It has been suggested that the VACS-I encompasses many features routinely associated with frailty, although it has not been validated against other established frailty measures.[157-160]

As treated HIV patients age, many will be at risk of becoming frail, which contributes to the development of other non-AIDS comorbidities. It remains to be determined how best to determine frailty in this vulnerable group and investigate how interventions may prevent and reverse frailty.

CONCLUSIONS

HIV/AIDS affected predominantly young adults at the start of the epidemic, although its potential to affect older adults was recognized early on by experienced geriatricians.[161] Effective therapy has transformed HIV into a chronic illness, with many features familiar to health providers caring for older patients. Concurrent with this changing clinical profile, management strategies have evolved. The imperative for an interdisciplinary approach for very ill patients was also realized early in the epidemic. Care units have often included social workers, psychologists, dietitians, pharmacists, and members of the clergy, in addition to traditional medical providers, all interacting with community support networks. The emphasis on patient-centered care models for patients with multimorbidity was aggressively adopted out of necessity. Thus, elements have been in place to transition HIV teams to the changing clinical landscape, focusing on chronic conditions common to older adults. As before, patients are at the center of the increasing awareness that the specialized needs of aging HIV patients must be urgently addressed.

HIV has demanded much of society in the past 30 years and, in return, there have been benefits accruing from an open and informed approach to health care delivery. This model adds to the similar path that geriatrics has successfully implemented. An active interaction between the two disciplines will surely reward all stakeholders.

KEY POINTS

- The survival rate of treated HIV patients currently approaches that of the general population.
- Chronic inflammation and immunosenescence underlie clinical features of aging HIV and older patients.
- Frailty is a common outcome in aging HIV and older adults with multiple health deficits.
- Non–AIDS-defining, age-related comorbidities predominate in the clinical landscape.
- Biologic and functional profiles of aging HIV patients are similar to those of older patients.
- Interdisciplinary patient-centered care of aging HIV patients is required.

For a complete list of references, please visit www.expertconsult.com.

KEY REFERENCES

3. Deeks SG, Lewin SR, Havlir DV: The end of AIDS: HIV infection as a chronic disease. Lancet 382:1525–1533, 2013.
6. Maartens G, Celum C, Lewin SR: HIV infection: epidemiology, pathogenesis, treatment, and prevention. Lancet 384:258–271, 2014.
10. Gunthard HF, Aberg JA, Eron JJ, et al: Antiretroviral treatment of adult HIV infection: 2014 recommendations of the International Antiviral Society-USA Panel. JAMA 312:4410–4425, 2014.
11. Samji H, Cescon A, Hogg RS, et al: Closing the gap: increases in life expectancy among treated HIV-positive individuals in the United States and Canada. PLoS ONE 8:e81355, 2013.
33. Cevenini E, Monti D, Franceschi C: Inflamm-ageing. Curr Opin Clin Nutr Metab Care 16:114–120, 2013.
36. Larbi A, Franceschi C, Mazzatti D, et al: Aging of the immune system as a prognostic factor for human longevity. Physiology 23:64–74, 2008.
41. De Biasi S, Pinti M, Nasi M, et al: HIV-1 Infection and the aging of the immune system: facts, similarities and perspectives. J Exp Clin Med 3:4143–4150, 2011.
46. Effros RB, Fletcher CV, Gebo K, et al: Aging and infectious diseases: workshop on HIV infection and aging: what is known and future research directions. Clin Infect Dis 47:542–553, 2008.
47. Pathai S, Lawn SD, Gilbert CE, et al: Accelerated biological ageing in HIV-infected individuals in South Africa: a case-control study. AIDS 27:2375–2384, 2013.
52. Barrett L, Fowke KR, Grant MD: Cytomegalovirus, aging, and HIV: a perfect storm. AIDS Rev 14:159–167, 2012.
57. Triant VA: HIV infection and coronary heart disease: an intersection of epidemics. J Infect Dis 205(Suppl 3):S355–S361, 2012.
66. Falutz J: Management of fat accumulation in patients with HIV infection. Curr HIV/AIDS Rep 8:200–208, 2011.

74. Shasha D, Walker BD: Lessons to be learned from natural control of HIV—future directions, therapeutic, and preventive implications. Front Immunol 4:162, 2013.
76. Falutz J: HIV infection, body composition changes and related metabolic complications: contributing factors and evolving management strategies. Curr Opin Clin Nutr Metab Care 14:255–260, 2011.
78. Cutrell J, Bedimo R: Non-AIDS-defining cancers among HIV-infected patients. Curr HIV/AIDS Rep 10:207–216, 2013.
87. Miro JM, Cofan F, Trullas JC, et al: Renal dysfunction in the setting of HIV/AIDS. Curr HIV/AIDS Rep 9:187–199, 2012.
91. Walker Harris V, Brown TT: Bone loss in the HIV-infected patient: evidence, clinical implications, and treatment strategies. J Infect Dis 205(Suppl 3):S391–S398, 2012.
106. Greene M, Steinman MA, McNicholl IR, et al: Polypharmacy, drug-drug interactions, and potentially inappropriate medications in older adults with human immunodeficiency virus infection. J Am Geriatr Soc 62:447–453, 2014.
111. Pathai S, Lawn SD, Weiss HA, et al: Increased ocular lens density in HIV-infected individuals with low nadir CD4 counts in South Africa: evidence of accelerated aging. J Acquir Immune Defic Syndr 63:307–314, 2013.
116. Scherzer R, Heymsfield SB, Lee D, et al: Decreased limb muscle and increased central adiposity are associated with 5-year all-cause mortality in HIV infection. AIDS 25:1405–1414, 2011.
118. Erlandson KM, Allshouse AA, Jankowski CM, et al: Relationship of physical function and quality of life among persons aging with HIV infection. AIDS 28:939–943, 2014.
123. Erlandson KM, Allshouse AA, Jankowski CM, et al: Risk factors for falls in HIV-infected persons. J Acquir Immune Defic Syndr 61:484–489, 2012.
129. Clifford DB, Ances BM: HIV-associated neurocognitive disorder. Lancet Infect Dis 13:976–986, 2013.
130. Hellmuth J, Milanini B, Valcour V: Interactions between ageing and NeuroAIDS. Curr Opin HIV AIDS 9:527–532, 2014.
148. Brothers TD, Kirkland S, Guaraldi G, et al: Frailty in people aging with human immunodeficiency virus (HIV) infection. J Infect Dis 210:1170–1179, 2014.

114 Palliative Medicine for the Older Patient

Margred M. Capel

This chapter will define palliative care and consider it in the context of the older patient. In addition, it will briefly consider the impact of age and frailty on the illness, its social impact, and the strategies available. The second part of this chapter will concentrate on symptom control.

INTRODUCTION

The hospice movement arose out of religious orders in the late nineteenth and early twentieth centuries, although arguably it has been practiced by medical practitioners in some form throughout history.[1,2] However, it was Cicely Saunders pioneering work that brought the advances in pain and symptom control, leading to the special skills known as modern palliative care.

Death is an inevitable consequence of life; increasing life expectancy and altered disease trajectories mean that death from disease occurs more commonly in older adults. In developed countries, older adults may be affected by multiple coexisting acute and chronic illnesses. The annual number of worldwide deaths is expected to rise by 2030, an increase that is expected to occur through conditions related to organ failure and physical and cognitive frailty.[3] In the twenty-first century, palliative medicine aims to ensure that the dying process itself does not have to be the excruciating struggle that many older adults remember from when their grandparents died.

Palliative medicine can have an important role when patients are entering their last days of life, but it also can contribute to ameliorating the quality of life of patients suffering from chronic or intractable disease.[1,2] Palliative care is defined by the World Health Organization (WHO) as follows: "Palliative care is an approach that improves the quality of life of patients and their families facing the problems associated with life-threatening illness, through the prevention and relief of suffering by means of early identification and impeccable assessment and treatment of pain and other problems, physical, psychosocial, and spiritual."[4]

The Aging Process

Illnesses and coexisting morbidities encountered in older adults differ from those encountered in the young. The consequence of the aging process can mean that patients have coexisting cardiac, metabolic, and rheumatologic disorders (e.g., ischemic heart disease, diabetes, arthritis) in addition to developing illnesses associated with age itself (e.g., neurodegenerative disorders [dementia, Parkinson disease], stroke, cancer). The prevalence of failing organ function, such as heart failure and renal failure, can impose significant physical and psychological distress on the individual, restricting activities and quality of life of the patient and caregiver. In addition, the abnormal health state of frailty will contribute significantly to general weakness and fatigue. Frailty in this context refers to those who demonstrate progressive weakness and deterioration in their overall functional ability. Their decline may not correlate with their comorbidities, but they often lack the reserve to tolerate stressors such as intercurrent illness, examination, or hospital admission. This group of individuals, however, may experience a significant impact on their quality of life, undergo multiple hospital admissions, and incur significant amounts of health care and direct and indirect social care costs.[5,6]

Providing palliative care to older patients with frailty or chronic illness may mean that at different stages of the illness, the patient may require preventive or life-prolonging intervention, rehabilitation, or purely comfort measures, depending on the needs of the individual that are identified and their place along the illness journey. Recognition and shifting emphasis of care toward a goal-directed care may require sensitive communication with the patient and their care providers.[7,8]

The aging process alters organ function, which affects the pharmacokinetics of drug metabolism.[6,7] Pharmacodynamic processes are also affected by age, with some receptors (e.g., benzodiazepine, opiates) demonstrating greater sensitivity and others (e.g., insulin) having comparative insensitivity. The presence of coexisting disease risks compounding this through the consequences of polypharmacy.[7,9-11]

Care Providers

Cultural, ethnic, and social differences exist within communities, affecting the availability of support and expectations of care for the patient. The burden of home care falls mainly on female members of the family, and the intensity and economic costs can compare with those incurred by formal care provision.[2,12-15] A minority of care of older adults is from paid caregivers. In addition to spouses providing care for their partners, in the absence of spouses or in the event of their ill health, children often provide care for their older parents. This role reversal affects relationships and caregivers' physical and psychological health and has economic consequences.[12-15] Care providers have an increased risk factor for death, significant physical ill health, and depression.

Care providers of the older patient need increased support from the medical team during episodes of acute illness of the patient and ongoing support during chronic stages, which may require them to provide care over many years.[12-16] Care providers need full explanations of the disease processes to help manage their expectations and help them cope with the uncertainty that ill health brings.

The umbrella of palliative care may entitle patients and care provider's access to financial and social resources to help alleviate the economic and social burdens of care provision. Access to a day center or sitting service may provide some respite to the care provider. Respite care should be considered if the care provider has acute health needs and at planned regular intervals to provide a break from the work of caring. Unrelieved stress and the burden of care can otherwise result in a breakdown in the relationship between the care provider and patient, potentially spiraling down into situations of neglect, abuse, and worsening health in both parties.[14,15]

Care providers frequently have concerns and feeling of guilt when the patient is being cared for in a nursing or residential home environment so they need to be listened to and, when necessary, reassured of the reasons for the appropriateness of place of care. Often, those who have cared for a patient for a long time want to continue to provide some care when the patient is transferred to a nursing home or hospice facility. Helping them do this can relieve the burden of guilt and worry that they feel from relinquishing care in the home environment.

Following the death of the patient, the care provider may experience severe grief for the profound loss they have experienced and for their loss of this role in addition to readjusting to life and organizing funeral arrangements and financial affairs. Such individuals are at risk of prolonged or complicated bereavement and referral to bereavement support groups and counselors may be beneficial, depending on the individual's support network and coping strategies.

Future Planning

The importance of forward planning with older patients and their families or care providers cannot be underestimated. This can prevent considerable distress and disagreement if family members or care providers have to make decisions concerning health and social care when the patient is unable to do so. Many primary care practices and care facilities actively encourage Advance Care Planning (ACP) to explore, address, and record these discussions when patients are recognized to have significant comorbidities, frailty, or life-threatening illness. These discussions may require several meetings to cover all the relevant areas the patient wishes to explore and can benefit from the health practitioner who is most familiar with the individual taking the lead during the discussion and in future coordinated care delivery.

The Mental Capacity Act 2005 (England) directs medical teams to consider the information provided by individuals who are familiar with the patient in the event that the patient is unable to communicate her or his wishes. The responsibility for medical decisions that have to be taken on behalf of a patient who has lost capacity still ultimately rests with the medical team and not the family; an existing ACP can support and inform decision making. In the absence of family or friends, there is provision under the act for a court-appointed patient advocate who may provide input about aspects of social and medical care.[16]

An advanced decision to refuse treatment is legally binding and enables the patient to consider the recognized complications of his or her illness or dying process, explore treatment options, and communicate future preferred medical management in specific circumstances. The advance decision to refuse treatment can set limits on the interventions a patient would want to refuse in the future—for example, with respect to artificial feeding and nutrition, use of antibiotics, repeated venipuncture, resuscitation, and respiratory support. However, an advance decision cannot direct the clinical team to undertake an intervention if it is not clinically indicated in the patient's best interest.

The four ethical principles of autonomy, beneficence, nonmaleficence, and justice create a framework within which all clinical decisions should be considered. Autonomy or self-governance requires respect for the individual's right to determine her or his own well-being; however, to do this, patients require information in a comprehensible format to make informed choices concerning the future. The principle of nonmaleficence means that patients should not be burdened with futile investigations, treatments, or useless information that does not enhance their life. Attempts at cardiopulmonary resuscitation may fall into this category in certain circumstances. Beneficence dictates that the anticipated benefits must outweigh the anticipated risks and burdens of intervention or treatment. Justice implies that all patients may have similar access to investigations and treatments, without prejudice. It also implies that they may have the best possible care with the resources available, but these have to be fairly allocated and divided among their community.

The use of ethical frameworks can be applied to decisions regarding withdrawal of active treatment to achieve the appropriate choice for the individual and prevent unethical blanket policies.

Place of Care

The preferred place of care throughout life and when dying should be explored sensitively and honestly, making the older patient aware of feasible options and their limitations. Inequalities of access to home care nursing exists throughout the United Kingdom and can preclude care at home. Patients are recognized as being able to change their preferences during their illness journey. Factors recognized to influence decision making or preferred place of care are outlined in Figure 114-1.[17,18] Primary care teams who keep palliative care registers can use the trigger for completing DS1500 and/or the question: "Would you be surprised if the patient died within the next 6 months?" to identify patients for such a register. The DS1500 is the medical report outlining the terminally ill individual's condition and enabling him or her to access other financial benefits under special rules. This obviates the requirement of proving what care is needed, having a medical examination, and waiting for a mandatory period of time. In addition to this question, various tools exist to identify patients with palliative care needs, including the Gold Standards Framework (GSF)[19] and Supportive and Palliative Care Indicators Tool (SPICT).[20] A register can be used to inform out-of-hours services of the patient's condition and tailor provision of health care to prevent unwanted or unnecessary admissions to the hospital via the emergency or out-of-hours services.[19,20] Use of the GSF in care homes can reduce crisis hospital admissions, decrease the percentage of residents dying in the hospital, and facilitate patient-centered care. ACP should be offered to individuals included in any of these criteria.

Many hospices offer short-term admissions but cannot accommodate people for a prolonged period of terminal illness, which may mean that the individual experiences several admissions throughout the course of the terminal part of their illness. Use of individualized care plans or care priorities can support end-of-life care, encouraging care delivery to be of the highest standard, irrespective of location, and enhance communication.[15,17,19]

Patients can be considered terminally ill when they are likely to die within the foreseeable future from a specific progressing disease. Older patients often suffer from one or more chronic illnesses and/or frailty, in addition to experiencing progressive disease or receiving a terminal diagnosis, and can benefit from care with a palliative approach, apart from those who are actively dying and within their last days of life. Whenever symptoms occur, the potential cause of the symptom should be identified to guide treatment. Appropriate treatment of the cause may resolve the symptom and improve quality of life, even in the presence of concurrent terminal illness, such as treatment of hypothyroidism, Parkinson disease, or intercurrent infection. Problem-oriented clinical notes prove particularly useful in patients with multiple comorbidities.

SYMPTOM CONTROL

Pain

"Pain is what the patient says it is," and the same principle apply to treating pain in older adults as in younger patients.[2] Each pain should be identified, characterized (including site, duration intensity) and separately recorded, and precipitating and relieving factors identified. Application of the simplistic pneumonic PQRST[23] (see later, Key Points) may aid this process. This detailed history may suggest the underlying pathophysiology, which may determine pain treatments and possible disease-modifying interventions. Meticulous physical examination is essential; for example, abdominal pain from urinary retention compared with pain from acute abdomen or a tumor mass may give a similar history but have very different signs. The pain should be considered in holistic terms, including considering the impact this has on the individual because effective control of the physical aspect of symptom control requires consideration and intervention to the social, emotional, and spiritual dimensions of the individual. Pain assessment should include mood and

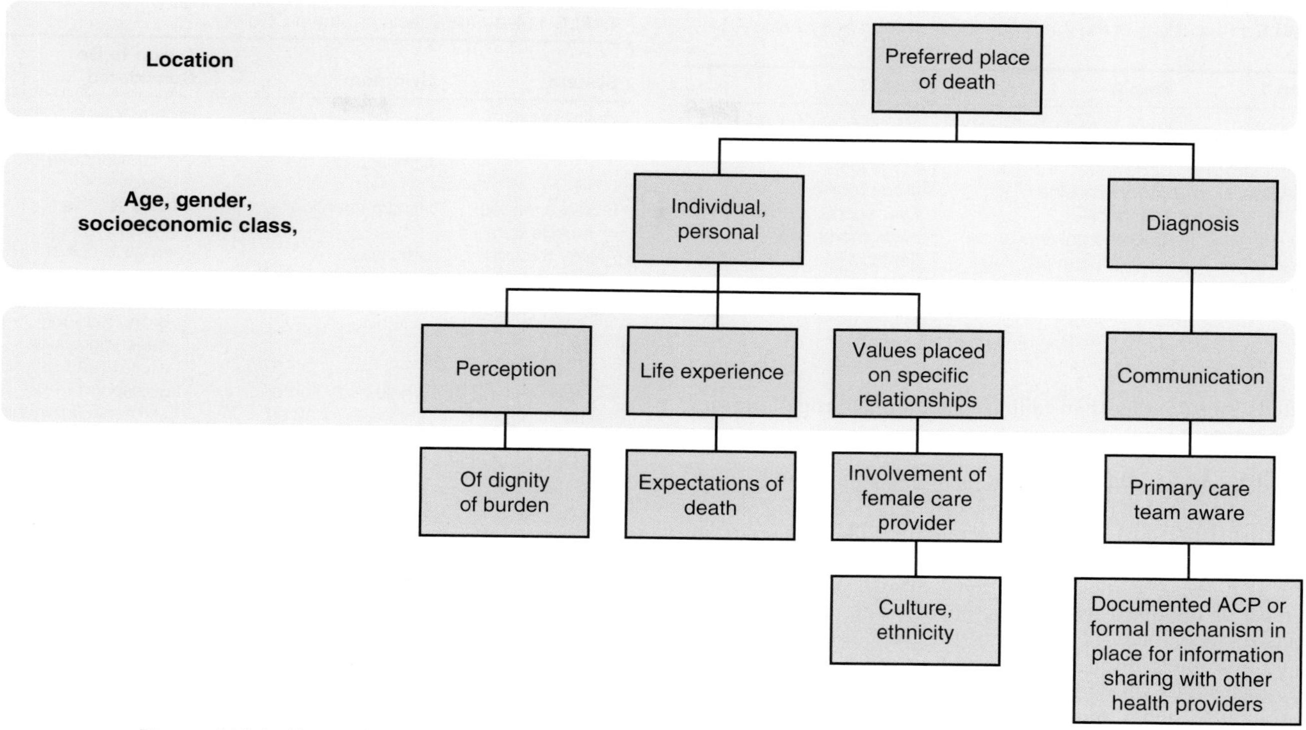

Figure 114-1. Personal and external influences concerning preferred place of care. *ACP,* Advance care planning.

emotional, functional, and cognitive assessment because these are recognized to affect pain perception and, unless addressed, may continue to be manifested as physical pain unresponsive to analgesia. Older patients, in comparison to their younger counterparts, are more likely to experience musculoskeletal, leg, and foot pain and less likely to experience headache and visceral pain (Box 114-1).[10,11,24]

After a baseline assessment of the pain, the situation should be evaluated every 24 hours until pain is controlled. A variety of tools can be used to assess pain, including the Simple Descriptive Pain Intensity Scale, Numeric Pain Intensity Scale, and Visual Analogue Scale. The Functional Pain Scale has been validated for use in older adults.[2,25] Altered behavior or agitation may be a manifestation of pain in patients with impaired communication; there are tools to support accurate monitoring of behavior and, through, this the impact of the introduction or titration of analgesia. Preferably, the tool should be accessible and applicable to the individual, family, and caregiver or staff using it.

Analgesic Titration

Analgesia can be titrated in accordance with the WHO analgesic ladder (Table 114-1), and, depending on the underlying pathophysiology of the pain, appropriate adjuvants can be included in the regimen. Consideration of tablet burden, medication compliance, and comorbidity may indicate that the most simplistic regimen is appropriate, or a blister pack or pill organizer box may need to be considered for a patient at home, with support from the appropriate community services.

Paracetamol is appropriate for osteoarthritis or musculoskeletal pains; the dose should be reduced in patients with liver impairment or probable malnutrition. Codeine is a prodrug of morphine. Co-codamol (paracetamol and codeine), 30/500, is an effective analgesic administered every 6 hours; however, variations in metabolism through cytochrome P4502D6 may significantly impair the analgesia available for use. Analgesia should be

BOX 114-1 Causes of Pain Reported by 500 Patients on Admission to Marie Curie Hospice Unit

- Aches associated with debility (but not attributable to malignancy)
- Angina
- Arthritis
- Bone, metastases, and pathologic fractures
- Concomitant infection: pleuritic chest pain, mouth discomfort, bladder spasm
- Cystitis
- Diaphragmatic pain, varying with respiration, from liver and diaphragmatic metastases
- Headache from raised intercranial compression
- Herpes zoster (shingles)
- Increased tone in paralyzed limb
- Infected pressure sores
- Intrinsic and extrinsic esophageal tumor mass
- Nerve compression
- Neuropathic pain
- Oral herpes simplex
- Organ capsule stretching, including liver capsule pain
- Pain not directly attributable to malignancy:
- Peptic ulcer pain manifested as abdominal pain, referred pain to shoulder tip from perforation
- Pleuritic pain from tumor nodules
- Radicular pain from spinal cord compression
- Rectal tenesmus
- Reflux esophagitis or dyspepsia
- Skin burning following radiotherapy
- Skin metastases
- Tumor bulk
- Visceral, caused by compression of adjacent structures

TABLE 114-1 Steps of the WHO Classification System for Analgesic Use

Step 1	Step 2	Step 3
Nonopioid ± adjuvant Paracetamol NSAIDs	Weak opioids ± adjuvant ± nonopioid Codeine Dihydrocodeine Tramadol (Buprenorphine is a mixed agonist-antagonist)	Strong opioids ± adjuvant ± nonopioid Morphine Diamorphine Oxycodone Hydromorphone Fentanyl Alfentanil Methadone

titrated upward rather than adding an additional drug of the same class or step.

Opioid Analgesia. Morphine is a recommended first-line step 3 analgesic (see Table 114-1); the dose can be titrated in increments of 30% to 50% until analgesia is achieved.[26] There is no ceiling dose for step 3 analgesics; rather, these should be titrated stepwise if the pain responds (i.e., can be demonstrated on assessment to diminish or disappear with analgesia use). The presence of side effects or incomplete resolution of the pain despite opioid use should prompt addition of an adjuvant, if not already begun. In frail older adults whose pain severity indicates that they should go straight to step 3, morphine (Oramorph, 2.5 mg), may be an appropriate starting dose of a step 3 opioids given on a regular 4-hour basis, reflecting the half-life of the drug.

Patients and care providers should be warned about the potential side effects of medication used and, where, possible these should be minimized; these are outlined in Table 114-2. For example a regular stimulant or mixed stimulant-softener laxative is almost always indicated when commencing step 3 strong opioids; about one third of patients will experience opioid-induced nausea, so an antiemetic such as haloperidol may be indicated for the first 7 to 10 days on the drug. Reassurance and explanation is often needed for those patients and care providers who think that the use of opioids could lead to the patient becoming a drug addict or becoming tolerant to the analgesic effect. The dosing interval or choice of opioids is influenced by coexisting organ failure. Persistence of side effects, including drowsiness, may be an indication for opioid rotation. Opioids that are extensively metabolized in the liver and do not accumulate during renal failure, such as fentanyl and alfentanil, would be drugs of choice for patients with analgesic requirements and renal impairment. Fentanyl is poorly orally absorbed and subject to extensive first-pass metabolism but is well absorbed from the oromucosal, transdermal, intranasal and subcutaneous routes. However, the patch or transdermal route is a comparatively inflexible route of drug delivery and is not suitable for a patient with unstable pain or rapidly escalating requirements; in such situations, subcutaneous administration may be needed.

The signs of fentanyl excess in older adults can initially be more subtle than those typically associated with morphine excess. In fentanyl toxicity, care providers may report that the patient is quieter and more sedentary than usual, whereas morphine toxicity usually causes drowsiness, confusion, hallucinations, grimacing, pinpoint pupils, slowed respiratory rate (respiratory depression), twitching, and myoclonus. Allodynia and hyperalgesia, are occasionally seen as a paradoxic hyperalgesia, but often their presence indicates a neuropathic pain that is only partly opioid-sensitive. Comparisons of equivalent doses of steps 2 and 3 opioids are available, and they should be applied when switching opioids.[26,27]

The route of drug delivery depends on the patient's condition and ability to ingest, retain, and absorb oral medication. Potential routes of drug delivery in frail palliative care patients include the oral, rectal, buccal, transdermal, and subcutaneous routes. Subcutaneous routes (including infusions and injections) are less painful than intramuscular injections and attenuate the rapid tolerance that may develop with repeated use of the intravenous route, making the subcutaneous route the parenteral route of choice. In cachectic patients, several drugs can be combined with use of a syringe driver; compatibility tables demonstrate which medication and concentrations can be combined safely.[28,29]

TABLE 114-2 Side Effects of Strong Opioids

System	Symptom	Action to Be Considered
Gastrointestinal	Nausea and vomiting Hiccup Constipation	Prophylactic antiemetic Prokinetic antiemetic Concomitant use of laxative
Increase smooth muscle tone	Urinary retention	Monitor for this symptom
Allergy through histamine release	Urticaria, bronchoconstriction and dyspnea, itching	Alternative opioid preparation, or antihistamine and bronchodilator depending upon context and severity
Centrally mediated phenomenon of itch	Whole body itch or can be localized with spinal morphine	May respond to use of serotonin antagonist
CNS	Multifocal myoclonus Cognition, sedation, vivid dreams Delirium and hallucinations	Exclude other causes, consider dose reduction use of benzodiazepine, or alternative opioid May resolve within few days of starting Check renal and liver function, consider dose reduction or alternative opioid Consider dose reduction, use of haloperidol or use of alternative opioid
Respiratory	Antitussive	

Diamorphine is preferred in the United Kingdom for subcutaneous administration because it is highly soluble, so a high concentration can be given in a small volume. However, in many countries, it is not available, and morphine is the drug of choice. When analgesia is obtained that controls ongoing or background pain, provision must still be made for short-acting analgesia to be available to ameliorate any breakthrough pain.

Types of Pain

Breakthrough Pain. Breakthrough pain is any pain that occurs over and above a background of well-controlled pain. This is a different entity from that in patients who have an increasing analgesic requirement that increases over time because of underlying disease progression, rather than tolerance.[29] Oral transmucosal fentanyl citrate (OTFC) lozenges or dispersible tablets can be applied to the patient's moist oral mucosa to provide rescue analgesia for breakthrough pain as the drug is absorbed transmucosally. Fentanyl or alfentanil preparations are also available via an inhaler or nasal delivery system, but specialist supervision is suggested for the initial test dose. This is because drug delivery is rapid but comparatively short-lived, making this useful for pain associated with movement or dressing changes. Theoretically, any short-lived opioid may be given in advance if the pain is predictable in nature. Pain that occurs unpredictably requires accurate diagnosis of the cause of the pain and interrupting the pathologic process, when possible; if not possible, adding an adjuvant medication or increasing the background dose of opioids may be helpful.

Bone Pain. Bone and joint pain may respond to adjuvant analgesia, including nonsteroidal antiinflammatory drugs (NSAIDs), which have a synergistic effect with paracetamol. NSAIDs should be prescribed with caution for patients already taking aspirin, steroids, or selective serotonin reuptake inhibitors (SSRIs; increased risk of gastrointestinal bleeding), diuretics, or angiotensin-converting enzyme (ACE) inhibitors, among others, because these increase the risk of renal failure.

In malignant disease, bone metastases can erode the bone cortex. This can be identified on plain radiographs. Prophylactic surgical intervention may prevent subsequent pathologic fracture. Radiotherapy provides analgesia in 80% of patients with pain from bone metastases and can be considered for frail individuals.[1,2] Patients with multiple bone metastases, in the absence of spinal cord compression and with a prognosis longer than 6 weeks, may benefit from radioactive isotope injection (e.g., strontium). Bone pain, particularly from breast, myeloma, or prostate primary, may respond to infusions of intravenous bisphosphonates, despite a normal calcium level, and there is some evidence that bisphosphonates protect against bone metastases in certain cancers (e.g., breast).[30,31] Fractured bones should always be immobilized, if possible. If immobilization is not possible, local injection into the fracture site with Depo-Medrone (methylprednisolone acetate), 80 mg, and bupivacaine hydrochloride, 0.5%, may provide sufficient relief to allow the patient to be turned in the last days of life. An alternative would be an interventional anesthetic procedure and nerve block to the area.

Musculoskeletal Pain. Topical capsaicin cream has been advocated for mild musculoskeletal and neuropathic pain. However, repeated applications are required to prevent substance P reaccumulating and pain recurring. Because the capsaicin is a strong irritant, it can cause a burning sensation on initial application, and care must be taken to prevent any contamination of the eyes and mucous membranes. Topical analgesic preparations or lignocaine patches may be useful alternatives in select circumstances.[32,33] Massage and heat therapy (if sensation is intact) may ameliorate musculoskeletal pain. Physiotherapy may prevent contractures developing in paralyzed limbs, and the patient and care providers should also be taught maintenance therapy exercises. Skeletal muscle relaxants such as baclofen may relieve discomfort caused by stiffness under these circumstances, but the dose has to be titrated against the sedative side effects.[27]

Neuropathic Pain. Neuropathic pain is characterized by pain with a burning or electric shock quality or pain in an area of altered sensation and may occur as a result of any part of the central or peripheral nervous system being subject to compression, destruction, or infiltration. Patients may describe this pain in limbs affected by cerebrovascular events, especially if the thalamus is involved. The pain can be severe and associated with altered sensations, including allodynia. Relief of nerve compression may be attempted through radiotherapy to diminish tumor size and high-dose steroids (up to 16 mg dexamethasone in divided doses, to be reduced over time) to reduce any peritumor edema. In certain circumstances, surgical intervention may be appropriate.

Tricyclic antidepressants in low doses, such as amitriptyline, 10 to 25 mg at night, are useful adjuvant medications for neuropathic pain; the mode of action occurs through potentiation of opioids, serotonin reuptake inhibition, and reduction in pain perception.[27,29] In older adults, the use of tricyclic antidepressants, even in low doses, may be limited by anticholinergic side effects, including constipation, dry mouth, urinary retention, confusion, and tachycardia. The use of membrane-stabilizing anticonvulsants such as carbamazepine and valproate are also limited by side effects, the most significant of which in older adults is drowsiness; their use in neuropathic pain has been largely overtaken by gabapentin. Gabapentin has been approved for use in neuropathic pain but the dose must be tapered against the side effects of drowsiness and impaired renal function. Its precursor, pregabalin, is also marketed for neuropathic pain but its advantage seems relatively small (tolerability), and the cost is generally higher.

Ketamine, an anesthetic agent, has a role in the control of difficult neuropathic pain. It is effective in low-dose subcutaneous infusions, 50 to 200 mg/24 hr, combined with low-dose midazolam or an antipsychotic medication to combat the side effects of dysphoria and hallucinations. It is a cardiovascular stimulant so it may be of use in combination with opioids because it counteracts their hypotensive effects and can be used in patients with renal failure.[27,33] Emerging case reports have suggested that it may have a toxic effect on the urinary tract in some individuals, so it should be used under specialist supervision only. Methadone can provide useful analgesia. However, its unpredictable half-life makes it difficult to use routinely because it tends to accumulate in older adults and has been associated with a prolonged QT interval on electrocardiograms (ECGs).

Nerve Blocks

Nerve blocks have a role in the management of pain from malignant and nonmalignant causes. Celiac plexus blocks, in particular, are useful for pain associated with pancreatic cancer, liver capsule stretch, and intraperitoneal and retroperitoneal structures. The block can be repeated after several months, as required. Psoas compartment blocks can provide relief from hip pain. Epidural injections or indwelling catheters can provide relief from spinal nerve infiltration or compression. The medication used depends on local policy and preference but tends to involve opioids and local anesthetics; steroids may also have a place. Complex pain with sympathetic involvement may also respond to sympathetic nerve blockade. Suprascapular nerve blocks may relieve pain arising in the shoulder joint, intraarticular injections may also be effective in providing analgesia and relieving the systemic analgesic burden.

Nausea and Vomiting

To treat nausea and vomiting effectively, it is essential to identify the underlying cause and target the intervention accordingly. For example, vomiting can be an indication of hypercalcemia, renal failure, or bowel obstruction, each of which requires specific interventions in addition to tailored antiemetic therapy.

In the older patient, causes related to comorbidity should always be considered, such as benign positional vertigo, gastroparesis related to diabetes, and constipation. Nausea and vomiting can be an unwanted side effect of opioids and many other drugs. The opportunity to review an individual's medication with the general practitioner and discontinue any inappropriate medication(s) to prevent polypharmacy should always be taken.

Vomiting is initiated by the stimulus of different receptors on brain stem nuclei. Antiemetics can be selected to target different receptors, depending on the cause of the stimulus identified.[34] The specific neurotransmitters involved include dopamine, acetylcholine, histamine, and serotonin. Attention should be paid to comorbidities, such as Parkinson disease, when selecting specific antiemetics to prevent exacerbating these conditions. Toxins, drugs, and metabolic abnormalities stimulate the chemoreceptor trigger zone lying next to the vomiting center on the floor of the fourth ventricle. Central dopamine antagonists, including low-dose haloperidol, 1.5 to 3 mg, or metoclopramide, 10 to 80 mg orally or subcutaneously, are effective. Buccal or rectal prochlorperazine has limited use because it can cause confusion in older adults as a side effect.

Cyclizine is an antihistamine anticholinergic drug that may be used in combination with drugs acting at the central dopamine receptors to increase receptor blockade. It can be given orally; subcutaneous injections can be painful and associated with inflammation at the injection site. It may precipitate with certain drugs at high concentration in a syringe driver (syringe pump).

Prokinetics, such as metoclopramide or domperidone (available as tablets or suppositories, respectively), are useful if the individual has delayed gastric emptying as a consequence of extrinsic pressure from liver metastases, a duodenal, mesenteric, or pancreatic tumor, or ascites. Domperidone is of particular use because it does not readily cross the blood-brain barrier and therefore does not precipitate central dopamine loss.

Patients with ascites caused by malignant pathology can receive symptomatic relief from nausea, vomiting, dyspnea, and discomfort from paracentesis. This can be performed in established centers on an outpatient basis. It is not always appropriate or necessary to perform paracentesis against the intravenous administration of fluids.[27,35] Consideration should be given to the pathologic and physiologic processes contributing to the formation of ascites in the individual and to avoiding dehydration by removing excessive amounts of ascites while continuing diuretics or ACE inhibitors. Patients on a therapeutic trial of diuretics aimed at reducing the accumulation of ascites should be monitored for hypotension and the drugs discontinued if no discernible benefit is observed.

Nausea from liver metastases may respond to low-dose dexamethasone, 2 to 4 mg daily. Serotonin receptor antagonists, such as ondansetron or granisetron, have a role in the short-term management of vomiting related to chemotherapy, radiotherapy, or nausea related to bleeding within the gastrointestinal tract. There is a transdermal preparation effective for 7 days that can be administered prior to chemotherapy and subsequently removed. Constipation, headache, and expense limits prolonged use.

Hiccups can be distressing. Again, drug management must be tailored to the identified cause; for example, gastric distention through stasis may respond to prokinetic agents. Tumors involving the diaphragm or brain stem can respond to centrally acting drugs, including nifedipine,[34,36] baclofen,[37] and low-dose chlorpromazine.

Constipation

Constipation is a very common problem among older adults. Chronic conditions that predispose to constipation include Parkinson disease, hypothyroidism, diabetes mellitus, depression, diverticular disease, and hemorrhoids.[2] Immobility and medication also contribute significantly to constipation. Constipation is a common side effect of opioid medications, and all patients started on opioids should be co-prescribed laxatives. Nonopioid medications that predispose to constipation include iron and calcium supplements, calcium channel blockers, antihistamines, tricyclic antidepressants, and diuretics.

Assessment of constipation should include frequency, normal habit, consistency, pain, and diet. A rectal examination is useful to exclude impaction. High-fiber preparations should be avoided because they may exacerbate constipation if used without adequate fluid intake. It may be prudent to avoid, or use with caution, stimulant medication in patients with known colonic lesions. Lactulose is an effective stool softener in large divided doses (60 to 90 mL daily) but can produce a lot of flatus.[1,5,23,38]

Unless contraindicated, a stimulant (e.g., senna) and sodium docusate or magnesium hydroxide softener are appropriate combinations to use. Co-danthramer (dantron, poloxamer) has a mixed action. The liquid preparation is still available but the tablets are no longer manufactured. It is approved for use in terminally ill patients only and can discolor urine and feces. It can cause severe skin irritation in patients with fecal incontinence. In cases of severe constipation, high-dose polyethylene glycol 3350 (e.g., Movicol or Laxido, up to eight sachets daily for up to 3 days) or sodium picosulfate 5-10 mg od may be needed. Fecal impaction can be treated with high-dose polyethylene glycol 3350, enemas, or manual disimpaction with suitable analgesia cover. In countries where this is still available, peanut (arachis) oil retention enemas (in patients who are not allergic to peanuts) followed by a phosphate enema the next morning can be successful. Constipation should be actively prevented in those who suffer from shortness of breath because the effort of defecating can exacerbate dyspnea.

Bowel Obstruction

Surgery is often not indicated in patients with bowel obstruction at multiple sites. This situation usually arises in ovarian and colon cancers. Patients who are identified to be at risk benefit from preventive management with stool softeners. Bowel obstruction is associated with vomiting, which can become feculent; additional late signs include pain and distention. The diagnosis can be made on clinical grounds; plain abdominal films may be surprisingly unremarkable early.

Medical management of acute obstructive episodes requires antispasmodics such as hyoscine butylbromide for colic, with an opioid to relieve abdominal pain. An antiemetic acting at the vomiting center, such as cyclizine, should be considered. In case of obstruction, the oral route is unreliable, so medication is often best delivered via a syringe driver (pump), but cyclizine cannot be mixed in the same syringe with hyoscine butylbromide.

Corticosteroids sometimes are of benefit in obstruction, but unfortunately the factors that determine patients who will benefit have not been elucidated.[39] It may be appropriate to try high-dose dexamethasone for a few days and discontinue this if there is no discernible improvement. Octreotide may reduce the volume of intestinal secretions, but should be used under specialist supervision.[40] There is no evidence to support drip and suck regimens in most patients with intestinal obstruction. Patients can usually take oral fluids and even light meals, but may have to contend with a minimal number of vomit episodes during the day.

Diarrhea

Diarrhea can result in dehydration, electrolyte imbalance, exhaustion, and loss of dignity. It can be exhausting and distressing for care providers who have to assist patients to the bathroom or change pads, clothing, and bed clothes for the bedridden patient.

Identifying the cause is essential. Radiotherapy, antibiotics, malabsorption, stress, and gastrointestinal bleeding are recognized precipitants. Rectal examination can exclude fecal impaction and overflow leakage, which are all too common; see earlier ("Constipation") for treatment. A stool specimen will exclude *Clostridium difficile* infection. Once reversible causes have been excluded, patients can be managed with rehydration, bulking agents, loperamide, or codeine-based products. Patients with fistulae, high-output stomas, or secretory diarrhea as a consequence of underlying pathology can benefit from octreotide.[40,41] Early referral to a local continence service is essential.

Problems With Oral intake

Dysphagia and disordered swallowing may occur as part of end-stage dementia, other neurodegenerative diseases, stroke, and some malignancies, predisposing the individual to malnutrition and aspiration pneumonia. Changing the texture of food and fluid, use of thickeners, and careful positioning of the individual when eating supports safe swallowing. Patients should be reassessed by speech and language therapists as their disease progresses and swallowing changes so that appropriate advice can guide care.

Eating is a social activity; altered diets or exclusion of the individual from family meals can lead to social isolation and diminish quality of life.[42] Providing food and drink can be a source of stress between patients and their care providers, with patients turning their heads away or clenching their teeth and refusing to eat carefully prepared meals, so care providers need support and explanation. Anorexia can be part of the natural dying process; in this situation, artificial nutrition will not prolong life and may be burdensome and distort the focus of care. However, this matter must be explained and understood by care providers via a sensitive explanation to avoid the perception that the patient is being starved to death and food or fluid is forced into the mouth of someone unable to swallow. Symptoms of thirst can be relieved with good oral hygiene, artificial saliva, and sips of water or ice cubes. These are practical interventions, easily undertaken by the nurse or care provider. If this does not appear adequate, subcutaneous fluids can be considered in the community or inpatient environment.

Artificial and supplemental feeding may need to be considered, depending on the stage of the illness or acute intercurrent illness, with the patient's consent, particularly in the preterminal stages. However, subcutaneous fluid rehydration may provide comfort to some patients, even in the last days of life. Nasogastric feeding should not be considered a long-term option because it is uncomfortable and may require frequent replacement, with risk of pulmonary placement, nasal irritation, and aspiration pneumonia. For long-term nutrition, gastrostomy and jejunostomy tubes should be considered. These confer their own risks related to the procedure and infection and do not prevent the risk of aspiration if they are used with the patient in a supine position; diarrhea is a potential complication. Parenteral feeding predisposes to infection and loss of integrity of the intestinal lumen. Patients should be considered as individuals and options tailored accordingly, rather than adhering to a single policy.

Anosmia is a frequent concomitant of advancing years, particular in those who have smoked; lack of smell aggravates lack of appetite because taste is impaired. Good dentition is essential to eating, so oral hygiene is key. The loss of dentures should be considered an emergency because it immediately restricts the individual's diet, oral intake, communication, and socialization. Good dental care is increasingly important in those on bisphosphonates or the monoclonal antibody targeted to ligand receptor activator of nuclear factor κB (RANKL) because osteonecrosis of the jaw is a devastating potential complication.

Medication commonly causes dry mouth. In addition to discontinuing medication, where possible, symptomatic relief can be achieved by sucking crushed ice, sips of fluid, artificial saliva, or fresh or frozen pineapple pieces.[1,2] Oral *Candida* infection is a relatively frequent finding because the fungi adhere to denture plastic, but oral candidiasis does not necessarily correlate with oral symptoms.[2,42,43] Dysphagia is an indication for systemic antifungals. However, radiologic imaging is indicated if the dysphagia does not resolve rapidly because other pathology may be concurrent. Oral ulcers can be systematically managed with a coating gel or mouthwash with topical lidocaine, steroid-based cream, or coating agents, but the underlying cause—often ill-fitting dentures or poor nutrition—must be sought.[1,2]

Dyspnea

Shortness of breath is a subjective sensation, which can be experienced despite normal pulse oximetry and respiratory rate. It is a common symptom in malignant and nonmalignant disease, which increases in prevalence in the last weeks of life.[2,44] Patients with nonmalignant disease but clear deteriorating health and recurrent hospital admissions should be encouraged to discuss their perceptions and fears; they may want to regain control of their condition through ACP or an advance decision to refuse treatment should they suddenly deteriorate again.

Elucidating the cause of breathlessness requires a detailed history and examination. Often, modification of the disease process concurrently with palliation of symptoms is the most effective approach. Steroids, bronchodilators, diuretics, β-blockers, and ACE inhibitors have a place in the management of chronic obstructive pulmonary disease (COPD) and cardiac failure, respectively. Acute cardiac failure may need intravenous frusemide, nitrates, and parenteral diamorphine. Uncontrolled arrhythmias should be identified and managed appropriately. Antibiotics have a place in symptom management, even in the terminally ill, to resolve pleuritic pain and the sensation of systemic ill health associated with pneumonia and infection. Draining pleural effusions can provide prompt symptom relief. In selected individuals, endobronchial stents may relieve the dyspnea resulting from airway collapse and tumor occlusion.[1,2]

Patients with anemia rarely benefit from iron supplementation. Transfusion of packed cells may achieve the most rapid improvement, particularly when the hemoglobin level is below 10 g/L.

Long-term oxygen therapy may improve exercise tolerance and longevity in patients with COPD but, unless humidifiers are used, can produce nasal irritation and dryness. The mask and tubing are cumbersome. Relief from dyspnea can often be achieved simply through use of a fan or open window to cool the patient's face.[44,45]

Opioids reduce the symptoms of dyspnea.[45-48] There have been case reports and studies on small series of patients involving the administration of various opioids via different routes, but the most robust evidence exists for the use of morphine. Research has demonstrated that in the dosages used for symptom control, there is no significant adverse effect on respiratory rate, oxygen, or carbon dioxide concentration.[47] In the opioid-naïve patient, 1 mg to 5 mg of oral morphine every 4 hours may suffice. In patients already receiving regular opioids, an increase in the background dose of 25% to 30% may provide similar relief.[45,46] In patients unable to swallow, subcutaneous administration of diamorphine can be used to achieve the same effect. Patients in whom anxiety and fear are prominent may benefit from the administration of benzodiazepine, either low-dose oral diazepam or subcutaneous midazolam.

Dyspnea clinics incorporating the principles of activity pacing, relaxation, breathing control, and efficient mobilization can improve symptoms for patients able to attend them.[48]

Cough

Persistent cough can be an irritating and tiring symptom in malignant and nonmalignant disease. Common nonmalignant causes include esophageal reflux, postnasal drip, COPD, cardiac failure, pneumonia, and side effects of medication. The treatment should target the underlying pathology. Cough assist devices can have a role in individuals with identified neuromuscular weakness. Treatment of cough resulting from malignant pathology may include steroids and radiotherapy. Oxygen should be humidified if the cough results from dry airways, or regular saline nebulizers can be used. Mucolytics, expectorants, bronchodilators, and chest physiotherapy may be useful in the management of productive coughs. Cough syrup containing preparations of codeine or methadone or regular low-dose opioids, including morphine, can have an antitussive effective.

Patients entering their last days of life with a weak or absent cough reflex are unable to clear their airways and may develop the so-called death rattle, the sound of air passing over fluid in the trachea. The sound can be distressing to families who need reassurance and an explanation from staff. Anticholinergics, including hyoscine hydrobromide, hyoscine butylbromide, atropine, and glycopyrronium, can reduce secretions and can be administered subcutaneously.[1,2,49] If it is important to prevent the sedative side effects and propensity to cause confusion or delirium, then glycopyrronium or hyoscine butylbromide should be used because they do not cross the blood-brain barrier.

Dizziness

Dizziness is commonly reported by older patients and is recognized as a syndrome in its own right. Unfortunately, there is rarely a single cause for this distressing symptom, which may result in falls, syncope, functional disability, residential or nursing home placement, or death.[50] Medication, cardiac arrhythmias, vascular disease, vestibular disorders, diabetic neuropathy, and altered proprioception may all contribute. In the absence of reversible causes, management involves educating the patient and care providers to prevent triggers and create a safe home environment. Medication should be reviewed and rationalized.

TABLE 114-3 Common Causes of Confusion

Comorbidity	Cognitive impairment Neurodegenerative conditions Dementia Cerebrovascular disease Poor vision Hearing loss
Drugs	Anticholinergics Benzodiazepines Withdrawal from medication Withdrawal from alcohol Opioids
Systemic	Infection Urinary retention Constipation
Metabolic	Hypoxia Uremia Organ failure Hypercalcemia Hyperglycemia, hypoglycemia
Malignancy-related	Cerebral metastases Paraneoplastic syndromes

Fatigue

Fatigue is a common and distressing symptom experienced as a consequence of many diseases, including malignancy and end-stage cardiac and respiratory failure. This symptom results in a loss of independence of the patient; the dependence on care providers can have a profound psychological impact on the patient, who may think that he or she is becoming a burden. Reversible causes are worth excluding; these include anemia, depression, thyroid disease, hypokalemia, hypocalcaemia, and magnesium deficiency. Drugs that cause daytime somnolence, such as anxiolytics, antipsychotics, and β-blockers, should be minimized or discontinued. Antihypertensives should be reviewed with respect to the patient's current cardiovascular and fluid status.

Optimizing physical fitness, pacing activities, and sleeping routine, and working with the patient and care providers to set realistic and achievable goals, can help the patient maximize his or her quality of life.

Anorexia-cachexia syndrome commonly occurs in patients with end-stage illness, often leading to protein undernutrition. The syndrome is caused by altered equilibrium and disrupted metabolism of inflammatory cytokines.[51] Communicating this information to the patient and care provider may help in understanding and acceptance. Treatment of nausea and altered taste, maximizing oral hygiene, and ensuring that dentures fit properly are essential. There are various protein and calorie supplements but they should not be forced on the patient if they are found to be unpalatable. Frequent small meals of favorite foods may be an acceptable alternative. Steroids are often used to augment appetite but the effect is short lived; long-term steroid therapy may exacerbate myopathy and fatigue.[1,2]

Depression and Adjustment Disorder

Patients may undergo a bereavement process themselves as they become aware of their terminal illness and loss of independence and future. Patients may experience and express a range of emotions. These feelings can be exacerbated by unresolved bereavements or losses. Allowing time to explore a patient's past may reveal these losses and provide support to enable patients to reconcile themselves to events.

Estimates vary about the number of terminally ill patients with depression, perhaps 7% to 30%. Antidepressants may be appropriate for patients with early morning waking, anxiety states, lack of reactivity, feelings of pessimism toward others, or anhedonia or those who are socially withdrawn. Symptoms including weakness, tiredness, loss of appetite, or pessimism concerning oneself are recognized manifestations of the terminal illness process and are not necessarily indicators of depression.[52-55]

Confusion

Cognitive impairment, unfortunately, can accompany some chronic diseases and, as noted earlier, patients should be encouraged to participate in advance preparation and share their wishes and preferences for future care. Older patients are particularly at risk of acute confusion states. The risk of delirium has been demonstrated to increase with age, cognitive impairment, infection, organ failure, certain drugs, polypharmacy, and fracture.[56] Common causes of confusion are listed in Table 114-3.[1,2]

Management of acute confusion involves treating reversible causes and minimizing sensory impairment by restoring hearing aids and glasses. The individual should be cared for in a well-lit room, with minimal background noise, and spoken to calmly and reassuringly.[27,56,57] Short-term low-dose antipsychotic medication may be helpful in treating the agitated confused individual who is expressing paranoid thoughts or experiencing hallucinations. Benzodiazepines can exacerbate symptoms. Care providers require explanation and reassurance for a symptom that can be distressing to observe in a loved one.

The causes of confusion specifically related to malignancy include cerebral metastases and hypercalcemia. Paraneoplastic syndromes are uncommonly encountered and respond to modification of the disease process where possible.[57,58] Cerebral metastases may respond to high-dose dexamethasone (16 mg).[56-58] If there is no response after 5 days, the steroid can be stopped abruptly.

Hypercalcemia is a reversible cause of confusion. In the context of solid malignancy, it usually confers a poor prognosis. It can occur in patients with mainly osteolytic bone metastases that release cytokines, which stimulate osteoclast-activating factors, tumors secreting a parathyroid-like hormone or tumors producing 1,25-dihydroxyvitamin D. Rehydration with intravenous fluid, 0.9% sodium chloride, should be commenced, followed by intravenous bisphosphonate. Pamidronate can be effective or zoledronic acid, a more effective but expensive alternative, may be considered.[1,2] Treatment for hypercalcemia may need to be repeated periodically, and the calcium monitored on discharge into the community. The new monoclonal therapies, which reduce osteoclastogenesis through action at the RANKL (e.g., denosumab), may have a role.

Advanced illness can often be complicated by infection. Reduction of risk factors through maintenance of good skin care, individual nursing care to ensure appropriate toileting, repositioning of the immobile patient, and careful feeding to minimize aspiration are necessary. Symptom relief measures, including antipyretics and analgesics, should be commenced if infection is identified. Antibiotics can be prescribed for symptom relief but may not be appropriate or confer any benefit in certain circumstances; advance planning with the patient and care providers is essential to identify the goals of care in the presence of the changing needs of the patient. For example, antibiotics in advanced dementia do not improve survival benefit.[59,60] Disadvantages of antibiotic therapy include allergic reactions, development of resistant infections, *C. difficile* infection, diarrhea, bone marrow impairment, seizures, renal failure, and vomiting. Patients with severe cognitive impairment may not be able to rationalize the administration of intravenous antibiotics or accept painful intramuscular antibiotics.

Pressure Ulcers

Immobility, incontinence, cachexia, malnutrition, and comorbidity contribute to the formation of decubitus pressure ulcers, which should be managed according to standard wound care guidelines.[58,59] The presence of a wound is an indicator of advanced disease and poor prognosis, but is not in itself an independent risk factor for death.[8-10]

Depending on local access and availability, it may be appropriate to refer patients incapacitated from lymphedema to local lymphedema services to reduce its size and restore function to limbs. General management of lymphedema includes careful skin hygiene and prevention of acute inflammatory episodes.

Those at risk of pressure sores require an appropriate level of nursing intervention to turn and adjust the position of the patient regularly and systematically, whether the patient is at home or in a long-term care facility. Caregivers need instructions on how to protect vulnerable pressure points.

In the context of end-of-life care, when a pressure sore is present, it may be more appropriate to focus on comfort, including relief of pain and control of odor, bleeding, or discharge because healing may be an unrealistic goal. Pressure-relieving measures are essential for wound management, and dressings have a role in the relief of pain. Short-acting analgesia can be administered to the patient before painful dressing changes. There is some evidence that the application of a topical analgesia in the form of diamorphine or morphine sulfate mixed in a medium or lubricating gel (e.g., Instillagel) to a painful wound can cause local relief without the disadvantage of incurring systemic side effects.[61] Odor can be limited through the use of adequate cleaning, frequent dressing changes, and use of topical metronidazole or silver sulfadiazine. Appropriate topical dressings such as charcoal dressings can contain odors. If the patient is not suffering from nausea, lemon or vanilla oils or a filtering or air purifier can be used to mask smells in the immediate environment. A short prognosis should not preclude a patient from referral to local wound care services if their input could ameliorate suffering from a wound.

Spiritual Suffering

The religious or spiritual beliefs of older patients are important. Faced with a debilitating or terminal illness, patients may question their self-identity, meaning and purpose of their life, and prior decisions or actions undertaken during their lives.[62,63] Faith leaders or religious customs may support the individual patient and care providers, particularly during stressful periods, and enable them to reconcile events.

Specific requests for euthanasia should be dealt with sympathetically and the request should be considered an opportunity to explore the deep distress that the patient may be experiencing. The request may be associated with untreated physical or psychological symptoms, fear of the future, including fear of becoming a burden, anger and guilt concerning the effect of the disease on their life, and lack of an appropriate environment or dignity in their care delivery.[52,53,62-64]

Terminal Stage

Accurately predicting an individual's prognosis is difficult and fraught with misinterpretation by the patient and care providers.[1,2] Dying can be difficult to diagnose in patients who have been significantly unwell for a period of time because of chronic ill health. Reflecting and comparing the individual's current condition and performance with that acknowledged 6 or 12 months previously may enable the patient and caregivers to achieve perspective.

In general, the prognosis is likely to be measured in days when the patient's condition is deteriorating on a daily basis to the extent that they are unable to take oral medication or tolerate more than sips of water and are bedridden or semicomatose.[1,2,17] Sensitive communication of this information enables the patient and care providers to prepare for death, but it can provoke various emotional responses in a situation where caregivers have looked after patients through various stages of health and illness.[63,65] This may be an opportunity for resolution of any outstanding family or interpersonal conflict, apologies, and reconciliations and to express feelings and love. Poor communication surrounding dying underpins over half of the complaints received in the National Health Service.[65-68] Missed opportunities can result in bitterness, anger, and unresolved grief in care providers following the bereavement.

Realistic goals can then be set for care, which encompass the maintenance of dignity and comfort rather than prolonging the dying phase. This should be discussed with the care providers and, where appropriate, with the individual. Care providers may find that knowing that death will be allowed to occur naturally is far more acceptable than being told that their loved one will not be resuscitated. Explanations should include what to expect during the dying process (including the potential for death rattle and a Cheyne-Stokes breathing pattern) and what to do after death occurs if the patient is dying at home.

Medication can be reviewed and many drugs omitted without detriment to the individual. Regular or routine monitoring of blood test results and other observations (e.g., blood pressure) can be discontinued, although it can be useful sometimes to monitor respiratory rate to reassure relatives that the patient has not been oversedated. Medications essential for symptom control can be given as subcutaneous injections or via infusion using a syringe pump (driver).[27] If repeated subcutaneous injections are needed, a small subcutaneous butterfly cannula can be sited for administration. Fluid intake can be poor, but careful oral care (see earlier) may relieve the sensation of thirst. Occasionally, patients will benefit from subcutaneous hydration to maintain comfort when dying and prevent dehydration; subcutaneous fluids can be given at home.

Preemptive planning allows medication to be prescribed and obtained in the patient's home to be administered to maintain symptom control, if needed.[2,8,19] Medication should include opioids to administer for pain and dyspnea, antiemetics, anticholinergics for the death rattle, and sedatives (e.g., midazolam) if the individual becomes agitated. Restlessness may have several potential causes, including urinary retention, constipation, metabolic abnormalities, pain, fear, and unresolved spiritual distress.

Once reversible causes have been addressed, the patient may benefit from sedative medication administered subcutaneously via a syringe pump. Realistic goals for monitoring and interventions in diabetes management should be agreed on and documented in the individual's care plan, recognizing that hyperglycemia, even during end-of- life care, can add to symptom distress.[20,67,68]

Care providers should be encouraged to talk to the patient and each other. They should also be shown how to participate in caregiving if they wish to, including mouth care and physical turning if the patient is dying at home, in particular. Any religious ceremony or customs surrounding death should be undertaken. Many of these goals are embodied in the care pathway, and individual care plans should strive for these standards at a minimum.[1,2,19,27]

Many deaths in patients with chronic disease follow recognized patterns or illness trajectories.[19,59] Occasionally, a sudden catastrophic event, such as a massive hemorrhage, stridor, or pulmonary embolism, occurs, and death can take place in a few moments.[2,58] Staff are encouraged to maintain a calm and reassuring manner for the patient and any care providers present. If this situation has been foreseen and time permits, the patients can be rendered unconscious and unaware through the use of anxiolytic medication, which has an amnesic effect. Care providers will require reassurance and explanation after the event to understand why the event occurred and that their loved one did not experience any distress.

CONCLUSION

Palliative care for older patients focuses on preserving function, dignity, and quality of life to enable individuals to live their life actively. Recognition of illness trajectories, including cancer, organ failure, and frailty, may enable service coordination to support the individual with goal-directed care and preemptive planning. Preparation and open discussion of the future, including end-of-life care and death, enable patients to regain control over their lives and relieve the stress that caregivers experience from decision making. Attention should be paid to identifying and relieving care provider stress.

KEY POINTS: ELICITING THE CAUSE OF EACH PAIN USING "PQRST"

For each type of pain, identify the following:

- Precipitating or relieving factors
- Quality of the pain (e.g., burning in an area of altered sensation may point to neuropathic pain)
- Radiation of the pain (e.g., radicular pain)
- Severity (often rated using visual analogue or numeric on 0-10 scale)
- Temporal factors (how long it has been present/how long it lasts if intermittent; whether worse at particular times of day)

PALLIATIVE MEDICINE FOR THE OLDER PATIENT

- The definition of palliative medicine and its application along with the different stages of the illness journey of the elderly population
- Supporting decision making and future planning, a place for the Mental Capacity Act and ethical frameworks
- The origin of pain and the therapeutic management options
- Palliation of gastrointestinal and respiratory symptoms
- Confusion, depression, and spiritual suffering
- Identifying the terminal phase in patients with chronic illness and end of life care for common symptoms

For a complete list of references, please visit www.expertconsult.com.

KEY REFERENCES

2. Doyle D, Hanks GWC, MacDonald N, editors: Oxford textbook of palliative medicine, ed 4, Oxford, England, 2011, Oxford University Press.
9. Stansby G, Avilal L, Jones K, et al: Prevention and management of pressure ulcers in primary and secondary care summary of NICE guidance. BMJ 348:31–34, 2014.
16. Shickle D: The Mental Capacity Act 2005. Clin Med 6:169–173, 2006.
17. Capel M, Gazi T, Vout L, et al: Where do patients known to a community palliative care service die? BMJ Support Palliat Care 2:43–47, 2012.
19. Gold Standards Framework www.goldstandardsframework.org.uk.
20. SPICT www.spict.org.uk.
24. Helme RD, Gibson SJ: The epidemiology of pain in elderly people. Clin Geriatr Med 17:417–431, 2001.
25. Kovach CR, Weissman DE, Griffe J, et al: Assessment and treatment of discomfort for people with late stage dementia. J Pain Symptom Manage 18:412–419, 1999.
27. Twycross RG, Wilcox A, Howard P, et al: Palliative care formulary, ed 4, Oxford, England, 2013, Radcliffe Medical Press.
29. Portenoy RK: Pharmacologic management of cancer pain. Semin Oncol 22:160–170, 1995.
35. Stephenson J, Gilbert J: The development of clinical guidelines on paracentesis for ascites related to malignancy. Palliat Med 16:213–218, 2002.
46. Brown D: Palliation of breathlessness. Clin Med 6:133–135, 2006.
63. Chochinov HM: Dignity and the essence of medicine: the ABC and D of dignity conserving care. BMJ 335:184–187, 2007.
69. End of Life Diabetes Care, Clinical Care Recommendations, Second Edition October 2013. Commissioned by Diabetes UK.

115 Ethical Issues in Geriatric Medicine

Søren Holm

In one sense, there are no ethical issues or principles that are specific to geriatric medicine. Our moral status as persons do not change when we grow old, and older adults are due the same measure of respect and attention as the young.[1] The clinical situations in which ethical issues arise are also, in most cases, very similar to clinical situations that may arise in other areas of medical practice.

In another sense, there are specific ethical issues in geriatric medicine caused by the following: (1) a stereotypical social image in many Western societies of older adults as less competent and less worthy of attention than younger individuals; (2) the complexities introduced because of the increased frailty that comes with older age; (3) the tendency in many health care systems to underfund geriatric medicine in comparison to other specialties; and (4) the complex interface between health care and social services for older adults.

This chapter will briefly review some core general elements of medical ethics as they relate to geriatric medicine before considering some of the ethical problems that occur frequently in geriatric medicine. These include decision making for incompetent patients, advanced decision making and the use of health care proxies, and research involving the incompetent and end-of-life issues. The final section will be concerned with resource allocation and the health care claims of older adults.

RESPECT FOR AUTONOMY

The cornerstone of clinical medical ethics is respect for autonomy or self-determination.[2] Competent patients who are informed about the available treatment options can decide which of the treatment options they prefer and can also decide not to have any treatment at all. It is generally accepted in ethics and law that competent patients can refuse treatment even if that treatment is simple and lifesaving.

The main reason that we ought to respect autonomy in health care is that the decisions are about the life of the patient, and she or he has a right to be able to shape that life according to his or her own values and ideas about the good life.

In most health care systems, respect for autonomy is institutionalized in clinical practice through a requirement for valid, informed consent for diagnostic and therapeutic procedures. And, in research ethics, there is even stronger protection of autonomy through much more explicit informed consent requirements.

However, respect for autonomy entails more than just respecting the decisions people make; it also entails respecting them as the primary decision maker in relation to their own life. This means the following: (1) patients have to be involved in decision making processes at a point where there is real choice and before a default decision has already been made; (2) they should not be forced to make decisions before they are ready to make them; and (3) they have to be given the information that they require to make a decision, not only the information that a health care professional thinks is relevant.

Taking patients seriously as decision makers may therefore have implications for the way decision making processes are designed and structured at the ward or department level to ensure that patients are involved at the right time and that there is time enough for them to be properly informed. In a broader perspective, respect for self-determination also creates an obligation to promote people's abilities to make decisions by promoting their autonomy. If there is something we can do which will enable a person to make autonomous decisions, we should do it. This may include clinically relatively trivial interventions (e.g., rehydrating a dehydrated and confused patient to bring her back to competence), but may also include patient education or the use of modern patient decision support programs.

Two common misunderstandings of what respect for self-determination means need to be mentioned. The first is that respect for autonomy entails that patients have to make all decisions themselves and that they cannot delegate decision making to other people—but delegating decision making is a perfectly autonomous thing to do. We all do it on a regular basis. There is nothing ethically problematic in a patient asking a physician to make the decision if the patient trusts that the physician is able to make a better decision, or in a patient involving a trusted relative or friend in the decision making. Forcing patients to make decisions they do not want to make is not respecting the patient's self-determination.

The other common misconception is that people's autonomy is respected by giving them what they want; for example, this means that if a person wants something, such as a specific treatment, there is a moral obligation to help her or him get it. Respect for autonomy only, strictly speaking, implies a negative duty of noninterference. Any positive duty to help cannot be derived from respect for self-determination. It has to be justified differently—for example, through some account of the professional obligations that flow from an established physician-patient relationship.

PATERNALISM

Paternalism is the term used for actions taken or decisions made for another person with the intention of benefiting that person. The word is derived from the Latin word for father; the idea is that a paternalist decision is like the decision a good father would make for his child.

It is important to note that an action can only count as paternalist if it is done to benefit the other person. Actions chosen and performed to benefit the physician or health care system, or with mixed intentions, are not paternalistic but simply coercive.

Paternalistic decision making is not problematic if the person in question is incompetent (see later). This situation is sometimes referred to as genuine paternalism. However, paternalistic decision making is problematic if the person is competent and wants to make her or his own decisions. In that case, the paternalistic action overrides the autonomy of the person. Paternalistic decision making can be justified in emergency situations, in which there is no time to consult the patient and it can sometimes be justified in a public health context, but it is rarely, if ever, justified in non-emergency interactions with individual patients. Patients may be frail and vulnerable, but as long as they want to make their own decisions, they are their decisions to make.

An increasingly common form of paternalism is what can be called informational paternalism. Informational paternalism occurs when a patient has clearly signaled that he or she does not want some piece of information about the condition (e.g., does not want to know the precise prognosis) but is sometimes given this information because the health care team thinks that … "it is best for him [or her] to know. …" This is sometimes supported by the claim that health care professionals have a duty to tell the truth to their patients. However, it does not follow that there is a duty to impress the truth on people who do not want to hear it. This is easily seen if we consider a parallel example. All of us have a duty to tell the truth to our friends, but this does not generate an obligation to provide unsolicited evaluations of their dress sense or latest haircut, even if those evaluations are true.

DIGNITY

In the context of geriatric medicine, respecting and preserving the dignity of patients is the second ethical consideration that takes center stage. Respect for autonomy and for the decisions of a person can be seen as part of preserving and respecting the dignity of that person, but dignity is a complex concept that is not exhausted by respect for self-determination.[3]

To treat someone in a dignified manner is to treat them in a way that recognizes that they are a complete person, with personal integrity and worth and a protected zone of privacy. Exactly what this means will vary from culture to culture and from time to time, but everyone in a culture will be able to identify a core set of behaviors that is undignified and disrespectful behavior. This is also an area where research focusing on the experiences of patients can play a role in making it clear when they experience care that is impinging on their dignity. It should come as no surprise that many older adults think it is undignified if they are shabbily dressed or if they are exposed naked or half-naked to the gaze of others.[3]

In this context, it is important to remember that some of the largest problems in relation to the protection of dignity are brought about by the numerous, small routine violations of dignity that may erode a person's sense of personal worth and the staff's sense of what is right and proper. Although the actions are done by individual health care professionals, the solution to this type of problem is often organizational.

FRAILTY, CLINICAL COMPLEXITY, AND ETHICAL DECISION MAKING

Respecting the autonomy and dignity of patients, and involving them in decision making about diagnosis and treatment is simple in principle, but becomes complicated for patients who are frail and may already have significant comorbidities. Hospitalization and treatment may trigger new problems and lead to loss of function, and our knowledge about the effectiveness of treatments and their side effects have often come from studies in patients specifically selected not to be frail or have major comorbidities. The risks that frailty creates need to be taken into account by the health care professionals in their decision making about appropriate treatment options and in communication and shared decision making with patients, families, and caregivers about these treatment options. This entails the following: (1) physicians need to have frailty in mind and not just the current problems, and (2) much more time may need to be spent in communicating the risks and benefits of available treatment options.[4]

Incompetent Patients

Not all patients are competent to make decisions about health care matters. Patients may become temporarily incompetent during an acute illness episode or become permanently incompetent, such as in the later stages of dementia. Health care and other decisions still have to be made, even when patients cannot make these decisions themselves.

The concept of incompetence initially seems to be straightforward. The normal adult is the paradigm case of an individual who is competent to make decisions, and that competence is lost if the person becomes unconscious, is very inebriated, or develops late-stage Alzheimer disease, in which almost all memory and most reasoning capacities are gone. Between the extremes of full competence and complete incompetence there is, however, a very wide range of situations in which a person is partially competent (competent to make certain decisions but not others) or where a person's competence is questionable. This gray area is created by two complicating factors: (1) competence always entails competence to make a specific decision; and (2) we do not have a good account of exactly what it takes to be competent and how far you can deviate from the norm before you become incompetent.

That competence is always competence to make a specific decision is obvious in the case of children. It is not the case that one day they are completely incompetent to make decisions, and the next day they become fully competent. Even a 3-year-old is competent to decide which ice cream he or she wants when given the choice on a warm day at the beach. In the same way, people with dementia may be incompetent to make decisions about their treatment without being incompetent to make decisions about what to eat for dinner, what to wear, or when to get up in the morning.

The second complicating factor in decisions about competence is that it is unclear how rational and how informed a decision has to be to count as competent. Most decisions that people make do not conform to strict rules of rationality and are made in a situation of at least partial ignorance. Just think of how most of us decide on important matters, such as applying to medical school, buying a house, marrying, or starting to save for a pension. We do not seek all the information that we could have sought, and we do not always think through all the options carefully. This means that unless we want to rule most decision making as incompetent, and therefore possibly open to being overruled by others, we have to have a less stringent standard of competent decision making than full rationality and complete information.

We could try to say that what matters is not how the decision was made, but its content—that is, what decision that was made—but this is a problematic argument because we generally allow people to make foolish choices, even about very important things. The fact that a decision is not one that we would have made does not, on its own, make it an incompetent decision.

Here it is important to note that questions about incompetence are often only raised when patients make decisions that we don't agree with. As long as the patients agree with us, we do not question their competence, and take their informed consent to treatment and diagnosis to be valid. This is in itself problematic. There are probably as many patients who make decisions that we do agree with, but for which we could have challenged their competence to make these decisions.

Decision Making for the Incompetent

In a situation in which one person has to make important decisions for another, often called proxy decision making, there are in principle two different ways in which such a decision can be made. These are commonly referred to as the substituted judgment standard and the best interest standard.[5]

According to the substituted judgment standard, the task of the decision maker is to try to make the decision that the incompetent person would have made, if competent. This might involve empathic identification with the patient to discern what the patient would have decided. The problem with this standard for proxy decision making is that it is not obvious which of the incompetent person's characteristics should play a role. For example, should someone make rash decisions for a patient who was a rash decision maker all his or her life, or should the patient's needle phobia be taken into account? Because of these problems, the substituted judgment standard has fallen out of favor.

The best interest standard specifies the task of the proxy decision maker as making the decision that is in the patient's best interest—the decision that is most likely to benefit the patient. This is the standard that is accepted in most jurisdictions for legal decision making for the incompetent. The conception of best interest that is at play here varies widely. A patient's best interest is not confined to his or her medical best interest (e.g., determining which treatment that is medically optimal) but also encompasses social issues. It is furthermore generally accepted that what is in a patient's best interest is at least partly determined by the patient's prior values and life goals. What is in the best interest of a Muslim patient may be different from what is in the best interest of a Christian patient. If understood in this broad way, and drawing on knowledge about the patient's values, decision making guided by best interest will often become close to decision making guided by substituted judgment.

The term *best interest* seems to imply that there is one, and only one, decision and course of action that will promote the patient's best interest, and that our task is to find that course of action, but this view rests on a mistake. There are many situations in which we will be unable to decide which course of action will benefit the patient most because of uncertainties about the clinical situation and/or uncertainties about the patient's values.[6] We are often able to identify some decisions that are clearly not in someone's best interest without being able to specify one of the remaining options as the one that clearly best serves the patient's interest. This means that there can be legitimate disagreements within health care teams or between health care professionals and families or caregivers about best interest judgments, without any of the parties clearly being wrong.

Advanced Decision Making

Many jurisdictions now allow people to make legally valid advance decisions about health care that come into force if and when the person becomes incompetent. This can be in the form of advance directives, the appointment of a designated proxy decision maker, or a combination of the two. Advance directives allow a person to specify what treatment he or she wants or does not want in specific future circumstances and are most useful for those suffering from a disease process with at least a somewhat predictable future course. In that situation, it is also possible to help patients clarify their wishes for future treatment by outlining the range of likely scenarios.

Advance directives formulated in more general statements such as "If I become unable to take care of myself I do not want. . . ." will always require a considerable amount of interpretation to decide whether they apply to the situation at hand and whether they should still be considered valid. The problems in writing sufficiently specific advance directives have led to a move toward combining advance directives with the appointment of a designated proxy decision maker.

The task of the designated proxy is to make decisions on behalf of the patient when the patient is no longer competent to make those decisions. These decisions have to be made in the best interest of the patient (see earlier concerning best interest), just as decisions for patients who do not have a designated proxy. The advantage of having a proxy is that patients can appoint someone who knows them and their values and preferences well and who is therefore more likely to evaluate best interest in the same way as the patient. In jurisdictions in which it is possible to designate a proxy, it is usually the case that health care professionals can only override the proxy's decisions if they can show that they are clearly not in the patient's best interest.

Role of the Family in Decision Making

In most Western countries, family members have no formal role in making decisions as family members. There may be a requirement to consult them before decisions are made concerning an incompetent patient, but there is usually no legal requirement to follow their advice unless they are the patient's legally designated proxy decision maker.

In reality, families justifiably play a larger role in decision making in many circumstances. Many competent patients want to involve their family members in the decisions, and some may want to leave decisions to the family or caregiver.

In relation to incompetent patients, families often have a better understanding of the patient's value system than the health care team. Furthermore, the family often has to care for the patient outside the health care context. This means that it will almost always be appropriate to consult the family or caregiver before important decisions are made about an incompetent patient. It is also important to realize that the interests of the patient, and the family or caregiver can be involved in complicated ways that may make it difficult for them to see clearly what is best for the patient. There may also be conflicting views among family members or caregivers as to what should be done.

Research and Incompetent Persons

The traditional research ethics problem discussed in connection with dementia is the problem of research involving persons who are incapable of giving valid informed consent. This problem has been extensively analyzed and, at the regulatory level of research ethics, a consensus has been developed about the requirements that have to be fulfilled for such research to be deemed ethically acceptable. These requirements are as follows: (1) consent must be sought from the person's representative (proxy); (2) if the person is able to assent or dissent, although unable to consent, the person's assent must be obtained; (3) the research must be directly beneficial to the person or must be beneficial to the patient group to which the person belongs, and it must be impossible to perform the research in a group of patients who can consent; and (4) the risk to the person must be minimal in those circumstances in which there is no direct benefit.

This consensus is expressed in the most recent revision of the Helsinki Declaration from the World Medical Association.[7] The restriction on types of research for which an incompetent person can be included can be justified in three different ways:

1. The first line of argument is based on the historical fact that vulnerable groups have often been used in ethically problematic research, and that if the incompetent could be used as research participants in ordinary projects there is a risk that they would become an easy source of research material.
2. The second focuses on the intersection of interests between the person with a specific condition and the group of sufferers with that condition. The argument is that even if a person does not realize a personal benefit from the research, he or she benefits indirectly through the benefits accruing to the group.
3. The third possible justification is the pragmatic one; unless we allow some types of research without consent into conditions where all sufferers are incompetent, very little progress will be made in the treatment of such conditions (the so-called golden ghetto argument). However, such research should be limited to those projects that cannot be performed in any other way to minimize the infringements caused by research without consent.

END-OF-LIFE ISSUES

Three types of end-of-life issues are currently under discussion in medical ethics: (1) withdrawing and withholding treatment; (2) physician-assisted suicide; and (3) active euthanasia. There is no doubt that a physician can withdraw or withhold any treatment if a competent patient refuses the treatment, or the treatment is futile (i.e., cannot benefit the patient).

Withdrawing and Withholding Treatment

There are still three open questions in relation to withdrawing and withholding treatment:

- Is there a moral difference between withdrawing and withholding?
- What about treatments that are not completely futile or are not futile from all points of view?
- Is the provision of nutrition and hydration considered as treatment?

Physicians often think that there is a difference between withdrawing and withholding a given treatment. It might seem more difficult to stop an ongoing treatment than not to start a treatment, but it is very difficult to find any good justification for this. The consequences of stopping and not starting are often the same—for example, think of stopping and not starting respiratory support for a patient who needs it. Also, the reasons for the decision are almost always very similar (e.g., it is not in the patient's best interest to continue or initiate this treatment). This has meant that there is a growing consensus that despite the phenomenologic difference, the difference in how it feels, there is no real ethical difference between decisions to withdraw and decisions to withhold.

When thinking of withdrawing or withholding a treatment from a patient, it is not difficult to reach a decision if the treatment in question is completely futile, if it has no chance of benefiting the patient in any way. However, there are many situations in which the treatment is not completely futile. It may have a small chance of being successful, or it may be likely to prolong the patient's life but raise the subsequent question of whether this longer life is worth living, as seen from the patient's point of view. A typical situation in which these issues arise is when contemplating cardiopulmonary resuscitation and the appropriateness of a "do not resuscitate" decision. If the patient is competent, all this can be discussed with him or her, and the patient can decide, but, in the case of the noncompetent patient, others must decide what is in the best interests of the patient. It is not possible to give a percentage figure for when a treatment could be regarded as futile, but it is generally agreed that a mere theoretical chance that something will work does not make it a worthwhile treatment.

The final controversial issue in relation to withdrawing and withholding treatment is whether nutrition and hydration, or food and water, should be defined as treatment or as basic humane care that can never be withdrawn or withheld. Part of this controversy has involved a discussion of whether withdrawal of nutrition and hydration leads to suffering and whether such suffering (e.g., thirst) can be relieved, but this discussion is in some sense a red herring. The core issue in the controversy is not suffering but whether it can ever be justified not to provide this basic level of care. Legally, the position has now been settled in many jurisdictions by explicit legal judgments that it is acceptable to withdraw nutrition and hydration. However, the ethical discussion is still not over, partly because it involves the thorny question of whether it is ever better for a person to be dead than alive. This links the withdrawing and withholding issue to the discussion of physician-assisted suicide and euthanasia.

A common scenario where the issue of withholding treatment occurs is when a patient with dementia begins to develop problems with swallowing, and the question arises as to whether some artificial means of providing nutrition and hydration should be started. Many physicians, patients, families, and caregivers think that the answer to this question is "no" because they see the treatment as being futile in the long run. Some patients, families, and caregivers take a different view, however, often because they believe that every day of life is a benefit, even for a person with severe dementia. This can lead to conflict between health care professionals and families and caregivers; although such conflicts can sometimes be resolved, this is not always the case, and a disagreement about what is in the patient's best interest may persist. In some jurisdictions, the physicians' decision prevails, in some the decision of the families and caregivers, and in some the issue has to be resolved by the courts. This illustrates that the way in which we resolve hard ethical issues in practice is influenced by local tradition and context.

Physician-Assisted Suicide and Euthanasia

Physician-assisted suicide (PAS) is the situation in which a physician provides a patient with the means to commit suicide—for example, by issuing a prescription for a lethal combination of drugs but the patient performs the physical act of actually taking the drugs.

Active euthanasia is the situation in which a physician actively ends the life of a patient—for example, by injecting a lethal combination of drugs. In relation to active euthanasia, it is possible to distinguish among voluntary euthanasia, where the patient has requested euthanasia; nonvoluntary euthanasia, where the patient is incompetent and nothing is known about his or her wishes; and involuntary euthanasia, where a patient is killed against his or her will. Involuntary euthanasia is murder, and nonvoluntary euthanasia raises a host of complex ethical and legal problems. Thus, the discussion about euthanasia is usually focused on whether or notvoluntary active euthanasia should be legalized.

PAS and/or voluntary active euthanasia has been legalized in a few countries. PAS is legal in Switzerland, the Netherlands, Luxembourg, the state of Oregon and some other U.S. states, and active euthanasia is legal in the Netherlands, Luxembourg, and Belgium. In all cases, except in Switzerland, there are extensive procedural safeguards in place to try to ensure that the decision to ask for PAS or euthanasia is well considered and fully voluntary. The ethical justification of PAS and/or euthanasia proceeds along two dimensions.

Respect for Autonomy

The first line of justification relies on respect for autonomy. If people have a strong interest in leading their life according to their own values, it is plausible that they also have a strong interest in how that life ends and that their choice should be respected. A hypothetical example, which is often discussed in this line of argument, is the successful academic with the first symptoms of Alzheimer disease who does not want his life to end in severe dementia and who claims that such an end would make a mockery of his life's achievements and would furthermore be undignified. Proponents of this line of argument often claim that it is the individual person who has to decide whether he would be better off dead, and that only he can make that evaluation.

Suffering

The second line of justification focuses on suffering. It is based on the claim that if a person is in great pain, has breathing difficulties or severe psychological suffering, and there is no way to relieve the suffering, then PAS or euthanasia may be justified to end the suffering.

The two lines of justification come together in the core case of severe irremediable suffering in a person with terminal illness who wants the suffering to end. The opposition toward legalizing PAS and/or euthanasia may be opposition to the two practices as such (e.g., based on the view that suicide or killing is never right), or it may be opposition to legalization of these practices. It is common for some to agree that there are specific cases in which active voluntary euthanasia is justified, but still argue that it should not be legalized.

The arguments against legalization are primarily of two types. One claims that it is important that the law symbolically upholds the view that taking the life of another human is always wrong. The second line of argument is worried about slippery slopes and a gradual expansion from a core cases to one that is less so. Here, the argument is that even if we write a law that only allows PAS or euthanasia for people with terminal illness and irremediable suffering who wish to die, we will over time also allow euthanasia in cases in which the voluntary element is less clear, or the suffering is not present but merely predicted for the future. Some also worry that we will allow euthanasia in situations in which the decision is formally voluntary but based on motivations that are perceived as problematic—for example, if a patient wants euthanasia so as not to be a burden to the family or an economic drain on the health care system. Would it not be better if these problems were solved in another way, such as by appropriate allocation of resources to health and social care for older adults?

PRIORITY SETTING AND OLDER ADULTS

Until this point, this chapter has mainly been concerned with decision making in relation to specific identifiable patients, but resource allocation decisions between groups of patients also raise ethical issues. No health care system has the resources to provide medically optimal treatment to everyone who is ill. There is always a mismatch between the available resources and the claims on the health care system. This means that priority setting between patients and patient groups is a reality in all health care systems. Politicians may want to deny this, but it is nevertheless a fact.

This raises the question of how the health care claims of older adults should be prioritized. Should the claims of older adults be given the same, greater, or lesser weight than the claims of those who are younger?

It is obvious that unreflective opinions on this issue vary according to how it is framed. We generally and rightly agree that older adults have the same worth and importance as younger people, and that there should be no difference in how we treat severe pain in older adults and younger individuals. However, many people might express the opposite opinion if the issue is to decide who should receive a kidney transplant, and the hypothetical choice is between someone who is young and someone who is very old. People's views are often further complicated by considerations of merit and past contributions to the development of the welfare state. Those who are old now did not have access to the type of health care we have today when they were young and may therefore have a stronger claim now.

It is difficult to devise a resource allocation system that takes all these views into account concerning the relevance of age to priority setting. It is far beyond the scope of this chapter to try to settle which, if any, is correct, but it is important to note that some views on this issue raise considerable ethical concerns.

Some of the major tools of health economics directly institutionalize the discrimination of older adults. A number of methods can determine the benefit of an intervention in terms of the increase in welfare and health or decrease in suffering and illness it produces and when the patient experiences this benefit. However, because older adults have a shorter life expectancy than younger individuals, this has the consequence that a given curative treatment counts for less if given to an older adult than to a younger person, simply because the older adult is likely to have less life left in which to benefit.[1] This is clearly unjust and against all principles of respecting every person equally. The same is true of any type of resource allocation that primarily bases itself on future contribution to society because that will also systematically discriminate against older adults.

KEY POINTS

- Older adults have the same moral status and importance as anyone else.
- The health care claims of older adults should be treated with the same attention as the health care claims of everyone else.
- Decision making for persons who are incompetent to make their own decisions have to be guided by what is in their best interest.
- The concept of best interest covers a wider range of considerations than merely medical best interest.
- Advanced decision making is most useful for patients with a predictable clinical course.

KEY REFERENCES

1. Harris J: The age-indifference principle and equality. Cambridge Q Health Care Ethics 14:93–99, 2005.
2. Beauchamp TL, Childress JF: Principles of biomedical ethics, ed 6, New York, 2009, Oxford University Press.
3. Woolhead G, Calnan M, Dieppe P, et al: Dignity in older age: what do older people in the United Kingdom think? Age Ageing 33:165–170, 2004.
4. Mallery LH, Moorhouse P: Respecting frailty. J Med Ethics 37:126–128, 2011.
5. Buchanan AE, Brock DW: Deciding for others—the ethics of surrogate decision making, Cambridge, England, 1989, Cambridge University Press.
6. Holm S, Edgar A: Best interest: a philosophical critique. Health Care Anal 16:197–207, 2008.
7. World Medical Association: World Medical Association Declaration of Helsinki—ethical principles for medical research involving human subjects. http://www.wma.net/en/30publications/10policies/b3. Accessed November 10, 2015.

116 Managing Frailty: Roles for Primary Care

Steve Iliffe

INTRODUCTION

The aging population in industrialized societies is a challenge for primary care. Older people with multimorbidity, disabilities, cognitive impairment, and frailty are not well served by brief encounters with practitioners whose working style is reactive rather than proactive. In a competition for attention and clinical assessment, the complex patient is at a disadvantage compared with the younger, more articulate patient with a single problem to solve.

The clinical task is made more difficult because population aging is a diverse and complex process, with older individuals moving along a spectrum of fitness to frailty at different speeds. Identifying those individuals most likely to benefit (and least likely to experience harm) from interventions to delay their progress along this spectrum is becoming a priority for primary care practitioners,[1] but it is not clear how to do it. The evidence base for interventions to limit or even reverse frailty and pre-frailty is shallow.

The overarching task is to overcome the obsolescence of the current health and social care systems, but there is a pressing need for primary care practitioners to acquire the skills needed to manage clinical complexity and frailty. This chapter describes how primary care needs to reconfigure itself to manage an increasingly frail population, focusing on promoting healthy aging; case finding, case management, and interventions for frailty; understanding patients' perspectives on frailty; working with care home residents; and providing end-of-life care.

WHAT IS FRAILTY AND WHO IS FRAIL?

Frailty as a state of heightened and disproportionate vulnerability resulting from multisystem failure and is distinct from multimorbidity and disability.[2] One quarter to one half of people older than 85 years is frail, and these people have significantly increased risk of disability, hospitalization, long-term care, and death.[3] Frailty, however defined, is more common in women and some ethnic minorities, increases in prevalence with age, and is associated with poor survival.[4]

However, up to three quarters of people older than 85 years might not be frail; frailty is not synonymous with being among the oldest old.[2] It is a dynamic process that evolves over time, offering opportunities for prevention and remediation.[5] The dependency oscillations observed in older people who are frail reflect the often marked changes in functional ability seen in clinical practice. However, at present, progression of frailty is more common than improvement, and the onset of frailty frequently results in a spiral of decline.[6]

Frailty also has psychological and social dimensions. It is associated with worse well-being, taking into account depression and functional limitations, while financial resources may act as a partial buffer against the psychological effects of frailty.[7] Maintaining a stronger sense of psychological well-being in later life may protect against the development of physical frailty, although the mechanisms underlying this are unclear.[8] There appears to be a social gradient in frailty, with educational level, income adequacy, and income satisfaction being associated with frailty.[9] Older adults who are poor and live in deprived neighborhoods are those most likely to develop frailty.[10]

Frailty provides a conceptual basis for moving away from organ- and disease-based medical approaches toward a more integrative model of health, and therefore it fits the biopsychosocial model of generalism very well.[11] Its identification and management in general practice is, then, a test of the claims made for the biopsychosocial model.

The concept of frailty, and measures based on it, may also provide a more user-centered approach to developing services that cuts across unidisciplinary preoccupations and definitions of clinical effectiveness. It also has potential in the identification of individuals requiring integrated care, in the planning of care packages, and in the monitoring of the health status of patients and service users. A caveat here: most frail older adults report that they receive sufficient help for their physical needs but not for their psychosocial needs.[12] A wide variety of frailty measures are available, and further work is required to establish which are the most suitable for these different applications.[13]

PROMOTING HEALTHY AGING

In most people, multimorbidity, disability, and frailty develop slowly over decades and may be difficult to distinguish. For example, the duration of unhealthy behaviors in mid-life, particularly poor diet and physical inactivity, increases the likelihood of frailty features like slow walking speed and reduced grip strength emerging in later life,[14] but these features will coexist with other consequences of inactivity and poor nutrition such as heart disease, obesity, and diabetes, among others. Aging well may therefore depend in part on changing behaviors and modifying risks for disability and frailty earlier in life.

Unfortunately, refocusing attention "upstream" does not solve the problem because we do not yet know how to maximize the uptake of preventive activities in mid-life across the population. Prevention holds the promise of maintaining good health by testing, diagnosing, and treating conditions before they cause symptoms. However, prevention can harm as well as help when tests or treatments for asymptomatic conditions cause immediate complications. "Lag time to benefit" is defined as the time between a preventive intervention (when complications and harms are most likely) to the time when improved health outcomes are seen. Just as different interventions have different magnitudes of benefit, different preventive interventions have different lag times to benefit, ranging from 6 months for statin therapy for secondary prevention to more than 10 years for prostate cancer screening. Many standardized measures, such as relative risk, odds ratio, and absolute risk reduction, quantify the magnitude of benefit ("How much will it help?"). The measures and methodologies to calculate a lag time to benefit ("When will it help?") are underdeveloped and often not reported.[15] So, for example, the promotion of physical activity in community settings (which has been a disappointing experience, to date) may be resisted because the benefits, including the postponement of disability and frailty, are distant while the disadvantages are immediate.

Interventions in later life are therefore more attractive because of the shorter time scale to demonstrate effectiveness and because of the proximity of benefit. In primary care such interventions take the form of health maintenance (e.g., through weight control, smoking cessation, and exercise promotion) and "anticipatory care," a broader approach to case finding and case management of long-term conditions. Unfortunately, and despite substantial research efforts over decades, health maintenance and anticipatory care for older people in the community have not yet been shown to be clinically effective or cost-effective.[16] Their history provides a salutary lesson for researchers as well as those developing services. Health promotion trials for older people in the United States, United Kingdom, and Denmark up to 1990[17] showed a rise in patient morale, increased referrals to all agencies, reduced duration of inpatient stay (sometimes), increased inpatient rates (mostly because of respite care), reduction in mortality (in some trials), but no improvement in functional ability and increased workload for general practitioners unless alternative services bypassed primary care.

Subsequent studies were essentially negative, and only recently has research begun to show more promising outcomes. For example, the largest community-based study in the United Kingdom, the MRC 75+ assessment trial, showed little or no benefits to quality of life or health outcomes.[18] Similarly, a systematic review of 15 trials of preventive home visits published in 2000 showed no clear evidence of effectiveness,[19] and the ProAge study in 2006 showed no change in health risk behaviors in older people.[20] There are now some grounds for thinking that interventions can have a positive impact. Comprehensive geriatric assessment (CGA) followed by tailored case management is beginning to show an impact on function.[21] One clinical trial showed that health educators doing preventive home visits can improve older people's functional mobility.[22] Another study provided evidence that nurse-led case management impacts positively on functional ability, caregiver burden, and satisfaction.[23]

CASE FINDING METHODS

Given that preventive interventions have limited impact on the development of disability or frailty, primary care practitioners are left to manage the impact of these states on their older patients. Whereas disability may be evident, identifying frailty can be more difficult; practitioners may need help in recognizing and responding to it. The point about recognition is not that it is diagnostic of frailty but rather that it helps physicians identify patients who may benefit from more detailed assessment. Primary care would be well placed for the early identification and management of frailty in older adults if a simple, easy-to-use measure to identify frailty specifically in primary care settings were available.[24-26] A recent review recommends a two-step approach to identifying individuals who would benefit from a further detailed assessment.[27]

However, there are a number of problems that complicate the task of recognition. The validity and diagnostic accuracy of instruments for frailty have not been tested in well-defined community-based longitudinal studies. Several of the frailty instruments are also derived from small-scale studies, including some that are cross-sectional and not primary care based. There is a need for a simple screening tool for frailty for use in general practice based on large prospective studies of community-dwelling older populations.

Despite their scientific validity, the "Fried frailty phenotype" (capturing a syndrome) and the "frailty index" (capturing a state) are difficult to apply in routine clinical practice in primary care, because they rely on objective measures such as grip strength (in the frailty phenotype) or the number of different deficits (in the frailty index).

Most studies have assessed screening tools for frailty that are not directly applicable for use by general practitioners as first-stage screening instruments, but recently developed instruments have been assessed for use in primary care; these include the SHARE (Survey of Health, Ageing and Retirement in Europe) frailty instrument, the Groningen Frailty Indicator, the Tilburg Frailty Indicator, and the Edmonton Frail Scale. These measures also are extensive (approximately 15 to 20 items) and/or include objective measures (such as the timed get-up-and-go test) and therefore may not be suitable as brief, first-stage screening tools; they may be more useful as second-stage assessment instruments.

A single-item assessment would be an ideal first stage in frailty case finding. Gait speed is the most predictive single factor associated with frailty,[2] whereas fatigue that restricts activity, although common, is often episodic and of short duration and is a less accurate predictor of frailty.[28] The second stage of case finding could then include use of a validated instrument such as the Edmonton Frail Scale, a multidimensional assessment instrument that includes the timed get-up-and-go test and a test for cognitive impairment. It is quick to administer (less than 5 minutes) and is valid, reliable, and feasible for routine use by nongeriatricians.[29] There are alternatives, and the properties of some are compared in Table 116-1.[25]

Complex interventions based on CGA delivered to older people in the community can increase the likelihood of them continuing to live at home, principally through a reduced need for care home admission and through fewer falls. However, effect sizes in trials of CGA and other complex interventions are small[30] and are likely to decline further once interventions are deployed in routine care. Because CGA is time consuming and requires expertise, referral of older patients with suspected frailty to specialist services is appropriate.[30,31] Referral decisions should be qualified by the knowledge that categorization of frailty by severity is important, since those who are most frail appear to receive least benefit. CGA is not a practical tool for primary care clinicians to screen individuals for frailty,[32] even as a second-stage tool.

INTERVENTIONS FOR FRAILTY AND CASE MANAGEMENT

If recognition can be managed in a two-step process, how can primary care practitioners respond to frailty? One approach is to focus on common clinical features of frailty and seek specialist help with those features that may be tractable. For example, sarcopenia is a feature of frailty in older people and a major determinant of adverse health outcomes such as functional limitations and disability. Resistance training and adequate protein and energy intake are plausible strategies for the management of sarcopenia. Management of weight loss and resistance training could be the most relevant protective countermeasures to slow down the decline of muscle mass and muscle strength, with additional potential gain from correcting vitamin D deficiency.[33] The critical role of micronutrients in frailty suggests the need to improve the quality (and not just the quantity) of food eaten by older people.[34] Specialist services should include dietary expertise and experience in increasing physical activity in older people.

Frailty and late-life depression are comorbid conditions, but frailty also increases the risk of developing depression[35] and vice versa.[36] Distinguishing between the two is not always easy. Frail older people may be diagnosed as experiencing depression during bouts of physiologic low mood and receive inappropriate antidepressant treatments that can increase risks of sedation and falls.[37]

TABLE 116-1 Comparison of Four Frailty Scales

	Groningen Frailty Indicator (GFI)	Frailty Staging System	Frailty and Autonomy Scoring Instrument Leuven (FRAIL)	Edmonton Frail Scale
ADLs	✓	✓	✓	✓
IADLs	✓	✓	✓	✓
Activities outside	✓	✓	✓	✓
Sensory functions	✓	✓	✓	
Medication	✓		✓	✓
Memory	✓	✓	✓	✓
Orientation		✓	✓	✓
Behavior	✓		✓	✓
Social contacts	✓		✓	
Familial functioning	✓		✓	
Ability to plan things			✓	
Finances			✓	
Feeling fit/health status	✓			✓
Weight loss	✓			✓
Continence		✓	✓	✓

ADLs, Activities of daily living; *IADLs,* instrumental activities of daily living.

Further studies are needed to investigate whether multimodal interventions targeting depression symptoms, functional deficits, and fatigue can reduce the morbidity and improve the quality of life of older people with frailty, but the opinion of an old age psychiatrist may clarify treatment options.

Frailty is associated with a twofold to threefold risk of cardiovascular disease[38] and is a strong predictor of mortality in patients with cardiovascular disease independent of age, disease severity, comorbidity, and disability.[39] This is likely to be due to strong associations between cardiovascular disease risk factors (including dyslipidemia, obesity, poor lung function, poor renal function, increased white blood cell counts, low albumin and sodium levels, and altered liver function) and both frailty and pre-frailty, independently of established cardiovascular disease.[40] Management of cardiovascular risk factors and established cardiovascular disease may help limit some of the symptoms of frailty, but medication effects can exacerbate them; thus, specialist advice should be sought.

The question for primary care is how best to manage complex patients. Case management as a new care coordination role within nursing has become a popular response to clinical complexity, but expectations that it would reduce hospital admission rates for frail older people have not been met,[41] and there is some evidence that introduction of case managers can disrupt established nursing teams and informal, collaborative "communities of practice" in primary care.[42] Multidisciplinary interventions for frail older people in community settings are attractive but of unproven value. For example, a recent study of an interdisciplinary primary care approach designed for frail older people in the Netherlands failed to show a beneficial effect on disability or other clinical outcomes.[43] Overall, home-based interventions for older adults do not reduce mortality or increase independent living, and no specific program produces benefit (although this may be because of poor reporting of intervention components).[44] Until the evidence base deepens, we are left with the task of enhancing the skills of primary care practitioners in recognizing frailty and responding to it by seeking expert advice on symptom management.

AVOIDING CRISES IN FRAIL OLDER PEOPLE

One way to measure the impact of primary and secondary care on older people with frailty is to observe their use of emergency medical care. Frailty is an underlying state in approximately one third of critically ill adults aged 50 and older who are admitted to hospitals.[45] There are multiple drivers for hospital admission in the frail older population,[46] including overwhelming clinical need, the concentration of expertise and technology in hospitals, patient preference (to reduce burden on families), the ease of admission compared to the effort of orchestrating home care, and, in some cases, perverse financial incentives for hospitals to admit patients.

Older people are more likely to be admitted to hospital as an emergency if they live in deprived areas where the quality of primary care is poor; 45% of variation in admissions between practices is attributable to deprivation. Similarly, admission risks are higher for those who experience limited continuity of care or who encounter general practitioners who default to hospital admission, especially out-of-hours; there is a fivefold variation among general practitioners in admission rates.[47]

There are different views about how to avoid crisis admissions of frail older people. In a selective review, Purdy[47] proposes combining multiple methods to reduce them. These include using predictive modeling of older populations to identify those at greatest risk of emergency admission, promoting continuity of care in general practice, tackling modifiable clinician factors, providing hospital-at-home services, integrating health and social care and general practitioner and hospital services, and deploying senior geriatricians in emergency departments.

Predictive modeling is work in progress. The Fried phenotype of frailty appears to be of limited value for risk stratification of older people admitted to hospital,[48] and the predictive properties of other frailty rating scales is poor, at best, for medical inpatients.[49] The FORECAST tool predicts outcomes for frail older people undergoing cardiac surgery,[50] and prediction tools are under development in primary care.

A review of reviews by Philp and colleagues[51] advocates targeted preventive health checks (in the younger old), care coordination (case management) for frail older people, and care home liaison by clinicians, but dismisses multifactorial falls prevention services and community-based medicines reviews as ineffective. By contrast, two geriatricians recently argued in a forthright editorial in the *British Medical Journal* that there is no evidence that managing frail older people in the community using case management, integrated care teams, hospital outreach, or CGA reduces admissions.[52]

PATIENTS' PERSPECTIVES ON FRAILTY

The debates about recognizing and responding to frailty in primary care all too often exclude the views of frail older people. Frailty can be perceived by older people as a state of powerlessness, dependency, and cognitive decline, all feared aspects of aging.[53] Not surprisingly, the frailty label may be rejected or resisted as individuals struggle to maintain a positive self-regard and postpone an identity crisis.[54] Some frail older people distinguish between "being frail" and "feeling frail," with the former an imposed medical category and the latter a reflection of the emotional consequences of traumatic events (like bereavement).[55]

Hospital-at-home services may help circumvent the frail older patient's fears by providing short-term hospital-standard care for some acute episodes (especially infections) in the familiar setting of home. For selected patients, hospital at home is as safe as admission to a hospital ward (in terms of mortality over following months) but may have slightly higher readmission rates[56]; studies of hospital-at-home services have not characterized participants by frailty status.

FRAILTY IN CARE HOMES

The care home sector in the United Kingdom has three times as many beds as all National Health Service (NHS) hospitals and provides care for the most disabled and frail people in the population, but this care is variable in quality and lacks a standard, evidence-based package of medical support. The typical care home resident is female, 85 years or older, in the last phase of her life, living with cognitive impairment, and in receipt of seven or more medications. Median survival time following a move to a care home is approximately 2 years for care homes without on-site nursing and slightly more than 1 year for care homes with nursing. A substantial proportion live with depression, impaired mobility, and persistent pain.[57,58] Care home residents are high users of primary care resources and are perceived to be at heightened risk of emergency admission to hospital.

The care home sector in the United Kingdom is diverse, varying in size, ownership, funding sources, focus, organizational culture, and presence or absence of nursing on site.[59,60] Arrangements between care homes (90% of which are commercial or charitable) and the NHS differ greatly geographically. As a result of this diversity, some care home residents may have unequal access to NHS services, particularly those that offer specialist expertise in dementia, rehabilitation, and end-of-life care.[61,62]

A patchwork of service arrangements allows experimentation and innovation, but at some point these natural experiments need to coalesce into a small number of models of best practice. A 2011 British Geriatrics Society report on the quality of health care support for older people in care homes concluded that there was a need to clarify NHS obligations to care home residents. The United Kingdom has no specific training or accreditation for general practitioners, community nursing staff, allied health professionals, or secondary care physicians working with care home residents. There is no professional organization specifically for these practitioners and no published care standard for health care provision. Because general practitioners are the main source of medical care for care home residents, the optimal management of frailty will be tested out by them in care homes.

SUPPORT AT THE END OF LIFE

Specialist palliative care has developed from within oncology and has struggled to include those dying with other conditions. Forty percent of deaths are attributable to "progressive dwindling" (i.e., the combination of frailty and dementia) compared with 20% from cancer and another 20% from other long-term conditions. It seems unlikely that existing specialist palliative care services could expand to include those with "progressive dwindling," and it may not be necessary for them to do so if basic palliative care skills are available in general practice and community nursing. Expansion of generalist palliative care skills will be a necessary part of the change needed in primary care.

KEY POINTS

- Frailty in older people is a growing problem that needs to be managed, even though the tools available to identify frailty have limitations and the evidence underpinning interventions is sparse.
- Improving the quality of primary care by enhancing clinical skills in the recognition of and response to frailty, optimizing continuity of care, and supporting systematic, proactive management of the pre-frail and frail patient is fundamental to containing the challenge of frailty.
- Upstream interventions to delay the onset of disability and the progression of frailty are still in the development phase and cannot be relied on to reduce the scale of the problem.
- Primary care practitioners can recognize frailty using a two-stage process, beginning with a simple assessment (gait speed) and following this, where appropriate, with a more complex assessment using a tool such as the Edmonton Frail Scale.
- Expert advice should be sought about potentially tractable features of frailty, such as sarcopenia, cardiovascular disease and risk factors, and depression.
- Case management approaches and multidisciplinary interventions in the community have yet to show substantial benefits. Hospital-at-home services may be helpful, especially as a way of reducing the stigma of frailty.
- Care homes are the test-bed for primary care engagement with the problem of frailty.

For a complete list of references, please visit www.expertconsult.com.

KEY REFERENCES

1. Romero-Ortuno R, O'Shea D: Fitness and frailty: opposite ends of a challenging continuum. Age Ageing 42:279–280, 2013.
2. Clegg A, Young J, Iliffe S, et al: Frailty in older people. Lancet 381:752–762, 2013.
4. Shamliyan T, Talley C, Ramakrishnan R, et al: Association of frailty with survival: a systematic literature review. Ageing Res Rev 12:719–736, 2013.
6. Fried LP, Tangen CM, Walston J, et al: Frailty in older adults: evidence for a phenotype. J Gerontol A Biol Sci Med Sci 56:M146–M156, 2001.
7. Hubbard RE, Goodwin VA, Llewellyn DJ, et al: Frailty, financial resources and subjective well-being in later life. Arch Gerontol Geriatr 58:364–369, 2014.
8. Gale CR, Cooper C, Deary IJ, et al: Psychological well-being and incident frailty in men and women: the English Longitudinal Study of Ageing. Psychol Med 44:697–706, 2014.
9. Hoogendijk EO, Muntinga ME, van Leeuwen KM, et al: Self-perceived met and unmet care needs of frail older adults in primary care. Arch Gerontol Geriatr 58:37–42, 2014.
14. Sabia S, Elbaz A, Rouveau N, et al: Cumulative associations between midlife health behaviours and physical functioning in early old age: a 17 year prospective cohort study. J Am Geriatr Soc 62:1860–1868, 2014.
26. Lacas A, Rockwood K: Frailty in primary care: a review of its conceptualization and implications for practice. BMC Med 10:4, 2012.
28. De Rekeniere N, Leo-Summers L, Han L, et al: Epidemiology of restricting fatigue in older adults: the precipitating events project. J Am Geriatr Soc 62:476–481, 2014.
30. Beswick AD, Rees K, Dieppe P, et al: Complex interventions to improve physical function and maintain independent living in elderly people: a systematic review and meta-analysis. Lancet 371:725–735, 2008.
32. Pialoux T, Goyard J, Lesourd B: Screening tools for frailty in primary health care: a systematic review. Geriatr Gerontol Int 12:189–197, 2012.

35. Feng L, Nyunt M, Yap K, et al: Frailty predicts new and persistent depressive symptoms among community-dwelling older adults. J Am Med Dir Assoc 15:76e7–76e12, 2014.
37. Collard RM, Comijs HC, Naarding P, et al: Physical frailty: vulnerability of patients suffering from late-life depression. Aging Ment Health 18:570–578, 2014.
40. Ramsay S, Ariyanagam DS, Whincup P, et al: Cardiovascular risk profile associated with frailty: cross-sectional results from a population-based study of older British men. Heart 101:616–622, 2015.
43. Metzelthin S, van Rossum E, de Witte LP, et al: Effectiveness of an interdisciplinary primary care approach to reduce disability in community dwelling frail older people. BMJ 347:f5264, 2013.
44. Mayo-Wilson E, Grant S, Burton J, et al: Preventive home visits for mortality, morbidity and institutionalisation in older adults: a systematic review and meta-analysis. PLoS One 9:e89257, 2014.
45. Bagshaw SM, Stelfox T, McDermid RC, et al: Association between frailty and short- and long-term outcomes among critically ill patients: a multicentre prospective cohort study. CMAJ 186:E95–E100, 2014.
51. Philp I, Mills KA, Thanvi B, et al: Reducing hospital bed use by frail older people: results from a systematic review of the literature. Int J Integr Care 13:e048, 2013.
53. Grenier A: Constructions of frailty in the English language, care practice and the lived experience. Ageing Soc 27:425–445, 2007.
54. Fillit H, Butler R: The frailty identity crisis. J Am Geriatr Soc 57:348–352, 2009.
55. Grenier A: The distinction between being and feeling frail: exploring emotional experiences in health and social care. J Soc Work Pract 20:299–313, 2006.

117 Geriatric Emergency and Prehospital Care

Jacques S. Lee, Judah Goldstein

EMERGENCY MEDICINE IN CONTEXT

The arrival of the aging baby boomers has been anticipated for over a decade. The consequences are now beginning to be clear in emergency departments (EDs; British equivalent is accident & emergency [A&E]) worldwide. These aging baby boomers are challenging our North American preconceptions of what a typical older emergency patient looks like. Although the stereotype of the depression generation emergency patient has been characterized by increased risk for disease due to lifestyle and diet, stoicism that sometimes bordered on self-neglect, deference for the medical profession, and lack of comfort with technology, aging baby boomers challenge all these stereotypes. They may be very involved in fitness, resulting in sports-related injuries not previously seen among older adults. They can be extremely comfortable with technology and are more likely to have higher expectations and challenge physicians unlike previous generations. Currently, they often present accompanying their aging parent rather than as a patient, but may have young children in tow from a second or third marriage. Nonetheless, despite their improved lifestyle and diet, there is no evidence that these trends will eliminate disease or frailty. As a consequence, it is likely that older ED patients will show increasing variability from extremely fit to severely frail over the next 2 decades. Treating a stereotype instead of the patient in front of you has always been ill advised, and this increased variability among older patients poses an additional challenge for clinicians.

Just as older patients will change dramatically over the next 20 years in character and in number, the approach of emergency and paramedic services to older patients must also change.

The classic approach to emergency medicine was focused on the rapid assessment and treatment of otherwise healthy patients with a single-system problem. Emergency physicians can safely see up to three patients/hour, although they are sometime compelled to see more. Psychosocial issues were often considered outside the scope of emergency medicine. The ultimate goal of resuscitation and prolongation of life at any cost was never questioned. Emergency physicians typically make patient care decisions alone.

In contrast, geriatric medicine involves the care of patients for whom multiple comorbidities are the norm, and challenging social circumstances are common. Their problems typically involve multiple systems, and psychosocial assessments are routinely needed. Extending the quantity of life may not be the overarching goal, focusing instead on quality. Also, geriatric medicine has pioneered the incorporation of an interprofessional and interdisciplinary team approach into decision making and care of such patients.

The emergency management of older adults begins in the community, often with a request for paramedic assistance. Paramedics are among the only health providers that currently attend to most of their patients in the patient's own home, which offers them the opportunity for unique insights into the home environment and clues to a patient's functional status. Whether this information is gathered, how it is communicated, and how it might best be leveraged without duplication remain pragmatic challenges in most jurisdictions.

In the typical case, patients who call emergency medical services are then transported to the ED. Even so, a large proportion of patient encounters do not result in transport to hospital (see later, "Epidemiology of Emergency Department and Paramedical Services Use"). Once in the ED, care is provided by the emergency providers and, depending on the presentation, a decision is made to discharge home or admit to the hospital. For those discharged, follow-up can be highly variable, ranging from instructions to return to the ED, if necessary, to proactive case management models by specialized geriatric emergency management professionals. These programs provide targeted interventions or alternatives to traditional care, with the goal to ensure the patients get the right care in the right place by the right provider at the right time.

We will discuss some creative approaches to the challenges faced by older patients in the ED (see later, "Innovative Approaches to Older Patients in the Emergency Department").

Paramedical Services

In North America, paramedics typically staff emergency medical services (EMS) systems, with nurses present in some critical care transport models. In consequence, there has been a move to refer to paramedic services (PS) as opposed to emergency medical services. Other agencies throughout the world have varying staffing configurations, including physicians, nurses, and other allied health professionals. Paramedicine has been protocol-driven and focuses on targeted assessments, skills and interventions, and making decisions, often with medical oversight. As the education and professionalism of paramedicine evolves,[1] more emphasis is being placed on clinical decision making and increased integration into the health care system. This chapter will primarily focus on the paramedic model, so will refer to these services as paramedical services.

Paramedical services are a community-based resource, initially established to minimize morbidity and mortality from cardiac arrest (cardiovascular disease) to major trauma.[2] The time it takes for a paramedic crew to arrive at the scene of a cardiac arrest has been shown to affect survival rates.[3] As a result, paramedical services are designed to minimize response times to all patients in their geographic catchment area. This may result in relative underutilization of paramedic crews in rural settings with a low population density. In urban centers, paramedics may have extended wait times in hospital prior to patient handover to ED staff, known as off-load delay (see later). Paramedics provide care to the most vulnerable in society. In geriatrics, this would encompass the frail older adult. For these reasons, paramedics are uniquely positioned to play an important role in geriatric community-based care by merging primary and acute care services when there is a service request. Paramedics can serve as a conduit between primary and acute care to enable system integration and continuity of care, with the goal to improve the overall quality of care for this demographic and potentially improve system efficiencies.

The term *prehospital care* is becoming a misnomer when considering the changes that are occurring in the realm of EMS. Services are evolving from the traditional transport service to more of an integrated health care service. Traditional paramedical services involved patient treatment and stabilization on scene, with subsequent transport, typically to the closest emergency department. Nontraditional paramedic roles can be referred to as expanded-scope paramedical services. In these nontraditional roles, paramedics assess patients and transport them to the most appropriate facility (e.g., trauma center, stroke center), provide referral services, or treat in place, in addition to the traditional idea of transport to the ED.

Paramedics are caring for older adults for longer durations due to offload delay—the period of time between arrival at a health care facility and completing the handover to in-hospital staff—and, more frequently, with the closure of smaller health care facilities and regionalization of care (longer transports). Optimizing this care should be a priority for medical directors, EMS leadership, and other clinicians who may have a stake in care provision for older adults, including geriatricians. Paramedics receive little specific geriatrics training in their educational programs. Also, there is often a mismatch between the expectations of the job (e.g., classic expectations of trauma or cardiac arrests) and the reality, in which older adults with complex presentations comprise the bulk of care. This role dissonance might stem from paramedics identifying as rescuers but acting as care providers[4] and can be a source of stress for EMS providers, especially in the traditional model of transport to the closest ED, with little thought regarding where the patient would be best managed. This is changing.

Epidemiology of Emergency Department and Paramedical Services Use

In North America, close to 50% of paramedic emergency responses are for people 65 years and older.[5,6] This is even higher in the United Kingdom, where 65% of older adults come to the ED by ambulance, compared with 20% of those who are younger age.[7] Older adults comprise 12% to 24% of ED visits and this leads to high ED bed occupancy among this demographic.[8,9] Older adults are often more acutely ill on arrival.[9] They tend to have more medical tests performed in the ED, and this contributes to a longer length of stay in the department.[9] Older adults also have more hospitalizations and intensive care unit (ICU) admissions.[10] Adverse events are common in older adults discharged from the ED.[10] In a study of U.S. Medicare beneficiaries, 32.9% of older adults discharged from the ED experienced an adverse event (e.g., readmission, hospitalization, institutionalization, death) within 90 days of the visit.[11] Older adults are also more likely to be admitted to a nursing home following an encounter with emergency services.[10] Paramedical services and ED use are expected to rise, especially in the oldest old.[12]

Older age is a major predictor of paramedical services and ED use.[13] Even so, age does not fully explain these trends.[14] Other contributors include the fact that older adults are living alone in their own home more often and there is reduced capability of caregivers and often difficulties accessing primary care.[14] In addition, many chronic illnesses become more common with increasing age, increasing the likelihood of acute illness.[15] Realizing that age is not the full contributor means that interventions or innovative models of care can be developed to serve this demographic in the community better. The need for less reliance on acute care services and a larger role for paramedics, emergency services, and intermediate and community-based care has been recognized,[16] but moving away from acute care services is a challenge. Emergency medicine can play a role in facilitating this change.

Frailty in Acute Care

Frailty is an important predictor of adverse outcomes in the ED[11,17]; however, it is not well recognized as an important concept in this setting. Various approaches have been used to operationalize a definition of frailty within the context of emergency services. The prevalence of frailty, using the phenotype, was 20% in a cohort of older adults discharged from the ED.[18] This was thought to be the "floor" of frailty because only discharged patients willing to participate were included.[18]

The frailty index (FI), a score based on the proportion of deficits or health problems of an individual, can predict adverse outcomes in patients seen in the ED and can be determined based on questionnaires completed by care partners.[11,17] The FI likewise predicts outcomes in major trauma patients.[19] Another approach uses the clinical frailty scale (CFS), which describes categories of increasing frailty and reduced function. Patients are placed in the category that best describes their current health.[20] The CFS predicts adverse events in ICU patients[21] and across a variety of other hospital settings[22-27] and may represent a means to evaluate frailty in ED patients quickly. Different settings may require differing approaches that match the constraints of the setting. It is evident that frailty has been receiving more attention but more research is required to determine best practices. Novel programs to improve care for older adults should aim to include methods for improving the care for the frailest. Frailty is one of the predictors of emergency services use that can be better managed prior to ED arrival, in the ED, and during discharge.

NEW APPROACHES TO GERIATRICS IN PARAMEDICAL SERVICES AND THE EMERGENCY DEPARTMENT

Here we outline existing, more progressive approaches, organized as before, during, and after. If emergency services are thought of as an episode of care, it can be further delineated in terms of decision points. When emergency services are accessed, it is possible to intervene during various nodes of the emergency episode of care continuum (Figure 117-1). When patients decide to access emergency care, there has typically been an acute change in condition or difficulties accessing other services (e.g., primary care).[28] Calls for service are processed through dispatch centers, with ambulances dispatched as per local policies. The structured information obtained at this point determines the nature of the response. In addition, callers can be advised to initiate medical care. In most cases, the traditional paramedic response involves an ambulance, with varying paramedic configurations. In a number of locations worldwide, there are nontraditional paramedical services in the form of community paramedic responses that are often non–transport-capable. The responding paramedics conduct assessments and initiate treatment in the field. A decision to transport (or not) is made in consultation with the patient, family, and potentially medical oversight. In most cases, patients are still transported to the ED.

The next transition point is the patient handover, or offload, period. In the ED, patients are assessed, treated, and discharged or referred for consultation within the department. Many older adults (≈20%) will be admitted.[8] There are opportunities to improve the discharge process or transition of patients back into the community for the group not admitted. This is a group at high risk for further health decline immediately following the ED discharge.[11] Throughout the continuum of care, there are opportunities to change how care is provided to address the individual's unique needs. Paramedical services can be flexible, adaptable, and responsive to the demands of the system. We will highlight some of the ways the emergency system of care has changed to improve care provision for older adults. This often means using health care professionals in nontraditional ways.

Paramedical Service Care before the Emergency Department

Paramedics are frequently requested to respond when a health crisis occurs in the community. Paramedics have been providing more care within the community that does not necessarily result

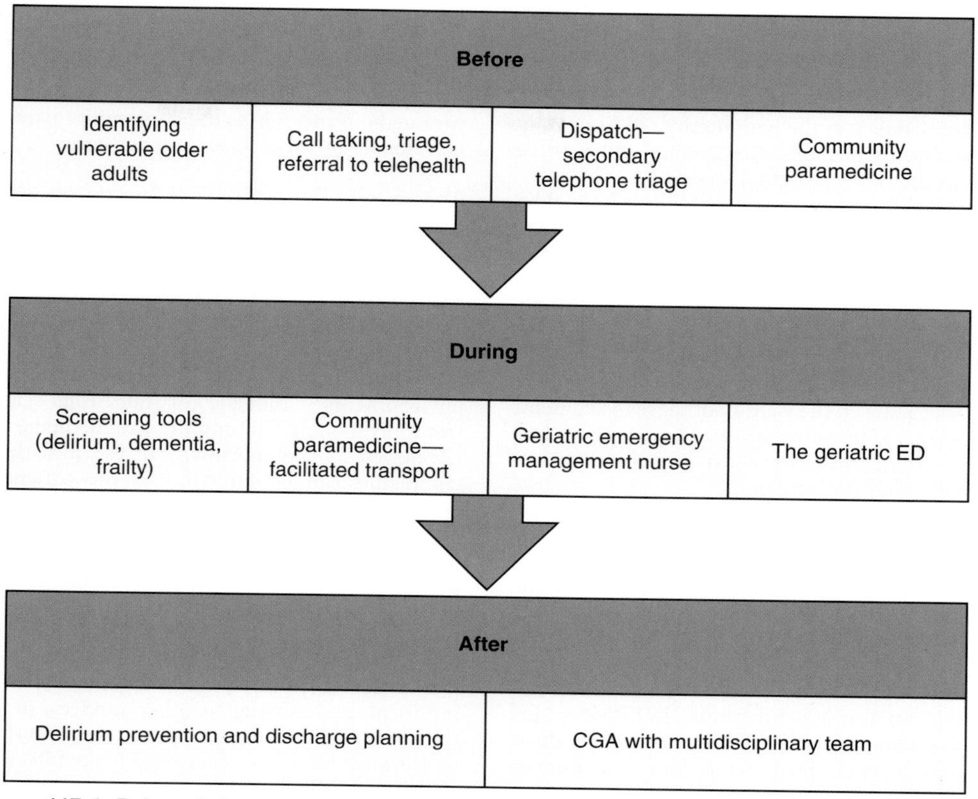

Figure 117-1. Before, during, and after approaches to geriatrics in paramedical services and the emergency department.

in transport to the ED or, if it does, is described as a facilitated transport. Some of these programs span the continuum of emergency care and have an impact prior to ED arrival, within the ED, and on discharge. The goal of such programs is often ED diversion; however, care should also be patient-centric. Programs should focus on providing rational care that aligns with the patient's (and care provider's) preidentified goals of care. Some older adults are frail but not acutely ill and could benefit from community-based care, as opposed to direct transport to the ED, whereas others may be acutely ill and would benefit from the specialized knowledge, diagnostics, and treatments afforded by acute care. Discerning between these groups is a challenge. The subsequent section will describe promising programs at various points of the emergency continuum of care that aim to direct patients to the most appropriate resource or provide care differently.

Accessing Emergency Services: Communications and Dispatch

The first point of contact with the emergency system is with ambulance communication or dispatch centers. During primary telephone triage call takers triage calls, prioritizing them for dispatch using computer-based priority dispatch systems.[29] Dispatch algorithms have been developed, such as the internationally used Medical Priority Dispatch System (MPDS). This system aims to identify high- and low-acuity patients so that the appropriate resources can respond. Dispatch centers may be staffed by civilian call takers and dispatchers or by paramedics or other health care staff. For this reason, health care knowledge can be variable. High-acuity conditions include cardiac arrest and major trauma. Low-acuity conditions may be more difficult to identify, especially in older adults. Nevertheless, programs are being developed to divert lower acuity calls to other services.

Secondary Telephone Triage

In some systems, low-priority calls (omega priority) are transferred for secondary triage with a nurse or other advanced health care practitioner.[30] Secondary telephone triage has been suggested as a mechanism to divert lower acuity calls by determining who might benefit from alternatives to ambulance transport. Secondary telephone triage appears safe; however, there are questions regarding its organization and impact on resource use.[31] Up to 50% of low-acuity calls may be helped by medical advice alone,[32,33] but this may be dependent on system-level factors. In a recent study, successful transfer to nurse triage without an ambulance response occurred in 12.3% of cases.[30] There is also no information on how secondary telephone triage might work in the context of geriatrics specifically.

Traditional Paramedical Services

In the traditional paramedical service, the focus is on a rapid response, focused assessment, identification of the chief complaint, and transport decision, with the idea to treat life-threatening conditions, provide symptom relief, and mitigate further deterioration in the patient's condition. The definition, scope, and role of paramedics can vary among countries. For example in Canada, four levels are recognized (http://paramedic.ca/wp-content/uploads/2012/12/2011-10-31-Approved-NOCP-English-Master.pdf). The paramedic levels differ in degree of medical knowledge and types of delegated medical acts. At the advanced levels, there is enhanced assessment skills and the ability to implement invasive treatments and medications. Paramedics are differentiated from other health care practitioners by their degree of mobility, accessibility in the community (24 hours/day, 7 days/week), and ability to manage emergencies and provide comprehensive care in the out-of-hospital setting.[34]

Traditional paramedical services must be able to assess older adults competently, accessing emergency services and making sound decisions regarding care. In caring for older adults, studies have focused on identifying vulnerability via the development of risk screening measures and screening for cognitive impairment, depression, falls, immunization status, and frailty.[35-37] Many of these programs have demonstrated that it is feasible for traditional paramedical services to screen for a variety of health care conditions, but few have assessed the validity of these instruments or follow-up interventions to improve health. There is also a lack of valid EMS measures to screen for mobility impairment, functional impairment, and caregiver burden.

Paramedics often respond to older adults who have suffered a fall. A falls protocol has been evaluated for use in assisted living facilities to determine which patients might safely remain at home.[38] This protocol uses the patient history and examination findings to recommend transport versus nontransport with primary care follow-up. Ground-level falls were broken down by tiers. Those in tier 1 include uncontrollable hemorrhage, lacerations requiring suture repair, acute medical conditions (e.g., ST-segment elevation myocardial infarction [STEMI]), and others that would necessitate transport. Tier 2 cases include those with borderline abnormal vital signs, acute pain, and injuries requiring splinting. In these cases, a physician would be consulted, and then the decision to transport or provide care in place is made. Tier 3 cases (e.g., simple contusions or skin tears, no complaint, no hip pain and otherwise normal examination, no obvious injury) are recommended for no transport. The falls protocol had a sensitivity of 96%, specificity of 54%, and negative predictive value of 97% for predicting time-sensitive injuries.[38] This is one example of a tool that can be used to support decision making in this setting. Safety and appropriate medical follow-up are key components to ensuring programs are successful.

One of the biggest research priorities facing emergency services in relation to caring for older adults is whether critical illness can be diagnosed and treated effectively in a prehospital setting.[39] Discerning between the frail older adult who is acutely ill and an older adult with a health care need but no acute illness is a challenge. Often, presenting complaints appear benign and are described as nonspecific[40] (e.g., weakness, sudden onset immobility, falls) but, in the context of frailty, are indications of serious life-limiting, illness. Recently, a prehospital FI was found to have similar predictive properties as an in-hospital assessment (FI and comprehensive geriatric assessment [CGA]; FI-CGA).[17]

Determining frailty in the EMS setting, where there are often competing priorities and time constraints, is a challenge. The care partner FI-CGA (CP-FI-CGA) may be an efficient approach that captures the knowledge of care partners for frailty assessment. In this study, care partners were asked questions about the patients' comorbidities, mobility, function, sensory impairment, and social supports.[17] Responses were used to calculate an FI. This FI predicted 1-year mortality and demonstrated similar properties to other FIs. Whether the CP-FI-CGA can help guide care requires further evaluation. It may be possible to use this tool to discern among those who may benefit from community services versus those who would benefit in the ED.

Once issues are identified, it may be possible to transport to the most appropriate non-ED provider, treat in place, or transport to the ED. In the context of other single acute conditions, systems of care have developed whereby paramedics use the assessment to determine the most appropriate health care facility for care. For major trauma, STEMI, and stroke, transport is usually to a tertiary care facility that specializes in providing care to these populations. A similar system of care may be beneficial for frail and acutely ill older adults. An emerging role within the paramedic profession is the community paramedic, and this may be valuable in geriatric emergency care.

Community Paramedicine: Nontraditional Paramedical Services

There are a number of terms used to describe the expanded-scope paramedic model; however, the one endorsed by clinical and operational leaders is the term *community paramedic*.[34] A community paramedic is "a model of care whereby paramedics apply their training and skills in non-traditional community-based environments"[1] (outside of the usual emergency response/transport model). Community paramedicine programs have been developed to take advantage of the idea that many presenting complaints can be cared for in the patient's home or can be referred to other non–ED-based services, with potentially better outcomes, improved resource use, and patient satisfaction.[34] Community paramedics should have the skill set to assess older adults within the community while operating within new models of care. These include more referral or transport options beyond the closest ED, additional resources, and improved linkages with other services, including primary care. The goal of such programs is to intervene prior to the emergency department visit by treating in place, referring to other services, or possibly facilitating transport to the emergency department. In the United Kingdom, conveyance rates have decreased from 58% to 90% over the past decade, and this has been associated with the development of community paramedic programs.[41] Community paramedic programs appear safe, with better patient outcomes for certain populations.[42,43] We will review examples of such programs, focusing on care provision for older adults.

Extended-Care Paramedic Program

One community paramedic program that specifically addresses the needs of long-term care (LTC) residents is the extended-care paramedic (ECP) program in Halifax, Nova Scotia.[44] LTC residents represent a unique group of ED attendees who often have worse health outcomes. The ECP program was initiated in February 2011. Seven experienced, advanced-care paramedics were provided additional training on extended-care roles, including geriatric assessment, end-of-life care, primary wound closure techniques, and point-of-care (bedside) testing.[44] ECPs work alone in nontransport-capable vehicles that respond to predesignated LTC facilities within the region. The goal of the program is to provide care on site with medical direction (emergency and LTC physician advisors). Disposition for ECP patients includes treat and release, facilitated transport (e.g., transport for x-ray, with return to residence), or immediate emergent transport. This type of program spans the entire spectrum of care, including the before, during, and after stages. The ECP-LTC program provides care in nursing homes, but also aims to facilitate transfer to the ED for diagnostics and treatment when necessary. In some cases, it can help with discharge in that follow-up care will be provided that is typically not available in the LTC setting or can take time to implement.

There have been a number of important attributes to the program that may improve emergency care provision in this setting. ECP responses involve more collaboration among LTC facility staff (physicians, nurses), patients, and families,[45] thus promoting better communication among these groups during a health crisis. Another important aspect of this program was the identification of the role that ECPs could play in end-of-life care,[45] during which patients could be provided with comfort care in their own residence, negating the need for transport if that was the ultimate goal of the patient. In the ECP cohort, 70% of patients enrolled in the study were treated in the residence, with 24% being facilitated transport and 6% urgent transport to the ED, compared to an 80% transport rate for traditional EMS during the time frame.[44] Whether such a program is adaptable to other settings requires further investigation.

Collaboration with Primary Care (Referral Services)

EMS referral programs are being established as an alternative to ED transport or what is known as treat and release. Referral programs aim to identify safe alternatives to ED transport for those with less urgent conditions. However, there is controversy over whether paramedics can determine medical necessity.[46] Referral programs have been successful for specific conditions. For example, referrals to falls teams have demonstrated positive results for high-risk patients.[47] In this program, the referral was generated following the response by administrative staff. Community referrals by EMS (CREMS), based in Toronto, Canada, was launched in 2006 (Solutions East Toronto Health Collaborative) with the goal to make efficient use of resources and generate referrals to community-based care. These services require more rigorous evaluation. Paramedics were traditionally not points of referral, but this is changing.

Other models aim to evaluate decision support systems for referrals.[48,49] Vicente and colleagues have investigated a decision support system to determine whether frail older adults with certain complaints can be safely referred to geriatric services.[49] Another example is the paramedic pathfinder.[48] This is an algorithmic approach to decision making based on symptom discriminators from the local triage system. Two pathways have been created for use by ground ambulance paramedics; these include the trauma and medical pathways.[48] These systems use symptom-related findings rather than diagnostics to discern disposition, with acceptable levels of sensitivity and specificity observed.[48]

Emergency Care Practitioner Model

In the United Kingdom, paramedics have expanded their assessment, triage, and treatment skills to manage the growing demand for paramedic services. The emergency care practitioner (ECP) model involves having a paramedic or nurse respond in nontransport-capable vehicles to provide care to patients in their own home. Services were initially established to provide care to older adults with seemingly minor complaints.[50] If necessary, paramedics can facilitate transport to the ED for diagnostics. Education typically entails an brief period of intensive specialized training (3 weeks) focused on obtaining histories, physical assessments, and ordering diagnostics. A portion of the training is also spent in supervised practice.

In a randomized controlled trial (RCT) of the paramedic practitioner model, those treated by paramedic practitioners were less likely to have attended an ED during the initial episode or in the next 28 days. Patients were also less likely to require a hospital admission and were more likely to report that they were very satisfied with their care.[29,42] The authors concluded that the service reduced resource use (ED conveyance) and appeared safe.[51] The emergency care practitioner's role can have varying effects that are dependent on the setting in which they are deployed.[52] The role should be used to supplement existing roles rather than replacing existing services.

The goal of community paramedic programs is to reduce emergency department visits while also providing safe and effective care that is in accord with the patient's wishes. These models might ensure that frail older adults get the care that they need by the right provider in the right place; however, more research is required to understand the role of these services.

Emergency Department Care

Challenges

Care in the ED involves a number of specific challenges.

Emergency Department Visits. Would you normally trust your life to someone you just met? In essence, this unexamined reality is faced by patients every day in the ED. As opposed to a primary care physician, who may have a lifelong relationship with the patient, intimate knowledge of the patient's past medical history, and developed a therapeutic alliance. Emergency physicians typically treat patients they have never seen before and too often lack access to needed medical history. Also, by definition, patients seek the care of emergency physicians for their most serious health events. The encounter can happen at any time of day or night, during a weekend, or while on vacation. This may be why emergency medicine has been described as unbounded in scope, unpredictable and potentially unlimited in demands.[52a]

Crowding and Older Adults. In contrast with other health care settings, in which appointments can be scheduled, EDs have no control of the timing and volume of patients arriving. When this highly unpredictable inflow of patients peaks and is coupled with reduced outflow of admitted patients to inpatient units, EDs can become crowded.[53-56] The understanding that ED crowding is primarily due to restriction in flow or the rate at which patients exit the ED is relatively new and supplants the prior understanding that only ED factors were associated with long ED waits. ED crowding is a global phenomenon increasingly reported in Canada,[57,58] Australia,[59] United Kingdom,[60] and the United States.[61]

ED crowding worsens quality of care and increases hospital mortality.[57,61-63] Patients admitted to hospital from a crowded ED were recently shown to have increased 7-day hospitalization and mortality rates.[64]

Unfortunately, studies have suggested that older patients are adversely[65-68] and disproportionately[69-71] affected by ED crowding. Older patients consistently have longer ED wait times when controlling for disease severity.[69-71] A population-based study has shown that older patients in the province of Ontario, Canada, had wait times in the ED that were 2.7 times longer compared to younger patients with the same illness severity.[71] Of particular concern is the fact that one U.S. study has found that older patients with an ED wait time longer than 12 hours had double the risk of developing delirium.[72]

In addition, studies have shown that older patients experience worse care during ED crowding. One study has shown delayed analgesic treatment for older patients with hip fractures.[67] A recently published single-center Canadian study has indicated that ED crowding is associated with a 3% increase in adverse events by older patients for each hour spent in the ED.[68] McCusker and colleagues found that ED crowding increased health service utilization for older adults following ED discharge—that is, an increased rate of return to the ED and unplanned hospital readmission.[66]

Emergency Department Screening Tools

Given the high volume of decisions that emergency physicians must make under time and pressure constraints, emergency medicine has focused a significant amount of research on developing clinical decision rules (CDRs) to assist in the management of high-risk groups such as older patients.

A clinical decision or prediction rule is a simple algorithm that uses a combination of clinically sensible variables[73] or variables that are available and can be feasibly collected by front-line clinicians in real time to identify high-risk individuals. Decision rules standardize clinical assessment, can identify high risk patients, and have been shown to improve decision making compared to unaided clinical judgment.[74-79]

However, the higher prevalence of disease, greater variability in health, and atypical presentations among older adults have reduced the predictive accuracy of CDRs for targeting older adults. The highest sensitivity reported for a CDR targeting older adults is 72%, compared to a sensitivity of 99% to 100% for many CDRs targeting younger populations.[76,80-82] We have shown that the predictive accuracy of the Canadian cervical spine and computed tomography head CDR degrade substantially when applied to older patients.[83,84] The same prognostic challenges that reduce the sensitivity of CDRs also impair clinical judgment, resulting in missed diagnoses, unplanned return ED visits, and worse outcomes among older adults following an EMS or ED encounter.[10,85-88] Despite suboptimal predictive performance, research is needed to establish whether CDRs targeting older adults can identify high-risk individuals better than unaided clinical judgment and whether their use can reduce adverse outcomes in this vulnerable population.[85]

Triage Risk Stratification Tool. The five-item triage risk screening tool (TRST) is completed by ED triage nurses and has a sensitivity of 55% to predict ED revisits, hospitalization, or institutionalization within 120 days. The specificity of the TRST tool was found to be 66%.[89,90] TRST predictors were chosen based on expert opinion only and not empirically derived.[75,77-79] The predictive performance of the TRST was found to have a lower predictive ability in a direct comparison to the Identifying Seniors at Risk (ISAR) screening tool.[85] One meta-analysis found low predictive ability of the TRST in six studies with over 3233 patients enrolled.[91]

Identifying Seniors at Risk Screening Tool. McCusker and associates followed rigid methodologic standards in developing the ISAR screening tool.[92-94] This tool was originally designed to identify people older than 70 years who present to the ED and are at highest risk for an adverse outcome, defined as functional decline,[92] hospitalization,[93] institutionalization,[94] or death within 6 months. An ISAR score of 2 is 72% sensitive for identifying patients who experience one of these adverse outcome within 120 days and has a specificity of 58%.[95] The most common adverse event observed was functional decline (54%), followed by death (35%), and then by nursing home admission (10.8%).

This six-item ED screening tool was meant to be completed by older patients, family members, or caregivers while in the waiting room of the ED. However, in actual practice, it was found that many patients, families, and caregivers required the assistance of someone familiar with the screening tool to complete it.

The data from the original study was subsequently used to assess the ability of the ISAR to predict return to the ED within 30 days, although the predictive performance for early return to ED was substantially lower (AUC [area under the curve], 0.63).[94,96,97] Other studies have shown difficulties in identifying or preventing return visits to the ED, and some have questioned whether this is a worthwhile goal, since most ED visits are appropriate.

McCusker and associates subsequently performed a systematic review 72 of studies predicting return to the ED.[96] It was found that most return ED visits were appropriate in that they were due to need factors, but concluded that when controlling for need, factors associated with increased access to primary care were associated with reduced return ED visits.

Currently, ISAR is the best tool to identify older patients at highest risk for the adverse outcomes outlined earlier. It has been translated and validated in several other languages. The value of these tools, given a lack of evidence as to the effectiveness of interventions, has recently been challenged.[98]

Screening for Dementia and Delirium. Unfortunately, multiple studies have found that cognitive impairment is poorly recognized in the ED. Delirium is unrecognized by ED staff in 60% to 80% of cases, and up to one third of patients with unrecognized delirium are sent home.[99-103] One study found that 100% of patients sent home with delirium returned within 4 days of discharge.[102] Also, the consequences of unrecognized delirium can be more severe. Kakuma and coworkers have completed a retrospective secondary analysis of outcomes in a cohort of 107 ED patients in which patient disposition decisions were left to the emergency physician. They found that patients who were sent home with unrecognized delirium had a mortality rate of 31% at 6 months, compared to 6% among all other patients.[104]

Similarly, dementia is also poorly recognized. Hustey and associates have found that only 46% of patients with dementia were recognized by ED staff.[100-102] Failure to recognize cognitive impairment has important consequences because discharge planning and follow-up instructions need to be modified in these patients.

Although the use of previously validated screening tools, such as the Mini Mental State Exam (MMSE) or Montreal Cognitive Assessment (MoCA) have been advocated, the time they take to administer, plus the requirement for pen and paper to complete elements of these tests, have led to low adoption rates in the ED. As a result, a number of cognitive screening tools that can be completed in less than 3 minutes have been proposed for use in the ED (Table 117-1).[105-107] These include the six-item screener, Brief Alzheimer Screen (BAS), Short Blessed Test (SBT), Ottawa 3 Date and Year (O3DY), caregiver-completed eight-item interview to differentiate aging and dementia (C-AD8), six-item screener, Mini-Cog, confusion assessment method (CAM), and confusion assessment method for the intensive care unit (CAM-ICU). Carpenter and colleagues have compared the performance of four brief screening tools (O3DY, BAS, SBT, C-AD8) against the MMSE and concluded that the SBT has high sensitivity and maximum specificity among the four tests they compared.[105]

Of note, longer cognitive screening methods only marginally add to sensitivity for cognitive impairment, although they do improve specificity (Table 117-2). Therefore, one possible strategy would be to use one of the brief screening tests in the ED listed earlier and to verify any positive results with one of the longer screening tests.

Innovative Approaches to Older Patients in the Emergency Department

We have outlined significant challenges faced in providing high-quality care to older patients in the ED. However, thanks to a wave of research outlining the nature of these challenges, we have also witnessed significant and innovative attempts to improve the care of geriatric patient in the ED. Next, we will describe some of these progressive approaches to geriatrics in the ED.

TABLE 117-1 Brief Cognitive and Delirium Screening Tools for the Emergency Department[105-108]

Test	Sensitivity (%)	Specificity (%)	Time (Minutes)
Short Blessed Test	95	65	2
Brief Alzheimer Screen	95	52	2
Ottawa 3DY	95	51	2
Six-item screener	89-94	86-88	2
Mini-Cog	75-99	91-93	3
CAM-ICU	76	98	3-5
C-AD8	83	63	3-5

C-AD8, Caregiver-completed eight-item interview to differentiate aging and dementia; *CAM-ICU,* confusion assessment method for the intensive care unit.

TABLE 117-2 Cognitive Assessment Methods for the Emergency Department

Test	Sensitivity (%)	Specificity (%)	Time (Minutes)
Montreal Cognitive Assessment (MoCA)	100	87	10
St. Louis University Mental Status (SLUMS) examination	100	81	10
MMSE	71-95	76-100	8
Confusion assessment method (CAM)			8

Geriatric Consultation Services

Evidence that comprehensive geriatric assessments (CGAs) of older patients admitted to the hospital results in reduced functional decline and loss of independence and mortality[109] raises the question as to whether CGA could improve outcomes among patients discharged from the emergency department. One obvious barrier to CGA in the emergency department is the time it takes to perform.[110] Although a CGA team may take an entire day to assess a patient, holding patients all day to complete a lengthy assessments would be a barrier to implementation in many EDs.

Caplan and coworkers[111] have described the Discharge of Elders from the Emergency Department (DEED) program, whereby patients older than 75 years were discharged home following an ED visit. In this RCT, intervention patients received a 30- to 60-minute interview in the ED. Any urgently needed referrals for care were initiated immediately by an advanced practice nurse in discussion with the primary care physician. Patients also received case management for 4 weeks and a full case review by an interdisciplinary panel within 1 week of discharge. Intervention patients had 1.7 new problems identified by the CGA and received 2.3 home visits, on average, in the month following ED discharge. The rate of subsequent hospitalization was decreased by 5.7% in the intervention group compared to control patients who had all their discharge planning arranged by the ED physician, typically a junior house staff in the Australian care model.

Graf and associates[110] have carried out a systematic review of CGAs in the ED and identified eight RCTs of use of CGA in the ED. They found four clinical trials that demonstrated a reduction in functional decline.[29,111-113] However, impact on service use, and return to the ED in particular, have been less consistent.[114,115]

Geriatric Emergency Management Nurse

Given the difficulties with conducting a full CGA in the ED, and the relative scarcity of geriatricians, the potential impact of a geriatric discharge coordinator was first examined in Montreal.[112] Subsequently, the geriatric emergency management (GEM) nursing role, which combined specialized geriatric knowledge and an understanding of emergency care processes, was introduced to Ontario at Sunnybrook Health Sciences Center in 1995.[116] Having knowledge and skills in geriatric and emergency care is important to function effectively in this role.[117] The GEM model began to be implemented in Ontario in 2004. Currently, there is a network of 103 GEM nurses working in 60 hospital EDs; the Ontario GEM network covers an area of over 123 million acres (0.5 million km^2).[117,118] GEM nurses thus provide a variety of services to improve the care of ED patients, including the following:

- Geriatric case finding
  - Liaising with community services, agencies, primary care, and specialized geriatric services to obtain information relevant for the current ED visit
- Modified ED geriatric comprehensive assessments
  - Liaising with community services, agencies, primary care and specialized geriatric services to plan for discharge and follow-up following the current ED visit
  - Telephone follow-up of patients discharged on weekends or outside of GEM nurse hours
  - Case management—longitudinal follow-up and interventions to provide patients with the right care in the right place at the right time
  - Geriatric capacity building in the ED by acting as an educational resource for ED front-line staff

The four most common presenting problems assessed by GEM nurses in Ontario include many of the so-called *geriatric giants*, each covered elsewhere in this text:

1. Falls
2. Mobility problems
3. Delirium, acute confusion
4. Breakdown of social supports

The median number of hours that GEM nurses are typically staffed is 75 hours/week, and GEM nurses are currently assessing an average of 800 older patients/year.[118] Despite this, GEM nurses are still only able to assess one third of eligible ED patients. Thus, building geriatric capacity among front-line ED staff is a very important role performed by GEM nurses to leverage and maximize their impact on improving the care of older ED patients. Currently, the impact of the GEM nurses' role is undergoing process evaluations across Ontario. Well-designed clinical trials to examine immediate and downstream impacts of the GEM nurse role are needed.

Geriatric Emergency Department

Given the challenges to delivering high-quality care to older patients, another proposed model is to establish specialized geriatric emergency departments[119,120] parallel to specialized pediatric hospitals. Hwang and colleagues[120] have described modifications to the care processes and to the physical design and furnishings of the ED. The increased costs of such EDs could be offset by potential savings associated with improved care, such as improved soundproofing, diurnal lighting systems, reduced catheter use leading to reduced delirium, and improved mattresses to increase patient comfort and skin integrity. Several such geriatric EDs have been established in the United States and Italy. The impact of these new designs and processes of care on patient outcomes has yet to undergo extensive evaluation and will be an important focus of future research.

Emergency Department Avoidance and Diversion

Another attempt to address the concerns regarding the care of older adults is the possibility of bypassing the ED for older patients whose needs would not be best met in the ED. The ECP model for paramedics outlined earlier is one example. Geriatric nurse practitioners have provided outreach to nursing homes to attempt ED avoidance. In this model of care, nurse practitioners with geriatric expertise consult on patients when transfer to the ED is being considered. Possible scenarios in which ED avoidance may be achieved include patients requiring feeding tube re-insertion. Because these fluoroscopy-guided procedures are not typically available overnight in the ED, many centers have developed rapid next-day protocols with their local interventional radiology colleagues. Overnight intravenous (IV) hydration or hypodermoclysis may be used as a bridging technique.

In addition, much work has been done on avoiding ED transfers for patients whose self-identified goals of care do not include resuscitation or acute care to prolong life. Ongoing efforts have been made to improve the documentation of palliative goals of care and do not resuscitate (DNR) directives.

Code Silver: Holistic System-Wide Approach

Banerjee and coworkers have examined a system-wide, quality improvement approach to the care of older patients treated in the A&E departments in the Sheffield region.[121] An interdisciplinary committee including ambulance service directors, College of Emergency Medicine, British Geriatrics Society, Chartered Society of Physiotherapists, College of Occupational Therapists, Royal College of Nursing, and patient advocacy groups developed standards of care for older people to receive with the first 24 hours of presentation to an A&E department. The Silver Book[121] advocates for "respect for the autonomy and dignity of older persons" and suggests that a systemic integrated approach be taken toward improving care of older adults during an urgent care episode.

In addition, the Silver Book standards include ensuring that all patients have the following issues assessed within 24 hours of presentation:

- Pain
- Delirium and dementia
- Depression
- Nutrition and hydration
- Skin integrity
- Sensory loss
- Falls and mobility
- Activities of daily living
- Continence
- Vital signs
- Safeguarding issues
- End-of-life care issues

Some other recommendations include the following:

1. CGAs for older patients with frailty
2. Use of clinical decision units for older adults who can be discharged but who will need ongoing treatment in the community
3. Availability of multidisciplinary teams to assist with discharge planning for older patients, including social services and mental health
4. Creation of a 24-hour single access point for community services to facilitate discharge of stable older adults who do not require hospital admission

Planning for After Discharge

ED visits by older adults are indicative of changing health care needs. A return visit to the ED is likely for many older adults shortly after the initial encounter. Adverse events (e.g., repeat visit, hospital admission, death, LTC placement) following discharge from the ED occurred in 33% of attendees.[11] In older adults, past ED use predicts future use.[122] Almost 73% of people aged 65 years and older have a low to average risk of subsequent return to the ED; the other 27% have a higher than average risk of return and may be most likely to benefit from postdischarge follow-up.[122]

EMS systems require methods for integrating care and ensuring health care providers have a platform for communicating. The Physician Orders for Life-Sustaining Treatment (POLST) is an effective method for sharing advanced care plans with paramedics. This communication tool may help with changing treatment decisions in the pre-hospital setting in the context of cardiac arrest.[123] This has been confirmed by identifying that 6.4% of patients with "comfort measures only" directives died in hospital versus 44.2% with full treatment orders.[124] This is an example of a platform that is shared among providers.

Delirium Prevention—Interprofessional Prevention of Delirium

Inouye and colleagues have carried out fundamental work to establish the determinants of delirium among older medical inpatients.[65,125] They first showed that in patients admitted to a medical inpatient ward, a prolonged ED stay, lasting 12 hours or longer, was independently associated with a twofold increased odds of developing incident delirium as an inpatient.[29] When this study was performed in the eastern United States, only 23% of eligible patients had an ED stay as long as 12 hours. Currently, in the Canadian health care system, as many as 75% of older patients stay in the ED longer than 12 hours prior to admission to the ward.[29]

Inouye and coworkers subsequently developed a multicomponent intervention known as the hospital elder life program (HELP) to prevent delirium.[126] The HELP program uses volunteers to assist the clinical staff in promoting ambulation, adequate hydration, and nutrition, having meaningful orienting conversations with patients, and avoiding psychoactive medications and use of physical restraints; it was shown to reduce delirium by 50%.[65] Although this program has been successfully implemented in over 50 countries, ensuring that patients receive the interventions at least 75% of the time were found to be important predictors of the success of the intervention.[126,127]

The HELP program was subsequently modified for use in the ED at Sunnybrook Health Science Center. Volunteers and ED staff received training on the importance of mobility, hydration, and nutrition, starting conversations, medication use, and avoidance of physical restraints.[128] The use of Foley catheters was discouraged; this was described as an effective single-point restraint system because they reduce mobility and increase urinary tract infections.

To stress the importance of having all team members committed to prevention, the program was called the interprofessional prevention of delirium (IPPOD) program; it involved paramedics, security guards, orderlies, and clerical staff in addition to those in the traditional health care professions. Once staff members were comfortable with the IPPOD protocol, a pamphlet describing the risk factors and signs of delirium was created for patients and families. The pamphlet also led to accountability for the ED staff because it stressed the importance of implementing the IPPOD interventions to reduce delirium (e.g., adequate hydration and mobilization at least every 8 hours).

CONCLUSIONS

The care of older adults during crises currently presents special challenges to paramedic and emergency personnel, as well as patients, families, and caregivers, and these challenges are likely to increase over the next 2 decades. Understanding these challenges will be important for future research and the design and implementation of potential solutions.

We have also catalogued a large number of novel and innovative approaches for improving the care of older ED patients. Although many of these have not been evaluated, they provide a substantial tool chest for those interested in improving the care of older patients in the future. Clearly, older adults who need emergency care will benefit if emergency personnel have a better understanding of geriatric medicine and if geriatricians have a better understanding of emergency services.

KEY POINTS

- Because paramedic and emergency personnel provide care for older adults for longer and longer periods, efforts to optimize this care are needed.
- Prehospital care and emergency rooms are misleading terms because they fail to describe the full range of services provided by paramedics and emergency staff.
- Community paramedicine is an important evolving concept whereby the role or scope of paramedic practice is expanded in the community, often including proactive care or referrals to improve care and prevention of avoidable transport to the hospital.
- Determining whether a frail older patient's symptoms are the effects of multiple chronic comorbidities or an acute medical condition is challenging. Systems to ensure the communication of baseline function during emergency health crises are thus critical.
- Innovations are being implemented to improve the care of older people by paramedics and emergency personnel. Evaluations of these interventions are needed.

For a complete list of references, please visit www.expertconsult.com.

KEY REFERENCES

1. International Roundtable on Community Paramedicine: 12th Annual International Roundtable on Community Paramedicine. http://ircp.info. Accessed May 4, 2015.
5. Goldstein J, Jensen J, Carter AJ, et al: The epidemiology of prehospital emergency responses for older adults in a provincial EMS. CJEM 17:491–496, 2015.
10. Aminzadeh F, Dalziel WB: Older adults in the emergency department: a systematic review of patterns of use, adverse outcomes, and effectiveness of interventions. Ann Emerg Med 39:238–247, 2002.
14. Lowthian JA, Jolley DJ, Curtis AJ, et al: The challenges of population ageing: accelerating demand for emergency ambulance services by older patients, 1995-2015. Med J Aust 194:574–578, 2011.
16. Andrew MK, Rockwood K: Making our health and care systems fit for an ageing population: considerations for Canada. Can Geriatr J 17:133–135, 2014.
17. Goldstein J, Hubbard RE, Moorhouse P, et al: The validation of a care partner-derived frailty index based upon comprehensive geriatric assessment (CP-FI-CGA) in emergency medical services and geriatric ambulatory care. Age Ageing 44:327–330, 2015.
20. Rockwood K, Song X, MacKnight C, et al: A global clinical measure of fitness and frailty in elderly people. CMAJ 173:489–495, 2005.
27. Wallis SJ, Wall J, Biram RW, et al: Association of the clinical frailty scale with hospital outcomes. QJM 108:943–949, 2015.
29. Mion LC, Palmer RM, Meldon SW, et al: Case finding and referral model for emergency department elders: a randomized clinical trial. Ann Emerg Med 41:57–68, 2003.
31. Eastwood K, Morgans A, Smith K, et al: Secondary triage in prehospital emergency ambulance services: a systematic review. Emerg Med J 32:486–492, 2015.
34. Bigham BL, Kennedy SM, Drennan I, et al: Expanding paramedic scope of practice in the community: a systematic review of the literature. Prehosp Emerg Care 17:361–372, 2013.
35. Lee JS, Verbeek PR, Schull MJS, et al: Paramedics assessing elders at risk for independence loss (PERIL): derivation, reliability and comparative effectiveness of a clinical prediction rule. Can J Emerg Med 2016. (In Press).
36. Shah MN, Brooke Lerner E, et al: An evaluation of paramedics' ability to screen older adults during emergency responses. Prehosp Emerg Care 8:298–303, 2004.
42. Mason S, Knowles E, Colwell B, et al: Effectiveness of paramedic practitioners in attending 999 calls from elderly people in the community: cluster randomised controlled trial. BMJ 335:919, 2007.
51. Mason S, Knowles E, Freeman J, et al: Safety of paramedics with extended skills. Acad Emerg Med 15:607–612, 2008.
54. Viccellio A, Santora C, Singer AJ, et al: The association between transfer of emergency department boarders to inpatient hallways and mortality: a 4-year experience. Ann Emerg Med 54:487–491, 2009.
55. Khare RK, Powell ES, Reinhardt G, et al: Adding more beds to the emergency department or reducing admitted patient boarding times: which has a more significant influence on emergency department congestion? Ann Emerg Med 53:575–585, 2009.
68. Ackroyd-Stolarz S, Read Guernsey J, Mackinnon NJ, et al: The association between a prolonged stay in the emergency department and adverse events in older patients admitted to hospital: a retrospective cohort study. BMJ Qual Saf 20:564–569, 2011.
85. Lee JS, Schwindt G, Langevin M, et al: Validation of the triage risk stratification tool to identify older persons at risk for hospital admission and returning to the emergency department. J Am Geriatr Soc 56:2112–2117, 2008.
90. Meldon SW, Mion LC, Palmer RM, et al: Does a simple emergency department (ED) screening tool correlate with functional impairments among older adults? Acad Emerg Med 11:448, 2004.
93. McCusker J, Bellavance F, Cardin S, et al: Prediction of hospital utilization among elderly patients during the 6 months after an emergency department visit. Ann Emerg Med 36:438–445, 2000.
98. Carpenter CR, Shelton E, Fowler S, et al: Risk factors and screening instruments to predict adverse outcomes for undifferentiated older emergency department patients: a systematic review and meta-analysis. Acad Emerg Med 22:1–21, 2015.
102. Hustey FM, Meldon SW, Smith MD, et al: The effect of mental status screening on the care of elderly emergency department patients. Ann Emerg Med 41:678–684, 2003.
105. Carpenter CR, Bassett ER, Fischer GM, et al: Four sensitive screening tools to detect cognitive dysfunction in geriatric emergency department patients: brief Alzheimer's Screen, Short Blessed Test, Ottawa 3DY, and the caregiver-completed AD8. Acad Emerg Med 18:374–384, 2011.
117. Flynn D, Jennings J, Moghabghab R, et al: Raising the bar of care for older people in Ontario emergency departments. Int J Older People Nurs 5:219–226, 2009.
118. Ryan D, Splinter Flynn D, Wilding L: An overview of geriatric emergency management nursing practices in Ontario. J Emerg Nurs 2015.
119. Hwang U, Morrison RS: The geriatric emergency department. J Am Geriatr Soc 55:1873–1876, 2007.
124. Inouye SK, Charpentier PA: Precipitating factors for delirium in hospitalized elderly persons. Predictive model and interrelationship with baseline vulnerability. JAMA 275:852–857, 1996.

118 Acute Hospital Care for Frail Older Adults

Simon Conroy

INTRODUCTION

Hospitalization of an older adult can be a sentinel event that heralds an intensive period of health and social care service use.[1-3] This is especially the case for frail older adults—here referring to people with multiple comorbidities, polypharmacy, often cognitive impairment (delirium and/or dementia)—many of whom present nonspecifically. Such patients are not always well served by the increasingly specialized, protocol-driven care provided in acute hospitals, but can benefit more from a more nuanced and holistic approach to their care.

The literature on acute care of (frail) older adults points toward comprehensive geriatric assessment (CGA) being more effective than usual care.[4-6] This chapter will offer examples of why CGA might work in the acute care context, critique the evidence base, and finally describe a systems-based approach to the care of frail older adults in acute hospitals.

Why Comprehensive Geriatric Assessment Works in Acute Care

CGA is defined as "a multidimensional, interdisciplinary diagnostic process to determine the medical, psychological, and functional capabilities of an older person in order to develop a coordinated and integrated plan for treatment and long-term follow-up."[7] Why this is important will be addressed in this section.

Multidimensional Process

This highlights the importance of taking a holistic overview. In this cohort of patients, it is not sufficient to focus simply on one domain. For example, an approach to chest pain that simply states that the troponin level is negative and a coronary angiogram is not required, but fails to test for and identify the cognitive impairment that led to the individual not taking analgesia for arthritis (the true cause of the pain), is doomed to fail. Also, a purely functional approach to falls that seeks to provide only rehabilitation and not identify the underlying reasons for a fall, of which there are many, including serious disorders such as aortic stenosis, will not succeed. It is the integrated assessment of all the domains of the CGA that allows an accurate problem list to be generated.

Interdisciplinary Diagnostic Process

In a mature CGA service, the hierarchy should be flattened so that all staff members should feel empowered to put forward a constructive challenge within and without their particular area of expertise. For example, the option to admit for rehabilitation by a therapist concerned about falls at home might be challenged by pointing out that admission often increases the risk of falls and that home-based rehabilitation may offer substantial benefits.[8] Equally, therapists will bring useful information to the diagnostic process; for example, the patient who is fit to return home but develops new dyspnea on mobilization might prompt a reevaluation of respiratory function and identify potentially new diagnoses, such as pulmonary embolus. That this assessment is a process and not a discrete event is also key; the process should continue in an iterative manner over the course of the acute stay, and the diagnostic elements should be sensitive to deviations from the anticipated pathway. For example, if the initial treatment plan for an older adult with a fall and hip pain but no fracture was to "increase analgesia, reduce antihypertensives, and aim to return home once able to walk 5 m unaided using a frame," yet after 14 hours, pain remains a problem, the diagnosis may need to be revisited and further imaging considered.

Coordinated and Integrated Plan for Treatment

This reinforces the idea that the team caring for an older adult needs to know and respect each other's roles and know and understand what each is doing, and understand how medical treatment will affect the rehabilitation goals, and vice versa. For example, although therapists would not need to know the detailed intricacies of the management of acute heart failure, it is important that they know that intravenous diuretics might be required for the first few days and result in polyuria and then be able to incorporate continence needs into the rehabilitation plan. Similarly, physicians will need to appreciate that just because a patient has grade 5 power on the Medical Research Council (MRC) grading system, this does not necessarily translate into useful functional ability.

Follow-Up

Because many older adults have multiple long-term conditions, they usually require some form of ongoing care and support. How this is delivered will vary among regions worldwide, but there is little point in providing excellent acute care if conditions are only going to be allowed to decline because of a lack of ongoing support. For example, a 2-week admission, during which Parkinson disease medications are carefully titrated and optimized in conjunction with the multidisciplinary rehabilitation process, can easily be reversed if there is no ongoing titration of L-dopa once the patient returns home. So, while integrating the standard medical diagnostic evaluation, CGA emphasizes problem solving, teamwork, and a patient-centered approach.

How Should Comprehensive Geriatric Assessment be Delivered in Acute Care?

What Does the Evidence Suggest?

Multiple systematic reviews have suggested that discrete units or wards are more effective than a dispersed or liaison-type service; the most recent reviews on liaison services offering CGA suggest limited or no effect in acute care.[9,10] However, the trials used in the Ellis meta-analysis that led to this conclusion are somewhat dated, with the most recent being reported in 2007. In the more recent review on liaison services, Deschodt and colleagues[10] reported on studies up until 2012 in a range of settings, but also found limited evidence of benefit from liaison services. The perceived wisdom is that liaison services are thought to be less effective because there is less control over the care that patients receive.[11] This has been supported by process evaluations that indicate that only about two thirds of all recommendations are implemented.[12] It is equally possible that usual care is improving, reducing the absolute benefit from CGA, and it is noteworthy that the United Kingdom's Future Hospitals Commission has emphasized generic care over geriatric care.[13]

This raises some important issues. Do you need a geriatrician to deliver CGA or just the geriatric competencies applied well? The only logical answer is that it is the application of the competencies that is key, not who applies them. As Coni noted, "Geriatrics is too important to be left to geriatricians. We are all geriatricians now, and geriatric medicine should be like a caretaker government-self-appointed to instruct others how to do it, and then to preside over its own demise."[14] However, at the heart of this, is the difference between knowing and doing. Most physicians are taught the principles of geriatric medicine,[15] but not all practice them. This has been suggested in more recent service developments, in which geriatric medicine is incorporated into the care of frail older adults in new settings.[16-18] Surely, if usual care were so good at providing geriatric competencies, wouldn't such service developments show limited benefit?

Establishing Integrated Pathways

Vertical Integration. Where resources permit, it seems sensible that conventional CGA services focus their efforts on frail older adults. This would mean streaming patients into dedicated services and ensuring that they are vertically integrated, which requires simple, clear, and locally acceptable criteria for defining frail older adults. Ideally, these criteria can be applied quickly in the emergency department or acute medical unit so that patient streaming can occur as soon as possible. It also requires CGA to be delivered at each stage of the patient journey—including the emergency department, acute medical unit, base ward, and rehabilitation setting—with the opportunity to transfer into community services at each point, where CGA should also be available (Figure 118-1).

Given that discrete geriatric units or wards will not be able to cater to the needs of all frail older adults in the acute care context, alternative approaches are required. Liaison services are generally considered to be ineffective, as noted earlier, so how can the principles of CGA be best applied in nongeriatric ward settings? This will include diverse areas such as surgery, oncology, and other areas of specialized medicine, such as cardiology, for whom geriatric medicine has not traditionally been a strong component of training. Clearly, the longer term solution is to ensure that all clinicians are competent in the delivery of basic CGA in the same way that all clinicians should be competent in managing common cardiologic or respiratory or other common conditions. In the United Kingdom, at least, this is slowly becoming a reality, with more recent undergraduate and postgraduate curricula starting to contain CGA principles. However, the long-term goal of generalizing geriatrics is some way off.

In the meantime, the preferred model appears to be developing liaison-plus services, learning from the hip fracture journey over recent years. Initially, hip fracture care models involved geriatric medicine support to orthopedic surgeons but, over the years, the preferred model of care has emerged as geriatric medicine embedded within the orthopedic team, offering pre- and postoperative care.[19] In some cases, geriatricians have taken on the entire unit and reversed the roles, so that the orthopedic team provides liaison and surgical input only, leaving the holistic medical care to geriatricians. This might be achievable in the short term but, given the aging demographic, unless there is a radical change in the number of geriatricians and other gerontologic clinicians being trained, it is clearly not sustainable. Moreover, so-called geriatric takeover of the hospital does not really help in countries where geriatric medicine is less well developed.

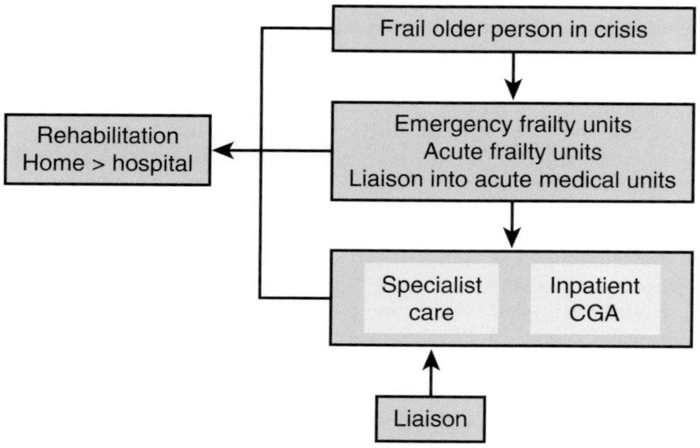

Figure 118-1. Examples of integrated acute care pathways.

PRACTICAL ISSUES FOR FRAIL OLDER ADULTS IN ACUTE CARE

Thinking about what can be done now is pertinent, given the complexity of issues related to the care of frail older adults. It is not possible to provide a complete approach here, but some useful principles can be outlined. More details on individual issues are covered in other chapters in this text.

Use the urgent care scenario as a trigger to offer a holistic assessment and address any potential unmet needs. Not all of these will need to be addressed in the acute care setting but, once identified, they can be flagged for those in charge of ongoing care. A holistic assessment should cover the following domains:

- Pain
- Cognition
- Depression
- Nutrition and hydration
- Skin integrity
- Sensory loss
- Falls and mobility
- Activities of daily living
- Continence
- Vital signs
- Safeguarding issues
- End-of-life care issues

Also, the presence of frailty syndromes should be specifically assessed (Box 118-1).[20-23]

For a more comprehensive review of approaches to caring for frail older adult with urgent care needs, see the Silver Book (http://www.bgs.org.uk/campaigns/silverb/silver_book_complete.pdf).

CLOSING THOUGHTS

Research is under way to explore if there are alternative approaches to caring for frail older adults. Meanwhile, the practical and evidence-based approach is to focus the flow of frail older adults through core CGA wards and services that can influence immediate decision making and provide support in the form of education, training, leadership, and role modeling to other areas. Importantly, the reader should be reminded that what happens during acute hospital care, although important and potentially hugely influential on future events, it is but a small part of an overall journey. Strong links with community services and primary care are required pre- and postadmission to optimize outcomes for frail older adults with urgent care needs.

BOX 118-1 Frailty Syndromes: A 30-Second Guide

Older adults tend to present to clinicians with nonspecific presentations or frailty syndromes, in contrast to the typical presentation seen in younger people. The reasons for nonspecific presentations include the presence of multiple comorbidities, disability, and communication barriers. The ability to recognize and interpret nonspecific syndromes is key because they are markers of poor outcomes.

FALLS

Distinguish between syncopal factors (e.g., cardiac, polypharmacy) and nonsyncopal factors (e.g., strength, balance, vision, proprioception, vestibular and environmental hazards), which all should be assessed.

IMMOBILITY

"Off-legs" can mask many diagnoses, ranging from cord compression to end-stage dementia. A comprehensive assessment is needed to focus on the urgent and important issues to be addressed.

DELIRIUM AND DEMENTIA

These are closely interrelated, but each requires clinically distinct management. A collateral history is key for detecting a recent change in cognition; it is common for delirium to be superimposed on preexisting dementia. Delirium can be hyperactive, hypoactive, or mixed.

POLYPHARMACY

Adverse drug events lead to increased hospital stay, morbidity, and mortality.[20] Consider a medication review focusing on identifying inappropriate prescribing as well as drug omissions (e.g., STOPP/START[21]). Consider also medicine reconciliation.

INCONTINENCE

This is an unusual acute presentation, but is a marker of frailty and a risk factor for adverse outcomes. More common is abuse of urine dipstick testing leading to erroneous diagnosis of infection, inappropriate antibiotics, and increased risk of complications, such as clostridial diarrhea.

END-OF-LIFE CARE

Mortality rates for frail older adults in the year following discharge from hospital are high (25% in one series[3]), which suggests that for some patients, it is reasonable to consider advance care planning.[22]

KEY POINTS

- Hospitalization of an older adult can be a sentinel event that heralds an intensive period of health and social care service use.
- Comprehensive geriatric assessment (CGA) is more effective than usual care, and ward-based CGA services are more effective than liaison services.
- Disjointed service provision is problematic, so integration within and without the hospital (e.g., with community or social care providers) to create an integrated care pathway is critical.
- Embedding CGA competencies in all services likely to manage frail older adults is key.
- Further work is required to determine optimal models of care for these patients outside of conventional geriatric ward settings
- The presence of one or more frailty syndromes should trigger a detailed CGA in the community, person's own home, or outpatient clinic, or as an inpatient, according to individual needs.
- Do not delay, defer, or delegate the collateral history. A 10-minute conversation with a caregiver can rapidly reveal the diagnosis and direct ongoing management.
- Ensure that clinicians can readily distinguish delirium from dementia and that aids to communication are readily available (e.g., hearing aid batteries, visual aids).
- Pain can be difficult to assess in older adults who have communication barriers; consider using a structured pain scale.[23]
- Multidisciplinary assessments will take time, but this is time well spent early on in the admission—for example, facilitating early discharge. Make provisions for multidisciplinary assessments so that they are expected, planned, and orderly.
- Do not assume that hospitals are safe places for older adults; consider carefully what needs to be done in the hospital and what might better be achieved in the community setting.

KEY REFERENCES

1. Krumholz HM: Post-hospital syndrome—an acquired, transient condition of generalized risk. N Engl J Med 368:100–102, 2013.
2. Sager MA, Franke T, Inouye SK, et al: Functional outcomes of acute medical illness and hospitalization in older persons. Arch Intern Med 156:645–652, 1996.
3. Woodard J, Gladman J, Conroy S: Frail older people at the interface. Age Ageing 39(Suppl 1):i36, 2010.
4. Ellis G, Whitehead M, O'Neill D, et al: Comprehensive geriatric assessment for older adults admitted to hospital. Cochrane Database Syst Rev (7):CD006211, 2011.
5. Fox MT, Persaud M, Maimets I, et al: Effectiveness of acute geriatric unit care using acute care for elders components: a systematic review and meta-analysis. J Am Geriatr Soc 60:2237–2245, 2012.
6. Baztan JJ, Suarez-Garcia FM, Lopez-Arrieta J, et al: Effectiveness of acute geriatric units on functional decline, living at home, and case fatality among older patients admitted to hospital for acute medical disorders: meta-analysis. BMJ 338:b50, 2009.
7. Rubenstein LZ, Rubenstein LV: Multidimensional assessment of elderly patients. Adv Intern Med 36:81–108, 1991.
8. Shepperd S, Doll H, Broad J, et al: Early discharge hospital at home. Cochrane Database Syst Rev (1):CD000356, 2009.
9. Bakker FC, Robben SHM, Olde Rikkert MGM: Effects of hospital-wide interventions to improve care for frail older inpatients: a systematic review. BMJ Qual Saf 20:680–691, 2011.
10. Deschodt M, Flamaing J, Haentjens P, et al: Impact of geriatric consultation teams on clinical outcome in acute hospitals: a systematic review and meta-analysis. BMC Med 11:48, 2013.
11. Allen CM, Becker PM, McVey LJ, et al: A randomized, controlled clinical trial of a geriatric consultation team. Compliance with recommendations. JAMA 255:2617–2621, 1986.
12. Deschodt M, Braes T, Broos P, et al: Effect of an inpatient geriatric consultation team on functional outcome, mortality, institutionalization, and readmission rate in older adults with hip fracture: a controlled trial. J Am Geriatr Soc 59:1299–1308, 2011.
13. Royal College of Physicians. Future hospital: caring for medical patients. http://www. nhsconfed.org/~/media/Confederation/Files/public%20access/Dalton%20review%20roundtable_RCP%20presentation_110714.pdf. Accessed December 15, 2015.
14. Coni N: The unlikely geriatricians. J R Soc Med 89:587–589, 1996.

15. Gordon AL, Blundell A, Dhesi JK, et al: UK medical teaching about ageing is improving but there is still work to be done: the Second National Survey of Undergraduate Teaching in Ageing and Geriatric Medicine. Age Ageing 43:293–297, 2014.
16. Conroy SP, Ansari K, Williams M, et al: A controlled evaluation of comprehensive geriatric assessment in the emergency department: the 'Emergency Frailty Unit.' Age Ageing 43:109–114, 2014.
17. Harari D, Hopper A, Dhesi J, et al: Proactive care of older people undergoing surgery ('POPS'): Designing, embedding, evaluating and funding a comprehensive geriatric assessment service for older elective surgical patients. Age Ageing 36:190–196, 2007.
18. Ellis D, Spiers M, Coutts S, et al: Preoperative assessment in the elderly: evaluation of a new clinical service. Scott Med J 57:212–216, 2012.
19. Darowski A: The care of patients with fragility fracture, London, 2007, British Orthopaedic Association.
20. Mannesse CK, Derkx FH, de Ridder MA, et al: Contribution of adverse drug reactions to hospital admission of older patients. Age Ageing 29:35–39, 2000.
21. Gallagher P, Baeyens J-P, Topinkova E, et al: Inter-rater reliability of STOPP (Screening Tool of Older Persons' Prescriptions) and START (Screening Tool to Alert doctors to Right Treatment) criteria amongst physicians in six European countries. Age Ageing 38:603–606, 2009.
22. Conroy S, Fade P, Fraser A, et al: Advance care planning: concise evidence-based guidelines. Clin Med (Lond) 9:76–79, 2009.
23. Royal College of Physicians: Pain: assessment of pain in older people, London, 2007, Royal College of Physicians.

119 Intensive Care Medicine in Older Adults: A Critical Age?

Richard Pugh, Chris Thorpe, Christian Peter Subbe

INTRODUCTION

Care for the critically ill demands prompt diagnosis and early initiation of treatment to allow the best chance for patients to recover without complications. Once a patient has been assessed as at risk, the flow of care from low to high dependency should be prompt, with a response that involves both general and critical care physicians. Not all patients are necessarily suitable for all levels of therapy. Older patients may have particular needs and vulnerabilities that need to be taken into account when delivering effective and appropriate care. This chapter provides an overview of current intensive care medicine practice in the management of the critically ill and discusses areas of particular relevance to frail and older populations.

Defining Critical Care

The term *critical care medicine* is used to describe the practice of caring for the critically ill. In this context, it has been defined by the Society for Critical Care Medicine as "the multidisciplinary health care specialty that cares for patients with acute, life-threatening illness or injury."[1] Critical illness is distinguished by the failing of single or multiple organs, sequentially or simultaneously, and the extent of care needed can be separated into four levels based on this aspect (Box 119-1).[2] These levels of critical care needs have been defined so as to be independent of the location of a patient. The term *critical care unit* is used to describe the space in which level 2 and level 3 care is usually delivered and may comprise an intensive care (level 3) unit and/or a high dependency (level 2) unit. In most hospitals, level 2 and level 3 care is provided in dedicated units, but it is possible to set up advanced support outside intensive care, at least temporarily, if capacity in a unit is severely restricted. Many hospitals may also provide single organ support in dedicated wards outside of the critical care unit, for example, noninvasive ventilation to patients with an exacerbation of chronic obstructive pulmonary disease who meet very specific criteria. Provision of critical care capacity differs by a factor of 8 between western countries,[3] but direct comparison of care provided in different health care settings can be difficult.

Critically Ill Older Patients

Meeting the needs of older adult patients is an increasingly important issue for intensive care medicine. Patients aged 65 to 80 years are those most commonly represented in critical care. However, as the global population ages, increasing numbers of older patients will be referred and admitted to critical care; in some regions in the very near future it is anticipated that 1 in 4 patients in the intensive care unit (ICU) will be 80 years or older. Furthermore, expectations among clinical teams, patients, and their families are changing. The historical pessimism associated with admitting older adults to critical care appears to be less well-grounded, at least among certain patient groups, and the threshold for introducing certain levels of organ support appears to be declining. Given the disparity in critical care bed resources worldwide, some regions will feel the need to predict the likelihood of an acceptable outcome following older adult admission to intensive care particularly keenly. Furthermore, under these circumstances, the intensive care team will want to know that the patient in question is likely to benefit more than any other patient referred to, or treated in, the local ICU.

Predisposition of Older Adults to Developing Critical Illness

The detrimental effects of aging on organ systems have been described elsewhere in this textbook. These effects mean that although comorbidity is frequently present among older adult patients admitted to critical care, subclinical disease and a vulnerability of organ systems to acute illness are particularly common in older critically ill patients. The concept of frailty as a reflection of a disproportionate susceptibility to stressors[4,5] is relatively new to intensive care medicine, although the importance of physiologic age as opposed to chronologic age in determining outcome has long been appreciated. With aging, fewer people have just one active illness. In consequence, how aging challenges health care is not so much by the rising rates of cancer, stroke, heart disease, or other common age-related illnesses; instead, the key challenge is that many age-related illnesses arise in the same people. Crucially, these people have other challenges in addition to their illnesses. People with more diseases also have more deficits—"subclinical," age-related problems, such as motor slowing, or abnormal lab test results, or less initiative. These deficits add to the risk and thus it is the whole package of health deficits (and not just diseases or disabilities) that makes people frail. The combination of more damage and less efficient damage repair gives rise to frailty. These clearly interact: more deficits increase recovery time from damage and thereby give rise to additional deficits. This chapter specifically looks at the potential use of frailty measurement in anticipating outcomes in, and the needs of, critically ill older adults. Furthermore, the importance of sepsis is highlighted in this chapter, an example of a situation where older individuals may be more susceptible to an acute stress (e.g., a urinary tract infection), which may then be more likely to overwhelm homeostatic mechanisms and result in multiple system impairment (e.g., severe sepsis and multiple organ failure).[6]

PRE–INTENSIVE CARE UNIT CARE

Recognition of Critical Illness

Patients who develop critical illness vary in their clinical presentation. Some are in extremis and need immediate life-saving intervention (e.g., those in cardiac or respiratory arrest), but most follow a path of gradual deterioration. This deterioration may happen at home or in the hospital. Wider appreciation of the deteriorating patient in the community has come from campaigns to raise awareness about specific problems, such as meningococcal disease and cerebrovascular disease, but detecting the point where hospital admission is needed in those with chronic medical conditions remains a challenge.

In the hospital environment, there is the potential for close monitoring of the sick patient and use of this information to trigger escalation of care. Changes in vital signs are probably the most significant warning for impending critical illness. Extensive research into the antecedents of cardiac arrests and unscheduled critical care admissions shows that the majority of patients show abnormalities in vital signs, particularly in respiratory and mental

TABLE 119-1 Modified Early Warning Score*

	3	2	1	0	1	2	3
Systolic blood pressure (mm Hg)	<70	71-80	81-100	101-199		≥200	
Heart rate (bpm)		<40	41-50	51-100	101-110	111-129	≥130
Respiratory rate (bpm)		<9		9-14	15-20	21-29	≥30
Temperature (°C)		<35		35-38.4		≥38.5	
AVPU score				*Alert*	Reacting to *Voice*	Reacting to *Pain*	*Unresponsive*

*Scores for single parameters are added to obtain a summary score. If the summary score exceeds a predefined level, then escalation to more senior staff should be triggered. Improvements in Early Warning Scores also allow teams to track progress of a patient.

BOX 119-1 Levels of Critical Care

Level 0: Patients whose needs can be met through normal ward care in an acute hospital setting.

Level 1: Patients at risk of their condition deteriorating, or those recently relocated from higher levels of care, whose needs can be met on an acute ward with additional advice and support from the critical care team.

Level 2: Patients requiring more detailed observation or intervention, including support for a single failing organ system or postoperative care, and those "stepping down" from higher levels of care.

Level 3: Patients requiring advanced respiratory support alone or basic respiratory support, together with support of at least two organ systems. This level includes all complex patients requiring support for multiple organ failure.

From Bagshaw SM, McDermid RC: The role of frailty in outcomes from critical illness. Curr Opin Crit Care 19:496–503, 2013.

TABLE 119-2 Sample Escalation Protocol NHS Wales

Level of EWS	Minimum Monitoring: Observations	Alert	Review
0-2	q12h	If concern	
3-5	q4-6h unless otherwise stated	Nurse in charge	Check in 1 hour. Then document: Observation frequency; Need for fluid balance chart; Presence of sepsis; Plan for escalation
6-8	q1-2h	+ Doctor of patient's parent team and rapid response team	Within 30 min concern or failure to improve: SBAR senior
9+	q30min	+ Experienced doctor with intensive care skills	Within 15 min inform consultant and intensive care

EWS, Early Warning Score; *NHS*, National Health Service; *SBAR*, situation, background, assessment, recommendation.

Note of caution: Frequency of observations can be increased at your discretion. If you are concerned about a patient, please escalate regardless of the score!

function, but that the patient's care teams can take up to 72 hours before the need for escalation is realized. A lack of decisive action in the face of obvious abnormalities is described in the literature as "failure to rescue." To reduce failure-to-rescue events, a systematic assessment of bedside observations with the aid of track and trigger systems can improve reliability; this concept has been described by Smith as a "chain of prevention"[7] and by Subbe and Welch as a "chain of survival."[8] Early Warning Scores (Table 119-1) are standardized assessments of abnormalities whereby each vital sign is scored by its degree of abnormality (usually between 0 and 3) and the summary score of all parameters (the Early Warning Score) is compared with a predefined threshold to trigger an alert to the patient's primary care team or a dedicated specialist team[9-11] (Table 119-2). These teams have been named rapid response teams, medical emergency teams, or critical care outreach teams, depending on the make-up and country of residence.

Other aspects of assessment are particularly relevant for older people. A detailed past medical history will help define areas of vulnerability and organs most likely to be affected by acute illness. Hematologic and biochemical laboratory tests highlight both preexisting illness such as chronic renal or liver disease and also changing values that reflect deteriorating organ function. Electrocardiographic abnormalities are more common in older patients, and changes are highly significant in predicting poor outcomes. The side effects of medication can be magnified in acute illness, for example, the increased nephrotoxic effect of drugs in hypovolemic patients. An awareness of older adult patients' individual vulnerabilities helps facilitate earlier recognition of the need for intervention.

Deciding Whom to Admit to Intensive Care

There are two crucial questions to consider when deciding whether a patient should be admitted to a critical care unit:

1. Is the condition that drives the deterioration reversible?
2. Will the patient derive overall benefit from critical care management for an actual or potential illness?

If the patient is not at risk or the condition is not reversible, then admission to a critical care bed is unlikely to be of benefit. The Society of Critical Care Medicine states that ICUs should be reserved for patients with "reasonable prospect of substantial recovery."[12] Only in extraordinary circumstances would a patient without a reversible condition be admitted to intensive care to facilitate high intensive palliative or end-of-life care. In some cases the acute nature of deterioration requires physiologic stabilization without definitive proof of an underlying reversible cause.

The clinical assessment is the cornerstone of decision making with regard to escalation of care. Obtaining an accurate medical and social history is paramount in coming to an appropriate conclusion; however, the patient may not be able to give an accurate history, and relatives or caregivers may need to be interviewed to assimilate the information needed. For example, it may become clear that the patient has no desire for escalation of therapy or has such limitation of function that the aggressive pursuit of reversing organ failure is deemed inappropriate. Patients and relatives may not have an appropriate picture of the benefits and drawbacks of intensive care management. Although most understand that the patient may not survive, other drawbacks that may not be understood include increased risk of infections, sleep deprivation and delirium, discomfort from invasive care, and, in particular, decreased functional capacity in survivors.[13] Communication between the ward team, the critical care team, and the patient and family is essential in forming a robust plan; however, inevitably in some patients there remains a degree of uncertainty when making a decision about whether to escalate care.

Who gets admitted to critical care units varies depending on the country, hospital, and clinical team. The reasons for this variation are complex, but financial limitations and political imperatives play a role.[3] Among developed health care systems there is a large disparity in the number of critical care beds available for a given population. Germany and the United States have just under 30 ICU beds per 100,000 population, whereas the United Kingdom has approximately 4 ICU beds per 100,000.[14,15] Inevitably this will affect decision making regarding what represents unacceptable risk of catastrophic deterioration and the threshold for effecting placement in a higher level care environment.

Sepsis: Diagnosis and Initial Management

The incidence of septic shock has increased in recent years and now kills approximately 37,000 patients a year in the United Kingdom. It is likely that at least some of this increase is related to improved recognition and diagnosis of the disease.[16] Research into therapies targeting the complex systemic inflammatory response that results in organ failure has so far been disappointing. The current best management of sepsis therefore comprises early diagnosis and antibiotic administration accompanied by expert support and management of organ dysfunction. The Surviving Sepsis Campaign has increased awareness of the disease and produces updated best practice guidelines that incorporate diagnostic aids.[17] Sepsis diagnostic criteria require a combination of suspected or confirmed infection and signs of physiologic deterioration. Worsening septic illness is referred to as *severe sepsis* when acute organ dysfunction develops and *septic shock* when there is persistent hypotension despite adequate fluid resuscitation.

Once sepsis has been diagnosed, timely management is essential. Application of best practice has been helped by the introduction of ward-level care bundles that detail the elements of initial treatment needed. These care bundles provide a consistent framework for prompt treatment and can greatly shorten the time taken for new evidence to become standard practice. An example of an intervention bundle is the Sepsis Six, which comprises six elements of care to be introduced within the first hour of diagnosing sepsis (Box 119-2).

This bundle is an example of interventions that target both initial organ support and treatment of the cause. Sepsis leads to changes in peripheral blood flow through changes in arterial and venous vascular tone, leakage of volume into the extracellular space through changes in permeability of the endothelial basement membrane, and changes in myocardial contractility. The resuscitation elements in the bundle are therefore aimed at maintaining oxygen delivery to vulnerable cells. The treatment of the cause is through appropriate antibiotic use. Prompt treatment of sepsis with antibiotics is crucial. Delay in administering antibiotics worsens mortality from 24.6% if given within the first hour to 33.1% if given after 6 hours.[19]

Sepsis is most common at extremes of age, and 50% of cases of severe sepsis occur in those aged older than 65 years.[6] Unfortunately, mortality associated with severe sepsis also increases with age; this probably reflects the loss of resilience and disproportionate susceptibility to organ dysfunction that may occur with aging. This clearly underlines the importance of recognizing sepsis in older adult patients promptly and to intervene early to avoid decline into multiple organ failure.

BOX 119-2 The "Sepsis Six"*

1. Administer high-flow oxygen.
2. Take blood cultures and consider infective source.
3. Administer intravenous antibiotics.
4. Give intravenous fluid resuscitation.
5. Check hemoglobin and serial lactates.
6. Commence hourly urine output measurements.

Modified from Daniels R, Nutbeam T, McNamara G, Galvin C: The sepsis six and the severe sepsis resuscitation bundle: a prospective observational cohort study. Emerg Med J 28:507–512, 2011.

*To be applied within the first hour.

Care in the Intensive Care Unit

Organizational factors within the ICU are thought to be an important determinant of outcome, although observational studies have provided conflicting evidence on the best way to deliver intensive care. Aspects that could improve outcome within ICUs include high patient volume, round-the-clock intensivist cover, and a closed rather than open model of intensive care cover. In a comparison of hospitals in the United States, hospitals with a higher volume of patients requiring mechanical ventilation had better risk-adjusted mortality, with those ICUs ventilating more than 400 patients/year having better survival figures than those ventilating fewer than 150 patients/year.[20] Intensivist cover has been shown to improve outcome; high-level daytime presence of an intensivist seems to reduce both risk-adjusted mortality and length of stay, although resident night-time intensivist cover does not convincingly add value.[21,22] A recent international observational study of organizational differences suggested that outcomes can be improved with nurse-to-patient ratios of higher than 1 : 1.5.[23] Furthermore, multidisciplinary ward rounds appear to improve patient outcomes, increase team member satisfaction, and reduce costs.[24] There are many confounding factors when comparing outcomes from different ICUs, however, and caution must be used when interpreting observational results across units, hospitals, or health care systems. In particular, it must be remembered that critical care medicine is a rapidly changing specialty and historical data can be misleading.

Organ Support in Critical Illness

The treatment of critically ill patients demands a fine balance between proactive measures and supportive care. Over the past 20 years, evidence has slowly accumulated that many aggressive treatments thought to improve the chances of survival are not effective and may even worsen outcome. For example, altering elements of the host response to sepsis has been a target for improving survival, but this physiologic response is a complex, incompletely understood process. The main targets for intervention have been the balance between proinflammatory and antiinflammatory processes, and although individual elements of this process can be targeted, the domino effects of this intervention are often unpredictable. To date, research has failed to find a "magic bullet." Other examples include the aggressive approach to improve cardiac output, which has been hampered by subsequent research casting doubt on the benefit of this goal-directed approach, and the realization that treating anemia with blood transfusions is not necessarily helpful in the critically ill population.

Where modern intensive care medicine has proved invaluable is in delivery of supportive care to patients with organ failure. The delivery of critical care has benefitted from a worldwide push to produce clear guidance on the minimum standards required to provide an effective safe service. Guidance on both structural and personnel requirements is available from a number of sources, for example, the Intensive Care Society and the Faculty of Intensive Care Medicine in the United Kingdom. In addition to providing guidance on setting up a safe environment for critically ill patients, the introduction of ICU care bundles into practice has helped to ensure that the best available evidence is incorporated into routine care (e.g., prophylaxis against deep vein thrombosis and stress ulcers). These packages of protocolized care help to accelerate incorporation of published evidence into everyday practice and have been widely adopted by many hospitals, with encouraging results.[25]

Once admitted to the ICU, patients frequently require support for several organs. The following paragraphs discuss support for respiratory, circulatory, and renal failure in the critically ill.

Respiratory Failure

Patients admitted to intensive care with respiratory failure frequently need intubation and ventilation, which is a life-saving therapy. However, intermittent positive pressure mechanical ventilation (IPPV) is not a physiologic process, and it reverses the usual negative pressure drive of lung expansion. Long-term outcome improves if the pathophysiologic effects of IPPV are kept to a minimum.

Two of the main determinants of this ventilator-induced injury are thought to be excessive tidal volumes, which cause volutrauma by damaging the alveoli, and a lack of positive end-expiratory pressure, which allows repeated shearing forces to damage the surfactant-depleted alveolar walls.[26,27] There is a balance between limiting the damage done to the lungs by the physical act of repeated inflation and maintaining a permissible level of abnormal gas exchange. Hypercapnia and a degree of hypoxia are therefore often tolerated in respiratory failure to allow low tidal volumes, and studies have shown improved outcomes in patients with tidal volumes of 6 mL/kg despite worse gas exchange in the first days of IPPV.[26]

Intubation and ventilation increase the risk of infection, and immobility as a result of sedation worsens neuromuscular function. Patients are therefore weaned as soon as possible from IPPV, and other methods of respiratory support (e.g., continuous positive airway pressure and noninvasive ventilation) are used to minimize the need for invasive ventilation. When weaning is prolonged, a tracheostomy may be performed to increase patient comfort and reduce the need for sedation. This procedure is in common use, and although helpful in managing slow-to-wean patients, it has not been shown to improve survival. Unfortunately, among the very old, a prolonged period of ventilation is associated with a very low probability of recovering sufficiently to achieve discharge home.[28]

Circulatory Failure and Shock

Shock can be defined as inadequate delivery of oxygen to the cells as a result of circulatory failure. Shock manifests as low blood pressure and signs of reduced tissue perfusion such as oliguria, impaired consciousness, poor skin perfusion, and elevated lactate. The six major causes of shock are cardiogenic, septic, hypovolemic, anaphylactic, neurogenic, and obstructive. Support of the patient with circulatory failure requires an appropriate diagnosis. The two main treatment options are fluids and inotropes/vasopressors, but the balance of use will depend on the diagnosis and response.

A trial of fluid resuscitation is the first step in the treatment of a patient with shock of unknown cause. Assessment of fluid responsiveness is an important part of treatment; this can be achieved through bedside monitoring of parameters such as pulse, blood pressure, and jugular venous pressure, together with assessment of the effect on organ function, for example, improved urine output, improved conscious level, or improved skin perfusion. There is no evidence that gelatins or albumin have any advantage over crystalloids, which remain the first choice for a fluid challenge. An initial volume of 300 to 500 mL is reasonable, and this can be repeated if there is a positive response. Another way to assess fluid responsiveness is to raise the patient's legs.[29] This increases venous return, and if the blood pressure rises as a result, it suggests that fluid resuscitation will be of benefit. Observing the transient rise is better achieved with invasive monitoring, however.

Fluid resuscitation may not be enough to treat the shocked patient alone, and the use of inotropes and vasopressors to support blood pressure may be required. In general, vasopressors are used for vasodilatory shock, such as septic shock, and noradrenaline is the first choice. Inotropes such as dobutamine are preferred when treating cardiogenic shock. Adrenaline is a useful drug in resuscitation, particularly when the cause of shock is unknown. The choice of vasoactive drug beyond this division is dependent on the preference of the clinician, as there is limited evidence that demonstrates superiority of one drug over another. Dopamine causes an increase in dysrhythmias compared with noradrenaline (24.1% vs. 12.4%).[30] Vasopressin may have some benefit as a noradrenaline-sparing agent,[31] but there has been no clear evidence supporting one drug over another, and often drugs are titrated against response using invasive monitoring as a guide.

Several invasive monitoring techniques are employed on the ICU. Examples include arterial and central venous lines, cardiac output monitoring, and echocardiography. These techniques are widely used and are helpful in providing a standardized approach to guide treatment, but they have not been shown to improve survival.[32]

Renal Failure

Among the many causes of renal failure, the most common cause of acute renal failure in the critically ill is acute tubular necrosis resulting from ischemic injury. The importance of this is that acute tubular necrosis is recoverable, and support with renal replacement therapy can allow the time for the kidneys to recover function. Early diagnosis and resuscitation of the sick patient can limit the development of acute kidney injury. A target mean arterial blood pressure of greater than 65 mm Hg is an acceptable initial goal to prevent initial insult to the kidney and to prevent worsening of function in established acute kidney injury.[30] The use of diuretics can aid fluid management but does not improve the renal recovery profile.[33] It is very important not to use nephrotoxic drugs such as nonsteroidal antiinflammatory drugs in vulnerable patients with deteriorating renal function.

Illness Severity Scores

Critical care units use a number of scoring systems that facilitate case-mix adjustment for purposes of benchmarking and comparison of clinical outcomes. Examples of these systems are APACHE II,[34] SAPS,[35] SOFA,[36] and MDM.[37] Although these scores usually combine vital signs, laboratory parameters, and features of the acute and chronic illnesses of a patient, it is worth noting that they are unsuitable for prognostication of individual patients and are not usually helpful in deciding whether a patient might benefit from admission to critical care or initiation of a particular therapy.

Critical Care Support in Older Adults

Historically, the oldest critically ill patients have received a lower intensity of therapy than the younger, particularly with respect to initiation of mechanical ventilation and renal replacement therapy.[38] Recent reports suggest that such a difference still exists,[39] although it appears that ICU clinicians' threshold for introducing therapy (e.g., vasopressors and/or renal replacement therapy) is decreasing.[40] This may perhaps help explain the decrease in risk-adjusted mortality that has been observed in some centers among the very old.[41]

OUTCOME FROM CRITICAL ILLNESS

Unfortunately age remains an independent predictor of poor short-term and long-term outcomes following critical illness, and the impact of age and age-related processes inevitably will influence expectations with regard to the appropriateness of ICU admission and initiation of organ support. Given this, there is clearly variation in resilience to acute stress among cohorts of older patients, and the mortality difference between those admitted to intensive care and those declined appears to be greatest among the oldest critical care referrals.[42]

Mortality

Mortality increases with age following development of critical illness. In patients followed up for 3 years after ICU discharge, cumulative mortality was worse in those aged 65 or older (57%) compared with those younger than 65 years (40%).[43] Among those that survive ICU, the majority of deaths in those older than 65 years occur within the first month of discharge.[43] With advancing age, short- and long-term mortality figures worsen. Approximately half of those aged 80 years and older admitted to ICU do not survive to hospital discharge, and at 12 months mortality among unselected patients older than 80 years rises to 70% and at 24 months to 80%.[44,45] Strikingly, among very old patients (aged older than 85 years), use of vasopressor therapy in ICU is associated with 97% mortality at 12 months.[46]

Sustained Vulnerability

A significant proportion of patients die after a "successful" episode of critical care. This is a reflection of the complexity of the multiple organ failure insult, persistent physiologic instability, and the continued vulnerability of a recovering patient to further stresses, particularly when premorbid frailty has been apparent. Among frail patients, recovery may be more protracted and incomplete, and a number of patients will be referred to intensive care for a second or further episode of treatment (Figure 119-1).

Readmission may be linked to premature discharge from critical care in a proportion of patients. The latter can be caused by clinical misjudgment or a response to scarcity of intensive care beds. The risk of readmission can be reduced, in part, by critical care outreach teams who improve the continuity of care on transition between ICU and general ward teams.[48] Follow-up intervention after hospital discharge probably has less effect on long-term recovery.[49,50]

Readmission to intensive care is associated with reduced chances of surviving a hospital stay[51] and returning to a premorbid status. The discharge from intensive care and hand-over to a general ward would therefore seem an eminently suitable time to review with patients and their relatives the possible outcomes of their illness and to agree on the type of issues that require extra attention, including a discussion about the type of treatments or outcomes that might not be seen as achievable or desirable.

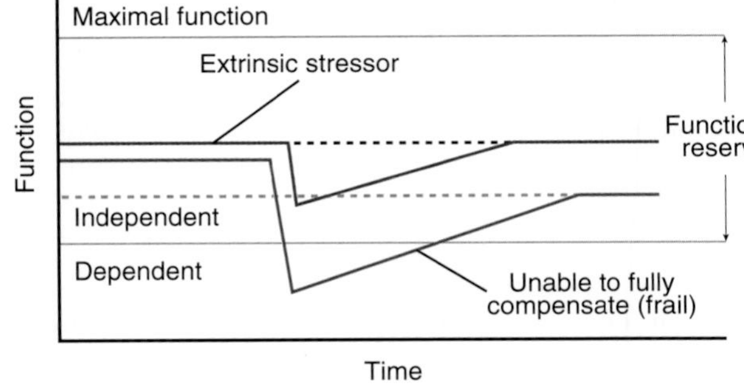

Figure 119-1. The relationship between frail state and recovery from extrinsic stress. *(Modified from Bagshaw SM, McDermid RC: The role of frailty in outcomes from critical illness. Curr Opin Crit Care 19:496–503, 2013.)*

Recovery from Critical Illness

Many patients will leave intensive care profoundly weakened and with sensory and mental health problems. After protracted critical illness, long-term complications of critical care become the rule rather than the exception. The persistence of features is highly variable and the mechanisms of the illness are still not entirely clear, but a consensus conference in 2012 agreed to categorize these physical, cognitive, or psychologic impairments arising following critical illness as "post–intensive care syndrome."[52] Baldwin and colleagues suggested recently that frailty may be acquired, unmasked, or accelerated through exposure to critical illness and may be identified in the majority of ICU survivors older than 65 years approaching hospital discharge.[53]

Among older patients, the bulk of intensive care literature has used chronologic age to describe the profile of the recovering patient population. With the recent work in frailty, this might be no longer appropriate. Recovery from critical illness can take prolonged periods of time and is often associated with setbacks that require patience and perseverance from both health care teams and patients. The author's own experience and that of others would suggest that increasing frailty is particularly associated with increased length of hospital stay, indicating the need for prolonged period of recovery and rehabilitation.[54]

Intensive Care Unit–Acquired Weakness

There are a number of known risk factors for ICU-acquired weakness[55] (Box 119-3). Drugs contributing to this phenomenon (e.g., prolonged use of paralyzing agents or corticosteroids) are increasingly avoided in critical care medicine, but disease-related risk factors must be accepted. Physical inactivity is recognized as a significant risk factor, and there is some indication that early mobilization can attenuate this process and indeed promote better glycemic control.[56] In intensive care, sedation is therefore reduced at the earliest possible time, and the patient's circulation is challenged by sitting up, standing up, and walking, even while

BOX 119-3 Factors Associated With Development of ICU-Acquired Weakness

Drugs (e.g., paralyzing agents, corticosteroids, antibiotics, sedative agents)
Muscle inactivity (including prolonged ventilation)
Multiple organ failure (e.g., severe sepsis)
Suboptimal nutrition/poor substrate utilization
Electrolyte imbalance/hyperglycemia

ICU, Intensive care unit.

still on a ventilator. The process of muscle protection can involve stationary cycles that can be used in bed. These processes are important to slow pathologic muscle breakdown and psychological problems of feeling powerless while encouraging patients to take an active part in their recovery.

Posttraumatic Stress Syndrome

Posttraumatic stress syndrome is a complex syndrome that can occur in up to one third of intensive care survivors. The National Institute for Health and Care Excellence (NICE) clinical guideline 83[57] describes the syndrome as consisting of flashbacks; avoidance of people, situations, or circumstances; anxiety; depression; substance misuse; anger; and unexplained physical symptoms resulting in repeated attendance and other symptoms. These symptoms can develop with a significant delay from the triggering admission. Symptoms might be less pronounced in older adults[58] and more frequent in patients with prolonged usage of benzodiazepines, episodes of delirium in ICU, and preexisting mental health problems.[59]

Depression and Anxiety States

Depression is frequent in survivors of critical illness[60]: a quarter to a third of patients will suffer with anxiety or depression as indicated by the Hospital Anxiety and Depression Scale.[61] Anxiety and depression correlate to a degree with social security and may or may not correlate with severity of illness.[62] Depression impacts negatively on health-related quality of life[62,63] and can be assessed with simple tools.[64]

Function and Disability After Critical Illness

Critical illness can lead to profound and long-lasting effects in older adults, to the extent that many older ICU survivors may not regain their independence. Older patients who have been mechanically ventilated during hospitalization have a demonstrably higher level of disability 12 months after discharge, compared with hospitalized patients who did not require this level of support.[65] Similarly, comparing older patients who have been hospitalized because of sepsis with patients hospitalized for other reasons, there is evidence of persistent cognitive and functional disability for several years after their episode.[66] Especially when cognitive impairment is present at baseline, there appears to be a high risk of poor cognitive outcomes. Even so, the evidence for this is sparse.[67-69] The oldest-old (those 80 years and older) are especially likely to have impaired cognitive and functional status before hospital admission.[68,70] In this, the detrimental effects of sleep deprivation may play an important role.[71]

Quality of Life After Critical Illness

The experience of survivors of critical illness after they are discharged from the hospital is extremely varied; however, quality of life may be comparable to that of patients from age-matched controls: emotional well-being and social functioning often return to the expected range, although physical functioning is impaired.[72,73] Older patients appear to experience limitations differently compared with younger patients; they tolerate decline better[74] and retain better mental health following their critical illness.[43] In this context it might be worth remembering that physicians often misjudge the quality of life of their patients[75] and that proxies of patients in ICU only show moderate correlation with quality-of-life estimates of patients: "proxies tended to overestimate quality of life when patient scores were low and underestimate the quality of life when patient scores were high."[76]

Frailty Measurement as a Predictor of Outcome in Critical Illness

Studies that have explored frailty among those admitted to critical care have tended to measure outcomes in one of two situations: risk stratification of patients undergoing high-risk surgery and frailty assessment in unselected patients after the onset of critical illness. This distinction is probably important, since long-term outcomes among older patients admitted to critical care following elective procedures are generally much better than for admission after emergency surgery or medical admission.[77]

Nevertheless, major surgery can represent a significant insult and can result in physiologic phenomena that resemble acute illness with activation of inflammatory cells, cytokine cascade, and clinical features commonly observed in sepsis. Approaches to preoperative frailty measurement have been far from uniform and have included measures of fitness (e.g., gait speed), cognitive ability, and physiologic measurement (such as spirometry). However, identification of frailty in older adult patients before major surgery (particularly cardiac surgery), is associated with subsequent occurrence of delirium, adverse events, prolonged length of stay, increased mortality, and a higher likelihood of institutional discharge.[78,79]

For nonselected patients in whom frailty measurement occurs at the time of critical care admission or after admission, the range of reported frailty measurements to date has been restricted to the Canadian Study of Health and Aging Clinical Frailty Scale (CFS)[80] or assessment of frailty phenotype.[81] Applied to medical, surgical, and trauma patients aged 65 years and older in Canadian and in French critical care units, 20% to 40% patients were considered to be at least moderately frail before ICU admission depending on which measurement was used.[54,82] The CFS might be superior for the prediction of resource utilization and clinical outcomes.[83]

Identifying frailty among acutely ill older patients is of clinical significance. Frail patients admitted with an acute medical problem tend to demonstrate more abnormal physiology; conversely, patients demonstrating abnormal vital signs and/or signs of deterioration are likely to have identifiable premorbid frailty. In trauma, frailty appears to be a better predictor than age of in-hospital complications among trauma patients aged 65 years and older. Among critically ill older patients, identification of frailty is associated with increased ICU, short-term, and 12-month mortality; increased hospital length of stay; and greater disability and dependence following hospital discharge.

DECISION PROCESSES SPECIFIC TO OLDER ADULTS

Age may predispose toward development of critical illness and remains an independent poor predictor of short-term and long-term outcomes following critical care admission. Resource constraints are apparent in most modern health care settings. However, many other factors are important in determining outcome, and age should not be relied on too heavily during triage and escalation decision making. Furthermore, as the relationships between the risks and benefits of critical care support change with age, an appreciation of the spectrum of perspectives and expectations of patients and their relatives is essential.

Patient and Family Considerations

Acute illness will prevent many older patients from taking part in meaningful discussion about escalation decisions, and often older patients appear not to know of a clinical team's decision to refer to critical care. The ETHICA study sought to find preferences regarding life-sustaining intensive care interventions among older patients living in the community.[84] After viewing films of scenarios designed to portray the administration of critical care interventions to older patients, a quarter of individuals surveyed stated they would not want to undergo noninvasive ventilation, nearly one half would not want to undergo invasive ventilation, and nearly two thirds would not wish for the combination of invasive ventilation and renal replacement therapy. Unfortunately, advance directives with regard to life-sustaining interventions appear to be very uncommon among this age group.

The anticipated decline in cognitive and physical function after critical illness is an important issue raised for discussion at point of referral (or re-referral) to critical care. As mentioned earlier, several authors have found that quality of life is relatively preserved after critical illness among older adults, and when interviewed several months after hospital discharge, most indicated that they would wish to be considered for readmission to ICU if required in future.[44,85]

"Do Not Resuscitate" Decisions

Issues relating to critical care admission and escalation of organ support in frail older patients are mirrored in the decision allow or forego cardiopulmonary resuscitation (CPR). Hospital survival following in-hospital cardiopulmonary arrests has recently been reported as 18.4% in the United Kingdom[86] and 19.2% in the United States.[87] Although "successful" resuscitation is often a prelude to a significant period of critical care support, and despite these low survival figures, as a therapy, cardiopulmonary resuscitation can arguably achieve numbers-needed-to-treat that would be acceptable for most other treatments of chronically ill patients.

Among older patients, in the United Kingdom more than 40% of in-hospital cardiac arrests occur in those aged 80 years and older, after which hospital survival is approximately 11%.[86] Unfortunately, identification, before cardiac arrest occurs, of patients likely and not likely to benefit from CPR is currently poor. Evaluating a consecutive series of unselected in-hospital cardiac arrest cases in the United Kingdom, the National Confidential Enquiry into Patient Outcome and Death advisors recently suggested that "do not resuscitate" decisions should probably have been broached in 85% cardiac arrests.[88] Undoubtedly, advanced age is a negative predicator of survival after cardiac arrest,[89] and older patients at risk of cardiac arrest may have a range of personal views about the appropriateness of CPR.[90] However, this is another area in which assessment of underlying frailty could usefully inform decision making and discussions regarding appropriateness of a highly invasive therapy.

CONCLUSIONS

Older patients have a particular vulnerability to critical illness. They have an increased incidence of chronic disease and frailty, both of which worsen outcome following critical illness. Not all patients will benefit from management in a critical care environment, but age in itself is not a barrier to escalation of care. The basic principles of critical care management apply to old and young alike, focusing on prompt diagnosis and treatment of the deteriorating patient and expert management of organ support.

There are many uncertainties in treating critically ill older patients, and there is an ongoing struggle to improve long-term outcomes in survivors. Setbacks are commonplace: continual support and explanation provide the backbone to caring for patients and relatives who are frequently distressed and exhausted. It is important that health care professionals are aware of the strengths and limitations of the care available to older patients and that this information is communicated effectively from the point of deterioration through to rehabilitative care once patients are discharged and return home.

KEY POINTS

- Older adults are particularly vulnerable to critical illness.
- Chronic disease and frailty are associated with poorer outcome in critically ill patients.
- Track and trigger systems prompt timely recognition of, and response to, acute physiologic deterioration on general floors.
- Despite long-term physical and cognitive sequelae of critical illness, quality of life appears to be relatively preserved among older survivors.
- The expectations and wishes of older adults in critical care and their families are particularly important in deciding the overall benefit of initiating or continuing organ support.

For a complete list of references, please visit www.expertconsult.com.

KEY REFERENCES

5. De Vries NM, Staal JB, van Ravensberg CD, et al: Outcome instruments to measure frailty: A systematic review. Ageing Res Rev 10:104–114, 2011.
8. Subbe CP, Welch JR: Failure to rescue: using rapid response systems to improve care of the deteriorating patient in hospital. Clin Risk 19:6–11, 2013.
12. Task Force of the American College of Critical Care Medicine: Guidelines for intensive care unit admission, discharge, and triage. Crit Care Med 27:633–638, 1999.
13. Herridge M, Cameron JI: Disability after critical illness. N Engl J Med 369:1367–1369, 2013.
28. Feng Y, Amoateng-Adjepong Y, Kaufman D, et al: Age, duration of mechanical ventilation, and outcomes of patients who are critically ill. Chest 136:759–764, 2009.
38. Boumendil A, Aegerter P, Guidet B: Treatment intensity and outcome of patients aged 80 and older in intensive care units: a multicenter matched-cohort study. J Am Geriatr Soc 53:88–93, 2005.
43. Kaarlola A, Tallgren M, Pettilä V: Long-term survival, quality of life, and quality-adjusted life-years among critically ill elderly patients. Crit Care Med 34:2120–2126, 2006.
45. Roch A, Wiramus S, Pauly V, et al: Long-term outcome in medical patients aged 80 or over following admission to an intensive care unit. Crit Care 15:R36, 2011.
46. Biston P, Aldecoa C, Devriendt J, et al: Outcome of elderly patients with circulatory failure. Intensive Care Med 40:50–56, 2014.
47. Bagshaw SM, McDermid RC: The role of frailty in outcomes from critical illness. Curr Opin Crit Care 19:496–503, 2013.
52. Needham DM, Davidson J, Cohen H, et al: Improving long-term outcomes after discharge from intensive care unit. Crit Care Med 40:502–509, 2012.
53. Baldwin MR, Reid MC, Westlake AA, et al: The feasibility of measuring frailty to predict disability and mortality in older medical intensive care unit survivors. J Crit Care 29:401–408, 2014.
54. Bagshaw SM, Stelfox HT, McDermid RC, et al: Association between frailty and short- and long-term outcomes among critically ill patients: a multicentre prospective cohort study. CMAJ 186:E95–E102, 2014.
68. De Rooij SE, Abu-Hanna A, Levi M, et al: Factors that predict outcome of intensive care treatment in very elderly patients: a review. Crit Care 9:R307–R314, 2005.
69. De Rooij SEJA, Govers AC, Korevaar JC, et al: Cognitive, functional, and quality-of-life outcomes of patients aged 80 and older who survived at least 1 year after planned or unplanned surgery or medical intensive care treatment. J Am Geriatr Soc 56:816–822, 2008.
74. Rockwood K, Noseworthy TW, Gibney RT, et al: One-year outcome of elderly and young patients admitted to intensive care units. Crit Care Med 21:687–691, 1993.
79. Makary MA, Segev DL, Pronovost PJ, et al: Frailty as a predictor of surgical outcomes in older patients. J Am Coll Surg 210:901–908, 2010.
80. Rockwood K, Song X, MacKnight C, et al: A global clinical measure of fitness and frailty in elderly people. CMAJ 173:489–495, 2005.
81. Fried LP, Tangen CM, Walston J, et al: Frailty in older adults: evidence for a phenotype. J Gerontol A Biol Sci Med Sci 56:M146–M156, 2001.

82. Le Maguet P, Roquilly A, Lasocki S, et al: Prevalence and impact of frailty on mortality in elderly ICU patients: a prospective, multicenter, observational study. Intensive Care Med 40:674–682, 2014.
83. Pugh R, Subbe C, Thorpe C: A critical age: the influence of frailty measurements on prognosis and management in intensive care. ICU Manag 14:30–33, 2014.
85. Montuclard L, Garrouste-Orgeas M, Timsit JF, et al: Outcome, functional autonomy, and quality of life of elderly patients with a long-term intensive care unit stay. Crit Care Med 28:3389–3395, 2000.
89. Ebell MH, Jang W, Shen Y, et al: Development and validation of the Good Outcome Following Attempted Resuscitation (GO-FAR) score to predict neurologically intact survival after in-hospital cardiopulmonary resuscitation. JAMA Intern Med 173:1872–1878, 2013.

120 Geriatric Medicine in Europe

Peter Crome, Joanna Pleming

AGING IN EUROPE

In common with more developed countries throughout the world, population demographics throughout Europe will change dramatically in the next 50 years (Figure 120-1).

In 31 countries (European Union plus the countries of the European Free Trade Association), the overall population of those aged 65 years and older was 16.0% in 2010 and is predicted to rise to 29.3% by 2060.[1] The comparable figures for those aged 80 years and older are 4.1% and 11.5%, respectively, representing an almost tripling of the very old population. These differences are due to reduced fertility and increasing life expectancy; however, there remain differences in life expectancy between European countries. For example, the lowest projected life expectancy for males born in 2012 is 68.4 years in Lithuania compared to the highest of 81.6 years in Iceland. The differences between countries for women are not as great but still substantial at 79.6 years and 84.3 years for Lithuania and Iceland, respectively.[2]

The rationale for public policies to adapt to meet this population change is similar in all European countries. The need for specialized services for older people has also been recognized. Geriatric medicine as a distinct specialty has developed at different rates in different countries despite the needs of older people being relatively similar. This chapter summarizes the state of geriatric medicine in Europe and the work of organizations whose focus is improving the health of older people.

HEALTH CARE IN EUROPE

The requirement that all citizens should have access to good-quality health care has been one of the principal features of European public policy. Different models have emerged based on state-funded systems, work-based or independent compulsory health insurance, or various combinations of the two. Some countries require co-payments, whereas others do not. There has also been recognition that older people are disadvantaged in terms of burden of illness, disability, frailty, and poverty in relation to the rest of the community. Special arrangements have been introduced in most countries to try and reduce these disadvantages. For example, in England all those older than 60 years do not pay for prescription medication. Citizens of the European Union are also entitled to health care in every EU country. However, the specific way health care is funded, and what services are provided and by whom, is a matter for national and, in some countries, regional determination.

THE DEVELOPMENT OF GERIATRIC MEDICINE

It is generally recognized that the definition of geriatric medicine as a distinct specialty resulted from the publications of Nascher in the United States.[3,4] However, the development of a national geriatric medicine service has been credited to the United Kingdom and the pioneering work of Marjorie Warren, who implemented her service at the West Middlesex Hospital.[5,6] Fortuitously, this interest coincided with the introduction of a new universal British National Health Service (NHS) in 1948, which incorporated from its foundation a network of hospitals that provided care for the chronically disabled, most of whom were older people.

The history of the development of the specialty has been described in a previous edition of this textbook,[7] and further information can be found in the excellent articles of Barton and Mulley [8] and of Morley.[9] Therefore, only an abbreviated account is given here. Until the reformation, care for older disabled and sick people was provided under the auspices of the monasteries. These were closed during the reign of Henry VIII (1509-1547), and responsibility for this group of people passed to the civil authorities, who, as time went on, built institutions for their incarceration in what were called workhouses. The basic principle was that of "less eligibility," with life being worse than that of the poorest laborer. The scandal of the workhouse, drawn to public attention through the work of Charles Dickens (in *Oliver Twist*, e.g.), led toward the end of the nineteenth century to the establishment of Poor Law Infirmaries, which in turn were transferred to the management of county and city municipalities in the 1920s. These hospitals became the first geriatric medicine hospitals in 1948. The arrangements of the NHS allowed for services to develop in accordance with local needs and the existing hospital structures. Three types of service were developed. The integrated model had geriatricians working alongside general internal medicine physicians, often sharing wards and support medical staff.[10] Under the age-related model, medical emergency patients were admitted to geriatric medicine or general medicine services according to age, with those 75 years and older more frequently admitted to geriatric medicine services.[11] The third model, the "needs-related" service, had geriatric medicine services taking responsibility for older people with complex needs but often not until their acute needs had been treated. In practice, many services were not so rigidly demarcated.

GERIATRIC MEDICINE IN THE UNITED KINGDOM

The NHS came into being in July 1948 based on the principles of universality, and care was provided on the basis of need rather than the ability to pay. Devolution of political power to the nations of the United Kingdom (England, Scotland, Wales, and Northern Ireland) has produced differences in organizational structures, financial arrangements for medical staff, and some patient co-payments for medication and dental services, but the underlying premise of "free at the point of use" remains. Private sector medicine is essentially geared to provide services for simple one-off conditions, whereas the management of chronic disease remains essentially within the NHS.

All people are eligible to register with a general practitioner (GP), who now usually works in small groups or practices although "single-handed" practices remain. There is a right to register with a GP of one's choice, but in practice this may be difficult for those in rural areas and those who live in underdoctored areas and with those doctors whose "list" might be closed. The range of services provided by the primary care team varies but might include therapy, minor surgery, and specialist outpatient clinics. In rural areas, they might dispense drugs.

GPs undergo a 5-year training program after qualifying as a doctor. This 5-year program includes a 2-year foundation program, common to all physicians, followed by 3 years in a GP training program that comprises 2 years in hospital posts and 1 year in general practice as a trainee registrar. This may change to a 5-year training program in line with most other medical

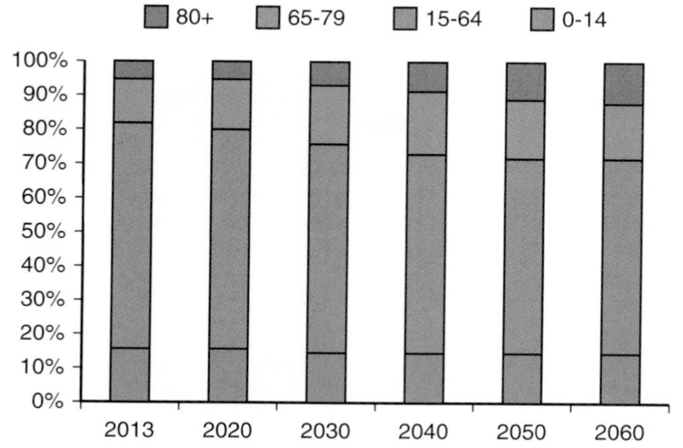

Figure 120-1. Projected population structure by age group in Europe. *(Modified from http://ec.europa.eu/eurostat/documents/3433488/5578868/KS-SF-11-023-EN.PDF/882b8b1e-998b-454e-a574-bb15cc64b653. Accessed September 1, 2013.)*

specialist trainee programs. There is, however, no obligatory requirement to have a placement in geriatric medicine or old age psychiatry, although this is a major part of general practice.

Most GPs are independent contractors, who are paid by a combination of basic allowances, capitation fees, meeting specific service targets (e.g., identifying patients with hypertension), and fees per item of service. Other GPs are salaried, employed by the practice partners or by the local health service. Medical consultations involve no direct payment for all patients, and medications for people older than 60 years are free.

GPs may have their competence in the specialty of geriatric medicine recognized through a diploma examination organized by the Royal College of Physicians in London and in Glasgow. A few GPs who undertake some degree of specialist work (e.g., falls investigation, care home medicine) may be employed as a General Practitioner with a Special Interest (GPwSI). They have to undergo specific training supervised by the local geriatrician.

Specialists

The training program for geriatricians lasts 9 years and has three components: the 2-year common foundation program, 2 years of core medical training, and 5 years of training in geriatric medicine and general (internal) medicine. Entry into training is competitive, and various assessment methods are used to monitor and confirm progress. Successful completion of training renders a physician eligible to apply for a consultant post. In addition, many hospitals will employ a number of physicians who have not completed the full training program and who work as assistants to consultants. Training takes place in the main teaching hospitals associated with medical schools, in smaller district general hospitals, and in the community. Responsibility for the organization and delivery of postgraduate training rests with the NHS rather than the university, which is only responsible for the first year of the foundation program. Full details of training can be obtained from the Joint Royal Colleges Training Board website (www.jrcptb.org.uk).

Consultant Numbers

The Federation of the Royal Colleges of Physicians of the United Kingdom undertakes an annual census of the numbers and work practices of consultants in the medical specialties in the United Kingdom. Geriatric medicine is the largest of the medical specialties, with 1252 consultants in post in 2012. Geriatric medicine is the largest of the medical specialties, with 1332 consultants in post in 2014 (Table 120-1). It should be noted that only a minority of physicians practice general or acute medicine as a stand-alone specialty although it is expected that this will rise in the next few years with the reintroduction of acute medicine as a specialty. In contrast, in 1993 there were only 658 consultant geriatricians and the growth has been steady over the past couple of decades. Approximately one third of the consultant workforce is female, but it is expected that this proportion will also increase. Women form the majority of geriatricians younger than age 40 and the majority of trainees.

TABLE 120-1 Number of Consultants in the Larger Medical Specialties in the United Kingdom (2014)

Specialty	Number of Consultants
Geriatric Medicine	1332
Gastroenterology	1170
Cardiology	1167
Respiratory	1135
Haematology	929
Endocrinology and Diabetes Mellitus	833
Neurology	783
Rheumatology	756
Dermatology	729
Renal medicine	610
Acute Internal Medicine	564

Data from Federation of the Royal Colleges of Physicians of the UK: Census of consultant physicians and higher specialty trainees in the UK, 2014–15: data and commentary. London, 2016, Royal College of Physicians.

The Work of a Geriatrician

The majority of geriatricians work as part of a multidisciplinary team based within an acute hospital. Geriatric medicine (often called care of the elderly or similar) is in turn usually placed within a medical division alongside specialties such as diabetes and respiratory medicine. Some geriatricians work in smaller community hospitals as community geriatricians. Referral to geriatricians is usually via the patient's GP, from other consultants, or via emergency admissions. Local arrangements may now allow direct referral from community nurses, therapists, and social services. Typically there will be six or more consultant geriatricians in each acute hospital, with support provided by doctors at different stages of training. The standard care pathway is for emergency admissions to be transferred either directly to the most appropriate inpatient service or to an acute all-specialty assessment unit. Patients no longer needing the services of an acute hospital may be transferred to a range of step-down (now often called intermediate care) facilities in community hospitals and care homes. A range of enhanced home care services are also usually available for the first month or so after discharge from hospital. A list of important recent documents on health policy relevant to older people is contained in Table 120-2.

Most geriatricians have a subspecialty interest, such as orthogeriatrics, stroke, continence care, or falls investigation, and a few may practice exclusively or almost exclusively in this subspecialty. The training of geriatricians in acute care and in rehabilitation has made them ideally suited to lead the development of stroke care in separate acute stroke units. Most patients admitted to hospital with a stroke are now treated by geriatricians. Stroke has become a recognized subspecialty of geriatrics, neurology, general medicine, clinical pharmacology, and cardiovascular disease, although the number of physicians who have undergone the required extra training in stroke care is small.

More than 80% of geriatricians take part in unselected medical emergency work, and geriatricians are the largest specialty providing this work apart from those working exclusively in acute

TABLE 120-2 Recent United Kingdom Policy Documents Relevant to Geriatric Medicine

Document	Author	Outline of Contents	URL
NSF for Older People 2001	Department of Health	Sets quality standards for health and social care for older people	https://www.gov.uk/government/uploads/system/uploads/attachment_data/file/198033/National_Service_Framework_for_Older_People.pdf (Accessed Oct 27, 2015)
National Service Framework (NSF) for Older People in Wales 2006	Welsh Assembly Government	Adapted from the NSF for England, sets national standards to ensure that older people are enabled to maintain their health, wellbeing and independence and receive prompt, seamless and quality treatment and support when necessary.	http://www.wales.nhs.uk/documents/NSF%20for%20Older%20People.pdf (Accessed Oct 27, 2015)
Better Health in Old Age Resource Document 2004	Professor Ian Philp, National Director for Older People's Health	A report highlighting progress following implementation of the NSF for Older People highlighting positive outcomes for older people in the United Kingdom	http://webarchive.nationalarchives.gov.uk/+/www.dh.gov.uk/en/Publicationsandstatistics/Publications/PublicationsPolicyAndGuidance/DH_4092840 (Accessed Oct 27, 2015)
A New Ambition for Old Age: Next Steps in Implementing the National Service Framework for Older People 2006	Professor Ian Philp, National Director for Older People's Health	The second phase of the government's 10-year NSF for Older People set out in three broad headings: (1) dignity in care, (2) joined up care, (3) healthy aging	http://library.nhsggc.org.uk/mediaAssets/dementiasp/A_new_ambition_for_old_age_12-Nov-07.pdf (Accessed Oct 27, 2015)
National Dementia Strategy 2009	Department of Health	A government strategy with 17 recommendations to improve dementia care services centered around three key themes: (1) raising awareness and understanding, (2) early diagnosis and support, (3) living well with dementia	https://www.gov.uk/government/publications/living-well-with-dementia-a-national-dementia-strategy (Accessed Oct 27, 2015)
National Stroke Strategy 2008	Department of Health	A government framework for action in stroke medicine outlining strategies for prevention, acute care, and rehabilitation	http://clahrc-gm.nihr.ac.uk/cms/wp-content/uploads/DoH-National-Stroke-Strategy-2007.pdf (Accessed Oct 27, 2015)
Managing the Care of People with Long-term Conditions. Second Report of Session 2014-2015	House of Commons Health Committee	An inquiry into NHS management of long-term conditions Recommends integration of health and social care for greater personalization of health services to the individual, moving care of long-term conditions from hospitals into primary care with the goal of reducing unplanned admissions	http://www.publications.parliament.uk/pa/cm201415/cmselect/cmhealth/401/401.pdf (Accessed Oct 27, 2015)
Ageing in the Twenty-First Century: A Celebration and A Challenge 2012	United Nations Population Fund (UNFPA), New York, and HelpAge International, London	A 10-year review report assessing global progress after adoption of the Madrid International Plan of Action on Ageing in 2002, looking at three priority areas: development, health, and well-being Recommendations made, including action to be taken to eliminate age discrimination in employment and training, to consider older women in particular as a vulnerable group when developing social policy, and to provide adequate access to older people in health and social care and transport	http://www.unfpa.org/publications/ageing-twenty-first-century (Accessed Oct 27, 2015)
BGS Commissioning Guidance: High Quality Health Care for Older Care Home Residents 2013	British Geriatrics Society	A two-page document outlining the clinical and service priorities for meeting the needs of care home residents Report detailing desired outcomes from commissioned services, providing guidelines, and giving practical advice on monitoring and evaluation of outcomes	http://www.bgs.org.uk/campaigns/2013commissioning/Commissioning_2013.pdf (Accessed Oct 27, 2015)
Specialty Training Curriculum for Geriatric Medicine Curriculum 2010, Amendments 2013	Joint Royal Colleges of Physicians Training Board	Geriatric Medicine Specialty training curriculum for all higher specialty trainees in Geriatric Medicine in the UK covering all areas of specialist medical care of older people in the UK. Produced using standards provided by the GMC.	http://www.gmc-uk.org/geriatric_curriculum_2010.pdf_32486221.pdf_43566788.pdf (Accessed Oct 27, 2015)
UK Study of Abuse and Neglect of Older People Prevalence Survey Report 2007	National Centre for Social Research and King's College London Commissioned by Comic Relief and the Department of Health	Report of survey of 2100 adults older than 66 years. Of those surveyed, 2.6% reported either abuse or neglect by a family member, close friend, or care worker, a figure increasing to 4.0% when including neighbors or acquaintances. The report calls for early intervention, more choice for older people, reduced inequalities, improved access to community services, and more support for people with long-term needs.	http://assets.comicrelief.com/cr09/docs/older_people_abuse_report.pdf (Accessed Oct 27, 2015)

TABLE 120-2 Recent United Kingdom Policy Documents Relevant to Geriatric Medicine—cont'd

Document	Author	Outline of Contents	URL
Making Integrated Out-of-Hospital Care a Reality 2012	Royal College of General Practitioners and NHS Confederation	Paper aiming to provide a set of principles to deliver effective integrated out-of-hospital care promoting risk profiling systems, creation of new incentivizing tariffs, and wider information sharing	http://www.nhsconfed.org/resources/2012/12/making-integrated-out-of-hospital-care-a-reality (Accessed Oct 27, 2015)
The Mid Staffordshire NHS Foundation Trust Public Inquiry, 2013 Also known as the "Francis Report"	Chaired by Robert Francis QC	An inquiry into failing of care at Mid Staffordshire NHS Foundation Trust between 2005 and 2009. The report makes 209 recommendations highlighting openness and transparency within the health service and improving support for compassionate care and strong leadership within the NHS.	http://www.midstaffspublicinquiry.com/report (Accessed Oct 27, 2015)
Counting the Cost Caring for People With Dementia on Hospital Wards 2009	Alzheimer's Society	A report amalgamating data from questionnaires applied to caregivers, nursing staff, and managers and researching quality and cost-effectiveness of care for patients with dementia in the acute hospital settings	http://www.alzheimers.org.uk/countingthecost (Accessed Oct 27, 2015)

TABLE 120-3 Outline of Roles of Consultant Geriatricians in a Tertiary Center in London, United Kingdom

Consultant Number	Special Responsibilities	Activities
1	Acute geriatrics and surgical liaison lead	Acute and rehabilitation geriatrics—allocated acute medical ward; responsible for all patients older than 80 years Proactive liaison service for all older or complex postoperative patients
2	Acute geriatrics Clinical director Dementia lead	Acute and rehabilitation geriatrics—allocated acute ward of 32 patients older than 80 years; ward shared with another consultant Participates in multidisciplinary community meetings to discuss patients with frailty who are living at home
3	Stroke consultant Senior clinical lecturer	Patients with stroke Academic post Infection control
4	Falls lead	Acute and rehabilitation geriatrics Falls clinic
5	Admission avoidance and ambulatory care geriatrics Clinical governance lead	Lead and run admission avoidance service and ambulatory care clinic—direct referrals from general practitioners (GPs) and proactive identification of patients from emergency department who can be discharged with specialist nursing support in the community
6	Acute geriatrics Orthogeriatrics lead	Acute and rehabilitation geriatrics Proactive liaison service for all complex older patients undergoing elective and emergency surgery Comprehensive geriatric assessment of all patients with fractured neck of femur before and after surgery
7	Acute geriatrics Admission avoidance and ambulatory care geriatrics Care home medicine Cardiology liaison	Acute and rehabilitation geriatrics Admission avoidance and ambulatory care geriatrics Monthly consultation service in each of four nursing homes supporting GPs and reviewing patients requiring specialist input
8	Acute geriatrics Community dementia lead Admission avoidance and ambulatory care geriatrics	Acute and rehabilitation geriatrics Admission avoidance and ambulatory care geriatrics Once-weekly memory clinic based in the hospital
9	Acute geriatrics Community frailty clinic Admission avoidance and ambulatory care geriatrics	Acute and rehabilitation geriatrics Admission avoidance and ambulatory care geriatrics Home visits of geriatric patients identified by GPs as in need of comprehensive geriatric assessment but unable to attend hospital

and general medicine. Table 120-3 summarizes the specific responsibilities of a team of geriatricians working in one U.K. teaching hospital. More information on the work of U.K. geriatricians can be found in the report by Wykro.[12]

GERIATRIC MEDICINE IN OTHER EUROPEAN COUNTRIES

The continent of Europe is generally considered as extending from the Atlantic Ocean to the Ural Mountains. However, for largely political reasons other countries are often considered as part of Europe and of its organizations. Almost all countries on the continent are members of the Council of Europe, whereas a smaller number of countries are members of the European Union.

There has not been a comprehensive review of the state of geriatric medicine in each of the countries of Europe. However, national societies have produced summaries of their own activities, key features of training, and the current state of development of the specialty for the websites of the European Union Geriatric

Medicine Society (EUGMS) (www.eugms.org) and the European Union of Medical Specialists (UEMS) (www.uemsgeriatricmedicine.org). Principal features are described here.

Austria. The Austrian Society for Geriatrics and Gerontology is involved in research on the aging process and diseases in old age, the production of guidelines, and the organization of scientific meetings alone and in collaboration with other German-speaking countries. Undergraduate medical education in geriatrics occurs mainly as noncompulsory lectures and seminars within other subjects. Geriatric medicine was established in July 2011 as a subspecialty of internal medicine, neurology, psychiatry, rehabilitation medicine, and general practice (www.em-consulte.com/en/article/765978). In 1999 the Austrian Federal Institute for Health Care (OBIG) commissioned an expert panel to address whether specialist geriatric departments were required in hospitals where previously older patients had been cared for under general medical teams. This report led to the proposal that a network of specialist geriatric treatment units (geriatric acute care and remobilization units) be required in the acute sector. This proposal was adopted in 2000. To date, 40 such units have been established in 61 hospitals (http://geriatrie-online.at/english/). The society publishes two journals: *Geriatrie Praxis Österreich* and *Zeitschrift für Gerontologie und Geriatrie*.

Belgium. Geriatric medicine has been recognized as a full specialty since 2005. Approximately 330 geriatricians serve a population of 10 million people living in Belgium. There is a geriatric department in each of the 120 general hospitals in Belgium which equates to approximately 6 geriatric beds per 1000 patients (http://www.eugms.org/our-members/national-societies/belgium.html; http://www.uemsgeriatricmedicine.org/uems1/belgium1.asp). The Belgian Society of Gerontology and Geriatrics organizes two conferences a year.

Bulgaria. Bulgaria's health expenditure as a percentage of gross domestic product is one of the lowest in Europe. Much of the care of older people following hospital admission is still provided by families. The difficulties in providing postacute care have been discussed since the change of government in 2009, and the most recent health care provider contract contains an earmarked portion for selected postacute conditions. The Bulgarian Association on Aging was founded in 1997 although there were other societies previously. The association holds regular meetings for its multidisciplinary membership. With regard to training, optional geriatric training courses for undergraduates have been instituted in Sofia Medical School, although the uptake among medical students has been poor (http://www.uemsgeriatricmedicine.org/uems1/bulgaria1.asp; http://www.eugms.org/our-members/national-societies/bulgaria.html).

Czech Republic. In the Czech Republic, geriatric medicine is a separate subspecialty within internal medicine. It is included in the undergraduate curriculum. Postgraduate medical training has been restructured twice, first in 2004 and again in 2009. Since 2006, approximately 20 centers have been accredited for a specialist geriatric training program, which lasts 4 years (http://www.uemsgeriatricmedicine.org/uems1/czech1.asp).

The Czech Society of Gerontology and Geriatrics (CGGS) is involved in the development of clinical practice, education, research, and national and regional government policies. It organizes scientific conferences and publishes the *Česká Geriatrická Revue*. Geriatric medicine in the Czech Republic still faces a number of challenges, including low numbers of acute geriatric beds and long waiting lists for institutional care, but it has made progress recently in community geriatrics (http://www.uemsgeriatricmedicine.org/uems1/czech1.asp). The National Action Plan Supporting Positive Ageing for the period 2013-2017, adopted by the Czech Republic in February 2013, aims to support senior citizens to remain independent and in their own homes through coordination of health and social care.[13]

Denmark. In Denmark geriatric medicine developed as part of the assessment for care home admission. Today, however, geriatricians are involved in all aspects of the care of older people, including care of older adult patients within the emergency department. Geriatric medicine is one of nine internal medicine specialties. All three medical schools in Denmark have a geriatric medicine curriculum. Geriatric medicine encompasses the spectrum of health care with specialist geriatric units offering acute care of older patients and geriatric teams providing evaluation and treatment at home, collaborating with primary care doctors and nursing staff (http://www.eugms.org/our-members/national-societies/denmark.html). In a shift from an early focus on institutional care in the late twentieth century, Danish health care now aims to keep older people in their own homes for as long as possible. Services that facilitate this include a 24-hour public health nurse service, day care centers, respite care for caregivers, and a "Seniors Help Seniors" volunteer program aiming to create social networks and combat loneliness among the older population (http://www.globalaging.org/elderrights/world/densocialhealthcare.htm).

Estonia. The Estonian Association of Gerontology and Geriatrics was founded in 1997 and has a multidisciplinary membership. Its mission includes geriatric training, raising the profile of older people, and organizing scientific conferences. In 2007 a training course in geriatric medicine was organized, supported by the Estonian Ministry of Social Affairs and the European Social Fund. The course trained 24 doctors to be the first geriatricians in the country. These doctors founded the Estonian Society of Geriatrics (EGERS) (http://www.eugms.org/our-members/national-societies/estonia.html).

Finland. Finland has one of the oldest geriatrics societies (founded in 1948), which organizes an annual conference and other symposia. Geriatric medicine is a recognized independent specialty previously having been a subspecialty of internal medicine, neurology, and psychiatry. Most geriatricians in Finland today work in primary health care settings although larger city hospitals have well-developed geriatric services. Only 25% of district hospitals surveyed in 2012 had a separate geriatrics department. There are professors of geriatric medicine in all Finnish medical schools, and geriatrics is a compulsory part of the undergraduate medical curriculum. Finland has a national exam that must be completed prior to entry into Finnish geriatric medicine higher specialty training. Postgraduate training was standardized in 2012, and specialization takes 5 years. Additionally, the Finnish universities recommend that, after specialization, an additional 10 days a year be spent training in a site external to the physicians' usual place of work (http://www.eugms.org/our-members/national-societies/finland.html). In early 2012 there were 239 practicing geriatricians with 171 trainees registered in the specialty (http://www.uemsgeriatricmedicine.org/uems1/finland1.asp).

France. Geriatric medicine has been a standalone subspeciality since 2004. It is possible to specialize as a geriatrician from any medical discipline but the most common route is through internal or family medicine with the training lasting 4 years from medical specialties and 3 years from family medicine.[21] The French geriatric society is the Société Française de Gériatrie et Gérontologie (SFGG) and it combines both geriatic medicine and gerontology. It is open to geratricians as well as professionals from allied fields including public health and psychology. There are 17 regional geriatric medicine societies and four daughter societies linked to the SFGG and there is an annual scientific meeting in December of each year. The SFGG publishes guidelines within geriatrics and is involved in national policy-making around the care of older people in France. SFGG's published journal is *La Revue de Gériatrie* (www.sfgg.fr, http://www.eugms.org/our-members/national-societies/france.html).

Germany. The first German Gerontology Society was founded in 1938, reconstituted after both World War II and the reunification of Germany. A separate medical geriatric society was founded in 1995. Geriatric medicine is recognized as a subspecialty of internal medicine, family medicine, neurology, and psychiatry, although there are variations in each of the Länder. The German Geriatrics Society favors a training program that graduates joint internal medicine–geriatrics specialists. Although geriatric medicine is a compulsory part of the curriculum, academic departments have only been established in a minority of medical schools. The German Geriatrics Society organizes scientific meetings and publishes two journals and a newsletter: the *European Journal of Geriatrics* (bilingual), the *Geriatrie Journal* (German), and *Geriatrie online*, the newsletter (http://www.eugms.org/our-members/national-societies/germany.html).

Greece. The Hellenic Association of Gerontology and Geriatrics (HAGG) was founded in 1977. Its main goal is the enhancement of the quality of life and well-being of older people. It focuses on research and international collaboration with other gerontological societies and works with political and social bodies (e.g., the Greek Ministry of Health) and local authorities to advise on health and social care matters. HAGG organizes a national congress every two years.

Hungary. The first Hungarian congress on gerontology as held in 1937 and the fifteenth World Congress of Gerontology was hosted in Budapest in 1993. Recognition of the specialty occurred only in 2000. In 2011, the Hungarian Association of Gerontology (HAGG), together with the National College of Geriatrics and Chronic Care, created a health initiative that would set up "active" geriatric units first in university hospitals and then in all major regions. This process was initiated in 2012. Specialization in geriatric medicine requires 5 years of dedicated subspecialty training, and the exit examination has both practical and theoretical components (http://www.eugms.org/our-members/national-societies/hungary.html).

Iceland. The Icelandic Health Care System is a tax-funded national health insurance with weighted contributions based on age; younger taxpayers fund two thirds and older people fund one third. Geriatrics is recognized as a subspecialty of internal medicine and is being considered as a subspecialty of family medicine. Although it is possible to train in geriatric medicine entirely in Iceland, trainees are encouraged to train overseas. Geriatrics is taught in the medical school, and the Icelandic Geriatrics Society was founded in 1989. In 2013 there were 17 fully specialized geriatricians. Geriatricians manage both acute and postacute inpatient wards, ambulatory care, and memory clinic outpatient services (http://www.eugms.org/our-members/national-societies/iceland.html). The Gerontological Research Institute, established in 1999, has been involved in genetic and environmental research in collaboration with the U.S. National Institute on Aging (http://www.uemsgeriatricmedicine.org/uems1/iceland1.asp).

Ireland. Ireland has traditionally spent less on health compared with other Western European countries, and this is reflected in generally lower numbers of specialists. The development of geriatric medicine in Ireland has in many ways paralleled that in the United Kingdom, although the first geriatrician was not appointed until 1969. These similarities include the presence of geriatricians in all general hospitals, the involvement of geriatricians in acute medicine on-call duties, and dual training in geriatric and general medicine. In 2003 O'Neill and O'Keeffe[14] reported that there were 41 geriatricians in the country, the largest specialty within internal medicine. Two models of care existed: an age-related service in the major teaching hospitals and an integrated approach in smaller hospitals where there might be a solo geriatrician working alongside four or five other medical specialists. The pattern of postgraduate training is very similar to that in the United Kingdom, and there is cross-representation on many postgraduate training bodies. The Membership of the Royal College of Physicians (MRCP) in Ireland examination is recognized as equivalent to that of the MRCP UK. Most Irish geriatricians will have undertaken part of their postgraduate training in the United Kingdom or other countries. The Irish Society of Physicians in Geriatric Medicine was founded in 1979, but geriatricians are also active in the Irish Gerontological Society, whose membership extends into Northern Ireland, part of the United Kingdom.

Italy. There are 34 specialist geriatric departments within universities in Italy. The national geriatric society, Società Italiana di Gerontologia e Geriatria (SIGG), was founded in 1950 and has a biogerontology, nursing, and sociobehavioral section in addition to its large clinical section. SIGG is one of the largest geriatric societies in the world, with 1872 registered members in 2013. It has conducted large-scale national studies and publishes a number of journals, including *Aging Clinical and Experimental Research* and *Giornale di Gerontologia*. It organizes an annual scientific meeting and a summer school for fellows.

Luxembourg. The Luxembourg Society of Gerontology and Geriatrics was founded in 1985. It holds an annual conference and produces a journal, *Journée de Gérontologie et Gériatrie*, annually in October (http://www.eugms.org/index.php?id=126).

Malta. Health care in the Maltese Islands is divided between the public and private sectors. All medical postgraduate training in Malta is undertaken overseas. There is one Department of Geriatrics with 11 consultant geriatricians working in this small island country. The Geriatric Medicine Society of Malta (GMSM), set up in 2006, represents the specialty of geriatrics in discussions and decisions surrounding training and links the geriatric community of Malta with the European geriatric community (http://www.gmsmalta.com/index.php). In 2013, GMSM had 24 members. In Malta, the department of geriatrics is primarily hospital based. Geriatricians also conduct several dedicated outpatient services, including falls and memory clinics, and provide a consultation service to care home residents. Orthogeriatric beds were set up in 2012 within the acute hospital setting for joint care management of patients with neck of femur fractures (http://www.eugms.org/our-members/national-societies/malta.html).

The Netherlands. Geriatric medicine was recognized as a specialty in 1982. The Dutch Geriatrics Society was founded in 1999 and publishes the *Tijdschrift voor Gerontologie en Geriatrie (Journal of Gerontology and Geriatrics)* and holds an annual congress, Geriatriedagen. Geriatric departments exist in most hospitals in the Netherlands. In January 2013 there were 201 practicing geriatric consultants. All health care is funded publically, and health insurance is compulsory. Medical care in nursing homes is provided by specialists in chronic care and rehabilitation medicine (http://www.eugms.org/our-members/national-societies/the-netherlands.html).

Norway. In Norway geriatrics remains a subspecialty of internal medicine. Geriatrics is part of the undergraduate curriculum, and there are professors in Oslo, Bergen, Trondheim, and Tromsø. The precise functioning of the geriatric medicine department varies from hospital to hospital. Recently, the Norwegian government legislated that every acute hospital should have an acute geriatric unit, and this is currently being implemented nationally (www.eugms.org/our-members/national-societies/norway.html). The Norwegian Geriatrics Society holds a scientific meeting every other year but also takes part in pan-Nordic congresses.

Poland. The number of geriatricians in training is not keeping pace with the rise in the number of older people in Poland. A study in 2013 estimated that the ratio of geriatricians to citizens was 0.16 : 10,000 and that there would be an insufficient number of specialists in post to meet the needs of a growing older population. The need to improve GPs' knowledge of geriatric medicine was stressed.[15] The Geriatric Society in Poland promotes development of care of older people in Poland, supports research, and promotes education in geriatric medicine in undergraduate teaching and in the specialist curriculum. It has a journal, *Geriatria*. There are approximately 650 geriatric beds around the country with most districts having a geriatric unit. There is one geriatric hospital in Poland, in Katowice, which houses both acute and rehabilitation units. Geriatric medicine is taught in undergraduate curricula but is only compulsory in three universities, with optional classes provided in five other universities (http://www.eugms.org/our-members/national-societies/poland.html).

Portugal. Geriatric medicine is not yet recognized as an independent medical specialty in Portugal. Until 2010, there were no specialist geriatricians or specialist geriatric units within the country. Geriatric medicine teaching in Lisbon and Coimbra medical schools began in 2010, and the first geriatric unit was opened in Lisbon Medical University Hospital in the same year (http://www.eugms.org/our-members/national-societies/portugal.html).

Romania. The Romanian Society of Gerontology and Geriatrics (SRGG) was founded in 1957. It holds an annual scientific meeting that includes specialist programs for multidisciplinary teams. It supports an affiliate organization, the Association of Young Geriatricians, which aims to support junior colleagues by offering scholarships and prizes for outstanding achievements in research. These scholarships and prizes are presented at the annual congress.

Spain. The Spanish Society of Geriatrics and Gerontology (Sociedad Española de Geriatría y Gerontología; SEGG) was founded in 1948 and has clinical, biological, and behavioral-social sections. In February 2013, SEGG had 2358 members; 70% of these were doctors from various specialties and the remaining 30% comprised allied health professionals, scientists, patients, and caregivers. In addition to a national conference, the society publishes *Revista Española de Geriatría y Gerontología* bimonthly. A second society, the Sociedad Española de Medicina Geriátrica (SEMEG) was founded in 2000 and holds biennial scientific meetings and has published a number of books. SEGG has significant e-media presence; it posts regularly on Twitter (@seggeriatira) and publishes an online newsletter e-mailed to members and available on the website (https://www.segg.es). A survey conducted in 2003 revealed that there were no acute geriatric care units in seven of the country's regions amounting to two thirds of the country's acute hospitals. This does not seem to have improved significantly, as a further study in 2009 revealed that only 12% of Spanish hospitals had an acute geriatric unit.[16]

Slovakia. Geriatric medicine is recognized as a specialty in Slovakia with training following European guidelines. Since the first four doctors gained geriatric specialization in 1983, more than 150 doctors have become specialists (http://www.eugms.org/index.php?id=132). The Slovakian Society of Geriatrics and Gerontology includes among its roles the dissemination of knowledge about older people to physicians and other health care workers, policy development, activities aimed at ending age discrimination, and organizing scientific meetings. Its journal, *Geriatria*, is published four times a year.

Slovenia. Geriatrics is not yet recognized as a specialty in Slovenia. Older patients are cared for within family medicine, a branch of medicine containing a special working group for care of older adults and care within nursing homes. With regard to training, several specialties (including internal medicine, family medicine, and psychiatry) contain modules on geriatrics within their curricula. The Institute of Gerontology and Geriatrics was founded in 1966 but, with the death of its founder, Bojan Accetto, in 1988, the focus of the society moved from care of older adults toward vascular medicine. A multidisciplinary sister organization, the Slovenian Society of Gerontology, has taken on the role of older patients' health advocacy, promoting gerontological research, participation in health and social care, legislation development, and public health information on age-related issues (http://www.eugms.org/our-members/national-societies/slovenia.html).

Sweden. Geriatrics is recognized as a full specialty in Sweden. Most geriatricians work in specialist services for older people with a minority working in primary care or internal medicine. The Swedish Society for Geriatrics and Gerontology organizes three scientific conferences each year and publishes the journal *Geriatrik*. There are six chairs of geriatric medicine within Sweden (in Stockholm, Gothenburg, Malmö, Linköping, Uppsala, and Umeå), and all departments are very active in geriatric research (http://www.eugms.org/our-members/national-societies/sweden.html; http://www.slf.se/Foreningarnas-startsidor/Specialitetsforening/Svensk-Geriatrisk-Forening/In-English/).

Switzerland. Geriatric medicine was recognized as a specialty in 2000, and the Swiss Geriatrics Society was founded shortly after that in 2002. Before this time, geriatricians had formed a section of the Swiss Gerontological Society. The two societies share the same administrative office and are now collectively known as the SFGG-SPSG. Most geriatricians initially train in internal medicine before undertaking geriatric medicine specialization, but a small number first become family physicians. Specialist training comprises 2 years in geriatric medicine and 1 year in old age psychiatry after the 5 years in either internal medicine or family medicine. Training in geriatric medicine has improved in recent years, with seven hospitals now accredited to provide postgraduate training. The four university hospitals (Basel, Berne, Lausanne, and Geneva) have chairs in geriatric medicine (http://www.eugms.org/our-members/national-societies/switzerland.html). Geriatricians face the additional ethical challenge of assisted suicide, which is legal in Switzerland for Swiss nationals and foreigners (http://www.slf.se/Foreningarnas-startsidor/Specialitetsforening/Svensk-Geriatrisk-Forening/In-English/). (Assisted death is also legal in Belgium and the Netherlands but is restricted to nationals within these countries.) The SFGG-SPSG participates in meetings of the Swiss Society of Internal Medicine and participates in scientific meetings in French- and German-speaking neighboring countries.

Turkey. In February 2013, Turkey had 47 geriatricians working in 14 geriatric medicine departments. There are two national geriatrics societies. The Turkish Geriatrics Society organizes conferences, arranges training courses for doctors and nurses, and participates in national and international events through its affiliation to outside bodies (http://www.turkgeriatri.org/index_en.php). The Academic Geriatrics Society, an organization founded in 2005, publishes the journal *Akademik Geriatri Dergisi*. The society's aims include the promotion of health of older people, teaching about their health care needs, public education, and the organization of scientific meetings. Two regular meetings take place: the Rational Usage of Medications and Nutritional Products Symposium and the National Education for Nursing Home Personnel meeting (www.turkgeriatri.org and http://www.eugms.org/our-members/national-societies/turkey-turkish-geriatrics-society-observer-status.html, http://www.eugms.org/our-members/national-societies/turkey-academic-geriatrics-society-observer-status.html).

GERIATRIC MEDICINE ORGANIZATIONS IN EUROPE

There are three major European organizations whose principal *raison d'être* is the advancement of the specialty of geriatric medicine and the improvement of health care for older people. These are

- International Association of Gerontology and Geriatrics (IAGG) (http://www.iagg.info) and The International

Association of Gerontology and Geriatrics (IAGG) -European Region (http://www.iagg-er.net)

- The European Union Geriatric Medicine Society (EUGMS) (www.eugms.org)
- Union of Medical Specialists -Geriatric Medicine Section (UEMS-GM) (http://www.uemsgeriatricmedicine.org/uems1)

International Association of Gerontology and Geriatrics

The IAGG is a worldwide learned society for all those interested in the health and welfare of older people:

> *The mission of the International Association of Gerontology and Geriatrics is to promote the highest levels of achievement in gerontological research and training worldwide, and to interact with other international, intergovernmental and nongovernmental organizations in the promotion of gerontological interests globally and on behalf of its member associations. The Association pursues these activities with a view of enhancing the highest quality of life and well being of all people as they experience ageing at individual and societal levels. (www.iagg.info)*

Its 73 member organizations come from 65 countries with a combined total membership of more than 45,000. It has consultative status with the United Nations and its subsidiary bodies, including the World Health Organization, participating in various task forces and committees and responding to consultations on a broad range of subjects relating to older people. Founded in 1950, it has held 20 World Congresses and plans to hold the 21st in San Francisco in 2017. In addition to these major conferences, IAGG organizes training in countries where geriatrics and gerontology are developing. It has three standing committees: the International Council of the Gerontology Student Organization, the International Network for the Prevention of Elder Abuse, and the International Society for Gerontechnology. Its official journal is *Gerontology—International Journal of Experimental, Clinical and Behavioural Gerontology*.

The IAGG is organized into five regions: Africa, Asia/Oceania, North America, Latin America and the Caribbean, and Europe (ER). The latter region, IAGG-ER (http://www.iagg-er.net), is organized into three sections: clinical, biologic, and sociobehavioral science. Its affairs are coordinated by an executive board elected every 4 years by delegates from European societies affiliated with IAGG. Some countries have more than one member organization (Table 120-4). For example, the United Kingdom has three societies affiliated to IAGG: the British Geriatrics Society (clinical), the British Society of Gerontology (social science), and the British Society of Research on Ageing (biologic).

The principal activity of the IAGG-ER is to organize scientific conferences, which are held every 4 years. The conferences comprise plenary sessions, symposia, and free communications organized by the three sections together with some cross-sectional events. The clinical section has held 10 separate congresses, the first being in Berlin in 1992 and most recent in Prague in 2013 in association with the annual meeting of the Czech Society of Geriatrics and Gerontology. A joint symposium with the British Geriatrics Society was held in April 2009. The clinical section has its own president and secretary-general, but only the president is a member of the board of IAGG-ER. Membership of the IAGG-ER includes countries outside the European Union and some outside the traditional boundary between Europe and Asia (e.g., Georgia, Israel). Ribera Casado has reviewed the history of the clinical section.[17]

European Union Geriatric Medicine Society

The EUGMS was founded in 2000. It held its first congress in Paris in 2001. Individuals are members of the EUGMS on the basis that their national society is a member. As the European Union has enlarged to encompass countries from Middle and Eastern Europe, the number of affiliated societies and overall membership have steadily increased. It is possible that all national geriatric medicine societies in Europe will eventually affiliate. The current countries represented on the EUGMS are shown in Table 120-4. Its affairs are coordinated by a full board consisting of representatives of all member organizations and others. The full board meets once a year and elects an executive board. The secretariat is based in Vienna, having previously been housed in the British Geriatrics Society headquarters in London.

The goals of EUGMS include continuing professional development, representation of the specialty to the European Union, guideline development, and the promotion of research and education. However, its most obvious visible activity has been the organization of major international conferences, which now take place annually. The society has now established a number of Special Interest Groups that meet at or between EUGMS conferences, and Task and Finish Groups. Their activities encompass a broad range of subjects, including emergency care, nutrition, palliative care, vaccines, education, pharmacology, sarcopenia, and comprehensive assessment. Details of the work of these committees are posted on the EUGMS website (www.eugms.org). A position paper setting out EUGMS' priorities is abridged in Box 120-1.

TABLE 120-4 Countries Represented on European Bodies (IAGG, EUGMS, and UEMS-GM) as Full or Associate Members or as Observers

Country	IAGG	EUGMS	UEMS-GM
Albania		Observer	
Austria	Member	Member	Member
Belgium	Member	Member	Member
Belarus	Member		
Bulgaria	Member	Member	Member
Czech Republic	Member	Member	Member
Denmark	Member	Member	Member
Estonia	Member	Member	Member
Finland	Member	Member	Member
France	Member	Member	Member
Georgia	Member		
Germany	Member	Member	Member
Greece	Member	Member	Member
Hungary	Member	Member	Member
Iceland		Member	Member
Ireland	Member	Member	Member
Israel	Member	Observer	Member
Italy	Member	Member	Member
Kazakhstan	Member		
Lithuania			Member
Luxembourg	Member	Member	
Malta	Member	Member	Member
Netherlands	Member	Member	Member
Norway	Member	Member	Member
Poland	Member	Member	Member
Portugal	Member	Member	Member
Romania	Member	Pending	Member
Russia	Member		
San Marino	Member		
Serbia	Member	Member	Member
Slovakia	Member	Member	Member
Slovenia	Member	Member	
Spain	Member	Member	Member
Sweden	Member	Member	Member
Switzerland	Member	Member	Member
Tunisia	Member		
Turkey	Member	Observer	Member
Ukraine	Member		
United Kingdom	Member	Member	Member

EUGMS, European Union Geriatric Medicine Society; *IAGG,* International Association of Gerontology and Geriatrics; *UEMS-GM,* European Union of Medical Specialists–Geriatric Medicine.

BOX 120-1 Key Points from a Position Paper on the State of Geriatric Medicine in Europe

- Geriatric medicine is involved in the medical care of older people with acute, rehabilitation, and long-term health conditions in the community, care homes, and hospitals.
- There is a need to harmonize geriatric medicine throughout Europe.
- Geriatricians are able to undertake a comprehensive assessment of the patient with cognizance of atypical presentation, comorbidity, and functional state.
- Undergraduate medical students and postgraduate physicians need training in geriatric medicine from suitably qualified teachers.
- There is a need to develop an objective-based curriculum for specialists.
- There is a need to increase research capacity in aging research.
- Guidelines on ethical issues related to caring for older adults should be developed.
- There is a need for geriatricians to collaborate with other medical specialties and with allied health professionals to improve the health of older people.

Modified from Duursma S, Castleden M, Cerubini A, et al: European Union Geriatric Medicine Society. Position statement on geriatric medicine and the provision of health care services to older people. J Nutr Health Aging 8:190–195, 2004.

BOX 120-2 The Undergraduate Curriculum in Geriatric Medicine: UEMS-GM Policy

- Respect for patients regardless of age
- Knowledge and understanding of normal and abnormal structure and function, natural history of diseases, body's defense mechanisms, disease presentation, and responses to illness
- Knowledge of common medical conditions in older people
- Ability to conduct a history and physical assessment in an older person
- Ability to treat older people, including effective and safe use of medications
- Understanding of responses to disease; ability to provide help toward recovery and reducing and managing impairments, disabilities, and handicaps
- Understanding of the main ethical and legal issues in both international and national contexts
- Understanding of the roles of other health and social care professionals
- Ability to provide care for older people in different settings
- Knowledge about specific aspects of health and social care relevant to one's region or country

Modified from Masud T, Blundell A, Gordon AL, et al: European undergraduate curriculum in geriatric medicine developed using an international modified Delphi technique. Age Ageing 43:695–702, 2014.
UEMS-GM, European Union of Medical Specialists–Geriatric Medicine.

Other activities include the publication of guidelines (e.g., on type 2 diabetes mellitus and syncope). On the political front, EUGMS interacts with both the European Commission and the European Parliament. EUGMS also has an official scientific journal (*European Geriatric Medicine*). In addition to publishing research and clinical papers, the journal also produces a series on the same topic in various countries (e.g., elder abuse[18]) and a second series on geriatric care in different countries (e.g., Malta, Sweden, and Austria).[19]

The desirability of having two separate clinical societies in Europe has been questioned, particularly as many organizations are members of both societies and several geriatricians hold or have held office in both organizations.[17]

Union of Medical Specialists–Geriatric Medicine Section

One of the basic tenets of the European Union is the free movement of workers between its countries with each nation's qualifications being recognized in all member countries of the European Union. In relation to the medical field, this means that undergraduate and postgraduate diplomas and certificates are accepted in all EU member countries without the need for further examinations. The UEMS, which has been in existence for more than 50 years, is the body charged with coordinating specialist education within the European Union.

Responsibilities for specialist training are divided between national authorities and UEMS. National bodies are responsible for the duration and contents of training, quality control, determination of entry procedures, assessment, and control of numbers. UEMS is allowed to set minimum standards, which have to be met in each country.

UEMS is organized into numerous specialist sections, including one for geriatric medicine, UEMS-GM. The activities of the section are coordinated through a board, the current president of which is Tahir Masud of the United Kingdom. Countries represented on the board are shown in Table 120-4. National representation is via the recognized national medical body in each country. In the case of the United Kingdom, this is the British Medical Association although this is then delegated to each specialty society. UEMS-GM works collaboratively with the other European organizations and has recently established a European Education Board, which has subgroups developing proposals for undergraduate, postgraduate, and interdisciplinary training in geriatric medicine. The proposals for undergraduate training are summarized in Box 120-2. The overall goals of the section are to promote the recognition of geriatric medicine in all countries of the European Union, to standardize training standards and requirements, and, as a consequence, to ensure that all older people in Europe have access to adequately trained geriatric medicine specialists. It is tackling these issues through a wide range of activities (Box 120-3).

BOX 120-3 Achievements and Activities of the UEMS-GM

- Producing standards and curricula for postgraduate training in geriatric medicine
- Producing an agreed curriculum for undergraduate training for medical students
- Producing a system for the inspection of training posts
- Contributing to a master's program
- Contributing to the European Union manual of internal medicine
- Producing a database of training opportunities in Europe
- Disseminating information about the organization and practice of geriatric medicine in Europe and issues such as revalidation and continuous professional development
- Producing and updating a website with links to member websites

Data from the Geriatric Medicine Section of the UEMS: http://www.uemsgeriatricmedicine.org. Accessed October 27, 2015.
UEMS-GM, European Union of Medical Specialists–Geriatric Medicine.

GERIATRIC MEDICINE TRAINING IN EUROPE

Undergraduate Education in Europe

There is general acceptance that undergraduate medical students are inadequately trained to manage the growing number of older people that almost all of them will encounter in routine medical practice. Using a Delphi process, UEMS-GM has published a comprehensive new syllabus for undergraduate medical students.[20] There was wide consensus across Europe on the substance of what graduates should be able to do and understand. Reference to national and regional differences in relation to ethics, law, and the provision of services has been included using the statement "ethical and country specific legal issues." It is hoped that this curriculum can be used by individual medical schools and national bodies to benchmark what they do against a Europe-wide agreed standard.

Specialist Training

One of the features of the European Union is the mutual recognition of specialty status within its member countries. Geriatric medicine is recognized as a specialty or subspecialty in Belgium, Denmark, Finland, France, Germany, Ireland, Italy, the Netherlands, Spain, Sweden, and the United Kingdom. However, it is not recognized in Greece or in Portugal. The situation in the "new" European countries in Central and Eastern Europe is in transition, with the specialty being recognized in the Czech Republic, Hungary, and Slovakia.

The UEMS-GM has produced a curriculum that should serve as a basis for those produced by national bodies. In summary, specialist training should take place over a 4-year period preceded by 2 years in general internal medicine. One of the 4 years may be in research. Training should take place predominately in hospitals. Training institutions should be capable of delivering training and have a broad range of high-quality services. Research ethics and therapeutics committees should be in place. The director of training should be a specialist of at least 5 years standing, although it is recognized that exceptions may be needed. Training should comply with all national and international requirements, and each trainee should have a named educational supervisor. Trainees should keep a personal logbook or other record of training. Following both national and EU regulations is stressed.

The duration of training varies slightly from country to country. In the United Kingdom those wishing to become a geriatrician undertake the 2-year foundation program that all physicians must complete. This is followed by 2 years of core medical training and then 5 years further training in both geriatric medicine and acute medicine. This qualifies physicians to work in both geriatric medicine and acute medicine. This pattern is similar to that of other medical specialists (e.g., respiratory medicine, diabetes) who also undertake acute medicine. In other countries, different routes exist. For example, for those wishing to practice as geriatricians in the Netherlands, there is a common trunk of 2 years in general medicine, 2 years in geriatrics, and 1 year in old age psychiatry. Consultants in general medicine with a special interest in geriatric medicine have to undertake 4 years in general medicine and 2 years in geriatrics, of which 6 months must be in old age psychiatry. In Belgium, trainees have to complete 3 years in general medicine and 3 years in geriatric medicine.

A more recent update review by Reiter and colleagues summarized the differences in training to become a geriatric medicine specialist in 14 EU member countries and in Switzerland and Turkey.[21] In 8 of the 16 countries, geriatric medicine is a "stand-alone specialty"; in 6 countries it is a subspecialty of internal medicine and, in 3 cases, of other specialties as well; whereas in 2 of the countries it is not recognized as a specialty at all. Training in geriatric medicine lasted between 1.5 years (Germany) and 7 years (United Kingdom). Total training time after qualification to become a geriatrician is shortest in Spain and France (4 years) and longest in the United Kingdom (9 years). The authors of this survey attribute these differences in training length principally to the status of the specialty. Other differences include the requirement to undertake research, to make a presentation at a national society, and to complete a specialist examination. Such differences in training must draw into question the equivalency of specialist qualifications over European borders.

European Academy for Medicine for Ageing

The need for a concerted effort to increase academic capacity in geriatric medicine in Europe has long been recognized. The linking of the development of the specialty to the state of academic geriatrics was identified by the Group of European Professors in Medical Gerontology (GEPMG).[22] This group suggested a number of concerted activities, including training junior faculty, developing a core curriculum at both undergraduate and postgraduate levels, and establishing a professorship in medical gerontology in every medical school. One of the outputs from this report was the establishment of the European Academy for Medicine of Ageing, which graduated its first cohort of potential geriatric medicine leaders in 1996.[23] The program comprised four 1-week sessions held in Switzerland which covered a broad range of biologic and clinical topics. A subsequent evaluation reporting on the first 10 years of the program[24] identified a number of important factors, including the involvement of international leaders, the intense interactive nature of the course, and the international nature of the student body, which now includes younger geriatricians from outside Europe. A large proportion of the students were able to advance their careers, but whether they would have done so without their involvement in this program is not clear. The 10th course, in 2015-2016, offered modules in principles of geriatric care, evidence-based medicine in geriatrics, cognitive behavior, and ways to provide geriatric care. Further information about the European Academy for Medicine for Ageing is available from its website (http://www.eama.eu/mvc/index.jsp).

The European Master's Program in Gerontology

This interdisciplinary program was coordinated by the Free University of Amsterdam and was designed for professionals from both health and social science backgrounds. Modules were offered in different countries, and students could study individual modules or undertake the whole course. The program closed in 2012, but an international master's degree is offered by the University of Malta (http://www.um.edu.mt/eurgeront/listofcourses).

COLLABORATIVE RESEARCH IN EUROPE

The European Union fosters collaborative international projects through its Framework programs. The current program (Framework 7) includes a number of projects relevant to the needs of older people. These have included PREDICT: Increasing the participation of older adults in clinical trials; SMILING: Self mobility improvement in older adults by counteracting falls; RESOLVE: Resolve chronic inflammation and achieve healthy aging by understanding nonregenerative repair; CAPSIL: International support of a common awareness and knowledge platform for studying and enabling independent living; and HERMES: Cognitive care and guidance for active aging. Current projects include SENATOR: Development and clinical trials of a new software engine for the assessment and optimization of drug and nondrug therapy in older persons; IMPACT: Impact of quality indicators in palliative care study; and CHROMED: Clinical trials for older adult patients with multiple diseases. Basic and translational research is also funded by the European Research Area. More information on European geriatric medicine research is available on the European Commission's Community Research and Development Information Service website (http://cordis.europa.eu/search/result_en?q=geriatric+medicine).

Other European Activities

National nongovernmental organizations have also formed European collaborations aimed at influencing European policy and offering mutual support. The European Older People's Platform AGE has as its aim "to voice and promote the interests of older people in the European Union and to raise awareness of the issues that concern them most" (http://www.age-platform.eu). The year 2012 was designated as the year of healthy aging by the European Union. The website (http://www.healthyageing.eu/) details activities of the EuroHealthNet in this area.

CONCLUSION

As has been described, the development of the specialty of geriatric medicine has progressed at varying paces in different European countries despite the demographic needs being relatively similar. A number of organizations have been established whose aim is to advance the health care of older people by professional development within the specialty of geriatric medicine and related disciplines. Several geriatricians hold office in more than one of these organizations, and it is therefore not surprising that calls have been made for working in close collaboration.[17,25]

The demographic and technologic changes that are taking place are having similar effects on the development of policy regarding health care of older people with the move to the provision of more care in the home and ever shorter hospital stays. This will have an impact on the role of the geriatrician with an increased presence outside of the hospital and a continued key role in general hospitals. It is of interest that a majority of leading European geriatricians opted for a division of geriatrics into a community and a hospital branch.[26] However, there is consensus that older people, particularly those with physical and mental health comorbidity, in whatever setting they are, need to be treated by doctors and allied health care practitioners who have received specific training in older adult care medicine.

KEY POINTS

- Geriatric medicine is an established medical specialty in the majority of countries in Europe either as a specialty in its own right or as a subspecialty.
- There are three main European organizations (European Union Geriatric Medicine Society, International Association of Gerontology and Geriatrics, and European Union of Medical Specialists–Geriatric Medicine) that support the development of the specialty of geriatric medicine through scientific conferences, policy initiatives, and publications.
- There is mutual recognition of specialist training of geriatric medicine throughout the European Union, although the duration and details of training vary from country to country.
- The European Union funds research in geriatric medicine, which requires collaboration across Europe.

For a complete list of references, please visit www.expertconsult.com.

KEY REFERENCES

8. Barton A, Mulley G: History of the development of geriatric medicine in the UK. Postgrad Med J 79:229–234, 2003.
9. Morley JE: A brief history of geriatrics. J Gerontol A Biol Sci Med Sci 59:1132–1152, 2004.
13. Skampova V, Rogalewicz V, Celedova L, et al: Ambulatory geriatrics in the Czech Republic: a survey of geriatricians' opinions. Kontact 16:e119–e131, 2014.
14. O'Neill D, O'Keeffe S: Health care for older people in Ireland. J Am Geriatr Soc 51:1280–1286, 2003.
15. Koziarska-Rościszewska K: Improving the care of older people by family physicians in Poland. New Med 1/2013, s.:9–13, 2013. http://www.czytelniamedyczna.pl/4360,improving-the-care-of-older-people-by-family-physicians-in-poland.html. Accessed January 1, 2014.
16. Romero Rizos L, Sánchez Jurado PM, Abizanda Soler P: Elderly in an acute geriatric unit. Rev Esp Geriatr Gerontol 44(Suppl 1):15–26, 2009.
17. Ribera Casado JM: Point of view IAGG/ER clinical section congresses: a brief history (remembering the past/regarding the future). J Nutr Health Aging 10:432–433, 2006.
18. Crome P, Moulias R, Sanchez-Castellano C, et al: Elder abuse in Finland, France, Spain and United Kingdom. Eur Geriatr Med 5:277–284, 2014.
19. Akdahl A, Fiorini A, Maggi S, et al: Geriatric medicine care in Europe—the EUGMS survey Part II: Malta, Sweden and Austria. Eur Geriatr Med 3:388–391, 2012.
20. Masud T, Blundell A, Gordon AL, et al: European undergraduate curriculum in geriatric medicine developed using an international modified Delphi technique. Age Ageing 43:695–702, 2014.
21. Reiter R, Diraoui S, van den Noortgate N, et al: How to become a geriatrician in different European countries. Eur Geriatr Med 5:347–351, 2014.
22. Group of European Professors in Medical Gerontology (GEPMG), Stahelin HB, Beregi E, et al: Teaching medical gerontology in Europe. Age Ageing 23:179–181, 1994.
23. Verhaar HJ, Becker C, Lindberg OI: European Academy for Medicine of Ageing: a new network for geriatricians in Europe. Age Ageing 27:93–94, 1998.
24. Bonin-Guillaume S, Kressig RW, Gavazzi G, et al: Teaching the future teachers in geriatrics: the 10-year success story of the European Academy for Medicine of Aging. Geriatr Gerontol Int 5:82–88, 2005.
25. Duursma S, Overstall P: Quality control and geriatric medicine in the European Union. Age Ageing 34:104–106, 2005.
26. Duursma SA, Overstall PW: Geriatric medicine in the European Union: future scenarios. Z Gerontol Geriatr 36:204–215, 2003.

121 Geriatric Medicine in North America

David B. Hogan

INTRODUCTION

In this chapter we examine the history and current state of geriatric medicine in Canada (2014 estimated population 35.5 million) and the United States (2014 estimated population 319 million). Although geriatric medicine developed in response to similar demographic pressures, it evolved in differing manners within the two countries.

DEMOGRAPHIC IMPERATIVE

As seen in other high-income nations, the absolute number and relative proportion of older individuals in Canada and the United States are increasing. Although a chronological age of 65 is typically used to demarcate the start of old age, this is arbitrary and not driven by a strong biologic or clinical rationale. If the intent is to describe the oldest segment of the age pyramid, the lower age cutoff should have been continuously moved upward over the past 50 years. Thirty years ago, those individuals 65 years or older made up a tenth of the Canadian population, whereas today it is nearly one in six.[1] Because of large post–World War II baby booms in the United States and Canada, the pace of societal aging will accelerate over the coming decades. In 2012 approximately 43.1 million Americans were 65 or older (13.7% of the population).[2] By 2060 the number of older individuals is projected to grow to 92.0 million. Just over one in five Americans will be 65 years or older.[2] Similar changes will be taking place in Canada, where by 2016 seniors will for the first time outnumber children younger than 15 years of age. In 2063 it is estimated that 24% to 28% of the population will be 65 years or older.[3] In 2012 life expectancy in the United States was 79 years (76 for men and 81 for women) and 82 (80 for men and 84 for women) in Canada.[4]

Although the majority of North American seniors are in good health, their per capita health cost, on average, is three to five times higher than that of younger adults.[5] Seniors currently account for approximately one fourth of physician office visits and one third of both acute care stays and consumption of prescribed medications.[6] With the projected increase in the number of seniors, health care use and costs are expected to increase. Aging, though, is less important than other drivers of rising expenditures such as increases in per capita utilization rates or the introduction of promising but costly technologies.[5] The health care workforce required to deal with the anticipated increase in demand has to be recruited, trained, and efficiently deployed.[7,8] Another issue is the financing of retirement. Rather than putting aside sufficient funds to deal with retirements that might last for 30 years or longer, Americans are now saving less for old age than in any decade since the Great Depression.[9] The average working household has virtually no retirement savings.[10] Finally, there are concerns about the potential impact on family caregiving. Already up to 40% of North American adults are caregivers to family members.[11,12] With the projected rise in the number of seniors with cognitive and functional impairments, the demand for this already strained resource will likely increase.

All of these factors have led to considerable angst about the cost and care implications of our aging population.[13] As an extreme example of this, in 1984 the governor of Colorado, Richard D. Lamm, was inaccurately but widely reported as saying older Americans had "a duty to die and get out of the way."[14] These worries are widespread. In a nationally representative survey of middle-aged and older (45 years and older) Canadians conducted in 2014, more than one fourth stated they were caring for an aging relative or friend, 6 in 10 were concerned about their financial situation during their retirement years, most lacked confidence in the ability of the health care system to provide for seniors in the future, and nearly all (95%) agreed that a national strategy on seniors' health care was needed.[15]

As will become evident, the burgeoning number of seniors hasn't been paralleled by similar growth in the number of North American subspecialists in geriatric medicine. (Note: In North America, geriatric medicine is more appropriately viewed as a subspecialty than a specialty because it is an area of focused and advanced practice that builds on prior training and/or experience in broader disciplines such as family or internal medicine.)

HISTORICAL DEVELOPMENT

Geriatric medicine deals with the study, understanding, prevention, and management of disease, disability, and frailty in later life. The rise in the number of older people during the twentieth century led to increasing interest in their care. In 1909 a New York physician, Ignatz Leo Nascher, coined the term *geriatrics*. He wrote that old age was as "distinct [a] period of life … as … childhood" and deserved "a special branch of medicine" to deal with its unique challenges.[16] In 1914 Nascher authored *Geriatrics: The Diseases of Old Age and Their Treatment* but failed in making it an enticing field of medical practice partially because, as noted in a contemporary review of the textbook, he was "inclined to dwell on the darker lines of the picture."[17,18]

During the first half of the twentieth century, medical care in Canada and the United States was organized and financed in a similar manner, leading to a good deal of cross-border movement. A number of Canadian physicians and researchers who immigrated to the United States, such as Sir William Osler whose departure from Johns Hopkins was marred by the "Fixed Period" controversy,[19] played an important role in shaping the attitudes and approaches taken by American medicine toward older persons.[17] The birth of gerontology as a scientific discipline is dated from 1939 when *The Problems of Ageing* was published.[20] This book was edited by Edmund Vincent Cowdry, who was born in Canada but spent most of his professional career in the United States, principally at Washington University in St. Louis.[17,21] The founding of the American Geriatrics Society (AGS) in 1942 predated that of the Medical Society for the Care of the Elderly (renamed the British Geriatrics Society in 1959) in the United Kingdom.[21] Canadian physicians joined the AGS in large numbers (approximately 400 were members of the AGS in 1970), with five serving as its president.[17] One of them, Willard O. Thompson, was the founding editor of the *Journal of the American Geriatrics Society*.[17,21]

Early North American geriatricians were part-time specialists with "other duties to perform from which they generally earn[ed] a living."[22] Although aging well was felt to be dependent on adhering to the advice of an experienced and sage physician,[23] no unique diagnostic or therapeutic approaches were linked to the field. The development of geriatrics as a recognized area of full-time practice in North America lagged behind the United Kingdom. As noted by John Grimley Evans, while "Nascher invented the word, Marjory Warren created the specialty."[24]

William R. Hazzard was mostly correct when he wrote that before 1978 in the United States, "there were no trained geriatricians … no geriatrics faculty … no recognition [of the field] as a specialty … [and] no designated training programs."[25] Barriers to the acceptance of geriatric medicine as a legitimate field of practice found in a number of countries include skepticism that there is a unique body of knowledge and skills, the sense that the diseases of old age are inevitable and incurable, and the relative lack of public interest in the plight of older patients compared to other patient populations (e.g., children).[26] Other issues delaying recognition in the United States included organizational ones (i.e., the multidisciplinary nature of aging societies detracted from their ability to lobby effectively within organized medicine, lack of representation within the upper reaches of the power structure of academic medicine), slow development of clinical research in aging, ageism and the unspoken fear of aging, the unwillingness of established specialties and subspecialties to share resources, and the fear within these fields that geriatric medicine would encroach into their area of practice.[27-29] There was also uncertainty about the specific form recognition should take.[30,31] It was not until 1988 that the first American certifying examination in geriatric medicine was held.[28]

Things moved more rapidly in Canada. The Council of the Royal College of Physicians and Surgeons of Canada (RCPSC) formally recognized geriatric medicine as a subspecialty of internal medicine in 1977 with the first certifying examinations held in 1981.[17] This took place in spite of persistent opposition from within organized medicine as shown by the reaction of the RCPSC Specialty Committee for Internal Medicine. They had not been consulted before the decision was taken to recognize the field. Once informed, they expressed strong disapproval and, on two separate occasions (1978 and 1979), passed motions "deploring" the recognition of geriatric medicine by the RCPSC. In their meeting minutes, recorded comments included "geriatrics is the business of internists… [And] segregation [of older patients is] not in their best interests." British geriatricians were described as "curators of parking lots" with the field a "refuge for failed internists … [where] the elderly receive very indifferent care in settings apart from other medical patients." The practice of geriatrics was stated to be "very depressing" and physicians were thought to be "more likely to perform well with a broad spectrum of patients."[17] The RCPSC committee held that geriatrics had no specific knowledge base and that advances in the care of older patients were not being made by geriatricians but by clinicians and researchers in other fields. An inescapable conclusion is that, within at least this corner of organized medicine, geriatric medicine, like its patients, was both disrespected and marginalized.[5] Another important take-home message is to never assume support and always be able to cogently make the case for the discipline.

A particular strength of American medicine is the breadth and depth of its research activities. At the close of World War II, the federal government in the United States became the world's leading funder of medical research, including that on aging.[20] Americans authored over half (53.9%) of the articles published in gerontology and/or geriatric journals in 2002.[32] This compares to 9.7% and 6.7% for contributors from the United Kingdom (the nation that ranked second) and Canada (ranked third), respectively. Important contributions to geriatric medicine[33] include work on frailty[34,35] and the creation of innovative, effective models of care for older patients.[36,37]

CARE OF OLDER PATIENTS

There are important differences between older and younger adults. Seniors typically have diminished physiologic reserves. Chronic conditions such as cardiovascular disease, stroke, diabetes, cancer, chronic obstructive airway disease, musculoskeletal conditions, and dementia are common and, when present, often severe. Of even greater note is the frequent presence within an aging patient of multiple morbidities occurring in varying combinations. Geriatric syndromes (e.g., delirium, falls, incontinence, frailty), malnutrition, sensory impairments, impaired mobility, and disability are frequently encountered. The physical and social environment of the older patient is an important consideration in the planning of their care. Polypharmacy (the consumption of many drugs together) to deal with the multiple symptoms, diseases, and risk states (e.g., hypertension, hypercholesterolemia, osteoporosis) is the rule rather than the exception. This in turn can lead to problems like adverse drug effects, prescribing cascades, disease-drug and drug-drug interactions, and nonadherence. The inherent complexity of older patients all too often leads to fragmented, uncoordinated care provided by an array of practitioners working in isolation.

In 2008 the Institute of Medicine released the report *Retooling for an Aging America*, which warned of the need to plan for the growing number of older adults.[8] Recommendations included increasing the number of geriatric specialists, redesigning how care is delivered, expanding the role of other providers, and enhancing the competency of the entire health care workforce in the care of older patients. With regard to the latter point, physicians without advanced training in geriatric medicine provide most of the medical care received by older patients in North America. A study of a representative sample of Medicare beneficiaries showed that general internists and family physicians are responsible for much of this care.[38] Specialists in geriatric medicine ranked only 38th among providers of ambulatory medical services to these patients. This will not change in the foreseeable future. The physicians (and other health care providers) providing this care require sound training about health and illness in older patients.[8] *Geriatricizing* (or *gerontologizing*) is the awkward sounding term used to describe the introduction within the various fields of medicine the principles required to successfully care for older patients.[24,25] A number of medical and surgical specialties in the United States have committed themselves to defining the specific competencies needed by practitioners in their field of practice to deal with older patients and incorporating them within both their training programs and examinations.[39]

Research shows ample room for continued improvement in the provision of care to older patients across all settings. For example, within the community, the quality of care offered for geriatric syndromes (e.g., falls, urinary incontinence, dementia, osteoporosis, hearing impairment, malnutrition) is generally worse than that provided for medical conditions (e.g., hypertension, coronary artery disease, cerebrovascular disease, diabetes, heart failure, atrial fibrillation).[40] The overall incidence of adverse events (defined as unintended injuries or complications resulting in death, disability, or prolonged hospital stay arising from the care provided) during hospitalization of adult patients in Canada is approximately 7.5/100 hospital admissions, with increasing age a statistically significant risk factor for its occurrence.[41] Finally, a recent study showed widespread use of medications with questionable benefits in nursing home residents with advanced dementia.[42]

The need to deal with the unique characteristics of seniors has to be recognized within the broader context of health care planning and delivery for the entire population. An example of this is emergency care. Hurricane Katrina and other natural disasters consistently show that older persons are at particular risk for adverse outcomes during such events. Emergency planning has to take this into account as well as the difficult ethical issues that might arise.[43-45] It is also clear that the care provided within emergency departments will have to be modified if the pending influx of aging baby boomers is to be dealt with effectively, efficiently, and humanely.[46,47]

Given that improving the care of all older patients must be a goal of our respective health care systems, how do subspecialists in geriatric medicine contribute to this overarching aspiration?

GERIATRIC MEDICINE TODAY

In the United States, the American Board of Family Medicine and the American Board of Internal Medicine jointly offer a certificate of added qualifications in geriatric medicine. After completion of a residency in either family medicine or internal medicine, trainees can take additional accredited training in geriatric medicine followed by a certifying examination. About 80% of residents are from internal medicine. Few take more than one year of training in the field. It was initially thought that physicians with subspecialty training in geriatric medicine would be principally concerned with the medical care of residents in long-term care facilities. Over time this view has evolved. Some view geriatricians as consultants called on to help with complex cases, whereas others believe that geriatricians' true calling is the provision of primary medical care to seniors.[48] Early on, and more recently as well, it has been argued that an academic model should be embraced with practitioners focusing on training other physicians, conducting research, and providing medical leadership.[48-50] In 2011 there were 7162 active board-certified geriatricians. This leads to a ratio of approximately 3.8 geriatricians per 10,000 individuals 75 years and older in the United States.[51] By 2030 the ratio is expected to drop to 2.6 per 10,000 because of the projected increase in the number of older Americans coupled with poor recruitment (and retention) of specialist physicians.[51]

There are two recognized training options available for Canadian physicians interested in geriatric medicine. Physicians who have completed their training in family medicine can enroll in a 6- or 12-month residency program in Care of the Elderly accredited by the College of Family Physicians of Canada. There is no national certifying examination for this option. Training is intended to equip graduates with the skills required to provide primary medical care to older individuals, work within specialized geriatric programs, and/or function as a medical resource for their community in the care of older patients. The second training option is restricted for those with at least 3 years of prior training in internal medicine. They can enroll in a 2-year training program accredited by the RCPSC. A national certifying examination administered by the RCPSC can be taken after first passing the specialty examination in internal medicine and successfully completing a residency in geriatric medicine. Graduates function as consultants. While physicians from either option can be involved in academic activities, graduates of the RCPSC stream are the ones principally involved in research, teaching, and program development. In 2012 there were 404 (326.15 full-time equivalents [FTEs]) Canadian specialists in geriatrics (i.e., defined as physicians with advanced clinical training or equivalent practice experience in geriatrics who work as consultants).[52] Nationally this translates to a ratio of 1.4 FTE geriatricians per 10,000 individuals 75 years or older.

It is important to mention another age-defined medical specialty, geriatric psychiatry. This field deals with the assessment and management of mental disorders in later life. Notwithstanding the field's long history in Canada,[17] the RCPSC did not recognize geriatric psychiatry as a subspecialty of psychiatry until 2009.[53] After completion of psychiatry training, a candidate can be accepted into a 2-year approved residency. As with geriatric medicine, a certifying examination is offered after successful completion of training. The first examination was held in 2013. In 2013-2014 there were nine residents in training nationally.[54] Based on reported professional society membership and the number of specialists listed in the RCPSC directory, there are more than 200 geriatric psychiatrists practicing in Canada. The American Board of Psychiatry and Neurology recognized geriatric psychiatry as a subspecialty in 1989. A certifying examination is offered at the end of successful completion of a year of postgraduate training. In 2011 there were 1751 board-certified geriatric psychiatrists in the United States.[51] A total of 63 residents were enrolled in geriatric psychiatry training programs in 2013-2014.[55] This compares to 817 in child and adolescent psychiatry training. Unfortunately the specific issues relating to geriatric psychiatry in North America are beyond the scope of this chapter.

TABLE 121-1 Number of Trainees Enrolled in Postgraduate Training Programs in Care of the Elderly (6- to 12-Month Program) and Geriatric Medicine (2-Year Program) in Canada (2004-2014)*

	Care of the Elderly	Geriatric Medicine	Total
2004-2005	10	15	25
2005-2006	12	15	27
2006-2007	10	19	29
2007-2008	14	24	38
2008-2009	13	25	38
2009-2010	9	23	32
2010-2011	11	19	30
2011-2012	13	27	40
2012-2013	17	29	46
2013-2014	19	43	62

*Data from annual reports of the Canadian Post-M.D. Education Registry.

A critical issue on both sides of the border is the recruitment and retention of physicians. Table 121-1 shows data on the number of trainees in Canada over time. The 62 Care of the Elderly and geriatric medicine trainees in 2013-2014 made up only 0.5% of all Canadian postgraduate trainees that year.[54] Trainees in pediatrics that year numbered 669 (4.3% of the total). The problem is not insufficient training positions, as annually there are unfilled ones (e.g., 14 of 27 [51.9%] training positions were unfilled in 2014).[56] In 2013, 14 Care of the Elderly and 8 geriatric medicine trainees, a total of 22, entered practice,[54] well less than what is needed to correct the current physician resource deficit, deal with population growth, and replace retirees.[52] Retention is a particular issue for physicians who received Care of the Elderly training, as slightly over 50% end up in a general family medicine practice rather than focusing on the care of older patients.[52]

Between 1988 and 1994 the U.S. certifying examination in geriatric medicine could be taken based on practice experience. After this pathway closed, there was a marked decline in the number of physicians seeking certification. In an attempt to recruit more trainees, the initial 2-year training program was shortened to a single required year in 1998. Notwithstanding this change, the number of trainees remained static. To maintain certification, an American geriatrician has to meet a number of requirements, which include passing an examination every 10 years. The "first time" recertification rate for geriatric medicine was 53.8% for those with previous internal medicine training (59.1% among those with previous family medicine training). This is substantially lower than the approximately 80% seen for other medical subspecialties.[6,51] It has been argued that those not recertifying were "closet geriatricians" who knew enough to pass the examination but lacked the commitment to make this their field of practice.[48] The low recruitment and recertification rates mean that the total number of active certificates in geriatric medicine has slowly declined since 1996.[51]

Table 121-2 provides data on the number of residents in training for the United States. In 2013 there were 146 training programs in geriatric medicine with a total of 319 (52 family medicine, 267 internal medicine) trainees. They represented less than 0.3%

TABLE 121-2 Number of Trainees from Family Medicine and Internal Medicine Enrolled in Postgraduate Training (1-Year Program for Most) in Geriatric Medicine in the United States (2004-2014)*

	Family Medicine	Internal Medicine	Total
2004-2005	46	288	334
2005-2006	50	301	351
2006-2007	44	243	287
2007-2008	46	246	292
2008-2009	64	256	320
2009-2010	54	242	296
2010-2011	64	237	301
2011-2012	56	219	275
2012-2013	65	246	311
2013-2014	52	267	319

*Data from annual *JAMA* issue on medical education.

of all residents in training compared to the 8529 (7.3%) in pediatrics. Of the 488 first-year positions, 306 (62.7%) were filled.[55] Geriatric medicine is an unpopular career choice for U.S. medical school graduates. Most of those in a training program attended a medical school outside the United States (201/319 [63.0%] in 2013-2014).[55] Assuming current rates of recruitment and retention, the predicted number of geriatricians in the United States in 2030 will be 7750, which is less than a quarter of the need for 36,000 projected by the Alliance for Aging Research.[8]

Whereas there has been a modest absolute increase in the number of Canadian trainees, there is no evidence of an increase in the U.S. figures. An important barrier to recruitment is the relatively poor pay within a fee-for-service financial model earned by geriatricians compared to most other fields of medical practice.[57] In the United States, physicians with additional training in geriatric medicine training end up making less money on average than those who don't have any such training.[58] As noted by Robert L. Kane, the "prospect of working hard for less money is not a strong recruitment device."[48] In 2010 the median salary of an American geriatrician in private practice (US$183,523) was US$5,879 less than that of a family physician not doing obstetrics and US$21,856 less than a general internist.[51] The lower average income is probably explained by the lack of financially rewarding interventions associated with the discipline, lower overall patient volumes because of the additional time required to assess and coordinate the care of complex older patients, and poor reimbursement for much of the additional work (e.g., care coordination) done to provide good care.[59,60] An area where geriatricians can command a higher salary is functioning as a hospitalist (a physician whose primary professional role is the general medical care of hospitalized patients) for older adults.[50] Hospital medicine has grown rapidly in the United States with many more practitioners than in geriatric medicine. In 2009 there was an estimated 27,600 to 29,700 active hospitalists in the United States.[61] Other reasons given for the unpopularity of geriatric medicine are similar to those that delayed its acceptance as a field of practice and include its low prestige and the perceived futility of caring for older patients.[62]

Recommendations have been made to improve recruitment in both countries, but it is uncertain how effective they will be in the long run.[8,50,63,64] The failure to recruit more trainees is particularly disheartening considering geriatricians have significantly greater career satisfaction than most other physicians in both the United States[65] and Canada.[66] As a group, geriatricians have not marketed themselves well. Negatives (e.g., relatively poor pay) tend to be accentuated while the benefits of a career in geriatric medicine (e.g., job satisfaction, life-work balance) are not highlighted. They also hide their light under a bushel with others given credit for observations such as the risks of hospitalization for older patients long known to geriatricians.[67]

FUTURE DIRECTIONS

In 2002 Robert Kane described a number of possible directions for geriatric medicine in the United States.[48] He thought if the status quo were maintained, the subspecialty could survive as a marginal academic field primarily involved in teaching others to care for older patients. Another option would be focusing on primary care with geriatricians either directly providing this to older patients with complex needs (possibly combined with providing hospital care for them when admitted) or supporting geriatric nurse practitioners who would do the bulk of the work. Practitioners might retrench within long-term care facilities, although recently nursing home medicine as a specialty separate from geriatric medicine has been proposed.[68] Geriatricians could become end-of-life specialists, but this might be in direct competition with the emerging subspecialty of hospice and palliative care.[69] Kane's preference was for practitioners to concentrate on developing and providing exemplary chronic disease care to patients defined by need rather than age.[48,70] The invited responses to Kane's article were united only in their opposition to Kane's favored option.[71-76] Most advocated holding fast, taking a "generalist strategy" and avoiding "premature narrowing" of the available options for the field.[71-73,75] A number advised placing increased emphasis on acute care,[74,76] although Leslie Libow, in a perspective published a few years later, argued that geriatrics would "lose its way if its resources are disproportionately devoted to acutely ill, hospitalized patients."[29] Although its important role in hospital-based care has been suggested as a reason for the success of geriatrics in the United Kingdom,[24] there has been a call to shift from "high-cost, reactive and bed-based care to care that is preventive, proactive and based closer to people's home."[77]

The lack of any discernible growth in the number of active geriatricians in the United States is an issue of great concern to the leaders of the field. Chris Langston (program director of the John A. Hartford Foundation, whose current mission is to improve the health of older Americans) has authored a series of posts with gloomy titles on the foundation's website about the failure to recruit more physicians into geriatric medicine ("Can Geriatrics Survive?" [August 11, 2009], "The Operation Is a Success but the Patient Has Died, Part 1 and Part 2" [March 22 and 24, 2011],"Falling Leaves, Falling Numbers" [September 15, 2011], and "Decline in Geriatric Fellows Defies Pay Boost: +10% = −10%" [December 20, 2012]). Adam G. Golden and colleagues suggested that the subspecialty is heading toward extinction in the United States.[62] They argue that it isn't a necessary branch of medicine, noting that most older patients receive care from other practitioners. In fact the majority of Americans appear to have never even heard of the term *geriatricians*.[78] The value of certification for the practitioner is questioned, and Golden holds that the care provided by geriatricians has not been shown to lead to improved outcomes. Even if an academic role could be justified, the 1-year training program was felt insufficient for developing the skills needed for this.[62] Golden argues that the discipline's limited resources should not be spent on trying to create more subspecialists but rather should be reallocated to teaching students, residents, and practicing physicians about the principles of geriatric medicine coupled with training nongeriatrician educators to assume more of this role.

Respondents to Golden and colleagues' article[62] noted the accomplishments of geriatricians and the need to retain a cadre of committed subspecialists.[79,80] National leaders believe that focusing on teaching, research, medical leadership, and caring for those most in need of their expertise will ensure that geriatric medicine plays a key role in the response of organized medicine to the aging of American society. End-of-training entrustable professional activities describe the specific expertise of a medical discipline and can help differentiate it from other fields of practice.[81] Those recently developed for geriatric medicine in the

BOX 121-1 American Geriatrics Society and Association of Directors of Geriatric Academic Programs End-of-Training Geriatrics Entrustable Professional Activities

1. Provide patient-centered care that optimizes function and/or well-being.
2. Prioritize and manage the care of older patients by integrating the patient's goals and values, comorbidities, and prognosis into the practice of evidence-based medicine.
3. Assist patients and their families in clarifying goals of care and making decisions.
4. Prevent, diagnose, and manage geriatric syndromes (broadly defined as falls and dizziness; cognitive, affective, and behavioral disorders; pressure ulcers; sleep disorders; hearing and vision disorders; urinary incontinence; weight loss and nutritional concerns; constipation and fecal incontinence; and elder abuse).
5. Provide comprehensive medication review to maximize benefit and minimize number of medications and adverse events.
6. Provide palliative and end-of-life care for older adults.
7. Coordinate health care and health care transitions for older adults with multiple chronic conditions and multiple providers.
8. Provide geriatric consultation and co-management.
9. Skillfully facilitate a family meeting.
10. Collaborate and work effectively as a leader or member of an interprofessional health care team.
11. Teach the principles of geriatrics care and aging-related health care issues to professionals, patients, families, health care providers, and others in the community.
12. Collaborate and work effectively in quality improvement and other system-based initiatives to ensure patient safety and improve outcomes for older adults.

Modified from Leipzig RM, et al: What is a Geriatrician? American Geriatrics Society and Association of Geriatric Academic Programs Ennd-of-Training Entrustable Professional Activities for Geriatric Medicine. J Am Geriatr Soc 62:924-029, 2014.

United States are shown in Box 121-1.[82] They provide a degree of clarity on the desired attributes of trainees completing 1 year of accredited training in geriatric medicine and their future role in the health care system. To fulfill the desired leadership role in academic medicine, a portion of these trainees will have to extend their residency to 2 or more years in order to acquire advanced skills in teaching, research, and/or administration.[49,50,60]

To deal with the growing gap between demand and supply in the United States, changes are required. As noted previously, suggestions have been made to enhance recruitment and retention.[8,50] Alternative pathways to subspecialty recognition are likely required.[49,60] Help from others in meeting even the core components of the discipline's mission will be needed. For example, the important role of nongeriatricians in teaching has long been acknowledged,[83] and major strides have been made in developing more clinician-educators both within the discipline and outside.[84] There is a need to refine the clinical role of the field.[50] It is clear that the number of subspecialists will be insufficient for the provision of primary and secondary medical care to all seniors. American geriatrics has been accused of trying to sit on two chairs at once by attempting to maintain both a primary care role and a consultant role.[85] Choosing one or the other would have a moderating effect on projected physician resource needs.[86] Whether in primary care or as a consultant, those with advanced training will have to restrict their clinical work to those most likely to benefit from their involvement.

BOX 121-2 Suggested Roles for Canadian Physicians with Additional Training Caring for Older Patients

A. Advocacy for older persons and their care
B. Clinical
   a. Primary clinical role was seen as providing consultations on older patients with complex needs (e.g., multiple chronic medical conditions requiring multidisciplinary care, polypharmacy) and/or geriatric syndromes (e.g., delirium, dementia, falls, frailty, impaired mobility, incontinence)
   b. Potential secondary clinical roles included
      i. Supervision of geriatric rehabilitation
      ii. Provision of medical care in long-term and supportive care settings
      iii. Acute hospital care of older patients
      iv. Provision of end-of-life care
C. Medical leadership
   a. Health policy and system development as it relates to the care of older patients
   b. Program leadership and administration
D. Academic
   a. Education
      i. Primary education roles would be on the training of
         1. Physicians (including undergraduate, general and specialty postgraduate training, and continuing medical education)
         2. Other health care providers
      ii. Secondary education roles would be targeted at
         1. Older individuals and their caregivers
         2. General public
   b. Research
      i. Primary research areas
         1. Clinical
         2. Health systems and services
      ii. Secondary research areas
         1. Biomedical
         2. Social, cultural, and environmental factors that affect the health of populations
         3. Knowledge translation

Modified from Hogan DB: Proceedings and recommendations of the 2007 Banff Conference on the future of geriatrics in Canada. Can J Geriatrics 10:133-48, 2007.

Directors of geriatric academic programs in the United States suggest that functionally impaired, medically complex very old (i.e., 85 years and older) patients with frailty, other geriatric syndromes, an unexplained decline in health, or in need of end-of-life care would be the most appropriate target population.[87] The editor in chief of the *Journal of the American Geriatrics Society*, Thomas T. Yoshikawa, wrote that formally trained geriatricians should restrict clinical services to the very old (i.e., those 80 years of age and older).[88] These target groups make up an estimated one quarter to one third of the older population. Approximately 26,000 geriatricians would be required by 2030 solely to provide primary medical care to them.[89] To reach this number, more than 850 would have to be trained on a yearly basis between now and 2030. From 2004 to 2014, the average number of residents per year entering geriatric medicine training in the United States was 309 (see Table 121-2).

There isn't a sense among Canadian geriatricians that the field is facing as severe an existential threat.[90] Possibly this is because of greater consensus on the clinical role and future direction of the field. At the 2007 Banff Conference on the future of Canadian geriatrics, participants were surveyed about the roles of practitioners.[64] Box 121-2 summarizes the responses receiving the most support. Clinical service was the most noted responsibility followed by education, research, medical leadership and administration, and advocacy. An arguable advantage of Canadian training compared to U.S. training is the 2-year program duration for internal medicine trainees, as this allows more time for acquiring the skills needed for the enumerated nonclinical roles. The overwhelming majority (93%) of the Banff Conference participants felt geriatricians were not responsible for the primary medical care of unselected older persons, with nearly two thirds (64%) in favor of restricting clinical activities to consultations. The target population of older patients would be those with complex needs and/or geriatric syndromes. Strategies to deal with the challenges facing the subspecialty endorsed at the Banff meeting included combating ageism, which is the most tolerated form of social prejudice in Canadian society[91]; better marketing of the field; improved remuneration; developing a renewed commitment to medical education (e.g., gerontologize undergraduate and postgraduate medical education, actively recruit medical students and residents, make subspecialty training more flexible, secure additional funds for training positions, and develop more continuing medical education opportunities); and reforming medical practice (e.g., explore different models of care, promote interdisciplinary collaboration, and "inoculate" protocols, guidelines, and quality improvement initiatives with geriatric principles). Others have noted the importance of advocacy, better defining the role of the field in Canada, working with primary care to develop proactive and collaborative models of service delivery, lobbying key decision makers and organizations about the importance of disseminating the principles of geriatric care within the health care system, and developing alliances with older adults and their organizations.[92,93]

CONCLUDING REMARKS

In both Canada and the United States, for the field to move forward, stakeholders within and outside the discipline will have to agree on the desired (and feasible) roles for geriatricians. This will entail the courage to make hard decisions about what not to do.[94] Although those in the subspecialty cannot personally look after all seniors, they can strive to directly care for those most likely to benefit and ensure that the needs of all seniors are being met by the health care system. The latter means that geriatricians must play important roles in advocating for seniors, training other practitioners, and taking a lead in devising innovative models of care. A sufficiently numerous and skilled cadre of committed practitioners able to accomplish these tasks will have to be recruited, retained, and supported. All this cannot be done without effective and mutually beneficial collaborations with other medical disciplines, health professions, and older persons and their families.

Although unlikely that geriatric medicine will disappear entirely as a subspecialty, it has happened in other health professions. The American Nurses Credentialing Center of the American Nurses Association formerly had two certifications in gerontological nursing: gerontological nurse practitioner (GNP) and gerontological clinical nurse specialist (GCNS). The GNP certification will not be offered after 2016, and the GCNS has already been retired. They are being replaced by credentials in caring for adults that include, but are not specific to, older individuals.[95] Although a number of factors went into this decision, one can speculate that an underlying factor was the belief that there is nothing unique about the care of older patients and that much of it is just "common sense" although, unfortunately, not common practice.[96] Striking the appropriate balance between carving out an essential, attainable, and attractive role for geriatricians while working with (and through) other practitioners to improve the care of all seniors will be the greatest challenge facing the field over the coming decades.

KEY POINTS

- Physicians without advanced training in geriatrics will provide most of the medical care received by seniors. Geriatricians have an important role to play in ensuring that these physicians receive appropriate training in the principles of effective care of older patients.
- In both Canada and the United States, the recruitment and retention of geriatricians has been relatively poor. With the anticipated growth in the number of seniors, the projected shortfall in physician resources will be significant.
- In each country, steps are needed to clarify the desired roles and responsibilities of geriatricians within the health care system, to determine the number required to fulfill these obligations, and to put into place a comprehensive strategy for the recruitment and retention of these physicians.

For a complete list of references, please visit www.expertconsult.com.

KEY REFERENCES

8. Institute of Medicine (IOM): Retooling for an aging America, Washington, DC, 2008, National Academies Press.
49. American Geriatrics Society Core Writing Group of the Task Force on the Future of Geriatric Medicine: Caring for older Americans: the future of geriatric medicine. J Am Geriatr Soc 53:S245–S256, 2005.
52. Hogan DB, Borrie M, Basran JFS, et al: Specialist physicians in geriatrics—report of the Canadian Geriatrics Society Physician Resource Work Group. Can Geriatr J 15:68–79, 2012.
60. Leipzig RM, Hall WJ, Fried LP: Treating our societal scotoma: the case for investing in geriatrics, our nation's future, and our patients. Ann Intern Med 156:657–659, 2012.
62. Golden AG, Silberman MA, Mintzer MJ: Is geriatric medicine terminally ill? Ann Intern Med 156:654–657, 2012.
63. Torrible SJ, Diachun LL, Rolfson DB, et al: Improving recruitment into geriatric medicine in Canada: findings and recommendations from the geriatric recruitment issues study. J Am Geriatr Soc 54:1453–1462, 2006.
64. Hogan DB: Proceedings and recommendations of the 2007 Banff Conference on the future of geriatrics in Canada. Can J Geriatr 10:133–148, 2007.
82. Leipzig RM, Sauvigné K, Granville LJ, et al: What is a geriatrician? American Geriatrics Society and Association of Directors of Geriatric Academic Programs end-of-training entrustable professional activities for geriatric medicine. J Am Geriatr Soc 62:924–929, 2014.
84. Helfin MT, Bragg EJ, Fernandez H, et al: The Donald W. Reynolds Consortium for Faculty Development to Advance Geriatrics Education (FD–AGE): a model of dissemination of subspecialty educational expertise. Acad Med 87:618–626, 2012.
94. Patterson C, Hogan DB, Bergman H: The choices facing geriatrics. Can Geriatr J 15:24–27, 2012.

122 Geriatrics in Asia

Jean Woo

There is varying information about older adults in countries other than Europe and North America. In general, characteristics of older adults in Asia are similar, depending on the degree of economic development; however, health and social care systems are different. This chapter describes the impact of demographic and economic changes on life expectancy, morbidity, disability, and frailty and responses of health care systems to these changes.

LIFE EXPECTANCY, MORBIDITY, DISABILITY, AND AGING WELL

According to the Organisation for Economic Co-operation and Development (OECD) 2012 health data[1] from selected Asian countries, life expectancy at birth ranges from 79.6 years for men and 86.4 years for women in Japan to 52.7 years for men and 65.8 years for women in Myanmar (Figure 122-1). Men in Hong Kong, China, enjoy the highest life expectancy among the world, 79.7 years. At the same time, the rate of population aging for many Asian countries is higher than in many developed economies. For example, the projected growth of population aged 60-plus years between 2012 and 2050 is projected to increase 2.7 times in China and 3.0 times in Indonesia.[2] As for Europe and the United States, chronic diseases is the major morbidity burden for high-income as well as lower middle income countries in Asia, such as Japan, Republic of Korea, Singapore, Hong Kong, Thailand, Malaysia, and the Philippines. Although China is not considered a low-income country overall, nevertheless, in some rural areas, there is a double burden of communicable and noncommunicable diseases (NCDs). Heart disease, stroke, and diabetes are the major NCDs. Disability-adjusted life years (DALYs), expressed as rate per 100,000 population, range from the lowest in Singapore (14,354) to the highest in Myanmar (48,793; Figure 122-2).[3]

Statistics of particular relevance to aging populations relating to dependency in activities of daily living (ADLs) are not widely available. The largest data set has been provided by the China Health and Retirement Longitudinal Study carried out in 2000, consisting of a sample of 11,199 older Chinese from 22 provinces of China. Among those aged 60 years and older, 38% reported difficulty with ADLs, 24% reported needing help with ADLs, 40% showed symptoms of depression, and 23% lived in poverty (http://charls.ccer.edy.cn/en). Two disorders were major contributors to disability—chronic pain and depression; 33% (39% women, 28% men) of older adults aged 60 years had chronic pain. The suicide rate per 100,000 for those older than 70 years was 51.5 in China, 25.5 in Japan, and 25.4 in Hong Kong, compared with 6.3 in the United Kingdom and 16.5 in the United States. This difference may be a reflection of cultural and service provision differences.

Political and economic factors play a contributory role. In China, market transition, as defined by the proportion of non–state-owned sector employees among the total number of employed persons, was shown to be positively associated with an individual's likelihood of aging successfully, independent of socioeconomic status, social support, and lifestyle factors.[4] This finding highlights the fact that the health of older adults is a function of medical, social, and political factors, so that strategies for improvement should adopt an integrated approach, as indicated by the Global Age Watch Index. The overall index is calculated as a geometric mean of four domains, of which health status is one; the others are income security, employment, and education, and enabling environment.[2] The health status domain is constructed from data on life expectancy and healthy life expectancy at 60 years and psychological well-being. For Asian countries with available data, among a total of 91 countries, Japan ranked 10, China 35, Thailand 42, Philippines 44, Vietnam 53, South Korea 67, Indonesia 71, and Cambodia 80. For the health domain, Japan ranked 5, South Korea 8, Vietnam 36, Thailand 46, China 51, Indonesia 65, Philippines 70, and Cambodia 88. It can be seen that the health of older adults should not be considered in isolation but should be considered together with other domains for achieving the goal of aging well.

TRENDS IN PREVALENCE AND INCIDENCE OF COMMON CHRONIC DISEASES AND GERIATRIC SYNDROMES

It is important to document temporal age-specific trends in common chronic diseases and geriatric syndromes affecting older adults to assess the impact on health care and social services in terms of care burden and economic costs to inform service planning. However, few countries collect such data. An example of the type of data required for health and social care planning for aging populations is provided from data recently compiled in Hong Kong, as noted in the following sections.

Diabetes

Data on incidence among Asian populations are sparse, but there is a suggestion that incidence is higher among Chinese. A population survey carried out among Hong Kong Chinese estimated the incidence of self-reported diabetes to be 55.6/1,000 people aged 65 years and older in 2003-2004.[5] At the same time, the age-adjusted mortality rates from diabetes has shown a declining trend in the past decade, from 90 to 50/100,000 population. These figures are comparable to those for Japan, with both lower than those for the urban population in mainland China, as well as available data from the United Kingdom, United States, and Australia (Table 122-1).[6-8] The self-reported prevalence in the Chinese population is similar to those reported for whites—12% for those older than 75 years and 14% for 65- to 74-year-olds. However, the prevalence based on glucose measurements is higher at 23% and 20% for women and men aged 65 to 84 years. Diabetes in older adults increases the risk of functional limitations from 1.5- to 4-fold and predisposes to poorer health-related quality of life and depressive symptoms. The attributable medical costs of diabetes in the public sector for older adults have been projected to be U.S. $0.46 billion in 2036.

Ischemic Heart Disease

Disease burden is a function of disease incidence and case fatality rate. Trends in these figures for any population will be useful in planning preventive and hospital service programs. However,

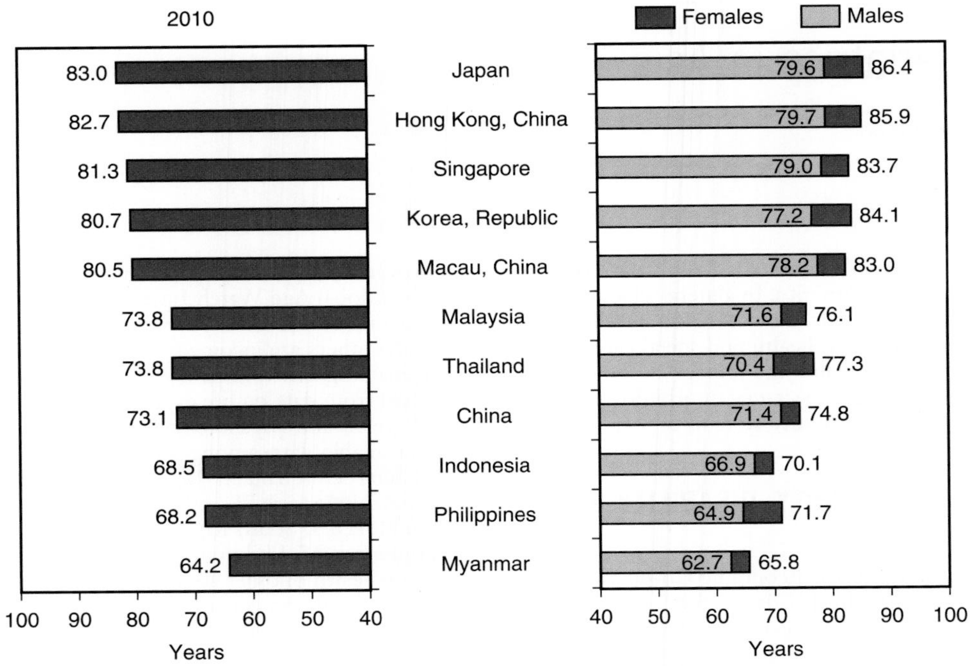

Figure 122-1. Life expectancy at birth in selected Asian countries (2010) by gender. *(From World Bank: Life expectancy at birth, total [years]. http://data.world bank.org/indicator/SP.DYN.LE00.IN. Accessed December 28, 2015.)*

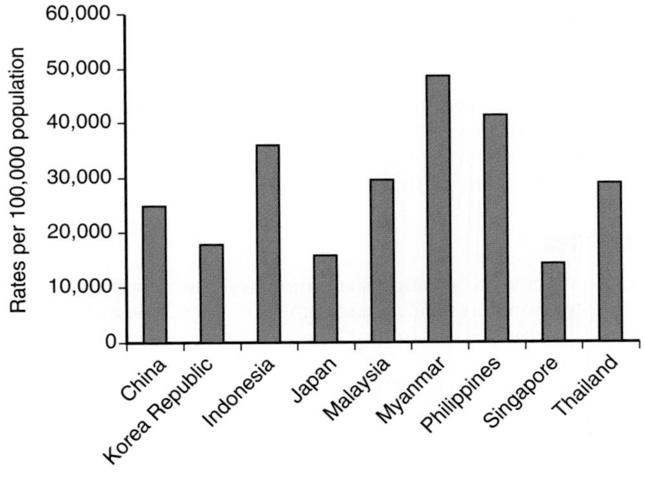

Figure 122-2. Disability-adjusted life-years in selected Asian countries. *(From World Health Organization: Chronic diseases and health promotion. http://www.who.int/chp/chronic_disease_report/en. Accessed August 29, 2014.)*

such data are not readily available. For white populations, incidence and case fatality rates have shown diverse trends, with a slow decline in the United States and a trend toward increase among certain age groups in England and Wales. Between 2000 and 2009, no overall decline in incidence was observed among a Chinese population in Hong Kong. However, the incidence for men 15 to 24, 35 to 44, and older than 85 years has shown an increasing trend, whereas those for other age groups have shown a decreasing trend. Case fatality rates remained have unchanged except for men aged 55 to 64 and 75 to 84 years and women 65 years and older. The increasing prevalence of hypertension may account for this observation.[9]

TABLE 122-1 Mortality Rates from Diabetes in Hong Kong, China, and Japan

Study	Country	Year	Age (yr)	Mortality Rate (Per 100,000 Population)
Healthy HK, Department of Health of Hong Kong, Special Administrative Region[6]	Hong Kong	2007	65-74	22.6
			75-84	64.1
			85+	141.0
Ministry of Health, Labour and Welfare of Japan, 2010[7]	China (urban areas)	2007	65-69	51.6
			70-74	106.9
			75-79	198.2
			80-84	268.5
			85+	361.6
Ministry of Health, Labour and Welfare of Japan, 2008[8]	Japan	2006	65-69	18.0
			70-74	27.9
			75-79	41.6
			80-84	62.6

Stroke

Available data during 1999 to 2007 has shown that the trend for age-adjusted ischemic stroke incidence declined in a Hong Kong Chinese population, similar to observations for white populations, although the incidence is higher. However, the overall incidence of hemorrhagic stroke remained static, except for those 35 to 44 years of age.[10] Although the incidence of stroke was lower in women, the case fatality rate was higher in women 85 years of age and older.[11] Spatiotemporal variations in incidence and case fatality rate were also observed.[12] Among older Chinese stroke survivors, poor health-related quality of life, depression, social participation, loss of self-esteem, loss of functional independence, and poor self-rated health have all been documented.

Chronic Obstructive Pulmonary Disease

Chronic obstructive pulmonary disease (COPD) is an important cause of functional limitation and dependence among older adults. Psychosocial consequences include poorer health-related quality of life and depression. Data for the incidence of COPD are sparse. In Japan, the incidence rate of clinically diagnosed COPD/1000 person-years among those aged 65 to 69 years was 27.5 for men and 16.9 for women; among those aged 70 to 74 years, the rates were 49.5 for men and 20.5 for women. Rates were lower among Hong Kong Chinese, based on self-reported data only.[13] The mortality rate/100,000 population is highest in mainland China (approximately 130), compared with much lower rates in Hong Kong and Singapore (≈20). The difference is likely to be a consequence of smoking and air pollution.

Hip Fracture

From the 1960s until 2000, hip fracture incidence increased in the Hong Kong Chinese population. From 2001 to 2009, the age-adjusted incidence rate per 100,000 population of hip fracture among those aged 65 years and older in Hong Kong started to decline, from 381.6 for men and 853.3 for women to 341.7 for men and 703.1 for women, with no significant changes in post-fracture mortality trends.[14] This follows the pattern of economically developed countries, which initially showed an increasing trend that declined following a peak.

Dementia

The percentage of community-dwelling people aged 60 years and older in Hong Kong with dementia[13] increased from 0.6% in 2009 to 1.1% in 2004 and remained stable until 2008. The percentage of older adults aged 70 years and older with clinically diagnosed dementia increased from 4.5% in 1995 to 9.3% in 2005 to 2006 and approximately doubled every 5 years until 90 years of age; the prevalence was higher in women compared with men. Approximately 30% of people aged 60 years and older living in residential care homes have dementia. Age-adjusted mortality rates for dementia (per 100,000 population) for those aged 60 years and older have shown an increasing trend from 2001 (23.3 for men and 47.3 for women) to 2009 (45.6 for men and 62.0 for women). These figures are comparable to those of mainland China, lower than among whites in the United Kingdom, United States, and Australia, but higher than Japan and Singapore. Increasing awareness and diagnosis may account for the increasing trend. However, increasing trends of prevalence of midlife risk factors, such as low physical activity, hypertension, and diabetes, may also contribute to the increase in late-life dementia.[15] These trends represent considerable challenges to long-term care in community and residential care settings and highlight the need for capacity building and adaptations in health care settings when caring for those with dementia.

Frailty

The concept of frailty has been recognized among geriatricians in Asia. Frailty has primarily been a topic of epidemiologic research using the phenotypic model developed by Fried and colleagues[16] as well as the multiple deficit model proposed by Rockwood and associates.[17] Studies using both definitions have been carried out in the Hong Kong Chinese population and showed the ability of this measure to predict mortality, functional, and cognitive decline, as well as the susceptibility of those with frailty syndrome to social and environmental factors.[18-22] This is in accord with the concept of frailty being multidimensional. Similar studies on population prevalence and risk factors have been carried out in Malaysia[23] and community-dwelling older adults in Beijing, China.[24] A frailty index was constructed using the multiple deficit model for the Beijing Longitudinal Study of Aging II Cohort. Using an empirical cutoff value of 0.25 or higher, the overall prevalence of frailty was 13%. The prevalence was higher in women and higher in those 85 years of age and older (33% for women and 18.5% for men). Urban living, being single, daily exercise less than 30 minutes, daily sleep less than 6 hours, having three or more chronic diseases, and taking four or more medications were risk factors for frailty. At 12 months, frailty increased the risk of falls, hospital admission, ADLs, dependency, and mortality. In Japan, the Kihon Checklist, an assessment of frailty, is used routinely in long-term care management plans.[25]

The incorporation of some assessment of frailty into everyday clinical practice has been limited as a result of the need to operationalize the criteria. The FRAIL score,[26] a brief assessment consisting of five questions, may be suitable for clinical practice or population screening. It has been shown to have similar predictive characteristics as other scales. It is quick and may be applied by non–health care professionals. Recently, it has been used in frailty screening of community-living older Chinese aged 65 years and older in Hong Kong. The score was initially determined by volunteers—12.5% were identified as frail, 52% as prefrail, and 35% as robust. These proportions were similar to those from large-scale epidemiologic studies.[23,24]

Sarcopenia

Similarly, the concept of sarcopenia has been gathering momentum, as in other parts of the world, spearheaded by research studies. Of the 97 articles published on sarcopenia between January and November in 2013, 18% were from Asia. Much research effort has been concentrated in the definition. Currently, there appears to be worldwide consensus that the diagnosis should encompass measurements of muscle mass, muscle strength, and muscle function.[27-30] However, the need to use cutoff points has raised the question of whether those derived from whites, who have a larger body size, could be applied to Asians. Preliminary data have shown that there are differences between whites and Asians, even within Asian populations.[31] The Asian Working Group has published Asian criteria and cutoff points: 6-m walking speed, 0.8 m/second; grip strength, less than 26 kg for men and less than 18 kg for women; dual-energy x-ray absorptiometry (DXA) height-adjusted appendicular mass (ASM) of 7.0 kg/m^2 for men and 5.4 kg/m^2 for women.[29] However, these values are from a consensus panel and there are uncertainties due to lack of data. For example, the walking speed cutoff may be higher, at 1.0 m/second. Ideally, cutoff values should be derived from longitudinal data using mobility limitation as the key outcome for these values to be related to. Such an exercise has been carried out in the United States. Cutoff values were determined using incident mobility limitation (gait speed < 0.8 m/second) as the key outcome. Interestingly, grip strength was less than 26 for men and less than 16 for women, values similar to Asian Working Group for Sarcopenia (AWGS) criteria. The ratio of ASM to weight was also proposed to take into account the adverse impact on muscle function as a result of obesity. Further research to establish cutoff values for the measures described for Asians using longitudinal study data is indicated.

A collection of studies representing the current status of sarcopenia research in China, Hong Kong, Taiwan, Japan, Thailand, and Korea has been summarized in a special issue of *Geriatrics and Gerontology International.*[32] Age-related changes in anthropometric measures used in sarcopenia definition, methodologic problems, sarcopenia as a reversible state, prevalence, and risk factors are described.

Multimorbidity, Dependency, and Frailty

Although the concept of frailty has begun to be accepted among geriatricians from research and practical clinical perspectives, the views regarding the needs of aging populations in primary care settings predominantly center on multimorbidity and perhaps dependency. These factors were examined concurrently among 4000 Chinese older adults aged 65 years and older living in the community to determine whether they are interchangeable or whether they need to be considered separately with respect to adverse outcomes.[33] Only 15% had none of these syndromes, whereas all three were present in 11%. Of the remainder, there were various degrees of overlap between the three states: frailty and multimorbidity, 28.2%; frailty and dependency, 2.8%; multimorbidity and dependency, 4.5%. Different states had different associations with adverse outcomes; 9-year mortality was associated with the frail state alone and combinations that included the frail state. Only a combination of all three states, and age per se, increased the risk of depressive symptoms at 4-year follow-up. Multimorbidity, but not frailty or dependency, and all combinations that included multimorbidity, were associated with polypharmacy (use of four or more medications). These emerging concepts would be important in prevention, management, and design of service delivery models, as well as intervention research using randomized trials.

IMPACT OF THE LIVING ENVIRONMENT

Although there is a large volume of research on the influence of personal factors, such as lifestyle, socioeconomic, and psychosocial factors on health among older adults, there have been comparatively few studies on the health impact of the living environment. This dimension could be equally important from a preventive perspective if attributable risk from environmental factors is of a comparable magnitude to personal factors. Furthermore, few studies have used outcome indicators of relevance to older adults, such as quality of life and frailty, in addition to the traditional outcomes, such as mortality and morbidity.

Spatial and temporal variations in incidence and case fatality have been documented for stroke and hip fracture for older adults aged 65 years and older, even within the 18 districts of Hong Kong, which covers a total area of only 1070 km^2. Furthermore, regional variations occur in health-related quality of life, frailty, and 4-year mortality. These variations are independent of socioeconomic and lifestyle risk factors, and the magnitude of direct regional effects is comparable to those of socioeconomic and lifestyle factors. These observations suggest that there are as yet unidentified environmental factors that should be identified in efforts to reduce health disparities in older adults.[21]

With respect to the neighborhood environment, studies carried out among white populations have shown that it influences physical and mental health. Characteristics of a so-called desirable neighborhood for older adults have been listed under eight domains by the World Health Organization Age-Friendly City initiative.[34] However, there are few data regarding how neighborhood factors affect health of older people in Asia. In a comparative study of older adults living in Hong Kong and Beijing, the higher level of happiness among Beijing older adults was attributed to their larger social networks.[35] A telephone survey of 814 people living in two contrasting districts in Hong Kong has shown that older adults rated leisure facilities, hospitals, and social facilities lower compared with younger age groups. Adjusting for individual sociodemographic characteristics, walkability was the strongest factor associated with the physical component of health-related quality of life, particularly in the older age groups. A study has shown that the ideal neighborhood for older adults using user-oriented and participatory approaches indicates that the optimum location of facilities should be clustered together and within 15 minutes walking distance from home, with covered walkways and close to green spaces.[36] Such information would be important for age-friendly urban design.

It is well documented that older adults are more susceptible to stress induced by temperature extremes. This phenomenon occurs even in temperate climates in Asia, because it is the extremes of a temperature range to which the body adapts, rather than absolute values. For example, in a subtropical climate such as Hong Kong, where the average monthly minimum and maximum temperatures range from 14.1° to 31.3° C (57° to 88° F), mortality and hospital admissions from ischemic heart disease and stroke increase at both temperature extremes among older adults aged 65 years and older.[37] The number of falls that result in going to the Accident and Emergency Department also increases during winter months, which is more likely to be related to the effect of cold on muscle function rather than on ice- or snow-related accidents.[38] The lack of indoor heating in homes and residential care homes for older adults likely contributed to hospital admissions for hypothermia, as well as increased admissions for ischemic heart disease.[39] Thus, even in a subtropical climate, there is a need to maintain an optimum indoor temperature.

SELF-MANAGEMENT OF CHRONIC DISEASES

The increasing prevalence of chronic diseases and multimorbidity with population aging highlights the need to develop self-management and coping skills to mitigate the impact. Raising health literacy is a first step, followed by acquiring self-management skills in coping and living with chronic disease. A behavioral therapy approach to self-management has been developed to be a key feature of self-management programs, and the first model for single chronic diseases has been promoted in the United States.[40] Problem-solving skills and the ability to make action plans are core features of self-efficacy, which is an essential feature of self-management. However, it is uncertain whether these principles can be applied to older adults with multimorbidity coexisting with various geriatric syndromes. This model was explored in a case-control study of Chinese adults aged 65 years and older. The intervention group underwent a 6-week Chronic Disease Self-Management Program (CDSMP) based on the Lorig program, consisting of 2.5-hour weekly group sessions. Because the desired effect is change in behavior, assessment was also carried out after 6 months to determine whether there were any long-lasting changes. Those in the intervention group achieved better self-efficacy, better health status in terms of reduced social and role activity limitation, reduced depressive symptoms, less health distress, pain, and discomfort, and better self-rated health. Age, education level, and frailty did not affect outcomes. Self-management principles incorporated into group programs for chronic obstructive pulmonary disease, congestive heart failure, and arthritis have also been evaluated and shown to produce beneficial outcomes.

AGE-FRIENDLY SERVICE DELIVERY

The increasing prevalence of multimorbidity, dependency, and frailty in aging populations described above results in heterogeneous service needs. Health care systems need to be redesigned to match the needs of older adults across a declining continuum, from a robust state to living with chronic disease to a frail state, followed by disability, dependency, and end-of-life stages, requiring care in diverse settings. Key features include coordination of care across conditions, health care providers, and settings, enhancement of knowledge and information among patients and providers, and medical social service integration. The cornerstone of care for older adults is primary care, covering preventive, supportive, rehabilitative, and maintenance of physical and cognitive functions. Hospital care is essentially episodic and covers end-of-life care. In most parts of Asia, the needs of frail older adults are beginning to be understood, so that community services are being redesigned. For the most part, primary care services are still modeled on clinic-based physician consultation and drug prescription, as for the general adult population. Efforts toward long-term care of older adults are being undertaken in various countries.

Primary Care

Preventive care is an important part of primary care. One performance measure of the effectiveness of preventive services is avoidable mortality. Cardiovascular diseases and malignancies were the largest contributors to avoidable mortality in Hong Kong. A comparison with other cities worldwide has shown that the avoidable mortality rate is similar to that in New York, higher than in Paris, and lower than in inner London. However, taking into account ethnic and lifestyle differences among these populations by using avoidable mortality proportion, derived by dividing the avoidable mortality rate by the total mortality rate, Hong Kong has the highest avoidable mortality proportion.[41] This is likely a reflection of primary care being largely out of pocket, and there is no universal medical insurance system in Hong Kong.

The Department of Health runs 18 older adult health care centers that provide screening at low cost; however, there are long waiting lists of more than 1 year. The Hospital Authority also provides community outreach geriatric and psychogeriatric teams to support people who have just been recently discharged from hospital. There are also geriatric day hospitals that may be used for comprehensive geriatric assessment by multidisciplinary teams for frail older adults, as well as for rehabilitation.

Various community models involving multidisciplinary teams have been piloted and evaluated. One example is the Hong Kong Jockey Club Cadenza Hub, which seeks to integrate health activities into social settings. The spectrum of activities mirrors the changing states experienced by older adults in a downhill trajectory and includes health promotion activities through lifestyle change, health maintenance, and chronic disease self-management, rehabilitation, and day care for the very frail. In such settings, screening for various domains can be carried out covering physical, psychological, functional, nutritional, and social domains. Frailty screening may also be carried out using simple tools such as the FRAIL score.[22] Such centers can complement medical consultations and facilitate one-stop nonmedical management plans, such as muscle-strengthening exercises and nutrition advice.

Care in Hospitals

In Hong Kong, as well as in mainland China, many hospitals function as the first stop for people seeking health care. In Hong Kong, many older people use the Accident and Emergency Department for any health problems because it is free for those who cannot afford to pay. The demands for hospital services are greater than the available supply, and the duration of stay in acute hospitals is about 4 days, on average. Patients may be transferred to nonacute hospitals if stable for further management; the average duration of stay in these hospitals ranges from 14 to 21 days. As in other parts of the world, these limitations constitute considerable challenges to managing frail older adults unless there are well-developed, long-term, community care support systems. Lack of training among health care professionals, in addition to staff shortages, results in a large proportion of older adults being placed in restraints and a nasogastric (Ryles) tube inserted. On the whole, delirium, dementia, incontinence, and falls are poorly managed.

Long-Term Residential Care

Largely as a result of suitable community services to enable frail older adults to live at home, especially for those with dementia, the proportion of those aged 65 years and older living in long-term residential care settings is highest compared to Japan, Singapore, Taiwan, and mainland China, as well as Europe, the United States, and Canada. It is approximately 5% for those aged 60 years and older, rising to 21% for women and 11% for men aged 80 years and older.[42] About 80% of these are privately run. Costs constraints such as high rent and a trained staff shortage render it difficult for most institutions to provide high-quality care. Affordability is also an issue, so that homes without government funding may have vacancies and government-supported homes have long waiting lists. Dementia is the most common precipitating factor for residential care.

End-of-Life Care

Services for end-stage noncancer chronic diseases have lagged behind the development of palliative services for cancer patients in many Asian countries. In recent years, geriatricians have been spearheading the development of such services in some hospitals in Hong Kong as well as in Singapore. In Hong Kong, a series of continuous quality improvements (CQIs) were first carried out in a nonacute hospital; a new model was tested and evaluated and then applied to the acute hospital and residential care settings. First, the gap between service needs from the patient's perspective and service provisions was documented.[43] The hospital survey showed that patients with end-stage chronic diseases have a high prevalence of symptoms, similar to those dying of cancer. The CQI consisted of education through seminars, ward-based meetings, role play aiming at culture change and identification of barriers toward change, using community support services, and improving the caregiver's experience. The CQI resulted in reductions in length of stay, number of unnecessary investigations, and hospital readmissions. Applying this model to the residential care setting facilitated direct admission to nonacute hospitals for predefined categories of residents enrolled in the end-of-life care program, bypassing waiting and unnecessary investigations at the Accident and Emergency Department.[44,45] At the same time, the promulgation of advanced directives facilitated such developments.

Development of Gerontechnology

The development of technology that may benefit older adults to delay dependence or facilitate care in Asia has largely been driven by industry. Industry has developed products thought to be of use from the developers' point of view. Few products are developed together in consultation with end users or older adults themselves. The result is that the huge potential of the so-called silver market has been frequently promoted, but has not yet been realized. Japan, Korea, and Taiwan lead Asia in the development of such products.[46]

The use of robots in social and personal care settings in Japan is particularly impressive. Tracking and monitoring devices are also increasingly used. Over a decade ago, Hong Kong started medical and multidisciplinary support of residential care homes by the hospital geriatric team using teleconferencing for medical and nursing assessment and consultation, physiotherapy and occupational therapy assessment and treatment, psychiatric consultation, and podiatry evaluation and treatment using the camera function to monitor progress.[47]

Recently, a housing complex for older adults has incorporated smart features such as movement sensors and physiologic monitoring, with signals monitored centrally by health care staff. Multisensory gadgets are being increasingly used for dementia patients in hospitals for behavior disturbance as alternatives to drugs. In community settings, the use of toys, social robots such as the baby seal PARO, and computer gaming in various types of rehabilitation are increasing. A pilot study using PARO for people with dementia has been found to improve mood and social interaction.[48]

Training and Research

Asian countries have formed a close relationship with the International Association of Gerontology and Geriatrics (IAGG) by participating in master classes held in Taiwan, Hong Kong, Beijing, Kyoto, and Seoul. Participants from Thailand, Malaysia, Singapore, and India also attended. Apart from talks on common geriatric diseases and syndromes, the master classes also incorporated a research element, in which participants presented a project and international and regional teachers provided critique and encouragement. Through such settings, the Asian Group on Sarcopenia Research was started, culminating in the consensus panel definition for sarcopenia among Asians[29] and the participation of members from Hong Kong, Taiwan, and Japan in the International Sarcopenia Initiative.[49]

There are also various collaborative geriatric training programs in institutions from the United States, Europe, and Asian hospitals and universities, such as the Johns Hopkins–Peking Union Medical College in Beijing. The British Geriatrics Society has regular teaching sessions in Taiwan. Through such activities, mutual learning and research may flourish.

KEY POINTS

- Populations in Asia are aging, accompanied by an increasing prevalence of morbidity and disability. The Global Age Watch Index has introduced a four-domain model to monitor whether countries are aging well.
- There is an increasing burden from diabetes, stroke, ischemic heart disease, fracture, and dementia, from an increasing incidence rate or decreasing mortality rate, or both.
- Frailty and sarcopenia are syndromes that are receiving increasing attention, with efforts to incorporate screening and management into clinical practice.
- Physical and social living environments affect the well-being of older adults.
- Primary care and chronic disease self-management are becoming increasingly important in health care for older adults.
- Health care systems need to adapt to the long-term care needs of aging populations in the provision of acute care, residential care, end-of-life care, and role of gerotechnology. In parallel, training and research needs to be reinforced.

For a complete list of references, please visit www.expertconsult.com.

KEY REFERENCES

2. HelpAge International: Global Age Watch Index 2013: insight report. http://reports.helpage.org/global-agewatch-index-2015-insight-report.pdf. Accessed December 23, 2015.
9. Chau PH, Wong M, Woo J: Trends in ischaemic heart disease hospitalization and case fatality in the Hong Kong Chinese population 2000-2009: a secondary analysis. BMJ Open 3:e002963, 2013.
10. Chau PH, Woo J, Goggins WB, et al: Trends in stroke incidence in Hong Kong differ by stroke subtype. Cerebrovasc Dis 31:138–146, 2011.
13. Yu R, Chau PH, McGhee SM: Trends in prevalence and mortality of dementia in elderly Hong Kong population: projections, disease burden, and implications for long-term care. Int J Alzheimers Dis 2012:406852, 2012.
14. Chau PH, Wong M, Lee A, et al: Trends in hip fracture incidence and mortality in Chinese population from Hong Kong 2001-09. Age Ageing 42:229–233, 2013.
15. Woo J, Wong M: Targeting mid-life risk factors to reduce late-life dementia. Public Health 128:952–954, 2014.
16. Fried LP, Tangen CM, Walston J, et al: Frailty in older adults: evidence for a phenotype. J Gerontol A Biol Sci Med Sci 56:M146–M156, 2001.
17. Rockwood K, Fox RA, Stolee P, et al: Frailty in elderly people: an evolving concept. CMAJ 150:489–495, 1994.
18. Goggins WB, Woo J, Sham A, et al: Frailty index as a measure of biological age in a Chinese population. J Gerontol A Biol Sci Med Sci 60:1046–1051, 2005.
19. Woo J, Goggins W, Sham A, et al: Social determinants of frailty. Gerontology 51:402–408, 2005.
20. Woo J, Goggins W, Sham A, et al: Public health significance of the frailty index. Disabil Rehabil 28:515–521, 2006.
21. Woo J, Chan R, Leung J, et al: Relative contributions of geographic, socioeconomic, and lifestyle factors to quality of life, frailty, and mortality in elderly. PLoS One 5:e8775, 2010.
29. Chen LK, Liu LK, Woo J, et al: Sarcopenia in Asia: consensus report of the Asian Working Group for Sarcopenia. J Am Med Dir Assoc 15:95–101, 2014.
30. Studenski SA, Peters KW, Alley DE, et al: The FNIH sarcopenia project: rationale, study description, conference recommendations, and final estimates. J Gerontol A Biol Sci Med Sci 69:547–558, 2014.
34. World Health Organization: Global age friendly cities: a guide, Geneva, Switzerland, 2007, World Health Organization.
41. Chau PH, Woo J, Chan KC, et al: Avoidable mortality pattern in a Chinese population—Hong Kong, China. Eur J Public Health 21:215–220, 2011.
44. Woo J, Cheng JO, Lee J, et al: Evaluation of a continuous quality improvement initiative for end-of-life care for older noncancer patients. J Am Med Dir Assoc 12:105–113, 2011.
49. Cruz-Jentoft AJ, Landi F, Schneider S, et al: Prevalence of and interventions for sarcopenia in ageing adults—a systematic review report of the international Sarcopenia Initiative (EWGSOP and IWGS). Age Ageing 43:748–759, 2014.

123 Geriatrics in Latin America

Fernando Gomez, Carmen-Lucia Curcio

Most older people live in less developed countries, and these countries will experience the most rapid aging compared with other countries. For example, in Latin American and Caribbean (LAC) countries, population aging will be the most significant demographic trend of the coming decades. From the mid-twentieth century to the present, the region has shown an accelerated aging of its population: from the 561 million people living in this region, about 5.7% are 65 years or older. The proportion of the population aged 60 years or older increased from 6% in 1950 to 10% in 2010. It is expected to reach 21% in 2040 and nearly 36% by 2100.[1] LAC populations are aging at a faster rate than the population in North American and European countries. Most developed nations have had decades to adjust to their changing age structures. For example, it took more than 100 years for the share of France's population aged 65 years or older to rise from 7% to 14%, whereas in Latin America the same percentage increase took only 50 years.[2] Furthermore, many countries of the region are experiencing a rapid increase in the number and percentage of older people, often within a single generation. By 2025, the number of people older than 60 years in LAC countries will be increased twofold to threefold, from 43 million to 100 million. Fertility and mortality decline have occurred in less than half the time observed in industrialized countries. In Latin America, older persons are predicted to outnumber children for the first time by around 2036, and their numbers will continue to grow until 2080.[2]

In conclusion, by the mid-twenty-first century, the region may be at the same stage of the aging process as the developed countries now are, with 1 in 5 people aged 60 years or older.

As a consequence, the demographic transition has taken place rapidly, although there is still some diversity among countries. Within these countries, at the regional level, two major changes have taken place: a reduction in demographic dependency and population aging.[1] For example, in countries with old and very old populations (Cuba, Barbados, Argentina, and Uruguay), a drastic situation is expected to arise during the second half of the twenty-first century, comparable with that of Europe in terms of the age structure of the population.[3] Thanks to medical and health care advances, life expectancy indices are at levels that were unimaginable just a few decades ago. Over the past 25 years, the life expectancy in LAC countries has increased: 79% of the population will reach old age and at least 40% will live until 80 years. Life expectancy at 60 years varies across the region: it is 19 years for men and 22 years for women.[2] However, this phenomenon of rapid aging has not been accompanied by social and health policy reforms that appropriately address the needs of an aging country.[4]

The Economic Commission for Latin America and the Caribbean (ECLAC) has classified LAC countries into four stages of demographic transition according to life expectancy and fertility rates.[3] Cuba and Barbados have been classified as being at a very advanced stage of demographic transition; both countries have seen the mortality rate decline more slowly than the fertility rate. Among the countries at an advanced stage of demographic transition are Argentina, Uruguay, and Chile; all three countries saw an early drop in their vital rates with growth rates lower than 1%. Unlike other countries at an advanced stage of transition, Brazil, Colombia, Costa Rica, and Mexico have growth rates between 1.3% and 1.4%. Brazil and Colombia have achieved the least in terms of increasing life expectancy (72.4 years and 72.8 years, respectively). In full demographic transition are Venezuela, Dominican Republic, Ecuador, El Salvador, Panama, and Peru; their fertility rates had declined considerably in the past two decades. Finally, the countries at a moderate stage of demographic transition are Bolivia, Guatemala, and Haiti.[3]

With respect to epidemiologic transition, LAC countries are characterized as a "prolonged polarized model," with high incidence of communicable and noncommunicable diseases. High death rates from infectious diseases are commonly associated with poverty, poor diets, and limited infrastructure found in the region. Most LAC countries have passed the epidemiologic transition, and the main causes of mortality and morbidity in these countries have shifted from infectious diseases to degenerative diseases, including disability-causing disorders such as osteoarthritis. However, the characteristic of LAC countries is heterogeneity in the epidemiologic transition between social groups and geographic areas within each country and among the countries. For example, death caused by communicable diseases has a rate of less than 10% in Uruguay, Costa Rica, Cuba, and Chile, whereas it is higher than 30% in Peru, Bolivia, Guatemala, and Haiti. Behind apparent uniformity, LAC countries are extremely diverse, reflecting a long history of human settlement.[5]

Although the demographic peculiarity described in this chapter makes the aging process in developing countries unique, it is by no means the only one that stands out. Indeed, the demographic process takes place within the boundaries of institutional arrangements, political organization, and cultural superstructure that are, to say the least, in contrast to those that hosted the aging process in Europe and North America. The blend of unique demography with contrasting economic, institutional, political, and cultural contexts can result in very large diversity of aging processes, diversity that, if identified and suitably taken into account, can go a long way toward explaining observed regularities.[6]

HEALTH OF OLDER ADULTS IN LATIN AMERICA AND THE CARIBBEAN

The major study on the health of older adults in LAC countries is the Salud, Bienestar y Envejecimiento en América Latina y Caribe (SABE) study (Survey on Health, Well-being and Aging in Latin America and the Caribbean), a multicentric project conducted by the Pan-American Health Organization (PAHO).[6-9] It included 10,891 people aged 60 years and older, living in seven big cities of the region (Bridgetown, Buenos Aires, Havana, Mexico City, Montevideo, Santiago, and Sao Paulo). SABE was based on a probabilistic, stratified, multistage, cluster-sampling design of the noninstitutionalized older adult population of the seven participating cities. The SABE study represented a milestone in the field of population aging in the region and could provide enough information to study the phenomena of aging in detail. Results of SABE increased understanding of the aging process and the formulation of public policy toward the well-being of LAC populations and provided a solid base for a second generation of studies in the region.[7]

Data from the SABE study showed that a high percentage of old people have a poor self-perception of their health. The cities with the highest proportions of individuals in bad self-reported health were found in Santiago (21%), Mexico City (20%), and

Havana (13%), whereas those with the lowest were found in Buenos Aires, Bridgetown, and Montevideo (5% to 7%). The poor self-reported health was higher in women and old age groups. The mean number of self-reported chronic conditions increased with age and is higher for females than it is for males. Of all chronic conditions highlighted in the SABE survey, arthritis, heart disease, obesity, and diabetes are the most salient across all LAC regions.[8] The prevalence of self-reported diabetes in this study ranged from 12.9% (Santiago) to 21.6% (Mexico City); diabetes is directly related to diet and obesity and has a strong association with disability. This study also documented that the prevalence of difficulties in activities of daily living (ADLs) fluctuated between 14% in Bridgetown and 23% in Santiago (the mean for the LAC region was 19%). Difficulties with instrumental activities of daily living (IADLs) ranged from 12% in Montevideo to 40.3% in Sao Paulo. There are strong age gradients and important gender differences in self-reported limitations in ADLs and IADLs. The SABE study also focused on basic problems, such as falls and mental health. The prevalence of falls varied from 21.6% in Bridgetown to 34.0% in Santiago. The prevalence of cognitive decline evaluated by the Mini Mental State Examination (MMSE) was 1.1% in Montevideo and 12% in Sao Paulo, and depression oscillated between 21.5% and 33.2%.[4]

In conclusion, the most important findings of SABE include all LAC countries differ in self-reported health but exhibit much less difference in terms of functional limitations. The number of chronic conditions increases with age and is higher among females than among males. On average, SABE countries display levels of self-reported diabetes (and obesity) that are as high as if not higher than those found in the United States. Furthermore, there is evidence suggesting deteriorated health and functional status in the region, and there is important evidence pointing toward rather strong inequalities (by education and income) in selected health-related outcomes.[4]

At least 40 papers from the SABE study have been published in the past decade on topics such as gender,[10] chronic conditions,[11,12] hypertension,[13] diabetes mellitus,[14,15] obesity,[16] cancer,[17] anthropometric measures,[18] mobility,[19] frailty and sarcopenia,[20-23] disability,[24-28] falls,[29] depression,[30,31] cognitive function,[32] and caregivers.[33]

After the SABE study was conducted in Latin America, several cross-sectional studies were carried out in the region. Between 2009 and 2010 in Ecuador, a similar study with emphasis on the aborigine population (10.4% of total population), SABE Ecuador, was conducted.[34] As expected, ethnicity was found to be a critical factor in poverty, inequity, and social exclusion for aborigines in the region. Data from this study showed that at least half of the aborigine older people live in extreme poverty situation, with no access to health services and high vulnerability status due to socioeconomic conditions and ethnicity.[35] Recently, with a similar methodology of SABE study, a cross-sectional survey including 2044 people of 60 years and older, living in the urban zone of Bogota (Colombia), was conducted.[36] A SABE Colombia study with a similar methodology of original study is in progress.

Longitudinal Studies

In the past decade, several population longitudinal studies in aging have been conducted in the LAC region.

The **Costa Rican Study on Longevity and Healthy Aging**, known by its Spanish language acronym CRELES, is a longitudinal study of a nationally representative sample of adults born before 1945 (aged 60 years and older in 2005), a total 2900 respondents, residing in Costa Rica, with oversampling of the oldest old.[37] One of the most important findings of this study is that organ-specific functional reserve biomarkers (hand grip strength, walking speed, and pulmonary peak flow), along with C-reactive protein, hemoglobin A_{1c}, and DHEAS, have been found to be suitable biomarkers for improving the identification of vulnerable individuals in an older adult population of the developing world.[38] Several papers of this study have been published with emphasis on cardiovascular risk factors,[39] hypertension,[40] socioeconomic status,[37,41] and neuroendocrine system dysfunction.[42]

Another longitudinal study in the region is **REDE FIBRA** (Frailty in the Brazilian Elderly Study). The REDE FIBRA study was carried out in 17 Brazilian cities, designed to identify conditions of frailty in relation to social, demographic, health, cognitive, functional, and psychosocial variables in community-dwelling older adults.[43] The aim of this study was to determine the traits, prevalence, and associated biologic, psychological, and environmental factors related to the frailty syndrome. At this time, the study continues with only the Rio de Janeiro sample (FIBRA-SJ) with 847 individuals aged 65 years or older. This study has three phases, the first related with frailty and risk factors,[44] the second with cognitive impairment,[45] and the third (ongoing) with sarcopenia. Results of this longitudinal study have revealed identifying characteristics of Brazil's older people with respect to frailty, cognitive impairment, and sarcopenia.

A Mexican population-based cohort study, the **Mexican Study of Nutritional and Psychosocial Markers of Frailty** (also referred to as the **"Coyoacan cohort"**), was designed to assess the nutritional and psychosocial determinants of frailty and its consequences on the health of Mexican older adults living in Coyoacan, one of the 16 districts of Mexico City. A total of 1124 noninstitutionalized men and women aged 70 years and older participated.[46] Papers based on results from the Coyoacan cohort study cover topics such as normative data for the MMSE and Isaacs Set Test to use in the Mexican older population,[47] the close relationship between self-perception of oral health and the probability of being frail,[48] the importance of urinary incontinence as a factor in decreased health-related quality of life,[49] and the influence of writing and reading skills of older people with no formal education on their cognitive performance.[50]

The **Mexican Health and Aging Study** (**MHAS** or **Estudio Nacional sobre Salud y Envejecimiento en México**) is a prospective two-wave panel study of health and aging in Mexico with 7000 older adults who represent 8 million subjects nationally; with a representative cohort of Mexicans born before 1951 (aged 50 years and older). The survey has national and urban/rural representation. The study was designed with a field protocol and content similar to the Health and Retirement Survey conducted in the United States.[7] MHAS recorded detailed information on individual health, migration history, socioeconomic status, family transfers, kin availability and attributes, and household composition of Mexicans. The most important findings of this longitudinal study included explaining the unique health dynamics of Mexico within a wide socioeconomic context with a life-course perspective approach[51] and how the epidemiologic transition in LAC countries adds to the mortality health burden experienced by older people in Mexico and how the inequalities based on socioeconomic status are important mortality risk factors.[52]

Another longitudinal study, the **Sao Paulo Aging and Health Study (SPAH),** conducted between 2005 and 2007, involved 1025 participants aged 65 years or older who lived in sectors with the lowest human development index in the borough, including numerous shantytowns.[53] This study showed a high incidence of vertebral fracture in older Latin Americans[54] and a high prevalence of 25-hydroxyvitamin D insufficiency in Brazilian community-dwelling older adults.[55] With respect to the prevalence of dementia, one survey of this study showed how nearly 50% of this prevalence could be potentially attributed to the combination of two or three of the socioeconomic adversities during the life span: illiteracy, nonskilled occupations, and lower income.[56]

One of the most recent ongoing longitudinal cross-cultural studies in the region is the **International Mobility in Aging Study** (**IMIAS**), which aims at understanding the mobility differences between men and women by comparing mobility disability in populations that differ widely in gender norms and values. The primary objective of IMIAS is to measure the magnitude of the sex/gender gap in mobility and to increase the understanding of sex/gender differences in life course exposures related to mobility. IMIAS is ongoing at five sites: Tirana (Albania), Natal (Brazil), Manizales (Colombia), Kingston (Ontario, Canada), and Saint-Hyacinthe (Quebec, Canada). The study population is composed of community-dwelling older people between 65 and 74 years of age. The sample was stratified by sex with an aim to recruit 200 men and 200 women at each site. The total sample size of the study at the five research sites is 1995.[57]

In conclusion, Latin American nations have begun to develop appropriate data systems and research capacity to monitor and understand aging accompanied by a longer period of good health, a sustained sense of well-being, and extended periods of social engagement and productivity, specifically with longitudinal studies that incorporate measures of health, economic status, family, and well-being. As a consequence, in addition to demographic information, more detailed information about the aging process in LAC countries is becoming increasingly available in English-language journals.

Self-Rated Health

As a powerful predictor of mortality, disability, and health care utilization, self-rated health (SRH) has been regarded as a key indicator of health status.[58,59] Information from the SABE study showed high percentages of poor SRH in the region. Environmental factors related to poor SRH have been explored in the region. For example, in a cross-sectional study to determine the association between urban and environmental characteristics in the city of Bogota (Colombia) with SRH and quality of life related to health, a positive association was found between the perception of neighborhood safety with good SRH and quality of life related to health. Likewise, the availability of recreational spaces such as safe parks that promote social interaction and recreational activities was associated with good SRH and quality of life in the mental health domain. On the contrary, zones with high levels of noise were associated with bad SRH and poor quality of life.[60] Other studies based on Brazil SABE data determined the relationship between SRH and demographic, social, and economic factors along with the presence of chronic diseases and functional ability. It was found that the presence of a chronic disease in relation to gender had the greatest association with SRH; males presenting four or more chronic illnesses had 10.53 times greater opportunity for bad SRH; similarly, for females, it was 8.31 times. Likewise, educational level, income, and functional capacity were related to SRH.[61] For older people, an LAC religiosity is associated with SRH; in other studies with data from SABE study, it was found that most (90%) participants reported having some religious affiliation and that those who considered religion very important in their lives had better SRH compared with those who considered religion less important.[62] Another recent paper from the Coyoacan cohort insisted that poor SRH shares common correlates and adverse health-related outcomes with frailty syndrome and remains associated with it even when possible confounders are taken into account. They concluded that SRH as an option for frailty syndrome screening could be further explored.[63]

GERIATRICS CONDITIONS

Dementia

The major study on dementia in older adults in LAC countries is the 10/66 population-based study.[64] It investigated the prevalence and severity of dementia in sites in low-income and middle-income countries according to two definitions of dementia diagnosis. This cross-sectional study had a target sample size of 2000 to 3000 participants for every country, in total more than 12,800 individuals. It included five countries: Cuba, Dominican Republic, Venezuela, Mexico, and Peru. The main finding was that the prevalence of dementia (as defined in the *Diagnostic and Statistical Manual of Mental Disorders*, fourth edition [DSM-IV]) in urban Latin America is similar to that previously recorded in Europe and other developed country settings. However, the prevalence of DSM-IV dementia in rural Latin America was very low, a quarter or less than that typically seen in Europe. The researchers concluded that the DSM-IV dementia criteria might substantially underestimate the true prevalence of dementia, especially in the least developed regions, because of difficulties in defining and ascertaining decline in intellectual function and its consequences.[65] However, other studies in the region have shown higher prevalence of cognitive impairment than that found by population-based studies, for example, in Brazil (16.1%)[45] and Mexico (28.7%).[66]

In another cohort survey of the 10/66 study, the independent effects of age, sex, socioeconomic position, and indicators of cognitive reserve (educational level, occupational attainment, literacy, and executive function) on dementia incidence were investigated. Results provided supportive evidence for the cognitive reserve hypothesis for dementia in LAC older people.[67] Other related findings were about awareness of dementia being lower than in high-income countries, probably because in the region, older adults are routinely supported in many basic and instrumental activities of daily living.[67]

In the Coyoacan cohort referred to earlier, cognitive impairment is suggested as a very important component of frailty because of its strong association with prevalent disability in the Mexican population. This study showed that, as in other regions of the world, the life course socioeconomic indicators and current wealth are important predictors of cognitive impairment.[68] In the SABE study, respondents who experienced disadvantaged conditions (lived in rural areas during childhood, perception of poor health during childhood, illiteracy, unskilled occupation or being a farmer or housewife, and reporting insufficient income) presented the highest prevalence of cognitive impairment.[32]

Frailty

A few studies on frailty in older adults have been conducted in Latin America. The first epidemiologic study on the prevalence of frailty in the region was the SABE.[20] In this study, the prevalence of frailty ranged from 30% to 48% in women and from 21% to 35% in men, rates that were much higher than those of their American and European counterparts. In 2009, a frailty index using 34 variables was developed, which allows stratifying older Mexicans into several groups according to the degree of the risk of mortality.[69] The prevalence of frailty using modified Fried criteria has been reported in several studies in the region: Peru, 7.7%[70]; Mexico, ranging from 13.9% to 37%[68]; Colombia, 12.1% frail and 53% prefrail[71]; and Brazil, ranging from 9.1% to 17.1% frail and 47.3% to 60.1% prefrail.[44,72,73] In these studies, multiple factors were identified with frailty, including advanced age, lower education, presence of comorbidity, poor SRH status, dependence in basic and instrumental activities of daily living (ADLs and IADLs, respectively), depression, and cognitive impairment. Data from SABE showed that age, schooling, sedentary lifestyle, and screening positive for depression were associated similarly with more than one component of frailty in Brazilian older men and women. These associations were more similar between the following components of frailty: weakness and slowness (MMSE $\leq$ 18 points in men and schooling in women); weakness, slowness, and low physical activity level (LPAL) (age in both genders and stroke in men) or weakness, slowness, and exhaustion (schooling in men and sedentary lifestyle in both genders).[21] Furthermore, another Mexican study determined that phenotype of frailty was a predictor for adverse health-related outcomes (including mobility, ADL, and IADL disability).[73] Finally, several studies in the region also support the idea that cognitive functioning must be considered as part of the phenotype of frailty and can contribute to a more accurate profile of frailty in older adults.[68,72]

Sarcopenia is considered as a key component of frailty and has also been evaluated in the region. Based on the European Working Group on Sarcopenia in Older People (EWGSOP) with data from the second wave of the SABE study in Brazil, sarcopenia prevalence was established. Sarcopenia was present in 16.1% of women and 14.4% of men. Advanced age, cognitive impairment, lower income, smoking, undernutrition, and risk for undernutrition were factors associated with sarcopenia.[22]

Fewer studies have been carried out in the region related with other geriatric conditions and syndromes.

Falls and Fear of Falling

There is a poor understanding of the scope of falls among older people in developing countries. Falls are often a marker for underlying, preventable problems relating to an older person's health, environment, behavior, and socioeconomic conditions. In LAC countries, the prevalence of falling (in the previous year) ranged from 22% to 37%.[29] The range that we found was close to that reported in other countries around the world (27% to 36%).[74] Among fallers, 30.6% reported a fall-related injury, which increased with age and was higher among women older than 70 years.[34] As a consequence of falling, 28% reported functional restrictions on basic or instrumental ADLs. Advanced age, female gender, previous falls, cognitive impairment, previous stroke, medications such as benzodiazepines, urinary incontinence, and environment were risk factors referred in falling in hospital settings in the region.[74] Of the 83.3% of people aged 60 years and older living in the Colombian Andes Mountains who reported fear of falling, 52.2% reported activity restriction. Independent factors for activity restriction because of fear of falling were low income, functional difficulty, falling or decreasing physical activity, polypharmacy, poor self-perceived health, and depression.[75]

Dizziness

Dizziness is a frequent and prevalent symptom among older people. Several epidemiologic studies have been carried out in the region. A population-based cross-sectional study with 1692 community-living people aged 60 years and older living in four rural and suburban areas of villages in coffee-grower zones in the Colombian Andes Mountains showed a prevalence of 15.2% of dizziness with age, number of chronic conditions, visual impairment, polypharmacy, poor self-perceived health, cognitive impairment, and depression independently associated. Health and psychological factors accounted for 85% of dizziness.[76] Another cross-sectional, population-based study derived from REDE FIBRA, with 391 older adults (65 years and older) reported dizziness associated with depressive symptoms, perceived fatigue, recurrent falls, and excessive drowsiness. The discrimination of the final model was AUC = 0.673.[77] Dizziness is common in older people, and its association with poor physical health, comorbidities, and sensory impairment factors has been established. These factors are known markers of future incident disability, and these studies confirmed the association of dizziness with other common geriatric conditions in Latin American and Caribbean older adults.

Urinary Incontinence

Urinary incontinence is a common clinical condition that occurs frequently in older adults. The estimated prevalence of urinary incontinence ranges from approximately 35% for those who reside in the community to more than 60% for those who live in long-term care facilities. Data from SABE Brazil determined that the prevalence of self-reported urinary incontinence was 11.8% among men and 26.2% for women in Sao Paulo (16.5% among older people between 60 and 74 years old and 33.3% among those aged 75 years and older). The associated factors found were advanced age, female gender, depression, and important functional limitation.[78] Another study of the same cohort showed a significant positive association between caregiver burden and urinary incontinence, demonstrating that urinary incontinence in older patients produced greater caregiver burden.[79] In Mexico, prevalence of urinary incontinence was 18%, and it was severe in 29.3% of cases. Severely incontinent subjects were older and had worse self-perceived health status, greater disability, and more depressive symptoms in comparison with continent participants or with those affected to a lesser degree.[80]

DISABILITY

The World Health Organization reports that 80% of persons with disabilities live in low-income nations and most are poor, as is the case in LAC countries.[81] Data from the SABE study showed higher prevalence of diseases and comorbidity (presence of at least one, and at least two, of seven chronic diseases/conditions, respectively) and disability (difficulty with at least one ADL) in the region. For every 100 persons older than 60 years in LAC countries, 77 had at least one disease, 44 had at least two diseases, 19 had a disability, 17 had both disability and at least one disease, 12 had disability and at least two diseases, and only 21 had neither disability nor disease.[24] An analysis based on SABE data aimed to identify the relationship between chronic diseases and the presence of disability expressed in ADL and IADL difficulties. The variables that showed a direct association with difficulty in carrying out ADLs and IADLs were suffering from a higher number of noncommunicable diseases, from cerebrovascular diseases, from osteoarthritis, or from depression; being older; being female; poor SRH; and experiencing cognitive impairment. In general, the strongest associations were between difficulty in carrying out IADLs and depression, being older, reporting one's health as bad, and the presence of cerebrovascular diseases, osteoarthritis, or cognitive impairment.[11] Other studies based on SABE data show the association between disability and sociodemographic variables (age, women, and fewer years of schooling), lower body mass index (BMI < 20), and high number of medical conditions were independently significantly associated with IADL and ADL difficulties.[25] Another study about functional limitation in Chilean prospective community-dwelling older people showed a clear socioeconomic gradient: older adults with low socioeconomic status remained functionally limited whereas those with high socioeconomic status remained nonlimited in the follow-up period. The researchers insist on the importance of social stratification and functional status and the importance of reducing inequalities to prevent disability in older age.[82] Accordingly, in LAC countries, poor social conditions at childhood, low education, unskilled occupations, and low wages still coexist, and with greater prevalence of functional impairments during retirement years.[11,25] One study about self-reported stroke diagnosis, disability, care needs, and caregiver burden in LAC countries, India, and China showed that the prevalence is nearly as high as in industrialized countries, with high levels of disability and dependence in the other, mainly rural and less developed sites.[83]

The higher incidence and prevalence of obesity in the LAC region is correlated with the higher prevalence of diabetes, hypertension, stroke, and heart attack in older people.[5] Thus, the trend of increasing incidence of obesity in LAC countries would produce a corresponding rise in chronic disease and disability, and the relation between disability and obesity is well recognized. Based on data from SABE, a study showed that the proportion of participants with a BMI greater than 30 ranged from 13.3% (Havana) to 37.6% (Montevideo). A significant odds ratio for ADL limitation of 1.63 for persons with a BMI greater than 35 was shown. Authors insisted that controlling obesity should be a priority in the region.[16] With data from the two waves (2000 and 2006) of the SABE cohort study conducted in Sao Paulo, Brazil, a study examined the impact of obesity on disability and mortality. Obesity was associated with higher incidence of ADL and IADL limitations and with lower recovery from Nagi limitations. When compared with those who maintained their weight, those who gained weight experienced higher incidence of ADL and Nagi limitations, even after controlling initial BMI.[84] Thus, further research on obesity in LAC older adults is warranted.

Owing to a lifelong history of social and economic hardship, disability rates among older adults in LAC countries are high.[19,20,26] Socioeconomic status at individual and contextual levels as well as chronic medical conditions have been found to contribute to the occurrence of disability in these populations.[85] Results of various studies suggest a multifaceted relation with disability involving age, gender, obesity, city, and other health conditions in older people who live in LAC countries.[16] Thus, there is a growing interest in appropriately assessing disability transition among older adults in LAC populations and in identifying the determinants that will help prevent disability and maintain quality of life among members of the aging population.[86]

EDUCATION

A recent dramatic increase in the older adult population has not been accompanied by a parallel increase in the number of specialized health care professionals in Latin America. However, during the past two decades, an interest in postgraduate gerontology training has developed in Latin America. Presently, there are programs of specialization (geriatric/gerontology training) in Mexico, Costa Rica, Colombia, Venezuela, Peru, Chile, Argentina, Ecuador, Paraguay, Panama, and Brazil. A common characteristic of these programs is their focus on the life course. This approach considers aging and old age as constructions in historical and sociocultural contexts in which multiple variables converge, requiring an interdisciplinary viewpoint.[87] Interdisciplinary health care programs provide integral, effective, constant, and high-quality care for older people, stressing the importance of the family as part of the approach, with shared decision making and care centered on patients' needs.[88]

A survey about the state of geriatrics teaching for undergraduate and graduate medical levels in LAC countries was recently developed. The authors surveyed geriatricians from 16 countries: 8 from South America and 8 from Central America. Among 308 medical schools, 35% taught undergraduate geriatrics, ranging from none in Uruguay, Venezuela, and Guatemala to 82% in Mexico. The authors identified 36 programs in 12 countries with graduate medical education in geriatrics, ranging from 2 to 5 years of training. The authors conclude that although the population is aging rapidly in Latin American countries, there has been a slow development of geriatrics teaching at undergraduate and postgraduate levels in the region.[89]

Moreover, global approaches to defining core competencies for students in geriatrics medical training programs have been identified.[90] The Academia Latinoamericana de Medicina del Adulto Mayor defined minimal competencies for medical students in South America based on knowledge and skills. These highlight the need for future doctors to adopt a positive attitude toward older people and that the curriculum can be delivered in a horizontal or vertical way. Their report also specifies the resources needed to achieve this, such as adequate teachers, teaching materials, and assessment methods.[91]

In conclusion, despite the limitations to better development of geriatrics and gerontology education in the region, an increasing number of innovative approaches for teaching at the undergraduate and postgraduate levels will ensure a basic teaching of geriatrics for all medical students.

LIFE COURSE APPROACH: FUTURE PERSPECTIVES

The concept of health capital and aging proposed by Guimarães highlighted that health status in old age reflects lifetime events, including genetics, socioeconomic factors, formal education, and health support. Thus, the health condition of older people who survive in adverse conditions in many developing Latin American countries reveals a low health capital, with a low functional reserve and high prevalence of disability, as a consequence of a lifetime of deprivation.[92]

The SABE study provided a unique opportunity to explore gender differences in health and function in LAC older people from a life course perspective.[10] Thus, gender and early life conditions are significantly and consistently associated with many geriatric conditions. For example, across five cities from the SABE study, women and those who had experienced impoverished childhoods were more likely to be frail. Lack of schooling, working a manual occupation, being a housewife, and perceived economic hardship later in life were related to greater likelihood of frailty. In the same study, significant differences between women and men were observed in the relationship between chronic conditions, BMI, and frailty.[20] Life course socioeconomic indicators and current wealth are important predictors of cognitive impairment. In the Latin American context, another study based on SABE data showed that early exposure to rural environments may reflect poor living conditions, leading to low educational attainment and a lifelong occupation in farming as a day laborer (*peon*), both of which are widely recognized risk factors for dementia and cognitive impairment. Additionally, in this study, childhood health remained an important predictor of cognitive function later in life, with those reporting fair or poor health during childhood being more mentally impaired than those who enjoyed good health.[32] Another study that used the Geriatric Depression Scale corroborated the evidence that cumulative exposure to social and material disadvantage and current material, social, and health conditions explain the higher frequency of depression in women in LAC countries.[31] Life course exposures predict mobility; in a study mentioned earlier with data originating from SABE, exposures in childhood such as hunger, little education, and insufficient income were associated with prevalence of low extremity limitations for both men and women. Authors concluded that life course exposures, cognitive impairment, depression, and chronic conditions are important predictors of mobility in LAC older individuals, but the gender differential in mobility remains largely unexplained by these risk factors.[19]

In conclusion, these findings increase our understanding of the role of socioeconomic inequalities with respect to health and functional status in LAC older adults, especially those inequalities that are determined early in life, such as childhood deprivation, lack of education, and low occupational status. These life course exposures influence physical and mental health in later life; thus, prevention of social disadvantage may result in improvement of functional status within the older adult population. Further research into the health status of LAC older people needs to take into account differences between older men and women and needs to consider a life course approach to analyzing the findings. Thus, future research should test the hypotheses of differential exposure and differential vulnerability by gender in older people living in LAC countries. In addition, it should emphasize the importance of understanding health inequalities in Latin America for research on Latino health patterns in the United States and other developed countries where the Latin American population is a significant percentage of the total population.[93]

KEY POINTS

- The major study on health of older adults in Latin America and the Caribbean is the Salud, Bienestar y Envejecimiento en América Latina y Caribe (SABE) study (Survey on Health, Well-being and Aging in Latin America and the Caribbean), a multicentric project conducted by the Pan-American Health Organization (PAHO).
- Several population-based longitudinal studies in aging have been conducted in the region, including the Costa Rican Study on Longevity and Healthy Aging, REDE FIBRA (Frailty in the Brazilian Elderly Study), Mexican Study of Nutritional and Psychosocial Markers of Frailty (also called the "Coyoacan cohort"), Mexican Health and Aging Study (MHAS), Sao Paulo Aging and Health Study (SPAH), and the International Mobility in Aging Study (IMIAS).
- Older age–related topics of research conducted in the region include self-rated health (SRH), dementia, frailty and sarcopenia, falls and fear of falling, dizziness, urinary incontinence, and disability from a life course approach.

For a complete list of references, please visit www.expertconsult.com.

KEY REFERENCES

4. Palloni A, McEniry M: Aging and health status of elderly in Latin America and the Caribbean: preliminary findings. J Cross Cult Gerontol 22:263–285, 2007.
7. Wong R, Peláez M, Palloni A, et al: Survey data for the study of aging in Latin America and the Caribbean: selected studies. J Aging Health 18:157–179, 2006.
11. Menéndez JA, Guevara MA, Arcia N, et al: Chronic diseases and functional limitation in older adults: a comparative study in seven cities of Latin America and the Caribbean. Rev Panam Salud Publica 17:353–361, 2005.
20. Alvarado BE, Zunzunegui MV, Béland F, et al: Life course social and health conditions linked to frailty in Latin American older men and women. J Gerontol A Biol Sci Med Sci 63:1399–1406, 2008.
25. Reyes-Ortiz CA, Ostir GV, Pelaez M, et al: Cross-national comparison of disability in Latin American and Caribbean persons aged 75 and older. Arch Gerontol Geriatr 42:21–33, 2006.
32. Nguyen CT, Couture MC, Alvarado BE, et al: Life course socioeconomic disadvantage and cognitive function among the elderly population of seven capitals in Latin America and the Caribbean. J Aging Health 20:347–362, 2008.
37. Rosero-Bixby L, Dow WH: Surprising SES gradients in mortality, health and biomarkers in a Latin American population of adults. J Gerontol Soc Sci 64:105–117, 2009.
43. Sousa AC, Dias RC, Maciel ÁC, et al: Frailty syndrome and associated factors in community-dwelling elderly in Northeast Brazil. Arch Gerontol Geriatr 54:e95–e101, 2012.
46. Ruiz-Arregui L, Ávila-Funes JA, Amieva H, et al: The Coyoacan cohort study: Design, methodology and participants characteristics of a Mexican study on nutritional and psychosocial markers of frailty. J Frailty Aging 2:68–76, 2013.
52. González-González C, Samper-Ternent R, Wong R, et al: Mortality inequality among older adults in Mexico: The combined role of infectious and chronic diseases. Rev Panam Salud Publica 35:89–95, 2014.
53. Scazufca M, Menezes PR, Vallada HP, et al: High prevalence of dementia among older adults from poor socio-economic background in Sao Paulo, Brazil. Int Psychogeriatr 20:394–405, 2008.
64. Prince M, Ferri CP, Acosta D: The protocols for the 10/66 Dementia Research Group population-based research programme. BMC Public Health 7:165, 2007.
67. Prince M, Acosta D, Ferri CP, et al: Dementia incidence and mortality in middle-income countries, and associations with indicators of cognitive reserve: a 10/66 Dementia Research Group population-based cohort study. Lancet 380:50–58, 2012.
71. Curcio CL, Henao GM, Gomez F: Frailty among rural elderly adults. BMC Geriatr 14:2–9, 2014.
76. Gomez F, Curcio CL, Duque G: Dizziness as a geriatric condition among rural community-dwelling older adults. J Nutr Health Aging 15:490–497, 2011.
80. Aguilar-Navarro S, Navarrete-Reyes AP, Grados-Chavarría BH, et al: The severity of urinary incontinence decreases health-related quality of life among community-dwelling elderly. J Gerontol A Biol Sci Med Sci 67:1266–1271, 2012.
89. López JH, Reyes-Ortiz CA: Geriatric education in undergraduate and graduate levels in Latin America. Gerontol Geriatr Educ 9:1–11, 2014.

124 Medical Care for Older Long-Term Care Residents in the United Kingdom

Finbarr C. Martin

INTRODUCTION

Care homes are a major part of the health care system in the United Kingdom. The majority of the frail older people occupying publicly funded beds in the United Kingdom are in care homes, not in hospitals. The specialty of geriatric medicine started with such patients. In contrast, most geriatric medicine services currently have little or no involvement with care home residents. Indeed, the responsibilities and arrangements for their health care are ill-defined, inconsistent, and, in some places, chaotic. Hence knowledge of what high-quality medicine for care homes residents should consist of, and how it might best be organized, lags behind the progress made for the acute care of older people. But change is afoot: the last decade has seen growing momentum in policy and practice not evident when the corresponding chapter was written for the previous edition of this book. This chapter describes this journey and the clinical and contextual challenges of providing high-quality care, with an account of recent trends in service innovations and clinical interventions. Finally, it ends with recommendations for future progress and research priorities.

A BRIEF HISTORY OF LONG-TERM CARE IN THE UNITED KINGDOM

In 1948, the National Health Service (NHS) inherited a disorderly array of chronic sick wards in municipal hospitals, workhouse infirmaries, former infectious disease hospitals, and sanatoria; many of these poorly funded institutions were derived from Poor Law origins. The pioneering work of Marjory Warren in one such institution is credited with the birth of geriatric medicine as a specialty.[1] Essentially it was about addressing decades of neglect. This meant discharging some long-term residents and reducing the influx of new residents through comprehensive clinical and social assessment, improving access to conventional medicine, and developing a rehabilitative approach. This constituted the core of geriatric practice through the 1950s and 1960s. It was facilitated by the gradual emergence of community and domiciliary support from the NHS or local government.

Simultaneously, however, new long-term care facilities were being created. Part III of the National Assistance Act of 1948 [2] set out the legal responsibilities of local councils to provide accommodation for frail and financially insecure older people. Over time, the residents were increasingly those with mental and/or physical reasons for losing capacity for independence, but the details of their ongoing clinical and social needs and care did not receive much attention or investment. In 1962 Townsend published *The Last Refuge*, a study of residential institutions and homes for the aged in England and Wales.[3] This study concluded that communal homes were "not adequately meeting the physical, psychological, and social needs of the elderly people living in them, and that alternative services and living arrangements should quickly take their place."

Diagnosis was not part of the social care offer, although by the 1980s it was clear that the resident profile in dependency terms was becoming similar to the remaining hospitalized older residents in geriatric or old-age psychiatry NHS long-stay wards. The next period saw major policy changes and resulted in transformation of both sectors with a massive expansion of the independent (private, voluntary, not for profit, etc.) sector care home capacity, which became the major provider, albeit mostly enabled by public finance. The number of geriatric beds in the NHS had remained fairly constant from 1959 to 1985, with improved and new treatments, rehabilitation, and community care counterbalancing increasing numbers of older people. But from the mid-1980s, the numbers declined as old, inadequate, often Victorian accommodations were closed, and the geriatric medical services took their place in the expanding district general hospital sector. There was scant room for the long-term care wards, and, increasingly, the NHS and geriatricians looked to the independent sector to offer the alternative. By 1990s, care homes had become a major component of the welfare system's provision of care for vulnerable and clinically unstable older people, many providing specialized services (e.g., services for older people with dementia).

CURRENT PROVISION AND FUTURE TRENDS

Between 3% and 4% of the older (older than 65 years) population live in care homes. In the 2011 census,[4] more than a quarter of a million (291,000) people aged 65 and older were living in care homes in England and Wales, representing 3.2% of the total population of this age group. This is slightly less than the European average. The census data showed a geographic range across local government districts from 1.0% to 6.1% (median 3.1%) of adults older than 65 years and from 3.5 to 22.8% (median 13.7%) of those older than 85 years.[4] This variation is partly due to new residents migrating to where the care homes exist (e.g., the south coast of England). But it also reflects differential use of NHS and local government resources. For example, across England there was a more than twofold difference in the proportion of adult social care spending allocated to fund care home residence, and this variation appeared unexplained by differences in local demographics, deprivation levels, or indeed the local NHS bedpool, suggesting that genuine and major differences in practice exist.[5]

Current projections for an increase in life expectancy have been predicted to create the need for many more residential care home places, a rise overall by perhaps 150% over the next 50 years.[6] The percentage of people aged 65 years and older entering care homes is expected to increase 20% by 2028.[7] The prediction of future need for care home places is difficult. Future levels of dependency will depend on the changing nature and prevalence of multiple morbidities, the increasing prevalence of dementia, and the growing importance of frailty in the very old. The availability of informal caregivers, the paid caregiver workforce, and preferences among older people add to the complexity. A detailed assessment of factors affecting projections was provided by a Royal Commission in 1999.[8]

Recent trends illustrate that the picture is indeed complex and changing. According to the most recent census data (2011), the number of residents has remained almost stable since 2001, increasing by just 0.3%, whereas the older population grew by 11% over that decade. Women have always outstripped men, but the trend during this period was for slightly fewer women and 15.2% more men, although the ratio remains at around 2.8

women for each man. The resident care home population is aging: in 2011, people aged 85 and older represented 59.2% of the older care home population compared to 56.5% in 2001. Although residents of care homes with nursing services have higher levels of morbidity and disability, surveys have shown that there is considerable overlap. There is likely to be an increasing need for specialist dementia skills and specialized care home places.

An additional challenge is the increasing diversity of the older population in terms of ethnicity, religion, and culture. This affects catering and communication between caregivers and residents, but more fundamentally it will bring a range of complexities to health care and technologic approaches, from eating and drinking to death and dying. A resident-centered approach to care is required, keeping up with the population as it becomes more diverse and anticipating requirements for interpretation, advocacy, and other appropriate resources.

REGULATION, FUNDING, AND STANDARDS

Each nation of the United Kingdom has a regulatory body, overseeing a statutory requirement for providers to register and then comply with certain standards. In England, a care home has been defined as social care residential accommodation where people live, but do not own or rent, and are in need of nursing services, personal care, or both.[9] Within that broad definition, registration can identify specific services providing care for people with learning disabilities, people with mental health conditions, adults older than 65 years. In all cases, the registration (and associated regulations and standards) must specify whether or not the care includes nursing. Other nations of the United Kingdom use these terms with slight differences: Northern Ireland continues to use the terms *nursing homes* and *residential homes*[10]; in Scotland and Wales the general term *care home* is used to include those with or without nursing care.[11,12]

There is a mixed economy of provision. In England, for example, ownership of care homes in 2010 was described as 73% independent, 14% voluntary sector, 11% local council, 1% NHS, and 1% "other."[7] Care homes vary enormously in size from small, family-run "residential homes" to major chains with tens of thousands of beds. In 2012 in England across all ownership sectors, the average size was 18.5 places for residential care homes and 46.6 places for nursing homes.[13]

Successive laws and regulations have refined the funding arrangements and entitlements of individuals for financial support. The underlying legal framework has been the 1948 historic separation of obligations of the NHS, free at the point of use, and those of local government, means tested with some details locally determined. Changes in patterns of provision resulted in significant geographic variation and major anomalies in access and funding, sometimes resulting in legal challenges to clarify interpretations of law.

The current arrangements in all four U.K. nations require a rigorous assessment of individual care needs as a condition of accessing public funding. Those deemed to have needs resembling those for which hospital-type care would have been the traditional option are entitled to "NHS continuing health care" funded by the local NHS body with no personal contribution. This is a small proportion of current residents. For the remainder, the bulk of the costs are treated as personal "social care" resources and therefore means tested according to criteria of wealth laid out by government in ongoing regulations. The component of care deemed to be nursing must, by law, be funded by the NHS and is paid at the same rate across England: for 2013/14, the standard rate was £109.79 a week. The provision of nursing care can affect the individual resident's entitlement to NHS services usually available when living at home, such as general district nursing.

The exception to these funding arrangements is in Scotland, where personal care is also publically funded for residents needing 24/7 nursing. Throughout the United Kingdom, older individuals may opt to fund their own care in total, obviating the need for any statutory assessment. This accounts for perhaps a quarter of residents in some regions. In 2012, the total value of the care home market in England was estimated at £22 billion,[14] 73% of which was state funding, the rest being self-funded. The sustainability of this public funding continues to occupy the attention of politicians and policy makers with a succession of inquiries and official reports, while the professions have been more concerned with issues of care and quality.

The Care Quality Commission (CQC) in England combines the regulatory and inspection functions and provides publically available grading of care homes on its website.[9] Until 2014 the CQC inspections produced ratings (inadequate, requires improvement, good, or outstanding) with respect to five domains: respect and dignity; care and welfare; suitability of staffing; safeguarding and safety; and monitoring quality. These judgments are now made in response to the following considerations: Are they safe? Are they effective? Are they caring? Are they responsive? Are they well-led? In Wales and Northern Ireland, these functions are also combined, whereas in Scotland, National Care Standards exist that provide the basis for the work of the Care Inspectorate as an independent scrutiny and improvement body for care services.

TRENDS IN QUALITY AND THE SPECTER OF ELDER ABUSE

On quality indicators, the standards of care provided appear to have improved consistently over the past decade. For example, since 2003 in England, more care homes each year have met National Minimum Standards up to 93% by 2011 and the proportion achieving safe working practices doubled to 80%.[15] The percentage of older people living in care homes rated "good" or "excellent" rose from 75% to 86%. For care, compliance rates rose each year to 2014, but the trends were mixed for the other domains.[16] Certainly, some poor standards of care persist and examples continue to attract media attention, focusing on personal care and dignity.

At its extreme, poor care amounts to elder abuse, whether it is caused by ignorance, inadequate staffing, or willful harm. The incidence of abuse is difficult to establish. The most definitive study, Prevention of Abuse and Neglect in the Institutional Care of Older Adults (PANICOA),[17] was reported in 2013. It comprised a linked set of eight primary research studies and three secondary analyses and included more than 2600 hours of observation and approximately 500 interviews in 43 care homes (and 32 acute hospitals), predominantly across England and Wales. This study provided valuable insight into the context, nature, and frequency of different types of abuse likely to be broadly indicative of the situation in care homes generally.

The results of the PANICOA study showed that the risk of physical assault to residents from care staff was low, but residents were potentially at risk of assault from others' challenging behavior if this was not managed effectively by care staff. Overall, the weakest areas related to the maintenance of dignity and privacy in personal care (e.g., in using the toilet), although care homes were slightly better in this regard than hospital wards. Supporting social engagement and facilitating a sense of meaning and purpose in residents' lives were other important weaknesses. PANICOA identified key attributes affecting the experiences of residents around leadership, staff training and support, the care culture, and the relationship between care homes and their surrounding health and social care communities.

The PANICOA report made 100 recommendations for several audiences. Key recommendations are highlighted in Box 124-1.

The research community (funders and researchers) were encouraged to investigate organizational change and behaviors that affect the wider culture of caring and to identify markers of

BOX 124-1 Key Recommendations from PANICOA for Government, Health Education England, and Care Home Employers

Developing a strategy to improve the capability of the workforce should include the following:

- Consideration of a national system to register and regulate the workforce
- A common career development framework and revised pay structure for health care assistants
- A national body to support the professional development and standing of care home managers

Data from Key Recommendations from PANICOA for Government, Health Education England and Care Home Employers.
PANICOA, Prevention of Abuse and Neglect in the Institutional Care of Older Adults.

organizational "fragility" that can be used to identify risk of institutional abuse.

These data give little indication of the standard of medically related care, but an important finding was the relative isolation of care homes from the wider sector. This is consistent with previous research showing that care homes and their residents are frequently denied the levels of health care support that would be expected for individuals living at home. A number of policy, financial, and cultural factors have contributed to this, and the result is a lack of a collaborative model of care in which the NHS could provide consistent support.

Taking a more positive perspective, care homes have the potential to improve people's lives socially, physically, and psychologically, more so if relationship-centered approaches to care are employed, allied to understanding the resident's attitude toward living in care homes.[18]

This approach is exemplified by the My Home Life project (http://myhomelifemovement.org/), which has worked with care homes to support them in improving daily care and the experience of both staff and residents. These developments have demonstrated the appetite in care homes to gain recognition as an integral and specialist resource for the future health and social care of older people.

HEALTH AND HEALTH CARE NEEDS OF RESIDENTS

The majority of older care home residents need help with some aspect of personal care in daily life. A survey in 2003 of 16,043 people residents in 244 care homes across the United Kingdom (25% residential and 75% nursing) [19] identified that

- 78% had at least one form of cognitive impairment,
- 71% were incontinent,
- 76% required assistance with their mobility or were immobile, and
- 27% were immobile, confused, and incontinent.

Multiple physical and mental health issues are the norm.[20] There is considerable overlap in dependency between residential and nursing care. Depression is also common, as is malnutrition at the time of admission. Many report pain,[21] particularly associated with arthritis, limb stiffness, or immobility. Chronic conditions such as chronic obstructive pulmonary disease (COPD) and heart failure contribute to fatigue and immobility, albeit often undiagnosed and perhaps not producing the classic symptoms seen in a more active population.[22]

Although only a minority of care homes are registered to provide dementia care, a survey conducted by the Commission for Social Care Inspection (CSCI) of 657 care homes in England found that 40% of residents had particular needs as a result of dementia, and over 84% of homes in the survey had at least one resident with dementia.[23] In England, approximately 208,000 people with dementia live in care homes, with 91,000 of those in dedicated dementia care beds.[24]

It is becoming more common for care homes to provide more technical care aspects. For example, survey data for 2009 reported 9000 care home residents were receiving tube feeding, mostly via a percutaneous endoscopic gastrostomy (PEG) tube feed.[25] Unsurprisingly, many care home residents are on multiple medications. The most definitive recent survey in 2009 found that residents were prescribed an average of 7.2 medicines, with inappropriate prescribing evident in 50% to 90% of patients.[26]

The clinical course of residents is highly variable. Some move in to receive palliative care for a short, final phase of life, but others who are admitted following disabling injury or illness may stabilize for long periods. A primary care–based database study including 9772 care homes in 293 English and Welsh general practices reported 26.2 % one-year mortality among residents older than 65 years (an approximately 10-fold higher rate than community dwellers). Both age and number of comorbidities were weaker predictors than for community dwellers.[27] Age, gender, activities of daily living functioning, and health stability were predictive of the 28.8% of residents who died within a year of admission to nursing homes in Iceland from 1996 to 2006.[28] Mortality rates among residents of nursing care homes are generally higher. From a total of 2444 resident deaths in 38 homes in England over a 3-year period, 56% were within 12 months of admission.[29] In general, the more frail the population is, the less predictive for death are these factors, chance playing a greater part as reserves are lost.

Thus, clinical expertise is required in recognizing the final phase of life, for example, the feature characteristics of late-stage dementia. Proactive care also involves anticipating health-related events likely to occur in the last year or so of life.[30]

ARRANGEMENTS FOR MEDICAL CARE

Provision of NHS health care in the context of an independent care home provider presents particular challenges. With or without nursing supervision, the bulk of care for residents with complex needs is provided by an unregulated low-paid workforce, with limited access to training. Thus, effective collaboration is key to success. There are no specific national standards or models for provision of appropriate health care: provision is highly variable. There is no separate specialty of care home physicians, as exists in the Netherlands. In the United Kingdom, all residents have right of access to a general medical practitioner (GP), but the General Medical Services (GMS) contract is not considered to encompass what care home residents may need. Some care homes (or their local primary care organizations) have secured an agreement with a single GP practice to register all residents on admission. Clearly this infringes on the individual's freedom to choose a GP and, for some, disrupts continuity, but the alternative approach of maintaining continuity is impractical for most residents, as even relatively short moves will render them too far away. In any case, care homes report that working with numerous GPs is counterproductive to effective collaboration.[31,32]

Whatever pattern of primary care exists, it is unusual for it to be tailored to the specific challenges of the care home context. To address these issues, some primary care organizations have funded a higher than usual level of care through a Local Enhanced Service (LES) agreement or other device. There is some evidence that this may have clinical and resource advantages.[33] In some areas of urban density, or where there is a lack of GP provision, care home–specific practices have been set up so that the GPs and nurses working in these practices are employed to work solely for care home residents.[7]

BOX 124-2 Key Positive Features of National Health Service Involvement with Care Homes

- Service interventions are explicitly specified and monitored through systems such as contracting, incentive payments to general practitioners, or audit.
- Interventions are designed to be age appropriate and provided by specialists in the health care of older people (e.g., care home support teams, care home therapy teams, community geriatricians, or specialist mental health nurses).
- Interventions are supported by approaches that foster improved collaborative working relationships between National Health Care Service professionals and care home staff, such as through joint educational and training initiatives or service codesign.

There is compelling evidence of the limited medical, multiprofessional, and specialist geriatric input into care homes,[34,35] and this is perceived to negatively affect the quality of life for residents.[36]

In response to this, guidance on commissioning health care has been published.[37] Numerous small-scale innovations have been reported concerning aspects of care such as medication management, but conclusive evidence of effectiveness is lacking.[38] Conversely, improvements in end-of-life care have been achieved, increasing the chance that residents can die with dignity in the care home. The experience of the Gold Standards Framework (http://www.goldstandardsframework.org.uk/), along with other end-of-life initiatives, have shown what a proactive planned care approach can achieve. With NHS generalists, specialists and care homes' staff and management working collaboratively, dramatic improvements have been made to the experiences of residents and their families, alongside increased staff satisfaction.[39]

There is no direct evidence about a model of care in which this best clinical practice can be sustained. There is considerable evidence, however, about the features of health care provision that care home providers, residents, and residents' families believe to be conducive to good care[40] (Box 124-2).

Studies are ongoing to investigate whether models of health care incorporating one or more of these features result in better experience or outcomes for residents and/or more efficient use of health care resources.[41]

COMMON CLINICAL CHALLENGES AND RESPONSES

What are the overall objectives of high-quality health care in this context? Arguably, from the individual's viewpoint, it is the same as elsewhere: optimizing day-to-day quality of life, limiting functional dependency, and preventing avoidable death. But the balance of these three goals may change over time in a patient whose complex multimorbidity is causing significant dependency toward the end of life. Conventional long-term condition management may or may not contribute to any of these three objectives. Each situation needs individual consideration and judgment. There is no place for the lazy assumption that "active treatment" is not indicated. The medical challenge for the clinician is to gauge the attributable contributions of various, usually numerous factors to these outcomes and then gauge the potential of clinical interventions to alter them. Evidence-based clinical practice guidance may help. The clinical course of most patients includes a degree of predictability, for example, in the risks of contractures, skin damage, depression, or aspiration pneumonia. The communication challenge is to explain these clearly so that the patient can weigh the potential advantages and burdens in light of their overall objectives. The patient's challenge is to reflect on what matters most to them. Does a bit more dependency matter? Are a few extra months of life important? What mental or physical symptoms are the most troublesome?

In practice, many care home residents lack the capacity for much of the detail and sometimes cannot participate at all. In this context, as elsewhere, and guided by the Mental Capacity Act,[42] discussions with relevant others (such as family) is vital to ascertain what might be in the patient's best interests, taking into account any stated view, legal advance directives, and cultural factors if necessary. Thus, based on a comprehensive assessment, a set of health care objectives for each individual can be determined. For example, in the context of a short life expectancy, the target blood sugars in a diabetic person might be set to avoid ketosis, if relevant, to avoid hypoglycemic episodes, and to minimize the burden of treatments and monitoring. Relief of pain and spasticity will be more important for some individuals than being sufficiently alert to complete every meal. The social and sensory pleasures of eating and drinking may be worth a risk of occasional coughing, if a patient has irreversible dysphagia.

There is also need for reactive care, responding to concerns of the resident but in practice more often to the concerns of family or staff. Subtle changes in behavior, alertness, or facial expression are usually evident to those closest to the resident, but they may lack the confidence or the language to articulate them. Thus, relationship building and trust is an essential requisite for effective reactive care. Detailed conversation with caregivers generally pays dividends. The task then is to distinguish new events or illnesses from the anticipated trajectory for the patient. For example, patients approaching end-stage dementia do not stop eating overnight, but they may do so if they develop thrush or a tooth abscess. Agitated behavior may be induced by hallucination but is more likely to be pain related and treatable.[43] Fecal incontinence rarely precedes urinary incontinence in patients except when impaction or primary gut problems supervene.

The work is clearly dissimilar from routine primary care or the work that geriatricians do in wards or clinics. The scope of the medical responsibility is shown in Box 124-3.

There is a small but growing body of relevant evidence about how best to perform these activities. In England, the National Institute of Health and Care Excellence (NICE) has issued guidance covering older people in care homes on oral nutrition support, including enteral tube feeding (CG32); medication management; promotion of mental well-being, generally, and specifically through occupational therapy and physical activity interventions; delirium; dementia; falls prevention; prevention of health care–acquired infections; and end-of-life care.[44] Guidance on oral health is set to appear in 2016.[45] Other relevant guidance, such as on nutritional assessment and support, is available from specialist professional sources.[46]

Weight loss toward the end of life is a common but difficult challenge. A diagnostic assessment, including assessment of swallowing difficulties, is essential. It is important to identify potentially treatable causes such as mouth ulcers, poor dentition, or painful presbyesophagus but also to recognize the features of cognitive dysphagia and its significance in advanced dementia. This would prompt a review of health care goals toward avoidance of distressing choking during pleasure-oriented feeding and away from maintenance of body weight or perfect hydration. Discussion between families and care providers can be challenging; to some extent, this is because the various parties come to the discussion with different understandings and knowledge. For example, it is not unreasonable for a lay person (or unqualified care provider) to believe that inadequate fluid intake must cause distress and that this can best be alleviated by fluid in a drip. Thus, information, as well as sensitivity to culture and family values, is necessary.

BOX 124-3

- Agree to health care goals before or soon after admission. This is achieved through a full comprehensive geriatric assessment taking into account the resident's psychosocial resources, preferences, and culture.
- Identify the key clinical challenges likely to impact the resident's quality of life, dependency, or survival, such as swallowing difficulties or contractures developing as a result of spasticity and/or immobility.
- Provide guidance on regular observations and assessments and the management of these clinical challenges, including pain control, weight loss, difficulties eating and drinking, skin integrity, sleep quality, continence, constipation, nonparticipation, and challenging and distressing behaviors.
- Create anticipatory clinical plans based on the agreed health care goals and clinical challenges, incorporating decisions about end-of-life care.
- Plan regular reviews of residents and their medications in the light of health care goals and clinical changes.
- Be proactive in providing medical care. For instance, identify people at risk for falls and support a care plan to minimize risk that is consistent with the resident's preferences.
- Provide reactive medical care based on a system of communication between the care home and medical staff, setting out mutual expectations about seeking help.
- As part of an enablement approach, support needs-based access to community health services, including specialist nursing and allied health professionals, to minimize the impact of sensory, cognitive, and physical function impairment.
- Medically manage long-term conditions in the context of health care goals, taking into account the impact of frailty and multimorbidity on the benefits and risks of conventional treatments.
- Support a clinical governance framework in partnership with care home staff and involving multidisciplinary clinicians to maintain and improve clinical care and quality of life of residents. This might review specific clinical challenges or use a reflective practice approach in response to events such as injurious falls or repeated hospital admissions.

PROSPECTS FOR THE FUTURE

It is likely that the care home sector and the quality of care it provides will grow in social and health policy importance. Expectations of residents and families are likely to grow with the postwar baby boom generation. The Equality Act 2012 specifically outlawed age-based discrimination of health care and emphasized that this included explicit criteria not simply about access but also about suitability. Clearly the current patterns in most regions would fail at this hurdle. There is also the economic consideration that inadequate care results in greater acute hospital use and that this is a potential impetus for improved and more focused commissioning in the NHS.

The current U.K. model is essentially primary care–based GPs, with variable degrees of specialist support. Building on this model is the predominant view of relevant professional groups. This might incorporate the role of a medical director, which, in the United States, is considered to have promoted more consistency in care,[47] although the development of more precisely defined specialists also has some support.[48]

There is need for ongoing research on models of care as well as clinical details. Key findings from a two-stage Delphi process among international care home clinical researchers suggested the topics shown in Box 124-4.[49]

BOX 124-4 International Consensus of Key Priorities for Nursing Homes Research

- Prioritization of research to underpin the care of people with cognitive impairment/dementia and of the management of the behavioral and psychological symptoms of dementia within the nursing home
- End-of-life care
- Nutrition
- Polypharmacy
- Developing new approaches to putting evidence-based practices into routine practice in nursing homes
- Research into innovative educational approaches, addressing why best practices are difficult

KEY POINTS

- Geriatric medicine has its origins in long-term care institutions.
- Despite demographic change, the importance of care homes in the overall health and social care provision is not increasing.
- The morbidity and dependency of the care home resident population has increased in recent decades.
- A social care model, rather than a health care model, has predominated in the United Kingdom.
- Regulation and inspection, rather than professional standards, have been the main drivers for quality.
- The importance of specialist knowledge and skills has been underplayed in policy and provision.
- Increasing research in recent years has highlighted the key clinical challenges and some successful approaches.
- There is no consensus on the optimal model of health care for care home residents in the United Kingdom.
- There is a need for geriatricians and other specialists to join primary and social care to improve the quality of health care provision in the United Kingdom.

For a complete list of references, please visit www.expertconsult.com.

KEY REFERENCES

7. British Geriatrics Society: Quest for quality—an inquiry into the quality of healthcare support for older people in care homes: a call for leadership, partnership and improvement, London, 2011, British Geriatrics Society.
8. Royal Commission on Long Term Care: With respect to old age: long-term care—rights and responsibilities, Rep. no. CM4192, London, 1999, Royal Commission on Long Term Care.
17. Department of Health: Protect and respect: The experience of older people and staff in care homes and hospitals. The PANICOA report, 2013. http://www.panicoa.org.uk. Accessed January 1, 2015.
18. Bradshaw SA, Playford ED, Riazi A: Living well in care homes: a systematic review of qualitative studies. Age Ageing 41:429–440, 2012.
20. Gordon AL, Franklin M, Bradshaw L, et al: Health status of UK care home residents: a cohort study. Age Ageing 43:97–103, 2014.
29. Kinley J, Hockley J, Stone L, et al: The provision of care for residents dying in U.K. nursing care homes. Age Ageing 43:375–379, 2014.
32. Donald IP, Gladman J, Conroy S, et al: Care home medicine in the UK—in from the cold. Age Ageing 37:618–620, 2008.
37. British Geriatrics Society: Commissioning for excellence in care homes, London, 2013, BGS. http://www.bgs.org.uk/index.php/commissioning2013-2. Accessed January 2, 2015.
38. Alldred DP, Raynor DK, Hughes C, et al: Interventions to optimise prescribing for older people in care homes. Cochrane Database Syst Rev (2):CD009095, 2013.
48. Katz PR, Karuza J, Intrator O, et al: Nursing home physician specialists: a response to the workforce crisis in long-term care. Ann Intern Med 150:411–413, 2009.
49. Morley JE, Caplan G, Cesari M, et al: International survey of nursing home research priorities. J Am Med Dir Assoc 15:309–312, 2014.

125 Institutional Long-Term Care in the United States

Joseph G. Ouslander

OVERVIEW

The purpose of this chapter is to give readers a brief perspective on institutional long-term care (LTC) in the United States. The focus will be on assisted living facilities (ALFs) and nursing homes (NHs). In the United States, NHs are also commonly referred to as nursing facilities and skilled nursing facilities (SNFs). For ALFs, most states use the term *assisted living*, but some use residential care or other similar terminology. Other types of LTC facilities exist, and some care for younger patients but, given the focus of this text, the care of the geriatric population in ALFs and NHs will be highlighted.

ALFs and NHs provide health, social, and recreational services to chronically ill people who, for medical, functional, psychological, and/or social reasons, choose not to live in their own homes. Most ALFs and NHs are for-profit businesses and operate independently of each other. However, in many areas of the United States, there are campuses with independent living units, an ALF, and a NH in close proximity, and home care services are also commonly available. In these continuing care retirement communities (CCRCs), individuals pay an up-front entry fee (or purchase a unit) and live the rest of their lives on the campus, guaranteed a higher level of care when they need it. Because of the community nature and resulting high quality of care common in CCRCs, this is becoming an increasingly popular choice for older adults who can afford it.

There are several fundamental differences between U.S. ALFs and NHs (Table 125-1). First, ALFs are generally more like senior housing based on a social model, as opposed to the predominant health care focus of NHs. Although ALFs care for relatively well and functionally impaired older adults, and many have dementia units, the level of functional disability in NHs is generally higher, and medical acuity is higher in NHs that have a high volume of patients admitted immediately after an inpatient hospital stay (referred to subsequently as postacute care). NHs also care for medically complex and disabled younger people, a population that comprises 10% to 15% of the NH population. Thus, the availability of licensed nurses is highly variable in ALFs, whereas a minimum number are required in NHs. Similarly, physicians are not required or frequently present in ALFs, but NHs are required to have a medical director, and those admitted to NHs are required to be certified for this level of care and have a primary care physician of record. Residents of ALFs generally go to a physician's offices for their primary care, although some ALFs have established clinics, and physicians and other health care professionals can provide services on site. ALFs generally have limited access to on-site pharmacy services and diagnostic testing, whereas NHs are required to have pharmacy consultants, generally have ready access to medications through an on-site or contracted pharmacy, and have ready availability of a variety of diagnostic tests (e.g., blood work, electrocardiography, x-rays and, in some cases, other imaging procedures). ALFs are generally smaller and vary in size more than NHs; the average bed capacity of a NH is close to 100 beds, and some are much larger. State and federal regulations that oversee care in ALFs are generally less stringent than those in NHs. NHs are subject to an extensive code of federal regulations related to safety and clinical care. Finally, care is paid for very differently in the ALF versus the NH setting, as will be discussed.

Despite the growth of community-based, long-term care programs that strive to maintain older adults in their own homes, the need for institutional LTC continues to grow in the United States. This is in large part because of the increasing longevity and corresponding functional disability among those who live to extreme old age, decreasing number and geographic proximity of children (especially daughters, who provide the most support to functionally impaired older Americans and who are increasingly joining the work force, thus limiting their caregiving abilities), and economic factors. Although the number of NHs has stayed the same or decreased slightly over the last decade, the number of ALFs has grown substantially, and care for many functionally impaired older adults who would have previously been admitted to NHs. Economic factors are also critical in determining the need for institutional LTC, and are very different in countries with a national health program combined with more ready availability of in-home social support. Thus, to understand the role of institutional LTC in the U.S, one must understand how LTC is financed.

FINANCING OF LONG-TERM CARE

Health care for older Americans is funded in one of four basic ways: (1) private health insurance; (2) Medicare; (3) Medicaid; and (4) out-of-pocket expenditures. Although many insurance companies sell long-term care policies, private insurance still plays a relatively small role in paying for LTC at the present time. Medicare is a federally administered health insurance program for those aged 65 years or older and for a smaller number of younger people who are severely medically disabled and/or who have end-stage renal disease requiring renal replacement therapy. The vast majority of older Americans qualify for basic Medicare coverage by contributions that they or a spouse have made during their working years. Most older Americans still incorrectly believe that Medicare will pay for LTC. It is not until they or a relative needs LTC services that reality sets in. Less than 10% of overall Medicare expenditures go to LTC. Medicare does not pay for in-home support for assistance with activities of daily living (ADLs) on an ongoing basis and does not pay for care in an ALF. Medicare will pay for time-limited skilled services (nursing, rehabilitation therapy) at home or in an ALF after a hospitalization for people who are home-bound. Medicare will also pay for up to 100 days of care in a NH after an acute illness (20 days are fully covered, and thereafter there is a substantial co-payment), but only in certain situations. To qualify for Medicare reimbursement, admission to the NH must follow a 3-day stay in an acute-care hospital, and the patient must require continuous skilled nursing care and/or active rehabilitation with carefully documented potential and progress to achieve a lower level of care. This so-called 3-day rule is highly controversial and incentivizes hospitalizing older people so that they can receive the Medicare benefit for postacute care. This rule is waived for some types of managed care programs (see later).

Patients recovering from surgery, hip fracture, or stroke with good rehabilitation potential, patients with unstable medical conditions (e.g., those requiring intravenous medications), and patients with multiple chronic illnesses who have become deconditioned in the hospital resulting in new functional disability are examples of patients who will qualify for Medicare coverage for

TABLE 125-1 Characteristics of Assisted Living Facilities (ALFs) and Nursing Homes (NHs)

Characteristics	Assisted Living Facilities	Nursing Homes
Model of care	Residential with supportive services	Nursing, rehabilitative, and medical care
Residents	Close to 95% > 65 yr, most with impairments in instrumental activities of daily living (ADLs) and some with impairment of basic ADLs Many ALFs have dementia units	85% to 90% > 65 yr, almost all with impairments in basic ADLs Population is heterogeneous depending on characteristics and goals of care (short vs. long stayers; see Figure 125-1)
Payment for care	Almost all private pay In some states, Medicaid will support ALF care for the poor. Medicare will pay for home care for a temporary period of time after an acute illness.	Medicare will pay for up to 100 days of skilled care after acute illness for patients who meet specific criteria. Medicaid pays for close to two thirds of care in U.S. NHs. The remainder is private pay.
Size	Most <25 beds, about one third have 26-100 beds, only 5% have >100 beds	Average size is 100 beds; one third larger than 100 beds
Ownership	About 80% are for profit.	About two-thirds for profit
Staff	Key staff are residential care coordinators and aides. Availability of licensed nurses variable Other clinical staff usually not on site	Availability of registered nurses and licensed practical nurses mandated at specific levels Most hands-on care provided by certified nursing assistants Other interdisciplinary team members usually on site (e.g., social worker, rehabilitation therapists, etc.)
Availability of clinical services	On-site diagnostic testing and pharmacy services uncommon	Most, especially in urban areas have on-site availability of diagnostic testing and pharmacy services.
Medical care	Physicians usually not present on site No requirement for medical director	Physicians and physician extenders (NPs, PAs) usually present > once/wk Medical director required
Regulations	Federal regulations not as stringent as for nursing homes; state regulations vary considerably	Subject to extensive code of federal regulations focused on safety, environment, and clinical care

TABLE 125-2 Characteristics of Short-Stay Postacute Patients in Nursing Homes

- Skilled nursing observation and care of congestive heart, chronic obstructive pulmonary disease, renal failure, diabetes, stroke
- Physical, occupational, and/or speech therapy five times/wk
- Acute and chronic pain management
- Intravenous or central line–administered antibiotics
- Injectable medications daily or more often
- Weaning oxygen requirement with pulse oximetry
- Respiratory therapy treatment once daily or more frequently
- Frequent capillary blood glucose level monitoring
- Wound care daily for pressure ulcers
- Enteral tube feedings
- Laboratory monitoring required
- Renal dialysis with monitoring
- Bladder and bowel training protocols

postacute care in an NH (Table 125-2). However, the average coverage period is approximately 25 days because patients have reached their maximum medical and rehabilitative benefits, and Medicare will no longer pay for their care. Patients with dementia and other chronic functional disabilities, on the other hand, are viewed as requiring custodial institutional LTC and do not qualify for Medicare coverage.

Thus, the vast majority (>60%) of funding for institutional LTC comes from out-of-pocket expenditures or Medicaid. Medicaid is a state-administered medical welfare program for the poor; one has to have very limited income and assets to qualify, and benefits vary among the 50 states. This has created a phenomenon termed *spend down*—older Americans must spend down their assets to pay for institutional and noninstitutional LTC until they become poor enough to qualify for Medicaid, which will then cover LTC costs. Because private pay rates for most LTC facilities are in the range of $4,000 to $10,000/month (and in some cases higher), spend down occurs relatively quickly for most older Americans who enter an institutional LTC setting.

In many areas of the United States, the growth of managed capitated systems of care is also substantially affecting LTC. Nationally, approximately one third of older Americans have opted into a Medicare Advantage plan, which is a managed capitated program administered by an insurance company. In these managed capitated systems of care (previously known as a health maintenance organization [HMO]), the insurance company receives a fixed rate for a Medicare beneficiary each month. One of the main ways of saving money in this system is to reduce the number of acute hospitals days. As a result, patients in these health plans are being discharged rapidly from acute hospitals into NHs while still subacutely ill. In addition, because in most capitated systems there is no 3-day acute hospital requirement for Medicare reimbursement of postacute care in a NH, some acutely ill patients may completely bypass the acute hospital. For example, patients in a Medicare Advantage program with deep vein thrombosis or mild pneumonia or cellulitis requiring intravenous antibiotics may be directly admitted to a NH, without an acute hospital stay. These economic incentives are driving the growth of a higher level of skilled care in NHs and are resulting in an unmet need for more highly trained nurses and physicians in this setting.

Assisted Living Facilities

ALFs are a growing entity in the continuum of LTC in the United States. In 2011 to 2012, there were over 700,000 residents of over 22,000 ALFs and similar residential facilities. Almost 80% of ALFs are owned and operated by a for-profit business. Most ALFs have a 25-bed capacity or less, about one third have 26 to 100 beds, and about 5% have more than 100 beds. ALFs are residential units that can provide additional services to residents, including meal preparation, laundry, housekeeping, incontinence care, and medication management. The vast majority of ALF residents need assistance with several instrumental ADLS and with at least one basic ADL. In general, the more assistance a resident needs, the higher the monthly payment. Older adults needing skilled nursing care, intensive rehabilitation, and/or who have complex multimorbidity and functional impairments generally require placement in a NH. Many ALFs have, however, adopted an aging in place philosophy, which has led to many very impaired individuals continuing to live in an ALF. Many also have locked dementia units. This has in turn created concerns over safety issues and quality of care. Preventable and treatable conditions may not be optimally identified, evaluated, and managed in the ALF setting.[1-3]

Most ALFs are managed by a full-time care coordinator and a number of nursing assistants. ALFs may have one or more licensed nurses present during daytime hours or who are available on-call for emergencies. Because ALFs do not receive Medicare funding, they are outside the purview and regulation of federal laws and are regulated in varying degrees on a state-by-state basis. The vast majority of ALFs do not have on-site medical oversight by a physician or a so-called physician extender (e.g., nurse practitioner [NP], physician's assistant [PA]). Medical care is provided by a resident's primary care physician and, usually, transportation to and from the physician's office must be arranged.

Although ALF costs are on average substantially less than NH care, this cost remains unaffordable to many low- and moderate-income older adults. Medicare does not pay for care in an ALF unless the resident qualifies for an episode of skilled care after an acute illness. In this situation, a home health agency can come into the ALF and provide nursing and rehabilitation therapy on a temporary basis. Medicaid only pays for ALF care on a limited basis and only in some states. Thus, ALF care is an out-of-pocket personal expense for older adults choosing to live in this setting.

Nursing Homes

In the United States, there are many more NH beds than acute-care hospital beds. There are between 6,000 and 7,000 acute-care hospitals, with a total of approximately 1 million beds, and there are close to 16,000 NHs, with over 1.5 million beds. The average size of a NH is close to 100 beds, and about one third are larger than 100 beds. Two thirds are run for profit, and a large proportion of these are run by organizations that own several or a chain of NHs. The federal and state governments also operate some NHs, including over 120 in the Veterans Administration system, which serves veterans of the U.S. Armed Forces who are eligible for LTC placement.

Because of how health and social services are funded, and the extensive regulations imposed on NHs by the federal and state governments, these facilities tend to follow a medical rather than a social model. Thus, most U.S. LTC facilities look like and are administered in a manner similar to small acute-care hospitals, rather than residential homes, in which skilled nursing, medical, and other services are available. A growing movement for culture change in U.S. NHs has advocated for more homelike environments and for more person-centered care.[4]

Oversight of medical care in NHs is provided by a physician medical director. This federally mandated position allows input by the medical director into policy and procedure development and is a valuable liaison to the administrator and director of nursing. The medical director is also required to provide, or arrange for, emergency medical coverage when a resident's primary care physician of record cannot be reached.

At any one time about 5%, or 1.6 million, of the U.S. population aged 65 years and older is in an NH. However, this is a deceiving statistic for several reasons. First, the rate of NH use varies considerably with age and gender. Among those 65 to 74 years of age, less than 3% are in a NH; among those 85 years of age and older, about 15% of men and 25% of women are in a NH, and close to 50% in this age group die there or shortly after discharge from an NH to an acute-care hospital. Second, a subgroup of NH residents resides in the NH for only a short time period. Thus, this lifetime risk of entering a NH is underestimated by the prevalence data cited above. It is now estimated that Americans who were 65 years old in 1990 have a 43% chance of spending some time in an LTC facility; the chance is greater for women (≈50%) than for men (≈33%). Third, for every older U.S. adult in an NH, there are two or three with a similar clinical and functional status living at home or in an ALF. The primary factors that determine whether an older U.S. adult enters an NH include their medical and functional status, availability and accessibility of family, friends, and other noninstitutional, community-based, long-term care services, and financial resources.

Nursing Home Staff

The key staff members in a U.S. NH are the administrator, who is responsible for the daily operation of the facility, and the director of nursing, who supervises the bulk of the facility's employees. Although there are federal staffing standards, most NHs have relatively few registered and licensed nurses; staff ratios average about one registered nurse for each 50 beds and one licensed practical nurse for each 25 to 30 beds. Over 90% of the hands-on care in U.S. NHs is provided by certified nursing assistants (CNAs), who are generally poorly educated, may not speak English (especially in some areas), and earn low wages. This staffing ratio makes caring for an increasingly complex and subacutely ill population being discharged from hospitals very challenging. Moreover, CNA turnover rates exceed 50%/year in many facilities, and there is also a relatively high turnover of licensed nurses and NH leadership in some NHs. This makes staff education and consistent implementation of clinical care programs very challenging. In addition, the high rate of turnover makes person-centered care challenging and also results in a failure to recognize changes in a resident's condition, resulting in potentially preventable progression of illness and hospitalizations.

The interdisciplinary team is critical to high-quality care in NHs. Most members of the team are required by federal regulation. However, in some NHs, members of the interdisciplinary team, including rehabilitation therapists, social workers, activity therapists, pharmacists, clergy, and dietitians, are part-time and/or work under contract, rather than as employees of the NH. Ancillary services, such as laboratory, x-ray and other imaging studies, dentistry, and podiatry, are provided by outside contractors. In U.S. urban areas, these professionals and services are generally readily available.

Nursing Home Residents

NH residents are generally characterized as predominantly older women with impaired mobility and dementia. Although it is true that close to 75% of NH residents are women older than 75 years, over 50% are nonambulatory and need assistance in transferring, and over 50% are incontinent of urine and have some degree of dementia, this type of characterization masks the heterogeneity of the NH population. NH residents can also be broadly characterized based on their length of stay: short stayers (e.g., <100 days) versus long stayers. Short-stayers can be subdivided into two groups—patients who enter a NH for short-term rehabilitation after an acute illness (e.g., hip fracture, stroke) and those who are medically unstable or terminally ill who are quickly discharged to an acute hospital or will eventually die in the NH. Table 125-2 lists the types of conditions that are prevalent among short stayers and those for which Medicare will pay for postacute care. The proportion of NH residents who are short stayers is growing because patients are being rapidly discharged from acute hospitals and, as mentioned earlier, some acutely ill patients in capitated systems of care are admitted directly to NHs to avoid costly acute hospital stays. Short stayers account for about 15% to 20% of NH residents at any one time but probably outnumber long stayers because of their rapid turnover. Long stayers can be subdivided into three groups: (1) those with primarily cognitive impairment (e.g., the ambulatory wandering resident with Alzheimer disease or related dementia); (2) those with primarily impairments of physical function (e.g., the resident with severe arthritis or end-stage heart or lung disease); and (3) those with cognitive and physical impairments. Figure 125-1 illustrates this

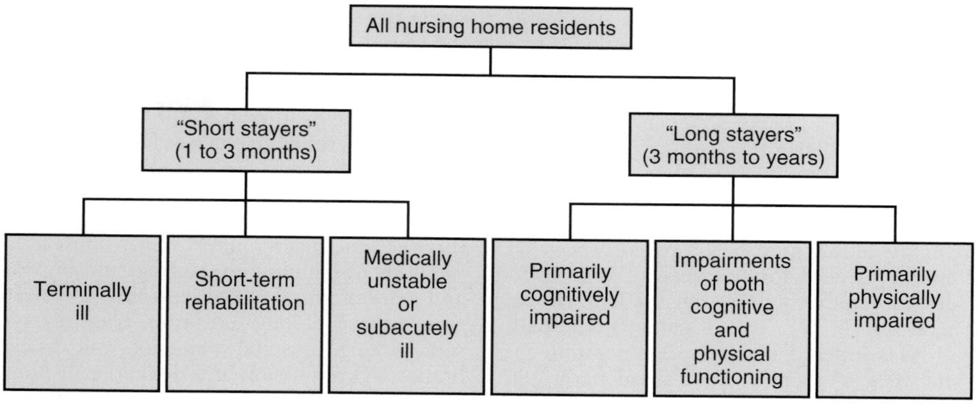

Figure 125-1. Different types of residents in nursing homes. *(From Kane RA, Ouslander JG, Abrass IB, Resnick B: Essentials of clinical geriatrics, ed 7, New York, 2013, McGraw-Hill.)*

subgrouping of the NH population.[5] Obviously, residents may move from one subgroup to another when acute illnesses intervene, chronic illness develops or worsens, or cognitive or physical function declines.

Conceptualizing NH residents in this manner has important implications for the goals of care, evaluating the quality of care, and structure of the NH environment. The goals of caring for a previously healthy patient undergoing rehabilitation after a hip fracture are obviously very different from the goals of caring for a resident with advanced dementia and related behavioral disorders or the goals of caring for someone with a terminal malignancy. Similarly, from the perspective of quality, processes and outcomes of care relevant for one subgroup of NH residents may be inappropriate or irrelevant to another subgroup. Many NHs geographically separate different subgroups of residents by creating specialized units. This approach offers many potential advantages when it is feasible—the physical environment can be modified for certain types of residents (e.g., those are at risk of elopement), the staff can be trained and develop expertise in managing specific types of care (e.g., palliative or hospice-type care, rehabilitative care), and residents are often more comfortable when they are around others to whom they can relate. The latter is especially true for cognitively intact patients who are often very distressed by constant interaction, especially at mealtimes, with residents who have dementia and associated behavioral disorders. In a typical 100 to 120 bed NH, 10 to 30 beds are occupied by those needing short-term, skilled, postacute care, and the remainder are occupied by long stayers. Many NHs try to maximize the number of short stayers because of the relatively high Medicare payments for post-hospital care. Such NHs have a substantially higher medical acuity level than other NHs and require more trained and skilled nurses and physicians to provide safe, high-quality care.

Medical Care in Nursing Homes

The goals of medical care in U.S. NHs are listed in Table 125-3. Although these goals appropriately focus on several nonmedical aspects of care, the increasing acuity of medical conditions of NH residents and the influence of these conditions on function and quality of life demand that well-trained physicians be integrally involved in NH care. The American Medical Directors Association (AMDA; the Society for Post-Acute and Long-Term Care Medicine) has developed numerous clinical practice guidelines, standards, and competencies for medical care in NHs.[6]

Each NH resident is required to have a primary care physician. Often, an individual's usual primary care physician does not provide care in the NH and, in this situation, newly admitted residents are assigned a primary physician. This role is commonly fulfilled by the medical director, especially in rural areas of the United States. The vast majority of NHs are too small to have a full-time medical staff or even a full-time medical director, although a small proportion of the larger facilities have both. Most facilities have a loosely organized medical staff supervised by a medical director who works part-time for the NH and is paid on an hourly, monthly, or annual basis. Because most NHs are run for profit and have an open medical staff, numerous primary care physicians may be involved in a single facility. This situation can make it difficult for the nursing staff to develop effective communication and rapport with the medical staff, as well as making it more difficult for the medical director to monitor policies, procedures, and standards for medical care.

The role of the primary attending physician is to perform a comprehensive medical evaluation at the time of admission, periodically reassess the resident's progress, and assess acute changes in condition when they occur. In general, residents must be seen by a physician within 72 hours of admission, every 30 days for the first 90 days and then every 60 days thereafter. Thus, physicians are usually in the NH only once or twice a month, depending on the number of residents they care for in a given NH. The lack of physician presence in NHs results in many unnecessary phone calls and the overuse of acute-care hospital emergency departments for evaluation of acute changes in condition. One successful approach to this issue is the involvement of physician extenders (NPs and PAs). They are trained in basic patient care assessment techniques and generally manage acute conditions using standard protocols under the supervision of a physician. They may be hired by a physician or group of physicians and

TABLE 125-3 Goals of Medical Care in Nursing Homes

- Provide a safe and supportive environment for chronically ill and dependent people.
- Restore and maintain the highest possible level of functional independence.
- Preserve individual autonomy.
- Maximize quality of life, perceived well-being, and life satisfaction.
- Provide comfort and dignity for terminally ill patients and their loved ones.
- Stabilize and delay progression, whenever possible, of chronic medical conditions.
- Prevent acute medical and iatrogenic illnesses, and identify and treat them rapidly when they do occur.
- Provide rehabilitation-oriented interdisciplinary care to postacute patients.
- Prevent iatrogenic illness and adverse events.

spend a substantial amount of their time in the facility. Medicare pays NPs and PAs 85% to 90% of a physician's allowable fee for such care. Several studies have demonstrated that physician-NP teams provide a high quality of care and reduce the number of hospital transfers.[7,8]

QUALITY OF CARE

Although many U.S. LTC facilities provide excellent care, the overall quality of care in this setting must be improved, especially given the projected enormous need for and costs of LTC over the next several decades. In a study conducted by the U.S. Office of the Inspector General (OIG), 22% of 650 patients admitted to a national sample of NHs suffered an adverse event within 35 days of admission, and 50% of these events caused harm.[9] A review of these events by expert clinicians has suggested that 59% are preventable. The most common adverse events were medication-related (e.g., altered mental status, bleeding, falls, constipation), infections, falls, dehydration, and omissions in care. The annual costs of these adverse events were estimated to be close to $3 billion.

At least four approaches are required to improve institutional LTC in the United States: (1) changes in the way that LTC is financed; (2) improvements in regulations and the survey and certification process; (3) education and training in the use of clinical practice tools; and (4) research. The Patient Protection and Affordable Care Act (ACA; commonly called Obamacare) includes provisions for Medicare to shift reimbursement from a fee-for-service–based system that incentivizes more care to a system that incentivizes quality of care and coordination of care between acute care hospitals and LTC. These changes are intended to reduce the unnecessary use of diagnostic and therapeutic interventions that have higher risks in the LTC population and lack evidence of benefit. A major focus is on reducing unnecessary hospital admissions and the associated incidence of hospital-acquired conditions and costs. The Centers for Medicare & Medicaid Services (CMS) has funded numerous demonstration projects to develop and test new and innovative models of care that meet these goals.[10]

From a regulatory standpoint, quality indicators have been developed that are derived from the federally mandated resident assessment the minimum data set (MDS),[11] and are used to post the incidence of these measures publicly on the CMS website, along with a five-star rating derived in part from these quality indicators. Despite improvements in the MDS (version 3.011), the quality indicators and five-star rating system remain imperfect and require substantial improvement. Although NHs are highly regulated in the United States and must adhere to an extensive code of federal regulations, the survey and certification process that assesses adherence to these regulations remains challenging. Improvements in the interpretive guidance that surveyors use to assess adherence could make an impact on the quality of the surveys and the quality of care. The ACA has also mandated that NHs have a system of Quality Assurance and Performance Improvement (QAPI). CMS has developed tools and resources for NHs to use in meeting this requirement.[12] However, more than financial changes and regulations will be necessary to improve care in U.S. LTC institutions. Education in geriatric medicine, gerontology, and LTC must increase for physicians, nurses, and all other health care professionals who care for LTC residents. AMDA's clinical practice guidelines, other clinical practice tools, continuing education programs, and the certification process for medical directors have made important contributions in this regard, as have other professional organizations. A comprehensive curriculum and related resources on NH care targeting an international audience has recently been published.[13]

Although research in the LTC setting is challenging,[14] there is a critical need to increase research in NHs and ALFs. A broad range of research is needed.[15] Basic studies will help determine the causes, treatment, and prevention of conditions that lead to institutional LTC admission, such as Alzheimer disease, stroke, and osteoporosis. Clinical trials can also assist in identifying the most effective strategies for managing common conditions among LTC residents, such as falls, incontinence, depression, and behavioral disorders associated with dementia. More research is also needed to address issues of quality of life and ethics, which are so important in the institutional LTC population. Health services and quality improvement research will help identify methods of defining, measuring, and improving quality of care and determining the most cost-effective strategies for managing many aspects of long-term care. Transitions of care between care settings (e.g., hospital admission and discharge to the NH or home, NH admission and discharge to home) has evolved as a major focus of such research, examining the nature, incidence, and prevention of hospitalizations that may be unnecessary.[16-20] Such research will improve care, reduce morbidity from hospital-acquired conditions, and save billions of dollars that can be reinvested in high-quality care programs. Only through this type of multifaceted research will we learn more about caring for the millions of people who will spend some time in a U.S. LTC facility. Additionally, research can help identify methods of improving quality of care, which may decrease the risk of litigation against LTC facilities seen during the last decade.

KEY POINTS

- Institutional long-term care in the United States is largely provided in assisted living facilities (ALFs), other residential care facilities, and nursing homes (NHs), also called nursing facilities or skilled nursing facilities.
- There are substantial differences between ALFs and NHs in terms of the model of care, size, resident population, reimbursement, availability of clinical staff, medical care, and ancillary services and how the settings are regulated.
- ALFs provide a residential setting with supported services, with limited on-site nursing staff, clinical services, and physician availability.
- NHs care for a heterogeneous group of patients, including short stayers (e.g., <100 days) and long stayers, and specified nursing staffing levels and a medical director are required.
- Most ALF care is paid for out of pocket, whereas most NH care is supported by Medicaid for those poor enough to qualify. Medicare pays for postacute care in an NH, but only under specific circumstances.
- Regulations for ALFs vary state by state, whereas NHs are subject to an extensive code of federal regulations focused on safety, the environment, and clinical care.
- Adverse events are common within the first month of admission to an NH and most are preventable. Multifaceted approaches are needed to improve the quality of institutional LTC in the United States.

For a complete list of references, please visit www.expertconsult.com.

KEY REFERENCES

1. AGS Health Care Systems Committee: Assisted living facilities: American Geriatrics Society position paper. J Am Geriatr Soc 53:536–537, 2005.
2. Rosenblatt A, Samus QM, Steele CD, et al: The Maryland Assisted Living Study: prevalence, recognition, and treatment of dementia and other psychiatric disorders in the assisted living population of central Maryland. J Am Geriatr Soc 52:1618–1625, 2004.
3. Young HM, Gray SL, McCormick WC, et al: Types, prevalence, and potential clinical significance of medication administration errors in assisted living. J Am Geriatr Soc 56:1199–1205, 2008.

4. Advancing Excellence Long-Term Care Collaborative: Advancing excellence in America's nursing homes campaign. https://www.nhqualitycampaign.org. Accessed October 16, 2014.
5. Kane RA, Ouslander JG, Abrass IB, et al: Essentials of clinical geriatrics, ed 7, New York, 2013, McGraw-Hill.
6. AMDA Foundation: Clinical practice guidelines in the long-term care setting. http://www.amda.com/tools/guidelines.cfm. Accessed October 16, 2014.
7. Rueben D, Buchanan J, Farley D, et al: Primary care of long-stay nursing home residents: a comparison of 3 HMO programs with fee-for-service care. J Am Geriatr Soc 47:131–138, 1999.
8. Konetzka RT, Spector W, Limcangco MR: Reducing hospitalizations from LTC settings. Med Care Res Rev 65:40–66, 2008.
9. Office of Inspector General, Department of Health and Human Services: Adverse events in skilled nursing facilities: national incidence among Medicare beneficiaries. http://oig.hhs.gov/oei/reports/oei-06-11-00370.pdf. Accessed October 16, 2014.
10. Centers for Medicare & Medicaid Services: The CMS Innovation Center. http://innovation.cms.gov. Accessed October 16, 2014.
11. Saliba D, Jones M, Streim J, et al: Overview of significant changes in the minimum data set for nursing homes. J Am Med Dir Assoc 13:595–601, 2012.
12. Centers for Medicare & Medicaid Services: Quality assurance and performance improvement. http://www.cms.gov/Medicare/Provider-Enrollment-and-Certification/QAPI/nhqapi.html. Accessed October 16, 2014.
13. Morley J, Tolson D, Ouslander J, et al: Nursing home care: a core curriculum for the International Association for Gerontology and Geriatrics, New York, 2013, McGraw Hill.
14. Ouslander JG, Schnelle JF: Research in nursing homes: practical aspects. J Am Geriatr Soc 41:182–187, 1993.
15. Morley JE, Caplan G, Cesari M, et al: International survey of nursing home research priorities. J Am Med Dir Assoc 15:309–312, 2014.
16. Ouslander JG, Lamb G, Perloe M, et al: Potentially avoidable hospitalizations of nursing home residents: frequency, causes, and costs. J Am Geriatr Soc 58:627–635, 2010.
17. Walsh EG, Wiener JM, Haber S, et al: Potentially avoidable hospitalizations of dually eligible Medicare/Medicaid beneficiaries from nursing facility and home and community-based services waiver programs. J Am Geriatr Soc 60:821–829, 2012.
18. Ouslander JG, Maslow K: Geriatrics and the triple aim: defining preventable hospitalizations in the long-term care population. J Am Geriatr Soc 60:2313–2318, 2012.
19. Ouslander JG, Lamb G, Tappen R, et al: Interventions to reduce hospitalizations from nursing homes: evaluation of the INTERACT II collaborative quality improvement project. J Am Geriatr Soc 59:745–753, 2011.
20. Berkowitz RE, Fang Z, Helfand BK, et al: Project ReEngineeing Discharge (RED) lowers hospital readmissions of patients discharged from a skilled nursing facility. J Am Med Dir Assoc 14:736–740, 2013.

126 Education in Geriatric Medicine

Adam L. Gordon, Ruth E. Hubbard

Midway through the second decade of the twenty-first century, geriatric medicine finds itself at an interesting crossroads. There seems to be a "know-do" gap. Although we *know* about the aging population and how to deliver evidence-based care to achieve the best outcomes, most health and social care economies continue to struggle to *do* so. Recruitment crises afflict geriatric medicine in North America[1,2] and Australia,[3] while the availability of geriatricians varies considerably across Europe.[4] Outside developed economies, the specialty frequently does not exist.[5] Internationally, the specialist nursing skills required to support older people are underrecognized, with implications for recruitment and retention in services for these patients.[6] Medical students, although increasingly appreciative of the emotional and intellectual rewards associated with geriatric medicine, continue to recognize financial and status-related limitations associated with a career in the specialty.[7]

Comprehensive reviews of medical training in the United Kingdom,[8] United States,[9] and Australia,[10] among other countries, have stated that the identification and management of frailty and functional dependency are integral to effective training in general (internal) medicine. However, as countries work out how to operationalize recommendations, a number of tensions have been identified. In some health economies, there are powerful specialties with historical responsibility for generalist practice, examples being general (internal) medicine and general practice. In other countries, emergent specialties have developed to fill the gap left as organ specialists have become ever more removed from general practice by subspecialization such as hospitalism[11] in the United States and acute medicine in the United Kingdom.[12] At best, these traditional or emerging power-bases have recognized the knowledge and skill sets required to care for older patients, and they are up-skilling appropriately. At worst, they exert control and moral authority over the care of older people with frailty ("We're all geriatricians now"[13]) without recognizing the important lessons from the literature around comprehensive geriatric assessment (CGA) or realizing the skill sets required to deliver it.

A further set of tensions has emerged from the tendency of hospital-based, single-organ or single-system doctors to become ever more subspecialized; this has resulted in two contrary lines of argument. The first states that the needs of those with multiple pathologies would best be met by ensuring that all older patients have access to an appropriate array of subspecialists[14]; the second states that, in order to maintain a subspecialist skill set, single-organ specialists must retreat from the demands of the acute unselected medical take, as continued involvement will make disproportionate demands on their time with the effective assertion that generalism is the preserve of hospitalists, acute physicians, general practitioners, and geriatricians.[15]

Clearly these dichotomies will play out differently in different countries, depending on historical power bases, models of health care funding, and prevailing assumptions among doctors, policy makers, and the population at large. However, while the policy and service delivery context differs between nations, the basic fundamentals of what doctors and other health care professionals need to deliver good care remain the same. That is to say, effective education in the core knowledge, skills, attitudes, and competencies in the care of older people is a banner behind which geriatricians around the world can effectively rally to drive up the standards seen by patients.

This chapter presents a summary of recent progress in key areas of education about health care of older people under four main headings: (1) what doctors need to know, (2) innovations in how we teach doctors what they need to know, (3) the importance of multidisciplinarity and interprofessional education, and (4) facilitators and barriers to effective educational interventions.

WHAT DOCTORS NEED TO KNOW ABOUT AGING

All doctors need to know something about aging. Older people make up the largest proportion of health and social care users. In the United Kingdom, two thirds of acute hospital admissions are aged older than 65[16] and the highest general practice consultation rates are for people aged 85 to 89.[17] In the United States outpatient visits from adults older than 65 years comprise 56% of the workload in ophthalmology, 54% in cardiology, and 46% in urology.[18] The Council on Resident Education in Obstetrics and Gynecology predicts that one fifth of women cared for by obstetricians and gynecologists will be older than age 65 by 2030.[19] The average age and number of comorbidities of elective surgical patients are increasing.[20] Given these statistics, the service and resource implications of caring effectively for older patients are such that even those very few doctors who don't interact at all with older adults in their clinical practice, such as pediatricians, will need to know enough about the core issues to effectively contend a place for their own discipline within the broader medical endeavor.

Clearly, though, the level of knowledge required by pediatricians is different from that required by general physicians, who are likely to see older patients as a routine part of their daily work. General physicians need to have competencies enabling them to safely provide basic care to older patients, while identifying opportunities for more specialized intervention. Specialist geriatricians, meanwhile, need to have competencies in frailty identification and management, in the coordination and facilitation of CGA, and in commonly presenting conditions of later life (e.g., falls, syncope, fractures, stroke, movement disorders, incontinence, cognitive impairment, and end-of-life care) to augment upon and support the work of more generalist colleagues. This leads to a three-tiered competency model as summarized in Figure 126-1.

Competencies Required by All Doctors

International agreement about the specifics of what should be taught is most advanced at the undergraduate level—the competencies required by all doctors—where a number of international curricula have been published.[21] The International Association of Geriatrics and Gerontology (IAGG), through consultation with its 73 member organizations representing 65 countries, produced a guideline comprising 15 statements specifying minimum requirements for geriatric medical education in 2008. These guidelines are no longer available in print or online. There are, however, English language curricula specified by a number of national specialist societies; these organizations and links to curricula are given in Table 126-1.

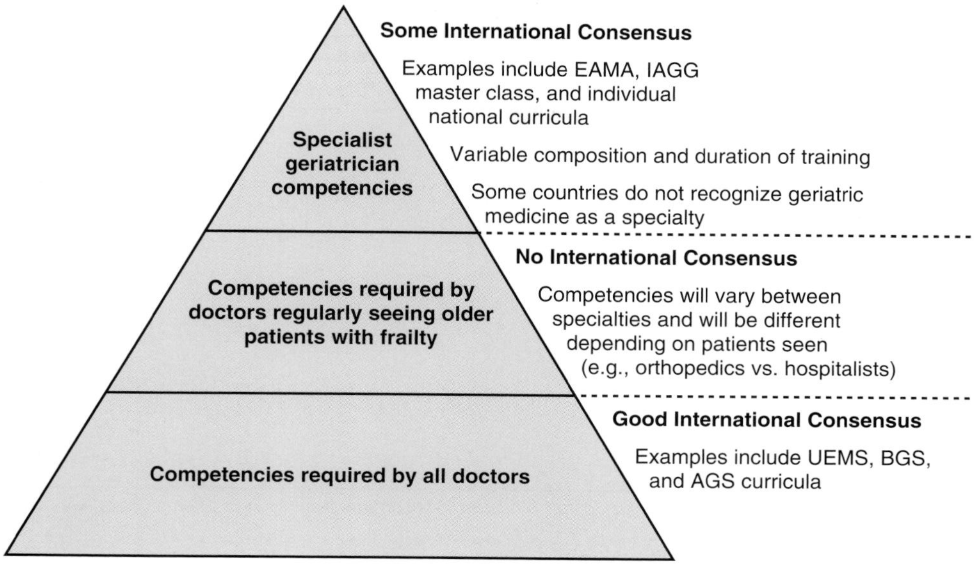

Figure 126-1. The "three-tiered" competency model of care of older people. *AGS,* American Geriatrics Society; *BGS,* British Geriatrics Society; *EAMA,* European Academy for Medicine of Ageing; *IAGG,* International Association of Geriatrics and Gerontology; *UEMS,* European Union of Medical Specialists.

TABLE 126-1 English Language Undergraduate Curricula in Geriatric Medicine

Organization	Web Link to Curriculum
Association of American Medical Colleges	http://www.pogoe.org/Minimum_Geriatric_Competencies
Australia and New Zealand Society for Geriatric Medicine	http://www.anzsgm.org/documents/PositionStatementNo4-Revision.pdf
British Geriatrics Society	http://www.bgs.org.uk/index.php/medicalstudentstop/959-undergraduatecurriculum8
Canadian Geriatrics Society	http://www.canadiangeriatrics.ca/default/assets/File/CGS_Competencies.pdf
Union of European Medical Specialists	http://ageing.oxfordjournals.org/content/43/5/695

TABLE 126-2 English Language Curricula for Postresidency Training in Geriatric Medicine

Organization	Web Link to Curriculum
American Geriatrics Society and Association of Directors of Geriatric Academic Programs	http://onlinelibrary.wiley.com/doi/10.1111/jgs.12821/full
Joint Royal Colleges of Physicians Training Board and British Geriatrics Society	http://www.jrcptb.org.uk/specialties/geriatric-medicine
Royal Australasian College of Physicians	https://www.racp.edu.au/page/specialty/geriatrics
Royal College of Physicians and Surgeons of Canada	http://www.royalcollege.ca

In the United States, a consortium of geriatrician educators used an iterative multistage approach to develop a list of core competencies for foundation-level doctors called the "keeping granny safe" competencies.[22] Starting from a literature review of U.S. curricula in geriatrics, they identified 52 non–mutually exclusive geriatric competency domains. They then conducted an iterative process with four stages: experts and broader stakeholders in geriatric medicine were asked to score domains in order of importance, and the top eight were selected; core competencies were written by the steering group to match the selected domains; an electronic survey further reduced the list; and final agreement on 26 competencies was made at a national stakeholder conference.

In the United Kingdom, a literature review identified English language curricula in geriatric medicine and gerontology, which were then presented at a consensus conference involving the national societies for geriatric medicine, biogerontology and social gerontology, and a research collaboration representing gerontechnologists.[23] A core curriculum was agreed and then mapped to the core specifications stipulated in Tomorrow's Doctors, the generic statutory guidance about undergraduate medical training in the United Kingdom. The resulting curricular map became the Recommended Curriculum for Undergraduate Teaching specified by the British Geriatrics Society (BGS).[24]

The European Union of Medical Specialists (UEMS) used the BGS curriculum as the basis for a modified Delphi consensus procedure in 2013. Three Delphi rounds were conducted, involving 49 experts from 29 countries, and complete agreement was reached following the third round. The final curriculum consisted of detailed objectives grouped under 10 overarching learning outcomes.[25]

By nature of their evolution, the U.K. and EU curricula map closely to each other and to previously published guidelines from Australasian and U.S. specialty societies. Work has yet to be undertaken to compare these to the more recent 26 U.S. competencies or to the Canadian curriculum. It may be, though, that the basis of international consensus lies in comparing the EU and U.S. recommendations and identifying core overarching themes.

Competencies Required by Specialist Geriatricians

Consensus is more limited about the core skill set required for doctors to become specialists in geriatric medicine. Freely available English language postresidency training curricula are available from a number of nations; links to these are provided in Table 126-2.

A recently published review of postgraduate training in geriatric medicine across 16 European countries[26] revealed that programs vary substantially in duration, from 1.5 to 7 years, and that

TABLE 126-3 Features of Specialty Training in Geriatric Medicine Across 16 European Countries

Country	Duration of Geriatric Medicine Training (Years)	Clinical Rotations during Geriatric Medicine Training ±				
		Internal Medicine	*Geriatrics*	*Old Age Psychiatry*	*Neurology*	*Community Geriatrics*
Belgium	6	+	+	−	−	−
Denmark	5	+	+	−	−	−
Finland	5	+	+	+	+	+
Italy	5	+	+	+	+	+
Netherlands	5	+	+	+	−	−
Spain	4	+	+	+	+	+
Sweden	5	+	+	+	+	+
United Kingdom	7	+	+	+	−	+
Austria	3	−	+	+	+	−
France	3	−	+	−	−	−
Germany	1.5	−	+	−	−	−
Norway	2	−	+	−	−	−
Switzerland	3	−	+	+	−	−
Turkey	3	−	+	+	+	+
Greece	Specialty not recognized					
Portugal	Specialty not recognized					

Modified from Reiter R, Diraoui S, Van Den Noortgate N, Cruz-Jentoft AJ: How to become a geriatrician in different European countries. Eur Geriatr Med 5:347–351, 2014.

geriatric medicine remains unrecognized in a number of developed health care economies (Table 126-3). The UEMS–Geriatric Medicine Section has set an objective of coordinating consensus regulations for specialist training but recognizes "significant challenges" in doing so, given the considerable variability across member nations.

International training programs have emerged through the European Academy for Medicine of Ageing (EAMA),[27] established under the aegis of professors from Switzerland, Germany, the Netherlands, and United Kingdom in the 1990s and running regular courses since then, and the five master classes run by the IAGG in Asia between 2011 and 2014.[28] However, these have focused very much upon establishing a cadre of international leaders, researchers, and teachers in geriatric medicine rather than equipping a large number of doctors with specialist skills to substantively move forward service developments in their respective regions. Clearly opportunities exist to replicate the consensus exercises undertaken around undergraduate teaching. Although one size is unlikely to fit all, the needs of patients are likely to be relatively similar across most settings and are unlikely to be served by broad variation in what it means to be a specialist geriatrician.

Competencies Required by Doctors Seeing Frail Older Patients

The area of greatest uncertainty is represented by the middle tier of the pyramid in Figure 126-1. There is no doubt that doctors in specialties other than geriatrics require core skills in the management of frail older patients. This has been acknowledged in statements by the U.K. Royal College of Surgeons[29] and American College of Obstetricians and Gynecologists,[19] among others. It is also clear that the skill set required by each of these specialties will overlap, but there will also be areas of mutual exclusivity. One way to engage with these varying requirements has been to develop "bolt on" modules allowing nonspecialists with an interest in developing core knowledge in aging to explore the subject in a way that meets their individual needs, with support and input from expert geriatricians. Important examples of this approach are the Chief Resident Immersion Training (CRIT) in Geriatrics scheme,[30] developed by the Association of Directors of Geriatric Academic Programs (ADGAP) in the United States and the Diploma in Geriatric Medicine run by the Royal College of Physicians of London in the United Kingdom. These schemes remain voluntary, however, and to develop a medical profession truly fit for purpose, individual specialties should be encouraged to develop curricula around aging and frailty that fit their own needs. This should be undertaken with input from specialist geriatricians, given that the convergent knowledge bases will minimize the risk of overlooking "unknown unknowns" (Figure 126-2). Examples of how such programs might proceed come from the pioneering work to develop consensus-based competencies for internal, family, and emergency medicine residents in the United States.[31,32]

INNOVATIONS IN HOW WE TEACH DOCTORS WHAT THEY NEED TO KNOW

The temptation, with an ever-increasing array of novel educational interventions, particularly those focusing on technological advances, is to use interventions for their novelty alone. Educational innovations need to be used where they can logically enhance teaching in geriatric medicine. The literature around novel teaching interventions in the specialty suggest that educators have sought to use them for three main reasons: to free up teacher time, to ensure a reproducible learning experience, or to help develop skills and attitudes in medical students who will care for older patients.

Freeing Up Teacher Time

Some areas of geriatric practice require consideration of challenging concepts that require detailed reflection and discussion. Examples are mental capacity, end-of-life care, elder abuse, and age discrimination. Some of these offer medical students and doctors the opportunity to develop competencies related to more generic learning outcomes that are transferrable to other situations.[33] The consideration of medical principlism in the context of mental capacity, for example, allows application of concepts that can otherwise seem dry and esoteric to real-world scenarios that bring them to life. To teach such complex topics well requires methods that are recognized as promoting discursiveness, dialectic tension, and depth learning—particularly small-group, tutorial-based, and problem-based teaching.[34] These take time from curricula that are already overfilled with medical facts and details. Small-group teaching is more resource intensive: moving a traditional didactic lecture for 70 students to small-group teaching in groups of seven will require a faculty 10 times as large and six

	Known to Geriatricians	Not known to Geriatricians
Known to topic specialists	Geriatric subspecialty competencies included in topic specialty (e.g., syncope in cardiology, stroke in neurology, continence in urology) **Sharing perspectives**	Topic-specific competencies
Not known to topic specialists	Evidence base, skills, and competencies underpinning CGA Geriatric subspecialty competencies not included in topic specialty **Sharing expertise**	**Unknown unknowns** Objective of collaboration is to ensure that core skill sets don't end up in this window pane—important role for allied health professions in minimizing oversights

Figure 126-2. The Johari window of collaboration with "middle-tier" specialties. *CGA,* Comprehensive geriatric assessment.

additional teaching rooms. Canceling seven moderately effective large-scale didactic lectures to make space for one small-group teaching session of uncertain benefit requires that the information conventionally taught at lectures is imparted by alternative modalities that are at least as effective as the conventional methods.

Learning using electronic media, "e-learning," is increasingly popular as a way of taking core information-dense subjects out of lecture format and allowing students to learn in their own time and at their own pace.[35] The Consortium of E-Learning in Geriatrics Instruction (CELGI)[36] was established in the United States to exploit these opportunities, and the Association of Directors of Geriatric Academic Programs (ADGAP) has developed a free online portal of geriatric medicine resources, the Portal of Online Geriatrics education (POGOe), which houses evidence-based teaching resources and curricula.[37]

The main disadvantage of e-learning is the potential isolation of the learner, and some courses have sought to mitigate against this by using interactive discussion boards or blended learning approaches (e-learning combined with more traditional techniques). A U.K. study[38] considered blended learning—traditional ward-based and didactic teaching combined with a computer-aided learning package—and demonstrated improvement in geriatric medicine exam results, when compared with traditional teaching methods. Despite the initial time burden of setting up computer-aided learning, it freed up time for teachers in the long term. The computer-aided learning packages developed as part of this study comprise a suite of freely available open-source learning objects available online[39] and are now in use in four U.K. medical schools.

Ensuring Reproducible Student Experiences

Some geriatric syndromes are, by their definition, evanescent. Delirium is an obvious example. Others, such as behavioral symptoms in dementia, can place students or patients in scenarios where they can feel threatened if they are used as the focus for structured teaching. While the value of hands-on clinical apprenticeship in these scenarios cannot be overstated, the challenge to educators is to ensure that students across large academic years address learning outcomes in broadly comparable ways.

Technology has been used to reduce variability in student experience in domiciliary visits. Home visits represent an opportunity for students to see patients in their home environment and to consider interactions between environment, social supports, and physical, mental, and functional impairments. Teaching that is structured around such interactions can improve student attitudes toward older patients.[40] A collaborative of Australian and Canadian researchers developed a video game that simulated a patient's house that students were able to explore, looking for hazards to health and well-being. This provided a fun and standardized learning experience, student satisfaction levels were high, and their knowledge improved following the intervention.[41]

Simulation, using computer-enhanced simulation mannequins or actors as patients, is another way to provide students with a safe and reproducible clinical experience[42,43] and has been exploited for some time to teach about high-stakes critical care scenarios. It has only recently been explored in the context of geriatric medicine. A U.K.-based group developed and delivered a simulation session on delirium, falls, elder abuse, and breaking bad news—scenarios that can be managed inconsistently in ward settings and that students can find threatening. Teachers used a combination of simulation mannequins, professional role players, and simulated clinical documentation. Students showed improved knowledge and perceptions of geriatric medicine.[44]

Developing Skills and Positive Attitudes in the Management of Older Patients

There is strong evidence from both lay and scientific literature of ageism within the health care sector.[45] The constructs underpinning negative attitudes are relatively poorly explored and are likely to be complex. Detailed interviews with 25 U.K. doctors and medical students with assorted specialty backgrounds[46] found that their perceptions, both positive and negative, regarding health care for older people were clearly separated into two discrete domains: (1) attitudes toward older patients and (2) attitudes toward the work of caring for older patients. In teaching to encourage attitudinal change, it is likely that both need to be considered.

Attitudinal change was the most common outcome measure used in a systematic review of teaching interventions in geriatric medicine published in 2010.[47] Although this review found that teaching can improve attitudes toward care of older people, it also found that 9 of 19 interventions targeting attitudes failed to make a difference; this was a significantly lower success rate than in studies that aimed to improve knowledge as an outcome. A more detailed review,[48] focusing only on the studies that aimed to improve attitudes, found success to be more likely where teaching involved experiential learning, which delivered insights into the lives of older patients—senior mentoring and instant aging were cited as examples.

Instant aging (a form of simulation focusing on reproducing the patient experience) has been cited as a technological innovation,[49] although many teachers who use it do so in a decidedly "low tech" way. It simulates what it might feel like to have functional impairments and asks students to reflect on how these would impact daily living. Joints might be bandaged to reproduce stiffness, glasses smeared with petroleum jelly to simulate visual impairment, and rubber gloves donned to simulate peripheral neuropathy. Modern aged simulation suits can reproduce the same effects with less preparation and effort but at greater expense.[50] A group based in Minnesota[51] packaged instant aging into a game, with different "rounds" comprising managing medication, independent living, and living in an institutional setting. A cohort of 77 students wore instant aging equipment and were asked to conduct tasks appropriate for each setting, followed by a period of reflection. They showed improvement in attitudes toward older patients.

Involving older people, as either patients or citizens, in teaching has been the focus of innovative teaching to improve attitudes. A John A. Hartford Foundation senior mentor program in the United States matched all students with an individual or couple aged 65 years or older. This was reported to drive attitudinal change.[52] Although innovative programs of this type have been explored elsewhere, they remain underused and underevaluated. The challenges of engaging frail and cognitively impaired patients in prolonged contact with undergraduates as part of a structured educational intervention are likely to be part of the reason for this underuse and underevaluation.

THE IMPORTANCE OF INTERPROFESSIONAL EDUCATION

Interprofessional education has been defined as two or more professions learning with, from, or about each other to improve collaboration and quality of care[53] and has intuitive appeal in the context of geriatric medicine, which is multidisciplinary and collaborative. The most widespread, concerted, and sustained effort to roll out interprofessional education in the context of care of older people was through the Geriatric Interdisciplinary Team Training programs funded by the John A. Hartford Foundation in the United States. These programs delivered training across eight centers, teaching medical undergraduates alongside master's students in nursing and social work.[54] They showed that interprofessional education was feasible in the context of care of older people and that student attitudes toward other professions and patients improved as a consequence. Skills in interdisciplinary working also improved.

Given the intuitive advantages of such programs, it is striking that they are not used more widely. However, the organizational challenges of establishing interprofessional education are considerable, have been well described, and should not be underestimated. They include differential commitment between the professions; perceived differences in status between professions, leading to conflict and competition for resources between professional groupings historically organized in silos; and practical considerations about timetabling students and faculty.

Recent international collaborations supported by the World Health Organization[55] and the Bill and Melinda Gates Foundation[56] have advocated interprofessional education as a means to establishing a set of transferable competencies, which are not profession specific and can be delivered by different professional groupings depending upon the prevailing health care setting. Thus, in developing countries, where doctors are less available, more competencies might be undertaken by nurses or allied health professionals. These collaborations have outlined programs of change that are ambitious and require innovations from the level of higher education policy through to everyday teaching. It is striking, though, that the visionary changes identified as providing health care education fit for a developing world could afford geriatricians an opportunity to deliver health care fit for an aging population in more developed health care economies. Educators in aging and geriatric medicine should remain focused on developing initiatives in this area.

FACILITATORS AND BARRIERS TO EFFECTIVE EDUCATIONAL INTERVENTIONS IN GERIATRIC MEDICINE

To deliver effective education in geriatric medicine, adequate resources (both financial and human) are clearly essential. It is no coincidence that many of the innovations described in this chapter occurred under the auspices of the John A. Hartford[57] and Donald W. Reynolds[58] foundations, both of which provided substantial cash injections into geriatric medicine training initiatives in the United States. A cadre of adequately trained lecturers to lead teaching in medicine of older people was a central part of the proposition of the EAMA and IAGG master class initiatives. Much has been said in the past about the importance of a professorial class, and of academic units, in the specialty to spearhead change; however, pan-European studies have not shown a clear correlation between the number of professors in geriatric medicine and the amount of teaching devoted to geriatrics in a given jurisdiction.[59]

The presentation of geriatric medicine as a specialty founded on utilitarian values ("our interventions work") may have compromised its appeal. Modern concepts of frailty have the potential to provide a scientific framework, helping us understand and explain why these interventions work and for whom.[60] Fifty years ago, "senile dementia" was viewed as an inevitable consequence of aging, but "Alzheimerization" has changed public perceptions and motivated enhanced research endowments.[61] A clear description of clinical features, insights into pathogenesis, and development of modifying interventions have been essential components in this transformation. The "frailterization" of decrepitude and decline through comparable investigative steps is a tantalizing prospect.

Perceptions of prestige also contribute to negative attitudes. In one survey,[62] medical students and junior and senior doctors consistently ranked neurosurgery and thoracic surgery as the highest prestige specialties. Only dermatovenerology rivaled geriatric medicine for the lowest prestige rating. Highest prestige conditions, such as myocardial infarction, leukemia, and brain tumor, seem to share an acute onset, definitive diagnostic strategies, high-tech interventions, and the possibility of complete cure. They reinforce the doctor's role as healer (anticipated by medical students as "Your job is to make the person better and help them live"[63]). Low prestige conditions, such as fibromyalgia and anxiety neurosis, often require a shift in philosophy from cure to care and demand communication skills rather than procedural finesse. Indeed, the knowledge and skills required to manage such conditions are the very ones that physicians report the most difficulty in mastering.[64,65]

Medical student beliefs are shaped not just by their own experiences but by the attitudes of wider society, which is, arguably, fundamentally ageist. All threats represent possible opportunities, however, and by exploring and confronting ageist attitudes head on, important learning outcomes can be realized.

CONCLUSION

Educational interventions lie at the heart of improving care for older people and spreading the message of the good that can be achieved by adopting geriatrician models of working more widely. Technological innovations, the recognition of the increased importance of patient involvement in health care education, and the interprofessional education agenda may afford educators opportunities to have an impact on curricula in ways that have evaded them to date.

There is now wider consensus than ever before, at a policy and service delivery level, that expertise in aging and care of older patients is central to effective and sustainable service delivery: international consensus documents are gradually moving us close to agreement about how to achieve this by educational means. However, the challenges posed by inflexible professions and ageist attitudes remain as real as ever. If ever there was a time for expert educators in geriatric medicine, that time is now.

KEY POINTS

- What doctors need to know about aging can be considered in a three-tiered competency model: competencies required by all doctors, competencies required by doctors seeing frail older patients, and specialist geriatrician competencies.
- Educational innovations (such as computer-aided learning packages, simulation modeling, and senior mentorship programs) can free up teacher time, ensure a reproducible learning experience, and help doctors develop skills and attitudes that will help them care for older patients.
- Interprofessional education has intuitive appeal in the context of geriatric medicine and should be the focus of further initiatives.
- Barriers to change in medical schools include negative attitudes of students, an overcrowded curriculum, and lack of motivated teachers.
- Charismatic educators with geriatric knowledge and teaching skills have the potential to increase recruitment of geriatricians and improve standards of care across all specialties.

For a complete list of references, please visit www.expertconsult.com.

KEY REFERENCES

4. Kolb G, Andersen-Ranberg K, Cruz-Jentoft A, et al: Geriatric care in Europe—the EUGMS survey part I: Belgium, Czech Republic, Denmark, Germany, Ireland, Spain, Switzerland, United Kingdom. Eur Geriatr Med 2:290–295, 2011.
5. Mateos-Nozal J, Beard JR: Global approaches to geriatrics in medical education. Eur Geriatr Med 2:87–92, 2011.
7. Robbins TD, Crocker-Buque T, Forrester-Paton C, et al: Geriatrics is rewarding but lacks earning potential and prestige: responses from the national medical student survey of attitudes to and perceptions of geriatric medicine. Age Ageing 40:405–408, 2011.
21. Oakley R, Pattinson J, Goldberg S, et al: Equipping tomorrow's doctors for the patients of today. Age Ageing 43:442–447, 2014.
22. Leipzig RM, Granville L, Simpson D, et al: Keeping granny safe on July 1: a consensus on minimum geriatrics competencies for graduating medical students. Acad Med 84:604–610, 2009.
24. Forrester-Paton C, Forrester-Paton J, Gordon AL, et al: Undergraduate teaching in geriatric medicine: mapping the British Geriatrics Society undergraduate curriculum to Tomorrow's Doctors 2009. Age Ageing 43:436–439, 2014.
25. Masud T, Blundell A, Gordon AL, et al: European undergraduate curriculum in geriatric medicine developed using an international modified Delphi technique. Age Ageing 43:695–702, 2014.
26. Reiter R, Diraoui S, Van Den Noortgate N, et al: How to become a geriatrician in different European countries. Eur Geriatr Med 5:347–351, 2014.
31. Williams BC, Warshaw G, Fabiny AR, et al: Medicine in the 21st century: recommended essential geriatrics competencies for internal medicine and family medicine residents. J Grad Med Educ 2:373–383, 2010.
32. Hogan TM, Losman ED, Carpenter CR, et al: Development of geriatric competencies for emergency medicine residents using an expert consensus process. Acad Emerg Med 17:316–324, 2010.
33. Tullo E, Gordon A: Teaching and learning about dementia in UK medical schools: a national survey. BMC Geriatr 13:29, 2013.
46. Samra R: Medical students' and doctors' attitudes toward older patients and their care: what do we know and where do we go from here? 2013. http://eprints.nottingham.ac.uk/14107/. Accessed January 9, 2016.
47. Tullo ES, Spencer J, Allan L: Systematic review: helping the young to understand the old. Teaching interventions in geriatrics to improve the knowledge, skills, and attitudes of undergraduate medical students. J Am Geriatr Soc 58:1987–1993, 2010.
48. Samra R, Griffiths A, Cox T, et al: Changes in medical student and doctor attitudes toward older adults after an intervention: a systematic review. J Am Geriatr Soc 61:1188–1196, 2013.
53. Thistlethwaite J: Interprofessional education: a review of context, learning and the research agenda. Med Educ 46:58–70, 2012.
56. Frenk J, Chen L, Bhutta ZA, et al: Health professionals for a new century: transforming education to strengthen health systems in an interdependent world. Lancet 376:1923–1958, 2010.
58. Reuben DB, Bachrach PS, McCreath H, et al: Changing the course of geriatrics education: an evaluation of the first cohort of Reynolds geriatrics education programs. Acad Med 84:619–626, 2009.
59. Michel J-P, Huber P, Cruz-Jentoft AJ: Europe-wide survey of teaching in geriatric medicine. J Am Geriatr Soc 56:1536–1542, 2008.

127 Improving Quality of Care for Older People in England

Jim George, Henry J. Woodford, James M. Fisher

A nation's greatness is measured by how it treats its weakest members.

Mahatma Gandhi

Measuring and monitoring quality of care in the National Health Service (NHS) in England has attracted sustained attention over the past several years. The 2008 Darzi report ("High Quality Care for All") was designed to place the focus of the NHS firmly on quality.[1] However, few could have anticipated the two Francis inquiries[2,3] in 2010 and 2013, the Keogh mortality review[4] and the Berwick report,[5] all of which profoundly influenced the Care Quality Commission (CQC) inspection regimes that are designed to improve the quality of care in the NHS, particularly for older people. The most vulnerable patients are older adults: people older than 85 years account for only 8.3% of admissions to hospital but 21% of patient safety incidents.[6] Standards for care for older people act as an overall barometer for quality of care in the NHS. The aim of this chapter is to take readers through the experience of the NHS in England over the past several years so that they can learn from the mistakes and successes and, hopefully, be in a better position to continue their own quality improvement journey.

WHAT IS QUALITY?

There is no universally accepted definition of *quality*. A broad understanding is "doing the right things well." Donabedian made the classic distinction between the structure, processes, and outcomes of health care and argued that processes and outcomes should be assessed seperately.[7] Donabedian also emphasized that quality of health care not only includes technical excellence but also the manner and humanity in which it is delivered—hence the importance of processes or systems. Maxwell took this further by defining six dimensions of quality: (1) access, (2) relevance to need, (3) effectiveness, (4) equity, (5) social acceptability, and (6) efficiency and economy.[8] It is interesting that safety does not feature in Maxwell's list of quality dimensions. It was not until 1999 with the publication of the Institute of Medicine's report "To Err Is Human"[9] that it was generally realized that health care can sometimes be harmful, and safety was put at the forefront of quality. This is particularly relevant to older people among whom adverse events, such as falls, delirium, pressure ulcers, deconditioning, and medication errors, are so common.[6] The more recent Institute of Medicine definition of quality includes six domains[10]: safety, effectiveness, patient centeredness, timeliness, efficiency, and equity. For older people in the NHS, a seventh domain needs to be added: continuity and coordination of care.[11]

NHS STRATEGY TO IMPROVE QUALITY

The Darzi Next Stage Review was commissioned by the government to set a vision for the NHS in the twenty-first century. (Professor Darzi is an eminent colorectal surgeon and a former health minister.) The report "High Quality Care for All" was issued in June 2008. The key theme was there should be no new central targets; instead, clinicians would be expected to lead, and not just manage, a service and create a shared vision to drive improvements in safety and quality.[1] This led to the NHS Outcomes Framework, which targeted three distinct areas of quality (Figure 127-1):

1. The effectiveness of the treatment and care provided to patients measured by both clinical outcomes and patient reported outcomes
2. The safety of the treatment and care provided to patients
3. The broader experience patients have of the treatment and care they receive

The NHS Outcomes Framework is supported by the development of quality standards by the National Institute of Health and Care Excellence (NICE); the introduction of best practice tariffs (e.g., for stroke and neck of femur fracture) to encourage hospital trusts to provide the best possible care by paying them more if it is achieved; and the *C*ommissioning for *Qu*ality and *In*novation (CQUIN) framework in which trusts are penalized for not achieving best quality standards (e.g., for dementia care and prevention of thromboembolism).

The Francis Inquiries (2010 and 2013)

In 2009 the Health Care Commission (the NHS regulator prior to the CQC) published the findings of an investigation into the reported widespread care failures at Mid Staffordshire NHS Foundation Trust. The focus was on poor quality of care of older patients in Stafford Hospital, a district general hospital in England. It is troublesome that the Mid Staffordshire NHS Foundation Trust had achieved coveted "foundation status" while the problems were ongoing. A local campaign group, Cure the NHS, lobbied for an inquiry.

The First Francis Inquiry (2010)[2]

The first Francis inquiry was designed to identify the key failures in Mid Staffordshire and make recommendations. It was led by Robert Francis, QC, an eminent lawyer. Key failures identified were the following:

1. Too great a focus on finances. To save 10 million pounds, the Mid Staffordshire NHS Foundation Trust set out to make cuts, including losing 150 staff. Wards were reorganized with separate floors for surgery and medicine without any risk assessment. Numbers of beds were cut, and patient care was compromised.
2. Poor governance with little clinical audit, poor investigation of complaints and serious incidents, and not overseen by the trust governing board.
3. The trust board "buried its head in the sand," concentrating only on strategic matters and ignoring operational issues.
4. Poor care of older patients; lack of attention to patient dignity (e.g., incontinent patients left in a degrading condition). Failure to recognize dementia and delirium and treat appropriately (see quote).
5. Poor communication with lack of compassion, friends and relatives ignored, and lack of involvement of patients and caregivers in decisions.
6. Poor diagnosis and management, especially in acute emergency patients.

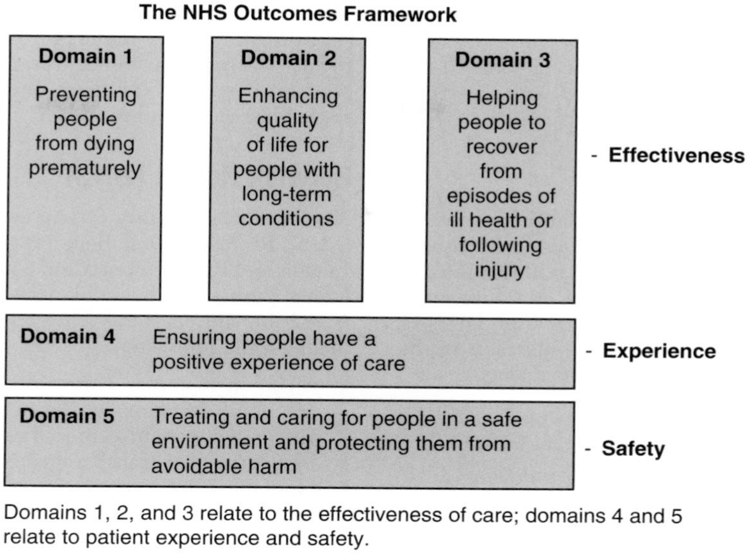

Figure 127-1. The NHS outcomes framework. *NHS*, national health service.

7. A bullying culture, target focused and needs of patients ignored.
8. Constant change of management with poor leadership and the doctors and nurses isolated from management.

Quote from Francis inquiry (2010):

It appears from the evidence presented at oral hearings that many patients suffered from acute confusional states: this occurs in a high proportion of older people admitted to hospital with serious illness. The evidence suggests that some medical staff did not understand this diagnosis and its importance, and in some instances treated it as "bad behaviour," rather than a valid medical condition.

The Second Francis Inquiry (2013)[3]

The second Francis inquiry looked at wider NHS issues and focused on why the serious failings in Mid Staffordshire were not recognized earlier by inspection, commissioning, supervision, and regulation of the hospital. The inquiry highlighted the following further issues relevant to the quality of care of older people:

1. Emphasis on targets and finances and not on quality and patient outcomes; failure to put patients first
2. Doctors (particularly consultants) failed to speak up for patients
3. Defensiveness, secrecy, and complacency; ignoring basic standards of care
4. Poor monitoring arrangements
5. Poor accountability with "diffusion" of responsibility
6. Lack of nurse training (particularly in older adult care) and lack of compassion
7. "Blind trust" in the hospital management and lack of external checks

The second Francis inquiry made more than 200 recommendations, including the following:

1. Patient safety should be the number one priority.
2. Quality accounts should be published in a common format and made public.
3. The profession of health care assistants should be regulated.
4. For older adults, one person should be made responsible for individual care and maintain continuity.
5. Patient involvement should be increased.
6. Staff and hospitals should speak up and be honest about mistakes.
7. Oversight of education and training and care must be nationally coordinated, and education and training bodies and regulators should share information.

The recommendations of the second Francis inquiry have been accepted by the government.[12] Both inquiries recognized the crucial importance of improving quality of care for older people and that this requires specialist skills and training. Subsequently, the government made the care of older people and, in particular, people with dementia central to NHS policy. Although the findings of the Francis inquiries were very distressing to many who work in the care of older people, the specialty of geriatric medicine has become more prominent in the NHS. Older patients and their caregivers and relatives are now much more encouraged to comment on the services provided, and the leadership and management skills of geriatricians are consequently more appreciated.

The Keogh Report[4]

Following the publication in February 2013 of the second Francis inquiry, Sir Bruce Keogh (National Medical Director) led a review of 14 trusts in July 2013, purposely selected because they had higher than average mortality rates. The Keogh report[4] found key issues in the 14 trusts, all relating to quality.

Patient Experience

The review team talked directly to patients and also received written feedback. There was a tendency in many of the hospitals to view complaints as something to be managed rather than to inform and be acted upon.

Patient Safety

Safety is a key indicator of overall quality of care. National indicators measuring safety and harm are included in the NHS Safety Thermometer (see later). In particular, infection rates and pressure ulcer rates were measured, as well as mortality rates. The review teams found there was scope for improvement in the use of early warning scores to anticipate and prevent acute deterioration of patients. It also found there was room for improvement in organizational learning from safety incidents. In some of the hospitals, multiple serious events had occurred with the same theme, indicating that lessons had not been learned.

Workforce

Many of the hospitals had medical and nurse staffing problems with difficulties in recruitment, high sickness rates, and frequent use of locums and agency staff. There was a statistical relationship between inpatient staff ratios and standardized mortality rates. All of the hospitals reviewed were functioning at high levels of capacity. Much of the pressure was due to large increases in the number of older patients with complex health problems.

Leadership and Governance

The Keogh review teams found evidence of the following:

1. There was poor articulation of strategy to improve quality.
2. Many of the trusts could not show a comprehensive and consistent approach to learning from safety reviews.
3. There was a significant disconnect between what the clinical leadership said were the key risks and issues and what was actually happening on the wards.

The Keogh report of 14 trusts confirmed that many of the quality deficiencies found in the Francis reports were not unique. A common factor in all 15 trusts (Keogh 14, plus Mid-Staffordshire) were workforce, training, safety, quality, and governance issues, exacerbated by the pressures caused by an increase in older adult acute emergency admissions. The findings of the Keogh Review led to immediate changes in the CQC hospital investigation process.[13]

Junior Doctors' Response and Involvement in the Francis and Keogh Reports

The Francis report[1] highlights the unique perspective junior doctors possess with regard to patient safety, describing them as "the eyes and ears" of the United Kingdom's NHS. The junior doctors' comparative lack of experience relative to more senior colleagues can be seen as beneficial, because they are less likely to be "infected" by any unhealthy local cultures. Furthermore, junior doctors in training regularly move between clinical sites. This provides a unique perspective on potential variance of quality between institutions. Consequently, it has been suggested that junior doctors are perhaps more likely to perceive practice to be unacceptable than staff who have worked in the same clinical environment for a much longer period. The Francis report also highlighted that, in a number of instances, concerns regarding suboptimal care had been raised by junior doctors but not acted upon. The report recommends that such concerns should be rigorously explored and not discounted simply on the basis of a lack of experience or seniority. The importance of providing appropriate forums for junior doctors to voice concerns is also highlighted. Suggested methods include trainee surveys and face-to-face feedback during visits that relate to approval or accreditation of training placements.

The Keogh report[4] directly acknowledges the contribution junior doctors can make to patient safety, describing them as "potentially our most powerful agents for change." Junior doctors were included in each of the rapid responsive review teams that were assembled to collect data in trusts. Junior doctor involvement is now integrated into the team employed by the CQC to undertake a hospital trust inspection. The Keogh report calls upon medical directors to consider how the latent energy of junior doctors can be "tapped" rather than "sapped" and also issues a call to arms to junior doctors themselves, citing them as "not just the clinical leaders of tomorrow, but clinical leaders of today." With this in mind, trusts should be encouraging junior doctors to act as conduits through which good practice can be shared between institutions.

Berwick Report (2013)[5]

The National Advisory Group on Safety in Patients in England led by Professor Don Berwick gathered information from the Francis and Keogh reports and combined it with additional statements from patients and experts. The Berwick report concentrated on the cultural changes required. Recommendations included the following:

1. Abandon blame as a tool for change and trust the goodwill and good intentions of the staff.
2. Emphasize patient-centered care.
3. Recognize that transparency is essential.
4. Give the NHS career staff training in quality improvement methods.
5. Culture change is more important than rules and regulations for a safer NHS.

Care Quality Commission

The CQC is an independent care regulatory body and describes its functions as ensuring that the care provided by hospitals, dentists, ambulances, care homes, and home-care agencies meet government standards of quality and safety.[14] Recent radical changes have been made to the CQC inspection methodology.[15] Moving away from inspecting individual aspects of care, the CQC now aspires to inspect a health care provider as a whole. Rather than just trying to establish and identify problems, the CQC wants to be able to get under the skin of the organization to understand the cause of problems. To use the analogy of an unwell patient, it aims not only to determine symptoms and signs but also reach a diagnosis.[15] In acute trusts, eight core services will always be inspected: accident and emergency, medicine (including older adult care), critical care, maternity, pediatrics, end-of-life care, and outpatients. The assessment is divided into three parts: preinspection, inspection, and postinspection. In the preinspection phase, data are collected from national data sources, the trust, and stakeholders. During the inspection, the CQC seeks to assess five questions, each related to a quality domain:

1. Is it safe (are people protected from harm)?
2. Is it effective (do patients have good outcomes)?
3. Is it caring (do staff look after people well)?
4. Is it responsive (does the trust organize its services in a patient-centered manner)?
5. Is it well led?

A large team, comprising clinical experts, lay people, junior doctors, and nurses, are brought together to undertake an inspection over a 2- to 4-day period (Box 127-1). Trusts are rated on a 4-point scale identical to that used by Ofsted (the education regulator); the ratings are outstanding, good, requires improvement, or inadequate. Informal feedback suggests that this new approach to inspection by the CQC represents a significant improvement.[15] The hope is that it will eventually result in improvements to the quality of care for older people.

The Future Hospital Commission

The Royal College of Physicians (RCP) report "Hospitals on the Edge"[16] highlighted services having to cope with increasing numbers of older patients with complex needs and difficulties in providing continuing care to these patients and the challenges

BOX 127-1 Typical Composition of a Team for Inspection of a Hospital Trust by the Care Quality Commission

1 Team chair (senior clinician or health care worker)
1 Team leader (Care Quality Commission [CQC] head of hospital inspectors)
3 Senior managers
5 Doctors (junior and senior) and nurses
5 CQC inspectors
5 Experts (trained lay people)
2 Analysts
1 Inspection planner
1 Recorder

BOX 127-2 Care Priorities Identified by the Future Hospital Commission

- Safe, effective, and compassionate medical care for all who need it as hospital inpatients
- High quality, sustainable 24 hours a day, 7 days a week
- Continuity of care as a norm, with seamless care for all patients
- Stable medical teams that deliver both high-quality patient care and an effective environment in which to educate and train the next generation of doctors
- Effective relationships between medical and other health and social care teams
- An appropriate balance of specialist care and care coordinated expertly and holistically around patient's needs
- Transfer of care arrangements that are realistic

From Future Hospital Commission: Future hospital: caring for medical patients, London, 2013, Royal College of Physicians.

maintaining medical services after hours and on weekends. The RCP convened an independent group, The Future Hospital Commission, to discuss potential remedies to this crisis in care.[17] The solution proposed was that care oriented around the patient's needs should be achieved by increasing the proportion of generalists (e.g., geriatricians). The report went further by suggesting more integration of health and social care teams and that acute care should be coordinated better beyond the hospital walls. The care priorities identified by the Future Hospital Commission are summarized in Box 127-2.

QUALITY IMPROVEMENT

In the past, clinically led improvement methods (clinical audit, guidelines, clinical governance) were differentiated from so-called management-led performance management. This is now an outmoded separation, as both of these approaches are valid and not exclusive. The process of improvement is more important than the method, and leading health care organizations operate within a definition of quality that covers both clinical and management domains.[18] In this section, we briefly describe the most frequently used quality improvement tools, which are guidelines audit and the model for improvement.

Guidelines

The emphasis on evidence-based practice has led to the development of clinical guidelines. Guidelines are described as "systematically developed statements to assist practitioner and patient decisions about specific clinical circumstances."[19] The National Institute for Health and Care Excellence (NICE) produce clinical guidelines for England and Wales[20] and also produce national quality standards to help deliver high quality care and treatment. The Scottish Intercollegiate Guidelines Network (SIGN) produces guidelines for Scotland.[21] Particularly relevant to the care of older people are the NICE guidelines on dementia, delirium, osteoporosis, falls, and incontinence, and quality standards for delirium.[20] Despite the massive investment in guideline development, their impact on actual practice and patient outcomes is variable.[18]

Clinical Audit and Clinical Governance

Audit was formally introduced into the NHS in 1989 and was the main quality improvement method used by clinicians in the 1990s.[18] Clinical audit is a review of current health practices compared against agreed standards and is designed to ensure that, as clinicians, we provide the best level of care to our patients and we constantly seek to improve our practice where it is matching those standards. Audit is one of the key elements of clinical governance and helps to ensure that the quality of care is maintained at an agreed standard. *Clinical governance* is an umbrella term that encompasses a range of activities, including audit, clinical effectiveness, risk management, and education and training, designed to improve and maintain the quality of care to patients and ensure accountability. At a national level, audit has been very successful in improving quality for older people in the United Kingdom (see later examples), but at a local level the results of audit are variable. For example, in one study only 27% of audits were complete, only 22% were re-audited, and only 5% of audits led to change in practice.[22]

The Model for Improvement

Leading on from the Donabedian systems of care approach are a multitude of tools for improving quality of systems (e.g., Lean Six Sigma),[18] but the most tried and tested for frontline medical care is the model for improvement, the Plan, Do, Study, Act (PDSA) method. This was originally developed by Deming.[23] PDSA are small tests of cyclical change that are evaluated as part of a continuous improvement approach. A plan of change is devised (Plan), the change is carried out (Do), the result is evaluated (Study), and the plan is acted on (Act) in the next cycle of change. Examples of this approach in health care are given later in this chapter. The PDSA approach is often combined with a collaborative approach in which groups of hospitals addressing the same problem learn from each other's experience. It is suggested that the PDSA approach is more cost effective than other quality improvement methods, but the longer term impact in terms of sustainability and spread has not yet been evaluated.[18]

EXAMPLES OF QUALITY INITIATIVES IN THE UNITED KINGDOM

These examples of quality initiatives represent a very broad definition of quality improvement. Some are very clinical and some are both clinical and managerial. Some have been more successful than others and many are still ongoing. They have been included as potential sources of learning and inspiration for clinicians and managers inside and outside the United Kingdom.

The Silver Book[24]

The Silver Book is an intercollegiate document scoped by the National Clinical Directors for Urgent Care, for Older People, and for Dementia. It arose from a growing concern about the quality of care and safety of the increasing number of frail older people admitted to acute hospitals as emergencies. Importantly, for the first time it sets standards for the emergency care of older people similar to the standards previously set for children.

The recommendations made include the following:

1. An initial primary care response to an urgent request within 30 minutes and a multidisciplinary response (comprehensive geriatric assessment) within 2 hours (14 hours overnight), 24 hours a day, 7 days a week
2. Routine multidisciplinary assessment for pain, depression, delirium and dementia, falls and mobility, continence, nutrition and hydration, activities of daily living, vital signs, end-of-life care, and safeguarding issues
3. A prompt structured medication review within the first 24 hours of the older, frail person presenting with an acute crisis

National Audit of Dementia

The National Audit of Dementia was set up in 2008 to assess the quality of care provided to people with dementia admitted to general hospitals in England and Wales. This was as a result of concerns over the quality of inpatient care that patients with dementia receive.[25] Over a third of people in hospital beds in the United Kingdom have cognitive impairment, either delirium or dementia.[26] The audit was commissioned by the Healthcare Quality Improvement Partnership (HQIP) and carried out by the Royal College of Psychiatrists Centre for Quality Improvement in partnership with other organizations. The 2013 audit was a cross-sectional audit of the key physical and psychological assessments carried out in 7934 patients with dementia in 206 general hospitals.[27] Most people had a standardized assessment of their cognitive state (56.8%). Information from caregivers was documented in 39% of cases. Compared to a previous audit in 2011, there had been a 10% drop in the overall number of prescriptions of antipsychotic drugs and patients were more likely to receive an assessment of their nutrition. There was considerable variation between hospitals. Key assessments were less likely when dementia patients were admitted to surgical wards. Patients with dementia are very vulnerable in the hospital and need special consideration.[28] The audit highlighted the lack of liaison psychiatry services and the lack of training of staff in dementia. The hospitals that took part in the audit were asked to produce an action plan to tackle any deficiencies. It is hoped that a repeat audit will demonstrate further improvement.

National Confidential Enquiry Into Patient Outcomes and Death (NCEPOD): An Old Age Problem[29]

This is a national audit of all patients aged 80 years and older who died within 30 days of a surgical procedure between April 1, 2008, and June 30, 2008. The report makes depressing reading with the primary finding that older surgical patients received good care in hospital in only one third of cases. At present in the United Kingdom approximately 40% of all surgical inpatients are older than 65 years, and this proportion will increase as the population ages.[30] There was insufficient recognition of the complexity of patients presenting to surgical wards. Cognition was only assessed in half the patients, but most often by clinical assessment rather than using a formal mental test score. There was lack of knowledge regarding the management of medical complications in surgical patients; for example, acute kidney injury (1 in 4 patients) and fluid status imbalance (1 in 3) were poorly recognized. The report recommended early multidisciplinary input and early involvement of geriatricians to improve the quality of care of older people after surgery.[31] Since 2008, geriatricians have made significant progress with joint cooperation between the British Geriatrics Society and the British Orthopaedic Association (e.g., the hip fracture database) and the recognition of orthogeriatrics and surgical liaison as an important subspecialty.[31] An important advance has been implementation of new models of care, such as POPS (Proactive care of Older People undergoing Surgery).

National Hip Fracture Database[32]

The National Hip Fracture Database (NHFD) is the largest hip fracture database in the world. It was originally developed in 2004 and supported by the British Orthopaedic Association and British Geriatrics Society. The first national report was in 2009. The latest report in 2013 gives an average 30-day mortality rate for hip fracture as 8.02% compared to 8.10% in 2011, which corresponds to 300 fewer people dying within 30 days of hip fracture as a result of better quality care. Improvements are shown in the time it takes for hip fracture patients to get to surgery, and more patients are seen by an orthogeriatrician (81.6% of patients compared with only 25% in 2009). Regular publication of the figures broken down by hospital trust is a potent stimulus for continuous improvement. Hospital outliers are notified and asked to check data and are offered a visit by an improvement team.

NHS Safety Thermometer[33]

The NHS Safety Thermometer is part of the national CQUIN scheme designed to incentivize providers of NHS care to take snapshot measures of four common harms affecting older people; these harms are pressure ulcers, falls, urinary infections (in patients with catheters), and venous thromboembolism. An estimated 750,000 patients per quarter are screened for harm.[33] It is well known that patients who suffer from one harm (e.g., catheter-associated urinary infection) are at much higher risk of developing another (e.g., a pressure ulcer). By measuring these four harmful events, it is possible to derive the frequency of "harm-free care" and make comparisons between different hospitals using the national database. Organizations that are exceptionally poor or variable are encouraged to examine their data and look for underlying causes (e.g., nurse staffing levels). The data are scrutinized by the CQC as part of regular inspections.

FallSafe Improvement Project[34]

Over a quarter of a million falls are reported by U.K. hospitals each year, predominantly harming older patients whose vulnerability to falls arises from a complex interaction of risk factors, including impaired mobility, dementia, delirium, medications, and acute illness.[35] Hospital falls can have serious consequences and approximately 30% result in serious injury, including approximately 200 fractures annually.[35] Even falls with minor or no injury can cause anxiety and distress to patients and their families and result in loss of confidence and increased dependency.

In the FallSafe quality improvement project, nine FallSafe units were compared to nine control units. The FallSafe project was run by the Royal College of Physicians Clinical Effectiveness and Evaluation Unit in partnership with the Royal College of Nursing, the National Patient Safety Association, the Association for Victims of Medical Accidents, and South Central Regional Health Authority and was funded by the Health Foundation. The FallSafe intervention included the training and inspiring of 17 registered nurses from acute rehabilitation and mental health wards to lead their local multidisciplinary teams to reliably deliver a falls assessment and intervention through a care bundle approach (Box 127-3). The FallSafe project resulted in a substantial improvement in care, including a doubling of patients who received a lying and standing blood pressure assessment, medication review, and being asked about fear of falling. The project delivered around a 25% reduction in hospital falls.[34]

Improving Patient Flow in Sheffield for Older Emergency Medical Patients[36]

The biggest challenge to quality care faced by emergency services is the increasing number of older people presenting with

BOX 127-3 FallSafe Bundle

Cognitive assessment
Call bell in sight and within reach
Asked about fear of falling
History of falls
Lying and standing blood pressure
Medication review
Night sedation not given
Safe footwear
Urine dip test

nonspecific presentations.[16] Delay in their assessment prolongs hospital stay and compromises safety, increasing costs and increasing stress on staff and systems. This study, funded by the Health Foundation, used a quality improvement approach to improve the flow of emergency geriatric patients in an NHS trust. The key constraints in the emergency pathway for older patients in Sheffield before the intervention will be familiar to most geriatricians. Two thirds of frail older patients did not "arrive" on the medical assessment unit (MAU) until after 6 PM (many had waited in the accident and emergency department before being transferred to MAU). The traditional model of "post-take" meant that many of these patients were not assessed by a specialist geriatrician for 24 hours. After discussion and involvement of all the staff involved, a series of test changes (PDSA cycles) were introduced to improve flow of patients by reducing delays in decision making and discharge for older emergency patients.

These interventions included:

1. Changing consultant working patterns from "post-take" to "on-take." Earlier specialist geriatric assessment increased the chance of early supported discharge with the associated reduced risk of health care associated adverse effects.
2. Pooling of junior doctors so that more doctors were available at the busiest times.
3. Establishing a separate MAU focused on the needs of frail older people. Other hospitals have found that establishing a specialist frail older adult unit increases quality and efficiency.
4. Merging inpatient and outpatient care.
5. Establishing a multidisciplinary team for early comprehensive geriatric assessment (CGA). This prevents older people from becoming deconditioned in the hospital, resulting in poorer outcomes and longer lengths of stay.

The results of these interventions were reductions in bed occupancy and mortality without affecting readmission rates or requiring extra resources.[36]

Junior Doctors and Quality Improvement

As highlighted earlier in the chapter, concerns have been raised about the efficacy of clinical audit as a tool to drive up local standards of care. For junior doctors specifically, a number of barriers to high quality audit have been recognized.[37] First, for junior doctors in training, clinical audit is now mandatory and forms part of their annual assessment of progression. Mandating clinical audit risks disempowering junior doctors. They may be less motivated to produce a clinically meaningful piece of work that might influence quality of care and may be more likely to undertake a cursory data collection task or "box-ticking exercise." Second, the issue may be further compounded among junior doctors because of a lack of time. The standard duration of a junior doctor's clinical placement is 4 months, which this leaves little time to identify an area of interest and complete an entire audit cycle. Consequently, there have been calls for junior doctors to focus instead on quality improvement projects. It has been argued that data collection should no longer be seen as the endpoint but instead should be reframed as the resource that can directly inform and drive the process of clinical change.

The Health Foundation document "Involving Junior Doctors in Quality Improvement"[38] outlines factors that have been recognized as catalysts for junior doctors' participation in quality improvement projects. The importance of support from senior clinicians and demonstration of the importance of quality improvement is highlighted. Factors at an organizational level include the cultivation of a local environment that values improvement and proactively supports change and the provision of appropriate resources to enable improvements to be implemented.

Older People in Acute Care (OPAC) Improvement Program in Scotland

In 2012 Healthcare Improvement Scotland was asked by the Scottish Government to "improve acute care for older people" by March 2014. The older people in acute care (OPAC) improvement program was set up.[39] The program has two themes:

1. Think frailty. Ensure frail older people who need to stay in hospital receive prompt CGA and input from a specialist team within 1 day of admission.
2. Think delirium. Improve the identification and early management of delirium in acute settings through the use of the 4AT tool[40] and through the development and testing of a care bundle.

These initiations have already led to improvements—for example, in the Grampian area where front door triage with CGA and fast track to a specialist geriatric assessment unit has improved outcomes and resulted in an 18% reduction in emergency bed days. Further details of the OPAC program are available on its website.[41] The program was completed with a final report in June 2015.

British Geriatrics Society and Quality Initiatives

The British Geriatrics Society (BGS) is a professional association of doctors practicing old age medicine or old age psychiatry, general practitioners, nurses, therapists, scientists, and others with a particular interest in the medical care of older people and in promoting better health in old age. It has more than 2500 members worldwide and is the only society in the United Kingdom offering specialist medical expertise in the wide range of health care needs of older people. The BGS, as well as having regular scientific meetings, has produced a compendium of good practice and practical clinical guidelines on common conditions affecting older people. In particular, the BGS has produced an important document making recommendations to improve the commissioning of care, especially the medical care, of residents in care homes,[42] and this has been included in the new NHS 5-year plan.[43] The BGS has also produced best practice guidelines for management of frailty in the community.[44] A list of the achievements of the BGS in quality improvement following the Francis report is given in Box 127-4.[45] Most notable are the recommendations to improve both undergraduate and postgraduate training in geriatrics[46] and also the Frailsafe initiative.[47] Frailsafe is a breakthrough series collaborative designed to help hospitals learn from each other and make improvements in a specific area (i.e., improvements in the quality of care, especially safety of frail older patients). Common harms for older people were identified from the literature; they include delirium, equipment-related harms, reduced mobility, falls, pressure ulcers, poor advance care planning, and adverse drug reactions. The intervention is to reduce these harms by the use of an agreed checklist of actions. The rate of harm, mortality, and length of stay will be measured using time series data. This important project has been facilitated by the BGS with funding from the Health Foundation.

BOX 127-4 Quality Achievements of the British Geriatrics Society after Francis[45]

1. Raising the profile of geriatric medicine on the agenda of regulators and providers
2. Best practice guidelines for the management of frailty in the community and outpatient settings and recommendations to improve the quality of medical care for older people in care homes
3. The Frailsafe quality initiative
4. Recommendations to improve training in geriatrics at both undergraduate and postgraduate levels
5. Experienced geriatricians are involved with the Care Quality Commission inspections on a regular basis, and in Scotland, BGS Scotland has given expert advice to NHS Health Improvement Scotland

BOX 127-5 Ward-Level Quality Assurance Measures

1. Routine cognitive assessment of patients
2. Ask about previous falls routinely
3. Ensure adequate nutrition and hydration; ensure drinks are within easy reach
4. Protected meal times
5. Ensure call bells are within easy reach and easy access to toilets
6. Good communication—staff always introduce themselves to patients and relatives
7. Encourage patient and caregiver feedback. Involve caregivers as part of the team
8. Regular monitoring of number of falls, pressure ulcers, and hospital-acquired infections
9. Regular ward staff meetings to discuss complaints, serious incidents, deaths, and lessons learned

Recruitment Challenges and Junior Doctor–Led Educational Initiatives

The importance of ensuring that doctors are better trained to care for older patients has been highlighted in a number of recent high-profile policy documents, including the Shape of Training report [48] and the Francis report.[3] Serial survey data has demonstrated that although the number of U.K. medical schools teaching and assessing geriatric medicine has increased, a comparatively short period of time is dedicated to teaching on the specialty.[49,50] Similar shortcomings in the content and amount of undergraduate teaching have been reported in a number of international surveys.[46] Evidence also exists that suggests some students perceive the specialty of geriatric medicine to lack prestige[51] and that some hold negative attitudes toward older people.[52]

Oakley and colleagues[46] cite a need to develop novel teaching approaches for geriatric medicine that target attitudinal change and suggest that incorporating new technologies may further enhance delivery of geriatric medicine teaching. An example of the application of new technologies to geriatric medicine teaching is provided by a recent trainee-led educational program for medical students that used simulation mannequins and actors to provide teaching on delirium, falls, and elder abuse.[53] This work demonstrated an improvement in knowledge and perceptions of the specialty. The use of e-learning in geriatric medicine has also been described. Mini-GEMs (Geriatrics E-learning Modules) are short, focused online video presentations, each covering a specific clinical topic within geriatric medicine.[54] These modules are aimed at junior doctors and allied health professionals who care for older patients. Each presentation is a maximum of 7 minutes and thus provides a more consumable alternative to the existing longer online learning resources that already exist. This trainee-led initiative now comprises a library of 15 modules, which have been accessed over 4500 times in more than 90 countries.

In a postgraduate context, concerns have been raised about whether the geriatric medicine workforce of the future will be adequately staffed given the aging population and increased need for geriatricians, the changing medical workforce, and a rising number of unfilled posts.[55] The 2013 Royal College of Physicians document, "The Medical Registrar: Empowering the Unsung Heroes of Patient Care"[56] highlighted that many junior doctors were deterred from exploring a career as a hospital physician because of negative perceptions surrounding the medical registrar role. Another example of a trainee-led educational initiative is the Association for Elderly Medicine Education (AEME), which was founded in 2012 by three U.K. geriatric medicine trainees in response to the recruitment challenges highlighted earlier. AEME organized a targeted educational event, Geriatrics for Juniors, that provided teaching to junior doctors on the subspecialty areas of geriatric medicine. The event also included a dedicated session allowing junior doctors to explore their concerns about the medical registrar role with a panel of existing registrars. The conference sold out in 2013 and 2014, highlighting the appetite for such education among junior doctors. Serial survey data arising from the 2013 event demonstrated a positive influence on attitudes toward the specialty and on perceptions about the role of the medical registrar.[57]

THE FUTURE

Many geriatricians in the United Kingdom have been somewhat daunted by the recent multiple reorganizations of the NHS, particularly in England and Wales. This has contributed to a possible decline in the quality of care for older people, as evidenced by the Francis reports, with an emphasis on finance rather than quality and diffusion of responsibility. However, we should now gain encouragement from the recent new emphasis on quality and safety, particularly the genuine moves to improve care for patients with dementia and frailty and the new emphasis on integration. Sustained quality improvement is more likely to be achieved by quality initiatives within the specialty than through government targets and regulations.[58] Working in hospitals and increasingly in the community, geriatricians are ideally placed to use their skills to improve quality by influencing colleagues, NHS managers, and hospital governors. On most governing boards of hospitals, it is possible to find at least one ally, often someone caring for an older frail relative. Also, perhaps more importantly, geriatricians can influence at the ward and patient levels, ensuring that the service they provide is patient centered, with quality of care considered more important than cost. (There is evidence that high quality care is more cost effective.) This necessitates regular data collection, audit, participation in quality improvement projects, and setting a good example for nurses and junior doctors (Box 127-5).

The Future Hospital Commission sets an agenda for more integration and cooperation between primary and secondary care and provides a direction for the future. Finally, attracting new enthusiastic doctors to the specialty of geriatrics and encouraging them to improve the quality of care for older people will provide the necessary sustainability for high quality care for older people in the United Kingdom.

SUMMARY

Quality improvement is a journey rather than a destination. The Darzi report and the NHS reforms put quality of care at the center of the NHS. However, the Francis and Keogh reports demonstrated that lofty aims are not always translated into real action and benefit for patients. In fact, successive, well-intentioned reorganizations, and financial and clinical targets paradoxically can reduce quality of care rather than improve it. This has led to a radical rethink. The CQC has been rejuvenated with a new inspection regime, and the Berwick report has pointed the way to cultural change in the NHS. Improving quality for older people encompasses safety, effectiveness, and patient centeredness. Collaboration and continuity and the move toward more integration of health and social services are a welcome development. Encouragingly, there are many examples in the United Kingdom of promising clinically led initiatives to improve quality of care for older people. There is a lot we can learn from the U.K. experience. Improving quality of care for older people is an enormous challenge, and to be sustainable it needs to be clinician led. There has never been a better time to be a geriatrician in the United Kingdom. We need to encourage many more young doctors to train in the specialty to ensure continued quality improvement for older people in both hospitals and the community.

KEY POINTS

- Quality in care for older people encompasses collaboration and continuity, as well as safety, effectiveness, and patient-centeredness.
- Improving quality cannot be achieved by regulation alone but needs a clinician-led quality improvement culture.
- Physicians can learn not only from bad examples of where quality of care for older people has been compromised (e.g., Mid Staffordshire Hospital Trust) but also from the many good examples of quality improvement initiatives (e.g., OPAC, Frailsafe, and the National Dementia Audit).
- Geriatricians are ideally placed to promote quality "from board to ward" and lead on quality improvement initiatives for older people.
- A major contribution to improving quality of care for older people will be to improve education, training, and recruitment in geriatric medicine. Junior doctors have a vital role to play in quality improvement for older people.

For a complete list of references, please visit www.expertconsult.com.

KEY REFERENCES

6. Long SJ, Brown KF, Ames D, et al: What is known about adverse incidents in older medical hospital inpatients? A systematic review of the literature. Int J Qual Health Care 25:542–554, 2013.
11. Oliver D, Foot C, Humphries R: Making our health and care systems fit for an ageing population, London, 2014, King's Fund.
17. Future Hospital Commission: Future hospital: caring for medical patients, London, 2013, Royal College of Physicians.
27. Souza R, Gandesha A, Hood C, et al: Quality of care for people with dementia in general hospitals: national cross-sectional audit of patient assessment. Clin Med (Lond) 14:490–494, 2014.
28. George J, Long S, Vincent C: How can we keep patients with dementia safe in our acute hospitals? A review of challenges and solutions. J R Soc Med 106:355–361, 2013.
36. Silvester KM, Mohammed AM, Harriman P, et al: Timely care for frail older people referred to hospital improves efficiency and reduces mortality without the need for extra resources. Age Ageing 43:472–476, 2014.
44. Turner G, Clegg A: Best practice guidelines for the management of frailty: a British Geriatrics Society, Age UK and Royal College of General Practitioners report. Age Ageing 43:744–747, 2014.
46. Oakley R, Pattinson J, Goldberg S, et al: Equipping tomorrow's doctors for the patients of today. Age Ageing 43:442–447, 2014.
57. Fisher JM, Hunt K, Garside MJ: Geriatrics for juniors: tomorrow's geriatricians or another lost tribe? J R Coll Physicians Edinb 44:106–110, 2014.
58. Ham C: Reforming the NHS from within, London, 2014, King's Fund.

128 Quality Initiatives Aimed at Improving Medicare

Richard G. Stefanacci, Jill L. Cantelmo

Quality combined with cost is now a central component of a value-based system which is quite different from the priorities when Medicare was first introduced. When Medicare started, quality and costs were easily managed. In 1966, the year Medicare went into effect, expenses were limited by the scarce availability of, and demand for, services. The total number of Medicare beneficiaries was only around 10 million, with a life expectancy for a Medicare older adult at that time averaging about 4 years. Nearly a half-century later, the impact of the aging baby boomer generation, increasing life expectancy, rising health care costs, and an almost unlimited array of innovative and expensive services is challenging Medicare's ability to provide health services in a financially sustainable manner to the 45 million subscribed beneficiaries, a number growing by 10,000 daily as baby boomers receive their Medicare cards.

As Medicare has expanded to become the single largest payer in the U.S. health care system, politically difficult restriction of benefits does not provide a valid approach for extending the viability of Medicare for future generations. Instead, a wealth of accumulating evidence has demonstrated the variations in care quality that exist across the nation, as well as numerous opportunities to increase the efficiencies of services provided. Although Medicare has a history of innovative program development, especially with regard to different payment approaches, it was not until 2010, when the Patient Protection and Affordable Care Act (PPACA; commonly referred to as the Affordable Care Act [ACA]) was signed into law—the largest piece of Medicare legislation since the Medicare Modernization Act (MMA) in 2003—that a centralized, nationwide effort was put forth, with various provisions to strengthen the integrity of the program through improvements in quality and efficiency.

Although the range of program initiatives specified as part of the ACA do not apply solely to Medicare, many of these have a direct impact on the health care providers that treat Medicare beneficiaries, Medicare beneficiaries themselves, and reimbursement of services that are covered by Medicare.

In broad terms, the main objectives of the ACA are to expand health care access, improve the quality and safety of care provided, and control costs through increased care efficiency.[1] The various initiatives specified can be grouped into several main categories, according to their ultimate goals: quality and safety, including more extensive use of performance reporting on quality measures and disease prevention programs; health care delivery reform, including adjustments to hospital reimbursement for readmissions related to potentially preventable conditions and development of new models of reimbursement, such as bundled payments; and regulatory oversight and program integrity, including enhanced screening of providers and suppliers that wish to participate in Medicare and additional funding for antifraud activities.[1]

A rationale for the comprehensive mobilization of efforts to develop these programs and initiatives can be found in the wealth of evidence demonstrating important gaps in the current system[2-5]:

- Failure to receive indicated care at least 30% of the time, potentially leading to poor outcomes, complications, and unnecessary costs
- Overuse of unnecessary care, increasing costs directly and incrementally when complications occur
- Misuse of services and poor safety, with approximately 210,000 in-hospital deaths associated with preventable events among Medicare beneficiaries
- Enormous variations in the delivery of health care nationally, regionally, and locally
- Disparities in the quality of care provided, especially among certain races and ethnicities
- High costs of health care based on volume of services provided, without equally high rates of care quality
- Limited use of screenings and programs to prevent complications of chronic diseases

This evidence indicates the need for new systemic improvements to the health care provided to Medicare beneficiaries. Although Medicare has been active in implementing programs for measuring and reporting quality of care, introducing innovative payment models, and ensuring that regulations are in place to prevent fraudulent activities, the comprehensive and enhanced approach to which these will be undertaken through the ACA will provide greater traction for the initiatives to have a meaningful impact on quality and efficiency and, ultimately, to preserve Medicare for the benefit of future generations. To this end, ACA created the Center for Medicare and Medicaid Innovation, commonly referred to as the Innovation Center, for the purpose of testing "innovative payment and service delivery models to reduce program expenditures…while preserving or enhancing the quality of care" for those who receive Medicare, Medicaid, or Children's Health Insurance Program (CHIP) benefits.

QUALITY MEASUREMENT AND REPORTING

In the first 3 decades of Medicare, public data reporting rarely occurred. Even in the commercial world, data was limited to information available in HEDIS (Health Plan Employer Data and Information Set). Centers for Medicare & Medicaid Services (CMS) started collecting and using data through peer review organizations (PROs), now referred to as Quality Improvement Organizations (QIOs). QIOs systematically promoted improvements in quality measures tracked using voluntary, collaborative, and educational approaches.

Initially, reporting of quality measures was viewed as a way to promote self-improvement among providers through comparison with their peers. Over time the role has evolved, enabling patients to review performance data to select high-quality providers in a model of "consumer-directed health care." Companies such as Healthgrades, a leading health care ratings organization, provide ratings and profiles of hospitals, nursing homes, and physicians to consumers, corporations, health plans, and hospitals. Consumer access to physician performance measures has helped move health care toward a more demand-type system, with patients selecting higher quality providers over lower quality providers, thus creating incentives for physicians to provide a higher quality of care.

Quality measurement and reporting in health care are recognized as crucial for identifying areas in need of improvement, monitoring progress, and providing consumers and purchasers with comparative information about health system performance. Spurred by rising costs and lagging quality improvement, large purchasers, health plans, and others began to implement approaches for rewarding high performance and creating incentives for quality improvement. An early example of these types of approaches was the pay-for-performance programs implemented by health plans with physicians. These programs provided important examples to assess the impact of quality reporting on the effectiveness and efficiency of a health care system and were the building blocks of subsequently developed programs, which have continued to evolve into the initiatives being implemented through the ACA.

Physicians

The vast majority of Medicare payments for physician services are made directly on the basis of a fee schedule, which has been in place since 1992. The Medicare fee schedule is intended to relate payments to the actual resources used in providing the health care services. In 2006, the Tax Relief and Health Care Act (TRHCA; P.L. 109-432) required the establishment of a physician quality reporting system, including an incentive payment for eligible professionals who satisfactorily reported data on quality measures for covered services furnished to Medicare beneficiaries during the second half of 2007. CMS named this program the Physician Quality Reporting Initiative (PQRI). In 2007, the Medicare, Medicaid, and State Children's Health Insurance Program (SCHIP) Extension Act of 2007 (MMSEA) was enacted, authorizing CMS to make PQRI incentive payments for satisfactorily reporting quality measures data; eligible professionals would earn an incentive payment of 2% of the total allowed charges for Physician Fee Schedule (PFS)–covered professional services furnished during that same period. In 2008, the PQRI consisted of 119 quality measures, including two structural measures; one of these reported whether a professional had or used electronic health records (EHRs) and the other electronic prescribing. To test the effectiveness of this early pay-for-performance system, CMS implemented the Physician Group Practice demonstration, which provided rewards to large, multispecialty group practices for improving the quality of care and reducing the cost increases for their patients. Although results of this demonstration showed that a number of groups did not earn performance payments due to the inability to generate savings to the Medicare program, consistent improvements in quality on various measures were observed across participants.[6] PQRI was developed as a pay-for-reporting program, designed to validate the utility of the clinical performance measures included, and serves as the foundation for future pay-for-performance programs.[7]

The PQRI was included as a key voluntary Medicare physician quality reporting initiative in the ACA, with penalties implemented in 2015 for all Medicare providers that failed to participate in the program. In 2011 the program underwent a name change, becoming the Physician Quality Reporting System (PQRS), with several other important changes to the program noted in response to requirements of the ACA, including the following[8]:

- Extension of the incentive payment program through 2014 for eligible practitioners who submit quality measure data
- Decrease in Medicare payment for practitioners not participating in 2015
- Requirement of reporting for 50% of Medicare patients, rather than 80%, for claims-based reporting of individual measures
- Update to the definition of a group practice from 200 to two or more practitioners
- Revision of measures available for reporting
- Establishment of an informal appeal process for practitioners

Participation in the PQRS allows Medicare physicians to assess the quality of care that they are providing to their patients, track their performance on various quality metrics, and enable comparison of performance compared with peers.[9]

Through 2014, eligible providers or group practices could receive an incentive payment of 0.5% of their total estimated Medicare Part B. PFS allowed charges for covered professional services furnished during that same reporting period for meeting the criteria for satisfactory submission of PQRS quality data, but unsatisfactory reporting would be subject to a 2% payment adjustment to their Medicare PFS amount for services provided in 2016.

Physicians and group practices must report their data through one of several methods to be eligible for incentive payments:

- Medicare Part B claims (physicians)
- Qualified PQRS registry (physicians and group practices)
- EHR using Certified EHR Technology (CEHRT; physicians and group practices)
- Web interface (group practices of 25+ only)
- CEHRT via a data submission vendor (physicians and group practices)
- Qualified clinical data registry (physicians)
- Clinician and Group Consumer Assessment of Healthcare Providers and Systems (CGCAHPS) CMS-certified survey vendor (for groups of 25+ only; group practices)

The program offers a selection of more than 200 separate quality measures that have been developed by provider associations, quality groups, and CMS and are typically applicable to patients based on combinations of Current Procedural Terminology (CPT) codes, international classification of disease (ICDs) codes, and patient age at the time of their interaction with the provider (Table 128-1).[7,9]

In keeping with the model of consumer-directed health care, CMS indicates on its Physician Compare website whether a physician is a successful participant in PQRS and may begin to publish each participating provider's individual performance ratings on specific quality measures—again, creating incentives for physicians to perform well to attract a higher proportion of patient consumers over their lower performing peers. The motivation is increased volume and higher reimbursement for improved performance.

Hospitals

Initially, CMS hospital quality measures came from information collected by hospitals that volunteered to provide data for public reporting. The information, collected through the hospital Inpatient Quality Reporting (IQR) program, is intended to illustrate how quality of care varies among hospitals, providing consumers with data for making informed decisions about their health care options and encouraging hospitals and providers to improve the quality of inpatient care, and coordinating care, for all patients. CMS first attempted to collect this information on a purely voluntary basis but could not garner sufficient interest from hospitals. When voluntary participation failed, CMS tied submission of quality data to payments for services administered to Medicare patients, resulting in almost 99% of U.S. hospitals providing data for comparative quality measures. Measures of hospital quality have been developed through the Hospital Quality Alliance (HQA), which consists of more than a dozen organizations, including the American Association of Retired Persons (AARP), American Federation of Labor and Congress of Industrial Organizations (AFL–CIO), Agency for Healthcare Research and Quality (AHRQ), American Heart Association (AHA), America's Health Insurance Plans (AHIP), American Medical Association (AMA), American Nurses Association (ANA), and The Joint Commission (TJC). Reported data is available to consumers on the Hospital Compare website.

Initially, available quality information related only to the care given to patients with three serious medical conditions that are

Text continued on p. 1063

TABLE 128-1 PQRS 2016 Measures

Measure Title	Measure Description
Diabetes: Hemoglobin A_{1c} Poor Control	Percentage of patients 18-75 years of age with diabetes who had hemoglobin A_{1c} > 9.0% during the measurement period
Diabetes: Low Density Lipoprotein (LDL-C) Control (<100 mg/dL)	Percentage of patients 18-75 years of age with diabetes whose LDL-C was adequately controlled (<100 mg/dL) during the measurement period
Heart Failure (HF): Angiotensin-Converting Enzyme (ACE) Inhibitor or Angiotensin Receptor Blocker (ARB) Therapy for Left Ventricular Systolic Dysfunction (LVSD)	Percentage of patients aged 18 years and older with a diagnosis of heart failure (HF) with a current or prior left ventricular ejection fraction (LVEF) < 40% who were prescribed ACE inhibitor or ARB therapy either within a 12-month period when seen in the outpatient setting OR at each hospital discharge
Coronary Artery Disease (CAD): Antiplatelet Therapy	Percentage of patients aged 18 years and older with a diagnosis of coronary artery disease (CAD) seen within a 12-month period who were prescribed aspirin or clopidogrel
Coronary Artery Disease (CAD): Beta-Blocker Therapy—Prior Myocardial Infarction (MI) or Left Ventricular Systolic Dysfunction (LVEF < 40%)	Percentage of patients aged 18 years and older with a diagnosis of coronary artery disease seen within a 12-month period who also have prior MI OR a current or prior LVEF < 40% who were prescribed beta-blocker therapy
Heart Failure (HF): Beta-Blocker Therapy for Left Ventricular Systolic Dysfunction (LVSD)	Percentage of patients aged 18 years and older with a diagnosis of heart failure (HF) with a current or prior left ventricular ejection fraction (LVEF) < 40% who were prescribed beta-blocker therapy either within a 12-month period when seen in the outpatient setting OR at each hospital discharge
Anti-Depressant Medication Management	Percentage of patients 18 years of age and older who were diagnosed with major depression and treated with antidepressant medication, and who remained on antidepressant medication treatment. Two rates are reported a. Percentage of patients who remained on an antidepressant medication for at least 84 days (12 weeks). b. Percentage of patients who remained on an antidepressant medication for at least 180 days (6 months).
Primary Open-Angle Glaucoma (POAG): Optic Nerve Evaluation	Percentage of patients aged 18 years and older with a diagnosis of primary open-angle glaucoma (POAG) who have an optic nerve head evaluation during one or more office visits within 12 months
Age-Related Macular Degeneration (AMD): Dilated Macular Examination	Percentage of patients aged 50 years and older with a diagnosis of age-related macular degeneration (AMD) who had a dilated macular examination performed that included documentation of the presence or absence of macular thickening or hemorrhage AND the level of macular degeneration severity during one or more office visits within 12 months
Diabetic Retinopathy: Documentation of Presence or Absence of Macular Edema and Level of Severity of Retinopathy	Percentage of patients aged 18 years and older with a diagnosis of diabetic retinopathy who had a dilated macular or fundus exam performed that included documentation of the level of severity of retinopathy and the presence or absence of macular edema during one or more office visits within 12 months
Diabetic Retinopathy: Communication With the Physician Managing Ongoing Diabetes Care	Percentage of patients aged 18 years and older with a diagnosis of diabetic retinopathy who had a dilated macular or fundus exam performed with documented communication to the physician who manages the ongoing care of the patient with diabetes mellitus regarding the findings of the macular or fundus exam at least once within 12 months
Perioperative Care: Selection of Prophylactic Antibiotic—First OR Second Generation Cephalosporin	Percentage of surgical patients aged 18 years and older undergoing procedures with the indications for a first OR second generation cephalosporin prophylactic antibiotic, who had an order for a first OR second generation cephalosporin for antimicrobial prophylaxis
Perioperative Care: Discontinuation of Prophylactic Parenteral Antibiotics (Non-Cardiac Procedures)	Percentage of non-cardiac surgical patients aged 18 years and older undergoing procedures with the indications for prophylactic parenteral antibiotics AND who received a prophylactic parenteral antibiotic, who have an order for discontinuation of prophylactic parenteral antibiotics within 24 hours of surgical end time
Perioperative Care: Venous Thromboembolism (VTE) Prophylaxis (When Indicated in ALL Patients)	Percentage of surgical patients aged 18 years and older undergoing procedures for which VTE prophylaxis is indicated in all patients, who had an order for low-molecular-weight heparin (LMWH), low-dose unfractionated heparin (LDUH), adjusted-dose warfarin, fondaparinux or mechanical prophylaxis to be given within 24 hours prior to incision time or within 24 hours after surgery end time
Communication With the Physician or Other Clinician Managing Ongoing Care Post-Fracture for Men and Women Aged 50 Years and Older	Percentage of patients aged 50 years and older treated for a fracture with documentation of communication, between the physician treating the fracture and the physician or other clinician managing the patient's ongoing care, that a fracture occurred and that the patient was or should be considered for osteoporosis treatment or testing. This measure is reported by the physician who treats the fracture and who therefore is held accountable for the communication
Stroke and Stroke Rehabilitation: Discharged on Antithrombotic Therapy	Percentage of patients aged 18 years and older with a diagnosis of ischemic stroke or transient ischemic attack (TIA) with documented permanent, persistent, or paroxysmal atrial fibrillation who were prescribed an antithrombotic at discharge
Screening for Osteoporosis for Women Aged 65-85 Years of Age	Percentage of female patients aged 65-85 years of age who ever had a central dual-energy X-ray absorptiometry (DXA) to check for osteoporosis
Osteoporosis: Pharmacologic Therapy for Men and Women Aged 50 Years and Older	Percentage of patients aged 50 years and older with a diagnosis of osteoporosis who were prescribed pharmacologic therapy within 12 months
Coronary Artery Bypass Graft (CABG): Use of Internal Mammary Artery (IMA) in Patients With Isolated CABG Surgery	Percentage of patients aged 18 years and older undergoing isolated CABG surgery who received an IMA graft
Coronary Artery Bypass Graft (CABG): Preoperative Beta-Blocker in Patients with Isolated CABG Surgery	Percentage of isolated coronary artery bypass graft (CABG) surgeries for patients aged 18 years and older who received a beta-blocker within 24 hours prior to surgical incision

TABLE 128-1 PQRS 2016 Measures—cont'd

Measure Title	Measure Description
Medication Reconciliation Post-Discharge	The percentage of discharges from any inpatient facility (e.g., hospital, skilled nursing facility, or rehabilitation facility) for patients 18 years and older of age seen within 30 days following discharge in the office by the physician, prescribing practitioner, registered nurse, or clinical pharmacist providing ongoing care for whom the discharge medication list was reconciled with the current medication list in the outpatient medical record. This measure is reported as three rates stratified by age group: • Reporting Criteria 1: 18-64 years of age • Reporting Criteria 2: 65 years and older • Total Rate: All patients 18 years of age and older
Care Plan	Percentage of patients aged 65 years and older who have an advance care plan or surrogate decision maker documented in the medical record or documentation in the medical record that an advance care plan was discussed but the patient did not wish or was not able to name a surrogate decision maker or provide an advance care plan.
Urinary Incontinence: Assessment of Presence or Absence of Urinary Incontinence in Women Aged 65 Years and Older	Percentage of female patients aged 65 years and older who were assessed for the presence or absence of urinary incontinence within 12 months
Urinary Incontinence: Plan of Care for Urinary Incontinence in Women Aged 65 Years and Older	Percentage of female patients aged 65 years and older with a diagnosis of urinary incontinence with a documented plan of care for urinary incontinence at least once within 12 months
Chronic Obstructive Pulmonary Disease (COPD): Spirometry Evaluation	Percentage of patients aged 18 years and older with a diagnosis of COPD who had spirometry results documented
Chronic Obstructive Pulmonary Disease (COPD): Inhaled Bronchodilator Therapy	Percentage of patients aged 18 years and older with a diagnosis of COPD and who have an FEV_1 less than 60% predicted and have symptoms who were prescribed an inhaled bronchodilator.
Asthma: Pharmacologic Therapy for Persistent Asthma—Ambulatory Care Setting	Percentage of patients aged 5 years and older with a diagnosis of persistent asthma who were prescribed long-term control medication
Emergency Medicine: 12-Lead Electrocardiogram (ECG) Performed for Non-Traumatic Chest Pain	Percentage of patients aged 40 years and older with an emergency department discharge diagnosis of non-traumatic chest pain who had a 12-lead electrocardiogram (ECG) performed
Appropriate Treatment for Children With Upper Respiratory Infection (URI)	Percentage of children 3 months through 18 years of age who were diagnosed with upper respiratory infection (URI) and were not dispensed an antibiotic prescription on or three days after the episode
Appropriate Testing for Children With Pharyngitis	Percentage of children 3-18 years of age who were diagnosed with pharyngitis, ordered an antibiotic and received a group A streptococcus (strep) test for the episode
Hematology: Myelodysplastic Syndrome (MDS) and Acute Leukemia: Baseline Cytogenetic Testing Performed on Bone Marrow	Percentage of patients aged 18 years and older with a diagnosis of myelodysplastic syndrome (MDS) or an acute leukemia who had baseline cytogenetic testing performed on bone marrow
Hematology: Myelodysplastic Syndrome (MDS): Documentation of Iron Stores in Patients Receiving Erythropoietin Therapy	Percentage of patients aged 18 years and older with a diagnosis of myelodysplastic syndrome (MDS) who are receiving erythropoietin therapy with documentation of iron stores within 60 days prior to initiating erythropoietin therapy
Hematology: Multiple Myeloma: Treatment With Bisphosphonates	Percentage of patients aged 18 years and older with a diagnosis of multiple myeloma, not in remission, who were prescribed or received intravenous bisphosphonate therapy within the 12-month reporting period
Hematology: Chronic Lymphocytic Leukemia (CLL): Baseline Flow Cytometry	Percentage of patients aged 18 years and older seen within a 12-month reporting period with a diagnosis of chronic lymphocytic leukemia (CLL) made at any time during or prior to the reporting period who had baseline flow cytometry studies performed and documented in the chart
Breast Cancer: Hormonal Therapy for Stage IC-IIIC Estrogen Receptor/Progesterone Receptor (ER/PR) Positive Breast Cancer	Percentage of female patients aged 18 years and older with Stage IC through IIIC, ER or PR positive breast cancer who were prescribed tamoxifen or aromatase inhibitor (AI) during the 12-month reporting period
Colon Cancer: Chemotherapy for AJCC Stage III Colon Cancer Patients	Percentage of patients aged 18 through 80 years with AJCC Stage III colon cancer who are referred for adjuvant chemotherapy, prescribed adjuvant chemotherapy, or have previously received adjuvant chemotherapy within the 12-month reporting period
Prevention of Central Venous Catheter (CVC)-Related Bloodstream Infections	Percentage of patients, regardless of age, who undergo central venous catheter (CVC) insertion for whom CVC was inserted with all elements of maximal sterile barrier technique, hand hygiene, skin preparation and, if ultrasound is used, sterile ultrasound techniques followed
Hepatitis C: Ribonucleic Acid (RNA) Testing Before Initiating Treatment	Percentage of patients aged 18 years and older with a diagnosis of chronic hepatitis C who started antiviral treatment within the 12-month reporting period for whom quantitative hepatitis C virus (HCV) ribonucleic acid (RNA) testing was performed within 12 months prior to initiation of antiviral treatment
Hepatitis C: Hepatitis C Virus (HCV) Genotype Testing Prior to Treatment	Percentage of patients aged 18 years and older with a diagnosis of chronic hepatitis C who started antiviral treatment within the 12-month reporting period for whom hepatitis C virus (HCV) genotype testing was performed within 12 months prior to initiation of antiviral treatment
Hepatitis C: Hepatitis C Virus (HCV) Ribonucleic Acid (RNA) Testing Between 4-12 Weeks After Initiation of Treatment	Percentage of patients aged 18 years and older with a diagnosis of chronic hepatitis C who are receiving antiviral treatment for whom quantitative hepatitis C virus (HCV) ribonucleic acid (RNA) testing was performed between 4-12 weeks after the initiation of antiviral treatment
Acute Otitis Externa (AOE): Topical Therapy	Percentage of patients aged 2 years and older with a diagnosis of AOE who were prescribed topical preparations
Acute Otitis Externa (AOE): Systemic Antimicrobial Therapy—Avoidance of Inappropriate Use	Percentage of patients aged 2 years and older with a diagnosis of AOE who were not prescribed systemic antimicrobial therapy
Breast Cancer Resection Pathology Reporting: pT Category (Primary Tumor) and pN Category (Regional Lymph Nodes) with Histologic Grade	Percentage of breast cancer resection pathology reports that include the pT category (primary tumor), the pN category (regional lymph nodes), and the histologic grade

Continued

TABLE 128-1 PQRS 2016 Measures—cont'd

Measure Title	Measure Description
Colorectal Cancer Resection Pathology Reporting: pT Category (Primary Tumor) and pN Category (Regional Lymph Nodes) with Histologic Grade	Percentage of colon and rectum cancer resection pathology reports that include the pT category (primary tumor), the pN category (regional lymph nodes) and the histologic grade
Prostate Cancer: Avoidance of Overuse of Bone Scan for Staging Low Risk Prostate Cancer Patients	Percentage of patients, regardless of age, with a diagnosis of prostate cancer at low risk of recurrence receiving interstitial prostate brachytherapy, OR external beam radiotherapy to the prostate, OR radical prostatectomy, OR cryotherapy who did not have a bone scan performed at any time since diagnosis of prostate cancer
Prostate Cancer: Adjuvant Hormonal Therapy for High Risk or Very High Risk Prostate Cancer	Percentage of patients, regardless of age, with a diagnosis of prostate cancer at high or very high risk of recurrence receiving external beam radiotherapy to the prostate who were prescribed adjuvant hormonal therapy (GnRH [gonadotropin-releasing hormone] agonist or antagonist)
Adult Major Depressive Disorder (MDD): Suicide Risk Assessment	Percentage of patients aged 18 years and older with a diagnosis of major depressive disorder (MDD) with a suicide risk assessment completed during the visit in which a new diagnosis or recurrent episode was identified
Rheumatoid Arthritis (RA): Disease Modifying Anti-Rheumatic Drug (DMARD) Therapy	Percentage of patients aged 18 years and older who were diagnosed with rheumatoid arthritis and were prescribed, dispensed, or administered at least one ambulatory prescription for a disease-modifying anti-rheumatic drug (DMARD).
Osteoarthritis (OA): Function and Pain Assessment	Percentage of patient visits for patients aged 21 years and older with a diagnosis of osteoarthritis (OA) with assessment for function and pain
Preventive Care and Screening: Influenza Immunization	Percentage of patients aged 6 months and older seen for a visit between October 1 and March 31 who received an influenza immunization OR who reported previous receipt of an influenza immunization.
Pneumonia Vaccination Status for Older Adults	Percentage of patients 65 years of age and older who have ever received a pneumococcal vaccine.
Breast Cancer Screening	Percentage of women 50 through 74 years of age who had a mammogram to screen for breast cancer within 27 months
Colorectal Cancer Screening	Percentage of patients 50-75 years of age who had appropriate screening for colorectal cancer
Antibiotic Treatment for Adults With Acute Bronchitis: Avoidance of Inappropriate Use	Percentage of adults 18 through 64 years of age with a diagnosis of acute bronchitis who were not prescribed or dispensed an antibiotic prescription on or 3 days after the episode
Diabetes: Eye Exam	Percentage of patients 18-75 years of age with diabetes who had a retinal or dilated eye exam by an eye care professional during the measurement period or a negative retinal or dilated eye exam (no evidence of retinopathy) in the 12 months prior to the measurement period
Coronary Artery Disease (CAD): Angiotensin-Converting Enzyme (ACE) Inhibitor or Angiotensin Receptor Blocker (ARB) Therapy—Diabetes or Left Ventricular Systolic Dysfunction (LVEF < 40%)	Percentage of patients aged 18 years and older with a diagnosis of coronary artery disease seen within a 12-month period who also have diabetes OR a current or prior left ventricular ejection fraction (LVEF) < 40% who were prescribed ACE inhibitor or ARB therapy
Diabetes: Medical Attention for Nephropathy	The percentage of patients 18-75 years of age with diabetes who had a nephropathy screening test or evidence of nephropathy during the measurement period
Adult Kidney Disease: Laboratory Testing (Lipid Profile)	Percentage of patients aged 18 years and older with a diagnosis of chronic kidney disease (CKD) (stage 3, 4, or 5, not receiving renal replacement therapy [RRT]) who had a fasting lipid profile performed at least once within a 12-month period
Adult Kidney Disease: Blood Pressure Management	Percentage of patient visits for those patients aged 18 years and older with a diagnosis of chronic kidney disease (CKD) (stage 3, 4, or 5, not receiving renal replacement therapy [RRT]) with a blood pressure < 140/90 mm Hg OR ≥ 140/90 mmHg with a documented plan of care
Diabetes Mellitus: Diabetic Foot and Ankle Care, Peripheral Neuropathy—Neurological Evaluation	Percentage of patients aged 18 years and older with a diagnosis of diabetes mellitus who had a neurological examination of their lower extremities within 12 months
Diabetes Mellitus: Diabetic Foot and Ankle Care, Ulcer Prevention—Evaluation of Footwear	Percentage of patients aged 18 years and older with a diagnosis of diabetes mellitus who were evaluated for proper footwear and sizing
Preventive Care and Screening: Body Mass Index (BMI) Screening and Follow-Up Plan	Percentage of patients aged 18 years and older with a BMI documented during the current encounter or during the previous six months AND with a BMI outside of normal parameters, a follow-up plan is documented during the encounter or during the previous six months of the current encounter Normal parameters: Age 65 years and older BMI ≥ 23 and < 30 kg/m^2; age 18-64 years BMI ≥ 18.5 and < 25 kg/m^2
Documentation of Current Medications in the Medical Record	Percentage of visits for patients aged 18 years and older for which the eligible professional attests to documenting a list of current medications using all immediate resources available on the date of the encounter. This list must include ALL known prescriptions, over-the-counters, herbals, and vitamin/mineral/dietary (nutritional) supplements AND must contain the medications' name, dosage, frequency and route of administration.
Pain Assessment and Follow-up	Percentage of visits for patients aged 18 years and older with documentation of a pain assessment using a standardized tool(s) on each visit AND documentation of a follow-up plan when pain is present
Preventive Care and Screening: Screening for Clinical Depression and Follow-Up Plan	Percentage of patients aged 12 years and older screened for clinical depression on the date of the encounter using an age-appropriate standardized depression screening tool AND if positive, a follow-up plan is documented on the date of the positive screen
Melanoma: Continuity of Care—Recall System	Percentage of patients, regardless of age, with a current diagnosis of melanoma or a history of melanoma whose information was entered, at least once within a 12-month period, into a recall system that includes: • A target date for the next complete physical skin exam, AND • A process to follow up with patients who either did not make an appointment within the specified time frame or who missed a scheduled appointment

TABLE 128-1 PQRS 2016 Measures—cont'd

Measure Title	Measure Description
Melanoma: Coordination of Care	Percentage of patient visits, regardless of age, with a new occurrence of melanoma who have a treatment plan documented in the chart that was communicated to the physician(s) providing continuing care within 1 month of diagnosis
Age-Related Macular Degeneration (AMD): Counseling on Antioxidant Supplement	Percentage of patients aged 50 years and older with a diagnosis of age-related macular degeneration (AMD) or their caregiver(s) who were counseled within 12 months on the benefits and/or risks of the Age-Related Eye Disease Study (AREDS) formulation for preventing progression of AMD
Primary Open-Angle Glaucoma (POAG): Reduction of Intraocular Pressure (IOP) by 15% OR Documentation of a Plan of Care	Percentage of patients aged 18 years and older with a diagnosis of primary open-angle glaucoma (POAG) whose glaucoma treatment has not failed (the most recent IOP was reduced by at least 15% from the pre-intervention level) OR if the most recent IOP was not reduced by at least 15% from the pre-intervention level, a plan of care was documented within 12 months
Oncology: Medical and Radiation—Pain Intensity Quantified	Percentage of patient visits, regardless of patient age, with a diagnosis of cancer currently receiving chemotherapy or radiation therapy in which pain intensity is quantified
Oncology: Medical and Radiation—Plan of Care for Pain	Percentage of visits for patients, regardless of age, with a diagnosis of cancer currently receiving chemotherapy or radiation therapy who report having pain with a documented plan of care to address pain
Radiology: Exposure Time Reported for Procedures Using Fluoroscopy	Final reports for procedures using fluoroscopy that document radiation exposure indices, or exposure time and number of fluorographic images (if radiation exposure indices are not available)
Radiology: Inappropriate Use of "Probably Benign" Assessment Category in Mammography Screening	Percentage of final reports for screening mammograms that are classified as "probably benign"
Nuclear Medicine: Correlation with Existing Imaging Studies for All Patients Undergoing Bone Scintigraphy	Percentage of final reports for all patients, regardless of age, undergoing bone scintigraphy that include physician documentation of correlation with existing relevant imaging studies (e.g., x-ray, MRI, CT, etc.) that were performed
Falls: Risk Assessment	Percentage of patients aged 65 years and older with a history of falls who had a risk assessment for falls completed within 12 months
Falls: Plan of Care	Percentage of patients aged 65 years and older with a history of falls who had a plan of care for falls documented within 12 months
Oncology: Radiation Dose Limits to Normal Tissues	Percentage of patients, regardless of age, with a diagnosis of breast, rectal, pancreatic or lung cancer receiving 3D conformal radiation therapy who had documentation in medical record that radiation dose limits to normal tissues were established prior to the initiation of a course of 3D conformal radiation for a minimum of two tissues.
HIV/AIDS: *Pneumocystis jiroveci* Pneumonia (PCP) Prophylaxis	Percentage of patients aged 6 weeks and older with a diagnosis of HIV/AIDS who were prescribed *Pneumocystis jiroveci* pneumonia (PCP) prophylaxis
Diabetes: Foot Exam	Percentage of patients aged 18-75 years of age with diabetes who had a foot exam during the measurement period
Coronary Artery Bypass Graft (CABG): Prolonged Intubation	Percentage of patients aged 18 years and older undergoing isolated CABG surgery who require postoperative intubation > 24 hours
Coronary Artery Bypass Graft (CABG): Deep Sternal Wound Infection Rate	Percentage of patients aged 18 years and older undergoing isolated CABG surgery who, within 30 days postoperatively, develop deep sternal wound infection involving muscle, bone, and/or mediastinum requiring operative intervention
Coronary Artery Bypass Graft (CABG): Stroke	Percentage of patients aged 18 years and older undergoing isolated CABG surgery who have a postoperative stroke (i.e., any confirmed neurological deficit of abrupt onset caused by a disturbance in blood supply to the brain) that did not resolve within 24 hours
Coronary Artery Bypass Graft (CABG): Postoperative Renal Failure	Percentage of patients aged 18 years and older undergoing isolated CABG surgery (without pre-existing renal failure) who develop postoperative renal failure or require dialysis
Coronary Artery Bypass Graft (CABG): Surgical Re-Exploration	Percentage of patients aged 18 years and older undergoing isolated CABG surgery who require a return to the operating room (OR) during the current hospitalization for mediastinal bleeding with or without tamponade, graft occlusion, valve dysfunction, or other cardiac reason
Rheumatoid Arthritis (RA): Tuberculosis Screening	Percentage of patients aged 18 years and older with a diagnosis of rheumatoid arthritis (RA) who have documentation of a tuberculosis (TB) screening performed and results interpreted within 6 months prior to receiving a first course of therapy using a biologic disease-modifying anti-rheumatic drug (DMARD)
Rheumatoid Arthritis (RA): Periodic Assessment of Disease Activity	Percentage of patients aged 18 years and older with a diagnosis of rheumatoid arthritis (RA) who have an assessment and classification of disease activity within 12 months
Rheumatoid Arthritis (RA): Functional Status Assessment	Percentage of patients aged 18 years and older with a diagnosis of rheumatoid arthritis (RA) for whom a functional status assessment was performed at least once within 12 months
Rheumatoid Arthritis (RA): Assessment and Classification of Disease Prognosis	Percentage of patients aged 18 years and older with a diagnosis of rheumatoid arthritis (RA) who have an assessment and classification of disease prognosis at least once within 12 months
Rheumatoid Arthritis (RA): Glucocorticoid Management	Percentage of patients aged 18 years and older with a diagnosis of rheumatoid arthritis (RA) who have been assessed for glucocorticoid use and, for those on prolonged doses of prednisone ≥ 10 mg daily (or equivalent) with improvement or no change in disease activity, documentation of glucocorticoid management plan within 12 months
Elder Maltreatment Screen and Follow-Up Plan	Percentage of patients aged 65 years and older with a documented elder maltreatment screen using an Elder Maltreatment Screening Tool on the date of encounter AND a documented follow-up plan on the date of the positive screen
Functional Outcome Assessment	Percentage of visits for patients aged 18 years and older with documentation of a current functional outcome assessment using a standardized functional outcome assessment tool on the date of encounter AND documentation of a care plan based on identified functional outcome deficiencies on the date of the identified deficiencies

Continued

TABLE 128-1 PQRS 2016 Measures—cont'd

Measure Title	Measure Description
Hepatitis C: Hepatitis A Vaccination	Percentage of patients aged 18 years and older with a diagnosis of chronic hepatitis C who have received at least one injection of hepatitis A vaccine, or who have documented immunity to hepatitis A
Colonoscopy Interval for Patients with a History of Adenomatous Polyps—Avoidance of Inappropriate Use	Percentage of patients aged 18 years and older receiving a surveillance colonoscopy, with a history of a prior adenomatous polyp(s) in previous colonoscopy findings, who had an interval of 3 or more years since their last colonoscopy
Stroke and Stroke Rehabilitation: Thrombolytic Therapy	Percentage of patients aged 18 years and older with a diagnosis of acute ischemic stroke who arrive at the hospital within 2 hours of time last known well and for whom IV t-PA was initiated within 3 hours of time last known well
Cataracts: 20/40 or Better Visual Acuity within 90 Days Following Cataract Surgery	Percentage of patients aged 18 years and older with a diagnosis of uncomplicated cataract who had cataract surgery and no significant ocular conditions impacting the visual outcome of surgery and had best-corrected visual acuity of 20/40 or better (distance or near) achieved within 90 days following the cataract surgery
Cataracts: Complications within 30 Days Following Cataract Surgery Requiring Additional Surgical Procedures	Percentage of patients aged 18 years and older with a diagnosis of uncomplicated cataract who had cataract surgery and had any of a specified list of surgical procedures in the 30 days following cataract surgery which would indicate the occurrence of any of the following major complications: retained nuclear fragments, endophthalmitis, dislocated or wrong power IOL, retinal detachment, or wound dehiscence
Radiology: Stenosis Measurement in Carotid Imaging Reports	Percentage of final reports for carotid imaging studies (neck magnetic resonance angiography [MRA], neck computed tomography angiography [CTA], neck duplex ultrasound, carotid angiogram) performed that include direct or indirect reference to measurements of distal internal carotid diameter as the denominator for stenosis measurement
Ischemic Vascular Disease (IVD): Use of Aspirin or Another Antithrombotic	Percentage of patients 18 years of age and older who were discharged alive for acute myocardial infarction (AMI), coronary artery bypass graft (CABG) or percutaneous coronary interventions (PCI) in the 12 months prior to the measurement period, or who had an active diagnosis of ischemic vascular disease (IVD) during the measurement period and who had documentation of use of aspirin or another antithrombotic during the measurement period
HIV/AIDS: Sexually Transmitted Disease Screening for Chlamydia, Gonorrhea, and Syphilis	Percentage of patients aged 13 years and older with a diagnosis of HIV/AIDS for whom chlamydia, gonorrhea and syphilis screenings were performed at least once since the diagnosis of HIV infection
Functional Deficit: Change in Risk-Adjusted Functional Status for Patients with Knee Impairments	Percentage of patients aged 18 or older that receive treatment for a functional deficit secondary to a diagnosis that affects the knee in which the change in their risk-adjusted functional status is measured
Functional Deficit: Change in Risk-Adjusted Functional Status for Patients with Hip Impairments	Percentage of patients aged 18 or older that receive treatment for a functional deficit secondary to a diagnosis that affects the hip in which the change in their risk-adjusted functional status is measured
Functional Deficit: Change in Risk-Adjusted Functional Status for Patients with Lower Leg, Foot or Ankle Impairments	Percentage of patients aged 18 or older that receive treatment for a functional deficit secondary to a diagnosis that affects the lower leg, foot or ankle in which the change in their risk-adjusted functional status is measured
Functional Deficit: Change in Risk-Adjusted Functional Status for Patients with Lumbar Spine Impairments	Percentage of patients aged 18 or older that receive treatment for a functional deficit secondary to a diagnosis that affects the lumbar spine in which the change in their risk-adjusted functional status is measured
Functional Deficit: Change in Risk-Adjusted Functional Status for Patients with Shoulder Impairments	Percentage of patients aged 18 or older that receive treatment for a functional deficit secondary to a diagnosis that affects the shoulder in which the change in their risk-adjusted functional status is measured
Functional Deficit: Change in Risk-Adjusted Functional Status for Patients with Elbow, Wrist or Hand Impairments	Percentage of patients aged 18 or older that receive treatment for a functional deficit secondary to a diagnosis that affects the elbow, wrist or hand in which the change in their risk-adjusted functional status is measured
Functional Deficit: Change in Risk-Adjusted Functional Status for Patients with Neck, Cranium, Mandible, Thoracic Spine, Ribs, or Other General Orthopedic Impairments	Percentage of patients aged 18 or older that receive treatment for a functional deficit secondary to a diagnosis that affects the neck, cranium, mandible, thoracic spine, ribs, or other general orthopedic impairment in which the change in their risk-adjusted functional status is measured
Melanoma: Overutilization of Imaging Studies in Melanoma	Percentage of patients, regardless of age, with a current diagnosis of stage 0 through IIC melanoma or a history of melanoma of any stage, without signs or symptoms suggesting systemic spread, seen for an office visit during the one-year measurement period, for whom no diagnostic imaging studies were ordered
Radiology: Reminder System for Screening Mammograms	Percentage of patients undergoing a screening mammogram whose information is entered into a reminder system with a target due date for the next mammogram
Preventive Care and Screening: Tobacco Use: Screening and Cessation Intervention	Percentage of patients aged 18 years and older who were screened for tobacco use one or more times within 24 months AND who received cessation counseling intervention if identified as a tobacco user.
Controlling High Blood Pressure	Percentage of patients 18-85 years of age who had a diagnosis of hypertension and whose blood pressure was adequately controlled (<140/90 mm Hg) during the measurement period
Use of High-Risk Medications in the Elderly	Percentage of patients 66 years of age and older who were ordered high-risk medications. Two rates are reported. a. Percentage of patients who were ordered at least one high-risk medication. b. Percentage of patients who were ordered at least two different high-risk medications.

TABLE 128-1 PQRS 2016 Measures—cont'd

Measure Title	Measure Description
Weight Assessment and Counseling for Nutrition and Physical Activity for Children and Adolescents	Percentage of patients 3-17 years of age who had an outpatient visit with a primary care physician (PCP) or obstetrician/gynecologist (OB/GYN) and who had evidence of the following during the measurement period. Three rates are reported. — Percentage of patients with height, weight, and body mass index (BMI) percentile documentation — Percentage of patients with counseling for nutrition — Percentage of patients with counseling for physical activity
Childhood Immunization Status	Percentage of children 2 years of age who had four diphtheria, tetanus and acellular pertussis (DTaP); three polio (IPV), one measles, mumps and rubella (MMR); three H influenza type B (HiB); three hepatitis B (Hep B); one chickenpox (VZV); four pneumococcal conjugate (PCV); one hepatitis A (Hep A); two or three rotavirus (RV); and two influenza (flu) vaccines by their second birthday
Ischemic Vascular Disease (IVD): Complete Lipid Profile and LDL-C Control (< 100 mg/dL)	Percentage of patients 18 years of age and older who were discharged alive for acute myocardial infarction (AMI), coronary artery bypass graft (CABG) or percutaneous coronary interventions (PCI) in the 12 months prior to the measurement period, or who had an active diagnosis of ischemic vascular disease (IVD) during the measurement period, and who had each of the following during the measurement period: a complete lipid profile and LDL-C was adequately controlled (< 100 mg/dL)
Coronary Artery Disease (CAD): Symptom Management	Percentage of patients aged 18 years and older with a diagnosis of coronary artery disease (CAD) seen within a 12-month period with results of an evaluation of level of activity and an assessment of whether anginal symptoms are present or absent with appropriate management of anginal symptoms within a 12-month period
Cardiac Rehabilitation Patient Referral from an Outpatient Setting	Percentage of patients evaluated in an outpatient setting who within the previous 12 months have experienced an acute myocardial infarction (MI), coronary artery bypass graft (CABG) surgery, a percutaneous coronary intervention (PCI), cardiac valve surgery, or cardiac transplantation, or who have chronic stable angina (CSA) and have not already participated in an early outpatient cardiac rehabilitation/secondary prevention (CR) program for the qualifying event/diagnosis who were referred to a CR program
Barrett's Esophagus	Percentage of esophageal biopsy reports that document the presence of Barrett's mucosa that also include a statement about dysplasia
Radical Prostatectomy Pathology Reporting	Percentage of radical prostatectomy pathology reports that include the pT category, the pN category, the Gleason score and a statement about margin status
Quantitative Immunohistochemical (IHC) Evaluation of Human Epidermal Growth Factor Receptor 2 Testing (HER2) for Breast Cancer Patients	This is a measure based on whether quantitative evaluation of Human epidermal growth factor receptor 2 testing (HER2) by immunohistochemistry (IHC) uses the system recommended in the current ASCO/CAP Guidelines for human epidermal growth factor receptor 2 testing in breast cancer
Ultrasound Determination of Pregnancy Location for Pregnant Patients with Abdominal Pain	Percentage of pregnant female patients aged 14 to 50 who present to the emergency department (ED) with a chief complaint of abdominal pain or vaginal bleeding who receive a transabdominal or transvaginal ultrasound to determine pregnancy location
Rh Immunoglobulin (Rhogam) for Rh-Negative Pregnant Women at Risk of Fetal Blood Exposure	Percentage of Rh-negative pregnant women aged 14-50 years at risk of fetal blood exposure who receive Rh-Immunoglobulin (Rhogam) in the emergency department (ED)
Statin Therapy at Discharge After Lower Extremity Bypass (LEB)	Percentage of patients aged 18 years and older undergoing infra-inguinal lower extremity bypass who are prescribed a statin medication at discharge
Rate of Open Repair of Small or Moderate Non-Ruptured Abdominal Aortic Aneurysms (AAA) without Major Complications (Discharged to Home by Postoperative Day #7)	Percent of patients undergoing open repair of small or moderate sized non-ruptured abdominal aortic aneurysms who do not experience a major complication (discharge to home no later than postoperative day #7)
Rate of Endovascular Aneurysm Repair (EVAR) of Small or Moderate Non-Ruptured Abdominal Aortic Aneurysms (AAA) Without Major Complications (Discharged to Home by Postoperative Day #2)	Percent of patients undergoing endovascular repair of small or moderate non-ruptured abdominal aortic aneurysms (AAA) that do not experience a major complication (discharged to home no later than postoperative day #2)
Rate of Carotid Endarterectomy (CEA) for Asymptomatic Patients, Without Major Complications (Discharged to Home by Postoperative Day #2)	Percent of asymptomatic patients undergoing CEA who are discharged to home no later than postoperative day #2
Referral for Otologic Evaluation for Patients With Acute or Chronic Dizziness	Percentage of patients aged birth and older referred to a physician (preferably a physician specially trained in disorders of the ear) for an otologic evaluation subsequent to an audiologic evaluation after presenting with acute or chronic dizziness
Image Confirmation of Successful Excision of Image–Localized Breast Lesion	Image confirmation of lesion(s) targeted for image guided excisional biopsy or image guided partial mastectomy in patients with nonpalpable, image-detected breast lesion(s). Lesions may include: microcalcifications, mammographic or sonographic mass or architectural distortion, focal suspicious abnormalities on magnetic resonance imaging (MRI) or other breast imaging amenable to localization such as positron emission tomography (PET) mammography, or a biopsy marker demarcating site of confirmed pathology as established by previous core biopsy
Preoperative Diagnosis of Breast Cancer	The percent of patients undergoing breast cancer operations who obtained the diagnosis of breast cancer preoperatively by a minimally invasive biopsy method
Sentinel Lymph Node Biopsy for Invasive Breast Cancer	The percentage of clinically node negative (clinical stage T1N0M0 or T2N0M0) breast cancer patients who undergo a sentinel lymph node (SLN) procedure

Continued

TABLE 128-1 PQRS 2016 Measures—cont'd

Measure Title	Measure Description
Biopsy Follow-up	Percentage of new patients whose biopsy results have been reviewed and communicated to the primary care/referring physician and patient by the performing physician
Epilepsy: Counseling for Women of Childbearing Potential With Epilepsy	All female patients of childbearing potential (12-44 years old) diagnosed with epilepsy who were counseled or referred for counseling for how epilepsy and its treatment may affect contraception OR pregnancy at least once a year
Inflammatory Bowel Disease (IBD): Preventive Care: Corticosteroid Sparing Therapy	Percentage of patients aged 18 years and older with a diagnosis of inflammatory bowel disease who have been managed by corticosteroids greater than or equal to 10 mg/day of prednisone equivalents for 60 or greater consecutive days or a single prescription equating to 600 mg prednisone or greater for all fills that have been prescribed corticosteroid sparing therapy within the last 12 months
Inflammatory Bowel Disease (IBD): Preventive Care: Corticosteroid Related Iatrogenic Injury—Bone Loss Assessment	Percentage of patients aged 18 years and older with an inflammatory bowel disease encounter who were prescribed prednisone equivalents greater than or equal to 10 mg/day for 60 or greater consecutive days or a single prescription equating to 600 mg prednisone or greater for all fills and were documented for risk of bone loss once during the reporting year or the previous calendar year
Inflammatory Bowel Disease (IBD): Testing for Latent Tuberculosis (TB) Before Initiating Anti-TNF (Tumor Necrosis Factor) Therapy	Percentage of patients aged 18 years and older with a diagnosis of inflammatory bowel disease (IBD) for whom a tuberculosis (TB) screening was performed and results interpreted within 6 months prior to receiving a first course of anti-TNF (tumor necrosis factor) therapy
Inflammatory Bowel Disease (IBD): Assessment of Hepatitis B Virus (HBV) Status Before Initiating Anti-TNF (Tumor Necrosis Factor) Therapy	Percentage of patients aged 18 years and older with a diagnosis of inflammatory bowel disease (IBD) who had Hepatitis B Virus (HBV) status assessed and results interpreted within 1 year prior to receiving a first course of anti-TNF (tumor necrosis factor) therapy
Sleep Apnea: Assessment of Sleep Symptoms	Percentage of visits for patients aged 18 years and older with a diagnosis of obstructive sleep apnea that includes documentation of an assessment of sleep symptoms, including presence or absence of snoring and daytime sleepiness
Sleep Apnea: Severity Assessment at Initial Diagnosis	Percentage of patients aged 18 years and older with a diagnosis of obstructive sleep apnea who had an apnea hypopnea index (AHI) or a respiratory disturbance index (RDI) measured at the time of initial diagnosis
Sleep Apnea: Positive Airway Pressure Therapy Prescribed	Percentage of patients aged 18 years and older with a diagnosis of moderate or severe obstructive sleep apnea who were prescribed positive airway pressure therapy
Sleep Apnea: Assessment of Adherence to Positive Airway Pressure Therapy	Percentage of visits for patients aged 18 years and older with a diagnosis of obstructive sleep apnea who were prescribed positive airway pressure therapy who had documentation that adherence to positive airway pressure therapy was objectively measured
Dementia: Staging of Dementia	Percentage of patients, regardless of age, with a diagnosis of dementia whose severity of dementia was classified as mild, moderate or severe at least once within a 12-month period
Dementia: Cognitive Assessment	Percentage of patients, regardless of age, with a diagnosis of dementia for whom an assessment of cognition is performed and the results reviewed at least once within a 12-month period
Dementia: Functional Status Assessment	Percentage of patients, regardless of age, with a diagnosis of dementia for whom an assessment of functional status is performed and the results reviewed at least once within a 12-month period
Dementia: Neuropsychiatric Symptom Assessment	Percentage of patients, regardless of age, with a diagnosis of dementia and for whom an assessment of neuropsychiatric symptoms is performed and results reviewed at least once in a 12-month period
Dementia: Management of Neuropsychiatric Symptoms	Percentage of patients, regardless of age, with a diagnosis of dementia who have one or more neuropsychiatric symptoms who received or were recommended to receive an intervention for neuropsychiatric symptoms within a 12-month period
Dementia: Counseling Regarding Safety Concerns	Percentage of patients, regardless of age, with a diagnosis of dementia or their caregiver(s) who were counseled or referred for counseling regarding safety concerns within a 12-month period
Dementia: Counseling Regarding Risks of Driving	Percentage of patients, regardless of age, with a diagnosis of dementia or their caregiver(s) who were counseled regarding the risks of driving and the alternatives to driving at least once within a 12-month period
Dementia: Caregiver Education and Support	Percentage of patients, regardless of age, with a diagnosis of dementia whose caregiver(s) were provided with education on dementia disease management and health behavior changes AND referred to additional sources for support within a 12-month period
Parkinson's Disease: Annual Parkinson's Disease Diagnosis Review	All patients with a diagnosis of Parkinson's disease who had an annual assessment including a review of current medications (e.g., medications that can produce Parkinson-like signs or symptoms) and a review for the presence of atypical features (e.g., falls at presentation and early in the disease course, poor response to levodopa, symmetry at onset, rapid progression [to Hoehn and Yahr stage 3 in 3 years], lack of tremor or dysautonomia) at least annually
Parkinson's Disease: Psychiatric Disorders or Disturbances Assessment	All patients with a diagnosis of Parkinson's disease who were assessed for psychiatric disorders or disturbances (e.g., psychosis, depression, anxiety disorder, apathy, or impulse control disorder) at least annually
Parkinson's Disease: Cognitive Impairment or Dysfunction Assessment	All patients with a diagnosis of Parkinson's disease who were assessed for cognitive impairment or dysfunction at least annually
Parkinson's Disease: Querying about Sleep Disturbances	All patients with a diagnosis of Parkinson's disease (or caregivers, as appropriate) who were queried about sleep disturbances at least annually
Parkinson's Disease: Rehabilitative Therapy Options	All patients with a diagnosis of Parkinson's disease (or caregiver(s), as appropriate) who had rehabilitative therapy options (e.g., physical, occupational, or speech therapy) discussed at least annually
Parkinson's Disease: Parkinson's Disease Medical and Surgical Treatment Options Reviewed	All patients with a diagnosis of Parkinson's disease (or caregiver(s), as appropriate) who had the Parkinson's disease treatment options (e.g., non-pharmacological treatment, pharmacological treatment, or surgical treatment) reviewed at least once annually

TABLE 128-1 PQRS 2016 Measures—cont'd

Measure Title	Measure Description
Cataracts: Improvement in Patient's Visual Function within 90 Days Following Cataract Surgery	Percentage of patients aged 18 years and older in sample who had cataract surgery and had improvement in visual function achieved within 90 days following the cataract surgery, based on completing a pre-operative and post-operative visual function survey
Cataracts: Patient Satisfaction within 90 Days Following Cataract Surgery	Percentage of patients aged 18 years and older in sample who had cataract surgery and were satisfied with their care within 90 days following the cataract surgery, based on completion of the Consumer Assessment of Healthcare Providers and Systems Surgical Care Survey
Initiation and Engagement of Alcohol and Other Drug Dependence Treatment	Percentage of patients 13 years of age and older with a new episode of alcohol and other drug (AOD) dependence who received the following. Two rates are reported. a. Percentage of patients who initiated treatment within 14 days of the diagnosis. b. Percentage of patients who initiated treatment and who had two or more additional services with an AOD diagnosis within 30 days of the initiation visit.
Cervical Cancer Screening	Percentage of women 21-64 years of age, who received one or more Pap tests to screen for cervical cancer
Chlamydia Screening for Women	Percentage of women 16-24 years of age who were identified as sexually active and who had at least one test for chlamydia during the measurement period
Use of Appropriate Medications for Asthma	Percentage of patients 5-64 years of age who were identified as having persistent asthma and were appropriately prescribed medication during the measurement period
Use of Imaging Studies for Low Back Pain	Percentage of patients 18-50 years of age with a diagnosis of low back pain who did not have an imaging study (plain X-ray, MRI, CT scan) within 28 days of the diagnosis.
Preventive Care and Screening: Cholesterol—Fasting Low Density Lipoprotein (LDL-C) Test Performed AND Risk-Stratified Fasting LDL-C	Percentage of patients aged 20 through 79 years whose risk factors* have been assessed and a fasting LDL test has been performed AND percentage of patients aged 20 through 79 years who had a fasting LDL-C test performed and whose risk-stratified fasting LDL-C is at or below the recommended LDL-C goal. *There are three criteria for this measure based on the patient's risk category. 1. Highest level of risk: coronary heart disease (CHD) or CHD risk equivalent OR 10-year Framingham risk >20% 2. Moderate level of risk: multiple (2+) risk factors OR 10-year Framingham risk 10-20% 3. Lowest level of risk: 0 or 1 risk factor OR 10-year Framingham risk <10%
Preventive Care and Screening: Screening for High Blood Pressure and Follow-Up Documented	Percentage of patients aged 18 years and older seen during the reporting period who were screened for high blood pressure AND a recommended follow-up plan is documented based on the current blood pressure (BP) reading as indicated.
Falls: Screening for Fall Risk	Percentage of patients 65 years of age and older who were screened for future fall risk at least once during the measurement period.
Appropriate Follow-Up Interval for Normal Colonoscopy in Average Risk Patients	Percentage of patients aged 50 to 75 years of age receiving a screening colonoscopy without biopsy or polypectomy who had a recommended follow-up interval of at least 10 years for repeat colonoscopy documented in their colonoscopy report
CAHPS for PQRS Clinician/Group Survey	• Getting timely care, appointments, and information; • How well providers Communicate; • Patient's Rating of Provider; • Access to Specialists; • Health Promotion & Education; • Shared Decision Making; • Health Status/Functional Status; • Courteous and Helpful Office Staff; • Care Coordination; • Between Visit Communication; • Helping Your to Take Medication as Directed; and • Stewardship of Patient Resources
Cardiac Stress Imaging Not Meeting Appropriate Use Criteria: Preoperative Evaluation in Low-Risk Surgery Patients	Percentage of stress single-photon emission computed tomography (SPECT) myocardial perfusion imaging (MPI), stress echocardiogram (ECHO), cardiac computed tomography angiography (CCTA), or cardiac magnetic resonance (CMR) performed in low risk surgery patients 18 years or older for preoperative evaluation during the 12-month reporting period
Cardiac Stress Imaging Not Meeting Appropriate Use Criteria: Routine Testing After Percutaneous Coronary Intervention (PCI)	Percentage of all stress single-photon emission computed tomography (SPECT) myocardial perfusion imaging (MPI), stress echocardiogram (ECHO), cardiac computed tomography angiography (CCTA), and cardiovascular magnetic resonance (CMR) performed in patients aged 18 years and older routinely after percutaneous coronary intervention (PCI), with reference to timing of test after PCI and symptom status
Cardiac Stress Imaging Not Meeting Appropriate Use Criteria: Testing in Asymptomatic, Low-Risk Patients	Percentage of all stress single-photon emission computed tomography (SPECT) myocardial perfusion imaging (MPI), stress echocardiogram (ECHO), cardiac computed tomography angiography (CCTA), and cardiovascular magnetic resonance (CMR) performed in asymptomatic, low coronary heart disease (CHD) risk patients 18 years and older for initial detection and risk assessment
Adult Major Depressive Disorder (MDD): Coordination of Care of Patients With Specific Comorbid Conditions	Percentage of medical records of patients aged 18 years and older with a diagnosis of major depressive disorder (MDD) and a specific diagnosed comorbid condition (diabetes, coronary artery disease, ischemic stroke, intracranial hemorrhage, chronic kidney disease [stages 4 or 5], end stage renal disease [ESRD] or congestive heart failure) being treated by another clinician with communication to the clinician treating the comorbid condition
Atrial Fibrillation and Atrial Flutter: Chronic Anticoagulation Therapy	Percentage of patients aged 18 years and older with a diagnosis of nonvalvular atrial fibrillation (AF) or atrial flutter whose assessment of the specified thromboembolic risk factors indicate one or more high-risk factors or more than one moderate risk factor, as determined by CHADS2 risk stratification, who are prescribed warfarin OR another oral anticoagulant drug that is FDA approved for the prevention of thromboembolism

Continued

TABLE 128-1 PQRS 2016 Measures—cont'd

Measure Title	Measure Description
Pediatric Kidney Disease: Adequacy of Volume Management	Percentage of calendar months within a 12-month period during which patients aged 17 years and younger with a diagnosis of end stage renal disease (ESRD) undergoing maintenance hemodialysis in an outpatient dialysis facility have an assessment of the adequacy of volume management from a nephrologist
Pediatric Kidney Disease: ESRD Patients Receiving Dialysis: Hemoglobin Level < 10 g/dL	Percentage of calendar months within a 12-month period during which patients aged 17 years and younger with a diagnosis of end stage renal disease (ESRD) receiving hemodialysis or peritoneal dialysis have a hemoglobin level < 10 g/dL
Adult Kidney Disease: Catheter Use at Initiation of Hemodialysis	Percentage of patients aged 18 years and older with a diagnosis of end stage renal disease (ESRD) who initiate maintenance hemodialysis during the measurement period, whose mode of vascular access is a catheter at the time maintenance hemodialysis is initiated
Adult Kidney Disease: Catheter Use for Greater Than or Equal to 90 Days	Percentage of patients aged 18 years and older with a diagnosis of end stage renal disease (ESRD) receiving maintenance hemodialysis for greater than or equal to 90 days whose mode of vascular access is a catheter
Adult Sinusitis: Antibiotic Prescribed for Acute Sinusitis (Overuse)	Percentage of patients, aged 18 years and older, with a diagnosis of acute sinusitis who were prescribed an antibiotic within 10 days after onset of symptoms
Adult Sinusitis: Appropriate Choice of Antibiotic: Amoxicillin With or Without Clavulanate Prescribed for Patients With Acute Bacterial Sinusitis (Appropriate Use)	Percentage of patients aged 18 years and older with a diagnosis of acute bacterial sinusitis that were prescribed amoxicillin, with or without clavulanate, as a first-line antibiotic at the time of diagnosis
Adult Sinusitis: Computed Tomography (CT) for Acute Sinusitis (Overuse)	Percentage of patients aged 18 years and older with a diagnosis of acute sinusitis who had a computed tomography (CT) scan of the paranasal sinuses ordered at the time of diagnosis or received within 28 days after date of diagnosis
Adult Sinusitis: More Than One Computed Tomography (CT) Scan Within 90 Days for Chronic Sinusitis (Overuse)	Percentage of patients aged 18 years and older with a diagnosis of chronic sinusitis who had more than one CT scan of the paranasal sinuses ordered or received within 90 days after the date of diagnosis
Maternity Care: Elective Delivery or Early Induction Without Medical Indication at ≥ 37 and < 39 Weeks	Percentage of patients, regardless of age, who gave birth during a 12-month period who delivered a live singleton at ≥ 37 and < 39 weeks of gestation completed who had elective deliveries or early inductions without medical indication
Maternity Care: Post-Partum Follow-Up and Care Coordination	Percentage of patients, regardless of age, who gave birth during a 12-month period who were seen for post-partum care within 8 weeks of giving birth who received a breast feeding evaluation and education, post-partum depression screening, post-partum glucose screening for gestational diabetes patients, and family and contraceptive planning
Tuberculosis Prevention for Psoriasis, Psoriatic Arthritis and Rheumatoid Arthritis Patients on a Biological Immune Response Modifier	Percentage of patients whose providers are ensuring active tuberculosis prevention either through yearly negative standard tuberculosis screening tests or are reviewing the patient's history to determine if they have had appropriate management for a recent or prior positive test
HIV Viral Load Suppression	The percentage of patients, regardless of age, with a diagnosis of HIV with a HIV viral load less than 200 copies/mL at last HIV viral load test during the measurement year
Prescription of HIV Antiretroviral Therapy	Percentage of patients, regardless of age, with a diagnosis of HIV prescribed antiretroviral therapy for the treatment of HIV infection during the measurement year
HIV Medical Visit Frequency	Percentage of patients, regardless of age with a diagnosis of HIV who had at least one medical visit in each 6-month period of the 24-month measurement period, with a minimum of 60 days between medical visits
Pain Brought Under Control Within 48 Hours	Patients aged 18 and older who report being uncomfortable because of pain at the initial assessment (after admission to palliative care services) who report pain was brought to a comfortable level within 48 hours
Screening Colonoscopy Adenoma Detection Rate Measure	The percentage of patients age 50 years or older with at least one conventional adenoma or colorectal cancer detected during screening colonoscopy
Rate of Carotid Artery Stenting (CAS) for Asymptomatic Patients, Without Major Complications (Discharged to Home by Postoperative Day #2)	Percent of asymptomatic patients undergoing CAS who are discharged to home no later than postoperative day #2
Rate of Postoperative Stroke or Death in Asymptomatic Patients Undergoing Carotid Artery Stenting (CAS)	Percent of asymptomatic patients undergoing CAS who experience stroke or death following surgery while in the hospital
Rate of Postoperative Stroke or Death in Asymptomatic Patients Undergoing Carotid Endarterectomy (CEA)	Percent of asymptomatic patients undergoing CEA who experience stroke or death following surgery while in the hospital
Rate of Endovascular Aneurysm Repair (EVAR) of Small or Moderate Non-ruptured Abdominal Aortic Aneurysms (AAA) Who Die While in Hospital	Percent of patients undergoing endovascular repair of small or moderate abdominal aortic aneurysms (AAA) who die while in the hospital
HRS-3: Implantable Cardioverter-Defibrillator (ICD) Complications Rate	Patients with physician-specific risk-standardized rates of procedural complications following the first time implantation of an ICD
Total Knee Replacement: Shared Decision-Making: Trial of Conservative (Non-surgical) Therapy	Percentage of patients regardless of age or gender undergoing a total knee replacement with documented shared decision-making with discussion of conservative (non-surgical) therapy (e.g. clavulanate anti-inflammatory drugs [NSAIDs], analgesics, weight loss, exercise, injections) prior to the procedure
Total Knee Replacement: Venous Thromboembolic and Cardiovascular Risk Evaluation	Percentage of patients regardless of age or gender undergoing a total knee replacement who are evaluated for the presence or absence of venous thromboembolic and cardiovascular risk factors within 30 days prior to the procedure (e.g. history of deep vein thrombosis (DVT), pulmonary embolism (PE), myocardial infarction (MI), arrhythmia and stroke)

TABLE 128-1 PQRS 2016 Measures—cont'd

Measure Title	Measure Description
Total Knee Replacement: Preoperative Antibiotic Infusion with Proximal Tourniquet	Percentage of patients regardless of age or gender undergoing a total knee replacement who had the prophylactic antibiotic completely infused prior to the inflation of the proximal tourniquet
Total Knee Replacement: Identification of Implanted Prosthesis in Operative Report	Percentage of patients regardless of age or gender undergoing a total knee replacement whose operative report identifies the prosthetic implant specifications including the prosthetic implant manufacturer, the brand name of the prosthetic implant and the size of each prosthetic implant
Anastomotic Leak Intervention	Percentage of patients aged 18 years and older who required an anastomotic leak intervention following gastric bypass or colectomy surgery
Unplanned Reoperation within the 30-Day Postoperative Period	Percentage of patients aged 18 years and older who had any unplanned reoperation within the 30-day postoperative period
Unplanned Hospital Readmission within 30 Days of Principal Procedure	Percentage of patients aged 18 years and older who had an unplanned hospital readmission within 30 days of principal procedure
Surgical Site Infection (SSI)	Percentage of patients aged 18 years and older who had a surgical site infection (SSI)
Patient-Centered Surgical Risk Assessment and Communication	Percentage of patients who underwent a non-emergency surgery who had their personalized risks of postoperative complications assessed by their surgical team prior to surgery using a clinical data-based, patient-specific risk calculator and who received personal discussion of those risks with the surgeon
Optimizing Patient Exposure to Ionizing Radiation: Utilization of a Standardized Nomenclature for Computed Tomography (CT) Imaging Description	Percentage of computed tomography (CT) imaging reports for all patients, regardless of age, with the imaging study named according to a standardized nomenclature and the standardized nomenclature is used in institution's computer systems
Optimizing Patient Exposure to Ionizing Radiation: Count of Potential High Dose Radiation Imaging Studies: Computed Tomography (CT) and Cardiac Nuclear Medicine Studies	Percentage of computed tomography (CT) and cardiac nuclear medicine (myocardial perfusion studies) imaging reports for all patients, regardless of age, that document a count of known previous CT (any type of CT) and cardiac nuclear medicine (myocardial perfusion) studies that the patient has received in the 12-month period prior to the current study
Optimizing Patient Exposure to Ionizing Radiation: Reporting to a Radiation Dose Index Registry	Percentage of total computed tomography (CT) studies performed for all patients, regardless of age, that are reported to a radiation dose index registry AND that include at a minimum selected data elements
Optimizing Patient Exposure to Ionizing Radiation: Computed Tomography (CT) Images Available for Patient Follow-up and Comparison Purposes	Percentage of final reports for computed tomography (CT) studies performed for all patients, regardless of age, which document that Digital Imaging and Communications in Medicine (DICOM) format image data are available to non-affiliated external health care facilities or entities on a secure, media free, reciprocally searchable basis with patient authorization for at least a 12-month period after the study
Optimizing Patient Exposure to Ionizing Radiation: Search for Prior Computed Tomography (CT) Studies Through a Secure, Authorized, Media-Free, Shared Archive	Percentage of final reports of computed tomography (CT) studies performed for all patients, regardless of age, which document that a search for Digital Imaging and Communications in Medicine (DICOM) format images was conducted for prior patient CT imaging studies completed at non-affiliated external health care facilities or entities within the past 12 months and are available through a secure, authorized, media free, shared archive prior to an imaging study being performed
Optimizing Patient Exposure to Ionizing Radiation: Appropriateness: Follow-up CT Imaging for Incidentally Detected Pulmonary Nodules According to Recommended Guidelines	Percentage of final reports for computed tomography (CT) imaging studies of the thorax for patients aged 18 years and older with documented follow-up recommendations for incidentally detected pulmonary nodules (e.g., follow-up CT imaging studies needed or that no follow-up is needed) based at a minimum on nodule size AND patient risk factors
Hemoglobin A_{1c} Test for Pediatric Patients	Percentage of patients 5-17 years of age with diabetes with a HbA_{1c} test during the measurement period
ADHD: Follow-up Care for Children Prescribed Attention-Deficit/Hyperactivity Disorder (ADHD) Medication	Percentage of children 6-12 years of age and newly dispensed a medication for attention-deficit/ hyperactivity disorder (ADHD) who had appropriate follow-up care. Two rates are reported. a. Percentage of children who had one follow-up visit with a practitioner with prescribing authority during the 30-day initiation phase. b. Percentage of children who remained on ADHD medication for at least 210 days and who, in addition to the visit in the initiation phase, had at least two additional follow-up visits with a practitioner within 270 days (9 months) after the initiation phase ended
Bipolar Disorder and Major Depression: Appraisal for Alcohol or Chemical Substance Use	Percentage of patients with depression or bipolar disorder with evidence of an initial assessment that includes an appraisal for alcohol or chemical substance use
HIV/AIDS: Medical Visit	Percentage of patients, regardless of age, with a diagnosis of HIV/AIDS with at least two medical visits during the measurement year with a minimum of 90 days between each visit
Pregnant Women That Had HBsAg Testing	This measure identifies pregnant women who had a HBsAg (hepatitis B) test during their pregnancy
Depression Remission at 12 Months	Adult patients age 18 and older with major depression or dysthymia and an initial PHQ-9 score > 9 who demonstrate remission at 12 months defined as PHQ-9 score less than 5. This measure applies to both patients with newly diagnosed and existing depression whose current PHQ-9 score indicates a need for treatment
Depression Utilization of the PHQ-9 Tool	Adult patients age 18 and older with the diagnosis of major depression or dysthymia who have a PHQ-9 tool administered at least once during a 4-month period in which there was a qualifying visit
Maternal Depression Screening	The percentage of children who turned 6 months of age during the measurement year, who had a face-to-face visit between the clinician and the child during child's first 6 months, and who had a maternal depression screening for the mother at least once between 0 and 6 months of life
Hypertension: Improvement in Blood Pressure	Percentage of patients aged 18-85 years of age with a diagnosis of hypertension whose blood pressure improved during the measurement period
Closing the Referral Loop: Receipt of Specialist Report	Percentage of patients with referrals, regardless of age, for which the referring provider receives a report from the provider to whom the patient was referred

Continued

TABLE 128-1 PQRS 2016 Measures—cont'd

Measure Title	Measure Description
Functional Status Assessment for Knee Replacement	Percentage of patients aged 18 years and older with primary total knee arthroplasty (TKA) who completed baseline and follow-up (patient-reported) functional status assessments.
Functional Status Assessment for Hip Replacement	Percentage of patients aged 18 years and older with primary total hip arthroplasty (THA) who completed baseline and follow-up (patient-reported) functional status assessments
Functional Status Assessment for Complex Chronic Conditions	Percentage of patients aged 65 years and older with heart failure who completed initial and follow-up patient-reported functional status assessments
Children Who Have Dental Decay or Cavities	Percentage of children, aged 0-20 years, who have had tooth decay or cavities during the measurement period
Primary Caries Prevention Intervention as Offered by Primary Care Providers, Including Dentists	Percentage of children, aged 0-20 years, who received a fluoride varnish application during the measurement period.
ADE Prevention and Monitoring: Warfarin Time in Therapeutic Range	Average percentage of time in which patients aged 18 and older with atrial fibrillation who are on chronic warfarin therapy have international normalized ratio (INR) test results within the therapeutic range (i.e., TTR) during the measurement period
HIV/AIDS: RNA Control for Patients With HIV	Percentage of patients aged 13 years and older with a diagnosis of HIV/AIDS, with at least two visits during the measurement year, with at least 90 days between each visit, whose most recent HIV RNA level is <200 copies/mL
Child and Adolescent Major Depressive Disorder (MDD): Suicide Risk Assessment	Percentage of patient visits for those patients aged 6 through 17 years with a diagnosis of major depressive disorder with an assessment for suicide risk
Adherence to Antipsychotic Medications for Individuals With Schizophrenia	Percentage of individuals at least 18 years of age as of the beginning of the measurement period with schizophrenia or schizoaffective disorder who had at least two prescriptions filled for any antipsychotic medication and who had a PDC of at least 0.8 for antipsychotic medications during the measurement period (12 consecutive months)
Adult Primary Rhegmatogenous Retinal Detachment Surgery: No Return to the Operating Room Within 90 Days of Surgery	Patients aged 18 years and older who had surgery for primary rhegmatogenous retinal detachment who did not require a return to the operating room within 90 days of surgery
Adult Primary Rhegmatogenous Retinal Detachment Surgery: Visual Acuity Improvement Within 90 Days of Surgery	Patients aged 18 years and older who had surgery for primary rhegmatogenous retinal detachment and achieved an improvement in their visual acuity, from their preoperative level, within 90 days of surgery in the operative eye
Amyotrophic Lateral Sclerosis (ALS) Patient Care Preferences	Percentage of patients diagnosed with amyotrophic lateral sclerosis (ALS) who were offered assistance in planning for end of life issues (e.g. advance directives, invasive ventilation, hospice) at least once annually
Annual Hepatitis C Virus (HCV) Screening for Patients Who Are Active Injection Drug Users	Percentage of patients regardless of age who are active injection drug users who received screening for HCV infection within the 12-month reporting period
Cataract Surgery With Intraoperative Complications (Unplanned Rupture of Posterior Capsule Requiring Unplanned Vitrectomy)	Percentage of patients aged 18 years and older who had cataract surgery performed and had an unplanned rupture of the posterior capsule requiring vitrectomy
Cataract Surgery: Difference Between Planned and Final Refraction	Percentage of patients aged 18 years and older who had cataract surgery performed and who achieved a final refraction within +/- 1.0 diopters of their planned (target) refraction.
Hepatitis C: Discussion and Shared Decision Making Surrounding Treatment Options	Percentage of patients aged 18 years and older with a diagnosis of hepatitis C with whom a physician or other qualified health care professional reviewed the range of treatment options appropriate to their genotype and demonstrated a shared decision making approach with the patient. To meet the measure, there must be documentation in the patient record of a discussion between the physician or other qualified healthcare professional and the patient that includes all of the following: treatment choices appropriate to genotype, risks and benefits, evidence of effectiveness, and patient preferences toward treatment
Follow-up After Hospitalization for Mental Illness (FUH)	The percentage of discharges for patients 6 years of age and older who were hospitalized for treatment of selected mental illness diagnoses and who had an outpatient visit, an intensive outpatient encounter or partial hospitalization with a mental health practitioner. Two rates are reported: — The percentage of discharges for which the patient received follow-up within 30 days of discharge — The percentage of discharges for which the patient received follow-up within 7 days of discharge.
HRS-12: Cardiac Tamponade and/or Pericardiocentesis Following Atrial Fibrillation Ablation	Rate of cardiac tamponade and/or pericardiocentesis following atrial fibrillation ablation This measure is reported as four rates stratified by age and gender: • Reporting age criteria 1: females less than 65 years of age • Reporting age criteria 2: males less than 65 years of age • Reporting age criteria 3: females 65 years of age and older • Reporting age criteria 4: males 65 years of age and older
HRS-9: Infection within 180 Days of Cardiac Implantable Electronic Device (CIED) Implantation, Replacement, or Revision	Infection rate following CIED device implantation, replacement, or revision
Immunizations for Adolescents	The percentage of adolescents 13 years of age who had the recommended immunizations by their 13th birthday
Lung Cancer Reporting (Biopsy/Cytology Specimens)	Pathology reports based on biopsy and/or cytology specimens with a diagnosis of primary nonsmall cell lung cancer classified into specific histologic type or classified as NSCLC-NOS with an explanation included in the pathology report
Lung Cancer Reporting (Resection Specimens)	Pathology reports based on resection specimens with a diagnosis of primary lung carcinoma that include the pT category, pN category and for non–small cell lung cancer, histologic type
Melanoma Reporting	Pathology reports for primary malignant cutaneous melanoma that include the pT category and a statement on thickness and ulceration and for pT1, mitotic rate

TABLE 128-1 PQRS 2016 Measures—cont'd

Measure Title	Measure Description
Optimal Asthma Control	Patients ages 5-50 (pediatrics ages 5-17) whose asthma is well controlled as demonstrated by one of three age appropriate patient reported outcome tools
Postprocedural Optimal Medical Therapy Composite (Percutaneous Coronary Intervention)	Percentage of patients aged 18 years and older for whom PCI is performed who are prescribed optimal medical therapy at discharge
One-Time Screening for Hepatitis C Virus (HCV) for Patients at Risk	Percentage of patients aged 18 years and older with one or more of the following: a history of injection drug use, receipt of a blood transfusion prior to 1992, receiving maintenance hemodialysis OR birthdate in the years 1945-1965 who received a one-time screening for HCV infection
Hepatitis C: Screening for Hepatocellular Carcinoma (HCC) in Patients with Cirrhosis	Percentage of patients aged 18 years and older with a diagnosis of chronic hepatitis C cirrhosis who underwent imaging with either ultrasound, contrast enhanced CT or MRI for hepatocellular carcinoma (HCC) at least once within the 12-month reporting period
Tobacco Use and Help With Quitting Among Adolescents	The percentage of adolescents 12 to 20 years of age with a primary care visit during the measurement year for whom tobacco use status was documented and received help with quitting if identified as a tobacco user
Adult Kidney Disease: Referral to Hospice	Percentage of patients aged 18 years and older with a diagnosis of end-stage renal disease (ESRD) who withdraw from hemodialysis peritoneal dialysis who are referred to hospice care
Anesthesiology Smoking Abstinence	The percentage of current smokers who abstain from cigarettes prior to anesthesia on the day of elective surgery or procedure
Appropriate Follow-up Imaging for Incidental Abdominal Lesions	Percentage of final reports for abdominal imaging studies for asymptomatic patients aged 18 years and older with one or more of the following noted incidentally with follow-up imaging recommended: • Liver lesion ≤ 0.5 cm • Cystic kidney lesion < 1.0 cm • Adrenal lesion ≤ 1.0 cm
Appropriate Follow-Up Imaging for Incidental Thyroid Nodules in Patients	Percentage of final reports for computed tomography (CT) or magnetic resonance imaging (MRI) studies of the chest or neck or ultrasound of the neck for patients aged 18 years and older with no known thyroid disease with a thyroid nodule < 1.0 cm noted incidentally with follow-up imaging recommended
Appropriate Treatment of Methicillin-Sensitive *Staphylococcus aureus* (MSSA) Bacteremia	Percentage of patients with sepsis due to methicillin-sensitive *Staphylococcus aureus* (MSSA) bacteremia who received beta-lactam antibiotic (e.g., nafcillin, oxacillin or cefazolin) as definitive therapy
Opioid Therapy Follow-up Evaluation	All patients 18 and older prescribed opiates for longer than 6 weeks' duration who had a follow-up evaluation conducted at least every three months during opioid therapy documented in the medical record
Clinical Outcome Postendovascular Stroke Treatment	Percentage of patients with a mRs score of 0 to 2 at 90 days following endovascular stroke intervention
Psoriasis: Clinical Response to Oral Systemic or Biologic Medications	Percentage of psoriasis patients receiving oral systemic or biologic therapy who meet minimal physician- or patient-reported disease activity levels. It is implied that establishment and maintenance of an established minimum level of disease control as measured by physician- and/or patient-reported outcomes will increase patient satisfaction with and adherence to treatment
Depression Remission at 6 Months	Adult patients age 18 years and older with major depression or dysthymia and an initial PHQ-9 score > 9 who demonstrate remission at 6 months defined as a PHQ-9 score less than 5. This measure applies to both patients with newly diagnosed and existing depression whose current PHQ-9 score indicates a need for treatment
Documentation of Signed Opioid Treatment Agreement	All patients 18 and older prescribed opiates for longer than 6 weeks' duration who signed an opioid treatment agreement at least once during opioid therapy documented in the medical record
Door to Puncture Time for Endovascular Stroke Treatment	Percentage of patients undergoing endovascular stroke treatment who have a door to puncture time of less than 2 hours
Evaluation or Interview for Risk of Opioid Misuse	All patients 18 and older prescribed opiates for longer than 6 weeks' duration evaluated for risk of opioid misuse using a brief validated instrument (e.g. Opioid Risk Tool, SOAAP-R) or patient interview documented at least once during opioid therapy in the medical record
Emergency Medicine: Emergency Department Utilization of CT for Minor Blunt Head Trauma for Patients Aged 18 Years and Older	Percentage of emergency department visits for patients aged 18 years and older who presented within 24 hours of a minor blunt head trauma with a Glasgow Coma Scale (GCS) score of 15 and who had a head CT for trauma ordered by an emergency care provider who have an indication for a head CT
Emergency Medicine: Emergency Department Utilization of CT for Minor Blunt Head Trauma for Patients Aged 2 through 17 Years	Percentage of emergency department visits for patients aged 2 through 17 years who presented within 24 hours of a minor blunt head trauma with a Glasgow Coma Scale (GCS) score of 15 and who had a head CT for trauma ordered by an emergency care provider who are classified as low risk according to the Pediatric Emergency Care Applied Research Network prediction rules for traumatic brain injury
Rate of Open Repair of Ascending Abdominal Aortic Aneurysms (AAA) Where Patients Are Discharged Alive	Percentage of patients undergoing open repair of abdominal aortic aneurysms (AAA) who are discharged alive
Osteoporosis Management in Women Who Had a Fracture	The percentage of women age 50-85 who suffered a fracture and who either had a bone mineral density test or received a prescription for a drug to treat osteoporosis
Overuse of Neuroimaging for Patients With Primary Headache and a Normal Neurological Examination	Percentage of patients with a diagnosis of primary headache disorder for whom advanced brain imaging was not ordered

Continued

TABLE 128-1 PQRS 2016 Measures—cont'd

Measure Title	Measure Description
Varicose Vein Treatment With Saphenous Ablation: Outcome Survey	Percentage of patients treated for varicose veins (CEAP C2-S) who are treated with saphenous ablation (with or without adjunctive tributary treatment) that report an improvement on a disease specific patient reported outcome survey instrument after treatment.
Appropriate Assessment of Retrievable Inferior Vena Cava Filters for Removal	Percentage of patients in whom a retrievable IVC filter is placed who, within 3 months post-placement, have a documented assessment for the appropriateness of continued filtration, device removal or the inability to contact the patient with at least two attempts
Performing Cystoscopy at the Time of Hysterectomy for Pelvic Organ Prolapse to Detect Lower Urinary Tract Injury	Percentage of patients who undergo cystoscopy to evaluate for lower urinary tract injury at the time of hysterectomy for pelvic organ prolapse
Perioperative Anti-platelet Therapy for Patients Undergoing Carotid Endarterectomy	Percentage of patients undergoing carotid endarterectomy (CEA) who are taking an anti-platelet agent (aspirin or clopidogrel or equivalent such as aggrenox/tiglacor, etc.) within 48 hours prior to surgery and are prescribed this medication at hospital discharge following surgery
Perioperative Temperature Management	Percentage of patients, regardless of age, who undergo surgical or therapeutic procedures under general or neuraxial anesthesia of 60 minutes' duration or longer for whom at least one body temperature greater than or equal to 35.5 degrees Celsius (or 95.9 degrees Fahrenheit) was recorded within the 30 minutes immediately before or the 15 minutes immediately after anesthesia end time
Photodocumentation of Cecal Intubation	The rate of screening and surveillance colonoscopies for which photodocumentation of landmarks of cecal intubation is performed to establish a complete examination
Post-Anesthetic Transfer of Care Measure: Procedure Room to a Post Anesthesia Care Unit (PACU):	Percentage of patients, regardless of age, who are under the care of an anesthesia practitioner and are admitted to a PACU in which a post-anesthetic formal transfer of care protocol or checklist which includes the key transfer of care elements is utilized
Post-Anesthetic Transfer of Care: Use of Checklist or Protocol for Direct Transfer of Care from Procedure Room to Intensive Care Unit (ICU)	Percentage of patients, regardless of age, who undergo a procedure under anesthesia and are admitted to an intensive care unit (ICU) directly from the anesthetizing location, who have a documented use of a checklist or protocol for the transfer of care from the responsible anesthesia practitioner to the responsible ICU team or team member
Pelvic Organ Prolapse: Preoperative Assessment of Occult Stress Urinary Incontinence	Percentage of patients undergoing appropriate preoperative evaluation for the indication of stress urinary incontinence per ACOG/AUGS/AUA guidelines
Pelvic Organ Prolapse: Preoperative Screening for Uterine Malignancy	Percentage of patients who are screened for uterine malignancy prior to surgery for pelvic organ prolapse.
Prevention of Postoperative Nausea and Vomiting (PONV)—Combination Therapy	Percentage of patients, aged 18 years and older, who undergo a procedure under an inhalational general anesthetic, AND who have three or more risk factors for postoperative nausea and vomiting (PONV), who receive combination therapy consisting of at least two prophylactic pharmacologic antiemetic agents of different classes preoperatively or intraoperatively
Preventive Care and Screening: Unhealthy Alcohol Use: Screening and Brief Counseling	Percentage of patients aged 18 years and older who were screened at least once within the last 24 months for unhealthy alcohol use using a systematic screening method AND who received brief counseling if identified as an unhealthy alcohol user
Proportion of Patients Sustaining a Bladder Injury at the Time of Any Pelvic Organ Prolapse Repair	Percentage of patients undergoing any surgery to repair pelvic organ prolapse who sustains an injury to the bladder recognized either during or within 1 month after surgery
Proportion of Patients Sustaining a Major Viscus Injury at the Time of Any Pelvic Organ Prolapse Repair	Percentage of patients undergoing surgical repair of pelvic organ prolapse that is complicated by perforation of a major viscus at the time of index surgery that is recognized intraoperative or within 1 month after surgery
Proportion of Patients Sustaining a Ureter Injury at the Time of Any Pelvic Organ Prolapse Repair	Percentage of patients undergoing a pelvic organ prolapse repair who sustain an injury to the ureter recognized either during or within 1 month after surgery
Quality of Life Assessment for Patients With Primary Headache Disorders	Percentage of patients with a diagnosis of primary headache disorder whose health related quality of life (HRQoL) was assessed with a tool(s)* during at least two visits* during the 12-month measurement period AND whose health related quality of life score stayed the same or improved.
Radiation Consideration for Adult CT: Utilization of Dose Lowering Techniques	Percentage of final reports for patients aged 18 years and older undergoing CT with documentation that one or more of the following dose reduction techniques were used: • Automated exposure control • Adjustment of the mA and/or kV according to patient size • Use of iterative reconstruction technique
Rate of Surgical Conversion from Lower Extremity Endovascular Revasculatization Procedure	Inpatients assigned to endovascular treatment for obstructive arterial disease, the percent of patients who undergo unplanned major amputation or surgical bypass within 48 hours of the index procedure
Statin Therapy for the Prevention and Treatment of Cardiovascular Disease	Percentage of the following patients—all considered at high risk of cardiovascular events—who were prescribed or were on statin therapy during the measurement period: • Adults aged ≥ 21 years who were previously diagnosed with or currently have an active diagnosis of clinical atherosclerotic cardiovascular disease (ASCVD); OR • Adults aged ≥21 years with a fasting or direct low-density lipoprotein cholesterol (LDL-C) level ≥ 190 mg/dL; OR • Adults aged 40-75 years with a diagnosis of diabetes with a fasting or direct LDL-C level of 70-189 mg/dL
Age-Appropriate Screening Colonoscopy	The percentage of patients greater than 85 years of age who received a screening colonoscopy from January 1 to December 31

Adapted from Centers for Medicare & Medicaid Services. PQRS fact sheet. Updated measures can be found at the following location: https://www.cms.gov/Medicare/Quality-Initiatives-Patient-Assessment-Instruments/PQRS/MeasuresCodes.html. Accessed May 25, 2014.
ASCO/CAP, American Society of Clinical Oncology/College of American Pathologists; *FDA,* U.S. Food and Drug Administration.

common in people with Medicare—myocardial infarction (i.e., heart attack), congestive heart failure (CFH), and pneumonia. In 2009, measures for hospital readmission of Medicare patients within 30 days of discharge for these same three conditions were added.

Hospital readmission occurring a short time after discharge may be an indicator of poor quality of care in the hospital or a lack of appropriate coordination of postdischarge care. The number of readmissions to the hospital within 30 days after a discharge has become an increasingly important quality measure for hospitals.[10] Additionally, data have indicated that readmissions are common, with about one in five Medicare patients discharged from a hospital being readmitted within 30 days. Although various factors can influence a readmission, a Medicare Payment Advisory Commission (MedPAC) report of 2005 Medicare data concluded that approximately 75% of readmissions within 30 days were likely preventable. These potentially avoidable events were found to represent about $12 billion in Medicare spending. Statistics such as these have helped make reducing preventable hospital readmissions another important objective of the ACA and led to the creation of the Medicare Hospital Readmissions Reduction Program (HRRP), which provides incentives for hospitals to lower their rates.[10]

Because Medicare pays most hospitals using the inpatient prospective payment system (IPPS), which pays a fixed average amount per admission according to patient diagnosis, regardless of actual resources used, the payment scheme neither discouraged the occurrence of hospital readmissions nor provided any additional reimbursement to cover the costs of interventions, such as after-discharge follow-up, that could potentially prevent readmissions. Thus, it was not until the implementation of the HRRP that hospitals were financially incentivized to reduce preventable readmissions. HRRP was first implemented in October 2012, with financial penalties applied to all general hospitals paid under the Medicare IPPS that were found to have excess Medicare readmissions, defined as admission to the same or another hospital within 30 days of a discharge, for three diagnoses—acute myocardial infarction, heart failure, and pneumonia.[11] To ensure that the program was being implemented appropriately, certain readmissions were excluded from the HRRP, including transfers to other IPPS hospitals and readmissions designated as "planned," such as chemotherapy or rehabilitation. Penalties for hospitals found to have excess readmissions, defined as those exceeding the expected readmission rate (as calculated by the national mean readmission rate, risk-adjusted for demographic characteristics and illness severity of the hospital's patients), are capped at 1% of the aggregate IPPS base payments for the first year, 2% for the second year, and 3% each year thereafter. In October 2014, these conditions assessed in the program expanded to include elective hip or knee replacement and chronic obstructive pulmonary disease.[10]

Reports from CMS and MedPAC in 2013 have suggested that the HRRP has already had a positive effect on lowering readmissions. The all-cause Medicare readmission rate dropped from 19% to 17.8%, indicating about 70,000 fewer readmissions, with an even greater reduction in rates of the focused areas of acute myocardial infarction, CHF, and pneumonia.

According to MedPAC recommendations, several improvements will be made to the HRRP program, including adjustments in the computation approach for penalties, adjustment of penalties based on a patient's socioeconomic status, and additional CMS funding for strategies to reduce readmissions, including discharge planning and follow-up. The expansion of this effort is expected to improve quality and, at the same time, reduce costs.

Nursing Homes

With 3 million of the frailest older Americans relying on services provided by nursing homes at some point during the year—and, of them, 1.5 million staying long enough to consider the nursing home their main residence[12] —it should come as no surprise that nursing homes are heavily governed to ensure quality care. However, despite heavy oversight, one in five nursing homes nationwide have been cited for serious deficiencies that caused actual harm or placed residents in immediate jeopardy.[13] Some major areas of focus identified by nursing home medical directors include telephone conversations, transitional care, falls and hip fracture, warfarin (Coumadin) use, pressure ulcers, inappropriate medications, pain control, urinary incontinence, weight loss, and exercise.[14]

Quality standards and requirements for nursing homes were established under the Omnibus Budget Reconciliation Act (OBRA) of 1987, which mandated that nursing homes participating in Medicare and Medicaid programs monitor residents using the Resident Assessment Instrument (RAI). The RAI consists of the Minimum Data Set (MDS) for nursing home resident assessment and care screening, which assesses functioning on activities of daily living (ADLs), cognition, continence, mood, behaviors, nutritional status, vision and communication, activities, and psychosocial well-being. Problems or risks for decline identified through the MDS assessment trigger further assessment on one or more of the RAI's 18 resident assessment protocols, which are used to identify treatable causes of problems common to nursing home residents.[15] OBRA 1987 requirements became federal law in 1990 after widespread evidence of poor quality of care in nursing homes, demonstrated through prevalent use of physical restraints, inappropriate use of psychotropic medications, overuse of urinary catheters, and inadequate treatment of incontinence, pressure ulcers, nutritional problems, and behavioral problems. Various studies have shown that implementation of the RAI led to improvements.

In 2002, CMS launched two important programs to help drive quality improvements in nursing homes. The first was the Medicare.gov Nursing Home Compare website, developed to improve public access to quality information on long-term care facilities. It contains data that includes facility ratings, selected results from survey and certification inspections, and staffing information on all Medicare and Medicaid nursing homes and skilled nursing facilities (SNFs). The second program was the national Nursing Home Quality Initiative, developed to improve the quality of nursing home care, including posting the performance of every nursing home on a set of various quality indicators.[16] As with other quality reporting, public access to these performance results has enabled consumers to make informed decisions while simultaneously motivating providers to improve their care. This CMS quality initiative marked a major redirection toward a more resident-centric focus on clinical care needs, instead of the historical focus on process of care. In 2008, a five-star rating system was added to the Nursing Home Compare website, with each nursing home having a rating from one star (much below average quality) to five stars (above average quality), based on health inspections, staffing, and performance on physical and clinical quality measures.[17]

Additional Quality Measures

In recognition of the importance of monitoring the quality of care provided in the long-term care (LTC) setting and driving further improvements, provisions of the ACA require further refinements and updates to the Nursing Home Compare website, including the incorporation of additional quality measures. Currently, there are 13 different quality measures for long-stay residents and five for short-stay residents.[16,18]

Long-Stay Quality Measures. These refer to the percentage of long-stay residents experiencing the following:

- One or more falls with major injury
- Urinary tract infection

- Moderate to severe pain (self-reported)
- Pressure ulcers
- Loss of control of their bladders
- Catheter inserted and left in their bladders
- Physical restraint
- Increased need for help with ADLs
- Excessive weight loss
- Depressive symptoms
- Appropriate administration of the seasonal influenza vaccine
- Appropriate administration of the seasonal pneumococcal vaccine
- Administration of antipsychotic medication

Short-Stay Quality Measures. These refer to the percentage of short-stay residents experiencing the following:

- Moderate to severe pain (self-reported)
- New or worsened pressure ulcers
- Appropriate administration of the seasonal influenza vaccine
- Appropriate administration of the seasonal pneumococcal vaccine
- New administration of antipsychotic medication

Quality measures can produce improvements in care and cost as designed, but unintended consequences can also occur. A report by Konetzka and colleagues[19] found that the public reporting of physical restraint use had the unintended consequences of increasing the use of antipsychotics in nursing home residents. This example highlights the importance of monitoring quality initiatives to guard against unintended consequences, which could actually decrease quality and increase cost.

In addition to the continued use of quality measures, provisions of the ACA also call for disclosure of ownership and organizational relationships of LTC facilities, implementation of ethics and compliance programs, direct care staff expenditure reports, development and dissemination of a standardized complaint form, implementation of a national independent monitor demonstration program, and assessment of the CMS Five-Star Quality Rating System. Additionally, civil financial penalties may be imposed on LTC facilities found to be jeopardizing residents' health and safety due to deficient care practices.[17] Finally, beyond simply reporting these quality measures, payment will be directly tied to achieving these outcomes.

Managed Care Plans

Medicare beneficiaries began enrolling in Medicare MCOs in 1985 under provisions of the Tax Equity and Fiscal Responsibility Act (TEFRA). However, it would be more than a decade later that the Medicare program would begin ongoing review of health care quality in Medicare MCOs. In the interim, comprehensive evaluations of quality performance were conducted under contract with CMS by Mathematica Policy Research for both the Medicare HMO demonstrations and the Medicare MCOs contracting in the first 5 years of the TEFRA risk-contracting program.[20] The evaluations compared measures of process and outcomes for beneficiaries receiving care in Medicare MCOs versus Medicare fee-for-service (FFS), demonstrating similar levels of quality performance. However, the standards for measures of quality performance and improvement used in commercial MCOs-those other than Medicare and Medicaid-such as HEDIS and NCQA accreditation, were in notable contrast to the lack of comparable quality performance standards applied to Medicare HMOs.

As a result, in 1998, CMS implemented requirements for HEDIS reporting by Medicare MCOs as well as submission for auditing of the beneficiary-level data used in the computation of the HEDIS measures. Over time, additional requirements were added, including measurement of clinical performance in the prevention or treatment of acute and chronic conditions, high-volume services, high-risk services, and continuity and coordination of care. Measurements of performance in nonclinical areas were also added, including the availability of and accessibility to care, quality of provider encounters, and resolution of appeals, grievances, and other complaints. As the number of measures grew, standards were applied to the measures themselves to ensure these were unambiguous, based on current clinical knowledge or health services research, and measured outcomes such as health status, functional status, beneficiary satisfaction, or valid proxies of the measures. Importantly, requirements for Medicare managed care organizations (MCOs) to develop and implement interventions for improving performance and tracking quality improvements over time were also enacted.

In 2003, Medicare Part C was renamed Medicare Advantage (MA) with the passing of the Medicare Modernization Act (MMA), providing Medicare patients who enroll in this type of plan the opportunity to receive benefits at least as extensive as those provided by traditional FFS Medicare, which typically includes prescription drug coverage. In return, CMS pays these private health plans to fund their benefit offerings to Medicare older adults. The often lower out of pocket costs and more generous benefits associated with MA plans drove substantial enrollment of Medicare patients into MA plans. Similarly, the higher reimbursement payments by CMS to private plans versus the traditional FFS plan drove an increase in the number of MA plans available, providing an enormous option for seniors nationwide. In recognition of the need to help Medicare beneficiaries make informed health care choices, CMS adopted a Five-Star Rating system in 2007 to allow comparison of options.[21] CMS created plan ratings that indicate the quality of Medicare plans on a scale of one to five stars, with five stars being the highest rating. The overall star rating is determined through numerous performance measures across several domains of performance. Each measure is awarded a star rating, and the individual measure stars are then aggregated at the domain and summary level. Only a small number of plans receive a five-star summary rating from CMS, with most plans receiving three to three-and-a-half stars.

Since 2007, plans have been awarded between one (poor) and five (excellent) stars based on 36 measures across five separate categories, including Staying Healthy, Managing Chronic Conditions, Plan Responsiveness, Members' Complaints and Appeals, and Telephone Customer Service, based on data from four different sources—HEDIS, Consumer Assessment of Healthcare Providers and Systems (CAHPS), Health Outcomes Survey (HOS), and CMS administrative data sets.[22] The rating for each plan, provided in a single summary score for easy comparison, is posted on the Medicare website.[23] A Kaiser Family Foundation analysis of the CMS Star Ratings of 2010 MA plans found the following[24]:

- 62% of plans received star ratings; 38% were not rated.
- 86% of MA plan members were in rated plans.
- Average rating was 3.32 stars.
- 24% of enrollees were in a plan with four or more stars.
- 17% of enrollees were in plans with fewer than three stars.

As part of the PPACA, in 2012, five-star ratings were begun to tie quality performance to bonus payments. In 2012, benchmarks for plans receiving four or more stars were increased by 1.5%, which was further increased to 3% in 2013 and estimated to increase to 5% in 2014 and beyond. Plans that earn fewer than four stars are not eligible for these increases, and plans consistently earning fewer than three stars over a 3-year period will be designated as low-quality on the Medicare website.[25] Encouraging plan competition based on quality performance ratings and financial incentives is thought to help drive quality improvement in the benefits and services offered to Medicare older adults.

Beyond monitoring against unintended consequences of quality measures, it is necessary to ensure that the measures being reported are accurate. Without this assurance, false reporting could mask poor quality. Such was the case in the 2014 Veterans Administration scandal, in which the quality measure of wait time for a consultant visit was falsely reported. The result was the failure to recognize provider access limitations that could result in poor-quality care. The issue was so severe that several deaths were attributed to this failure. It is thought that accurate reporting of this quality measure would have identified this failure. This highlights the need to ensure that quality measures are reported accurately.[26]

Prescription Drug Plans

Evidence for the need of improved medication management comes from data indicating the following:

- Medication mismanagement accounts for approximately 30% of all hospitalizations and 45% of readmissions among older adults.[27]
- One in four Americans, or approximately 75 million people, do not follow directions when taking their prescribed medications.[28]
- An estimated $290 billion is spent each year on hospital admissions, extra physician visits, laboratory tests, and nursing home admissions as a result of adverse drug events due to inappropriate use of medications.[28]

Quality measures and reporting involve all areas of Medicare, including the prescription drug benefit, or Medicare Part D. Since its inception in 2006, Medicare Part D plans have been responsible for providing medication therapy management (MTM). MTM encompasses programs developed through a collaboration of licensed and practicing pharmacists and physicians to help ensure that medications are used optimally to achieve improved therapeutic outcomes and reduce the risk of medication-related adverse events; they can be administered by pharmacists or other qualified providers.[29] MTM is viewed by CMS as an opportunity for prescription drug plans (PDPs) to improve the health outcomes of their patients. Although the structure of MTM had originally largely been left to the discretion of specific plans, including factors such as determining qualification criteria for beneficiaries and type of services provided, this lack of standardization created substantial variation across plans, creating the need for more extensive standards.

In recognition of the scope of the issue from clinical and economic perspectives, as well as the need for more consistent implementation of the MTM across plans, provisions in the ACA specified that starting in 2013, plans must offer, at a minimum, MTM services to targeted beneficiaries that include strategies for improving adherence to prescription medications or other associated goals. Specifically, MTM must include services and processes to achieve the following objectives[30]:

- Annual comprehensive medication review by a licensed pharmacist or other qualified provider
- Follow-up interventions, as warranted, based on the findings of the annual medication review or targeted medication enrollment
- Quarterly or more frequent assessment of medication use by at-risk individuals not enrolled in the MTM program, such as patients experiencing a recent transition in care, if this information is available to the PDP
- Automatic enrollment of targeted beneficiaries, such as those identified through a quarterly assessment
- Permission for beneficiaries to opt out of MTM enrollment

More consistent and standardized implementation of MTM programs across MA plans will help reduce medication-related adverse events, optimize therapeutic outcomes, and reduce resource use associated with medication mismanagement.

CMS has increasingly established prescription management standards beyond the MTM program, with the help of organizations such as the Pharmacy Quality Alliance (PQA), as well as the expectations that plans will adhere to them. Specifically, the PQA is tasked with improving the quality of medication management and use across health care settings, with the goal of improving patients' health through a collaborative process to develop and implement performance measures and recognize examples of exceptional pharmacy quality.

The PQA has assisted CMS in developing multiple components to evaluate medication-related quality across the Medicare prescription drug program through PDPs and MA plans. MA plans that include drug benefits (MA-PDs) are rated on performance measures for Parts C and D. For Part C, a subset of the HEDIS measure set from the National Committee for Quality Assurance (NCQA) is used for evaluation. Medicare Part D stars are applicable to MA-PDs and stand-alone PDPs. The stars are assigned based on performance measures across four domains:

1. Drug plan customer service
2. Member complaints, problems getting services, and choosing to leave the plan
3. Member experience with drug plan
4. Drug pricing and patient safety

Like other quality measures, those for Medicare prescription drug benefits, along with the MTM program, are meant to identify and promote higher quality plans, which, in turn, should improve outcomes for Medicare beneficiaries and reduce costs.

PREVENTION FOCUS

Although historically the focus of CMS has been on providing coverage for acute services, there has been an increasing realization that to provide substantial improvements to the health of older adults and the quality of their health care, initiatives aimed at encouraging wellness and prevention need to become more robust. An added benefit of programs that effectively help prevent the onset or progression of conditions would be the preservation of Medicare through a reduction in health care resource use associated with a healthier older adult population.

Statistics have demonstrated that chronic diseases are an enormous problem facing the U.S. health care system, In 2012, nearly 50% of all adults, or approximately 117 million people, had at least one chronic health condition, with 25% suffering from two or more.[31] Additionally, many of these conditions are preventable or could have been more effectively managed earlier in the disease progression—conditions such as diabetes, cancer, heart disease, and asthma, which can be caused by obesity, smoking, failure to follow medical directives, and alcohol abuse—and are estimated to cost from $303 to $493 billion annually.[32]

Recognition of the substantial impact of chronic, often preventable, diseases on the U.S. health care system has made efforts aimed at preventing disease and encouraging wellness another key objective of the ACA, several of which pertain to Medicare beneficiaries.[32] The first of these, implemented in 2011, included expansion of the preventive care benefits covered under Medicare Part B, establishing an annual wellness visit (AWV) for a personal prevention plan of service (PPPS) in addition to the existing Welcome to Medicare Visit (or Initial Preventive Physical Examination, IPPE) already in place for new Part B beneficiaries.[33] The AWV is available to Medicare beneficiaries with no copayment or deductible required and is aimed at proactive identification of conditions to prompt appropriate management and, potentially, prevention of negative clinical and economic consequences. Components of the AWV include the collection of medical and family histories, patient vital signs, list of the patient's medical providers, screens for cognitive impairment and depression, and functional status evaluation. The AWV also includes development of a personalized prevention plan to include identification of risk factors and recommendations for preventive screenings.[17,34] Additionally, the ACA established that co-insurance and deductible requirements would be waived for most preventive services, with 100% of costs being covered by Medicare, as well as modification of coverage for any Medicare-covered preventive services for consistency with recommendations of the U.S. Preventive Services Task Force.[17] Finally, the ACA also required CMS to implement the Senior Risk Reduction Demonstration (SRRD) project in Medicare beneficiaries aged 67 to 74 years to assess the ability of health promotion, health management, and disease prevention programs to reduce Medicare beneficiaries' health risk factors, improve overall health, and reduce health care expenditures for Medicare. The demonstration will also assess beneficiaries' participation rates and collect feedback from beneficiaries on their opinion of the programs.

By applying Benjamin Franklin's adage that "an ounce of prevention is worth a pound of cure," these ACA-inspired efforts by CMS are likely to improve the health and quality of life of older adults while simultaneously reducing health care expenditures for Medicare.

Coordinated Care Models

A nascent example of coordinated care emerged in the early 1970s in San Francisco through efforts to help Asian American and other non–English-speaking community members care for older adults in their own homes, because the use of nursing homes for frail older family members was not a culturally acceptable solution for these groups. PACE (Program of All-inclusive Care for the Elderly) evolved when On Lok Senior Health Services created an innovative way to offer a comprehensive array of medical supervision, physical and occupational therapies, nutrition, transportation, respite care, socialization, and other needed services to these older adults. The benefits for these groups living outside the nursing home have been demonstrated in several studies, including a 1996 study that concluded that expansion of home- and community-based services were a cost-effective alternative to institutional care of older adults eligible for nursing home placement in several states.[35]

The development of coordinated care approaches is also not something entirely new for Medicare. In 1987, United Healthcare launched Evercare, a program that used nurse practitioners in nursing homes to increase the on-site primary care of residents. This program aimed to reduce the need for emergency room evaluations and increase preventive care and timely acute care assessment and treatment, all of which help reduce avoidable admissions. More recently, the Medicare MMA has allowed for the development of a Medicare Advantage Coordinated Care Plan (CCP), designed to provide targeted care to patients with special needs, including residents of nursing homes, dual-eligible older adults (those entitled to Medicare Part A and/or Part B and eligible for some form of Medicaid benefit), or those suffering from multiple chronic illnesses. These plans were referred to as special needs plans (SNPs), and aimed to improve health outcomes for older adults with special needs through improved coordination and continuity of care, thereby avoiding preventable hospitalizations.[36]

In 2006, the concept that would come to be known as an accountable care organization (ACO) was introduced as a collaboration of a group of health care providers to provide better care at lower costs while also assuming financial responsibility for the health outcomes of their patients.[5] Support for the ACO model of care developed over time, perhaps in part as a result of positive findings from the first years of the CMS Physician Group Practice Demonstration—the first pay-for-performance initiative for Medicare physicians—that showed improvements in quality of care and provider-shared savings.[37,38] In recognition of the improvements in health care quality and costs that could be achieved with an ACO model of care, the ACA authorized the creation of a new, voluntary ACO program, beginning in 2012, in which ACOs could contract directly with Medicare.[39] Typically, the providers involved in the ACO model, which may include primary care physicians, specialists, and occasionally hospitals, agree to a budget for managing the health and long-term care of a specific population of patients based on their overall health. ACOs can then share in the savings if costs fall below the prespecified budget, provided that quality of care standards are met in several areas, including the following[24,39]:

- Patient and caregiver care experiences
- Care coordination
- Patient safety
- Preventive health
- At-risk population and frail older adult health

If ACOs exceed the prespecified care budget, they may also share in the losses, creating a true model of accountability for the quality and efficiency of services provided to patients.

Medicare currently offers several different ACO programs:

- Medicare Shared Savings Program for FFS beneficiaries
- Advance payment ACO model for specific eligible providers that are already participating or are interested in the Medicare Shared Savings Program
- Pioneer ACO model for health care organizations and providers already experienced in coordinating care for patients across care settings

Some of the quality improvements that may be associated with the use of ACOs include reducing rates of unnecessary hospital admissions and preventable readmissions, eliminating unnecessary emergency department visits, reducing the need for office visit–based care, and improving transitions in care.[40] Improving the efficiency of care transitions is an important objective, especially for older adults, with an average of 20% of Medicare FFS beneficiaries who are discharged from the hospital being readmitted within 30 days and 34% readmitted within 90 days, at an approximate cost of $12 billion annually.[41] In recognition of the substantial opportunity to improve care quality and reduce unnecessary costs, the ACA established the 5-year Community-Based Care Transitions Program Demonstration Project (CCTP), which began in 2011. The goal of the CCTP is to test modes for improving care transitions from the hospital to other settings and reduce the number of hospital readmissions.[42] Providers that elect to participate are paid based on a per eligible discharge basis for Medicare patients at high risk for readmission, such as those who have multiple chronic conditions, depression, or cognitive impairment, and will receive a set payment for every patient they follow after hospital discharge.[42] Currently, 102 sites nationwide are participating in the CCTP program.[43] The Innovation Center develops new payment and service delivery models organized into seven categories, including accountable care. The other six categories are as follows:

1. Bundled payments for care improvement
2. Primary care transformation
3. Initiatives focused on the Medicaid and CHIP population
4. Initiatives focused on the Medicare-Medicaid enrollees
5. Initiatives to speed the adoption of best practices
6. Initiatives to accelerate the development and testing of new payment and service delivery models

Through the Innovation Center, ACOs and other coordinated care delivery models aim at improving quality while reducing costs.

Health Information Technology

Electronic prescribing (e-prescribing) and the use of EHRs are often discussed as being core elements of health information technology (HIT). HIT, as defined by as the Health and Human Services Office of the National Coordinator for Health Information Technology, is "the application of information processing involving both computer hardware and software that deals with the storage, retrieval, sharing, and use of health care information, data, and knowledge for communication and decision making."[44] Although potential benefits of HIT include improvements in health care quality due to medication or medical errors and increasing the efficiency of care due to reducing unnecessary tests and increasing the exchange of information among providers, the full impact of HIT has yet to be realized.[45]

E-prescribing can help avoid medication errors that stem from difficulties in deciphering handwritten prescriptions, reduce rates of adverse drug events by alerting prescribers of the potential for drug interactions or contraindications at the time of prescription preparation, and improve patient adherence to therapy.[44,46] To encourage physicians to adopt the use of e-prescribing, CMS established standards in 2009 for Medicare Part D requiring e-prescribing system compliance with regard to factors such as medication history, fill status notification, and formulary and benefits information.[46]

Later the same year, to drive the adoption of e-prescribing further, a 5-year program authorized by the Medicare Improvement for Patients and Provider Act of 2008 (MIPPA) introduced incentives for eligible professionals who were successfully using e-prescribing systems. Another incentive program, authorized by Division B of the Tax Relief and Health Care Act of 2006–Medicare Improvements and Extension Act of 2006 (MIEA-TRHCA), known as the PQRI (now PQRS), provided an e-prescribing incentive based on the covered professional services furnished by the eligible professional during the reporting years 2009 through 2013. The MIPPA also required that quality measures used to qualify for the PQRI incentive payment could not include e-prescribing measures.

E-prescribing incentives started at 2.0% during reporting years 2009 to 2010 and decreased to 1.0% and 0.5% for reporting years 2011 to 2012 and reporting year 2013, respectively. Physicians who were eligible for incentives but failed to participate faced penalties of 1.0% and 1.5% in 2012 and 2013, respectively. In 2014, incentive payments were discontinued, and penalties increased to 2.0%.[46]

Full implementation and use of EHRs have resulted in several important improvements, including the quality and convenience of patient care, patient participation in care, accuracy of diagnoses and health outcomes, care coordination, and practice efficiencies and cost savings.[47] In an effort to encourage the use of EHRs, the American Recovery and Reinvestment Act (ARRA) and Health Information Technology for Economic and Clinical Health Act (HITECH), passed in 2009, included a requirement for the adoption of EHR use by 2014 for 70% of the primary care provider population.[48] The act also included approval for a CMS EHR Incentive Program, authorizing payments starting in 2011 and continuing through 2014 for physician and hospital providers that successfully become "meaningful users" of EHRs.[48] In 2015, providers not actively using an EHR in compliance with the meaningful use definition will be subject to financial penalties under Medicare. Meaningful use under the CMS EHR Incentive Program is determined when eligible professionals, hospitals, and critical access hospitals (CAHs) meet established measurement thresholds.[49]

Three stages of meaningful use are in place, with increasing requirements for participation. Participation begins when stage 1 requirements are met for a 90-day period in the first year of meaningful use and a full year in the second year of meaningful use. After providers meet stage 1 requirements, they must then meet stage 2 requirements for 2 years.[49] Providers must demonstrate meaningful use every year to receive an incentive and avoid a Medicare payment adjustment.[50] In stages 1 and 2, a number of meaningful use objectives must be met—those from a core set and a menu set—the number of which varies according to whether the participant is an eligible professional, eligible hospital, or CAH. In addition to meeting the core and menu objectives, eligible professionals, eligible hospitals, and CAHs are also required to report clinical quality measures, including those pertaining to health outcomes, clinical processes, patient safety, efficient use of health care resources, care coordination, patient engagements, population and public health, and adherence to clinical guidelines.[50]

CMS has also worked to ensure that providers have the support they need to take advantage of HIT to lower costs and improve quality, including working with the Veterans Administration to adapt their VISTA (Veterans Health Information Systems and Technology Architecture) system for EHR use and providing technical support through state-based QIOs. QIOs will assist providers in using evidence-based approaches to achieve measurable quality improvements and get the most benefit from quality-based payment systems. One important method for achieving this is to help them choose and implement HIT systems using advice and support that has worked well for similar providers and that is well coordinated with other administration efforts to support effective, interoperable IT systems. These IT systems help physician offices and other providers improve coordination of care and measure quality of care and improve it.

RESOURCES: QUALITY ORGANIZATIONS

Several government and nongovernmental organizations are dedicated to quality. They work to ensure quality through identification and analysis of quality issues and via resources to address these quality issues, including providing accreditation to notate quality organizations.

There are a few key organizations dedicated to identification and analysis of quality issues. The most influential, at least to the public, is the Institute of Medicine (IOM); the most influential to Congress is MedPAC, which is tasked with advising Congress on issues involving Medicare, including quality. CMS has given QIOs with the job of helping health care providers, whereas other organizations work with the federal government to place a stamp of quality on organizations and products (Table 128-2).

Identification and Analysis: Institute of Medicine

With a focus on quality, the IOM in 1996 launched a concerted ongoing effort focused on assessing and improving the nation's quality of care, which is now in its third phase. The first phase of this quality initiative documented the serious and pervasive nature of the nation's overall quality problem, concluding that "the burden of harm conveyed by the collective impact of all of our health care quality problems is staggering."[51]

The initial phase was built on an intensive literature review conducted by Dr. Mark A. Schuster at the Rand Corporation (Research and Development) to understand the scope of this issue. A framework was established that defined the nature of the problem as one of overuse, misuse, and underuse of health care services. During the second phase, spanning 1999 to 2001, the Committee on Quality of Health Care in America laid out a vision for how the health care system and related policy environment must be radically transformed to close the gap between what we know to be good quality care and what actually exists in practice. Phase 3 of the IOM's Quality Initiative has focused on operationalizing the vision of a future health system as described in the Quality Chasm report.

TABLE 128-2 Quality Organizations

Agency	Purpose
AGENCY WITHIN THE CENTERS FOR MEDICARE & MEDICAID SERVICES (CMS)—IDENTIFICATION AND ANALYSIS	
Center for Medicare and Medicaid Innovation (Innovation Center)	Established for the purpose of testing "innovative payment and service delivery models to reduce program expenditures … while preserving or enhancing the quality of care."
AGENCY WITHIN THE DEPARTMENT OF HEALTH AND HUMAN SERVICES (HHS)—IDENTIFICATION AND ANALYSIS	
Agency for Healthcare Research and Quality (AHRQ)	Supports health services research initiatives that seek to improve the quality of health care in America. AHRQ's mission is to improve the quality, safety, efficiency, effectiveness, and cost-effectiveness of health care for all Americans.
INDEPENDENT CONGRESSIONAL AGENCY—IDENTIFICATION AND ANALYSIS	
Medicare Payment Advisory Commission (MedPAC)	Established to advise Congress on issues affecting the Medicare program, such as payments to private health plans participating in Medicare and providers in Medicare's traditional fee-for-service program, and analyzing access to care, quality of care, and other issues affecting Medicare.
PRIVATE 501(C) NONPROFIT ORGANIZATION—ACCREDITATION	
National Committee for Quality Assurance (NCQA)	Dedicated to improving health care quality. The NCQA seal is a widely recognized symbol of quality. Organizations incorporating the seal into advertising and marketing materials must first pass a rigorous comprehensive review and must report on their performance annually. For consumers and employers, the seal is a reliable indicator that an organization is well managed and delivers high-quality care and service.
Utilization Review Accreditation Commission (URAC)	A leader in promoting health care quality through its accreditation and certification programs. URAC offers a wide range of quality benchmarking programs and services that keep pace with the rapid changes in the health care system and provide a symbol of excellence for organizations to validate their commitment to quality and accountability. Through its broad-based governance structure and an inclusive standards development process, URAC ensures that all stakeholders are represented in establishing meaningful quality measures for the entire health care industry.
The Joint Commission (TJC)	Works continuously to improve the safety and quality of care provided to the public through the provision of health care accreditation and related services that support performance improvement. TJC accredits and certifies more than 15,000 health care organizations and programs in the United States. TJC accreditation and certification is recognized nationwide as a symbol of quality that reflects an organization's commitment to meeting certain performance standards.
PRIVATE 501(C) NONPROFIT ORGANIZATION—IDENTIFICATION AND ANALYSIS	
Pharmacy Quality Alliance (PQA)	Tasked with improving the quality of medication management and use across health care settings, with the goal of improving patients' health through a collaborative process to develop and implement performance measures and recognize examples of exceptional pharmacy quality.
PRIVATE 501(C) NONPROFIT ORGANIZATION—RESOURCES	
Institute of Medicine (IOM)	Asks and answers the nation's most pressing questions about health and health care for the purpose of providing unbiased and authoritative advice to decision makers and the public so that these organizations can make informed health decisions.
Institute of Healthcare Improvement (IHI)	Works to accelerate improvement by building the will for change, cultivating promising concepts for improving patient care, and helping health care systems put those ideas into action.
Quality improvement organization (QIO)	Improves quality of care for beneficiaries and protects the integrity of the Medicare Trust Fund by ensuring that Medicare pays only for services and goods that are reasonable and necessary and that are provided in the most appropriate setting. QIO protects beneficiaries by expeditiously addressing individual complaints.

The IOM report, *Leadership by Example: Coordinating Government Roles in Improving Health Care Quality* (2002), has encouraged the federal government to take full advantage of its influential position as purchaser, regulator, and provider of health care services to determine quality for the health care sector. The vision for each of these distinct federal roles is very much in agreement with ideas laid out in the Quality Chasm report. Other efforts in this area include *Envisioning the National Healthcare Quality Report* (2001) and *Guidance for the National Healthcare Disparities Report*.

The IOM continues to be highly active in the area of quality and patient safety, performing assessments at the request of government agencies on various initiatives to understand challenges better and determine how to implement improvements.[52]

Quality Improvement Organizations

Since the inception of the Medicare program, the quality of care received by beneficiaries has been monitored. The earliest organizations responsible for quality performance measurement were the professional services review organizations (PSROs), local review boards that reviewed care received by a limited number of beneficiaries during an inpatient hospital stay. The jurisdiction of PSROs was typically for one or several counties within a state and had its primary focus on whether the health care received was medically necessary.

In 1984, PSROs were replaced by PROs, with jurisdiction for an entire state and, for several of the 43 PROs, jurisdiction for more than one state. Initially, PROs monitored inpatient care by selecting random samples of inpatient admissions from computerized Medicare hospital claims records. The initial review of medical necessity and quality of care for the sampled admissions was performed by nurse reviewers. Admissions identified with problems were then looked at by physician reviewers, who requested medical records for review if they concurred with the initial case review. Admissions judged to have problems after the review of medical records resulted in denial of payment for the admission.

By the end of the 1980s, PROs extended their review beyond inpatient care to include skilled nursing facilities, outpatient hospital departments, ambulatory surgery centers, and home health agencies. In addition, the reviews by PROs increasingly focused on quality performance measures. By the early 1990s, the effectiveness of PROs in successfully monitoring quality performance and improving quality was questioned. The reliability of physician reviews by PROs was questioned in some influential studies. In particular, one study showed that the agreement between reviews of PRO reviewers compared with reviewers at Johns Hopkins were no better than what would be expected by chance. The effectiveness of a retrospective review in identifying the source of quality problems and preventing them was also questioned, given the lapse in time since specific cases were reviewed. Also, in contrast to provider profiling, in which quality performance is based on some or all of the provider's patients, a PRO's retrospective review of a random sample of cases will identify, at most, very few cases per provider subject to review and no cases for many providers. Under the PRO system of review, this paucity of cases for any given provider invites attribution of quality problems for a specific case to random variation in outcomes, rather than systemic problems with a physician or health care facility.[53]

In light of this criticism of PROs, their activities were redefined under the Health Care Quality Improvement Program in 1993. Under this initiative, retrospective case review was replaced by collaborative initiatives with hospitals and physicians to improve quality so that it would be closer to the model of continuous quality improvement (CQI). Although the aggregate impact of this new initiative has been difficult to assess, case studies have suggested success in specific settings. For example, results from one quality improvement initiative for patients with CHF has shown that evaluation of left ventricular function improved from 53% to 65% and that appropriate use of angiotensin-converting enzyme (ACE) inhibitors improved from 54% to 74%.[54]

The mission of these organizations has been to improve the effectiveness, efficiency, economy, and quality of services delivered to Medicare beneficiaries. Based on this statutory charge, and CMS's program experience, CMS has identified the core functions of the QIO program as follows:

- Improving quality of care for beneficiaries
- Protecting the integrity of the Medicare Trust Fund by ensuring that Medicare pays only for services and goods that are reasonable and necessary and that are provided in the most appropriate setting
- Protecting beneficiaries by expeditiously addressing individual complaints, such as beneficiary complaints, provider-based notice appeals, violations of the Emergency Medical Treatment and Labor Act (EMTALA), and other related responsibilities, as articulated in QIO-related law

CMS relies on QIOs to improve the quality of health care for all Medicare beneficiaries. Furthermore, QIOs are required under Sections 1152-1154 of the Social Security Act. CMS regards the QIO program as an important resource in its efforts to improve quality and efficiency of care for Medicare beneficiaries. Throughout its history, the program has been instrumental in advancing national efforts to motivate providers in improving quality and measuring and improving outcomes of quality.

The Medicare QIO Program (formerly known as the Medicare Utilization and Quality Control Peer Review Program) was created by statute in 1982 to improve the quality and efficiency of services delivered to Medicare beneficiaries. In its first phase, which concluded in the early 1990s, the program sought to accomplish its mission through peer review of cases to identify cases in which professional standards were not met for the purpose of initiating corrective actions. In the second phase, quality measurement and improvement became the predominant mode of program operation. As a result of significant changes that have occurred in our understanding of how to improve quality, as well as changes in the environment to promote public reporting of provider performance and development of performance-based payment programs, the QIO is now positioned as an agent of change.

CMS views the QIO program as a cornerstone of its efforts to improve quality and efficiency of care for Medicare beneficiaries. The program has been instrumental in advancing national efforts to measure and improve quality, and it presents unique opportunities to support improvements in care in the future. Consequently, CMS is undertaking these activities to ensure that the program is focused, structured, and managed so as to maximize its ability for creating value. These improvements support broader initiatives to provide transparency for beneficiaries and create performance-based payment programs for providers. Most health care providers deliver care to Medicare beneficiaries and patients insured by commercial insurers. Recent efforts to improve quality reflect the idea that shared quality improvement goals and consistent quality measures for all patients will result in fewer burdens to providers and an opportunity to identify and achieve meaningful performance improvements. Thus, to achieve demonstrable and significant improvement in care for Medicare beneficiaries, the program is supporting partnerships that engage a broad group of stakeholders for the purpose of improving quality of care for all patients, based on common goals and measures. This approach facilitates leveraging private sector resources and expertise at the local and national levels, with a potentially more significant impact on the quality and efficiency of the health care system.

QIOs completed their eighth Statement of Work (SOW) between 2005 and 2008, focusing on improvements in quality through organizational transformations—including nursing homes, home health agencies, hospitals, and physician practices—with the aim of achieving more rapid and measurable improvements in care. This SOW included efforts to redesign provider care processes through systemic changes, including adoption and implementation of health information and communication technologies.

In 2011, CMS initiated a series of projects with the QIO program that ran through July 2014 and has focused on improved patient care, improved population health, and reduced health care costs as a result of these improvements. QIOs aimed to redesign health care processes to increase safety and patient centricity, with a focus on the following[55]:

- Review of beneficiary complaints and encouragement of beneficiaries and their families to take an active role in quality improvement and prevention activities
- Use of evidence-based change packages and other improvement tools to improve patient safety and health outcomes through partnership with CMS and the Patient Safety and Clinical Pharmacy Services Collaborative from the Health Resources and Services Administration
- Reduction of pressure ulcers in nursing homes
- Reduction of central line bloodstream infections
- Enhanced population health through improved EHR use to increase implementation of preventive services, such as flu and pneumococcal immunizations and colorectal and breast cancer screenings
- Reduction of 30-day readmissions by 20% over 3 years by changing processes of care at community levels, including hospitals, home health agencies, dialysis facilities, nursing homes, and physician offices

THE FUTURE OF QUALITY

The foundation for CMS quality improvement is focused on the vision of the right care for every person every time. This notion is based on CMS seeking to make care safe, effective, efficient, patient-centered, timely, and equitable.

To achieve this goal, CMS has strengthened its quality council, which meets regularly and has created workgroups in the areas of HIT, performance measurement and pay for performance, technology and innovation, prevention, Medicaid SCHIP, long-term care, cancer care, and methods for breakthrough improvement (e.g., the CMS QI Roadmap). These groups, with membership drawn from across CMS, report to the quality council, which reviews, approves, and tracks its work plans. The quality coordination team supports the quality council by managing this tracking and planning process and providing a variety of technical support measures to the workgroups. Accountability for individual tasks remains with the CMS unit that carries them out, but accountability for overall integration and for adjusting the plan in response to events remains with the workgroup and the quality council to which it reports.

The cross-cutting nature of the quality council workgroups has already been mentioned, but the same principles can produce clinical breakthroughs. For example, promoting influenza immunization in nursing homes might involve a partnership with stakeholders (by the CMS Long-Term Care Task Force), addressing the payment for administering vaccines (Center for Medicare Management), requiring that vaccines be offered to every patient (Office of Clinical Standards and Quality), enforcing that requirement (Center for Medicaid and State Operations), including immunization status in information that nursing homes report to the CMS (Office of Clinical Standards and Quality), publishing each home's immunization rate (Center for Beneficiary Choices), and providing technical assistance and promoting staff immunization (Office of Clinical Standards and Quality). These actions rarely require new organizational units because existing units of CMS already have responsibility for most of the needed activities, but strong planning and coordination are necessary to make activities of so many CMS components come together to change care.

The goal with regard to all quality measures is safe, efficient, effective, patient-centered, timely, and equitable care. The strategies critical to getting there will be carried out through systematic efforts that span all parts of the CMS, because all parts of our agency can and must support quality improvement.

Furthermore, through key initiatives of the ACA, including expansion of affordable health care, increased quality measurement, increased provider accountability, improved patient safety, focused approaches to disease prevention, and widespread use of health technology, the health status and quality of care for all Americans, especially Medicare beneficiaries, has the potential to achieve marked improvements, enabling important reductions in health care expenditures and the preservation of Medicare for the benefit of future generations.

KEY POINTS

- Preserving Medicare for future generations is an important objective that requires an increased focus on quality.
- Although early Medicare programs assessed quality of care and tested innovative payment models, larger-scale initiatives were not implemented until the PPACA was passed in 2010 and the Innovation Center established.
- Widespread use of quality measures, with bonus payments and penalties meant to encourage adoption of high-quality, evidence-based care across physicians, hospitals, nursing homes, and managed care plans.
- Greater focus on medication management will help to avoid the substantial clinical and economic burden associated with medication errors and adverse events.
- Increased use of prevention and wellness initiatives will help to reduce the burden of disease and lower health care resource utilization.
- Expansion of coordinated care models will help to improve care transitions and increase provider accountability for critical quality measures.
- Nationwide implementation of EHR and e-prescribing will affect a wide range of benefits, including improved quality of care through enhanced provider communications and improved patient safety.

For a complete list of references, please visit www.expertconsult.com.

KEY REFERENCES

1. Groszkruger D: Perspectives on healthcare reform: a year later, what more do we know? J Healthc Risk Manag 31:24–30, 2011.
2. Agency for Healthcare Research and Quality: 2012 National Healthcare Quality Disparity Report. http://www.ahrq.gov/research/findings/nhqrdr/nhdr12. Accessed May 25, 2014.
9. Centers for Medicare & Medicaid Services: PQRS fact sheet. http://www.cms.gov/Medicare/Quality-Initiatives-Patient-Assessment-Instruments/PQRS/Downloads/PQRS_OverviewFactSheet_2013_08_06.pdf. Accessed May 25, 2014.
10. James J: Pay-for-performance. New payment systems reward doctors and hospitals for improving the quality of care, but studies to date show mixed results. http://www.healthaffairs.org/healthpolicybriefs/brief.php?brief_id=78HealthPolicyBrief. Accessed December 11, 2015.
11. Centers for Medicare & Medicaid Services: Hospital readmission reduction program. http://www.cms.gov/Medicare/Medicare-Fee-for-Service-Payment/AcuteInpatientPPS/Readmissions-Reduction-Program.html. Accessed May 25, 2014.
16. Nursing Home Compare: Medicare: the official U.S. government site for people with Medicare. http://www.medicare.gov/nursinghomecompare/search.html. Accessed May 25, 2014.
18. Centers for Medicare & Medicaid Services: Quality measures. https://www.cms.gov/Medicare/Quality-Initiatives-Patient-Assessment-Instruments/QualityMeasures/index.html?redirect=/QUALITYMEASURES. Accessed December 11, 2015.
22. MedPac: The Medicare Advantage Program: status report. http://www.medpac.gov/chapters/Mar13_Ch13.pdf. Accessed May 25, 2014.
23. Centers for Medicare & Medicaid Services: Five star plan ratings. http://www.cms.gov/Outreach-and-Education/Training/CMSNationalTrainingProgram/Downloads/2013-5-Star-Enrollment-Period-Job-Aid.pdf. Accessed May 25, 2014.
26. Centers for Medicare & Medicaid Services: 2013 Medicare Part D Medication Therapy Management (MTM) Programs. Fact sheet. Summary of 2013 MTM programs. http://www.cms.gov/Medicare/Prescription-Drug-Coverage/PrescriptionDrugCovContra/Downloads/CY2013-MTM-Fact-Sheet.pdf. Accessed May 25, 2014.
30. American Pharmacists Association: Health care reform—the Affordable Care Act. http://www.pharmacist.com/health-care-reform-affordable-care-act. Accessed May 25, 2014.
31. Centers for Disease Control and Prevention: Chronic diseases and health promotion. http://www.cdc.gov/chronicdisease/overview/index.htm. Accessed May 25, 2014.
36. Centers for Medicare & Medicaid Services: Special needs plans. http://www.cms.gov/Medicare/Health-Plans/SpecialNeedsPlans/index.html?redirect=/specialneedsplans/. Accessed May 25, 2014.
38. Centers for Medicare & Medicaid Services: Medicare Physician Group Practice Demonstration. https://www.cms.gov/Medicare/Demonstration-Projects/DemoProjectsEvalRpts/Medicare-Demonstrations-Items/CMS1198992.html. Accessed May 25, 2014.
40. Agency for Healthcare Research and Quality: The state of accountable care organizations. http://www.innovations.ahrq.gov/content.aspx?id=3919. Accessed May 25, 2014.
47. About Health: The benefits of electronic health records (EHRs). http://patients.about.com/od/electronicpatientrecords/a/EMRbenefits.htm. Accessed December 11, 2015.
50. Centers for Medicare & Medicaid Services: Meaningful use. http://www.cms.gov/Regulations-and-Guidance/Legislation/EHRIncentivePrograms/Meaningful_Use.html. Accessed May 25, 2014.
55. Centers for Medicare & Medicaid Services: Quality improvement organizations: current work. http://www.cms.gov/Medicare/Quality-Initiatives-Patient-Assessment-Instruments/QualityImprovementOrgs/Current.html. Accessed May 25, 2014.

129 Managed Care for Older Americans

Richard G. Stefanacci, Jill L. Cantelmo

Managed care is thought by many to be the answer to the question of how to improve access to, and the quality and cost of, health care for older Americans. This is an especially critical issue given the number of aging baby boomers and the increasing availability of expensive new diagnostics and treatments, all in the context of limited Medicare resources.

In response to these significant challenges, Medicare and others are turning to managed care. Specifically, the Centers for Medicare and Medicaid Services (CMS) is moving from the use of traditional Medicare fee-for-service (FFS) programs, which are still used by about 70% of Medicare beneficiaries, to managed care within Medicare. Medicare managed care differs from FFS in the types of delivery and payment models utilized, and it offers more opportunities to increase the quality of care provided to patients while aligning financial incentives more closely with the quality of care, as opposed to the volume of services, provided.[1,2] The traditional FFS model is increasingly believed to contribute to suboptimal health care quality and higher costs because it encourages providers to use more—and potentially more expensive—services without any link to quality of care, patient outcomes, or coordination of care.[2]

Conversely, a managed care system aims to deliver value (i.e., quality tied to the investment in cost) through access to quality, cost-effective health care.[3] In its broadest sense, managed care refers to a system where a payment is made to a provider or health plan that is then responsible for a group of services. A more traditional and focused view of managed care refers only to health plans that are responsible for providing all of the services available under the entire Medicare program, with the exception of hospice services. These services can be provided either directly through a closed system of providers or through an open system using contracted community providers. The closed system uses a full complement of employed providers. Medicare managed care plans, referred to as Medicare Advantage (MA), were established by the CMS in 2003 as part of the Medicare Modernization Act (MMA). Prior to 2003, these plans, which fell under Medicare Part C, were referred to as Medicare+Choice or simply as a health maintenance organization (HMO).

Medicare managed care plans have several potential advantages over the traditional Medicare FFS program. These advantages include lower deductibles and co-payments, as well as benefits that are not part of Medicare FFS coverage, such as payments for preventive care, including reimbursement for eyeglasses and hearing aids; health education; and health promotion programs such as case management and disease management. Managed care plans can also provide discounts on, or improved access to, transportation, day care, respite care, or assisted living. MA plans are also not restricted by Medicare FFS rules such as the requirement for 3 hospital days plus a discharge day to qualify for subacute services. Instead, MA plans can admit members directly to skilled nursing facilities, thus avoiding hospitalizations and their associated costs, both financial and health-related. This subacute level of care is for services requiring skilled nursing care, such as intravenous therapy or rehabilitation.

The important benefits that MA plans offer over traditional Medicare FFS have led to increasing enrollment; 30% of Medicare beneficiaries were enrolled in an MA plan as of March 2014.[4] The number of MA plans offered is substantial, with the average urban- or suburban-dwelling beneficiary having a choice of approximately 20 plans and rurally located beneficiaries having about 11 plans to choose from. The average unweighted premium for an MA plan in 2014 was $49. This is far below the Medicare FFS premium, which was estimated to be $140.90 for Part B in 2016[4a] and does not include the supplemental insurance, Medigap, that many FFS beneficiaries add on to cover other costs (e.g., catastrophic hospital expenses) and which adds an additional average of $183 to their premiums.[5]

Although coverage for pharmaceutical costs has historically been a major reason why older adults have enrolled in Medicare managed care, the introduction of free-standing prescription drug plans under Medicare Part D, which started January 1, 2006, removed this differential from FFS in traditional Medicare. As a result of Medicare Part D, both Medicare FFS and Medicare managed care plans provide the opportunity for coverage of prescription medications.

Thus, principles of managed care are moving beyond MA plans and are increasingly being introduced into portions of Medicare FFS through such programs as pay-for-performance and various delivery and payment reform models. Medicare is applying the principles of managed care so older adults in traditional Medicare can also benefit.

MANAGED CARE TIMELINE

The modern era of managed care was heralded by a new law enacted by the U.S. Congress in 1974. This law permitted the establishment of HMOs, whose purpose was to encourage the development of prepaid health plans. From the mid-1970s until the late 1990s, managed care saw a slow and consistent growth. Participation in Medicare managed care increased steadily in the 1990s, reaching a peak of 6.3 million beneficiaries (16%) in 2000.

In 1997, revisions enacted by Congress that increased administrative burden and reduced payments to the health plans resulted in many plans exiting the market or limiting their enrollment.[4] Enrollment declined between 2000 and 2003 because of plan withdrawals from some areas, reduced benefits, and higher premiums.

A rebirth of managed care for Medicare beneficiaries occurred in 2003 with the passing of the MMA, which established MA and added different managed care options such as demonstration programs and special needs plans (SNPs). The MMA also increased payments to MA plans, which were used to raise payments to providers, decrease enrollee premiums, enhance existing benefits, and increase stabilization funds. As a result of these changes, enrollment in MA plans rose slightly from 2003 to 2004 and has steadily increased each year since, with 15.7 million Medicare beneficiaries enrolled in 2014[5] (Figure 129-1).

As part of the 2010 Patient Protection and Affordable Care Act (PPACA), reductions in the rates that CMS pays for MA plans were proposed in order to bring them more in line with the rates paid in traditional Medicare. The proposed cuts caused a backlash among insurers, who stated that the reduction in rates would lead to fewer plan options and increases in premiums for seniors to make up for the differences. Despite rate reductions introduced in 2013, enrollment in MA plans continued to increase, rising 9%.[6] In April 2014, CMS reversed its plan to implement further cuts to MA plan rates and actually increased these by 0.4%, citing changes in risk factor assessments for plans, a decrease in spending for Medicare health services, and changes to plans' payment formulas.[7]

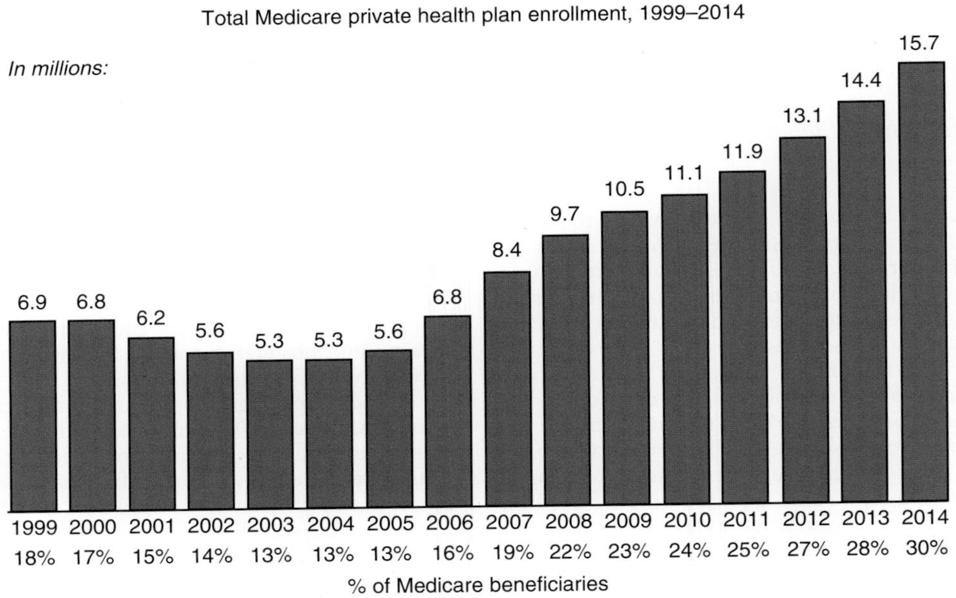

Figure 129-1. Total Medicare private health plan enrollment, 1999-2014. *(From Kaiser Family Foundation: Medicare Advantage 2014 spotlight: enrollment market update. http://kff.org/medicare/issue-brief/medicare-advantage-2014-spotlight-enrollment-market-update. Accessed January 26, 2016.)*

Today, Medicare managed care exists beyond traditional MA plans through delivery models such as accountable care organizations (ACOs), the patient-centered medical home (PCMH), and bundled payments arrangements. These and other models force the application of managed care principles to improve health outcomes for older Americans in addition to increasing access and quality and decreasing costs.

Many of these new models are being developed and tested under the Centers for Medicare and Medicaid Innovations. The Innovation Center was created by Congress for the purpose of testing "innovative payment and service delivery models to reduce program expenditures …while preserving or enhancing the quality of care" for those individuals who receive Medicare, Medicaid, or Children's Health Insurance Program (CHIP) benefits.

The Innovation Center is currently focused on the following priorities:

- Testing new payment and service delivery models
- Evaluating results and advancing best practices
- Engaging a broad range of stakeholders to develop additional models for testing

Congress provided the Secretary of the Department of Health and Human Services with the authority to expand the scope and duration of a model being tested through rulemaking, including the option of testing on a nationwide basis. In order for the Secretary to exercise this authority, a model must either reduce spending without reducing the quality of care or improve the quality of care without increasing spending, and it must not deny or limit the coverage or provision of any benefits. These determinations are made based on evaluations performed by the CMS and the certification of CMS's Chief Actuary with respect to spending.

Some of the Innovation Center models being tested include the following.

- **Advance Payment ACO Model**
  The Advance Payment ACO model is providing upfront and monthly payments to 35 ACOs participating in the Medicare Shared Savings Program (MSSP).
- **Comprehensive End-Stage Renal Disease (ESRD) Care Initiative**
  The Comprehensive ESRD Care initiative is designed to improve care for beneficiaries with ESRD while lowering Medicare costs.
- **Medicare Health Care Quality Demonstration**
  The Medicare Health Care Quality Demonstration is testing major changes to improve quality of care while increasing efficiency across an entire health care system.
- **Nursing Home Value-Based Purchasing Demonstration**
  The Nursing Home Value-Based Purchasing Demonstration provides incentive payment awards to participating nursing homes that perform the best or improve the most in terms of quality.
- **Physician Group Practice Transition Demonstration**
  A precursor to the MSSP, the Physician Group Practice Transition Demonstration rewarded groups for efficient and high-quality care.
- **Pioneer ACO Model**
  The Pioneer ACO model is rewarding 23 groups of health care providers experienced in working together to coordinate care.
- **For-Profit Demo Project for the Program of All-Inclusive Care for the Elderly (PACE)**
  This demonstration is studying the quality and cost of providing PACE program services under the Medicare and Medicaid programs.
- **Rural Community Hospital Demonstration**
  The Rural Community Hospital Demonstration is testing the feasibility and advisability of providing reasonable cost reimbursements for small rural hospitals.
- **Bundled Payments for Care Improvement (BPCI) Model 1: Retrospective Acute Care Hospital Stay Only**
  The BPCI initiative bundles payments for an episode of care. In BPCI model 1, retrospective bundled payments are made for acute care hospital stays only.
- **BPCI Model 2: Retrospective Acute and Post-Acute Care Episode**
  In BPCI model 2, retrospective bundled payments are made for acute care hospital stays plus post-acute care.

- **BPCI Model 3: Retrospective Post-Acute Care Only**
  In BPCI model 3, retrospective bundled payments are made for post-acute care only.
- **BPCI Model 4: Prospective Acute Care Hospital Stay Only**
  In BPCI model 4, prospective bundled payments are made for acute care hospital stays only.
- **BPCI: General Information**
  The BPCI initiative evaluates four different models of bundled payments for a defined episode of care to incentivize care redesign.
- **BPCI Medicare Acute Care Episode Demonstration**
  The Acute Care Episode Demonstration is testing the effect of bundling Part A and B payments for episodes of acute care.
- **BPCI Medicare Hospital Gainsharing Demonstration**
  This demonstration is testing arrangements between hospitals and physicians that are designed to govern the utilization of inpatient hospital resources and physician work and improve operational hospital performance with the sharing of remuneration.
- **BPCI Physician Hospital Collaboration Demonstration**
  The Physician Hospital Collaboration Demonstration is examining the effects of gainsharing aimed at improving the quality of care being delivered.
- **BPCI Specialty Practitioner Payment Model Opportunities: General Information**
  The CMS is seeking input on two areas related to initiatives surrounding innovative models of payment for specialty care.
- **Primary Care Transformation: Comprehensive Primary Care Initiative**
  The Comprehensive Primary Care initiative is a multipayer initiative providing financial support to primary care practices in seven markets.
- **Primary Care Transformation: Federally Qualified Health Center (FQHC) Advanced Primary Care Practice Demonstration**
  The FQHC Advanced Primary Care Practice Demonstration is testing the efficiency of PCMHs among FQHCs.
- **Primary Care Transformation: Graduate Nurse Education Demonstration**
  The Graduate Nurse Education Demonstration is supporting hospitals for the reasonable cost of providing clinical training to advanced practice registered nursing training.
- **Primary Care Transformation: Independence at Home Demonstration**
  The Independence at Home Demonstration is supporting home-based primary care for Medicare beneficiaries with multiple chronic conditions.
- **Primary Care Transformation: Medicare Coordinated Care Demonstration**
  The Medicare Coordinated Care Demonstration is testing whether providing coordinated care services to Medicare beneficiaries with complex chronic conditions can yield better patient outcomes without increasing program costs.
- **Primary Care Transformation: Multi-payer Advanced Primary Care Practice Demonstration**
  In the Multi-payer Advanced Primary Care Practice Demonstration, CMS is joining in multipayer primary care initiatives that are currently being conducted within states.
- **Primary Care Transformation: Transforming Clinical Practices Initiative**
  The CMS is seeking input on opportunities to help promote the transformation of clinical practices to improve health and health care across the country.
- **Initiatives Focused on the Medicaid and CHIP Population: Medicaid Emergency Psychiatric Demonstration**
  The Medicaid Emergency Psychiatric Demonstration is supporting treatment for psychiatric emergencies at private psychiatric hospitals in 11 states and the District of Columbia.
- **Initiatives Focused on the Medicaid and CHIP Population: Medicaid Incentives for the Prevention of Chronic Diseases Model**
  The Medicaid Incentives for the Prevention of Chronic Diseases model is supporting 10 states that are providing incentives for Medicaid beneficiaries to participate in prevention programs and demonstrate changes in health risks and outcomes.
- **Initiatives Focused on the Medicaid and CHIP Population: Strong Start for Mothers and Newborns Initiative: Effort to Reduce Early Elective Deliveries**
  The Strong Start effort to reduce early elective deliveries supports providers and mothers-to-be in their efforts to decrease the number of early elective deliveries and improve outcomes for mothers and infants.
- **Initiatives Focused on the Medicaid and CHIP Population: Strong Start for Mothers and Newborns Initiative: Enhanced Prenatal Care Models**
  This initiative will test three evidence-based maternity care service approaches that aim to improve the health outcomes of pregnant women and newborns.
- **Initiatives Focused on the Medicaid and CHIP Population: Strong Start for Mothers and Newborns Initiative: General Information**
  Strong Start supports reducing elective deliveries prior to 39 weeks and offers enhanced prenatal care to decrease preterm births through awards to 27 organizations.
- **Initiatives Focused on the Medicare-Medicaid Enrollees: Financial Alignment Initiative for Medicare-Medicaid Enrollees**
  This initiative enables states to integrate care and payment systems for Medicare-Medicaid enrollees and better coordinate their care.
- **Initiatives Focused on the Medicare-Medicaid Enrollees: Initiative to Reduce Avoidable Hospitalizations Among Nursing Facility Residents**
  This initiative offers enhanced clinical services to beneficiaries in extended-care nursing facilities.
- **Initiatives to Accelerate the Development and Testing of New Payment and Service Delivery Models: Frontier Community Health Integration Project Demonstration**
  This demonstration aims to develop and test new models of integrated, coordinated health care in the most sparsely populated rural counties.
- **Initiatives to Accelerate the Development and Testing of New Payment and Service Delivery Models: Health Care Innovation Awards**
  The Health Care Innovation Awards are funding competitive grants to compelling new ideas that deliver health care at lower costs to people enrolled in Medicare, Medicaid, and CHIP.
- **Initiatives to Accelerate the Development and Testing of New Payment and Service Delivery Models: Health Care Innovation Awards Round Two**
  The Health Care Innovation Awards Round Two are funding competitive grants to compelling new ideas that deliver health care at lower costs to people enrolled in Medicare, Medicaid, and CHIP.
- **Initiatives to Accelerate the Development and Testing of New Payment and Service Delivery Models: Maryland All-Payer Model**
  This model is a partnership between CMS and the state of Maryland to modernize Maryland's unique all-payer rate-setting system for hospital services.
- **Initiatives to Accelerate the Development and Testing of New Payment and Service Delivery Models: Medicare Care Choices Model**
  The Medicare Care Choices model aims to develop innovative payment systems to improve care options for hospice-eligible

beneficiaries by allowing greater beneficiary access to comfort and rehabilitative care in Medicare and Medicaid.

- **Initiatives to Accelerate the Development and Testing of New Payment and Service Delivery Models: Medicare Intravenous Immune Globulin Demonstration**
This demonstration is being implemented to evaluate the benefits of providing payment and items for services needed for in-home administration of intravenous immune globulin for the treatment of primary immune deficiency disease.
- **Initiatives to Accelerate the Development and Testing of New Payment and Service Delivery Models: State Innovation Models Initiative: General Information**
The State Innovation Models initiative is a $275 million competitive funding opportunity for states to design and test multipayer payment and delivery models that deliver high-quality health care and improve health system performance.
- **Initiatives to Accelerate the Development and Testing of New Payment and Service Delivery Models: State Innovation Models Initiative: Model Pre-testing Awards**
Three states are further developing their state-based models for multipayer payment reform and health care delivery system transformation.
- **Initiatives to Accelerate the Development and Testing of New Payment and Service Delivery Models: State Innovation Models Initiative: Model Testing Awards**
Six states are implementing, testing, and evaluating a multipayer health system transformation model that aims to deliver high-quality care and improve health system performance for state residents.
- **Initiatives to Speed the Adoption of Best Practices: Community-Based Care Transitions Program**
The Community-Based Care Transitions Program supports community-based organizations in reducing readmissions by improving transitions of high-risk Medicare beneficiaries from the inpatient hospital setting to home or other care settings.
- **Initiatives to Speed the Adoption of Best Practices: Innovation Advisors Program**
The Innovation Advisors Program is supporting dedicated, skilled individuals in the health care system who can test new models of care delivery in their own organizations and work locally to improve the health of their communities.
- **Initiatives to Speed the Adoption of Best Practices: Medicare Imaging Demonstration**
This demonstration collects data regarding physician use of advanced diagnostic imaging services to determine the appropriateness of services in relation to medical specialty guidelines.
- **Initiatives to Speed the Adoption of Best Practices: Million Hearts**
Million Hearts is a national initiative to prevent 1 million heart attacks and strokes over 5 years.
- **Initiatives to Speed the Adoption of Best Practices: Partnership for Patients**
The Partnership for Patients is a nationwide public-private partnership that offers support to physicians, nurses, and other clinicians working in and out of hospitals to reduce hospital-acquired conditions and readmissions.

MEDICARE MANAGED CARE UNDER FEE-FOR-SERVICE

Of course, several of these and previous attempts to manage Medicare were applied within the Medicare FFS model. Under the Medicare Part A benefit, also referred to as hospital insurance, providers are paid a defined amount for providing a bundle of services. Medicare Part A providers include acute care hospitals, skilled nursing facilities, subacute care, and hospice. It is important to note that while Medicare Part C (Medicare Advantage) includes Medicare Part A, Part B, and in most cases Part D, hospice is still provided as a separate benefit. Because Medicare Part A providers are paid a capitated payment, they are encouraged to use managed care principles to control cost and improve outcomes.

Medicare Part B, also known as medical insurance, covers physician provider services. Although, historically, these services were paid simply on the basis of the number and type of services provided, CMS is applying managed care principles to this program, as well. The 2006 Tax Relief and Health Care Act required the establishment of a physician quality reporting system, including an incentive payment for eligible professionals who satisfactorily report quality measure data for covered services furnished to Medicare beneficiaries. CMS named this program the Physician Quality Reporting Initiative (PQRI), which by 2008 consisted of 119 quality measures and 2 structural measures—one related to whether a professional has and uses electronic health records and the other related to the use of electronic prescribing.[8] The PQRI was included as a key voluntary Medicare physician quality reporting system in the PPACA, with extension of the incentive payment program through 2014 for eligible practitioners who submit quality measure data and implementation of penalties in 2015 for all Medicare providers who fail to participate in the program. In 2011, the program underwent a name change, becoming the Physician Quality Reporting System (PQRS). Participation in the PQRS allows Medicare physicians to apply the use of managed care principles to the Medicare FFS program by assessing the quality of care they are providing to their patients, tracking their performance on various quality metrics, and enabling comparison of their performance with that of their peers.[9]

Prescription drug plans, as previously mentioned, are authorized under the Medicare Part D program. In addition to general managed care principles to ensure appropriate medication use, prescription plans are required by CMS to provide medication therapy management (MTM) programs.[10] CMS's objectives with regard to MTM programs, which are provided by pharmacists and other qualified providers, are to control costs and improve quality and outcomes through optimized medication use and reduction in the risk of adverse drug events.[10] MTM programs were expanded as part of the PPACA, in part to increase the consistency with regard to Medicare beneficiaries' eligibility for MTM programs. Currently, Part D enrollees who have two or more chronic diseases must be targeted for MTM, and the following disease states must specifically be targeted: hypertension, heart failure, diabetes, dyslipidemia, respiratory disease, bone diseases and arthritis, and mental health diseases. Additionally, those beneficiaries who are taking multiple Part D drugs and are likely to incur annual costs for covered Part D drugs exceeding a predetermined level are targeted for MTM programs.[11,12]

Chronic illnesses, such as heart disease and diabetes, are a major detriment to beneficiaries' quality of life, and care for these beneficiaries is a major expense to the Medicare program. Furthermore, the number of beneficiaries who have multiple chronic illnesses is increasing dramatically. The proportion of Medicare beneficiaries with five or more chronic conditions increased from 30% in 1987 to 50% in 2002.[13] Having multiple chronic illnesses compounds the complexity and cost of care required, impacting beneficiaries' ability to perform regular activities of daily living (e.g., bathing, eating, and dressing), increasing rates of hospital readmissions and emergency room visits, and leading to longer lengths of stay.[13,14] Recent data show that almost half of the total of Medicare spending is attributable to the 14% of beneficiaries who have six or more chronic conditions.[14] Coordinating the care of patients with multiple chronic conditions is also a challenge for various reasons, including an increasing number of treating physicians (ranging from 4 physicians for a patient with one condition to 14 physicians for a patient with five or more conditions) and polypharmacy, and the related impact on adherence, compliance, and adverse drug events (such as drug-drug interactions).[12]

The CMS conducts and sponsors a number of innovative demonstration projects to test and measure the effect of potential program changes. The CMS demonstrations study the likely impact that new methods of service delivery, coverage of new types of service, and new payment approaches have on beneficiaries, providers, health plans, states, and the Medicare Trust Funds. Evaluation projects validate CMS research and demonstration findings and help CMS monitor the effectiveness of Medicare, Medicaid, and the State Children's Health Insurance Program.

Many of the demonstration projects are focused on managing care for those Medicare beneficiaries suffering from chronic illnesses. The following are examples of some of the many demonstration projects that CMS has funded in the past and continues to fund.

Independence at Home Demonstration[15]

The Independence at Home Demonstration was created to test the effectiveness of medical practices in delivering comprehensive primary care services at home and to assess whether this delivery model improves care for Medicare beneficiaries with multiple chronic conditions. The demonstration will also examine the impact of home-based care on hospitalization needs, patient and caregiver satisfaction, and Medicare costs. Providers will be rewarded for demonstrating improved care and lowered costs.

Community-Based Care Transitions Program[16]

This demonstration was established to test models for improving transitions of Medicare beneficiaries from the inpatient hospital setting to other care settings, to improve care quality, and to reduce readmissions for high-risk beneficiaries.

Comprehensive End-Stage Renal Disease Care Initiative[17]

The Comprehensive ESRD Care initiative was established to identify, test, and evaluate approaches for improving care for Medicare beneficiaries with ESRD through CMS's partnerships with groups of health care providers and suppliers, referred to as ESRD Seamless Care Organizations.

Program of All-Inclusive Care for the Elderly (PACE)[18]

Some demonstration programs that have proven their value have gone on to become permanent programs. PACE is such a program. The PACE model is centered on the belief that it is better for the well-being of seniors with chronic care needs and their families to be served in the community whenever possible.

PACE serves individuals who are aged 55 years or older and who are certified by their state to need nursing home care, are able to live safely in the community at the time of enrollment, and live in a PACE service area. Although all PACE participants must be certified to need nursing home care to enroll in the program, only about 7% of PACE participants nationally reside in a nursing home. If a PACE enrollee does need nursing home care, the PACE program pays for it and continues to coordinate the enrollee's care.[19]

PACE programs have had a beneficial impact on a long list of important outcomes, including greater use of adult day health care, fewer skilled home health visits, fewer hospitalizations, fewer nursing home admissions, greater contact with primary care providers, longer survival rates, an increased number of days in the community, better overall health, better quality of life, greater satisfaction with overall care arrangements, and better functional status.[20]

Managed Care Principles

- **Screen** enrolled population to identify individuals with special needs.
- **Coordinate** the actions of all providers across the continuum of enrolled beneficiaries' care.
- Ensure **medication self-management** by educating patients about medications, and have a medication management system.
- Implement a **dynamic patient-centered record** by educating patients about their personal health records (PHRs) and how to use them to facilitate communication and ensure continuity of their care plans across providers and settings.
- Emphasize appropriate **follow-up** by encouraging patients to schedule and complete a follow-up visit with the primary care physician or specialist physician and ensuring patients are empowered to be active participants in these interactions.
- Identify **red flags** by educating patients about signs that their condition is worsening and about how to respond.
- Offer effective **health promotion**, disease prevention, and self-management programs.
- Make available the services of **interdisciplinary** health care professionals, including physicians, nurses, social workers, pharmacists, and rehabilitation therapists.
- Use **geriatric expertise** available for designing and administering geriatric programs and for consultation with primary care physicians, case managers, and other providers.
- Enable timely **primary care provider access** to improve health and avoid emergency room services.
- Ensure **end-of-life management** plans are in place to prevent use of resources against a patient's wishes.
- Incorporate programs that offer **caregiver support** in acknowledgment of the critical role that the caregiver plays in overall patient management.

The PACE model of utilizing a health care team combined with managed health care services and care coordination has demonstrated the ability to improve health outcomes and reduce health care expenses over time, even within debilitated, frail population where health care expenses are expected to be high. This example demonstrates the potential large-scale clinical and economic improvements that are gained from improved methods of organized and coordinated care.[20]

Social/Health Maintenance Organization[21]

A similar program to PACE that did not achieve permanent status but instead was terminated because of the lack of demonstrated effectiveness was the social/health maintenance organization (S/HMO).

An S/HMO is an organization that provides the full range of Medicare benefits offered by standard HMOs, plus additional services that include care coordination, prescription drug benefits, chronic care benefits covering short-term nursing home care, a full range of home and community-based services such as homemaker, personal care services, adult day care, respite care, and medical transportation. Other services that may be provided include eyeglasses, hearing aids, and dental benefits. The demonstration was terminated due to the lack of convincing evidence that outcomes for S/HMO enrollees overall were better than enrollees who had not participated, with the exception of a reduction in hospital utilization in a very small subgroup of high-risk enrollees.[21]

Some of these same principles from S/HMOs are being applied in the development of ACOs. ACOs are groups of doctors, hospitals, and other health care providers, who come together voluntarily to give coordinated high-quality care to their Medicare patients. The goal of coordinated care is to ensure that patients, especially the chronically ill, get the right care at the right time, while avoiding unnecessary duplication of services and preventing medical errors. When an ACO succeeds in both delivering high-quality care and spending health care dollars more wisely, it will share in the savings it achieves for the Medicare program.

Medicare offers several ACO programs.

- MSSP—a program that helps Medicare FFS program providers become ACOs
- Advance Payment ACO model—a supplementary incentive program for selected participants in the MSSP
- Pioneer ACO model—a program designed for early adopters of coordinated care (no longer accepting applications)

FFS Medicare patients who see providers that are participating in a Medicare ACO maintain all their Medicare rights, including the right to choose any doctors and providers that accept Medicare. Whether or not a provider chooses to participate in an ACO, their Medicare patients may continue to see them. So unlike S/HMOs, ACOs currently do not have the level of control that could restrict patients to stay within their provider network.

Recently, the CMS released interim data on the two ACO initiatives, both of which showed somewhat mixed results. First-year data from the MSSP that was launched in 2012 showed that[7]

- 54 of the 114 MSSP participants had lower than projected expenditures in their first 12 months,
- 29 out of these 54 generated enough savings to benefit from bonus payments, and
- Several ACOs withheld their quality data and did not receive bonus payments, even though they qualified to share in the savings they achieved.

Similarly, a preliminary assessment of the Pioneer ACO program showed

- 9 of the 32 organizations exited the program after the first year, and
- 9 of the remaining 23 organizations had significantly reduced spending growth in the first year while maintaining high-quality care.

Although CMS was pleased with the results, particularly in the improvements in quality scores, others believe the initial data are not overwhelmingly positive enough to make other providers eager to participate in an ACO.[7]

MANAGED CARE PRINCIPLES

Managed care can be an efficient approach for Medicare to finance high-quality, cost-effective geriatrics. The American Geriatrics Society wrote in its position statement on managed care that to realize the potential flexibility and creativity inherent in capitated financing, managed care organizations (MCOs) should develop special processes for providing high-quality health care to enrollees who need complex health services.[22]

The starting point is identifying those members most at need for special attention by screening the enrolled population to identify individuals with special needs. Plans should use valid and reliable instruments to screen their enrollees regularly. They should assess the clinical needs of high-risk enrollees for both functional status and quality of life. The rationale for this approach is that about 14% of beneficiaries, most of whom have several chronic conditions, account for approximately 50% of Medicare's annual payments for health care. Early identification of those who are at highest risk for requiring expensive care—and assessing their clinical needs—would facilitate coordination of care and timely preventive interventions designed to improve the clinical and financial outcomes of care.[14,23]

Assessment for risk is typically accomplished through a health risk assessment. Two of the tools used for identifying members are the Pra and PraPlus.[24] Many organizations use the Pra or the PraPlus to screen older populations to identify individuals who are at risk for using health services heavily in the future. MCOs can then offer special forms of health care, such as case management, comprehensive geriatric assessment, or geriatric evaluation and management, to these at-risk individuals.

Coordinating the actions of all of the providers across the continuum of the enrolled beneficiary's care is critical for quality care. The rationale is that coordination improves the quality and the outcomes of health care, including safety, cost, and satisfaction with care. The coordination of care can be made more efficient and effective by using integrated medical records and improved communication tools.[25,26] Offering effective health promotion, disease prevention, and self-management programs can prevent or delay the progression of disease, resulting in better patient outcomes and lower costs of health care. In addition, programs that educate patients and their caregivers about the patient's condition and offer self-management initiatives empower both patients and the caregivers to be proactive and choose wise alternatives.[27-29] For example, medication self-management, whereby patients are knowledgeable about the medications they are taking and have a system in place to ensure that they are taking their medications as required and instructed by their physician, can help to ensure compliance and ensure that patients are achieving the full benefits of their therapy.[30] Similarly, patient use of a personal health record can help to ensure that critical health information is recorded by the patient and facilitate communication across providers and ensure continuity of care.[30] Furthermore, educating the patient about any "red flags" or signs of a worsening of his or her condition can ensure that patients are proactive participants in ensuring prompt care for their changing needs.[30] Patient participation is also critical for ensuring appropriate follow-up after a visit with a primary care provider or specialist.[30]

The services of health care professionals from several disciplines, including physicians, nurses, social workers, pharmacists, and rehabilitation therapists, must be available as needed. These professionals should function as interdisciplinary teams in managing not only the medical conditions but also social factors that affect the well-being of high-risk beneficiaries. The interdisciplinary team approach allows for comprehensive, coordinated assessment and management of beneficiaries' medical, psychological, social, and functional needs and those of their unpaid caregivers.[31-34] Geriatric expertise should be available for designing and administering geriatric programs and for consultation with primary care physicians, case managers, and other providers. MCOs would be well served by using a geriatrician in a medical director role to help guide the development and management of programs necessary for success in caring for seniors. Geriatricians have the background necessary in efficiently and effectively managing patients in teams and managing the care of complex patients with multiple problems across the continuum of care.[35,36] Additionally, access to a primary care provider, in the form of a geriatrician or a nurse practitioner, is critical to improving overall health and avoiding unnecessary use of emergency room services.[37] End-of-life management planning is important for preventing overuse of resources beyond the patient's wishes and is often best accomplished with the support of a participating caregiver who can assist the patient and ensure that he or she is aware of the patient's intentions. Finally, caregiver support is critical, as so many of the aforementioned aspects of care require caregiver attention and participation. For this reason, it is important that caregivers understand their important role and are appropriately supported with the education, resources, and tools to assist them in day-to-day management.[37]

Finally, the quality of the health care provided to beneficiaries by MCOs should be measured consistently and reported regularly to the plans' executives and providers, to CMS, and to the public. New instruments designed to measure the quality of outpatient care and coordination of care must be developed and tested for reliability and validity. Credible, understandable information about the quality of health care is essential to organizations' processes for improving quality and to consumers' efforts to make informed choices from among the available health plans and providers.[38]

PLAN REIMBURSEMENT

For payment purposes, there are two categories of MA plans: local plans and regional plans. Local plans may be any of the available plan types and may serve one or more counties. Medicare pays them based on their enrollees' counties of residence. Regional plans, however, must be preferred provider organizations and must serve all of one of the 26 regions established by CMS. Each region comprises one or more entire states.

Under the MA program, Medicare buys insurance coverage for its beneficiaries from private plans with payments made monthly. The coverage must include all Medicare Part A and Part B benefits except hospice. These payments are based on a number of factors, including age, geographic variations in health care costs, and health status of enrollees.[39] Since 2006, Medicare payments to plans have been according to a bidding process in which plans submit their bids based on the estimated per-enrollee costs for services covered under Medicare Parts A and B. Bids are compared with benchmark amounts that vary by county or region, which indicate the maximum amount that Medicare will pay a plan in a given area.[39]

Recommendations to Medicare on payments, including changes to the MA program, are made by the Medicare Payment Advisory Commission (MedPAC), the official, independent federal advisory body to Congress on Medicare payment policy. Increasing pressure to decrease reimbursement to Medicare managed care is based on a belief that private plans, which were initially brought into the Medicare program to reduce costs, have actually increased costs.[39,40] In 2009, CMS payments to private plans were 13% greater than corresponding costs to traditional Medicare to cover the same beneficiaries, equating to about $1138 for each beneficiary enrolled in a private plan, or about $11.4 billion.[40]

In a June 2005 report, MedPAC recommended various changes in how Medicare pays managed care plans under MA to reduce inefficient and wasteful Medicare payments. As estimates began to indicate the magnitude of the extra payments to MA plans, Congress's perspective on these payment polices shifted and led to the passing of the Medicare Improvements for Patients and Providers Act of 2008, which included many reductions in MA reimbursement.[40] This trend continued with the PPACA in 2010, which called for a reduction in federal payments to MA plans over time, bringing them in closer alignment to the average costs of care under traditional Medicare.[39] Based on this, benchmarks will be reduced over 2 to 6 years between 2012 and 2016, with new benchmarks fully phased in by 2017. These are expected to range from 95% of traditional Medicare costs for counties in the top quartile with relatively high per capita Medicare costs to 115% of traditional Medicare costs in the counties at the bottom quartile with relatively low Medicare costs.[39]

Additional adjustments are also made to the benchmark payments that CMS makes to MA plans. For instance, CMS uses a hierarchical conditions categories (CMS-HCC) model to adjust the payments to MA plans based on the health expenditure risk of their enrollees so that plans receive the appropriate payments based on their expected costs. The CMS-HCC model therefore helps to ensure that plans with a disproportionate number of healthy enrollees are paid less (because of fewer expected services used) compared with plans with a higher number of sick beneficiaries, who will have a much higher expected utilization of health care resources and therefore require higher payments from CMS.[41] Recent adjustments were made to the CMS HCC model, based on requirements of the 2010 PPACA, to improve the predictability of the model and to bring the risk scores for MA beneficiaries more in line with those for Medicare FFS beneficiaries.[42]

As part of the PPACA, CMS payments to plans are also based on quality measure performance. Starting in 2012, the 5-star plan ratings related to quality performance were linked to bonus payments, such that benchmarks for plans receiving 4 or more stars were increased by 1.5%. This percentage was further increased to 3% in 2013 and is estimated to increase to 5% in 2014 and beyond. Plans that earn fewer than 4 stars are not eligible for these increases, and plans consistently earning fewer than 3 stars over a 3-year period will be designated as low-quality plans on the Medicare website.[43]

Another change implemented as part of the PPACA relates to the amount of enrollee's premiums that MA plans can use for nonclinical services. MA plans, like commercial plans, use a large proportion of enrollee premiums to fund administrative expense and profits, including the salaries of executives and marketing expenses. The PPACA requires insurers to submit data on the proportion of premiums that are spent on clinical services and quality improvement; this is referred to as the medical loss ratio. The PPACA also requires insurers to issue rebates to enrollees if this percentage does not meet minimum standards. In 2014, this standard was increased such that plans must spend at least 85% of premium dollars on medical care.[39,44]

Finally, MA plans are being asked to collect encounter data so that CMS can be assured that payments to MA plans are appropriate. The rationale is that even with HCC risk adjustments and 5-star bonus payments, MA plans may actually be using significantly fewer resources that they are budgeted. In order to accurately assess this difference, CMS is requiring MA plans to submit claims to account for the actual services they are rendering to Medicare beneficiaries. These claims will be used to make adjustments in payments to MA plans such that CMS is assured of paying these plans appropriately.

In the case of prescription drug plans, which operate under the Medicare Part D program, payment is made for providing prescription drug coverage for those Medicare beneficiaries that enroll in that specific plan. Overall, for prescription drug plan payments, Medicare subsidizes premiums by about 75% and provides additional subsidies for beneficiaries who have low levels of income and assets (referred to as the low-income subsidy).[45] Medicare's payments to prescription drug plans are determined through a competitive bidding process, and enrollee premiums are also tied to plan bids. Payments from Medicare to these prescription drug plans are risk-adjusted based on the likely drug spending for that specific enrollee.[46] The prescription plan is responsible for paying the costs of medications (excluding the member's responsibility) and administrative overhead, which include MTM services.[47]

Health systems that are more integrated, such as the MA plans, typically offer greater pharmaceutical benefits because they benefit from pharmaceutical use that reduces hospitalization and use of medical services.

In 2010, important changes to Medicare prescription drug coverage were introduced as part of the PPACA, the most notable of which is gradual closure of the prescription drug "donut hole," or coverage gap—the range of time after the initial coverage limit is reached as part of the standard Medicare Part D prescription benefit, when enrollees are responsible for the total cost of their drugs, plus their plan premiums, until they reach a certain spending limit, at which time catastrophic coverage begins.[45] In recognition of the substantial cost burden that the coverage gap placed on seniors, the PPACA implemented a reduction of the coverage gap each year, starting in 2011 through 2020, at which time the gap would be eliminated entirely and beneficiaries will pay 25% coinsurance for prescriptions.[47] Other notable PPACA changes to Medicare Part D include reductions in the Part D subsidy for high-income beneficiaries and inclusion of all covered Part D drugs in a category or class within the plan formulary.[47]

CAPITATION AND PAY-FOR-PERFORMANCE

Capitation rates in all regions of the country should be sufficient for providing high-quality health care for all Medicare beneficiaries, regardless of the intensity of their clinical needs. Specifically, CMS should provide capitation that reflects the probable cost of caring for each enrolled beneficiary. This should be accomplished by risk-adjusting capitation payments according to individual beneficiaries' diagnosis, functional status, and use. Capitation payments that acknowledge that beneficiaries with chronic conditions require more health care than those who are healthy would encourage MCOs to enroll beneficiaries who have chronic conditions and to provide them with special services designed to address their needs for complex care. In contrast, inadequate risk-adjustment of capitation payments is a disincentive for plans to enroll frail or medically complex beneficiaries or to offer special services that might encourage such beneficiaries to enroll.[48-50]

Beyond capitation, there are a variety of different payment models that are being implemented in what is an increasing movement toward models that tie provider payments to quality of care and outcomes. This is based on recognition that the traditional FFS model pays providers based on the number and complexity of services provided to patients without regard to quality, efficiency, or impact on health outcomes. Pay-for-performance models, which have the potential to improve patient care and outcomes, have been proposed as one strategy designed to correct this deficiency.

It is important to note that a pay-for-performance program applied to a commercial population may not be entirely appropriate for Medicare beneficiaries who have multiple chronic conditions, are frail, are of advanced age, or require palliative care.[51] For these older beneficiaries, measures should account for comorbidities and assess aspects of health that are common to multiple conditions (e.g., cognitive status, functional status, and pain.) Measures should be constructed so that providers are not penalized when they honor patients' preferences for care or their cultural or religious beliefs.

In addition, the older adult population served by Medicare is extremely heterogeneous. Many people are healthy and functional, but up to one third of the Medicare population is vulnerable, with multiple comorbidities and geriatric conditions (functional and cognitive impairment, falls, and frailty). In addition, some older adults will place different values on participation in self-management and adherence to medical recommendations, especially in the setting of multiple comorbidities and health status vulnerability. Some older adults may put more emphasis on improved functioning and quality of life rather than traditional indicators of clinical care quality.

It is essential that a pay-for-performance program not unwittingly lead to a decrease in quality for vulnerable older adult patients or those who may have different clinical care goals. Failing to take this important policy concern into account could adversely affect access to primary and specialty care among those Medicare beneficiaries who might benefit the most from high-quality care.[52-55] Effective pay-for-performance systems support and stimulate the structural capabilities necessary for the provision, documentation, measurement, and continuous improvement of high-quality care. The need for different provider settings to care for unique patient populations must also be considered when designing and implementing payment based on performance. For example, larger practices may have more resources to implement quality care processes. Such resources include providing patient education materials for patients and their caregivers, language translation services, and other outreach activities to facilitate good patient care. A smaller practice may have fewer resources to measure and report quality, yet be an essential care provider, such as a rural care provider or care team for homebound older adults. Certain practices may be focused on a population subset for which no performance measures exist. Payment reform should lead to improved practice design without eliminating essential care providers.

An example of a pay-for-performance model within Medicare is the Hospital Value-Based Purchasing (VBP) program, established by the PPACA, that applies to the largest share of Medicare spending, that is, inpatient hospital stays.[56] Starting in fiscal year 2013, the VBP program began adjusting a portion of payments to hospitals based on how well the hospital performed on a set of about two dozen quality measures compared with other hospitals and the degree to which hospitals are able to improve their performance versus a prior baseline period. Among hospitals that are included in the VBP program for 2014, 1231 will see their payments increase, while 1451 will be paid less based on quality measure performance.[57]

Another type of pay-for-performance model that is currently being tested as part of the PPACA is the Bundled Payments for Care Improvement (BPCI) initiative. The bundled payments model is based on aggregation of a collection of related services for a specific patient—instead of the traditional payment for an individual service—such that payment is made as a single lump sum, independent of the number of services actually provided.[2] The bundled payment model provides strong incentives for providers (hospitals, post-acute care providers, physicians, and other practitioners), allowing them to work closely together across all specialties and settings, not only to improve the coordination of care during an episode, likely increasing the quality of care, but also to control the costs of the episode. Using this approach, if the cost of the bundle is less than the amount of the payment, the providers generally keep all of the savings; however, if the cost of the bundle exceeds the payment, providers must also bear much of the overage.[2,58]

The BPCI initiative includes four broadly defined models of care that link payments for multiple services provided to a beneficiary during an episode of care:

- Model 1 focuses on an episode of care related to an acute care inpatient hospitalization.
- Models 2 and 3 involve a retrospective bundled payment arrangement whereby actual expenditures are reconciled against a target price for an episode of care.
- Model 4 is a prospective bundled payment arrangement, in which a lump sum payment is made to a provider for the entire episode of care.

CMS will work with participating organizations to assess whether these models result in improved patient care and lower costs to Medicare over the 3-year length of the initiative.

MEASURING QUALITY OF CARE

The current reform of payment models marked by a transition from paying for the volume of services rendered toward paying for value and outcomes makes the measurement of care quality an increasingly critical element of our evolving health care system. Recognition of this need has led to the rapid expansion of performance assessment programs in the private sector as well as within Medicare, such as the Physician Quality Reporting System and the Hospital Value-Based Purchasing Program.[2]

Studies have demonstrated the positive impact that measurement has on care quality. One such study showed that although sharing hospital quality data internally within the organization had limited effects, public reporting of the data led to improvement, potentially as a result of patients switching from lower to higher performing providers or based on hospital revisions to practice patterns with the goal of improving their ranks and retaining patients.[2]

Although it is established that performance measurement is important for ensuring that and for providing value-based reimbursement to providers, a substantial barrier to performance measurement is suboptimal use of health information technology in the form of electronic health records (EHRs).[2] A recent survey indicated that this information infrastructure is beginning to be implemented in a more widespread fashion: 70% of health care providers indicated that they had an effective EHR system in place in 2012, up from just 35% in 2011.[2] The increase in adoption of EHR use has been driven by the financial incentives offered by CMS, starting in 2011, to providers who demonstrate meaningful use of EHRs. These incentive payments will be in place through 2014, but after 2015, providers not actively using EHRs in compliance with meaningful use will be subject to financial penalties.[59]

The increased use of EHRs is critical because unless a majority of providers use EHRs, data on patients' health, treatments, outcomes, and other key data cannot be shared across the broad health care system.[59] As quality becomes increasingly tied to reimbursement, EHRs provide the common platform for capturing and sharing these performance measurement data to serve the interconnected needs of policy makers, payers, purchasers, consumers, and providers.[60]

Structure, process, and clinical outcomes measures used must be valid and relevant for the unique care needs of frail or vulnerable older adults. These measures should be evidence based, be clinically relevant, have clear association with improved outcomes of care, and be applicable to all patients whose care they assess.

Technical specifications for numerators and denominators of measures should be constructed so that measures are not applied to special populations for which evidence of linkage between performance of care processes and improved outcomes is lacking. These populations include persons of very advanced age and those with multiple comorbidities, limited life expectancy, or moderate to severe dementia.

More importantly, specific measures are needed to assess the quality of care of persons aged 75 years and older, those who are vulnerable and/or frail, and those who are receiving palliative care near the end of life. There are three types of clinical performance measures relevant to the Medicare population:

1. Structure measures are used to recognize systems of care associated with improved health outcomes. Multidisciplinary teams for care, capacity for patient education in self-care management, disease registries, EHRs, systems to support the use of intervisit interval patient contacts, and monitoring are important aspects of the chronic care model. Important processes of care are difficult to deliver absent such structure(s). Initial reward systems should recognize investment in such delivery structure.[61]
2. Process measures are used to determine whether care that is known to be effective is provided.[62] The American Geriatrics Society believes that specific measures are needed to assess the quality of care of persons aged 75 years and older, those who are frail or vulnerable, and those who are receiving palliative care near the end of life. The Assessing Care of Vulnerable Elders (ACOVE) measures were developed by the RAND Corporation in response to the needs of persons at risk for frailty or persons aged 75 years and older. They have been tested in cohorts of community-dwelling vulnerable older adults.[63] Adoption of some or all of these indicators in addition to disease- and prevention-based measures appropriate for the younger population will greatly enhance the possibility of attaining the goal that quality of care can be measured for all Medicare beneficiaries and that the providers who care for these patients have measures of accountability.
3. Clinical outcome measures track the morbidity and mortality resulting from a disease and must be appropriate to the usual health care needs and goals of the patient population in which they are used.[62] Many of these measures are disease-specific, were originally developed in commercially insured populations, and do not account for other comorbidities. If not previously tested in the heterogeneous Medicare population, such measures may be particularly problematic. In frail or vulnerable older persons, the goals of treatment for chronic disease are more variable than in younger adults, and the linkage between process of care delivered and clinical measures is often imperfect. High-quality geriatric care requires providing services to a heterogeneous population with varied health care service needs and goals of care, including many with multiple chronic illnesses and geriatric conditions. Fundamental to the definition of quality is that the standard of care being measured is applicable to the individual to whom it is applied. Many available clinical performance measures have been developed in the middle-aged commercial population. Some of these measures have been tested in older adult populations, but some have not, so the applicability of untested measures to older adult, heterogeneous populations is not known. The complexity of delivering high-quality care to this population can only be guided by rigorous scientific testing of performance indicator measures. Such testing can allow us to adapt measures to the specific needs of vulnerable patient populations. These measures need to be developed and validated by individuals with expertise in the care of frail older adults. Measurement development and testing is a dynamic process, so even in the setting of value-based purchasing there should be an established process for continual evolution of performance indicator measures. Key stakeholders should remain involved.[64-67]

Pay-for-performance models must provide positive reinforcement for quality performance and improvement and not promote the avoidance of patients for whom providing high-quality care will be more challenging. When applied to individual providers, these measures should be constructed so that both achievement of target thresholds (excellence) and progress toward achievement of targets (improvement) can be positively reinforced. In addition, the collection of data that are used to evaluate performance should not be burdensome to providers and should accurately reflect the performance of care processes on an individual patient basis. Failure to consider these factors may unduly penalize providers who practice in small groups or care for special populations.

Linking a portion of payments to valid measures of quality and effective use of resources will result in providers having direct incentives and financial support to implement the innovative approaches that result in improved outcomes. All monies that are set aside for pay-for-performance should be distributed to providers achieving the quality criteria. Savings from improved care are likely to accrue to Medicare funds that are not part of the

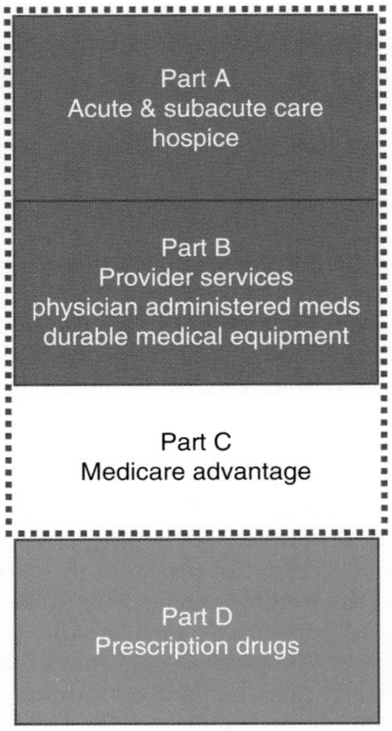

Figure 129-2. Medicare benefits.

physician resource pool. Performance-based funds should not be used in a withhold approach or a Medicare Part B budget-neutral manner. To the fullest extent possible, norms should be established for like populations and risk adjustment should occur. Although it is recognized that value-based purchasing should not be delayed while such adjustments are refined, such an approach will minimize the risk of providers avoiding patients (e.g., the frail and medically complex) who present the greatest challenge in meeting quality indicators used in for pay-for-performance[68,69] (Figure 129-2).

A VISION FOR CARE IN THE FUTURE

Managed care for older adults continues to evolve in the path originally laid out by the Institute of Medicine. The three key principles identified by the Institute of Medicine to form the basis of an improved system of care delivery for older Americans are in alignment with the six aims of quality defined in the report *Crossing the Quality Chasm*[70] and supported by several of the initiatives cited in PPACA.

First and foremost, the health needs of the older population need to be comprehensively addressed, and care needs to be patient-centered. For most older adults, care needs to include preventive services (including lifestyle modification) and coordinated treatment of chronic and acute health conditions. For frail older adults, social services may also be needed to maintain or improve health. These social services need to be integrated with health care services in their delivery and financing. Furthermore, efforts need to be made to reduce the wide variation in practice protocols among providers, which should further enhance the quality of care for older adults.

The principle of comprehensive care also includes taking into account the increasing sociodemographic diversity of older adults. The number and percentage of ethnic minorities in the older population is increasing dramatically, and even within ethnic groups, there is tremendous cultural diversity. Health care providers need to be sensitive to the wide variety of languages, cultures, and health beliefs among older adults. Other segments of the older population face additional challenges. For example, older adults in rural areas often face isolation and barriers to access for some services.

The second principle underlying the vision of care in the future is that services need to be provided efficiently. Providers need to work in interdisciplinary teams, and financing and delivery systems need to support this interdisciplinary approach. Care needs to be seamless across various care delivery sites, and all clinicians need to have access to patients' health information and population data, when needed. Health information technology, such as interoperable EHRs, need to be used to support the health care workforce by improving communication among providers and their patients, building a record of population data, promoting interdisciplinary patient care and care coordination, facilitating patient transitions, and improving quality and safety overall. Giving providers immediate access to patient information, especially for patients who are cognitively impaired and unable to provide their own clinical history, may reduce the likelihood of errors, lower costs, and increase efficiency in care delivery.

This vision for the future is being tested through use of the PCMH model of care, which includes pay-for-performance style bonuses based on quality performance metrics and a care management fee from CMS per beneficiary to support organizations' investment in patient care and infrastructure that enables specific changes in processes of care designed to produce better outcomes.[2]

This PCMH model was developed to transform the current model of primary care to address the health care needs of patients and to improve patient and staff experiences, outcomes, safety, and system efficiencies. Core principles of the PCMH are the following[71]:

- Use of wide-ranging, team-based care
- Patient-centered orientation toward the whole person
- Coordination of care across all elements of the health care system and the patient's community
- Enhanced access to care that uses alternative methods of communication
- Use of a systems-based approach to quality and safety

Reports on the impact of PCMH have been encouraging, with a recent analysis of the first four PCMH pilots implemented by United Healthcare demonstrating gross reductions in medical spending of between 4.0% and 4.5% over 2 years, with a 2-to-1 return on investment and improvement in quality measures.[2]

Efficiency can be further improved by ensuring that health care personnel are used in a way that makes the most of their capabilities. Expanding the scope of practice or responsibility for providers has the potential to increase the overall productivity of the workforce and at the same time promote retention by providing greater opportunities for specialization (e.g., through career lattices) and professional advancement. Specifically, this would involve a cascading of responsibilities, giving additional duties to personnel with more limited training to increase the amount of time that more highly trained personnel have to carry out the work that they alone are able to perform. Although the necessary regulatory changes would likely be controversial in some cases, the projected shortfall in workforce supply requires an urgent response. This response will most likely have to involve expansions in the scope of practice at all levels while, at the same time, ensuring that these changes are consistent with high-quality care.

Ultimately, the U.S. system of caring for older adults will rely on improving the effectiveness and efficiency of our current system. Many of the principles for efficient and effective care are already being applied through today's evolving managed care programs and initiatives. The key will be further applying and expanding managed care principles so that more older Americans can be served, including those covered in the larger FFS Medicare programs. Successful application of managed care principles will depend on properly identifying the right patient and providing him or her with the right services at the right time. Through application of the correct who, what, where, when, and how, managed care principles will successfully answer the question of how best to provide care to older Americans.

KEY POINTS

- Managed care shares some common goals and processes with geriatric medicine.
- Managed care principles are being applied outside of traditional managed care organizations in Medicare fee-for-service programs in greater numbers.
- Despite the benefits of managed care, there continues to be pressure to decrease reimbursement to these plans.
- Managed care principles include a focus on screening, coordination, health promotion, and interdisciplinary health care professionals with geriatric expertise
- The future success of older adult care in the United States depends on the application of managed care principles for efficiency and effectiveness beyond managed care organizations.

For a complete list of references, please visit www.expertconsult.com.

KEY REFERENCES

8. Centers for Medicare and Medicaid Services: Changes to PQRI reporting: alternative reporting periods and alternative criteria for satisfactorily reporting for 2008: measures groups and registry-based reporting (PQRI fact sheet). https://www.cms.gov/Medicare/Quality-Initiatives-Patient-Assessment-Instruments/PQRS/downloads/2008PQRIFactSheetMay.pdf. Accessed June 17, 2014.
9. Centers for Medicare and Medicaid Services: Physician Quality Reporting System overview (PQRS fact sheet). http://www.cms.gov/Medicare/Quality-Initiatives-Patient-Assessment-Instruments/PQRS/Downloads/PQRS_OverviewFactSheet_2013_08_06.pdf. Accessed June 17, 2014.
10. Centers for Medicare and Medicaid Services: 2013 Medicare Part D medication therapy management (MTM) programs (fact sheet). http://www.cms.gov/Medicare/Prescription-Drug-Coverage/PrescriptionDrugCovContra/Downloads/CY2013-MTM-Fact-Sheet.pdf. Accessed June 17, 2014.
25. Kane RL: Managed care as a vehicle for delivering more effective chronic care for older persons. J Am Geriatr Soc 46:1034–1039, 1998.
30. The Care Transitions Program: The four pillars. http://caretransitions.org/. Accessed June 17, 2014.
37. Stefanacci RG, Reich S, Casiano A: Application of PACE principles for population health management of frail older adults. Popul Health Manage 18:367–372, 2015.
45. Kaiser Family Foundation: Medicare Part D prescription drug benefit (fact sheet). http://kaiserfamilyfoundation.files.wordpress.com/2013/11/7044-14-medicare-part-d-fact-sheet.pdf. Accessed June 17, 2014.
56. Centers for Medicare and Medicaid Services: Linking quality to payment. http://www.medicare.gov/hospitalcompare/linking-quality-to-payment.html. Accessed June 17, 2014.
58. Centers for Medicare and Medicaid Services: Bundled Payments for Care Improvement (BPCI) initiative: general information. http://innovation.cms.gov/initiatives/bundled-payments/. Accessed June 17, 2014.
60. Conway PH, Mostashari F, Clancy C: The future of quality measurement for improvement and accountability. JAMA 309:2215–2216, 2013.
61. Agency for Healthcare Research and Quality: Selecting structure measures for clinical quality measurement. http://www.qualitymeasures.ahrq.gov/tutorial/StructureMeasure.aspx. Accessed June 17, 2014.
62. Centers for Medicare and Medicaid Services: Roadmap for quality measurement in the traditional Medicare fee-for-service program. http://www.cms.gov/Medicare/Quality-Initiatives-Patient-Assessment-Instruments/QualityInitiativesGenInfo/downloads/QualityMeasurementRoadmap_OEA1-16_508.pdf. Accessed June 17, 2014.
63. Rand Health: Assessing Care of Vulnerable Elders (ACOVE). http://www.rand.org/health/projects/acove/. Accessed June 17, 2014.
69. Agency for Healthcare Research and Quality: Strategies to support quality-based purchasing: a review of the evidence. Technical Reviews 10. Pub. No. 04–P024, Rockville, MD, 2004, AHRQ.
70. Institute of Medicine: Crossing the quality chasm. http://iom.edu/~/media/Files/Report%20Files/2001/Crossing-the-Quality-Chasm/Quality%20Chasm%202001%20%20report%20brief.pdf. Accessed June 17, 2014.

130 Telemedicine Applications in Geriatrics

Leonard C. Gray

BACKGROUND

Telemedicine is the delivery of health care and the exchange of health care information across distance.[1] Related terms, often used interchangeably, are *telecare* (the provision of nursing and community support services at a distance) and *telehealth* (the delivery of public health services at a distance).[1] *Mobile health* is a concept that embraces the notion of health services supported by mobile communication devices, including wireless monitoring devices, smartphones, and tablet computers.[2] *Telegeriatrics* is a term that refers to the application of telemedicine to geriatric medicine and aged care.

Telemedicine may subserve any branch of medical or health service delivery, depending on the nature of the service and the available systems to support delivery at a distance. It is dependent predominantly on communication technologies and software, including traditional telephony, video-conferencing, e-mail, and other forms of messaging. These depend, in turn, on available infrastructure, which, if suboptimal, will preclude use of the technology. For example, inadequate Internet bandwidth may preclude the use of video-conferencing.

The suitability of particular health care activities to a telemedicine strategy depends critically on the nature of the delivery systems. As new technologies emerge, additional telemedicine approaches will continuously evolve.

Telehealth interactions are broadly classified as synchronous (or real time) and asynchronous (or store and forward). Synchronous interactions are less efficient and thus more expensive. They are best suited to processes where considerable interaction is required, such as complex diagnostic interviews or provision of counseling to patients. Asynchronous interactions have the advantage that interacting individuals do not need to be available simultaneously. This approach works well for review of images and complex investigative materials. Telemonitoring is the most frequently reported form of telemedicine in the literature. This usually involves retrieval of physiologic parameters to support monitoring, but it may also involve diagnosis or therapy.

Health services often use combinations of synchronous and asynchronous approaches to deliver a service. For example, telemonitoring of patients with heart failure may be supplemented by telephone or video-conferencing when parameters move out of an acceptable range.

ACCESS TO HEALTH CARE CHALLENGES FOR OLDER PEOPLE

From its inception, the primary driver of telemedicine has been the need to deliver health care services to individuals who cannot easily access them. Therefore, the early focus of telemedicine was on communities in rural or remote locations, where health services that are usually available in larger cities are not easy to access. Access is most problematic when acute health care problems arise and emergency services or expertise is not readily available. However, as telemedicine has developed, the array of problems for which solutions have been constructed has broadened to include chronic illness and care of older adults.

The trend to home care and the impetus to substitute in-home for hospital services have led to a range of increasingly complex health services being delivered outside of hospitals. Most of these services require health professionals to visit the home. On-road time becomes an important cost penalty, with large periods of time spent traveling. Safety concerns arise when patients have potentially unstable conditions. Therefore, telemedicine strategies are also increasingly important in major cities.

Older patients often have physical or cognitive disability, which limits their ability to travel to health services. Therefore, in their circumstance, it is not only the distance from health services that precludes access but also the logistics of securing and affording transportation. For frail individuals, journeys to health care providers may become a challenge to their health stability. Cognitively impaired individuals experience greater confusion. Physically disabled individuals may sustain a fall, develop deep vein thrombosis, or simply be exhausted. They often require a caregiver to accompany them to appointments. Caregiver availability is declining in many societies where more people live alone, family size is declining, and children are more likely to live at a distance. To complicate matters, pressure on health professionals' time (related to declining workforce availability or constrained financial support) has reduced the capacity to visit patients at home. In many societies, the trend away from institutional care has led to the need for increasing travel time for health professionals.

These challenges create a situation where, ironically, some people with high needs have the least access to services. Conversely, it is apparent that telemedicine may have enormous advantages for older people, perhaps more so than for other age groups.

Thus, the impetus for telemedicine application is, broadly, threefold: (1) to overcome barriers to access to health services for people who live in rural communities or are disabled, (2) to improve health outcomes for all people, and (3) to reduce costs of health care delivery (Box 130-1). With population aging and its consequent challenge to health care demand and cost, telemedicine represents an important opportunity for both older people and the health services that serve them.

TELEMEDICINE MODALITIES

Health services may be delivered using a variety of modalities, alone or in combination.

Video-Conference

The prevalent form of synchronous telemedicine is generally considered to be video-conferencing. However, the use of the conventional telephone for communication between health professionals and patients, and for peer-to-peer communication, is long-standing and ubiquitous. However, this is usually regarded as an "adjunct" to clinical practice rather than a substitute. In most jurisdictions, telephone conversations are not formally recognized as health interactions, and there is rarely any payment system from health funders to reinforce their value. On the other hand, video-consultation is now increasingly regarded as a definitive health service, with governments and health funding agencies providing funding to support such interactions on a fee-for-service basis or through program funding.[3]

BOX 130-1 Potential Advantages of Telemedicine Systems

- Access to health services in rural and remote communities
- Reduction in travel time, inconvenience, and expense for patients
- Reduction in travel time for health professionals
- Improved follow-up and monitoring in home care
- Greater efficiency of service delivery in hospital and nursing home settings
- Improved autonomy for older patients and caregivers in accessing health care
- Reduced rate of admission to hospital and long-term care

The advent of video-conferencing equipment was associated with the emergence of video-consultation as a potential substitute for conventional consultation. This equipment depends on specialized hardware, is relatively expensive, and therefore, until recently, its use has been limited to institutionally based consultations (e.g., from hospital to hospital). However, the potential of video-conferencing is accelerating with the emergence of low-cost software-based systems. These systems are generally proprietary and are not interoperable with other systems, thus requiring end users to have the same software product. Because their performance is heavily reliant on the prevailing Internet infrastructure, they are subject to inconsistency of vision and sound and to dropout. This lack of quality interferes with the flow of consultations and reduces the value of vision to appreciate clinical signs and the subtleties of patient gestures and conversation.

Recently, the availability of low-cost software applications that are interoperable with conventional hardware-based systems has created the potential for interactions between larger and smaller institutions and patients' homes, paving the way for a large range of potential interactions using telemedicine.

The application of video-conferencing as a substitute for face-to-face encounters has been most successful in psychiatry. Because, in psychiatry, the use of physical examination is usually not required (other than perhaps for an initial encounter) and because the majority of follow-up interactions are based on conversation, it is well suited to this modality. In other disciplines, the suitability of video-conferencing practice often depends on the need for physical examination. Many practitioners are reticent to use video-consultation if they are unable to conduct a complete physical examination. A variety of work-arounds have been developed, including a requirement for a medical practitioner to be present at the patient end (when a specialist is consulting), the use of a specifically trained assistant, or the adoption of a protocol stating only follow-up consultations are conducted by video-conference.[4]

In emergency situations, in spite of potential compromises, telephone and video-consultation may be the only means of interaction. In the case of older people with less severe or chronic problems, an important consideration is whether a consultation, with a partial physical examination (i.e., visual inspection without palpation and auscultation), is preferable to no consultation at all. Most health systems will not support travel of frail older people to regional centers for consultation, unless there is a major, discrete indication (e.g., for a surgical procedure or medical procedure such as dialysis). As a result, in many regions, access to services for older people is suboptimal when compared to usual city-based practice.

Most studies that have examined the reliability of clinical assessment performed by synchronous telehealth have produced positive results. For example, the accuracy of dementia diagnosis by video-conference is similar in precision to conventional face-to-face assessment, and physical examination has little or no influence on the diagnosis.[5,6]

Store-and-Forward Telemedicine

There are two broad applications of asynchronous telemedicine: consultation online, (1) where a practitioner reviews clinical information and provides diagnostic and management advice, usually to another health professional, and (2) where continuous or intermittent monitoring is used to enhance patient management.

Store-and-forward applications are most developed in the areas of radiology, dermatology,[7] and wound care.[8] In these disciplines, the majority of clinical decision making depends on the inspection of images, supplemented by a small amount of clinical history and observations. In dermatology, telemedicine-mediated diagnostic accuracy has been shown repeatedly to be similar to in-person appraisal.[9,10] A similar approach has been adopted for wound management.[8] With the diagnosis secured and initial advice provided to the patient, further management can often be delivered by another practitioner. This approach is particularly valuable when the patient lives in a rural setting. In some disciplines, store-and-forward telemedicine may be used to supplement a conventional consultation or video-consultation.

Recent interesting developments are beginning to challenge conventional health care practice, wherein software applications interpret images and suggest diagnoses on downloadable applications for smartphones (e.g., in skin cancer diagnosis).[11] This development is a reflection of a continuous movement toward self-diagnosis and management made possible by the Internet and associated wealth of information repositories and low-cost applications. Even traditional medical devices (such as sphygmomanometers and glucometers) are operated by patients, often at their own instigation. These devices can be connected to mobile computers, with low-cost applications available to enable patients to interpret and respond to trends and to upload recordings to health practitioners.

Remote monitoring (or telemonitoring) is a technologic response to the burgeoning prevalence of chronic disease, which, in turn, is related to population aging and lifestyle trends. Various devices are available to monitor and transmit parameters such as pulse, blood pressure, blood glucose levels, movements, and even falls. Conditions that have been most commonly involved include diabetes mellitus, heart failure, and chronic obstructive pulmonary disease. Remote monitoring serves to either alert health professionals to impending deterioration or to assist in compliance with diagnosis or treatment. Health system objectives include reduction in demand on health professional travel and on hospital admission. Several large-scale studies have shown positive results in improving clinical outcomes, but there remains doubt about cost effectiveness.[12] However, as telemedicine systems become less expensive and more readily available, the cost-benefit balance is likely to move in favor of deployment of these approaches.

APPLICATION OF TELEMEDICINE FOR OLDER PEOPLE

The application of telemedicine to the health care of older people has been a relatively late development. As a result, its application around the world is patchy, characterized by a series of small-scale demonstrations, few of which are entrenched in practice across entire states or systems.

In this section, the use of telemedicine applications for older people is reviewed. Descriptions are organized according to care setting: hospital care, home care, and long-term (institutional) care. The descriptions pertain generally to care of older adults, but where relevant, there is specific reference to the use of

BOX 130-2 Telemedicine Applications in Geriatric Medicine and Aged Care

Hospital Care
- Emergency assessment and management (telestroke)
- Hospital avoidance (through remote monitoring and video-consultation)
- Inpatient geriatric consultation by video-conference
- Supervision of geriatric evaluation and management and rehabilitation programs by video-conference

Home Care
- Telemonitoring (hypertension, chronic obstructive pulmonary disease, diabetes mellitus, heart failure, falls)
- In-home consultations, management and advisory services (via e-mail and video-conference)

Long-Term Care
- Specialist consultations by data review or video-conference, ongoing management, remote monitoring during illness exacerbations

telemedicine in geriatric medical practice. A summary list of reported applications is provided in Box 130-2.

Hospital Care

Specialist aged care services are available in many hospitals, including acute geriatric units, geriatric consulting teams, and hybrid models such as acute care for elders (ACE) units.[13,14] Many hospitals operate or have direct access to post-acute geriatric and rehabilitation services.

Comprehensive geriatric assessment (CGA) is a key process in geriatric medicine and aged care. It requires the contribution of a specialist geriatrician and multidisciplinary team. The effectiveness of CGA is most apparent in the hospital setting.[15,16] However, in many nations there is a paucity of geriatricians. The process of CGA is often absent or underdeveloped, except in major hospitals or academic centers. In some jurisdictions, geriatricians travel to regional and rural hospitals to contribute to geriatric care. In smaller rural hospitals, or even small metropolitan community hospitals, there is insufficient work to sustain a geriatrician, so a visiting arrangement is unavoidable or absent. Such visits are inevitably infrequent, so that the geriatrician's ability to provide advice in acute cases is limited. In less acute cases, there are inevitable delays in securing advice, which is usually unacceptable in the hospital setting because of occupancy and financial pressures.

Geriatrician involvement in CGA can be facilitated by telemedicine. A method of providing specialist geriatric assessment (based on the ACE model) using a combination of shared electronic medical records (configured to present information to the geriatrician operating at a distance) and twice-weekly teleconferences appeared to improve some aspects of care in a group of hospitals in the U.S. state of Wisconsin.[17]

An Australian model uses a combination of online and video-conference to support geriatric consultation and to participate in post-acute programs of care for rural hospitals.[18] Cases are prepared by onsite nurse assessors using a web-based structured assessment system.[19] The assessment can be viewed online by the specialist and a diagnostic and treatment review prepared. This process seems to be reliable in making key triage decisions even without direct interaction with the patient.[20] Further assessment is conducted by video-conference using wireless mobile devices at the bedside. Weekly team meetings are conducted to facilitate care planning.

Many hospitals lack inpatient rehabilitation facilities, and many patients require ongoing rehabilitation beyond the inpatient phase of care. Telemedicine applications have been used to support post-acute rehabilitation programs, including for stroke,[21,22] joint replacement,[23] and speech therapy.[24] These programs rely mainly on video-consultation, into patients' homes or to rural ambulatory centers. There is growing evidence for feasibility, acceptability, and reliability, but clinical effectiveness and costing studies tend to be preliminary and small scale.

Hospital Avoidance and Emergency Care

Some telemedicine programs use a hospital avoidance strategy, explicitly targeting individuals. In some cases, the intervention has a largely preventive approach. However, some programs are designed to react to emergency situations, where immediate hospital admission is likely. A demonstration project offered urgent health assessment and primary care practitioner consultation to residents of a senior living community in the United States.[25] Cases were prepared by a trained telemedicine assistant, who visited the patient, recorded basic physiologic parameters (pulse, blood pressure, pulse oximetry) and facilitated a telephone or video-consultation. This approach seemed to result in the majority of patients being treated in situ, thus avoiding transfer to an emergency department. Similar approaches may be a component of telehealth interventions offered to nursing homes, but these elements are not explicitly evaluated.[26-28]

Telemedicine strategies are increasingly used to support early assessment and management of acute stroke, including the administration of thrombolysis. Preliminary evidence suggests the potential for improving clinical outcomes and for cost-effectiveness.[29,30]

Home Care

A growing body of evidence suggests that care coordination supported by regular monitoring of biometric data can improve patient outcomes and reduce hospitalizations among patients with chronic conditions such as heart failure and diabetes. However, such services demand significant on-road time from health professionals. Telemedicine is a logical response to improve compliance and efficiency in such programs.

Although the reported telemedicine models and evaluations are targeted on a diagnostic paradigm, most individuals with these problems are older persons. Typically, these programs install devices that can collect physiologic measures in the person's home and transfer them to a monitoring service. These measures can be used to assist in subsequent management consultations, or they may be used as alerts to deterioration or poor disease control. In some instances, the service is supplemented by telephone or video-conference support.

A large U.K. pragmatic randomized trial (the "Whole System Demonstrator") involving more than 3000 subjects offered remote monitoring for patients with chronic obstructive pulmonary disease, diabetes, or heart failure.[31] The majority of the cohort was older than 65 years. Measures were customized to the individual and included, at a minimum, pulse oximetry, random blood glucose, and weight. Predetermined protocols were applied by community nurses, who responded to information derived by telemonitoring according to specified protocols. The trial demonstrated statistically significant but modest reductions in hospital utilization and mortality among the intervention group.[32] However, the patterns of other social service use were unaffected,[33] and the overall program was found not to be cost-effective.[34]

A similar U.S.-based study also provided biometric monitoring, symptom reporting, and video-consultation to a very old population of community-dwelling individuals who were considered at high risk of hospitalization.[35,36] There was no effect on hospital visits or admissions, but an increased mortality rate was observed in the telemedicine group.

A retrospective analysis, repeated on two separate occasions, using matched control techniques of a large-scale telehealth-facilitated care coordination program operated by the Veterans Health Administration in the United States demonstrated significant cost savings in the telehealth group.[35,37] There were considerably fewer emergency room, hospital, and long-term institutional care admissions.

These three studies, with apparently contradictory findings, characterize the uncertainty surrounding the efficacy of home telemonitoring and associated services for older people. Differences might be explained by a host of factors, such as the format of the program, training of staff, the program infrastructure (e.g., electronic medical records), or methodologic issues.

Long-Term Care

Many long-term care facilities are small in size, are located at a distance from hospitals, have only intermittent access to onsite medical staff, and rarely have direct access to specialists. Residents have cognitive and functional deficits that limit their ability to access external services. Access may require a professional escort and specialized transport. In many jurisdictions, the rate of transfer to emergency departments appears high, and many visits are probably avoidable.[38,39] The use of telemedicine in this environment would seem highly advantageous, yet reports of its application are very limited.[40]

The major services reported to long-term care facilities are allied health, dermatology, and psychiatry.[40] Only two studies report links with geriatricians.[28,41] Several reports describe links between facilities and primary care physicians, including for out–of-hours consultation.[42] Both store-and-forward and videoconferencing strategies, and sometimes a combination of the two, are used to support evaluation and management.

Most studies are descriptive or evaluate acceptability, reliability, or safety.[40] Few examine the outcomes of improved clinical care or reduced costs of care. A Hong Kong project at a single nursing home offered a range of clinical services and found that there were reductions in hospital transfers.[43] A study of a videoconference–mediated telemedicine service to support out-of-hours primary care services to a chain of Massachusetts nursing homes demonstrated a small (4%) but potentially important reduction in hospitalizations over a 13-month trial period.[42] The study suggested that the greater the engagement was of the facility in the telemedicine program, the greater was the effect, and concluded that significant potential savings to the funding agency (Medicare) were possible.

Overall, although there is definite appeal for the application of telemedicine to long-term care facilities, and although the available evidence for acceptability, reliability, and efficacy is encouraging, uptake seems limited.

CHALLENGES TO TELEHEALTH IMPLEMENTATION

Although, in theory, telehealth has the potential to solve many problems around access and health care quality for older people, the uptake has been quite limited worldwide. Nevertheless, several large-scale sustainable implementations serve as examples for other jurisdictions. A notable example is the widespread use of care coordination supported by telehealth within the U.S. Veterans Affairs service system.[44]

Discussion about the uptake challenge is ongoing in the literature and telemedicine industry media.[45] The reasons for slowness of uptake can be broadly characterized as either issues pertaining to telehealth implementation, in general, or issues specific to older people.

Potential barriers to the uptake of telemedicine include technology issues, lack of suitable and sustainable funding sources, resistance to change among health practitioners, and practitioner licensing restrictions among jurisdictions.[2,46-47] These barriers appear largely determined by local policy and financing arrangements rather than being intrinsic to the delivery of telehealth. Recent rapid advances in communication infrastructure, electronic medical records, and connected devices may result in acceleration of telemedicine uptake. The almost ubiquitous use of powerful mobile devices with associated health applications seem to be facilitating a consumer-led transformation of health care delivery.[2]

SUITABILITY OF TELEMEDICINE FOR OLDER PERSONS

Involvement in many forms of telehealth requires participants to interact in some way with the associated technology. Interactions range from passive engagement in a video-consultation, where the call has been established by another person, to situations where participants must undertake a series of tasks, including recording and transmitting biometric data such as blood pressure or random blood glucose readings. These tasks involve cognitive, sensory, and motor skills of varying degrees. Among older people, particularly those in receipt of aged care or geriatric medicine services, impairments in these skill sets are common. Potentially, this reduces the usefulness of telemedicine for older people.

These challenges indicate that telemedicine application must be customized to individuals, or at least to groups of individuals with common attributes. For example, telemedicine services involving persons with cognitive impairment must either be "hosted" by a caregiver or health professional or be configured with a high level of simplicity. Clinical consultation via videoconference with persons with cognitive impairment is highly feasible, provided that there is an appropriate setup and hosting function.

Visual and auditory impairment is common among older people. To conduct effective communication via video-consultation, attention is required to ensure sufficient video and audio fidelity. This demands sufficient screen size, bandwidth, frame rates, and transmission speeds. These cannot necessarily be achieved, at this time, with some software-based videoconferencing solutions in all jurisdictions.

A further important consideration in video-consultation is the manner in which the clinician presents himself to the patient. The clinician should position himself before the camera and microphone to ensure that facial expression is clear and sound is transmitted clearly. Extraneous noise and echo should be eliminated. The background should be uncluttered and professional. If, in spite of good setup, the patient cannot hear clearly, the use of a headset by the patient may be helpful.

Telehealth solutions that use desktop, tablet, or other mobile devices may present challenges for older people with visual or dexterity limitations. Some systems can be adjusted by manipulating software to compensate. However, use of a mouse and keyboard may be particularly challenging. Generally, highly interactive telemedicine applications are not suitable for people with cognitive impairment.

FUTURE DIRECTIONS

Telemedicine has the potential to improve access, effectiveness, and efficiency of health care for older people. This potential is yet to be fully realized. Currently, a revolution in new technologies seems likely to accelerate the delivery of health care at a distance. The widespread availability of intelligent connected devices among the general population is likely to change expectations of the mode of health care delivery. Whereas adoption is likely to be least rapid among frail older people, it will inevitably occur through their partners and children. Over a longer time frame, the current generation of middle-aged individuals will take their familiarity with mobile devices and computers, and the skills to operate them, into old age.

Health administrators and funders are cautious about transformation of the health care delivery system, except, perhaps, where obvious cost savings are identified. However, it is likely that consumer expectation will drive demand for reform.

Telemedicine was born out of attempts to deliver health services to individuals living in remote communities. However, its future lies in its ability to reengineer the health care delivery process to improve the effectiveness and efficiency of health care.

KEY POINTS

- Older people experience access problems to health care because of cognitive and physical disability. Telemedicine has the potential to overcome access barriers.
- Chronic illness is highly prevalent among older people, often requiring frequent interactions with health care providers. Telemedicine can eliminate some of the travel requirements of both patients and care providers, resulting in improved access and potentially better health care outcomes.
- Telemedicine offers a wide variety of formats. Examples include direct video-consultation, online consultation using e-mail, and remote telemonitoring of biometric information. The telemedicine "solution" must be customized to the clinical scenario.
- Telemedicine sets out to improve access by reducing the need for travel, but it also has the potential to transform the manner in which health care is delivered. It need not be simply an emulation of conventional health care delivery.

For a complete list of references, please visit www.expertconsult.com.

KEY REFERENCES

2. Weinstein RS, Lopez AM, Joseph BA, et al: Telemedicine, telehealth, and mobile health applications that work: opportunities and barriers. Am J Med 127:183–187, 2014.
5. Martin-Khan M, Flicker L, Wootton R, et al: The diagnostic accuracy of telegeriatrics for the diagnosis of dementia via video conferencing. J Am Med Dir Assoc 13:487.e19–e24, 2012.
17. Malone ML, Vollbrecht M, Stephenson J, et al: Acute Care for Elders (ACE) Tracker and e-Geriatrician: methods to disseminate ACE concepts to hospitals with no geriatricians on staff. J Am Geriatr Soc 58:161–167, 2010.
18. Gray LC, Wright OR, Cutler AJ, et al: Geriatric ward rounds by video conference: a solution for rural hospitals. Med J Aust 191:605–608, 2009.
21. Rubin MN, Wellik KE, Channer DD, et al: Systematic review of telestroke for post-stroke care and rehabilitation. Curr Atheroscler Rep 15:343, 2013.
32. Steventon A, Bardsley M, Billings J, et al: Effect of telehealth on use of secondary care and mortality: findings from the Whole System Demonstrator cluster randomised trial. BMJ 344:e3874, 2012.
36. Takahashi PY, Pecina JL, Upatising B, et al: A randomized controlled trial of telemonitoring in older adults with multiple health issues to prevent hospitalizations and emergency department visits. Arch Intern Med 172:773–779, 2012.
37. Darkins A, Kendall S, Edmonson E, et al: Reduced cost and mortality using home telehealth to promote self-management of complex chronic conditions: a retrospective matched cohort study of 4,999 veteran patients. Telemed J E Health 21:70–76, 2014.
40. Edirippulige S, Martin-Khan M, Beattie E, et al: A systematic review of telemedicine services for residents in long term care facilities. J Telemed Telecare 19:127–132, 2013.
44. Darkins A: The growth of telehealth services in the Veterans Health Administration between 1994 and 2014: a study in the diffusion of innovation. Telemed J E Health 20:761–768, 2014.
45. Bashshur RL, Shannon G, Krupinski EA, et al: Sustaining and realizing the promise of telemedicine. Telemed J E Health 19:339–345, 2013.

131 Gerontechnology

Alex Mihalidis, Rosalie Wang, Jennifer Boger

INTRODUCTION

We live in a world where technology is increasingly intelligent, pervasive, and connected. These extend to virtually every aspect of health and health care, such as enabling earlier and more accurate diagnosis, enhancing treatment and evaluation, enabling function and activity participation, and supporting general health and wellness. As populations age, the health changes associated with aging become more common. Technology promises to play a central role in enabling older adults to enhance or maintain their preferred lifestyles or adapt to age-related changes, and, more broadly, to manage the increasing demand on care providers and the health care system.

As the name suggests, gerontechnology is the intersection of the fields of gerontology and technology. Gerontechnology is a multidisciplinary field that aims to produce technology to support the needs of aging adults.[1] Technologies do not have to be specifically designed for older adults to be considered gerontechnology; a technology can be so considered if it is useful to older adults. As such, gerontechnology encompasses a broad range of applications, ranging from relatively simple devices, such as grab bars and walking aids, to complex systems, such as home-based semi-autonomous monitoring of vital signs. Other applications include devices and systems that foster social connectivity and participation in society, such as tablet computers and smartphones. Care providers are encouraged to think beyond what is typically considered to be a gerontechnology to encompass any technology that can support older adults, that is, to recommend a technological solution because it is a good match for the individual and the problem rather than choosing a technology that is classified as being "for older adults." Finally, gerontechnology also includes environmental design and "built environments" that support independence, healthy living, and inclusion (see chapter 132).

Developers are putting increasing efforts into creating technologies that are usable by, and useful to, older adults and their social and care networks.[2] Their needs and use of technology vary, reflecting variability in health status from active individuals living in their own homes to very frail individuals with health challenges that necessitate ongoing caregiver assistance in an institutional setting. Furthermore, older adults cannot be viewed as a single cohort with respect to their knowledge, use, or perceptions regarding technology. In a recent study of technology use (e.g., Internet and broadband) among Americans 65 years old and older, it was concluded that in general, younger older adults (i.e., less than 80 years of age) had experience and enthusiasm toward technology.[3] This trend toward technically literate older adults is likely to continue as technology becomes increasingly pervasive. Moreover, as the large baby boomer cohort ages, it is likely that more technologies will be developed that reflect their needs, desires, and abilities.

Whereas not all gerontechnology is geared toward care provision, much of it specifically focuses on the prevention, detection, monitoring, and support of individuals with acute and chronic health conditions. These types of technologies may have one or more users, which can include the older adults themselves and, if required, their family, friends, and caregivers. Family and friends may interact with a technology as a peer (i.e., working and sharing the experience together with the older adult) or may be an informal (unpaid) caregiver, who is using the technology to provide support to the older adult. Formal caregivers, such as health care professionals and paid support workers, may also be users. Both formal and informal caregivers may be responsible for initializing and maintaining the technology but also may find the technology supports their role in enabling older adults in their care to live where they choose and can mitigate informal caregivers' emotional stress or physical injury.[4] Informal caregivers of older adults are often older themselves, and technology is often useful to address some of their own care concerns. As such, gerontechnologies represent part of a solution to address the current trend of decreasing caregiver numbers for older adults with chronic health conditions associated with the global population aging.

This chapter begins with a discussion of the role of health care professionals in gerontechnology, followed by considerations regarding the provision of gerontechnology. Examples of gerontechnologies are then given before the chapter concludes with thoughts regarding future trends in the field.

ROLES OF HEALTH CARE PROFESSIONALS

While many consumer technologies and some assistive technologies are privately and independently procured, health care professionals usually play a central role in the provision of appropriate technologies to support the often complex health and care needs of older adults. Ideally, health care professionals will work closely with older adults and others in their care network to determine treatment plans that may include technology recommendations. Provision typically entails (1) identification of need; (2) general and/or specialist assessment; (3) prescription, acquisition, training and/or education; and (4) follow-up and/or ongoing monitoring. It is the role of health care professionals, within the scope of their practice, to collaborate with older adults and, if necessary, their caregivers (who may be responsible for seeking out, procuring, using, maintaining, or otherwise managing the technologies) to make informed decisions in the selection and use of suitable technologies. Active involvement of older adults and their care network in the provision process helps to increase the likelihood that the person-technology fit is a good one and offers people who will be using the technology a chance to participate in the process. This can result in improved outcomes and can increase the likelihood that users will adopt recommended technologies.[5] Several disciplines are involved in the provision of gerontechnology, and the extent, duration, and stage of their involvement depends on the specific activities that an older adult or caregiver needs to carry out, the technology options, the training of specific professionals, the jurisdiction, and the individual's health care coverage.

Several health care professionals can be involved in technology recommendation, procurement, and implementation and can include physicians (including various specialists such as geriatricians, physiatrists, and others), physical therapists, occupational therapists, speech and language pathologists, audiologists, nurses, and social workers. In some specialized clinics, rehabilitation engineers and technologists are involved as well. In many care settings, such as acute care, community/home care, rehabilitation, and residential care, interdisciplinary teams work together in different permutations in the provision process. As with a transdisciplinary approach, there may be significant overlap and interchangeability in roles depending on the complexity of the technology and setting.[6] For example, when dealing with a reduced mobility case in community practice, a physician or nurse may be the first to identify the need for a walker or wheelchair and write a referral for a patient to rent or purchase standard equipment. In more complex cases, the referral may go to a specialist wheelchair clinic where an occupational therapist and a rehabilitation engineer may be involved in the acquisition of customized wheelchair seating equipment. In these situations, the occupational therapist and rehabilitation engineer involved will require substantial background information from medical professionals (including diagnoses, prognosis, contraindications, medications, and other therapies), social workers (including social history, living environment and supports, financial information and funding sources), and physical therapists (including physical functioning and current treatment programs). Equipment vendors can be important as well, particularly with highly specialized and customized technologies.

Health care professionals can also play an invaluable role in gerontechnology development. Gerontechnologies may address complex needs from a broad spectrum of users whose abilities, resources, and intended applications vary considerably. Creating a useful and usable technology requires a cross-discipline effort, where experts from relevant fields combine their knowledge to develop effective solutions. This approach involves expert knowledge regarding the problem that needs to be addressed, the probable way the technology will be used, and the features and functions that could be useful to a range of users. Health care professionals have a first-hand understanding of the physiologic changes, functional changes, and social issues of older adults as well as the ability to identify successful intervention outcomes and ways to achieve them; this knowledge is invaluable to guiding how to build appropriate technology. Contingent on the need to be addressed and the complexity of the technology, disciplines that may be involved in development include gerontologists, psychologists, engineers (e.g., biomedical, human factors, mechanical, electrical, or robotics engineers), computer scientists, health economists, and social scientists. Similar to the provision process of involving older adults and their care networks, involving end users in a user-centered design approach often results in technology that better meets needs.[7] Many developers employ user-centered design practices that involve the active engagement of end users throughout the development process to ensure that requirements for features, functions, usability, and aesthetics are reflected in the final product.

Advocacy is another important way that health care professionals are involved in gerontechnology. Ongoing issues with respect to older adult care across many jurisdictions include the following: improving services or access to services for the provision of technology that improves health and well-being; improving access to, availability of, and funding for technologies that demonstrate effectiveness and potential effectiveness; ensuring standards are in place for manufacturing and testing of technologies to be available on the market; improving and supporting translation of innovative technologies in development to address unmet needs or improve health and economic outcomes. Furthermore, health care professionals can play critical roles in public education, improving awareness of the availability of gerontechnologies and their application; dispelling ageist attitudes and beliefs in the public and in policy that older adults do not like, cannot use, or do not benefit from new technologies; and supporting older adults, caregivers, and other health care providers in learning about gerontechnologies.

MATCHING TECHNOLOGY TO USERS

Considering the widespread marketing of technologies, health care professionals are important in helping consumers to navigate and investigate new technologies. For a technology to be useful and usable, it must match an individual's context, including their needs, abilities, resources, environment, and perceptions. In other words, the technology must address a problem a person is having; be something he or she is able to procure, implement, and operate; and be perceived as beneficial. Technologies that do not fulfill these criteria are of little use because they are inaccessible or will be abandoned by intended users. Moreover, it is important to recognize that an individual's context is dynamic; his or her needs, abilities, environment, resources, and perceptions are dependent on a myriad of factors and will change over time. Hence a technology that works well at one point may become unsuitable as the user's context evolves, such as changes in his or her health, living arrangements, or personal support network.

A primary focus in providing and developing gerontechnology is to match the technology to the user, rather than to match a user to a technology. Appropriately matching a technology to the user tends to result in better outcomes, achieving the user's goals, acceptance, and use. Several models or frameworks are relevant to the provision and development of gerontechnology, such as the Human Activity Assistive Technology (HAAT) model,[6] Matching Person and Technology (MPT) model,[8] Comprehensive Assistive Technology (CAT),[9,10] and the Canadian Model of Occupational Performance and Engagement.[11] These models typically involve the following domains: user, activity or goal, environment of use, and technology. In general, it is understood that users have a desired activity or goal, the environment may act as an enabler or disabler for users who may or may not have specific limitations for that activity or goal, and the matched technology can help to enable, modify, mediate, or otherwise allow users to carry out that activity or goal in that environment. Again, active involvement of the intended users in this process is critical.

Several considerations are necessary when examining the user domain. A technology not only will have a primary user but often may have one or more secondary user(s) as well. For example, a caregiver or health care provider (secondary users) may be involved in setting up and maintaining a fall detection system for an older adult (primary user). The multiple users' physical and cognitive abilities, subjective needs and preferences, belief systems, resources (including social and financial supports), and goals need to be understood for a good technology match. It may also be important to understand the desired treatment approach, such as whether intervention objectives are *remedial* or *compensatory* in nature. For example, remedial goals may be to improve general physical tolerance or to improve attention span. Compensatory goals may involve performing an activity in a different way, such as using a wheelchair to enable ambulation when walking is no longer possible. Accounting for developmental aging and the conditions associated with aging, it is also important to consider the progressions in abilities, whether deterioration, maintenance, or improvements are anticipated.

There are also multiple considerations related to the activity domain. The nature of the targeted activity, whether it be related to taking care of oneself in daily activities, engaging in paid or unpaid work, or participating in recreational and social activities, may be highly variable and range from comparatively simple (e.g., pulling up one's pants) to complex (e.g., managing finances). To be able to identify appropriate gerontechnology solutions, it is necessary to understand how the activity is typically carried out, how users prefer to carry out the activities, the necessary steps, the requirements to carry out the activity (e.g., cognitive load, time, and performance criteria), the contingencies, and the desired outcomes.

Within the environmental domain, it is useful to examine physical, social, cultural, and institutional factors.[11] Physical factors often entail structural features of the environment (e.g., stairs, width of doorways, textures of surfaces), lighting, noise, and smells. Characteristics in the physical environment may determine the need for technology and the types of technology that may be recommended. Social and cultural factors may include a group's beliefs and values about a particular subgroup, situation, or technology and how members of groups behave in relation to these perceptions. Institutional factors include policies and laws. Social and cultural factors can be enablers or disablers for subgroups or individuals, and are often reflected in how the physical and institutional environments are constructed and what affordances are provided to those considered outside the group's norms. For example, perceptions of older adults and individuals with disabilities can limit what services or technologies are offered and developed, can result in stigma perceived by older adults, and may influence the adoption or rejection of different interventions.

The assessment phase of provision described earlier informs the various stages that follow. Depending on the complexity of the technology, the next steps of provision may include selection, trials, education and training, acquisition, and/or follow-up or ongoing monitoring. The selection of an appropriate technology for the user depends on the assessment and several additional factors, such as the local availability and supports available for maintenance. Some technologies may also require an extensive trial, mock-up, and customization phase (e.g., power wheelchairs and environmental control units). Training and education in use are critical for ensuring users are actively involved in ongoing use of the technology by helping them to understand the rationale behind the recommendations and to ensure they are able to operate and use the technologies to achieve intended goals. Follow-up and ongoing monitoring phases evaluate the outcomes of the technology intervention to ensure that the specified goals of the users are achieved.

Some of the concerns with technology provision and development include issues of uptake, acceptance, use, and abandonment. Contrary to what may be believed, older adults are often accepting of using technology, if they believe that its use can be beneficial and it is easy to use.[12] Furthermore, age has not been found to be a good predictor of frequency of use of devices in the home.[13] Assistive technology use or non-use may be the result of multiple factors that are personal, environmental, and technological. Personal factors may include need or perceptions of need, functional abilities and limitations, and beliefs, feelings, and experiences with respect to disability and technology.[13] Often the goal of a technology may be to improve independence, but to its user it may also act as a reminder of their functional loss, which can discourage use. Environmental factors may include various characteristics of the environment or the activities within those environments that promote or deter use. Technology factors include features of the technology itself, such as its usability, aesthetics, and durability and overall match between the user and the environment.

Common reasons for using technology are that it makes activities easier, more comfortable, or more enjoyable to carry out; improves function and independence; and offers feelings of security and safety. When a user perceives that the benefits outweigh the costs for using the technology it is found to significantly increase continued technology use.[5] A recent review explored the acceptance of electronic or digital technologies (e.g., sensors in home for activity monitoring, detection of wandering and falls, and e-health applications) for older adults living in the community and found factors at the preimplementation stage that seem to be related to acceptance.[14] These factors included technology concerns, expected benefits, perceived need, alternatives to technology, social influence, and older adults' characteristics. At a postimplementation stage, perceived need and social influences were still concerns, with many older adults indicating that they did not feel that they needed technology. Various reasons have been cited for not using or abandoning recommended assistive technology, including that the user's functional abilities change, technology use depends on use of other technologies, education and training on how to use the technologies were insufficient, the technology is somehow changed (broken and not repaired/replaced or lost), the cost was high, the user prefers to be assisted by another person, or the person feels embarrassed.[13]

Abandonment of technology means that resources may not be used effectively or efficiently and user needs may not be adequately met. Ways of overcoming such challenges are to involve users in the development and provision of technologies. In the development of new technologies, the concerns for adoption and use need to be carefully considered and addressed in the design to minimize the potential for abandonment. Within the provision process, it has been found that satisfaction with the technology and sustained use were associated with whether or not the user was able to trial the technology before acquisition and if the users felt they were involved in the selection and decision-making process for technology acquisition.[15] If a user has professional support (such as with education and training regarding use and maintenance), consideration for financial and funding concerns, and appropriate follow-up, they are more likely to continue using the technology.[5] With regard to training in technology use with older adults, it is recommended that tasks be divided into smaller tasks to be learned in short sessions, skills are learned in the context in which they will be used, and ample time for practice and customization of devices is offered.[5]

EXAMPLES OF TECHNOLOGIES

The evolution of gerontechnologies has moved from aids that address specific functional limitations and goals to more complex or integrated environments and systems that can enable several goals through multiple functions, including ongoing assessment and intervention. As technologies continue to become increasingly intelligent, pervasive, and networked, gerontechnologies will become increasingly sophisticated and interconnected. Although the former common technologies are not likely to become obsolete, in the future they, too, may be connected and integrated. This will result in greater connectivity between the primary users of a technology and associated stakeholders, such as with telehealth applications, as well as networking and information sharing between different technologies.

Currently Available Technologies

The following sections describe currently available technologies that support aging. These technologies have been categorized into three areas: (1) technologies to support specific limitations affecting performance of functional goals; (2) technologies for enabling health, function, safety, and comfort; and (3) technologies for communication, social participation, and inclusion.

Technologies to Support Specific Limitations Affecting Performance of Functional Goals

Many gerontechnologies aim to address specific physical, sensory and perceptual, and cognitive and affective changes that impact the performance of functional goals in self-care, leisure, and work.

Aids that assist mobility focus on transfers, ambulation, and manipulation that have been affected by physical changes in balance, range of motion, strength, and coordination. Examples of these devices include handrails, grab rails, ceiling-to-floor poles, lift chairs, bath transfer boards and benches, tub lifts, floor and overhead lifting devices, canes, walkers, manual and powered wheelchairs and scooters, adaptive eating utensils, and assistive robotic arms (Figure 131-1).

Technologies that address sensory issues primarily address vision and hearing changes. Examples include various low vision adaptations such as the use of large print, talking devices (e.g., watches, clocks, and other household items), screen magnifiers, white canes, and video magnifiers or closed circuit television (Figure 131-2). Computer-based technologies, including

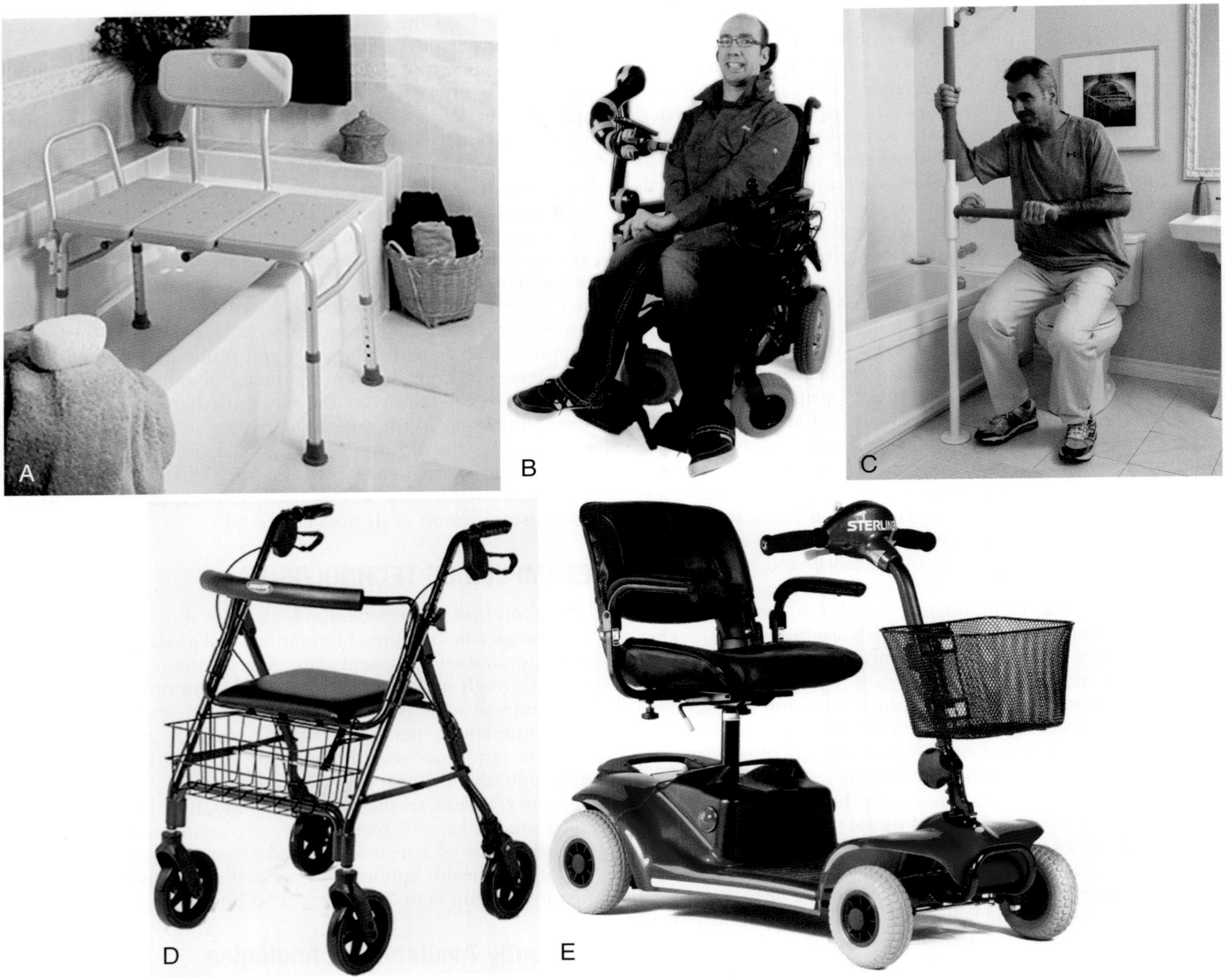

Figure 131-1. A, Bath transfer bench. **B,** Robotic arm on powered wheelchair. **C,** Ceiling to floor pole. **D,** Rollator walker. **E,** Mobility scooter. *(**A,** © Invacare Corporation. Used with permission. **B,** Robotic arm on powered wheelchair. **C,** Courtesy Health Craft. **D,** © Invacare Corporation. Used with permission. **E,** Sunrise Medical Limited.)*

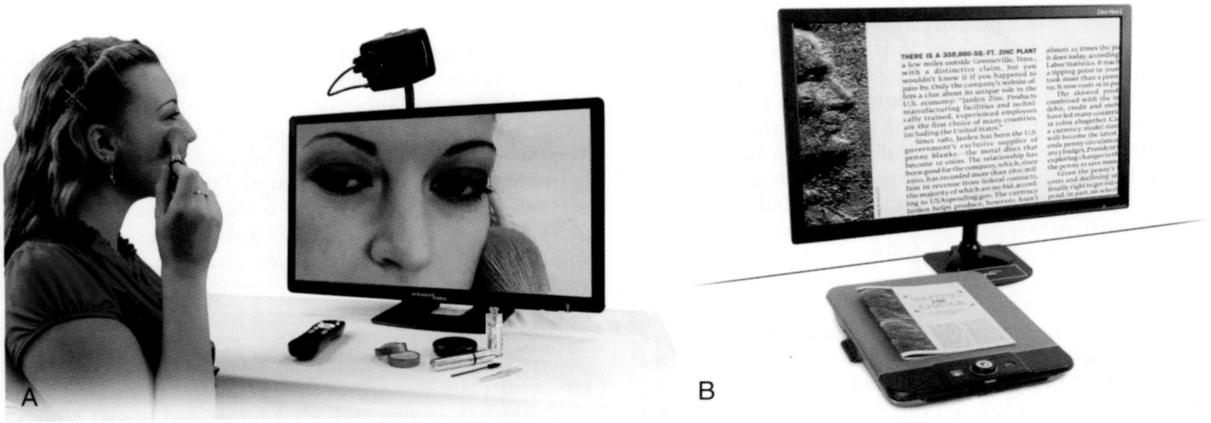

Figure 131-2. Examples of how a video magnifier (closed-circuit television) can be used for enabling tasks such as personal care **(A)** or reading **(B)**. *(**A** and **B** courtesy Optelec.)*

accessibility software that enables modifications to text size and text-to-speech software, are now standard features to facilitate computer use. Hearing may be enabled with common hearing aids, and adaptations include telephone typewriters, Internet, and mobile phone messaging. Devices with visual signals or vibrations can alert older adults to phone calls, text messages, e-mail messages, and fire alarms.

Many older adults experience decreased attention and reaction time, memory loss, and changes in executive functioning, with an increasing prevalence with age. Various gerontechnologies are available to support cognitive changes and/or improve affect and mood. Examples include electronic devices or smartphone applications that provide general reminders, medication reminders, and appointment scheduling, in addition to various technologically simpler tools such as paper calendars and notebooks. There are several computer-based cognitive training games that are designed to maintain and improve cognitive abilities in older adults; however, there is not yet substantive evidence to support measured improvements, and further research is necessary to determine the effects.[16] Novel approaches to cognitive and affective enhancement are becoming available, including robotic companions such as Paro the robotic seal, which is intended to provide the benefits of animal therapy in settings such as hospitals, long-term care facilities, or other settings where live animals would be problematic (Figure 131-3).

Technologies for Enabling Health, Function, Safety, and Comfort

Significant developments in consumer technologies now enable health, safety, and comfort, and many of these technologies are suitable for supporting older adults. In addition to systems that are embedded into a person's environment, smaller and cheaper sensors are driving the increasing use of mobile and wearable technologies to support older adults. Most smartphones (e.g., Apple iPhone, Android-based phones, etc.) are equipped with sensors such as accelerometers, gyroscopes, proximity sensors, and GPS, which can be used to infer user activity and mobility. Wearable physiologic and activity monitors are now commonly available, such as watches, clothing, or other on-person devices that collect data such as heart rate, galvanic skin response, temperature, sleep patterns, and other activities (Figure 131-4). Information gathered by devices such as these can be helpful in monitoring and implementing living habits that promote well-being, although currently this usually requires assistance with interpretation from qualified health care professionals.

Because falls are a common safety issue with older adults, fall detection and alerting systems are commonly recommended and used. These systems employ wearable push button sensors or accelerometers, smartphone accelerometers, or use sensors such as cameras embedded in the environment. When a fall is reported, either autonomously by the device or explicitly by the user, a chain of response events is set in place to determine the nature of the situation and to dispatch appropriate assistance, if necessary.

Environmental control units are available to improve safety, function, and comfort. For example, televisions, lights, and a host of other appliances may be controlled through a range of user interfaces and input methods (e.g., switches, voice) that may be stationary, portable, or mounted to a wheelchair. Many consumer products are available to automate functions in the home or to control the functions remotely through the Internet. Smart locks are available that enable door locks to be controlled through the Internet. There are thermostats that can learn residents' behaviors and determine the level of heating and cooling automatically (e.g., Nest Learning Thermostat). To track health information and provide various beneficial automated responses, various smart home components are available as well (e.g., Withings Aura

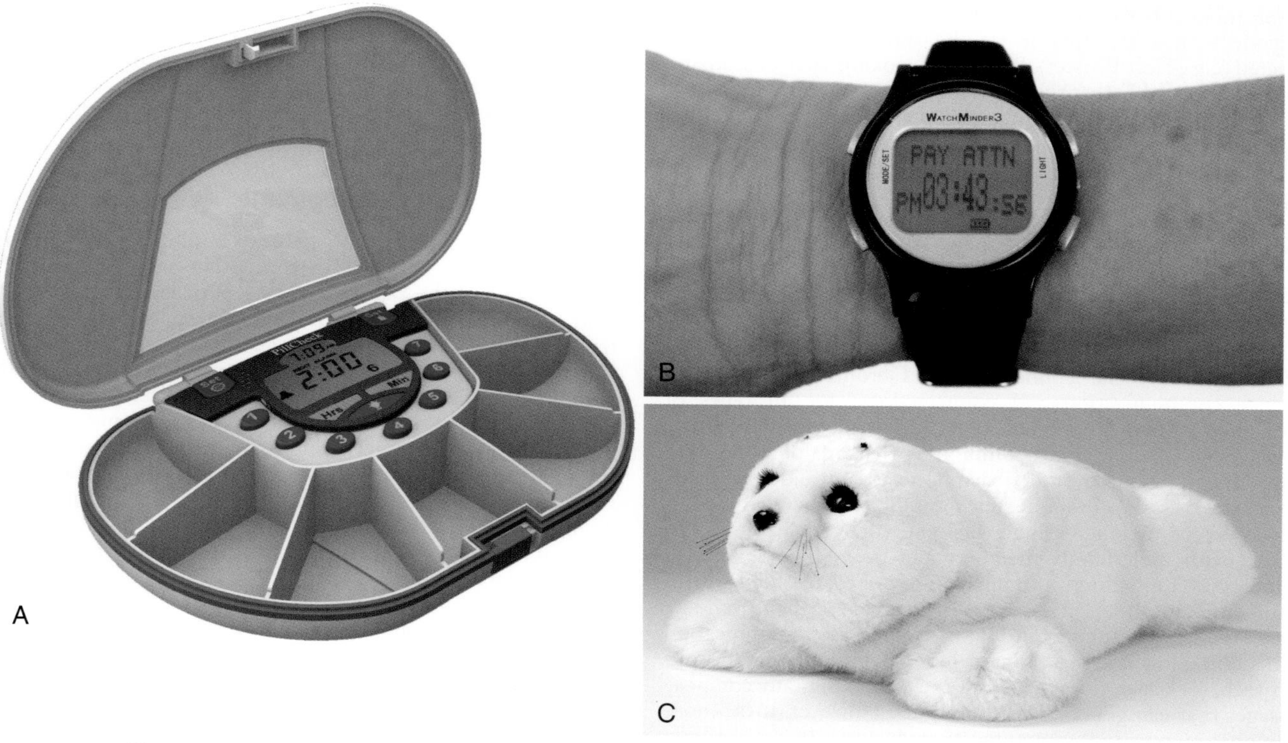

Figure 131-3. A, Pill dispenser with alarm reminder. **B,** Reminder watch. **C,** Companion robot, Paro. *(**B,** Courtesy Watchminder. **C,** Courtesy Paro, USA.)*

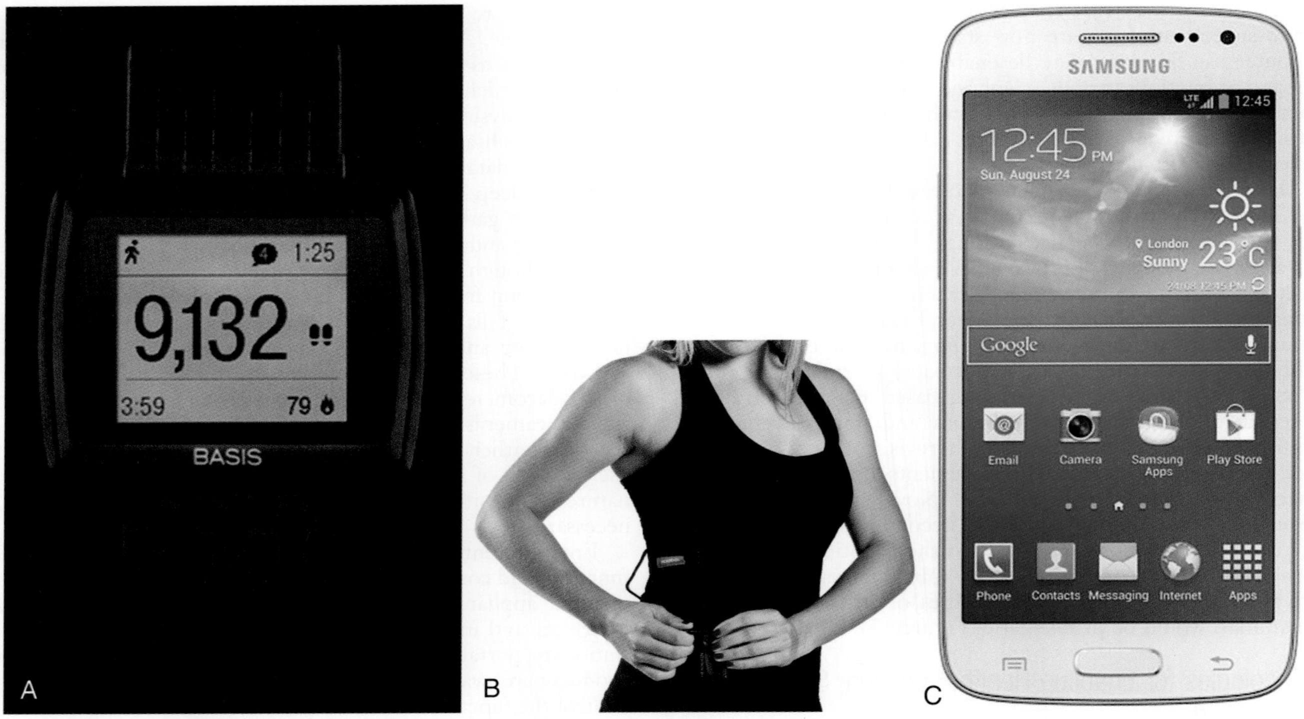

Figure 131-4. A, Smart watch (Basis). **B,** Heart rate monitoring clothing (HealthVest by SmartLife). **C,** Smartphone using various applications (iPhone). *(**A,** Courtesy Allison + Partners. **B,** Courtesy Hexoskin. **C,** Courtesy Samsung.)*

tracks sleep patterns using a mattress sensor and wakens the person with lights or music during a suitable point in the sleep cycle). To ensure home safety, sensors that detect smoke or carbon monoxide can be installed and can alert a call center or someone with a smartphone via the Internet if a problem is detected (e.g., Nest Protect). Related to cooking safety, automatic devices are available that turn the stove off when movement near the stove is absent. For older adults who wander, especially if they have dementia, wearable motion detectors with remote alarms are available to alert a caregiver when the person is outside a safe range.

Technologies for Communication, Social Participation, and Inclusion

An important aspect of well-being is the ability to communicate and engage in social connectedness. Gerontechnologies can enhance communication and connectedness for all types of older adults by providing a variety of flexible methods of getting in touch with people and communities that are of interest to them. General Internet and smartphone use by older adults is also on the rise.[3] For example, telecommunications technologies such as Skype are increasingly being used by older adults to connect with their family members and peers. There are also technologies for aiding communication for older adults with motor difficulties (e.g., dysarthria) or language difficulties (e.g., dysphasia), which range from low-tech, such as communication boards that allow users to point at letters, words, or pictures, to high-tech, such as devices that allow the user to digitally compose messages that can generate voice outputs. However, these more traditional augmented communication devices are increasingly being replaced by consumer technology such as tablet computers and mobile applications. In addition to enabling older adults to communicate more easily, the uptake of mainstream consumer computing technologies is making telehealth options more accessible (e.g., Internet and videoconferencing with health care professionals).

Central to the uptake of computer-based technologies is the ability for older adult users to learn what is available and how to use it. In addition to self-learning and relying on family and friends, organizations such as SeniorNet[17] provide education and training that is targeted toward older adult users.

Technologies in Development

The current direction of gerontechnology development is being shaped by advances in computing and communications technology and the rapidly growing population of older adults who are more comfortable with and keen to use technology than the previous generation.[18] These factors support technologies that are capable of more autonomous operation as well as technologies that actively involve older adult users, which can be beneficial for the self-management of health and well-being. These technologies are evolving to be more integrated and multifunctional to support specific limitations; enable health, safety, and comfort; and foster communication and social integration. As integrated systems, the technologies are increasingly incorporating functions for ongoing monitoring and assessment, diagnosis, and intervention.

Among the numerous technologies currently being developed in research institutions and labs around the world, we focus here on three specific categories: (1) mobile and wearable systems, (2) smart home systems, and (3) robotics. These categories represent those areas of research and development that have garnered the most attention within the gerontechnology community over the past several years and those technologies that have shown the most promise.

Mobile and Wearable Systems

Researchers have developed noninvasive sensors in the form of patches, small Holter-type devices, body-worn devices, and smart garments to monitor health signals. For example, blood glucose, blood pressure, and cardiac activity can be measured through wearable sensors using techniques such as infrared sensing, optical sensing, and oscillometrics. Smart garments or "e-textiles" promise the most noninvasive form of health monitoring. This fabric-sensor integration technology is categorized into several categories.[19] "Garment level" refers to a late-stage visible sensor integration, while "fabric level" refers to a more subtle sensor integration process during production. The ultimate goal is "fiber level" integration to achieve a seamless sensor-fiber integration where the material itself will be the sensor. It is envisioned that e-textiles will enable a host of monitoring activities through many interfaces, including clothing and furniture.

Smart Home Systems

A smart home is one that has been augmented with various types of sensors (to collect data) and actuators (that perform some kind of action, such as providing a reminder). These systems obtain data about the home's occupant through the use of multiple sensors (e.g., motion sensors, cameras, contact sensors) in order to understand the important contextual factors about the occupant that were described earlier in this chapter (see "Matching Technology to Users"). Most smart homes use such knowledge for automation, for providing more comfort for the residents, and for assessing the cognitive and physical health of the residents.

Many smart home projects around the world specifically focus on helping older adults to live healthy, productive, and safe lives. For example, the CASAS[20] project provides a noninvasive assistive environment for dementia patients at home. The Aging in Place project at the University of Missouri aims to provide a long-term care model for seniors in terms of supportive health.[21] The Aware Home project at Georgia Tech[22,23] employs a variety of sensors such as smart floor sensors, as well as assistive robots for monitoring and helping older adults. Other notable smart home test beds include DOMUS[24] at Université de Sherbrooke and the House_n project at MIT.[25] Finally, some smart home projects in Europe include iSpace,[26] Grenoble Health Smart Home (HIS),[27] Gloucester Smart House,[28] PROSAFE,[29] ENABLE,[30] and Assisted Living Lab.[31] These smart homes are able to perform a wide variety of monitoring, assessment, and supportive tasks, including real-time, step-by-step task reminders, tacking of vital signs, and automated environmental control. Many of these capabilities can be performed autonomously by the smart home, requiring little or no effort from its occupants.[32]

Robotics

Assistive robots are aimed to help older adults overcome various physical, cognitive, affective, and social challenges and enable functional performance in daily activities such as feeding, dressing, and grooming. Robots can also help older adults with using the telephone, taking medications, preparing food, managing finances, or engaging in social activities or hobbies. Most assistive robots help older adults compensate for decreased mobility by fetching objects.[33-36] For example, the Dusty robot retrieves dropped objects from the floor.[37] Care-O-bot is able to move safely among humans, to detect and grasp typical household objects, and to safely exchange them with humans.[33] RIBA robot realizes a series of patient transfer operations, including lifting up and transferring older adults from a bed or a wheelchair.[35] Other assistive robots mostly help with activities such as housekeeping,[38] meal preparation, medication management, laundry, shopping, and telephone use.[36] Robots such as uBot5[39] and PerMMA[40] use manipulator arms to compensate for older adults' impaired upper extremity function. In addition to providing physical assistance, robots might also compensate for cognitive changes in older adults by locating objects (e.g., Mamoru[41]), by helping with tasks such as taking medication (e.g., Pearl[42]), or by assisting with social communication and new learning.[36] Various companion robots are in development to facilitate cognitive and emotional stimulation, with the best known and commercialized one being Paro, the robotic seal.[43]

Besides assisting older adults with daily activities, robots may prove helpful in monitoring and assessing health[44] as well as interfacing with other technologies. Furthermore, robots may be integrated into a large system with a smart home. This integration enables information about the older adult and the environment to be exchanged between the robot and the embedded system to further enhance the technology's capabilities and reliability in understanding the older adult and his or her needs and activity patterns (e.g., CompanionAble[45]).

CONCLUSIONS AND FUTURE TRENDS

The role of gerontechnology in the support of older adults and in clinical practice will become more important as the older adult population grows and as the number of older adults with various conditions, such as dementia, increases. As discussed in this chapter, technologies need to be appropriately matched to the user's needs and requirements if they are to be useful. In response, advanced technologies are being developed that make use of concepts such as sensors and artificial intelligence to help these new systems better adapt to the needs of older adult users and to provide more clinically useful data to older adults' care networks. New and innovative approaches are not only used to develop new technologies like smart home systems and robotics but are also being incorporated into more "traditional" assistive technologies such as walkers and canes to help users maintain their balance and to help with way finding.

The future of gerontechnology will require work on the development and use of new clinical paradigms that include treatment approaches that are more inclusive of technological solutions, including new decision-making approaches and health care policies that will allow for the provision of new technologies. These approaches may include facilitating users' access to reimbursement for use of devices to support health and wellness and developing a stronger understanding and acceptance of the importance of these technologies in the prevention of health conditions. Important outcomes may be that older adults are able to remain in their own homes and communities with a higher quality of life and significant health care savings. This will require more effort in educating current health care professionals on the benefits (and limitations) of using technologies with their own clients and patients.

Finally, as gerontechnologies become more ubiquitous, more research on the social and ethical implications of these types of solutions needs to be completed. This population may not be similar to other typical technology users, due to the special considerations that often are needed with older adults because of various impairments and health conditions. For example, special considerations need to be taken in the design and use of these technologies when a cognitive impairment exists. In this instance, typically in practice, older adults with dementia are unable to provide their own consent for the use of these various technologies. This issue becomes even more problematic as more technologies are developed for private and personal activities and are installed in sensitive locations within a person's home (e.g., in the bathroom). Careful consideration needs to be taken in determining how consent will be obtained to use these new technologies and how users will be educated about the potential benefits and limitations of these systems in a fashion that is consistent with their cognitive abilities. These issues have not been fully addressed within the field of gerontechnology and hold the potential for new and fruitful areas of research and clinical consideration. Health care professionals play the central role in identifying how technology can be used to best serve older adults and will continue to be key players in shaping the landscape of gerontechnology.

KEY POINTS

- Gerontechnology is a multidisciplinary field that aims to produce technology to support the needs of aging adults.
- Any technology can be gerontechnology if it is useful to older adults.
- Health professionals have many roles in designing, promoting, adapting, and implementing gerontechnology.
- Technologies have a range of uses, including monitoring and interventions.
- Intervention technologies can be remedial (e.g., improving existing performance, such as walking devices) or compensatory (improving performance in a different way, such as a wheelchair).
- Many new vistas are opening, in areas such as robotics and smart homes.

For a complete list of references, please visit www.expertconsult.com.

KEY REFERENCES

1. Bouma H, Fozard JL, Bouwhuis DG, et al: Gerontechnology in perspective. Gerontechnology 6:190–216, 2007.
2. Lee C, Coughlin JF: PERSPECTIVE: Older adults' adoption of technology: an integrated approach to identifying determinants and barriers. J Prod Innovation Manage 32:747–759, 2015.
4. Mortenson W, Demers L, Fuhrer M, et al: How assistive technology use by individuals with disabilities impacts their caregivers: A systematic review of the research evidence. Am J Phys Med Rehabil 91:984–998, 2012.
6. Cook A, Polgar J, editors: Cook and Hussey's assistive technologies: principles and practice, St Louis, 2008, Mosby.
13. Gitlin L: Why older people accept or reject assistive technology. Generations 19:41–46, 1995.
14. Peek S, Wouters E, Van Hoof J, et al: Factors influencing acceptance of technology for aging in place: a systematic review. Int J Med Inform 83:235–248, 2014.
18. Fisk AD, Rogers WA, Charness N, et al: Designing for older adults: Principles and creative human factors approaches, Boca Raton, FL, 2012, CRC Press.
21. Rantz M, Skubic M, Koopman R, et al: Using sensor networks to detect urinary tract infections in older adults. In proceedings of 13th IEEE International Conference on e-Health Networking Applications and Services, Columbia, MO, 2011, pp 142–149.
22. Abowd G, Mynatt E: Designing for the human experience in smart environments. In Cook D, Das S, editors: Smart environments: technology, protocols, and applications, Hoboken, NJ, 2004, Wiley & Sons, pp 153–174.
24. Bouchard B, Giroux S, Bouzouane A: A keyhole plan recognition model for Alzheimer patients: first results. Appl Artif Intell 21:623–658, 2007.
32. Mihailidis A, Boger J, Hoey J, et al: Zero effort technologies: considerations, challenges and use in health, wellness, and rehabilitation. In Baecker RM, editor: Synthesis lectures on assistive, rehabilitative, and health-preserving technologies, San Rafael, CA, 2011, Morgan & Claypool Publishers.
42. Pineau J, Montemerlo M, Pollack M, et al: Towards robotic assistants in nursing homes: challenges and results. Robot Autonom Syst 42:271–281, 2003.
43. Shibata T: Therapeutic seal robot as biofeedback medical device: qualitative and quantitative evaluations of robot therapy in dementia care. P IEEE 100:2527–2538, 2012.

132 Optimizing the Built Environment for Frail Older Adults

June Andrews

This chapter focuses on practical actions to make the built environment accommodate the needs of frail older adults. New constructions or adaptations of older buildings can make the best of physical and mental strengths that continue, compensate for impairments, provide cues and supports for positive living, and create an aesthetically pleasing environment for frail older adults. Although many older frail people do not have dementia, it is clear that if the environment is designed to work well for those who do have dementia or a related cognitive impairment, it will work for other frail older people. Indeed, good design for people with dementia and people who are frail begins with good design principles in general. Planners and clinical staff who are advising on building and refurbishment projects must consider the following questions:

- What is dementia-friendly design as opposed to design for older frail adults?
- What can limit the positive effects of the built environment?
- Where are the greatest benefits to be had from these changes?
- What are the general features that can be considered anywhere?
- What are the special considerations for hospitals and acute care settings?
- What does a dementia-friendly care home or nursing home look like?
- What changes can be made in the domestic residence/patient's home?

WHAT IS DEMENTIA-FRIENDLY DESIGN AS OPPOSED TO DESIGN FOR OLDER FRAIL ADULTS?

Designing for dementia will make things right for most other people, because older people with dementia will have the common changes of aging but need additional help to adapt to those impairments. Thus "dementia friendly" could be described as an enhancement of compensations for disability. Advice on design for dementia is based on three levels of evidence: rigorous research, extrapolation from sensory and physical impairment, and international consensus on good practice.

Research on design in dementia in general and for frailty more broadly is not well funded, so the rigorous research evidence base for specific design features is limited. The Dementia Services Development Centre at the University of Stirling regularly commissions new literature searches to support the design advice given on its open access virtual environment and through its design publications.[1] Current advice consists of a blend of research, expert opinion, and international consensus because not enough original research has been done on what effect on dementia symptoms is created by key elements such as noise and light. However, it is important to start to make design changes immediately to try to improve lives, rather than waiting for absolute evidence. Unlike an untested pharmacologic intervention, the unwanted side effects of an experimental dementia design intervention are likely to be, at worst, an inoffensive wasted opportunity rather than a significant danger to older people, even if the proposed benefit is not achieved. However, some populist design ideas are, at face value, illogical and fanciful, and the absence of research is not a reason to follow those trends. One example is the use of retro-design. Some interior decorators choose a decade of design fashion (e.g., the 1950s) and use that as the theme of a care home environment. It is not sound to assume that all residents and future potential residents will have a common memory or recognize and be comfortable with design themes from the same historical decade. It may be an agreeable style for the care home provider to choose, but it should not be described as a therapeutic response to dementia.

Another challenge for environmental improvement in dementia care is potential conflict with regulators, such as inspectors from fire control, infection control, or food hygiene. Their advice that is aimed to reduce risks for the general population sometimes increases risks for older frail people with cognitive impairment. It is important for planners to be provided with briefings on key legislation, regulation, standards, and guidance with associated inspection and enforcement powers relating to buildings and to consider where these seem to be at variance with the optimal dementia design guidance so that a constructive way forward can be established once variances have been clarified.

This can be illustrated by the problem of fire exits in hospitals and care homes. Older adults with dementia may find the inside of the building tiresome and may observe through the glass panels of the fire door a much more eye-catching world. This might tempt them to go out and explore, oblivious to personal danger. In addition, there may be a sign on the fire door that says, "Push to exit"—this effectively acts as an instruction for cognitively impaired adults, who then make an undesirable, perhaps unobserved, departure. They may follow that incitement printed on the door 20 times a day, necessitating staff time to retrieve them because there may be a risk of falling down the fire escape stairs or walking into danger. Staff may resort to restraints or medication to reduce the exiting risk, even though restraints and medication present other risks to frail older people with dementia. It would be much more practical if the fire door were hidden. In particular, if personnel are trained to find the fire door in an emergency, when there may be no light and the room is filled with smoke and panic, there may be no need to highlight it continuously. Fire officers may have difficulty understanding this balance of risk for cognitively impaired older people and may resist a design change that would make the building less hazardous for dementia patients and make care less time-consuming for staff. These tensions in dementia-friendly design extend to infection control, food hygiene, health and safety at work, and other issues, and attempts have been made to bring together the conflicting advice that planners and builders may meet in order to start the discussion.[2] However, the main distinction between design for physical and sensory impairment and design for cognitive impairment is the extent to which the design compensates for the reduced capacity of people with dementia to avoid hazardous situations and reduces mental stress for all the people using the space.

WHAT CAN LIMIT THE POSITIVE EFFECTS OF THE BUILT ENVIRONMENT?

The best outcome cannot be achieved exclusively by shaping the built environment, because human behavior and systems have a huge impact on old frail people. Heroic health and social care staff, families, friends, and others may overcome many design flaws in a poor building, or people perversely at times may negate the benefit of a good design by not using the environment in the best way.

For example, food is extremely important in old age and ill health. For frail older people to eat well, it works best to have them eat in a leisurely way at an agreeably set table with others who are also enjoying the meal. In the absence of a patients' dining room, hospital staff can designate a quiet corner of the clinical area or ward and furnish it with a table and chairs where an attractive dining atmosphere can be created. On the other hand, even when there is a properly designed dining room, hurried or unthinking hospital personnel who decide to serve meals at the bedside fail to use this potential cue for eating well. Infection control and food hygiene processes may dictate a short mealtime "window" before food is cleared away, so even if the building design is optimal, the intended function is not fulfilled because the system does not give slower patients time enough to eat. There may not even be enough time for nurses to help the patients to get to the dining table. If staff do not understand the reason behind a design feature, it will lead to them failing to use it for the intended benefit.

WHERE ARE THE GREATEST BENEFITS TO BE HAD FROM THESE DESIGN IDEAS?

The overall aim of optimal design is to reduce dependency, and that means delaying or avoiding adverse incidents that might lead to older people needing more care or institutionalization. It is not currently feasible for the entire housing stock and all public buildings to be adapted to take dementia and frailty into account. The Disability Discrimination Act in the United Kingdom was passed as late as 1995, only then making it unlawful to discriminate against people with disabilities. This civil rights law outlawed building design that failed to take into account mobility and other physical and sensory impairments, so now this is expected as standard. It is conceivable that time will come when all buildings are required to take cognitive impairments into account; given the role of frailty as a risk for cognitive impairment, especially in very late life, a single set of design principles can be envisaged.[3] In the light of restricted resources in the meantime, it makes sense to prioritize dementia design ideas in the places where cognitively impaired frail older people are most likely to be, which is their own homes, hospitals, and care homes or specialist-supported housing that is dedicated to them.

Ideally, work on the domestic (home) environment should be completed when older people are still very fit and well and managing their daily lives. It is helpful to introduce changes before change itself becomes a problem. Individual families and homeowners can be given the advice that they need to make these alterations in their current home during routine maintenance of the property. Good design can be incorporated in new retirement housing schemes. As people start to be vulnerable or "slowed up" (as defined in the Dalhousie Clinical Frailty Scale),[4] the benefit of age-friendly or dementia-friendly design is more apparent. Before older people become dependent on others, good design and the use of assistive technology may help to delay any requirement for support, saving resources and supporting the desire of these people to remain independent and at home. If mild to moderate frailty settles in, older adults will require help with a range of issues, including housework, meal preparation, and self-care. Some of the aids and adaptations to support the strengths of frail older adults will also help to delay potential frailty and dementia symptoms in those who are managing well if used by them, because they reduce the possibility of an avoidable adverse incident, such as a fall, that would precipitate a hospital admission. Such accidents can put older individuals on a fast track to further adverse incidents, the unintended negative consequences of a hospital admission, leading to reduced capacity to care for themselves, and to increased dependency or unfortunately at times a faster track to institutionalization.

In the lifetime of a building, optimization of the environment can be undertaken at any stage, from the planning and construction phase of a new building to a makeover of an old property. There is increasing evidence that whole communities, towns, and cities aspire to be age-friendly or dementia-friendly.[5] Older adults' own homes can be adapted, and easy-to-read guidance is already available for families to make those changes.[6] Specialist housing must support predictable needs. Most people live at home until the end of life, and so it is rational to ensure that new general-purpose housing is designed in such a way that it can remain a "home for life" to prevent or delay the need for a move to new accommodation at a life stage when change and disruption are likely to be most disabling for frail older adults.

In the light of the aging demographic, public buildings and service structures such as shops and hotels should also take frailty into consideration. In general this can be approached by compliance with disability discrimination legislation and design regulations, with the addition of the elements that will support people with cognitive impairment. Although it is not yet a legal requirement, it is hoped that the cognitive support elements of design will become mandatory. Planners would do well to anticipate this future requirement in order to avoid trouble and expense later, and they will realize immediate benefits to themselves and their clients.

Dementia-friendly design is already seen as a quality mark in care homes and nursing homes because up to 90% of residents have dementia, even if they have not been formally diagnosed before admission and the care home is not designated as providing dementia care.[7] At least 30% of all older patients in general medical wards in acute hospitals have dementia or cognitive impairment from some related condition, and their care is not as good as that of other patients.[8] Attention to basic dementia design principles would alleviate that. Older people are the majority of other users, including visitors to hospitals, so these buildings must have the environment designed to be as supportive as possible for their identifiable needs. The greatest benefit to be achieved from dementia-friendly design is a reduction in care costs and an increase in independence and well-being toward the end of life.

WHAT ARE THE GENERAL FEATURES THAT CAN BE CONSIDERED ANYWHERE?

Older frail adults will develop impairment of their capacity to undertake activities of daily living independently. This is because they are easily tired and have reduced strength. A significant number of frail older people will have reduced capacity to learn new things and a reduction in short-term memory and capacity to work things out as a result of conditions that lead to dementia. Sensory impairment (including visual and auditory impairment) may add to the difficulty in making sense of the environment and undertaking self-care. Reduced mobility may be complicated by problems with balance and issues such as reduced depth perception that sometimes come with dementia. The environment can compensate for this in a number of ways.

It is important to remember that the needs of frail older adults, especially when accompanied by dementia symptoms, can be stressful and physically exhausting to both patients and caregivers. Stress can give rise to behavior that caregivers and care workers may find difficult to tolerate, and patients may be sedated or otherwise restrained as a result. Use of medication and physical restraint carry significant risks for patients, and at times it is counterproductive. It is vital that the design of the environment gives maximum support to the provision of a stress-free atmosphere. A calm and relaxed atmosphere can make a significant difference to the burden of care.

For example, staff working in care settings are often unaware of the level of unnecessary meaningless stressful noise (doors banging, alarms and phones sounding, clang of bin lids, crash of trolleys, and people talking loudly), and they become habituated to poor air quality and the absence of individualized temperature controls. Noise increases stress and damages concentration and can add to the difficulty in finding your way about a building, and this gives rise to frustration initially and eventually dependence. Particular attention is required to support people who have hearing loss. The use of auxiliary amplification devices is a useful alternative to the chaos caused by having everything very loud, and recognition should be given to the risk of social isolation that arises from hearing loss, because social isolation makes the experience of frailty and dementia worse, even in hospital. Access to fresh air and a comfortable temperature is vital for the avoidance of stress, and although this is common sense, it is often forgotten in the care of older frail people with cognitive impairment.

Good practice guidelines are available for the design of living spaces for people with dementia and sight loss, based on research undertaken by the University of Stirling with the support of the Thomas Pocklington Trust, which provides housing and support for people with sight loss.[9] There is also an auditory commentary for the guidelines. In summary, the general features that can be considered anywhere are those that minimize stress, bearing in mind those things that are most likely to cause stress for frail older people with dementia.

WHAT DESIGN FEATURES ARE REQUIRED IN HOSPITALS AND ACUTE SETTINGS?

This section outlines a number of practical responses to specific issues.

Toilets. An en suite toilet and shower/bath room can support continence and management of incontinence. The toilet pan should be visible by the patient when lying or sitting up in the bed, achievable at night with passive infrared sensors and lights. The seat should contrast with the porcelain, and a familiar flush mechanism should be used. Toilet paper can be made more visible with color and a portable dispenser that is placed in front of the user, to avoid the need for twisting around to the wall. Toilets for use in the day need highly visible doors and very obvious signage, including symbols and words. Wash hand basins need classic (cross head) taps (faucets), a sink plug, and familiar soap bars or soap dispensers, with towels as an alternative to air hand dryers. Grab bars should be in highly visible colors. Hard washable flooring should be similar in color and tone to the adjoining room with no threshold, non-slip, and not shiny or reflective. Discrete storage for incontinence products and clean underwear is required and preferably room for an attendant at either side of the pan. A shower to privately cope with consequences of incontinence reduces smell and prevents humiliation. Quiet extraction fans and automatic subtle air freshener help air quality.

Storage. Many hospitals were designed long before many modern useful walking and standing aids were available or hoists were needed as a result of new legislation about safe moving and handling of patients. As a result some spaces or corridors may be used as storerooms. It is vital to make sure that people not be confused about the function of a room, just because it is also being used for storage. Taking patients to a room that has a jumble of metal equipment and cardboard boxes full of continence products may make it hard for them to understand that this is a bathroom and that it is appropriate for you to attempt to undress them there.

Sound. It has been said that noise is as disabling to a person with dementia as stairs are to a person in a wheelchair. Many staff often are completely unaware of the soundscape around them, including noises of furniture, other conversations, central heating, nurse call systems, road traffic, and machinery. Particularly if they have sensory or cognitive impairment, many older adults have difficulty separating important and relevant auditory input from background noise. Changes that be made to the environment to reduce unnecessary noise include switching things off, using dampeners on doors and lids, and keeping people quiet. In addition, ceiling tiles, wall coverings, floor coverings, and curtains can reduce the reverberations in a space and thus reduce noise.

Skirting and walls. The color of walls has an important role in improving the light level in a room, but the junction between the wall and the floor needs to be well marked out to assist with problems of depth perception. Floor coverings that climb up the wall for decoration, or even for sealant for wet rooms, can exacerbate depth perception problems. Alternatives should be sought to prevent falls.

Signs. Way finding in hospitals is crucial for frail older patients, as well as for their spouses, friends, and relatives. It is not just a question of color contrast and size of print but also the use of illustrative pictures on signs and the height of positioning of signs on walls that make a difference. In addition, art objects can act as way-finding markers. For example, you may more helpfully instruct the patient to turn left at the painted lady and right beside the statue of a dog, rather than asking them to take first a left turn and then a right turn.

Outside spaces. Exercise is crucial for adults with dementia. Particularly if the air quality in the clinical area is poor, open-air exercise is beneficial. Exposure to bright daylight can help to reduce nocturnal wandering and assist with metabolism of vitamin D, which is essential for health and may be low in frail older people with poor appetite. In addition to supporting bone health to reduce fractures from falls, it is said to have a role in reducing falls themselves.

Nurses' stations. Nurses need a place to store notes and to update them. Increasingly this is done electronically. It is unnecessary to undertake this task in a central space in the clinical area. Pods can be arranged at intervals that allow nurses to be closer to patients, even when they have to attend to administrative tasks. This allows them to prevent incidents and to provide reassurance by their presence.

Nurse call systems. There is no parallel in most ordinary lives where we have used an audible call system to summon someone, except perhaps a door chime. The noise used in nurse call systems is not as gentle as a chime and usually sounds like an alarm. It can be set off at any time in the day and night and may cause distress over a long time, if routing does not limit the auditory signal to a restricted zone, but shatters the peace for everyone. Even if the care provider suspects that it is a person unnecessarily (often repeatedly) pressing the switch, she will be diverted from perhaps more critical tasks to check on the caller. Often, more than one care provider must interrupt what they are doing in order to check. This is completely unnecessary. In any building, provider call systems can be retrofitted that operate on a silent or vibrating paging system that assists responders to allocate and delegate responsibility for each call and prioritize the calls. Requiring frail older people to master and properly use an unfamiliar system is illogical, in particular if they have reduced capacity to learn as a result of dementia or other illness. Sleeping through such noise is impossible.

Notices and posters. Hospital and care home environments are often littered with notices, many very important and some out of date, and difficult to read. The environment should not be cluttered in this way. For example an environmental audit will tell you if the largely ineffective sign announcing a zero tolerance of violence to staff overshadows the useful and essential sign for the toilet. The environment must be seen from the patient's point of view, in the light of their challenges and impairments. There is a time and a place for other communications, but reducing the required reading for frail older people helps orientation.

Mirrors. Although availability of a mirror is vital for self-grooming, it is important that the mirror be concealed or removed. A frail older person with dementia might not recognize his own reflection and so may experience the illusion that the mirror is in fact a window, through which an unrecognized and perhaps angry or puzzled looking person is always peering. That is frightening or at times might cause the person to avoid the room, which is inconvenient if the mirror is in a bathroom.

Lighting. The aging eye needs much more light over time. It is advisable to take technical briefing on lighting that includes detail of issues such as the average daylight available in a room, color rendition (the effect that light has on the color appearance of objects), and advice on lamps. If lighting is to be used to help to avoid nocturnal wandering, refer to the recommendations for regulation of circadian rhythm for night shift workers that include exposure to bright light in the "day," an extremely dark sleeping environment, and an avoidance of light in the hours before trying to sleep.[10] Making these things possible is a building design issue.

Handrails. Handrails in corridors and bathrooms should have contrasting colors to the surrounding so that they are easily seen.

Furniture. It is vital that the furniture selected is visible and contrasts well with the surroundings. Beds must be low profile; that means they must be able to be lowered to the floor to avoid the use of cot sides as a falls prevention strategy. Classic simple designs are preferable to high fashion.

Floors. People with dementia and visual problems are likely to misplace their foot if the floor covering is confusing. Sources of confusion include highly polished reflective surfaces, patterns that are mistaken for hazards, door thresholds between rooms that contrast with the color of the floor in either room, which may be mistaken for steps. In slower and weaker patients, such a mistake may give rise to a stumble from which they are unable to recover, giving rise to a fall. Provide smooth matt self-colored floor coverings to reduce falls.

Enabling relatives to stay with the patient. A familiar face can reduce agitation and family or friends can encourage eating and drinking, with a view to decreasing the possibility of delirium or managing it. Relatives can ensure that medication is taken and reduce the burden of care that is carried by staff. The availability of single rooms for frail older patients with a fold-down couch beside the patient's bed can improve the patient's potential for rehabilitation and recovery. The presence of a relative or friend can be a great comfort at the end of life, and this is very important as 30% of hospital patients are in the last year of life. The single room itself will reduce the extent to which the patient disturbs others and will facilitate the creation of an individualized environment, with respect to light and temperature. Nurses' anxiety about observation can be overcome with movement sensors and other assistive technology.

Doors. Doors exclusively for staff use should be painted the same color as the wall so that they are less visible (or even invisible) to patients. This reduces the chance of patients going through the wrong door, making the environment less hazardous. On the other hand, doors that may need to be found in a hurry, such as bathroom doors, need to be very clearly contrasting and well signed. Signs that are high up are less likely to be read by smaller, more stooped older people so hospitals may choose to put staff-only signs much higher up.

Clocks and calendars. There is an increasing awareness of the advantage of clocks and calendars for orienting older people, but it is vital to make sure that they are low enough on the wall to be seen by older people who may have curved posture and have difficulty raising their eyes. It has been suggested that an analogue clock (a round face with numbers) is remembered and understood longer than a digital clock by the current generation of older people because this is how they learned to tell the time originally. In hospitals it may also be necessary to have a clock that distinguishes AM and PM, because of the disruptive routines that mean the patient may wake not knowing if it is night or day. Stress can reduce orientation, and support for orientation can reduce stress. Make sure that the times and dates displayed are always accurate.

Ceilings. Because light is crucial for the aging eye, ceilings should be light in color and reflect light back into the room. To help reduce noise, sound-absorbing ceiling tiles may be used. When positioning ceiling light fittings, lie on the bed and see whether the glare from the lamp will shine into the eyes of the patient. In the absence of single rooms, ensure that task lighting will allow one patient to have a task light to read at night, for example, without disturbing others by having a ceiling light on.

These special considerations are practical examples. More can be found at www.dementia.stir.ac.uk/design/virtual-environments/virtual-hospital.

WHAT DOES A FRAIL-FRIENDLY CARE HOME OR NURSING HOME LOOK LIKE?

For prospective developers or operators of care homes, profitability is important for survival, and it has been suggested that profitability is higher in buildings with 60 to 100 residents.[11] This will determine the size of care homes in the future as newer care homes outperform old care homes and new buildings are being created at the same rate as older substandard care homes are closing. The most pressing challenge for operators is staffing, including the cost of staff and the difficulties in recruiting and retaining them. Either because families are paying, or because local authorities allow choice in placement, the home has to be attractive to families who make choices for older frail people. As a result, design has to reflect competition in the market and has to provide the lowest care burden possible.

Austerity in the public sector means that local authorities restrict care home placement to those who are very frail and length of stay has been reduced to around 18 months, making a care home something like a dementia hospice. For affluent clients, care homes exist with private rooms and suites, access to gardens and private balconies, private dining rooms and room service, and laundry facilities in addition to the communal laundry services. These are very expensive and can be around £1500 ($2000) per week. This is almost three times what a local authority will pay and so state-funded clients are likely to be in more modest accommodations.

The ideal care home environment will provide the frail- and dementia-friendly design features that are described in the hospital setting, even though some of them may not be immediately attractive to commissioners. For example the bright light needed by the aging eye may seem harsh to younger family members or social workers who are arranging placements. Designers may favor modern bathrooms and toilets with infrared sensors for operating taps and toilet flushes, but older patients may not understand that type of plumbing and may fail to use it independently, so a balance has to be struck between style and function.

As the dependency of care home residents increases, the design must allow staff to provide end-of-life care, while at the same time offering a building where active and meaningful activity can take place, indoors and out, for people who are still relatively independent. New care homes offer en suite toilets and showers in individual rooms as standard, though many residents still share in older buildings. Even if the home has 70 to 100 or more beds, the residents should be sharing lounge and dining areas with a small group of others (perhaps 10), on a domestic scale.

The design and building of care homes is a big industry, and it will be increasingly unusual for people to live there as a lifestyle choice; rather, it will be where people go at the very end of life, if they are not able to stay at home. There are approximately half a million care home beds in the United Kingdom. Certification schemes for dementia friendliness are available[12] and short of that, care home developers should ensure that the architects and planners engaged on any new building can provide evidence of training (as opposed to experience) in dementia-friendly design.

Care homes look very different, depending on whether they are in converted older buildings or brand new buildings. In any case, the most important thing is that all the advice about dementia-friendly building is taken into account in the design.[13]

WHAT CHANGES CAN OLDER PEOPLE MAKE IN THEIR OWN HOME?

In general, most people at risk of the (further) loss of independence find it best to change as little as possible at home. Change is unsettling and even if the person approves the change, especially for people with sensory or cognitive impairment, they may forget it in subsequent days and feel uncomfortable or not recognize the introduced technology, or miss the rug that was the trip hazard, imagining that it was stolen. One strongly recommended change is to increase the light level. The prevalence of visual impairment increases exponentially with age.[14] The use of color contrast and tone rather than just color is needed to ensure that objects are visible. Increase in the light level can be achieved by increasing the lamps in the room and the power of those lamps. Cleaning windows and cutting back vegetation from around them, and painting exterior walls to reflect light back into the room can be helpful. Widen the curtain poles so that curtains can be pushed right back when open, not obscuring any part of the window aperture. All these practical measures will improve the situation without changing much; it will all just be a bit clearer and brighter to the resident.

In the domestic setting, assistive technology is particularly useful. Skype and FaceTime can be used for entertainment and communication to ward off boredom and loneliness. Sensors and alarms can be used to protect the person who may inadvertently leave the stove on or cause flooding. There are complications if the person is unable to understand what the alarm sound means, but this can be reinforced by telephone support. GPS tracking devices can be used to locate the person with dementia, inside or outside the house, allowing more freedom of movement and independence as long as possible. Biometric locks can overcome the problems of losing keys or having too many keys circulating in the community. Reminder devices can support the person in continuing to take medication or attend appointments. Even a simple product like the Magiplug, which empties the basin if you forget to turn the tap off, can make a huge difference to the confidence with which people with dementia can be supported to continue to live at home for as long as possible.

Seniors apartments advertise "age in place" design or remodeling of homes with features that support older frail people. These elements propose the use of drawers instead of shelves in the kitchen, including drawer-style dishwashers and fridges to reduce the need for stretching and lighting within drawers to make the contents more visible. Stoves with knobs on the front are easier to use from sitting-down positions, and motorized adjustable sinks and worktop counters allow kitchen work to be done from a sitting position, on a chair or wheelchair, before returning the work surface to the level required by others. Baths and showers are available with designs that allow independent self-care even if mobility and strength are limited, featuring threshold-free wet rooms with built-in seating. Wider corridors and doors allow access with any mobility aid. It is often described as "universal design" and can be aesthetically pleasing. Care needs to be taken with finishes. A hard floor surface that makes wheelchair access easier may be unforgiving on older bones in a fall, giving rise to fractures.

Older people who are well should consider introducing some of these ideas in their own homes before they are absolutely required, as familiarity with them will make it easier later, if they become essential. Health and social care workers need to keep themselves up to date with the latest inventions through attending exhibitions or browsing websites with useful information about assistive technology.*

CONCLUSIONS

Optimizing the built environment for older frail adults is an important element in their care and support. Failing to undertake the low-cost, practical measures that make a difference gives rise to unnecessary burden and dependence, increasing the cost of care and perhaps subjecting the patient or resident to unnecessary risk. In the long term it is to be expected that cognitive considerations will be added to those other elements of discrimination that are covered by human rights–based legislation and regulation. Enhancing the environment in order to make life easier for frail older people also makes life better for those who care for them, without whose work our health and care system would be unsustainable.

KEY POINTS

- Dementia-friendly design is a development beyond design for frail older people because it adds in elements that support older people with cognitive impairments in addition to sensory and physical impairments.
- The right design can reduce disability and make good care easier to achieve for people with dementia and their caregivers.
- The most important general dementia-friendly principles are enhanced light level and classic easy-to-understand furniture and fittings.

For a complete list of references, please visit www.expertconsult.com.

KEY REFERENCES

1. Dementia Services Development Centre: Virtual environments. http://dementia.stir.ac.uk/design/virtual-environments.
2. Fuggle E: Design for people with dementia: an overview of building design regulators (Scotland edition), Stirling, UK, 2014, Dementia Services Development Centre.
3. Robertson DA, Savva GM, Kenny RA: Frailty and cognitive impairment–a review of the evidence and causal mechanisms. Ageing Res Rev 12:840–851, 2013.
4. Geriatric Medicine Research, Dalhousie University: Clinical Frailty Scale. http://geriatricresearch.medicine.dal.ca/pdf/Clinical%20Faily%20Scale.pdf.
5. Dobner S: Bruges: a dementia friendly city. 2014. TheProtoCity.com. http://www.theprotocity.com/bruges-dementia-friendly-city/.
6. Andrews J: 10 Helpful hints for dementia design at home: practical design solutions for carers living at home with a person who has dementia, Stirling, UK, 2014, Dementia Services Development Centre.
7. Lithgow S, Jackson G, Brown D: Estimating the prevalence of dementia; cognitive screening in Glasgow nursing homes. Int J Geriatr Psychiatry 27:785–791, 2012.
8. Sampson EL, Gould V, Lee D, et al: Differences in care received by patients with or without dementia who died during acute hospital admission: a retrospective case note study. Age Ageing 35:187–189, 2006.
9. Dementia Services Development Centre: Good practice in dementia and sight loss. www.dementia.stir.ac.uk/design/good-practice-guidelines.
10. McNair D, et al: Light and lighting design for people with dementia, Stirling, UK, 2013, Dementia Services Development Centre.

*The website www.atdementia.org.uk/ is an excellent source of advice and information on assistive technology for domestic use.

11. Care homes trading performance review. 2014. www.knightfrank.co.uk/research/reports/care-homes-trading-performance-review-2014-2365.aspx.
12. Dementia Services Development Centre: Audit and accreditation. www.dementia.stir.ac.uk/design/audit-and-accreditation.
13. Dementia Services Development Centre: Virtual care home. www.dementia.stir.ac.uk/design/virtual-environments/virtual-care-home.
14. World Blind Union Elderly Working Group: Ageing and visual impairment. 2011. www.worldblindunion.org.

133 Transcultural Geriatrics

Alexander Lapin

INTRODUCTION

Our modern world is subjected to profound changes as never seen before in human history. Globalization of economics and communication and worldwide migration in all its forms bring new cultural confrontations during various moments of our daily lives. Moreover, extension of lifetime expectancy as a result of the achievements of modern medicine has produced the demographic phenomenon of population aging, which is not restricted to the developed countries but is recognized as an incipient global phenomenon. From the point of view of geriatric medicine, it means that situations of transcultural (or cross-cultural) confrontation, which would occur during an encounter between the physician and patient, can be expected to be occur more often and therefore should be considered with increased attention and competence.

This is particularly important in view of the current situation in Europe, which is characterized by the largest immigration movement since the Second World War. Most of these refugees are coming from Syria, Afghanistan and other Middle Eastern countries. They belong to different traditions of Islam, but also to various denominations of Eastern Christianity. Some of them are followers of the ancient religions of the Orient such as Yezidis or Druze.

In this chapter, general aspects of such transcultural encounters will be discussed. The focus will be on communication, acceptance, and medical compliance, especially when dealing with patients from another cultural background. Moreover, specific aspects of transcultural nursing will be presented, with examples from selected cultures.

DEMOGRAPHICS

Worldwide migration is a steadily growing phenomenon, especially in political, economic, social, and intercultural contexts. Refugees, seasonal workers, migrants with higher professional qualifications, and even short-time visitors such as tourists, transportation workers, and sometimes military personnel with their families. All these categories of migrants illustrate the complexity of the phenomenon, which is so characteristic for today's world.

At the same time, distinguishing between political and economic reasons for leaving one's homeland appears no longer to be valid, because both these aspects can play a role in any migrant's fate (Table 133-1). Even the type of integration into a new country has changed. The situation of a giving up one's own culture (e.g., language, customs, religion) is no longer required. This is also true for so-called multiculturalism, which for a long time has been considered as a promising model for coexistence of self-sufficient but mutually isolated cultural communities living in the same country.

What we find today is the transcultural type of coexistence, especially in the workplace, where people of different ethnic or cultural origins have to act together because of the same interests and goals. In the private sector, by contrast, the same people may maintain intensive contacts with their cultural community and even their home country. This is especially possible because of modern communication abilities and facile mobility. This is enabled by the Internet, cell phones and smartphones, tablets, and other technologic advances, as well as affordable long-distance flights. Incidentally, the best example of this transcultural coexistence can be observed among medical and nursing professions in many countries of today's world.

DILEMMA OF THE PHYSICIAN-PATIENT ENCOUNTER

Migrants especially know well from their own personal experience how bitter it can be if one is in a situation of illness and helplessness in a foreign country and in the middle of unfamiliar surroundings. For older adults, such a situation is particularly unpleasant—the hospital, room, bed, personnel, medical facilities—everything is new and unexpected. The misfortune of illness leads a person to think about the worst possible scenario regarding the immediate future. The patient is concerned about family and friends. At the same time, due to restriction of mobility and interference with privacy and intimacy, the person's mood can be changing between despair and hope.[1] All these aspects depend on the cultural and religious background of the patient and therefore affect the quality of life.

Despite actual demands for patient autonomy and consent for therapy, the encounter between the patient and physician still remains asymmetrical. Compared to the patient, the position of the physician during this encounter is quite different. Being in healthy condition, standing, and not being recumbent, as is the patient, the physician is in possession of medical knowledge; the patient depends on the physician's decision. Moreover, in contrast to the patient, the physician has to exclude any private interests from the work. Primary interest has to be focused on determining the right diagnosis and implementation of the most efficacious therapy. Often, such work has to be done under stress because of lack of time and sometimes limited material resources.

Finally, despite the distant positions of the physician and patient, there is an imperative to recognize the common interest of both. For this common aim—the improvement of the situation of the patient—complete understanding is indispensable. However, the transcultural aspect as a complication of this endeavor represents a special type of challenge here.

Culture Shock: Three Steps

The encounter with a person of apparently foreign origin leads to a psychological reaction, which is termed *cultural shock* and consists of three steps. The first is marked by curiosity and usually a positive euphoric attitude toward the unknown foreigner. The primary communication is initiated from preexisting assumptions and stereotypes concerning the not yet well-known culture or nation. The second step is the phase in which not only positive experiences have been made. It is the phase where a certain disillusionment, frustration, anxiety, and rejection take place. Under such a condition, stereotypes can easily turn into prejudices, with a negative emotional tint. Finally, the third step is marked by acquisition of some concrete knowledge about the individual and by confrontation with his or her problems. This in turn enables a more participative, and usually more objective, neutral and rational adjustment of the mutual relationship (Box 133-1). In this analogy, the encounter between the physician and patient is also a gradual process.

From the perspective of the physician, the first step is dominated by the question of personal motivation for becoming a geriatrician. This can be done individually—by professional

TABLE 133-1 Push-Pull Factors Affecting the Decision for Emigration

Push	Pull
Political or religious persecution	Political stability
Persecution	Democratic social culture
Economic crisis	Economic prosperity
Civil war	Better education
Natural catastrophe	Perspective for work and salary

Modified from Ravenstein EG: The laws of migration. J Statistics Soc London, 48:167-235, 1885.

BOX 133-1 Acquiring Knowledge About a Person

A confrontation between cultures can be characterized by the following terms:

- Enculturation—learning and acquisition of elements of another culture
- Acculturation—changing one's cultural elements as a result of a meeting between cultures
- Socialization—adoption of the moral views and behavior of the majority society
- Assimilation—giving up one's own culture in favor of another one

interest, one's moral duty, religious background, or simply by the desire to help older adults. What is always important is the empathy (if not to say love) toward the patient. Even this positive attitude, independently from the cultural and social background of the patient, is necessary to overcome negative prejudices. The second step is dedicated to the concrete acquisition of knowledge about the patient and her or his background. It is the evaluation of cultural status and the search for a common denominator of communication and cooperation. Finally, the third step is the phase of concrete integration of culture-specific measures and experiences into medical care and therapy.

Nonverbal and Formal Communication

The first contact of the physician with the patient is usually on a nonverbal level. There is abundant literature on this topic, which states that in this situation only 10% of the information is transmitted in textual form. The rest of the communication is done by body language and how one uses the voice. A major factor on which such a situation depends is also the ambiance and timing of the communication. The cultural and education level of both parts of the dialogue are equally decisive. In sum, because emotions play such a substantial role here, this situation is important for future understanding, confidence, and empathy between the physician and patient. It is therefore important to recognize the nonverbal signals during such a conversation correctly.[2]

Mimicking seems to be that part of body language that cannot be suppressed entirely by one's own will. Nevertheless, in a cultural context, there are some precautions that have to be considered. Direct eye contact in a Western context signals attention and sincerity. In the Middle East, the same attitude can be interpreted as overreaching and arrogance. When it happens between a man and woman, it can be interpreted ambiguously. Similarly, a smile in Europe or the United States signals friendship or a friendly attitude but, in the context of Chinese culture, it is rather an expression of uncertainty and defensive politeness.

Haptic refers to the type of bodily contact during a communication. In medicine and nursing, it includes so-called therapeutic touch, which is meant as a positive gesture of solace. Generally, in cultures of temperamental Mediterranean people, this approach is quite common and welcome. However, in the context of Islamic culture, it could be an understood as an offense, especially when ignoring the man-man and woman-woman principle.

The term *proxemic* refers to the distance between two individuals involved in a dialogue. Based on human anatomy, one can determine different proxemic zones:

- Intimate zone (hands): 15-30 cm
- Personal zone (talking): 120-210 cm
- Social zone (office): 210-360 cm
- Public zone (teacher): 360-760 cm

However, the cultural context here involves some corrections. In general, more temperamental Southern European cultures prefer shorter distances, whereas in Northern European cultures, these distances are longer.

Paralinguistics

This involves using the voice for the emotional part of communication—the fluency of the language and the loudness of the voice. In different cultures, such as Scandinavian (but not exclusively), slow speaking with pauses is not unusual. In other cultures, such as Hispanics or Italians, loud and fast language is quite normal. By contrast, for Vietnamese, loud speaking is considered to be rude.

Salutation

This is an important part of every communication. In different countries and cultures, it follows specific rituals. In Asian and Far Eastern cultural contexts, it is common to greet by prevention, but also by shaking hands longer. In Islamic countries, it is inappropriate for a man to shake the hand of a woman. Conversely, it is common that younger family members greet the grandfather, the head of the family, by kissing his hand. In Poland, it is still usual to greet an older lady by kissing her hand. In other middle European countries, especially for older adults, this requires a polite and noticeable greeting. Two cheek kisses are usual in France between two relatives or close girlfriends and three cheek kisses are done during at Easter between Orthodox Christians.

Address

In Europe, this is especially of considerable importance. In Central Europe (Germany, Austria) it is usual to greet someone using Mr., Mrs., or Miss with the family name—Herr Schmidt, Mrs. Robinson. It is also customary to use academic titles, such as Frau Doktor or Mr. President. The use of just a professional title is practiced in France and Italy—Commissario. In northern European countries, by contrast, it is customary to use only the family name—Johansson. In Anglo-Saxon cultures, it is common to address people only by their first name or nickname—Dick. In some countries, it is an expression of politeness to use the first name together with the father's name (so-called patronym). In Russia or Ukraine, for example, one uses the form Alexy Vladimirovich or Lydia Ivanovna. On the other hand, in Iceland, the patronym is generally used instead of the family name—Gunnar Petersen (son of Peter), Anna Pálsdóttir (daughter of Paul).

Another consideration is the use of "you" for familiar addressing. More precisely, in most languages, it is the second person singular: *"Toi, tu dois faire cela!"* (French). In English, by contrast, this aspect is not relevant, because one uses "you" in a general context. In southern European countries, to switch into the address by second-person singular is seen as harmless and regarded as a friendly offer of ease and friendship. However, especially in Middle European countries, when talking to older adults, it can be considered impolite, especially if the person is not asked if it's all right to be addressed in this way.

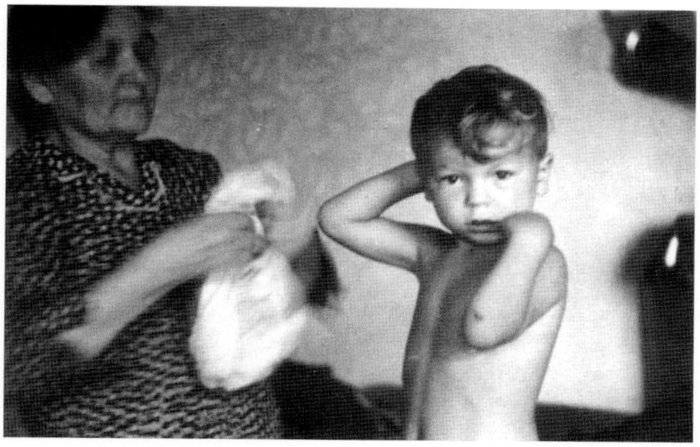

Figure 133-1. The mother tongue or "Grandma's Language" is learned in early childhood, where words and phrases are acquired through deep emotional perception of episodes and moments.

Not without interest is that in several languages, the family name of the woman has a special female form. This is the case especially in Slavonic languages—Jan Novák–Marie Nováková, Jacek Kowalski–Danuta Kowalska, Lev Tolstoy–Tatiana Tolstaya. In South America, it is the custom of a married woman to use both family names, that of the husband and her own maiden one—Isabella Rodríguez-Sanches–Miguel Rodríguez.

In this context, it has to be said that not only correct spelling of the name is important, but also the correct pronunciation, which usually has to be asked about. In any case, this signals interest and respect to the older patient.

LANGUAGE AS A SOURCE OF INFORMATION

How somebody uses language can reveal a lot of information—the history of the concerned person, original ethnicity, culture, sociologic and psychological status, and educational level. For this purpose, it is necessary to be aware of different forms of spoken language. In principle, one can distinguish three types of spoken language:

1. Mother tongue. This is better known as "grandma's language." It is derived from very deep and intimate emotions of childhood. It is not necessarily spoken for the rest of one's life but, as a person becomes older, because of an eventual cognitive reduction, this type of language can remain spoken when other linguistic knowledge has been suppressed or simply forgotten. This may sometimes occur with a focus on cultural stereotypes from childhood and reminiscences from youth (Figure 133-1).
2. Dominant language. This is the language of primary school and usually is formed before puberty. It is spoken in daily use and, in most cases, acquires the role and quality of the native language. Usually it is the language in which one speaks, thinks, and counts.
3. Secondary language. This is learned after puberty. It never reaches the level of the native language, and a foreign accent and minor grammatic errors remain. Thus, especially, this secondary language can indicate the country of origin and in which period of life he or she left that country—such as before or after going to school. Also, vocabulary and locution can reveal the person's level of education.

In sum, to communicate effectively with a patient from a foreign culture, one should follow some general guidelines (Box 133-2).

BOX 133-2 Points to be Considered During a Transcultural Encounter

- Schedule enough time.
  - Keep your own prejudices and biases under control.
  - Speak slowly and clearly.
  - If necessary, repeat and rephrase.
  - Do not use complicated phrases and terms.
  - Avoid shouting and emotion outbursts.
- Do not forget your own good manners.
  - Use professional forms of greeting and salutation.
  - Observe facial expression and body posture.
  - Show interest.
- Work in a quiet atmosphere.
  - Note the unifying aspects, but also what is divisive.
  - Always have paper or laptop ready, and also a dictionary.
  - Don't be arrogant and fawning but be friendly, accurate, and honest.

Modified from Ivanová K, Spirundová L, Kutnohorská J: Multikulturní osetrovatelství (multicultural care), Prague, 2005, Grada Publishing.

IMPORTANT CONSIDERATIONS

Transcultural Nursing

Probably the most systematic approach to the medical care of patients from other cultures was done by Madeleine Leininger (1925-2012). She was an American nurse, ethnologist, and anthropologist, and she dedicated her life's work to the problem of culture-specific nursing, She observed this during her work as a nurse for children of new immigrants to the United States shortly after World War II. Consequently, Leininger studied more than 60 different cultures around the world—for example, spending a long time studying native people in Papua–New Guinea. Based on her experiences, she created a system of working processes in transcultural nursing, with appropriate definitions and nomenclature. She defined nursing as a humanistic art and science that focuses on personal care behavior for improving living conditions and for the consideration of specific, culture-rooted needs of patients and professionals.[3] The founder of social anthropology, E.B. Taylor, applied the notion of culture, defining it as a complex of knowledge, beliefs, customs, morals, and laws.[4] In other words, culture involves, among other factors, intellect, tradition, history of bodily injury, type of communication, customs, expression of emotions, diet, relationships between genders and generations, family life, moral values, relationships and acceptance within and outside one's own culture and, finally, pride and shame (Box 133-3).

Nation and Ethnicity

In this context, an important concept is a person's ethnicity (from the Greek *ethnos*, the nation). Usually it is determined by two types of commonalities: (1) cultural—language, history, way of thinking, religion, and territory; and (2) biologic—skin color, physique, and temperament.

For an evaluation of the background of a specific person, it is not enough to consider all these factors in terms of the information or on the basis of self-generated stereotypes. It is at least equally important to consider the individual status of a person in view of the educational level, profession, and family situation, as well as life crises and crucial episodes of the person's life. Moreover, it is always valuable to obtain some additional basic information about the country and its history and culture. It is important to know if this person belongs to an ethnic minority or religious

BOX 133-3 Relevant Aspects in Transcultural Nursing

Obtain confidence and compliance through language, gestures, mindset, daily activities, clothing, appearance, adaptability to the environment, and relationship to technology.
Consider the person's spiritual and background beliefs, life experiences, religious faith, economic situation, education and profession, customs, tradition, and food and dietary considerations (fasting and celebrations).
Respect intimacy in regard to the following:
- Family, ethnicity, relationships between generations
- Religiosity, membership in a religious community, prayer practice, objects
- Male-female relationships, taboos, sexuality
- Illness and death (last things)

Modified from Ivanová K, Spirundová L, Kutnohorská J: Multikulturní osetrovatelství (multicultural care), Prague, 2005, Grada Publishing.

group that is a minority of the country of origin. For example, refugees from the Middle East do not necessarily belong to the majority of the Muslim Arab population. For example, they might belong to the Kurdish or other ethnic minority or they could be adherents of one of the Eastern Christian Churches.

It is also important to know under which political and/or sociologic circumstances the person has left the home country. Often, it may have been initiated by a specific political or economic situation that has mainly affected a particular sociologic group.[2] This, in turn, later formed the core of the resulting emigration waves. An example are the Russian emigrations of the twentieth century. Immediately after the Bolshevik Revolution, Russian emigration was dominated by aristocrats, intellectuals, and high-ranking military personnel. After World War II, it was mainly composed of the provincial and rural population of the Western part of the Soviet Union and, in the 1980s, many Russian emigrants were political dissidents and those in the arts, and their destinations were Israel and the United States.

Although these three waves of emigration remained emotionally connected to the home country, they showed some nuances in terms of awareness of cultural and spiritual values. Thus, although the first wave felt obligated to monarchist and traditional Christian Orthodoxy, the second was stigmatized by the experiences of World War II. It was more nationalistic and distinguished by its strong popular piety. The third wave by contrast, was marked by secular and cosmopolitan values.

Another important aspect represents the migration background of individuals and their descendants who live in a country after immigration. Here, it is not as important which ethnicity and generation represented by this background, but how much this person is integrated into the society of the country of residence. Obviously, first is the question of social status. In large cities, there are many descendants of former immigrant workers who, in spite of everything, lived for generations in their social and cultural ghettos. Sometimes, one hears of them in connection with excesses or radicalized youth. Usually, this is an expression of social frustration and a self-identification crisis, which can be projected into an overemphasis of their own culture.

Gender and Generations

The relationships between men and women and the younger and older generations are of central interest in every culture and civilization. In Western society, one can observe a certain liberalization of traditional relationships in the family and society. Moreover, one speaks about the crisis of family and the fall of taboos. The result is individualization of the society and the loss of social solidarity, which affects the relationships between men and women and the role of older adults in the society. In other, usually still more traditional cultures, even these two types of relationships are crucial. Respect toward older adults and the defined role of men in the family and society are central aspects of the most traditional cultures and religions.

In this context, usually one differentiates between patriarchal and matriarchal forms of social coexistence. A closer look at the culture reveals that this is somewhat of a stereotype; in reality, both are involved in the family and society, even with different affiliations.

In many cultures, special attention is given to the profession of physician. The physician is usually considered to be above traditional social relationships. However, physicians themselves should be self-aware enough to know that this occurs not because of their inner qualities, but is primarily affected by external circumstances.

A special question concerns the intimacy of the patient. In most cultures, the naked body or part of it can trigger an ambiguous situation. No less significant in a cultural context is the factor of body fluids, such as blood, urine, or feces. These should be handled tactfully and for as short a time as necessary in front of the patient.

Thus, in the case of mutual incomprehension between the physician and patient, if the language of one is not understood by the other, the assistance of an interpreter is indispensable. In most cases, such a role can be fulfilled by the spouse or by another relative, such as an adult child or niece or nephew.

However, one must be also aware of possibly delicate aspects of the conversation, which concerns the history of the patient or intimacy of bodily aspects. Topics such as pain or prognosis may not be expressed by a worried patient, and this can cause additional problems for the family.

Especially for patients of Far Eastern or Asian background, children or teenagers should never be used as as translators for their grandparent. In such a case, it is always better to use a professional or independent interpreter who belongs to a medical profession (Box 133-4).

Spirituality, Religion, and Religiosity

Because people can think in abstract terms, it is obvious that what occurs after the end of life will occupy their mind, especially in critical situations such as during an illness. To find final peace is not only the concern of those with a religious affiliation, but is simply a general feature of the human character.

On the question of religion, one should not be satisfied with only a statement of formal affiliation. It is far more important to learn how intensively the person is involved in this religion and what it means personally. It is important that religion should not be considered as a collection of rites, but as a sphere of spirituality of the person concerned. In this sense, it does not mean that if someone who has declared as being without faith has no need for spirituality.[6] Especially in emergency situations, such as illness in a foreign country, this need may be strongly expressed.

For religious people, religion is the center of their spiritual life. It is guidance in different moments of life, happy and sad, and the religious community is the secure harbor and home. Religion determines also the crucial moments of life, which also includes the last things, such as death and burial rituals.

Death is one of the natural taboos of human life. At the same time, death itself is a very important part of life for those who are concerned, family and friends. In every culture, it is the religion that determines the course of this process. In most cultures, it is important that someone at the end of life be surrounded by people who are closest to the partient. Similarly, the place where the end of the life occurs is very important. Traditionally, it was desirable that someone's death occurs at home. Today, it occurs mostly in hospitals, hospices, and nursing homes.

BOX 133-4 Culture-Related Differences in Communication

ORIENTATION

- By context:
  - Low context—accurate expression (Northern Europe)
  - High context—pictorial expression (Asia)
- By space—proxemic distance
  - Rather close (Southeast Europe)
  - Rather distant (Scandinavia)
- By angle of eye contact (in Arab and Asian–Far East countries)
- By time
  - Monochronic: doing just one thing at time; punctuality (Germany, Scandinavia, North America)
  - Polychronic: doing multiple things at the same time; flexibility (Latin America, Southern Europe)
  - Cyclic—oriented to seasons and events (Asians, Native Americans)

DISTANCE TO POWER (DISTANCE FROM AUTHORITY IN FAMILY, WORKPLACE)

- Large distance—Arab countries, Turkey, Southeast Europe
- Small distance—United States, the Netherlands.

INDIVIDUALISM VERSUS COLLECTIVISM

- United States, United Kingdom versus Japan, China

MEN VERSUS WOMEN (PERFORMANCE VS. FAMILY)

- Japan, Germany, United Kingdom versus The Netherlands, Portugal, France

Modified from Transkulturelle Pflege: Kulturspezifische Faktoren erkennen-verstehen-integrieren. (Transcultural Nursing. Culture specific factors to recognize, to understand, to integrate.) Vienna 2001, Facultas Verlag.

Another aspect is religiosity. It characterizes the type and intensity of participation in religious life. In general, it is a dynamic factor that evolves in the course of the lifetime. In this context, it is evident that the religiosity of a young or adult will be substantially different from that of an older adult.

On the other side, in each religious community, there are always followers who can be characterized as conservatives or liberals.[7] Even in our daily life, we know people who can be classified as churchgoers or even as bigots. At the same time, there are those whose attitude is anticlerical or who at least can be described as "seekers."

The question of the intensity and nature of each religion may be interesting for carrying out more effective medical interventions. It should therefore be helpful to inquire about dietary and fasting habits, prayer practices, and whether any help from the clergy is desired.

Details of religious observances, such as the presence of certain religious objects, compliance with religious rules, praying, celebration of holidays, and following fasting rules, can alleviate the time passed by older adults in the hospital. Because of the broad spectrum of traditions and rituals, it is advisable to consult the family or spiritual advisor of the religion (e.g., rabbi, pastor, imam, wise man) about all these questions to enable the comfort of the patient as much as possible.

All this is important to understand the way of thinking of the person being considered. This can provide valuable insight into customs, mood, and thought processes and into the spiritual and traditional needs of the person.

Biography and Life Story

Probably the most interesting aspect when dealing with older adults is their life story. Approaching the summit of life, an individual's lifelong acquired impressions and experiences are the most abundant and the most fulfilled.

In most cultures, the older adult is considered as a mediator and bridge to the past. At the same time, the older adult is someone who is at the threshold of death and possibly another life or more, the threshold of eternity. This is probably why, in many cultures, the older adult is regarded with authority, respect, and admiration. Unfortunately, in our times of fast living, it may be lost. An encounter with an older adult of another culture gives us a chance to rediscover this aspect as the precious experience of humanity.

Of practical interest may be the situation in which two older adults, who during a historical conflict or war were on opposite ends of the political spectrum, may not always have to get along. This consideration should be kept in mind—for example, when people are living together in a room in a nursing home.

Thus, exploring and trying to understand the depth of an individual's history can be very instructive and, at the same time, may allow us to know ourselves better. In the following discussion, we will present some examples of cultures and factors aspects relevant for transcultural care.

Some Cultures and Religions With Relevant Aspects of Clinical Geriatrics

About the half of the world's population belongs, at least culturally, to the monotheistic, so-called abrahamitic religions. Beyond the oldest of them, the Jewish religion, more than one third of the world's population are Christians and less than 25% belong to Islam. As for other religious affiliations, the major groups are Hindus, Buddhists, other Far East religions, and those who are nonreligious.

Judaism

The religion of the people of Israel and other Jewish people worldwide can be considered as the foundation for all other monotheistic abrahamitic religions.[8] Its basis is the Hebrew bible, which consists of the Torah, Five Books of Moses (Pentateuch), and other books of the scripture. Moreover, there is the Talmud, a very extensive compilation of interpretations and wisdom, as well as Halacha, the Jewish law, which regulates virtually all conceivable situations of human life.[7]

The history and theology of Judaism are very complex. Thus, one of the most important aspects of the Jewish religion is the liberation of the Israelites from slavery in Egypt and the Ten Commandments of Moses, which can be regarded as the ethical foundation of all humanity. The so-called Egyptian experience of the Jewish people determines not only their festivals and customs (e.g., Sabbath, Pesach [Passover]) but also the attitude toward life and even the ethics of the medical profession. In its center are prolife and this life references and the concept of the sanctity of life, which is the primary consideration in any medical or nursing situation. Hope is the central force. Thus, it is unthinkable to leave the very sick alone; the family always plays an important role.[7,8]

The feeling of being a member of the Jewish religion and culture is very important, but there is also a corresponding diversity—Orthodox, Conservative, Reform, Reconstructionist—as well as different local traditions. This has come about because of the long history of migration and the Diaspora. Beyond the very ancient Jewish religion and culture common to all Jewish people is the very painful Holocaust experience, which is is especially felt by the older generation.

In practical terms regarding a particular medical need, religious practices should be respected. One should respond to the request for kosher food, and the preparation of food must have been supervised by a rabbi. Also significant is the organization of festivals and celebrations, especially Pesach (in the spring). On the Sabbath, which begins on Friday afternoon, no activities should be performed, and pious believers will appreciate the lit Sabbath candles. It is equally pleasing for patients to enjoy visits from the family and their own rabbi. This may also be the most the source of information about the last things, and it is recommended that this may be the time to be in contact with members of the Jewish community to obtain relevant information.

Christianity

About half of Christians worldwide belong to the Catholic Church and consider the Pope of Rome as the head of Christianity. More than one third of Christians belong to Protestantism in the wider sense. The origin of the Lutheran, Reformed (Calvinist) and Anglican (Episcopal) goes back to the sixteenth century. Today, however, there are more than 2000 other Protestant denominations, such as Baptists, Methodists, Pentecostals, Mormons and others that have arisen later, especially in the Anglo-Saxon countries. Catholics and Protestants in a wider sense together represent Western Christianity. The rest of the Christian world consists of Orthodox and ancient Oriental Christians.[9] The separation between the Christian East and West dates back to 1054 AD, the year of the Great Schism, when the seat of Rome separated from other patriarchates of the East. Today, Orthodox Christians are members of 14 administratively independent, national, so-called autocephalous orthodox churches—Greek, Russian, Serbian, Antiochian, Bulgarian, Romanian. Together, Orthodox Christians form a uniform group, which has the same doctrines and liturgical tradition. Worldwide, there about 500 million adherents of Orthodox Christianity.

Finally, there are the ancient Oriental Christians, whose history goes back to ecclesiastical separations of the fifth and sixth centuries. Today, most of them are Ethiopians, Egyptian Copts, Syrians, Armenians, and some other smaller Christian churches of the Middle East and India.[10]

Despite a wide number of differences concerning doctrine, divine services, and traditions, the common feature of all Christians is the belief in Jesus Christ, the son of God, who was born more than 2000 years ago from the Holy Spirit and Virgin Mary. Later, in his adult life, he preached and healed the sick. He was crucified but became resurrected 3 days later. Thus, the person of Jesus Christ is the epitome of salvation and an eternal afterlife, giving hope to all Christians. Christmas and Easter, which are linked to the birth, death, and resurrection of Jesus Christ, are universal festivals of Christianity, but there are of other feasts such as the Pentecost feasts of various saints and others, depending on the denomination and tradition. For some Christians, the time before important feasts is preceded by period of fasting (lent), which is mostly vegan in nature.

The reading of the Holy Scripture, the Christian bible, is very important, especially for Protestants, and it takes the major place in most of their divine services. Some of these communities have no ordained priest, but only a pastor or preacher. By contrast, for Catholics, Orthodox, and ancient Oriental Christians, a priest is usually a person of major importance. Catholics and especially Christians of the East have a rich liturgical and sacramental tradition. Lent, the time before Easter, can be thought of as a time of deep spiritual importance. At the same time, sacraments and sacramental acts, such as confession, eucharistic Communion, or anointing of the sick, can be also of relevant importance, especially in critical moments of the life.

Some Christians, especially those of the East and in some Protestant communities, may have negative experiences from their previous life under the hostile rule of Islam or militant atheism during the communist regime. Migration and the Diaspora are very real to many individual's histories. In this case, the family's orientation can be very intensive and consideration of the person's the own religion can be a very intimate topic.

For most Christians, it is important to possess various religious objects. It can be a book, rosary, or small statue or icon. Very important is the visit of the person's own priest or pastor. He or she should preferably be not only of the same denomination, but also of the same ethnic origin. Finally, it has to be emphasized that some Christians, especially Eastern Christians, follow a different Church calendar. This is especially the case for different dates for the Orthodox or Oriental Easter.[10]

Islam

The word *Islam* means devotion to God, and a Muslim is one who has devoted himself or herself to God. Worldwide, there are about 1.4 billion followers of this religion,[9] consisting of a number of different nations, traditions, and views and beliefs. The world of Muslims represents a heterogeneous part of the world's population. For some of them, especially those from rural areas of traditionally Islamic countries, social and ethnic traditions may play a very important role. This can be strengthened by the self-maintained isolation of migrant ghettos. Conversely, many Muslims live very close to the Western way of life and has no problem in terms of integration and acceptance. Nevertheless, for better understanding, it is advantageous to know at least some of the basics of Islam.[7,11]

The Qur'an (Koran) and Sunna are considered the holy scriptures. The oral tradition is known by the terms *hadith* and *fatwa*, which stands for a concrete interpretation of certain practical questions of life. It is done by the Ulama, the Council of Wise Men, according to the country of origin. The fundamental doctrine of Islam is based on the *Five Pillars of Islam*:

- Shahada—confession ("There is no God except Allah; Muhammad is the Messenger of Allah.")
- Salat—prayer (five times per day)
- Zakat—giving alms
- Saum—fasting (Halal, Ramadan)
- Hadjj—pilgrimage (to Mecca)

From the medical point of view, one of the most relevant aspects of Islam is the fasting rule of Halal. It states that no pork or non–halal meat (obtained without ritual slaughtering) may be eaten. This may cause problems in some hospitals and care centers, but also with a consideration to address this issue. The strict prohibition of alcohol can lead to problems with the administration of tinctures. In such cases, other possibilities to administer drugs have to be considered. The highlight of the Muslim year is the month of Ramadan. Its onset is later by 11 days each year. During this time, there is total abstinence from food, from sunrise to sunset. However, these rules have exceptions, especially for sick people.

The family has the explicit duty to visit the sick and care for older adults, which has to be done primarily in the family. Thereafter, in most Islamic countries, residences for older adults, such as nursing homes, are still not common. This also explains visits of patients by a large number of friends and relatives at the same time.

A devout Muslim must perform daily prayers five times a day. For diabetics, as has recently been reported,[11] this can cause problems. One should know that for this purpose, the believer must take the shoes off, which may represent a healing obstacle in a diabetic foot. One way to get around this is simple—just prescribe slippers. Being ill means primarily an examination by God. In this context, the fatalistic and holistic consideration of the actual situation are always in the foreground.

A particularly sensitive issue concerns the patient's genital area. The general rule here is the principle of man-man and woman-woman. This means that female patient should be treated, whenever possible, by a woman physician, and vice versa.[12] Exceptions are possible in case of emergencies. As mentioned, it is fundamental to have a consultation with the family for each patient. In this case, a Muslim employee of the institution can provide a valuable service.[13]

Far Eastern and Asian Religions

Many of today's immigrants come from the Far East. Their culture and way of thinking may seem remote when considered from a Western perspective. Usually, their culture is rooted in religions such as Buddhism, Confucianism, and Taoism. From a Western viewpoint, these religions do not know the concept of a Creator or God, but have for many centuries a long tradition of rich and deep wisdom, as well as meditative elements. They have also a plethora of deeply religious aspects such as rituals, asceticism, priesthood, communities, and pastoral care. Thus, one finds in Buddhism the idea of rebirth and the cycle of life; Confucianism is characterized by a code of ethics, with very significant rendering of honor to the ancestors; Taoism invokes the creative principle and way of harmony and perfection.

Certainly, this statement is an oversimplification of what can be seen as a huge world cultural heritage. On the other hand, it should be recognized that large parts of the population are not religious—for example, in China, many continue to declare themselves as atheists. This is only partly a consequence of the ruling atheistic communist ideology. Many religious adherents consider their own religion not as such, but rather as a kind of philosophy of life.[7,14,15]

Generally speaking, it is always the family that plays a very important role for people from the Far East. From the Western point of view, the family is understood to be extremely hierarchical, with a great respect for older adults. Honor and harmony are therefore of great importance.

In terms of daily work in the hospital, it can mean that so-called great visits, with participation of almost all family members, have to be expected. As noted, another relevant fact may be the problem when children of these immigrants act as an interpreter for the older member of the family. This can stress the hierarchical structure of the family and, in turn, lead to restlessness.[14]

Another important aspect is the unwillingness to be a bearer of bad news. Even a very sick patient may intentionally not understand what is meant by consent for an operation. She or he may refuse to undergo a proposed medical intervention instead of burdening the rest of the family. Also noteworthy is the literal cyclic conception of the time, which is marked by periodically marking the returning reality, considered by some as reincarnation. Not only seasons of the year, but even birth and the death are closely related. In practical terms, this means that family events become more significance than the calendar (e.g., someone might say "I have this pain since the death of my cousin"). This can be problematic—for example, when agreement on an appointment with the physician has to be made.

Overall, the Asian concept of shame is often more complicated than that of the Western world. Much can be difficult to understand; the principle of saving face is important. Thus, for example, one might say nerve doctor, rather than psychiatrist.[14] In general, the concept of disease is far more comprehensive than in the West, with a large proportion of fatalism.

This, it is understandable that immigrants from the Far East and Asia can suffer profoundly from homesickness, without showing it. It is also evident that they prefer to live in ghettos, with close family relationships.

Roma

A remarkable "nation" of Europe includes the people of Roma,[2] which is known also by history and by a derogatory name such as gypsy, or Tsiganes. Its primary country of origin is India, notably the province of Punjab, which they left around the ninth century. Their language is therefore of very old origin, rooted in Sanskrit. The historic migration of Roma to the West in about the thirteenth century proceeded in two directions: The southern route went through Egypt (*Egyptiani*, gypsy), North Africa, and up to Spain, where the successive generations were responsible for Flamenco music. The more prominent part of the Roma migrants passed through Asia Minor and Southeast Europe. Going through the former Byzantine (East Roman) Empire, they acquired the privilege of naming themselves as Roma and, in Middle Europe, in the former Kingdom of Bohemia (today the Czech Republic), they were able to call themselves Bohemians.

Today's Roma live predominantly in the eastern part of Europe, but their tradition is to be a moving people. In many countries, such as Slovakia or Romania, the Roma people are on the lower lever of the social scale.

It is typical, however, for them to have a strong, cohesive, large family structure. Usually, four or five generations are living together, with a clear hierarchy in place. The man is the head of the family and the mother is mainly responsible for its nutritional sustenance. The children are always considered as great luck, but their life expectancy can be shorter than in the general population. Alcoholism, begging, insufficient education, and low-level criminality can be a big problem for them.

The Roma love humor, but do not understand irony. They revere their parents and are very sensitive to being judged by others and to angry criticism; they are very emotional.

During verbal communication, the generalization of terms can be understood with difficulty. Therefore, the physician should repeat the message several times, using a clear mode of expression.

Roma have some specific customs that can have medical implications. Thus, the preparation of food is a very important procedure—it has to be done in special vessels. No rewarmed food should be eaten, and mother should be in a good mood while doing cooking. The meal itself is a family ritual. In case of illness, Roma people may be quite independent. Sometimes they may be mistrustful and uncooperative. Separation from the family is very painful.

Finally, according to the culture of the Roma, there are three most important things in life. These are love, the family, and health.

CONCLUSION

During an encounter with an individual of a foreign culture, it is useful to get as much as information as possible about the country of origin. This is especially in regard to the geographic, ethnic, and religious composition of the country, as well as its historical and cultural characteristics. Therefore, a positive attitude and readiness to learn something new is important, especially as an interesting part of one's own education.

Especially in regard to current medical practice, purely somatic healing should be increasingly complemented by the holistic view. It is not enough merely to treat a sick body; one also has to be aware that older adults, especially, represent important witnesses of times past. In practical terms, one should instill a corresponding interest in the medical personnel and management staff of the geriatric institution.

KEY POINTS

- Aging and migration are two important factors that affect demographics. From a practical point of view, this means that older patients of foreign origin will be encountered more and more frequently in different geriatric institutions, such as nursing homes.

- Transcultural competence, such as a specific knowledge of different cultures, traditions, way of thinking, and religion, as well as the historical and geographic background, is of growing importance, even for those in the medical profession. It can enable more efficient communication, understanding, and compliance, especially in regard to older patients of foreign origin.
- Different aspects of nonverbal communication, such as haptic, proxemic, and mimicking, as well as man-women relationships, can be understood differently in different cultures.
- The type of use of a different spoken language, such as the mother tongue, dominant language, and secondary language, can provide valuable biographic information about a person.
- Migration occurs usually in waves. These are predominantly formed by social groups from the country of origin, such as an ethnic or religious minority, poor or rich, dissident or aristocrat, and from a rural area or town. The differentiation between economic and political emigration is not always correct.
- Spirituality seems to be a general human characteristic. Religion can also be considered as a spiritual base of a specific culture. Religiosity characterizes intensity of involvement and concrete practice in regard to a certain religion.
- Culture-specific aspects involve communication, patient intimacy, religious and spiritual needs, fasting and dietary considerations, and role of a spiritual person or member of the clergy (e.g., rabbi, priest, imam), as well as last things, were discussed in examples of five cultures: Judaism, Christianity, Islam, Roma, and Far East–Asian.

For a complete list of references, please visit www.expertconsult.com.

REFERENCES

1. Ravenstein EG: The laws of migration. J Statistics Soc London 48:167–235, 1885.
2. Ivanová K, Spirundová L, Kutnohorská J: Multikulturní osetrovatelství [multicultural care], Prague, 2005, Grada Publishing.
3. Leininger M: Culture care diversity and universality: a theory of nursing, New York, 1991, National League for Nursing Press.
4. Tylor EB: Die anfänge der cultur: untersuchungen über die entwicklung der mythologie, philosophie, religion, kunst und sitte. [The beginnings of civilization: studies on the development of mythology, philosophy, religion, art and custom], Leipzig, 1873, Hildesheim.
5. Transkulturelle Pflege: Kulturspezifische Faktoren erkennen-verstehen-integrieren. (Transcultural Nursing. Culture specific factors to recognize, to understand, to integrate.), Vienna, 2001, Facultas Verlag.
6. Giesinger C, et al: Seelsorge und spiritualität bei krankheit und pflege. [Pastoral care and spirituality in disease and nursing]. Osterr Arzteztg 15/16:28–29, 2007.
7. Neuberger J: Caring for dying people of different faiths, ed 3, Abingdon, England, 2004, Radcliffe Medical Press.
8. Clarfield MA, Gordon M, Markwell H, et al: Ethical issues in end-of-life geriatric care: the approach of three monotheistic religions—Judaism, Catholicism, and Islam. J Am Geriatr Soc 51:149–1154, 2003.
9. Barrett DB, Johnson TM, Crossing P: Missiometrics 2007: creating your own analysis of global data. Int Bull Missionary Res 31:1–8, 2007.
10. Lapin A: What is "psychotherapy" in context of the Orthodox Christianity? World Cult Psychiatry Res Rev 2:80–86, 2007.
11. Green V: Understanding different religions when carrying for diabetes patients. Br J Nurs 13:658–662, 2004.
12. Rispler-Chaim V: Islamic medical ethics in the 20th century. J Med Ethics 15:203–208, 2002.
13. Rohrmoser L: Wenn Muslime zum Arzt gehen. Der kleine unterschied von muslimischen und christlichen patientinnen. Ärzte Woche 21:4, 2007.
14. Tőtová V, Sedláková G: Problems of higher requirements in taking care of the Vietnamese minority. Osetrovatelstrví 8:36–43, 2006.
15. Hughes JJ, Keown D: Buddhism and medical ethics: a bibliographic introduction. J Buddhist Ethics 2:1, 1995.

Index

Note: Page numbers followed by "*f*" refer to illustrations; page numbers followed by "*t*" refer to tables; page numbers followed by "*b*" refer to boxes.

B

C

D

F

H

J

K

N

O

P

T

W